Blaustein's Pathology of the Female Genital Tract

Third Edition

Wonderful is he who can teach . . . and
wise is he who can be taught.

KATHA-UPANISHAD

Robert J. Kurman
Editor

Blaustein's Pathology of the Female Genital Tract

Third Edition

With 1176 Illustrations in 1355 Parts, 22 in Full Color

Springer-Verlag
New York Berlin Heidelberg London
Paris Tokyo Hong Kong Barcelona

Robert J. Kurman, M.D.
Departments of Pathology and Obstetrics and Gynecology
Georgetown University School of Medicine
Washington, DC 20007, USA

Library of Congress Cataloging in Publication Data
Pathology of the female genital tract.
Blaustein's pathology of the female genital tract.
Rev. ed. of: Pathology of the female genital tract / edited by Ancel Blaustein. 2nd ed. c1982.
Includes bibliographies and index.
1. Pathology, Gynecological. I. Blaustein, Ancel, 1919–1984. II. Kurman, Robert J. III. Title.
[DNLM: 1. Genitalia, Female—pathology. WP 100 P297]
RG77.P37 1987 618.1'07

Printed on acid-free paper.

Typeset by Arcata Graphics/Kingsport Press, Kingsport, Tennessee.
Printed and bound by Arcata Graphics/Halliday, West Hanover, Massachusetts.
Printed in the United States of America.

9 8 7 6 5 4 3

ISBN 0-387-96452-5 Springer-Verlag New York Berlin Heidelberg
ISBN 3-540-96452-5 Springer-Verlag Berlin Heidelberg New York

To my parents
and to my wife Carole

Preface to the Third Edition

The third edition of this textbook is a continuation of the work begun by Ancel Blaustein a decade ago. The text has been extensively revised to reflect the changes in the field of gynecologic and obstetric pathology since the previous edition. Pathology has not changed but our understanding of it has. New observations lead to the formulation of new criteria and terms that inevitably necessitate a revision of existing classifications. In this regard, the reader is reminded of a statement by Peter Gould[1] concerning the transient nature of what is considered the "truth" in science, "Whenever we observe and record information about the world around us, we must acknowledge the arbitrary nature of our choices and be aware of the way our choices change over time."

In the last five years application of immunocytochemical and molecular biological techniques to the study of premalignant and malignant lesions of the cervix and vulva has dramatically altered our concepts of neoplasia of the lower female genital tract. Identification of human papillomaviruses in these lesions has led to renewed interest in viral oncogenesis and this has had a major impact on the diagnosis and management of neoplasia in these organs. The chapters on the vulva, vagina, and cervix have been revised accordingly. The chapter on diseases of the vagina has also been expanded to include the changes induced by in utero diethylstilbestrol (DES) exposure, a subject that in the previous edition was considered separately.

The ovary and the endometrium undergo complex alterations as part of the aging process and during the menstrual cycle. The structural changes have been studied by pathologists using light, scanning, and transmission electron microscopy whereas the endocrinologic aspects have been studied by reproductive endocrinologists using biochemical techniques. The chapters on the anatomy and histology of the uterine corpus and ovary describe the morphologic changes in the light of serum hormone levels and tissue receptor concentrations, thereby providing a correlation of the physiology and morphology of these organs.

In recent years the endometrial proliferations that are precursors of endometrial carcinoma as well as lesions that mimic them, i.e., various forms of metaplasia, have been intensively investigated. The histologic features that distinguish the noninvasive precursor lesions from the biologically significant low-grade endometrial carcinomas are now well characterized. In addition, specific histologic types of endometrial carcinoma associated with favorable and unfavorable outcomes have been described and their behavior studied. The chapter in the previous edition entitled "Endometrial Neoplasia" has therefore been divided into two chapters, "Endometrial Hyperplasia and Metaplasia" and "Endometrial Carcinoma."

A new chapter entitled "Endometriosis, Lesions of the Secondary Müllerian System, and Pelvic Mesothelial Proliferations" is a unique contribution that presents an in-depth review of endometriosis and develops the concept of the peritoneum as a modified "müllerian-derived organ." This is useful to explain the presence of endometriosis and müllerian-related metaplasias in remote sites throughout the abdomen as well as multifocal extraovarian neoplasia in the absence of an ovarian tumor.

Clinicopathological studies of the common epithelial, sex cord–stromal, and germ cell tumors of the ovary in the last ten years have greatly influenced their diagnosis and management. The chapter entitled "Sex Cord–Stromal, Steroid Cell, and Other Ovarian Tumors with Endocrine, Paraendocrine, and Paraneoplastic Manifestations" not only summarizes our current understanding of functioning tumors but also describes a variety of ovarian neoplasms associated with paraendocrine and paraneoplastic disorders. Some of these entities, such as the small cell carcinoma, have only recently been described.

Gestational trophoblastic disease and germ cell tumors of the ovary represent areas where clinical management has been revolutionized by the use of tumor markers and multiagent chemotherapy. The highly malignant tumors in both of these categories were almost uniformly fatal as recently as fifteen years ago, but are now nearly always cured. It is therefore important for the pathologist to recognize these neoplasms and for the clinician to understand their management.

In addition to the content, the format of this edition has been modified to emphasize an integrated presentation of the clinical and pathologic aspects of disease in individual organ systems. Thus, except for the chapters on embryology, disorders of abnormal sexual development, endometriosis, cytology, and animal tumor models, all the other chapters embrace the spectrum of pathology for a particular organ. For example, infertility is discussed in the chapters on the uterus, fallopian tube, and ovary. Although seemingly fragmented, this approach more closely reflects the pathology of infertility which is commonly categorized into uterine, tubal, and ovarian factors. In instances where a particular disease crosses anatomic boundaries, liberal use of cross-referencing will lead the reader to other parts of the textbook where the subject is discussed. Adjunctive techniques such as electron microscopy and immunocytochemistry are considered in the context of conventional light microscopy and are included where they are useful in diagnosis or in elucidating pathogenesis.

The text is intended to provide an authoritative reference for the practicing obstetrician/gynecologist and pathologist. It is also designed to present a readable account of gynecologic pathology for medical students and residents in training. The emphasis is on pathophysiology since this provides the foundation for a rational approach to clinical diagnosis and treatment. Students will find that despite the immense accumulation of information in the field, research raises more questions than it answers. Nonetheless, as Esmond R. Long[2] stated in *A History of Pathology*, "An honest presentation of pathology compels the constant admission of uncertainty . . . which may lose the student's confidence, unless he is made to understand that the whole advancement of the science has been a conquest of similar uncertainties."

ROBERT J. KURMAN, M.D.

References

1. Gould P (1982) The Tyranny of Taxonomy. The Sciences May/June p 7–9
2. Long ER (1965) A History of Pathology. Dover Publications, Inc., New York p XIII

Preface to the First Edition

This text is written for the obstetrician, gynecologist, pathologist, and for residents training in these disciplines. It is a multiauthored book and the editor is aware of the problems this can create, but the expansion of information in the field of gynecologic pathology renders single authorship obsolete.

The format is largely traditional but the contents include topics that have not appeared in past texts. Clear cell adenocarcinoma of the vagina and vaginal and cervical adenoses are discussed in detail in a separate chapter. A chapter on embryology and congenital anomalies is written by an embryologist and the advantage of its inclusion is self evident. Ovarian neoplasms in childhood and adolescence are fortunately rare occurrences, but information concerning them is generally not readily available in existing texts. It is of sufficient importance to deserve a separate chapter. Amniotic fluid analysis for fetal viability is now commonly used and for this reason a detailed discussion of this subject is presented.

A chapter is included on gross description and preparation of gynecologic specimens. It contains the input and review of several directors of gynecologic-pathology laboratories.

The text contains many electron micrographs taken by transmission and scanning electron microscopy. Their inclusion is not an absolute necessity in gynecologic pathology, but is informative because they offer another perspective and are now a commonly used modality for studying tissue. The present day literature is replete with descriptions of specimens by electron microscopy, and it is hoped that the text will enable the readers to familiarize themselves with electron microscopy as used in this specialty.

Experimentation in the field of obstetrics and gynecology has become more sophisticated over the years and for this reason the chapter on animal models of tumors of the ovaries and uterus in included. The contributions that comparative pathology can make to understanding disease mechanisms justify the addition of the chapter on comparative uterine and ovarian tumors in the animal kingdom.

The authors include a mixture of clinicians, pathologists, and basic scientists, and it is hoped that this gives the book the balance between the experience of the clinician and the pathologist.

ANCEL BLAUSTEIN, M.D.

Acknowledgments

I was first introduced to gynecologic pathology by Dr. William B. Ober who I was fortunate to meet and work with during medical school. His influence led me to pursue a career in academic pathology and gynecology and I am grateful to him. My interest in gynecologic pathology was further stimulated during my residency training by Dr. John M. Craig and then by Dr. Robert E. Scully with whom I worked as fellow. To Dr. Scully I owe a debt of gratitude for his continued encouragement, support, and counsel in the succeeding years that I have known him. My association with Dr. Henry J. Norris as a collaborator and close friend has been a source of inspiration throughout my career.

I also wish to acknowledge my distinguished colleagues who contributed to this edition. They not only wrote the scholarly chapters which are the essence of this book but also provided helpful suggestions concerning its overall format and organization. Working closely with them has been an enjoyable and educational experience for me.

I am indebted to Ms. Gail Storey for both her secretarial assistance as well as her managerial skills in organizing the numerous tasks necessary in editing. I am also grateful to the photographic department of the Armed Forces Institute of Pathology, particularly Mr. Luther Duckett, for the excellent photomicrography that is evident in several of the chapters. The assistance of the staff at Springer-Verlag is also greatly appreciated.

Finally, I wish to pay tribute to the late Dr. Ancel Blaustein, whose vision and creativity led to the creation of *Pathology of the Female Genital Tract*. The standard of excellence that he set, as well as his wise counsel and infinite patience, were the intangible ingredients that contributed to the success of this book and represent the attributes to which we aspire.

ROBERT J. KURMAN, M.D.

Contents

Contributors

Rita Leff Blaustein, M.D.
Attending Cytopathologist
Department of Pathology
Booth Memorial Medical Center
Flushing, New York, USA

Philip B. Clement, M.D., F.R.C.P.(C)
Clinical Professor of Pathology
University of British Columbia
Consulting Pathologist
Vancouver General Hospital
Vancouver, British Columbia, Canada

Bernard Czernobilsky, M.D.
Professor of Pathology
Medical School of the Hebrew University and Hadassah
Jerusalem, Israel
Chief
Department of Pathology
Kaplan Hospital
Rehovot, Israel

Alex Ferenczy, M.D.
Professor of Pathology and Obstetrics and Gynecology
McGill University and The Sir Mortimer B. Davis Jewish General Hospital
Head
Gynecologic Pathology and Cytology and Colposcopy
The Sir Mortimer B. Davis Jewish General Hospital
Montreal, Quebec, Canada

Eduard G. Friedrich, Jr., M.D., L.L.D.
W.C. Thomas Professor
Department of Obstetrics and Gynecology
University of Florida School of Medicine
Gainesville, Florida, USA

Deborah J. Gersell, M.D.
Assistant Professor of Pathology
Washington University School of Medicine
Assistant Pathologist
Barnes Hospital
St. Louis, Missouri, USA

Frederick T. Kraus, M.D.
Professor, Pathology (Visiting Staff)
Washington University School of Medicine
Director
Laboratory Medicine
St. John's Mercy Medical Center
St. Louis, Missouri, USA

Robert J. Kurman, M.D.
Professor of Pathology and Obstetrics and Gynecology
Georgetown University School of Medicine
Director
Gynecologic Pathology
Georgetown University Hospital
Washington, D.C., USA

Joseph M. Lombardo, M.D., Ph.D.
Assistant Professor of Pathology
New Jersey Medical School
University of Medicine and Dentistry of New Jersey
Director of Clinical Immunovirology
University Hospital
Newark, New Jersey, USA

June Marchant, Ph.D.
Emeritus Senior Lecturer in the Biology of Cancer
University of Birmingham
Birmingham, England

Michael T. Mazur, M.D.
Associate Professor of Pathology
University of Alabama at Birmingham
Surgical Pathologist
University of Alabama Hospital
Birmingham, Alabama, USA

Henry J. Norris, M.D.
Clinical Professor of Pathology
Uniformed Services University of the Health Sciences
Bethesda, Maryland
Chairman
Department of Gynecologic and Breast Pathology
Armed Forces Institute of Pathology
Washington, D.C., USA

Tim Parmley, M.D.
Associate Professor of Gynecology and Obstetrics
Johns Hopkins University School of Medicine
Obstetrician and Gynecologist
Johns Hopkins Hospital
Baltimore, Maryland, USA

Maureen Burke Riffle, M.D.
Pathologist
De Paul Community Health Center
St. Louis, Missouri, USA

Stanley J. Robboy, M.D.
Chairman and Professor of Pathology
New Jersey Medical School
University of Medicine and Dentistry of New Jersey
Chief
Department of Pathology
University Hospital
Newark, New Jersey, USA

Robert E. Scully, M.D.
Professor of Pathology
Harvard Medical School
Pathologist
Massachusetts General Hospital
Boston, Massachusetts, USA

Alexander Sedlis, M.D.
Professor of Obstetrics and Gynecology
State University of New York, Health Science Center at Brooklyn
Director
Department of Gynecology
Kings County Medical Center
Health Science Center at Brooklyn
Brooklyn, New York, USA

Aleksander Talerman, M.D., Ph.D., F.R.C. Path.
Professor of Pathology and Obstetrics and Gynecology
University of Chicago
Chicago, Illinois, USA

William R. Welch, M.D.
Associate Professor of Pathology
Harvard Medical School
Chief
Gynecologic Surgical Pathology
Brigham and Women's Hospital
Boston, Massachusetts, USA

James E. Wheeler, M.D.
Professor
Departments of Pathology and Laboratory Medicine and Obstetrics and Gynecology
Hospital of the University of Pennsylvania
Philadelphia, Pennsylvania, USA

Edward J. Wilkinson, M.D.
Professor of Pathology and Obstetrics and Gynecology
University of Florida School of Medicine
Director of the Section of Gynecologic Pathology and Cytopathology
Shands Hospital
Gainesville, Florida, USA

Barbara Winkler, M.D.
Assistant Professor of Pathology and Obstetrics, Gynecology and Reproductive Sciences
University of California
Director
Obstetrical and Gynecological Pathology Service
Co-Director, Immunopathology Service
University of California at San Francisco Medical Center
San Francisco, California, USA

ROBERT H. YOUNG, M.D., M.R.C.PATH.
Associate Professor of Pathology
Harvard Medical School
Associate Pathologist
Massachusetts General Hospital
Boston, Massachusetts, USA

CHARLES J. ZALOUDEK, M.D.
Anatomic Pathologist
Alta Bates Hospital
Berkeley, California, USA

1

Embryology of the Female Genital Tract

Tim Parmley, M.D.

Embryologic Development

Early Embryogenesis

The fertilized ovum reaches the uterine cavity in about 4 days as a morula of 12 to 16 cells. After developing a blastocoele and losing the zona pellucida, it implants on approximately the sixth day after conception. By the eighth day, the blastocyst consists of a chorionic membrane containing within it a bilaminar embryonic disk, separating the amniotic and yolk sac cavities. By the 11th or 12th day, the trophoblastic portion of the chorionic membrane shows clear-cut differentiation into cytotrophoblast, intermediate trophoblast, and syncytiotrophoblast.[7]

At the end of the second week of embryonic life, the human embryo is a bilaminar, oval disk approximately 0.2 mm in its longest diameter. The two laminae are the first two germ layers. The dorsal layer is the ectoderm and the ventral layer is the endoderm (Fig. 1.1). The ectoderm is composed of columnar cells with vesicular oval-shaped nuclei and basophilic cytoplasm that are arranged perpendicularly to the plane of the embryonic disk. The ectoderm forms the floor of the amnionic space and is continuous at its edges with the amnion. This germ layer will give rise to the central nervous system, neural crest derivatives, and the epidermal layer of the skin as well as its appendages. In the human female external genitalia, the ectoderm contributes to the epithelium and appendages of the vulvar skin from the internal surface of the labia minora outward. Melanocytes in vulvar skin are migrants from the neural crest.

The endoderm is composed of smaller cells with dense nuclei and clear cytoplasm. It forms the roof of the yolk sac. Endodermal cells continue beyond the border of the disk to line the yolk sac. This germ cell layer will give rise to the gastrointestinal tract epithelium, the respiratory tract epithelium, liver, pancreas, parathyroid and thyroid glands, and several pharyngeal derivatives, as well as possibly to the germ cells. It also gives rise to the epithelium of the bladder, with the exception of the trigone, the epithelium of the anterior but not the posterior wall of the urethra, and the vestibule except for the hymen. Therefore, in the adult female, the epithelium of the vestibule from the urethra posteriorly including the fourchette and from the hymenal ring to the outer edges of the labia minora is endodermal in origin. The appendages of this epithelium are the minor and major vestibular glands.

The third embryonic layer, the mesoderm is derived from the ectoderm during the third week of embryonic life. Proliferating ectodermal cells crowd together in the

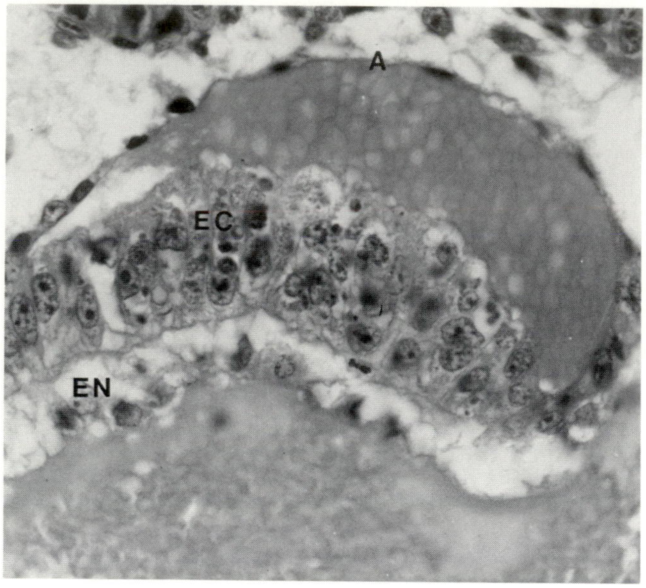

FIG. 1.1. The ectodermal layer (EC) appears multicellular because the section is slightly tangential. The endodermal layer (EN) is composed of small cells with clear cytoplasm. The amnion (A) is separated from the cytotrophoblast at the top of the photomicrograph by a few scattered mesodermal cells.

midline of the posterior portion of the bilaminar disk. At first bulging upward to form the primitive ridge, they subsequently descend into a space between the ectoderm and the endoderm, creating a linear groove called the *primitive streak*. The mesoderm continues to proliferate, separating the ectoderm and endoderm, except in the midline of the anterior portion of the disk at a site termed the *prochordal plate* and in the midline of the posterior portion of the embryo at a site termed the *cloacal plate*. The cloacal plate represents the site of the future anal and urogenital orifices.

The mesoderm gives rise to the musculoskeletal system and other connective tissues. In the genital tract, the mesoderm will give rise to the epithelium and supporting stroma of the coelomic cavity, the gonads (except for the germ cells), the fallopian tubes, the uterus, the cervix, the vagina, the hymenal membrane, the posterior wall of the urethra, and the trigone of the bladder.

During the latter part of the third week of embryonic life, an intramesodermal cavity develops in the lateral portion of the mesodermal layer on both sides of the disk. These bilateral intramesodermal cavities extend cephalad around the prochordal plate to meet in the midline, thus producing a continuous intramesodermal canal that extends around the anterior portion of the embryo. The mesodermal canal forms a cavity, the coelomic cavity, that is destined to become organized into the pericardial, pleural, and peritoneal cavities. The coelomic cavity is lined by flattened mesothelial cells that have epithelium-like features but have differentiated from the underlying stellate, stromal cells. The coelomic epithelium, i.e., the peritoneum, is therefore a mesothelial epithelium that is derived from the mesenchyme immediately beneath it (Fig. 1.2). This raises the possibility of a more intimate biologic relationship between epithelium and stroma in mesodermal systems than is the case where ectodermal or endodermal epithelia are supportd by mesodermal stroma.

By the end of the third week and during the fourth week of embryonic life, the trilaminar disk secondary to differential growth becomes folded into a three-dimensional tubular structure that is recognizable as an embryo (Fig. 1.3). The endoderm now lines an internalized tube that runs dorsally to the caudal pole of the embryo, where it turns ventrally to the umbilicus at the site of the cloacal plate. Thus, both the dorsal and ventral loops of the endodermal tube are separated from the ectoderm, which now surrounds the whole embryo by mesodermal tissue except at the cloacal plate, where the endodermal tube and the ectoderm are fused. The dorsal loop of the endodermal tube will become the lower gastrointestinal tract, and the ventral loop will become the urachus, the bladder, the urethra, and the vestibule. The site

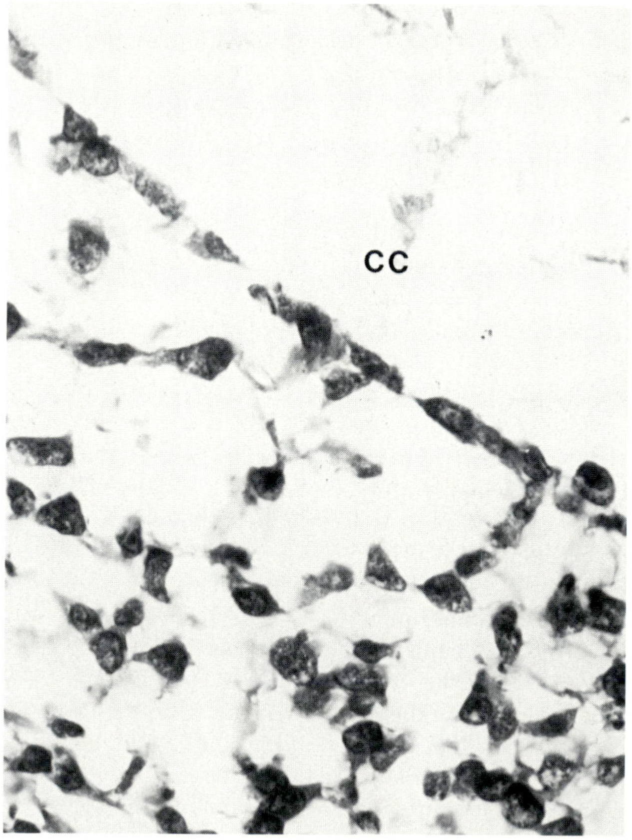

FIG. 1.2. The coelomic (peritoneal) cavity (CC) is lined by mesoderm. On the surface, the mesodermal cells are organized as an epithelium but are identical to the cells of the underlying stroma.

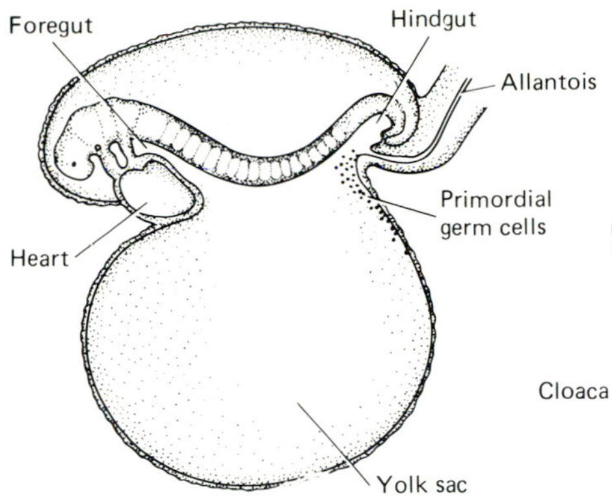

a

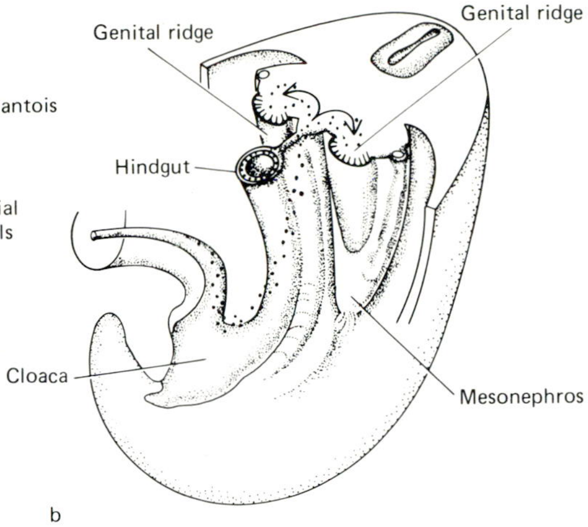

b

FIG. 1.3*a*. Drawing of a 3-week-old embryo showing curved embryo and the primordial germ cells in the wall of the yolk sac, close to the attachment of the allantois. (After Witschi, Ref. 18) *b*. The migration path of the primordial germ cells along the wall of the hindgut and the dorsal mesentery into the genital ridge is shown. Note the position of the genital ridge and mesonephros. (From Sadler TW: Langman's Medical Embryology, 5th ed. Copyright 1985, The Williams & Wilkins Company. Reproduced by permission.)

where the two loops meet is termed the *cloaca*. The coelomic or peritoneal cavity that developed earlier in the lateral mesoderm has now become internalized and lies in the mesoderm between the two endodermal loops. Subsequently, the mesoderm between the two loops, the urorectal septum, extends toward and fuses with the cloacal plate, separating the two loops entirely. The cloacal plate later disintegrates, and each of the loops opens separately onto the surface of the embryo. At this point, the ventral loop is termed the *urogenital sinus*.

In the latter part of the fourth week, a vertical ridge develops on each side of the posterior wall of the coelomic cavity. This ridge, the urogenital ridge (Figs. 1.4 and 1.5), begins cephalad and extends caudad. It is produced by the sequential development of the mesonephric tubules in the posterior wall mesoderm immediately beneath the coelomic epithelium. Whether the epithelium of these tubules is derived partially by invagination of the coelomic epithelium or whether some of it develops in situ is not known, but the result is a series of mesonephric glomeruli all emptying into a single mesonephric duct that runs vertically from cephalad to caudad, connecting the glomeruli at all levels. This duct opens into the urogenital sinus at the site that will eventually be the junction of the urethra and the vestibule.

Before entering the urogenital sinus, the mesonephric ducts give off the ureteric bud that migrates back into the posterior wall mesoderm and induces the development of the definitive kidney. As differential growth of the urogenital sinus occurs, more and more of the wolffian duct is incorporated into the posterior wall of the urogenital sinus (Fig. 1.6). The ureteric buds open separately into the sinus. The net effect is the insertion of a patch of mesoderm into the posterior wall of the urogenital

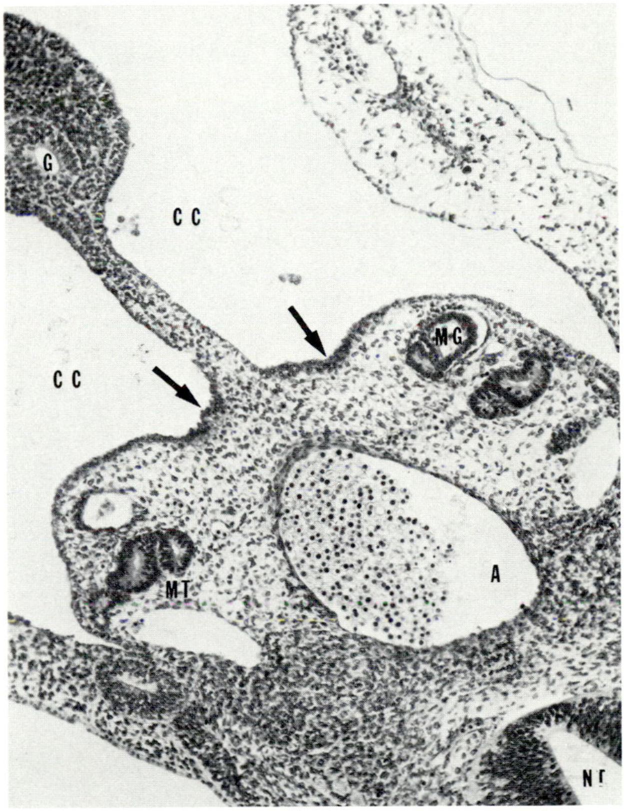

FIG. 1.4. Bilateral urogenital ridges lie in the posterior wall of the coelomic cavity (CC) in this 4-week embryo. In the midline from back to front lie the neural tube (NT), the dorsal aorta (A), and the hindgut (G) suspended in the coelomic cavity by its mesentery. At the angle of the mesentery with the urogenital ridge, the coelomic epithelium (*arrows*) is proliferating to form the indifferent gonad. This epithelium will subsequently invaginate into the urogenital ridge to form the müllerian duct. The mesonephric tubules (MT) and glomeruli (MG) lie within the ridge.

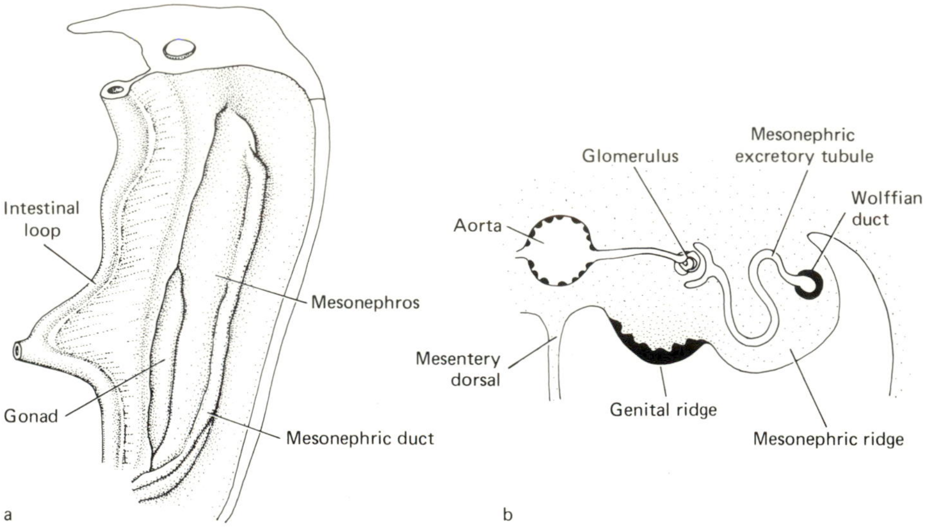

FIG. 1.5.*a*. Drawing of a 5-week embryo showing the relationship between the genital ridge and the mesonephros. Note the location of the mesonephric or wolffian duct. *b*. Transverse section through the mesonephros and genital ridge at a level indicated in *a*. (From Sadler TW, Langman's Medical Embryology, 5th ed. Copyright 1985, The Williams & Wilkins Company. Reproduced by permission.)

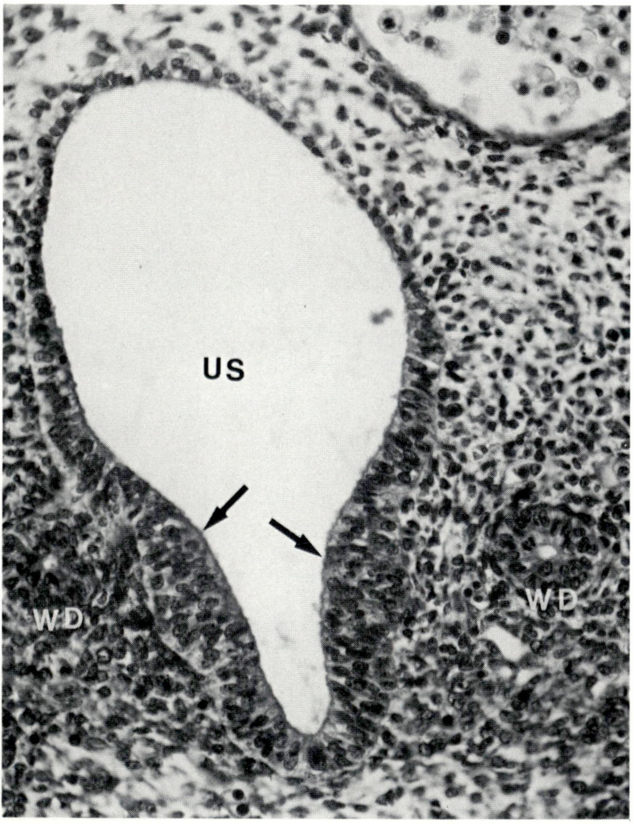

FIG. 1.6. The urogenital sinus (US) lies between the two umbilical arteries immediately behind the anterior abdominal wall outside of field at the top of the illustration. Note that its anterior and posterior walls are composed of different types of epithelium. The epithelium of the posterior wall (*arrows*) is similar to the epithelium of the wolffian duct (WD), which is entering the sinus on the left of the illustration.

sinus, which is elsewhere lined by endoderm (Fig. 1.7). The patch eventually encompasses the trigone of the bladder, the posterior wall of the urethra, and that portion of the vestibule that constitutes the hymenal membrane. This patch of mesodermal epithelium is distinctly different from the endoderm that lines the rest of the urogenital sinus, i.e., the future bladder, anterior urethral wall, and the vestibular epithelium peripheral to the hymen.

Gonadal Development

Late in the fourth week, the primordial germ cells characterized by large clear cells with vesicular nuclei may be identified in the wall of the yolk sac. During the fifth and sixth weeks of embryonic life, they migrate via the mesentery of the hindgut into the medial portion of the urogenital ridge[18] (Figs. 1.3 and 1.8). In conjunction with the arrival of the primordial germ cells into the site, the mesodermal epithelium on the medial surface of the urogenital ridge begins to proliferate (Fig. 1.9). This proliferation will produce the epithelium of the eventual gonad. In the presence of XY chromosomes, early in the sixth week of embryonic life, the proliferating surface cells differentiate into so-called sex cords, cords of epithelial cells that extend from the surface of the gonad into the medulla (Figs. 1.10 and 1.11). Subsequently, a capsule (tunica albuginea) develops and separates these epithelial cords from the surface. The cords become the testicular tubules as the epithelial cells differentiate into the tall, clear, flask-shaped Sertoli cells of the testis (Fig. 1.12). The gonadal stromal cells become the interstitial or Leydig cells (Fig. 1.12). In normal

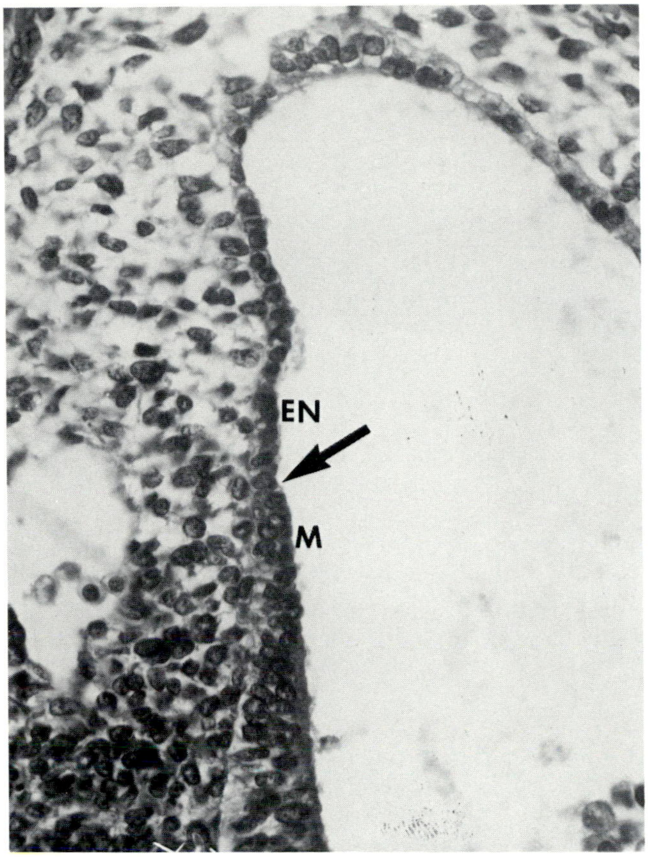

FIG. 1.7. The junction (*arrow*) between the mesodermal epithelium (M) and the endodermal epithelium (EN) in the posterior wall of the urogenital sinus is shown.

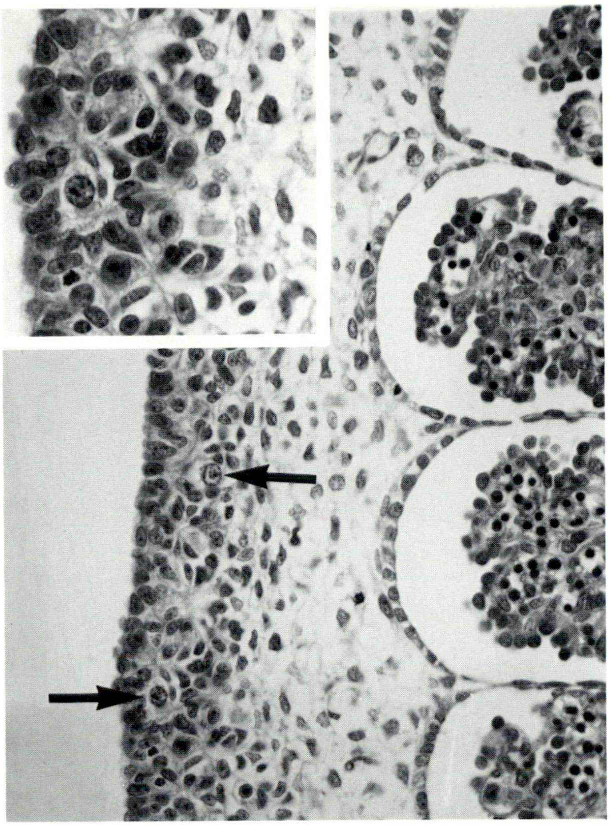

FIG. 1.8. The urogenital ridge. Beneath the surface epithelium is a thickened layer of cells investing two germ cells (*arrows*). The mesonephric glomeruli are below. *Inset*. Surrounding a germ cell is a compact layer of cells closely resembling the surface layer.

development, the germ cells are incorporated within the tubules.

If the genetic constitution is 46XX, the dividing germ cells become incorporated into a proliferating mass of surface epithelial cells (Figs. 1.13 and 1.14). This results in a thickened cortex presaging the organization of the adult ovary. From the second trimester to the early third trimester, this thickened cortical mass of proliferating epithelial and germ cells is divided into small groups by strands of stromal tissue extending from the medulla to the cortex. The small groups of germ cells and epithelial cells are further subdivided into primordial follicles composed of a single germ cell surrounded by a layer of epithelial cells, the primitive granulosa. In normal development, each germ cell is characteristically encapsulated in its own follicle. This is associated with entry into meiosis and no further proliferation.

If the genetic constitution is 46XY, some of the early epithelial proliferation will contribute to the connection between the sex cords and the mesonephric tubules. In the case of the gonad destined to become an ovary, early proliferation degenerates in the ovarian hilum, leav-

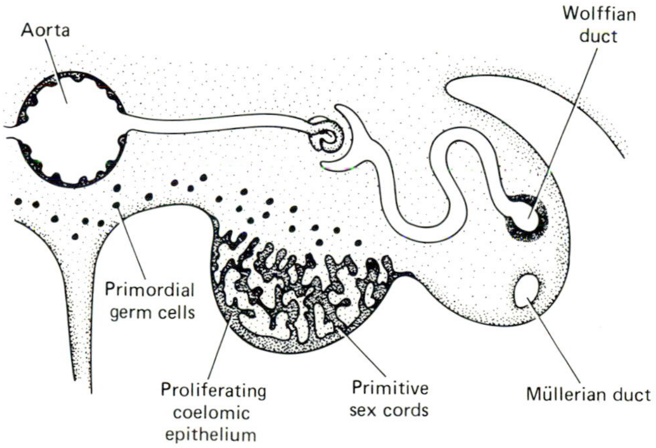

FIG. 1.9. Transverse section through the lumbar region of a 6-week embryo, showing the indifferent gonad with the primitive sex cords probably derived from proliferating coelomic epithelium. Some of the primordial germ cells are surrounded by cells of the primitive sex cords. (From Sadler TW, Langman's Medical Embryology, 5th ed. Copyright 1985, The Williams & Wilkins Company. Reproduced by permission.)

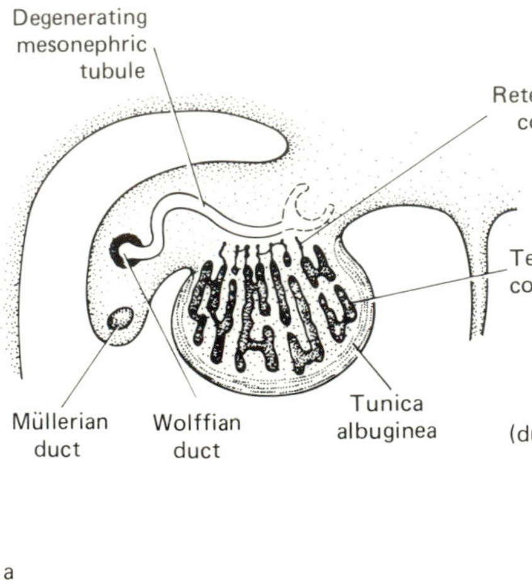

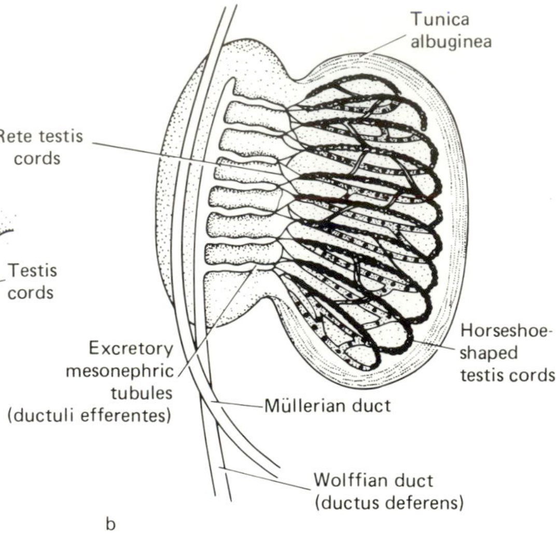

FIG. 1.10.*a*. Transverse section through the testis is in the eighth week of development. Note the tunica albuginea, the testis cords, the rete testis, and the primordial germ cells. The glomerulus and Bowman's capsule of the mesonephric excretory tubule are in regression. *b*. The testis and the genital ducts in the fourth month of development. The horseshoe-shaped testis cords are continuous with the rete testis cords. Note the ductuli efferentes (excretory mesonephric tubules), which enter the wolffian duct. (From Sadler TW, Langman's Medical Embryology, 5th ed. Copyright 1985, The Williams & Wilkins Company. Reproduced by permission.)

ing a few tubules, termed the *rete ovarii* (Fig. 1.15). Interstitial or Leydig cells develop extensively in the stromal tissue of the second-trimester female gonad but degenerate in most cases by term.[9] A few may be found in the hilum of the adult ovary, where they may be associated with the rete ovarii and are called *hilus cells*. Thus, the gonad develops primarily from mesodermal

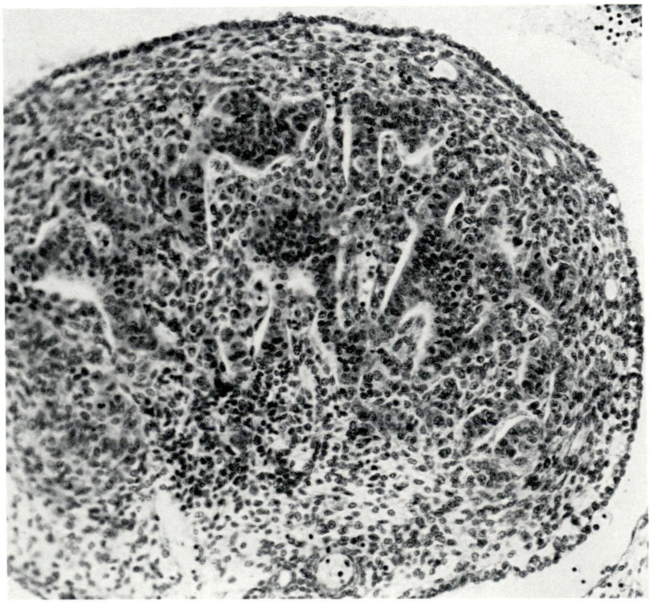

FIG. 1.11. Columns of epithelial cells form cords in this early testis.

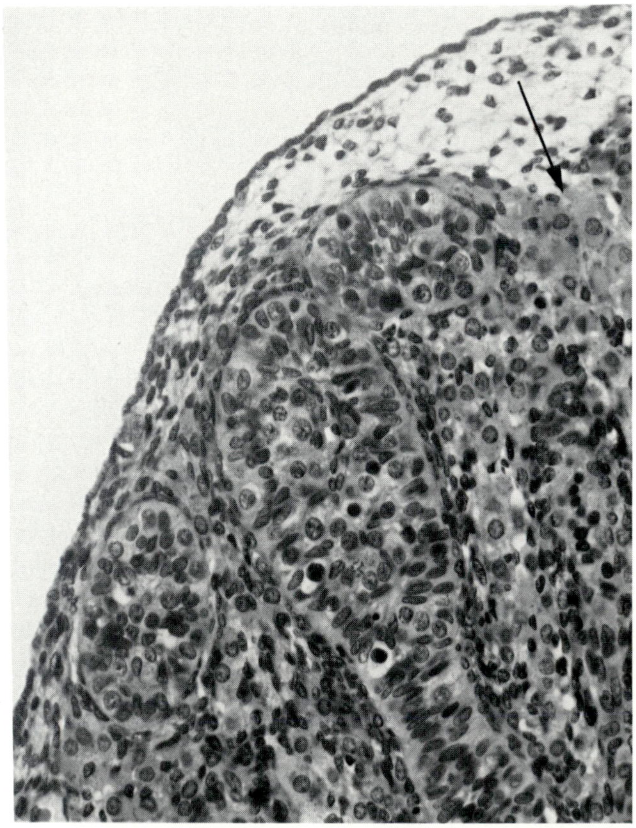

FIG. 1.12. The epithelial cords are destined to become the testicular tubules and contain the Sertoli cells. Between the cords are the interstitial cells, some of which contain abundant eosinophilic cytoplasm characteristic of Leydig cells (*arrow*). The surface is differentiating into a capsule.

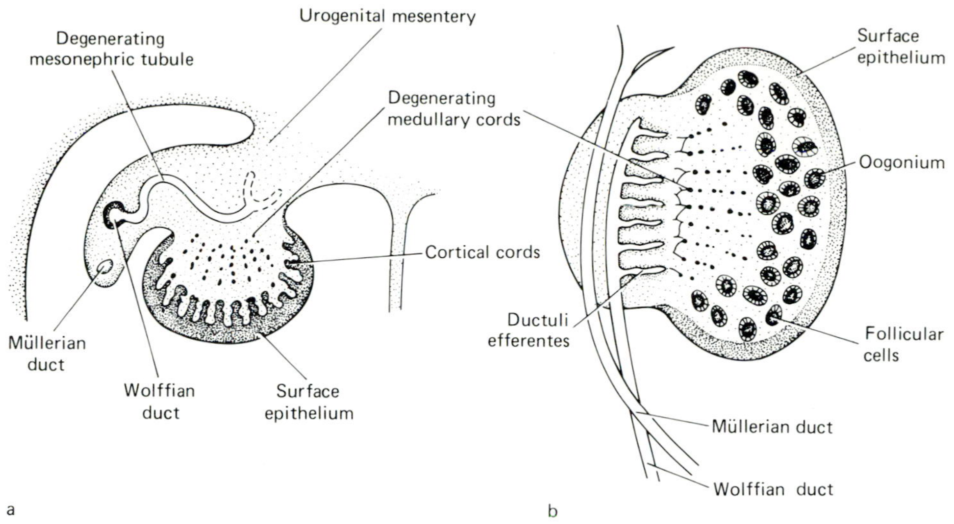

FIG. 1.13. *a*. Transverse section through the ovary at the seventh week of development, showing the degeneration of the primitive (medullary) sex cords and the formation of the cortical cords. *b*. The ovary and genital ducts in the fifth month of development. Note the degeneration of the medullary cords. The excretory mesonephric tubules (ductuli efferentes) do not communicate with the rete. The cortical zone of the ovary contains groups of oogonia surrounded by follicular cells. (From Sadler TW, Langman's Medical Embryology, 5th ed. Copyright 1985, The Williams & Wilkins Company. Reproduced by permission.)

tissues, with the exception of the germ cells, which are endodermal in origin.

Müllerian and Wolffian Duct Development

Late in the fifth to sixth week of embryonic life, the coelomic epithelium invaginates at several points on the lateral surface of the urogenital ridge, and coalesces to form a tube termed the *müllerian* or *paramesonephric*

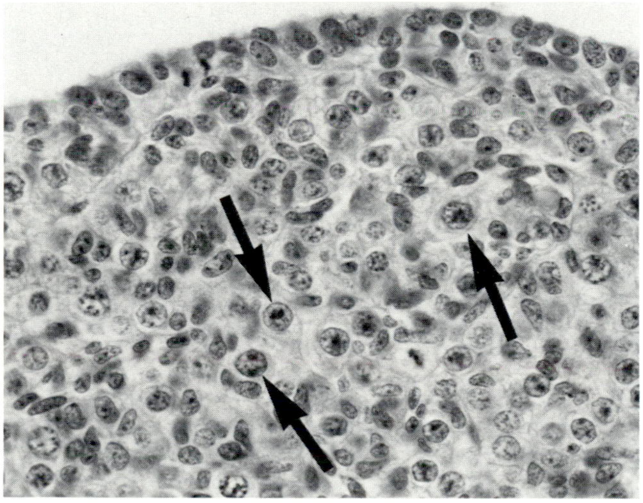

FIG. 1.14. There are no sex cords in this early ovary, only intermingled germ cells (*arrows*) and epithelial cells. The latter will eventually invest the germ cells to form individual follicles.

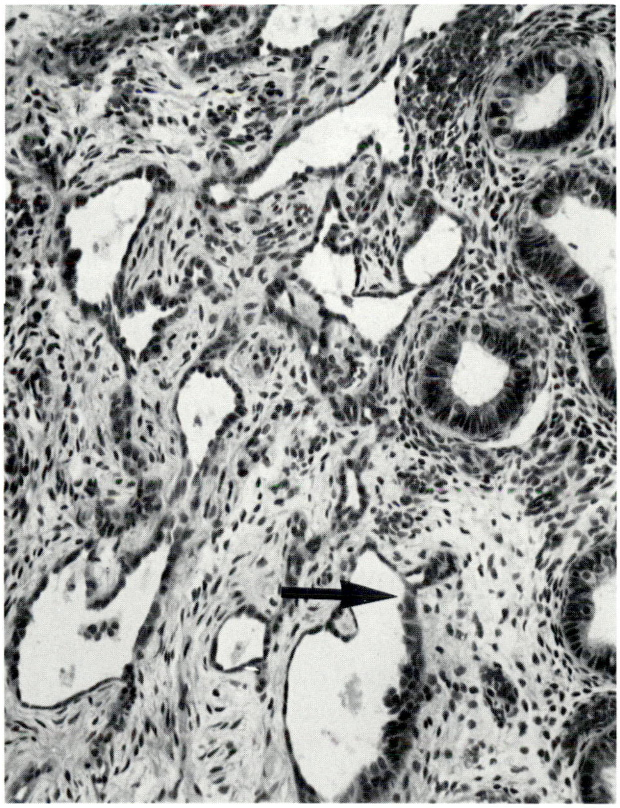

FIG. 1.15. This is the hilus of an ovotestis. Thin walled tubules at the top of the picture are of surface origin and correspond to the rete ovarii of the normal ovary. At the bottom are the mesonephric tubules, and a possible junction of the two is seen to the left (*arrow*).

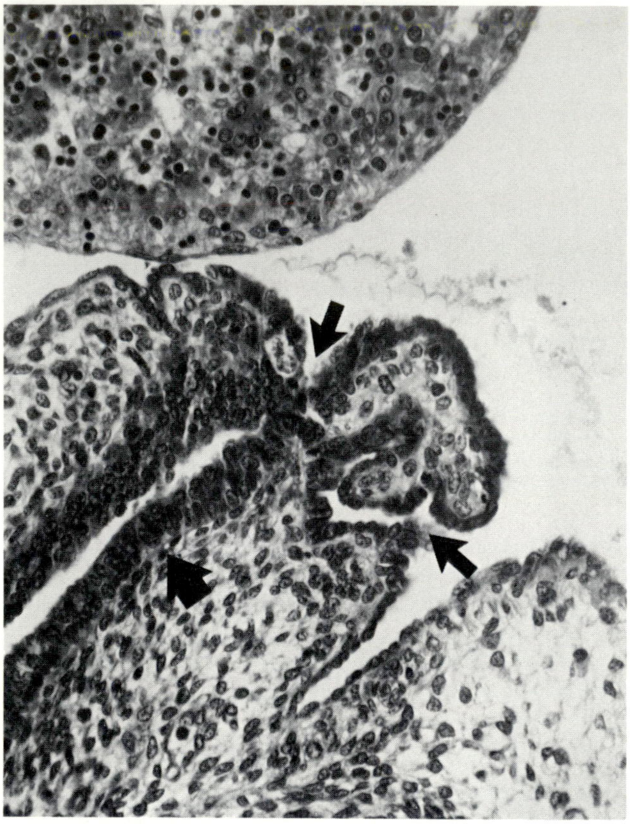

FIG. 1.16. The coelomic epithelium on the lateral surface of the urogenital ridge proliferates and forms several invaginations (*narrow arrows*), which coalesce to form the müllerian duct (*wide arrow*).

duct (Fig. 1.16). The duct extends caudally in the urogenital ridge immediately lateral to the wolffian duct (Fig. 1.17). The paired müllerian ducts give rise to the fallopian tubes, uterus, cervix, and upper vagina. The müllerian ducts follow the wolffian ducts so closely that some embryologists believe that the müllerian duct tip is actually within the basement membrane of the epithelium of the wolffian duct.[6] For proper müllerian duct migration to occur, it is essential that the wolffian duct be present.[11] At first lateral to the wolffian ducts, the müllerian ducts cross over to lie medial to them as they enter the pelvis (Figs. 1.17, 1.18, and 1.19). By the end of the seventh week of embryonic life, the müllerian ducts between the two wolffian ducts fuse to form a single structure (Fig. 1.20). The tip of the müllerian duct abuts upon the posterior wall of the urogenital sinus immediately between the two orifices of the wolffian ducts.[13] (Fig. 1.21). It is important that the point where the tip of the müllerian duct abuts on the posterior wall of the urogenital sinus is within the patch of mesoderm inserted into the wall of the sinus by the wolffian ducts. This point defines the site of the future vaginal orifice, the hymenal membrane.

The patch of mesodermal urogenital sinus epithelium lying between the orifices of the two wolffian ducts, in response to the apposition of the müllerian duct tip, begins to proliferate. A column of squamous epithelial cells is formed, termed the *vaginal plate*, which displaces the tip of the müllerian duct from the wall of the urogenital sinus. In contrast to previous opinions, recent studies suggest that the vaginal plate and müllerian duct are patent early in the second trimester. The vaginal plate will give rise to the lower two-thirds of the vagina[1,4] (Fig. 1.22). The fused müllerian duct will give rise to the upper third of the vagina, the cervix, and the fundus of the uterus (Fig. 1.23). Only in the vaginal portion is the columnar epithelium converted into squamous epithelium, probably as a result of stromal events.[8,13,16,17]

As early as the end of the first trimester,[13] there is a

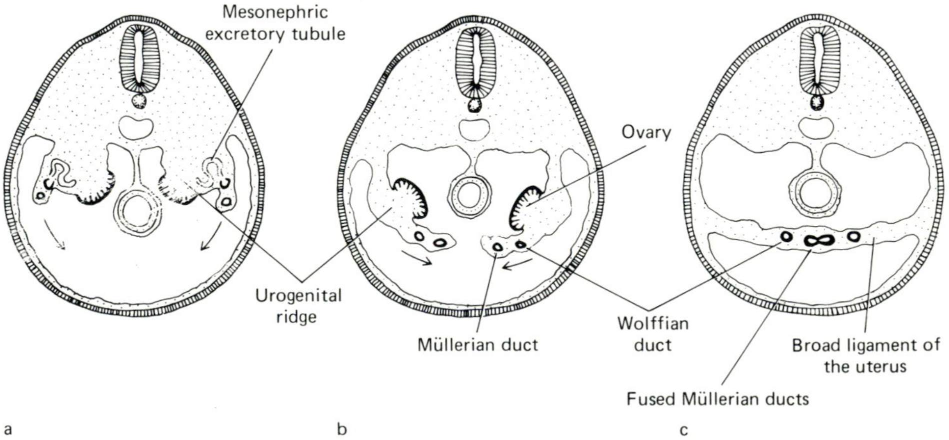

FIG. 1.17. Transverse sections through the urogenital ridge at progressively lower levels (*a*, *b*, *c*). Note that the müllerian ducts approach each other in the midline and fuse. As a result of the fusion of the ducts, a transverse fold, the broad ligament of the uterus, is formed in the pelvis. The gonads come to lie at the posterior aspect of the transverse fold. (From Sadler TW, Langman's Medical Embryology, 5th ed. Copyright 1985, The Williams & Wilkins Company. Reproduced by permission.)

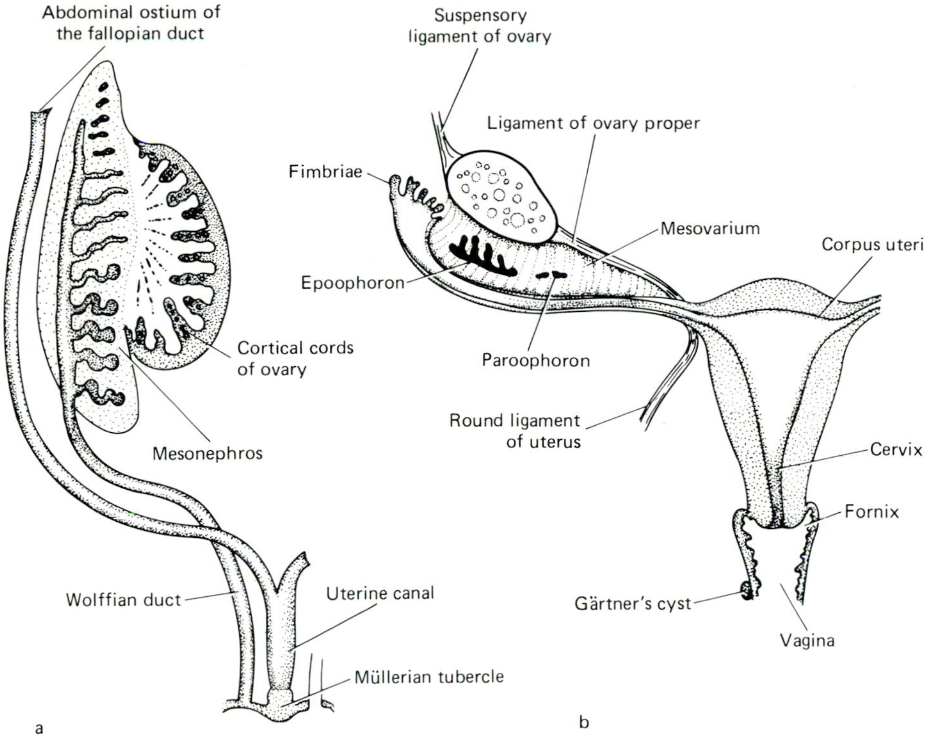

FIG. 1.18.*a*. The genital ducts in the female at the end of the second month of development. Note the müllerian tubercle and the formation of the uterine canal. *b*. The genital ducts after descent of the ovary. The only parts remaining of the mesonephric system are the epoophoron, the paroophoron, and Gartner's cyst. Note the suspensory ligament of the ovary, the ligament of the ovary proper, and the round ligament of the uterus. (From Sadler TW, Langman's Medical Embryology, 5th ed. Copyright 1985, The Williams & Wilkins Company. Reproduced by permission.)

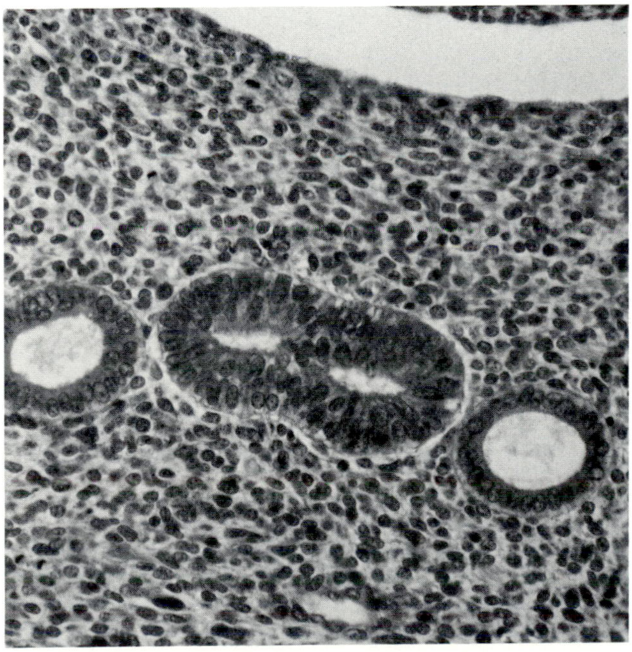

FIG. 1.19. The two müllerian ducts between the two wolffian ducts have met but have not yet fused.

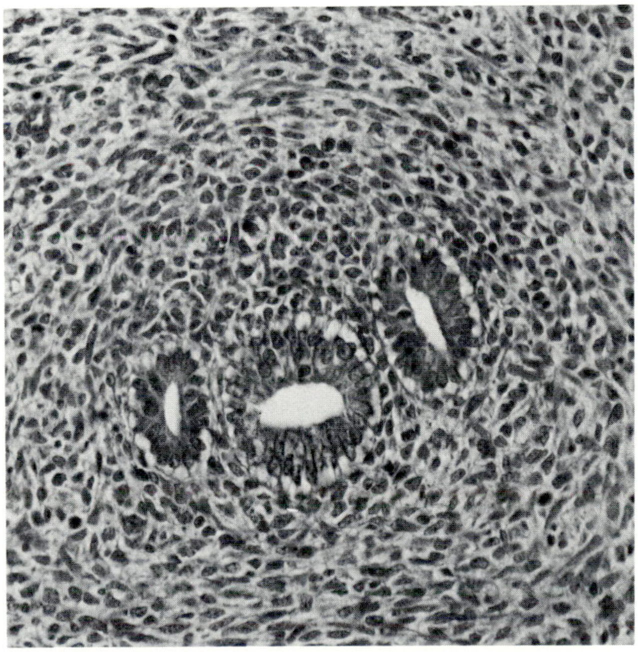

FIG. 1.20. The müllerian ducts have fused into a single structure lying between the two wolffian ducts.

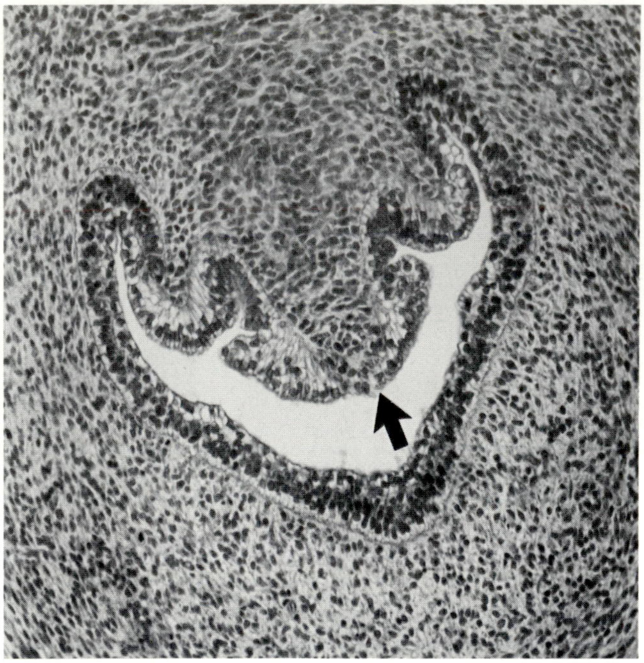

FIG. 1.21. The urogenital sinus at the level of the müllerian tubercle. The müllerian duct contacts the urogenital sinus at this site (*arrow*). The epithelium of the anterior and of the posterior walls of the sinuses is dissimilar.

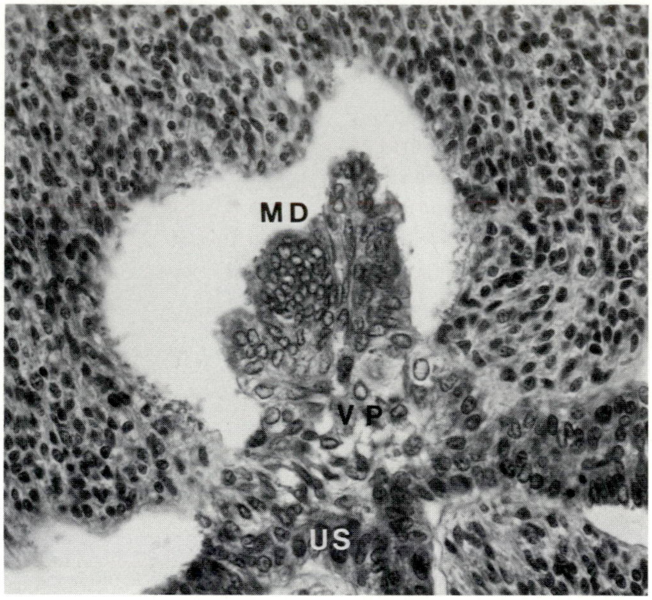

FIG. 1.22. At the bottom of the field is the posterior wall of the urogenital sinus (US). In the center, the cells are beginning to mature into squamous cells, the very early vaginal plate (VP). At the top, in the center of the vaginal plate, is a small collection of nuclei, which is the tip of the müllerian duct (MD).

mesenchymal thickening around that portion of the fused müllerian duct that is destined to become the endocervix. This mesenchymal thickening includes the wolffian ducts, so that remnants of the latter, which persist into adulthood, are found within the body of the cervix. At all other levels of the genital canal, remnants of the wolffian ducts are external to the wall of the adult müllerian derivative. By 26 weeks of gestational age, the cervix is about 20 mm in length, and the mesenchymal thickening that forms its wall is sufficiently rigid that it is no longer functionally patent when studied by silicone injection techniques.[16] It is tempting to speculate that this functional cervical barrier, by preventing any component of the external (amniotic fluid) environment from migrating into the endocervical canal, inhibits the transformation of the mucus-secreting epithelium of the endocervix into squamous epithelium and thereby determines the site of the squamocolumnar junction. Certainly, it is

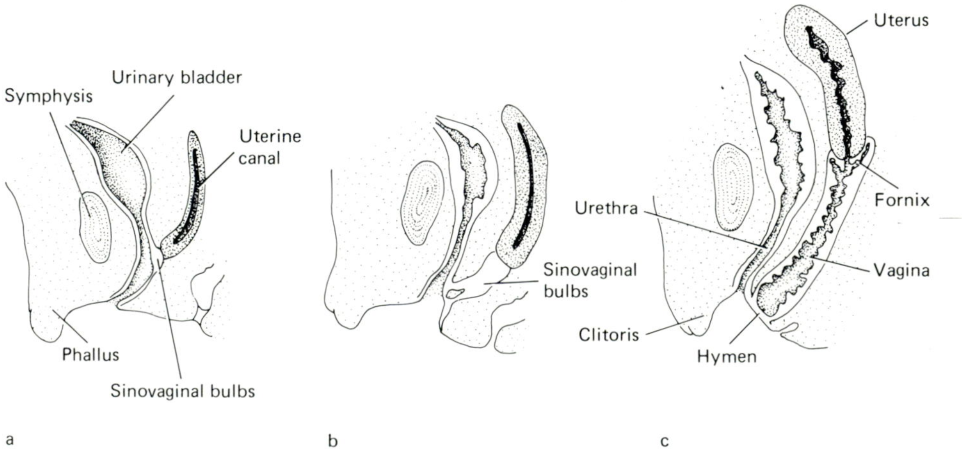

FIG. 1.23. Sagittal sections showing the formation of the uterus and vagina at various stages of development (*a*, *b*, *c*). (From Sadler TW, Langman's Medical Embryology, 5th ed. Copyright 1985, The Williams & Wilkins Company. Reproduced by permission.)

clear that in the adult, if at any point the mucus-secreting epithelium is everted into the vagina, it is converted to squamous epithelium.[10] Also, when complete transverse vaginal septae persist, the upper vagina remains lined by mucin-secreting epithelium (Fig. 1.24).

The development of the stromal component of the genital canal has not been well studied but is undoubtedly of major importance.[2,12,15–17] In addition to its role in the development of the walls of the tubular muscular organs, there is extensive experimental evidence to indicate that the stroma directs epithelial development as well.[12] Thus, the entire structure of the vagina, cervix, uterus, and tubes is determined by stromal–epithelial interaction.

Smooth muscle appears in the walls of the genital canal between 18 and 20 weeks, and by approximately 24 weeks, the muscular portion of the uterine wall is well developed.[13] Vaginal, uterine, and tubal muscular walls develop around the müllerian duct alone, so that the wolffian duct remnants are external to the true wall of the canal. Cervical glands appear at about 15 weeks and rudimentary endometrial glands by 19 weeks, but the endometrium is not well developed even at term in most infants.

External Genitalia Development

The urogenital sinus into which the vagina opens enlarges as the embryo grows, so that it becomes the vestibule

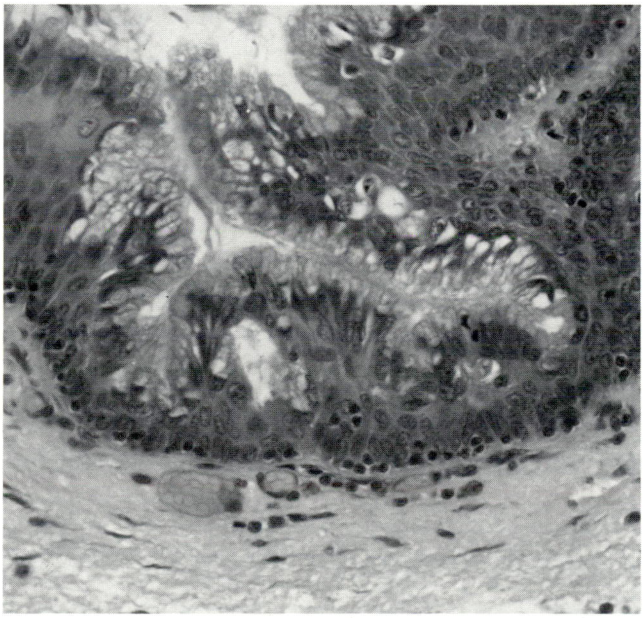

FIG. 1.24. The mucin-producing epithelium on the upper surface of this transverse vaginal septum is being replaced by metaplastic epithelium.

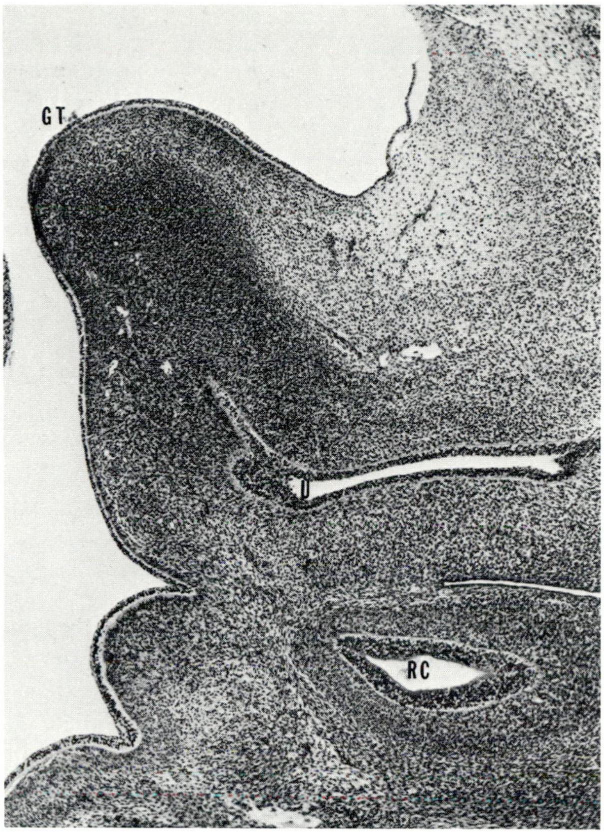

FIG. 1.25. This section, not quite in the midline, shows a portion of the rectal canal (RC) and a portion of the bladder and urethra (U). A tiny slit in the mesoderm between the two represents the coelomic cavity. The müllerian structures are not in the plane of the illustration but would lie in the mesoderm between the coelom and the bladder. The genital tubercle (GT) protrudes down.

of the adult external genitalia (Fig. 1.23). Consequently, the vestibule is lined, except for a variable portion anterior to the urethral orifice, by the endodermal epithelium of the urogenital sinus. This is clinically important in that endodermal-derived epithelium not only is different morphologically from either the mesodermal or ectodermal-derived epithelium but also responds differently to a variety of stimuli, notably sex steroids.

The form of the external genitalia results from events that began during the fourth embryonic week in the mesodermal stroma immediately lateral and ventral to the cloacal plate.[3] Just ventral to the plate, the stroma produces a rounded elevation of the ectoderm, the genital tubercle (Fig. 1.25). Immediately lateral to the cloacal plate, two parallel folds develop by the same mechanism (Fig. 1.26). The most medial is the urogenital fold that is destined to become the labium minus. The more lateral is the labioscrotal fold, which becomes the labium majus.

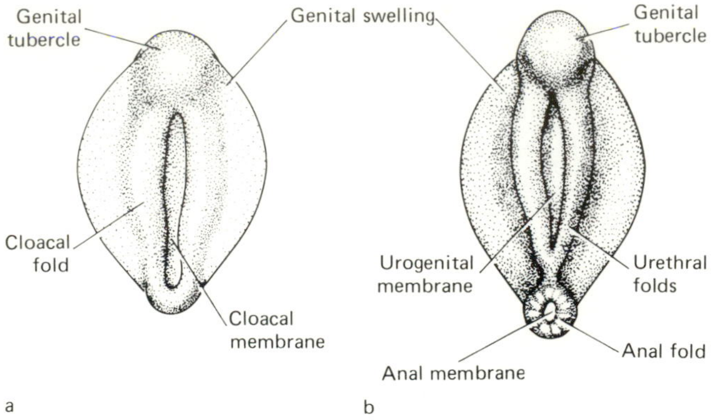

FIG. 1.26. The indifferent stage of the external genitalia (*a*) at approximately 4 weeks and (*b*) at approximately 6 weeks. (From Sadler TW, Langman's Medical Embryology, 5th ed. Copyright 1985, The Williams & Wilkins Company. Reproduced by permission.)

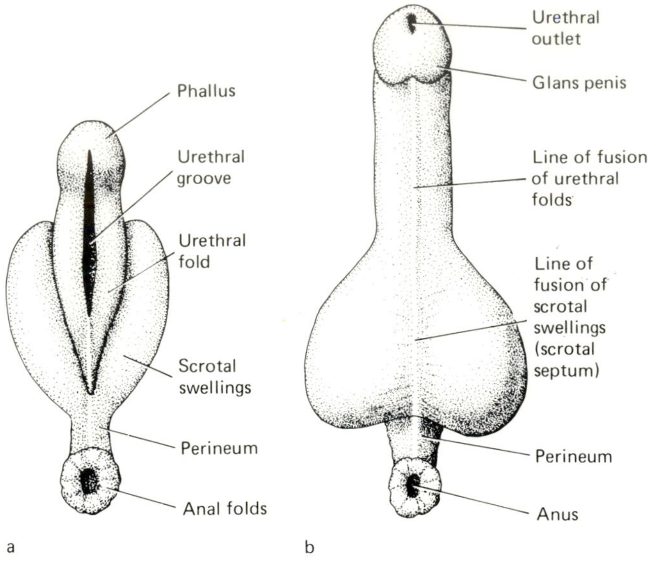

FIG. 1.27.*a*. Development of the external genitalia in the male at 10 weeks. Note the deep urethral groove flanked by the urethral folds. *b*. In the newborn. (From Sadler TW, Langman's Medical Embryology, 5th ed. Copyright 1985, The Williams & Wilkins Company. Reproduced by permission.)

The labioscrotal fold extends cranially around the genital tubercle and fuses with its partner on the other side, becoming the mons pubis. At the end of the sixth week, the urorectal septum fuses with the cloacal plate, thus dividing this structure into the anal membrane posteriorly and the urogenital membrane ventrally. The lateral folds are primarily distributed in relation to the urogenital membrane. In both the male and female, the lateral folds fuse across the midline in front of the anus. In the male, the fusion moves ventrally in zipper-like fashion. The urogenital folds fuse to form a portion of the wall of the penile urethra, and the labioscrotal folds fuse to form the scrotum (Fig. 1.27). As female differentiation is the absence of this fusion, it may be difficult to detect, although by the end of the first trimester, significant fusion should have occurred in a male fetus.

Clinical and Pathologic Implications of Embryologic Development

An appreciation of the embryologic development of the female genital tract permits an understanding of some of the clinicopathologic aspects of gynecologic diseases. These range from various types of congenital anomalies to neoplasms. The variable effects of steroid hormones on different parts of the genital tract, both in utero and in adulthood, can also be better understood in the context of embryologic events.

The most significant anomalies of the gonads are associated with failure of the germ cells to develop in the urogenital ridge. In general, the amount and type of gonadal tissue that develops is a reflection of the number and viability of the germ cells that reach this site. A spectrum of disease from streak or absent gonads to ovaries that lead to premature menopause may result. The normal migration of germ cells from the yolk sac epithelium involves their lateral displacement from the midline of the embryo to the urogenital ridges (Fig. 1.3) and their investment by gonadal epithelium. Failure to reach their normal location leaves them subject to premature death. An arrest in the normal migration may result in germ cells remaining in the midline of the embryo that may subsequently undergo neoplastic transformation. This accounts for the distribution of extragonadal germ cell tumors in midline structures, such as the retroperitoneum, mediastinum, and pineal region. Abnormal encapsulation even within the gonad, such as in gonadoblastoma, leaves them subject to abnormal proliferation.

The genital ducts and external genitalia develop as a result of circulating hormones in utero.[5] A nonsteroidal compound, termed *müllerian-inhibiting substance* (MIS), secreted by the fetal testes inhibits the development of the müllerian ducts and potentiates the development of the wolffian ducts. The fetal testes also secrete androgens that stimulate the development of the external genitalia as well as the central nervous system. If the fetal gonads are ovaries, MIS is not produced, and therefore the müllerian ducts develop and the wolffian ducts regress. In the absence of androgens, the indifferent external genitalia differentiate in a female direction.

Based on these considerations, the complex group of disorders related to abnormal gonadal development, so-called intersex disorders, can be understood. For example, patients with testicular feminization are phenotypic females but have a 46XY chromosome complement and testes. MIS is synthesized by the fetal testes, so the müllerian ducts are suppressed and the wolffian ducts are stimulated. Consequently, the uterus and fallopian tubes fail to develop but the ductus deferens is present. Although androgens are secreted by the testes, the genital end organ tissues are unresponsive to them, and therefore the external genitalia differentiate in a female direction. A detailed discussion of the various disorders related to abnormalities of sexual differentiation is presented in Chapter 2, Abnormal Sexual Development.

Other congenital abnormalities, unrelated to the action of hormones, arise from faulty morphogenesis and result in genital tract malformations, such as accessory tubal orifices, bicornuate uterus, or vaginal septae. These anomalies result from lack of fusion of the müllerian ducts or lack of degeneration of the solid vaginal plate and are discussed in greater detail in Chapter 10, Benign Diseases of Endometrium. Urinary tract abnormalities are also frequently associated with müllerian duct anomalies. Improper development of the wolffian ducts results in failure of proper migration of the müllerian ducts. Thus, the urinary tract anomaly is primary, and the genital tract anomaly is secondary.[11] Patients who are found to have müllerian duct-related abnormalities should, therefore, have an intravenous pyelogram performed in order to assess the status of the urinary tract.

The anatomic abnormalities induced by in utero diethylstilbestrol exposure can be understood based on the embryologic development of both the lower and upper genital tract.[8,14,15] Diethylstilbestrol inhibits the development of the vaginal plate, resulting in the müllerian duct component of the vagina being lower in the adult canal than is normally the case. This results in the presence of columnar, müllerian type epithelium as far down the vagina as the hymenal ring in extreme cases. Diethylstilbestrol also disorganizes the stromal differentiation, which is responsible for the gross structure of the cervix, uterus, and tubes. This accounts for the gross structural anomalies of the cervix, such as the cervical collar, pseudopolyp, and hood, as well as the uterine deformities, such as the T-shaped endometrial cavity, that may be encountered in these women.

Within broad limits, the embryologic development of a given tissue defines the spectrum of neoplastic and metaplastic variation seen within that tissue. For example, endocervical adenocarcinomas display a spectrum of histologic patterns that are similar to those observed in adenocarcinomas elsewhere in the upper genital canal, since all the primary tissues are of mesodermal origin. On the other hand, they do not resemble primary adenocarcinomas that arise in the ectodermal skin of the vulva, such as sweat gland tumors. Similarly, adenocarcinomas that arise in the Bartholin's gland are of endodermal origin and more closely resemble tumors of other endodermal sites, such as the salivary glands.

An awareness of the embryology of the peritoneal and müllerian duct epithelium is important in understanding the histogenesis of mesenchymal tumors of the uterus and the histologic features of the common epithelial tumors of the ovary. The müllerian duct develops as an invagination of coelomic epithelium, which in turn arises from the underlying mesenchyme. Thus, the epithelium and the stroma of the upper canal show a particularly intimate relationship not characteristic of epithelium and supportive tissues that are derived from two different germ layers. It is believed that not only during embryogenesis but also in adult life, epithelium may be generated from undifferentiated stromal cells in the endocervix and possibly in the endometrium.[10] Mesenchymal tumors presumably also arise from a stem cell that may display all the histologic features to which that stem cell gives rise in development. Examples are the biphasic tumors, such as adenosarcomas, carcinosarcomas, and mixed mesodermal tumors.

The development of the müllerian duct from the coelomic (peritoneal) epithelium also provides an embryologic basis for the histologic appearance and distribution of the common epithelial tumors of the ovary. Thus, the classification of these tumors into histologic types simulating müllerian-derived tissues, such as serous (tubal-related), mucinous (endocervical-related), and endometrioid (endometrial-related), is a reflection of the common origin of the peritoneal epithelium and the müllerian ducts. The multifocal origin of some ovarian carcinomas and the existence of extraovarian carcinomas extensively involving the peritoneum and omentum with only superficial involvement of the ovaries can be similarly explained (see Chapter 17, Endometriosis). The emerging realization that most tumor markers for ovarian epithelial neoplasia will be found in association with epithelial neoplasms at other sites in the canal is a predictable result in view of their common embryogenesis.

The various heterotopias or metaplasias are also reflections of the common origin of the genital tract. The differing adult histologic features of the vagina, endocervix, endometrium, tube, and peritoneal cavity are the result of local differentiation. Metaplasias, such as endocervical-type mucinous or tubal epithelium, in the endometrium are not unusual and are discussed more fully in Chapter 11, Endometrial Hyperplasia and Metaplasia. The most clinically important of the heterotopias is endometriosis (see Chapter 17, Endometriosis).

A variety of biologic features of the adult genital canal are understood better in a developmental context. For example, the bladder trigone and posterior urethra participate with the vagina both in the atrophy that follows estrogen deprivation and in the recovery that results from estrogen replacement. In contrast, the remainder of the bladder and the vestibule, which are of endodermal origin, do not respond.

References

1. Cunha GR (1975) The dual origin of vaginal epithelium. Am J Anat 143: 387
2. Cunha GR, Shannon JM, Neubauer BL, Sawyer LM, Fujii S, Taguchi O, Chung LWK (1981) Mesenchymal–epithelial interactions in sex differentiation. Hum Genet 58: 68
3. England MA (1983) Color atlas of life before birth. Chicago, Year Book Medical Publishers, Inc., pp 157–162
4. Forsberg JG (1973) Cervicovaginal epithelium: Its origin and development. Am J Obstet Gynecol 115:1025
5. Jost A (1971) Embryonic sexual differentiation (morphology, physiology, abnormalities). In: Jones H Jr, Scott WW (eds). Hermaphroditism, genital anomalies and related endocrine disorders, 2nd ed. Baltimore, Williams & Wilkins, p 16
6. Gruenwald P (1941) The relation of growing müllerian duct to the wolffian duct and its importance for the genesis of malformations. Anat Rec 81: 1
7. Hertig AT (1968) Human trophoblast. Springfield, Ill., Charles C Thomas
8. Kaufman RH, Adam E, Binder GL, Gerthoffer E (1980) Upper genital tract changes and pregnancy outcome in offspring exposed in utero to diethylstilbestrol. Am J Obstet Gynecol 137: 299
9. Konishi I, Fujii S, Okamura H, Parmley T, Mori T (1986) Development and regression of interstitial cells in the human fetal ovary: An ultrastructural study. J Anat 148: 121
10. Lawrence WD, Shingleton HM (1980) Early physiologic squamous metaplasia of the cervix: Light and electron microscopic observations. Am J Obstet Gynecol 137: 661
11. Marshall FF, Beisel DS (1978) The association of uterine and renal anomalies. Obstet Gynecol 51: 559
12. Mauger A, Demarchez M, Sengel P (1984) Role of extracellular matrix and of dermal–epidermal junction architecture in skin development. Prog Clin Biol Res (Matrices and Cell Differentiations) 151: 115
13. O'Rahilly R (1973) The embryology and anatomy of the uterus. In: Norris H, Hertig A (eds). The uterus. Baltimore Williams & Wilkins
14. Robboy SJ (1983) A hypothetic mechanism of diethylstilbestrol (DES)-induced anomalies in exposed progeny. Hum Pathol 14: 831
15. Robboy SJ, Taguchi O, Cunha GR (1982) Normal development of the human female reproductive tract and alterations resulting from experimental exposure to diethylstilbestrol. Hum Pathol 13: 190
16. Terruhn V (1980) A study of impression moulds of the genital tract of female fetuses. Arch Gynecol 229: 207
17. Valdes-Dapena MA (1973) The development of the uterus in late fetal life, infancy and childhood. In: Norris H, Hertig A (eds). Baltimore, Williams & Wilkins
18. Witschi E (1948) Migration of the germ cells of human embryos from the yolk sac to the primitive gonadal folds. Contrib Embryol 32: 67

2

Disorders of Abnormal Sexual Development

Stanley J. Robboy, M.D., Joseph M. Lombardo, M.D., Ph.D., and William R. Welch, M.D.

New insights into the biology of sexual development and advances in chromosome analysis have led to early identification and prompt treatment of the intersexual patient, which permit the person to lead a more normal life.[39] Based on these recent advances, we developed a classification of abnormal sexual development that correlates the gonadal and genital anatomy with the chromosomal findings and specific genetic or metabolic defects[69] (Table 2.1). This allows an integrated approach to this complex group of disorders according to the presenting signs as well as the pathophysiologic basis of the defect. The classification also groups patients who are at high risk for development of gonadal neoplasia.

Embryology of Sexual Development

Human genetic sex is established at conception; the homogametic state (XX) is considered female and the heterogametic state (XY) is considered male.[36] Table 2.2 details the chronologic development of the normal male and female genital tracts. Fig. 2.1 illustrates that the development is determined by several factors, all of which are time-specific during embryogenesis.

First, the sex chromosomes determine whether the indifferent gonad that develops in the urogenital ridge will differentiate into a testis or an ovary.[58] If the gonadal stroma is male, genes associated with the Y chromosome interact with other components of the somatic cells in the primitive gonad and initiate the development of seminiferous tubules.[22] Wachtel[67] identified an H–Y antigen complex. Testicular differentiation is partly dependent on the presence of a threshold titer of H–Y antigen that is secreted by Sertoli cells.[38] In the presence of beta-

TABLE 2.1. Classification of intersexual disorders.

Disorders associated with normal chromosome constitution
- Female pseudohermaphroditism
  - Adrenogenital syndrome (testosterone overproduction due to adrenocorticoid insufficiency)
    - 21-Alpha-hydroxylase deficiency
    - 11-Beta-hydroxylase deficiency
  - Maternal ingestion of progestins or androgens
  - Maternal virilizing tumors
- Male pseudohermaphroditism
  - Gonadal defects
    - Testicular regression syndrome (gonadal destruction)
    - Leydig cell agenesis
      - Defective hCG–LH receptor
    - Defects in testosterone synthesis
      - Testosterone and adrenocorticoid insufficiency
        - 20,22-Demolase deficiency
        - 3-Beta-hydroxylase dehydrogenase deficiency
        - 17-Alpha-hydroxylase deficiency
      - Testosterone insufficiency only
        - 17,20-Desmolase deficiency
        - 17-Beta-hydroxysteroid (17-ketosteroid reductase) dehydrogenase deficiency
    - Persistent müllerian duct syndrome (defect in müllerian-inhibiting system)
  - End-organ defects
    - Disordered androgen receptor binding
      - Androgen insensitivity syndrome (testicular feminization)
      - Incomplete androgen insensitivity syndrome (Reifenstein's syndrome)
    - Disordered testosterone metabolism
      - 5-Alpha-reductase deficiency

Disorders associated with abnormal sex chromosome constitution
- Sexual ambiguity infrequent
  - Klinefelter's syndrome
  - Turner's syndrome
  - XX Male syndrome
  - Pure gonadal dysgenesis (some forms)
- Sexual ambiguity frequent
  - Mixed gonadal dysgenesis (MGD)
    - Pure gonadal dysgenesis (some forms)
    - Dysgenetic male pseudohermaphroditism
  - True hermaphroditism

Idiopathic or *unclassified* conditions exist within each major category. We assume that each category of male pseudohermaphroditism with defects in specific protein products or receptors has forms where the abnormality is total or partial or where the defect results from a qualitatively abnormal structure.

microglobulin, the H–Y antigen binds to the membrane receptors of primitive gonadal cells, subsequently inducing testicular differentiation.[17] The precise site of the gene or genes for this antigen is not certain. Recent data suggest that the H–Y gene locus is, itself, autosomally located, and genes located on the X and Y chromosomes appear to have a regulatory influence on the expression of the H–Y gene.[72] This process is probably independent of whether the primordial germ cells, which migrate from the yolk sac to the urogenital ridge via the hindgut approximately 3 weeks after fertilization, are present or absent in the gonad or have proliferated normally.[33] The testis is anatomically distinct, with early tubular formation, by the 44th day. This contrasts with ovarian differentiation, i.e., development of primordial follicles, which occurs some weeks later.

Second, Sertoli cells produce müllerian-inhibiting substance (MIS) (see Table 2.3 for complete list of abbreviations), a polypeptide protein that causes the müllerian (paramesonephric) ducts to regress. In the absence of this substance, the müllerian ducts develop passively to form the fallopian tubes, uterus, and upper vagina. The exact timing of MIS secretion is uncertain. It is thought that MIS is first secreted in an effective amount 56 to 62 days after fertilization. Although the process of müllerian regression is normally completed by the end of the eighth week to around day 77, (after which time the müllerian tissue is no longer sensitive to MIS), the testis is capable of MIS production at progressively lower levels through the first 2 years of postnatal life. MIS has a local action, which inhibits development of the ipsilateral fallopian tube. To prevent development of the uterus and vagina, both testes must secrete adequate amounts of MIS. Thus, a patient with a testis and a contralateral streak, ovary, or ovotestis generally has a uterus and vagina and a single fallopian tube on the side with the streak or ovary.

Third, testosterone is required for the wolffian (mesonephric) duct to differentiate into epididymis, vas deferens, and seminal vesicle. The Leydig cells appear in the testis around day 54 to 64 and shortly thereafter begin to produce testosterone.[71] The activity of the Leydig cells is probably related to the increased production of human chorionic gonadotropin (hCG) from the placenta at that time. Testosterone acts locally on the ipsilateral wolffian duct. In the absence of a testis, inability of a testis to produce testosterone, or insensitivity of the wolffian duct anlage to testosterone, differentiation of the epididymis, vas deferens, and seminal vesicle does not occur. Only rarely are abnormally elevated testosterone levels reached early enough in embryogenesis in a female fetus to cause the wolffian duct to differentiate into definitive male organs (e.g., androgen administration to the mother during pregnancy or congenital adrenogenital syndrome).

Fourth, development of male external genitalia and differentiation of the prostate are dependent on the local conversion of testosterone (the prohormone) to dihydrotestosterone (DHT), which is mediated by the enzyme, 5-alpha-reductase. Dihydrotestosterone causes (1) the

TABLE 2.2. Chronologic development of normal male and female genital tracts.

Crown–rump (CR) (mm)	Week after ovulation	CR length, days	Description of event
		2.5 mm 24 days	Pronephric tubules form; pronephric (mesonephric) duct arises and grows caudad as solid cord
3	3.3		
		3–5 mm 27 days	Pronephros degenerated, but mesonephric duct reaches cloaca
7	4		
		7–9 mm 33 days	Cloaca divides into rectum and urogenital sinus (UGS)
12	5		
		8–11 mm 37 days	Müllerian ducts appear as funnel-shaped opening of coelomic epithelium Indifferent gonad bulges into coelom
18	6		
		17 mm/48 days 20–30 mm	Müllerian ducts about one-half distance to UGS Testis anatomically distinct, with seminiferous tubules
23	7		
		51+ days 51 days 23–28 mm/54 days 27–31 mm/56+ days	Müllerian ducts elongate and near UGS Ducts approach each other Ducts in apposition; sinus tubercle appears Ducts fuse and in contact with UGS
29	8		
		30? mm 56? days	So-called ambisexual stage ends; experimental data for dating müllerian duct regression unclear. Experimentally, the müllerian duct is sensitive to MIS through 25+ mm CR size; ducts in older embryos are not sensitive. Clinically, regression completed by 43–55 mm CR size. Leydig cells appear
43	9		
		50? mm	Testes and ovaries acquire capacity to secrete characteristic hormones at same stage of development; testosterone (T) coincides with histologic development of Leydig cells and immediately precedes virilization of genital tract; ovary not yet differentiated; rate-limiting step is appearance of 3-beta-OH-steroid-dehydrogenase, which is 50-fold more abundant in testis than ovary; ovary converts T to estradiol, which testis cannot do; later regulation shifted to pituitary–placenta gonadotropins where T → estradiol controlled by conversion of cholesterol to pregnenolone
		56 mm	Müllerian ducts completely fused (entire septum gone); caudal aspect proliferates; epithelium lining canal stratifies (2–3-cell layers thick)
		70 days	Anogenital distance lengthens
60	10		
		71 days	Testosterone synthesis sufficient to induce development of mesonephric duct into definitive structures (epididymis, vas deferens, and seminal vesicle) Subsequently, T converted peripherally into 5-alpha-dihydrotestosterone (5-DHT), which causes: UG sinus → prostate Genital tubercle → glans penis Genital folds → penis (only 3.5 mm long) Genital swelling → scrotum

TABLE 2.2 *Continued*

Crown-rump (CR) (mm)	Week after ovulation	CR length, days	Description of event
		72–74 days	Fusion of labioscrotal folds
			Closure of median raphe
			Closure of urethral groove
			Phallus in both sexes 3 mm long; thereafter grows in males 0.72 mm/week and females 0.20 mm/week
		75 days	Mesonephric ducts regress if not stimulated by T
		60+ mm	Vaginal plate first seen distinctly (complete at 140 mm; week 17)
			Initially, upper uterovaginal canal is large and oval in cross-section, mostly lined by pseudostratified columnar epithelium
			Extensive growth begins caudally; cells stratify
		68 mm	Uterovaginal canal occluded caudally, progresses cranially
71	11		
		77 mm	Extensive uterovaginal growth continues caudally
93	12		
		100–120 mm	Cervical glands appear; wavy, but undifferentiated
		105 mm	Vaginal rudiment approaches vestibule
			True ovarian organogenesis begins with onset of meiotic prophase
105	13		
116	14		
		126 mm	Primary folds of mucosa give uterine lumen W-shaped appearance on cross-section
		130 mm	Uterovaginal canal (15 mm total length) divisible into vagina (3/6), cervix (2/6), and corpus (1/6); boundaries ill-defined
			Uterine isthmus readily distinguishable
			Stromal layers of uterus begin definition
			Solid epithelial anlage of anterior and posterior vaginal fornices appear
			Vagina begins to show slight estrogen effect
130	15		
		139 mm	Fallopian tube begins active growth phase, begins to coil
		140 mm	Vaginal plate completed; lower end reaches vestibule; upper end extends into endocervical canal
			Female urogenital sinus becomes shallow vestibule
142	16		
		151 mm	Vaginal plate longest and begins to canalize
			Corpus glands appear as slight outpouchings
153	17		
		160 mm	Palmate folds of cervix appear (forerunner of adult cervix)
		162 mm	Mucoid development of cervix begins
			Smooth muscle of uterus appears
			Estrogen effect apparent throughout vagina
		162 mm	Cavitation of vaginal canal completed
164	18		
		170 mm	Fornices hollow
177	19		
		185 mm	Dramatic increase in growth and coiling of fallopian tube (about 3 mm/week to week 34)
186	20		
197	21		
208	22		

Table 2.2 *Continued*

Crown-rump (CR) (mm)	Week after ovulation	CR length, days	Description of event
		210 mm	Differentiation of muscular layer of uterus complete
		227 mm	Fundus well marked; uterus assumes adult form
230	24		
250	26		
270	28		
290	30		
328	34		
362	38	266 days	Birth

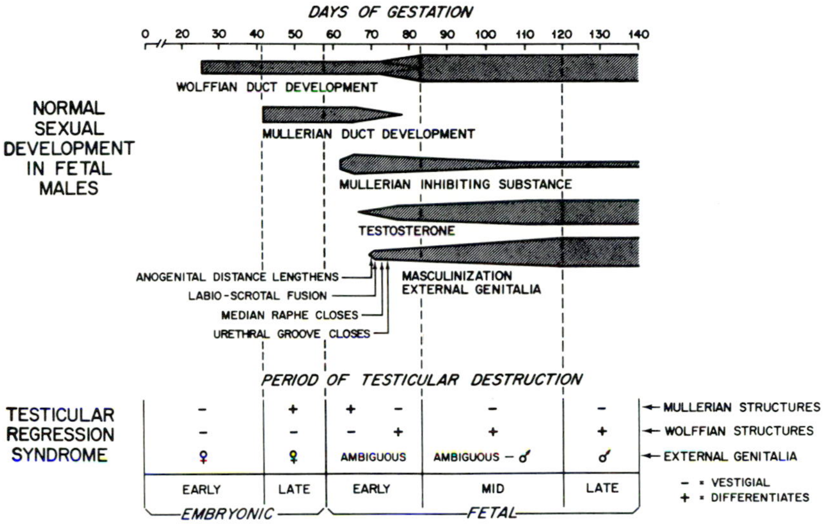

FIG. 2.1. Normal sexual development in the male and application in testicular regression syndrome. (Reprinted from Welch and Robboy, Ref. 69, with permission of Pediatric Andrology.)

genital tubercle to enlarge and form the glans penis, (2) the genital folds to enlarge and fuse to form the penile shaft, with migration of the urethral orifice along the lower border of the shaft to the tip of the glans, and (3) the genital swellings to fuse and form a scrotum. Dihydrotestosterone also causes the urogenital sinus tissues to differentiate into the prostate. Failure of male development of the external genitalia in the presence of testes may be due to a lack of adequate testosterone secretion into the systemic circulation, deficient enzyme (5-alpha-reductase) at the end-organ level to convert testosterone to DHT, or complete end-organ insensitivity (testicular feminization). Lesser degrees of deficiency or end-organ insensitivity may result in partial male development characterized by a small penis, hypospadias, deficient formation of the scrotum, or a persistent urogenital sinus (vaginal opening into urethra). The effects of DHT begin about day 70, with fusion of the labioscrotal folds and closure of the median raphe, and continue to day 74 with closure of the urethral groove. External genital development is complete by day 120 to 140 (18th to 20th week).

TABLE 2.3. Abbreviations and synonyms.

CR	Crown-rump
DHEA	Dehydroepiandrosterone
DHT	Dihydrotestosterone
hCG	Human chorionic gonadotropin
LH	Luteinizing hormone
MGD	Mixed gonadal dysgenesis
MIS	Müllerian-inhibiting substance
T	Testosterone
UGS	Urogenital sinus
Müllerian duct	Paramesonephric duct
Wolffian duct	Mesonephric duct

Fifth, female internal organs and external genitalia develop in the absence of hormones secreted by the fetal ovary and differentiate even when gonads are absent. Unless interrupted by the regressive influence of MIS, differentiation of the müllerian ducts proceeds cephalocaudally to form fallopian tubes, a uterus, and a vagina.[63] In the absence of the masculinizing effect of DHT, the undifferentiated external genital anlage develops into the vulva. The genital tubercle develops into the clitoris, the genital folds into the labia minora, and the genital swellings into the labia majora. Thus, the infant with ovaries or streak gonads has female internal and external genitalia at birth. Only if the female fetus has systemically elevated levels of androgens before 10th to 12th week of gestation does any degree of internal male development occur. In such cases, the external genitalia may appear ambiguous or may resemble those of a normal phenotypic male; the vagina in these instances opens into the membranous portion of the urethra. If the androgens are not elevated until after the 20th week, by which time the external genitalia have fully formed, the only male effect is an enlarged clitoris.

There are congenital anomalies that may be present on the genitalia of newborn females that, if present, should not be confused with virilization of the genitalia. Hymenal tags and hymenal bands (5.7% and 2.7%, respectively) are frequently found on female infants in the first 24 hours of life.[35,52] The tags usually regress spontaneously as the estrogen effect diminishes, but occasionally they may persist. The bands, if not superficial, may indicate the presence of a septate vagina or duplication of internal genitalia.

Disorders Associated with a Normal Chromosome Constitution

Intrauterine exposure of the fetus to virilizing hormones or specific genetic defects not detectable by the usual chromosome analysis are responsible for the developmental defects of people in this category. Female pseudohermaphrodites are 46XX and have grossly recognizable ovaries. Male pseudohermaphrodites are 46XY and, with the exception of the category testicular regression, have gonads recognizable as testes.

Female Pseudohermaphroditism

Female pseudohermaphroditism occurs as a result of an intrauterine state of relative androgen excess in an individual with two ovaries and two X chromosomes (46XX). The elevated level of androgen present during embryogenesis usually results in genital ambiguity and may result in the appearance of a phenotypic male.

Andrenogenital Syndrome

Of all conditions responsible for the appearance of ambiguous genitalia in the newborn, congenital adrenal hyperplasia is singular in that the lack of specific adrenal steroids may threaten the life of the patient. Prompt diagnosis and institution of appropriate therapy are therefore essential. With early treatment, normal external genitalia and fertility can be achieved. Conceptually, the manifestations of the adrenogenital syndrome in the XX person are most easily summarized through an understanding of the biosynthetic pathways of mineralocorticoid, glucocorticoid, and sex steroids (Fig. 2.2). Two enzymes, 21-hydroxylase and 11-beta-hydroxylase, participate in the formation of the glucocorticoid, cortisol, but not of testosterone or estrogen. Deficiency of either of these enzymes in the 46XX female causes elevated levels of androgenic intermediates, which may result in some cases of sexual ambiguity or marked virilization of the external genitalia in the newborn female.[34,41] Deficiency of 3-beta-hydroxysteroid dehydrogenase is associated with clitoral hypertrophy but not with labial fusion or anterior displacement of the urethral orifice. In these cases, the mild virilization has been attributed to dehy-

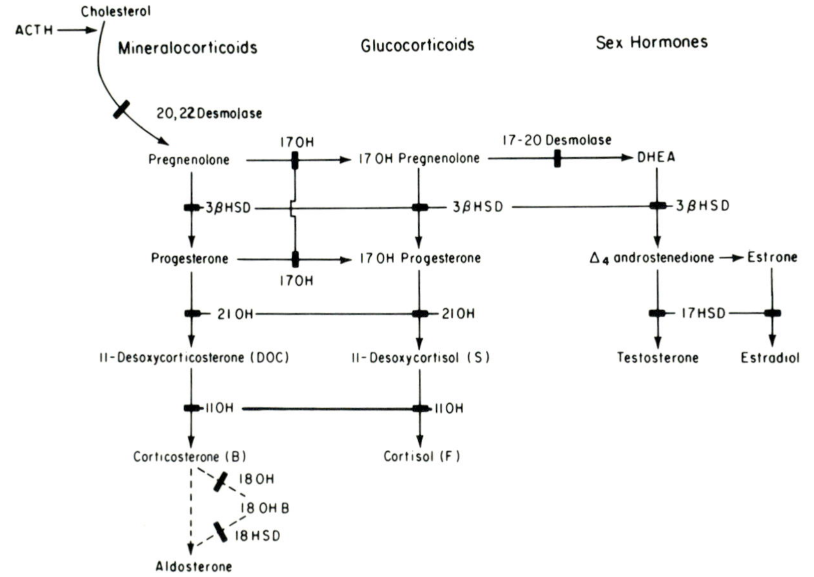

FIG. 2.2. Biosynthesis of mineralocorticoids, glucocorticoids, and sex steroids. (Reprinted from Saenger et al., Ref. 53, with permission of Pediatric Andrology.)

droepiandrosterone (DHEA), a weak androgen ($\frac{1}{20}$ the potency of testosterone) synthesized before the blockage point in the synthetic pathway.

21-Hydroxylase deficiency is inherited as an autosomal recessive trait and accounts for more than 95% of cases of congenital adrenal hyperplasia, occurring once in 50,000 births. Heterozygote carriers can be determined through the use of ACTH stimulation. Present data suggest that a series of allelic genes associated with many HLA markers code for the 21-beta-hydroxylase enzyme and that these allelic variants explain the occurrence of the wide variation in symptomatology observed in these patients.[28] Association of the gene for this enzyme with HLA loci[34] may lead to prenatal diagnosis and early therapy to avoid a salt-wasting crisis. In the female, the clitoris may be enlarged; if an excess of androgen is present earlier than the 16th week of gestation, the vagina and urethra may open into a common urogenital sinus. More marked clitoral enlargment and an opening of the urogenital sinus at the clitoral base may mimic penile hypospadias and suggest an even earlier temporal effect. On occasion, the changes have been of such severity that the female infants have been misdiagnosed as cryptorchid males with or without hypospadias. Virilization occurring in late childhood or pre- or postpuberty has been described in cases where 21-hydroxylase deficiency results in late-onset adrenal hyperplasia.

Males have no evidence of genital ambiguity but may have an enlarged phallus and a hyperpigmented rugated scrotum. Bilateral testicular nodules, composed of interstitial cells resembling Leydig cells or cells of adrenal rest origin, rarely may develop (Fig. 2.3).

The use of gas chromatography of urinary steroids to detect defects in 11-beta-hydroxylase has provided data indicating that the 11-beta-hydroxylase defect is more frequent than was previously assumed.[34] Indeed, two types of 11-beta-hydroxylase defects seem to exist: (1) when only the 17-beta-hydroxylated steroids cannot be 11-beta-hydroxylated, the patients are severely virilized, and (2) when both cortisol and deoxycorticosterone are reduced, the defect results in mild symptomatology.[74]

Maternal Ingestion of Progestins or Androgens

Maternal ingestion of synthetic progestins was implicated as a cause of female pseudohermaphroditism in the late 1950s when such treatment was used for threatened or habitual abortion; more recently, progestins have been implicated in the development of hypospadias in male offspring.[1] Most cases of female pseudohermaphroditism in this category developed after maternal ingestion of ethisterone (17-alpha-ethinyltestosterone) or Norlutin (17-alpha-ethinyl-19-nortestosterone), but occasionally after the ingestion of Enovid, diethylstilbestrol, androgens or the intramuscular administration of progesterone.

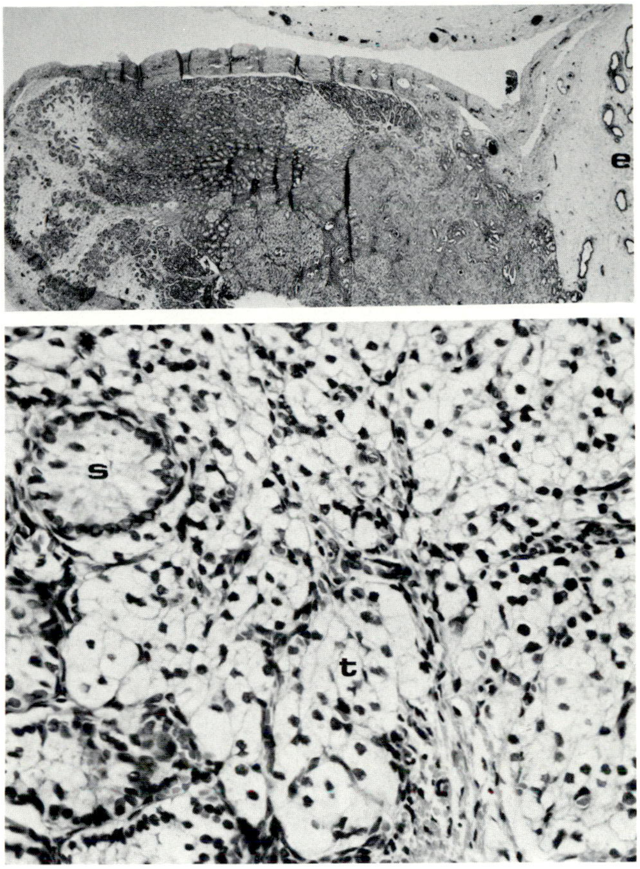

FIG. 2.3. Interstitial cell tumor of the testis in a 4-year-old infant with adrenogenital syndrome. The tumor cells (t), which are illustrated at high magnification adjacent to immature seminiferous tubules (s) in the inset, resemble adrenocortical cells more closely than Leydig cells. The epididymis (e) is adjacent to the testis. (Reprinted from Welch and Robboy, Ref. 69, with permission of Pediatric Andrology.)

Masculinization usually consists of phallic enlargement and variable degrees of labioscrotal fusion, depending on the time during gestation when the therapy was administered. Although the degree of masculinization is usually less than that associated with the adrenogenital syndrome, in some instances the sexual ambiguity in female infants has been of such severity as to result in male sex assignment. The degree of virilization does not progress with age. The gonads and internal genital organs are unaffected, and ovulation, menstruation, and normal secondary female characteristics appear at puberty.

Maternal Virilizing Tumors

Several benign and malignant tumors, both primary in and metastatic to the ovary have been associated with virilization of the mother and her female offspring.[23] The luteoma of pregnancy is the most common lesion that causes maternal virilization during pregnancy. The pregnancy luteoma is a benign hyperplastic lesion of the ovary (see Chapter 16, Nonneoplastic Lesions of Ovary) that is most often encountered as an incidental finding at the time of cesarean section or postpartum sterilization, usually in women who are multiparous. Elevated levels of hCG are thought to induce hyperplasia of theca–lutein or stroma–lutein cells. A small percentage of the female infants have become masculinized, with mild enlargement of the clitoris and occasionally minimal degrees of labioscrotal fusion or rugate, hyperpigmented (scrotal) labia. The nature of these changes indicates that the ovarian nodules do not function until the second half of gestation, which is in accord with the occasional onset of masculinization in the mother during the third trimester.

At operation, one and often both maternal ovaries are enlarged by soft, yellow-brown nodules that are well circumscribed but not encapsulated.[61] Although most are less than 2 cm in diameter, they may be as large as 20 cm in greatest dimension. On microscopic examination, the nodules consist of large, polygonal cells with granular, eosinophilic cytoplasm. These cells are smaller and more eosinophilic than the luteinized granulosa cells of the corpus luteum but larger than the theca–lutein cells. Intracellular lipid is sparse, if at all present. Mitoses may be observed, but only rarely are they numerous.

Elevated plasma and tissue levels of testosterone, DHT, androstenedione, and DHEA have been detected in virilized patients; the plasma levels return to normal once the tumor is extirpated. Even without treatment, the nodules regress and disappear shortly after delivery. One patient developed a second luteoma during a subsequent pregnancy. Other primary functioning tumors of the ovary that may lead to virilization of female offspring are considered in Chapter 19, Sex Cord–Stromal Tumors of Ovary, and metastatic tumors to the ovary that induce the stroma to function during pregnancy are discussed in Chapter 22, Metastatic Ovarian Tumors.

Male Pseudohermaphroditism

Male pseudohermaphroditism is characterized by apparently normal chromosomes (46XY), macroscopic testes or evidence that the testes were present during fetal development, and a state of relative or absolute androgen deficiency. The external genitalia are usually female or ambiguous, although in certain categories (e.g., testicular regression syndrome) they may appear as phenotypically male. The primary defect is in the gonad or the end-organs.

Gonadal Defects

These conditions are associated with regression (destruction) of the gonads or their anlage during intrauterine life, agenesis of Leydig cells, specific enzymatic defects in testosterone synthesis, or defects in elaboration or action of MIS.

Testicular Regression Syndrome. Testicular regression is a concept that unifies a variety of separate conditions in which both testes have regressed during prenatal life.[7,13] The various names given in the earlier literature to aspects of the syndrome (pure gonadal dysgenesis,* Swyer's syndrome, true agonadism, testicular dysgenesis, rudimentary testis, vanishing testis, complete bilateral anorchia) reflect the diverse findings in these patients. This heterogeneous group of disorders is a manifestation of the variable timing of gonadal regression in relation to the development of the urogenital ridge and müllerian ducts, the appearance of Sertoli cells and subsequent synthesis and secretion of MIS, and the development of Leydig cells capable of testosterone secretion. Regression of the testes during the critical periods of each of these events results in a slightly different phenotypic expression and spectrum of differentiation or atrophy of internal genital structures (Fig. 2.1).

At one end of the spectrum, the internal genitalia and gonads are absent, and the external genitalia are female. Presumably, the urogenital ridge was destroyed in its entirety during the embryonic period even before the müllerian ducts began to differentiate (i.e., before the sixth week). At the other end of the spectrum, which is close to the endpoint of normal genital development, the patients are phenotypic males with infantile to nearly normal male external genitalia, normally differentiated wolffian duct structures, and inhibited müllerian duct development. Testicular regression presumably occurred during the late fetal period (after 120 days) when müllerian structures had already atrophied under the influence of MIS and testosterone and DHT had exerted a major influence in the normal development of internal and external genitalia.

Intermediate in the spectrum are patients with genital ambiguity and various combinations of wolffian or müllerian duct development. Testes that regressed during the late embryonic period (days 43 to 59) will have secreted insufficient testosterone to affect the wolffian duct. The production of MIS will have been variable, resulting in poorly differentiated müllerian structures or rudiments thereof (incomplete inhibition). In the absence of systemic androgens, the external genitalia appear female. Regression of the testes during the early fetal period (days 59 to 84) after Sertoli cell (MIS) and Leydig cell (testosterone) function have begun or are about to begin results in ambiguous external genitalia and various combinations of wolffian and müllerian development depending on the duration of androgen secretion and müllerian inhibition. Regression of the testes during the midfetal

* Pure gonadal dysgenesis is a category that encompasses several distinct disorders.[3]

period (days 90 to 120) results in more advanced masculinization of the external genitalia, although degrees of ambiguity are usually present. Since müllerian duct inhibition is normally completed by day 80, the müllerian structures will have been suppressed and wolffian structures are developed.

Leydig Cell Agenesis. Leydig cell development in man is usually thought of as a biphasic pattern with two temporally discrete mature Leydig cell populations: fetal (correlated with the development of the male ductular system) and adult (correlated with pubertal development). Although the fate of fetal Leydig cells is controversial, examination of prepubertal and neonatal testicular tissue both ultrastructurally and for the presence of testosterone by immunoperoxidase techniques has resulted in the identification of immature Leydig cells, suggesting that regression and degeneration of fetal Leydig cells occur.

Leydig cell agenesis is a rare disorder described in only a few case reports.[2,55] In a 2-year-old child with ambiguous genitalia, biopsy specimens revealed Sertoli cells and spermatogonia but no evidence of Leydig cells, even after intensive hCG stimulation. Vasa deferentia and epididymides were present, however, indicating that some Leydig cells must have differentiated and functioned during early fetal life. It is unknown whether the defect lies in the Leydig cell itself or in a structural or functional hCG–luteinizing hormone (LH).

Defects in Testosterone Synthesis. Congenital deficiency of any enzyme involved in the production of testosterone in the testis or adrenal gland (Fig. 2.2) results in a state of relative estrogen excess. The histologic appearance of the testicular tissue has been variable. It has been described occasionally to be "normal," but the photomicrographs in some reports have disclosed large clusters of Leydig cells surrounding tubules lined only by Sertoli cells. In general, the number of gonads studied for any of the conditions and the range of ages studied (infancy, childhood, adulthood) have been limited. Müllerian structures are absent. Wolffian duct structures may be present. The degree to which the external genitalia develop abnormally depends on the type and severity of the defect.

Three inherited enzymatic defects involve both the synthesis of adrenal mineralocorticoid and glucocorticoid hormones as well as adrenal and testicular sex hormones. The most severe defect, which involves the conversion of cholesterol intermediates to pregnenolone (20–22-desmolase), almost always ends lethally from a salt wasting crisis if untreated by infancy.[53] Although the external genitalia in the male are ambiguous or female, sufficient testosterone must be secreted during embryogenesis since the internal genitalia are male. The testes in the infant shows immature seminiferous tubules presumably with spermatogonia (described as "normal");[4] by several years of age, the germ cells disappear.[27]

The deficiency of 3-beta-hydroxylase dehydrogenase, like the 20,22-desmolase deficiency, results in decreased synthesis of mineralocorticoid and glucocorticoid hormones as well as adrenal and testicular sex hormones, and may lead to life threatening salt wasting in infancy. DHEA, which is a weak androgen secreted in high amounts, results in slight clitoral enlargement in the female but rarely completely masculinizes the external genitalia in males. Hence, the male may be born with ambiguous genitalia and may resemble a virilized female. Males in whom the defect is partial may be born with hypospadias and develop gynecomastia at puberty. The testes in older boys generally are immature, exhibiting seminiferous tubules with spermatogenic arrest and diminished numbers of Leydig cells.[54]

In contrast to the early age of diagnosis in the two syndromes just discussed, the diagnosis in most patients with 17-alpha-hydroxylase deficiency has not been suspected until the anticipated time of puberty or later.[26,30] Recently, however, detailed steroid analysis of the urine of a newborn male with ambiguous genitalia led to the diagnosis of 17-hydroxylase deficiency.[8]

Deficiencies of two enzymes, 17–20-desmolase and 17-hydroxysteroid dehydrogenase (17-ketosteroid reductase), result in deficient testosterone synthesis but do not affect the production of either mineralocorticoids or glucocorticoids. The former defect (conversion of 17-hydroxypregnenolone to DHEA) is rare. This defect was described as a partial deficiency in only four patients, three of whom were related and one of whom was an "aunt," with an XY sex chromosomal constitution.[15,75] The patients with a 46XY karyotype had ambiguous external genitalia and inguinal or intraabdominal testes. Spermatogonia were present in the testes of infants but had disappeared in the biopsies of the older teenage patient. All had third-degree hypospadias but normal male internal ductal differentiation. Only one subject, the "aunt," had possible rudimentary müllerian structures (the slides from the rudimentary cervix and unilateral fallopian tube were not available for review). Defects in testosterone biosynthesis at puberty (resulting from hypothalamic–pituitary lesions) have been causally implicated in male transsexualism, prompting the biochemical examination of testicular tissue derived from transsexuals.[21] The ability of testicular tissue derived from transsexuals to synthesize DHEA has been assessed as a means of determining the presence of 17-alpha-hydroxylase and C-17,20-desmolase activity in such tissue and has been found to be qualitatively similar to that reported for testicular tissue derived from normal individuals.

Genetic males with 17-hydroxysteroid dehydrogenase deficiency have almost all been raised as females because of incomplete masculinization.[30] Most are diagnosed at or after puberty when signs of virilization, such as clitoromegaly and hirsutism, become apparent. Müllerian duct derivatives are absent, consistent with normal antimüllerian hormone action. Wolffian duct differentiation, indicative of testosterone secretion during embryogenesis, is normal. The testes, which are found in the inguinal canal or labia majora, contain only rare or no spermatogonia and may exhibit numerous Leydig cells. It has been stated that the diagnostic hallmark of 17-hydroxysteroid dehydrogenase (17-ketosteroid reductase) deficiency is the very high serum level of androstenedione relative to the low normal serum testosterone levels exhibited in the affected individuals.[29] Determination of steroid concentrations in the serum derived from the spermatic vein of a 13-year-old child with 17-ketosteroid reductase deficiency revealed elevated levels of androstenedione, estrone, and DHEA and subnormal levels of testosterone.[29] A lack of response to hCG revealed that this patient was producing testicular steroids at a maximal rate. The testicular tissue, which histologically exhibited Leydig cell hyperplasia and hypertrophy, contained high concentrations of androstenedione with relatively low testosterone concentrations. Occasionally, the enzymatic defects may be multiple and give rise to complex clinical and biochemical findings.[46]

Persistent Müllerian Duct Syndrome. The persistent müllerian duct syndrome, a defect in MIS also known as *hernia uteri inguinalis*, is a rare familial condition. The patients are 46XY phenotypic males with unilateral or bilateral cryptorchid testes and normal or almost normal male external genitalia. An inguinal hernia may be present into which prolapse an infantile uterus and fallopian tubes.[68] The pubertal development is normal, and a rare patient has been fertile. If a streak gonad or a tumor rather than bilateral testes is found at operation, the diagnosis of mixed gonadal dysgenesis should be considered.[50] The underlying defect in the persistent müllerian duct syndrome relates theoretically to deficient synthesis of MIS, synthesis of a biologically inactive compound, abnormality in the timing of its secretion, or end-organ resistance.

End-Organ Defects

The normal development of wolffian duct derivatives (epididymis, vas deferens, seminal vesicle) and the external genitalia requires that these structures be responsive to DHT and that the enzyme 5-alpha-reductase be present to convert testosterone to DHT. If the androgen-binding system is disordered, e.g., because of an unstable receptor or lack of a receptor (androgen insensitivity syndrome, or testicular feminization syndrome), neither internal nor external genital organs respond normally.[19] If only 5-alpha-reductase is absent or defective, the abnormalities in the reproductive tract are confined to the external genitalia and prostate.

Disordered Androgen Receptor Binding. Androgen insensitivity syndrome (testicular feminization). Testicular feminization, the most common form of male pseudohermaphroditism, is inherited as an X-linked trait and is due to a qualitative or quantitative deficiency of androgen receptor protein.[71] In the complete form, the external genitalia are phenotypic female. For this reason, the condition is rarely diagnosed before puberty unless an inguinal hernia or labial mass is encountered or unless the disease is known to be familial. Testicular feminization confirmed in a neonate with bilateral inguinal masses led to the evaluation of other siblings in the family, with the discovery of an older sibling (2 years old) similarly affected.[57] Knowledge of this familial tendency resulted in the prompt diagnosis of the disorder in still another asymptomatic sibling born 3 years later. Primary amenorrhea is, however, the most common complaint leading to evaluation and subsequent diagnosis. The medical history usually reveals that breast development occurred as expected at puberty. Pubic and axillary hair are scant, the vagina is shortened, the epididymides, vasa deferentia, seminal vesicles, and prostate are absent. As a rule, both the cervix and the uterus are absent, although there has been a case reported in which a person who exhibitied both complete testicular feminization (resulting from tissue insensitivity to androgen) and persistent müllerian duct structures (rudimentary bicornuate uterus-like tissue) was identified.[42] The testes are cryptorchid and located in the inguinal canal, the pelvis, or rarely the labia. In the complete or almost complete form of the testicular feminization syndrome, the individual exhibits a truly female consciousness gender identity, with "normal" extragenital erotogenic sensitivity and "normal" maternal attitude.[64]

The gonads in infants and young children are relatively normal, but by age 5 years, they show abnormalities.[37] By young adulthood, the gonad uninvolved by nodular growths is usually small and on section is tan to brown and traversed by thin white bands. A 1 to 2 cm firm, white nodule of hyalinized smooth muscle is present at one pole of the gonad and may represent an abnormally hypertrophied gubernaculum. Microscopic examination of the testicular parenchyma discloses immature seminiferous tubules usually sparsely distributed or clustered in small aggregates, sometimes on a background of stroma resembling ovarian stroma (Fig. 2.4). Spermatogonia may be present, but spermatogenesis is absent. Leydig cells may be abundant and resemble fetal Leydig cells.

Most testes contain multiple Sertoli cell adenomas that are discrete, firm, yellow to brown, and bulge above the sectioned surface (Fig. 2.4). Although the typical size varies from 1 mm to 1 cm, dimensions up to 25 cm have been recorded.[6] The bulk of the nodule is usually composed of seminiferous tubules lacking lumina; spermatogonia may be present. Leydig cells are frequently present in the interstitium. They may form relatively

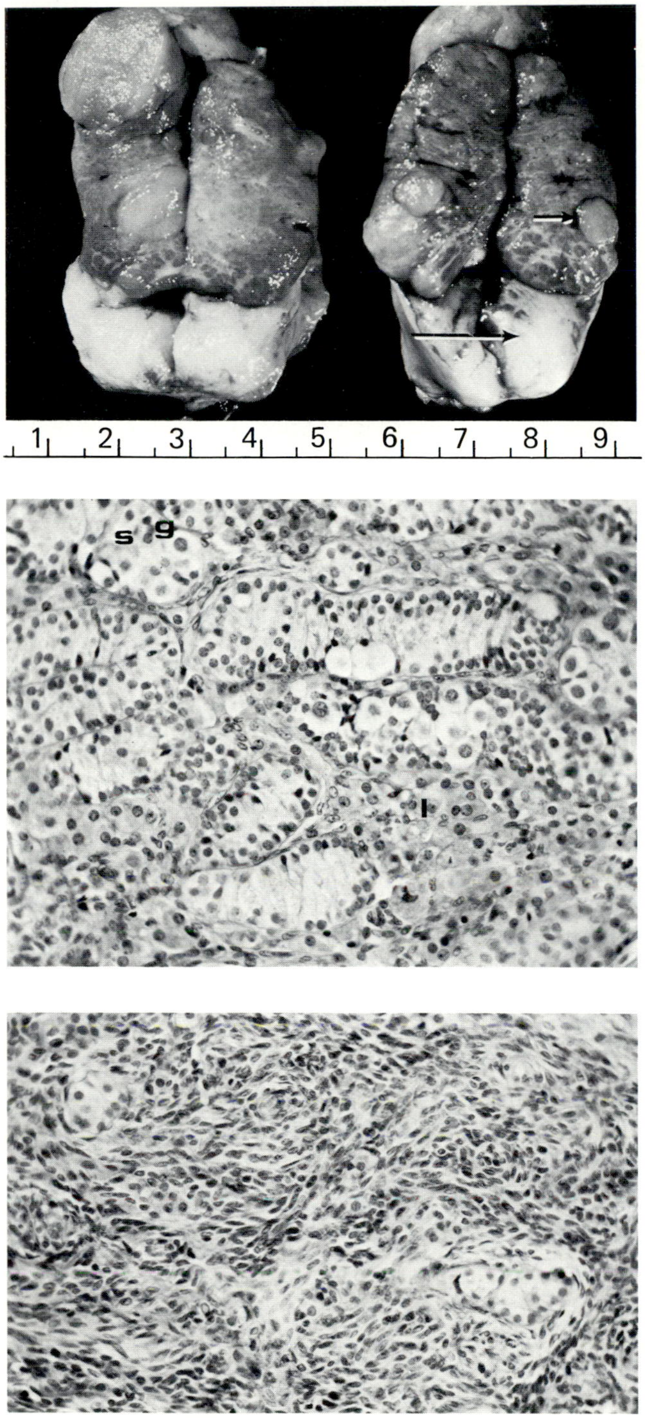

FIG. 2.4. *Top.* Testis in a 17-year-old with the complete form of androgen insensitivity (testicular feminization) syndrome. Numerous Sertoli cell adenomas (*short arrows*) are present in the parenchyma. The mass near one pole (*long arrow*) may represent an abnormally hypertrophied gubernaculum. *Middle.* Hamartoma with immature seminiferous tubules (s), numerous germ cells (g), and numerous Leydig cells in the interstitium (l). *Bottom.* Contralateral testis with scattered immature seminiferous tubules embedded in a dense ovarian type cortical stroma. Occasional interstitial cells are present. (Reprinted from Welch and Robboy, Ref. 69, with permission of Pediatric Andrology.)

pure stromal nodules that rarely exceed 1 cm in greatest dimension. Ultrastructural examination of the gonads removed from people exhibiting the testicular feminization syndrome reveal the presence of Leydig cells with features typically found in cells involved in active steroid hormone synthesis (many dilated cisternae of smooth endoplasmic reticulum and numerous mitochondria with tubular cisternae).[48] The Leydig cells examined have no Reinke crystals evident, indicating the fetal nature of the Leydig cells. Nonetheless, mature fetal Leydig cells are active hormone producers. These findings confirm that the pathologic defect in the testicular feminization syndrome is an end-organ defect and not due to a lack of hormone production by the testes. In addition, the interstitium may contain stroma resembling ovarian stroma. Depending on the type of components present, as well as their number (solitary versus multiple) and size, the nodules are classified as hamartoma, Sertoli cell adenoma, or rarely as Leydig cell tumor.

After the Sertoli cell adenoma, seminoma is the second most frequent neoplasm but the most common gonadal cancer in patients with testicular feminization. In addition, atypical germ cells and even seminoma in situ may be observed within the testicular tubules. Unlike mixed gonadal dysgenesis where tumors can develop in young people, the risk of malignancy in patients with testicular feminization is only 4% by the age of 25 years[32] but reaches 33% by 50 years. Since tumors rarely develop until after completion of puberty, castration can be delayed until after adolescence to permit the patients to undergo a normal pubertal spurt and develop feminine secondary sex characteristics.

Incomplete Androgen Insensitivity Syndrome (Reifenstein's Syndrome). About 10% of patients have partial expression of the androgen insensitivity syndrome (incomplete testicular feminization), which to date has been associated only with thermo-unstable receptor.[19] Patients vary in the degree of masculinization of external and internal organs. Since virilization may accompany breast development at puberty, gonadectomy should be performed before puberty. Various aspects of this syndrome, collectively called Reifenstein's syndrome, have been described. The range of features include hypospadias, breast development at puberty, female habitus, azoospermia, and sometimes absence or hypoplasia of wolffian duct structures. The mildest form of androgen insensitivity is represented by infertile males with gynecomastia but otherwise normal internal and external genitalia.

Reifenstein's syndrome, like the complete form of androgen insensitivity syndrome, is transmitted in an X-linked recessive pattern. Additional but as yet unidentified factors must act to affect the androgen receptor protein to modify the androgen action in vivo. Various members within a family can display a spectrum of clinical abnormalities and yet have the same degree of receptor abnormality in in vitro assays. The nosologic confusion between incomplete testicular feminization and Reifenstein's syndrome is discussed elsewhere.[59]

Disordered Testosterone Metabolism. 5-Alpha-Reductase Deficiency. Target organs in this familial form of male pseudohermaphroditism cannot reduce testosterone, the prohormone, to DHT, the hormone that masculinizes the indifferent urogenital sinus.[24] The disorder, transmitted as an autosomal recessive, is unique as an inherited disorder of steroid metabolism in that the carrier state is detectable.

Affected males have phenotypic female to ambiguous external genitalia at birth (pseudovaginal perineoscrotal hypospadias). The small clitoris-like phallus lacks a urethral orifice. In most affected individuals, the urogenital sinus opens on the perineum, and within the sinus an anterior orifice leads to the urethra and a posterior orifice to a blind vaginal pouch. The testes are in the inguinal canals or labia. The müllerian-derived structures are absent, whereas the wolffian structures (vas deferens, epididymis, and seminal vesicle), the anlage of which respond to testosterone, are developed normally.

At puberty, the penis lengthens, the bifid scrotum grows and becomes rugated and hyperpigmented, and the testes enlarge and descend. The prostate, however, remains impalpable. Erection, ejaculation, and orgasms are possible. The appearance of virilization at puberty and the lack of breast development contrast to the complete form of testicular feminization and defects of testosterone synthesis. Testicular biopsy specimens in three adults revealed spermatogenesis in one[45] and tubular atrophy, complete spermatogenic arrest, and Leydig cell hyperplasia in the others.[25,43]

Disorders Associated with an Abnormal Sex Chromosome Constitution

Additions, deletions, or mosaicism of the sex chromosomes characterize individuals in this category. The appearance of the gonads is variable and ranges from the presence of a streak gonad to a nearly normal female or male gonad on both gross and microscopic examination. These disorders are subdivided into two broad categories depending on the frequency with which sexual ambiguity occurs.

Sexual Ambiguity Infrequent

Klinefelter's Syndrome

Klinefelter's syndrome occurs in about 1 of every 600 newborn males. The karyotype is usually 47XXY or, occasionally, 47XXY/mosaic. Although a rare infant may have hypospadias or a congenital anomaly, such as hypoplasia of the middle phalanx of the fifth finger, the diagnosis is rarely suspected until adolescence, when the patient presents with gynecomastia, obesity, or signs of eunuchism. Sparsity of beard and body hair is common. Laboratory tests reveal low testosterone levels and azoospermia. Clinically, the patients are often limited in their economic striving and sexual drive. This may be due to the additional X chromosome (47XXY), which appears to be at least partially correlated with some intellectual deficits.[62]

In the Klinefelter testis, primary spermatogonia are already greatly reduced in number by late childhood. Shortly before the expected time of puberty, the seminiferous tubules begin to degenerate. The absence of elastic fibers in the tubular wall indicates that the process of atrophy began before puberty. The testes in adult 47XXY patients are small and rarely exceed 2 cm in maximal dimension (Fig. 2.5). On microscopic examination, they are largely atrophic, with hyalinized seminiferous tubules and a relative increase in the number of Leydig cells. Some of the tubules, however, may be preserved and lined only by Sertoli cells, and a rare one may even contain germ cells in varying stages of maturation. If sperm are detected, mosaicism, most likely of the 46XY/47XXY pattern, should be suspected.

The Leydig cells become pronounced in number some time after puberty. Although they appear hyperplastic relative to the atrophic appearance of the other elements, it is uncertain whether the absolute volume is greater than in normal testes. Functionally, the Leydig cells are abnormal, as evidenced by low levels of serum testosterone and a subnormal response to administration of hCG.

Testicular tumors of germ cell origin, including seminomas, teratomas, and embryonal cell carcinomas, have been reported to develop rarely in patients with Klinefelter's syndrome. Most germ cell tumors have occurred in extragonadal locations, especially in the mediastinum as choriocarcinoma.[60] Approximately 4% of males with breast cancer have Klinefelter's syndrome.

Turner's Syndrome

In the classic form, Turner's syndrome is a disorder in which sexually immature phenotypic females of short stature have various congenital anomalies and streak gonads. The cytogenetic hallmark is the 45X karyotype. About 98% of fetuses with a 45X karyotype abort; the incidence of Turner's syndrome is about 1:3000 in liveborn females.

In the newborn, the overt findings are related to lymph stasis, which is usually manifested as edema of the dorsum of the hands or feet or, less frequently, as swellings of the nape of the neck (cystic hygroma). Webbing of the

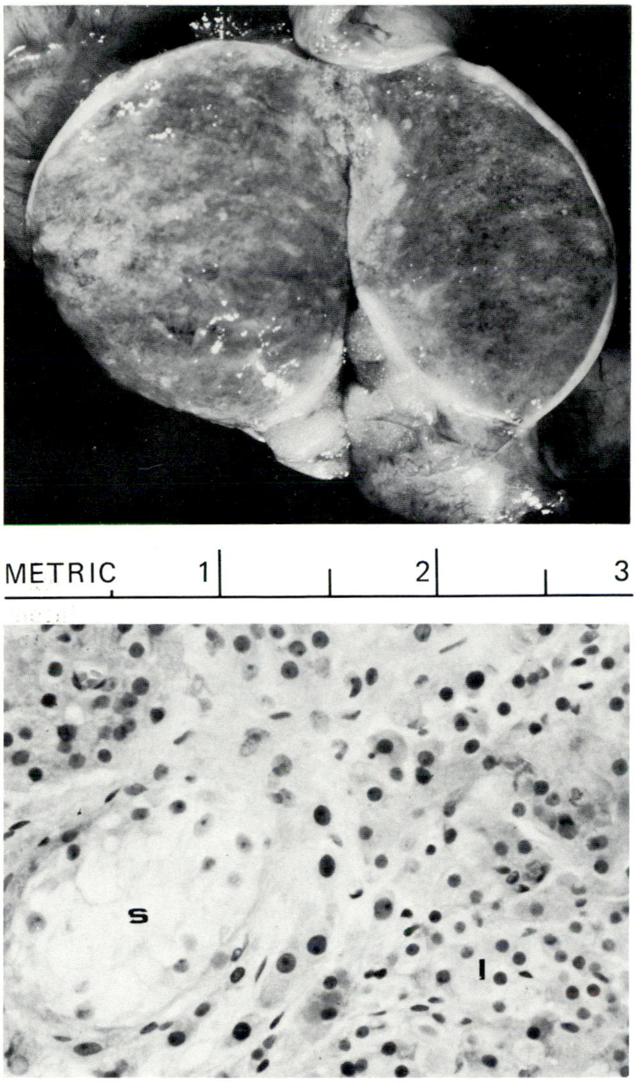

FIG. 2.5. Klinefelter's syndrome. *Top*. The parenchyma of the 2.5 cm testis is golden-yellow to slightly brown. *Bottom*. Clusters of Leydig cells (l) surround a seminiferous tubule (s). (Reprinted from Welch and Robboy, Ref. 69, with permission of Pediatric Andrology.)

neck and elevation of the distal portion of the nails are residua of more marked swellings present during fetal life and may provide a clue to the correct diagnosis. The full range of somatic anomalies is more than 40.

Patients who reach adolescence without a diagnosis often present with primary amenorrhea. Examination reveals undeveloped secondary sexual characteristics and a small uterus. Urinary gonadotropin excretion is always elevated, and the vaginal smear almost always reveals an absence of cornified cells. A buccal smear in the 45X individual will usually disclose few if any Barr bodies. One fifth of patients have a mosaic karyotype (usually 45X/46XX or 45X/47XXX), and in these instances the smear discloses a subnormal number of chromatin-positive cells (about 5 to 15%) for a female. The rare patient with Turner's syndrome who becomes pregnant should be suspected of having a 46XX cell line.[49]

At laparotomy, the internal genitalia are female and, although small, are in normal relation to one another. The gonads appear as white fibrous streaks, 2 to 3 cm long and 0.5 cm in diameter, and are located in the position normally occupied by the ovary (Fig. 2.6). On microscopic examination a streak consists of an attenuated cortex, a medulla, and a hilus. The cortex is composed of characteristic ovarian stroma in which the cells are elongate and wavy and are composed of conspicuous nuclei and scant cytoplasm. Rete tubules (rete ovarii) and hilar cells are typically present in the hilus region. The fact that oocytes are present in normal numbers in 45X embryos before the 12th week of gestation but reduced in older fetuses and almost always absent in adults has suggested that the second X chromosome controls granulosa cell development and primary follicular formation. In the absence of this X chromosome, granulosa cells fail to differentiate, and, as a result, the oocytes degenerate.[12]

Gonadal tumors are exceedingly rare. Tumors of germ cell origin are undoubtedly rare due to the paucity of germ cells. Individuals with phenotypic features of Turner's syndrome (short stature and primary amenorrhea) and a karyotype of 45X reported as having a gonadal tumor have been found to have an XO/XY mosaic chromosome constitution after rekaryotyping.[47] Development of neoplasms of the so-called common epithelial type in these patients suggests that the coelomic epithelium encapsulating the gonad can undergo malignant change even if the gonad is a streak.[40] Endometrial cancer may develop occasionally in those patients who have had long-term exogenous estrogen therapy to foster the appearance of the female secondary sexual characteristics.[51] Both natural estrogens and synthetic nonsteroidal estrogens have been implicated. The duration of usage usually

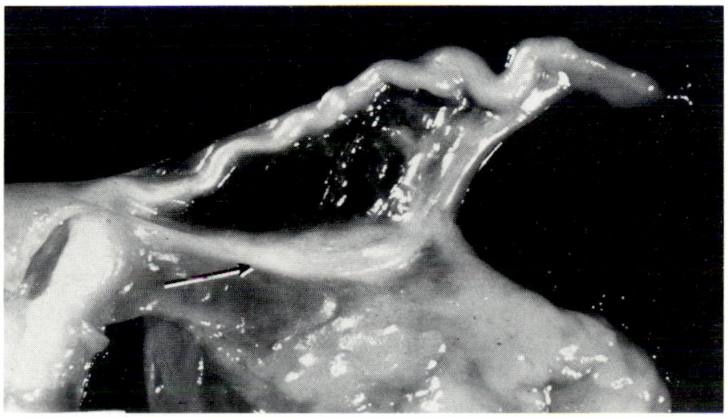

FIG. 2.6. Streak ovary (*arrow*) in Turner's syndrome. (Reprinted from Welch and Robboy, Ref. 69, with permission of Pediatric Andrology.)

exceeds 3 years. Extragonadal tumors, most often of neurogenic origin, have been reported in children and young adults.[70]

XX Male Syndrome

The XX male syndrome, which is one of the rarest sex chromosome anomalies, occurs in about 1 of every 24,000 newborn males.[9] XX males resemble people with Klinefelter's syndrome in their general masculine appearance and male psychosexual orientation. The XX male patients also exhibit normal to weak secondary sexual characteristics, azoospermia, normal or low androgen levels, small testes, prominent Leydig cells, and tubules lined only by Sertoli cells. Mild mental retardation, a common feature of Klinefelter's syndrome, is unusual in XX males. The most common reasons for referral are identical in both syndromes, namely, infertility or abnormal secondary sexual characteristics.

Dewald and Spurbeck[10] suggest that at least three possible mechanisms may account for the development of this syndrome. With the use of banding techniques, at least 70% of patients have been shown to have a small portion of the p (short) arm of the Y chromosome translocated to the p (short) arm of one of the X chromosomes. Even if no gross translocation is obvious, submicroscopic portions of the Y chromosome may still have translocated, based on the finding of H–Y antigen in some of these patients. It is also thought that about one sixth of 46XX males may owe their maleness to chromosome mosaicism or to chimerism. If a 47XXY zygote lost its Y chromosome by nondisjunction early during ontogeny, the 46XX cell line would persist; the 47XXY cell line may have persisted long enough to induce the male gonad.

Pure Gonadal Dysgenesis

Pure gonadal dysgenesis is a term that historically encompasses several diverse conditions, including testicular regression syndrome. In the context defined herein, pure gonadal dysgenesis refers to a phenotypic female without genital ambiguity in whom the internal genitalia include müllerian structures (uterus and fallopian tubes) and streak gonads. The patients may appear to be phenotypically normal or have hypoplastic external genitalia. Pure 46XX gonadal dysgenesis has been identified in identical twins whose primary complaint had been that of secondary amenorrhea. On examination, they were found to have bilateral streak gonads without any other identifiable somatic manifestations (pure gonadal dysgenesis).[73] This appears to be an example of heritable streak gonads associated with a 46XX karyotype. More commonly, heritable streak gonads are associated with a 46XY karyotype. One subgroup with an abnormal X chromosome has had a balanced translocation of the long to the short arm of the X chromosome.[5,18] In addition, there is a subgroup in which an X-autosome translocation is evident that disrupts the integrity and continuity of the X chromosome between bands q13 and q26, resulting in gonadal dysgenesis.[44]

Sexual Ambiguity Frequent

Patients in this category exhibit a wide range of phenotypic appearances and internal genitalia. A Y chromosome is often present, usually as part of a mosaic complement. Sexual ambiguity is a common finding.

Mixed Gonadal Dysgenesis

Mixed gonadal dysgenesis (MGD) is a syndrome characterized in most patients by a mosaic 45X/46XY karyotype, persistent müllerian duct structures, an abnormal testis, and a contralateral streak gonad. The functional deficit imposed by the abnormal testis is expressed as incomplete inhibition of müllerian development, incomplete differentiation of wolffian duct structures, and incomplete male development of the external genitalia. Often incomplete mediation of testicular descent occurs. This results in both internal and external asymmetry of the genitalia and a mixture of male and female features in a person in whom neither gonad is normal. Elsewhere, we have suggested[50] that the syndrome of MGD should be enlarged to incorporate some patients with bilateral streak gonads (included by others as one form of pure gonadal dysgenesis) or bilateral abnormal testes (dysgenetic male pseudohermaphroditism), since the clinical, pathologic, and chromosomal features of these syndromes closely resemble each other.

Mixed gonadal dysgenesis is detected in the neonate principally because of ambiguity of the external genitalia. Frequently, a palpable testis bulges through an indirect inguinal hernia or descends completely into the labioscrotal fold, resulting in asymmetry of the genital swellings. This clinical appearance has led some investigators to name the syndrome *Asymmetric gonadal dysgenesis.* If the gonads are intraabdominal, the labioscrotal folds may appear as normal labia or as empty scrotal sacs. The condition is likely to go unrecognized unless the clitoris is sufficiently enlarged to mandate investigation, which is common. The gonad that descends is almost always a testis, and the streak gonads are always intraabdominal unless dragged into a hernia uteri inguinale.

Mixed gonadal dysgenesis was detected in a neonate with apparently normal female external genitalia when phenotypic characteristics suggestive of Turner's syndrome (pedal edema and redundant skin folds) were recognized. Karyotypic analysis disclosed a predominantly XY karyotype with only a rare cell exhibiting an XO karyotype.[31] Laparotomy revealed a normal uterus with fallopian tubes and bilateral dysplastic ovaries with histologic features of gonadoblastoma. A partial deletion of the short arm of the Y chromosome was also present in this patient. Other individuals with XO/XY mosaicism have been found to have defects in their Y chromosome as well. Analysis of the Y chromosome in patients with XO/XY mosaicism who have normal-sized but nonfluorescent Y chromosomes by *Hae* III enzyme restriction has revealed loss of the male-specific Y fragments (3.4- and 2.1-Kb fragments of Y).[16]

Organs derived from the müllerian duct persist in 95% of cases (Fig. 2.7). The uterus is usually infantile or rudimentary. The fallopian tubes are frequently bilateral. If a testis is grossly near normal size and well differentiated, the fimbriated end of the ipsilateral tube may be absent. In only one-third of cases is the ipsilateral tube entirely absent. Organs of wolffian duct derivation may be present also, but the frequency is variable. The epididymis is identified in two-thirds of patients and is usually present on the side where there is a testis. The vas deferens is encountered less frequently. The seminal vesicle is only rarely identified probably because tissue near the bladder–prostate region is not usually removed.

The gonad may be a testis or streak. Streak gonads may be partially differentiated toward ovary or testis. Bilateral gross testes, frequently of an asynchronous de-

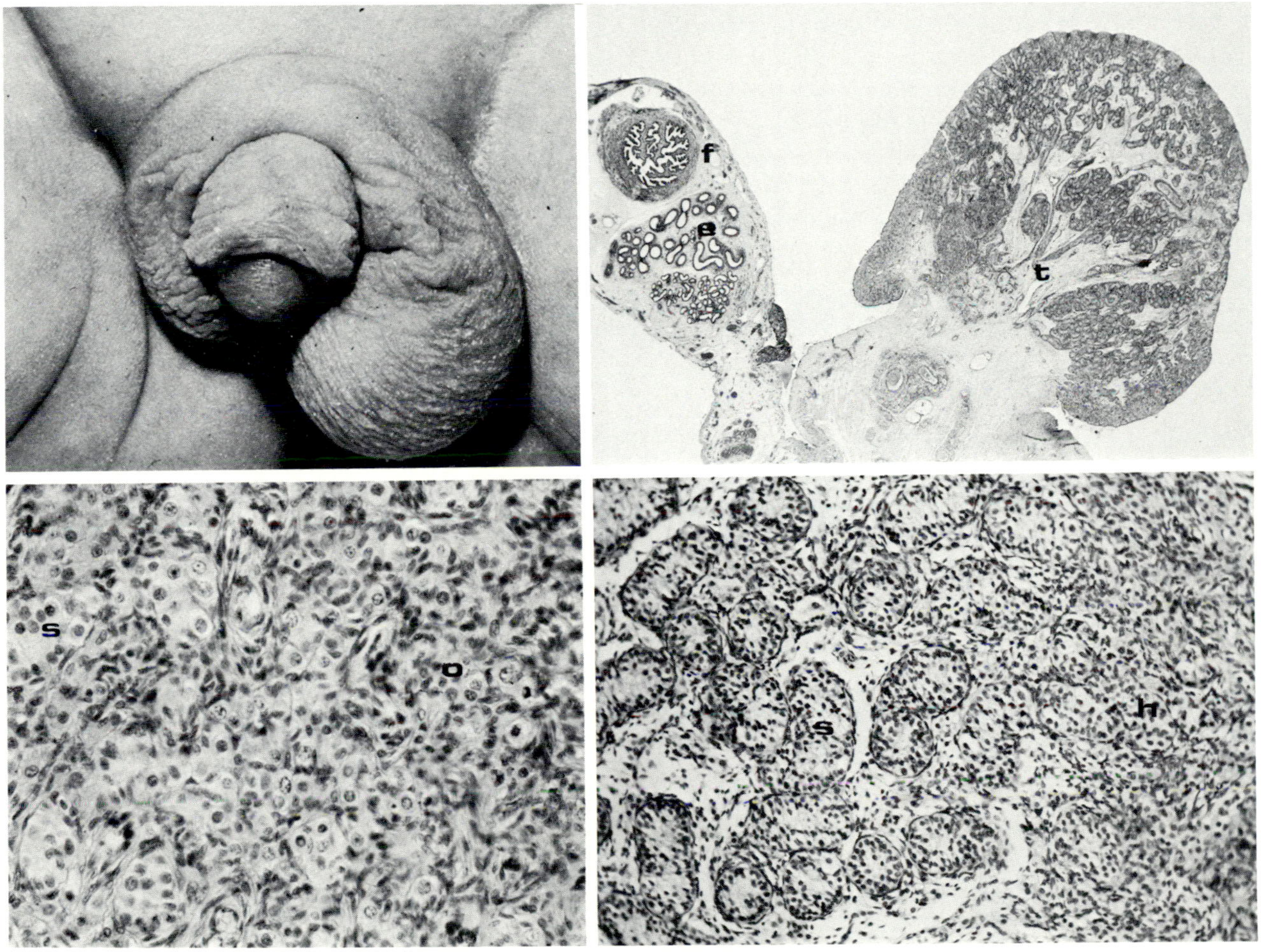

Fig. 2.7. Mixed gonadal dysgenesis. *Top left.* External genitalia in MGD. The left testis had descended into the scrotum; the right streak was in the abdominal cavity. Because of this characteristic appearance, some investigators prefer the name *asymmetric gonadal dysgenesis* rather than mixed gonadal dysgenesis. *Top right.* Testis (t) and adjacent fallopian tube (f) and epididymis (e). The medulla contains immature seminiferous tubules with germ cells and interstitial cells, whereas the region nearer the cortex resembles fetal ovary with immature sex cords and rare primordial follicles. *Bottom left.* Cortex of gonad in which testicular seminiferous tubules (s) merge into fetal type ovary (o). *Bottom right.* The medullary parenchyma of the testis is composed of normal immature seminiferous tubules (s) with germ cells and occasional interstitial cells, whereas the parenchyma in the region of the hilus (h) near the rete testis appears less committed as testis and is characterized by abnormal, pleomorphic seminiferous tubules. The photograph was taken at the junction of the two zones. (Reprinted from Robboy et al., Ref. 50, with permission of Human Pathology.)

gree of maturity, are found in about 15% of patients, whereas a unilateral gross testis is found in 60%. The testis is consistently abnormal architecturally, its organization being divided into three zones, each of which reflects the quantity and type of cellular components present. The three zones are: (1) the region of the tunica albuginea or cortex, which exhibits widely spaced seminiferous tubules or differentiation toward ovary, (2) the medulla, which is composed of normal or near-normal seminiferous tubules and interstitium, and (3) a hilar region with poorly differentiated seminiferous tubules that appears only partly differentiated toward testis.

The superficial cortex may contain seminiferous tubules that are often widely separated by edematous, undifferentiated stroma. Sometimes the tubules penetrate the incompletely formed tunica albuginea and open onto the serosa. Occasionally, broad zones of cortex differentiate slightly toward ovary, even displaying rare primordial follicles. It is of interest that mice that spontaneously develop chromosomal mosaicism as a result of nondisjunction often show gonads with ovarian tissue at the periphery and seminiferous cords centrally.[14]

The central zone (medulla) of the macroscopic infant testis is architecturally and cytologically normal. Narrow closed seminiferous tubules are lined by Sertoli cells with copious cytoplasm. The number of spermatogonia vary, and advanced forms of spermatogenic maturation are not observed. Leydig cells are present in small clusters of varying size. The nuclei of the Leydig cells contain finely dispersed chromatin. The cytoplasm varies from minimal and amphophilic or slightly basophilic to copious and eosinophilic.

The medulla is atrophic, and the tubules are lined only by Sertoli cells in older patients (Fig. 2.8). The basement membranes are often thickened. Prominent clusters of Leydig cells with copious eosinophilic cytoplasm fill the interstitium.

The architecturally disorganized hilar region discloses seminiferous tubules that are swollen by increased numbers of Sertoli cells and are lined by indistinct basement membranes. These tubules also merge with the surrounding stroma, imparting the appearance of a homogeneous blend of Leydig cells, germ cells, Sertoli cells, and an indeterminate type of interstitial stroma. The region resembles neither fetal ovary nor testis.

We have not observed a gonad that has been identifi-

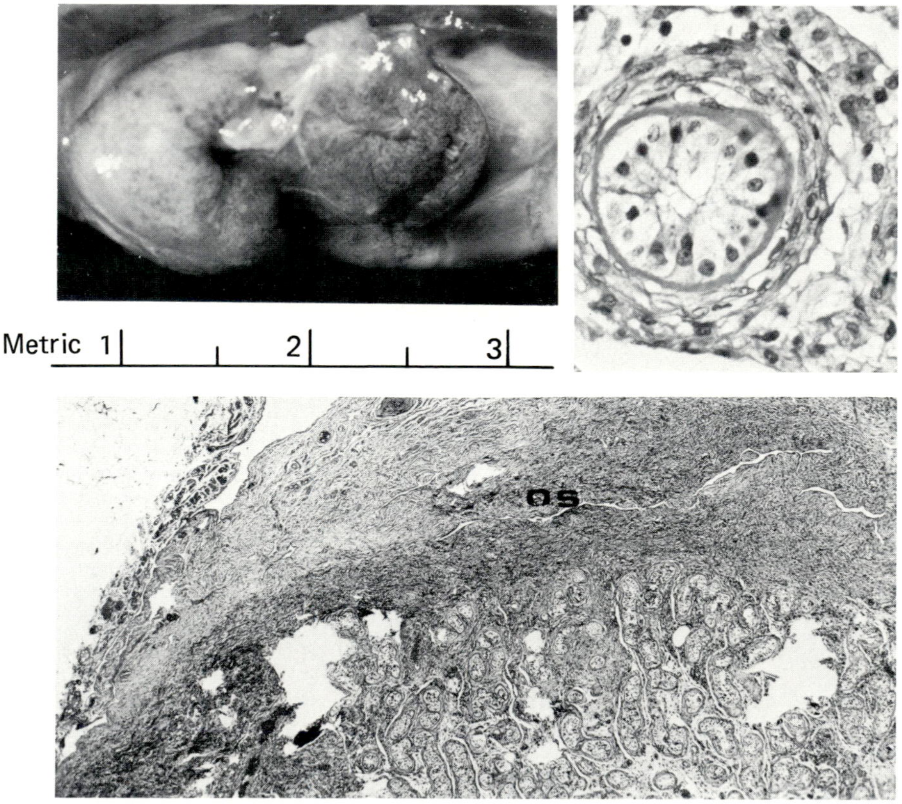

Fig. 2.8. Testis in a 35-year-old phenotypic male with mixed gonadal dysgenesis. *Top left.* The tunica albuginea is tan and maximally 1 mm thick; the parenchyma is golden yellow. *Bottom.* Cross-section of tunica albuginea, which is composed of stroma resembling the stroma of ovarian cortex (os) and medulla with seminiferous tubules. *Top right.* Detail of seminiferous tubules lined by only Sertoli cells. The interstitium is filled with Leydig cells. (Reprinted from Robboy et al., Ref. 50, with permission of Human Pathology.)

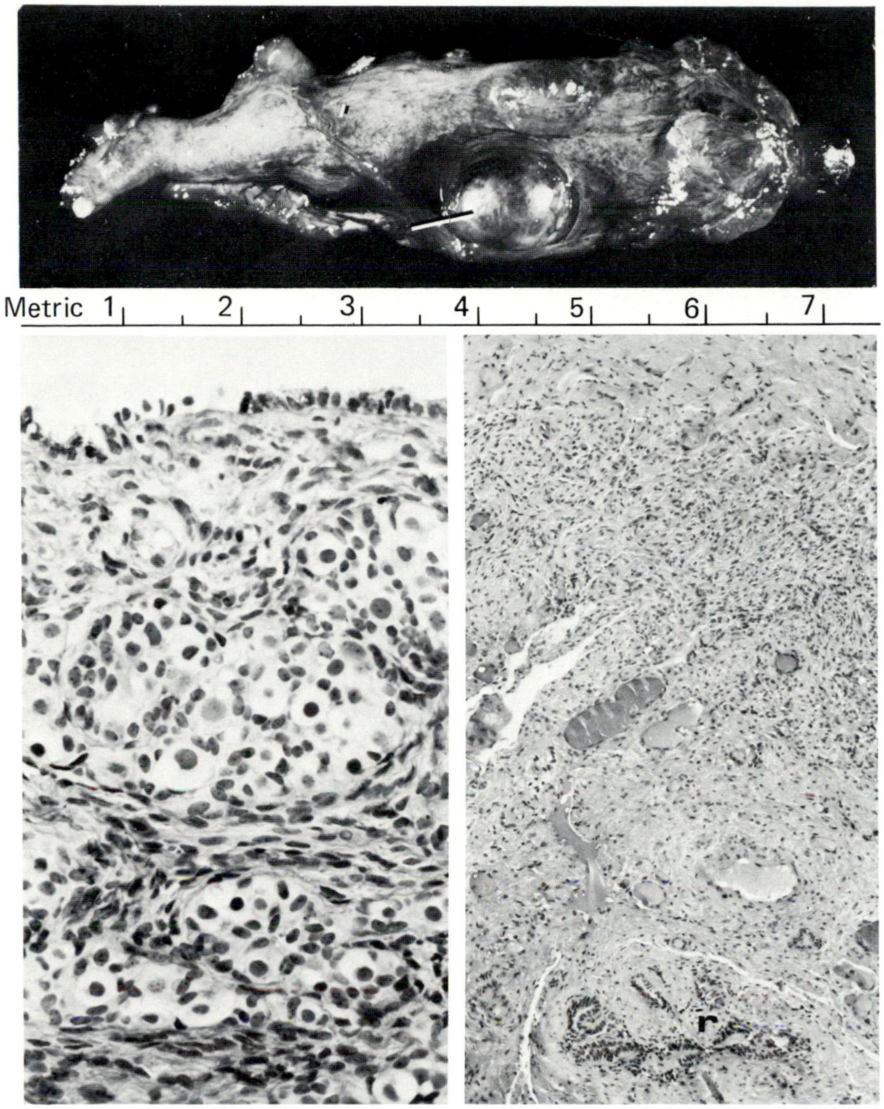

Fig. 2.9. Mixed gonadal dysgenesis. *Bottom left.* When the patient was an infant, the streak gonad resembled a fetal ovary with germ cells and immature sex cords. *Top.* When the streak gonad was removed in entirety 13 years later (*arrow*), it existed only as several microscopic areas of wispy ovarian type cortical stroma and rete ovarii (r) (*bottom right*). (Reprinted from Robboy et al., Ref. 50, with permission of Human Pathology.)

able grossly as an ovary or has been shown microscopically to contain graafian follicles, corpora lutea, or corpora albicantia. The presence of rare primordial follicles or, as in the fetal ovary, aggregates of germ cells partially surrounded by immature granulosa cells is evidence that a streak gonad can differentiate toward ovary.

Morphologic changes may occur over time in the gonads. Myriads of germ cells present in a streak of an infant may degenerate and disappear by puberty, resulting in a gonad composed exclusively of fibrous tissue and a few rete tubules (Fig. 2.9). Similar changes occur in the streak gonads of Turner's syndrome (45X karyotype).

Approximately one-third of patients with MGD develop gonadoblastoma (see Chapter 20, Germ Cell Tumors of Ovary.) Occasionally, gonadoblastoma occurs also in patients with true hermaphroditism. Many of the isolated reports of gonadoblastoma associated with other forms of hermaphroditism described clinically and pathologically may in actuality be examples of MGD-related gonadoblastoma.

The gross appearance of the gonad with gonadoblastoma varies according to the size of the neoplasm, the presence of calcification, and whether the gonadoblastoma has been overgrown by a malignant form of germ cell tumor (usually germinoma)[56] (Fig. 2.10). Approximately one fifth of gonadoblastomas are discovered solely because a streak gonad was examined microscopically

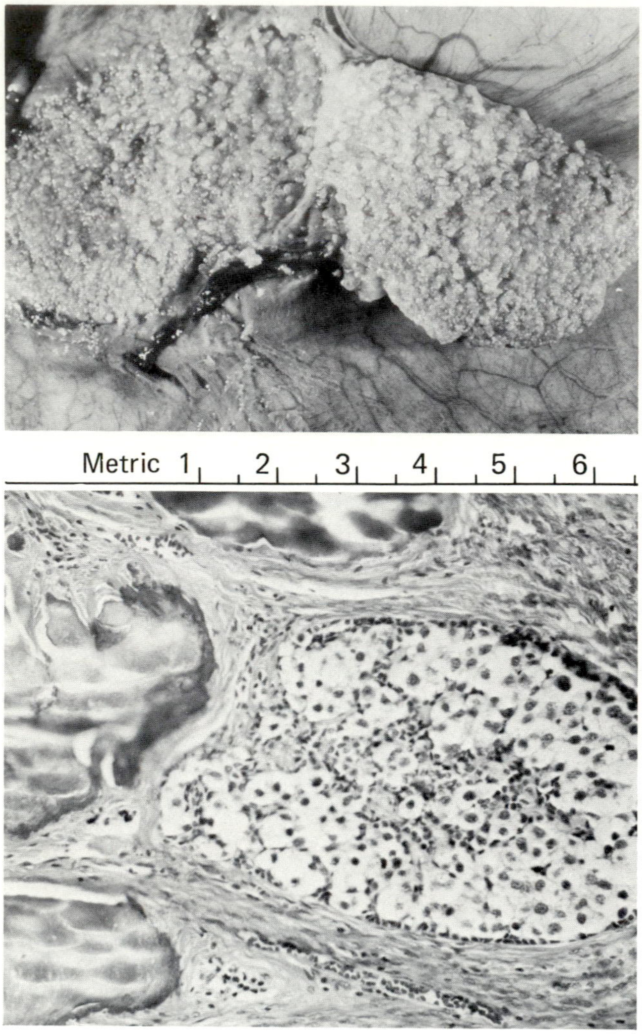

FIG. 2.10. Gonadoblastoma in mixed gonadal dysgenesis. *Top.* Gonadal tumor (15 cm) composed largely of dysgerminoma. At one pole is a 5 × 2 × 0.5 cm calcified gonadoblastoma. *Bottom.* Gonadoblastoma. Multiple mulberry-like calcific masses partially replace the tumor nests composed of germ cells surrounded by sex cord derivatives. (Reprinted from Welch and Robboy, Ref. 69, with permission of Pediatric Andrology.)

(Fig. 2.11). The contralateral gonad also contains a gonadoblastoma in over one third of patients.

On microscopic examination, the gonadoblastoma appears as circumscribed nests of neoplastic germ cells with the cytologic properties of germinoma (dysgerminoma and seminoma) (Fig. 2.10). The germinoma cells are encompassed individually or in groups by sex cord derivatives with inconspicuous cytoplasm and small round to oval nuclei resembling immature Sertoli or granulosa cells. Hyaline, composed of basement membrane material, is found along the margin or as nodules within the nests of tumors. In four-fifths of cases, the hyaline material is calcified, initially appearing as small, laminated spheres, which eventually fuse and coalesce into large mulberry-like masses. Not infrequently, the only evidence that a dysgerminoma originated in a gonadoblastoma is the presence focally of mulberry-like calcifications. Hormonally active cells that resemble lutein and Leydig cells are found interspersed among the nests of tumor in about two-thirds of cases. They are found least frequently in nonvirilized phenotypic females, more often in virilized females, and most frequently in phenotypic males. To some degree, their appearance may be related to the postpubertal age of the patient when the gonad is examined.

Approximately 30% of gonadoblastomas are overgrown by a malignant germ cell tumor, usually the germinoma; 8% are overgrown by endodermal sinus tumor, immature teratoma, embryonal carcinoma, or choriocarcinoma. Although the gonadoblastoma itself does not metastasize and therefore can be considered as an in situ malignancy, the typically malignant behavior of the other tumors makes early prophylactic removal of the gonads in all patients advisable. To avoid the consequences of onset of virilization if the patient is to be raised as a female, it is important that gonadectomy be performed before the patient reaches puberty.[12] Patients who have been treated with long-term administration of estrogen may on occasion develop endometrial carcinoma.[50]

True Hermaphroditism

True hermaphroditism is defined as the presence of both testicular and ovarian tissue in a patient. Because the wavy, cortical-type stroma typically seen in the female

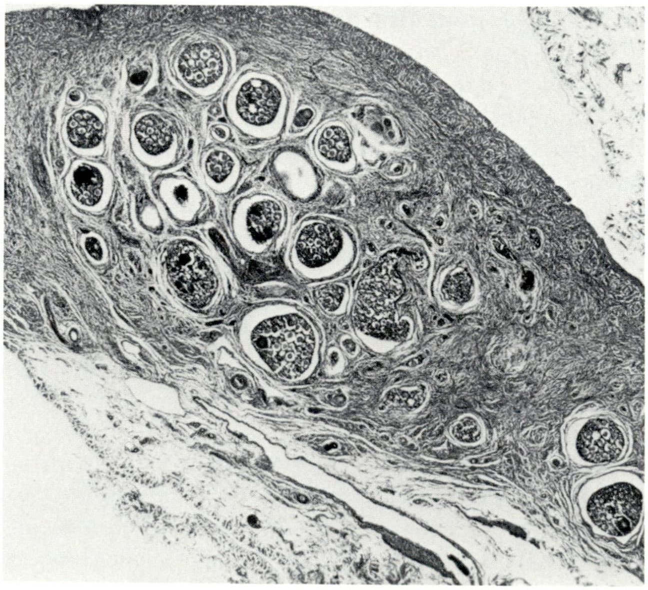

FIG. 2.11. Gonadoblastoma occupying a gonadal streak. (Reprinted from Scully, Ref. 56, with permission of Cancer.)

gonad can be found in both female and male gonads and therefore is nonspecific, follicular structures must be identified to classify gonadal tissue as ovarian. Seminiferous tubules must be identified to classify the tissue as testicular. In true hermaphrodites, the gonads may be ovary and testis separately or combined in an ovotestis.

The ovotestis is the most frequently encountered gonad in true hermaphroditism. In four-fifths of patients, the ovarian and testicular tissues are arranged in an end-to-end fashion. The ovarian portion of an ovotestis has a convoluted surface, whereas the testicular portion is smooth and glistening. Frequently, a distinct line demarcates the two tissues. The firm nature of the palpable ovarian tissue and the soft texture of the testis are a valuable clinical sign when evaluating the nature of a gonad in an infant with ambisexual external genitalia.[66]

An ovary, which preferentially develops on the left side, is the second most common gonad in true hermaphrodites. Every patient over 15 years of age in the series of van Niekerk[65] had either a corpus luteum or a corpus albicans. The testis, which is the gonad least often encountered, develops preferentially on the right. The location of the gonad is influenced by the type and quantity of gonadal tissue present. Increasing amounts of ovarian tissue increase the probability that the gonad will be in an ovarian position. When a gonad with the macroscopic features of an ovary is situated in the inguinal canal or in the labioscrotal fold, the possibility of its being an ovotestis should be seriously considered. The position of the testis is less constant. The majority (63%) reside in the scrotum, 14% in the inguinal region, 1% in the internal inguinal ring, and 22% in a normal ovarian position.

The nature of the genital organ adjacent to a gonad in true hermaphroditism is dependent on the nature of the gonad, which is in contrast to MGD, where a fallopian tube is often adjacent to the gonad regardless of whether it is a testis or streak. In true hermaphroditism, a fallopian tube is adjacent to an ovary and an epididymis or vas deferens is adjacent to a testis. Either a müllerian or a wolffian structure, but not both, is adjacent to an ovotestis. Müllerian-inhibiting substance appears to be functional. Ninety-five percent of fallopian tubes adjacent to ovotestes have closed ostia. Only 10% of uteri are normal; the other patients have absent uteri (13%), unicornuate uteri (10%), absent cervix (14%), or uterine hypoplasia (46%).

The most common karyotypes in true hermaphroditism are 46XX (60%), 46XY (12%), and mosaic (28%), usually 46XX/46XY, 46XY/47XXY, or least frequently 45X/46XY. Recent data have shown that even in some 46XX individuals the ovarian portion of the gonad is H–Y antigen-negative, whereas the testicular portion is H–Y antigen-positive,[67] implying that the hermaphroditic gonad may arise from a mosaic primordium regardless of the apparent karyotype. Patients with a Y chromosome have a two- to threefold increased frequency of having a testis as opposed to an ovotestis. Nearly 75% of true hermaphrodites with an ovary and ovotestis have a 46XX karyotype.

The clinical presentations of true hermaphrodites vary to some extent depending on the patient's age at the time of diagnosis.[11] Until recently, the condition often went undetected until adolescence, when phenotypic male patients were evaluated for gynecomastia and phenotypic female patients were evaluated for amenorrhea or failure to develop secondary sexual changes. Thus, in the series of van Niekerk and Retief,[66] 73% of patients were raised as males and 27% as females. Many patients, however, menstruated, and a few have become pregnant. With an increased awareness of intersex states, the condition is more often recognized in infants because of ambiguous genitalia, usually in the form of a small phallus (enlarged clitoris). Like MGD, the scrotum may be asymmetric, with the larger, more normal-appearing hemiscrotum containing a testis. Among 160 patients, the external genitalia were asymmetric in 76% (labioscrotal folds in 63% and hemiscrotums in 13%).

On microscopic examination, the gonadal tissue often appears normal if the patient is young. In infants, the ovarian tissue contains numerous follicles, and the testicular parenchyma discloses normal-appearing seminiferous tubules with spermatogonia. Patients in the reproductive years may have ovarian tissue with structures indicative of ovulation, but spermatogenesis is rare in the testicular portion.

At times, distinction between true hermaphroditism and MGD can be difficult. In the newborn, asymmetric ambiguous genitalia may be observed in both conditions. If a streak gonad from a patient with MGD is serially sectioned, a rare primordial follicle may be encountered in what otherwise appears to be a fetal type ovary admixed with testis with well-developed seminiferous tubules.[50] If the term *true hermaphroditism* is restricted to those patients in whom the ovarian and testicular tissue are both apparent grossly, it should be possible to segregate more clearly those individuals in whom the ovarian tissue may be functional.

Germ cell tumors, including gonadoblastoma, develop in 2.6% of gonads. Sertoli cell tumor may occur rarely in the testicular gonad and may be capable of ectopic production of gonadotropins.[20]

References

1. Aarskog D (1979) Maternal progestins as a possible cause of hypospadias. N Engl J Med 300: 75
2. Berthezene F, Forest MG, Grimaud JA, Clastrat B, Mornex R (1976) Leydig-cell agenesis. A cause of male pseudohermaphroditism. N Engl J Med 295: 969

3. Brogger A, Strand A (1965) Contribution to the study of the so-called pure gonadal dysgenesis. Acta Endocrinol 48: 490
4. Camacho CM, Kowarski A, Migeon CJ, Brough AJ (1968) Congenital adrenal hyperplasia due to a deficiency of one of the enzymes involved in the biosynthesis of pregnenolone. J Clin Endocrinol Metab 28: 153
5. Carpenter NJ, Say B, Browning D (1980) Gonadal dysgenesis in a patient with an X3 translocation: Case report and review. J Med Genet 17: 216
6. Case Records of the Massachusetts General Hospital (Case 8–1977) (1977) N Engl J Med 296: 439
7. Coulam CB (1979) Testicular regression syndrome. Obstet Gynecol 53:44
8. Dean HJ, Shackleton CHL, Winter JSD (1984) Diagnosis and natural history of 17-hydroxylase deficiency in a newborn male. J Clin Endocrinol Metab 59: 513
9. de la Chapelle A (1981) The etiology of maleness in XX men. Hum Genet 58: 105
10. Dewald GW, Spurbeck JL (1983) Sex chromosome anomalies associated with premature gonadal failure. Semin Reprod Endocrinol 1: 79
11. Donahoe PK, Crawford JD, Hendren WH (1978) True hermaphroditism: A clinical description and a proposed function for the long arm of the Y chromosome. J Pediatr Surg 13: 293
12. Donahoe PK, Crawford JD, Hendren WH (1979) Mixed gonadal dysgenesis, pathogenesis and management. J Pediatr Surg 14: 287
13. Edman CD (1983) Testicular regression syndrome. Semin Reprod Endocrinol 1: 129
14. Eicher EM, Beamer WG, Washburn LL, Whitten WK (1980) A cytogenetic investigation of inherited true hermaphroditism in BALB/cWt mice. Cytogenet Cell Genet 28: 104
15. Forest MG, Lecornu M, de Peretti E (1980) Familial male pseudohermaphroditism due to 17–20-desmolase deficiency. I. In vivo endocrine studies. J Clin Endocrinol Metab 50: 826
16. Ganshirt D, Pawlowitzki IH (1984) Hae III restriction of DNA from three cases with nonfluorescent Y chromosomes (45XO/46XYnf). Hum Genet 67: 241
17. Golimbu M (1984) H–Y antigen: Genetic control and role in testicular differentiation. Urology 24: 115
18. Grass FR, Schwartz RP, Deal JO, Parke J (1981) Gonadal dysgenesis, intra-X chromosome insertion, and possible position effect in an otherwise normal female. Clin Genet 20: 28
19. Griffin J, Wilson JD (1980) The syndromes of androgen resistance. N Engl J Med 302: 198
20. Gunasegaram R, Mathew T, Ratnam SS (1981) Sertoli cell tumour in a true hermaphrodite: Suggestive evidence for ectopic gonadotrophin production by the tumour. Br J Obstet Gynecol 88: 1252
21. Gunasegaram R, Loganath A, Peh KL, Kottegoda SR, Ratnam SS (1984) Steroid C-17,20-desmolase activity in testicular tissue of male transsexuals. IRCS Med Sci 12: 1151
22. Haseltine FP (1983) Defects in H–Y antigen expression and related gonadal failure. Semin Reprod Endocrinol 1: 113
23. Haymond MW, Weldon VV (1973) Female pseudohermaphroditism secondary to a maternal virilizing tumor. J Pediatr 82: 682
24. Imperato-McGinley J, Peterson RE, Gautier T, Sturla E (1979) Androgens and the evolution of male-gender identity among male pseudohermaphrodites with 5-α-reductase deficiency. N Engl J Med 300: 1233
25. Imperato-McGinley J, Peterson RE, Leshin M, Griffin JE, Cooper G, Draghi S, Berenyi M, Wilson JD (1980) Steroid 5-alpha-reductase deficiency in a 65-year-old male pseudohermaphrodite: The natural history, ultrastructure of the testes, and evidence for inherited enzyme heterogeneity. J Clin Endocrinol Metab 50: 15
26. Jones HW Jr, Lee Pa, Rock JA, Archer DF, Migeon CJ (1982) A genetic male patient with 17-alpha-hydroxylase deficiency. Obstet Gynecol 59: 254
27. Kirkland RT, Kirkland JL, Johnson C, Horning M, Librik L, Clayton GW (1973) Congenital lipoid adrenal hyperplasia in an eight-year-old phenotypic female. J Clin Endocrinol Metab 36: 488
28. Kohn B, Levine LS, Pollack MS, Pang S, Lorenzen F, Levy D, Lerner AJ, Pondanini GF, Dupont B, New M (1982) Late-onset steroid 21-hydroxylase deficiency: A variant of classical congenital adrenal hyperplasia. J Clin Endocrinol Metab 55: 493
29. Leinonen P, Dunkel L, Perheentupa J, Vihko R (1983) Male pseudohermaphroditism due to deficiency of testicular 17-ketosteroid reductase. Acta Pediatr Scand 72: 211–214
30. Madan K, Schoemaker J (1980) XY females with enzyme deficiencies of steroid metabolism. A brief review. Hum Genet 53: 291
31. Magenis RE, Tochen ML, Holahan KP, Carey T, Allen L, Brown MG (1984) Turner syndrome resulting from partial deletion of Y chromosome short arm: Localization of male determinants. J Pediatr 105: 916
32. Manuel M, Katayama KP, Jones HW Jr (1976) The age of occurence of gonadal tumors in intersex patients with a Y chromosome. Am J Obstet Gynecol 124: 293
33. McCoshen JA (1982) In vivo sex differentiation of congeneic germinal cell aplastic gonads. Am J Obstet Gynecol 142: 83
34. Mininberg DT, Levine LS, New MI (1982) Current concepts in congenital adrenal hyperplasia. Pathol Annu 2: 179
35. Mor N, Merlob P, Reisner SH (1983) Tags and bands of the female external genitalia in the newborn infant. Clin Pediatr 22: 122
36. Mosley JL, Stan EA (1984) Human sexual dimorphism: Its cost and benefit. Adv Child Devel Behav 18: 147
37. Muller J (1985) Morphometry and histology of gonads from 12 children and adolescents with the androgen insensitivity (testicular feminization) syndrome. J Clin Endocrinol Metab 59: 785
38. Muller U (1982) Identification and function of serologically detectable H–Y antigen. Hum Genet 61: 91
39. Muram D, Dewhurst J (1984) Inheritance of intersex disorders. Can Med Assoc J 130: 121
40. Murphy GF, Welch WR, Urcuyo R (1979) Brenner tumor and mucinous cystadenoma of borderline malignancy in a

patient with Turner's syndrome. Obstet Gynecol 54: 660
41. New MI, Dupont B, Pollack MS, Levine LS (1981) The biochemical basis for genotyping 21-hydroxylase deficiency. Hum Genet 58: 123
42. Oka M, Katabuchi HT, Munemura M, Mizumoto J, Maeyama M (1984) An unusual case of male pseudohermaphroditism: Complete testicular feminization associated with incomplete differentiation of the müllerian duct. Fertil Steril 41: 154
43. Okon E, Livni N, Rosler A, Yorkoni S, Segal S, Kohn G, Schenker JG (1980) Male pseudohermaphroditism due to 5-alpha-reductase deficiency. Arch Pathol Lab Med 104: 363
44. Perissel B, Geneix A, Mage B, Charbonne F, Bruhat M, Malet P (1984). Gonadal dysgenesis due to an Xq−;15q+ translocation. Rev Bras Genet 4: 799
45. Peterson RE, Imperato-McGinley J, Gautier T (1977) Male pseudohermaphroditism due to steroid 5-alpha-reductase deficiency. Am J Med 62: 170
46. Peterson RE, Imperato-McGinley J, Gautier T, Shackleton C (1985) Male pseudohermaphroditism due to multiple defects in steroid-biosynthetic microsomal mixed-function oxidases. A new variant of congenital adrenal hyperplasia. N Engl J Med 313: 1182
47. Pfeiffer RA, Tietze U, Krone HA, Schaaff A, Dhom G, Peter H (1983) Invasive dysgerminoma in a girl with 45,X/46,X:mar mosaicism. Arch Gynecol 233: 141
48. Pierre-Louis ML, Kovi J, Sampson CC, Worrell RG, Rosser SB (1983) Ultrastructure of the gonads in the testicular feminization syndrome. J Natl Med Assoc 75: 1177
49. Reyes FI, Koh KS, Faiman C (1976) Fertility in women with gonadal dysgenesis. Am J Obstet Gynecol 126: 668
50. Robboy SJ, Miller T, Donahoe PK, Jahre C, Welch WR, Haseltine FP, Miller WA, Atkins L, Crawford JD (1982) Dysgenesis of testicular and streak gonads in the syndrome of mixed gonadal dysgenesis: Perspective derived from a clinicopathologic analysis of twenty-one cases. Hum Pathol 13: 700
51. Rosenwaks Z, Wentz AC, Jones GS, Urban MD, Lee PA, Migeon CJ, Parmley TH, Woodruff JD (1979) Endometrial pathology and estrogens. Obstet Gynecol 53: 403
52. Roslyn JJ, Fonkalsrud EW, Lippe B (1983) Intersex disorders in adolescents and adults. Am J Surg 146: 137
53. Saenger P, Levine LS, New MI (1981) Male pseudohermaphroditism due to abnormal testosterone biosynthesis and metabolism. Clin Androl 7: 87
54. Schneider G, Genel M, Bongiovanni AM, Goldman AS, Rosenfield RL (1975) Persistent testicular isomerase 3-beta-hydroxysteroid dehydrogenase (3-beta-HSD) deficiency in the 3-beta-HSD form of congenital adrenal hyperplasia. J Clin Invest 55: 681
55. Schwartz M, Imperato-McGinley J, Peterson RE, Cooper G, Morris PL, MacGillivray M, Hensle T (1981) Male pseudohermaphroditism secondary to an abnormality in Leydig cell differentiation. J Clin Endocrinol Metab 53: 123
56. Scully RE (1970) Gonadoblastoma. A review of 74 cases. Cancer 25: 1340
57. Sheridan-Pereira M, O'Brien N (1983) Testicular feminization syndrome presenting in the newborn. Arch Dis Child 58: 380
58. Short RV (1979) Sex determination and differentiation. Br Med Bull 35: 121
59. Simpson JL, Golbus MS, Martin AO, Sarto GE (1982) Genetics in obstetrics and gynecology. New York, Grune & Stratton.
60. Sogge MR, McDonald SD, Cofold PB (1979) The malignant potential of the dysgenetic germ cell in Klinefelter's syndrome. Am J Med 66: 515
61. Sternberg WH, Dhurandhar HN (1977) Functional ovarian tumors of stromal and sex cord origin. Hum Pathol 8: 565
62. Stewart DA, Bailey JD, Netley CT, Rovet J, Park E, Cripps M, Curtis JA (1982) Growth and development of children with X and Y chromosome aneuploidy from infancy to pubertal age: The Toronto Study. Birth Defects 18: 620
63. Ulfelder H, Robboy SJ (1976) The embryologic development of the human vagina. Am J Obstet Gynecol 126: 769
64. Vague S (1983) Testicular feminization syndrome: An experimental model for the study of hormone action on sexual behavior. Hormone Res 18: 62
65. van Niekerk WA (1974) True hermaphroditism. Clinical, morphologic and cytogenetic aspects. Hagerstown, Md, Harper & Row.
66. van Niekerk WA, Retief AE (1981) The gonads of human true hermaphrodites. Hum Genet 58: 117
67. Wachtel SS (1979) The genetics of intersexuality: Clinical and theoretic perspectives. Obstet Gynecol 54: 671
68. Weiss EB, Kiefer JH, Rowlatt UF, Rosenthal IM (1978) Persistent müllerian duct syndrome in male identical twins. Pediatrics 61: 797
69. Welch WR, Robboy SJ (1981) Abnormal sexual development: A classification with emphasis on pathology and neoplastic conditions. Pediatr Androl 7: 71
70. Wertelecki W, Fraumeni JF Jr, Mulvihill JJ (1970) Nongonadal neoplasia in Turner's syndrome. Cancer 26: 485
71. Wilson JD, Griffin JE, Leshin M, George FW (1981) Role of gonadal hormones in development of the sexual phenotypes. Hum Genet 58: 25
72. Wolf U (1981) Genetic aspects of H–Y antigen. Hum Genet 58: 25
73. Youlton R, Michelsen H, Be C, Cruz-Coke R (1982) Pure XX gonadal dysgenesis in identical twins. Clin Genet 21: 220
74. Zachmann M, Tassinari D, Prader A (1983) Clinical and biochemical variability of congenital adrenal hyperplasia due to llb-hydroxylase deficiency: A study of 25 patients. J Clin Endocrinol Metab 56: 575
75. Zachmann M, Vellmin JA, Hamilton W, Prader A (1972) Steroid 17,20-desmolase deficiency. A new case of male pseudohermaphroditism. Clin Endocrinol 1: 369

3

Diseases of the Vulva

Edward J. Wilkinson, M.D., and Eduard G. Friedrich Jr., M.D.

Anatomy

The external female genitalia include the mons pubis, labia majora and minora, clitoris with its prepuce and frenulum, the vestibule into which open the orifices of Skene's and Bartholin's glands as well as those of the minor vestibular glands, and the urethral meatus (Fig. 3.1). After adrenarche, the mons pubis and lateral aspects of the labia majora acquire increased amounts of subcutaneous fat and develop the coarse curly surface hair characteristic of the adult. With maturation of the hair follicle apparatus, there is concomitant maturation and development of the sebaceous and apocrine glands in the hair-bearing regions, as well as in the labia minora and inner aspects of the prepuce. Other than the areola of the breast, these are the only areas in which sebaceous glands routinely develop without concomitant hair formation. During adolescence, the labia acquire a characteristic hyperpigmentation, and the clitoris undergoes some selective enlargement. The labia majora contain both smooth muscle and fat, whereas the labia minora are devoid of adipose tissue but are rich in elastic fibers and blood vessels.

The entire vulva is covered by a keratinized, stratified squamous epithelium. In addition to perspiration from the apocrine and eccrine sweat glands, significant transepidermal water loss occurs because of a relative inefficiency of the stratum corneum in the vulvar area. Thus, the vulva provides a consistently moist environment supportive of bacterial growth.[29] The quantitative microbiology of the human vulva has been studied, and diphtheroids, coagulase-negative staphylococci, and *Staphylococcus aureus* have often been found.[7] In the vestibule, as the vaginal introitus is approached, the epithelium becomes thinner, the rete ridges less prominent, and the keratin layer less pronounced. The hymen is thinly keratinized on its external surface but, on the vaginal surface, shows a nonkeratinized mucous membrane rich in glycogen. The epithelium of the vestibule merges with transitional epithelium at the urethral me-

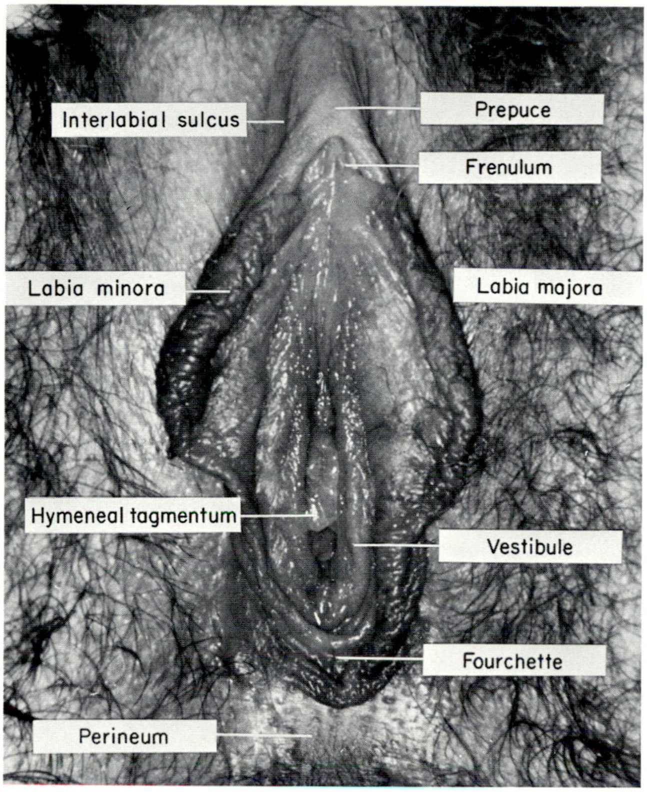

FIG. 3.1. Topography of the vulva.

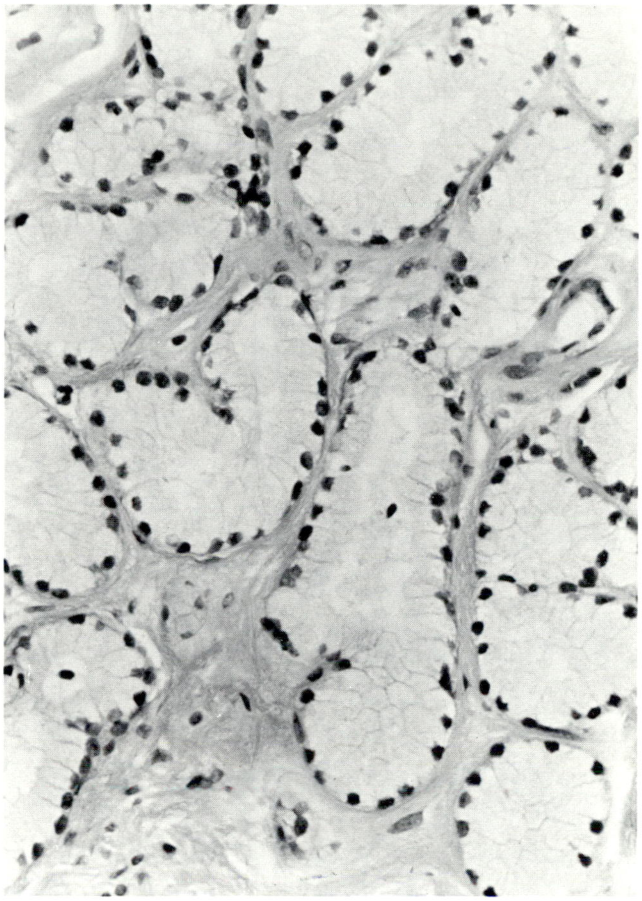

FIG. 3.2. Bartholin gland. Mucus-secreting acini in racemose arrangement.

atus and the duct openings of the paraurethral, minor, and major vestibular (Bartholin's) glands.

The apocrine glands of the majora, minora, and prepuce, like the apocrine glands of the axilla, develop their secretory function at adrenarche, whereas the eccrine sweat glands, primarily involved in heat regulation, function before puberty.[146] The apocrine glands are homologous to the scent glands of lower animals and secrete via a process of decapitation. The paired external openings of the paraurethral glands (Skene's) are found on either side of the urethral meatus, but these glandular structures are known to be distributed along the posterior and lateral aspects of the urethra itself.[145] The ducts are lined with cylindrical epithelium, whereas the glands are composed of pseudostratified mucus-secreting columnar epithelium. Involvement of these glands by inflammation or infection may contribute to the development of suburethral diverticula.

The major vestibular glands of Bartholin are racemose, tubular alveolar glands, with acini composed of simple columnar mucus-secreting epithelium (Fig. 3.2), drained by a duct measuring approximately 2.5 cm in length, and lined with transitional epithelium. The most superficial cells of the duct nearest the glands are of the mucus-secreting type.[291] The more distal duct has a transitional epithelium. The duct exits just external to the hymenal ring on the posterolateral aspect of the vestibule, where its lining is of squamous epithelium. Thus Bartholin's duct has three types of epithelial lining, depending on its location.

The minor vestibular glands are similarly composed of simple columnar lined mucus-secreting acini. These are shallow, within 2–3 mm of the superficial epithelium, and communicate with the vestibular surface via short ducts lined with transitional epithelium. Squamous metaplasia is often seen and may be confused with dysplastic change (Fig. 3.3). These minor glands ring the vestibule and are found from the frenulum anteriorly, downward on both sides of the meatus, around the external base of the hymenal ring, and in the fourchette.[100] Occlusion of their ducts results in mucous cysts. They may be involved in the chronic inflammatory process of vestibulitis (Fig. 3.4).[357,358] Vestibular adenomas arising from these structures, composed of nests of small glands with a tall, pale, mucus-secreting columnar epithelium, have also been reported.[12,91] The clitoris is a specialized structure covered with a stratified squamous epithelium that is thinly keratinized. No sebaceous, apocrine, or eccrine sweat glands are present. Within the stroma of the clitoris

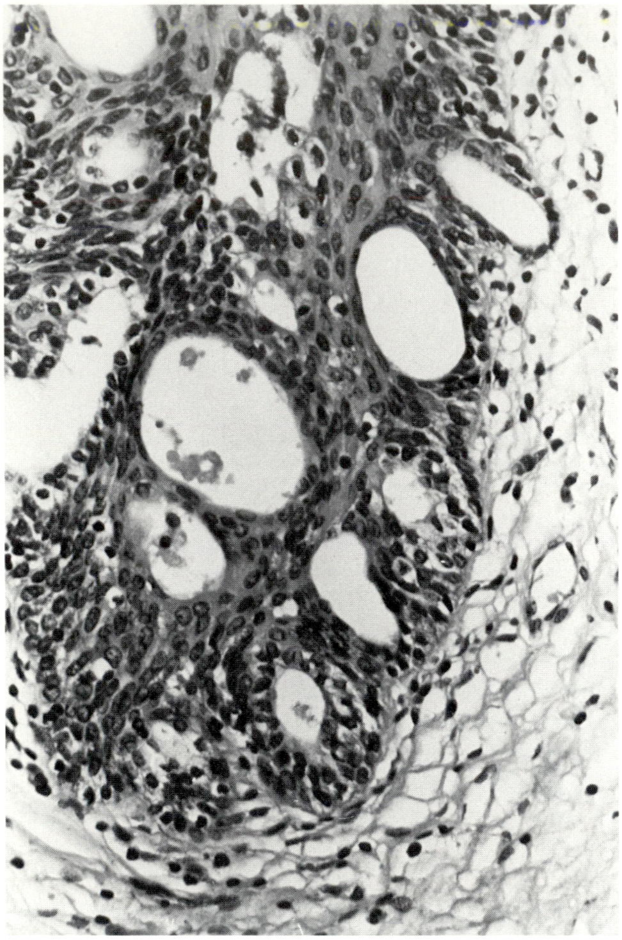

FIG. 3.3. Minor vestibular gland with squamous metaplasia. Some low columnar, mucus-secreting cells are seen lining gland lumens associated with metaplastic squamous epithelium.

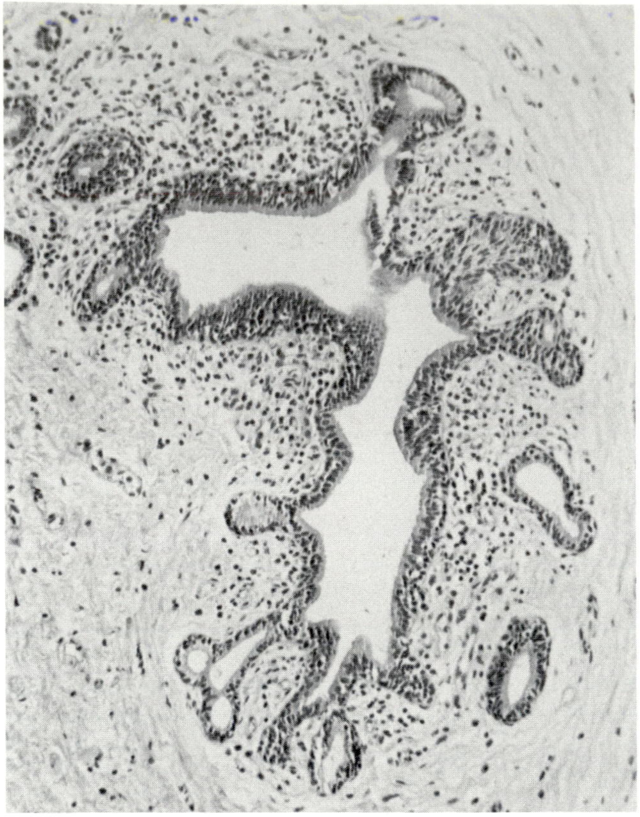

FIG. 3.4. Vestibulitis. A complex minor vestibular gland is seen in the superficial submucosa of the vestibule. A low cuboidal epithelium can be seen lining the gland. Note the chronic inflammatory cells within the adjacent submucosa. The inflammatory infiltrate consists predominately of lymphocytes and plasma cells, with some mast cells.

are two conjoined corpora cavernosa, which branch near the base of the clitoris and lie along the pubic rami as divided crura. They are invested in a loose fibrous tissue sheath with an incomplete center septum. At their insertion, the crura contain ischiocavernosus muscles. The clitoris is further supported bilaterally and dorsally by suspensory ligaments.

The superficial and deep external pudendal arteries branch from the femoral artery. The internal pudendal arteries branch from the internal iliac arteries. These major branches from the femoral and internal iliac arteries provide the major blood supply to the vulva via the anterior labial branches, from the external pudendal arteries, and posterior labial branches, from the internal pudendal. The clitoris, including the crura and corpora cavernosa, is separately supplied by the deep arteries of the clitoris, whereas the anterior vaginal artery supplies blood flow to the vestibule and Bartholin's glands. The venous return parallels the arterial supply.

The femoral and inguinal lymph nodes receive all the lymphatic drainage from the vulva, with the exception of the clitoris, which may have a minor secondary lymphatic pathway.[259,267] A multilayered diffuse meshwork of delicate intercommunicating lymphatic vessels extends over the labia minora, clitoral prepuce, and vulvar vestibule. The lymphatics from the anterior labia minora drain anteriorly and superiorly via three or four larger lymphatic channels that bypass the clitoris and join with the lymphatic channels draining the prepuce. The lymphatic vascular bed of the labia majora is composed of larger vessels than those of the labia minora and drains into lymphatic vessels that course in an anterior superior direction toward the mons. These anastomose with the lymphatic vessels draining the labia minora and prepuce and then course laterally, emptying into the ipsilateral inguinal and femoral nodes. Some contralateral lymphatic flow may also occur, draining into the superior medial nodes of the femoral group.[267] The superficial inguinal lymph nodes consist of 8 to 10 nodes on each side, which may be subdivided into a superior oblique and inferior ventral group. The superior oblique group is found about

Poupart's ligament. The inferior oblique group is found above the junction of the saphenous vein and fascia lata. The superficial inguinal lymph nodes are accepted as the major lymph node group that first receives lymphatic drainage from the vulva.[69,123] This nodal group is included in a radical vulvectomy specimen.[230]

Lymphatic drainage from the clitoris proceeds bilaterally, as does the lymphatic drainage of the midline perineum.[156] Lymphatic flow from other sites on the vulva usually proceeds to the ipsilateral groin and, subsequently, pelvic lymph nodes. In vivo, labial interstitial injection of ^{99m}Tc-colloid has demonstrated that the colloid will reach the lymph nodes within 5 hours of injection into the labia. Both ipsilateral and contralateral pelvic lymph nodes received lymphatic drainage from unilateral labial injection in over 67% of cases studied.[156]

A second, and apparently minor, lymphatic pathway from the glans clitoris proceeds with the lymphatic drainage of the urethra and dorsal vein of the clitoris to course inferior to the symphysis pubis. Traversing the urogenital diaphragm, it merges with the lymphatic plexus on the anterior surface of the bladder. Subsequently, the inferior trunks drain to the interiliac and obturator nodes, and the superior trunk terminates in the nodes of the femoral ring or the medial group of the external iliac nodes. No direct pathway of lymphatic flow from the clitoris to the pelvic nodes could be demonstrated by in vivo colloid injection.[156] It is a clinical fact that in cases of clitoral carcinoma if the inguinofemoral lymph nodes are free of tumor, it is highly unlikely that the pelvic nodes are involved.

The nerve supply to the vulva includes sensory nerves, special receptors, and autonomic nerves to the vessels and various glands. The major nerves of the vulva derive from the anterior (ilioinguinal) and posterior (pudendal) labial nerves. The clitoris is innervated by the dorsal nerve of the clitoris and the cavernous nerves of the clitoris, which also supply the vestibule.[191]

Developmental Defects

Clitoral enlargement may occur with or without associated hyperplasia of the remaining vulva. Clitoral enlargement in the newborn suggests either adrenogenital syndrome, exogenous maternal androgen therapy, or some form of hermaphroditism. A clitoral mass from an infant has been identified with chromosomal mosaicism where the clitoral skin had a hyperdiploid chromosomal abnormality, with normal chromosomes being found in the ovary. This is an example of ambiguous genitalia resulting from a somatic cell mutation with maldevelopment of the clitoris.[302] Clitoral enlargement has also been reported associated with Lawrence–Seip syndrome.[160] Granular cell tumors of the clitoris and leiomyomas may also be a cause of clitoral enlargement.[63,317] Such specimens may come to the attention of the pathologist after partial removal or surgical reduction of the clitoris in an attempt to return the cosmetic appearance of the vulva to normal.

Hypertrophy and asymmetry of the labia minora may occur without demonstrable etiology and, in some cases, may be associated with chronic irritation, as may be seen in women with indwelling urethral catheters. True hypoplasia occurs infrequently and may be a sign of defective steroidogenesis. Imperforate hymen is remarkably rare, with a reported frequency of 0.014%, and is usually discovered after the onset of expected menarche between ages 10 and 18. Slight fusion of the labia minora may be seen in infants without apparent cause. Labial fusion, like clitoral hypertrophy, may also be present with intersex disorders. In these situations, the defect is developmental, but such fusion may also be acquired secondary to inflammation with subsequent adhesion formation.[40] Duplication of the vulva is extremely rare and is usually associated with duplication of the internal müllerian system and rectum as well. The urethra may open into the vagina rather than into the vestibule. Ectopic urethral orifices are occasionally seen adjacent to the hymen.[66] In müllerian agenesis, the hymen and vagina are usually represented only by a depression in the vestibular area. Congenital absence of the clitoris[86] and external genitalia has also been described.[79]

Inflammatory Diseases of the Vulva

Infectious Diseases

The infectious lesions of the vulva prevalent in North American include condylomata acuminata, herpes genitalis, syphilis, and molluscum contagiosum. These and other infectious conditions of the vulva are listed in Table 3.1. It is accepted that the criteria for clinical diagnosis do not necessarily require specific organism characterization in all these conditions.

Human Papillomavirus Infection

Condylomata acuminata are contagious, usually sexually transmitted, polyclonal benign neoplasms that may involve the vulva, vagina, cervix, urethra, anal canal, and perianal skin and are caused by human papillomaviruses (HPV).[212,255] From 1966 to 1981, the estimated number of consultations for genital warts reported by office-based private physicians in the United States increased from 169,000 to 946,000, whereas in 1981, the number of consultations for genital herpes was 295,000.[43] If papillomavirus-associated dysplasias of the cervix are also considered, human papillomavirus infection may be the most

TABLE 3.1. Infectious diseases of the vulva.

Disease	Causative Microorganism	Salient Histopathologic Features	Diagnostic Methods
Condyloma acuminatum	Papillomavirus	Acanthosis, hyperkeratosis parakeratosis, papillomatosis perinuclear halo (koilocyte)	Histopathology Immunohistochemistry Molecular hybridization
Herpes genitalis	Herpes simplex hominis Type II	Intranuclear inclusions	Cytopathology, culture, serology
Syphilitic chancre	*Treponema pallidum*	Ulceration, chronic inflammation, vasculitis	Darkfield, fluorescence, silver stain, serology
Condyloma lata	*Treponema pallidum*	Like chancre, with epithelial hyperplasia	Same as syphilitic chancre
Molluscum contagiosum	DNA poxvirus group	Intracytoplasmic inclusions	Cytopathology, histopathology
Granuloma inguinale	*Calymmatobacterium granulomatis*	Donovan bodies, granulomatous reaction without caseation, pseudoepitheliomatous hyperplasia	Giemsa stain, silver stain
Lymphogranuloma venereum	*Chlamydia* (TRIC agent)	Granulomatous reaction without caseation	Serology
Tuberculosis	*Mycobacterium tuberculosis*	Acid-fast bacilli (AFB), granulomatous reaction with caseation	AFB stain, AFB culture
Chancroid	*Hemophilus ducreyi*	Granulomatous reaction without caseation	Culture, gram stain

common infection involving the lower female genital tract (see Chapter 7, Cervical Intraepithelial Neoplasia).

Clinically, condylomata acuminata present as papillary, verrucous, or papular lesions of the skin and mucous membrane that are nearly always multiple and frequently confluent (Fig. 3.5). Most lesions are asymptomatic unless secondarily infected. Pruritic vulvar squamous papillomatosis characterized by vestibular pruritus, which may be associated with burning, dyspareunia, and the subsequent presentation of multiple vestibular papillomas that contain HPV antigen, has been identified as a clinical complex.[125]

On gross inspection, typical condylomata acuminata usually are discrete verrucous or papillary growths, which may arise from a central stalk. Alternatively, they may involve a large area in a sessile fashion. Subclinical infection may also occur. Tiny, slightly raised, roughened areas located on the cervix, vagina, or vulva often represent foci of HPV infection. Such lesions are best appreciated through a colposcope, and their recognition is enhanced by dilute (3–5%) acetic acid lavage, which makes the lesions appear white (i.e., aceto-white).

Histologically, parakeratosis, acanthosis, and hyperkeratosis are evident with an associated chronic inflammatory infiltrate within the dermis. Typical perinuclear cytoplasmic halos are commonly seen in the more superficial epithelial cells (koilocytosis) (Fig. 3.6). Basilar hyperplasia with binucleated and multinucleated cells may be seen. Enlarged parabasal cells with a foamy nuclear

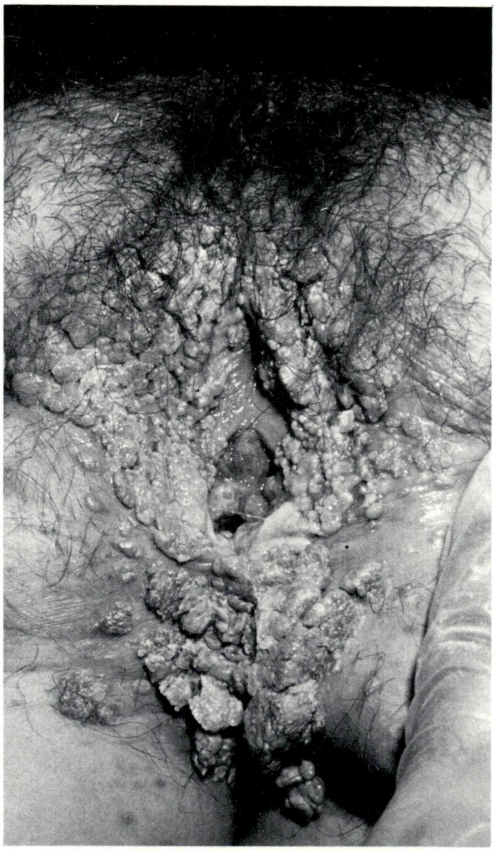

FIG. 3.5. Condylomata acuminata. Widespread involvement of vulva and perianal region.

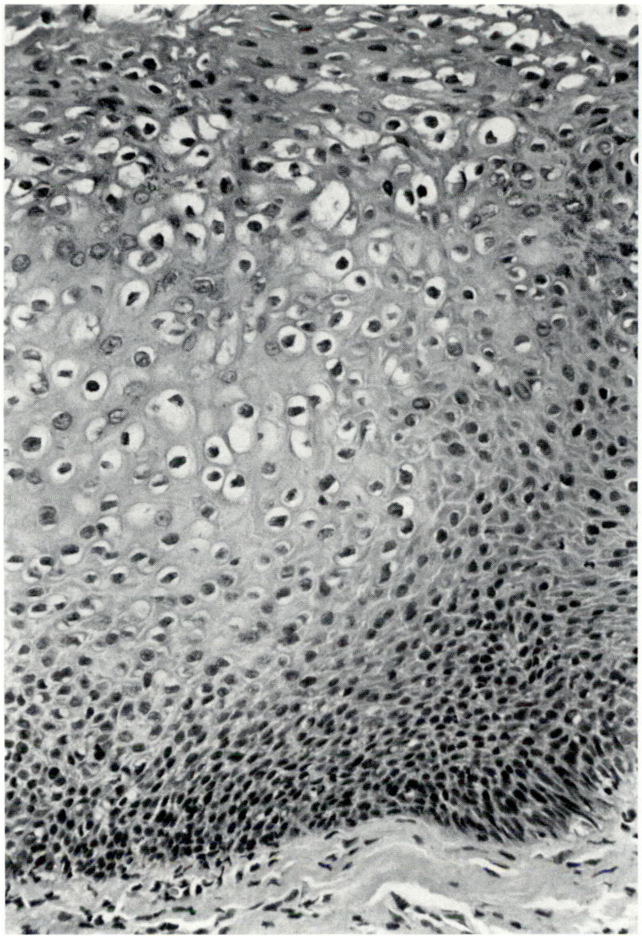

FIG. 3.6. Condyloma acuminatum. Basilar hyperplasia is seen with prominent intracellular bridges between some cells above the basilar layer. Koilocytotic cells with prominent perinuclear halos are found in the more superficial epithelium.

chromatin may be present. Intranuclear chromatin changes may also have a ground glass appearance in some cells. Electron microscopic studies have demonstrated the presence of the intranuclear viral particles in human warts. The number of identifiable particles is related to the age of the wart, reaching a peak after 6–12 months of growth and decreasing after 2–3 years.[254,255] Human papillomavirus has been identified in morphologically normal skin adjacent to condyloma acuminatum, and its presence in normal adjacent skin is associated with a significantly higher recurrence rate compared to patients without HPV in the adjacent normal skin.[88]

Condylomata acuminata are commonly associated with vaginitis, pregnancy, diabetes mellitus, oral contraceptive use, poor perineal hygiene, immunosuppression, and sexual activity with multiple partners.[254] Approximately 50% of women with vulvar condyloma acuminatum have associated cervical HPV infection.[340] The natural history of HPV infections of the vulva is usually one of a long protracted course. On the skin, the natural history may be influenced by immunologic factors.[335] Regression has been noted following pregnancy. The progression of HPV infections of the vulva to vulvar intraepithelial neoplasia (VIN) has been documented.[46,60,256] Invasive squamous carcinoma of the vulva arising in condylomata acuminata has also been reported.[190,306]

The topical application of dilute podophyllin resin in tincture of benzoin or the judicious application of halogenated acetic acid are common approaches to early vulvar condylomas. Success rates are poor, however, and the infection is often recurrent. Electrodesiccation and laser ablation[101,283] have both given good results. Cryosurgery has been used for condyloma in pregnancy.[16] Lesions of excessive size occurring during pregnancy can be managed by hot wire loop excision as well.[101] Removal is most safely performed during the second trimester. Highly vascular lesions on the cervix or vagina may respond to cryotherapy.

Approximately 40–60% of children with laryngeal papillomatosis are born of mothers with a history of genital HPV infection.[212,217,277] The true incidence of infection of the larynx of the newborn infant from a mother with genital papillomavirus infection is presently unknown but probably low. No correlation has been shown between volume of maternal wart tissue and occurrence of infantile laryngeal papillomas. Based on cytologic studies from prenatal clinics, the frequency of cervical human papillomavirus infection ranges from 1 to 3.5% (see Chapter 7, Cervical Intraepithelial Neoplasia).

Oncogenesis secondary to papillomavirus is well recognized in experimental animals. The giant condyloma of Buschke-Lowenstein, represents an example of the human transformation of a condyloma to a verrucous or squamous carcinoma. The earliest evidence of the transformation of genital condylomata into carcinoma is the observation, using DNA microspectrophotometry, of transition areas in condylomata wherein aneuploid neoplastic cell populations are found adjacent to the more normal polyploid cells of the condyloma.[159] The onconcogenic transformation of condylomata appears to be more common in immunosuppressed individuals.[42,344,352] The HPV type associated with VIN has been found to be predominately HPV-16.*

Using molecular hybridization with labeled HPV DNA, HPV-6 is the most common HPV type found in the usual genital condylomata acuminata, but Types 1, 6, 16, and 35 have been identified within vulvar intraepithelial neoplasia and vulvar squamous cell carcinomas[118,119] (A.T. Lorincz, personal communication) (see

---

* References 148, 222, 250, 309, 374, 375.

section Vulvar Intraepithelial Neoplasia). In addition, the condyloma of Bushke-Lowenstein, a locally aggressive, large, verrucoid lesion at present subclassified as a variant of verrucous carcinoma, has been identified as containing HPV-6.[118,251] HPV-11 has been found in approximately one-fourth of genital warts, as well as being found in cervical dysplasias and some cervical carcinomas.[119] HPV-16 has been found in seven of eight VIN III lesions (carcinoma in situ) of the vulva.[222] With DNA hybridization techniques, it has further been observed that approximately one-half of laryngeal papillomas contain HPV-11.[119] This finding has further supported the hypothesis that laryngeal papillomas of infancy and childhood may be acquired at the time of vaginal delivery.

Employing immunoperoxidase techniques for the localization of the papillomavirus antigens within vulvar epithelium, HPV antigens have been found in typical vulvar condyloma acuminatum in approximately 50% of patients.[200] The presence of human papillomavirus particles detected by electron microscopy has been associated with VIN.[264,344] In such cases, however, the virus particles are usually found in the adjacent, more typical condyloma acuminatum-appearing area and less commonly in the VIN area. Virus particles are usually not identifiable by electron microscopy in VIN. The association of vulvar and vaginal condyloma acuminatum with invasive squamous cell carcinoma has also been documented in two young women with Fanconi's anemia.[352] A woman with Hodgkin's disease, who had received radiation therapy, was subsequently found to have VIN and invasive squamous cell carcinoma associated with genital HPV infection.[209]

The possibility that the podophyllin effect on condylomas of the vulva can result in misinterpretation as vulvar carcinoma in situ is highly improbable, since changes associated with short-term podophyllin use are quite different from VIN. The mitotic arrest with cells in metaphase seen after podophyllin contrasts with the markedly abnormal mitotic figures seen in vulvar carcinoma in situ. Nuclear karyorrhexis is rarely present with in situ disease, whereas it can be found in at least 90% of condyloma patients.[187,337] In vulvar carcinoma in situ, the nuclear size is variable, and nuclear chromatin is usually coarse, with little cellular swelling. These changes are uncommon in the podophyllin effect. The cellular changes from a single application of podophyllin will regress within 1–2 weeks, whereas vulvar carcinoma in situ will persist. Consequently, although the histologic findings are not absolute, the education of physicians to avoid the use of podophyllin for at least 2 weeks before biopsy is the most expedient solution to this problem.[337]

It has been shown that those VIN lesions that are aneuploid infrequently have identifiable HPV virus antigen by immunoperoxidase methods, although DNA probes can detect the HPV DNA sequences (see Vulvar Intraepithelial Neoplasia). Atypia may also be seen within condyloma acuminatum not associated with intraepithelial neoplasia. This atypia is characterized by large polyploid cells with moderate nuclear pleomorphism and some degree of hyperchromasia, but rarely with abnormal mitosis. It is secondary to the tetraploidy and octoploidy (variate of normal polyploidy) that results in the cells having 26 × 4 or 26 × 8 chromosomes but does not reflect a premalignant process.[309] Condylomas that do not contain significant cytologic atypia are HPV antigen positive by immunoperoxidase techniques in approximately 50% of cases, whereas VIN tumors are immunoreactive in fewer than 10% of cases.[60] The presence of abnormal mitoses, cytologically atypical nuclei, marked nuclear variation in size and shape, and hyperchromasia are characteristics of VIN lesions. Such findings separate them from typical condylomas, which tend to show koilocytotic cells without the other features.[58–60]

There also exist lesions that are in a gray area of diagnosis or categorization. In a given case of VIN, a spectrum may be found from classic VIN III to adjacent changes that may have typical morphologic changes of condyloma acuminatum. As a matter of practice, the first diagnosis given on the pathology report is usually that of the most serious lesion identified, with subsequent diagnosis following, for example, with adjacent condyloma acuminatum. A comment relevant to the spectrum of changes may be appropriate in such cases. On occasion, foci of nonspecific cytologic atypia within what appears to be a condyloma acuminatum or a nonspecific hyperplastic process may be seen. There are some differences of opinion about how to identify such lesions. Some may classify them as VIN or bowenoid papulosis, whereas others may classify them as atypical condylomata acuminata or give a descriptive diagnosis only. The true nature of the lesions may be resolved with further biopsies or observation of the patient over time. However, in our present state of understanding, we must accept the possibility of associated VIN occurring adjacent to such nonspecific epithelial changes (see Vulvar Intraepithelial Neoplasia).

Herpes Virus Infection

Herpetic vulvitis is an infectious disease characterized by the sequential appearance of vesicles, pustules, and painful shallow ulcers often secondarily infected with bacteria. The causative agent is the herpes simplex virus (HSV) (var. hominis Type II), although in some instances the Type I virus may be involved. The patient with initial disease may have dysuria or urinary retention with vulvar pain that may be incapacitating. Systemic symptoms, including generalized malaise and fever, are

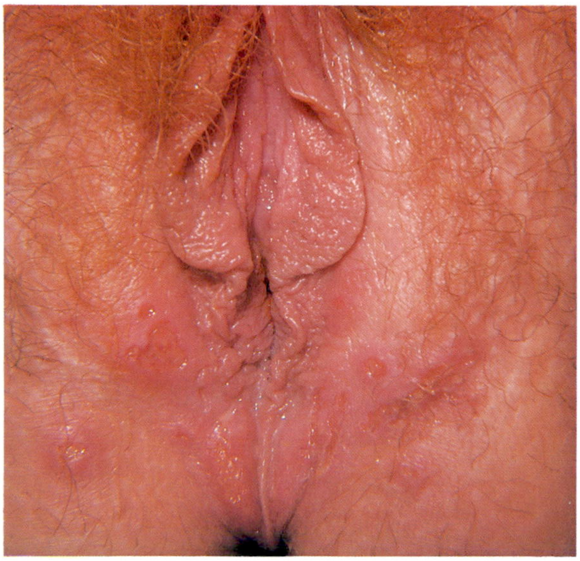

Fig. 3.7

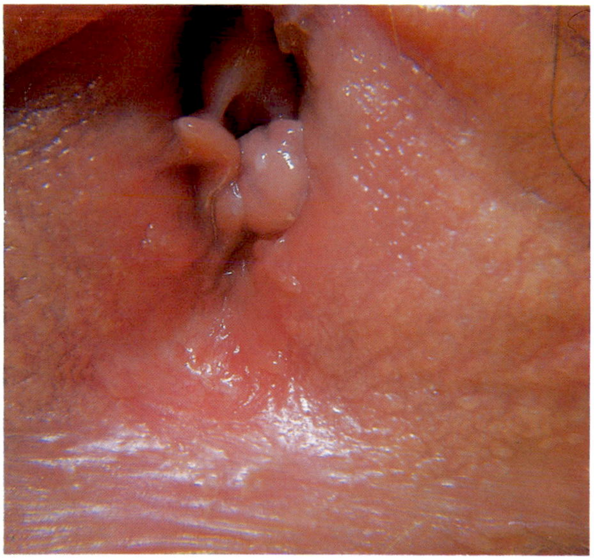

Fig. 3.19

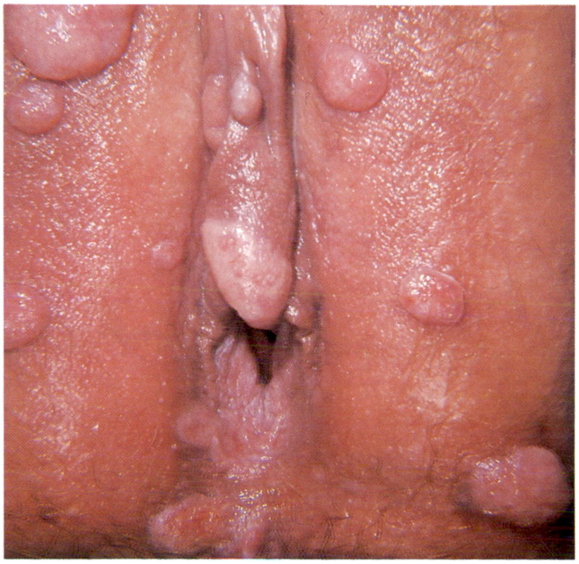

Fig. 3.9

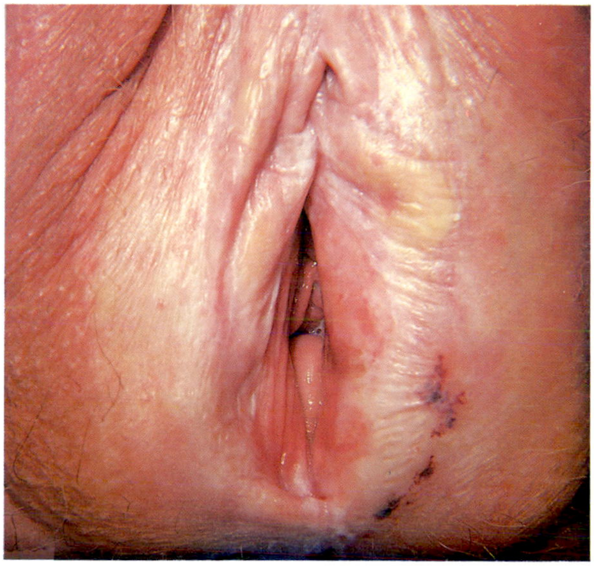

Fig. 3.23

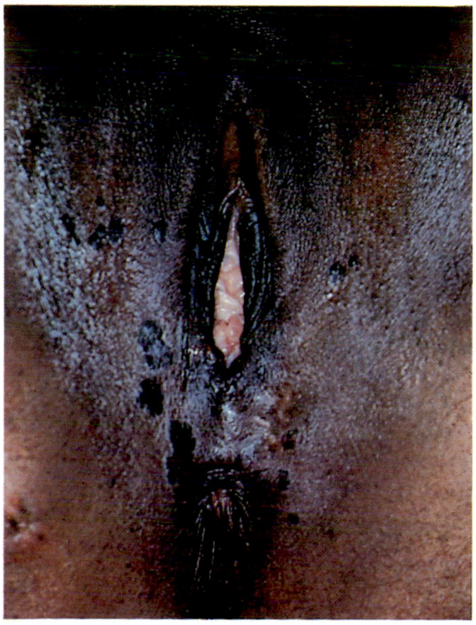

Fig. 3.38

Fig. 3.7. Herpes simplex ulcer. Herpes simplex virus infection, untreated, 7 days after the onset of symptoms. Multifocal ulceration is present.

Fig. 3.9. Condyloma lata. Multiple papules are present.

Fig. 3.19. Vestibulitis. There is marked inflammation adjacent and external to the hymenal ring. Point tenderness is present over these areas.

Fig. 3.23. Lichen sclerosus. White epithelium with focal subcutaneous ecchymoses is seen. The labia minora are somewhat atrophic.

Fig. 3.38. Vulvar intraepithelial neoplasia. Multiple pigmented macular areas are present about the vulva and perianal area.

Plate 2

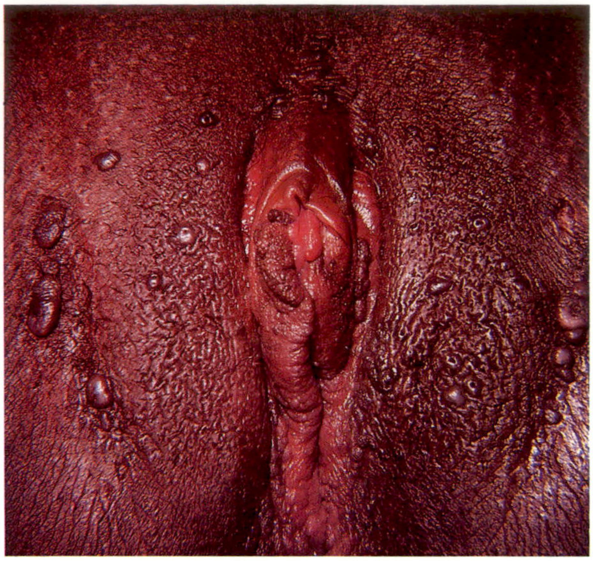

Fig. 3.39

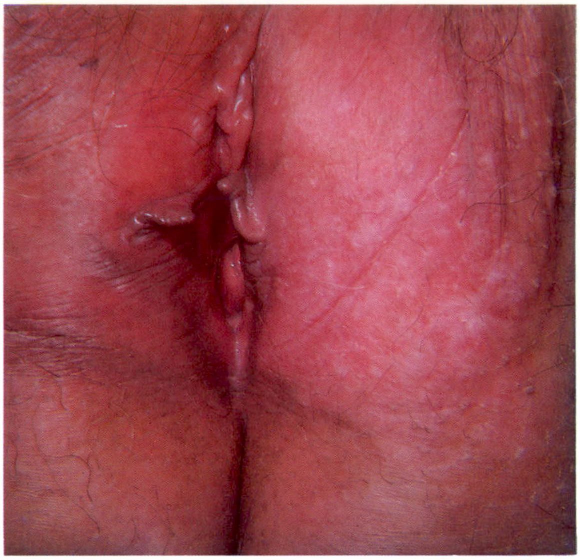

Fig. 3.47

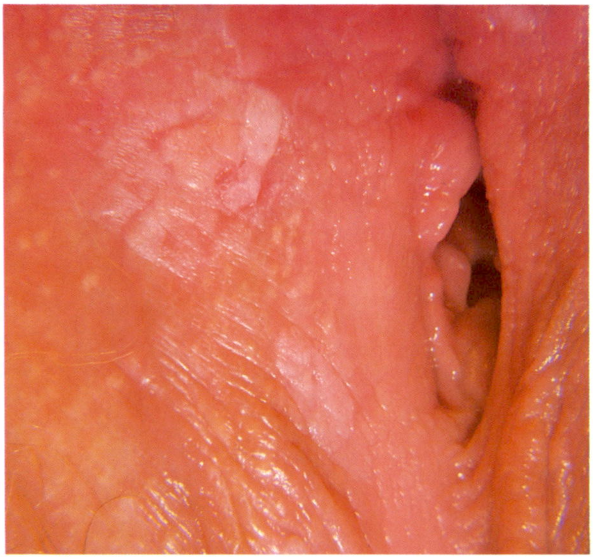

Fig. 3.40

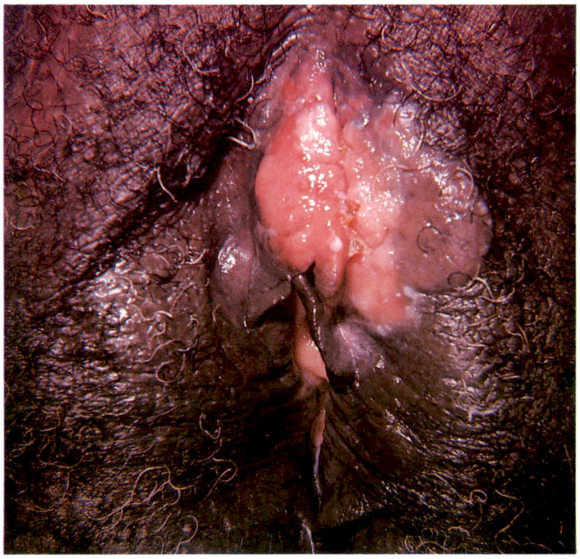

Fig. 3.50

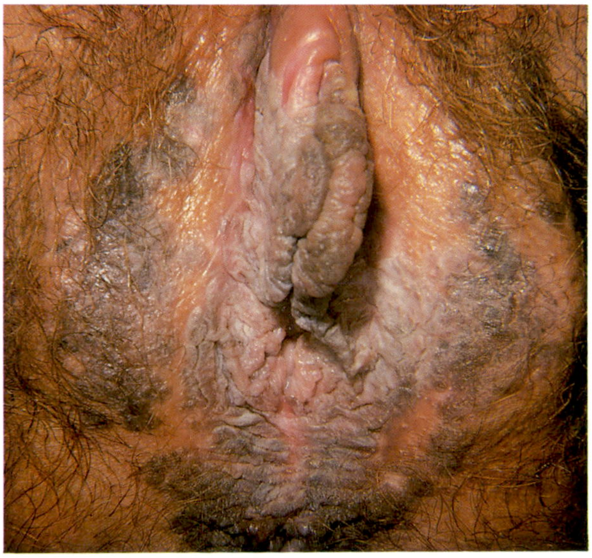

Fig. 3.41

Fig. 3.39. Vulvar intraepithelial neoplasia. Multiple pigmented papules are noted about the labia majora in this young pregnant woman. This finding is consistent with the clinical diagnosis of bowenoid papulosis.

Fig. 3.40. Vulvar intraepithelial neoplasia. Multiple macular and plaque-like white areas are seen about the labia majora.

Fig. 3.41. Vulvar intraepithelial neoplasia. Confluent distribution of pigmented, slightly raised, rough-surfaced areas are seen involving the labia majora and minora.

Fig. 3.47. Vulvar Paget's disease. An eczematoid, slightly raised area is noted on the medial anterior surface of the patient's left labia majora.

Fig. 3.50. Vulvar invasive carcinoma. Vulvar squamous cell carcinoma involving the medial aspect of the patient's left anterior labia majora and clitoris.

not infrequently seen along with a mild inguinal lymphadenopathy. The vesicles (Fig. 3.7, Plate 1) are usually asymptomatic, whereas the ulcers are extremely painful and may involve the urethra, bladder, cervix, and vagina, as well as the vulva.[117] The acute ulcers heal in approximately 16 days.[56]

Histopathologic examination of an early intact HSV vesicle demonstrates extension deep into the epidermis. The characteristic intranuclear inclusions are seen at the periphery of the lesion (Fig. 3.8). The histologic transformation of the HSV-infected epithelial cell begins with a homogenization of the nuclear chromatin, resulting in a ground glass appearance, which then progresses to the more typical eosinophilic intranuclear inclusion body. Subsequently, the cells undergo karyorrhexis and lysis. A biopsy taken in the late ulcerative phase, therefore, does not always show the characteristic intranuclear inclusions. Morphologic changes seen with HSV infection are not reliable in separating primary from secondary infection, or in distinguishing HSV Type I from Type II infection.

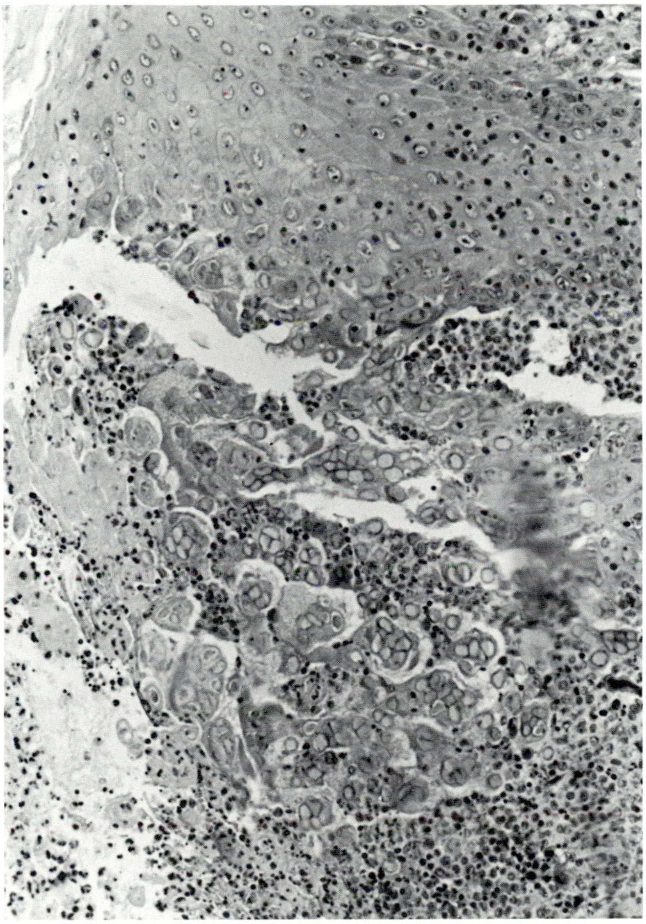

FIG. 3.8. Herpes simplex ulcer. Crater margin shows multinucleated clusters with distinctive intranuclear homogenization and inclusion bodies.

Cytologic evaluation or the scrapings of the base and edges of a fresh ulcer or scrapings from the base and sides of a freshly opened vesicle will usually show the multinucleated cells with viral cytopathic effects characteristic of herpes virus infection. Herpes zoster can involve the vulva and may have similar cytologic findings.[370] Moistening the ulcer with a saline-soaked sponge and then scraping the ulcer with a wooden spatula may improve the cell harvest. Whether the sample is from an ulcer or a freshly opened vesicle, the specimen should be smeared on a clean slide, rapidly fixed in 95% ethanol or with spray fixative, and stained with Papanicolaou stain. Herpes simplex virus-specific fluorescein-conjugated antiserum may be placed on such smears to identify HSV antigens. With monoclonal antibodies to HSV, Types I and II can be distinguished with reasonable accuracy by immunofluorescence. This distinction is usually unimportant, however, because it is clinically recognized that both types can infect the genital tract.

Isolation of HSV Types I or II can be achieved by the inoculation of tissue culture monolayers, such as WI-38 human embryonic lung fibroblasts or monkey kidney cells. Both types of HSV produce characteristic cytopathic changes on these cell lines, and virus isolation can be achieved within 4 days.[56,177] Rapid viral culture over 24 hours, followed by a search for HSV antigen using the immunoperoxidase technique can give results in less than 2 days. Most laboratories keep the culture at least 1 week to observe for the viral cytopathic effect of HSV. Culture swabs, obtained from opened vesicles or clean ulcers, can be transported and stored up to 24 hours in Stuart's transport medium, Amies Bactotransport medium, or Eagle's tissue culture medium. If a delay of more than 24 hours is anticipated before inoculation, the inoculated medium must be refrigerated, or a marked loss of live virus will occur.[177] Freezing is unnecessary; in fact, temperatures between −5 and −20°C may actually decrease the success of isolation. Rapid freezing at −70°C preserves the virus for extended periods of time for identification by culture or immunofluorescent techniques.

Serologic studies on acute and convalescent serum samples are of value, especially in distinguishing primary from recurrent infection. In primary infection, significant rises (over fourfold dilution) are found. In recurrent infection, the patient is seropositive at the time of acquisition of the acute sample, and antibody titers will not rise consistently. Serologic methods are not reliable in separating HSV Type I from Type II.[56] Cytologic examination of vesicular aspirate is an effective method of identifying the cytopathologic changes in HSV and is almost as sensitive as virus isolation.[238] Asymptomatic viral shedding of HSV has been documented in 1.5–3% of women who are seropositive for HSV Type II.[3,83,177,336]

Herpes virus infection may have some oncogenic potential, however, this relationship remains to be defined.[37,114,276,374,375]

Epstein–Barr Virus Infection

Epstein–Barr virus (EBV) has been cultured from painful ulcers on the labium minus that occurred during a primary infection of infectious mononucleosis. The ulcers slowly healed over 32 days.[270] EBV infection may be a sexually transmitted disease.[270]

Syphilis

Syphilis is a venereal disease caused by the spirochete *Treponema pallidum*. This organism measures up to 15 μm in length and 0.20 μm in thickness. The organism is spiral in shape, with 6–14 coils. Motility, characterized by flexion, rotation about the long axis, and random movement, is noted on dark-field examination of fresh exudate from an active lesion. The primary lesion is the chancre, a painless, shallow ulcer with raised edges. The chancre usually presents within 3 weeks after initial contact, with a range of 10–90 days. If secondarily infected, the chancre may become soft and painful and show an ulcerated surface. Although chancres are generally single, they may be multiple. Chancres may occur on inconspicuous surfaces, such as the cervix, anal mucosa, or oral pharnyx. In approximately 50% of females and 30% of males, the primary lesion is never seen. There is lymphadenopathy 3–4 days after the chancre. The nodes are nontender, freely movable, and rubbery.[78]

If syphilis is left untreated in the primary phase, the secondary stage of the disease will become evident within 6 weeks to 6 months. At this point, the patient may have a skin rash that often involves mucous membranes as well as the palms of the hands and soles of the feet.[355] On occasion, the secondary lesions are papular, especially about the vulva, presenting as elevated plaques up to 3 cm in diameter. These are known as *condylomata lata* (Fig. 3.9, Plate 1). Such lesions may also occur on other mucocutaneous borders. The tertiary gumma of syphilis is rarely seen on the vulva.

Chancres are not commonly biopsied on the vulva because the diagnosis can usually be made serologically or with the aid of dark-field or fluorescent methods if a lesion is seen. When a biopsy is performed, especially if syphilis was not considered in the clinical differential diagnosis, the diagnosis may be quite difficult from histologic material alone. The histologic picture of the primary chancre is one of ulceration of the epidermis, with acute and chronic inflammation within the dermis. There is a marked perivascular inflammatory response, and large numbers of plasma cells are seen within the tissue (Fig. 3.10). Histologic examination of condylomata lata indicates marked acanthosis, epithelial hyperplasia, and hyperkeratosis (Fig. 3.11). The inflammatory response within the dermis is similar to that in the primary chancre, with a marked chronic inflammatory cell infiltrate containing many plasma cells. The arteritis in both lesions may be sufficiently severe to result in obliteration of the smaller vessels. Dieterlie or Warthin-Starry silver stains for spirochetes are of value if there is any suspicion of syphilis.

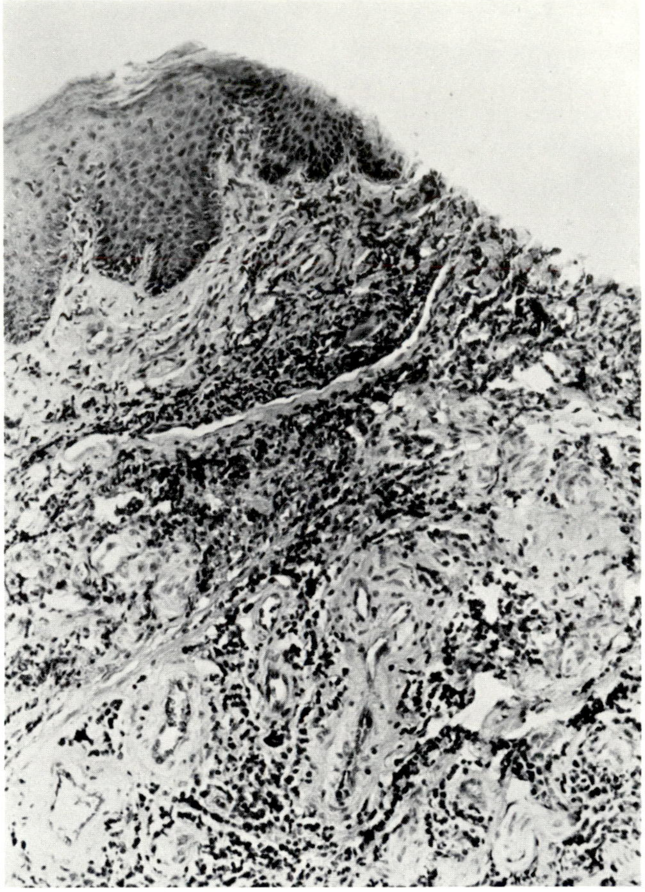

FIG. 3.10. Syphilitic chancre. Arteritis is present beneath the chancre margin.

The primary chancre, as well as the condyloma latum and other secondary lesions, are rich in spirochetes. Therefore, when a chancre or secondary lesion of syphilis is suspected, an attempt to identify spirochetes within the lesion should be made. This may be accomplished through either dark-field examination of fluid expressed from the base of the ulcer, or by the fluorescent conjugated antibody technique using a dried smear preparation. These methods are far more sensitive and specific than are silver stain methods with paraffin-embedded tissue.

The chancre may appear as early as the first week after exposure, and, therefore, it can be present for weeks before serologic tests become reactive. More than 70% of patients with dark-field-positive lesions have a reactive serology at the time of initial diagnosis. The most common

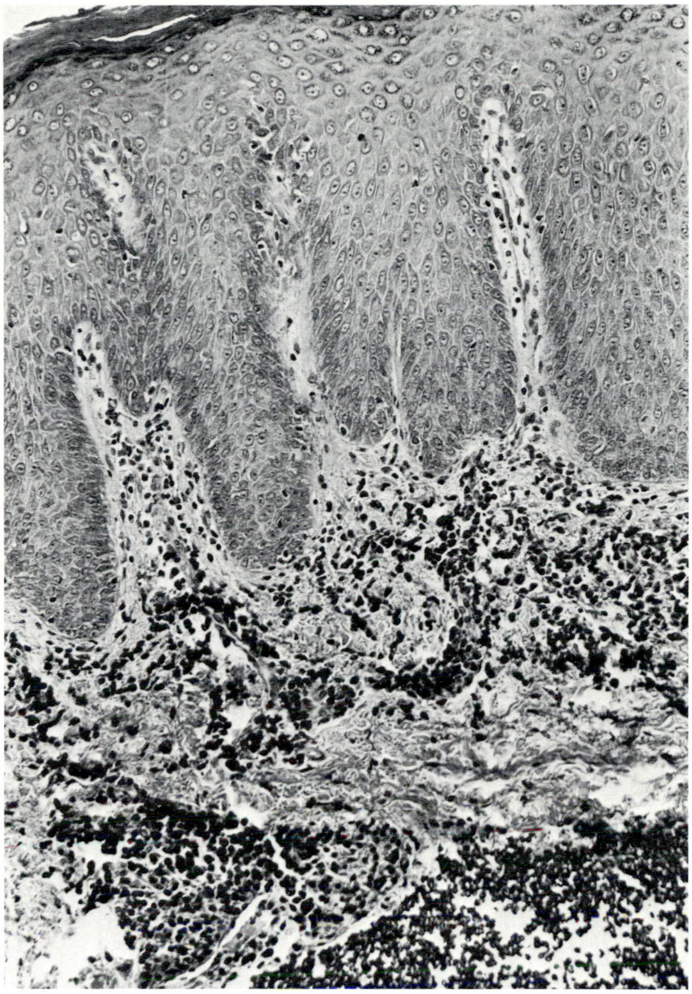

Fig. 3.11. Condyloma latum. Prominent acanthosis is present, with a marked dermal perivascular inflammatory cell infiltrate that consists primarily of plasma cells and lymphocytes, with some neutrophils. Vascular endothelial proliferation is present with associated arteritis. The lesion is rich in *Treponema pallidum* organisms, which can be demonstrated by Warthin–Starry or Dieterlie silver stain. ×160.

serologic testing methods are based on the identification of reagin, and these tests become positive approximately 1 month after the disease is contracted. Common reagin testing methods use microflocculation testing and include the Venereal Disease Research Laboratory (VDRL) and rapid plasma reagin (RPR) tests, which have similar specificity and can be quantitated to evaluate the course of the disease and response to therapy. The fluorescent treponemal antibody-absorbed (FTA-ABS) test is generally the next ordered if the VDRL or RPR test is nonreactive or weakly reactive or if there is a possibility of a false-positive VDRL or RPR. Biologic false positives can occur in lupus erythematosus, virus infection, cirrhosis of the liver, pregnancy, malaria, and other inflammatory or autoimmune diseases. The FTA-ABS is a more sensitive test early in the disease and can be used to evaluate weak reactions.[252] It is appreciated, however, that once the FTA-ABS becomes positive, it can remain so for the life of the patient. If the FTA-ABS is positive, spinal fluid serologic evaluation is necessary in order to rule out neurosyphilis. A false-positive FTA-ABS is rare and, if detected, requires *T. pallidum* immobilization (TPI) testing and careful follow-up.[310]

Approximately 30% of patients with primary syphilis will undergo spontaneous remission of the disease. Those who are not treated or who do not achieve spontaneous remission may progress to tertiary syphilis, with its well-recognized cardiovascular and central nervous system symptoms. Untreated syphilis may prove fatal in 10% of those afflicted.

Molluscum Contagiosum

Molluscum contagiosum is a moderately contagious viral disease that, in adults, is often related to intimate or sexual contact.[213] The lesions are small, smooth papules (3–6 mm in diameter) with a central punctum or umbilication. They are generally multiple and separate, although they may be single. Rare plaque formations, made up of 50–100 individual clustered lesions have also been described. The incubation period varies between 14 and 50 days.

Clinical diagnosis usually does not require biopsy. Cy-

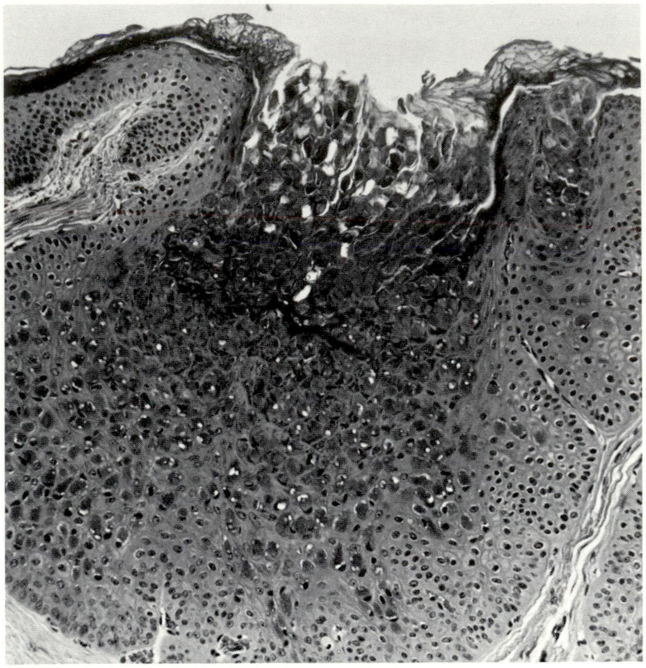

FIG. 3.12. Molluscum contagiosum. Cells within the acanthotic nest show increasing density of intracytoplasmic inclusions as the surface umbilication is approached.

tologic identification of the typical intracytoplasmic inclusion bodies within scrapings from the interior of the molluscum papule is adequate to confirm the diagnosis. When biopsies are submitted, histologic examination reveals a marked acanthosis, and the characteristic intracytoplasmic viral inclusions can be seen (Fig. 3.12). Young, recently infected cells show an eosinophilic cytoplasmic inclusion. With aging, the inclusion bodies take on a more basophilic appearance preceding lysis of the cell.[281] The central dimple of the lesion is often seen histologically if care is taken to bisect the lesion at the gross cutting table. Within the dermis, there is often a rather marked vascular response, with endothelial proliferation and moderate perivascular inflammation. Electron microscopy has demonstarted that the virus is brick-shaped and contains a DNA core with a two-layered protein coat measuring 300 nm × 210 nm.[20]

Molluscum contagiosum is usually asymptomatic, however, lesions about the anus frequently become pruritic or secondarily infected. Whereas most lesions will regress spontaneously, untreated lesions may persist for years, during which time they may be spread by close contact.

Granuloma Inguinale

Granuloma inguinale (donovanosis) is caused by *Calymmatobacterium granulomatis*, a gram-negative, heavily encapsulated rod in the bacterial family Enterobacteriaceae. Granuloma inguinale occurs with approximately equal frequency in men and women. Primary lesions may occur on the vulva, vagina, or cervix and may be painless papules or ulcers with rolled borders and a friable base. Inguinal adenopathy is usually absent.[76,292] The lesions usually appear within 2 weeks of exposure. Granuloma inguinale extends primarily by local infiltration, although lymphatic permeation may occur during later stages of the disease. Chronic lymphatic infiltration and fibrosis frequently result in a massive brawny edema of the external genitalia. There is some controversy about the true origin of the edema, as dye injection studies suggest that the lympathic drainage is intact. With involvement of the cervix, the disease may advance via the cervical lymphatics to involve parametrial tissues.[197]

The clinical diagnosis of granuloma inguinale is dependent on the identification of the Donovan bodies within the tissue. This is best accomplished by preparing smears of a biopsy specimen taken from the edge of the ulcer and pressing this biopsy tissue between two slides. These tissue imprints are then air-dried, fixed in methanol, stained with Giemsa stain, and examined.[303] Any antibiotic treatment may obscure the diagnosis, necessitating biopsy at a later date to confirm the diagnosis. Histologically, the main portion of the lesion consists of granulation tissue associated with an extensive chronic inflammatory cell infiltrate and endarteritis. The ulcer is usually covered with a fibrinous exudate, and necrosis may be present. Within its granulation tissue base, a dense mixed inflammatory cell infiltrate, consisting predominately of plasma cells and mononuclear cells with few lymphocytes, is seen that extends into the dermis. Large vacuolated histiocytes are found that contain the characteristic encapsulated bacilli, or Donovan bodies, within their cytoplasm (Fig. 3.13). They can be demonstrated with Warthin–Starry stain or Giemsa stain. The Donovan bodies may be found extracellularly, as well as intracellularly, and may appear coccoid, coccobacillary, or bacillary.[303] Ultrathin plastic-embedded sections, as well as electron microscopy, have been used to study these organisms in tissue.[197,292] The surface epithelium adjacent to the ulcer may show prominent pseudoepitheliomatous hyperplasia. Necrosis and microabscesses may be seen within the epidermis.[73,303]

Calymmatobacterium granulomatis may be cultured by special techniques. A complement-fixation test is available that is believed reliable in titers greater than 1:40.[76] The diagnosis depends on the clinical findings and documenting the organism within the tissue. Syphilis, chancroid, and HSV infection are usually included in the differential diagnosis.

Lymphogranuloma Venereum

Lymphogranuloma venereum (LGV) is caused by *Chlamydia* and occurs approximately three times more frequently in men than in women. This disease is character-

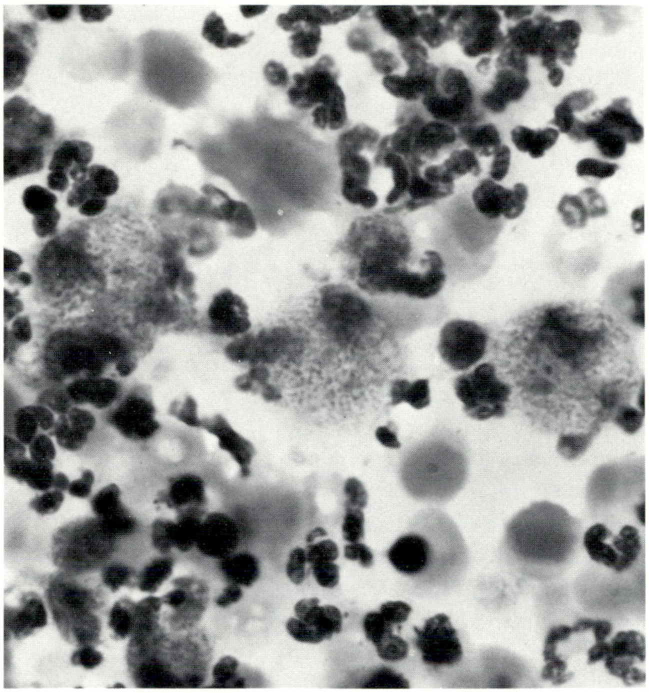

FIG. 3.13. Granuloma inguinale. Large histiocytes obtained by smear show numerous intracytoplasmic Donovan bodies.

ized clinically by three phases: phase one, erosion of the skin; phase two, adenitis; and phase three, fibrosis and destruction.[76] Lymphogranuloma venereum is primarily spread via the lymphatics. The initial ulcers, which are generally not tender or painful, are often ignored. Adenitis, which may evolve into painful superficial groin nodes, or buboes, frequently results in spontaneous rupture through the skin, accompanied by exudation of a purulent discharge. The third phase of the disease, the destructive phase, often results in stricture and fibrosis of the vagina and rectum.[355] During this phase, chronic lymphatic obstruction is responsible for the characteristic nonpitting edema of the external genitalia.

The histology of LGV is not diagnostic and reveals no characteristic viral inclusions or identifiable organisms by the usual modes of investigation. To establish a diagnosis, it is necessary to have the typical clinical presentation along with positive complement-fixation tests. Biopsy is often performed to rule out carcinoma. Smears of the base or the biopsy itself should be searched for organisms (e.g., spirochetes, Donovan bodies). Histologically, giant cells may be seen along with lymphocytes and plasma cells. Older lesions exhibit extensive fibrosis of the dermis, and sinus tracts may be seen.

Chancroid

The chancroid genital ulcer is usually tender and nonindurated and has a friable purulent erythematous base. The clinical differential diagnosis includes HSV infection and primary syphilis.[296] Primary lesions may be single or multiple and tend to be small, measuring approximately 1–2 mm in diameter. Coalescence of the lesions leads to ulcers approaching 3 cm in diameter. Tender inguinal adenopathy with flocculent nodes may be present. The incubation period may be as short as 10 days.[296]

Chancroid is caused by the organism *Haemophilus ducreyi*, a gram-negative, nonmotile bacillus, which in culture grows in pairs and parallel chains. This disease is relatively rare. Skin tests, biopsies, and antoinoculation may not be diagnostic. Selective agar medium has been developed for the organism, which has improved culture isolation, and identification of the organism by culture is necessary for accurate diagnosis.[246] Histologic examination of the tissue demonstrates a granulomatous-type reaction, with chronic inflammatory cells consisting primarily of lymphocytes and plasma cells.

Tuberculosis

Tuberculosis of the vulva is rare. When it occurs, it is usually associated with tuberculosis of other genital sites, primarily fallopian tube and endometrium. Autoinoculation by the hematogenous or direct spread is therefore the most common method of transmission to the vulva. Primary inoculation or sexual transmission of tuberculosis is most uncommon. The usual causative organism is *Mycobacterium tuberculosis*, however, atypical mycobacteria have also been incriminated. Diagnosis can usually be made by biopsy of the involved tissues. Caseating granulomas with Langhan's giant cells are found on histologic section (Fig. 3.14). Acid-fast stains usually reveal

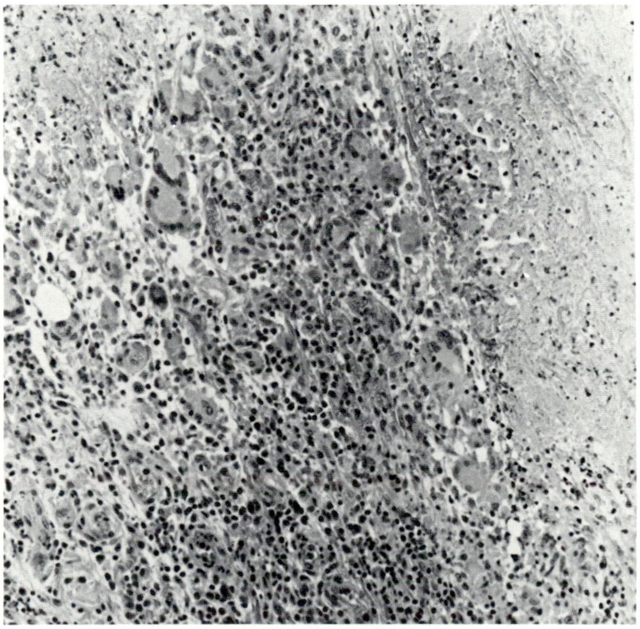

FIG. 3.14. Vulvar tuberculosis. Caseating granulomas with Langhan's giant cells.

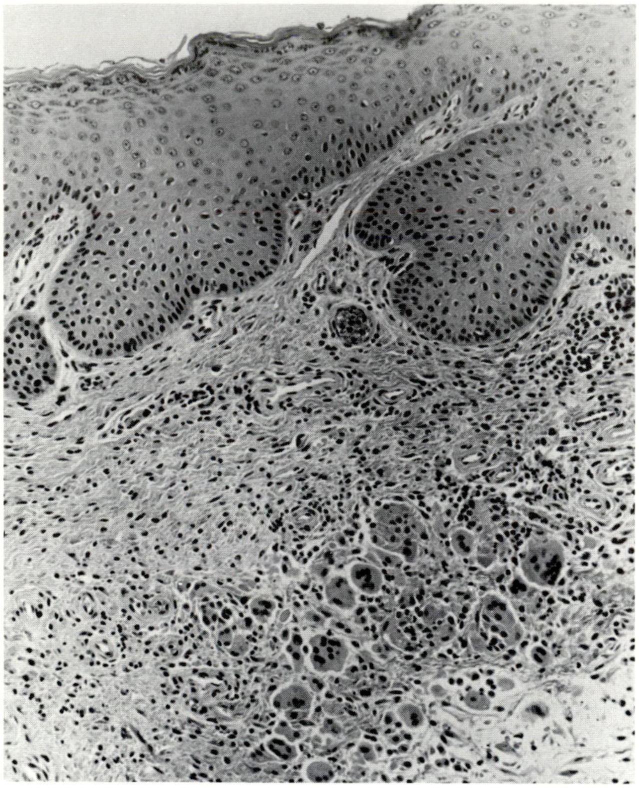

FIG. 3.15. Foreign body giant cell reaction. Multinucleated giant cells. Caseation is lacking.

the Mycobacterium, and identification can be confirmed by culture techniques.

Giant cells of the foreign body type are frequently encountered in vulvar tissues in which a previous biopsy has been performed (Fig. 3.15). These giant cells, associated with noncaseating granulomas, often result from embedded suture, occasionally seen in the biopsy area, and should not be confused with tuberculosis.

Vulvar ulceration secondary to sarcoidosis has been reported and should be included in the differential diagnosis of granulomatous ulcerations of the vulva.[241]

Miscellaneous Infectious Diseases

Chronic inflammatory conditions of the vulvar and perianal skin without concomitant ulceration are often caused by fungal infections, although a variety of vulvar irritants unrelated to infection are recognized.[28] *Candida* and dermatophytes are frequent pathogens. Such infections rarely require biopsy, and accurate diagnosis generally can be accomplished with microscopic examination of skin scrapings placed in 10% potassium hydroxide or through appropriate culture methods.

Bacterial infections may produce clinical findings similar to those seen with fungal infections. Erythrasma is a chronic bacterial infection of the genitocrural area that shows a coral-red fluorescence under Wood's light. The disease is most common in obese diabetics. Gram-stained scrapings of these lesions demonstrate the causative gram-positive bacterium, *Corynebacterium minutissimum,* in rods, filaments, and coccoid forms.[297]

A variety of mites are capable of producing local and limited chronic skin infections of the perineal area. Unless specifically considered, mites can be undetected because they are not demonstrable by the usual skin-scraping or culture techniques.[139] Mites, which belong to the order Acarina, cause scabies. Mites differ from lice, which are insects, in that they are small arachnids, having a fused head and thorax, devoid of primary segmentation, and having four pairs of legs. Mites burrow within the epidermis, inducing severe pruritus. The overt skin lesions are papular and, when examined under a magnifying lens, reveal an adjacent burrow. This burrow can be unroofed with a sharp knife blade coated with mineral oil. The scrapings, mixed in the oil, are then mounted on a glass slide.[234] If no papules are found, an alternative method of diagnosis is to shake out the patient's clothing into a plastic container to which is added an alcohol-ether-acetic acid-formalin mixture, which fixes the mites and facilitates their histologic identification.[139]

Lice are associated with irritation of the skin due to secondary infection of feeding sites. The pubic louse, *Phthirus pubis* of the class Insecta, is the usual offender and can be diagnosed by identifying the louse and nits on the hair shaft (Fig. 3.16).

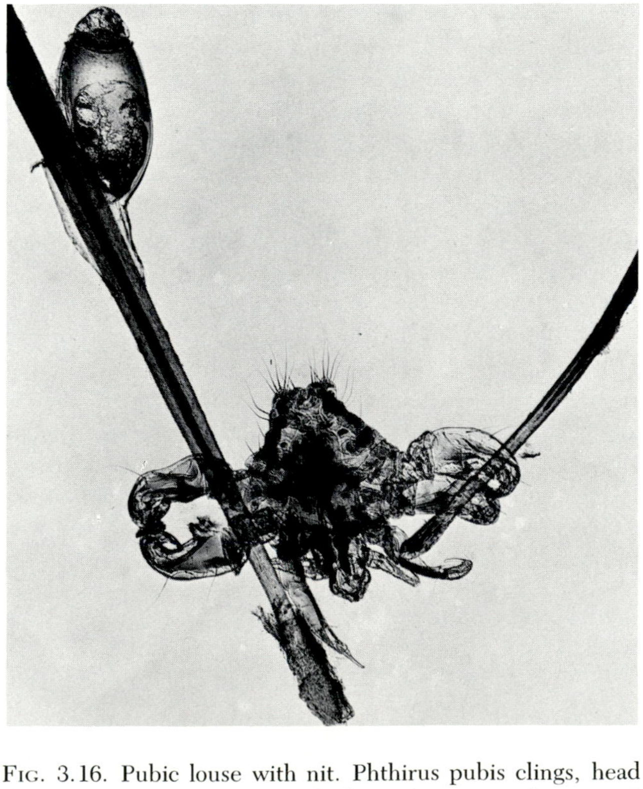

FIG. 3.16. Pubic louse with nit. Phthirus pubis clings, head down, to a hair shaft with attached egg. (Courtesy of G. Stout.)

A brown recluse (*Loxosceles reclusa*) spider bite on the vulva has been reported, associated with a protracted ulceration and infection of the vulva. Although secondary infection may occur with such ulcers, slow and progressive healing over several months is the usual clinical course.[215]

Enterobius vermicularis (pinworm, seatworm) is a relatively common intestinal parasite. The female worm measures 8–13 mm in length and 0.5 mm in diameter. The male is approximately one-fourth as long as the female and has the same diameter. Infected children frequently complain of severe vulvovaginal pruritus, which may awaken them at night. Other complaints include lower abdominal pains, diarrhea, restlessness, and nocturia. Studies for fungi and bacteria are not diagnostic, and examination of the vulvar vestibule and vagina reveal marked inflammation. Occasionally an adult female helminth found on the vestibule or perineal areas is brought to the laboratory. More commonly, the pathologist is presented with a cellulose tape–slide preparation for identification of the typical embryonated eggs of *E. vermicularis*.[101]

Vulvar schistosomiasis, usually caused by *Schistosoma mansoni* is well documented, and primary skin lesions on the vulva from penetration of the infective cercariae (second generation of the life cycle) may be seen. On biopsy, the parasite may be found within the epidermis.[223]

Noninfectious Diseases

Behçet's Syndrome

Behçet's syndrome is a triad of oral ulcers, genital ulcers, and various ophthalmologic inflammations.[137] Ocular changes may be absent in mild cases. Other findings include acne, cutaneous nodules, thrombophlebitis, encephalopathy, and colitis.[206,231,247] Histologically, necrotizing arteritis is frequently seen and can be considered a cardinal pathologic finding. A chronic inflammatory infiltrate is present about and within the vessel wall, with homogenization of the arterial media. Endothelial cell swelling also occurs and may result in arteriolar occlusion, as well as venous thrombosis. Behçet's syndrome causes deep ulcerations on the vulva that may result in fenestration of the labia. In one patient, this process was reported to have led to gangrene of the labia. These ulcerations characteristically relapse and are usually associated with simultaneous oral aphthosis.

Crohn's Disease

Crohn's disease is a chronic noncaseating granulomatous disease of unknown etiology that occurs more commonly in women. Although it usually involves the distal ileum and colon, it can involve any segment of the gastrointestinal tract, from the mouth to the anus. Cutaneous ulcerations occur in areas where there is close apposition of skin, such as the vulva and submammary areas.[175] When Crohn's disease involves the vulva, the resulting ulcers are often multiple, deep, and secondarily infected. Vulvar and perianal ulceration may be the presenting symptoms of Crohn's disease.[193] Involvement of the colon, rectum, or small bowel with ulcerative colitis is not always present when the vulva is involved. Perianal fistulas, as well as fistulas to other sites in the female genital tract, are, however, well recognized complications of Crohn's disease. When perianal draining sinuses and abscesses occur, the fluid released often resembles small bowel content.

Microscopic examination demonstrates a noncaseating granulomatous inflammation within the dermis. Tests for acid-fast bacteria and fungi are negative. A marked granulation tissue response is frequently seen about the ulcers, but significant lymphadenitis is rare. The differential diagnosis includes vulvar tuberculosis, actinomycosis, lymphogranuloma venereum, granuloma inguinale, and chronic inflammation of the skin appendages, as seen in hidradenitis suppurativa.

Pyoderma Gangrenosum

Pyoderma gangrenosum (PG) is a progressive necrotic and ulcerative condition of the skin of uncertain etiology. Most case reports of PG are associated with chronic ulcerative colitis. The dilemma of PG of the vulva is that it may appear some time after ileostomy and abdominal perineal resection of the colon and rectum. Antibiotic therapy is necessary, and wide local excision, with skin grafting, may be required.[365]

Synergistic Bacterial Infection and Necrotizing Fasciitis

Postoperative or posttraumatic synergistic bacterial infection and necrotizing fasciitis are life-threatening conditions that may develop following episiotomy or vaginal, vulvar, or abdominal surgery.[5,320] Diabetes mellitus predisposes to necrotizing fasciitis.[5] In both synergistic bacterial infection and necrotizing fasciitis, prompt radical excision of the infected tissue and broad-spectrum systemic antibiotic therapy may offer the only chance of cure.

Hidradenitis Suppurativa

Hidradenitis suppurativa is generally believed to be an apocrine gland disorder.[146] Deep-seated, painful, subcutaneous nodules are found in areas containing apocrine glands, especially the axilla and vulva. The lesions commonly progress subcutaneously, producing confluent masses that subsequently ulcerate the epidermis and result in draining sinuses and extensive scarring. The condition may coexist with Fox-Fordyce disease. Total excision of involved areas is necessary in advanced cases, although oral retinoid therapy is promising.[326] Histologically, during its early stages, hidradenitis suppurativa demonstrates a perifolliculitis, with an acute and chronic infiltrate within the dermis. The later stages of the disease result in destruction of the epithelial appendages and sinus tract formation.[206]

Fox–Fordyce Disease

Fox–Fordyce disease is a disorder of the apocrine glands; 90% of cases occur in women. The disease generally begins at puberty and presents as a pruritic, papular eruption usually involving the axillae, vulva, and perianal regions. The center of the papule often contains a hair follicle and apocrine sweat gland duct, plugged by hyperkeratosis. There is dilatation of the apocrine gland acini (Fig. 3.17). Chronic inflammatory changes in the dermis and epidermal acanthosis and spongiosis are also present. There may be an associated rupture of the inter-epithelial portion of the duct, with subsequent vesicle formation within the epidermis. These vesicles cannot be seen unless serial sections are performed.[146] Deposition of apocrine secretion may be found in the ducts and glands and in the tissues about the appendages.

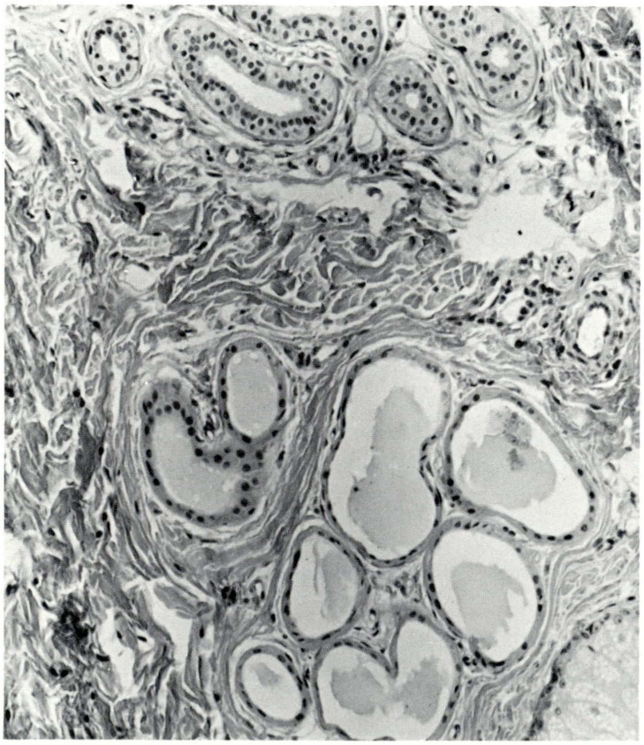

FIG. 3.17. Fox–Fordyce disease. Dilated apocrine glands show inspissated secretion.

Acute Idiopathic Vulvar Ulcer

An acute, single, painful ulcer of the medial portion of the labia minora has been described in women following within 24 hours of coitus.[24] Evaluation of these ulcerations shows no causative agent. Self-induced ulcers, usually secondary to scratching, may reflect some underlying cutaneous disease or have some neurotic basis. Such lesions are usually superficial and have no significant inflammatory reaction.[370]

Pemphigoid

Bullous pemphigoid has been reported on the vulva, usually as a result of drug sensitivity.[311] The clinical presentation may be one of moist, tender ulcers that involve the labia minora, majora, and perianal areas. At times, fluid-filled bullae are also noted. Biopsy of the ulcerated area at its advanced stage may show only granulation tissue. Biopsies, preferably of fresh lesions, that include normal adjacent skin as well as the ulcer may show the characteristic subepidermal bullae (Fig. 3.18).

Cicatricial pemphigoid has been reported secondary to drug hypersensitivity.[333] The symptoms are erosion, erythema, and small blisters of the vulva and perianal and anal mucosa, associated with chronic burning pain and painful ulcers. Severe cicatrization with shrinkage, suggesting advanced vulvar lichen sclerosus, characterizes the process. Small blisters, with a positive Nikolsky phenomenon, slippage of the more superficial epidermis from the underlying basal layer, or dermis, with sliding of the finger on the skin surface, may be helpful clinical findings in recognizing pemphigoid.

Biopsy shows subepithelial blister formation with a mixed inflammatory cell infiltrate within the dermis. Direct immunofluorescent slides for IgG show linear deposition along the basement membrane. Immunoglobulins IgA and IgM may or may not be present on the basement membrane. Linear deposition of complement C3 and C5 on the basement membrane may also be demonstrated by direct immunofluorescence.[311,333] Systemic corticosteroids and topical beta-methasone and 17-valerate may be of use. If the condition is drug related, the suspected medication should be discontinued.

Darier's Disease

Darier's disease, keratosis follicularis, is inherited as an autosomal dominant trait, although spontaneous cases are recognized. The disease frequently involves the vulva. It appears anytime after late childhood as crusted, hyperkeratotic papules that often seem darker than the surrounding skin and which may be secondarily infected.[206,285] Histologically, acantholysis of the suprabasal epithelial cells results in clefts that extend from the basal layer through the granular layer. Acantholytic cells are seen within the clefts. Corps ronds and nuclear

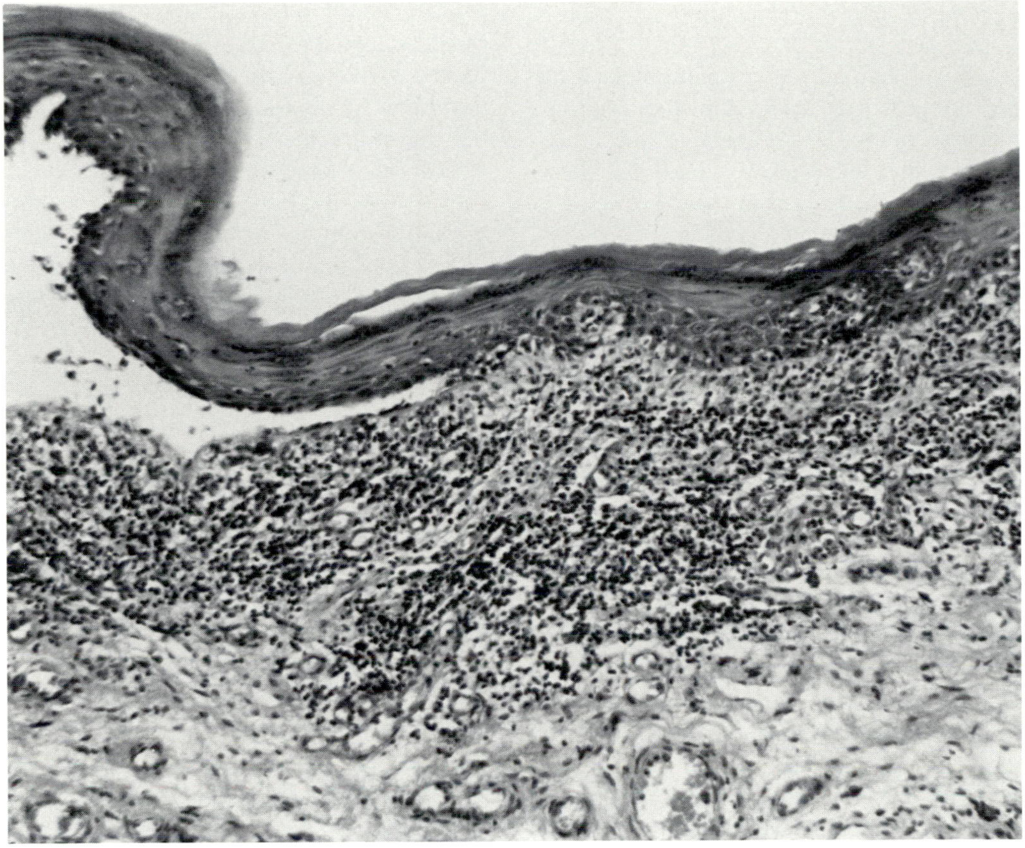

FIG. 3.18. Bullous pemphigoid. A subepidermal bulla is evident, with intact epithelium separated from the underlying dermis. An intense inflammatory infiltrate of lymphocytes, neutrophils, and eosinophils is seen within the dermis, with some inflammatory cells within the bulla. Linear deposition of IgM, IgG, and complement may be demonstrated about the basement membrane by immunofluorescence.

grains can be found in the granular layer, and individual cell keratinazation may be present, reflecting dyskeratosis. Hyperkeratosis, acanthosis, and papillomatosis are seen along with keratotic plugs. Rarely, epithelial cells proliferate into the dermis, with resultant basal budding. The inflammatory cell infiltration within the dermis is usually minimal unless the lesions are secondarily infected.[206]

Warty dyskeratoma of the vulva may have a histologic picture essentially identical to that of Darier's disease. An important clinical distinction is that Darier's disease is usually congenital, carried as an autosomal dominant, and dyskeratoma is not. In addition, Darier's disease is multifocal and may involve the trunk and extremities as well as the face. Warty dyskeratoma usually involves the head, neck, or vulva as a single lesion.[80]

Hailey–Hailey Disease

Hailey–Hailey disease, familial benign pemphigus, is inherited as an autosomal dominant trait, although approximately one-third of patients have no family history of the disease. The onset of the lesions often occurs during adolescence. Intertriginous areas are usually involved, and several cases confined exclusively to the vulva have been reported.[285] Presentation as an isolated white plaque on the labia majora may occur.[84] The usual clinical presentation is of recurrent clusters of vesicles that develop, rupture, and result in crusted, moist papules that later coalesce to form plaques. For diagnostic biopsy, early vesicles should be selected. Histologically, there is acantholysis with resultant suprabasalar lacunae. Unlike the case in Darier's disease, vesicles and bullae are also found.

Acantholytic cells, which maintain their nuclear detail, can be seen within the vesicles, and the acantholysis is more marked than in Darier's disease. Basal cells maintain their orientation to the basement membrane. Rarely, corps ronds are seen in the granular layer. There is minimal, if any, dyskeratosis in Hailey–Hailey disease, in contrast to Darier's disease. Strands of epidermal cells may proliferate into the dermis, but little dermal inflammatory infiltrate exists unless secondary infection is present.

Darier's disease and familial benign pemphigus must be distinguished not only from each other but also from pemphigus vulgaris, pemphigus vegetans, and warty dyskeratoma. These five acantholytic conditions must be considered whenever acantholysis with vesicles is found.[80,206]

Psoriasis

Psoriasis is inherited as a simple autosomal dominant trait with incomplete penetrance. Psoriasis affects approximately 2% of the population of the United States. On the vulva, the disease involves the lateral aspects of the labia majora and genitocrural areas.[285] The lesions are silvery-topped erythematous papules. When this loose, silvery scale is removed, several punctate bleeding points can be seen (Auspitz sign). Coalescence of papules results in plaque formation. The lesions are frequently symmetric and may persist for years. Koebner's phenomenon is the presentation of new psoriatic lesions at sites of trauma within 7–30 days of the trauma. Histologic findings include hyperkeratosis, parakeratosis, uniform acanthosis (elongation of the rete ridges to an even length), diminution of the granular layer, and collections of polymorphonuclear leukocytes within the epidermis (Monro's abscesses). Mitotic activity increases within the epidermis, reflecting the significantly increased rate of epithelial turnover. The dermal papillae are clubbed and edematous. Prominent vessels are seen within the papillae, and there is a minimal chronic inflammatory cell infiltrate within the dermis.[206]

Vulvar Vestibulitis

For many years, it was known that some women experienced severe dyspareunia on entry despite a relative lack of physical findings. An association of this symptom and exquisite tenderness of the minor vestibular gland-bearing area in the vestibule has now been described[100,358] and is recognized as vulvar vestibulitis. Slight inflammation of gland openings in the vestibule, associated with marked pinpoint tenderness to pressure on the inflamed area, is typical (Fig. 3.19, Plate 1).

Bacterial, chlamydial, and viral cultures from affected areas have not suggested an infectious agent, and antibiotics produce no response, nor can the symptoms be alleviated by corticosteroids. Laser ablation has not been helpful, but surgical excision of the involved mucosa and superficial submucosa has given relief to some.[357] Surgical specimens show areas of moderate to marked inflammatory response, often characterized by an abundance of plasma cells and lack of polymorphonuclear leukocytes. The stromal tissue beneath the vestibular epithelium is most prominently involved, and minor vestibular glands may also be surrounded by the process (see Fig. 3.4). Inflammatory cells are not found within the glandular epithelium or within the acini or ductal lumina. It is usually necessary to block in the entire vestibular specimen, making one slide per block, to identify these minor vestibular glands.

Vestibular adenomas, involving the minor vestibular glands, have been encountered in women undergoing vestibulectomy for symptomatic vestibulitis.[12] The adenomas are composed of tightly clustered, small, benign-appearing glands lined with mucus-secreting epithelium.

Pigmentation Disorders

Hypopigmented Conditions

The vulvar skin is usually more pigmented than the general body surface. Biopsies of the normal vulva show dendritic melanocytes scattered along the basal layer of the epithelium as well as squamous keratinocytes containing variable concentrations of melanin granules. Areas of the vulvar skin that appear hypopigmented are therefore clinically remarkable, and biopsies may be submitted from such areas. There are three basic conditions that result in vulvar hypopigmentation: vitiligo, albinism, and postinflammatory depigmentation (leukoderma).

Vitiligo is an inherited disorder in which the melanocytes are lost from areas of skin that were previously normally pigmented. This condition frequently affects the vulva, and biopsies from vitiliginous areas show a remarkable absence of both basilar melanocytes and melanin granules.

Albinism, also a genetic disorder, is characterized by an inability of the melanocytes to form melanin pigment. There is an absence of melanin granules in the keratinocytes, and, in addition, large pale cells may be present within the basal layer, representing the incompetent melanocytes. At times, this disorder is confined to small areas of ventral skin in a condition known as *piebaldism*.

Postinflammatory depigmentation, or leukoderma occurs in areas of previous ulcerative inflammation since recently healed skin will temporarily lack a normal population of melanocytes. This disorder is common following herpes infections and syphilitic ulcerations. Histologically, the skin appears somewhat thin, metabolically active, and lacking in the usual amount of pigment. On careful microscopic inspection, some degree of pigment formation will usually be evident.

Hyperpigmentated Lesions

Freckles

Freckles (ephelides) do not occur on the vulva, although they are certainly the most common hyperpigmented lesion in other areas of the skin. Freckles represent areas of epidermis in which a normal or decreased melanocytic population is stimulated to an excess of melanin production by actinic radiation. The vulvar skin, however, is rarely exposed to sunlight and, as such, does not exhibit common freckles.

Lentigo Simplex

The most common hyperpigmented lesion occurring on the vulva is that of lentigo simplex, which may occur on the mucous membranes as well as the skin. These lentigo consist of isolated areas of epidermis that contain a population of functioning melanocytes. Extreme degrees of epidermal pigmentation may be present, with numerous squamous cells exhibiting cytoplasmic melanin granules, usually in highest concentration near the epithelial–stromal junction (Fig. 3.20). There may be mild acanthosis and slight clubbing of the rete ridges, and heavily pigmented melanophages may be present in the upper dermis. At times, a minimal amount of inflammatory infiltration is noted, but this is by no means constant. Clinically, lentigines closely resemble junctional nevi and are, therefore, frequently biopsied. Except for the rare leopard syndrome, in which thousands of lentigines are present all over the body, lentigo simplex is essentially devoid of clinical significance. In contrast to lentigo simplex, actinic lentigines are usually seen on sun-exposed areas only.

Nevomelanocytic Nevi

Hamartomas of the skin are divided into two main types, congenital and acquired. Congenital nevi are found in approximately 10% of newborns and are usually under 4 mm in diameter. Giant nevomelanocytic nevi (over 20 cm in diameter) (garment type), although rare, carry an increased risk of developing malignant melanoma in prepubertal individuals. Vulvar melanocytic nevi may be junctional, compound, or intradermal. These nevomelanocytic types occur with nearly equal distribution.[106] As described by Pinkus and Mehregan, the typical nevus cell is characterized mainly by its negative attributes.[266] The cells are somewhat larger than melanocytes and have round or ovoid nuclei. Dendrites are not present, and intercellular connections are not visible. The cells may lie singly within the dermis, but more commonly, they tend to form nests. Unless they contain melanin, their cytoplasm is clear without granulations or fibrils.

In pure junctional nevi, the nevus cells are located within the epidermis and at the dermal epidermal junction. Individual cells, or cell nests, bulge downward from the tips of the rete ridges. There is no connective tissue noted between the nevus cells and the adjacent squamous keratinocytes. Such nevi are young and somewhat undifferentiated. With age, the basement membrane of the epidermis surrounding the nests disappears, and reticulum, collagen, and elastic fibers envelop the nests, pushing the epidermis upward. During this process, the lesion is clinically noted to be elevated above the level of the surrounding skin. Histologically, nevus cells are within both the epidermis and the dermis. Such lesions are called *compound nevi* (Fig. 3.21). Further

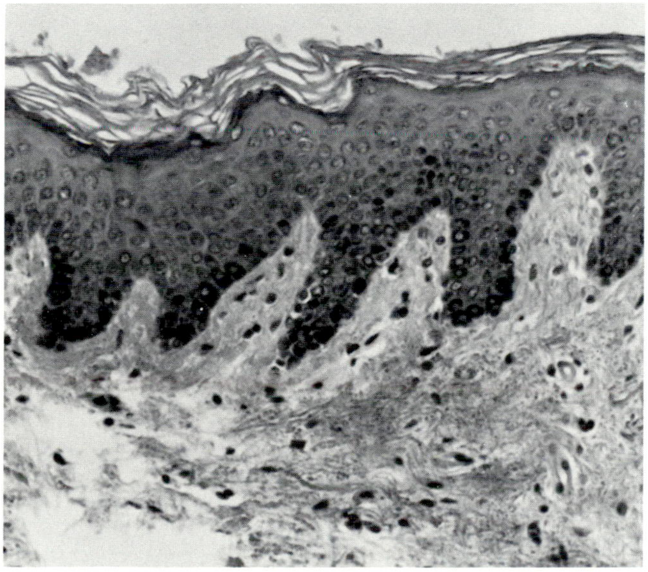

Fig. 3.20. Lentigo. Note the heavy concentration of deeply pigmented melanocytes at the tips of the accentuated rete ridges.

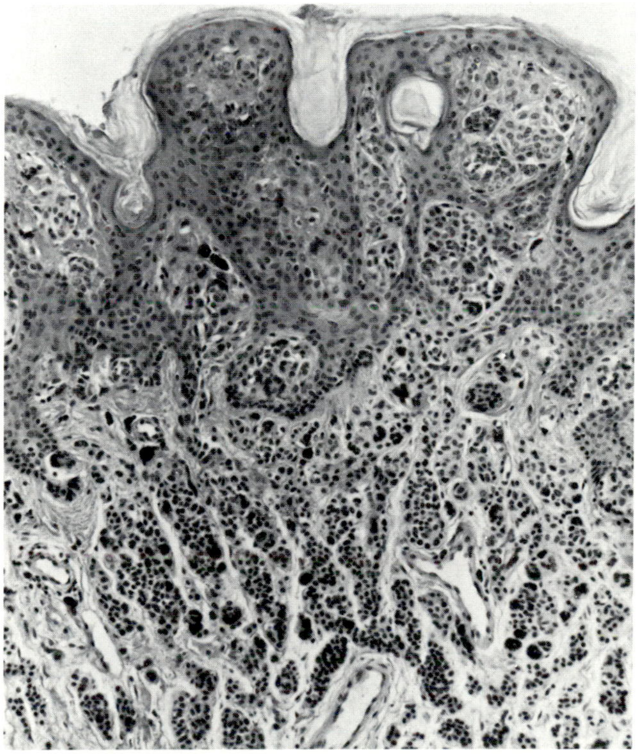

Fig. 3.21. Compound nevus. Nests of nevus cells are evident within the epithelium as well as within the dermis.

differentiation results in complete enclosure of the nevus cells and nests by connective tissue elements such that they lie wholly intradermal; no activity is seen at the dermoepidermal junction. With time, nevi may regress completely or may result in a fibrous papule or acrochordon.[263]

Atypical Nevomelanocytic Nevi

These are most commonly encountered in adolescent and premenopausal women and may be confused with malignant melanoma.[96] These nevi have cytologic atypia with nuclear pleomorphism and prominent nucleoli seen in some enlarged epithelial cells, with occasional spindle-shaped nevomelanocytes. These nevomelanocytic cells are often aggregated in nests. Features that distinguish atypical nevomelanocytic nevi from malignant melanoma include (1) symmetry of the nevus in both its side-to-side and top-to-bottom dimensions, (2) a progressive decrease in cell size and loss of cytologic atypia of the cells in the deeper levels (Fig. 3.22), and (3) a near absence of single nevus cells involving the upper third of the epidermis when pagetoid spread is present.[96,263]

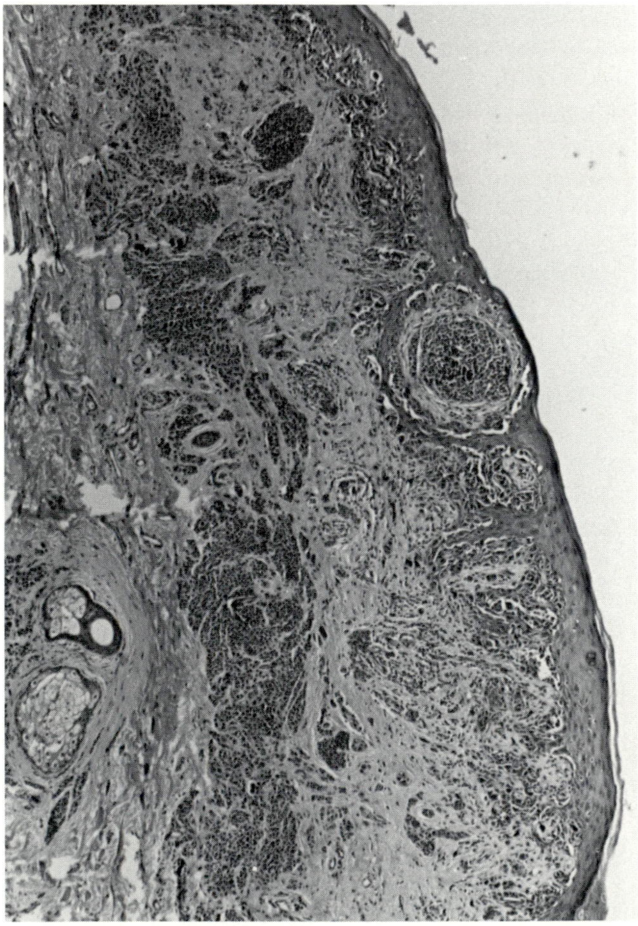

Fig. 3.22. Atypical vulvar nevus. This acquired atypical nevus has marked cytoatypia in the superficial and junctional areas with small, benign-appearing nevus cells within the dermis. (Photograph courtesy of K.K. Pierson, M.D.)

Dysplastic Nevomelanocytic Nevi

Dysplastic nevomelanocytic nevi generally exceed 0.5 mm in diameter, with a macular appearance and a somewhat roughened pebbly surface. Dysplastic nevi occur, on an average, 10 years later than typical acquired nevi and may often involve the breasts and buttocks, unusual sites for typical nevi. Dysplastic nevi should be excised if irregular darkening or depigmentation occurs or if there is a change in size.

Characteristics of dysplastic nevi include random focal cytologic atypia rather than atypia throughout the entire cell population, as is seen in malignant melanoma. The nevomelanotic cells of the dysplastic nevus may be spindle or epithelioid in appearance. The epithelioid cells may show focal nesting, whereas the spindled nevomelanocytic cells may show bridging between adjacent rete ridges.

Within the dermis there is a lymphohistiocytic inflammatory response that is irregular and scattered, unlike that of malignant melanoma, which is more band-like and regular. Associated dermal fibrosis is seen that may be delicate or more dense and fibrotic and is closely adherent to the tips and sides of rete ridges. Many of the features described in the dysplastic nevus are seen in the atypical vulvar nevus occurring in adolescent and premenopausal women.[263] Patients with dysplastic nevi have an increased risk of malignant melanoma, especially if they have a family history of malignant melanoma.

Nonneoplastic Epithelial Disorders

The vast majority of white lesions of the vulva have no premalignant potential. Both the clinician and the pathologist have been confused by such diagnoses as kraurosis vulvae, leukoplakia, and atrophic vulvitis.[116] Such vague terminology reflects an earlier age of gross morphologic description. A consolidating proposal was developed by the International Society for the Study of Vulvar Disease in an effort to establish a standardized system of nomenclature based on histopathologic findings that would allow the collection of comparable data.[151] This multinational group of pathologists, gynecologists, and dermatologists recommended that all such lesions be placed under the single heading of *dystrophy* and that the older terms be abandoned. The term *dystrophy* was first proposed by Jeffcoate and Woodcock in 1961 to group clinically those disorders of epithelial growth that usually present as white lesions of the vulva and have otherwise unclassified or mixed alterations of the epithelial and dermal architecture.[166,167] The dystrophy terminology was changed in 1987 (Table 3.2).

TABLE 3.2. Classification of vulvar nonneoplastic disorders.

1975–1986[a]	1987[b]
Lichen sclerosus	Lichen sclerosus
Hyperplastic dystrophy	Squamous hyperplasia
Mixed dystrophy	Other dermatoses

[a]Developed by the International Society for the Study of Vulvar Disease (ISSVD).
[b]Developed by the ISSVD and the International Society of Gynecological Pathologists.

It is not always possible to clinically distinguish the various forms of dystrophy on the basis of their gross appearance alone. All may be white, scaly, and fissured (Fig. 3.23, Plate 1). Such changes pose two basic problems for the clinician: "Is this now, or will it become, cancer?" and "What treatment will be effective?" Multiple representative biopsies must be obtained to sample the entire lesion. On the basis of the histologic findings, the pathologist can separate white lesions of a neoplastic type from dystrophic change and other dermatoses.

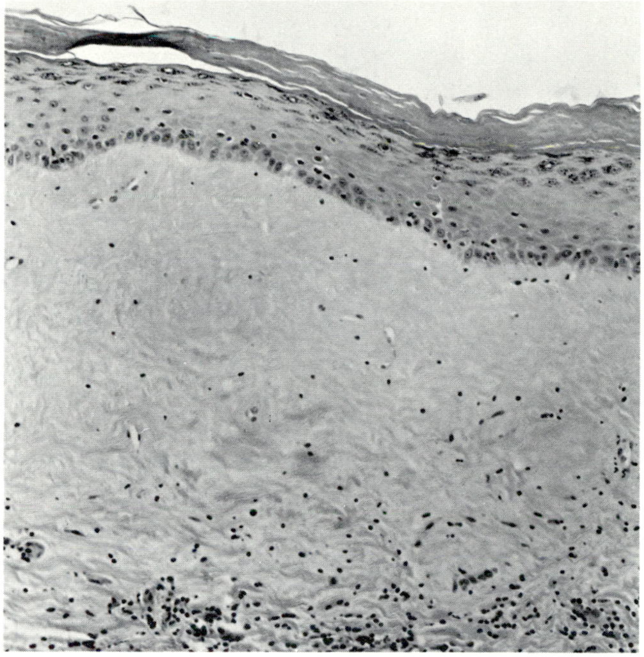

FIG. 3.24. Lichen sclerosus. Hyperkeratosis is present along with loss of rete pegs and homogenization of the dermis.

Lichen Sclerosus

Lichen sclerosus is the most common cause of dystrophic change of the vulva.[98,138] As a cutaneous disease, it may affect the trunk or extremities but is most frequently found on the genitalia. Wallace (1971) estimated the clinical frequency of the disease to be between 1:300 and 1:1000,[341] but the exact prevalence is unknown and awaits a definitive large-scale study. The disease is not racially confined, and although it is most commonly noted in postmenopausal Caucasian women, cases have been reported from South and Central Africa as well as from Japan.[39,101,341] Men may be affected, and the glans of the penis and prepuce are frequently involved and undergo phimosis. Under these circumstances, the condition is clinically known as *balanitis xerotica obliterans*. No age group is immune, and young children have been known to have the disease.[90,98] There is a genetic aspect to the disease. Fifteen families have now been recorded in which successive generations have manifested lichen sclerosus.[103] For the most part, these have been mother–daughter pairs, but in one instance both mother and father were affected, as was their young daughter. Within such families, there is a tendency toward a similar age at onset for affected individuals.

The principal histologic changes occurring in lichen sclerosus include blunting or loss of the rete ridges and the concomitant development of a homogeneous subepithelial layer of variable thickness of the dermis (Fig. 3.24). Hyperkeratosis is present in some cases. The homogeneous zone has been described as collagenized or edematous and usually shows a reduction or absence of elastic fibers. Beneath this layer, a band of scattered lymphocytes is usually seen. The number of cellular layers in the epidermis is decreased, and the basal cell layer is often disorganized and hydropic. There is both an absence of melanosomes in the keratinocytes and a disappearance of the melanocytes. This lack of pigment contributes to the white clinical appearance. Mitotic figures are rare or absent. In some cases, the mechanical trauma of rubbing and scratching will have produced bullous areas of lymphedema and lacunae filled with erythrocytes (Fig. 3.25). Areas of ulceration and acute inflammation may also be seen. Lichen sclerosus is sometimes associated with vulvar squamous carcinoma,[318] but it is not considered to be a premalignant lesion in the sense that an intraepithelial neoplasm is. In a large retrospective study, Hart et al. noted that carcinoma developed in only one patient, in whom it arose in an isolated area of hyperplasia.[132]

Ultrastructural studies have shown that collagen metabolism is abnormally active, and the number of capillaries is reduced. The basal lamina is thickened and discontinuous. Degenerate dermal and collagenous material can be found between the cells of the epidermis. An increased concentration of collagenase inhibitor has also been reported.[77] The presence of an elastase-type protease in vulvar fibroblasts from lichen sclerotic tissue has been reported, which may be responsible for the loss of elastic tissue so frequently seen.[120] The suffix *et atrophicus* was once applied to this condition, but studies

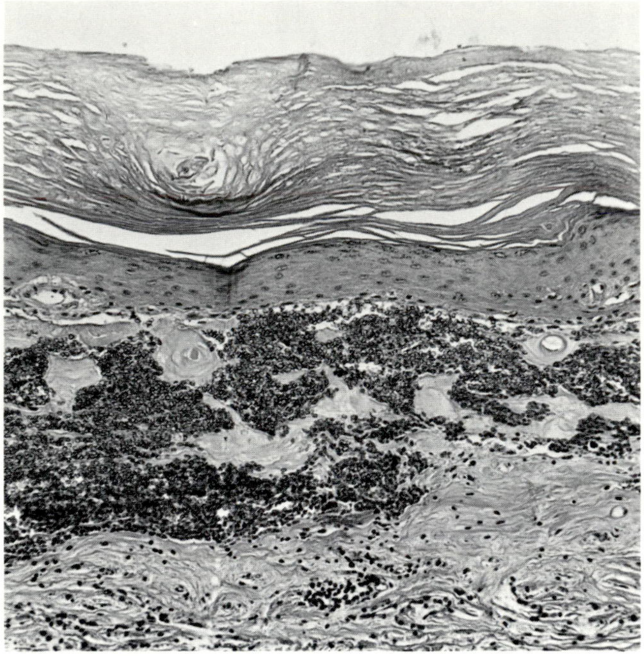

FIG. 3.25. Lichen sclerous. Marked hyperkeratosis with extravasation of blood in the dermis.

of the cellular kinetics involved suggest that this may no longer be appropriate. Tissue studies of glucose metabolism as well as alkaline phosphatase and adenosine triphosphatase have shown a surprisingly high rate of activity, equal to that seen in hyperplastic specimens and greater than that found in normal menopausal skin. These findings are consistent with other in vitro work that demonstrated that lichen sclerotic epithelium contained normal amounts of RNA and DNA and that the uptake of tritiated thymidine by such epithelium was even greater than normal despite the lack of mitoses.[107,361] An apparent premature maturation of all cells above the basal layer has been reported based on their high concentration of involucrin.[65]

There is a growing body of evidence that an autoimmune mechanism may be involved in the etiology. Patients with lichen sclerosus have been noted to have an increased number of organ-specific antibodies and more autoimmune disease than the unaffected population.[121,130] Histologically, direct immunofluorescence studies have shown a deposit of fibrin along the dermo-epidermal junction in 75% of the specimens studied.[35] An indirect fluorescent technique showed that IgM and C3 were heavily concentrated along the basal lamina of the epithelium.[67] A consistent systemic alteration was first noted in a group of 30 untreated women with lichen sclerosus who were found to have serum levels of dihydrotestosterone well below the normal values for their age.[102] This was true for patients in the reproductive age group as well as those in postmenopausal years. At the same time, their free testosterone levels were elevated, suggesting a block in the enzymatic conversion of testosterone to dihydrotestosterone. The pathophysiology of this disorder thus remains obscure, and curative therapy is not available. Current management consists in the topical application of testosterone or progesterone compounds, which have been successful in arresting the symptoms and progress of the disease.[101]

Squamous Hyperplasia

Squamous hyperplasia of the vulva is essentially a diagnosis arrived at by exclusion. It is believed to be a nonspecific response of the genital skin to a wide variety of irritants. When compared to the skin of the forearm, vulvar skin has an increased propensity to undergo some irritant reactions.[28] Hyperplastic reactions may occur at any time but are most commonly found in women between 30 and 60 years of age. There is no racial predilection. Clinically, the vulva appears pink or red, with an overlying gray-white keratin covering of variable thickness. The skin markings are often accentuated, a sign of intradermal edema, and excoriations and fissures frequently bear witness to the intensity of the itching. The condition is clinically indistinguishable from what has previously been called *neurodermatitis* or *eczema*. Psoriasis or lichen planus may be included in the differential diagnosis. However, these represent distinct dermotoses that are clinically and histologically identifiable.

The histopathologic features of squamous hyperplasia are nonspecific. Microscopic findings include elongation, widening, and clubbing of the rete ridges of the epidermis (acanthosis). Hyperkeratosis is usually present (Fig. 3.26). When this thickened layer of keratin is wet, it lends a white appearance to the vulvar tissues. As a rule, a chronic inflammatory infiltrate is noted within the dermis, which is otherwise normal or slightly edematous. At times, this infiltrate is predominantly perivascular in location; at other times, it is more diffuse. These features are similar to those seen in lichen simplex chronicus, which may be the preferred term when a prominent chronic inflammatory infiltrate is found within the dermis.[265] Chronic candidiasis of the vulva can usually be differentiated by silver stain for fungus or periodic acid-Schiff (PAS) stain for the organisms. The fungal organisms can be seen within the keratin layer. The dermal papillomatosis seen in condylomata acuminata or squamous papilloma is lacking. The individual squamous cells are regular, with distinct intercellular bridges. The nuclei are round to oval and contain finely distributed chromatin. Nucleoli may be prominent, and there is progressive maturation of the cells as they approach the superficial

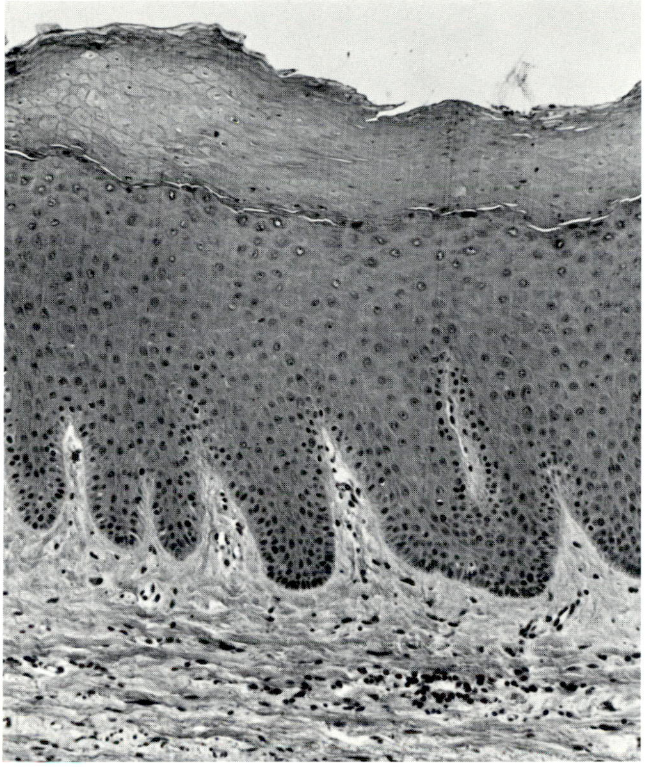

FIG. 3.26. Squamous hyperplasia. Hyperkeratosis, acanthosis, and mild inflammation characterize this entity.

layers. Mitotic figures are often quite numerous in the basal layers, and, occasionally, inflammatory exocytosis may be seen. Retention of nuclear material in the keratin layer, parakeratosis, is usually associated with loss of the granular zone, whereas in the presence of hyperkeratosis, this zone may be accentuated. Although parakeratosis may be present in otherwise typical areas of hyperplasia, its presence should prompt a careful search for signs of cellular atypicality deeper in the epithelium. In the absence of atypia, there is no evidence of risk of carcinoma from this process.[182]

Treatment is based on isolation of the vulva from potential irritants and the use of topical corticosteroids and antipruritics, which are usually quite successful. Occasionally, local excision, laser ablation, or alcohol injection may be required in unresponsive patients.

Mixed Dystrophy

Lichen sclerosus and squamous hyperplasia may affect different areas of the same vulva at the same time.[106] This finding is consistent with the spectrum of lichen sclerosus and therefore the term mixed dystrophy is no longer recommended (Table 3.2).

Benign Cystic Tumors

Cystic lesions of the vulva include Bartholin's cyst, keratinous cyst, mucous cyst, mesonephric cyst, and cyst of the canal of Nuck.

Bartholin Cyst

Bartholin's glands, first described by Bartholin in 1677, are tubular, alveolar, paired glands that produce a clear mucoid secretion thought to provide a continuous lubrication for the vestibular surface.[364] Secretion from the ducts occurs during the late excitement and early plateau stages of the sexual response.

Pain during sexual activity has been attributed to occlusion of Bartholin's duct.[298] Lined by transitional epithelium, the ducts of these glands are prone to obstruction at their vestibular orifice. Such obstruction results in subsequent accumulation of secretion and cystic dilatation of the duct.[291,364] The content of an uninfected Bartholin cyst is, therefore, a mucoid, liquid, which, when cultured, fails to grow bacteria. The Bartholin cyst secretion stains with mucicarmine and with PAS before and after diastase digestion. It stains with Alcian blue at pH 2.5. These properties are consistent with sialomucin. Such cysts generally show minimal, if any, inflammatory response within the stroma of the gland or about the dilated duct. Careful examination of the duct area, if available for study, may demonstrate variable degrees of synechia formation and duct occlusion. Bartholin cyst epithelium contains CEA on immunoperoxidase study.[235]

Such cysts may be recurrent and occasionally are associated with primary infection of Bartholin's gland. They may require marsupialization. In postmenopausal women, they should be surgically excised because of the possibility of associated carcinoma of Bartholin's gland. Bartholin adenocarcinomas, when present, tend to be in the tissues adjacent to the cyst wall. Fine needle aspiration of the Bartholin cyst and any adjacent nodule that may persist after drainage of the cyst may be of value in the identification of tumor within the glands or ducts of Bartholin's gland (K.J. Lohe, unpublished data, 1985).

Bartholin abscess is an acute process often associated with a *Neisseria gonorrhea* infection, although it may be related to staphylococci or to anaerobic organisms. The pathology of the Bartholin's duct abscess demonstrates a striking acute inflammatory reaction within the stroma about the ducts. A purulent exudate is present within the lumen of the abscess wall. Excision, drainage, and antibiotics are the treatments of choice. Occasionally, the infection subsides without abscess formation or becomes chronic. Bartholin's duct cysts, resulting from dilatation of the duct secondary to chronic inflammation and scarring, may be a late sequela of chronic infection.

Mucocele-like changes have been reported in Bartholin's glands. The patient has tenderness and swelling in the vulvar Bartholin's gland area, with nodularity or a deep cystic palpable mass. On gross examination, the tissue is nodular and may be partially cystic. Microscopically, dilated ducts with distended gland elements containing mucin-like material, which is also seen within the stroma, characterize the mucocele. Within the adjacent stroma, foamy histiocytes containing mucin-like material are seen.[95]

Keratinous Cyst

Keratinous cysts (epithelial inclusion cysts) are frequently seen on the vulva and are generally located on the labia majora. They also may be seen in the newborn.[227] Keratinous cysts usually contain a white to pale yellow grumose or cheesy material without hair. Giant cells may be seen in the tissue adjacent to the cyst wall. The lining of such cysts is characterized by a relatively flattened, stratified squamous epithelium that is immunoreactive for high-molecular-weight keratin.[235] Whether or not these cysts represent primary keratinous cysts, unrelated to sebaceous glands, or are actually occluded sebaceous glands that have undergone squamous metaplasia is debatable.[245] Step sections through those cysts, however, may show communication with the surface epithelium and underlying sebaceous glands in some cases (Fig. 3.27). An unusually high frequency of keratinous cysts has been reported in Nigerian children.[173] Such cysts are not considered premalignant, although carcinoma arising in keratinous cysts has been described.[245]

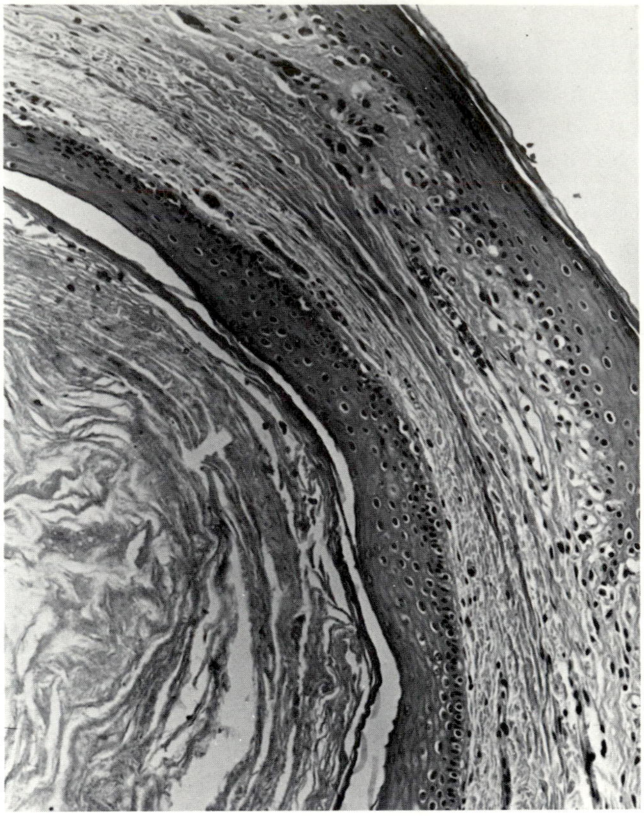

FIG. 3.27. Keratinous cyst. Stratified squamous epithelial lining is evident.

Mucous Cyst

Mucous cysts of the vulva are characterized by a lining of tall to cuboidal, mucus-secreting, columnar epithelium without peripheral muscle fibers or evidence of myoepithelial cells (Fig. 3.28). Squamous metaplasia may be present within the cyst lining. Mucous cysts are usually seen within the vestibule. Histochemical studies demonstrate that the cyst lining stains with both Alcian blue and Mayer's mucicarmine, whereas cysts of mesonephric origin do not exhibit these reactions.[104] Historically, these cysts have been related to müllerian anlage. However, it is now recognized that the müllerian system does not contribute to the formation of the vulvar vestibule. Rather, the cysts probably result from occlusion of minor vestibular glands, which have a similar mucinous epithelium (see Fig. 3.4).[100,104,286] Electron microscopic studies of mucinous cysts of the vestibule have demonstrated that these cysts have an epithelium consistent with an origin from urogenital sinus endoderm.[248] In that the vulvar vestibule arises embryologically primarily from the urogenital sinus, the origin of these cysts from minor vestibular glands is not inconsistent with a urogenital sinus origin.

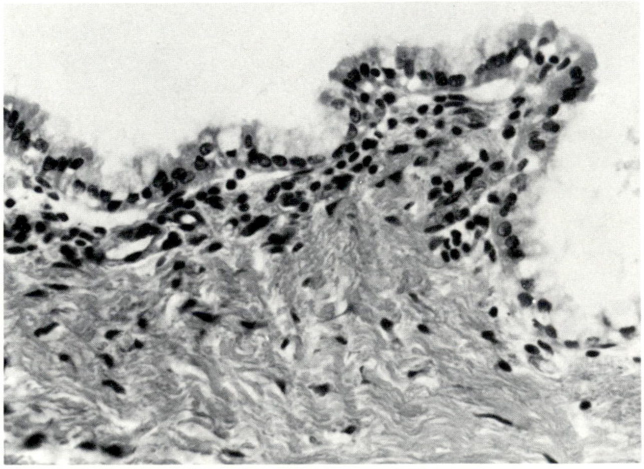

FIG. 3.28. Mucous cyst of the vestibule. Simple columnar mucus-secreting cells rest on the basement membrane. Note absence of underlying smooth muscle layer.

Mesonephric Cyst

Wolffian duct cysts, also known as *mesonephric cysts,* are usually encountered on the lateral aspects of the vulva and vagina. They are thin-walled, translucent, and contain a clear fluid. The lining epithelium is usually cuboidal, although it may be columnar. Histochemical techniques show smooth muscle in the submucosal areas.[161]

Cyst of the Canal of Nuck

Cysts of the canal of Nuck (peritoneal lined cysts) are generally found in the superior aspect of the labia majora or inguinal canal and are believed to arise from inclusions of the peritoneum at the inferior insertion of the round ligament into the labia majora. As such, they are analogous to the hydrocele of the spermatic cord. Such cysts can achieve substantial size and must be distinguished from inguinal hernias, with which they are associated in approximately one-third of cases.[198]

Benign Solid Tumors

The benign solid tumors of the vulva, although rare, comprise a complex group. For convenience, the lesions may be divided into those that arise from the vulvar soft tissue (mesenchyme) and those that are of epithelial origin.

Mesenchymal Tumors

The benign tumors arising from soft tissue include angioma, lymphangioma, angiokeratoma, hemangiopericytoma, and pyogenic granuloma. Fibroma, fibromyoma, leiomyoma, rhabdomyoma, and fibrous histiocytoma are also included, as are granular cell tumors, neurofibroma, schwannoma (neurilemmoma), lipoma, and hemangiofibrolipoma.

Vascular Tumors

Hemangiomas. The strawberry hemangioma (nevus vasculosis) and the cavernous hemangioma are rare on the vulva, although their occurrence in young children has been documented.[180] In children, as a rule, these lesions do not require therapy because they regress over time. Strawberry and cavernous hemangiomas may ulcerate and bleed, due to their superficial location, and on rare occasions may require therapy.[178] Far more common are the senile hemangiomas, which are small (1–3 mm), red to purple papules with no known clinical significance. Histologically, senile hemangiomas have numerous dilated capillaries in the intradermal tissue. These vascular spaces are lined with a single layer of endothelial cells and are separated by connective tissue that may show collagenization.[208] Hemangiomatous-like changes may be found on the vulva following radiotherapy.[371]

Angiokeratoma. The angiokeratoma is a variant of the hemangioma and occurs almost exclusively on the scrotum and vulva. Somewhat larger than senile angiomas, these lesions are often purple and occur primarily in women of childbearing age. Histologically, the dilated endothelium-lined channels are separated by strands and cords of squamous epithelial cells representing downgrowth from the overlying epithelium, which is often hyperkeratotic (Fig. 3.29). Varying degrees of acanthosis and papillomatosis are present along with a mild inflammatory reaction in the deep dermis. Their peculiar appearance often prompts excisional diagnostic biopsy, although they have no clinical significance.[19,150] Angiosarcomas and Kaposi's sarcoma are included in the differential diagnosis when reviewing vascular tumors of the skin.[208]

Pyogenic Granuloma. The pyogenic granuloma is a variant of hemangioma that may occur anywhere on the skin. It is analogous to the epulis tumor of pregnancy. Most of the pyogenic granulomas that occur on the vulva do so during gestation. Although previously thought to be secondary to a superficial wound infection, this tumor is a form of hemangioma characterized by rapid growth. Because the surface is easily traumatized, the lesion is often secondarily infected. Histologically, a thin ulcer-

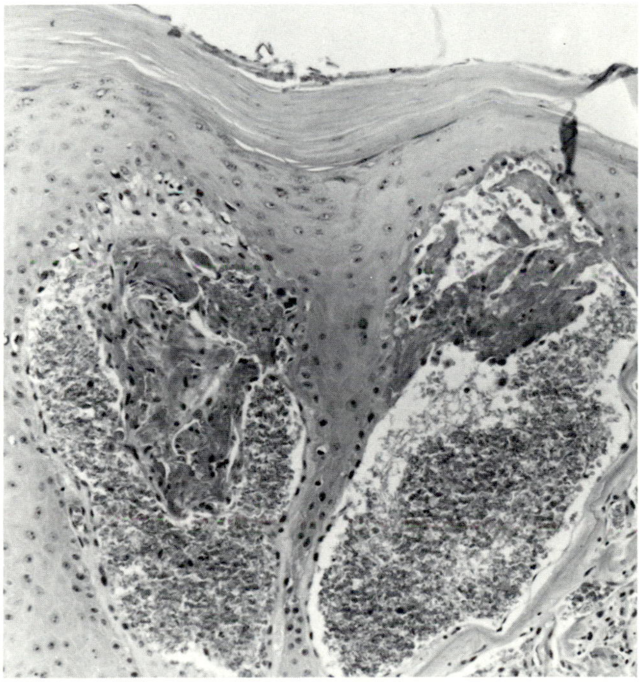

FIG. 3.29. Angiokeratoma. Strands of squamous epithelium surround endothelial lined vascular spaces.

ated epidermis is noted covering a mass of granulation tissue. Capillary proliferation is intense, and secondary inflammatory changes are frequently found within the stroma (Fig. 3.30). Around the periphery of the lesion, there may be a downward growth of the epidermis producing a collarette.

Hemangiopericytoma. The hemangiopericytoma is an extremely rare tumor, but its occurrence has been reported on the vulva.[61] Histologically, numerous small capillaries are seen separated by dense cords of spindle-shaped pericytes. Malignant variants of this tumor may occur. Although nuclear pleomorphism with numerous mitoses may characterize some aggressive lesions, clinical behavior is the most important determinant.[266] Differentiation from other malignant angiomatous tumors can be facilitated by the use of reticulum stains, which show the pericytes to be external to the reticulin network surrounding the individual blood vessels.[61,206,208] Tumors of endothelial cell origin are immunoreactive for factor VIII.[235]

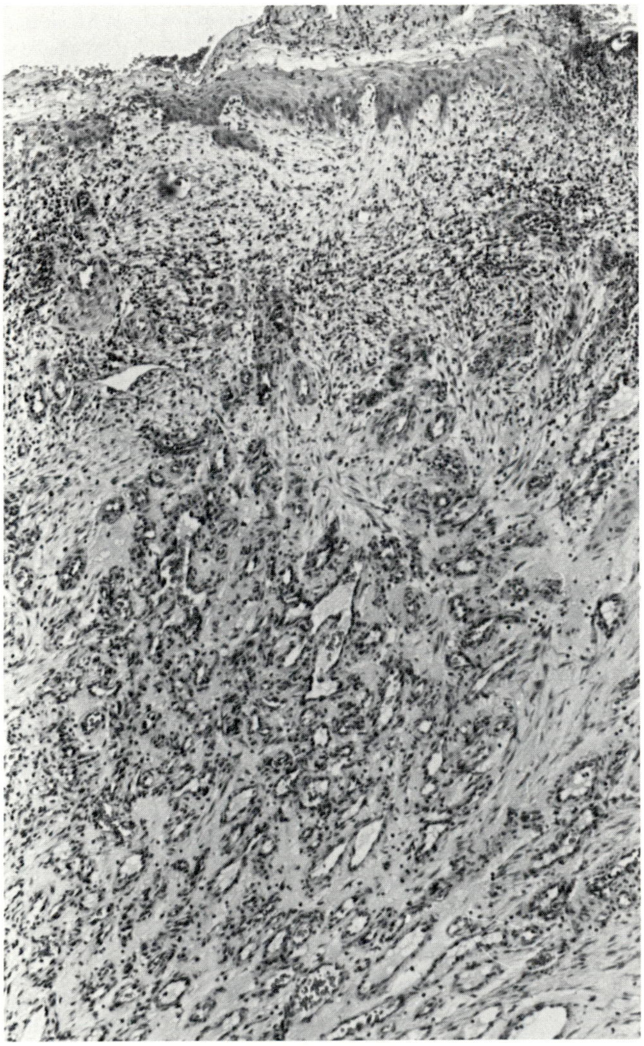

FIG. 3.30. Pyogenic granuloma. Superficial ulceration of the mucosa and a chronic inflammatory infiltrate is present. Within the submucosa, multiple endothelium-lined vascular spaces are seen, surrounded by a delicate fibrous stroma resembling granulation tissue.

Tumors of Muscle Origin

Leiomyoma. Benign leiomyomas have been reported to arise from the smooth muscle elements surrounding the crura of the clitoris.[180] They can be separated from leiomyosarcomas by their low or absent mitotic activity and lack of evidence of infiltration. Both are immunoreactive for desmin and do not contain myoglobin, as do rhabdomyosarcomas and rhabdomyomas.[208,235] Myxoid change may occur in pregnancy and must be distinguished from other tumors with myxoid stroma that may occur on the vulva[208] (Table 3.3).

Rhabdomyoma. Rhabdomyomas have been reported to involve the vulva in women of reproductive age.[72] Rhabdomyomas of the fetal myxoid type must be differentiated from embryonal rhabdomyosarcomas and benign sarcomatous polyps (see Table 3.3).

Neural Tumors

Granular Cell Tumor. Granular cell tumors in the vulva may occur at any age, presenting as painless, single or multiple, slow-growing subcutaneous masses.[186,204] They have also appeared as solitary enlargement of the clitoris, mimicking clitoral hypertrophy.[63] Granular cell tumors are not encapsulated, and unless they are treated with wide excision, local recurrences are common. Careful microscopic examination of the margins of the surgical specimen is, therefore, important. Histologically, irregular groups of large polyhedral cells with indistinct cell borders are noted. The cytoplasm of these cells is eosinophilic and granular, whereas the nuclei are generally small and hyperchromatic (Fig. 3.31). Granular cell tumors contain S100 protein and myelin basic protein, which can be demonstrated by immunoperoxidase techniques.[235] Carcinoembryonic antigen and myelin basic protein P0 and P2 have also been identified.[208,220]

In response to this tumor, the overlying squamous epithelium often exhibits remarkable pseudoepitheliomatous hyperplasia. Extreme degrees of acanthosis are noted, and the nests and cords of hyperplastic squamous cells may mimic the appearance of invasive squamous carcinoma.[180,245] Rapid enlargement of benign granular cell tumors may occur in pregnancy. Malignant granular cell tumors are extremely rare.[289]

Neurofibroma. Neurofibroma involving the vulva has been found in 18% of women with von Recklinghausen's

TABLE 3.3. Differential histopathologic features distinguishing tumors with myxoid change in the vulva.

	In children	Cambium layer	Sheets of immature cells	Gland elements	Prominent vascularity	Atypical fibroblasts	Nuclear pleomorphism	Mitotic figures	Cross-striations straplike muscle cells
Fetal myxoid rhabdomyoma	0	0	0	0	0	0	0	0	+
Aggressive angiomyxoma	0	0	0	+	+	0	0	±	0
Embryonal rhabdomyosarcoma (sarcoma botyroides)	+	+	+	0	+	0	+	+	+
Benign pseudosarcomatous polyps	0	0	0	0	+	+	±	0	0
Vulvar polyps with myxoid stroma	0	0	0	0	0	+	±	0	0
Leiomyoma with myxoid change (in pregnancy)	0	0	0	0	0	0	±	±	0
Nodular (pseudosarcomatous) fasciitis	±	0	0	0	0	±	0	+	0

+, present.
0, absent.
±, occasionally seen.

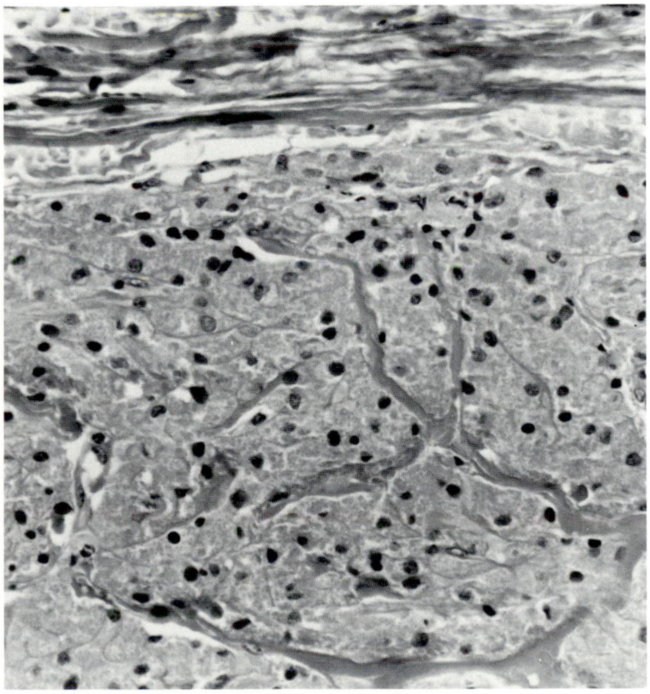

FIG. 3.31. Granular cell tumor. Note nests of polyhedral cells with granular cytoplasm separated by collagenous cords.

disease.[105,299] In patients with neurofibromatosis, the tumors are multicellular (polyclonal) in origin, unlike neurofibromas in normal individuals, where they are monoclonal in origin.[189] A giant solitary variant of neurofibroma of the labia has been reported.[334]

Occurrence of neurofibromata is rare before puberty; thereafter, they grow rapidly, and malignant degeneration to neurofibrosarcoma or malignant schwannoma may occur. Arising from the nerve sheath, these tumors are made up of whorls and wavy bundles of slender spindle cells that often exhibit a palisade arrangement of the nuclei. Special nerve stains show long, thin nerve fibers scattered throughout the tumors, and occasionally the intervening collagen may undergo a peculiar mucoid degeneration.[206] Neurofibromas contain S100 antigen.[235] Steroid receptors have been reported in some neural tumors in the pelvis and vulva.[47] People with hereditary neurofibromatosis also have an increased risk for other tumors, including glioma, ganglioneuroma, pheochromocytoma, meningioma, leukemia, Wilms' tumor, and rhabdomyosarcoma.[189]

Schwannoma. Schwannomas (neurilemmomas) rarely involve the vulva. However, the few cases reported have involved the clitoris. These benign tumors arise from the neuroectodermal nerve sheath and are usually solitary. Histologically, they contain both Antoni type A and type B tissue patterns (Fig. 3.32). A myxomatous matrix is usually present within which small vessels with prominent thickening of the vessel wall are seen. Local excision is the treatment of choice.[143]

Tumors of Fibroblastic Origin

Fibroma. Benign fibromas may appear as vulvar masses, but these tumors actually arise from the deeper connective tissues surrounding the vaginal introitus or adjacent to the perineal body. Rarely do such tumors undergo malignant degeneration. Left untreated, however, they can grow to substantial size. On cut section, fibromas are firm and smooth, with a white or grayish color. Yellow striae and a somewhat softer consistency signify the admixture of a lipomatous element, which is not uncommon. Histologically, parallel bundles of fibrocytes are seen. With large tumors, hyaline, cystic, and hemorrhagic degeneration have been described.[101,208]

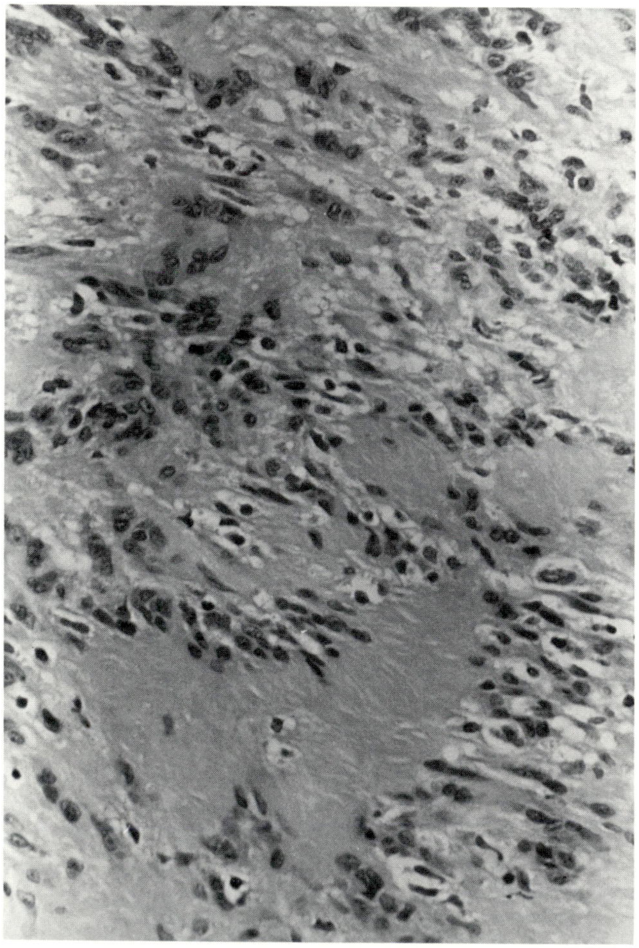

Fig. 3.32. Schwannoma. Densely packed spindle cells from Antoni type A areas are admixed with hypocellular Antoni type B areas.

Nodular Fasciitis. Although not a tumor, nodular fasciitis (pseudosarcomatous fasciitis, proliferative fasciitis) may present as a subcutaneous mass that clinically, as well as pathologically, mimics such sarcomas as leiomyosarcoma, rhabdomyosarcoma, fibrosarcoma, or liposarcoma. Pseudosarcomatous fasciitis may grow locally as a solid subcutaneous mass that may be attached to underlying tissues. The mass is usually solitary, sometimes tender, and may have been present for several years before medical assistance is sought.

The histopathologic features of nodular fasciitis show spindle cell-like growth without encapsulation. The mass is often infiltrated within fibrous cysts and may involve muscle within the collagenous or myxoid matrix. Prominent capillaries and chronic inflammatory cells are usually present. Although mitotic figures may be common in the fibroblasts, abnormal mitoses are not seen. Some cytolysis is usually present. Heterologous elements, such as bone and cartilage, as well as giant cells, have been reported (see Table 3.3).[112,224,288] Immunoperoxidase studies contribute only in that the spindle cells have no distinctive immunoreactive antigen and are negative for desmin and myoglobin, which distinguishes them from muscle tumors, which are immunoreactive for these antigens.[208,235]

Desmoid Tumor. Desmoid tumors (aggressive fibromatosis) are characterized by an infiltrating fibroblastic reaction without an associated inflammatory response.[185] Wide local excision is the treatment of choice.

Dermatofibroma. Dermatofibromas (benign fibrous histiocytomas) are rare on the vulva. However, they may appear as a slightly raised, nonpolypoid, pale brown to red, solitary subcutaneous mass. The term *dermatofibroma* is reserved for those lesions 1.5 cm in diameter or less. Masses that are larger or that are polypoid in appearance are referred to as *fibrous histiocytoma.*[280] These benign histiocytic tumors may have associated epithelial hyperplasia and lack stromal infiltration, unlike dermatofibrosarcoma protuberans, which usually has epithelial thinning and is characterized by infiltrative growth[22,208] (see Dermatofibrosarcoma).

Miscellaneous Tumors

Aggressive Angiomyxoma. Aggressive angiomyxomas may occur in the vulva, usually as large, gelatinous masses with superficial infiltration. These tumors typically occur in women under 40 years of age. Microscopic features include a prominent myxoid stroma with prominent vessels and associated collagen. Glandular elements may be seen (see Table 3.3). Local recurrence without metastasis has been reported. Wide local excision is adequate therapy.[208,313]

Lipoma. Lipomas arising from the vulvar fat pads appear as soft, lobulated growths generally attached to the labia majora by broad-based pedicles. Lipomas of the vulva at birth have been reported.[111] Histologically, mature fat cells are seen, often interspersed with strands of fibrous connective tissue. When the fibrotic element is prominent, the tumor should be called a *fibrolipoma.*[180]

Lymphoid Hamartoma. A benign lymphoid hamartoma has been described in the subcutaneous tissue of the labia majora as a symptomatic subcutaneous cystic mass.[183] The histologic features include lymphoid tissue within an apparent fibrous capsule in the subcutaneous tissue. Unlike a lymph node, no adjacent lymphoid sinusoids are seen. A whorled appearance to the epithelioid-like lymphoid element within the mass resembles Hassel's capsules. Chronic anemia with associated hypergammaglobulinemia has been reported with benign lymphoid hamartoma occurring in other sites but not within the female genital tract. Removal of the mass results in resolution of the laboratory findings and a benign clinical course.

Epithelial Tumors

Ectopic Tissue

Breast. Because the milk line extends into the vulva, the occurrence of breast tissue in this location is not strictly ectopic but rather accessory. The amount and character of breast tissue reported within the labia majora varies from small, isolated nodules of mammary duct epithelium to large, bilateral structures that have been observed to lactate during the puerperium. Clinically, ectopic breast tissue in the vulva usually is an amorphous enlargement of the labia, first noted in association with pregnancy.[115] Confusion with a periclitoral abscess may occur.[282] Histologically, accessory breast tissue is identical with that of mammary structures elsewhere. Adenocarcinoma of the accessory breast tissue of the vulva has been reported.[48] The complete removal of symptomatic ectopic breast tissue is advocated except when such tissue is discovered during pregnancy, in which case excision should be deferred until after puerperal regression is complete.

Salivary Gland. Ectopic salivary gland tissue has been observed in the vulva.[219]

Endometriosis. Vulvar endometriomas represent tumors caused by truly ectopic epithelium (see Chapter 17, Endometriosis). Decidua implanted in an episiotomy incision at the time of delivery and menstrual blood implanting in a small area of trauma have been implicated in the etiology of this condition. The clinical appearance is variable, ranging from bluish red cystic masses to amorphous, deep-seated nodules. Endometriomas of the vulva are usually located near the posterior fourchette. Cyclic enlargement and regression often are noted. Histologically, both endometrial glands and stroma are present, with a fibrotic response. A foreign body giant cell reaction and hemosiderin-laden macrophages may be noted in patients in whom the onset was preceded by recent surgery.

Acrochordon

The acrochordon, also known as a *fibroepithelial polyp* or *skin tag*, is a common benign tumor of the vulva, having both connective tissue and epithelial elements. These tumors vary in their clinical appearance from small, flesh-colored or hyperpigmented, papillomatous growths resembling condylomata to large, pedunculated tumors that are often hypopigmented on their apical surface. Small tumors may resemble nevi, and the larger lesions may present cosmetic problems; generally these tumors are clinically insignificant. Their origin is most probably from a regressing nevus.[263] On cut section, such tumors are soft and fleshy. Histologically, their epithelial surface varies from a thickened layer with papillomatosis, hyperkeratosis, and acanthosis to an attenuated, flattened layer exhibiting multiple primary folds. The connective tissue stalk is composed of loose bundles of collagen with moderate numbers of blood vessels.

Papillary Hidradenoma

Papillary hidradenoma of the vulva usually is a small tumor less than 2 cm in size. The lesion generally arises from the labia majora, interlabial sulci, or lateral surface of the labia minora. These tumors are usually asymptomatic. However, extrusion of the pulpy mass of adenomatous tissue through the center of the dome-shaped lesion or ulceration of the overlying surface may produce bleeding. Papillary hidradenomas have not been described before puberty, and almost all cases have occurred in Caucasian women.

Histologically, under low-power examination, an adenomatous pattern is seen, highly suggestive of adenocarcinoma (Fig. 3.33). Stromal compression often results in the formation of a pseudocapsule, although the epithelial cells may show infiltration into the surrounding connective tissue. An inflammatory reaction is unusual unless there is secondary infection. The tumor is composed of numerous tubules and acini lined with a single or double layer of cuboidal cells (Fig. 3.34). At times, the cells lining the lumen of the adenomatous structures are large and pale, exhibiting the morphologic and stain-

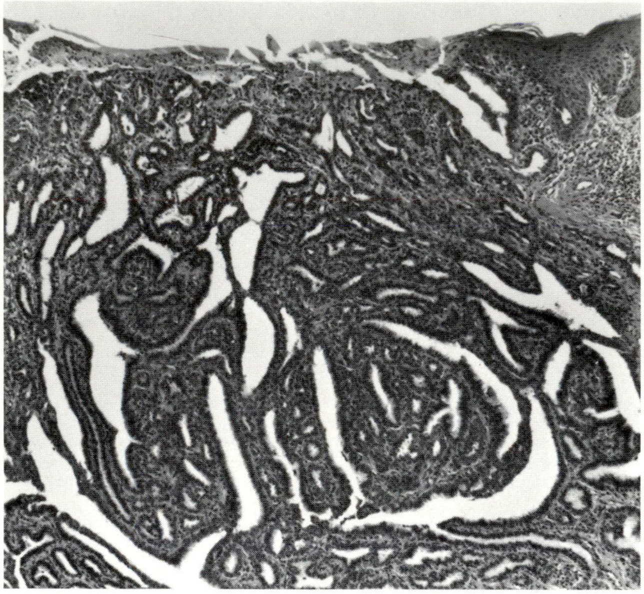

FIG. 3.33. Hidradenoma. Low-power pattern of this adenomatous tumor ulcerating through skin surface resembles adenocarcinoma.

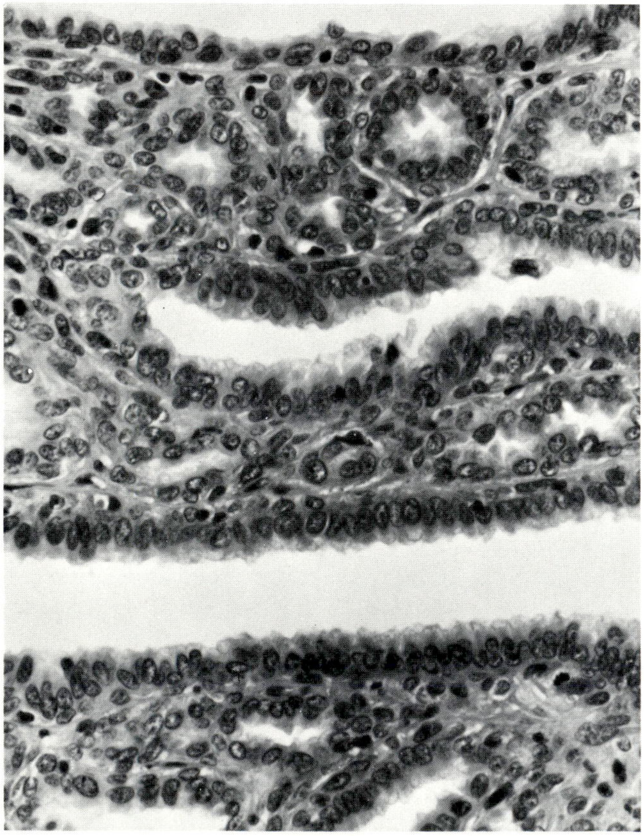

FIG. 3.34. Hidradenoma. High-power examination shows tubules and acini lined with a single or double layer of cuboidal to columnar cells.

ing characteristics of apocrine sweat gland secretory cells. When a double layer of cells is present, the outermost layer is thought to represent the myoepithelial cells, often demonstrable in apocrine gland structures.[363] Most authorities maintain that the tumor is of sweat gland origin, but the hidradenoma does not contain carcinoembryonic antigen as do sweat gland tumors.[235] Why these tumors have not been described in other areas of the body, equally rich in apocrine glands, is unknown.

Clinically, the hidradenoma is benign, but because of the complex glandular architecture, it can be misinterpreted as an adenocarcinoma. Careful high-power microscopy will show the two layers of cells covering the papillary structures, the outer myoepithelial cells, and the inner secretory cells. Mitotic figures are rare, and only mild degrees of cellular and nuclear pleomorphism are present. At the base of the mass, a well-defined junction between epithelium and stroma can be found, without evidence of infiltration. Local excision, including the base of the mass, is sufficient therapy.

Clear Cell Hidradenoma

The clear cell hidradenoma is not a variant of the papillary hidradenoma but rather represents a distinctive and unusual tumor of the epidermal adnexa, most often found on the face, scalp, thoracic wall, and abdomen. Isolated examples of this tumor have been found on the vulva; we have observed a single case in our own clinic. This tumor is believed to derive from the epithelial matrices in eccrine sweat gland primordia. Wide local excision is considered adequate therapy.[184]

Histologically, the clear cell hidradenoma is largely solid and does not resemble the papillary hidradenoma. Lobules or segments of large clear cells are divided by strands of reticular connective tissue. The characteristic cell is large and polygonal, and the cytoplasm appears transparent. The relatively small nucleus is round to oval and may exhibit an irregular outline. The chromatin is frequently clumped, and a single nucleolus is often seen. It is unusual to see mitotic figures (Fig. 3.35).

Syringoma and Mixed Tumor

The syringoma is assumed to be an adenoma of the eccrine ducts. These lesions occur on the vulva, as well as on the eyelids, cheeks, axillae, and abdomen. Clinically, multiple flesh-colored papules are noted within the deeper skin layers of the labia majora bilaterally. These are often asymptomatic, although pruritus may occur.[41,153,369]

Histologically, the tumor lacks a clearly defined border. Within the dermis, numerous small dilated duct spaces are seen. These spaces are usually lined by two rows of epithelial cells that appear flat secondary to pressure atrophy. The comma-like formation of these glandu-

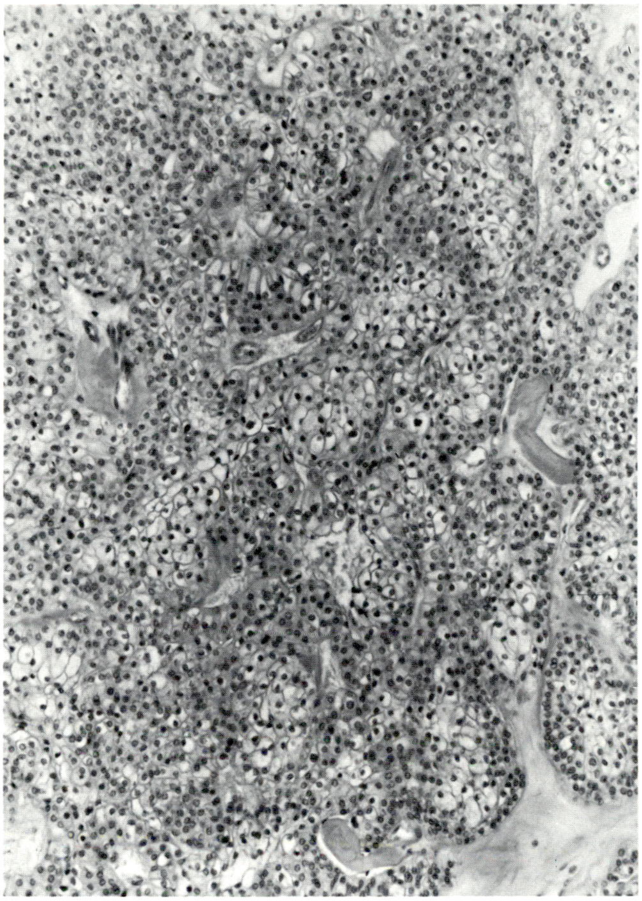

FIG. 3.35. Clear cell hidradenoma. The sheets of large clear cells are broken by occasional collagen bands and blood vessels.

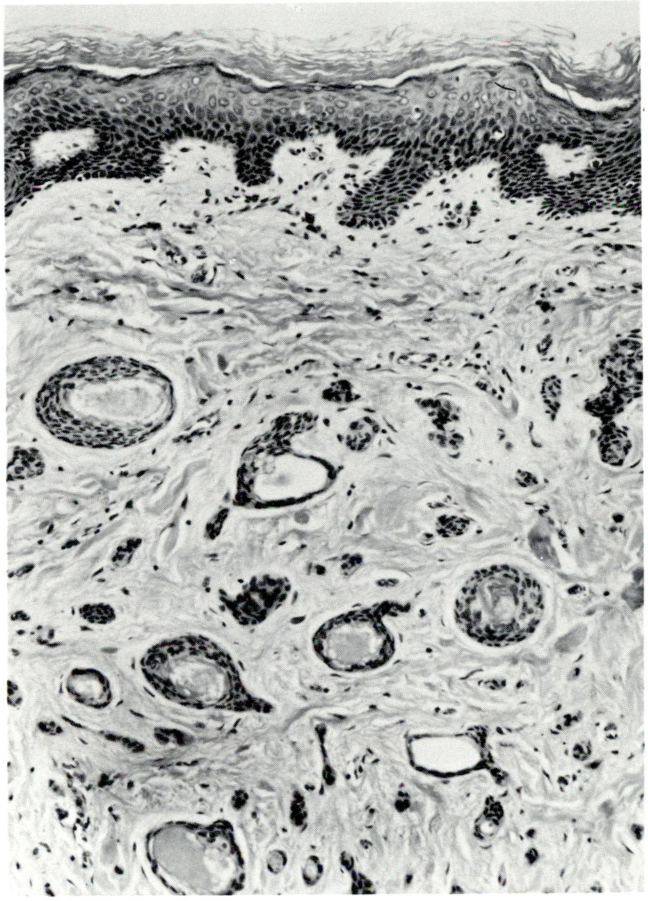

FIG. 3.36. Syringoma. The comma pattern of the eccrine structures is easily appreciated.

lar spaces is characteristic (Fig. 3.36). Although an apocrine origin has been suggested, histochemical and electron microscopic studies have established the syringoma as an eccrine derivative.

Mixed adnexoid tumors have been described on the vulva in which a mixture of syringomatous and pilosebaceous elements were noted.[126]

Mixed tumor of the vulva (pleomorphic adenoma) is a rare neoplasm that usually appears as a solid, subcutaneous tumor involving the labia majora or the Bartholin's gland area. The histopathologic findings are essentially those of the mixed tumors of the parotid and other salivary glands. The tumors consist of epithelial components, usually tubules or nests, mixed with a fibrous stroma with chondromatous, osseous, and myxoid elements. These stroma-like elements are believed to arise from the pluripotential myoepithelial cells, which, in the vulva, are found in the Bartholin's glands, sweat glands, and potentially in ectopic breast tissue.[290] Although these tumors are considered benign, variants of the tumor with local recurrence as well as metastasis may occur.[253]

When metastasis occurs from a malignant mixed tumor, it is usually composed of epithelial elements only. There are at present insufficient cases of vulvar mixed tumors to determine the natural history of this tumor in this site. Wide local excision, with free margins, is the recommended therapy for both primary tumors and local recurrences.

Squamous Papilloma

Benign tumors arising directly from the squamous epithelium of the vulva include the squamous papilloma, keratoacanthoma, and seborrheic keratosis. Squamous papillomas may be thought of as variants of common skin tags in which the epithelial element predominates. Histologically, papillomatosis, acanthosis, and varying degrees of hyperkeratosis are seen. Papillomas are usually single, and no viral etiology is suspected. They should be distinguished from condyloma acuminatum.

Keratoacanthoma

Keratoacanthomas are rapidly growing, self-limited proliferations of the squamous epithelium in which horny masses of keratin are pushed upward while tongues of squamous epithelium invade the dermis. These tumors may occur on any hairy cutaneous site[206] and have been reported on the vulva.[284]

Seborrheic Keratosis

Seborrheic keratoses are extremely common, raised lesions with irregular borders that may occur almost anywhere on the skin. Their color varies from pale brown to brownish-black, and they appear to be stuck onto the skin surface. Although clinically insignificant, their appearance often mimics that of a nevus or melanoma, and when present on the vulva, these tumors are often excised for diagnosis. Multiple seborrheic keratoses occurring over a short period of time may be associated with internal malignancy (Leser-Trelat syndrome).[280]

Histologically, hyperkeratosis, acanthosis, and papillomatosis are seen. On low-power examination, the entire keratosis appears to be above a straight line drawn from the normal epidermis at one side of the keratosis to the normal epidermis at the other side. Both mature squamous cells and basal type cells are noted in strands and cords surrounding numerous horny keratin cysts. Varying degrees of hyperpigmentation may be present (Fig. 3.37).

Vulvar Intraepithelial Neoplasia

(Dysplasia and Carcinoma In Situ)

Current terminology for VIN, as accepted by the International Society for the Study of Vulvar Disease (ISSVD), is listed in Table 3.4.[152] Typically, the lesions of VIN have a raised surface, and about two-thirds of them retain 1% toluidine blue when this dye is applied as a vital stain decolorized with 1% acetic acid. In the presence of an intact epithelium, retention of toluidine blue-O indicates parakeratosis.[51] One-third of patients have lesions that are hyperpigmented. Carcinoma in situ is, in fact, the second most common cause of vulvar dark lesions. The remainder may be pink, white, gray, or

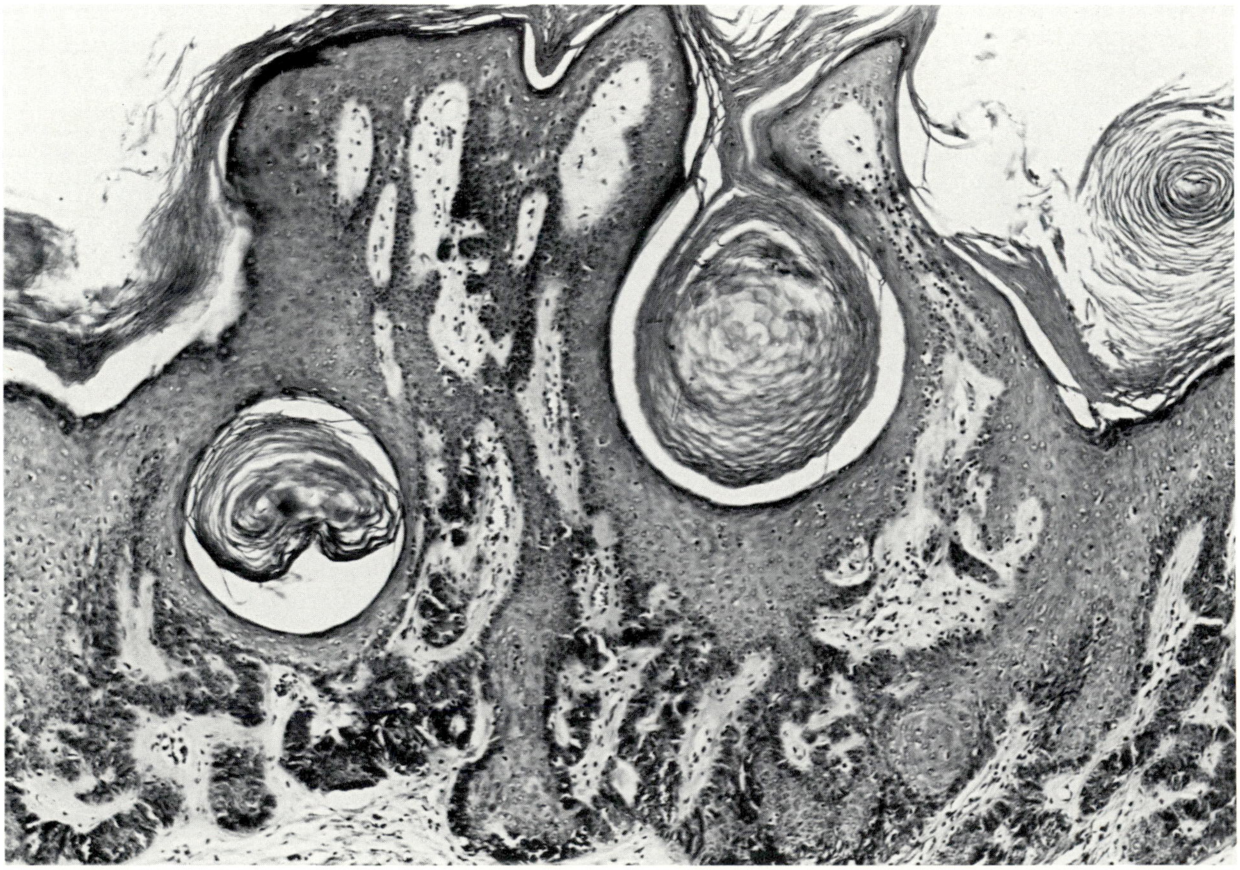

FIG. 3.37. Pigmented seborrheic keratosis. When pigmented, these lesions may mimic VIN or melanoma on the vulva. Note that the diameter of the lesion is substantially greater than its thickness. The melanocytic hyperplasia and hyperpigmentation is present primarily in the basal layers. Keratin pearls are present.

TABLE 3.4. International Society for the Study of Vulvar Disease classification of intraepithelial neoplasia.

Prior terminology 1976–1983	Present terminology 1985	
Mild atypia	VIN I	Mild dysplasia
Moderate atypia	VIN II	Moderate Dysplasia
Severe atypia	VIN III	Severe dysplasia
Carcinoma in situ	VIN III	Carcinoma in situ
Paget's disease	Paget's disease	

VIN, vulvar intraepithelial neoplasia.

red in color. The lesions may be macular (Fig. 3.38, Plate 1) or papular (Fig. 3.39, Plate 2), and they may be single or multiple. Confluent growth may be seen with plaques (Fig. 3.40, Plate 2), forming a diffuse pattern (Fig. 3.41, Plate 2).[108,275,351] Most patients are asymptomatic, although many complain of pruritus. The anal skin and squamous mucosa of the anal canal are the most frequently involved secondary sites.[62,108] Cytologic scraping from the surface of the lesion may be useful.[240]

The epidermal keratinocyte usually betrays the presence of an abnormal genome by a disturbance in the maturation process. The cell may retain the juvenile characteristics of mitotic capability, high nuclear/cytoplasmic ratio, and relative cytoplasmic basophilia as it progresses into the upper layers of the epithelium (Fig. 3.42). The cells may show evidence of altered maturation with nuclear pyknosis surrounded by keratinization of the individual cell cytoplasm while that cell is still well beneath the granular zone, or the formation of intraepithelial pearls within the acanthotic rete ridges may occur (Figs. 3.43 and 3.44). Multinucleation is indicative of the inability of cells to complete their cytoplasmic separation after nuclear reduplication has taken place. Atypical mitoses attest to a defect in the mitotic process. Radial dispersion of nuclear chromatin and coarse clumping of the chromatin are further suggestions of DNA abnormalities. Parakeratosis is seen when keratinocytes fail to form granules of prekeratin and retain basophilic nuclear material at the epithelial surface. When establishing the degree of change, one should consider the quality

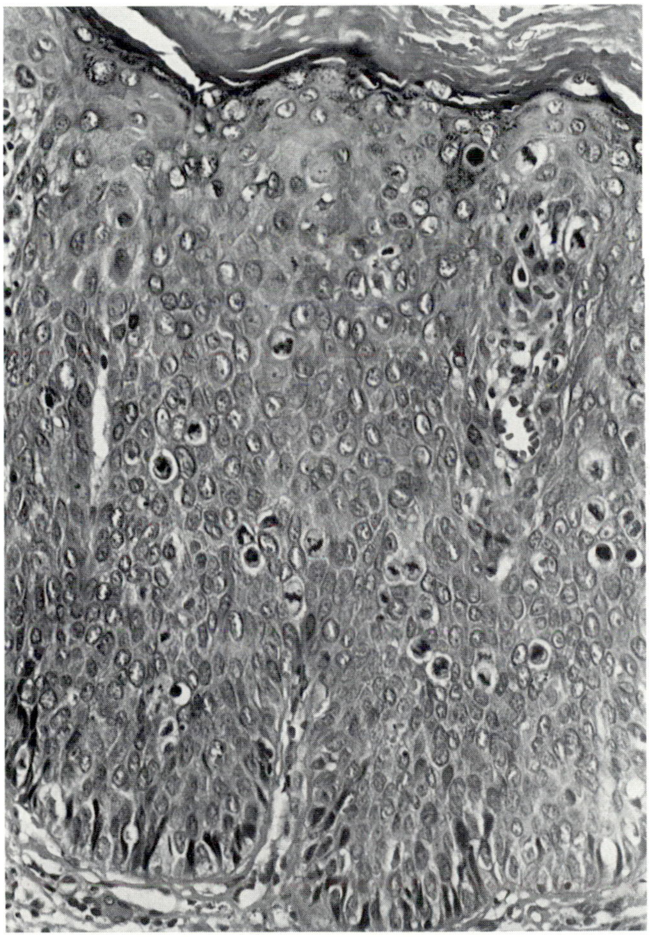

FIG. 3.42. Vulvar intraepithelial neoplasia (VIN II), moderate dysplasia. Hyperchromatic, pleomorphic cells are present in the lower two thirds of the epithelium that are crowded, vertically orientated, and show lack of maturation except near the surface. Many mitotic figures are present, some of which are abnormal. There is a hyperkeratotic surface.

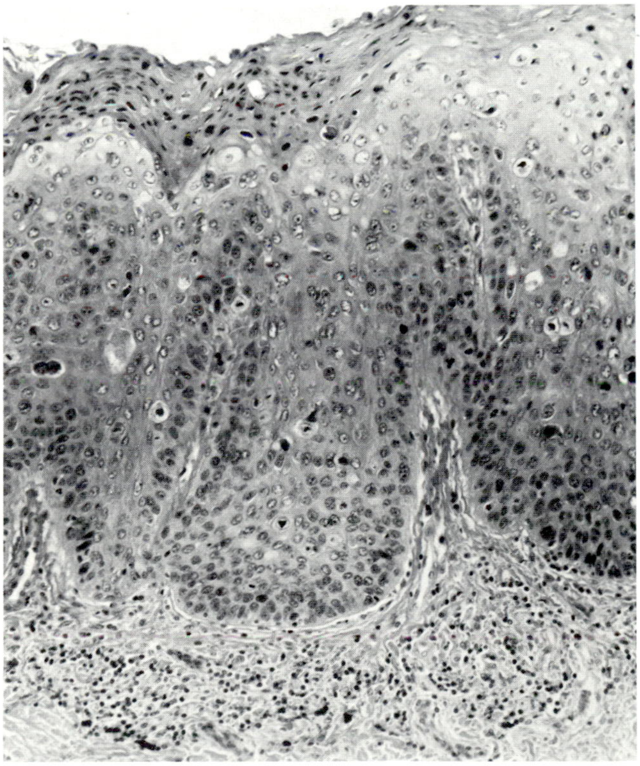

FIG. 3.43. Vulvar intraepithelial neoplasia (VIN III), carcinoma in situ. An area with parakeratosis, giant cells, dyskeratotic cells, and multinucleation.

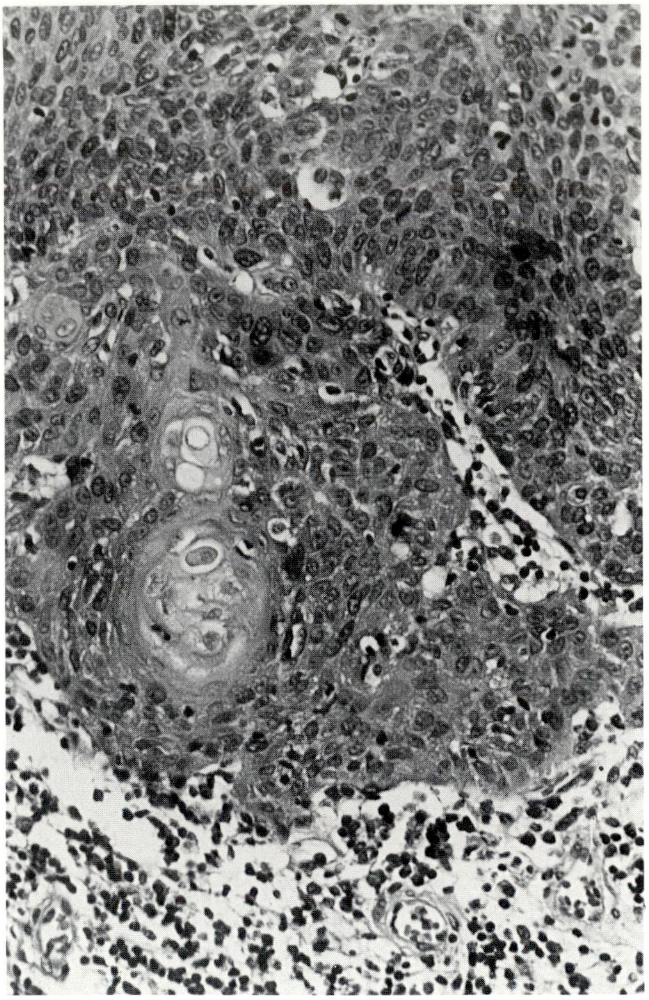

FIG. 3.44. Vulvar intraepithelial neoplasia (VIN III) with prominent eosinophilic cytoplasm and nuclear chromatin clearing noted in the cells near the basal layer with superficially invasive carcinoma; depth of invasion 1.2 mm.

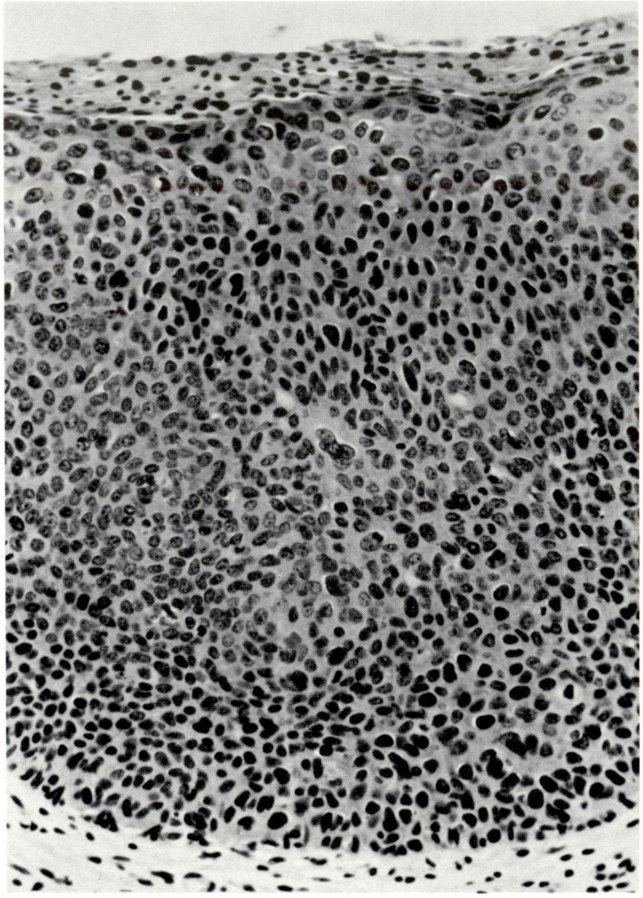

FIG. 3.45. Vulvar intraepithelial neoplasia, VIN III (carcinoma in situ.) Complete replacement of the epithelium with overlying parakeratosis resembling carcinoma in situ of the cervix. Note large multinucleated cell in the center.

and quantity of the individual cellular atypicalities along with the relative density of the cell population and overall architecture of the epithelium.

When such changes are few in number and confined to the lower third of the epithelium, VIN I (mild dysplasia) may be reported. This is a rare diagnosis. VIN II (moderate dysplasia) is recognized if such changes extend through approximately one-half to two-thirds of the epithelium, and individually keratinized cells and mitoses within this lower two-thirds of the epithelium may be seen (see Fig. 3.42). When cellular atypia involves more than two-thirds of the full thickness of the epithelium, disregarding the keratin layer, the diagnosis should be VIN III (severe dysplasia) or VIN III (carcinoma in situ) if the change is essentially full-thickness but does not necessarily include the surface layers above the granular zone (Figs. 3.43 and 3.45). Both intracellular and extracellular pigment granules may be seen distributed throughout the epidermis. Dermal melanophages are often prominent beneath the basal layer and within the dermal papillae. Squamous cell abnormalities are also found within the skin appendages in more than 50% of the cases studied.[225] Skin appendage involvement by VIN should not be confused with early invasion (Fig. 3.46).

Abnormal mitoses are nearly always present in VIN I, II, and III lesions and may be seen in all but the most superficial layers of the epithelium. Lack of abnormal mitoses should raise the question of whether or not a lesion belongs in the VIN category. A spectrum of epithelial changes may be seen extending from VIN I to VIN III, with variable degrees of hyperkeratosis. The subclassification of VIN may be somewhat arbitrary, and, in some cases, a diagnosis of VIN, not otherwise specified, may be sufficient. Nuclear size within VIN

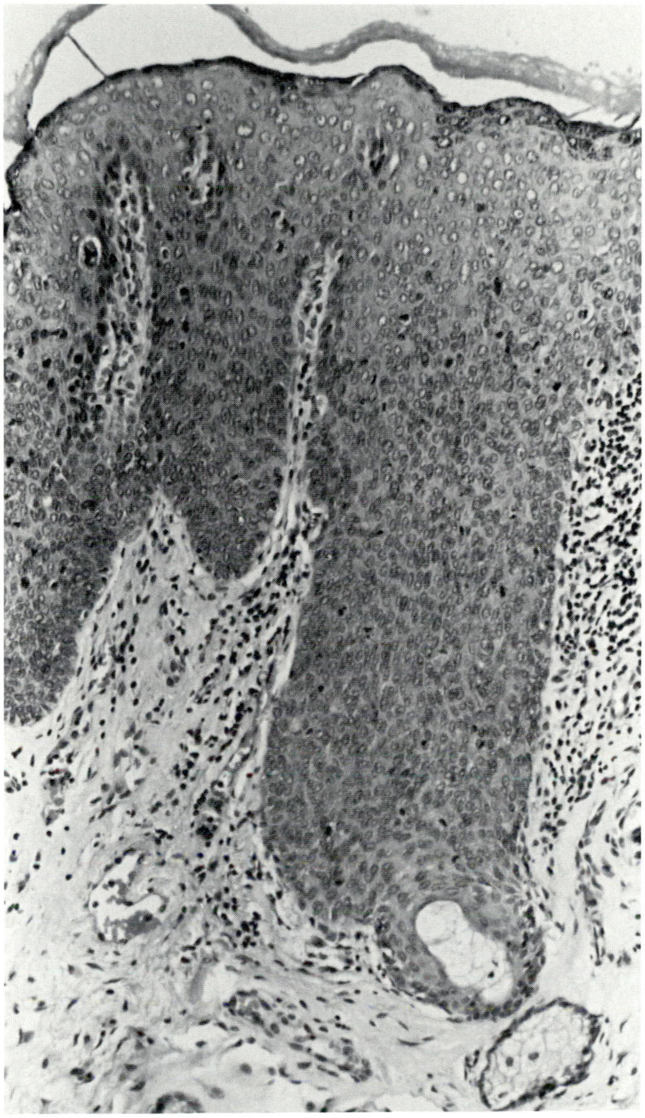

FIG. 3.46. Vulvar intraepithelial neoplasia (VIN III), severe dysplasia involving a skin appendage. Cellular disarray with lack of maturation is seen within the epithelium. The residua of a sebaceous gland element is seen at the base of the lesion.

may be large and pleomorphic (see Fig. 3.43) or relatively small and more uniform (see Fig. 3.45). Although such nuclear variations are striking, both are aneuploid populations of cells, that is, they contain a DNA content other than (23 × 2) or multiples of 23, i.e., 46, 69, 92, and so on. Aneuploidy is a characteristic of malignant neoplasia, although not all malignant neoplasias are aneuploid. The larger cells, being found in VIN lesions that have a higher cellular DNA content, are often aneuploid in the peritriploid (peritetraploid) range, whereas smaller cell lesions tend to be aneuploid in the peridiploid range.[108,351]

The coarse nuclear chromatin seen in the epithelial cells corresponds to an increased number of interchromatinic and perichromatinic granules that are sometimes clustered in globular structures.[176] The so-called individual cell keratinization seen within the epithelium is attributed to the presence of aggregated tonofilaments that may be produced in the process of abnormal cell division.[304] On rare occasions, cells particularly near the basal layer may show prominent eosinophilic cytoplasm with nuclear chromatin clearing, often with prominent nucleoli (see Fig. 3.44). This cellular change may be referred to as a *differentiated type* and has been referred to in the past as a carcinoma in situ of *simplex type,* a term rarely used.[2,32] This cellular change is commonly seen in invasive vulvar carcinoma.

In most cases, the lesions of VIN are multifocal. DNA analysis by microspectrophotometry suggests that separate lesions have arisen from separate stem cells, forming distinguishable clones. Large, spreading lesions may result from centrifugal growth from a single cell line or by confluence of separate and distinct clones.[351] With the same technique, it has been shown that most lesions are aneuploid.[60,108] Approximately half of single VIN lesions have been shown to have different stem cells by DNA microspectrophotometry, suggesting that such lesions may undergo clonal evolution.[351] A viral etiology now seems evident in a large number of cases. Herpes virus Type II nonstructural antigens have been identified in some specimens. Evidence for HPV in VIN and invasive carcinoma is based on immunohistochemistry demonstrating viral structural proteins and DNA hybridization studies that demonstrate the presence of HPV-DNA sequences.[124,148]

A number of studies* that have identified the common clinical features of this disease suggest that it is becoming more frequent in young women 20–35 years of age. Approximately 50% of these women will have other neoplasia involving the genital tract, most often carcinoma in situ or dysplasia (CIN) of the cervix.[31,362] Approximately one-half will exhibit a history of preexisting or concomitant sexually transmitted disease, of which condylomata acuminata is the most frequent.[36,108,140] Progression to invasive carcinoma is rare, occurring in approximately 6% of all reported series. Invasion, if present, usually occurs in postmenopausal women.[11,34,58,108,172,275] An equal number of women (6%) can be expected to show spontaneous regression, which appears to be most common in young women and in those who are pregnant.[97] Women of advanced age, as well as those who are severely immunosuppressed, are at greater risk for invasion.[42,352] Significantly lowered lymphocyte transformation re-

* References 9, 17, 38, 58, 108, 163, 181, 275.

sponses have been reported in unselected women with carcinoma in situ of the vulva as compared to control subjects.[305]

The differential diagnosis of VIN includes condyloma acuminatum, malignant melanoma, and Paget's disease. Immunoperoxidase methods to assist in distinguishing these are summarized in Table 3.5. Conservative therapy is now recommended, and most patients are managed with wide local excision, although laser ablation or shallow vulvectomy may also be appropriate for selected patients.[101,169,179,283;356] It is recognized that approximately 90% of VIN lesions will have evidence of HPV by DNA studies. Until more is understood about the relationship of viral disease to VIN, the diagnosis and therapy for VIN should not be influenced by the presence of condyloma acuminatum.

Lesions of the vulva that are distinctly papular or verrucoid have been clinically termed *bowenoid papulosis* by some authors, but they are histologically indistinguishable from other forms of intraepithelial neoplasia and behave in a similar fashion.[338,339] The separate term *bowenoid papulosis* is therefore not recognized by the ISSVD.

Paget's Disease

Paget's disease of the skin is a curious phenomenon generally confined to the integument along the milk line. It occurs most commonly on the nipple and areola, where its presence signifies an underlying adenocarcinoma of the breast. Extramammary lesions have been described in the genital, perianal, and axillary regions, as well as the ear canal, all of which contain abundant apocrine glands.

Clinically, vulvar Paget's disease appears as a red velvety area with white islands of hyperkeratosis and at times may be pinkish and eczematoid (Fig. 3.47, Plate 2). Pruritus is present in over half of the patients, and almost all are postmenopausal Caucasian women.[15,26] A single case of vulvar Paget's disease has been reported in a 24-year-old black woman.[312]

Paget cells often occur in nests surrounded by small hyperchromatic basaloid cells, considered to be Paget precursors by some investigators.[134,258] The individual cells within such a nest may surround a central clear area, giving an acinar appearance to the structure. Isolated Paget cells may file upward in the epithelium (pagetoid spread), where they are surrounded by squamous keratinocytes and are distinguished by an absence of intercellular bridges (Fig. 3.48). Hair shafts and sweat gland structures, deep in the dermis, may also contain Paget cells. Even in these locations, they must be considered intraepithelial as long as they are bordered by the basement membrane.

The typical Paget cell is large and round or oval. The cytoplasm is pale and occasionally vacuolated. The nuclei are variable in character; most are vesicular with finely

TABLE 3.5. The use of immunoperoxidase techniques in differentiating some vulvar diseases.

	Condyloma	VIN	Paget's disease	Melanoma
Human papilloma (HPV) antigen	+[a]	0/+[b]	0	0
Carcinoembryonic antigen (CEA)	0	0	+	0
S100 protein	0	0	0	+

+, immunoreactive.
0, negative.
[a] Detected in approximately 50% of cases.
[b] Detected in up to 10% of cases.

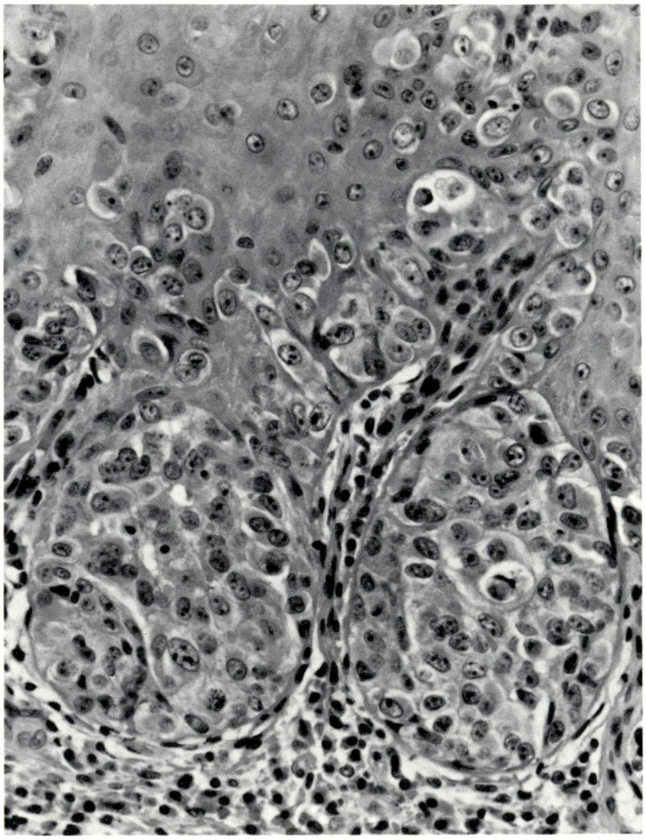

FIG. 3.48. Paget's disease. Paget cells are present singly and in nests. Their pale cytoplasm easily differentiates them from surrounding keratinocytes.

distributed chromatin, but others are more hyperchromatic and may be indented. The nucleoli are prominent but not markedly enlarged, and mitotic figures are infrequent. The cytoplasm of Paget cells contains neutral and acid mucopolysaccharides that account for their characteristic staining reactions: PAS-positive (diastase resistant), mucicarmine-positive, aldehydefuchsin-positive, and Alcian blue-positive.[134] The cells stain pink against a background of greenish blue with Movat stain. In addition, Paget cells, as well as the cells and secretions of normal eccrine and apocrine glands, are rich in carcinoembryonic antigen (CEA) demonstrable by immunoperoxidase methods.[237] These reactions distinguish Paget cells from the large pale cells sometimes seen in bowenoid types of carcinoma in situ or in superficial amelanotic melanomas (see Table 3.5). The 3,4-dihydroxyphenylalanine (dopa) reaction on fresh tissue has been studied and found to be negative in Paget's disease.[360] This indicates an inability of the cell to produce melanin and again distinguishes it from a melanoma cell. Paget cells, however, may contain granules of melanin, demonstrable with Fontana-Masson stain, but these are probably produced by neighboring melanocytes and are only secondarily engulfed by the Paget cell.

Extensive work on the ultrastructure of the Paget's cell has generally revealed features consistent with adenocarcinoma.[228,294] Some Paget cells contain the organelles associated with apocrine cells,[242] whereas others resemble eccrine cells,[87] and still others resemble squamous keratinocytes.[89,315] In some instances, more than one type of cell has been identified in the same patient. These findings are all consistent with the concept that the Paget cell represents an aberrant differentiation from a multipotent cell derived from the embryonic stratum germinativum of the epidermis. Primitive stem cells destined to form basal keratinocytes may differentiate into Paget cells with some of the ultrastructural characteristics of keratinocytes. Those stem cells that differentiate into apocrine anlage may form Paget cells with apocrine organelles, and so forth. Such an interpretation accounts for the observation that Paget cells are often first noted just above the basal layer of the epithelium and that they may be located within any of the skin adnexae.

The finding of Paget like cells in foci of metastatic tumors of either squamous or adenomatous origin may then indicate that the malignant tumor cell is still capable of aberrant differentiation into a Paget cell. Dermal invasion by previous intraepithelial Paget cells has been documented.[131,258] Vulvar Paget's disease is, therefore, properly classified as a form of intraepithelial neoplasia that may become invasive. Usually, it is a slowly progressive, indolent, superficial process. Not all involved areas are visibly altered on physical examination. In a careful topographic study, Gunn and Gallager (1980) demonstrated that the outline of the histologically involved area was highly irregular and of much greater extent than the visible lesion.[127] In addition, multicentric foci, some occurring in grossly normal appearing skin, were noted. These facts easily acccount for the frequent recurrences of disease despite seemingly adequate excision.

Of importance is the frequency with which epidermal changes are associated with separate invasive carcinomas. Early investigators noted underlying adnexal adenocarcinoma beneath the skin in the vicinity of the Paget's disease in many extramammary cases.[134] This led some to conclude that Paget cells in the epidermis represented an intradermal migration of neoplastic cells from an underlying tumor, as occurs in the breast. However, it now seems clear that Paget cells in extramammary sites arise de novo in the epidermis or epidermally derived adnexal structures, where their presence may or may not be associated with a separate and often subjacent independent carcinoma (Fig. 3.49).

Friedrich et al. found that 14% of reported cases of vulvar Paget's disease were associated with a carcinoma of the breast.[109] Urinary tract malignancy has been found with genital Paget's disease.[273] Patients with associated adenocarcinoma of the Bartholin's gland and squamous cell carcinoma of the vulva have also been reported.[359] Perianal involvement by Paget's disease is associated with a high incidence of adenocarcinoma of the rectum.[134] The treatment and prognosis of Paget's disease of the vulva, therefore, depend on whether an associated invasive carcinoma is present, and patients may be divided into two groups on this basis.[57,323] Consequently, it is incumbent on the pathologist to make a diligent search through all submitted tissue to identify or rule out an invasive carcinoma.

Invasive Carcinoma

Squamous Carcinoma

Vulvar squamous carcinoma has an incidence of approximately 1.5/100,000 women in the United States, which increases with advancing age.[136,373] An association has been reported with chronic granulomatous disease[133] (especially granuloma inguinale), exposure to carcinogens including cigarette smoking,[214,243,342] and suppressed immunocompetence.[42,352] Diabetes mellitus[243] and achlorhydria[343] have been associated with a slightly increased risk of vulvar carcinoma, and poor perineal hygiene has also been implicated. There is a recognized association between cervical and vaginal carcinomas and vulvar carcinomas.[31,168,214,375]

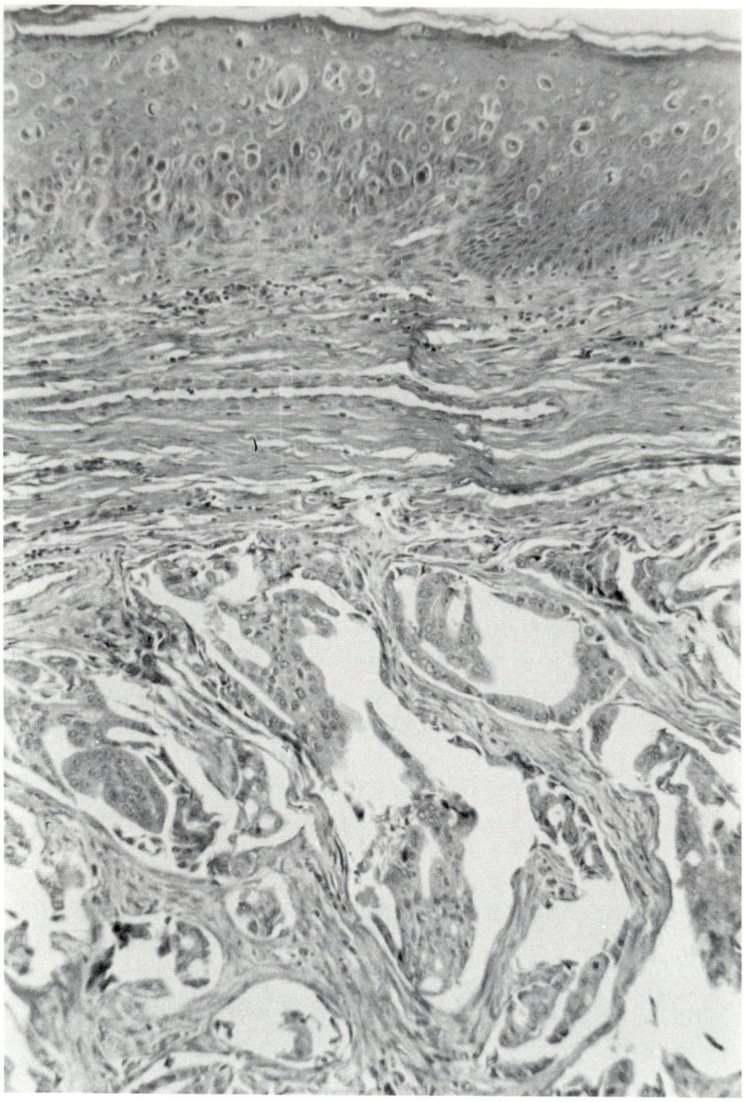

FIG. 3.49. Paget's disease of the vulva with underlying adeno carcinoma, an infrequent finding.

Vulvar squamous carcinoma may occur as an exophytic or papillomatous mass or an endophytic ulcer. The tumor is usually located on the labia minora or majora, however, the clitoris is primarily involved in approximately 5–15% of cases.[94,129,196] The tumor is usually solitary (Fig. 3.50, Plate 2), with less than 10% of patients having multifocal tumors (Figs. 3.51 and 3.52).[373] The clinical staging of vulvar carcinoma is summarized in Table 3.6.[92,195,196]

Vulvar carcinomas of squamous origin may be of several histologic types, including squamous cell,[271] giant cell,[343] spindle cell,[52,314] adenoid squamous,[203,331] verrucous,* basal cell,[1,27] adenoid basal cell,[1,266] and basosquamous (metatypical basal cell) carcinoma.[27,280] Histologically, invasive squamous cell carcinomas are usually well-differentiated tumors, but poorly differentiated varieties are found in 5–10% of patients (Figs. 3.53, 3.54, and 3.55).[157,216,271,342] Some investigators have noted an increased risk of node involvement with poorly differentiated tumors.[147,174] In Way's series,[342] 35% of differentiated tumors had positive nodes, whereas 62% of poorly differentiated tumors showed these metastases. Most authors, however, have not found any significant differences in node metastasis among different grades in superficially invasive tumors.[81,141,142,216,301] This may be because approximately 90% of squamous tumors are well differentiated or moderately well differentiated, a distinction that may be somewhat arbitrary. Poorly differentiated tumors are recognizable by the absence of keratin formation. Giant cell carcinoma of the vulva is a variant of squamous cell carcinoma characterized by multinucleated tumor giant cells, large nuclei with prominent nucleoli, and prominent eosinophilic cytoplasm (Fig. 3.56). This tumor

* References 11, 164, 192, 249, 260, 279, 316.

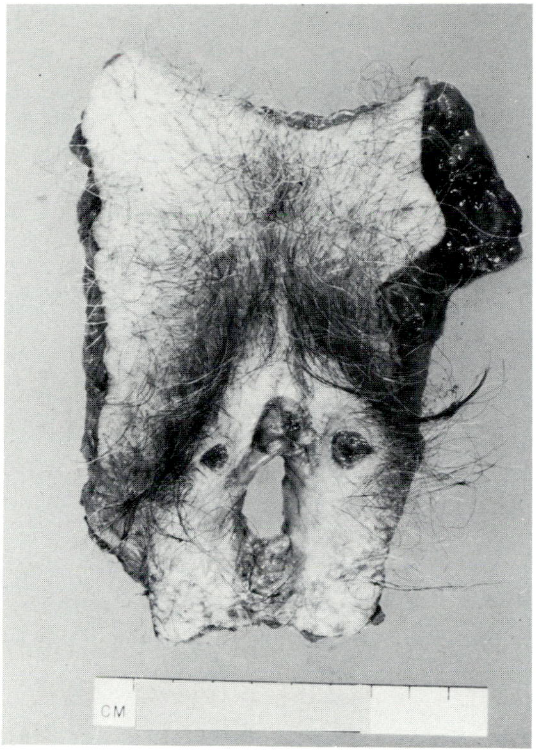

Fig. 3.51. Gross photograph of a total vulvectomy specimen with mirror-image squamous cell carcinomas on the medial aspects of the labia majora bilaterally.

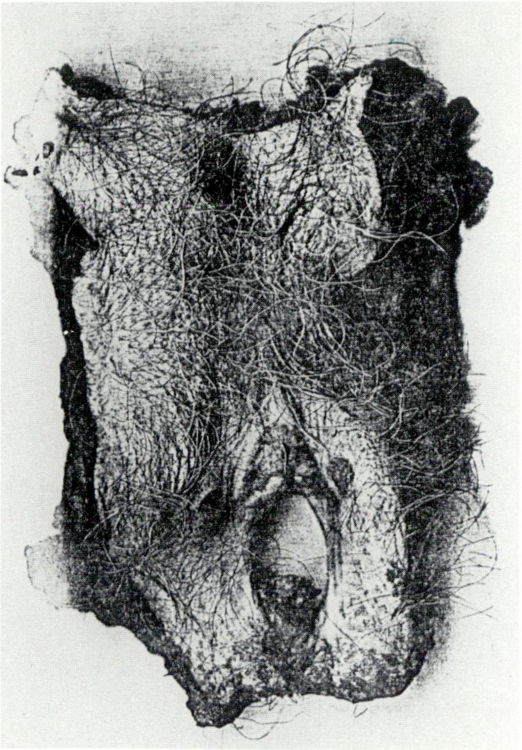

Fig. 3.52. A photocopy of the specimen in Figure 3.51 was made by placing the specimen, skin surface down, on a photocopy machine. Skin detail, with the bilateral tumors, is evident. This may be used in specimen preparation and may become part of the permanent record to document the source of a section.[127]

variant is relatively rare and is associated with a poor prognosis.[342,343]

More comprehensive grading methods incorporating keratinization, nuclear pleomorphism and hyperchromasia, mitotic rate, pattern of invasion, and inflammatory response remain to be tested.[373] The FIGO staging system makes no allowance for histologic grade. Nonetheless, it is clinically useful to differentiate those tumors that are well differentiated and moderately differentiated from those that are poorly differentiated since an increased risk of node involvement has been reported with poorly differentiated tumors.[147,174] Well-differentiated tumors show broad anastomosing masses of atypical squamous cells with prominent intercellular bridges and cytoplasmic inclusions of keratin (see Fig. 3.53). Whorls and nests of keratin (pearls) are almost constant features of the well-differentiated tumor. Nuclear pleomorphism and mitotic figures are not outstanding (see Fig. 3.54). In the poorly differentiated tumors, marked nuclear pleomorphism and low nuclear/cytoplasmic ratios are seen along with minimal or no keratin formation and numerous mitotic figures (see Fig. 3.55). Moderately well-differentiated tumors are of intermediate differentiation, showing some keratin formation. Spindle cell carcinoma of the vulva may mimic a sarcoma or be associated with sarcoma-like stroma,[52,314] however, malignant squamous cells are immunoreactive for keratin.[208,235,236]

Aberrant hormonal activity has been reported in some gynecologic tumors.[307,319] Gynecologic tumors were responsible for 20.5% of malignancy-associated hypercalcemia in one series.[319] After tumors of the ovary, those of the vulva are the second most common gynecologic tumor associated with hypercalcemia. Vulvar squamous

Table 3.6. Clinical staging of squamous carcinoma of the vulva.[a]

Stage	Description
I	Tumor confined to the vulva, 2 cm or less in diameter, without suspicious groin nodes
II	Tumor confined to the vulva, exceeding 2 cm in diameter, without suspicious groin nodes
III	Extension beyond the vulva, without suspicious groin nodes; or lesions of any size with suspicious groin nodes
IV	Grossly positive groin nodes, regardless of extent of primary; or evidence of other metastases

[a] Based on the International Federation of Obstetricians and Gynecologists (FIGO) classification.

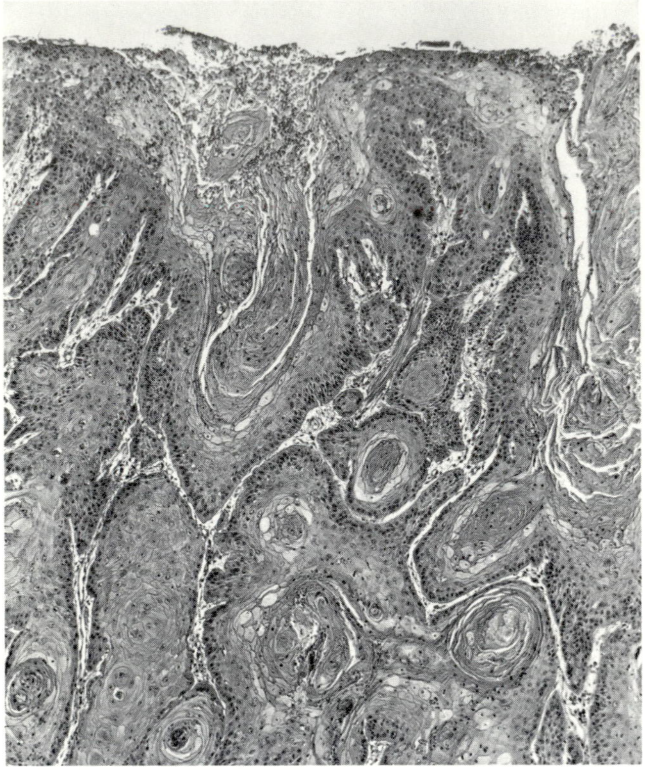

FIG. 3.53. Invasive well differentiated squamous carcinoma showing tongues and islands of keratin.

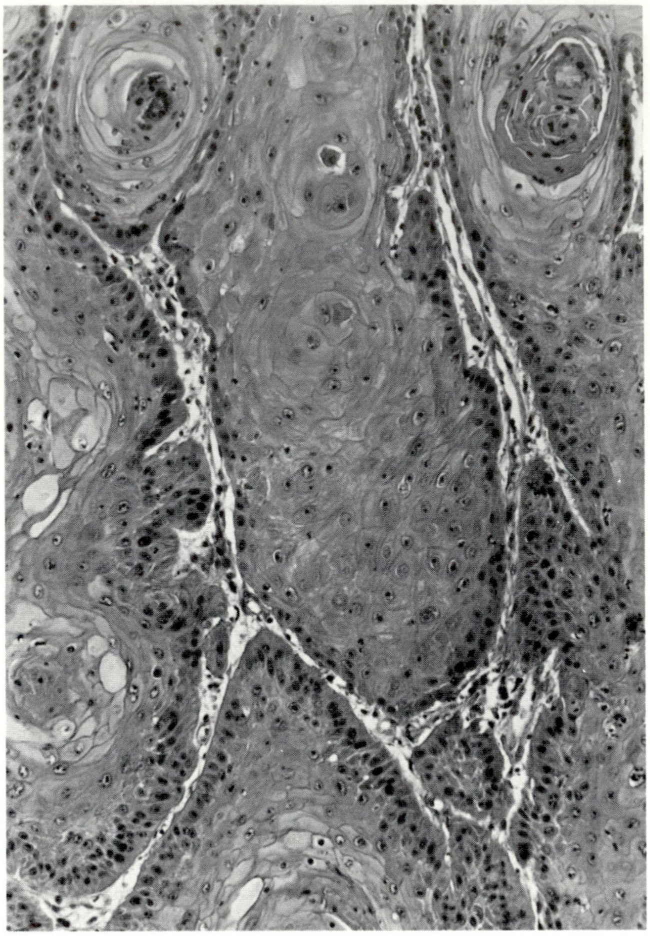

FIG. 3.54. Invasive squamous carcinoma, well differentiated. Tongues of disorganized squamous epithelium are seen and pearl formation is evident.

carcinomas, with associated hypercalcemia, are usually large, well differentiated, and without bony metastasis.[244] Surgical excision of the tumor results in the serum calcium levels returning to normal. The hypercalcemia results from a hormonal secretion by the tumor of a parathyroid hormone-like (PTH) substance. However, serum levels of parathyroid hormone area usually within normal limits in the patients, as are levels of 1,25-dehydroxyvitamin D and 29-hydroxyvitamin D.[319] Nevertheless, the hypercalcemia associated with a vulvar carcinoma that neither is metastatic nor involves bone may still be secondary to local production of PTH itself by the tumor. Parathyroid hormone has been demonstrated by immunoperoxidase techniques within carcinomas of the lung, bladder, and parotid gland associated with hypercalcemia even though the serum levels of PTH were reported within the normal range in these patients.[149]

Superficially Invasive Squamous Cell Carcinoma

Identification of a subset of superficially invasive vulvar squamous cell carcinomas that would not be at risk for metastasis to inguinal or regional lymph nodes has progressed through a series of definitions of microinvasion proposed by numerous investigators. Initial studies after studies on the cervix used 5 mm depth of invasion as the basis of separation.[93,346] Using this criterion, it has been found subsequently that 15.2% of these women will have inguinal lymph node metastasis (Fig. 3.57).* A 3 mm depth of invasion has been suggested, but this depth of invasion was found to be associated with inguinal lymph node metastasis in 12.1% of patients.† It is now becoming evident that to establish a depth of invasion that will not be associated with inguinal lymph node metastasis, the invasion cannot exceed 1 mm in depth.[353] With this depth of invasion, the frequency of inguinal lymph node metastasis is essentially zero.§

There are further problems related to vulvar microinvasive carcinoma relevant to the method of measurement

---

* References 10, 13, 25, 33, 62, 68, 70, 74, 81, 110, 128, 141, 157, 174, 188, 199, 216, 257, 301, 346, 349, 353.

† References 10, 25, 33, 49, 81, 129, 141, 157, 158, 174, 188, 239, 349, 353, 367, 368.

§ References 10, 33, 81, 129, 157, 174, 301, 349, 353.

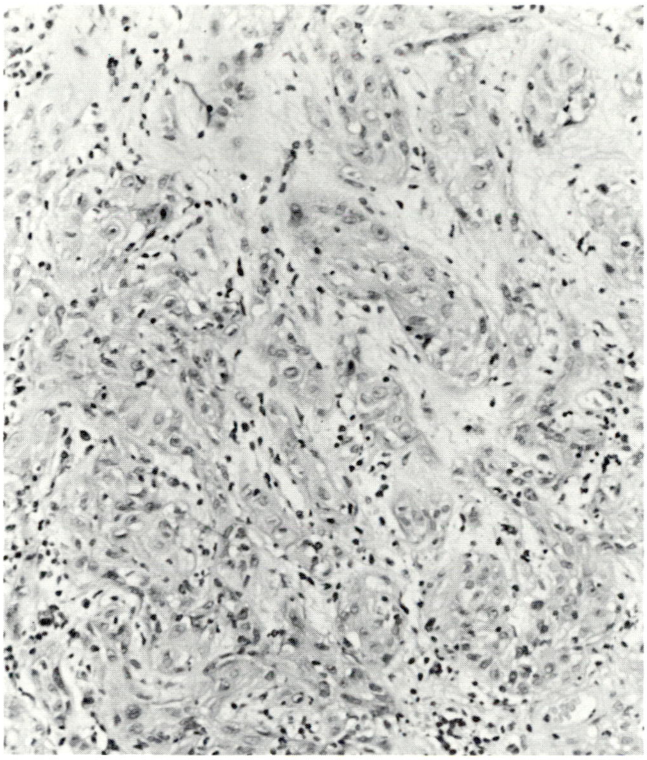

FIG. 3.55. Invasive squamous carcinoma, anaplastic. Small nests of invasive cells not clearly squamous in origin are seen.

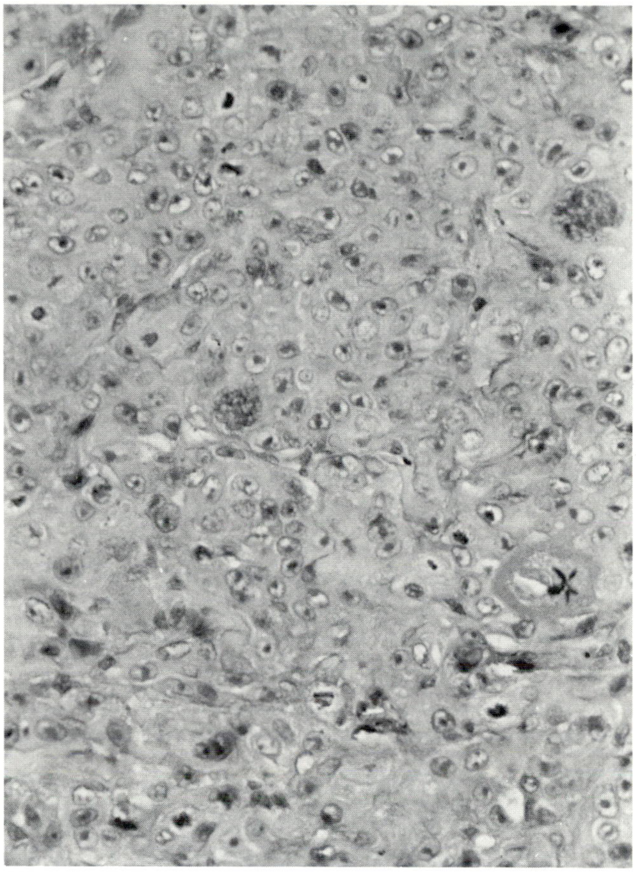

FIG. 3.56. Giant cell carcinoma of the vulva. Multinucleated tumor giant cells are evident. The cells contain nuclei with prominent nucleoli and abundant eosinophilic cytoplasm.

used to determine the depth of invasion. All investigators concur that the deepest point of invasion is the correct depth measurement. All pathologists further agree that a calibrated microscope, using a calibrated ocular, is necessary to make precise and accurate measurements. Differences of opinion exist about where the superficial point of measurement should be made to determine the depth of invasion. A variety of methods have been suggested, which are summarized in Fig. 3.58: Measurements from the epithelial stromal junction of the adjacent most superficial dermal papillae (A),[110,353] from the granular layer (B),[174] from the surface (C),[157,301] from the tip of the deepest rete ridge (D), and from the tip of the deepest adjacent tumor-free rete ridge (E),[33,81] have all been proposed. Alternatively, measurement of the surface of the tumor to the deepest point of invasion, and then subtraction of the thickness of the epithelium from the surface to the most superficial dermal papillae (F) has been suggested.[128,129] This method will give a measurement similar to the measurement from the epithelial stromal junction of the adjacent, most superficially dermal papillae (A = C − F).

The problem that occurs when measuring from the surface of an invasive lesion is that many squamous carcinomas of the vulva are ulcerated, and, therefore, measurement from the surface would not reflect a true depth but could seriously underestimate the depth of invasion. Marked hyperkeratosis may also cause underestimation. Measurement from the granular layer of the overlying epithelium would be possible only if the surface epithelium were intact and the granular layer present. The vestibule of the vulva does not have a well-defined granular layer. Thus, the granular layer could not be used in all sites on the vulva. Measurement from the tip of the deepest rete ridge or deepest adjacent rete ridge is complicated by the fact that the rete ridge itself may be involved in the neoplastic or a hyperplastic process. The same concern applies when attempting to find adjacent rete ridges not involved with the overlying neoplastic process. This may result in an underestimation of the depth of invasion. Measurement from the epithelial stromal junction of the adjacent, most superficial dermal papilla has the advantage that an adjacent dermal papilla can be found in all sites in the vulva, and it will not be significantly influenced by hyperkeratosis, tumor surface ulceration, or adjacent epithelial neoplasia or hyperplasia (Fig. 3.59). The major limiting factor is in dealing

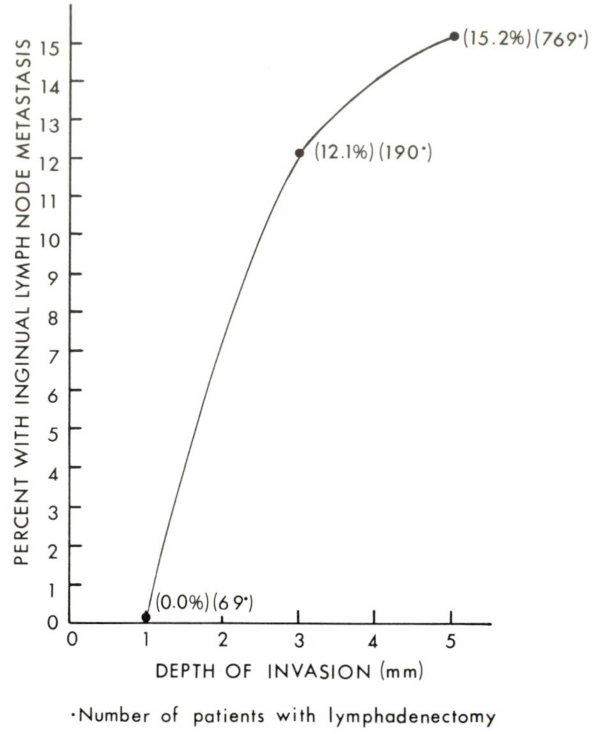

FIG. 3.57. The percentage of women who underwent lymphadenectomy with inguinal lymph node metastasis is plotted against the depth of invasion of their tumor. The frequency of lymph node metastasis rises rapidly with depth of invasion beyond 1 mm. (Reprinted by permission of Wilkinson, Ref. 349.)

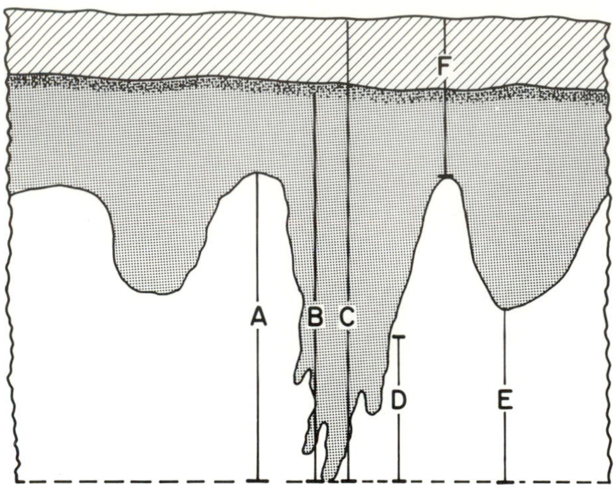

FIG. 3.58. Diagram of invasive squamous carcinoma, demonstrating reported methods of measurement for depth of invasion. All measure to the deepest point of invasion. A. Measurement from the epithelial–stromal junction of adjacent most superficial dermal papillae. B. Measurement from the granular layer. C. Measurement from the surface. D. Measurement from the rete ridge. E. Measurement from the tip's deepest adjacent rete ridge. F. Measurement (C) from the surface to the deepest point of invasion and then subtracting (F) the measurement from the surface to the epithelial stromal junction of the adjacent, most superficial dermal papillae. This measurement results in a measurement comparable to measurement (A). (A = C − F). (Reprinted by permission of Wilkinson, Ref. 349.)

with cases where there is no normal skin or mucous membrane adjacent to the tumor on the slide being used for measurement. This problem may occur in deeply invasive or large tumors but is rare with superficially invasive tumors. For the purpose of clarity of terms, the measurement from the surface of the tumor to the deepest point of invasion may be considered the *thickness of the tumor*, whereas the measurement from the epithelial stromal junction to the deepest point of invasion may be considered the *depth of invasion*. Other methods of measurement require a separate description along with the measurement.

In 1983, the ISSVD accepted the concept of superficially invasive squamous cell carcinoma of the vulva, and suggested that:[152] "Stage 1A carcinoma of the vulva be defined as a single lesion measuring 2 cm or less in diameter and with a depth of invasion of 1 mm or less." Patients with more than one site of invasion are not to be included.[152,188] This definition includes patients with capillary-like space involvement, provided that the tumor does not invade deeper than 1 mm.

In patients meeting the ISSVD criteria of Stage 1A carcinoma of the vulva, recommended therapy is wide local excision of the lesion, without vulvectomy. Sampling of the ipsilateral groin nodes, or bilateral groin nodes if the tumor is midline, has been suggested. However, with 1 mm or less of invasion, the probability of node metastasis is extremely small.

The Committee on Nomenclature of Vulvar Dystrophies and Tumors of the International Society of Gynecological Pathologists is of the opinion that when reporting the pathologic findings in superficial invasive carcinomas of the vulva the following information may be of value in the final pathology report, since it can influence therapeutic decisions:

1. The depth of invasion in millimeters
2. The thickness of the tumor in millimeters
3. The method of measurement of the depth of invasion and thickness
4. The presence or absence of vascular space involvement by tumor
5. The diameter of the tumor (as measured from the specimen
6. The clinical measurement of the tumor diameter, when available

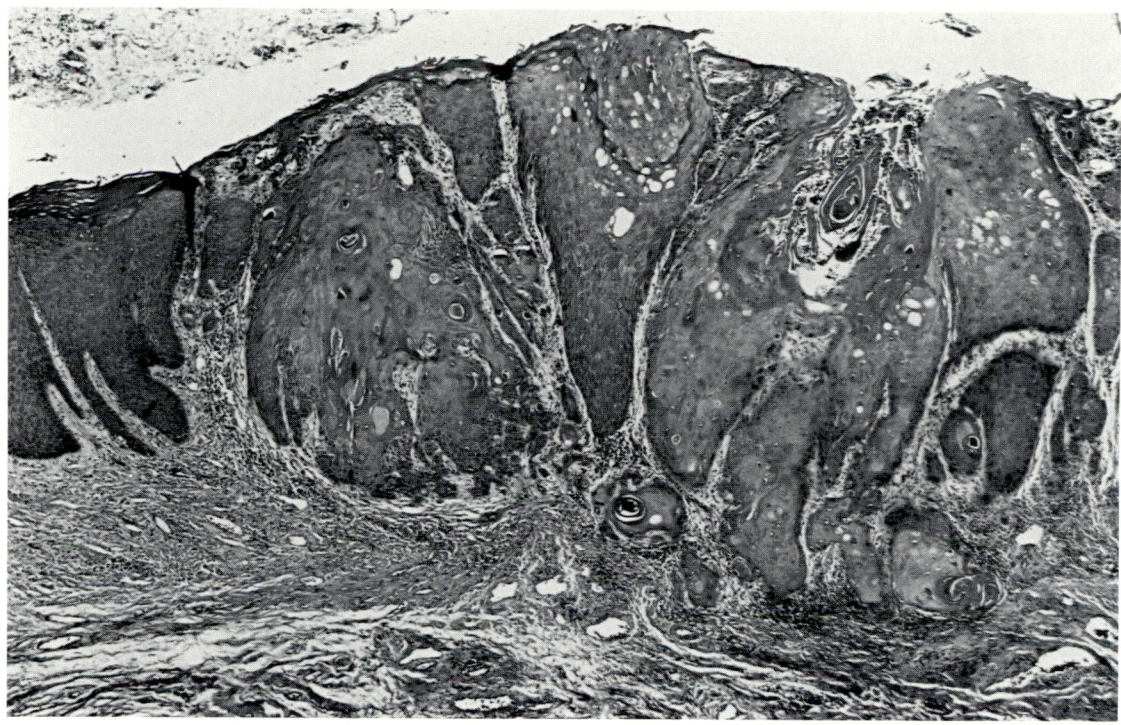

Fig. 3.59. Vulvar squamous carcinoma, depth of invasion 2.7 mm from the most superficial, adjacent dermal papilla to the deepest point of invasion. This is a frankly invasive carcinoma.

When there is a question of whether or not invasion is present and additional sectioning does not resolve the question, it is recommended that invasion not be diagnosed.

With more than 1 mm invasion, more extensive surgery can be planned, including groin node dissection.[70,92,129,342,343] The reliability of clinical evaluation of inguinal nodes in determining whether or not tumor is present is reviewed in Table 3.7. It is recognized that pathologic evaluation of lymph nodes for metastasis may be falsely negative approximately 15% of the time.[350,354] In assessing groin nodes, a fine needle aspiration may be the first step if suspicious nodes are present because the technique is rapid, safe, and cost effective and will detect gross metastasis. Current oncologic thought has become conservative, attempting to define high- and low-risk groups requiring individualization of therapy.[69,70,128,155,157,373] Many patients are now offered immediate reconstructive surgery as part of the initial procedure. Radiation techniques are now available that allow skin-sparing treatment of the groin nodes and have been used successfully in both primary and adjunctive treatment.[30,85]

Table 3.7. False-positive and false-negative clinical assessment of inguinal nodes.

	False-positive	False-negative
Way (1948)[343]	44%	61%
Franklin and Rutledge (1971)[93]	8%	21%
Boyce et al. (1985)[25]	6%	21%

Additional factors that may be of significance in prognosis and in the probability of lymph node metastasis include the diameter of the lesion, the presence of vascular channel invasion,[33,157,201] tumor ulceration,[201] the grade of the tumor[147] and confluent growth (defined as anastomosing cords or tumor (see Fig. 3.53), or tumor in the dermis exceeding 1 cu mm). Confluent growth, however, does not correlate with the occurrence of node metastasis in superficially invasive tumors[70,257] and is not found in tumors having 1 mm or less of invasion.[349] Until more definitive criteria are established for microinvasive cancer, it is suggested that this term not be used, instead reporting the diameter of the tumor, the depth of invasion, the presence or absence of vascular space involvement, and the status of surgical margins. These findings influence treatment options.

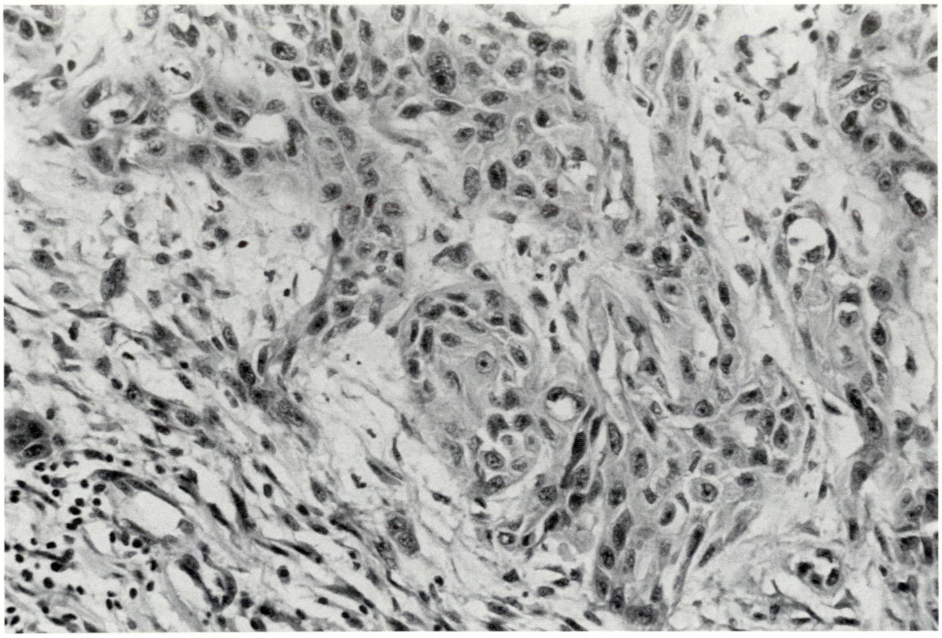

FIG. 3.60. Adenoid squamous carcinoma. Nests of poorly differentiated squamous carcinoma are seen that are arranged in a crude acinar manner. Some of the central acini are vacuolated.

Adenoid Squamous Carcinoma

Adenoid squamous carcinoma and verrucous carcinoma are two other varieties of squamous cell carcinoma of the vulva. The adenoid squamous type of tumor has rounded spaces, or pseudoacini, lined with a single layer of squamous cells.[203,331] Dyskeratotic and acantholytic cells are sometimes present in the central lumen (Fig. 3.60). These changes are focal in most cases and may occur within otherwise well-differentiated squamous tumors.[1] Although interesting, such foci of adenoid architecture do not appear to correlate with either the frequency of node involvement or the clinical course of the tumor.

Verrucous Carcinoma

Verrucous carcinoma is a distinct variant with a unique biologic course.[113,192] It is infrequent, rarely lethal, and often unrecognized by clinician and pathologist alike. Clinically, these lesions resemble large condylomata acuminata and are unresponsive to the usual methods of therapy. They are biopsied only after many attempts at eradication with topical podophyllin, local surgery, or other techniques (Fig. 3.61). With few exceptions, most patients with this disease are postmenopausal.

Verrucous carcinomas are well differentiated, with prominent acanthosis and parakeratosis (Fig. 3.62). The thin, supporting dermal papillae have a chronic inflammatory cell infiltrate. Squamous pearl formation is usually not present. Nuclear atypia is evident usually at the bases of the rete ridges, however, nuclear pleomorphism is usually not marked. Mitoses are rare, and abundant eosinophilic cytoplasm is retained. The tumor may be large, with local infiltration generally accompanied by an inflammatory response, and without nodal metastasis.[260] The association of this tumor with condylomata acuminata and HPV virus is supported by the identification of HPV DNA in the neoplasm.[249,251,279,306,329] HPV 6 variants are the most commonly identified. These lesions tend to remain locally infiltrative, however, more aggressive behavior of the neoplasm has been reported after radiotherapy.[192,210,274] The natural history of the untreated disease is one of local aggression amenable

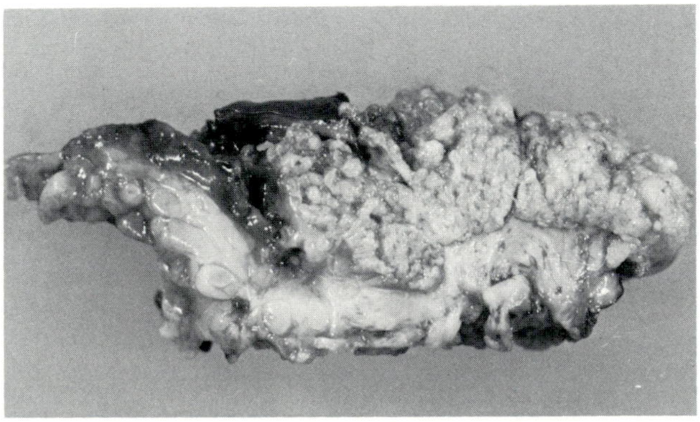

FIG. 3.61. Verrucous carcinoma of the vulva in cross-section. This tumor, 5 cm in diameter, has a broad, well-defined margin of infiltration involving the underlying fibrofatty tissue.

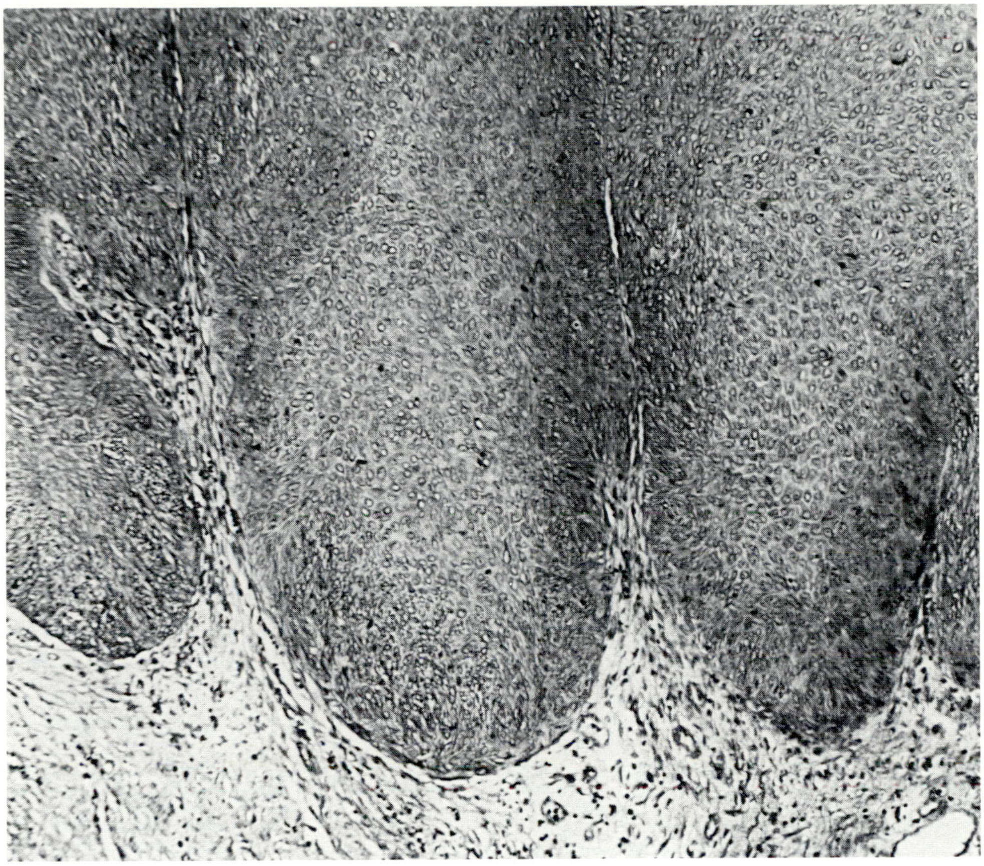

FIG. 3.62. Verrucous carcinoma of the vulva, a section from the specimen in Figure 3.59. There is a well-defined tumor–stromal interface. The cells are very well differentiated. A prominent chronic inflammatory infiltrate is present within the stroma.

to wide surgical excision.[11,164,192,210,316] Radiation is contraindicated.

Basal Cell Carcinoma

Although basal cell carcinomas of the skin are extremely common, they rarely occur on the vulva, a site not often exposed to actinic radiation. Breen et al. have shown that when such vulvar tumors do arise, they are primarily found in elderly white women whose symptomatology consists of itching or the presence of a mass.[27] Most lesions are confined to the labia majora, and a local recurrence rate of 20% is noted after wide local excision. The overall prognosis, however, is excellent, and no patients have died as a result of the disease. The histologic pattern resembles that of basal cell carcinomas occurring elsewhere on the skin. Small, elongated cells with deeply basophilic nuclei are present. A wide variety of architectural patterns can be recognized, ranging from slight pallisading of the basal layer of the epidermis to the formation of large, club-shaped masses of pleomorphic basal cells. In adenoid basal cell carcinoma gland-like growth and tubular formation may be seen, usually associated with solid areas of tumor growth.[226]

The connective tissue response frequently consists of a chronic inflammatory cell infiltrate and occasionally shows a mucoid or myxomatous change. Focal maturation of the malignant basal layer may occur, with the formation of mature squamous cells and keratin pearls. Such keratinization should be regarded as a sign of progressive maturation and not as dedifferentiation. Careful histologic study is necessary to distinguish the metatypical basal cell carcinoma, or basosquamous carcinoma, in which both squamous and basal elements show cytoplasmic and nuclear atypia (Fig. 3.63). The clinical significance of such change is unclear.[300] Basosquamous carcinoma is locally aggressive and may metastasize.[280]

Adenocarcinoma

Adenocarcinoma of the vulva is among the rarest of vulvar malignancies.[211] Many previous reports of this entity have been shown retrospectively to represent benign

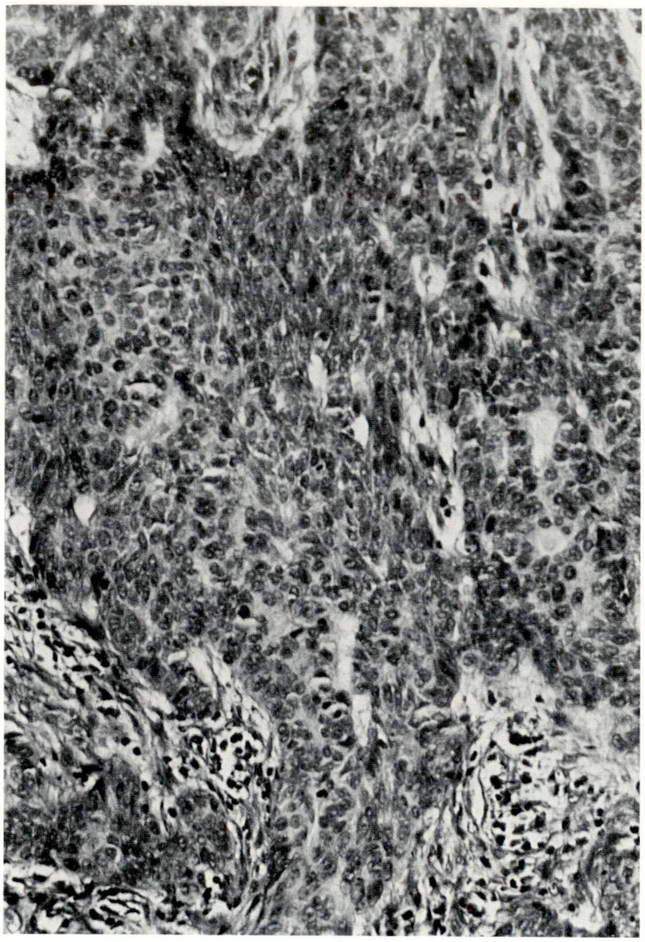

FIG. 3.63. Basosquamous carcinoma (metatypical basal cell carcinoma. Basal cell carcinoma in association with poorly differentiated squamous carcinoma. The cells show increased cytoplasm in the areas of squamous carcinoma.

hidradenomas or foci of adnexal Paget's disease. In fact, true adenocarcinoma of the underlying apocrine glands has been found in only 10–30% of the cases of vulvar Paget's disease (see Fig. 3.49).

Bartholin's Gland Adenocarcinoma

Most adenocarcinomas of the vulva arise as primary malignant tumors of the Bartholin's gland, although they may arise from the sweat glands.[348] Primary Skene's gland adenocarcinoma may also occur.[324] Criteria for establishing a diagnosis of adenocarcinoma or primary in the Bartholin's gland include (1) that an area of transition from benign to malignant Bartholin's gland elements be identified, (2) that the tumor found is consistent with a primary Bartholin's gland carcinoma, and (3) that the tumor is not a metastasis, that is, not histologically the same as a primary tumor found elsewhere.[44,373]

Adenocarcinoma and squamous cell carcinoma occur with nearly equal frequency in the Bartholin's gland and comprise approximately 80% of malignant tumors of Bartholin's gland (Table 3.8). Adenoid cystic carcinomas account for approximately 15% of all reported cases.[1,4,18,373] Although Bartholin's gland elements contain CEA, adenoid cystic carcinomas of the Bartholin's gland are immunoreactive for keratin and S100 antigen.[235] Electron microscopy may sometimes assist in establishing the diagnosis.[6,202]

Bartholin's gland malignancies carry a poor prognosis because of the rich lymphatic supply of the area, the deep, occult site of the primary tumor, and the tendency to dismiss enlargements of the Bartholin area as benign. The average age of patients with Bartholin's gland carcinoma is 50, with 67% of patients between the ages of 40 and 69. Accordingly, excision is recommended for all tumors of the Bartholin's gland in women over the age of 40 to obtain histologic documentation of the cause. Although the overall 5-year survival for patients with Bartholin's gland carcinoma is 30%, the survival following radical surgery is influenced by the presence or absence of inguinal node metastasis. If the groin nodes are negative, the 5-year survival is approximately 50%. If two or more groin nodes are involved with tumor, the overall survival is 18%.[44,205,347] Twenty percent of patients will have metastasis to the pelvic nodes. As with primary squamous carcinoma of the vulva, pelvic node metastases do not occur without inguinal–femoral node involvement.[44] Adenoid cystic carcinomas of the Bartholin's gland tend to recur locally, although distant metastasis and specifically pulmonary metastasis may occur. Wide, complete local excision, with ipsilateral inguinal lymphadenectomy, is recommended.[54]

Malignant lymphoma involving the Bartholin's gland has been reported.[268] Plasmocytoma has been observed occurring concurrently in the vulva and vagina.[75]

Sweat Gland Carcinoma

Carcinomas of the vulvar sweat glands are extremely rare, and symptoms are usually delayed until the formation of a painless vulvar mass.[348] In addition to undifferentiated sweat gland adenocarcinomas, ductal eccrine

TABLE 3.8. Classification of Bartholin's gland carcinoma.

Type	Percent of total
Squamous cell carcinoma	40
Adenocarcinoma	40
Adenoid cystic carcinoma	15
Adenosquamous carcinoma	Under 5
Transitional cell carcinoma	Under 5
Other carcinomas	Under 5

carcinoma, eccrine porocarcinoma, and eccrine hidradenocarcinoma have been reported.[228]

Sarcomas

Leiomyosarcoma

Sarcomas of the vulvar connective tissue are unusual tumors. Of these, the leiomyosarcoma is the most common type. In one series of 32 patients with vulvar leiomyosarcoma, the mean age was 35 years, with a range from 18 to 66 years. All patients had a mass in the vulva. None metastasized, and 4 recurred locally. Tumors 5 cm or larger with five or more mitosis per 10 high-power fields or with an infiltrating margin had a more aggressive behavior.[322] Recommended therapy is wide local excision. Malignant fibrohistiocytomas, neurofibrosarcomas, rhabdomyosarcomas, fibrosarcomas, angiosarcomas, and epithelioid sarcomas are among other sarcomas reported as occurring in the vulva.[71] Most sarcomas arise from the labia majora, and a wide age range (6–64 years) is noted.[55,71,208] The clinical course is unpredictable and is only somewhat dependent on the histologic type.

Rhabdomyosarcoma

Rhabdomyosarcomas of the vulva are rapidly growing tumors that metastasize early and may occur in infants as well as in young women.[55,71] Embryonal rhabdomyoblasts or cross-striated cells may be seen on light microscopy. Botryoid embryonal rhabdomyosarcoma (sarcoma botryoides) has been described arising from the labia majora and hymenal area in infants.[53,321] These tumors grow in a polypoid manner and, on light microscopy, reveal a myxomatous stroma and a denser cellular area beneath the epithelium, forming the cambium zone composed of spindle or round cells. Embryonal rhabdomyoblasts or cellular cross-striation may be found. These cells are immunoreactive for myoglobin. This characteristic and electron microscopy are of value in establishing the diagnosis.[208] Table 3.3 summarizes some of the differential diagnostic features found in myxoid soft tissue tumors that may occur in the vulva.

Dermatofibrosarcoma Protuberans

This locally aggressive tumor of histiocytic origin usually appears as a solitary, firm, brownish, subcutaneous nodule in postmenopausal women.[22] These neoplasms may be clinically confused with large nevi. Histologically, dermatofibrosarcoma protuberans is characterized by intradermal growth, with a broad junction with the adjacent epithelium, resulting in an elevated epithelial surface. The tumor is densely cellular, with the cells arranged in a characteristic storiform pattern. The cells, unlike those of malignant fibrous histiocytoma, show little cytologic atypia, rare mitotic figures, and no tumor giant cells.[208] In the base of the tumor, an infiltrative growth pattern may be seen. Wide local excision with a deep margin is necessary because recurrence may occur, although metastasis is rare. Apparent transformation to malignant fibrous histiocytoma has been reported.[208]

Malignant Fibrous Histiocytoma

Malignant fibrohistiocytomas may histologically resemble benign infiltrative dermatofibrosarcoma protuberans, however, tumor giant cells, mitosis, nuclear pleomorphism, and deep invasion are often seen. They may be extremely aggressive and result in early distant metastases.[135,325] Fibrohistiocytic tumors are immunoreactive for alpha-I-antitrypsin and alpha-I-antichymotrypsin.[232]

Epithelioid Sarcoma

The histogenesis of epithelioid sarcoma is obscure. These tumors occur in young people and are characterized by slow but progressive growth, with a marked tendency to recur after inadequate excision. Microscopically, they are composed of polygonal cells arranged in sheets and nests. The abundance of eosinophilic cytoplasm gives some cells an epithelial appearance. Nuclear pleomorphism and frequent mitotic figures are generally noted. Epithelioid sarcomas contain keratin, as shown by immunoperoxidase study.[45] Vascular space invasion has been associated with recurrence. Local recurrence with associated distant metatasis has been seen with unusual frequency in vulvar epithelial sarcoma.[330] Wide radical excision of the tumor is suggested.

Kaposi's Sarcoma

Among the malignant tumors of endothelial origin that may involve the vulva, Kaposi's sarcoma is of importance, because of its association with acquired immune deficiency syndrome (AIDS). Depending on the age of the tumor, the clinical presentation evolves from a skin patch to plaque to a nodular stage. Usually, more than one skin lesion is present. The early stage, a patch, reveals increased vascularity, with irregularly shaped vascular spaces within the dermis with surrounding mononuclear cells. Later stages show more irregularly shaped vessels associated with atypical spindle cells within the dermis (Fig. 3.64). The advanced, or nodular, stage reveals a highly vascular, spindle cell neoplasm. The differential diagnosis of Kaposi's sarcoma may include tumors of fibrohistocytic origin, benign vascular tumors, scar, and a variety of other skin changes.[21] Kaposi's sarcoma involving the vulva has been described.[208] Finally, lymphan-

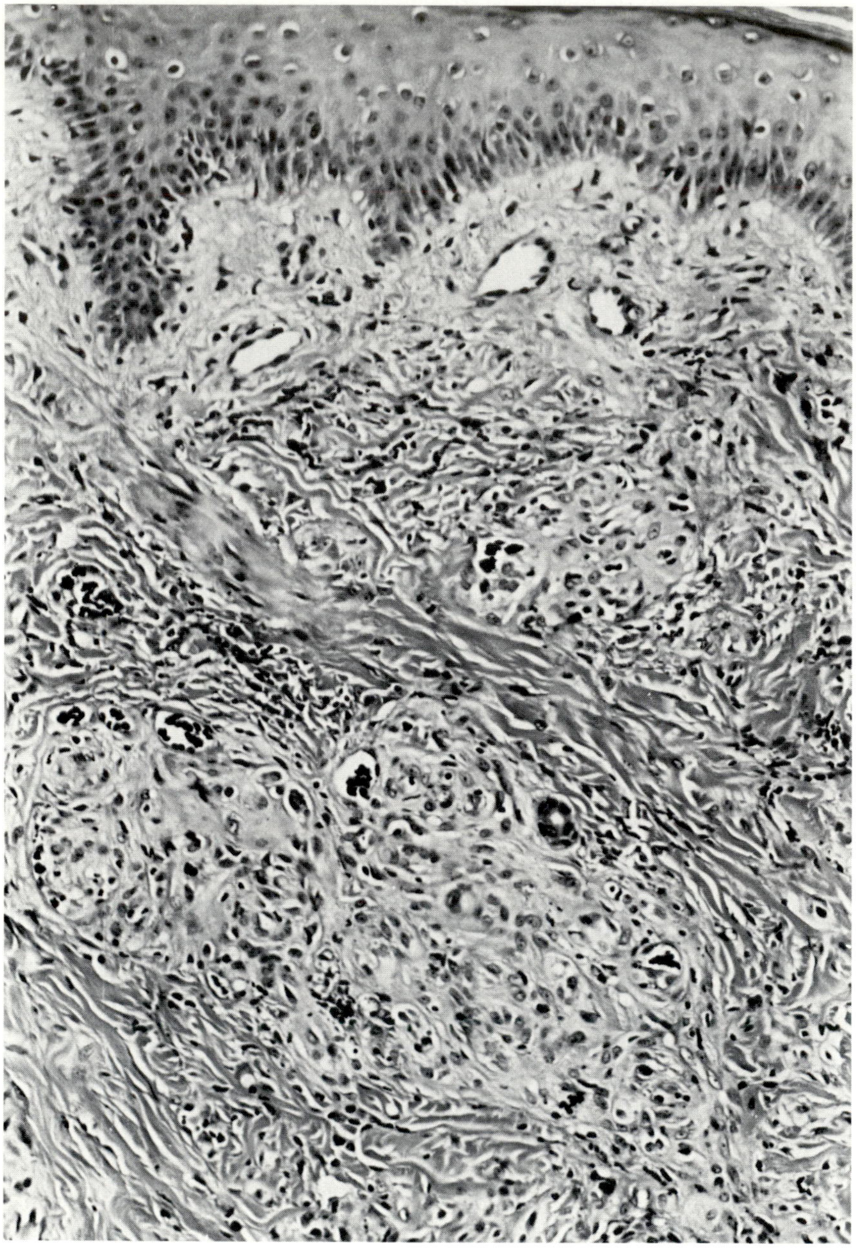

FIG. 3.64. Kaposi's sarcoma. Many vessels, some of which are irregularly shaped, are seen within the dermis. Atypical spindle cells are seen about the vessels within the dermis.

giosarcoma has been reported in the thigh after radiation therapy for vulvar carcinoma.[144]

Alveolar Soft Part Sarcoma

Alveolar soft part sarcoma arising in the right labium minus has been reported in a 62-year-old woman. Local recurrence is reported in 30–42% of patients, and the reported survival ranges from 30–50% in nonvulvar sites.[308] These tumors usually occur in the deep tissue of the extremities of young adults and may have an indolent course, although metastasis to lymph nodes and distant sites may occur.

The histopathology of the tumor is characterized by loosely arrayed polygonal cells with granular cytoplasm on delicate to thick fibrovascular and fibrocollagenous stalks. In some areas, the tumor cells form alveolar-like structures. No true glands or secretory products are seen, although the tumor cells do protrude into the tumor luminal spaces. Metastatic renal cell carcinoma or clear cell tumors may mimic this tumor.[208] Mitoses are rare, and the tumor tends to have a pushing border. Recommended therapy is wide local excision with resection of the regional lymph nodes. Radical surgery does not appear to improve survival, but chemotherapy or immunotherapy may be of value.[308]

Other Malignancies

Langerhan's Granulomatosis

Among the Langerhan's granulomatoses, histiocytosis X and eosinophilic granulomatosis have been described as involving the vulva.[154,208] Histocytosis X is immunoreactive for S100 antigen.[235] Eosinophilic granuloma may be localized to the vulva, although most cases reported have involved other sites as well, including the pituitary gland, resulting in diabetes insipidus.[154] Localized Langerhan's granulomatosis can usually be treated by radiation therapy, but more advanced disease may require chemotherapy.

Melanoma

Melanomas of the vulva comprise 2–9% of all malignant tumors of the vulva and account for approximately 3–5% of all melanomas of the skin.[211] Although this frequency is relatively high, it may be appropriate, taking into consideration that the vulva comprises approximately 1% of the total skin surface.[171,263] There are nearly 500 cases reported in the English literature. Although melanoma is a rare tumor, the highly aggressive behavior and low 5-year survival rate (30–50%) account for its clinical importance.*

The most common complaints are a vulvar mass, pruritus, and bleeding. Mucosal involvement is common, with the clitoris or labia majora being involved in approximately 75% of all cases.[171] The age range of patients with this tumor is wider than that of patients with squamous carcinoma. The mean age has been reported to be from 54 to 61 years of age. Most cases occur during the sixth and seventh decades, but up to 32% of patients are premenopausal.[233] Melanomas of the vulva occur predominately in white women. Primary vulvar melanomas appear to involve the clitoris, labia minora, and labia majora with nearly equal frequency.

Three major varieties of melanoma occur on the vulva: nodular melanoma (NM), superficial spreading melanoma (SSM), and acral lentiginous melanoma (ALM).[229] In the presence of invasive melanoma, vertical growth of an SSM can be separated from an NM by the finding of adjacent radial growth of SSM or atypical melanocytes, involving four or more rete ridges, adjacent to the invasive tumor (Figs. 3.65 and 3.66).[263] Acral lentiginous melanomas have both radial and vertical growth patterns, with atypical dendritic melanocytes (Fig. 3.67). Cell types include epithelioid spindle cell or mixed types. Pigmented (melanotic) and amelanotic variants of malignant melanomas may be seen on the vulva. In the series of Johnson et al. of 14 patients who died of vulvar melanoma NM comprised 65% of, SSM 21%, and ALM 14%.[171]

* References 162, 165, 171, 233, 263, 278, 366.

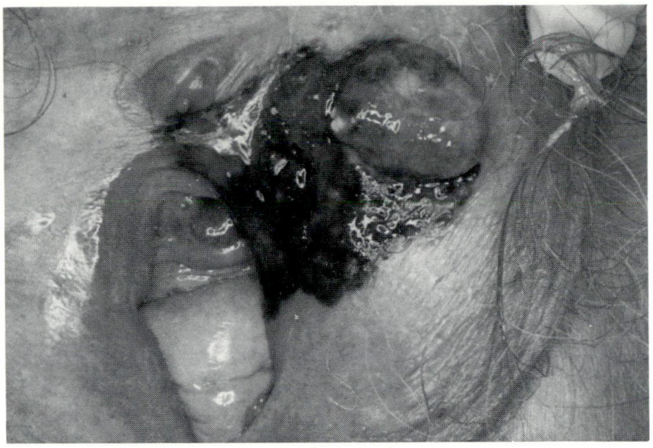

FIG. 3.65. Pigmented malignant melanoma on the vulva. This was a superficial spreading malignant melanoma with vertical growth within the field of the superficial tumor. (Photograph courtesy of Dr. Linda S. Morgan.)

Mihm et al.[229] have advocated that melanoma be staged according to the level of invasion; five levels are recognized. Chung et al.[50] have applied this system to the vulva (Fig. 3.68) and note that patients with Level I disease are extremely rare. Of those with Level II disease, all survived after adequate surgery. A 40–80% survival has been reported with Levels III and IV, whereas only a 20–28% survival is found after Level V has been reached. A microstaging system using both Clark's levels and Breslow's thickness measurements have been proposed.[262] Women with Stage II tumors, with a maximum tumor thickness of 1.3 mm, were the only survivors in Johnson et al.'s study.[171] Two of these women had SSM, and two had nodular melanomas. The clitoris is a common primary site of melanoma, and clitoral location is associated with a poor prognosis. Tumor thickness has been found to be inversely related to both survival and to length of survival.[171] Nodular melanomas are usually thicker than superficial spreading melanomas, with an early vertical growth. The increased thickness may explain, in part, the reason for the poorer survival seen in the vulvar nodular melanoma group. Nodular melanomas accounted for 50% of the Level V cases in one study.[269]

The tumor cell type does not appear to have an influence on survival, however, higher mitotic rates (10 per high-power field and higher) are found in tumors associated with poor survival.[171] Tumor ulceration, necrosis, and vascular space invasion may all be associated with a poorer prognosis in vulvar melanoma. Local recurrence on the vulva, urethra, vagina, cervix, and rectum may

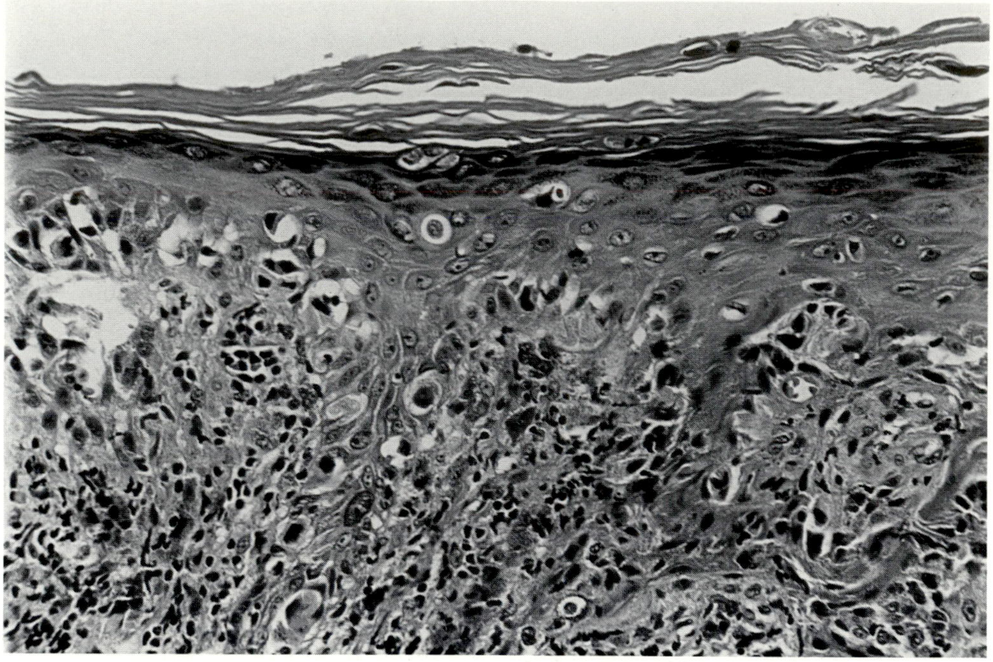

FIG. 3.66. Superficial spreading malignant melanoma. Pagetoid spread of the melanoma cells into the upper third of the epidermis is seen. Markedly atypical melanocytic cells are seen within the epithelial–stromal junctional area. No invasion is present. (Photograph courtesy of K. K. Pierson, M.D.)

be seen.[269] Approximately one-half of patients with recurrent vulvar melanomas will die of disease within 12 months of the recurrence. The 5-year survival after recurrence has been reported as 5%.[269] Patients who die of melanoma generally exhibit local lymph node involvement. Commonly, metastases occurs in the lungs and may be associated with metastasis to brain, bladder, bone marrow, and abdominal wall.[171] Regression may occur in malignant melanomas.[295]

Histologic sections from invasive areas of the superficial spreading variety of melanoma show relatively uniform, large, malignant melanocytes present in the epidermis. The dermis is not necessarily involved. The nuclei are relatively uniform, and there is usually an abundance of cytoplasm (see Fig. 3.66). In contrast, the nodular melanoma is a tumor in which intraepidermal growth is always associated with dermal invasion. Irregular junctional activity is frequent, and both spindle-shaped and polygonal epithelial cells are seen (Fig. 3.69). Epithelioid cells are large and usually contain a variable concentration of melanin granules. Mitotic figures are almost always present, but their absence does not preclude malignancy. Unlike benign nests of nevus cells, nests of melanoma cells are not surrounded by well-organized bundles of collagen. In addition, an inflammatory infiltrate of lymphocytes and plasma cells is often seen.[165,263] Melanoma cells can be distinguished from Paget's cells by immunoperoxidase methods. Melanoma cells contain S100 antigen, whereas Paget's cells do not.[232,235] In addition, Paget's cells contain CEA, which is not found in melanoma (see Table 3.5).[237]

Endodermal Sinus Tumor

Endodermal sinus tumor (EST) is a germ cell tumor occurring in the ovary and testis (see Chapter 20, Germ Cell Tumors of Ovary). Its occurrence in extragonadal sites is rare. In women, the vagina, pelvis, and vulva have been reported as primary sites.[194,293,332] The histopathologic features are well described, and there are several recognized patterns of growth. Characteristic Schiller-Duval bodies and intracytoplasmic alpha-fetoprotein demonstrated by immunoperoxidase techniques assist in distinguishing EST from a poorly differentiated adenocarcinoma. Recommended therapy for vulvar EST is radical vulvectomy with inquinal node lymphadenectomy and chemotherapy. Chemotherapy has markedly improved survival in patients with this tumor.

Metastatic Tumors

Metastatic tumors comprise approximately 8% of all tumors of the vulva. Squamous carcinoma of the cervix is the most frequent tumor metastatic to the vulva, followed by carcinomas of the endometrium, bladder, and urethra.[64,221] Other primary tumors that have metastasized to the vulva include carcinoma of the vagina, breast,

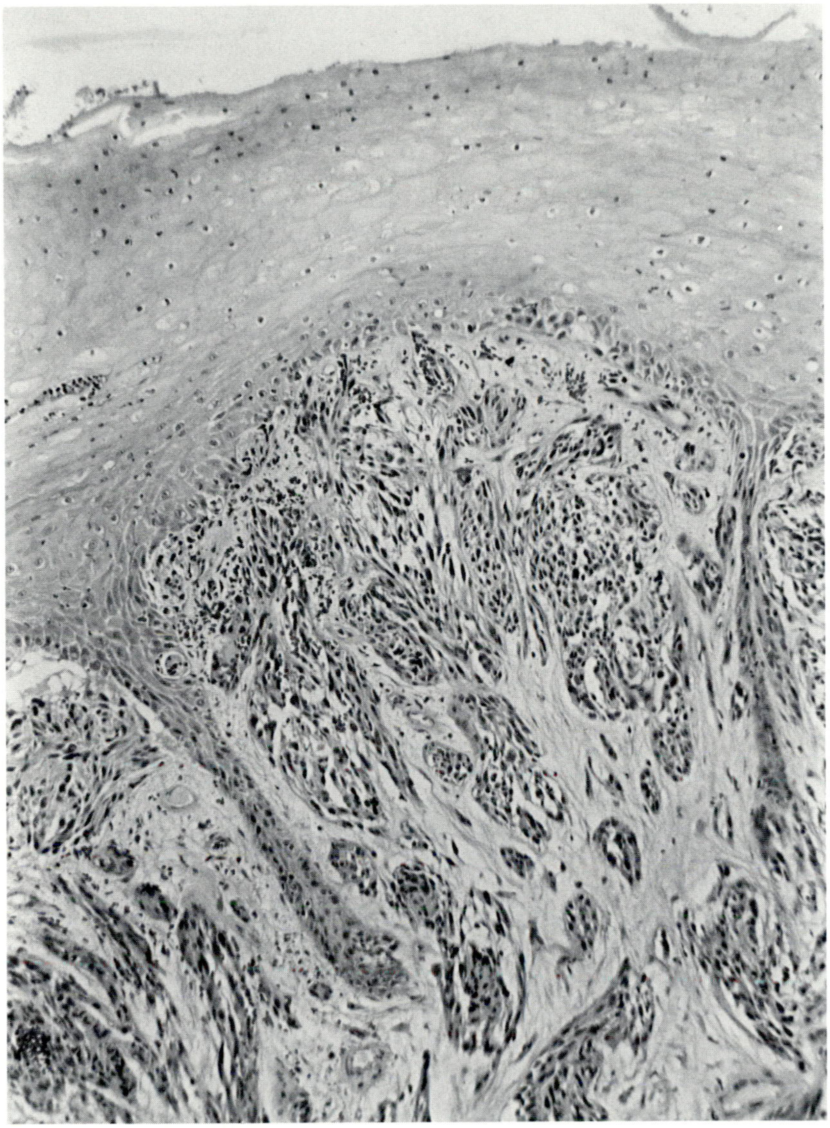

FIG. 3.67. Mucosal acral lentiginous melanoma of the vulva. This histologic variant of malignant melanoma is characterized by a radial component with a lentiginous pattern at the mucosal–stromal interface. In this case, spindle cells are seen within the submucosa near the junctional zone and within the deeper dermis with an associated desmoplastic response. The cytologic uniformity is characteristic. No pagetoid spread is evident. This type of malignant melanoma, when present on the vulva, is usually found within the vulvar vestibule. (Photograph courtesy of K.K. Pierson, M.D.)

ovary, kidney, and stomach, melanoma, gestational choriocarcinoma, and carcinoma of the lung.[221,272,278] Malignant lymphomas may also involve the vulva[82] and Bartholin's gland.[268,373]

Cloacogenic carcinoma usually arises from the anal transitional zone but may involve the vulva, although a primary adenocarcinoma arising in cloacal tissue has been reported.[327] These tumors are classified as transitional and basaloid types. A pleomorphic variant is also recognized. The basaloid and pleomorphic variants are believed to be differentiated variants of a tumor type that has a similar prognosis. The transitional type appears similar to urothelial carcinoma and has a relatively good prognosis. The basaloid type histologically resembles basal cell carcinoma and generally behaves aggressively. Both basaloid and pleomorphic variants have a poor prognosis.

Urethra

No discussion of vulvar pathology would be complete without mention of the lesions that afflict the female urethra. Prolapse of the urethral mucosa may occur at

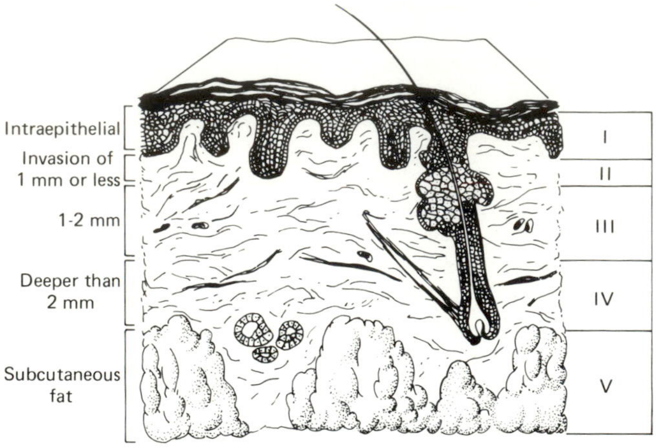

FIG. 3.68. Levels of vulvar melanoma invasion. [Reprinted with permission from The American College of Obstetricians and Gynecologists. (Obstetrics and Gynecology, 45: 638, 1975)]

any age, but it is most common in premenarchal children and in postmenopausal women.[14] Redundancy of the mucosa and laxity of the supporting periurethral fascia contribute to the formation of prolapse, which is aggravated by increased abdominal pressure. It may be related to a relative lack of estrogen. The prolapsing urethra may occur as a large, red, polypoid mass covered with urethral mucosa with edematous vascular submucosa, protruding from the urethra and mimicking a urethral neoplasm. Cryosurgery is an effective method of treatment.[99] Histologically, the urethral mucosa may exhibit ulceration, and the underlying connective tissue is generally filled with an inflammatory infiltrate. Vascular engorgement is usually present.

Caruncles are sessile or polypoid masses that arise at the urethral meatus in postmenopausal women. They may represent localized areas of prolapse and are by far the most common lesions of the urethra. Caruncles are often asymptomatic but may cause bleeding or dysuria. Clinical differentiation from urethral carcinoma may be impossible, therefore, excision, with hemostatic destruction of the base of the lesion, is the treatment of choice. Recurrences may be observed.[23] Histologically, the submucosa of the urethral caruncle may contain large venous channels that are often dilated and engorged. A myxomatous or granulomatous pattern may be present

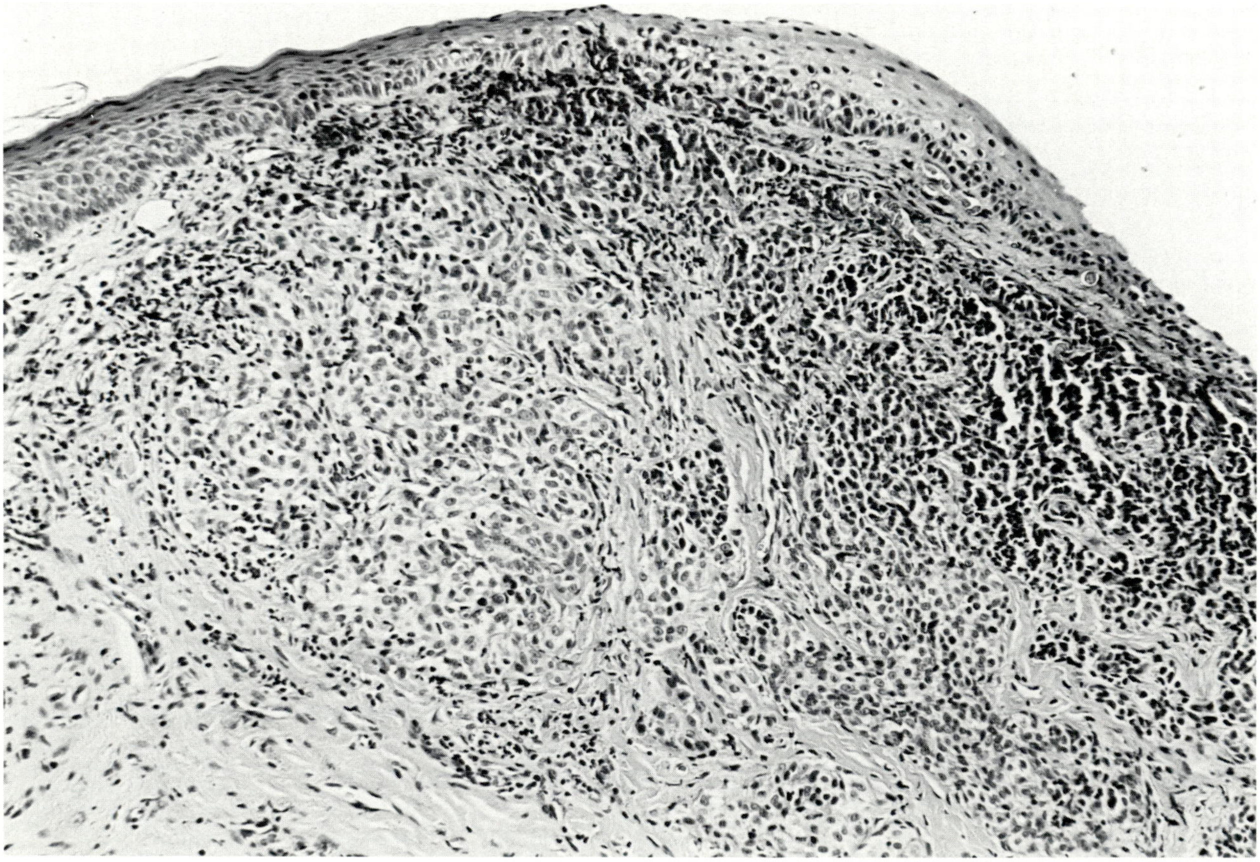

FIG. 3.69. Nodular melanoma of the vulva. The nodular melanoma is entirely within the dermis, with an elevated, intact epithelium overlying the tumor. The melanoma cells are large and polygonal, arranged in nests, sheets, and cords within the dermis. (Photograph courtesy of K. K. Pierson, M.D.)

in the supporting tissue, which is often densely infiltrated with chronic inflammatory cells.

Urethral condyloma acuminatum may resemble caruncle or urethral carcinoma. In children, urethral and periurethral condylomas may be polypoid and clinically suggest sarcoma botryoides.

Urethral carcinoma constitutes less than 1% of malignancies affecting the female genitalia and occurs in the elderly age group.[122] Urethral bleeding, frequency, and dysuria are the most frequent complaints.[207,328,345] The vast majority of these tumors are squamous in origin and arise form the distal urethra, where they usually cause symptoms early in their course.[8]

Transitional cell carcinomas may be seen in the distal as well as the proximal urethra. Adenocarcinomas may occur in the proximal urethra as well as within urethral diverticuli.[261,287] Both urethral squamous carcinomas and adenocarcinomas are immunoreactive for CEA.[236] Clear cell carcinoma, lymphoma, melanoma, and sarcoma have all been reported as arising within the urethra.[287,372,373] Although a staging system for tumors of the urethra has been proposed, none exists at present.[122,373]

The prognosis of urethral carcinoma is relatively poor, with a 5-year overall survival for anterior urethral tumor of 51% and for posterior or entire urethral involvement 6%. The overall survival has been reported at 22–27%, [122,373] Survival in urethral carcinoma is influenced by the fact that 20–50% of women with urethral carcinoma have metastasis to superficial or deep pelvic nodes when they are first seen by a physician.[122,207] Improved and individualized surgical and radiotherapy techniques may substantially increase survival rates.[345]

Suburethral diverticula originate from the upper two thirds of the posterior urethral wall and may extend cephalad to involve the region beneath the vesicle neck. Although a congenital etiology has been proposed for some cases, most are thought to begin as an infection in one of the tubular periurethral glands,[145] followed by abscess formation and eventual breakthrough into the urethral lumen. Adenocarcinomas have been described arising in urethral diverticula.[261]

References

1. Abell MR (1963) Adenocystic (pseudoadenomatous) basal cell carcinoma of vestibular glands of vulva. Am J Obstet Gynecol 86: 470
2. Abell, MR (1965) Intraepithelial carcinoma of epidermis and mucosa of vulvar and perineum. Surg Clin North Am 45: 1170
3. Adam E, Kaufman RH, Mirkovic RR, Melnick JL (1979) Persistence of virus shedding in asymptomatic women after recovery from herpes genitalis. Obstet Gynecol 54: 171
4. Addison A, Parker RT (1977) Adenoid cystic carcinoma of Bartholin's gland. Gynecol Oncol 5: 196
5. Addison WA, Livengood CH, Hill GB, Sutton GP, Fortier KJ (1984) Necrotizing fasciitis of vulvar origin in diabetic patients. Obstet Gynecol 63: 473
6. Advani H, Waldo ED, Bigelow B (1978) Bartholin's gland carcinoma: An ultrastructural study. Am J Obstet Gynecol 130: 362
7. Aly R, Britz MB, Maibach HI (1979) Quantitative microbiology of human vulva. Br J Dermatol 101: 445
8. Ampil FL (1985) Primary malignant neoplasm of the female urethra. Obstet Gynecol 66: 799
9. Andreasson B, Bock JE (1985) Intraepithelial neoplasia in the vulvar region. Gynecol Oncol 21: 300
10. Andreasson B, Nyboe J (1985) Predictive factors with reference to low risk of metastases in squamous carcinoma of the vulvar region. Gynecol Oncol 21: 196
11. Andreasson B, Bock JE, Strom KV, Visfeldt J (1983) Verrucous carcinoma of the vulvar region. Acta Obstet Gynecol Scand 62: 183
12. Axe S, Parmley T, Woodruff JD, Hlopak B (1986) Adenomas in minor vestibular glands. Obstet Gynecol 68: 16
13. Barnes AE, Crissman JD, Schellhas HF, Azoury RS (1980) Microinvasive carcinoma of the vulva: A clinicopathologic evaluation. Obstet Gynecol 56: 234
14. Bayonet-Rivera NP, Magoss I (1970) Vulvar tumor in children due to prolapse of urethral mucosa. Am J Obstet Gynecol 108: 572
15. Beecham CT (1976) Paget's disease of the vulva. Obstet Gynecol 47[Suppl]: 61
16. Bergman A, Bhatia NM, Broen EM (1984) Cryotherapy for treatment of genital condyloma during pregnancy. J Reprod Med 29: 432
17. Bernstein SG, Kovacs BR, Townsend DE, Morrow CP (1983) Vulvar carcinoma in situ. Obstet Gynecol 61: 304
18. Bernstein SG, Voet RL, Lifshitz S, Buchsbaum HJ (1983) Adenoid cystic carcinoma of Bartholin's gland. Case report and review of the literature. Am J Obstet Gynecol 147: 385
19. Blair C (1970) Angiokeratoma of the vulva. Br J Dermatol 83: 409
20. Blank H, Davis C, Collins C (1970) Electron microscopy for the diagnosis of cutaneous viral infections. Br J Dermatol 83: 69
21. Blumenfeld W, Egbert BM, Sagebiel RW (1985) Differential diagnosis of Kaposi's sarcoma. Arch Pathol Lab Med 109: 123
22. Bock JE, Andreason B, Thorn A, Holck S (1985) Dermatofibrosarcoma protuberans of the vulva. Gynecol Oncol 20: 129
23. Bolduan JP, Farah RN (1981) Primary urethral neoplasms: Review of 30 cases. J Urol 125: 198
24. Boyce DC, Valpey JM (1971) Acute ulcerative vulvitis of obscure etiology. Obstet Gynecol 38: 440
25. Boyce J, Fruchter RG, Kasambilides, E, Nicastri AD, Sedlis A, Remy JC (1985) Prognostic factors in carcinoma of the vulva. Gynecol Oncol 20: 364
26. Breen JL, Smith CI, Gregori CA (1978) Extramammary Paget's disease. Clin Obstet Gynecol 21: 1107
27. Breen JL, Neubecker RD, Greenwald E, Gregori CA

(1975) Basal cell carcinoma of the vulva. Obstet Gynecol 46: 122
28. Britz MB, Maibach HI (1979) Human cutaneous vulvar reactivity to irritants. Contact Dermatitis 5: 375
29. Britz MB, Maibach HI (1979) Human labia majora skin: Transepidermal water loss in vivo. Acta Derm Venereol 85[Suppl]: 23
30. Bryson SCP, Colgan TJ, Vernon CP (1986) Invasive squamous cell carcinoma of the vulva: Delineation of high-risk group requiring adjuvant radiotherapy. J Reprod Med 31: 976
31. Buchler DA (1975) Multiple primaries and gynecologic malignancies. Am J Obstet Gynecol 123: 376
32. Buckley CH, Butler EG, Fox H (1984) Vulvar intraepithelial neoplasia and microinvasive carcinoma of the vulva. J Clin Pathol 37: 1201
33. Buscema J, Stern JL, Woodruff JD (1981) Early invasive carcinoma of the vulva. Am J Obstet Gynecol 140: 563
34. Buscema J, Woodruff JD, Parmley TH, Genadry R (1980) Carcinoma in situ of the vulva. Obstet Gynecol 55: 225
35. Bushkell LL, Friedrich EG, Jordon RE (1981) An appraisal of routine direct immuofluorescence in vulvar disorders. Acta Derm Venereol 61: 157
36. Butler EB, Stanbridge CM (1984) Condylomatous lesions of the lower female genital tract. Clin Obstet Gynecol 11: 171
37. Cabral GA, Marciano-Cabral F, Fry D, Lumpkin CK, Mercer L, Gopelrud D (1982) Expression of herpes simplex virus type 2 antigens in premalignant and malignant human vulvar cells. Am J Obstet Gynecol 143: 611
38. Caglar H, Tamer S, Hreshchyshyn MM (1982) Vulvar intraepithelial neoplasia. Obstet Gynecol 60: 346
39. Calandra D, DiPaola GR, Gomez-Rueda N, Balina L (1979) Enfermedades de la vulva. Buenos Aires, Argentina, Panamericana
40. Capraro VJ (1971) Congenital anomalies. Clin Obstet Gynecol 14: 988
41. Carneiro SJC, Gardner HL, Knox JM (1971) Syringoma of the vulva. Arch Dermatol 103: 494
42. Caterson RJ, Furber J, Murray J, McCarthy W, Mahony JF, Shell AGR (1984) Carcinoma of the vulva in two young renal allograft recipients. Transplant Proc 16(2): 559
43. CDC (1983) Condyloma acumatum—United States 1966–1981. MMWR 23: 306
44. Chamlian DL, Taylor HB (1972) Primary carcinoma of Bartholin's gland. A report of 24 patients. J Obstet Gynecol 39: 489
45. Chase D, Enzinger F, Weiss SW (1984) Keratin in epitheloid sarcoma. An immunohistochemical study. Am J Surg Pathol 8: 435
46. Chaung T, Perry HO, Kurland LT, Ilstrup DM (1984) Condyloma acuminatum in Rochester, Minn., 1950–1978. II. Anaplasias and unfavorable outcomes. Arch Dermatol 120: 476
47. Chetkowski R, Sakamoto H, MacLusky N, Merino M, Schwartz PE (1985) Solitary pelvic neural tumors with high steroid receptor content. Gynecol Oncol 20: 43
48. Cho D, Buscema J, Rosenshein NB, Woodruff JD (1985) Primary breast cancer of the vulva. Obstet Gynecol 66[Suppl]: 79
49. Chu J, Tamimi HK, Ek M, Figge DC (1982) Stage I vulvar cancer: Criteria for microinvasion. Obstet Gynecol 59: 716
50. Chung AF, Woodruff JM, Lewis JL (1975) Malignant melanoma of the vulva. Obstet Gynecol 45: 638
51. Collins CG, Hansen LH, Theriot E (1966) A Clinical stain for use in selecting biopsy sites in patients with vulvar disease. Obstet Gynecol 28: 158
52. Copas P, Dyer M, Comas FV, Hall DJ (1982) Spindle cell carcinoma of the vulva. Diagn Gynecol Obstet 4: 235
53. Copeland LJ, Gershenson DM, Saul PB, Sneige N, Stringer CA, Edwards CL (1985) Sarcoma botyroides of the female genital tract. Obstet Gynecol 66: 262
54. Copeland LJ, Sneige N, Gershenson DM, Saul PB, Stringer CA, Sesk JC (1986) Adenoid cystic carcinoma of Bartholin's gland. Obstet Gynecol 67: 115
55. Copeland LJ, Sneige N, Stringer CA, Gershenson DM, Saul PB, Kavanagh JJ 1985) Alveolar rhabdomyosarcoma of the female genitalia. Cancer 56: 849
56. Corey L, Adams HG, Brown ZA, Holmes KK (1983) Genital herpes simplex virus infections: Clinical manifestations, course, and complications. Ann Intern Med 98: 958
57. Creasman WT, Gallager HS, Rutledge F (1975) Paget's disease of the vulva. Gynecol Oncol 3: 133
58. Crum CP, Liskow A, Petras P, Keng WC, Frick HC (1984) Vulvar intraepithelial neoplasia (severe atypia and carcinoma in situ). Cancer 54: 1429
59. Crum CP, Fu YS, Levine RU, Richart RM, Towensend DE, Fenoglio CM (1982) Intraepithelial squamous lesions of the vulva: Biologic and and histologic criteria for the distinction of condylomas from vulvar intraepithelial neoplasia. Am J Obstet Gynecol 144(1): 77
60. Crum CP, Braun LA, Shah KV, Fu YS, Levine RU, Fenoglio CM, Richart RM, Townsend DE (1982) Vulvar intraepithelial neoplasia: Correlation of nuclear DNA content and the presence of a human papillomavirus (HPV) structural antigen. Cancer 49: 468
61. Davos I, Abell M (1976) Soft tissue sarcoma of the vulva. Gynecol Oncol 4: 70
62. Dean RE, Taylor ES, Weisbrod DM, Martin JW (1974) The treatment of premalignant and malignant lesions of the vulva. Am J Obstet Gynecol 119: 59
63. Degefa S, Dhurandhar N, O'Quinn AG, Fuller PN (1984) Granular cell tumor of the clitoris in pregnancy. Gynecol Oncol 19: 246
64. Dehner LP (1973) Metastatic and secondary tumors of the vulva. Obstet Gynecol 42: 47
65. de Oliveira M, Saleiro V (1986) Involucrin expression in vulvar lesions. J Reprod Med 31: 828
66. Dewhurst CJ (1968) Congenital malformations of the genital tract in childhood. J Obstet Gynecol Br Commun 75: 377
67. Dickie RJ, Horne CH, Sutherland HW, Bewsher PD, Stankler L (1982) Direct evidence of localized immunological damage in vulvar lichen sclerosus et atrophicus. J Clin Pathol 35: 1395
68. DiPaola GR, Gomez-Rueda N, Arrighi L (1975) Relevance of microinvasion in carcinoma of the vulva. Obstet Gynecol 45: 647

69. DiSaia P (1985) Management of superficially invasive vulvar carcinoma. Clin Obstet Gynecol 28: 196
70. DiSaia PJ, Creasman WT, Rich WM (1979) An alternate approach to early cancer of the vulva. Am J Obstet Gynecol 133: 825
71. DiSaia PF, Rutledge F, Smith PJ (1971) Sarcoma of the vulva. Obstet Gynecol 38: 180
72. di Sant'Agnese PA, Knowles DM (1980) Extracardiac rhabdomyoma: A clinicopathologic study and review of the literature. Cancer 46: 780
73. Dodson RF, Fritz GS, Hubler WR, Rudolph AH, Knox JM, Chu LW (1974) Donovanosis: A morphologic study. J Invest Dermatol 62: 611
74. Donaldson ES, Powell DE, Hanson MB, van Nagell JR (1981) Prognostic parameters in invasive vulvar cancer. Gynecol Oncol 11: 184
75. Doss LL (1978) Simultaneous extramedullary plasmacytomas of the vagina and vulva. Cancer 41: 2468
76. Douglas CP (1962) Lymphogranuloma venereum and granuloma inguinale of the vulva. J Obstet Gynecol Br Commun 69: 871
77. Douglas CP (1984) Vulvar dystrophy: Preliminary investigations. J Reprod Med 29: 461
78. Drusin LM (1972) The diagnosis and treatment of infectious and latent syphilis. Med Clin North Am 56: 1161
79. Dunn JM (1970) Congenital absence of the external genitalia. J Reprod Med 4: 66
80. Duray PH, Merino MJ, Axiotis C (1983) Warty dyskeratoma of the vulva. Int J Gynecol Pathol 2: 286
81. Dvoretsky PM, Bonfiglio TA, Helmkamp BF, Ramsey G, Chuang C, Beecham JB (1984) The pathology of superficially invasive, thin vulvar squamous cell carcinoma. Int J Gynecol Pathol 3: 331
82. Egwuatu VE, Ejeckam GC, Okaro JM (1980) Burkitt's lymphoma of the vulva. Case report. Br J Obstet Gynaecol 87: 827
83. Ekwo E, Wong YW, Myers M (1979) Asymptomatic cervicovaginal shedding of herpes simplex virus. Am J Obstet Gynecol 134: 102
84. Evron S, Leviatan A, Okon E (1984) Familial benign chronic pemphigus appearing as leukoplakia of the vulva. Int J Dermatol 23: 556
85. Fairey RN, MacKay PA, Benedet JL, Boyes DA, Turko M (1985) Radiation treatment of carcinoma of the vulva, 1950–1980. Am J Obstet Gynecol 151: 591
86. Falk HC, Hyman AB (1971) Congenital absence of clitoris. Obstet Gynecol 38: 269
87. Ferenczy A, Richart RM (1972) Ultrastructure of perianal Paget's disease. Cancer 29: 1141
88. Ferenczy A, Mitao M, Nagai N, Silverstein SJ, Crum CP (1985) Latent papillomavirus and recurring genital warts. N Engl J Med 313: 784
89. Fetherston WC, Friedrich EG (1972) The origin and significance of vulvar Paget's disease. Obstet Gynecol 39: 735
90. Flynt J, Gallup DG (1979) Childhood lichen sclerosus. Obstet Gynecol 53: 79S
91. Fowler WC, Lawrence H, Edelman DA (1981) Paravestibular tumor of the female genital tract. Am J Obstet Gynecol 139: 109
92. Franklin EW (1972) Clinical staging of carcinoma of the vulva. Obstet Gynecol 40: 277
93. Franklin EW, Rutledge FD (1971) Prognostic factors in epidermoid carcinoma of the vulva. Obstet Gynecol 37: 892
94. Franklin EW, Rutledge FD (1972) Epidemiology of epidermoid carcinoma of the vulva. Obstet Gynecol 39: 165
95. Freedman SR, Goldman RL (1978) Mucocele-like changes in Bartholin's glands. Hum Pathol 9: 111
96. Friedman RJ, Ackerman B (1981) Difficulties in the histologic diagnosis of melanocytic nevi on the vulvae of premenopausal women. In: Pathology of malignant melanoma. New York, Masson
97. Friedrich EG (1972) Reversible vulvar atypia. Obstet Gynecol 39: 173
98. Friedrich EG (1976) Lichen sclerosus. J Reprod Med 17: 147
99. Friedrich EG (1977) Cryosurgery for urethral prolapse. Obstet Gynecol 50: 359
100. Friedrich EG (1987) Vulvar Vestibulitis Syndrome. J Reprod Med 32:
101. Friedrich EG (1983) Vulvar disease. Philadelphia, W.B. Saunders
102. Friedrich EG, Kalra PS (1984) Serum levels of sex hormones in vulvar lichen sclerosus, and the effect of topical testosterone. N Engl J Med 310: 488
103. Friedrich EG, MacLaren NK (1984) Genetic aspects of vulvar lichen sclerosus. Am J Obstet Gynecol 150: 161
104. Friedrich EG, Wilkinson, EJ (1973) Mucous cysts of the vulvar vestibule. Obstet Gynecol 42: 407
105. Friedrich EG, Wilkinson EJ (1985) Vulvar surgery for neurofibromatosis. Obstet Gynecol 65: 135
106. Friedrich EG, Burch K, Bahr JP (1979) The vulvar clinic: An eight-year appraisal. Am J Obstet Gynecol 135: 1036
107. Friedrich EG, Julian CG, Woodruff JD (1964) Acridine orange fluorescence in vulvar dysplasia. Am J Obstet Gynecol 90: 1281
108. Friedrich EG, Wilkinson EJ, Fu YS (1980) Carcinoma in situ of the vulva: A continuing challenge. Am J Obstet Gynecol 136: 830
109. Friedrich EG, Wilkinson, EJ, Steingraeber PH, Lewis DJ (1975) Paget's disease of the vulva and carcinoma of the breast. Obstet Gynecol 46: 130
110. Fu YS, Reagan JW, Townsend DE, Kaufman RH, Richard RM, Wentz WB (1981) Nuclear DNA study of vulvar intraepithelial and invasive squamous neoplasms. Obstet Gynecol 57: 643
111. Fukamizu H, Matsumoto K, Inouek K, Moriguchi T (1982) Large vulvar lipoma. Arch Dermatol 118(6): 447
112. Gaffney EF, Majmuder B, Bryan JA (1982) Nodular fasciitis (pseudosarcomatous fasciitis) of the vulva. Int J Gynecol Pathol 1: 307
113. Gallousis S (1972) Verrucous carcinoma. Obstet Gynecol 40: 502
114. Galloway DA, McDougall JK (1983) The oncogenic potential of herpes simplex viruses: Evidence for a "hit and run" mechanism. Nature 302: 21
115. Garcia JJ, Verkauf BS, Hochberg CJ, Ingram JM (1978) Aberrant breast tissue of the vulva. Obstet Gynecol 52: 225

116. Gardner HL, Kaufman RH (1969) Benign diseases of the vulva and vagina. St. Louis, Mo., Mosby
117. Gardner HL, Kaufman RH (1972) Viral infections in gynecology and obstetrics. Clin Obstet Gynecol 15: 856
118. Gissmann L, de Villers EM, Zur Hausen H (1982) Analysis of human warts (condylomata acuminata) and other genital tumors for human papilloma virus type 6 DNA. Int J Cancer 29: 143
119. Gissmann L, Wolnik L, Ikenberg H, Koldovsky V, Schnurch HG, Zur Hausen H (1983) Human papillomavirus types 6 and 11 DNA sequences in genital and laryngeal papillomas and in some cervical cancers. Proc Natl Acad Sci USA 80: 560
120. Godeau G, Frances C, Hornebeck W, Brechemier D, Robert L (1982) Isolation and partial characterization of an elastase-type protease in human vulva fibroblasts: Its possible involvement in vulvar elastic tissue destruction of patients with lichen sclerosus et atrophicus. J Invest Dermatol 78: 270
121. Goolamali SK, Barnes EW, Irvine WJ, Shuster S (1974) Organ-specific antibodies in patients with lichen sclerosus. Br Med J 4: 78
122. Grabstald H (1973) Tumors of the urethra in men and women. Cancer 32: 1236
123. Gray's textbook of anatomy (1984) 30th edn. Philadelphia, Lea & Febiger
124. Gross G, Hagedorn M, Ikenberg H, Rufli T, Dahlet C, Grosshaus E, Gissman L (1985) Bowenoid papulosis. Arch Dermatol 121: 858
125. Growdon WA, Fu Y, Lebherz TB, Rapkin A, Mason GD, Parks G (1985) Pruritic vulvar squamous papillomatosis: Evidence for human papillomavirus etiology. Obstet Gynecol 66: 564
126. Guindi SF, Silverberg BK, Evans TN (1974) Multifocal mixed adenxoid tumors of the vulva. Int J Gynecol Obstet 12: 138
127. Gunn RA, Gallager HS (1980) Vulvar Paget's disease: A topographic study. Cancer 46: 590
128. Hacker NF, Berek JS, Lagasse LD, Nieberg RK, Leuchter RS (1984) Individualization of treatment for stage I squamous cell vulvar carcinoma. Obstet Gynecol 63(2): 155
129. Hacker NF, Nieberg RK, Berek JS, Leuchter RS, Lucas WE, Tamimi HK, Nolan JF, Moore JG, Lagasse LD (1983) Superficially invasive vulvar cancer with nodal metastases. Gynecol Oncol 15: 65
130. Harrington CI, Dunsmore IR (1981) An investigation into the incidence of autoimmune disorders in patients with lichen sclerosus et atrophicus. Br J Dermatol 104: 563
131. Hart WR, Millman JB (1977) Progression of intraepithelial Paget's disease of the vulva to invasive carcinoma. Cancer 40: 2333
132. Hart WR, Norris HJ, Helwig EB (1975) Relation of lichen sclerosus et atrophicus of the vulva to development of carcinoma. Obstet Gynecol 45: 369
133. Hay DM, Cole FM (1970) Postgranulomatous epidermoid carcinoma of the vulva. Am J Obstet Gynecol 108: 479
134. Helwig EB, Graham JH (1963) Anogenital (extramammary) Paget's disease. Cancer 16: 387
135. Hensley GT, Friedrich EG (1973) Malignant fibroxanthoma: a sarcoma of the vulva. Am J Obstet Gynecol 116: 289
136. Henson D, Tarone R (1977) An epidemiologic study of cancer of the cervix, vagina, and vulva based on the Third National Cancer Survey in the United States. Am J Obstet Gynecol 129: 525
137. Hewitt AB (1971) Behcet's disease. Br J Vener Dis 47: 52
138. Hewitt J (1986) Lichen sclerosus. J Reprod Med 31: 781
139. Hewitt M, Barrow GI, Miller DC, Turk F, Turk S (1973) Mites in the personal environment and their role in skin disorders. Br J Dermatol 89: 401
140. Hilliard GD, Massey FM, O'Toole RV (1979) Vulvar neoplasia in the young. Am J Obstet Gynecol 135: 185
141. Hoffman JS, Kumar NB, Morley GW (1983) Microinvasive squamous carcinoma of the vulva: Search for a definition. Obstet Gynecol 61: 615
142. Hoffman JS, Kumar NB, Morley GW (1985) Prognostic significance of groin lymph node metastases in squamous carcinoma of the vulva. Obstet Gynecol 66(3): 402
143. Huang HJ, Yamabe T, Tagawa H (1983) A solitary neurilemmoma of the clitoris. Gynecol Oncol 15: 103
144. Huey GR, Stehman FB, Roth LM, Ehrlich CE (1985) Lymphangiosarcoma of the edematous thigh after radiation therapy for carcinoma of the vulva. Gynecol Oncol 20: 394
145. Huffman JW (1948) The detailed anatomy of the paraurethral ducts in the adult human female. Am J Obstet Gynecol 55: 86
146. Hurley HJ, Shelley WB (1960) The human apocrine sweat gland in health and disease. Springfield, Ill., Charles C Thomas
147. Husseinzadeh N, Zaino R, Nahhas WA, Mortel R (1983) The significance of histologic findings in predicting nodal metastasis in invasive squamous cell carcinoma of the vulva. Gynecol Oncol 16: 105
148. Ikenberg H, Gissmann L, Gross G, Grussenford-Conen EI, Zur Hausen H (1983) Human papillomavirus type 16 related DNA in genital Bowen's disease and in Bowenoid papulosis. Int J Cancer 32: 563
149. Ilardi CF, Faro JC (1985) Localization of parathyroid hormone-like substance in squamous cell carcinomas. An immunoperoxidase study with ultrastructural localization. Arch Pathol Lab Med 109: 752
150. Imperial R, Helwig EB (1967) Angiokeratoma of the vulva. Obstet Gynecol 29: 307
151. International Society for the Study of Vulvar Disease (1976) New nomenclature for vulvar disease. Obstet Gynecol 47: 122
152. Report of the ISSVD Terminology Committee. Proc. VIII World Congress (1986) Stockholm, Sweden, J Reprod Med 31: 973
153. Isaacson D, Turner ML (1979) Localized vulvar syringomas. J Am Acad Dermatol 1: 352
154. Issa PY, Salem PA, Brihi E, Azoury RS (1980) Eosinophilic granuloma with involvement of the female genitalia. Am J Obstet Gynecol 137(5): 608
155. Iversen T (1985) New approaches to treatment of squamous cell carcinoma of the vulva. Clin Obstet Gynecol 28: 204

156. Iversen T, Aas M (1983) Lymph drainage from the vulva. Gynecol Oncol 16: 179
157. Iversen T, Abeler V, Aalders J (1981) Individualized treatment of stage I carcinoma of the vulva. Obstet Gynecol 57: 85
158. Jafari K, Cartnick EN (1976) Microinvasive squamous cell carcinoma of the vulva. Gynecol Oncol 4: 158
159. Jagella HP, Stegner HE (1974) On the diagnosis of condylomata acuminata. Arch Gynaekol 216: 119
160. Janakiv JR, Dremalatha S, Raghuveera N, Thambiah AS (1980) Lawrence-Seip syndrome. Br J Dermatol 103: 693
161. Janovski NA, Weir JH (1962) Comparative histologic and histochemical studies of mesonephric derivatives and tumors. Obstet Gynecol 19: 57
162. Janovski NA, Marshall D, Taki I (1962) Malignant melanoma of the vulva. Am J Obstet Gynecol 84: 523
163. Japaze H, Garcia-Bunuel R, Woodruff JD (1977) Primary vulvar neoplasia: A review of in situ and invasive carcinoma. Obstet Gynecol 49: 404
164. Japaze H, van Dinh T, Woodruff JD (1982) Verrucous carcinoma of the vulva: Study of 24 cases. Obstet Gynecol 60: 462
165. Jaramillo BA, Ganjei P, Averette HE, Sevin BU, Lovecchio JL (1985) Malignant melanoma of the vulva. Obstet Gynecol 66(3): 398
166. Jeffcoate TNA (1966) Chronic vulval dystrophies. Am J Obstet Gynecol 95: 61
167. Jeffcoate TNA, Woodcock AS (1961) Premalignant conditions of the vulva, with particular reference to chronic epithelial dystrophies. Br Med J 2: 127
168. Jimerson GK, Merrill JA (1970) Multicentric squamous malignancy involving both cervix and vulva. Cancer 26: 150
169. Jobson VW, Homesley HD (1983) Treatment of vaginal intraepithelial neoplasia with the carbon dioxide laser. Obstet Gynecol 62: 90
170. Johnson DE, O'Connell JR (1983) Primary carcinoma of female urethra. Urology 21: 42
171. Johnson TL, Kumar NB, White CD, Morley GW (1986) Prognostic features of vulvar melanoma. Int J Gynecol Pathol 5: 110–118
172. Jones I, Buntine D (1978) Progression of vulval carcinoma in situ. Aust NZ J Obstet Gynaecol 18: 274
173. Junard TA, Thomas SM (1981) Cysts of the vulva and vagina: A comparative study. Int J Gynecol Obstet 19: 239
174. Kabulski Z, Frankman O (1978) Histologic malignancy grading in invasive squamous cell carcinoma of the vulva. Int J Obstet Gynecol 16: 233
175. Kao M, Paulson JD, Askin FB (1975) Crohn's disease of the vulva. Obstet Gynecol 46: 329
176. Karasek J, Smetana K, Oehlert W, Konrad B (1970) The ultrastructure of Bowen's disease: Nuclear and nucleolar lesions. Cancer Res 30: 2791
177. Kaufman RH, Faro S (1985) Herpes genitalis: Clinical features and treatment. Clin Obstet Gynecol 28: 152
178. Kaufman RH, Friedman K (1981) Hemangioma of the clitoris. Plast Reconstr Surg 62: 452
179. Kaufman RH, Friedrich EG (1985) The carbon dioxide laser in the treatment of vulvar disease. Clin Obstet Gynecol 28: 220
180. Kaufman RH, Gardner HL (1965) Benign mesodermal tumors. Clin Obstet Gynecol 8: 953
181. Kaufman RH, Gardner HL (1965) Intraepithelial carcinoma of the vulva. Clinic Obstet Gynecol 8: 1035
182. Kaufman RH, Gardner HL, Brown D, Beyth Y (1974) Vulvar dystrophies: An evaluation. Am J Obstet Gynecol 120: 363
183. Kernen JA, Morgan ML (1970) Benign lymphoid hamartoma of the vulva. Obstet Gynecol 35(2): 290
184. Kersting DW (1963) Clear cell hidradenoma and hidradenocarcinoma. Arch Dermatol 87: 91
185. Kfuri A, Rosenshein N, Dorfman H, Goldstein P (1981) Desmoid tumor of the vulva. J Reprod Med 26: 272
186. King DF, Bustillo M, Broen EN, Hirose FM (1979) Granular cell tumors of the vulva: A report of 3 cases. J Dermatol Surg Oncol 5: 794
187. King LS, Sullivan M (1947) Effects of podophyllin and of colchicine on normal skin, on condyloma acuminatum, and on verruca vulgaris. Arch Pathol 43: 374
188. Kneale BL (1984) Microinvasive cancer of the vulva: Report of the International Society for the Study of Vulvar Disease Task Force, VIIth Congress. J Reprod Med 29: 454
189. Knudson AG (1985) Hereditary cancer, oncogenes, and antioncogenes. Cancer Res 45: 1437
190. Kovi J, Tillman RL, Lee SM (1974) Malignant transformation of condyloma acuminatum: A light microscopic and ultrastructural study. Am J Clin Pathol 61: 702
191. Krantz KE (1958) Innervation of the human vulva and vagina. Obstet Gynecol 12: 382
192. Kraus FT, Perez-Mesa C (1966) Verrucous carcinoma. Cancer 19: 26
193. Kremer M, Nussenson E, Steinfeld M, Zuckerman P (1984) Crohn's disease of the vulva. Am J Gastroenterol 79: 376
194. Krishnamurthy SC, Sampat MB (1981) Endodermal sinus (yolk sac) tumor of the vulva in a pregnant female. Gynecol Oncol 11: 379
195. Krupp PJ, Lee FY, Batson HW, Allen PM, Collins JH (1973) Carcinoma of the vulva. Gynecol Oncol 1: 345
196. Krupp PJ, Lee FY, Bohm JW, Batson HW, Diem JE, Lemire JE (1975) Prognostic parameters and clinical staging criteria in epidermoid carcinoma of the vulva. Obstet Gynecol 46: 84
197. Kuberski T (1980) Granuloma inguinale (donovanosis). Sex Transm Dis 7: 29
198. Kucera PR, Glazer J (1985) Hydrocele of the canal of nuck: A report of four cases. J Reprod Med 30: 439
199. Kunscher A, Kanbour AI, David B (1978) Early vulvar carcinoma. Am J Obstet Gynecol 132: 599
200. Kurman RJ, Shah KH, Lancaster WD, Jenson AB (1981) Immunoperoxidase localization of papillomavirus antigens in cervical dysplasia and vulvar condylomas. Am J Obstet Gynecol 140: 9321
201. Kurzl RG, Messerer D, Baltzer J, Lohe KJ, Zander J (1986) Vulvar Carcinoma: a clinical, histologic and morphometric study of 197 patients with squamous cell carcinoma of the vulva. J Reprod Med 31: 980

202. Kuzuya K, Matsuyama M, Nishi Y, Chihara T, Suchi T (1981) Ultrastructure of adenocarcinoma of Bartholin's gland. Cancer 48: 1392
203. Lasser A, Cornog JL, Morris JM (1974) Adenoid squamous cell carcinoma of the vulva. Cancer 33: 224
204. Leib SM, Gallousis S, Freedman H (1979) Granular cell myoblastoma of the vulva. Gynecol Oncol 8: 12
205. Leuchter RS, Hacker NF, Voet RL, Berek JS, Townsend DE, Lagasse LD (1982) Primary carcinoma of the Bartholin gland: A report of 14 cases and review of the literature. Obstet Gynecol 60: 361
206. Lever WF, Schaumburg-Lever G (1983) Histopathology of the skin, 6th edn. Philadelphia, J.B. Lippincott
207. Levine RL (1980) Urethral cancer. Cancer 45: 1965
208. LiVolsi VA, Brooks JJ (1987) Soft tissue tumors of the vulva. In: Contemporary issues in surgical pathology. Pathology of the Vulva and Vagina. Vol. 9: 209 ed. Wilkinson, E.J. New York, Churchill Livingstone
209. Lowell DM, LiVolsi VA, Ludwig ME (1983) Genital condyloma virus infection following pelvic radiation therapy: Report of seven cases. Int J Gynecol Pathol 2: 294
210. Lucas WE, Benirschke K, Lebherz TB (1974) Verrucous carcinoma of the female genital tract. Am J Obstet Gynecol 119: 435
211. Lundwall F (1961) Cancer of the vulva. Acta Radiol (Stockholm) 208 [Suppl]
212. Lynch PJ (1985) Condylomata acuminata (anogenital warts). Clin Obstet Gynecol 28: 142
213. Lynch PJ, Minkin W (1968) Molluscum contagiosum of the adult. Arch Dermatol 98: 141
214. Mabuchi K, Bross DS, Kessler II (1985) Epidemiology of cancer of the vulva. A case-control study. Cancer 55: 1843
215. Magrine JR, Masterson BJ (1981) *Loxosceles reclusa* spider bite: A consideration in the differential diagnosis of chronic, nonmalignant ulcers of the vulva. Am J Obstet Gynecol 140: 343
216. Magrina JF, Webb MJ, Gaffey TA, Symmonds RE (1979) Stage I squamous cell cancer of the vulva. Am J Obstet Gynecol 134: 453
217. Majmudar B, Hallden C (1986) The relationship between juvenile laryngeal papillomatosis and maternal condylomata acuminata. J Reprod Med 31: 804
218. Mann PR, Cowan MA (1973) Ultrastructural changes in four cases of lichen sclerosus et atrophicus. Br J Dermatol 89: 223
219. Marwah S, Bergman ML (1980) Ectopic salivary gland in the vulva (choristoma): Report of a case and review of the literature. Obstet Gynecol 56: 389
220. Matthews J, Mason G (1983) Granular cell myoblastoma: An immunoperoxidase study using a variety of antisera to human carcinoembryonic antigen. Histopathology 7: 77
221. Mazur MT, Hsueh S, Gersell DJ (1984) Metastases to the female genital tract: Analysis of 325 cases. Cancer 53: 1978
222. McCance DJ In: Crawford L (1984) Papilloma viruses and cervical tumors. Nature 310: 16
223. McKee PH, Wright E, Hutt MSR (1983) Vulvar schistosomiasis. Clin Exp Dermatol 8: 189
224. Meister P, Buckmann FW, Konrad E (1978) Nodular fasciitis. Analysis of 100 cases and review of the literature. Pathol Res Pract 162: 133
225. Mene A, Buckley CH (1985) Involvement of the vulval skin appendages by intraepithelial neoplasia. Br J Obstet Gynaecol 92: 634
226. Merino MJ, LiVolsi VA, Schwartz PE, Rudnicki J (1982) Adenoid basal cell carcinoma of the vulva. Int J Gynecol Pathol 1: 299
227. Merlob P, Bahari C, Liban E, Reisner SH (1978) Cysts of the female external genitalia in the newborn infant. Am J Obstet Gynecol 132: 607
228. Michael H, Roth LM (1987) Paget's disease, skin appendage tumors, and congenital and acquired cysts of the vulva. In: Contemporary issues in surgical pathology. Pathology of the Vulva and Vagina. Vol. 9: 25 ed. Wilkinson, E.J. New York, Churchill Livingstone
229. Mihm MC, Clark WH, From L (1971) The clinical diagnosis, classification and histogenetic concepts of the early stages of cutaneous malignant melanomas. N Engl J Med 284: 1078
230. Milbrath JR, Wilkinson EJ, Friedrich EG (1975) Xerographic evaluation of radical vulvectomy specimens. Am J Roentgenol Radiat Ther Nucl Med 125: 486
231. Monacelli M, Nazzaro P (1966) Behcet's disease. Basel, Switzerland, S. Karger
232. Morales AR, Gould EW, Nadji M (1985) Immunocytochemistry in tumor diagnosis. Boston, Mass., Martinus Nijhoff
233. Morrow CP, Rutledge FN (1972) Melanoma of the vulva. Obstet Gynecol 39: 745
234. Muller G, Jacobs PH, Moore NE (1973) Scraping for human scabies. Arch Dermatol 107: 70
235. Nadji M, Ganjei P (1987) The application of immunoperoxidase techniques in the evaluation of vulvar and vaginal disease. In: Contemporary issues in surgical pathology. Pathology of the Vulva and Vagina. Vol. 9: 239 ed. Wilkinson, E.J. New York, Churchill Livingstone
236. Nadji M, Ganjei P, Penneys NS, Morales AR (1984) Immunohistochemistry of vulvar neoplasms: A brief review. Int J Gynecol Pathol 3: 41
237. Nadji M, Morales AR, Girtanner RE, Ziegels-Weissman J, Penneys NS (1982) Paget's disease of the skin: A unifying concept of histogensis. Cancer 50: 2203
238. Nahmias AM, Roizman B (1973) Infection with herpes simplex virus 1 and 2. N Engl J Med 289: 667
239. Nakao CY, Nolan JF, de Saia PJ, Futoran R (1974) Microinvasive epidermoid carcinoma of the vulva with an unexpected natural history. Am J Obstet Gynecol 120: 1122
240. Nauth HF, Boon ME (1983) Significance of the morphology of anucleated squames in the cytologic diagnosis of vulvar lesion. A new approach in diagnostic cytology. Acta Cytol 27: 330
241. Neill SM, Smith NP, Eady RA (1984) Ulcerative sarcoidosis: A rare manifestation of a common disease. Clin Exp Dermatol 9: 277
242. Neilson D, Woodruff JD (1972) Electron microscopy in in-situ and invasive vulvar Paget's disease. Am J Obstet Gynecol 113: 719
243. Newcomb PA, Weiss NS, Daling JR (1981) Incidence of

vulvar carcinoma in relation to menstrual, reproductive, and medical factors. JNCI 73: 391
244. Niebyl JR, Genadry R, Friedrich EG, Wilkinson EJ, Woodruff JD (1974) Vulvar carcinoma with hypercalcemia. Obstet Gynecol 45: 343
245. Novak ER, Woodruff JD (1979) Novak's gynecologic and obstetric pathology, 8th edn. Philadelphia, W.B. Saunders
246. Oberhofer TR, Back AE (1982) Isolation and cultivation of *Haemophilus Ducreyi*. J Clin Microbiol 15: 625
247. O'Duffy JD, Carney JA, Deodhar S (1971) Behcet's disease. Ann Int Med 75: 561
248. Oi RH, Munn R (1982) Mucous cysts of the vulvar vestibule. Hum Pathol 13(6): 584
249. Okagaki T (1981) "Warty carcinoma" of the vulva: A probable implication of human papilloma virus as the causative agent. Lab Invest 44: 49A
250. Okagaki T, Twiggs LB, Zachow KR, Clark BA, Ostrow RS, Faras AJ (1983) Identification of human papillomavirus DNA in cervical and vaginal intraepithelial neoplasia with molecularly cloned virus-specific DNA probes. Int J Gynecol Pathol 2: 153
251. Okagaki T, Clark BA, Zachow KR, Twiggs LB, Ostrow RS, Pass F, Faras AJ (1984) Presence of human papillomavirus in verrucous carcinoma (Ackerman) of the vagina. Arch Pathol Lab Med 108: 567
252. Olansky S (1972) Serodiagnosis of syphilis. Med Clin North Am 56: 1145
253. Ordonez NG, Manning JT, Luna MA (1981) Mixed tumor of the vulva: A report of two cases probably arising in Bartholin's gland. Cancer 48: 181
254. Oriel JD (1971) Natural history of genital warts. Br J Vener Dis 47: 1
255. Oriel JD, Almeida JD (1970) Demonstration of virus particles in human genital warts. Br J Vener Dis 46: 37
256. Oriel JD, Whimster IW (1971) Carcinoma in situ associated with virus-containing anal warts. Br J Dermatol 84: 71
257. Parker RT, Duncan I, Rampone J, Creasman W (1975) Operative management of early invasive epidermoid carcinoma of the vulva. Am J Obstet Gynecol 123: 349
258. Parmley TH, Woodruff JD, Julian CG (1975) Invasive vulvar Paget's disease. Obstet Gynecol 46: 341
259. Parry-Jones E (1963) Lymphatics of the vulva. J Obstet Gynaecol Br Commun 70: 751
260. Partridge EE, Murad T, Shingleton HM, Austin JM, Hatch KD (1980) Verrucous lesions of the female genitalia. I. Giant condylomata. Am J Obstet Gynecol 137: 412
261. Patanaphan V, Prempree T, Sewchand W, Hafiz MA, Jaiwatana J (1983) Adenocarcinoma arising in female urethral diverticulum. Urology 22: 259
262. Phillips GL, Twiggs LB, Okagaki T (1982) Vulvar melanoma: A microstaging study. Gynecol Oncol 14: 80
263. Pierson KK (1987) Malignant melanomas and pigmented lesions of the vulva. In: Contemporary issues in surgical pathology. Pathology of the Vulva and Vagina. Vol. 9: 155 ed. Wilkinson, E.J. New York, Churchill Livingstone
264. Pilotti S, Rilke F, Shah K, Torre GD, De Palo G (1984) Immunohistochemical and ultrastructural evidence of papilloma virus infection associated with in situ and microinvasive squamous cell carcinoma of the vulva. Am J Surg Pathol 8: 751
265. Pincus SH, Stadecker MJ (1987) Vulvar dystrophies and noninfectious inflammatory conditions. In: Contemporary issues in surgical pathology. Pathology of the Vulva and Vagina. Vol. 9: 11 ed. Wilkinson, E.J. New York, Churchill Livingstone
266. Pinkus H, Mehregan AH (1981) A guide to dermatohistopathology. New York, Appleton-Century-Crofts
267. Plentl AA, Friedman EA (1971) Lymphatic system of the female genitalia. Philadelphia, W.B. Saunders
268. Plouffe L, Tulandi T, Rosenberg A, Ferenczy A (1984) Non-Hodgkin's lymphoma in Bartholin's gland: Case report and review of literature. Am J Obstet Gynecol 148: 608
269. Podratz KC, Gaffey TA, Symmonds RE, Johansen KL, O'Brien PC (1983) Melanoma of the vulva: An update. Gynecol Oncol 16: 153
270. Portnoy J, Ahronheim GA, Ghibu F, Clecner B, Joncas JH (1984) Recovery of Epstein-Barr virus from genital ulcers. N Engl J Med 311(15): 966
271. Poulsen HE, Taylor CW, Sobin LH (1979) Histologic typing of female genital tract tumors. International Histologic Classification of Tumors, No. 13, Geneva, Switzerland, World Health Organization
272. Powell CS, Jones PA (1983) Carcinoma of the bladder with a metastasis in the clitoris. Br J Obstet Gynaecol 90: 380
273. Powell FC, Bjornsson J, Doyle JA, Cooper AJ (1985) Genital Paget's disease and urinary tract malignancy. J Am Acad Dermatol 13: 84
274. Powell JL, Franklin EW, Nickerson JF, Burrell, MO (1978) Verrucous carcinoma of the female genital tract. Gynecol Oncol 6: 565
275. Powell LC, Dinh TV, Rajaraman S, Hannigan EV, Dillard EA, Yandell RB, To T (1986) Carcinoma in situ of the vulva: A clinicopathologic study of 50 cases. J Reprod Med 31: 808
276. Prakash SS, Reeves WC, Sisson GR, Grenes M, Godoy J, Bacchetti S, de Britton RC, Rawls WE (1985) Herpes simplex virus type 2 and human papillomavirus type 16 in cervicitis, dysplasia and invasive cervical carcinoma. Int J Cancer 35: 51
277. Quick CA, Krzyzek RA, Watts SL, Faras AJ (1980) Relationship between condylomata and laryngeal papillomata. Clinical and molecular virological evidence. Ann Otol 89: 467
278. Radman HM (1981) Metastatic melanoma of the vulva. Md State Med J 30: 60
279. Rastkar G, Okagaki T, Twiggs LB, Clark BA (1982) Early invasive and in situ warty carcinoma of the vulva: Clinical, histologic, and electron microscopic study with particular reference to viral association. Am J Obstet Gynecol 143: 814
280. Reed RJ (1983) Neoplasms of the skin. In: Principles and practice of surgical pathology. New York, John Wiley & Sons
281. Reed RJ, Parkinson RP (1977) The histogenesis of molluscum contagiosum. Am J Surg Pathol 1: 161
282. Reeves KO, Kaufman RH (1980) Vulvar extopic breast

tissue mimmicking periclitoral abscess. Am J Obstet Gynecol 137: 509
283. Reid R (1985) Superficial laser vulvectomy: The efficacy of extended superficial ablation for refractory and very extensive condylomas. Am J Obstet Gynecol 151: 1047
284. Rhatigan RM, Nuss RC (1985) Keratoacanthoma of the vulva. Gynecol Oncol 21: 118
285. Ridley CM (1975) The vulva. Philadelphia, W.B. Saunders
286. Robboy SJ, Ross JS, Prat J, Keh PC, Welch WR (1978) Urogenital sinus origin of mucinous and ciliated cysts of the vulva. Obstet Gynecol 51: 347
287. Roberts TW, Melicow MM (1977) Pathology and natural history of urethral tumors in females. Review of 65 cases. Urology 10: 583
288. Roberts W, Daly JW (1981) Pseudosarcomatous fasciitis of the vulva. Gynecol Oncol 11: 383
289. Robertson AJ, McIntosh W, Lamont P, Guthrie W (1981) Malignant granular cell tumor (myoblastoma) of the vulva: Report of a case and review of the literature. Histopathology 5: 69
290. Rorat E, Wallach RC (1984) Mixed tumors of the vulva: Clinical outcome and pathology. Int J Gynecol Pathol 3: 323
291. Rorat E, Ferenczy A, Richart RM (1975) Human Bartholin gland, duct, and duct cyst. Arch Pathol 99: 367
292. Rosen T, Tschen JA, Ramsdell W, Moore J, Markham B (1984) Granuloma inguinale. J Am Acad Dermatol 11: 433
293. Roth LM, Panganiban (1978) Gonadal and extragonadal yolk sac carcinomas. A clinicopathologic study of 14 cases. Cancer 37: 812
294. Roth LM, Lee SC, Ehrlich CE (1977) Paget's disease of the vulva. A histogenetic study of five cases including ultrastructural observations and review of the literature. Am J Surg Pathol 1: 193
295. Sagabiel RW (1985) Regression and other factors of prognostic interest in malignant melanoma. Arch Dermatol 121: 1125
296. Salzman RS, Kraus SJ, Miller RG, Sottnek FO, Kleris GS (1984) Chancroidal ulcers that are not chancroid. Arch Dermatol 120: 636
297. Sarkany I, Taplin D, Blank H (1961) The etiology and treatment of erythrasma. J Invest Dermatol 37: 283
298. Sarrel PM, Steege JF, Maltzer M, Bolinsky D (1983) Pain during sex response due to occlusion of the Bartholin gland duct. Obstet Gynecol 62: 261
299. Schreiber MM (1963) Vulvar von Recklinghausen's disease. Arch Dermatol 88: 136
300. Schueller EF (1965) Basal cell cancer of the vulva. Am J Obstet Gynecol 93: 199
301. Sedlis A, Marshall R, Homesley H, Bundy B (1984) Positive groin lymph nodes in vulvar cancer with superficial tumor penetration. Society of Gynecologic Oncology, Miami, Florida, February 7
302. Seely JR, Bley R Jr, Altmiller CJ (1984) Localized chromosomal mosaicism as a cause of dysmorphic development. Am J Hum Genet 36: 899
303. Sehgal VN, Shyamprasad AL, Beohar PC (1984) The histopathological diagnosis of donovanosis. Br J Vener Dis 60: 45
304. Seiji M, Mizuno F (1969) Electron microscopic study of Bowen's disease. Arch Dermatol 99: 3
305. Seski JC, Reinholter ER, Silva J (1978) Abnormalities of lymphocyte transformations in women with intraepithelial carcinoma of the vulva. Obstet Gynecol 52: 332
306. Shafeek MA, Osman ME, Hussein MA (1979) Carcinoma of the vulva arising in condylomata acuminata. Obstet Gynecol 54: 120
307. Shane JM, Naftolin F (1975) Aberrant hormone activity by tumors of gynecologic importance. Am J Obstet Gynecol 121: 133
308. Shen JT, D'ablaing G, Morrow CP (1982) Alveolar soft part sarcoma of the vulva: Report of first case and review of literature. Gynecol Oncol 13: 120
309. Shevchuk MM, Richart RM (1982) DNA content of condyloma acuminatum. Cancer 49: 489
310. Sparling PF (1971) Diagnosis and treatment of syphilis. N Engl J Med 284: 642
311. Stage AH, Humeniuk JM, Easley WK (1984) Bullous pemphigoid of the vulva: A case report. Am J Obstet Gynecol 150: 169
312. Stapleton JJ (1984) Extramammary Paget's disease of the vulva in a young black woman. J Reprod Med 29: 444
313. Steeper T, Rosai J (1983) Aggressive angiomyxoma of the female pelvis and perineum. Am J Surg Pathol 7: 463
314. Steeper TA, Piscioli F, Rosai J (1983) Squamous cell carcinoma with sarcoma-like stroma of the female genital tract. Clinicopathologic study of four cases. Cancer 52: 890
315. Stegner HE (1986) Ultrastructure of preneoplastic lesions of the vulva. J Reprod Med 31: 815
316. Stehman FB, Castaldo TW, Charles EH, Lagasse LD (1980) Verrucous carcinoma of the vulva. Int J Gynaecol Obstet 17: 523
317. Stenchever MA, McDivitt RW, Fisher JA (1973) Leiomyoma of the clitoris. J Reprod Med 10: 75
318. Stening M (1980) Cancer and related lesions of the vulva. Balgowlah, Australia, ADIS Press
319. Stewart AF, Romero R, Schwartz PE, Kohorn EI, Broadus AE (1982) Hypercalcemia associated with gynecologic malignancies: Biochemical characterization. Cancer 49: 2389
320. Sutton GP, Smirz LR, Clark DH, Bennett JE (1985) Group B streptococcal necrotizing fasciitis arising from an episiotomy. Obstet Gynecol 66: 733
321. Talerman A (1973) Sarcoma botryoides presenting as a polyp on the labium majorus. Cancer 32: 994
322. Tavassoli FA, Norris HJ (1979) Smooth muscle tumors of the vulva. Obstet Gynecol 53: 213
323. Taylor PR, Stenwig JT, Klausen H (1975) Paget's disease of the vulva. Gynecol Oncol 3: 46
324. Taylor RN, Lacey CG, Shuman MA (1985) Adenocarcinoma of Skene's duct associated with a systemic coagulopathy. Gynecol Oncol 22: 250
325. Taylor RN, Bottles K, Miller TR, Braga CA (1985) Malignant fibrous histiocytoma of the vulva. Obstet Gynecol 66: 145
326. Thomas R, Barnhill D, Bibro M, Hoskins W (1985) Hidradenitis suppurativa: A case presentation and review of the literature. Obstet Gynecol 66: 592
327. Tiltman AJ, Knutzen VK (1978) Primary adenocarcinoma

of the vulva originating in misplaced cloacal tissue. Obstet Gynecol 51: 305
328. Turner AG, Hendry WF (1980) Primary carcinoma of the female urethra. Br J Urol 52: 549
329. Ubben K, Krzyzek R, Ostrow R, Bender M, Zelickson A, Faras A, Pass F (1979) Human papilloma virus DNA detected in two verrucous carcinomas. J Invest Dermatol 72: 195
330. Ulbright TM, Brokow SA, Stehman FB, Roth LM (1983) Epithelioid sarcoma of the vulva. Evidence suggesting a more aggressive behavior than extragenital epithelioid sarcoma. Cancer 52: 1462
331. Underwood JW, Adcock LL, Okagaki T (1978) Adenosquamous carcinoma of skin appendages (adenoid squamous cell carcinoma, pseudoglandular squamous cell carcinoma, adenoacanthoma of sweat glands of Lever) of the vulva. A clinical and ultrastructural study. Cancer 42: 1851
332. Ungerleider RS, Donaldson SS, Warnke RA, Wilbur JR (1978) Endodermal sinus tumor. The Stanford experience and the first reported case arising in the vulva. Cancer 41: 1627
333. Van Joost TH, Faber WR, Manuel HR (1980) Drug-induced anogenital cicatricial pemphigoid. Br J Dermatol 102: 715
334. Venter PF, Rohm GF, Slabber CF (1981) Giant neurofibromas of the labia. Obstet Gynecol 57: 128
335. Von Krogh G (1979) Warts: Immunologic factors of prognostic significance. Int J Dermatol 18: 195
336. Vontver LA, Reeves WC, Rattray M, Corey L, Remington MA, Tolentino E, Schweid A, Holmes KK (1979) Clinical course and diagnosis of genital herpes simplex virus infection and evaluation of topical surfactant therapy. Am J Obstet Gynecol 133: 548
337. Wade TR, Ackerman AB (1985) The effects of resin podophyllin on condyloma acuminatum. Am J Dermatopathol 6(2): 109
338. Wade TR, Kopf AW, Ackerman AB (1978) Bowenoid papulosis of the penis. Cancer 42: 1980
339. Wade TR, Kopf AW, Ackerman AB (1979) Bowenoid papulosis of the genitalia. Arch Dermatol 115: 306
340. Walker PG, Colley NV, Grubb C, Tejerina A, Oriel JD (1983) Abnormalities of the uterine cervix in women with vulvar warts. A preliminary communication. Br J Vener Dis 59(2): 120
341. Wallace HJ (1971) Lichen sclerosus et atrophicus. Trans St Johns Hosp Dermatol Soc 57: 9
342. Way S (1960) Carcinoma of the vulva. Am J Obstet Gynecol 79: 692
343. Way S (1982) Malignant disease of the vulva. Edinburgh, Scotland, Churchill Livingstone
344. Weed JC, Lozier C, Daniel SJ (1983) Human papilloma virus in multifocal, invasive female genital tract malignancy. Obstet Gynecol 62: 835
345. Weghaupt K, Gerstner GJ, Kucera H (1984) Radiation therapy for primary carcinoma of the female urethra: A survey over 25 years. Gynecol Oncol 17: 58
346. Wharton JT, Gallager S, Rutledge FN (1974) Microinvasive carcinoma of the vulva. Am J Obstet Gynecol 118: 159
347. Wheelock JB, Goplerud DR, Dunn LJ, Oates JF (1984) Primary carcinoma of the Bartholin gland: A report of ten cases. Obstet Gynecol 63: 820
348. Wick MR, Goellner JR, Wolfe JT, Su WPD (1985) Vulvar sweat gland carcinoma. Arch Pathol Lab Med 109: 43
349. Wilkinson EJ (1987) Superficially invasive carcinoma of the vulva. In: Contemporary issues in surgical pathology. Pathology of the Vulva and Vagina. Vol. 9: 103 ed. Wilkinson, EJ New York, Churchill Livingstone
350. Wilkinson EJ, Hause L (1974) Probability in lymph node sectioning. Cancer 33: 1269
351. Wilkinson EJ, Friedrich EG, Fu YS (1981) Multicentric nature of vulvar carcinoma in situ. Obstet Gynecol 58: 69
352. Wilkinson EJ, Morgan LS, Friedrich EG (1984) Association of Franconi's anemia and squamous-cell carcinoma of the lower female genital tract with condyloma acuminatum. J Reprod Med 29: 447
353. Wilkinson EJ, Rico MJ, Pierson KK (1982) Microinvasive carcinoma of the vulva. Int J Gynecol Pathol 1: 29
354. Wilkinson EJ, Hause LL, Hoffman RG, Kuzma JF, Rothwell DJ, Donegan WL, Clowry LC, Almagro UA, Choi J, Rimm A (1982) Occult axillary lymph node metastases in invasive breast carcinoma: Characteristics of the primary tumor and significance of the metastases. Pathol Annu 17(2): 67
355. Wisdom A (1973) Color atlas of venereology. Chicago Year Book
356. Woodruff JD (1985) Carcinoma in situ of the vulva. Clin Obstet Gynecol 28: 230
357. Woodruff JD, Friedrich EG (1985) The vestibule. Clin Obstet Gynecol 28: 134
358. Woodruff JD, Parmley TH (1983) Infection of the minor vestibular gland. Obstet Gynecol 62: 609
359. Woodruff JD, Richardson EH (1957) Malignant vulvar Paget's disease. Obstet Gynecol 10: 10
360. Woodruff JD, Williams TF (1959) The dopa reaction in Paget's disease of the vulva. Obstet Gynecol 14: 86
361. Woodruff JD, Borkowf HI, Holzman GB, Arnold EA, Knaack J (1965) Metabolic activity in normal and abnormal vulvar epithelia. Am J Obstet Gynecol 91: 809
362. Woodruff JD, Davis HJ, Jones HW, Recio RG, Salimi R, Park I (1969) Correlated investigative techniques of multiple anaplasias in the lower genital canal. Obstet Gynecol 33: 609
363. Woodworth H, Dockerty MB, Wilson RB, Pratt JH (1971) Papillary hidradenoma of the vulva: A clinicopathologic study of 69 cases. Am J Obstet Gynecol 110: 501
364. Word B (1968) Office treatment of cyst and abscess of Bartholin's gland duct. South Med J 61: 514
365. Work BA (1980) Pyoderma gangrenosum of the perineum. Obstet Gynecol 55: 126
366. Yackel DB, Symmonds RE, Kempers RD (1970) Melanoma of the vulva. Obstet Gynecol 35: 625
367. Yazigi R, Piver MS, Tsukada Y (1978) Microinvasive carcinoma of the vulva. Obstet Gynecol 51: 368
368. Yoonessi M, Goodell T, Satchidanand S, Fett W, Solis F (1983) Microinvasive squamous carcinoma of the vulva. J Surg Oncol 24: 315
369. Young AW, Herman EW, Tovell HMM (1980) Syringoma

of the vulva: Incidence, diagnosis, and cause of pruritus. Obstet Gynecol 55: 515

370. Young AW, Tovell HMM, Sadri K (1977) Erosions and ulcers of the vulva, incidence and management. Obstet Gynecol 50: 35
371. Young AW, Wind RM, Tovell HMM (1980) Lymphangioma of the vulva. NY State J Med 80: 987
372. Young RH, Scully RE (1985) Clear cell adenocarcinoma of the bladder and urethra. Am J Surg Pathol 9: 816
373. Zaino RJ (1987) Carcinoma of the vulva, urethra and Bartholin's gland. In: Contemporary issues in surgical pathology. Pathology of the Vulva and Vagina. Vol. 9: 119 ed. Wilkinson, E.J. New York, Churchill Livingstone
374. zur Hausen H (1982) Human genital cancer: Synergism between two virus infections or synergism between a virus infection and initiating events? Lancet 2: 1370
375. zur Hausen H, Gissman L, Schlehofer JR (1984) Viruses in the etiology of human genital cancer. Prog Med Virol 30: 170

4

Diseases of the Vagina

Alex Sedlis, M.D., and Stanley J. Robboy, M.D.

In this edition of the textbook, the pathologic changes related to in utero diethylstilbestrol (DES) exposure have been incorporated into the chapter on diseases of the vagina. This has been done in order to present an integrated review of various disease entities primarily affecting the vagina. However, for the sake of clarity, the DES pathology is presented in a separate section, as the various benign and malignant aspects of this entity are closely interrelated and involve other sites in the genital tract besides the vagina.

Anatomy

The vagina extends from the vestibule to the uterus, lying dorsal to the urinary bladder and ventral to the rectum. Its axis forms an angle of more than 90 degrees with that of the uterus (Fig. 4.1). It measures about 7 cm along its ventral wall and 9 cm along its dorsal wall. In early life, the vagina is constricted at its distal portion, dilated in the middle, and narrowed near the proximal end. The vagina surrounds the exocervix and forms vault-like vaginal fornices between its cervical attachment and the lateral wall. Several supports fix the vagina in position: the upper third is supported by the levator plate and indirectly through rectal attachments, the middle third is attached to the pelvic diaphragm and inferior aspects of cardinal ligaments, and the lower third is supported by the pelvic and urogenital diaphragm and the perineal body (Fig. 4.2).

Mucosa

The vaginal wall consists of three layers: mucosa, muscularis, and adventitia. The mucous membrane is thick and, on gross examination, shows a characteristic pattern of folds or rugae separated by furrows of variable depth. There are two longitudinal (anterior and posterior) and multiple transverse furrows (Fig. 4.3). The rugal pattern of the vaginal mucosa produces an undulating appearance on microscopic examination, in contrast to the flat surface of the cervix. The luminal surface is lined with nonkeratinized squamous epithelium, similar to cervical epithelium. The vaginal mucosa contains no glands. Its surface is lubricated by fluids that pass directly through the mucosa and by cervical mucus.

Vaginal epithelial cells proliferate and mature in response to stimulation by ovarian or exogenous estrogenic hormones. At the peak of estrogenic activity, e.g., the

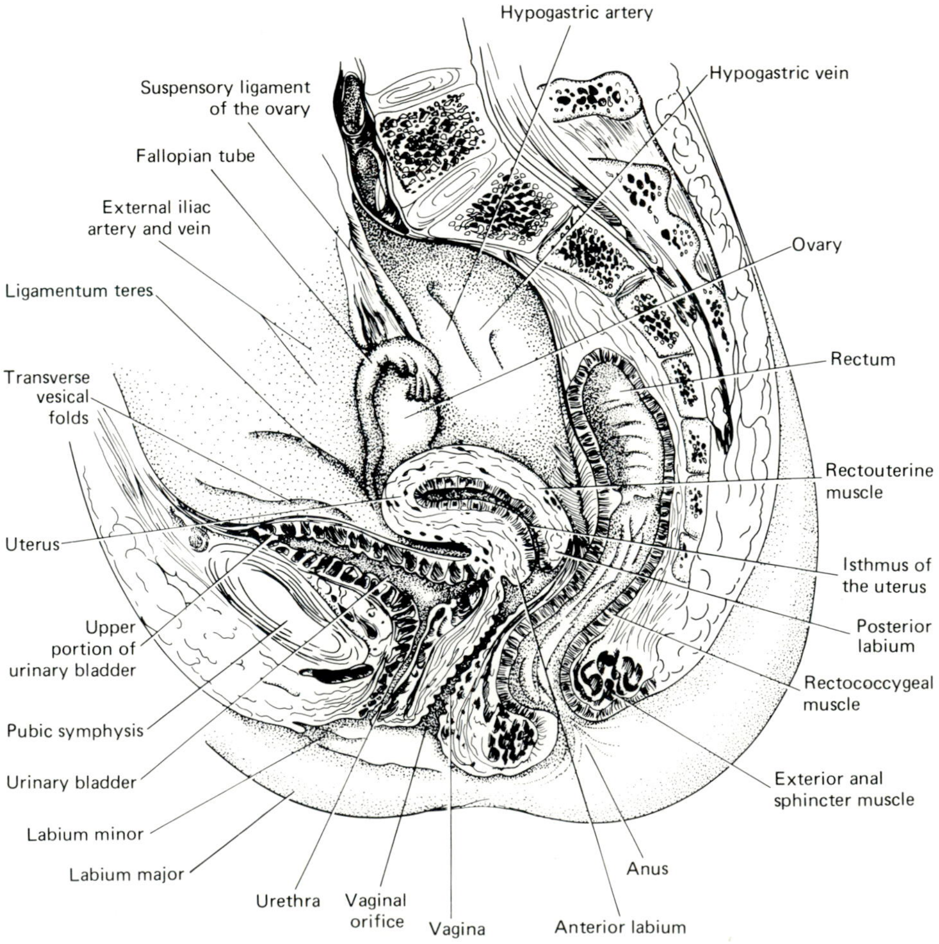

FIG. 4.1. Structural relationships of the vagina. Its axis forms an angle of more than 90 degrees with that of the uterus. [Modified from Clemente CD (ed) *Gray's Anatomy*, 30th ed., 1985. Courtesy of Lea & Febiger.]

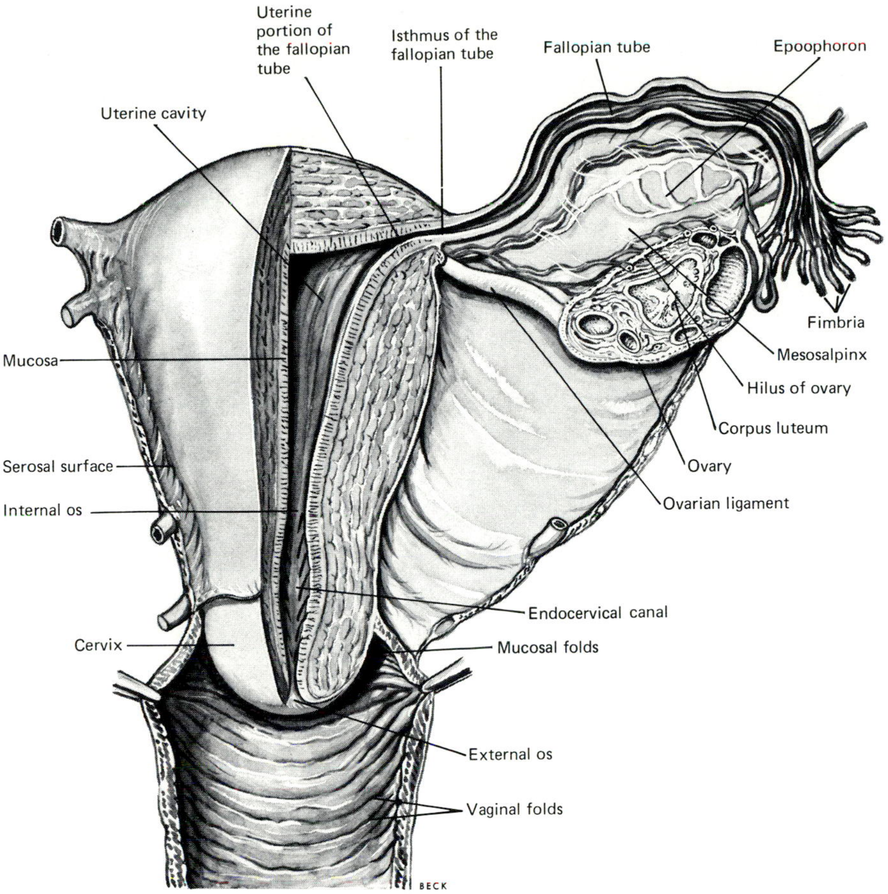

FIG. 4.2. Attachement of the vagina on the uterine wall, showing lateral process. [Modified from Clemente CD (ed) *Gray's Anatomy*, 30th ed., 1985. Courtesy of Lea & Febiger.]

preovulatory phase, the vaginal epithelium attains its maximum thickness, and superficial cells containing intracytoplasmic glycogen predominate in vaginal smears (Fig. 4.4) (see Chapter 25, Cytology). The glycogen is metabolized by *Lactobacillus Sp.*, normally present in the vagina, to lactic acid, which maintains a low vaginal pH, usually 4 to 5. An alternate view is that lactobacilli predominate in the acid environment by natural selection because they are acid resistant, however, their ability to produce acid is uncertain.[45] This view challenges the generally accepted notion that estrogen, glycogen, and lactic acid provide an effective barrier against colonization by pathogenic flora in the vagina.

Progesterone inhibits maturation of vaginal epithelium, consequently, the intermediate cells predominate in vaginal smears when the circulating levels of progesterone are high, e.g., during the postovulatory phase of the menstrual cycle or during pregnancy. Estrogenic activity is low or absent before puberty and after the menopause, and vaginal epithelium fails to mature and remains thin (Fig. 4.5). Parabasal and intermediate cells predominate in the vaginal smear. In the newborn child, the vaginal epithelium is frequently mature because of the influence of placental estrogens (Fig. 4.6).

Scanning electron microscopy shows the surface cells of the vaginal mucosa to be polygonal in outline and flattened. The surface of the cells is roughened, and terminal bars bridge adjacent cells (Fig. 4.7). The surface plasma membranes contain an intricate network of microridges (Fig. 4.8).

The submucosa, or lamina propria, is loosely textured and contains elastic fibers and a rich venous and lymphatic network. The muscular coats are composed of an outer longitudinal and an inner circular layer.

Vascular and Nerve Supply

The vaginal artery, which lies lateral to the vaginal axis, originates from the internal iliac, uterine, or other visceral branches of the internal iliac artery. It supplies the mucous membrane and wall of the vagina and anastomoses with the uterine, interior vesical, and middle rectal arteries. The branch of the uterine artery to the cervix

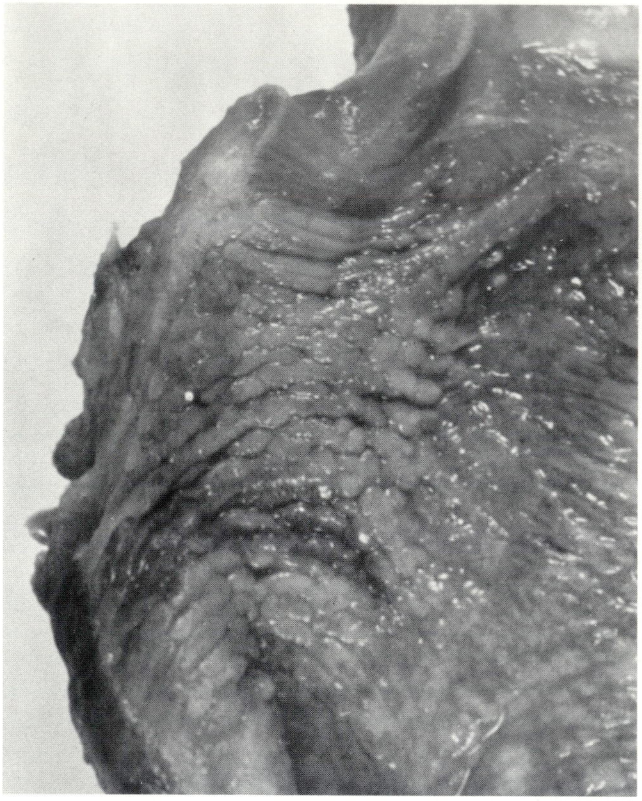

FIG. 4.3. Rugal folds of the vaginal mucosa.

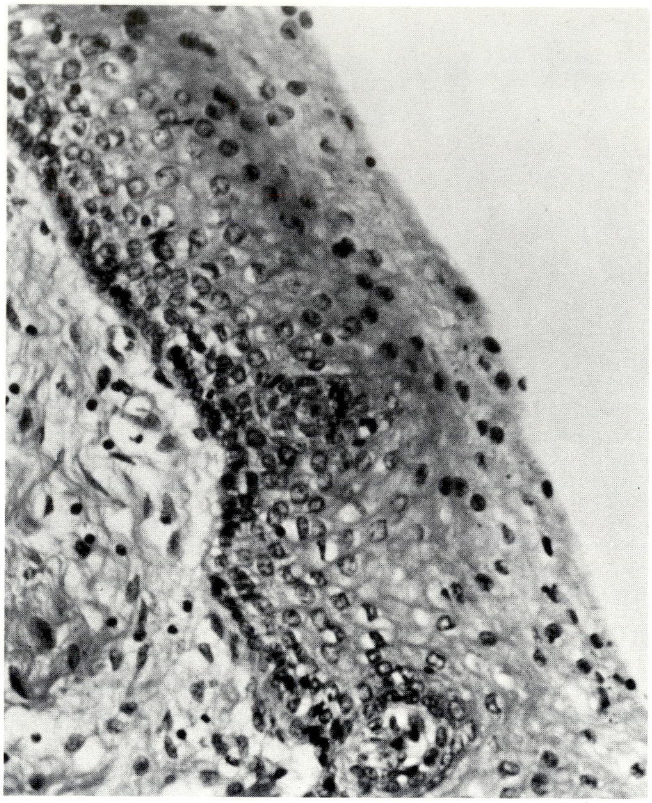

FIG. 4.5. Atrophic vagina with many layers of parabasal cells.

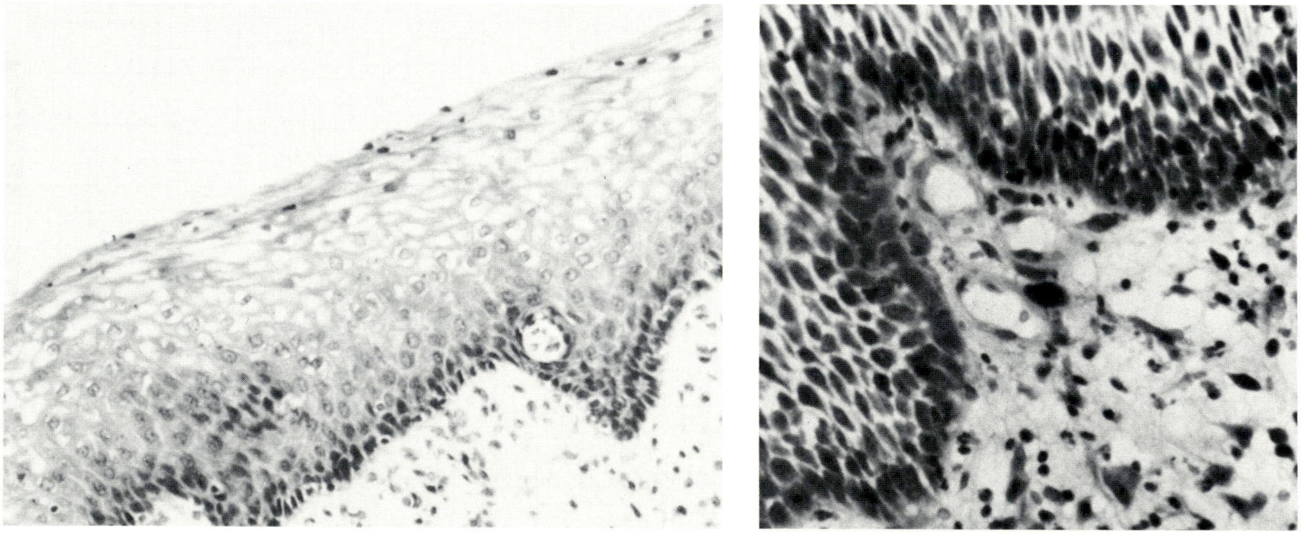

FIG. 4.4. Mucosa of the adult vagina. *Left:* Mature cells with glycogenic cytoplasm and pyknotic nuclei occupy most of the epithelial thickness. There is a single layer of dark basal cells and three to four layers of intermediate cells. *Right:* A high-power view of the basal and intermediate cells.

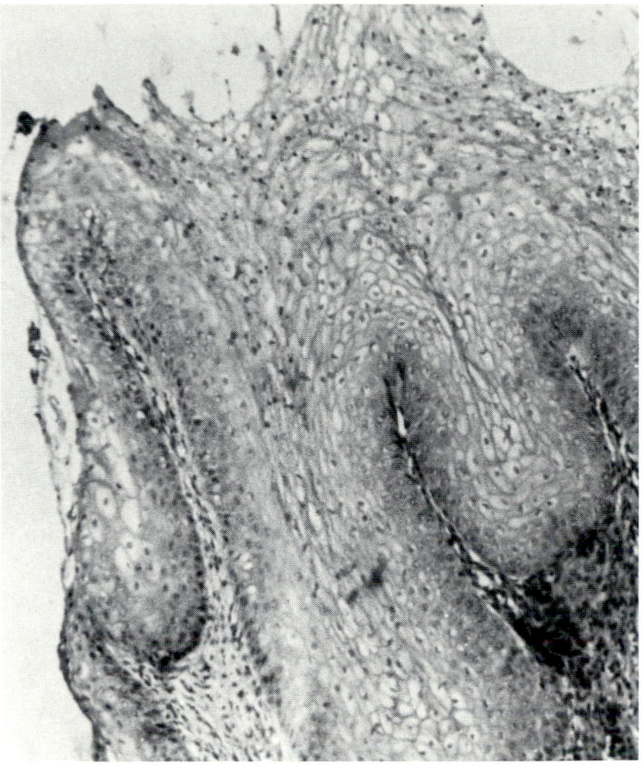

FIG. 4.6. Vaginal mucosa of a newborn. Mature cells predominate.

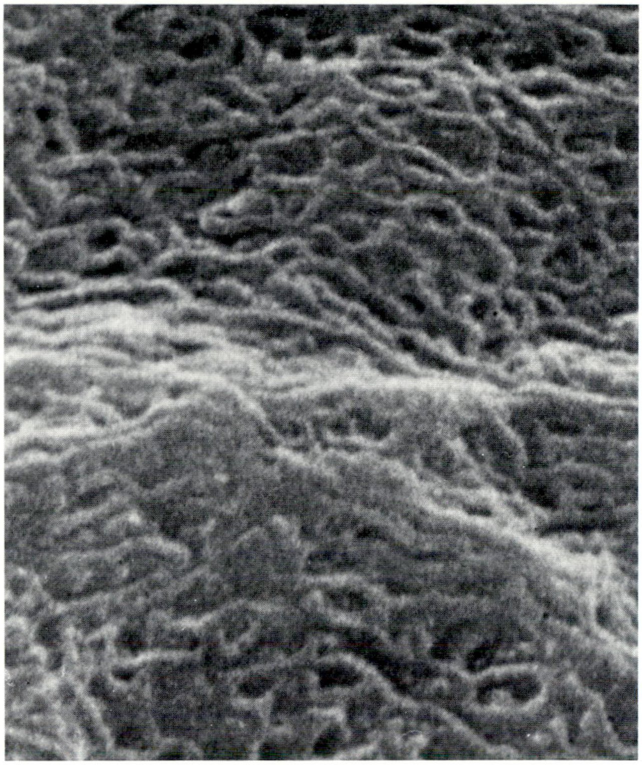

FIG. 4.8. Higher magnification of Figure 4.7, illustrating the surface of the most superficial squamous cells of the vaginal epithelium. The surface plasma membrane contains an intricate network of microridges. (Courtesy of A. Ferenczy, M.D.)

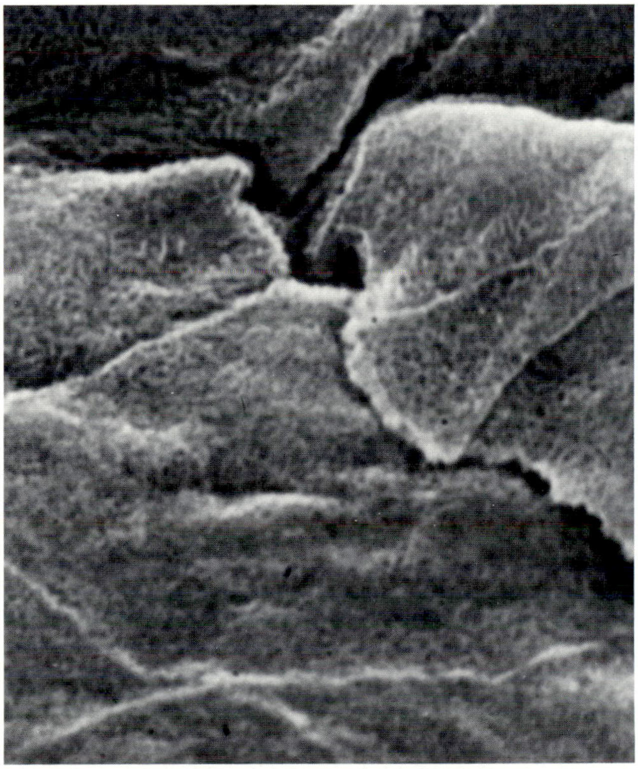

descends on the dorsal wall, forming the azygos artery of the vagina (Fig. 4.9).

The lower vagina is supplied by branches of the internal pudendal artery. The veins run along both sides, forming a plexus with the uterine, vesical, and rectal veins, ending in a branch that opens into the internal iliac vein (Fig. 4.10). The nerve supply derives from the lumbar plexus and pudendal nerve.

Lymphatic Drainage

The complex lymphatic drainage of the vagina proceeds through the perivaginal plexus at the lateral vaginal wall (Figs. 4.11 and 4.12) and is as follows:[70]

1. The lymphatic channels from the vaginal vault and upper anterior vagina communicate with the branches from the cervix uteri and drain into interiliac lymph nodes.

◁
FIG. 4.7. Scanning electron microscopy of normal vaginal epithelium. The most superficial cells have polygonal outlines and flattened cytoplasmic substance. Note the rough surface and well-developed terminal bars between adjacent superficial squamous cells. (Courtesy of A. Ferenczy, M.D.)

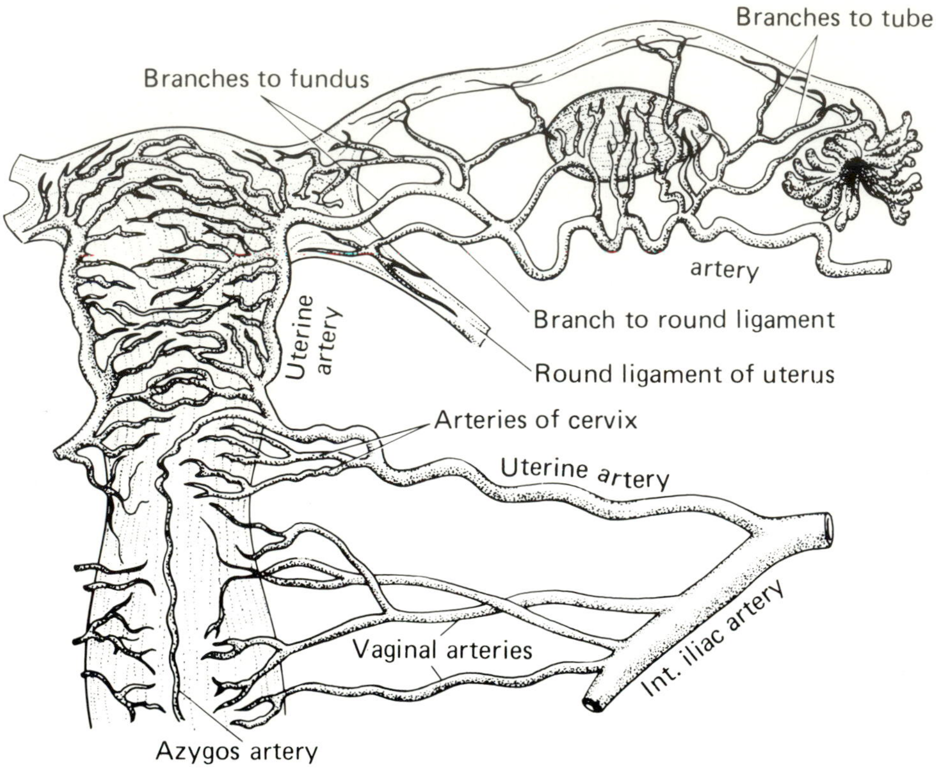

FIG. 4.9. Arterial blood supply of the vagina. [Modified from Clemente CD (ed) *Gray's Anatomy*, 30th ed., 1985. Courtesy of Lea & Febiger.]

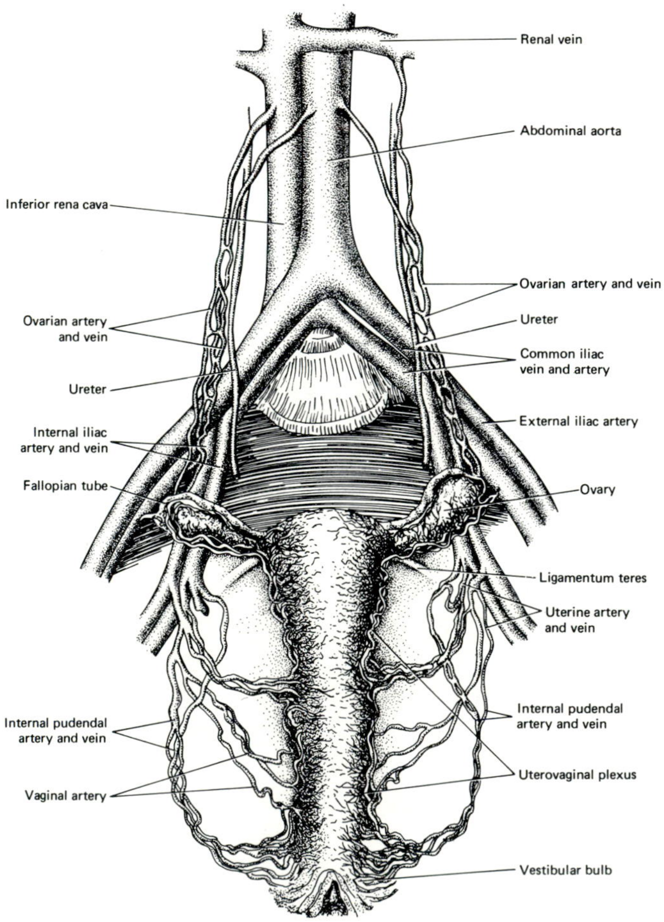

FIG. 4.10. Venous drainage of the vagina. [Modified from Clemente CD (ed) *Gray's Anatomy*, 30th ed., 1985. Courtesy of Lea & Febiger.]

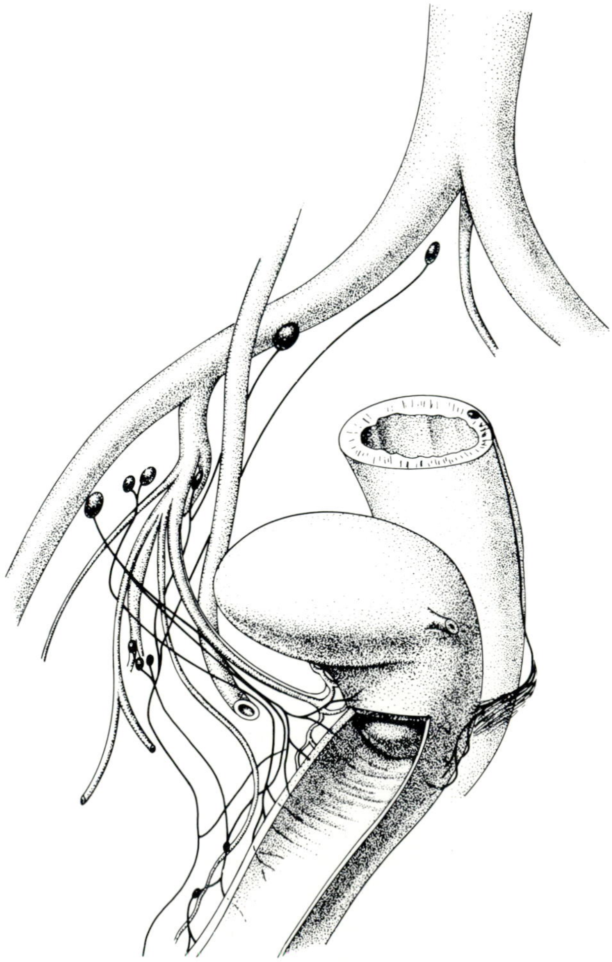

FIG. 4.11. Lymphatic drainage of the vagina. (Modified from Plentl and Friedman, Ref. 70.)

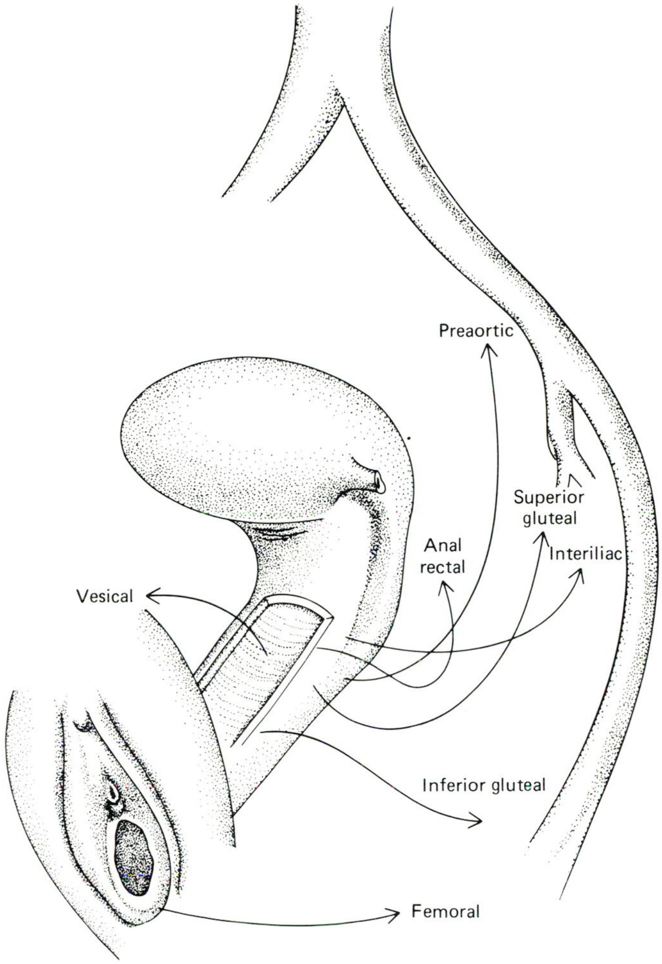

FIG. 4.12. Lymphatic drainage of the vagina. (Modified from Plentl and Friedman, Ref. 70.)

2. The lymph from the posterior aspect of the upper vagina drains into the inferior gluteal, sacral, and anorectal nodes.
3. The lowest portion of the vagina drains lymph to the femoral, inguinal, or pelvic nodes.
4. All pelvic lymph nodes as well as the nodes in the femoral triangle and anorectal region may be involved in lymphaic drainage of the vagina through anastamotic channels.

Congenital Anomalies

Congenital anomalies of the vagina include (1) complete or incomplete longitudinal vaginal septum, resulting from failure of müllerian (paramesonephric) duct fusion, (2) total atresia, and (3) transverse septum. (Double vagina and vaginal atresia are frequently associated with anomalies of the uterus and are described in Chapter 10, Benign Diseases of Endometrium.)

Transverse Septum

Transverse vaginal septum is one of the most frequent anomalies of the female genital tract. The septum may be complete, resulting in cryptomenorrhea and hematocolpos, or partial, with pinpoint openings allowing for drainage of menstrual flow. In the latter cases, the menstrual flow will be prolonged and scant. The location of the transverse septum is variable, occurring in the upper, middle, or lower third of the vaginal canal. The core of the septum is composed of stroma that contains smooth muscle bundles and blood vessels. The caudal side is lined by stratified squamous epithelium similar to the vaginal mucosa. The cranial side is often lined by mucinous columnar cells with squamous metaplasia, which resembles the normal lining of the endocervix (Fig. 4.13).

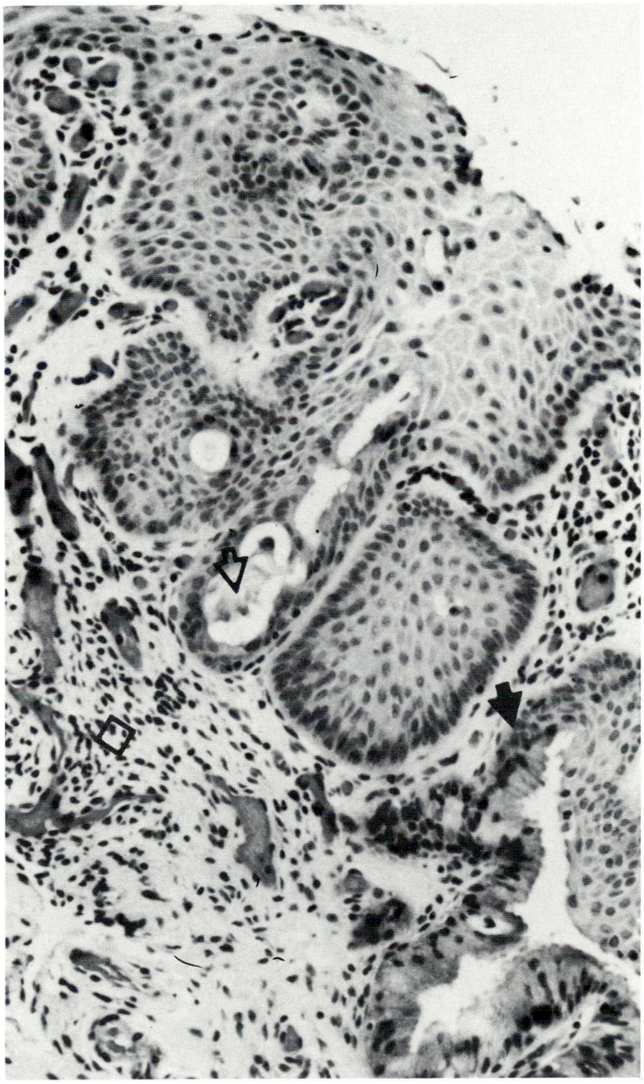

FIG. 4.13. Vaginal septum with adenosis. The cranial surface is lined by mucosa resembling the endocervix with mucinous cell-lined clefts and squamous metaplasia (*arrows*).

The origin of the glands in the transverse vaginal septum is thought to be similar to adenosis in diethylstilbestrol (DES)-exposed women. In both instances, the squamous epithelium of urogenital sinus origin is prevented from reaching the upper portion of the vagina during embryonic development (see Chapter 1, Embryology). According to one theory,[103] the vaginal wall derives from the müllerian (paramesonephric) duct, the mucosa of which eventually becomes replaced by squamous epithelium of endodermal origin, growing craniad from the urogenital sinus. The transverse septum blocks the craniad progression of the squamous epithelium; consequently, the upper vagina, including the upper surface of the transverse septum, retains the columnar epithelium of embryonic müllerian origin. The transverse septa that develop in relation to DES exposure are described later in this chapter.

Cysts of the Vagina

Gartner's duct cysts, vestigial remnants of the wolffian (mesonephric) duct, are common. They are located in the anterolateral or lateral wall of the vagina. The large cysts can protrude through the introitus; the small cysts are incidental findings. The cysts are lined by low cuboidal epithelium that is not ciliated (Fig. 4.14). A single case of adenocarcinoma presumably arising from a Gartner's duct cyst has been reported.[17] Inclusion cysts commonly follow birth trauma or surgery. The cyst wall is lined with squamous epithelium. The development of cysts related to adenosis that becomes cystic is described later in this chapter. Mucous cysts located in the vestibular area are presented in Chapter 3, Diseases of Vulva.

Adenosis

Most cases of vaginal adenosis have been linked to prenatal exposure to DES, however, adenosis may be unrelated to in utero DES exposure. Patients with adenosis unrelated to DES range in age from 25 to 62 years (median 39 years) and present with watery or mucoid discharge and pain or bleeding after intercourse. The lesions on clinical examination appear patchy or diffuse, red and stippled, granular or nodular, and as single or multiple cysts or ulcers. On occasion, the process extends onto the vulva. As adenosis has become a more recognized condition, increasing numbers of asymptomatic lesions have been encountered.

Microscopically, non-DES related adenosis is usually composed of mucinous columnar cells, but, occasionally, tuboendometrial cells are noted. Both types of cells have been found in association with clear cell adenocarcinoma, with atypical adenosis being present also in an occasional patient. The appearances of adenosis and clear cell adenocarcinoma are similar in both DES- and non-DES-exposed women. The major difference is that in DES-exposed women, the adenosis is more extensive and occurs at a younger age. The cancer also occurs at a younger age in DES-exposed women.[77]

Inflammatory Disorders

Infectious Diseases

Vaginitis, a common disorder, is caused by bacteria, viruses, fungi, and parasites.

Gonorrhea

The many-layered vaginal mucosa of the adult is resistant to *Neisseria gonorrhoeae*, but in children, the organism readily penetrates the thin vaginal mucosa and enters the submucosa. It produces edema, hyperemia, round cell infiltration, and clinical manifestations of purulent vaginitis.

Gardnerella

Gardnerella vaginalis[26] (formerly *Haemophilus vaginalis*) is the most common infectious agent in the vagina, accounting for 90% of nonspecific infections. Clinically,

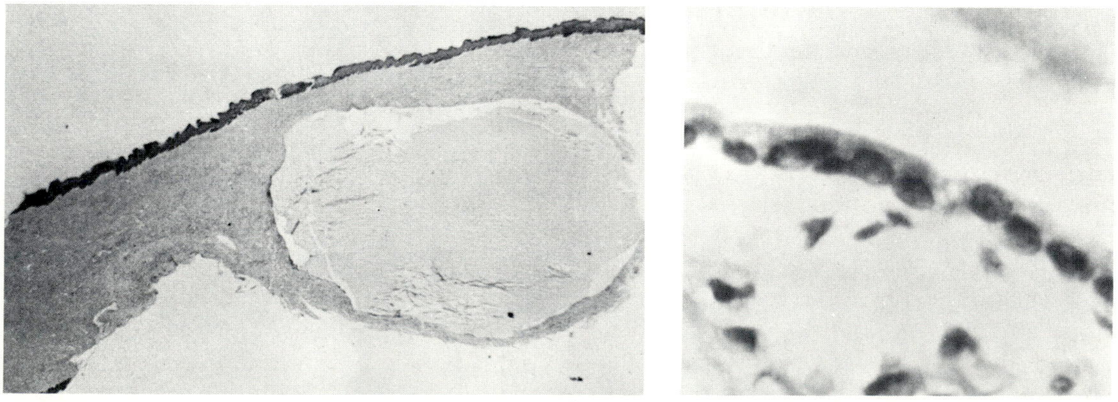

FIG. 4.14. *Left:* Gartner's duct cyst. *Right:* Lining epithelium of the cyst.

the infection is characterized by a nonirritating, malodorous vaginal discharge, a vaginal pH higher than 4.5, and elaboration of a fishy odor from the vaginal fluid after alkalinization with 10% potassium hydroxide. The organism is a minute, rod-shaped, gram-negative bacillus, transmitted by sexual intercourse. The diagnosis is made by examining wet mount preparations and identifying clue cells, epithelial cells in which the microorganisms are clumped over the cell's surface (see Chapter 25, Cytology). The organism does not penetrate the mucosa or evoke an inflammatory reaction.

It is now believed that several species of vaginal bacteria interact to produce the nonspecific vaginitis that is now termed, more appropriately, *bacterial vaginosis.*[95]

Candidiasis

Vaginal candidiasis manifests itself by vulvar pruritis and vaginal discharge. Inspection of the vagina reveals thrush, a thick, white, tree bark-like exudate that adheres to the vaginal mucosa in plaques. When the exudate is wiped away, the underlying vaginal mucosa appears red due to vascular congestion. *Candida albicans*, the causative organism, is a yeast-like fungus recognized readily on a wet smear preparation with normal saline or 10% potassium hydroxide. On microscopic examination, the organisms occur as blastospores, oval cells multiplying by budding, and as branching tubular hyphae. A complex of intertwining and branching hyphae is termed a *mycelium.* The fungus focally penetrates into the superficial layer of the vaginal epithelium, which can be demonstrated by performance of a biopsy before the thrush is wiped off.[53] Other microscopic changes observed in the mucosa are capillary congestion and inflammatory cell infiltration.

The diagnosis may be established either by demonstration of the fungus on wet smear preparation or on Sabouraud's medium. Approximately 3% of asymptomatic women harbor *Candida* in their vagina.[53] *Candida* becomes pathogenic when its growth is facilitated by immunosuppression or lack of inhibition by normal vaginal flora, e.g., after broad-spectrum antibiotic treatment. The role of sexual transmission is not clear.

Trichomoniasis

Trichomonas vaginalis has been recognized as a source of vaginal infection for nearly 150 years. The organism is a unicellular protozoan with prominent flagella that render it actively mobile. It is fusiform in shape and measures 15–30 μm (see Chapter 25, Cytology). The mobile protozoan may be recognized on wet smear preparations and in smears stained for routine cytology. Vaginal biopsies for *Trichomonas*, although rarely performed, disclose in hyperemic areas (so-called strawberry spots) edema, ulcerations, minute hemorrhages, and infiltration by leukocytes, lymphocytes, and plasma cells (Fig. 4.15). The infection is transmitted by sexual contact and, rarely, through contaminated clothes, towels, or bed linen.

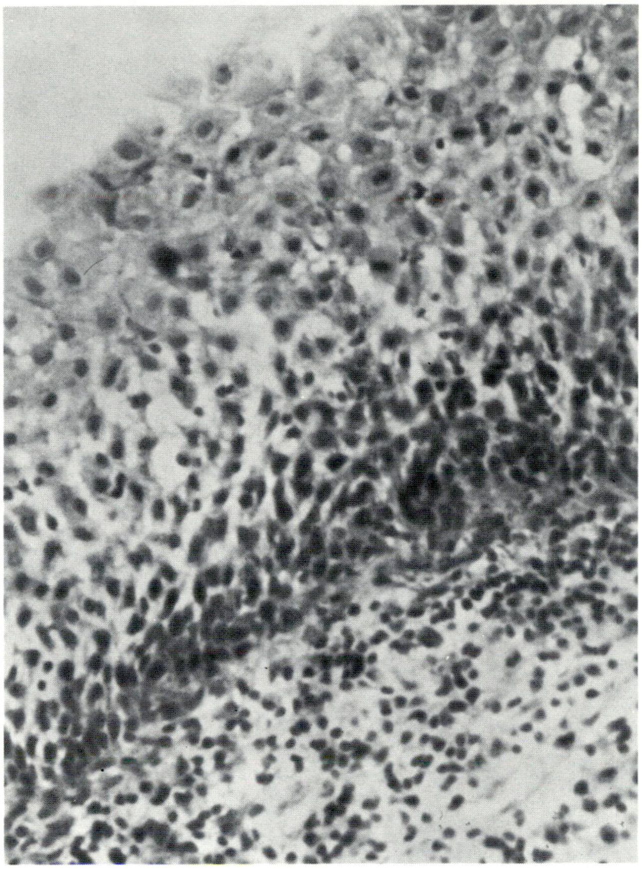

FIG. 4.15. Trichomoniasis. There is edema in the epithelial layer and leukocytic and lymphocytic infiltration in the submucosa.

Syphilis

The vaginal mucosa may manifest any stage of infection with *Treponema pallidum:* the primary chancre, condylomas of the secondary stage, and a gumma of the tertiary stage. The same histologic features are seen in the vagina as elsewhere (see Chapter 3, Diseases of the Vulva).

Parasitic Vaginitis

Entamoeba histolytica affects the colon primarily but secondarily may involve the upper vagina or cervix.[6] This is an uncommon occurrence and is found most often in tropical countries in areas where hygiene is poor. Genital schistosomiasis has been reported in Africa, South America, and the West Indies. It occurs in patients who have infestations of the pelvic venous plexuses by *Schistosoma mansoni* or *Schistosoma haematobium* (see Chapter 3, Diseases of Vulva).

Human Papillomavirus

The vaginal mucosa is a frequent site of human papillomavirus (HPV) infection. A detailed discussion of HPV infection, including pathology, virology, and its possible role in neoplasia, is found in Chapter 3, Diseases of Vulva, and Chapter 7, Cervical Intraepithelial Neoplasia.

The vaginal lesions have an appearance similar to those on the exocervix, both developing from the squamous epithelial mucosa. The basic alterations are excesive proliferation of the stromal papillae and the squamous epithelium. The affected squamous epithelial cells exhibit characteristic viral cytopathic effects: perinuclear vacuolization (koilocytosis), enlarged hyperchromatic nuclei with wrinkling of the nucleus, parakeratosis of superficial cells, and single cell dyskeratosis in deeper layers. The lesion, if macroscopically visible, appears as a raised growth with finger-like projections, the size being commensurate with the degree of hypertrophy of the stromal papillae. Surface keratinization imparts a pearly white appearance to the lesions. Early lesions are often macroscopically invisible. On colposcopic examination, the early lesions frequently have a granular surface and whiten upon application of 3% acetic acid. Both vaginal and cervical condylomas appear to be capable of undergoing neoplastic transformation, i.e., dysplasia and carcinoma in situ, manifested by nuclear pleomorphism, increased numbers of mitotic figures, and abnormal mitoses. The neoplastic changes are particularly frequent in immunosuppressed patients, e.g., the renal transplant patient (see section, Vaginal Intraepithelial Neoplasia).

Other Vaginitides

Staphylococcus aureus, *Streptococcus pyogenes*, *Escherichia coli*, *Mycoplasma*, and *Chlamydia* all have been cultured from the vagina of women with vaginitis. The exact role these organisms play in the causation of infection has not been determined. *Leptothrix* is usually found in association with trichomonas vaginitis, but this organism has not been identified as a sole cause of infection. Tuberculosis infection in the vagina is extremely rare. The appearance of the lesion is similar to that found in other sites, i.e., granulomas with or without caseation.

Noninfectious Diseases

Ulcers in Association with Uterine Prolapse

Keratinization, abrasions, and pressure ulcers may develop when the vaginal mucosa is exposed to repeated trauma. Deep ulcers also occur from pressure necrosis trauma caused by the use of vaginal pessaries.

Prolapsed Fallopian Tube

Prolapse of the fallopian tube into the vault of the vagina is an uncommon complication of vaginal surgery. The prolapse may become symptomatic because of bleeding after intercourse. Physical examination discloses a small, granular, bleeding mass in the apex of the vagina. Microscopically, the lesion may be confused with adenocarcinoma. Unlike carcinoma, however, the epithelial cells found in the prolapsed tube show no atypia or mitoses and are arranged in a single layer. Often, the structure of the fallopian tube may be recognized by its characteristic club-shaped mucosal fronds, which contain abundant connective tissue stroma (Fig. 4.16).

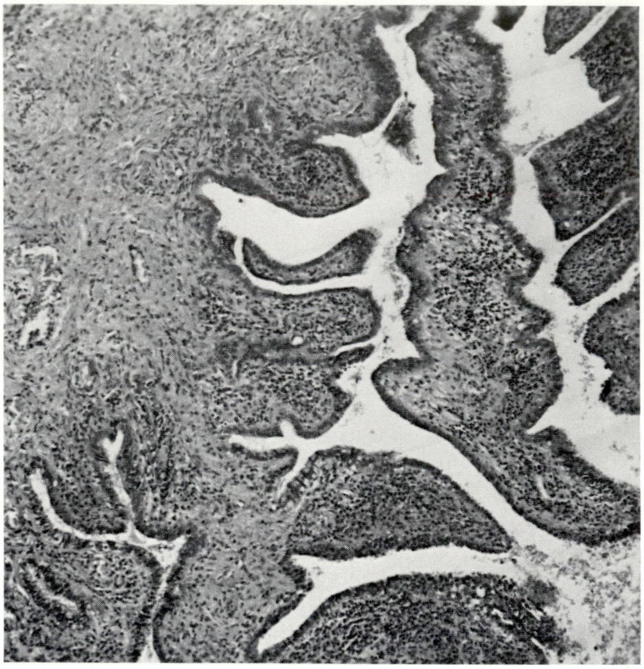

FIG. 4.16. Prolapsed fallopian tube.

Ulcers in Association with Use of Vaginal Tampons (Including Toxic Shock Syndrome)

Vaginal tampons may produce various lesions in the vaginal mucosa. Some lesions are grossly visible as shallow ulcers with smooth edges, but more subtle changes require colposcopy for their detection. These lesions are described as (1) layering produced by peeling of small sheets of superficial squamous epithelial cells from the underlying cell layers and (2) microulcerations that develop when the epithelial peeling reaches the underlying stroma.[19] The tampon lesions are transient and quickly disappear when the use of tampons is discontinued. The microscopic appearance reflects variable degrees of damage to the mucosa, ranging from epithelial peeling and congestion of stromal blood vessels to complete loss of epithelium, ulceration and replacement by granulation tissue.

Vaginal ulcerations in tampon users have been considered as a portal of entry for *S. aureus* and its toxic products in patients with toxic shock syndrome (TSS). Toxic shock syndrome, which was first described in 1978,[102] is characterized by fever, diffuse erythematous rash, and hypotension. In addition, there are symptoms involving at least three of the following organs and systems: gastrointestinal, muscular, mucous membranes, renal, liver, cardiovascular, and central nervous system. Serologic tests remain negative in patients with TSS. The desquamation of cutaneous lesions occurs in 1–2 weeks from the onset of illness.[104] It is now believed that the syndrome is caused by the release into the circulation of enterotoxin F and pyrogenic exotoxin C by the *S. aureus* phage group 1.

Over 1000 instances of TSS have been reported since 1978, with a fatality rate of 5.9%. The findings on postmortem examination include perivasculitis, predominantly in the skin, mucous membranes, lungs, and kidney. The vaginal mucosa shows edema, ulceration, and perivasculitis. The lungs are focally hemorrhagic and edematous, with hyaline membrane formation. The liver reveals periportal inflammation and microscopic fatty infiltration. The kidneys show acute tubular necrosis.[64] Toxic shock syndrome is not confined to female tampon users. Although 90% of reported patients with TSS have been females at or near the time of menstruation, most of whom used vaginal tampons, TSS occurs also in females using polyurethane vaginal contraceptive sponges and in males.

Emphysematous Vaginitis

The frequency of emphysematous vaginitis (vaginitis emphysematosa, colpocervicitis cystica, emphysema vaginae, colpocervicitis emphysematosa) is low, judging from the approximately 200 cases reported to date. No symptoms are produced in the majority of cases, although popping sounds have been described caused by release of gas from the cystic spaces. Vaginal examination may show gas-filled blebs projecting above the mucosal surface. They vary in size from pinhead to 2 cm in greatest dimension, may be few to extensive, and may be clustered or diffusely scattered on the exocervix or vagina (Fig. 4.17). The air-filled spaces may be visible on x-ray examination.[44]

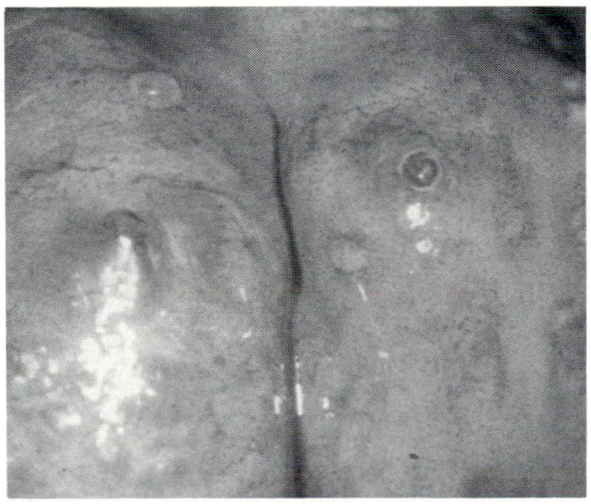

FIG. 4.17. Emphysematous vaginitis, colposcopic view. Note the air-filled blebs.

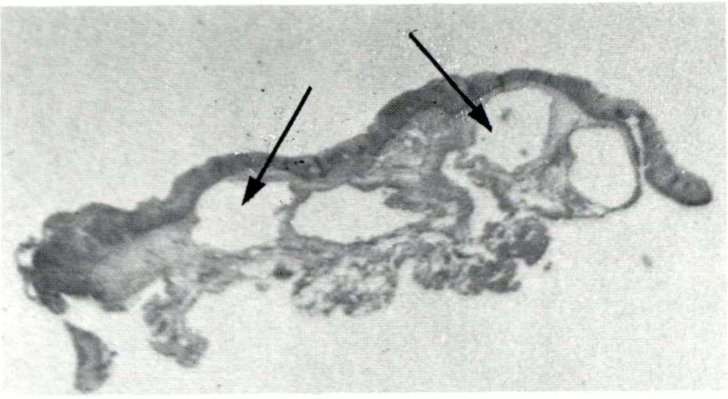

FIG. 4.18. Emphysematous vaginitis. Submucosal blebs (*arrows*).

On microscopic examination, the mucosa is usually intact, and the cystic spaces are found in the lamina propria (Fig. 4.18). Lymphocytes, histiocytes, and multinucleated giant cells surround the cysts (Fig. 4.19). The exact etiology of emphysematous vaginitis is not known. Although *Trichomonas vaginalis* is frequently associated with emphysematous vaginitis, its role in pathogenesis has not been documented.

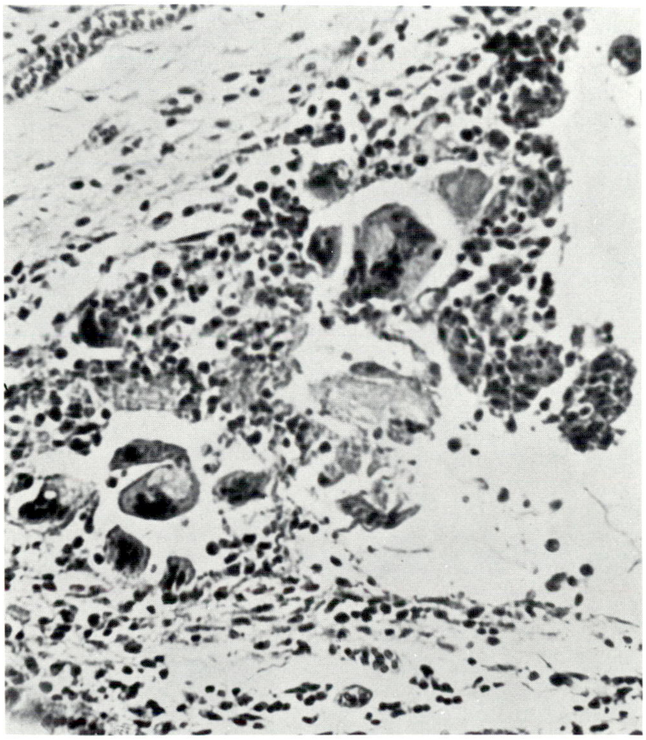

FIG. 4.19. Emphysematous vaginitis. Cystic spaces surrounded by histiocytes, multinucleate giant cells, and lymphocytes.

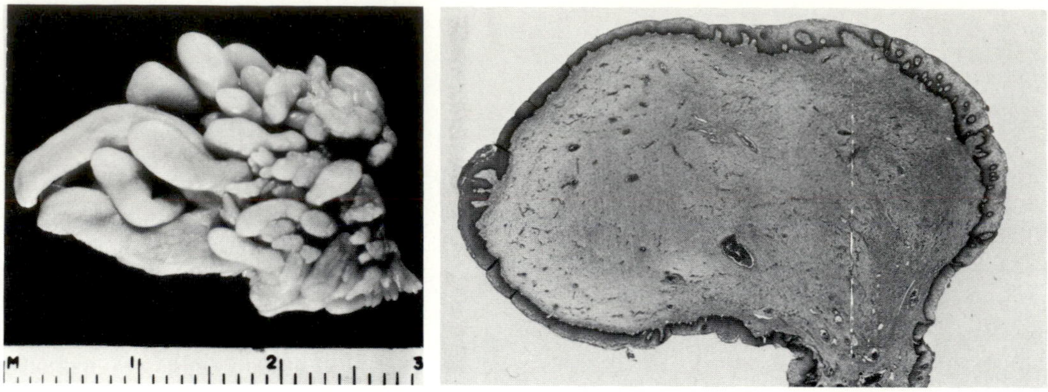

FIG. 4.20. Fibroepithelial polyp. *Left:* Gross; note finger-like projections. *Right:* Microscopic view; note squamous epithelial lining. (Courtesy of H. J. Norris, M.D.)

Benign Tumors and Tumor-Like Conditions

Fibroepithelial Polyp

Vaginal polyps, described initially in 1966,[61] are generally single, occasionally have multiple finger-like projections, and measure up to 1.5 cm in diameter (Fig. 4.20).[8,54] They are rubbery in consistency and usually have a pedicle. The surface is covered by squamous epithelium, and the stroma is composed of loose fibrous connective tissue. Large atypical stromal cells are present in about half of the patients[8] and are characterized by delicate pointed cytoplasmic processes and hyperchromatic, pleomorphic, sometimes triangular nuclei with occasionally prominent nucleoli (Fig. 4.21). Mitotic figures are uncommon and rarely exceed three per 10 high-power fields.

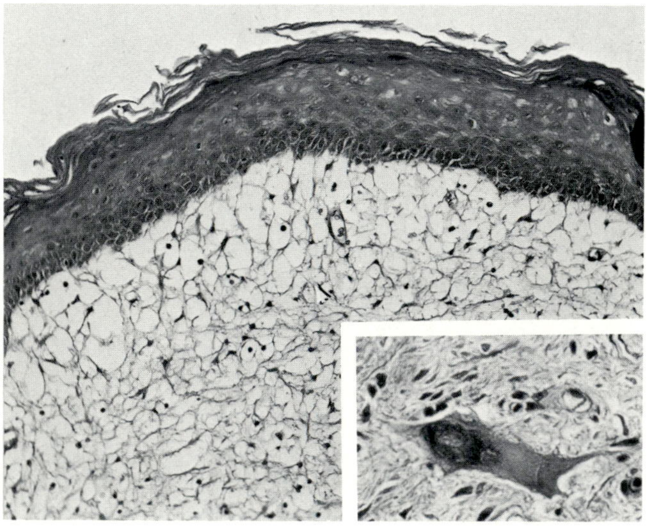

FIG. 4.21. Fibroepithelial polyp. High-power view of an atypical stromal cell. (Courtesy of H. J. Norris, M.D.)

According to Elliot and Elliot,[18] the polyps arise from a myxomatous zone of subepithelial mesenchyme that extends from the endocervix to the vulva. As atypical nuclei are frequently found in the myxomatous zone of the normal vaginal mucosa, the polyps may represent a focal hyperplasia of this zone. Fibroepithelial polyps are benign and do not recur after simple excision. These polyps are frequently confused with embryonal rhabdomyosarcoma (sarcoma botryoides) but may be differentiated because they lack the hypercellular cambium layer, the primitive round cells with mitotic figures, and the rhabdomyoblasts.

Leiomyoma

Leiomyomas arise in the submucosal layer and are usually located in the rectovaginal septum. They vary in size and, on occasion, can form pedunculated masses that project into the vaginal canal. The microscopic appearance is similar to that of leiomyomas elsewhere. Interlacing bundles of spindle-shaped, smooth muscle cells contain elongated nuclei with rounded ends (Fig. 4.22).

Variants of leiomyoma include the epithelioid leiomyoma, which is characterized by plump cells with abundant clear or eosinophilic cytoplasm. The mitotic count is important in differentiating leiomyomas from locally recurrent or metastatic leiomyosarcomas. Recurrences have not been found in tumors with less than five mitotic figures per 10 high-power fields.[100]

Fibroma

A fibroma is composed of fibroblasts that differ from leiomyoma in that they have more elongated and wavy nuclei with pointed ends. The cells of fibromas are

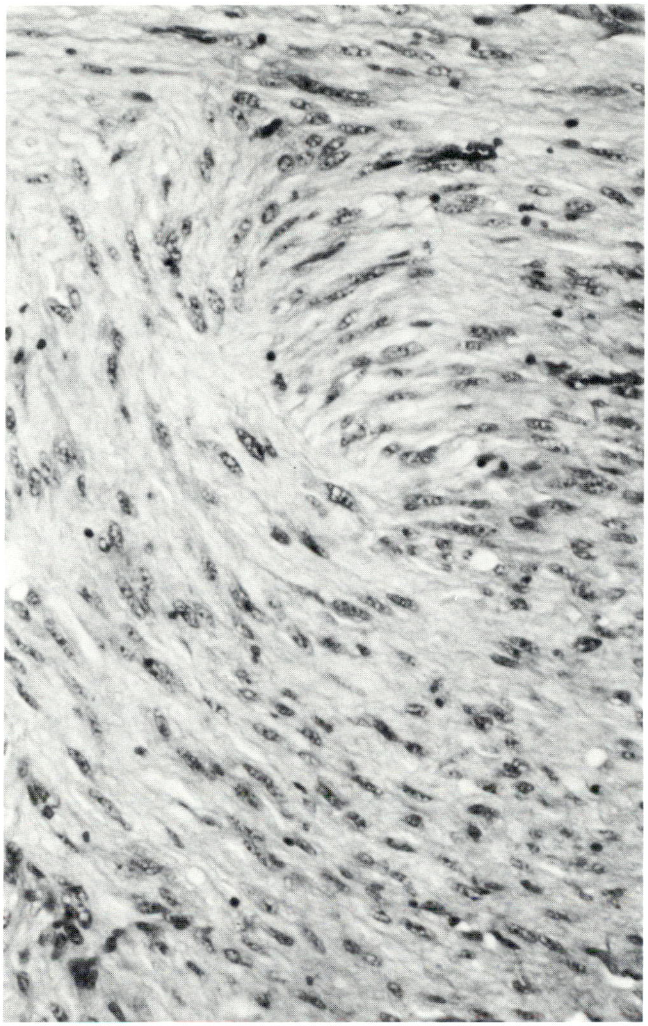

Fig. 4.22. Leiomyoma composed of interlacing bundles of smooth muscle. The cells are plump and fusiform.

smaller, and the intercellular substance contains abundant collagen fibers. The neurofibroma resembles the fibroma but contains serpentine cytoplasmic processes.[100]

Rhabdomyoma

Rhabdomyoma of the vagina is an extremely rare benign tumor.[24] The tumors are small (Fig. 4.23), multilobulated, pale tan, smooth, and glistening. Microscopically, they are nonencapsulated and poorly defined. The rhabdomyoma is composed of broad interlacing bundles of striated muscle cells in a dense connective tissue stroma and covered by an intact squamous epithelium. The tumor cells are uniformly large and vary from round to oval to an elongated strap form (Fig. 4.24). Usually only one nucleus with a large nucleolus is present in each cell, although two nuclei have been seen occasionally in the strap form. No nuclear atypia or mitoses are present. The abundant cytoplasm is eosinophilic, with longitudinal fibrils and cross-striations in many areas. The collagenous stroma contains mast cells and dilated, thin-walled vascular spaces. Electron microscopic examination shows rhabdomyocytes with sarcomeres containing A, I, and Z bands and M line (Fig. 4.25). Rhabdomyomas occurring in the female genital tract differ from fetal rhabdomyomas primarily in their more abundant intercellular stroma and their larger, more mature muscle cells.

Mixed Tumor

The mixed tumor of the vagina is a rare neoplasm located proximal to the hymen[7,94] (Fig. 4.26). The tumors are composed of three elements. The stroma consists of small bland cells with spindle-shaped nuclei, showing rare mitosis, and intercellular substance containing abundant collagen. Islands of glycogenated and sometimes keratin-

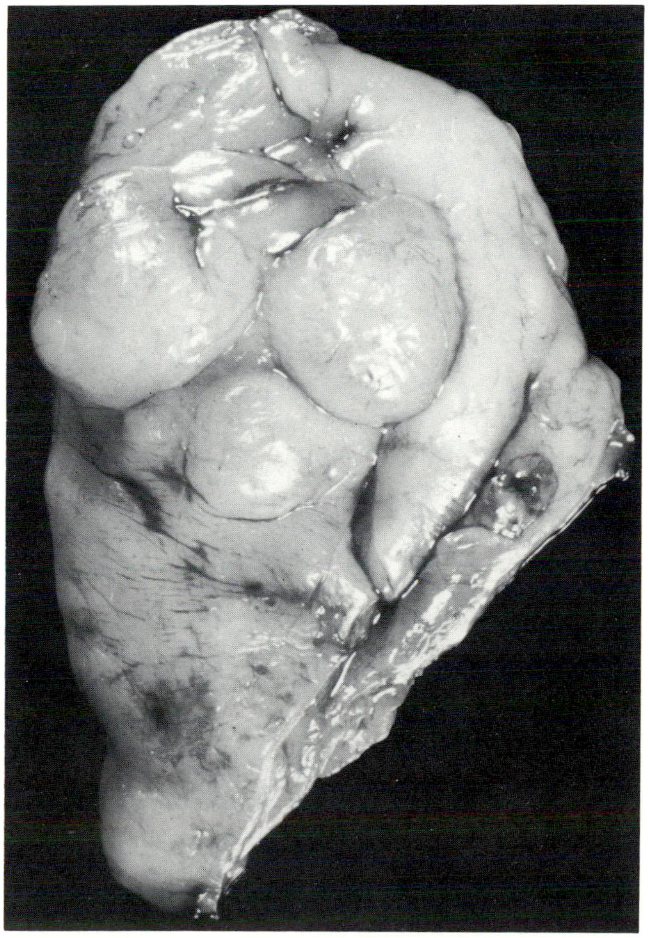

Fig. 4.23. Rhabdomyoma of vagina. The tumor is multilobulated and has a glistening cut surface. (Reprinted by permission of Gold and Bossen, Ref. 24.)

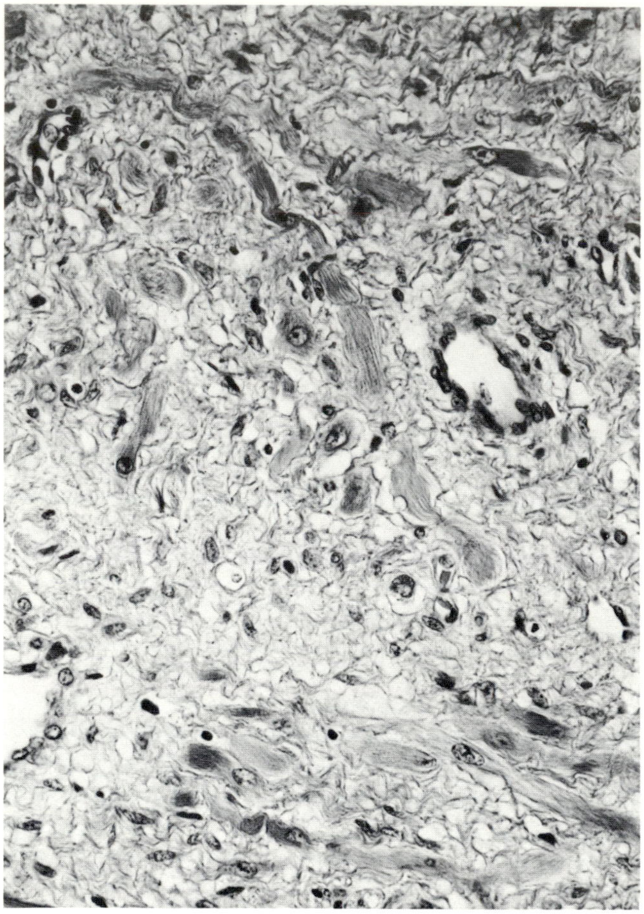

FIG. 4.24. Rhabdomyoma of vagina. The tumor cells are large and round, oval, or markedly elongated. (Reprinted by permission of Gold and Bossen, Ref. 24.)

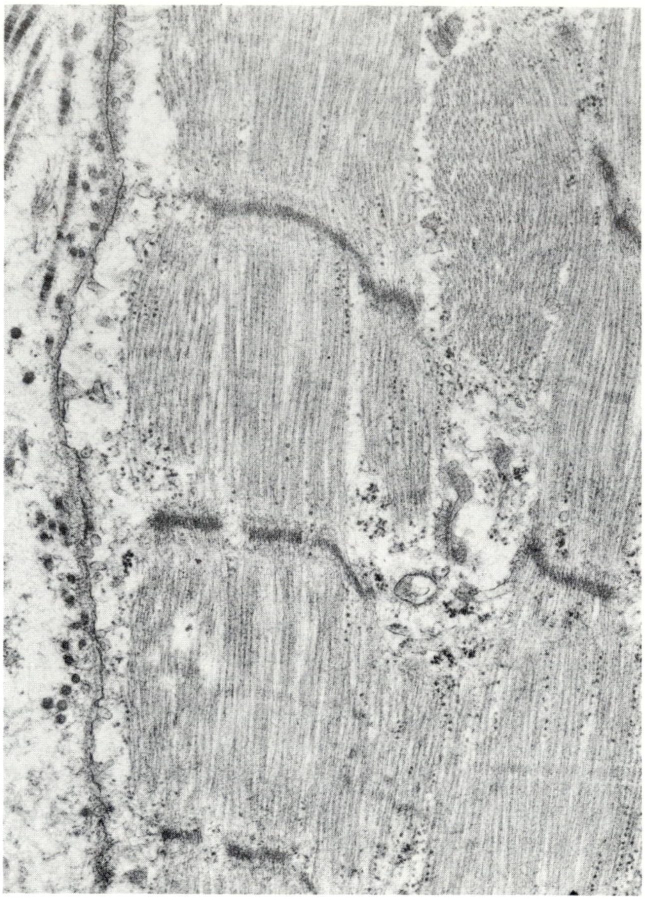

FIG. 4.25. Rhabdomyoma. Electron microscopic examination shows rhabdomyocytes, A, I, and Z bands, and M line. Microtubules and two membrane-bound sacs of various size filled with an electron-dense granular material are present. (Reprinted by permission of Gold and Bossen, Ref. 24.)

ized squamous epithelial cells constitute the second component (Fig. 4.27). The third component consists of mucinous cells occasionally forming glands. The squamous and mucinous epithelium resembles endocervical mucosa with squamous metaplasia. The most probable origin is the urogenital sinus. The tumors are benign and do not recur after local excision, even in those cases with atypia, infiltrating borders, or pseudopapillomatous structures.[94]

Granular Cell Tumor

The granular cell tumor, a tumor of Schwann cell origin, is a submucosal neoplasm that is usually small but can measure up to 5 cm in diameter. It is firm in consistency and has ill-defined borders. The tumor is composed of nests of large cells with characteristic granular cytoplasm (Fig. 4.28). The immunoperoxidase reaction for S100 protein is positive in the tumor cells, supporting the Schwann cell origin of this tumor.[96] The squamous epithelium overlying the tumor often discloses pseudoepitheliomatous hyperplasia, which at times has been incor-

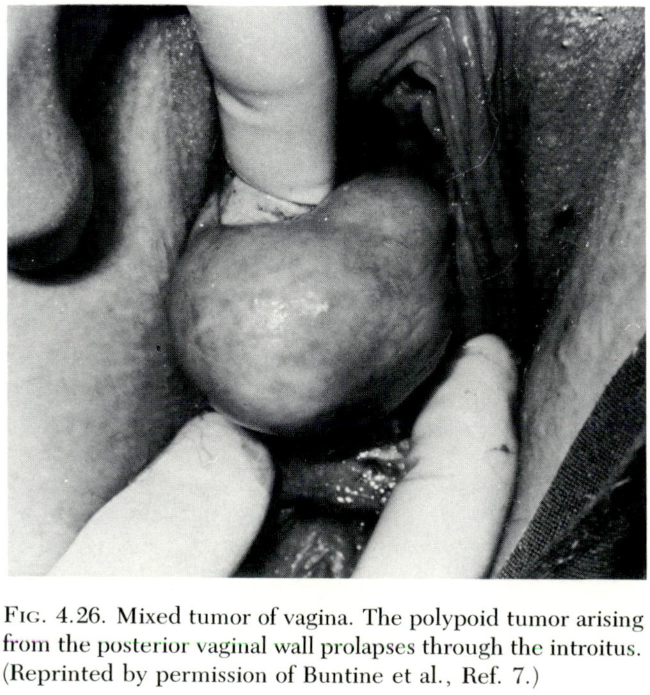

FIG. 4.26. Mixed tumor of vagina. The polypoid tumor arising from the posterior vaginal wall prolapses through the introitus. (Reprinted by permission of Buntine et al., Ref. 7.)

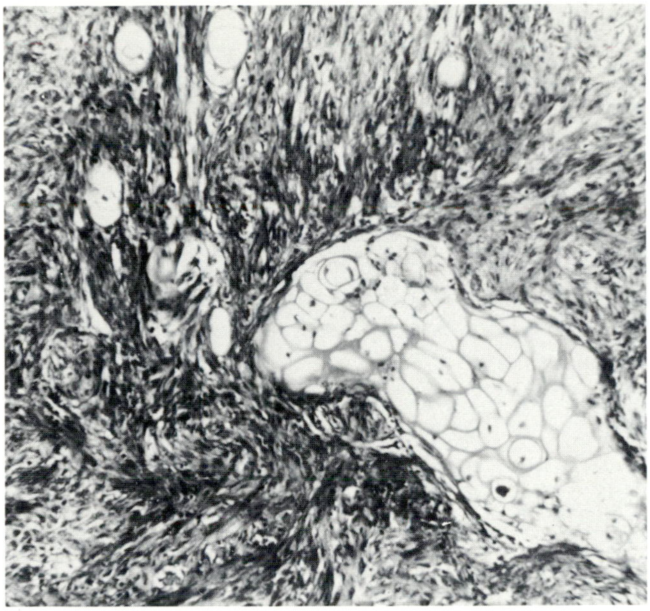

FIG. 4.27. Mixed tumor of vagina. The mass is composed predominantly of fibrous tissue in which nests of well-glycogenated squamous epithelium are scattered. (Reprinted by permission of Buntine et al., Ref. 24.)

rectly interpreted as cancer. Some granular cell tumors invade locally, which is suggested by the often irregular margin observed on microscopic examination and by the instances of local recurrence after excision. No deaths or metastases, however, have been reported from this tumor.

Endometriosis

This subject is discussed in Chapter 17, Endometriosis.

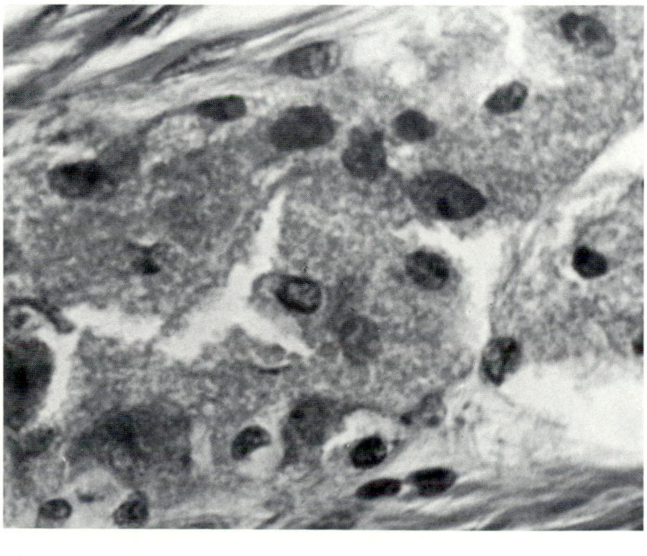

FIG. 4.28. Granular cell tumor. High-power view of tumor cells with prominent intracytoplasmic granules.

Vaginal Intraepithelial Neoplasia (Dysplasia and Carcinoma In Situ)

Vaginal intraepithelial neoplasia (VAIN) has been diagnosed more frequently during the last decade than in previous years because of the widespread use of cervical vaginal cytologic testing. Intraepithelial neoplasia is considerably less frequent in the vagina than in other sites. Vaginal carcinoma in situ (CIS) comprises only 0.4% of female genital tract in situ cancers, whereas the cervix accounts for 94.4% and the vulva 1.8%.[12] Also, the annual incidence of vaginal CIS is only 0.3 per 100,000 compared to 37.5 for cervical CIS.[12]

The epidemiology and etiology of VAIN have been inadequately studied. The major predisposing factor is probably the same as that of cervical intraepithelial neoplasia (CIN), namely, exposure to sexually transmitted carcinogenic microorganisms (see Chapter 7, Cervical Intraepithelial Neoplasia).[67] Furthermore, 80% of cases of VAIN are found in women previously treated for preinvasive or invasive cancer of the uterine cervix.[92] In the remaining 20%, VAIN is diagnosed following hysterectomy for benign disease. The ages of women with VAIN range from 19 to 86, with a mean of 54.12 years. The invasive potential of VAIN is similar to that of CIN.[23]

VAIN most commonly affects the upper vagina (in over three quarters of patients)[92] and is multifocal in half of patients. Although VAIN is asymptomatic and cannot be recognized on gross examination, it may be suspected on vaginal smear, detected on colposcopic examination, and diagnosed on biopsy of excised mucosa. The colposcopic appearance is similar to that of CIN, i.e., white discoloration of the affected epithelium and a mosaic or punctate pattern of subepithelial blood vessels (Fig. 4.29).

The microscopic changes of VAIN resemble those of CIN and include nuclear pleomorphism, loss of polarity, and the presence of abnormal mitoses. Grading has been variously expressed either as mild, moderate, or severe dysplasia and CIS or as VAIN, grades 1, 2, and 3. In CIS (VAIN 3), the neoplastic cells are undifferentiated and extend through the full thickness of squamous epithelium (Fig. 4.30). In mild or moderate dysplasia (VAIN 1 and 2), cytoplasmic atypia is mainly confined to the lower one third or two thirds of the epithelium (Fig. 4.31). Since there are no glandular crypts present in the vagina, any deep stromal extension of malignant epithelium must be viewed with suspicion.

Caution must be exercised when diagnosing VAIN from cytologic or histologic material from postmenopausal women and in patients following radiotherapy. Postmenopausal atrophic changes of vaginal epithelium may resemble VAIN, especially if inflammation is present. Atrophic immature epithelium retains enlarged nuclei throughout the entire thickness, and the inflammatory

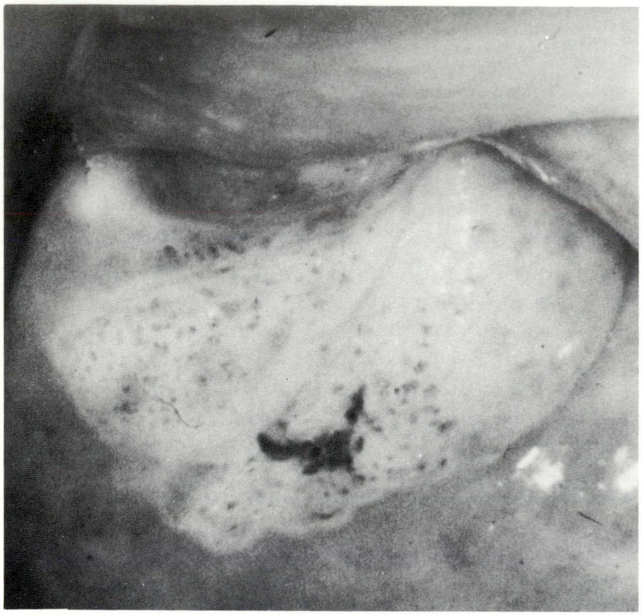

FIG. 4.29. Carcinoma in situ of the vaginal vault occurring after hysterectomy for cervical intraepithelial carcinoma, colposcopic appearance. The neoplasia appears as a raised white plaque with a punctate pattern produced by engorged subepithelial capillaries. (Reprinted by permission of Frederick Sillman, M.D.)

changes may simulate neoplastic nuclear pleomorphism. Also, the radiation effect usually persists for many years after treatment and may induce marked nuclear enlargement and bizarre nuclear shapes on cytologic smears. Local estrogen therapy before repeat cytologic or histologic evaluation may help clear the superimposed inflammatory changes and facilitate the interpretation.

Nearly three quarters of patients with VAIN have concomitant or prior neoplasia of other sites in the lower genital tract.[92] The cervix is the most frequent second site (68%), followed by vulva (3%), and synchronous involvement of both cervix and vulva (2%). Vaginal neoplasia developing in association with other sites of neoplasia, the so-called lower genital tract neoplastic syndrome (LGNS), may be due to the common embryologic origin of the cervical, vaginal, and vulvar squamous epithelia from the urogenital sinus and to exposure to a common carcinogen. Immunosuppressed individuals are at increased risk for LGNS by a factor of 14[71]. The epithelial neoplasia is not only more frequent but also more often multifocal, persistent, and aggressive.[93] In renal transplant patients, the frequency of lower genital tract neoplasia is 10 times higher than in the general population.[27] Multiple foci involving several sites in the lower genital tract have been found in 50% of renal transplant patients with intraepithelial neoplasia.[27] Multiple foci of neoplasia have been found also in half of immunosuppressed patients with systemic lupus erythematosus and sarcoidosis.[93]

Human papillomavirus may play a major role in the pathogenesis of intraepithelial neoplasia in immunosuppressed individuals. Koilocytosis and other cytopathic viral effects, e.g., multinucleation, have been found in every patient with intraepithelial neoplasia of the lower genital tract who has received immunosuppressive treatment as a result of renal transplantion, lupus erythematosus, sarcoidosis, or other causes. Papillomavirus capsid antigen has been identified in the tissues with the immunoperoxidase method in 60% of the tested patients.[93]

Malignant Tumors

Epithelial Tumors

Squamous Carcinoma

Primary squamous carcinoma of the vagina is infrequent and accounts for approximately 1% of all gynecologic malignancies. The age-adjusted incidence of squamous

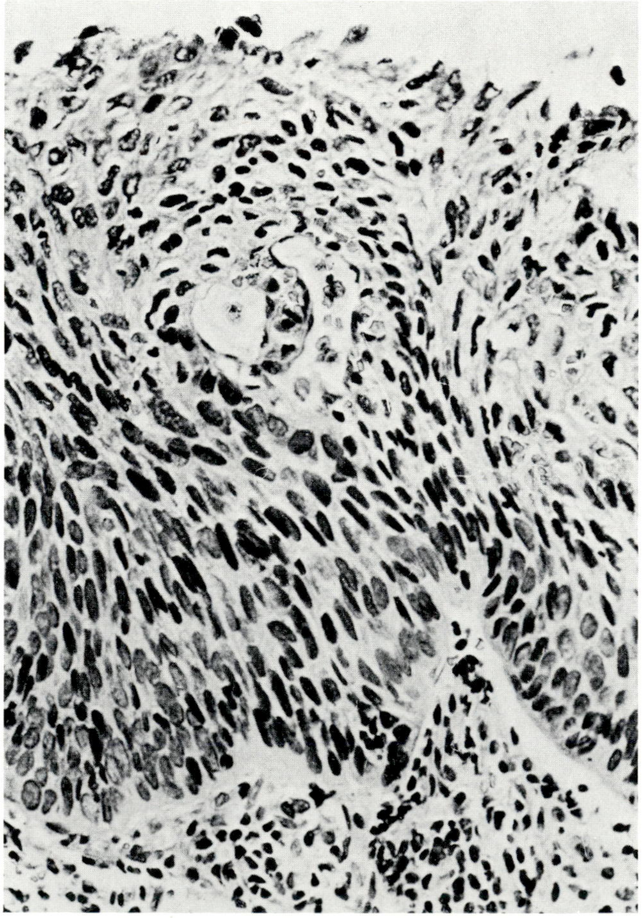

FIG. 4.30. Carcinoma in situ. Immature neoplastic cells are present throughout the full thickness of the epithelium.

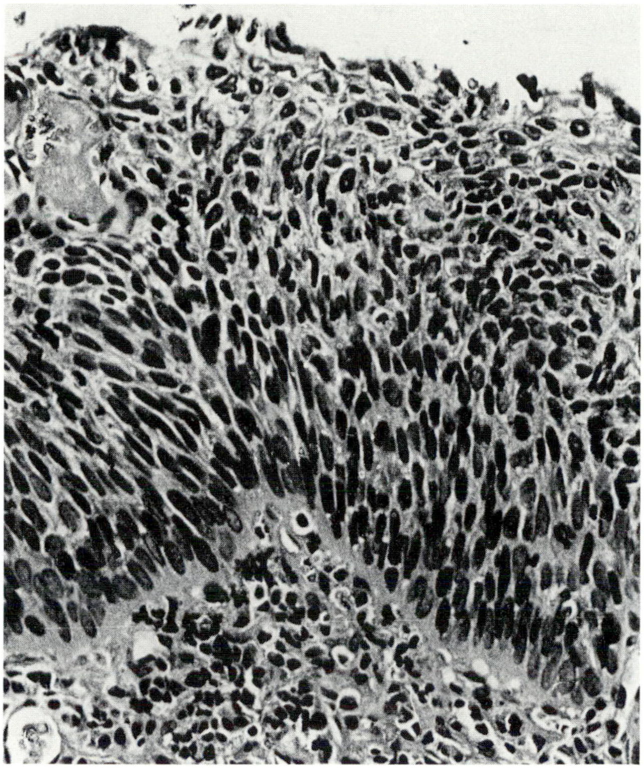

FIG. 4.31. Moderate dysplasia. Immature neoplastic cells occupy the lower two thirds of the epithelium.

carcinoma in the United States is 1/100,000 in black women and 0.6/100,000 in white women.[12] Squamous carcinoma of the vagina is characteristically a disease of older women. Seventy percent of cases occur in women after age 50, with the peak incidence between ages 60 and 70 years. Squamous carcinoma occurs at a considerably younger age, 25–35 years of age, in women with a neovagina after vaginal reconstructive surgery for congenital absence of the vagina or other reasons.[88]

Little is known about the epidemiology of vaginal carcinoma. There is some evidence for increased risk of vaginal cancer after radiotherapy given a decade earlier for other gynecologic malignancies.[72] These tumors have a better prognosis than tumors diagnosed soon after radiotherapy.[65] Tumors occurring late are primary cancers, probably related to the radiation. Chronic irritation resulting from the use of pessaries for the treatment of genital prolapse has been considered as one predisposing factor, although no statistically significant correlation has been established. Other risk factors include immunosuppression, papillomavirus infection, and the lower genital tract neoplastic syndrome (see section Vaginal Intraepithelial Neoplasia above).

Primary squamous carcinoma of the vagina must be differentiated from vaginal extension of cervical or vulvar cancer and from metastatic tumors. A valid diagnosis of primary vaginal cancer requires that there be no cancer in the cervix and vulva at the time of diagnosis and for 10 years or more before diagnosis.[9] The possibility of metastatic growth must also be excluded by survey of other organs.

The most common location of vaginal carcinoma is in the upper portion of the posterior wall: 51% of tumors arise in the upper third and 60% originate from the posterior wall.[70] The tumor occurs most frequently as an exophytic mass and, rarely, as an infiltrating or flat lesion. The microscopic appearance of squamous carcinoma of the vagina is similar to that of squamous cancer of the cervix. It is characterized by solid masses of neoplastic cells with pleomorphic nuclei and numerous mitotic figures, infiltrating the stroma in cords, masses, or isolated clusters of cells (Fig. 4.32). The well-differentiated tumor cells have abundant eosinophilic cytoplasm and may produce keratin either as the characteristic pearls or as individual cell keratinization. Poorly differentiated tumor cells are small and have scant cytoplasm and hyperchromatic nuclei.

Local extension of the tumor involves the paracolpos, parametria, bladder, and rectum. Involvement of pelvic lymph nodes occurs in approximately 20% of patients with stage I cancer. Inguinal node metastases increase in frequency when the tumor involves the lower vagina (25% of inguinal lymph node involvement).[70] The clinical

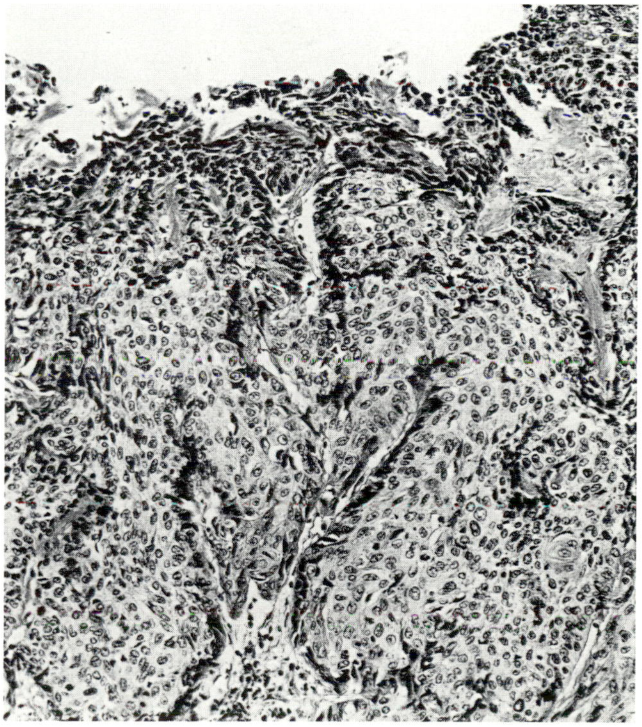

FIG. 4.32. Invasive squamous carcinoma of the vagina. Nests and cords of neoplastic cells invade the stroma in an irregular fashion.

TABLE 4.1. FIGO staging of vaginal carcinoma.

Stage	Clinical status
0	Intraepithelial
I	Limited to vaginal wall
II	Extends to subvaginal tissue but not to pelvic side wall
III	Extends to pelvic side wall
IV	Extends beyond the true pelvis or involves mucosa of the bladder or rectum (bullous edema does not consign the patient to stage IV)
IVa	Adjacent organs involved
IVb	Distant organs involved

staging for vaginal cancer was adopted by the International Federation of Gynecology and Obstetrics (FIGO) in 1974[9] (Table 4.1).

Survival figures for patients with vaginal squamous carcinoma are inconsistent, perhaps because vaginal cancer is infrequent and various authors have used different methods for diagnosis, staging, and treatment. The early literature emphasized high mortality probably because the cancer arose in unfavorable anatomic locations in close proximity to the bladder and rectum. With only a thin septum separating these structures from the tumor, the bladder and the rectum become invaded early and may be severely injured during radiotherapy. With earlier diagnosis and advances in radiotherapy technique, survival figures have improved and, stage for stage, are similar to those for cervical carcinoma.[65] The stage I 5-year survival is about 90%, stage II 50%, and stages III and IV, 20%.

Verrucous Carcinoma

Verrucous carcinoma of the vagina is rare.[39] It is characterized by epithelial proliferation resembling condyloma, with little cytologic atypia. Unlike condyloma, however, verrucous carcinoma lacks the central fibrous core and invades the underlying tissue with bulbous masses of neoplastic squamous epithelium. Verrucous carcinoma may recur after surgical therapy, but distant metastases are rare (see Chapter 3 Diseases of Vulva).

Basal Cell Carcinoma

Basal cell carcinoma is exceedingly rare. It is similar to basal cell carcinoma arising in the vulva, (see Chapter 3, Diseases of Vulva). In one reported case, the 8 mm tumor appeared in the upper posterior third of the vagina in a 42-year-old woman. She had not had any antecedent hormonal therapy.[55]

Adenocarcinoma

Before the DES era, both adenosis and clear cell adenocarcinoma (previously termed *mesonephroma* were recognized but extremely rare lesions (see Chapter 18, Epithelial Tumors of Ovary). Clear cell adenocarcinoma was encountered principally in women past the menopause.[77] Adenocarcinomas of the endometrioid or mucinous type are also rare but were the most common varieties of vaginal adenocarcinoma in the pre-DES era. They develop in older women and occur in any area of the vagina, most commonly in the upper third on the anterior or posterior walls. Mucinous adenocarcinomas may be associated with a mucous discharge.

Sarcomas

Sarcomas comprise less than 2% of all malignant vaginal neoplasms. Of these, embryonal rhabdomyosarcoma (sarcoma botryoides) is the most common type in infants and young adolescent girls. The leiomyosarcoma is the most frequent mesenchymal tumor in middle-age and older women. The rare types of sarcoma include malignant mixed mesodermal tumor, alveolar soft part sarcoma, synovial-like sarcoma, fibrosarcoma, neurofibrosarcoma, and angiosarcoma.

Leiomyosarcoma

Leiomyosarcomas are bulky lesions varying from 3 to 10 cm in diameter. They originate in the rectovaginal septum and as they expand may produce ulceration of vaginal mucosa or invasion into the rectum.[14] The microscopic appearance is similar to that of leiomyosarcoma in other sites, i.e., fascicles of spindle-shaped cells with fusiform, hyperchromatic, and pleomorphic nuclei and frequent mitoses (Fig. 4.33). The mitotic count per 10 high-power fields CHPF is an important diagnostic and prognostic indicator in all leiomyosarcomas, including the vagina. Tumors showing less than five mitoses per 10 HPF cause no mortality and, therefore, should be considered benign leiomyomas. A mitotic count of 16 or more per 10 HPF is associated with a fatal outcome in 100% of patients.[100] The majority of deaths occur within a 2-year period, usually from bloodborne metastases.[101]

Embryonal Rhabdomyosarcoma

Embryonal rhabdomyosarcoma (sarcoma botryoides) is the most common neoplasm of the lower genital tract in girls. Most of these tumors occur in children younger than 5 years old.[10] Almost two-thirds occur within the first 2 years of life (Fig. 4.34).[35] It is exceedingly rare in young girls and teenagers. The tumor arises in the lamina propria, originating from undifferentiated mesen-

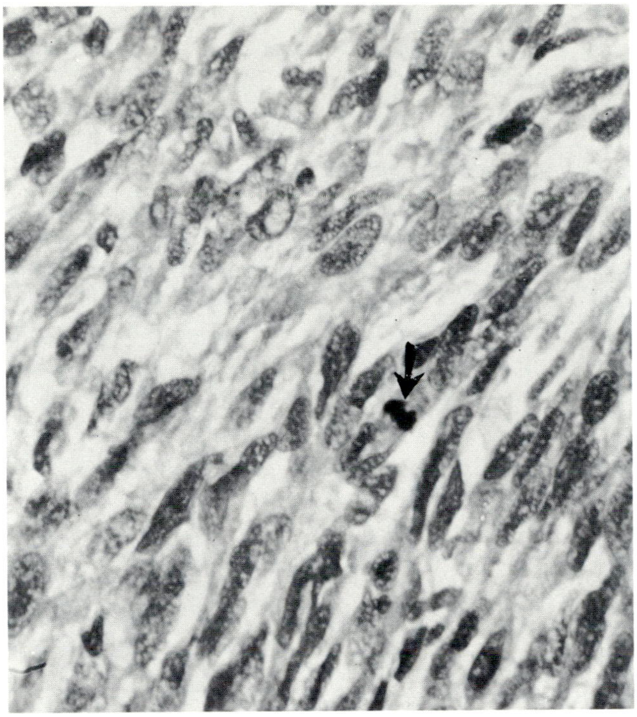

FIG. 4.33. Leiomyosarcoma of the vagina. Tumor is composed of plump, elongated cells with large nuclei. Note mitotic figure (*arrow*). (Reproduced by permission from: Rosai, Juan: Ackerman's Surgical Pathology, ed. 6, St. Louis, 1981, The C. V. Mosby Co.)

chyme, and infiltrates the vaginal wall and pelvic structures. The gross appearance is that of a confluence of polypoid masses resembling a bunch of grapes (Fig. 4.35 and 4.36). The polypoid masses may be hemorrhagic, myxoid, or both and are often ulcerated.

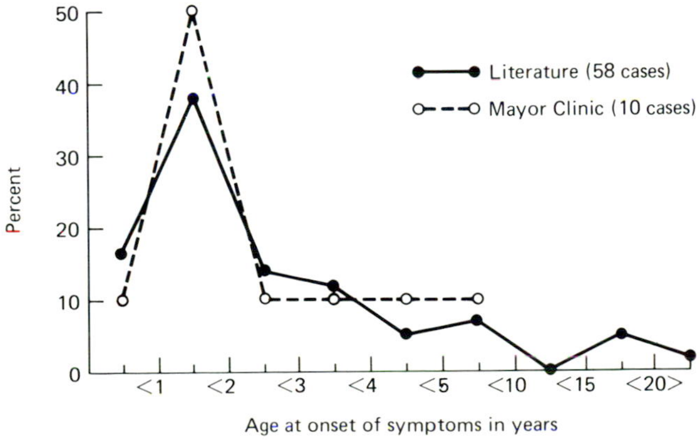

FIG. 4.34. Sarcoma botryoides of the vagina. Age distribution at onset of symptoms in years. [Reprinted by permission from Hilgers R, Malkasian GD Jr, Soule EH (1970) Embryonal rhabdomyosarcoma (botyroid type) of the vagina: A clinicopathologic review. Am J Obstet Gynecol 107:484.]

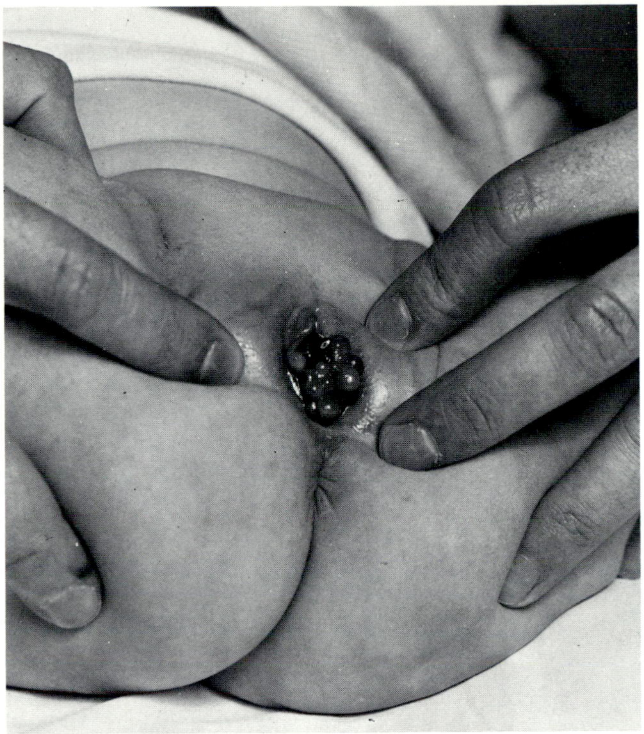

FIG. 4.35. Sarcoma botryoides of the vagina. The gross appearance is that of a polypoid mass protruding through the vaginal introitus and resembling a bunch of grapes. [Reprinted by permission from Hilgers R, Malkasian GD Jr, Soule EH (1970) Embryonal rhabdomyosarcoma (botyroid type) of the vagina: A clinicopathologic review. Am J Obstet Gynecol 107:484.]

Microscopically, the tumor is composed of polypoid masses containing poorly differentiated, round or spindle-shaped cells. The neoplastic cells are for the most part immature rhabdomyoblasts (Fig. 4.37) that frequently surround blood vessels. The typical rhabdomyoblast found in almost all tumors may be recognized

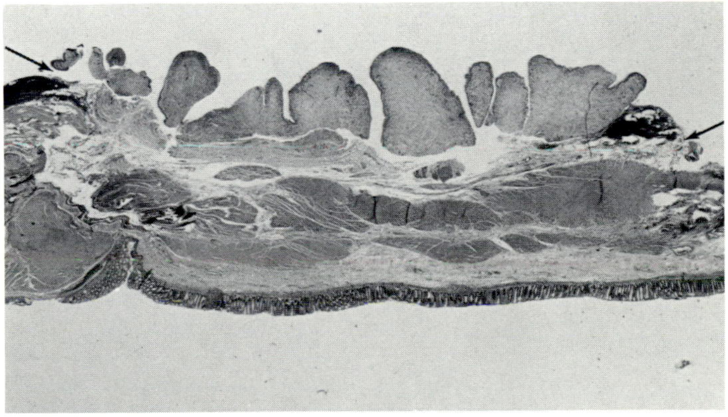

FIG. 4.36. Sarcoma botryoides of the rectovaginal septum. Note the polypoid appearance of the tumor outlined by *arrows*.

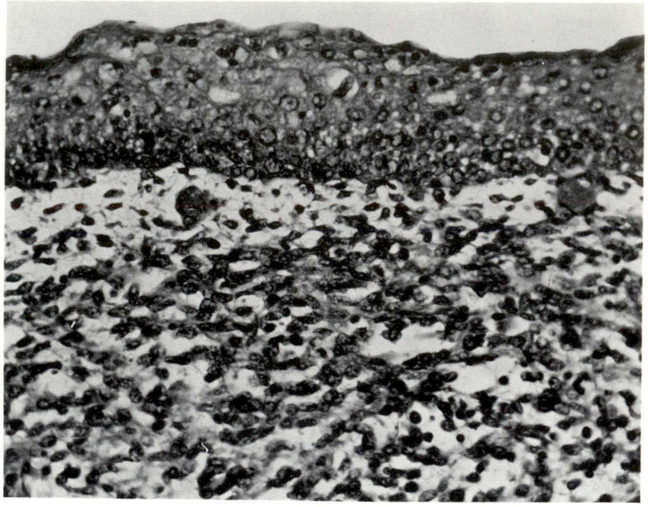

FIG. 4.37. Sarcoma botryoides. Cambium layer beneath the epithelium. [Reprinted by permission from Hilgers R, Malkasian GD Jr, Soule EH (1970) Embryonal rhabdomyosarcoma (botyroid type) of the vagina: A clinicopathologic review. Am J Obstet Gynecol 107:484.]

by its characteristic round, racket, or strap-shape, bright eosinophilic cytoplasm, and multinucleation. Cross-striations are present in the majority of rhabdomyoblasts (Fig. 4.38) and are usually prominent, but in some instances they may require prolonged search or special stains, e.g., immunoperoxidase stain for desmin or myoglobin. The stroma is usually myxoid. Crowding of undifferentiated tumor cells and rhabdomyoblasts beneath the vaginal epithelium results in a distinct subepithelial dense zone, referred to as the *cambium layer* (Fig. 4.37).

Embryonal rhabdosarcoma should not be confused

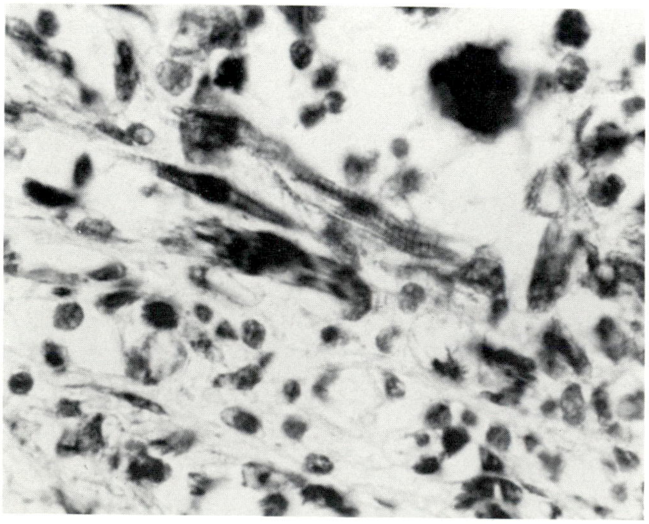

FIG. 4.38. Sarcoma botryoides. Rhabdomyoblast with cross-striations.

with benign vaginal polyps containing atypical stromal cells, with the benign rhabdomyoma, a mixed tumor, or with endodermal sinus tumor of the vagina. The tumor invades adjacent structures and metastasizes to the lymph nodes and distant sites, the latter by the hematogenous route. As reported by the Intergroup Rhabdomyoma Study No. 1, the frequency of lymph node metastases exceeds 25%.[50] The prognosis is poor, and the cause of death is by direct extension of the tumor, more often than by distant metastases.[35] The 5-year survival is between 10 and 35%, but in the series reported by Hilgers et al.,[35] the survival increased to almost 50% after pelvic exenteration, regional lymphadenectomy, and partial or total vaginectomy. Success has been reported with local excision followed by chemotherapy in patients with early stage disease.[10]

Malignant Mixed Müllerian Tumors

Malignant mixed müllerian tumors of the vagina are exceedingly rare.[66] The tumors are histologically similar to those seen in the uterus (see Chapter 13, Mesenchymal Tumors of Uterus). The tumors may be homologous,

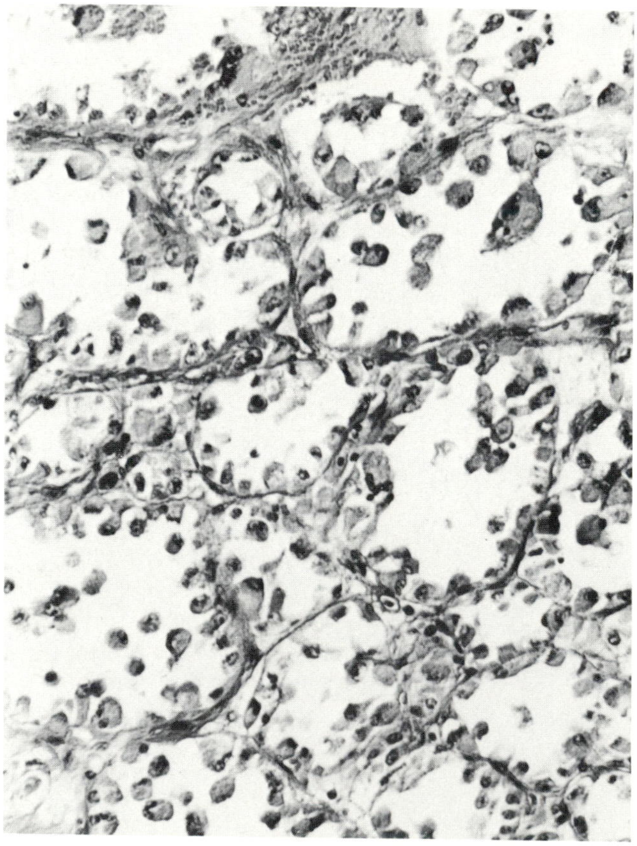

FIG. 4.39. Alveolar soft part sarcoma. Note the uniformity of the alveolar cells. (Reprinted by permission of Kasai et al., Ref. 40.)

consisting of adenocarcinoma, squamous carcinoma, stromal sarcoma, or leiomyosarcoma. Some are heterologous, containing chondrosarcoma or osteosarcoma. Previous irradiation is a frequent finding, an association reported earlier for the uterine counterpart. The mortality is high, with death occurring within 2 years after diagnosis.[66]

Alveolar Soft Part Sarcoma

Kasai et al.[40] described the first case of alveolar soft part sarcoma in the vagina of a 34-year-old Japanese patient. During a 6-year period of observation, the tumor grew from the size of an "index fingertip" to a "goose-egg" that extended outside the introitus. On gross examination, the mucosa covering the tumor mass was intact, and the mass was fixed. The cut surface was buff gray with yellow spots.

Microscopic examination revealed an alveolar arrangement of cell groups. Each alveolus (Fig. 4.39) was composed of 20–30 large, oval to polyhedral cells with distinct cell boundaries. The cytoplasm was light eosinophilic, finely granular, or reticulated. The cytoplasm also contained an amorphous, mucin-like substance, which was intensely PAS positive and diastase resistant and did not stain with Alcian blue. There were variations in nuclear size and shape, and an occasional cell was atypically binucleated and larger than usual. Transmission electron microscopy revealed aggregations of secretory granules possibly of glycoprotein nature in the cytoplasm. The individual granules were bounded by a limiting membrane (Fig. 4.40).

Synovial-Like Sarcoma

Okagaki et al.[62] described a malignant tumor of the vagina that resembled a synovial sarcoma in a 24-year-old woman. The main part of the tumor was epithelioid, forming a tubular or acinar pattern (Fig. 4.41). At the periphery, the tumor cells were more spindle-shaped and formed sheets resembling fibrosarcoma.

Electron microscopy revealed light cells with ovoid nuclei and darker cells with irregular nuclei and dense nuclear chromatin. There was no clear distinction be-

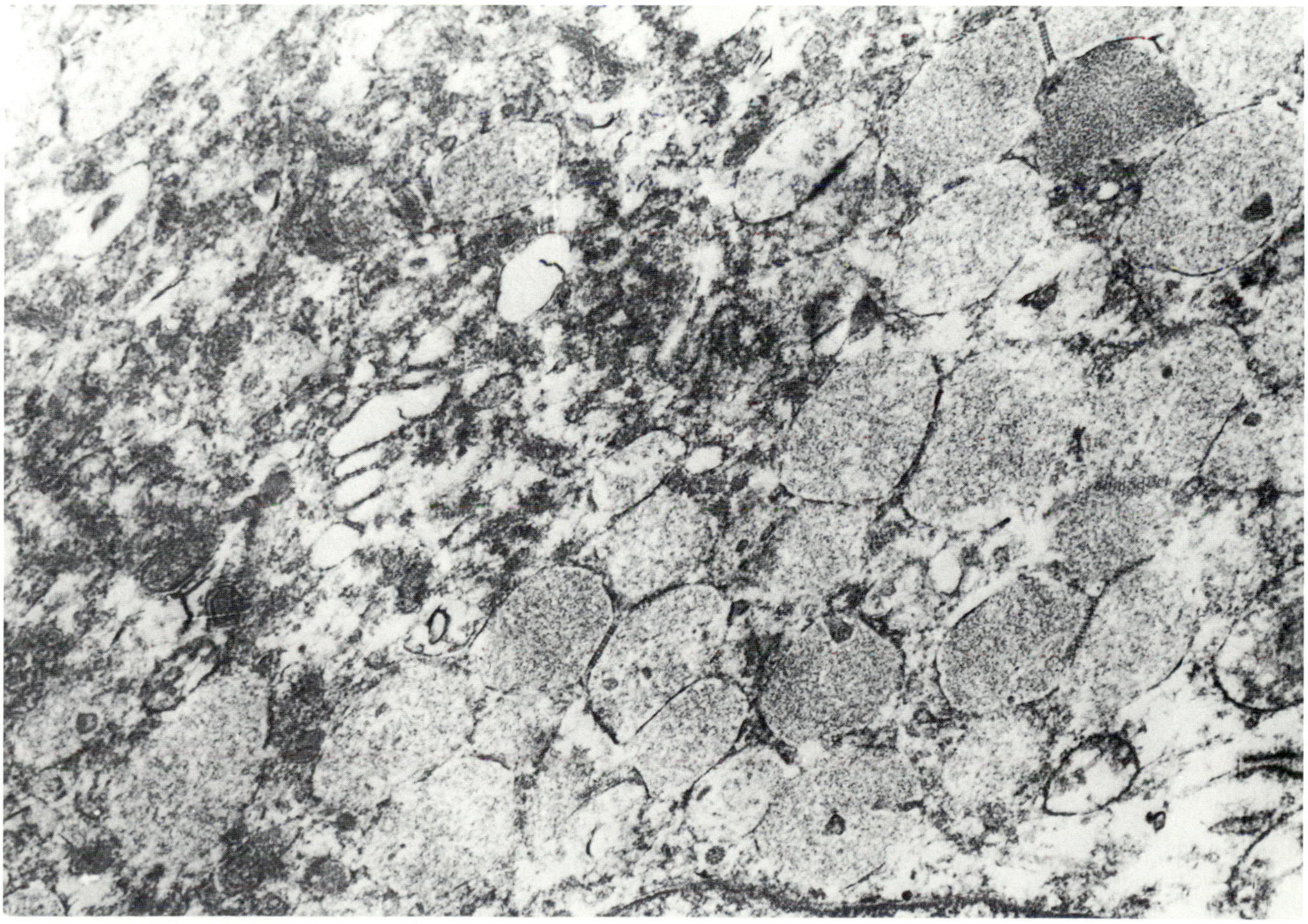

Fig. 4.40. Alveolar soft part sarcoma. PAS-positive and diastase-resistant granules adjacent to the golgi apparatus. (Reprinted by permission of Kasai et al., Ref. 40.)

tween the light and dark cells. However, cuboidal or flattened cells lined the glandular lumina, with slender nonfilamented microvilli projecting into the lumina (Fig. 4.42). The findings suggested that the tumor was of mesenchymal origin closely related to synovial sarcoma.

Other Sarcomas

Fibrosarcoma, rhabdomyosarcoma (adult type), neurofibrosarcoma, and angiosarcoma have been reported in the vagina.

Endodermal Sinus Tumor

Approximately 50 cases of endodermal sinus tumor of the vagina have been reported.[11,107] The tumor develops exclusively in children less than 3 years of age. The clinical presentation is blood-tinged vaginal discharge or bleeding. Vaginal examination demonstrates a polypoid lesion. Microscopically, the tumor resembles the ovarian endodermal sinus tumor with (1) a loose network of cystic spaces lined by flattened epithelial cells forming a reticular or honeycomb pattern (Fig. 4.43), (2) Schiller-Duval bodies (Fig. 4.44), (3) anastomosing channels and tubules lined by cuboidal epithelial cells with vacuolated cytoplasm and hyperchromatic nuclei, and (4) intra- and extracellular hyaline bodies that stain positively with PAS and are resistant to diastase digestion. Mitotic figures are numerous, and atypical forms are present. Alpha-fetoprotein and alpha-1-antitrypsin have been demonstrated with immunoperoxidase methods in the hyaline bodies and epithelial cells. Tumors that must be considered in the differential diagnosis include sarcoma botryoides, vaginal polyps, and clear cell adenocarcinoma.

The origin of endodermal sinus tumor remains speculative. Most of the evidence points to a derivation from extragonadal germ cells, e.g., the midline site, the histologic pattern, and the presence of alpha-fetoprotein. It is surprising that no other elements of a germ cell tumor, such as teratoma, have been found to date in association with endodermal sinus tumor of the vagina.

The median survival of patients is 11 months. Prolonged survival has been achieved by the use of extensive surgery (exenteration) or by combination chemotherapy with local excision.[11]

Melanoma

Melanoma is the second most common cancer of the vagina, accounting for 3% of vaginal malignancies[48] and 0.3% of all melanomas (see Chapter 3, Diseases of the Vulva). It is usually located in the caudal third of the

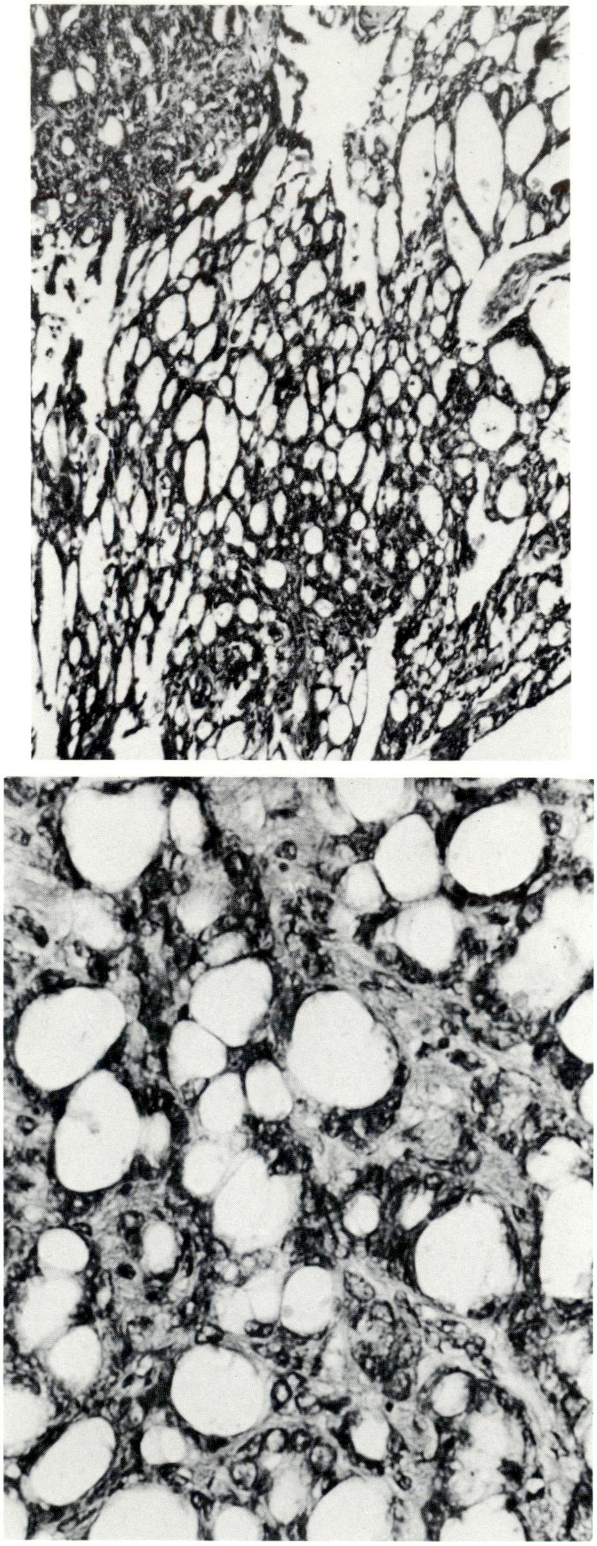

FIG. 4.41. *Top:* Malignant tumor of the vagina resembling synovial sarcoma. In this area, the tumor is predominantly acinar. Mucin stains showed positive reactions in inspissated material in lumina and in some of the cells. *Bottom:* High-power view of the acini. The nuclei of cells are prominent, whereas cytoplasmic borders are indistinct. (Reprinted by permission of Okagaki et al., Ref. 62.)

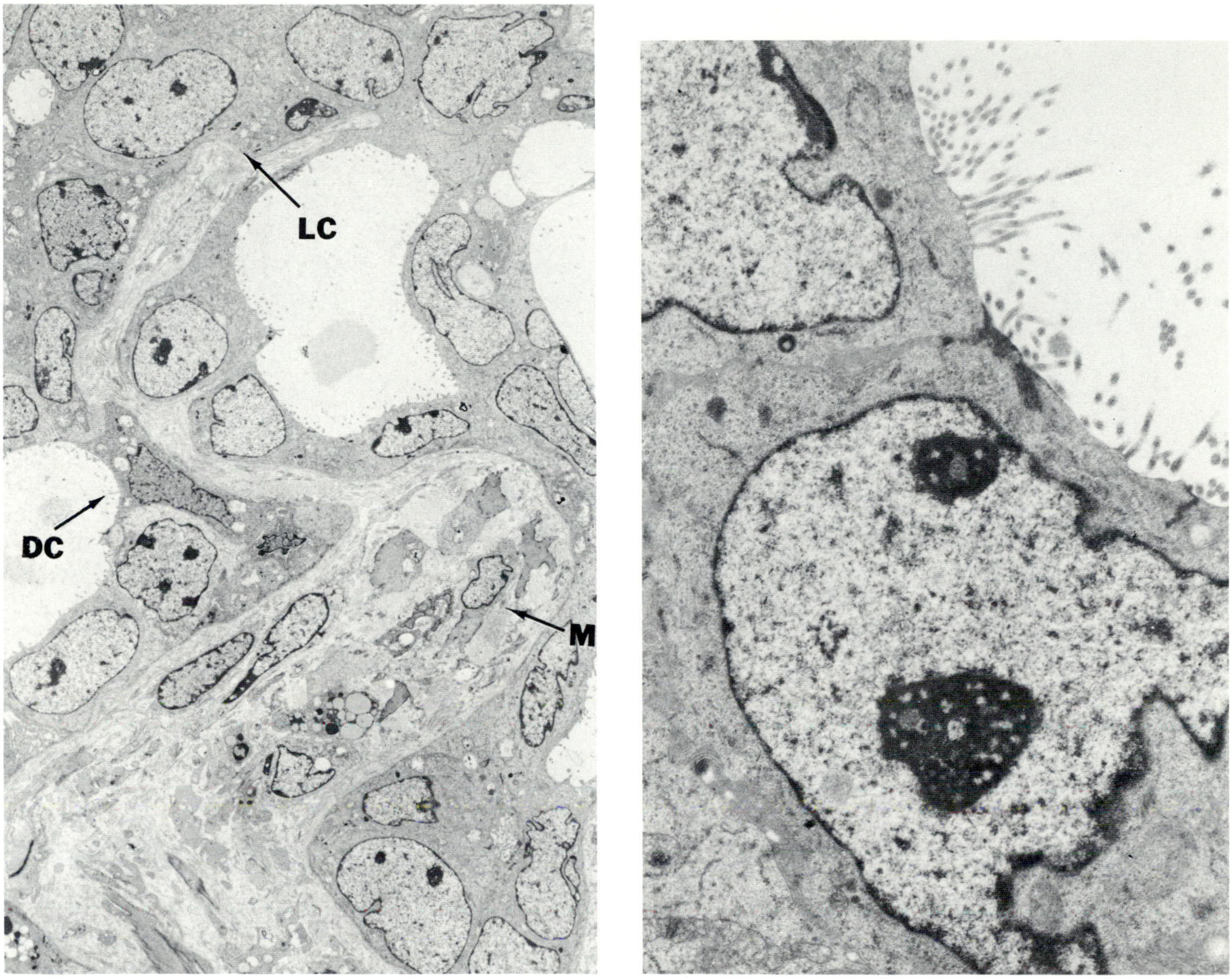

FIG. 4.42. Malignant tumor of the vagina resembling synovial sarcoma. *Left:* Low-magnification electron micrograph of acinar area. Note dark (DC) and light (LC) cell types and microvilli projecting into the lumina. Smooth muscle cells (M) are seen in the collagenous stroma. *Right:* Higher magnification of the epithelioid cells with long slender microvilli. (Reprinted by permission of Okagaki et al., Ref. 62.)

vagina and frequently exhibits a characteristic black or blue pigmentation (Fig. 4.45). The lesions are often ulcerated. On microscopic examination, vaginal melanoma reveals pleomorphic cells laden with melanin (Fig. 4.46). Pigmentation may be absent in the amelanotic variety of melanoma. Immunoperoxidase staining for S100 protein and electron microscopic examination may facilitate the diagnosis in these instances. The characteristic ultrastructural features include (1) premelanosomes, numerous membrane-bound sacs containing granules of varying intensity, and (2) absence of desmosomes.[5] Melanomas are thought to originate from melanosis, a melanocytic hyperplasia. Melanocytes are present in the vagina of 3% of women.[48] The prognosis is poor.

Metastatic Tumors

The endometrium and cervix are the most common sources of metastases. Tumors of the ovary, rectum, and kidney[60] may also metastasize to the vagina. Metastases from endometrial adenocarcinoma reach the vagina by submucosal lymphatics or implantation. They are usually seen in the upper third and on the anterior wall. The metastases may be small and at times can resemble granulation tissue. The microscopic appearance is similar to that of the original tumor.

Choriocarcinoma can metastasize to the vagina. Microscopically, the tumor is composed of cytotrophoblast and syncytiotrophoblast.

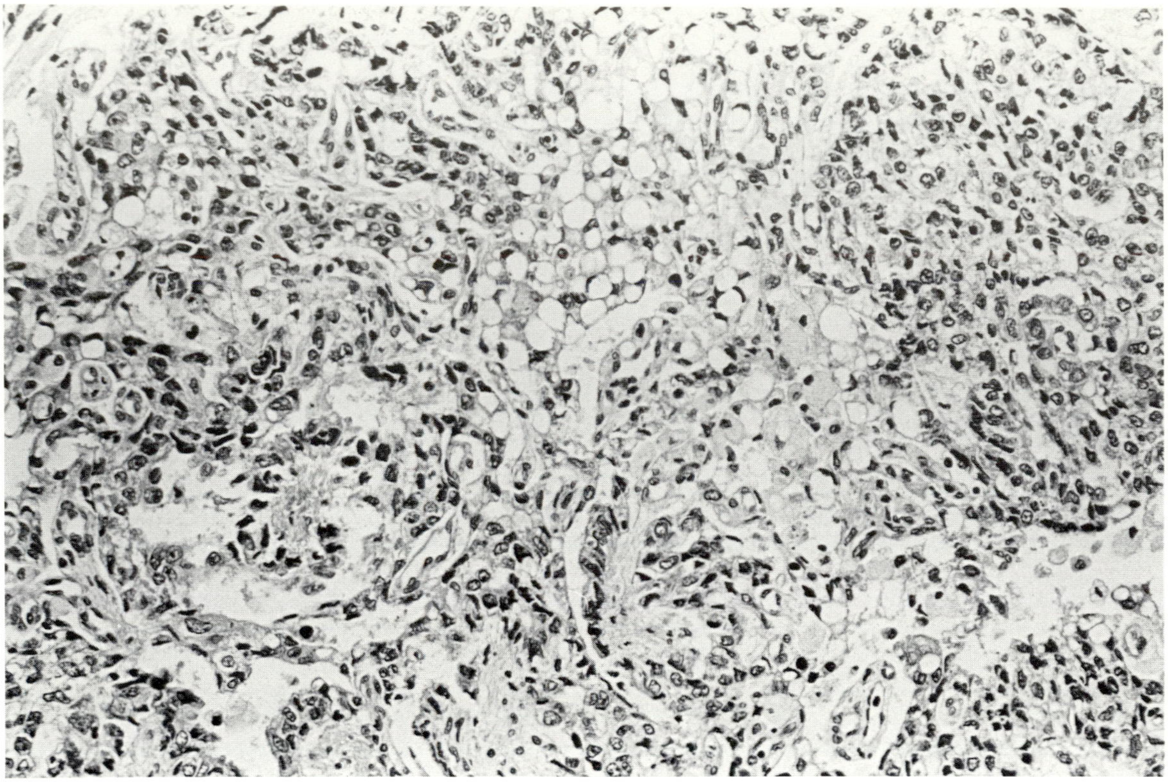

Fig. 4.43. Endodermal sinus tumor of the vagina. Loose network of cystic spaces (reticular or honeycomb pattern). (Courtesy of L. J. Copeland, M.D.)

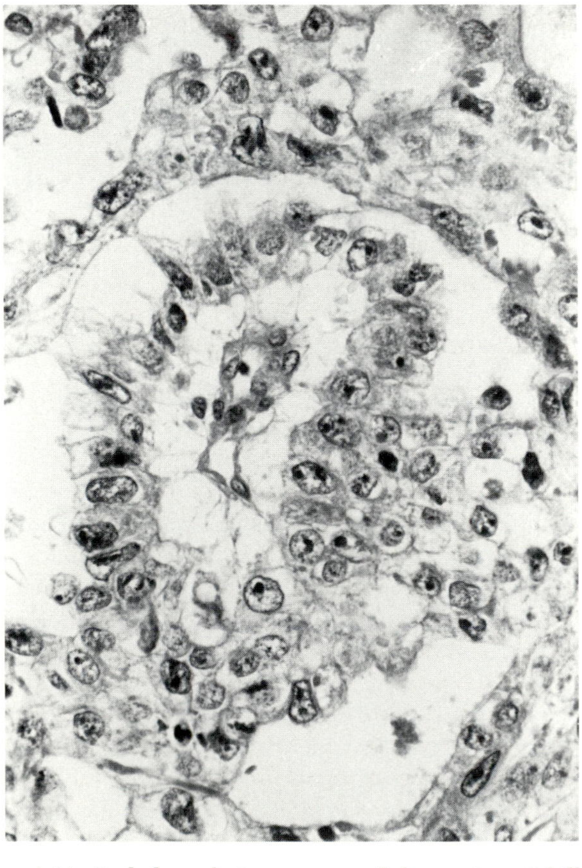

Fig. 4.44. Endodermal sinus tumor of the vagina. Schiller-Duval body. (Courtesy of L.J. Copeland, M.D.)

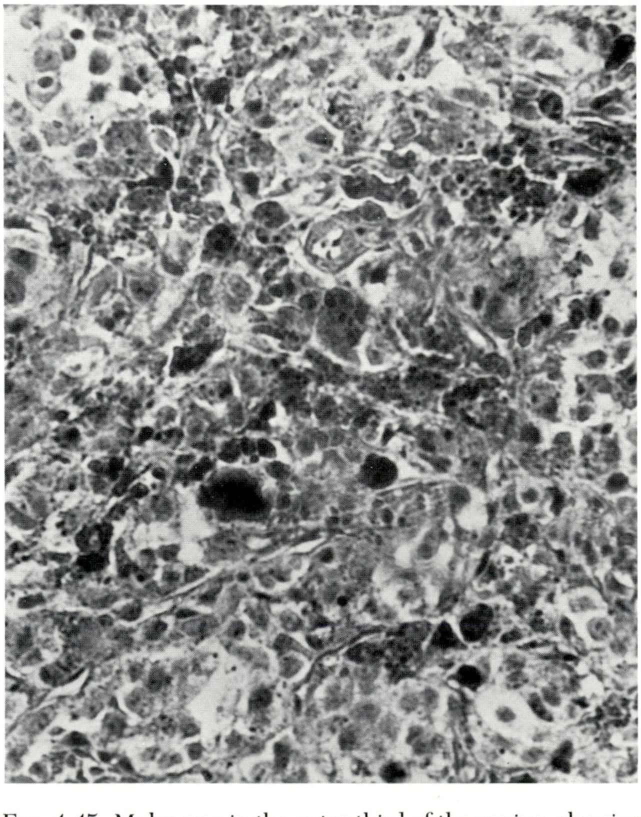

Fig. 4.45. Melanoma in the outer third of the vagina, showing melanin pigment.

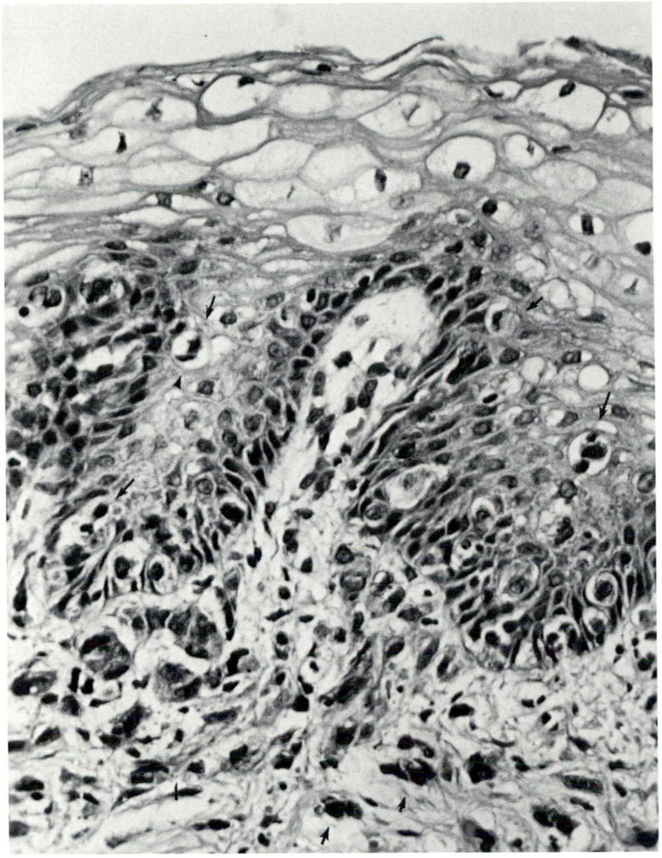

FIG. 4.46. Melanoma. Malignant melanocytes in stromae with invasion into epithelium (*arrows*).

Changes Related to Prenatal Diethylstilbestrol Exposure

Diethylstilbestrol and the chemically related drugs, hexestrol and dienestrol, are synthetic, nonsteroidal estrogens that were frequently administered to mothers for high-risk pregnancies during the 1940s through the 1960s.[58] In 1971, the rare development of clear cell adenocarcinoma of the vagina in young women was linked to their exposure in utero to these drugs.[30] Subsequently, a number of nonneoplastic changes were identified in the genital tract of DES-exposed daughters, such as adenosis (glandular epithelium or its secretory products in the vagina), cervical ectropion, various types of cervicovaginal ridges, and structural abnormalities of the uterine corpus and fallopian tube. This section is limited to a description of the pathology and pertinent clinical aspects of clear cell adenocarcinoma of the vagina and cervix as well as the nonneoplastic changes associated with, or possibly related to, DES exposure. Recommendations for the identification and management of exposed daughters,[82,83] possible sequelae in mothers,[25] and sons,[4,47,49,90,91] animal models for the study of DES exposure,* and general reviews[29] are presented elsewhere.

* References 13, 15, 51, 52, 56, 57, 68, 69, 76, 98, 99.

Neoplastic Changes

Clear Cell Adenocarcinoma

Clinical Aspects

More than 500 cases of clear cell adenocarcinoma of the vagina or cervix in young females had been accessioned by the beginning of 1986 by the Registry for Research on Hormonal Transplacental Carcinogenesis. Most patients were born in the United States; a few with documented exposure to DES were born in Mexico, Canada, Europe, Australia, or Africa. The median age at the time of diagnosis is 19 years (Fig. 4.47). Although a rare patient has been as young as 7 years of age, only after the age of 14 years does the age-incidence curve rise sharply. It plateaus between ages 17 and 21 and then declines rapidly. A rare DES-exposed woman has been over 30 years of age at the time of tumor diagnosis. Approximately 61% of the patients have had documented exposure in utero to DES, hexestrol or dienestrol; another 10% were exposed to an unknown form of medication, usually for a high-risk pregnancy. The records in

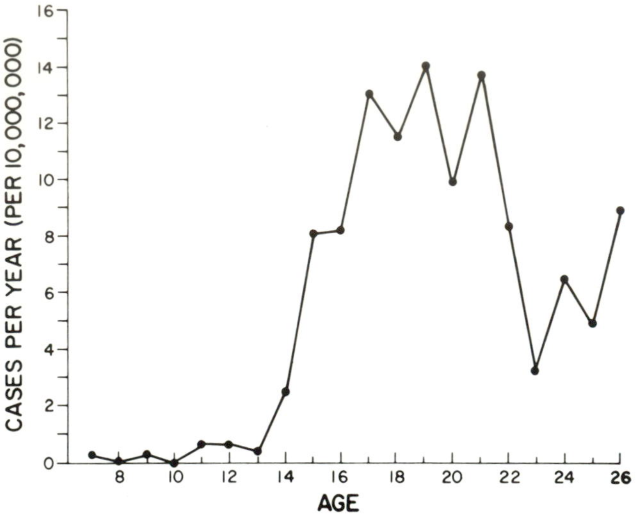

FIG. 4.47. Incidence of clear cell adenocarcinoma by age at diagnosis among native-born, white, resident female subjects. (Reprinted by permission of Herbst et al., Ref. 32.)

several cases indicate only exposure to steroidal estrogens or progesterone, but there is no evidence of an association of clear cell adenocarcinoma with prenatal exposure to these hormones.[41] The proportion of negative to positive histories of DES exposure is greater for cervical tumors than for vaginal tumors, a finding consistent with the observation that clear cell adenocarcinoma of the cervix in young women was a recognized but rare entity before the DES era, whereas clear cell adenocarcinoma of the vagina was exceedingly rare, limited only to a few case reports.

On the basis of the number of cases accessioned by the Registry, it has been established that clear cell adenocarcinoma develops in 0.014–0.14% of exposed women up to the age of 24 years.[31] Recent studies indicate that misdiagnosis of the cancer is common and the frequency may be double that previously suspected.[36] The overall low frequency has been confirmed by several studies in which no cancers were found in more than 3000 exposed women identified through review of their mothers' prenatal records.[63] Whereas recent data confirm that the cancer incidence is low, a note of caution is still necessary, as tumors are being discovered in several of the many thousands of DES-exposed women being followed. The greatest number of DES-exposed patients with these tumors were born between 1951 and 1953, the period during which the drug was most frequently prescribed for pregnancy support. The number of tumors that have developed in women born after 1953 has declined progressively. The risk of tumor development is higher in patients in whom the drug was started early in pregnancy.[32] In a rare case, the tumor developed in only one of two monozygotic twins,[89] suggesting that

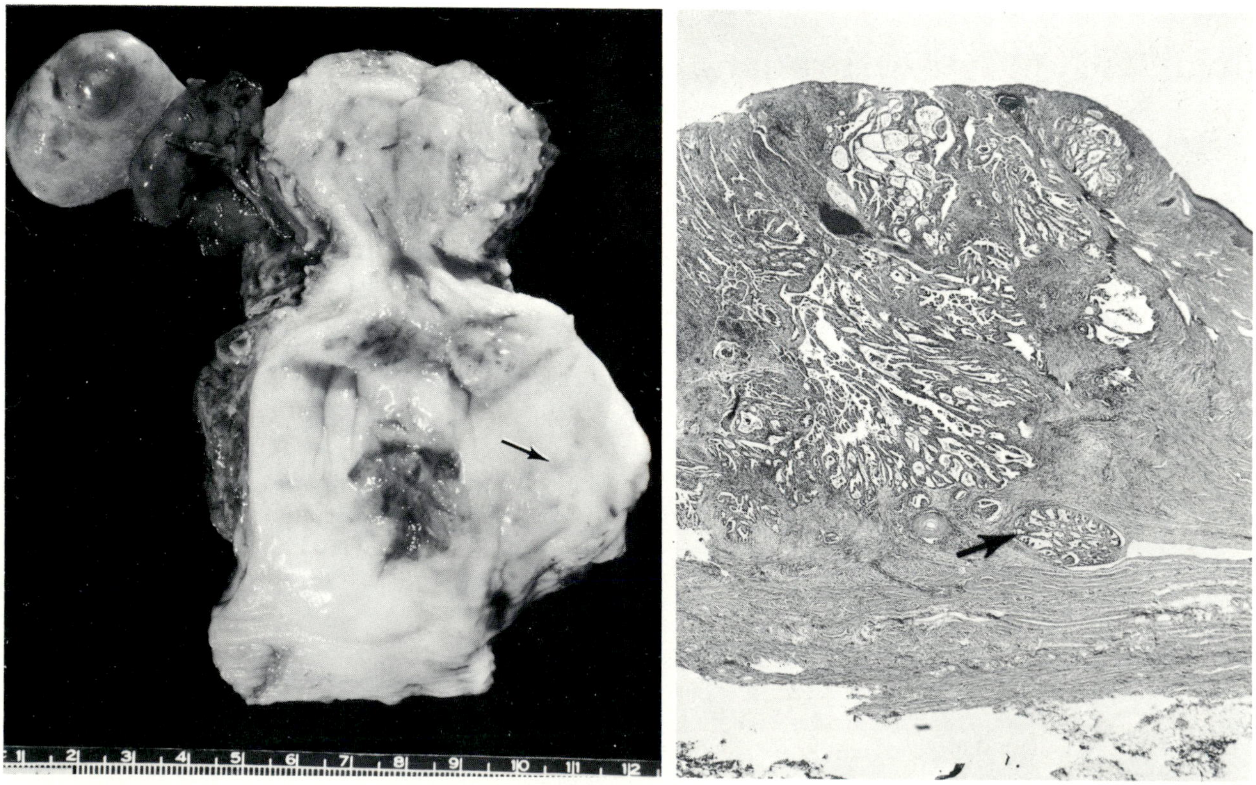

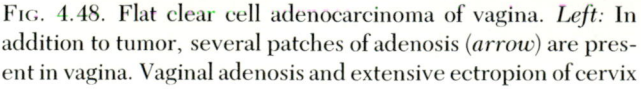

FIG. 4.48. Flat clear cell adenocarcinoma of vagina. *Left:* In addition to tumor, several patches of adenosis (*arrow*) are present in vagina. Vaginal adenosis and extensive ectropion of cervix appeared red in fresh state. *Right:* Cross-section of vagina with deeply invasive tumor and vascular invasion (*arrow*).

factors other than DES exposure play a role in carcinogenesis.

The tumor can involve any portion of the vagina or cervix, or both. Approximately 50% of lesions have been confined to the vagina (Fig. 4.48), with the rest limited to the cervix or involving both the cervix and vagina. Most vaginal tumors arise on the anterior wall, usually in the upper third, corresponding to the most frequent site of adenosis. The lateral and posterior walls and, occasionally, the middle and lower third of the vagina may also be involved. On occasion, multicentric tumors have been demonstrated on microscopic examination. Whereas a multicentric origin has been suspected grossly in some larger tumors, submucosal continuity has often been found on microscopic examination in these cases. Kissing lesions along the wall opposite the main tumor are also seen.

Gross Appearance

Tumors have varied in size from microscopic to more than 10 cm in greatest dimension. Most of the larger cancers are polypoid and nodular (Fig. 4.49), but some are flat or ulcerated, having a granular or indurated surface. Small tumors, currently being seen more frequently, are usually palpable. They may be invisible on colposcopic examination if confined to the lamina propria and if covered by intact, normal or metaplastic squamous epithelium. Although most cancers are superficial and invade only a few millimeters into the vaginal or cervical wall (Fig. 4.50), some penetrate far more deeply or extend more centrifugally than might be anticipated on gross examination. Unlike the larger tumors, which almost always cause such symptoms as vaginal bleeding or discharge, many small tumors are asymptomatic and have been detected only as more young women

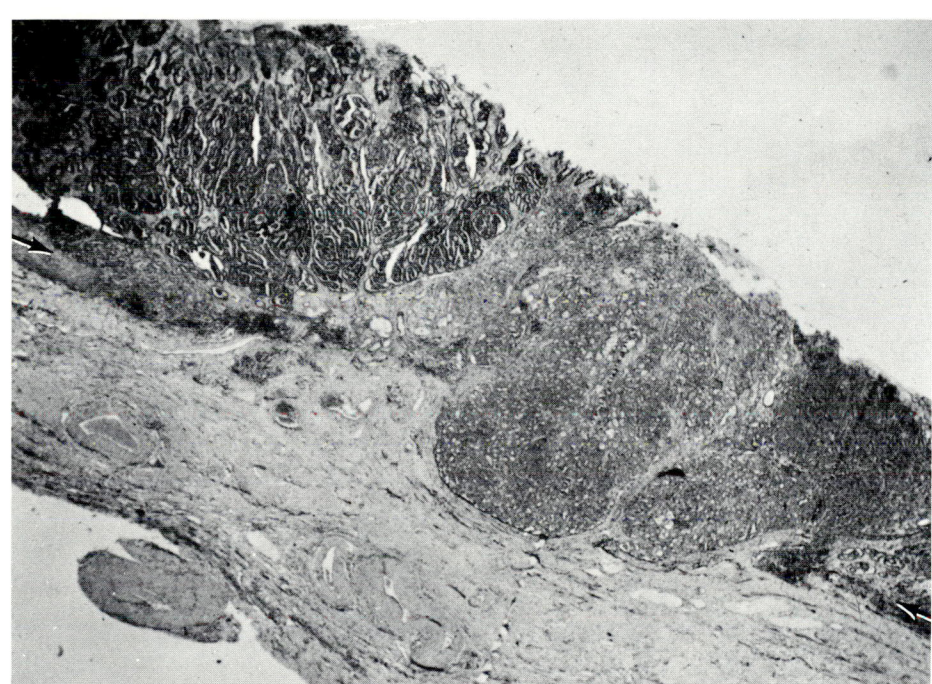

FIG. 4.49. Polypoid adenocarcinoma arising in vagina. Imaginary line drawn between borders of adjacent normal mucosa (*arrows*) illustrates superficial nature of many tumors.

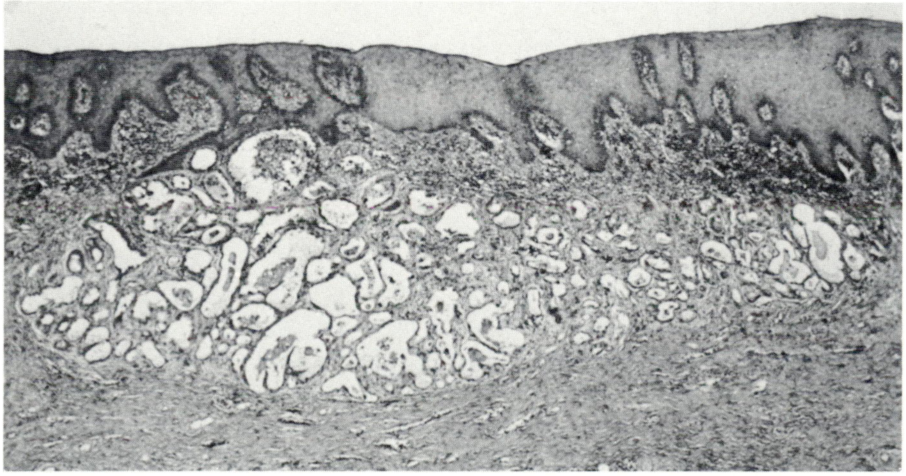

FIG. 4.50. Tumor confined to lamina propria. Tumor itself is palpable, cut cannot be seen with colposcope.

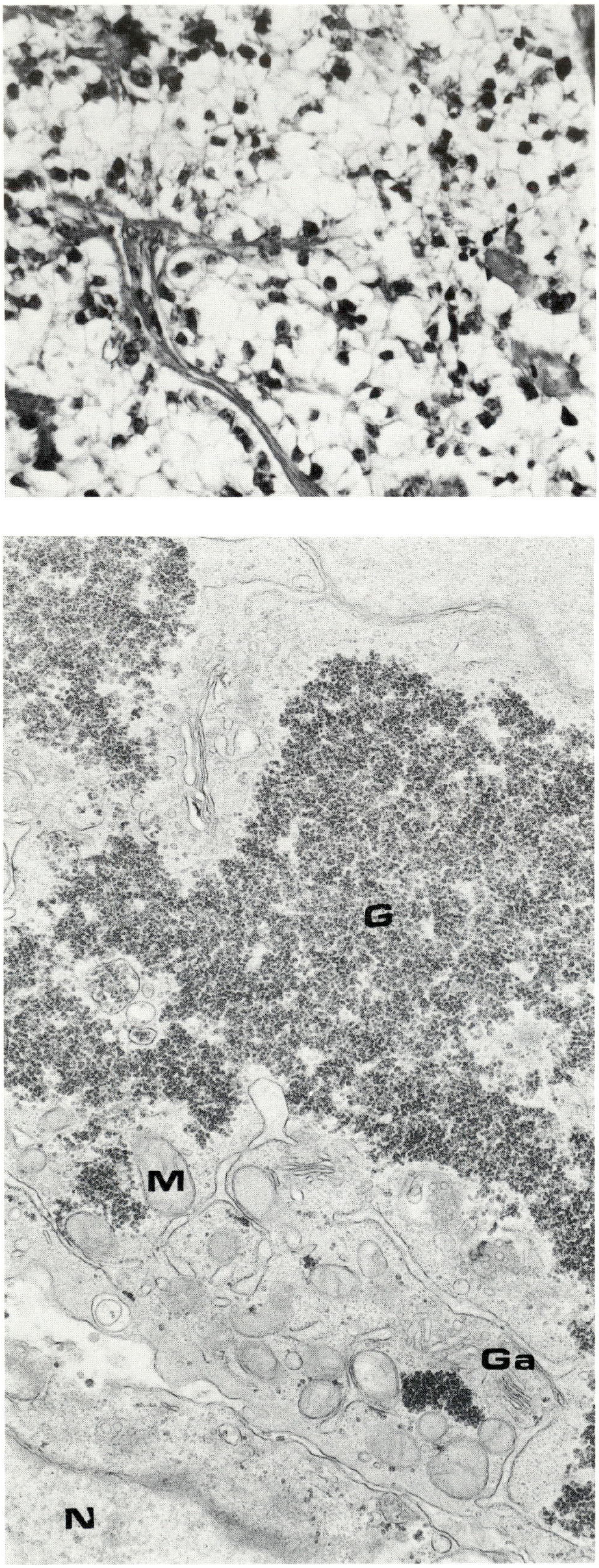

◁ FIG. 4.51. *Top:* Clear pattern of tumor, shown by light microscopy to resemble clear cell carcinoma of ovary and endometrium. *Bottom:* Special processing of specimen for electron microscopy demonstrates glycogen particles (G) in large collections in cytoplasm. Nuclei (N) and cytoplasmic organelles, such as mitochondria (M) and Golgi apparatus (Ga), are less electron dense by this technique. Osmium tetroxide. ×12,000. (Reprinted by permission of (*top*) Scully et al. Ann Clin Lab Sci 4:222–233, 1974; (*bottom*) Dickersin et al., Ref. 16.)

have sought examination because of their known exposure to DES.

Microscopic Appearance

By light and electron microscopy, the DES-associated clear cell adenocarcinoma is identical to the clear cell adenocarcinoma of the ovary and endometrium, which occur sporadically in older women. Several histologic patterns may be observed, either alone or in combination. A characteristic pattern, for which the tumor is named, consists of solid sheets of clear cells (Fig. 4.51), the clear appearance of the cytoplasm being caused by the dissolution of glycogen when the specimen is processed for microscopic examination. A second (and the most frequent) pattern, the tubulocystic pattern, is characterized by tubules and cysts lined by hobnail cells (Fig. 4.52), by flat cells (Fig. 4.53), or by cells that resemble to varying degrees the epithelium of the müllerian tract. The hobnail cell is characterized by a bulbous nucleus that protrudes into the lumen beyond the apparent cytoplasmic limits of the cell. Flat cells often appear innocuous. When only this type of epithelium is present in a small biopsy, it may be difficult to differentiate tumor from adenosis. Other patterns encountered include complex papillae (Fig. 4.54), an endometrioid pattern (Fig. 4.55), or cords of cells with eosinophilic cytoplasm (Fig. 4.56). Mitoses are usually rare. In any of these patterns, the lumen may contain mucin. The cytoplasm, however, is mucin free.

Ultrastructure

By electron microscopy the neoplastic cells from each of the patterns are of the same basic type, with glycogen and microvilli being prominent features (see Fig. 4.51).[16] Intracellular glycogen is abundant in clear cells in the solid areas and is present in varying but lesser amounts in the other cell types, including areas in which it is not apparent at the light microscopic level (Fig. 4.57).

Cytology

Clear cell adenocarcinoma can be detected cytologically. Occasionally, a suspicious or positive smear may be the first indication of a tumor in an asymptomatic woman.[97] With the use of circumferential vaginal and cervical

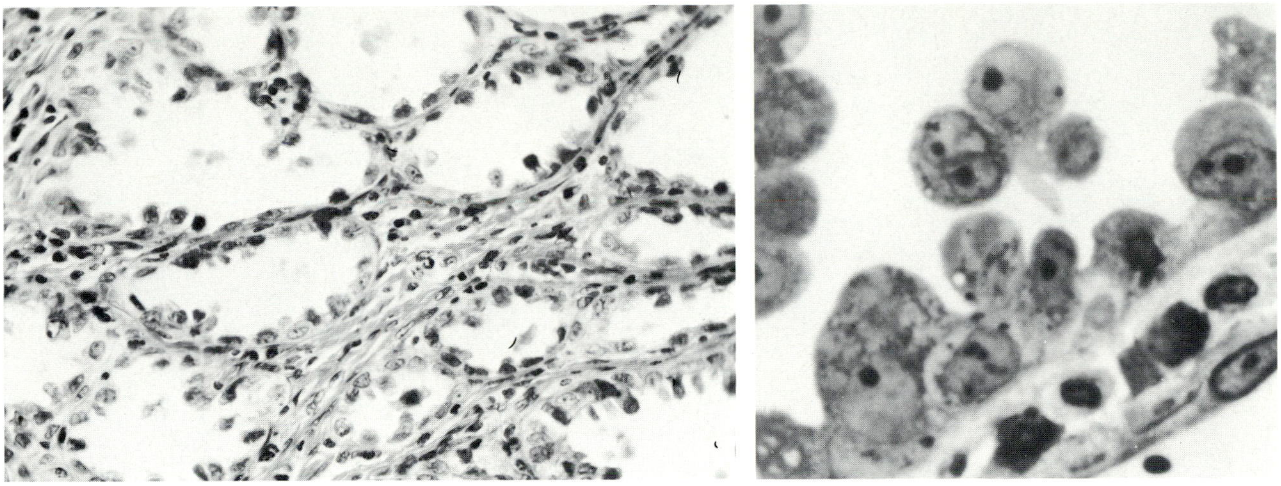

FIG. 4.52. *Left:* Tubulocystic pattern of tumor in which small tubules are lined by neoplastic hobnail, columnar, or cuboidal cells. *Right:* Detail of hobnail cells showing luminal protrusion of nucleus and scant apical cytoplasm. *Left:* Hematoxylin & eosin. *Right:* Giemsa. (Reprinted by permission of Dickersin et al., Ref. 16.)

scrapes and endocervical aspiration, a high percentage of tumors should be detected. Improved cytologic preparations are obtained if excess mucus is removed from the vagina and cervix with a soft swab. The tumor cells often resemble large endocervical cells or nonspecific adenocarcinoma cells (Fig. 4.58) but vary greatly and may appear even as undifferentiated carcinoma. False-negative results in one fifth of patients may be attributable to difficulty in distinguishing the tumor cells from endocervical cells, occasional confinement to the tumor to the lamina propria, a heavy overlay of polymorphonuclear leukocytes, and possibly the fact that some of the neoplasms may not shed cells.

Behavior and Treatment

The tumor spreads locally and also metastasizes via lymphatics and blood vessels. Approximately one-sixth of tumors confined clinically to the vagina or cervix (stage I) are discovered on exploration to have metastasized

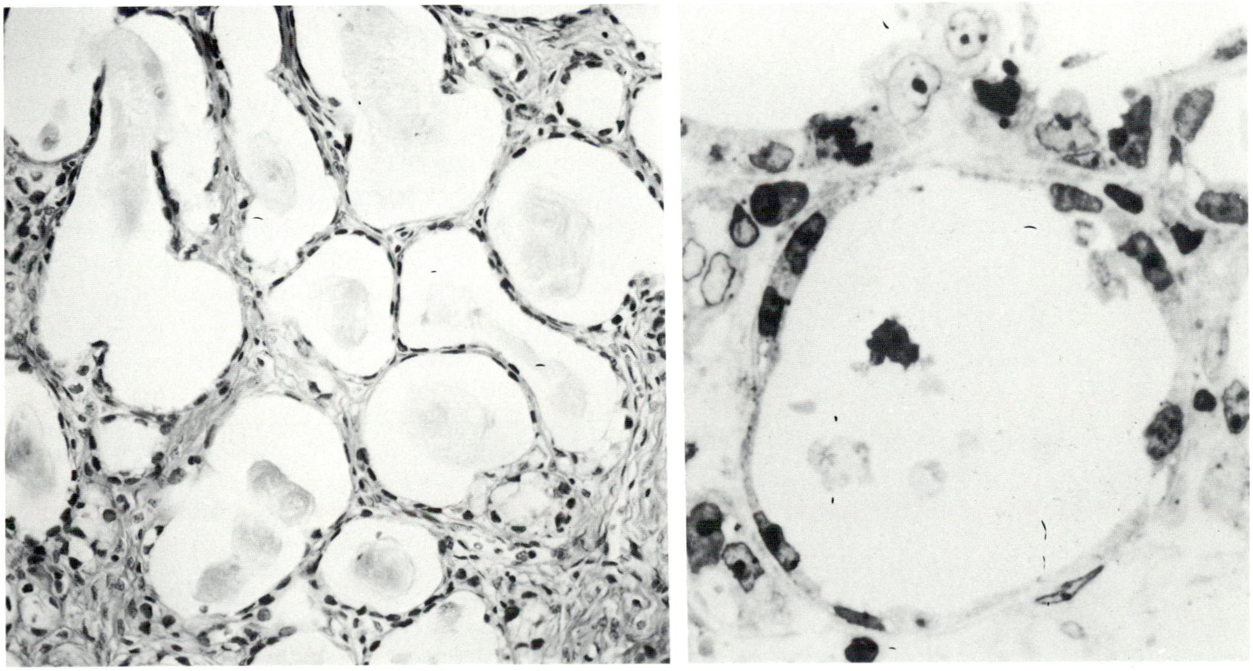

FIG. 4.53. *Left:* Dilated cysts lined by flat cells in clear cell carcinoma. *Right:* Detail of neoplastic flat cells, one of which has an atypical mitosis. Small clear spaces in cytoplasm are vestiges of glycogen. *Left:* Hematoxylin & eosin. *Right:* Giemsa. (Reprinted by permission of Dickersin et al., Ref. 16.)

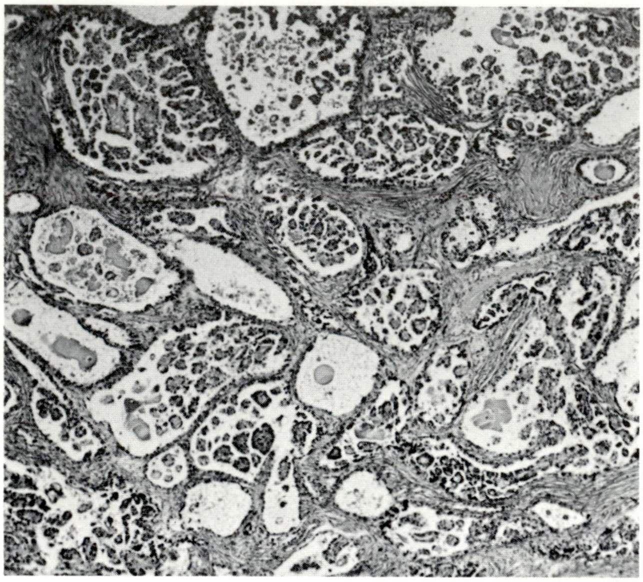

FIG. 4.54. Papillary pattern of tumor.

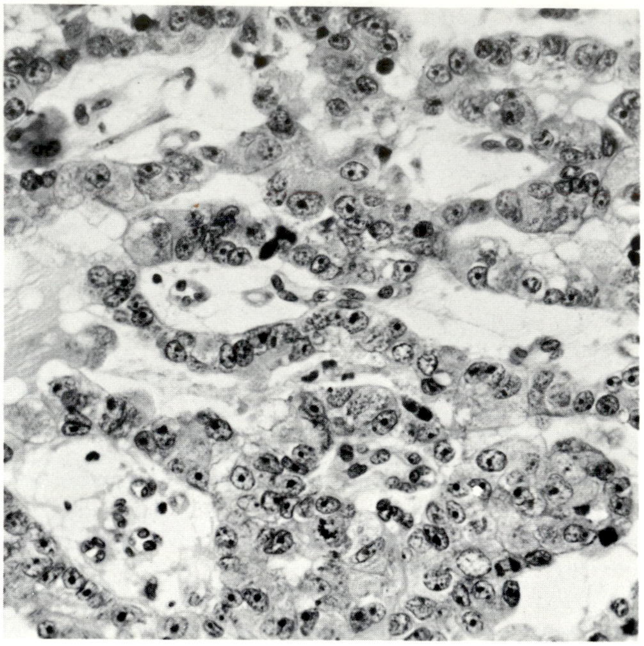

FIG. 4.56. Cords and solid masses of tumor with unusually deeply eosinophilic cytoplasm and nuclei with prominent nucleolus and delicate chromatin.

to the pelvic lymph nodes.[33,75] The frequency of nodal involvement reaches approximately 50% when stage II tumors are considered. Clear cell carcinoma extends outside the abdominal cavity more frequently than does squamous cell carcinoma of the vagina or cervix. Thirty-six percent of the initial recurrences of clear cell carcinomas are in the lung or a supraclavicular lymph node, in contrast to less than 10% for squamous cell carcinomas.[75]

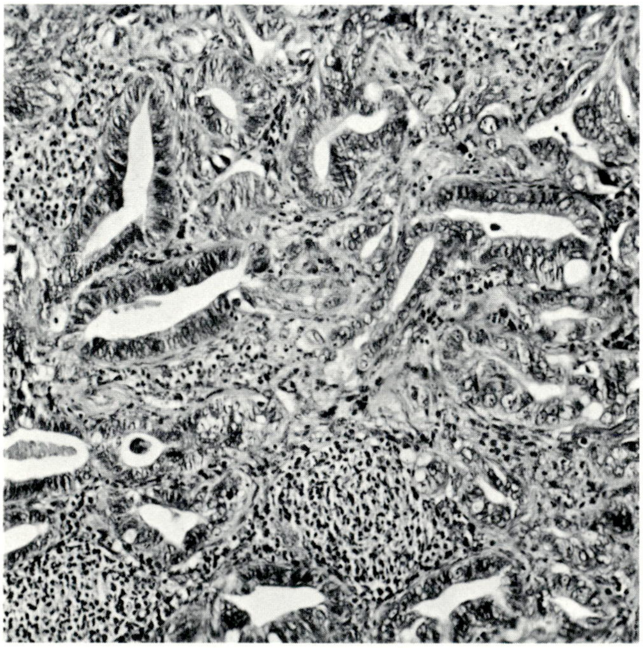

FIG. 4.55. Endometrioid pattern of tumor.

The 5-year actuarial survival for all patients with clear cell adenocarcinoma is 80%. For patients with a stage I tumor, survival increases to 88% (vagina) and 90% (cervix).[29] Factors associated with a better prognosis are an older age (19 years or older) at the time of diagnosis and a tubulocystic microscopic pattern. A factor associated with a worse prognosis is symptoms at the time the tumor was detected. Large size, deep invasion into the wall, or both are associated with a poorer prognosis, but small or superficial tumors may also recur or metastasize. The presence of aneuploidy appears to have no affect on prognosis.[105] Recurrences develop most often within 3 years after primary therapy. Following treatment of the recurrences, approximately one-fifth of the patients survive an additional 3 years or more. Several patients have survived 2 or more years after treatment of a second recurrence.

FIG. 4.58. Vaginal and cervical smears of adenocarcinoma. *a*. Clump of adenocarcinoma cells varies markedly in size; large cytoplasmic vacuoles are filled with polymorphonuclear leukocytes. *b*. Cluster of four tumor cells with prominent nucleoli. *c*. Clump of tumor cells with strikingly large nucleoli. Nuclei vary in size more than in shape. Borders are delicate and chromatin is granular. Cytoplasm is finely vacuolated with indefinite borders. *d*. Well-preserved adenocarcinoma cells with large nuclei, coarse chromatin, and multiple nucleoli. Cytoplasm is variable; several nuclei are naked. Papanicolaou stain. (Reprinted by permission of Taft et al., Ref. 97.)

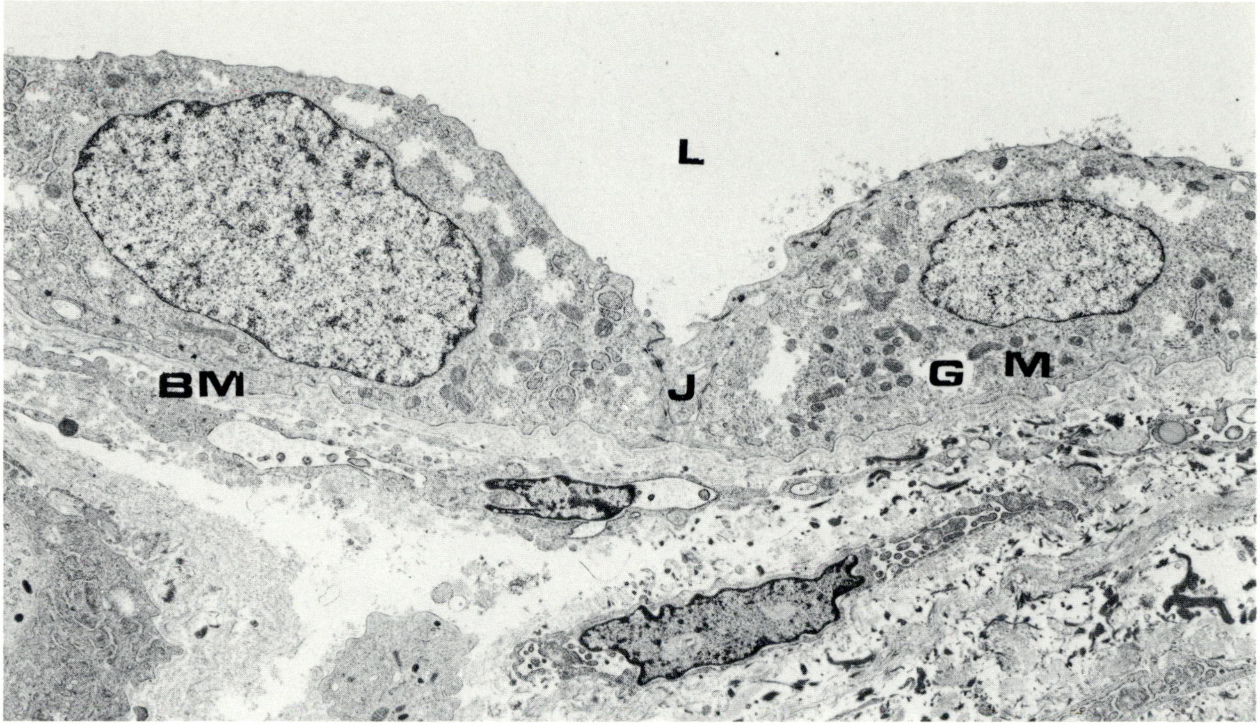

FIG. 4.57. Flat tumor cells lining a glandular lumen (L). Note empty spaces of glycogen (G), moderate numbers of mitochondria (M), distinct junctions (J), and discrete basement membrane (BM). ×4800. (Reprinted by permission of Dickersin, Ref. 16.)

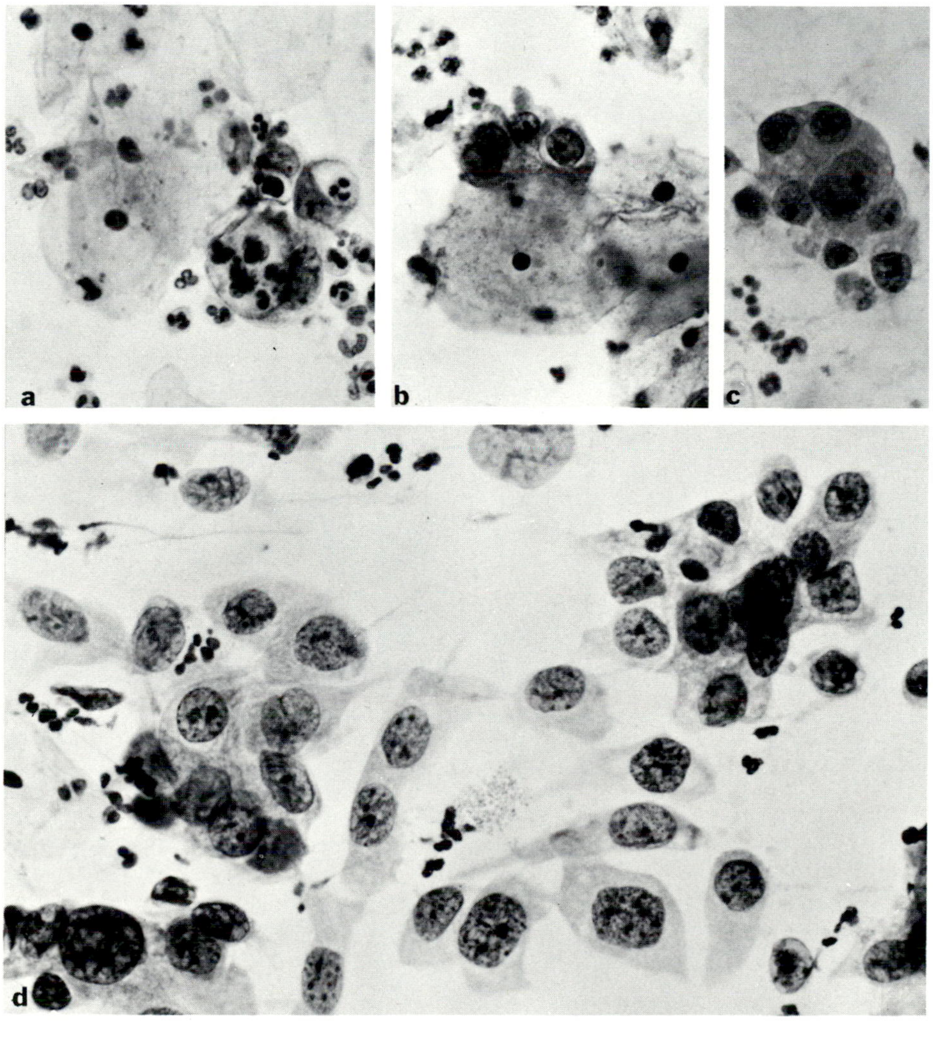

Nonneoplastic Changes

Gross Structural Changes of Vagina and Cervix

Gross structural abnormalities of the cervix or vagina occur in about one fifth of exposed women. Because they are only rarely encountered in unexposed women,[34,37] the presence of such abnormalities should always raise suspicion of DES exposure. In the cervix, their appearances vary, so that several descriptive designations have been given: cockscomb (hood), collar (rim), and pseudopolyp (Fig. 4.59). The pseudopolyp is caused by a peripheral concentric cervical band that gives the portio vaginalis central to it the appearance of a protruding cervical polyp, however, the presence of the external os at its center differentiates it from a true polyp. The cervix may be hypoplastic, the vaginal fornices may be obliterated, or the vagina may be traversed by a ridge (septum) composed of fibrous connective tissue (Fig. 4.60). The natural history of the structural anomalities is not yet well understood, although some ridges have been observed to disappear as the cervix and vagina undergo remodeling with age.[1]

Vaginal Epithelial Changes: Adenosis and Squamous Metaplasia

Vaginal adenosis and metaplastic squamous epithelium—vaginal epithelial changes (VEC)—are common in DES-exposed females. During the pre-DES era, vaginal adenosis was a clinical rarity, detected only occasionally in women, usually in their 30s or 40s, who often complained of an excessive mucous discharge from the vagina. Not surprisingly, it is found more frequently in autopsy studies in which the vagina is extensively sampled microscopically.[38,43] Recent studies have shown that the adenosis found in non-DES women is identical microscopically to that of young women who were so exposed in utero.[77] Clinically, adenosis should be suspected when

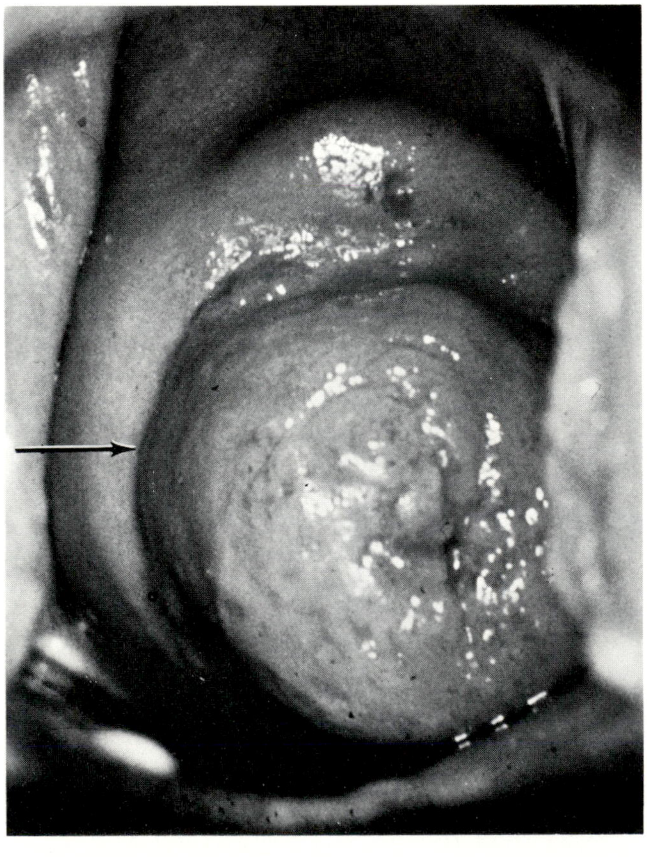

FIG. 4.59. Concentric ridge (*arrow*) in cervix creating appearance of pseudopolyp at center of which is the external os. Circular fold gives appearance of hood covering the cervix. (Reprinted by permission of Robboy et al., J Reprod Med 15: 13–18, 1975.)

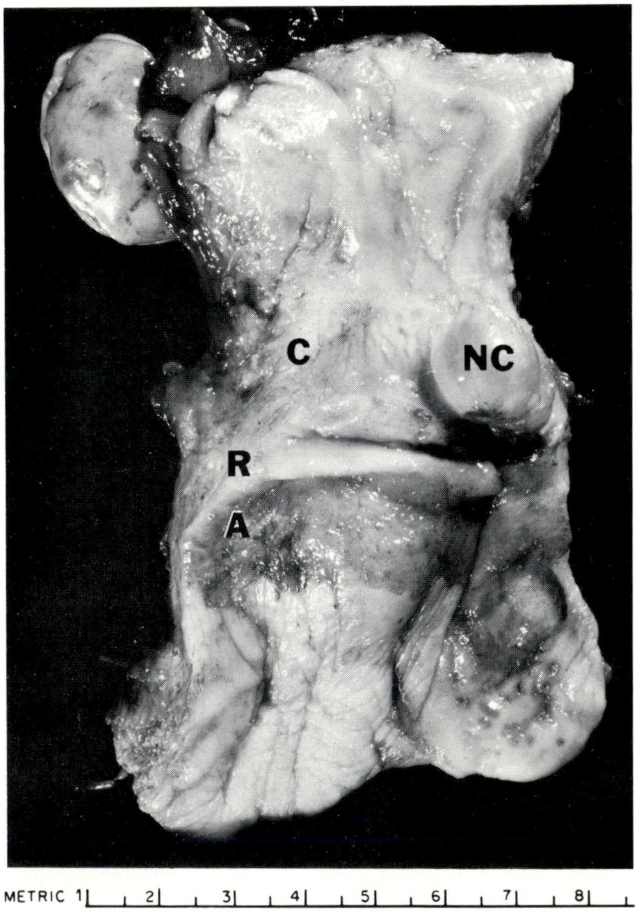

FIG. 4.60. Opened uterus and vagina with transverse vaginal ridge (R), cervix (C), and zone of adenosis (A) that macroscopically appears as patch of red granularity. Nabothian cyst (NC) of cervix is also visible along right margin of specimen. (Reprinted by permission of Herbst, N Engl J Med 287: 1259–1264, 1972.)

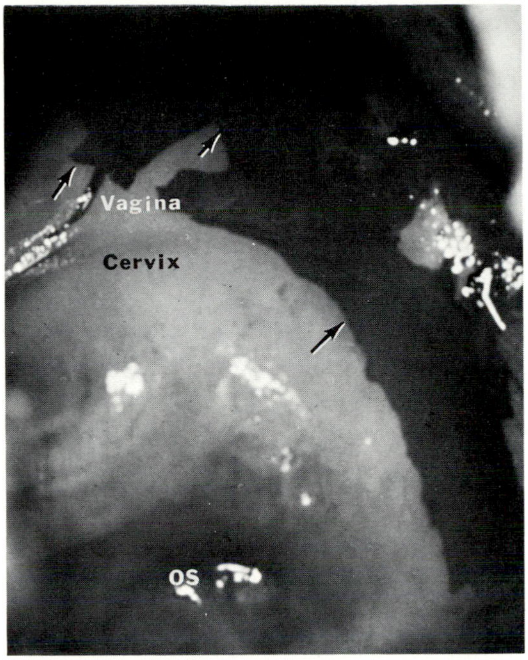

FIG. 4.61. Abnormal iodine (Schiller) stain in which aglycogenated (nonstaining) areas in both vagina and cervix appear white in photograph and represent the transformation zone. Glycogenated vaginal epithelium stains black. *Arrows* demarcate staining from nonstaining areas. (Reprinted by permission of Robboy et al., J Reprod Med 15: 13–18, 1975.)

the vaginal mucosa contains red granular spots or patches (Fig. 4.60) and does not stain with an iodine solution (Fig. 4.61). On colposcopy, adenosis appears as glandular or metaplastic epithelium replacing the native squamous epithelium of the vaginal mucosa. Punctation and mosaic pattern frequently accompany squamous metaplasia in adenosis. In 34% of all DES-exposed women, adenosis, with or without squamous metaplasia, involves the upper third of the vagina. The anterior wall is involved most frequently and the posterior wall least frequently.[80] These changes extend into the middle third of the vagina in 9% and the lower third in 2% of exposed women.

Mucinous columnar cells, which by light and electron microscopy resemble those of the normal endocervical mucosa, comprise the glandular epithelium most frequently encountered as adenosis (62% of biopsy specimens with vaginal adenosis).[80] This epithelium frequently lines the surface of the vagina and is the glandular epithelium most commonly seen by colposcopy (Fig. 4.62). Commonly, the mucinous columnar cells also appear lining glands in the lamina propria (Fig. 4.63).

Dark cells and light cells, often ciliated and resembling the lining cells of the fallopian tube and endometrium, are found in 21% of specimens with adenosis (Fig. 4.64). These cells are usually found in glands in the lamina propria and not on the surface of the vagina. Mucinous

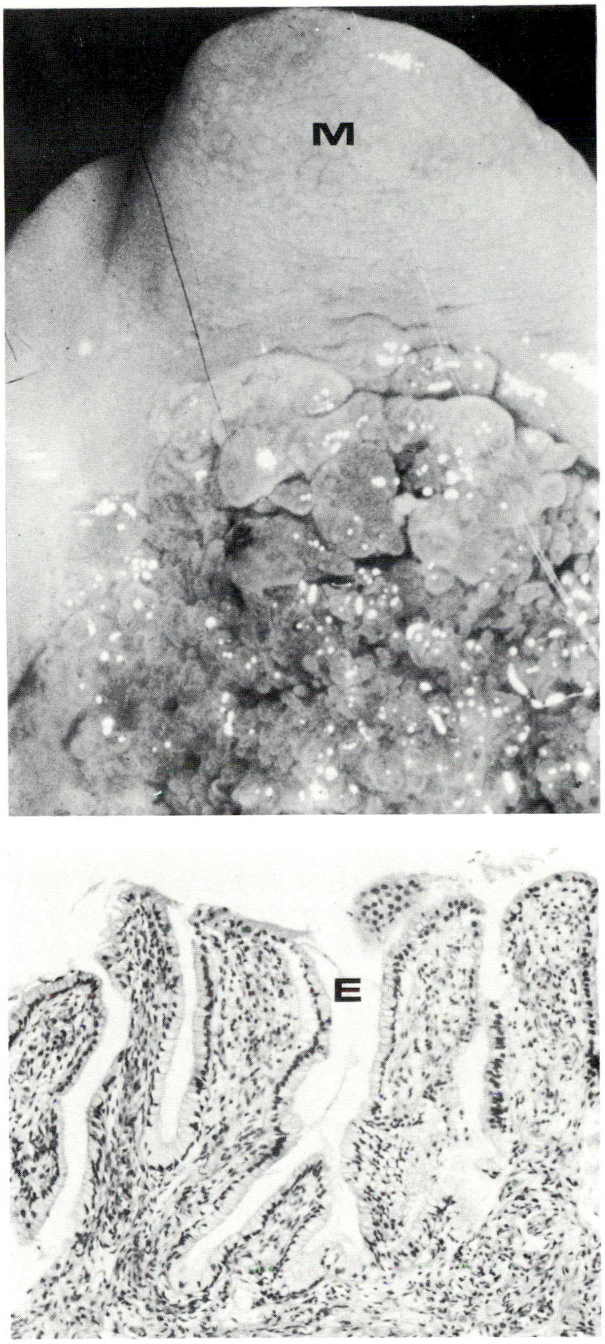

FIG. 4.62. Cervical ectropion. *Top:* Colpophotograph of anterior cervical cockscomb covered with metaplastic squamous epithelium in mosaic pattern (M). Grape-like structures along inner half of cervix are composed of fibrovascular cores covered by mucinous columnar epithelium (ectropion). *Bottom:* Photomicrograph of mucinous columnar cells (E) lining fibrovascular papillae. Same microscopical pattern in vagina is called *adenosis*.

glands and mucinous pools or droplets are encountered frequently in the same biopsy specimen; mucinous and tuboendometrial cells are found together only occasionally in biopsy material.

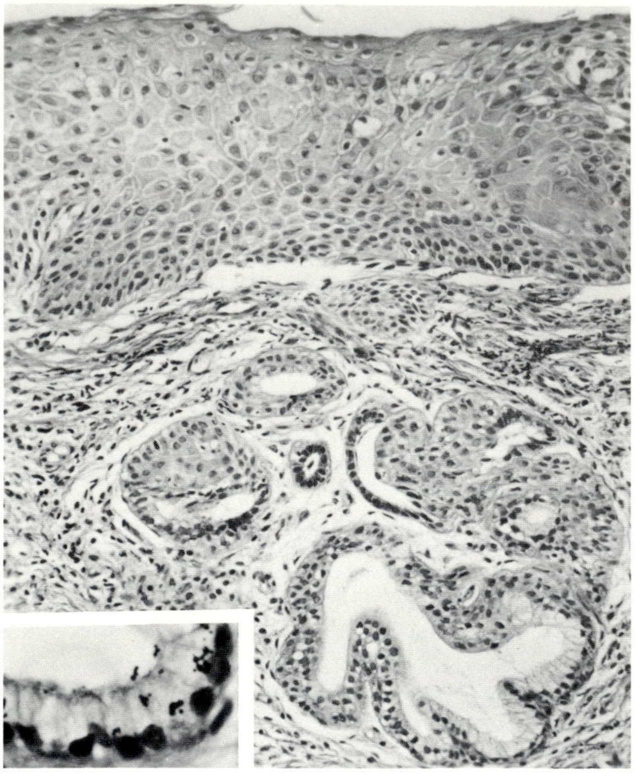

Fig. 4.63. Vaginal adenosis. Mucinous gland with focal squamous metaplasia in lamina propria. *Inset:* Detail of individual mucinous columnar cells.

In most biopsy specimens, adenosis is replaced to some degree by metaplastic squamous cells (Fig. 4.63), indicating the manner by which the adenosis regresses. Remnants of columnar cells, which appear as intercellular pools of mucin surrounded by metaplastic squamous cells (Fig. 4.65) or as intracellular droplets of mucin in metaplastic squamous cells (Fig. 4.66), constitute the evidence for adenosis in 48% of biopsy specimens with adenosis. Squamous metaplasia begins as reserve cell proliferation, then progresses through immature and mature stages. The glandular epithelium gradually disappears, and intercellular pools of mucin and droplets remain as the final vestiges of adenosis. When completely replaced by squamous epithelium, obliterated glands appear in the lamina propria as squamous pegs, which are continuous with the metaplastic squamous epithelium covering the surface (Fig. 4.67). Cytologically, the reparative process is indicated by an increase in the relative proportions of metaplastic squamous cells to mucinous columnar cells (Fig. 4.68).[85]

The paucity or total lack of glycogen in the earlier stages of squamous metaplasia often accounts for the failure of the epithelium to stain with iodine, whereas the increased vascularity, the tortuous arrangement of the vessels surrounding the pegs in the lamina propria, and the chronic inflammatory infiltrate are responsible for atypical colposcopic patterns, such as mosaicism and punctation, seen so often in patients with adenosis.[106] Hyperkeratosis accounts for the colposcopic findings of leukoplakia. Eventual maturation of the metaplastic squamous epithelium with acquisition of glycogen makes it indistinguishable from the normal (native) squamous epithelium.

Adenosis, squamous metaplasia, and cervicovaginal structural changes can disappear spontaneously. The regression of the changes is partly age related. In the National Collaborative Diethylstilbestrol Adenosis (DESAD) Project and other studies, the frequency of VEC (which includes both adenosis and squamous metaplasia) declined markedly in women 26 years of age or older, on the basis both of colposcopic examination[63] and cytologic analysis.[85] Follow-up studies in which the same subjects have been repeatedly examined over a period of several years have also indicated that the structural changes and VEC may regress spontaneously.[1,59] After 3 years of follow-up, the hoods had disappeared in more than half the participants (Fig. 4.69). The extent of VEC did not increase with time. Because VEC disappear spontaneously, they should not be treated.

Cytologic studies, in addition to their usefulness in the detection of malignancy, are helpful also in the detection of adenosis and associated squamous metaplasia, raising the strong suspicion that the patient might have been exposed in utero to DES. In smears obtained by scraping the middle and upper thirds of the entire circumference of the vagina after the excess mucus has been removed, columnar cells with mucinous cytoplasm (Fig. 4.70) or metaplastic squamous cells (Fig. 4.71) have been found in more than 22% of patients.[77,79] These cells have been found in 54% of scrapings of the exocervix and in 75% of specimens submitted together with an aspirate of the endocervical canal. Metaplastic cells may occasionally contain intracytoplasmic droplets of mucin (Fig. 4.71), and some contain keratohyaline granules. In some studies made up largely of referred patients, up to 78% of the smears have contained columnar cells. However, it is most important to recognize that columnar and metaplastic squamous cells are also found in the vagina in 11% of nonexposed subjects, in most of whom the vagina is colposcopically unremarkable, staining uniformly with an iodine solution.[85] This finding suggests either that the source of cells in the vagina may be those shed normally from the cervix or that the spatula used to obtain the vaginal smear might have touched an area of cervical ectropion, contaminating it. Endometrial-type cells found in scrape smears of the vagina rarely originate from the tuboendometrial type of adenosis but are true endometrial cells shed from the uterine corpus.

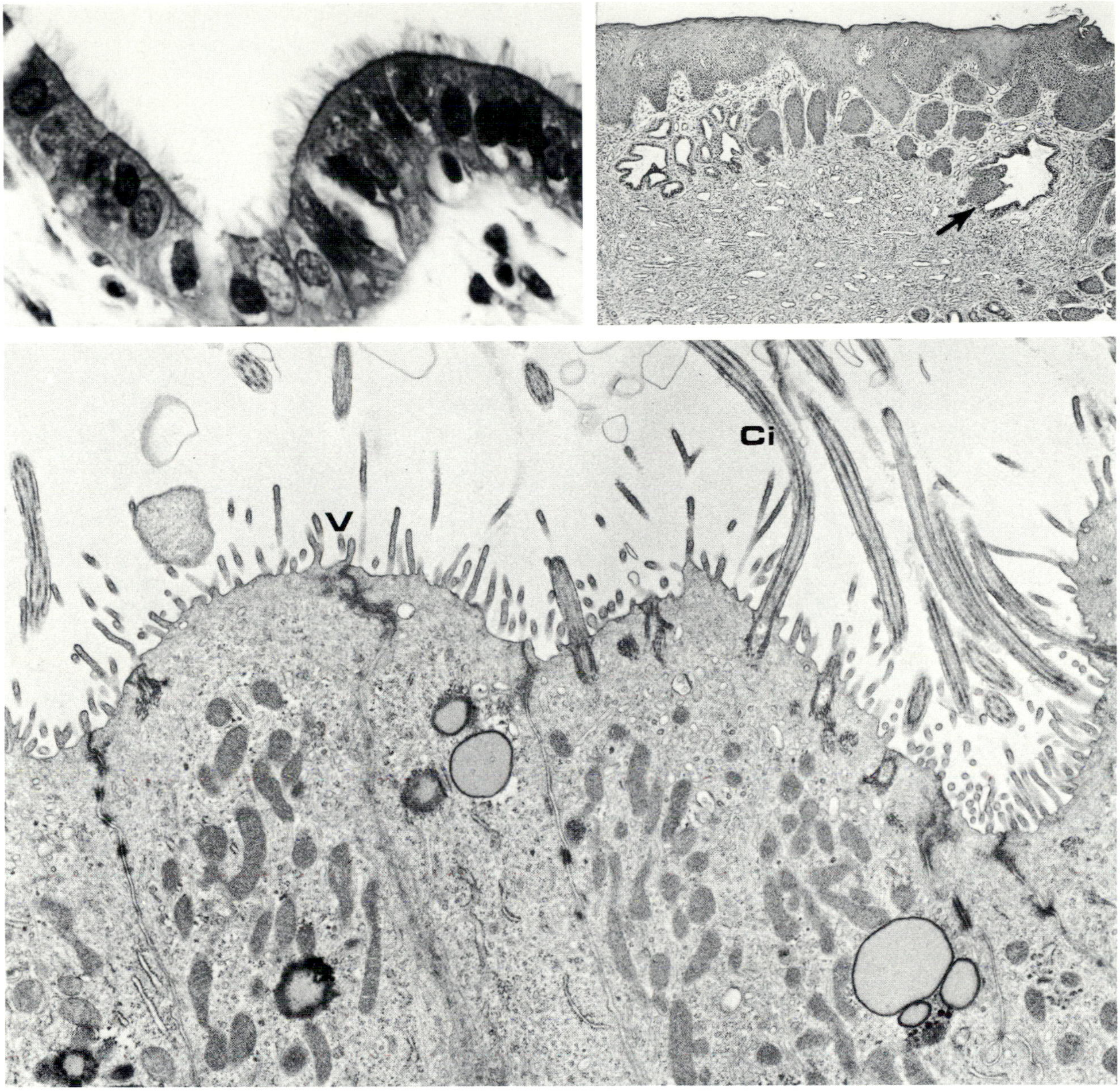

FIG. 4.64. Vaginal adenosis. *Upper right:* Glands lined by ciliated dark cells similar to tubal or endometrial epithelium are present in inflamed lamina propria and merge with squamous pegs (*arrow*). Surface epithelium is composed of glycogen-free squamous cells, accounting for abnormal iodine staining. *Upper left:* Detail of ciliated dark (tuboendometrial) cells. *Bottom:* Tuboendometrial cells are tall columnar and have orderly arrangement and distribution of organelles, some, e.g., mitochondria, in a supranuclear location. Many cilia (Ci) are in apex. Microvilli (V) are numerous and regularly distributed along luminal surface. (Reprinted by permission of Dickersin et al., Ref. 16.)

Embryologic Basis of Vaginal Adenosis and Cervical Ectropion

Ectropion and squamous metaplasia are found in the cervix in nearly all exposed women. Like adenosis and squamous metaplasia in the vagina, to which they are probably closely related, the cervical changes may be seen with the naked eye, on colposcopic examination, with iodine staining, or on microscopic study. Although many of the features described for adenosis are applicable to ectropion, important differences exist between these processes.[80] First, tuboendometrial type cells are found in only 3% of the cervical specimens with ectropion, in contrast to much higher frequencies in specimens

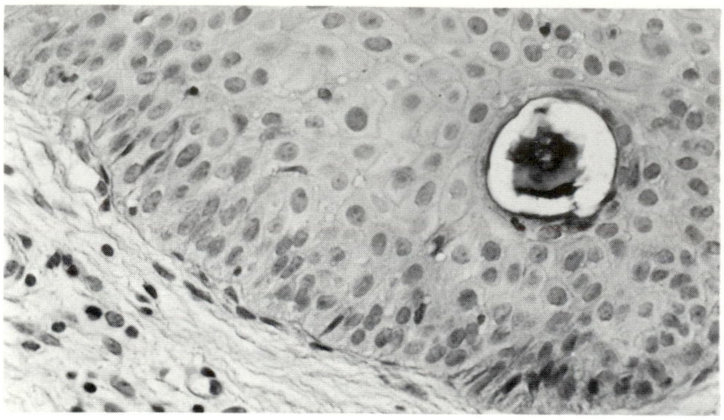

FIG. 4.65. Vaginal adenosis. Pool of mucin surrounded by flat cells with mucinous cytoplasm obvious only with mucin stains. Mucicarmine stain. (Reprinted by permission of Robboy et al., J Reprod Med 15: 13–18, 1975.)

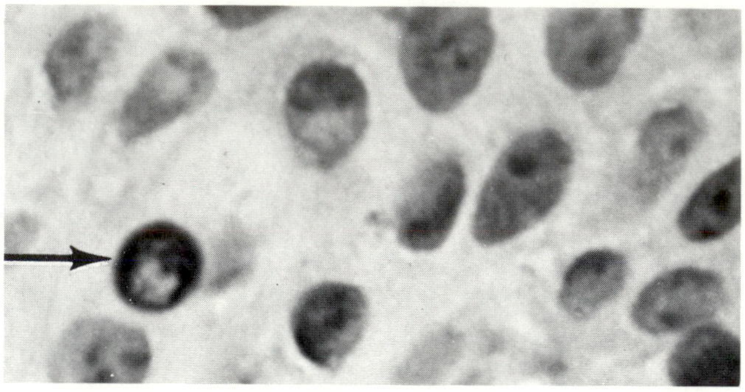

FIG. 4.66. Vaginal adenosis. Single mucin droplet (*arrow*) is bright red, nuclei of cells are brown-black, and the cytoplasm is pale yellow in tissue slide. Mucicarmine stain. (Reprinted by permission of Robboy et al., J Reprod Med 15: 13–18, 1975.)

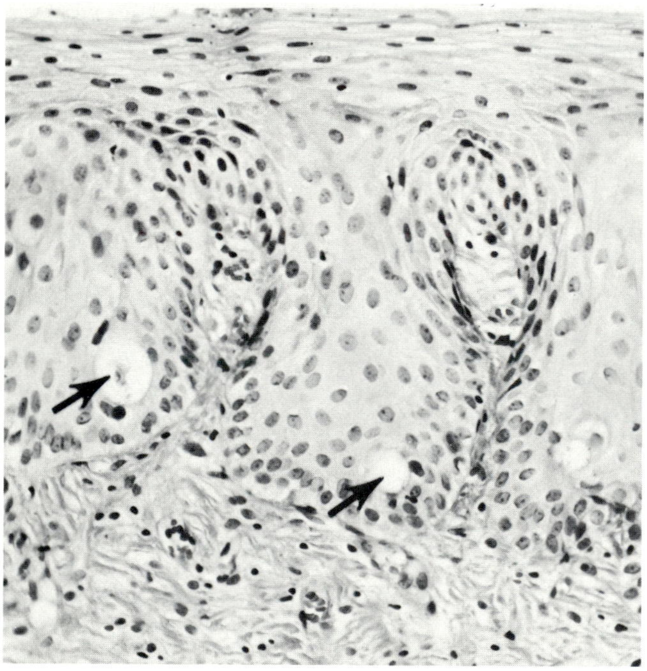

FIG. 4.67. Squamous pegs. Nests of metaplastic squamous cells are present in lamina propria and are continuous with surface epithelium. Intracellular droplets of mucin (*arrows*) represent final vestiges of healing process of adenosis. (Reprinted by permission of Robboy et al., Ref. 80.)

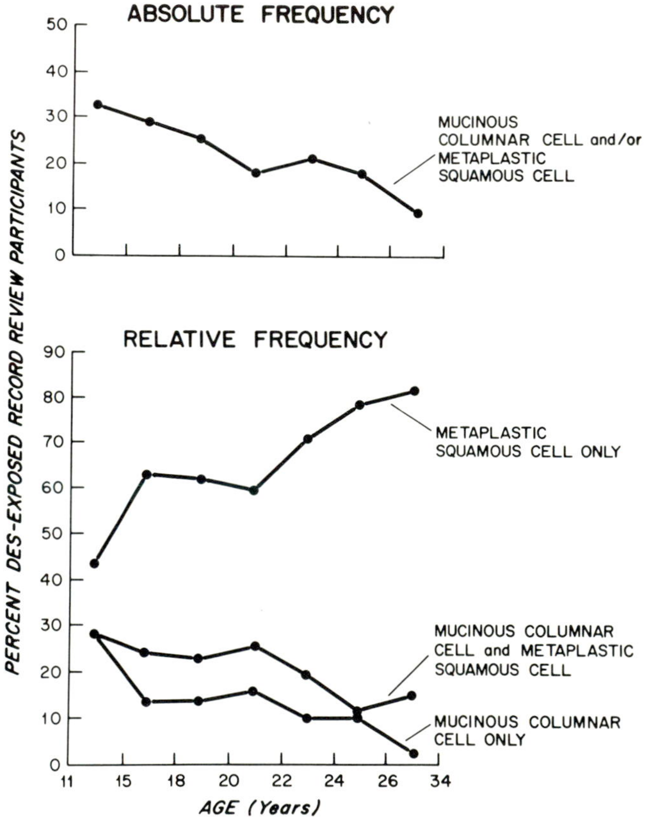

FIG. 4.68. Frequency of mucinous columnar cells and metaplastic squamous cells in vaginal scrape smears of DES-exposed women identified by review of prenatal records. (Reprinted by permission of Robboy et al., Ref. 85.)

that show adenosis from the upper (20%), middle (31%), and lower (100%) vagina. Second, adenosis occurs most often in the form of glands in the lamina propria with only occasional involvement of the surface, whereas in ectropion, the columnar epithelium commonly lines the surface of the cervix as well as the glands.

The DES experience and the new experimental studies it has fostered have provided new insights about the

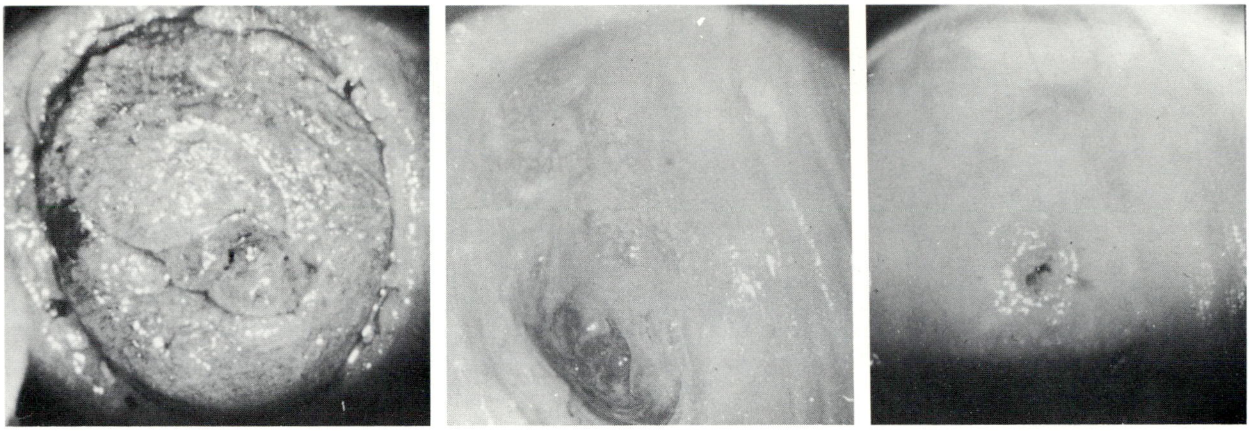

FIG. 4.69. Serial colpophotographs of cervix. *Left:* Portio of cervix displaying extensive ectropion. Cervical rim is circumferential and covered with columnar epithelium. Note prominent groove demarcating it from portio vaginalis. *Middle:* After 24 months, much of rim has disappeared and 70% of the ectropion has been replaced by metaplastic epithelium. Groove is obliterated between 9 and 4 o'clock. *Right:* Forty-two months after initial observation, entire portio vaginalis covered by metaplastic epithelium, with rim completely obliterated. (Reprinted by permission of Antonioli et al., Ref. 1.)

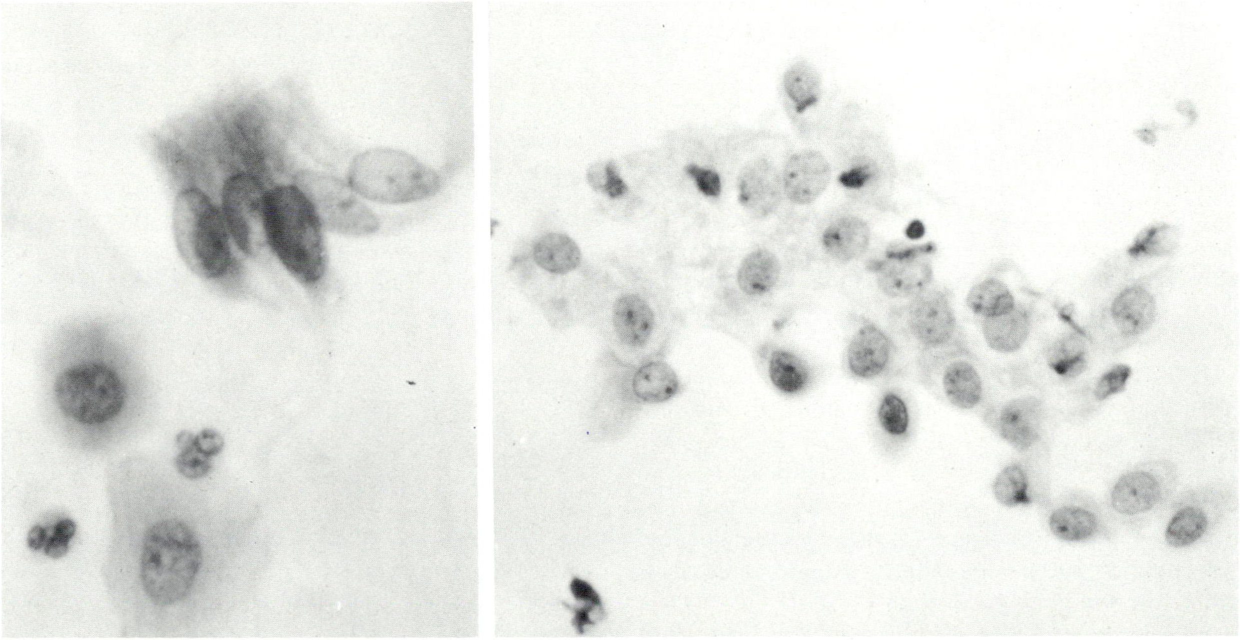

FIG. 4.70. Mucinous columnar cells, which occur singly (*left*), in strips or sheets (*right*), and sometimes as glandular groupings, are columnar in profile (*left*) and small and polygonal when viewed from end on (*right*). Cytoplasm is usually delicate and faintly eosinophilic but may be diffusely vacuolated or diminished by a single large vacuole. Round to oval nucleus is bounded by a thin, well-defined membrane, usually containing two to three chromocenters and a small nucleolus. Papanicolaou stain.

development of the normal lower genital tract and the effects caused by prenatal DES exposure.[73] In brief, the embryonic transitional-squamous epithelium of the urogenital sinus is now believed to grow up the vagina and exocervix, replacing the original columnar (müllerian) epithelium lining these organs. Estrogen appears to affect the stroma, which then inhibits the upgrowth, and hence leads to the development of adenosis from persistent residual embryonic glandular epithelium. The stroma of the vaginal wall (like the uterine corpus and fallopian tube) induces the growth of a tuboendometrial-type epithelium. The stroma of the superficial endocervix

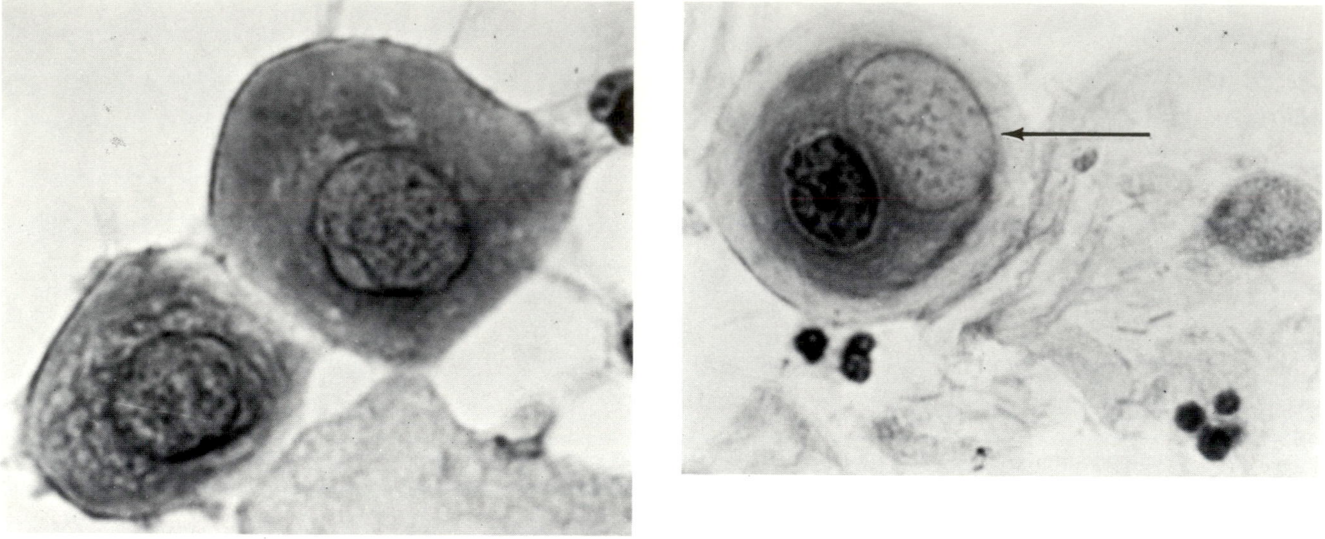

FIG. 4.71. Metaplastic squamous cells in vaginal scrape smear from patient with vaginal adenosis. *Left:* Nuclei are large, centrally located, and have finely granular and uniformly dispersed chromatin. Chromocenters are evenly distributed. Cytoplasm stains deeply pyranophilic and resembles that of normal intermediate cells, being oval to polygonal with flattened, sharply defined, angulated borders. Immature metaplastic cells resemble parabasal cells but are smaller. When nuclear:cytoplasmic ratio is slightly increased or the nuclear chromocenters are prominent, these cells may be conspicuous in a background of normal cells. *Right:* Intracytoplasmic mucinous droplet (*arrow*) is single, large, clear to amphophilic vacuole in the cytoplasm. Papanicolaou stain. (Reprinted by permission of Robboy et al., J Reprod Med 15: 13–18, 1975.)

favors mucinous columnar epithelium. In the DES-exposed woman, the embryonic müllerian epithelium that has not been replaced by sinus epithelium differentiates into predominantly mucinous epithelium in the upper vagina and predominantly tuboendometrial epithelium in the lower vagina.

In DES-exposed fetal organs, the stromal components of the uterine wall fail to segregate normally into an outer layer of smooth muscle and an inner layer of endometrial stroma.[76,98] The related clinical consequences, as the daughters mature, appear to be the gross abnormalities seen in the vagina and cervix and a functionally imperfect uterus (see section, Uterine Abnormalities and Reproductive Problems following).

Preneoplastic Changes

Atypical Adenosis

Atypical adenosis is characterized by one or more glands with cellular stratification, nuclear pleomorphism, and hyperchromasia and prominent nucleoli (Fig. 4.72). It has been identified near the periphery of most carcinomas in which the excised vagina has been serially blocked for microscopic examination. Atypical cells with nuclei that are larger and more irregular in outline than those seen in normal endocervical cells or the cells lining the glands of the adenosis have been identified in approximately 0.5% of cervical and vaginal smears from DES-exposed women.[79,85] The frequent finding of the tuboendometrial type of glandular cell and the rarity of the mucinous type of cell adjacent to the tumors suggest that the clear cell adenocarcinoma arises from the tuboendometrial cells.[86,87] Similarly, there are no mucinous

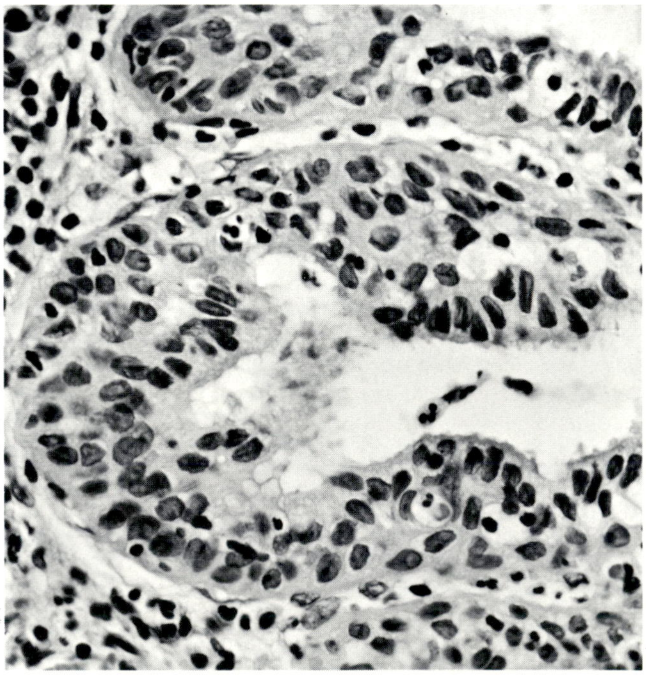

FIG. 4.72. Atypical adenosis of vagina. Nuclei vary both in size and shape; cells are stratified.

cells adjacent to clear cell carcinoma arising from the endometrium in elderly women. The studies of nuclear DNA content, show that (1) atypical forms of tuboendometrial-type cells have an aneuploid pattern, (2) tuboendometrial cells demonstrate greater proliferative activity (more often in a tetraploid state) than do endocervical-type cells, and (3) polyploid patterns are associated with active-appearing vaginal adenosis.[21] However, there has been no case yet where, over time, microscopically proven atypical adenosis has progressed to carcinoma, and, consequently, proof that atypical adenosis is a precursor of clear cell carcinoma is lacking.

Dysplasia

In the unexposed female, cervical ectropion is replaced by metaplastic epithelium, which eventually becomes mature and indistinguishable from normal squamous epithelium. Occasionally, immature metaplastic epithelia do not differentiate normally, instead evolving into dysplasia, CIS, or squamous cell carcinoma. During the past several years, multiple studies have shown that the prevalence rates of dysplasia are about the same in exposed and unexposed women (about 3%)[78] but that the incidence rates in exposed women are increased (15.9 versus 7.8 cases per 1000 patient-years of follow-up).[84] The dysplasia has been almost always mild and slightly more frequent in the cervix than in the vagina.

Several problems are of particular concern to the pathologist in the evaluation of dysplasia in DES-exposed women. First, immature metaplastic squamous cells may be misinterpreted for dysplastic cells. Whereas immature squamous metaplasia may demonstrate increased cellularity, scant cytoplasm, and occasional mitoses, the nuclei vary little in size and shape, abnormal forms are not encountered, and the chromatin is not coarsely clumped (Fig. 4.73). The DNA histogram of metaplastic squamous cells is one of euploidy or slight polypoidy.[20,22]

A second problem concerns discordance between cytology and biopsy specimens, which is commonplace in the detection and follow-up of dysplasia, especially in its milder forms.[81] Nuances in criteria among observers had been considered one cause of the discord, but in the DESAD project, repeated review conferences have shown this to be a negligible factor. A more likely cause may be intrinsic to the dysplastic cell itself and to an as yet undefined effect of DES exposure. Ultrastructural examination has demonstrated that the numbers of tonofibrils and well-developed desmosomes in dysplastic cells from DES exposed women are increased compared to dysplastic cells of the same degree of abnormality in an unexposed female.[46] Increased adherence of the cells to one another could explain the observation that dysplastic cells, especially in the lower grades, are often detected in sheets in exposed women rather than as single cells in vaginal and cervical scrape smears, as in unexposed women (Dr. James Reagan, unpublished observation).

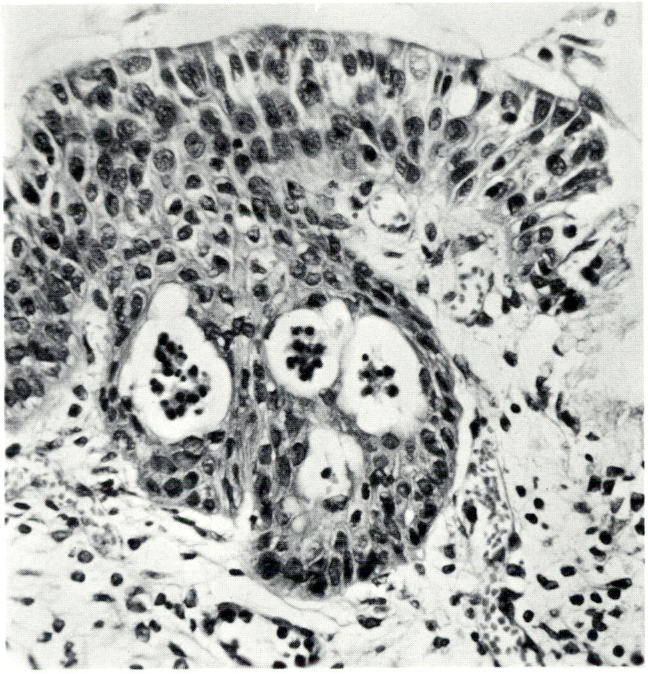

FIG. 4.73. Immature squamous metaplasia in vaginal adenosis. Although immature squamous cells have large nuclei, they are uniform in size and shape and have finely dispersed chromatin and should not be misdiagnosed as dysplastic. (Reprinted by permission of Herbst et al., Hosp Practice 10: 51–57, 1975.)

Other Entities

Microglandular Hyperplasia

Microglandular hyperplasia is a benign condition that can resemble a carcinoma on gross and microscopic examination. Usually associated with the use of oral contraceptives or occasionally with pregnancy, it is rarely observed in their absence. Although microglandular hyperplasia almost always develops in the cervix, eight cases have been described arising in foci of vaginal adenosis. Five of the young women had been exposed prenatally to DES.[74] Initially, each lesion was misinterpreted as a clear cell adenocarcinoma. Grossly, the lesion is soft, granular, tan-yellow, and usually flat. Occasionally, it may be cauliflower-like and multicentric (Fig. 4.74). Microscopic examination demonstrates many small, closely packed glands devoid of intervening stroma (see Chapter 6, Benign Lesions of Cervix). The presence of extensive nests of metaplastic squamous cells with pale eosinophilic cytoplasm may make the lesion difficult to distinguish from the solid pattern of clear cell carcinoma. A clue

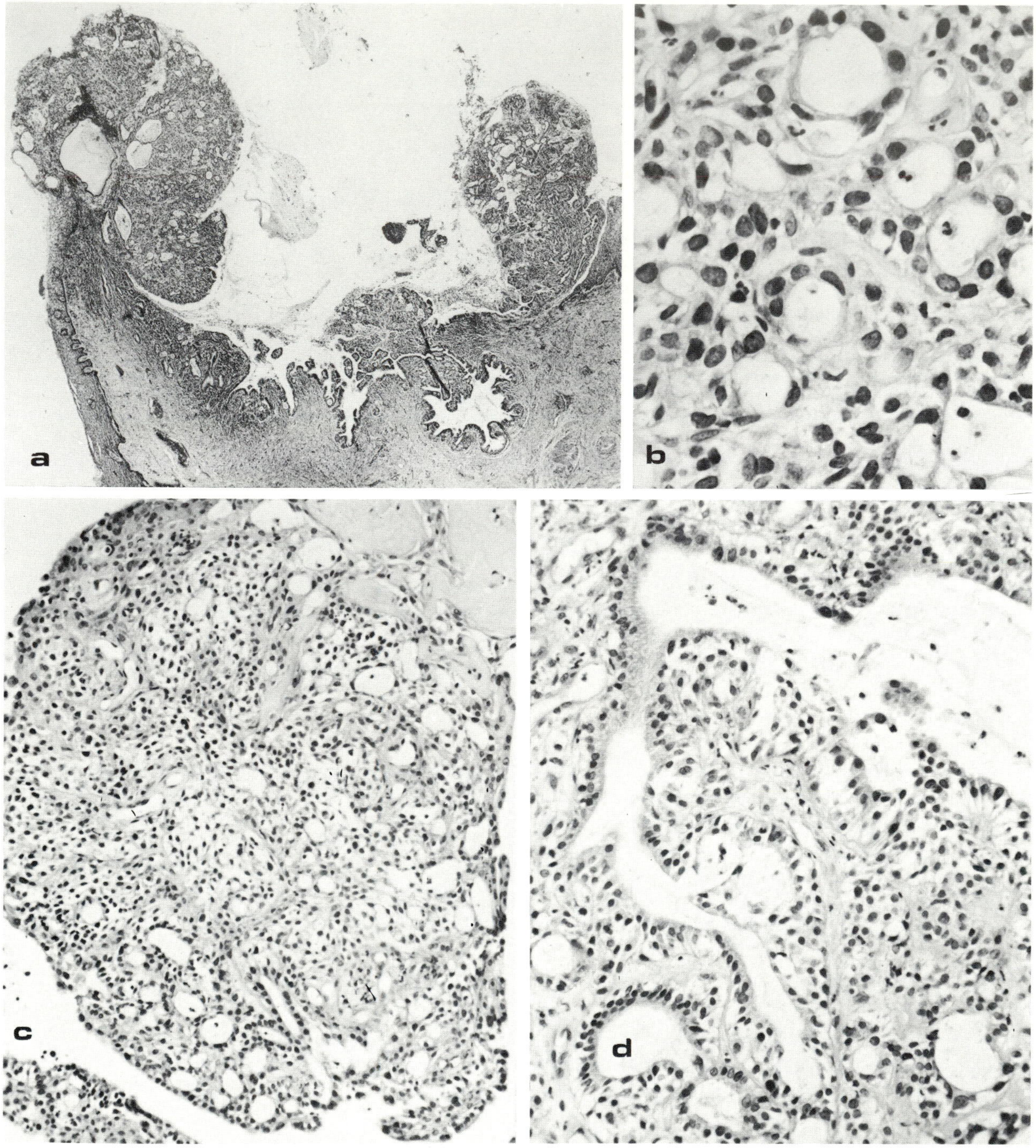

FIG. 4.74. Microglandular hyperplasia. *a*. Polypoid mass in which irregular clefts lined by mucinous columnar cells are continuous with mucinous glandular epithelium of adenosis in lamina propria of vagina. *b*. Detail of glands closely packed and separated by little or no stroma. Nuclei are uniform and have relatively fine, evenly dispersed chromatin. *c*. Nests composed largely of metaplastic squamous cells. *d*. Cleft lined by mucinous cells is continuous with the microglands. (Reprinted by permission of Robboy et al., Ref. 74.)

to the diagnosis is the presence of clefts lined by mucinous epithelium that course through the metaplastic squamous epithelium. The fact that the glands have been observed in continuity with the clefts suggests that the glands result from budding and arborization of the mucinous epithelium that constitutes one type of vaginal adenosis as well as the lining of the normal endocervix. Microglandular hvperplasia has not been shown to arise from the tuboendometrial type of adenosis. The lesion is generally reversed when oral contraceptives are discontinued.

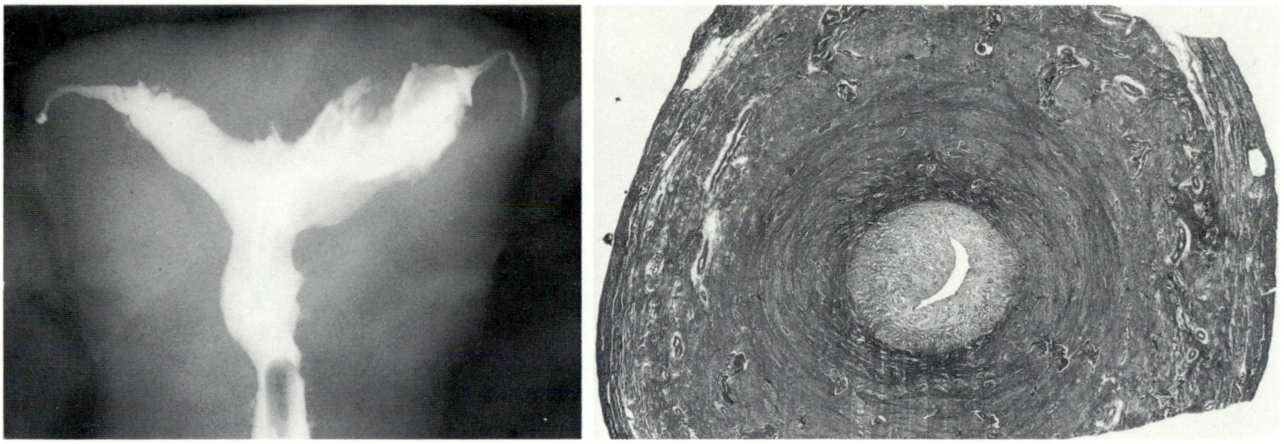

FIG. 4.75. *Left:* T-shaped appearance of uterus with circular constriction around proximal portion of horns. Polypoid mass in upper right horn is a 13-day intrauterine pregnancy. Lower uterus appears tapered and narrow. *Right:* Cross-section of tapered uterus. Trichrome Masson stain.

Arias–Stella Reaction

The Arias–Stella reaction (see Chapter 9, Uterine Corpus) usually occurs in pregnant women and must be distinguished from clear cell adenocarcinoma. Although usually seen in the endometrium, the Arias–Stella reaction has been observed in the endocervix and occasionally in vaginal adenosis of the tuboendometrial type. Characteristically, hypersecretory glands are lined by cells with markedly enlarged nuclei resembling hobnail cells. However, in clear cell adenocarcinoma, the presence of sheets of clear cells or prominent papillae should enable the two lesions to be distinguished. In addition, the hobnail-like nuclei in the Arias–Stella phenomenon are commonly smudged, lack mitotic activity, and appear to be degenerative.

Uterine Abnormalities and Reproductive Problems

Preliminary data about the frequency and extent of functional uterine disturbances in exposed daughters are conflicting. It now appears that exposed and unexposed women are similar in their frequency of menstrual irregularities and the ability to conceive.[2,3] However, the ability of an exposed daughter to give birth to a full-term, live infant is impaired. Unfavorable outcomes, including spontaneous abortion, ectopic pregnancy, premature birth, and stillbirth, are more frequent in exposed than in unexposed women. Possibly, the adverse risk is partly related to structural changes in the cervix or to the presence of an anatomically deformed uterine corpus. Detailed planometric measurements have documented that the endometrial cavity area, upper uterine segment, and endocervical canal measurements are one-third to two-thirds less in some exposed than unexposed women.[28] In a study of 267 DES-exposed daughters, abnormal hysterosalpingograms (Fig. 4.75) were found in 86% of those who had structural changes of the cervix (as against 56% for no changes) and in 82% of women with VEC (as compared with 44% when VEC were absent).[42] Normal term pregnancies were achieved in 87% of nonexposed women, 58% of exposed women with normal hysterosalpingograms, but in only 34% of exposed women with abnormal hysterosalpingograms.

References

1. Antonioli DA, Burke L, Friedman EA (1980) Natural history of diethylstilbestrol-associated genital lesions: Cervical ectopy and cervicovaginal hood. Am J Obstet Gynecol 137: 847
2. Barnes AB (1979) Menstrual histories of young women exposed in utero to diethylstilbestol. Fertil Steril 32: 148
3. Barnes AB, Colton T, Gundersen JH, et al. (1980) Fertility and outcome of pregnancy in women exposed in utero to diethylstilbestrol: Preliminary findings from the DESAD Project. N Engl J Med 302: 609
4. Beard CM, Melton LJ III, O'Fallon WM, et al. (1984) Cryptorchism and maternal estrogen exposure. Am J Epidemiol 120: 707
5. Berman ML, Tobon H, Surti U (1981) Primary malignant melanoma of the vagina: Clinical, light and electron microscopic observations. Am J Obstet Gynecol 139: 963
6. Braga CA, Teoh TB (1964) Amoebiasis of the cervix and vagina. J Obstet Gynaecol Br Commonw 71: 299
7. Buntine DW, Henderson PR, Biggs JS (1979) Mixed tumor of the vagina. Gynecol Oncol 8(1): 21
8. Chirayil SJ, Tobon H (1981) Polyps of the vagina: A clinicopathologic study. Cancer 47: 2904
9. Classification and staging of malignant tumors in the female pelvis. (1977) Am Coll Obstet Gynecol Tech Bull 47: 3

10. Copeland LJ, Gerschenson DM, Patton BS, et al. (1985) Sarcoma botryoides of the female genital tract. Obstet Gynecol 66: 262
11. Copeland LJ, Sneige N, Ozdones NG, et al. (1985) Endodermal sinus tumor of the vagina and cervix. Cancer 55: 2558
12. Cramer D, Cutler S (1974) Incidence and histopathology of malignancies of the female genital organs in the United States. Am J Obstet Gynecol 118: 443
13. Cunha GR, Fujii H (1981) Stromal–mesenchymal interactions on normal and abnormal development of the genital tract. In: Herbst AL, Bern H (eds). Developmental Effects of DES in Pregnancy. New York, Thieme Stratton, Inc., pp 179–183
14. Davos I, Abell MR (1976) Sarcomas of the vagina. Obstet Gynecol 47(3): 342
15. DeCherney AH, Cholst I, Naftolin F (1981) Structure and function of the fallopian tubes following exposure to diethylstilbestrol (DES) during gestation. Fertil Steril 36: 741
16. Dickersin GR, Welch WR, Erlandson R, Robboy SJ (1980) Ultrastructure of 16 cases of clear cell adenocarcinoma of the vagina and cervix in DES-exposed young women. Cancer 45: 1615
17. Dzikonski M, Raber G, Kohly A (1979) Gartner's duct carcinoma of vagina in pregnancy. Zentralbl Gynaekol 101: 24,1595
18. Elliot GB, Elliot JDA (1973) Superficial stromal reactions of lower genital tract. Arch Pathol 94: 100
19. Friedrich EG, Siegesmund SK (1980) Tampon-associated vaginal ulcerations. Obstet Gynecol 55: 149
20. Fu YS, Robboy SJ, Prat J (1978) Nuclear DNA study of vaginal and cervical squamous cell abnormalities in DES exposed progeny. Obstet Gynecol 52: 129
21. Fu YS, Reagan JW, Richart RM, Townsend DE (1979) Nuclear DNA and histologic studies of genital lesions in diethylstilbestrol-exposed progeny. I. Intraepithelial glandular abnormalities. Am J Clin Pathol 72: 515
22. Fu YS, Lancaster WD, Richart RM, et al. (1983) Cervical papillomavirus infection in diethylstilbestrol-exposed progeny. Obstet Gynecol 61: 59
23. Gallup DG, Morley G (1975) Carcinoma in situ of the vagina. Obstet Gynecol 46: 339
24. Gold JM, Bossen EH (1976) Benign vaginal rhabdomyoma. Cancer 37: 2283
25. Greenberg ER, Barnes AB, Resseguie L, et al. (1984) Breast cancer in mothers given diethylstilbestrol in pregnancy. N Engl J Med 311: 1393
26. Greenwood JR, Picket MJ (1980) Transfer of *Haemophilus vaginalis* Gardner and Dukes to a new genus, *Gardnerella: G. vaginalis* (Gardner and Dukes) comb. nov. Int J Syst Bacteriol 30: 170
27. Halpert R, Butt KMH, Sedlis A, et al. (1985) Human papillomavirus infection and lower genital neoplasia in female renal allograph recipients. Transplant Proc 17: 93
28. Haney AF, Hammon CB, Soules MR, Creasman WT (1979) Diethylstilbestrol-induced upper genital tract abnormalities. Fertil Steril 31: 142
29. Herbst AL, Bern H (1981) Developmental effects of DES in pregnancy. New York, Thieme Stratton, Inc.
30. Herbst AL, Ulfelder H, Poskanzer DC (1971) Adenocarcinoma of the vagina: Association of maternal stilbestrol therapy with tumor appearance in young women. N Engl J Med 284: 878
31. Herbst AL, Cole P, Colton T, et al. (1977) Age-incidence and risk of diethylstilbestrol-related clear cell adenocarcinoma of the vagina and cervix. Am J Obstet Gynecol 128: 43
32. Herbst AL, Cole P, Norusis MJ, et al. (1980) Epidermiologic aspects and factors related to survival in 384 Registry cases of clear cell adenocarcinoma of the vagina and cervix. Am J Obstet Gynecol 135: 876
33. Herbst AL, Norusis MJ, Rosenow PJ, et al. (1979) An analysis of 346 cases of clear cell adenocarcinoma of the vagina and cervix with emphasis on recurrence and survival. Gynecol Oncol 7: 111
34. Herbst AL, Poskanzer DC, Robboy SJ, et al. (1975) Prenatal exposure to stilbestrol: A prospective comparison of exposed female offspring with unexposed control. N Engl J Med 292: 334
35. Hilgers R, Malkasian GD Jr, Soule EH (1970) Embryonal rhabdomyosarcoma (botryoid type) of the vagina: A clinicopathologic review. Am J Obstet Gynecol 107: 484
36. Horwitz RI, Viscoli CM, Merino M, et al. Clear cell adenocarcinoma of the vagina and cervix. Incidence, misclassified disease, and diethylstilbestrol, submitted
37. Jefferies JJ, Robboy SJ, O'Brien PC, et al. (1984) Structural anomalies of the cervix and vagina in women enrolled in the diethylstilbestrol adenosis (DESAD) project. Obstet Gynecol 148: 59
38. Johnson LD, Driscoll SG, Hertig AT, et al. (1979) Vaginal adenosis in stillborns and neonates exposed to diethylstilbestrol and steroidal estrogens and progestins. Obstet Gynecol 53: 671
39. Jones MJ, Levin JH (1981) Verrucous carcinoma of the vagina. Case report. Cleve Clin Q 48: 305
40. Kasai K, Yoshida Y, Okumura M (1980) Alveolar soft part sarcoma in the vagina: Clinical features and morphology. Gynecol Oncol 9: 277
41. Katz Z, Lancet M, Skornik J, et al. (1985) Teratogenicity of progestogens given during the first trimester of pregnancy. Obstet Gynecol 65: 775
42. Kaufman RH, Adam E, Binder GL, Gerthoffer EA (1980) Upper genital tract changes and pregnancy outcome in offspring exposed in utero to diethylstilbestrol. Am J Obstet Gynecol 137: 299
43. Kurman RJ, Scully RE (1974) The incidence and histogenesis of vaginal adenosis: An autopsy study. Hum Pathol 5: 265
44. Laing FC, Shanser JD, Salmen BJ (1978) Vaginitis emphysematosa, importance of its radiologic recognition. Arch Surg 113: 561
45. Larsen B, Galask RP (1980) Vaginal microbial flora: Practical and theoretic relevance. Obstet Gynecol 55[Suppl]: 1005
46. Lawrence WD, Shingleton HM, Gore H, Soong SJ (1980) Ultrastructural and morphometric study of diethylstilbestrol-associated lesions diagnosed as cervical intraepithelial neoplasia III. Cancer Res 40: 1558
47. Leary FJ, Resseguie LJ, Kurland LT, et al. (1984)

Males exposed in utero to diethylstilbestrol. JAMA 252: 2984
48. Lee RB, Buttoni L, Dhru K, et al. (1984) Malignant melanoma of the vagina: A case report of progression from preexisting melanosis. Gynecol Oncol 19: 238
49. Loughlin JE, Robboy SJ, Morrison AS (1980) Risk factors for cancer of the testis. N Engl J Med 303: 112
50. Maurer HM, Moon T, Donaldson M, et al. (1977) The Intergroup Rhabdomyosarcoma Study: A preliminary report. Cancer 40: 2015
51. McLachlan JA, Newbold RR, Bullock BC (1980) Long-term effects on the female mouse genital tract associated with prenatal exposure to diethylstilbestrol. Cancer Res 40: 3988
52. McLachlan JA, Newbold RR, Shah HC, et al. (1982) Reduced fertility in female mice exposed transplacentally to diethylstilbestrol. Fertil Steril 38: 364
53. Merkus JMWM, Bisschop MPJM, Stolte LAM (1985) The proper nature of vaginal candidiasis and the problem of recurrence. Obstet Gynecol Rev 40: 493
54. Miettinen M, Wahlstrom T, Vesterinen E, et al. (1983) Vaginal polyps with pseudosarcomatous features: A clinicopathologic study of seven cases. Cancer 51: 1148
55. Naves AE, Monti JA, Chichoni E (1980) Basal cell-like carcinoma in the upper third of the vagina. Am J Obstet Gynecol 137: 136
56. Newbold RR, Bullock BC, McLachlan JA (1983) Exposure to diethylstilbestrol during pregnancy permanently alters the ovary and oviduct. Biol Reprod 28: 736
57. Newbold RR, Tyrer S, Haney AF, McLachlan JA (1983) Developmentally arrested oviduct—A structural and functional defect in mice following prenatal exposure to diethylstilbestrol. Teratology 27: 417
58. Noller KL, Fish DR (1974) Diethylstilbestrol usage: Its interesting past, important present, and questionable future. Med Clin North Am 58: 793
59. Noller KL, Townsend DE, Kaufman RH, et al. (1983) Maturation of vaginal and cervical epithelium in women exposed in utero to diethylstilbestrol (DESAD Project). Am J Obstet Gynecol 146: 279
60. Nordrum TA (1966) Vaginal metastases of hypernephroma: Report of three cases. Acta Obstet Gynecol Scand 45: 515
61. Norris HJ, Taylor AB (1966) Polyps of the vagina: A benign lesion resembling sarcoma botryoides. Cancer 19: 227
62. Okagaki T, Ishida T, Hilgers RD (1976) A malignant tumor of the vagina resembling synovial sarcoma. Cancer 37: 2306
63. O'Brien PC, Noller K, Robboy SJ, et al. (1979) Vaginal epithelial change in young women enrolled in the national cooperative diethylstilbestrol adenosis (DESAD) project. Obstet Gynecol 53: 300
64. Paris AL, Loreen AM, Blum D, et al. (1982) Pathologic findings in twelve fatal cases of toxic shock syndrome. Ann Intern Med 96: 852
65. Perez CA, Arneson AN, Dehner LP, Galakotos A (1979) Radiation therapy of carcinoma of vagina. Obstet Gynecol 44: 862
66. Peters WA III, Kumar NB, Anderson J, et al. (1985) Primary sarcoma of the adult vagina: A clinicopathologic study. Obstet Gynecol 65: 699
67. Petrilli ES, Townsend DE, Morrow CD, et al. (1980) Vaginal intraepithelial neoplasia: Biologic aspects and treatment with topical 5-fluorouracil and the carbon dioxide laser. Am J Obstet Gynecol 138: 321
68. Plapinger L (1981) Morphological effects of diethylstilbestrol on neonatal mouse uterus and vagina. Cancer Res 41: 4667
69. Plapinger L, Bern HA (1979) Adenosis-like lesions and other cervicovaginal abnormalities in mice treated perinatally with estrogen. J Natl Canc Inst 63: 507
70. Plentl A, Friedman EA (1971) Lymphatic system of the female genitalia. Philadelphia, W.B. Saunders Co.
71. Porreco R, Penn I, Droegmueller W, et al. (1975) Gynecologic malignancies in immunosuppressed organ homograft recipients. Obstet Gynecol 45: 359
72. Pride GC, Buchler DA (1977) Carcinoma of vagina 10 or more years following pelvic irradiation therapy. Am J Obstet Gynecol 127: 513
73. Robboy SJ (1983) A hypothetic mechanism of diethylstilbestrol (DES)-induced anomalies in prenatally exposed women. Hum Pathol 14: 831
74. Robboy SJ, Welch WR (1977) Microglandular hyperplasia in vaginal adenosis associated with oral contraceptives and prenatal diethylstilbestrol (DES) exposure. Obstet Gynecol 49: 430
75. Robboy SJ, Herbst AL, Scully RE (1974) Clear cell adenocarcinoma of the genital tract in young females. Analysis of 37 tumors that persisted or recurred after primary therapy. Cancer 34: 606
76. Robboy SJ, Taguchi O, Cunha GR (1982) Normal development of the human female reproductive tract and alterations resulting from experimental exposure to diethylstilbestrol. Hum Pathol 13: 190
77. Robboy SJ, Hill EC, Sandberg EC, Czernobilsky B (1986) Vaginal adenosis in women born prior to the diethylstilbestrol (DES) era. Hum Pathol 17: 488
78. Robboy SJ, Truslow GY, Anton J, Richard RM (1981) Role of hormones including diethylstilbestrol (DES) in the pathogenesis of cervical and vaginal intraepithelial neoplasia. Gynecol Oncol 12: S98
79. Robboy SJ, Friedlander LM, Welch WR, et al. (1976) Cytology of 575 young females exposed prenatally to diethylstilbestrol (DES). Obstet Gynecol 48: 511
80. Robboy SJ, Kaufman RH, Prat J, et al. (1979) Pathologic findings in young women enrolled in national cooperative diethylstilbestrol adenosis (DESAD) project. Obstet Gynecol 53: 309
81. Robboy SJ, Keh PC, Nickerson RJ, et al. (1978) Squamous cell dysplasia and carcinoma in situ of the cervix and vagina after prenatal exposure to diethylstilbestrol. Obstet Gynecol 51: 5628
82. Robboy SJ, Noller KL, Kaufman RH, et al. (1982) An atlas of findings in the human female after intrauterine exposure to diethylstilbestrol. DHEW publication No. 82-2344
83. Robboy SJ, Noller KL, Kaufman RH, et al. (1980) Prenatal diethylstilbestrol (DES-exposure): Recommendations of the Diethylstilbestrol Adenosis (DESAD) project for the

identification and management of exposed individuals. DHEW publication No. 80-2049
84. Robboy SJ, Noller KL, O'Brien P, et al. (1984) Increased incidence of cervical and vaginal dysplasia in 3,980 diethylstilbestrol (DES)-exposed young women: Experience of the National Collaborative DES-Adenosis (DESAD) Project. JAMA 252: 2979
85. Robboy SJ, Szyfelbein WM, Goellner JR, et al. (1981) Dysplasia and cytologic findings in 4,589 young women enrolled in diethylstilbestrol-adenosis (DESAD) project. Am J Obstet Gynec 140: 579
86. Robboy SJ, Welch WR, Young RH, et al. (1982) Topographic relation of adenosis, clear cell adenocarcinoma and other related lesions of the vagina and cervix in DES-exposed progeny. Obstet Gynecol 60: 546
87. Robboy SJ, Young RH, Welch WR, et al. (1984) Atypical (dysplastic) adenosis: Forerunner and transitional state to clear cell adenocarcinoma in young women exposed in utero to diethylstilbestrol. Cancer 54: 869
88. Rotmensch J, Rosenshein N, Dillon M, et al. (1983) Carcinoma arising in the neovagina: Case report and review of the literature. Obstet Gynecol 61: 534
89. Sandberg EC, Christian JC (1980) Diethylstilbestrol-exposed monozygotic twins discordant for cervicovaginal clear cell carcinoma. Am J Obstet Gynecol 137: 220
90. Schottenfeld D, Warshauer ME, Sherlock S, et al. (1980) The epidemiology of testicular cancer in young adults. Am J Epidemiol 112: 232
91. Schumacher GFB, Gill WB, Hubby MM, et al. (1981) Semen analysis in male exposed in utero to diethylstilbestrol (DES) or placebo. IRSC Med Sci 9: 100
92. Sillman FH, Sedlis A, Boyce JG (1985) A review of lower genital intraepithelial neoplasia and the use of topical 5-fluorouracil. Obstet Gynecol Surv 40: 190
93. Sillman FH, Stanek A, Sedlis A, et al. (1984) The relationship between human papillomavirus and lower genital intraepithelial neoplasia in immunosuppressed women. Am J Obstet Gynecol 150: 300
94. Sirota RL, Scully RE (1980) Mixed tumors of the vagina. Lab Invest 42(I) (Abstract)
95. STD Treatment Guidelines (1985) Morbidity and Mortality Weekly Report (Supplement) 34: 1045
96. Stefansson K, Wollman RL (1982) S100 protein in granular cell tumors (granular cell myoblastomas). Cancer 49: 1834
97. Taft PD, Robboy SJ, Herbst AL, et al. (1974) Cytology of the clear-cell adenocarcinoma of the genital tract in young females: Analysis of 95 cases from the registry. Acta Cytol 19: 279
98. Taguchi O, Cunha GR, Robboy SJ (1983) Experimental study of the effect of diethylstilbestrol (DES) on the development of the human female reproductive tract. Biol Res Prac 4: 56
99. Taguchi O, Cunha GR, Lawrence WD, Robboy SJ (1984) Timing and irreversibility of müllerian duct inhibition of the embryonic reproductive tract of the human male. Dev Biol 106: 394
100. Tavassoli FA, Norris HJ (1979) Smooth muscle tumors of the vagina. Obstet Gynecol 53: 689
101. Tobon H, Murphy A, Salazar H (1973) Primary leiomyosarcoma of the vagina: Light and electron microscopic observations. Cancer 32: 450
102. Todd J, Fishant M, Kappal F, et al. (1978) Toxic shock syndrome associated with phage group 1 staphylococci. Cancer 2: 1116
103. Ulfelder H, Robboy SJ (1976) The embryological development of the human vagina. Am J Obstet Gynecol 126: 769
104. Wagner JP (1983) Toxic shock syndrome: A review. Am J Obstet Gynecol 146: 93
105. Welch WR, Fu YS, Robboy SJ, Herbst AL (1983) Nuclear DNA content of clear cell adenocarcinoma of the vagina and cervix and its relations to prognosis. Gynecol Oncol 15: 230
106. Welch WR, Robboy SJ, Kaufman RH, et al. (1985) Pathology of colposcopic findings in 2,635 diethylstilbestrol-exposed young women. Gynecol Oncol 21: 277
107. Young RH, Scully RE (1984) Endodermal sinus tumor of the vagina: A report of nine cases and review of the literature. Gynecol Oncol 18: 380

5

Anatomy and Histology of the Cervix

Alex Ferenczy, M.D., and Barbara Winkler, M.D.

Gross Anatomy

The cervix (term taken from the Latin, meaning *neck*) is the most inferior portion of the uterus, protruding into the upper vagina. The vagina is fused circumferentially and obliquely around the distal part of the cervix, dividing it into an upper, supravaginal and lower, vaginal portion.[19] The cervix measures 2.5–3.0 cm in length in the adult nulligravida, and its normal position is slightly angulated downward and backward. The vaginal portion (portio vaginalis) of the cervix, also referred to as the exocervix, is delimited by the anterior and posterior fornices and has a convex elliptical surface. It is centered by the external os, a circular (in the nulligravida) or slit-like (in the parous woman) opening (Fig. 5.1). The portio may be divided into anterior and posterior lips, of which the anterior is shorter and projects lower than its posterior counterpart. The external os is interconnected with the isthmus (internal os) by the cervical canal. The canal is an elliptical cavity, measuring in its greatest width 8 mm, and contains longitudinal mucosal ridges, the plicae palmatae (Fig. 5.2). The area between the endocervical and endometrial cavity is called the *isthmus* or *lower uterine segment*. The latter term is used principally for descriptive purposes during gestation and labor. The use of the terms *anatomic* and *histologic internal os* seems arbitrary, as no convincing morphologic evidence is offered to support such a geographic subdivision. The uterus is best divided into corpus, isthmus, and cervix. The muscular layer in the region of the isthmus is less well developed than in the corpus, a feature that facilitates effacement and dilatation during labor.

The blood supply of the cervix is provided by the descending branches of the uterine arteries, reaching the lateral walls along the upper margin of the paracervical ligaments (cardinal ligaments of Mackenrodt). These ligaments and the uterosacral ligaments, which attach the supravaginal portion of the cervix to the second through fourth sacral vertebrae, are the main source of fixation, support, and suspension of the organ. The venous drainage parallels the arterial system, with communication between the cervical plexus and neck of the urinary bladder. The lymphatics of the cervix have a dual origin:[24] beneath the mucosa and deep in the fibrous stroma. Both systems collect into two lateral plexuses in the region of the isthmus and give origin to four efferent channels running toward (1) the external iliac and obturator nodes, (2) the hypogastric and common iliac nodes, (3) the sacral nodes, and (4) the nodes of the posterior wall of the urinary bladder. The innervation of the cervix is chiefly limited to the endocervix and peripheral deep portion of the exocervix.[19] This distribution is responsible for the relative insensitivity to pain of the portio vaginalis. The cervical nerves derive from

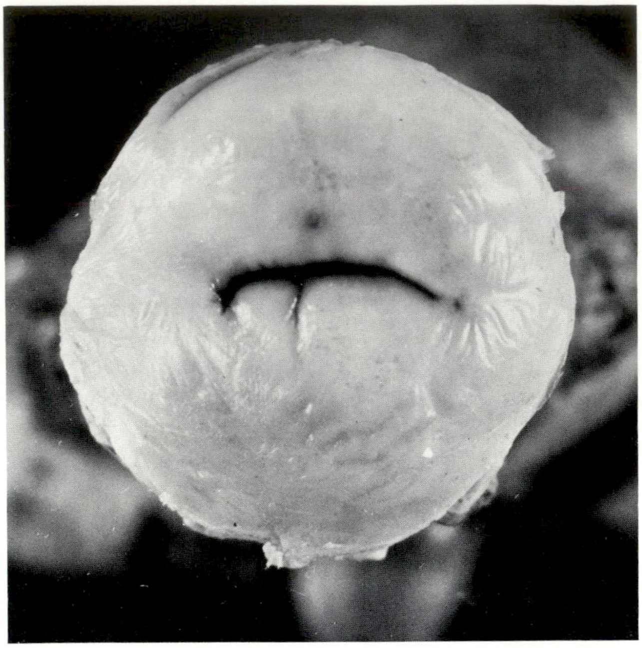

FIG. 5.1. Multiparous exocervix with slit-like external os.

the pelvic autonomic system, the superior, middle, and inferior hypogastric plexuses.

Normal Morphology and Physiology

The cervix is composed of an admixture of fibrous, muscular, and elastic tissue and is lined by columnar and squamous epithelium. The fibrous connective tissue is the predominant component. Smooth muscle, making about 15% of the substance, is mainly located in the endocervix, the portio vaginalis being virtually devoid of smooth muscle fibers.[19] By contrast, at the isthmus, 50–60% of the supportive tissue is made of muscular elements arranged in a concentric fashion, serving the function of sphincter.

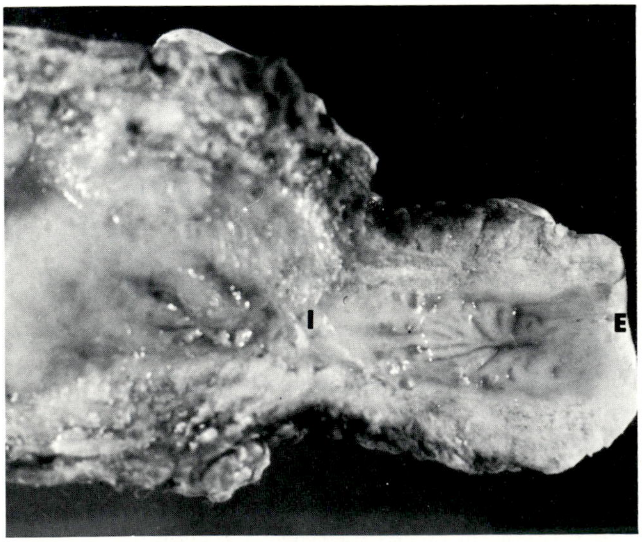

FIG. 5.2. Transected multiparous uterus. The endocervical canal is delimited by the isthmus (I) and external os (E). Note prominent muscosal folds of endocervical canal.

Squamous Epithelium

The exposed, or vaginal, portion of the cervix is generally lined by a nonkeratinizing, squamous stratified epithelium, which is referred to as *the native portio epithelium* (Fig. 5.3). The portio epithelium is remodeled by proliferation–maturation–desquamation during the reproductive period. The epithelium is completely replaced by a new population of cells every 4–5 days; the process of squamous epithelial maturation can be accelerated to 3 days by the administration of estrogenic compounds.[18,19] In general, estradiol-17 β stimulates epithelial proliferation, maturation, and desquamation, whereas progesterone inhibits maturation at the upper midzone level of the epithelium. As a result, the portio epithelium during the postnatal period is fully mature and contains large amounts of glycogen from the influence of maternal estrogens. Maturation ceases and glycogen

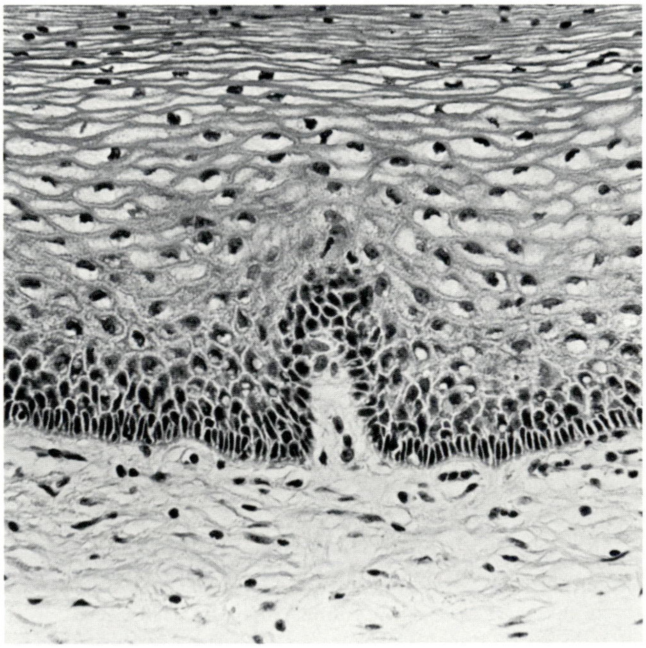

FIG. 5.3. Mature squamous epithelium of the portio of the cervix. Note gradual ascending maturation, vacuolization of midzone cells, and a single layer of basal cells in which the nuclei are perpendicularly oriented to the basal lamina. The stromal–epithelial junction contains a finger-like, fibrovascular stromal papilla penetrating the lower portion of the epithelium.

rapidly disappears as the serum hormone levels fall. The epithelium remains atrophic until the time of menarche when, under the stimulatory effect of ovarian hormones, maturation occurs again and glycogen reappears. During pregnancy, when progesterone levels are elevated, superficial cell maturation is absent.

The mature cervical squamous epithelium is similar to the vaginal epithelium but under normal circumstances lacks the rete pegs seen in the vagina. It is divided into three zones: (1) the basal or germinal cell layer, which is responsible for continuous epithelial renewal, (2) the midzone or stratum spinosum, the dominant portion of the epithelium, and (3) the superficial zone, containing the most mature cell population (Fig. 5.3). The basal zone is composed of one or two layers of elliptical cells, about 10 μm in diameter, with scant cytoplasm and oval nuclei oriented perpendicular to the underlying basal lamina (Fig. 5.3). Epithelial regeneration is the major function of the basal cells; their fine structural organization[8,14] and mitotic activity are those seen in an actively dividing cell population. The lower third of the midzone contains larger cells than the basal variety, with comparatively more abundant cytoplasm. Because of their geographic placement, they are called *parabasal cells*. They may occasionally exhibit mitotic divisions, and radioautographic studies[1] have demonstrated a high uptake of tritiated thymidine, a nucleoprotein precursor, suggesting that they also contribute to epithelial growth.

Ultrastructurally, the parabasal cells are attached by numerous tonofilament–desmosomal complexes, and there is some intracytoplasmic glycogen (Fig. 5.4). Phosphorylase and amylo-1,6-glucosidase, enzymes essential for glycogen synthesis, are localized in this region.[11] The upper portion of the midzone is occupied by cells that are involved in a process of ascending maturation, characterized by a gradual increase in the volume of the cytoplasm. Nuclear size, however, remains constant up to the most superficial cell level. These cells are referred to as *intermediate cells* when exfoliated. They do not divide. Intermediate cells have abundant PAS-positive, diastase-labile intracellular glycogen, which is responsible for the clear, vacuolated appearance of their cytoplasm (Fig. 5.3). The superficial zone forms the most differentiated compartment of the squamous epithelium. Here, the cells are flattened and have a larger area of cytoplasm (50 μm in diameter) and smaller pyknotic nuclei than the underlying intermediate cells (Fig. 5.5). The pink, eosinophilic, glycogen-rich cytoplasm has abundant intermediate filaments, which provide rigidity (Fig. 5.5, inset). Superficial cells also contain occasional membrane-bound keratinosomes. These structures are the source of protein-bound disulfide keratin precursors,[12] which are responsible for cornification and the complex network of microridges seen on the surface of the most superficial and mature cells.[8] The function of the cornified surface is to protect the underlying epithelial cells and subepithelial vasculature from trauma and infection. The microridges are believed to enhance surface adhesiveness (Fig. 5.6). The virtual lack of desmosomes between the upper superficial cells explains their loose attachment and easy desquamation (Fig. 5.5).

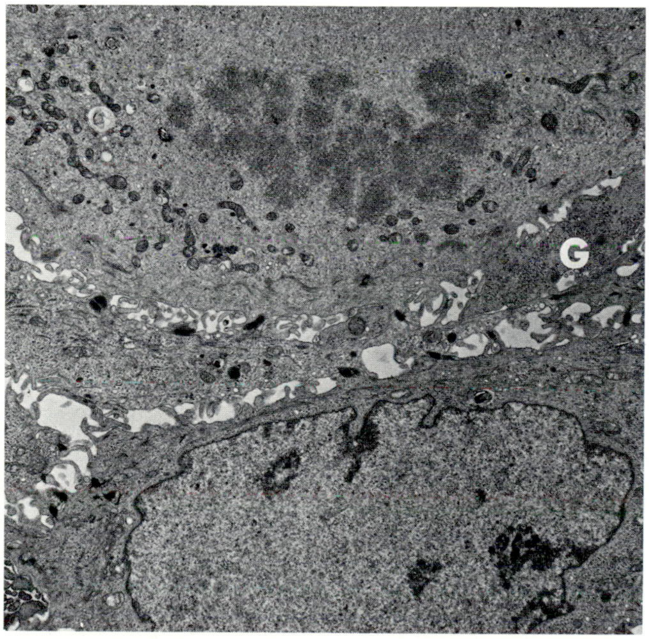

FIG. 5.4. Electron micrograph of parabasal cells, one of which is in mitosis. The organelle-rich cytoplasm contains small collections of glycogen granules (G). ×4250.

Biochemical and immunohistochemical analysis of the squamous epithelium of the cervical portio has demonstrated the presence of cytoplasmic proteins specific for terminally differentiated squamous cells, corresponding to the orderly vertical maturation process seen histologically and ultrastructurally. The keratin intermediate filaments of the native squamous epithelium of the portio are complex and heterogeneous, belonging to those types of high molecular weight keratins unique to maturing keratinized epithelia and absent from simple columnar epithelium and immature squamous metaplasia.[5,21] Involucrin, a precursor of envelope protein necessary for cross-linkage of intermediate and superficial squamous cells, is also diffusely present in the suprabasal layers of the squamous portio[27] (Fig. 5.7). It can serve as a marker of suprabasal differentiation unrelated to keratinization.

In postmenopausal women, who no longer produce ovarian hormones, the squamous epithelium is atrophic with little or no intracytoplasmic glycogen. Surface epithelial maturation and stromal papillae are absent (Fig. 5.8). These cellular alterations should not be confused with cervical intraepithelial neoplasia. The thin epithelial

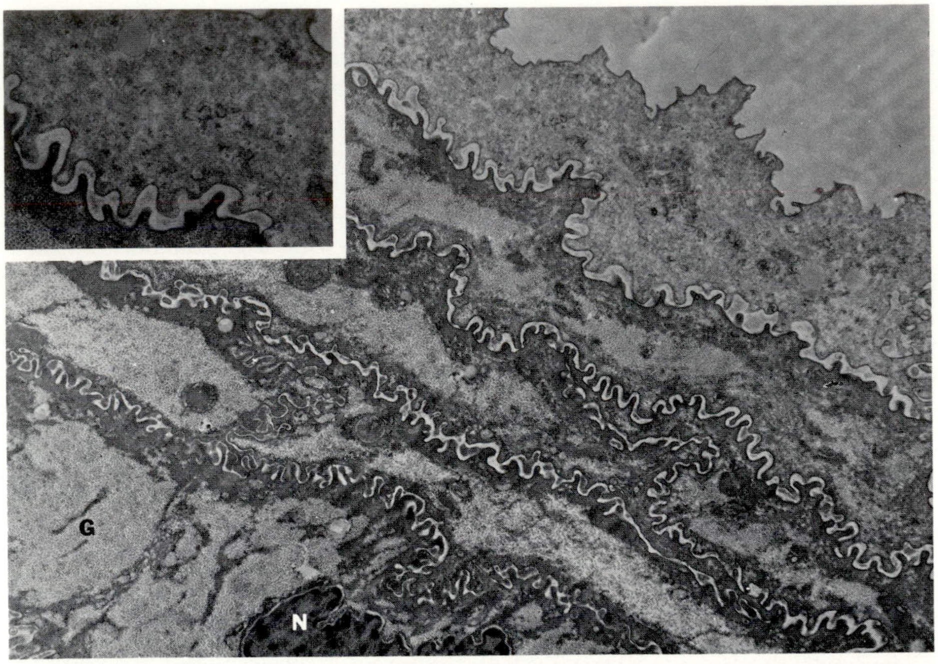

FIG. 5.5. Electron micrograph of superficial cells. The cells have pyknotic nuclei (N) and flattened cytoplasm packed with glycogen (G). The most superficial cells are rich in microfilaments and contain irregular surface membrane projections. Note the lack of desmosomal attachments between the most superficial cells, a feature facilitating desquamation. ×4795. *Inset:* Higher magnification of intracytoplasmic microfilaments in the most superficial cells. ×11,370.

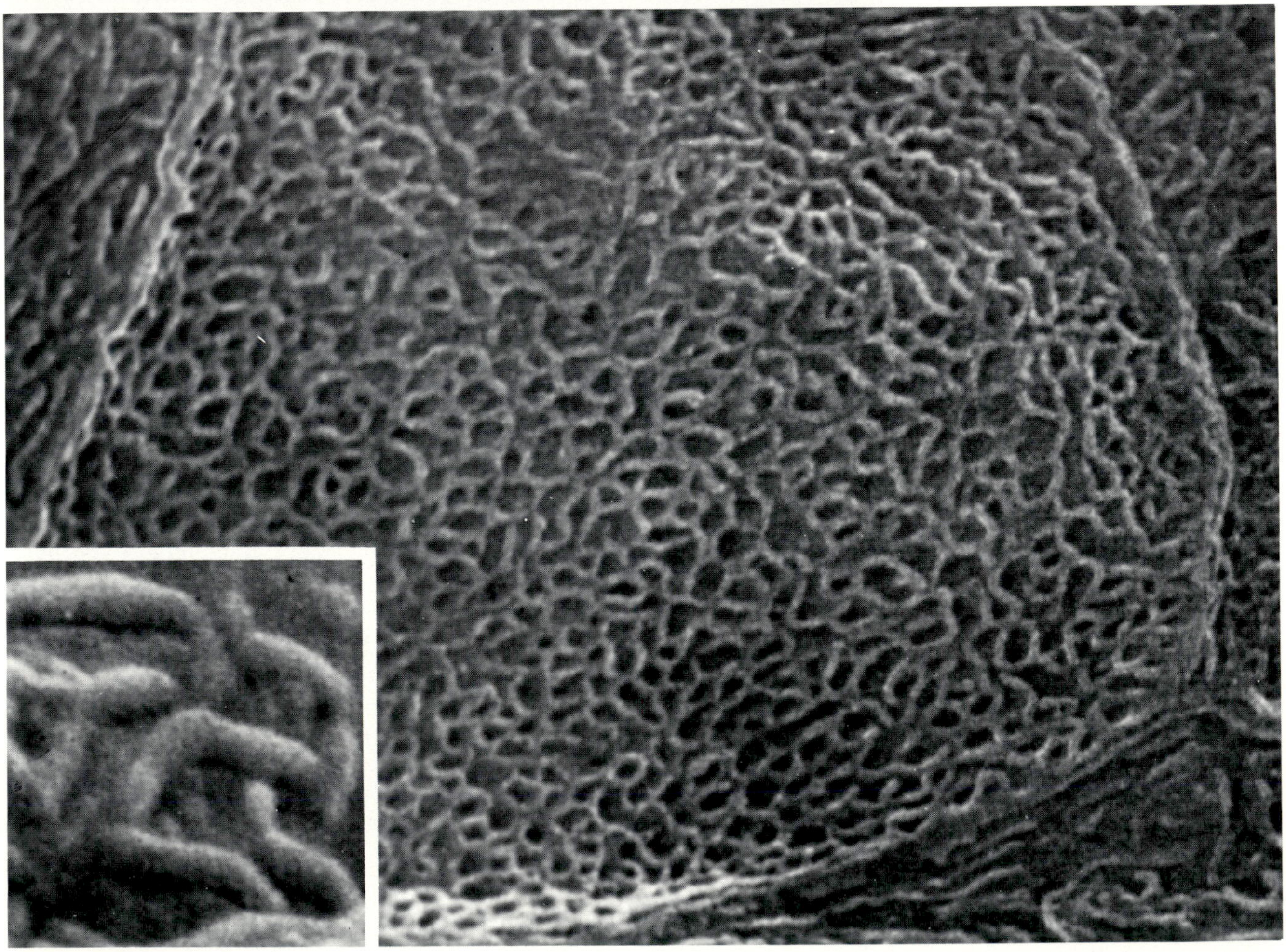

FIG. 5.6. Scanning electron micrograph of the most superficial cells of the native squamous portio epithelium. The surface contains an intricate system of microridges. ×8240. *Inset:* Higher magnification of microridges representing nodular evaginations of the surface plasma membrane. ×22,660.

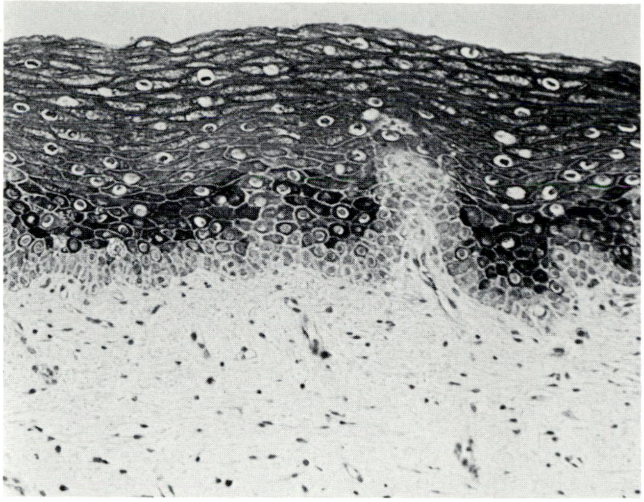

FIG. 5.7. Normal cervical epithelium, stained with anti-involucrin. Note intense staining in suprabasal stratum spinosum and absence of staining in the basal cells. (Courtesy of Dr. M. J. Warhol, Boston, Massachusetts.)

covering does not adequately protect the subepithelial vasculature against trauma, a situation that frequently leads to bleeding and inflammation. The squamous epithelium of the portio is supported by a fibrous connective tissue stroma, devoid of endocervical glands. There is a well-developed capillary network at the stromal–epithelial junction, with occasional finger-like extensions into the epithelium, the stromal papillae[17] (see Fig. 5.3). The penetrating vessels supply the epithelial cells with nutrients and oxygen. In addition to connective tissue fibers and capillaries, occasional free nerve endings are seen entering the stromal papilla.[19]

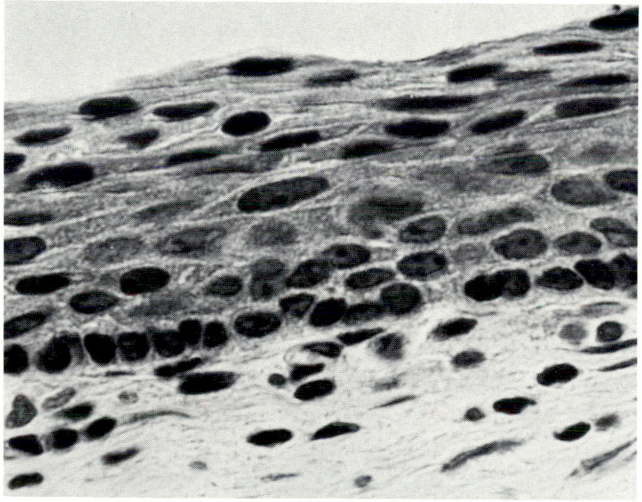

FIG. 5.8. Atrophic squamous portio epithelium. The epithelium is thin and devoid of glycogen-rich vacuolated cells. The cells in the lower half of the epithelium have prominent nuclei and nucleoi, but cellular cohesion is normal and cytologic atypia is absent.

Columnar Epithelium

The mucosa of the cervical canal (endocervix) is composed of a single layer of mucin-secreting, columnar epithelium, which lines both the surface and the underlying glandular structures. The latter are traditionally called *compound, tubular racemose, endocervical glands*. Fluhman,[10] however, using three-dimensional plastic reconstructions from serial histologic sections, demonstrated that the endocervical glands actually represent deep, uncrossed, cleft-like infoldings of the surface epithelium with numerous blind, tunnel-like collaterals (Fig. 5.9). Because of the complex organization of these clefts, or grooves, including oblique, transverse, and longitudinal arrangements, in histologic sections they often appear as isolated glandular units (Fig. 5.9). The epithelium lining the clefts is identical with that lining the surface, and consequently the endocervical mucin-producing apparatus is not considered glandular but a complex infolding mucinous membrane.

True glands, in contrast, have different epithelial lining in their secretory portions than in their secretory (ductal) or surface epithelial portions. The columnar epithelial

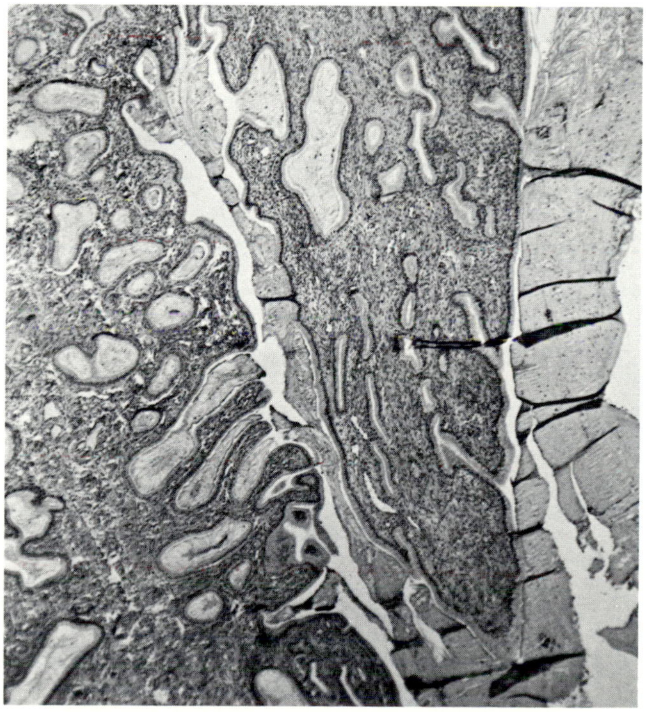

FIG. 5.9. Endocervical mucosa with cleft-like infoldings and tunnel-like collaterals. The neighboring gland-like structures represent tangentially sectioned cleft–tunnel complexes.

cells characteristically have basally placed nuclei and tall, uniform, finely granular cytoplasm filled with mucinous droplets (Fig. 5.10). The droplets have great affinity for Alcian blue stains, reflecting their sulfated, sialic acid mucopolysaccharide content.[6] Cells lining the luminal surface have been termed *picket cells* because of their resemblance to a picket fence (Fig. 5.10). Occasionally, nonsecretory cells with cilia are observed[15] (Fig. 5.10, inset), the main function of which appears to relate to the distribution and mobilization of endocervical mucus. Isolated neuroendocrine epithelial cells of argyrophil and argentaffin type may also be identified within the endocervical epithelium by histochemical stains.[9,13] The argentaffin-positive cells often contain serotonin, as demonstrated by immunoperoxidase techniques. The physiologic purpose of these rare endocrine endocervical cells is obscure. Biochemically and immunohistochemically, the columnar cells of the endocervix are characterized as simple epithelia by the presence of only a few, low molecular weight keratins.[5,21] Involucrin is not expressed.

Mitosis in the columnar epithelium is not seen under normal conditions. Whether epithelial renewal is generated from the underlying subcolumnar reserve cells,[15] which under normal circumstances are seldom seen even at the ultrastructural level, or from the persisting mature endocervical cells is unknown. Unlike the attenuated vascular stromal papillae of the original squamous portio epithelium, the subepithelial capillary network in the endocervical mucosa is well developed.

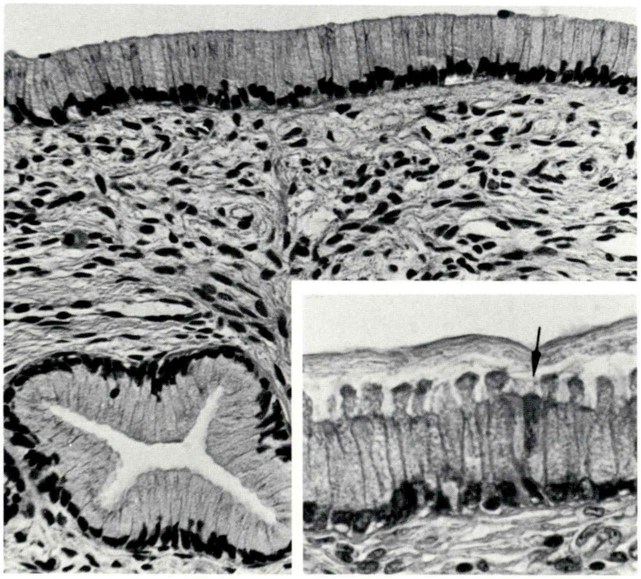

Fig. 5.10. Tall mucin-filled endocervical picket cells with basal nuclei. *Inset:* Endocervical cells engaged in apocrine secretion whereby portions of apical cytoplasm are expelled. Ciliated cells are present (*arrow*).

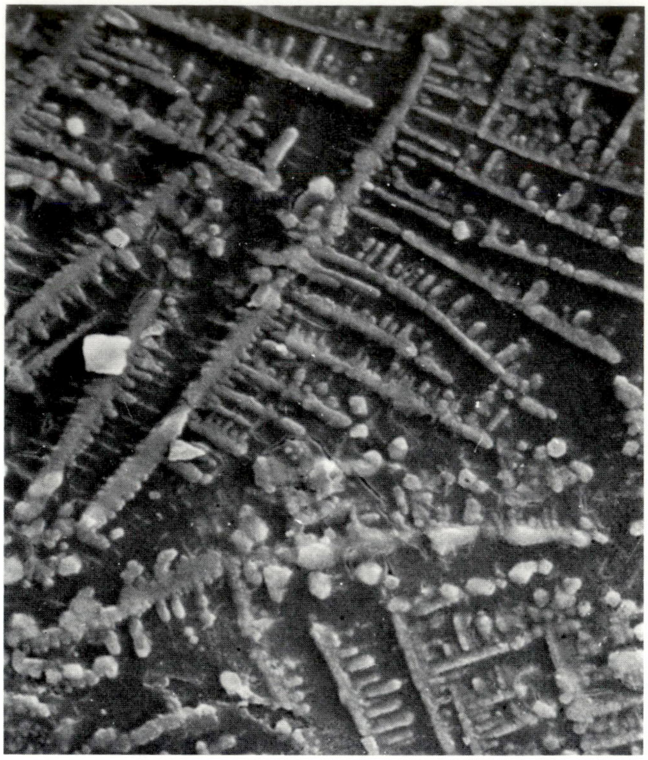

Fig. 5.11. Scanning electron photomicrograph of ferning reaction in cervical mucus during the ovulatory period.

Unlike the endocervical epithelium, its viscoelastic secretory product, the cervical mucus, is subject to profound cyclic changes. Under estrogenic stimulation, the endocervical secretions are profuse, watery, and alkaline, facilitating sperm penetration. During the postovulatory phase, secretions are scant, thick, and acid, contain numerous leukocytes, and act as a barrier for sperm penetration. Biochemical[23] and fine structural analyses[2] have shown that the cervical mucus gel is made of a heterogeneous micellar network of glycoproteins. The intermicellar space is occupied by cervical plasma rich in sodium chloride and potassium, the ions of which are responsible for the crystallization of mucus or ferning (arborization) reaction (Fig. 5.11). Under estrogenic influence, the glycoprotein micelles are arranged parallel to each other at a distance of 5–15 μm, creating a channel system that is favorable to sperm penetration. During progestogenic stimulation, the micellar channel system is replaced by a dense network composed of interlacing micellar fiber bridges that preclude sperm penetration (Fig. 5.12). Ultrastructurally,[8,14] endocervical secretory activity operates by both the apocrine and the merocrine type of expulsion of secretory products. In the former type, a portion of apical cytoplasm packed with secretory granules is detached (Figs. 5.10 and 5.13), whereas in the latter, secretory products are released from apical gran-

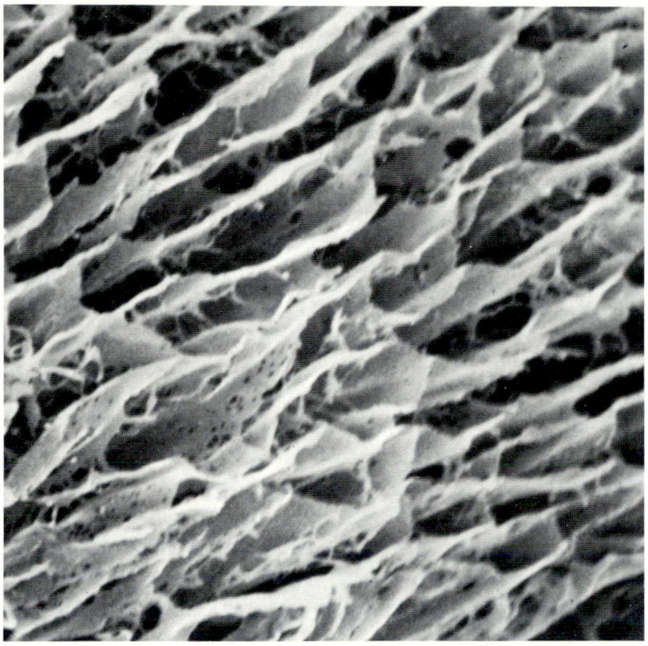

FIG. 5.12. Scanning electron microscopic appearance of unpurified cervical mucus in the secretory phase of the menstrual cycle. The mucoid material is made of an interlacing filamentous micellar meshwork, unfavorable for sperm migration. ×4000.

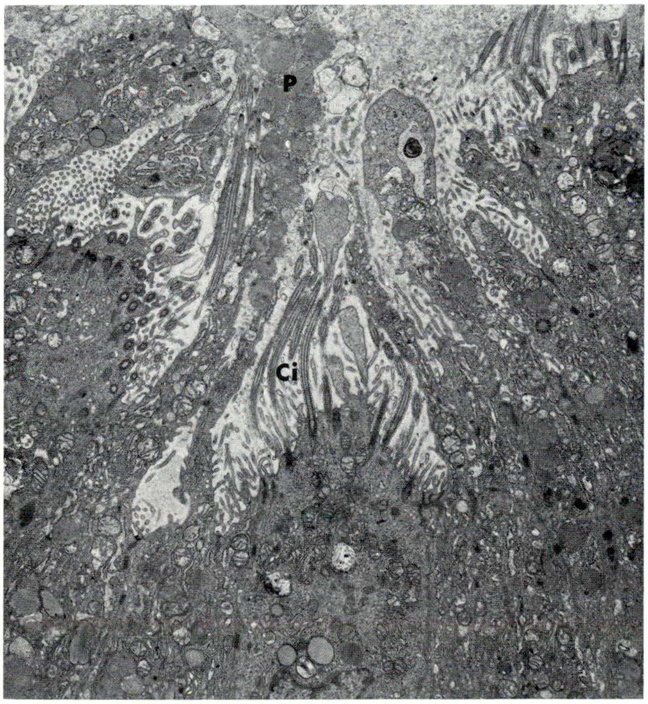

FIG. 5.13. Electron micrograph of mucin-containing endocervical cells alternating with ciliated cells (Ci). Secretion is of the apocrine type, as indicated by intraluminal protrusions (P) of apical cytoplasmic substance packed with mucinous droplets and various organelles. ×4030.

ules through pore-like openings of the surface cytoplasmic membrane (Fig. 5.14, inset). Synthesis of mucoproteins is initiated in the Golgi cisternae and perigolgian vesicles.[8,14] The coalescence of perigolgian vesicles leads to the formation of larger secretory units, which, by a similar process, form prominent granules with granulofilamentous content. The Golgi is associated with free ribosomes, granular endoplasmic reticulum, and mitochondria, providing the essential protein matrix and energy for mucoprotein synthesis (Fig. 5.14).

The stroma of the endocervix is comparatively better innervated than that of the portio vaginalis. The nerve fibers are found running parallel to muscle bundles, but sensory free endings have not been clearly demonstrated.[19] True lymphoid follicles, with or without germinal centers, are encountered in the subepithelial stroma of both the exocervix and the endocervix.

The Transformation Zone

The squamocolumnar junction of the cervix is the border between the stratified squamous epithelium and the mucin-secreting columnar epithelium of the endocervix. Morphogenetically, there are two types of squamocolumnar junctions (Fig. 5.15). One is termed the *original* squamocolumnar junction, where the native squamous covering of the portio vaginalis joins the columnar epithelium and is established between the newly formed squamous epithelium of the transformation zone and the endocervical columnar cells. The union between the two epithelia is a sharp one (Fig. 5.16). The second is called the *physiologic* or *functional* squamocolumnar junction and is established between the newly formed squamous epithelium of the transformation zone and the endocervical columnar cells. In this instance, the transition may be abrupt or gradual (Fig. 5.17). The transformation zone may be difficult to visualize with the naked eye. Its localization, however, is greatly enhanced with the application of 5% acetic acid and the use of the colposcope (see Chapter 7, Cervical Intraepithelial Neoplasia). The presence of squamous epithelium with circular openings and spherical bumps of 2–4 mm, which correspond to the underlying endocervical glands and nabothian cysts, respectively, represents the transformation zone (Fig. 5.18). Nabothian cysts are formed when the mouths of endocervical clefts become obliterated by the proliferating surface squamous epithelium. As secretion continues but excretion is blocked, the secretory products accumulate, leading to cystic glandular dilations, or nabothian cysts. Microscopically, the cystic spaces are lined by low columnar endocervical cells, supported by a distended basal lamina (Fig. 5.19).

In most women during the reproductive period, the mucin-secreting columnar epithelium of the endocervix is present on the cervical portio, forming the endocervical

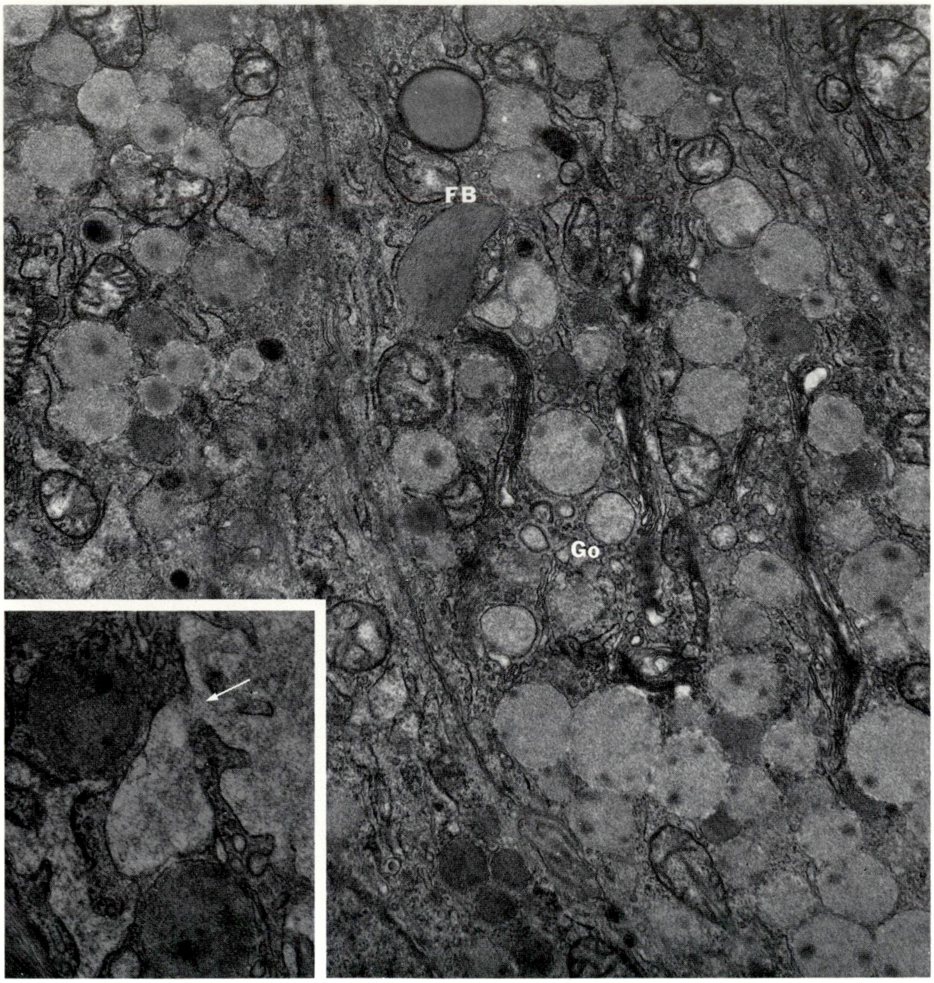

FIG. 5.14. Detail of endocervical mucinogenesis. The membrane-bound mucin-containing secretory granules derive from Golgi (Go) and mature through progressive stages of intercoalescence. The Golgi are associated with free and bound ribosomes and mitochondria, providing the protein matrix and energy for mucin synthesis. A characteristic feature of endocervical mucinous cells is the presence of fibrillar bodies (FB), presumably representing a fibrillar form of mucoprotein storage. ×19,320. *Inset:* Electron microscopic view of the merocrine type of secretion. Filamentous mucus is discharged through focal pore-like opening (*arrow*) of the surface plasma membrane. ×22,080.

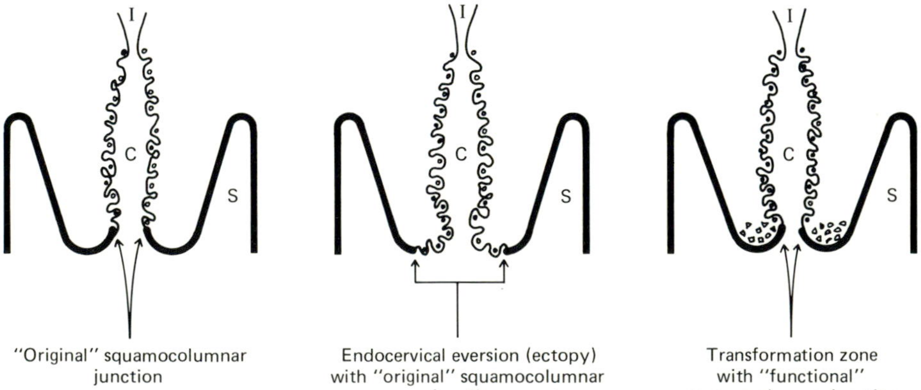

FIG. 5.15. Schematic representation of original and functional squamocolumnar junctions and three basic types of portios. *Left:* Diagram of a portio completely covered with native squamous epithelium. The squamocolumnar junction is at the external os. *Middle:* Denotes endocervical ectropion, with the squamocolumnar junction being located on the exocervix below the external os. *Right:* Indicates areas of ectropion covered with squamous epithelium. This area is the cervical transformation zone. The new, or functional, squamocolumnar junction of the transformation zone is at the external os. S, squamous epithelium; C, endocervical columnar epithelium; I, uterine isthmus.

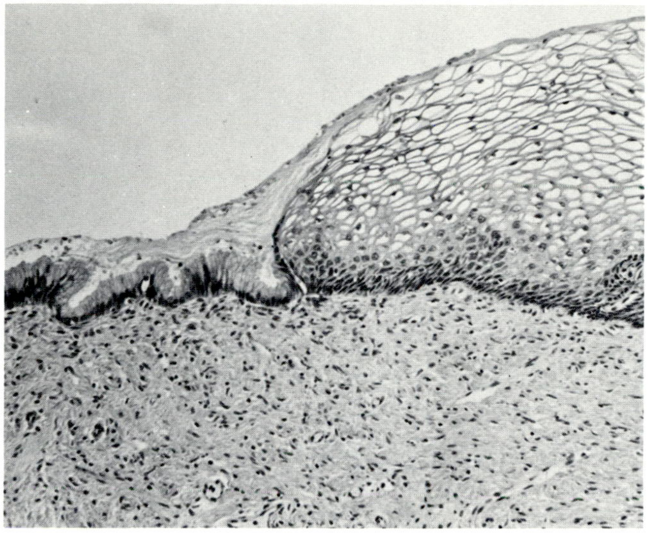

FIG. 5.16. Original squamocolumnar junction. Note the abrupt transition between the mature squamous epithelium of the portio and the endocervical mucosa. A similar sharp demarcation may be seen at the squamocolumnar junction of the mature transformation zone.

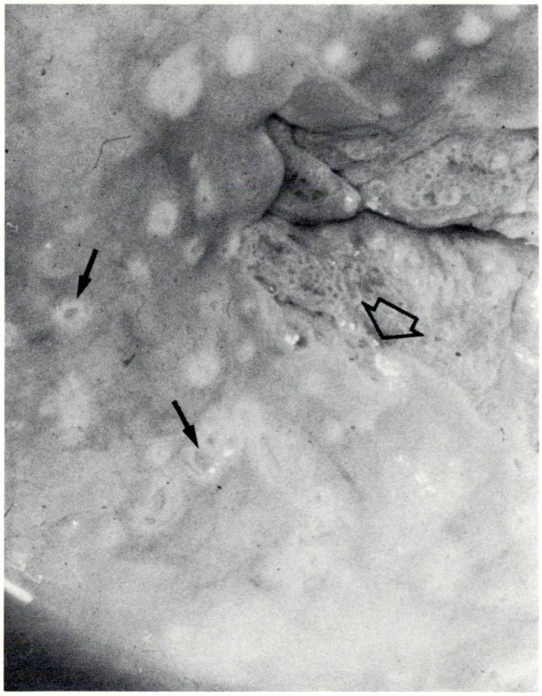

FIG. 5.18. Colposcopy of a mature transformation zone with endocervical gland openings (*small arrows*). The squamocolumnar junction of the transformation zone is just outside of the os (*large arrow*).

ectropion or cervical ectopy. This occurs twice as commonly on the anterior as on the posterior lip,[27] but both lips may be involved simultaneously. The endocervical mucosa appears as a red velvety zone, sharply contrasting with the neighboring pink and shiny squamous portio epithelium. Because of its gross appearance, the term *cervical erosion* is often used by clinicians. The term

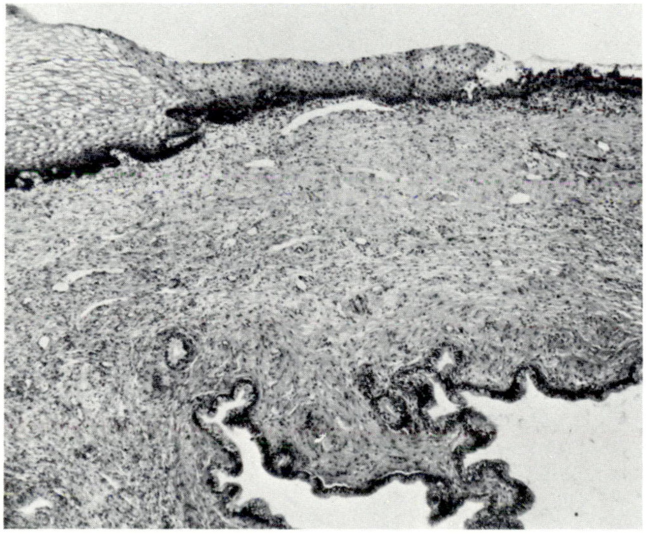

FIG. 5.17. Functional squamocolumnar junction of the immature transformation zone. Note the gradual transition between mature (*left*) and immature squamous epithelium (*right*). The latter is continuous with proliferating subcolumnar reserve cells. There are endocervical clefts in the subjacent area.

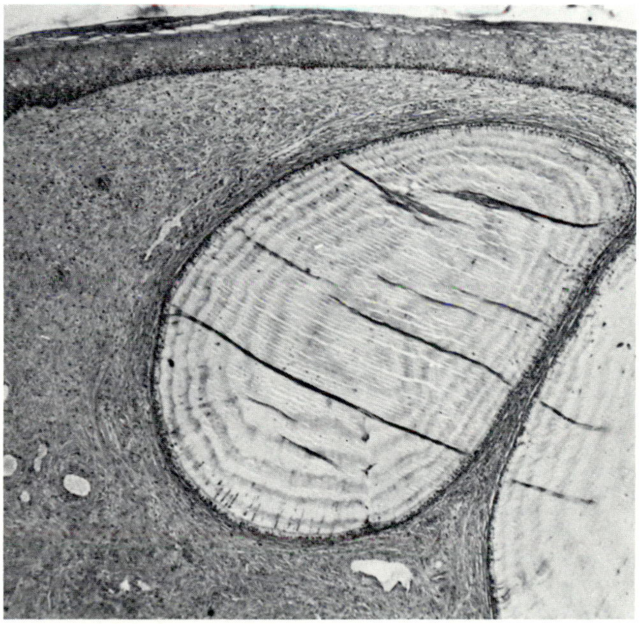

FIG. 5.19. Microscopic appearance of the outer portio limit of the transformation zone. Mature squamous epithelium covers underlying nabothian cysts filled with laminated mucin. In this case, the cysts represent the last glands of previously everted endocervical mucosa.

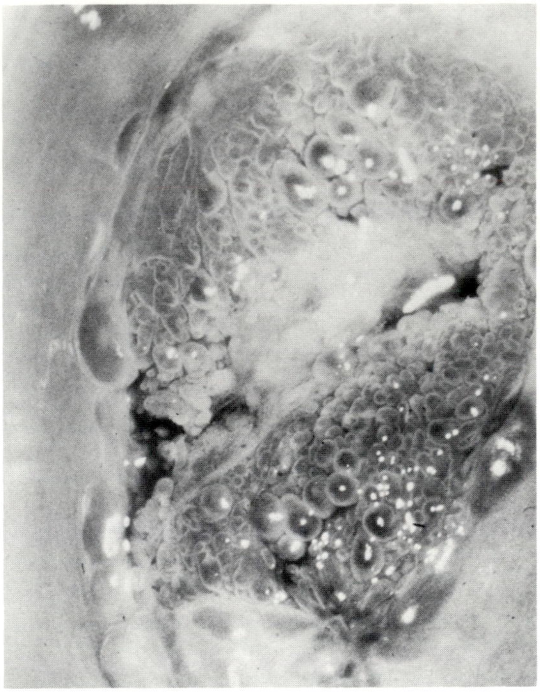

FIG. 5.20. Colpophotograph of endocervical eversion. Grape-like endocervical mucosa is everted on both the anterior and the posterior lip and surrounds the anatomic external os. The original squamocolumnar junction is displaced below the os.

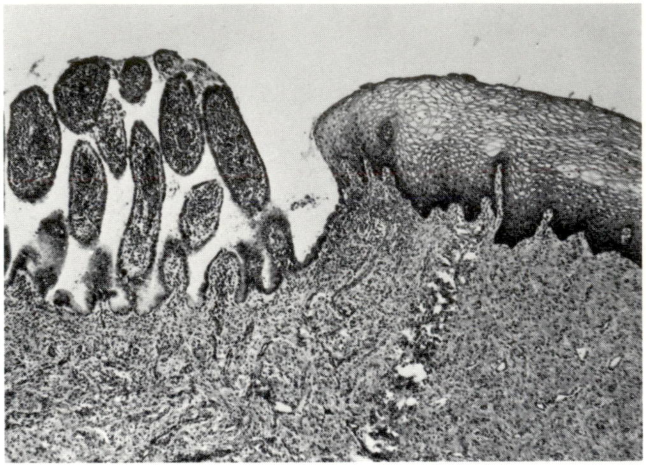

FIG. 5.21. Endocervical eversion meets the native squamous portio epithelium. The everted endocervical mucosa has a papillary configuration and the lamina propria is obscured by chronic inflammatory exudate.

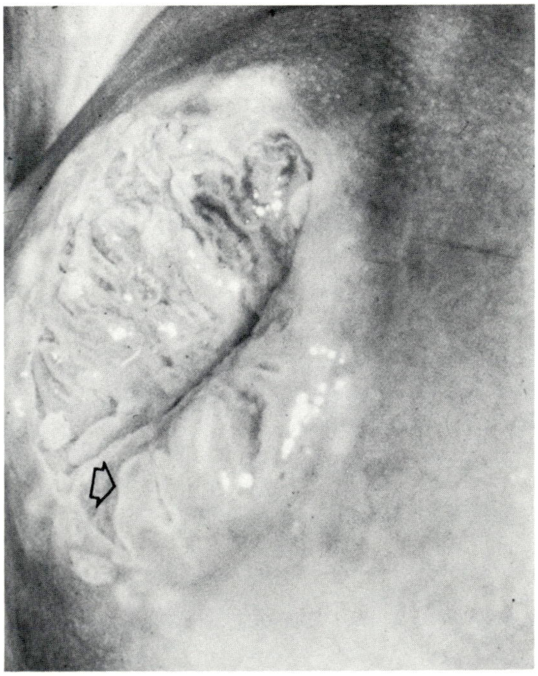

FIG. 5.22. Colpophotograph of early transformation zone. Everted endocervical mucosa with tongue-like ingrowths from the native squamous portio epithelium (*arrow*). Some of these tongues appear to interanastomose with whitish, immature squamous metaplastic epithelium, which covers the tip of endocervical villi. Note the irregular outline of the new squamocolumnar junction.

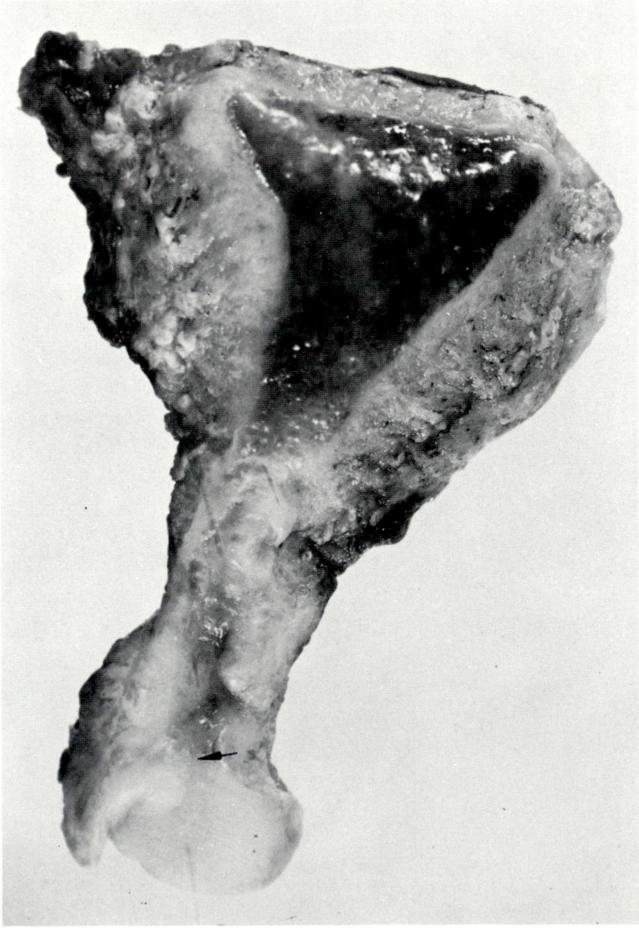

FIG. 5.23. Prolapsed, postmenopausal uterus. The cervix is atrophic and elongated and the squamocolumnar junction is visualized above the external os (*arrow*).

is incorrect, however, because there is no epithelial denudation (true erosion)[20] but numerous villi or papillary excrescences of varying size, resembling a bunch of grapes when viewed with the colposcope (Fig. 5.20). Histologically, these are blunt-ended papillae lined by endocervical columnar epithelium and supported by a fibrovascular stroma containing numerous chronic inflammatory cells (Fig. 5.21). The endocervical ectropion is a normal physiologic finding and should not be construed as a pathologic abnormality. The location of the orginal squamocolumnar junction and the distribution of the endocervical ectropion are determined embryologically when inward migration of squamous epithelium from the lower third of the vagina stops. The endocervical ectropion is most extensive in younger women (under 20 years of age), following the first pregnancy. It becomes reduced in size as remodeling of the transformation zone occurs with time.[3] In women exposed to diethylstilbestrol (DES) in utero, the normal migration of the squamous epithelium is prematurely halted and the original squamocolumnar junction is often located in the vagina rather than on the exocervix.[26] The columnar epithelium that composes the endocervical ectropion in both non-DES-exposed and DES-exposed women is gradually replaced by squamous epithelium, causing the functional (new) squamocolumnar junction to move centripetally toward the os. This results in the formation of the immature transformation zone[25] (Fig. 5.22). Subsequently, in older and postmenopausal women, the new squamocolumnar junction is virtually always located above the external os (Fig. 5.23). Hormonal and other physical factors influence the size and distribution of the endocervical ectropion by altering the shape and volume of the cervical lips. Ectopy may be particularly exaggerated with progestin therapy (as in oral contraceptive users) or during pregnancy.

There are two histogenetic mechanisms proposed by which the cervical epithelium is replaced by squamous epithelium (Fig. 5.24). The first and most important mechanism consists of the direct ingrowth from the native portio epithelium bordering the columnar epithelium. Histologic, colposcopic, colpomicroscopic, and electron microscopic observations[4,7] have shown that tongues of native squamous epithelium of the portio grow beneath the adjacent columnar epithelium and expand in between the mucinous epithelium and its basement membrane.

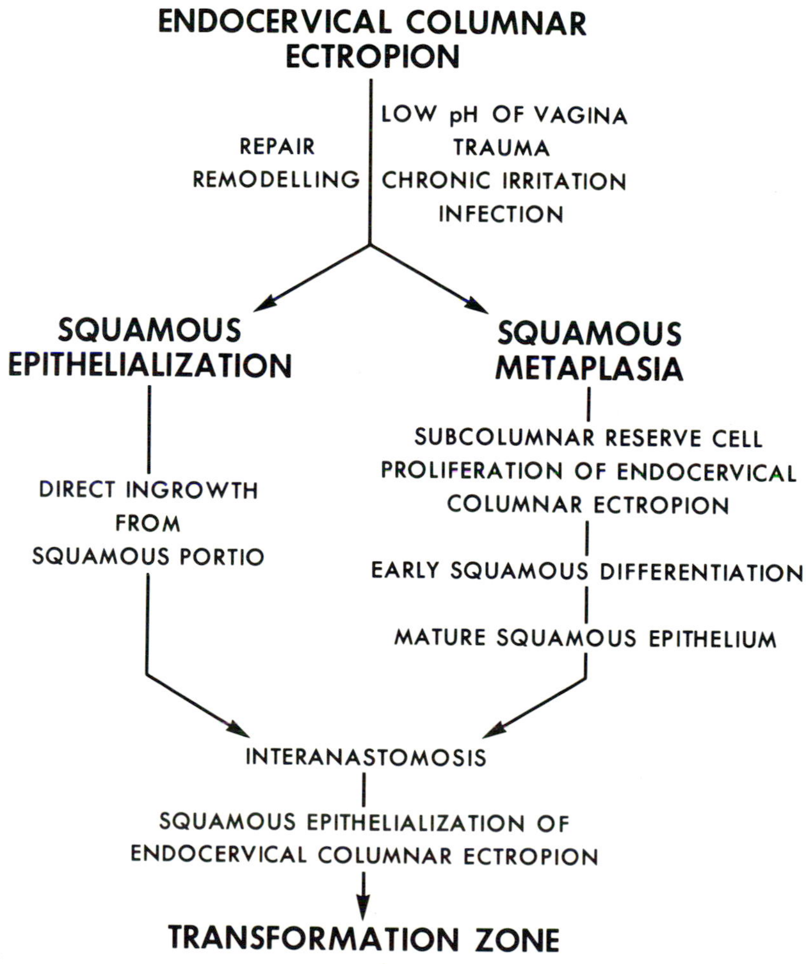

Fig. 5.24. Summary of the sequence of events in the histogenetic development of the transformation zone.

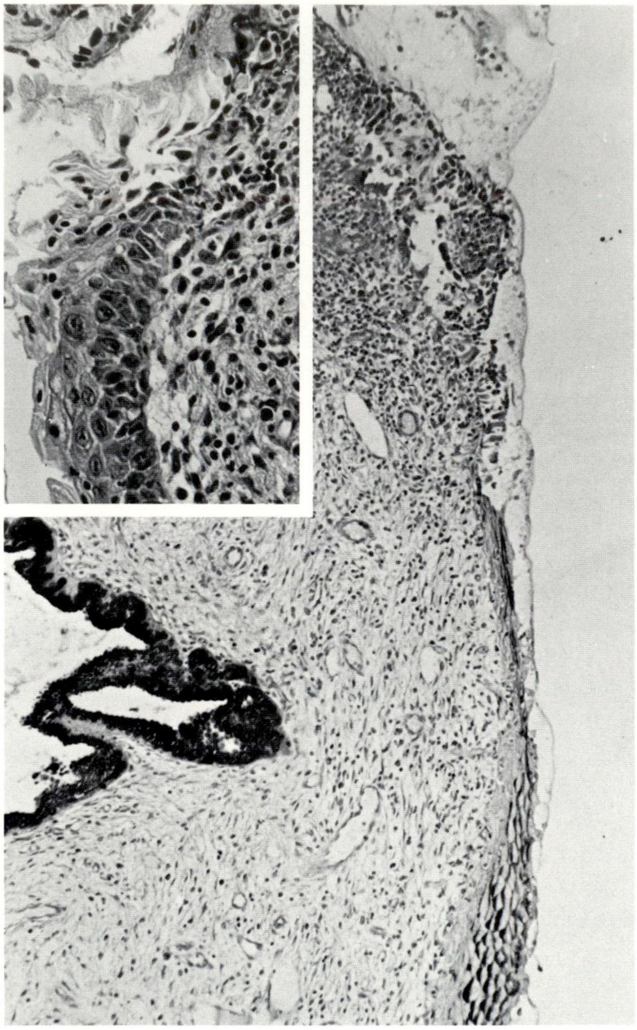

FIG. 5.25. Outer edge of the early transformation zone. A narrow tongue of glycogen-containing native squamous epithelium of the portio (*lower right*) grows onto everted endocervical mucosa. The underlying endocervical epithelium is rich in mucin. *Inset:* Detail of advancing edge of squamous cells growing beneath endocervical columnar cells, which are displaced upward. Nuclei and nucleolar enlargement in squamous cells are a reflection of epithelial hyperplasia associated with repair.

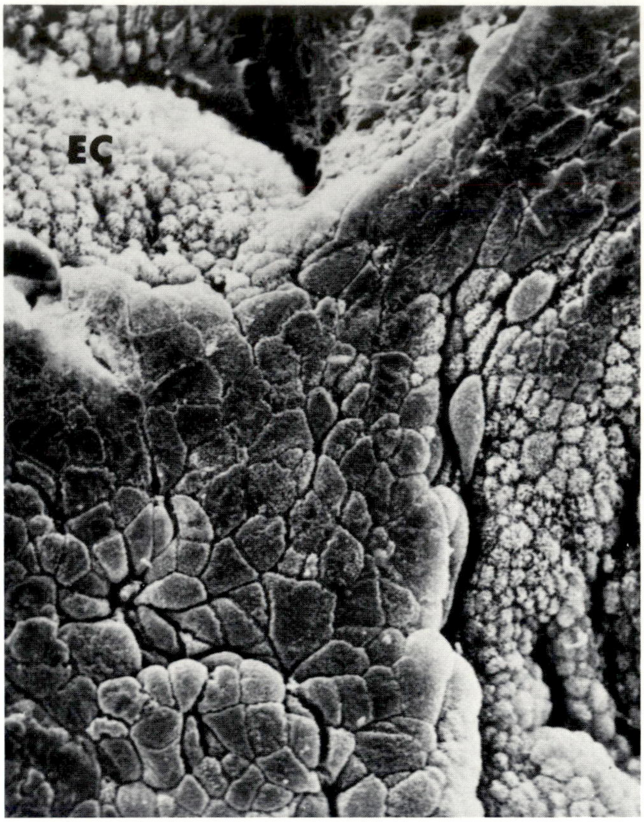

FIG. 5.26. Scanning electron microscopic appearance of the outer edge of the early transformation zone. Narrow tongues of squamous epithelium with a pavement-like surface pattern extend onto the everted endocervical mucosa (EC). ×4,280. (Reprinted by permission of Ferenczy and Richart, Ref. 8.)

As the squamous cells expand and mature, the endocervical cells are gradually displaced upward, degenerate, and eventually are sloughed (Figs. 5.25 and 5.26). A similar process is observed in the re-epithelialization of true pathologic erosion of the endocervix, the so-called ascending healing of Meyer.[20]

The progression of squamous transformation of the endocervical ectropion is primarily dependent on local (vaginal) environmental factors, with the initial stimulus being the low (acid) pH of the vagina after puberty.[3] Trauma, chronic irritation, or cervical infection also plays a role in development and maturation of the transformation zone by stimulating repair and remodeling; eventually the ectocervix is covered by a protective surface of mature squamous epithelium. The process of squamous epithelialization is thought to be responsible for the obliteration of the outer two-thirds of endocervical ectopy. Rapid squamous re-epithelialization of the columnar epithelium of the transformation zone may also be produced iatrogenically by electrocautery, cryosurgery, or laser surgery.

The second mechanism involved in the genesis of squamous epithelium of the transformation zone is most commonly termed *squamous metaplasia*, but such names as *epidermidization* and *squamous prosoplasia*[10] are also used. The latter term, derived from the Greek meaning *forward* and *to form*, was proposed by Fluhman[10] and is probably the most accurate one. It refers to a proliferation of undifferentiated subcolumnar reserve cells of the endocervical epithelium and their gradual transformation into a fully mature squamous epithelium. The morphogenetic development of squamous metaplasia (prosopla-

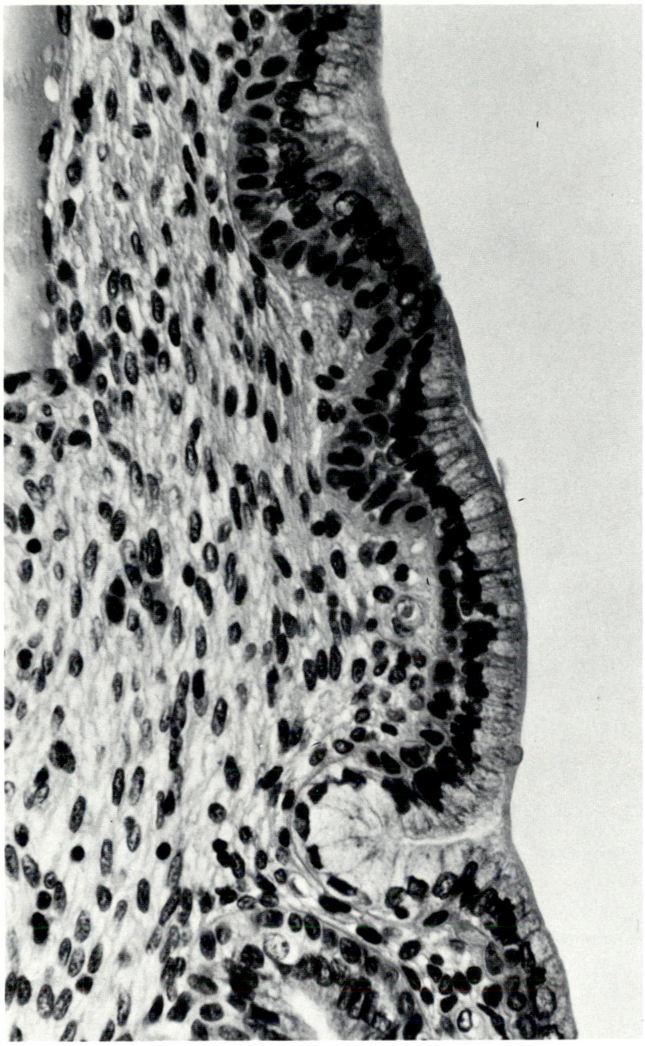

Fig. 5.27. A single layer of cuboidal to low, columnar reserve cells is seen between tall, columnar endocervical cells and basal lamina.

sia) has been thoroughly documented by Fluhman[10] and others.[4] The first stage of metaplasia is manifested by the appearance of small cuboidal cells beneath the columnar mucinous epithelium, the so-called subcolumnar reserve cells (Fig. 5.27). The cells have large nuclei that have an increased rate of nucleic acid synthesis when examined by autoradiography.[15] Their general, fine structural characteristics[7,15] are similar to those of the basal cells of the mature squamous portio epithelium (Fig. 5.28).

The origin of subcolumnar reserve cells is controversial. Some investigators suggest a direct derivation from columnar mucinous secretory cells,[10] and others favor the basal cells of the squamous portio epithelium, squamous basal cells, embryonal rests of urogenital origin, and stromal cells as possible sources.[3] In any event, the basic feature of these cells is their bipotency and ability to evolve into either columnar epithelium, including ciliated cells, or squamous epithelium.[15] The subsequent steps are characterized by a progressive growth and stratification of reserve cells (subcolumnar reserve cell hyperplasia), followed by differentiation into immature squamous (Fig. 5.29) and, ultimately, fully mature squamous epithelium indistinguishable from the native portio epithelium (Fig. 5.30). The immature squamous metaplastic epithelium is distinguished from its mature counterpart by lack of surface maturation and inconspicuous intracytoplasmic glycogen. It is, characteristically, sharply demarcated from the native portio epithelium by a perpendicular or oblique line to the surface (Fig. 5.31). As a result, the uninitiated observer may mistake immature squamous metaplasia for cervical intraepithelial neoplasia, particularly when the process also involves the underlying glands (Fig. 5.32). In contrast to neoplastic epithelium, in the immature squamous metaplastic epithelium, cell organization and cohesion are maintained, nuclear atypia is absent, and usually a single row of endocervical cells overlies the squamous cells. Fine structurally, the immature, squamous metaplastic cells resemble the parabasal cells of the portio epithelium (see Fig 5.4). The superficial cells of the immature transformation zone epithelium are covered by numerous microvillous projections rather than surface microridges[8] (Fig. 5.33). Unlike squamous epithelialization, which involves the peripheral regions of the endocervical tissue, squamous metaplasia has a random distribution within the ectropion, reflecting its asynchronous development. The patchy, uneven distribution of squamous metaplasia within the ectropion may be due to the presence of circumscribed, focal stimuli or to differing rates of cell transition and maturation.[7]

Biochemically and immunohistochemically, immature squamous metaplasia shares features of both the mature squamous epithelium and the columnar mucinous epithelium. The keratin intermediate filaments of metaplastic squamous cells are similar to those of terminally differentiated squamous cells but are less complex and fewer in number.[5,21] Involucrin expression is highly variable and is related to the amount of intermediate and superficial cell maturation present within an area of metaplasia.[27] Focal mucin production may be demonstrated by cytoplasmic mucicarmine positivity. The bipotential nature of immature metaplasia is further corroborated ultrastructurally by the finding of individual cells, within islands of metaplasia, that contain both squamous and columnar mucinous cytoplasmic organelles, including varying ratios of tonofibrils, glycogen with secretory granules, and glycocalyces. Cilia may occasionally persist in otherwise mature squamous cells.[7]

With the aid of the colposcope, islands of squamous metaplastic epithelium are seen on the summit of endo-

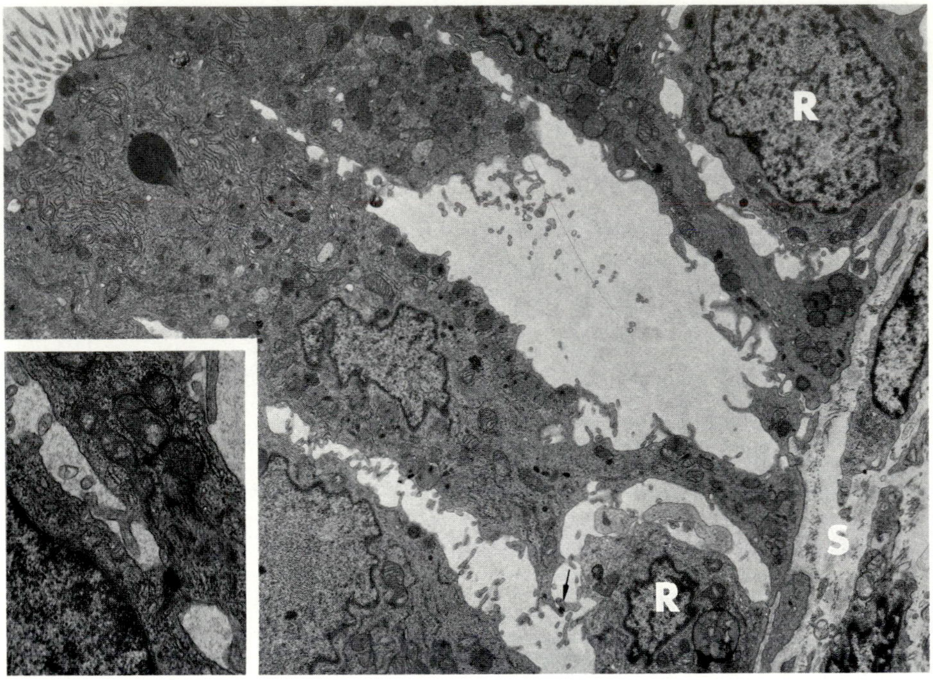

FIG. 5.28. Electron microscopy of subcolumnar reserve cells (R). The nucleocytoplasmic ratio is in favor of the nucleus, and the cells are attached to neighboring endocervical cells and underlying basal lamina by desmosomes (*arrow*) and hemidesmosomes, respectively. The stroma (S) contains spindle-shaped fibroblasts. ×4345. *Inset:* Cytoplasmic details of reserve cells containing bundles of tonofilaments, free and bound ribosomes, and mitochondria. Note the immature tonofilament–desmosome complex between two reserve cells. ×7170.

cervical papillae, expanding centripetally and developing delicate epithelial bridges that fuse with neighboring epithelial proliferations (see Fig. 5.22). Further growth, expansion, and interanastomosis between squamous epithelial islands eventually lead to complete obliteration of the underlying columnar mucosa (see Fig. 5.18). The clinical identification of the squamocolumnar junction

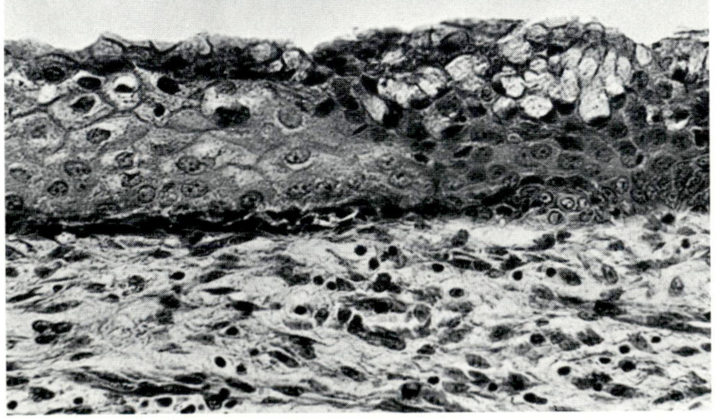

FIG. 5.29. Immature metaplastic squamous epithelium. Note the endocervical cells on top of the proliferating immature squamous cells.

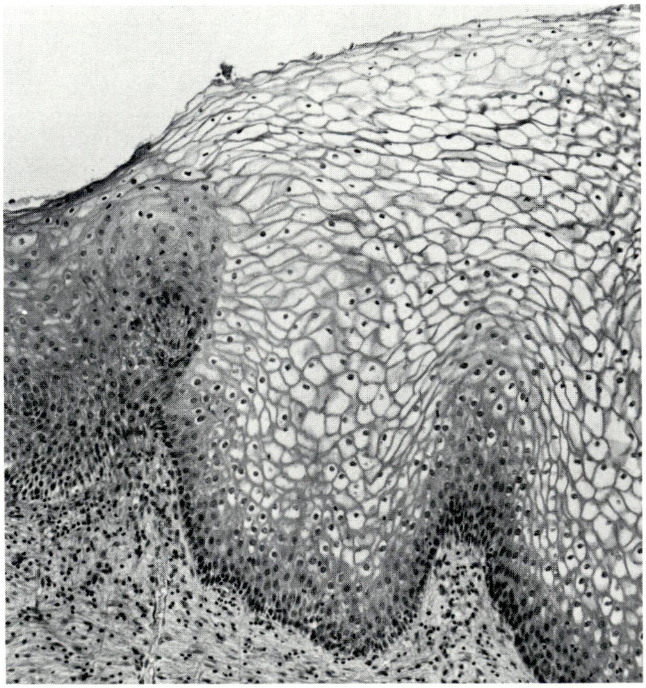

FIG. 5.30. Transformation zone epithelium. On the right, the epithelium has achieved full maturation and is identical with normal native portio epithelium, whereas on the left, squamous differentiation, including glycogenization, is incomplete.

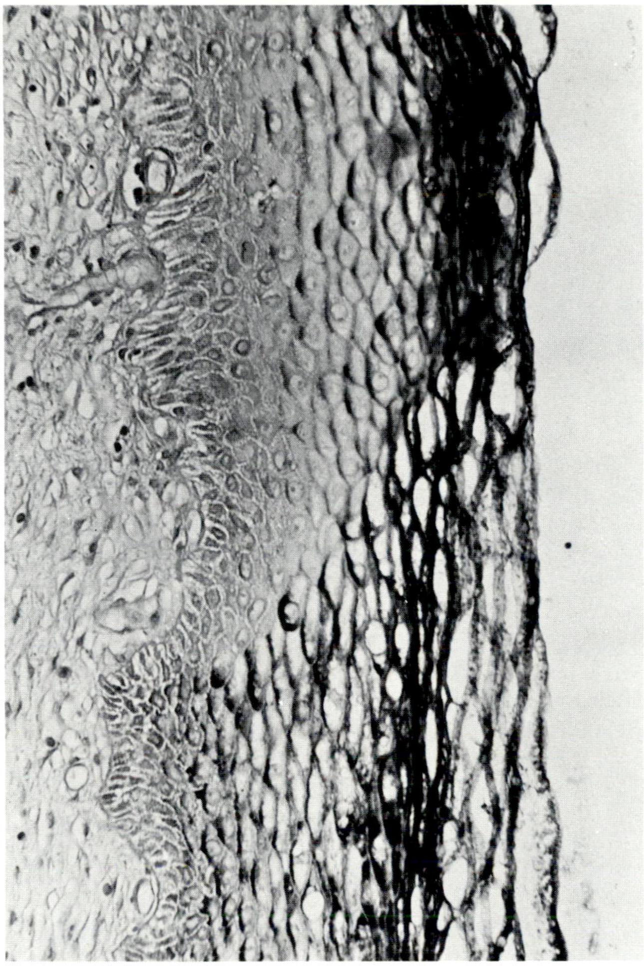

Fig. 5.31. PAS-stained squamous epithelium with a sharp demarcation between poorly glycogenized immature squamous epithelium (*top*) of the transformation zone and heavily glycogenized, mature native portio epithelium (*bottom*).

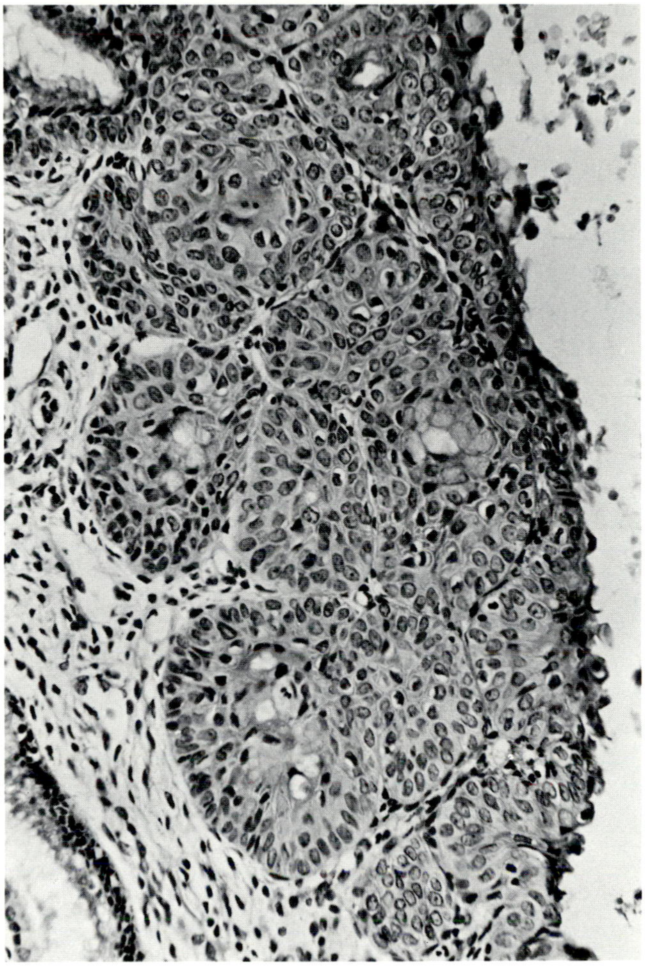

Fig. 5.32. Early squamous cell metaplasia involving both the surface and the deeper endocervical epithelium. Note trapped mucinous endocervical cells in the center of metaplastic foci. Unlike cervical intraepithelial neoplasia with gland involvement, in squamous cell metaplasia nuclear atypia is totally lacking and cellular cohesion is normal.

of the transformation zone is important because virtually all cervical squamous neoplasia begins at this junction and because the extension and limits of cervical intraepithelial neoplasia coincide with the distribution of the transformation zone.[25] It is also important to remember that during the childbearing ages and pregnancy, the transformation zone is located, in almost all instances, on the exposed portion of the cervix. Consequently, the vast majority of cervical neoplasias can be removed for histologic diagnosis by punch biopsy.

Pregnancy and Puerperium

The morphologic alterations that occur in the antepartum or postpartum cervix are not pathognomonic of pregnancy or parturition but are seen more commonly at these times than in the nonpregnant postpartum state. They are correlated with the stimulatory actions of elevated gestational hormones. The spongy enlargement of the pregnant cervix is caused by increased vascularity and edema of the stroma accompanied by acute inflammation.[22] The massive destruction of collagen fibers and accumulation of extracellular glycoproteinic ground substance before labor result in cervical softening and effacement, facilitating dilatation of the cervix to about 10 cm during labor. Decidualization of the stroma, either patchy or diffuse, occurs in about one-third of the patients examined histologically (Fig. 5.34) and disapears by 2 months postpartum.[16] It is presumably mediated by the high levels of progesterone during pregnancy.

The gestational cervical mucus is thick, tenacious, rich in leukocytes, and forms a mucous plug that obliterates the cervical canal, sealing the endometrial cavity from

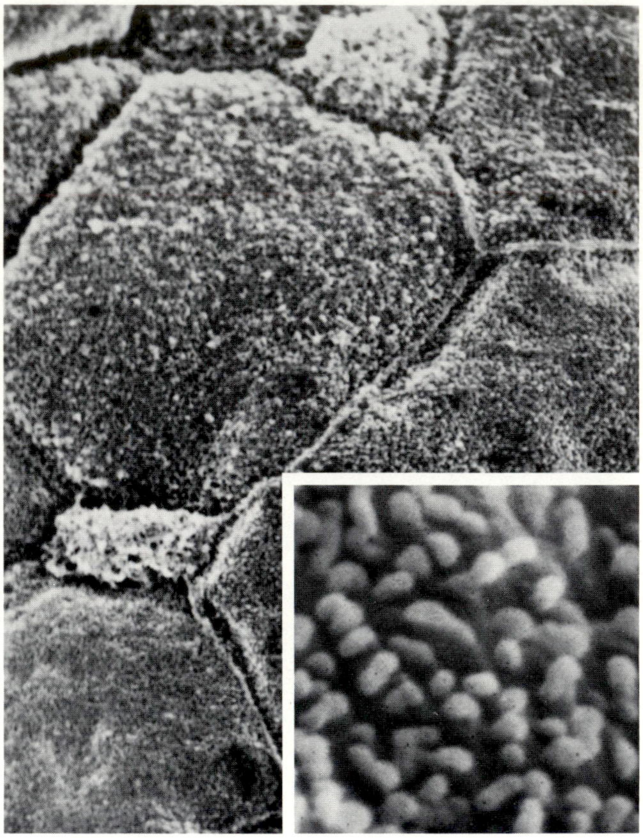

FIG. 5.33. Scanning electron microscopy of immature squamous metaplastic cells with well-developed terminal bars. In contrast to the superficial cells of the mature squamous epithelium, which are covered by microridges, the superficial cells of the immature transformation zone are covered by microvilli. Among the squamous cells is an entrapped endocervical cell (*lower left*). ×2500. *Inset:* Higher magnification of surface microvilli. ×15,000.

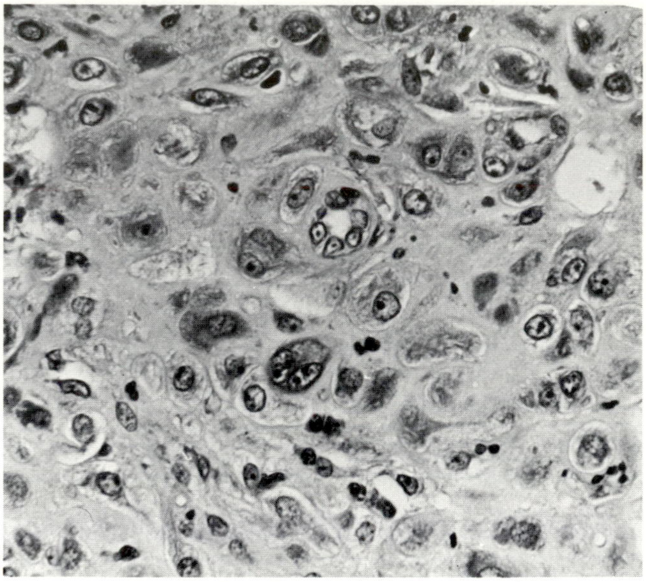

FIG. 5.34. Decidual reaction of cervical stromal cells during pregnancy. The cells are identical with gestational decidual cells of the endometrium. Decidual change in the cervix should be distinguished from poorly differentiated invasive squamous cell carcinoma or undifferentiated carcinoma.

the vagina and thus preventing bacterial invasion. Squamous metaplasia and lobules of tightly packed, small endocervical glandular units forming polypoid protrusions into the canal are often seen. The term *microglandular endocervical hyperplasia* is used for the latter type of lesion. Identical endocervical proliferation is seen in patients using oral contraceptives (see Chapter 6, Benign Lesions of Cervix). The intense proliferation of endocervical mucinous cells is associated with enlargement and softening of the portio during the course of gestation and leads to a more exaggerated protrusion of the endocervical ectropion onto the exposed portion of the cervix. It is rapidly replaced by immature squamous epithelium of both native portio and subcolumnar reserve cell origin.[3,10,16] As a result, in most primigravidas an immature cervical transformation zone is seen, which often persists for long periods of time. The squamocolumnar junction of the transformation zone is nearly always located distal to the external os. Subsequent active remodeling of the transformation zone occurs to a comparatively lesser extent in subsequent pregnancies.[10] True pathologic erosion during pregnancy is observed to involve the everted endocervix next to the native portio epithelium in about 10% of biopsies.[16] Postpartum injuries, such as lacerations produced during labor, are seen in most primiparous and half of multiparous patients,[16] with a distribution of 2:1 in favor of the anterior lip.[25] The denuded areas are subsequently re-epithelialized by ingrowing native squamous epithelium of the portio vaginalis.

Acknowledgment. This work was aided by grant MA 5137 from the Medical Research Council of Canada.

References

1. Averette HE, Weinstein GD, Frost P (1970) Autoradiographic analysis of cell proliferation kinetics in human genital tissues. I. Normal cervix and vagina. Am J Obstet Gynecol 108: 8
2. Chretian FC, Gernigon C, David G, Psychoyos A (1973) The ultrastructure of human cervical mucus under scanning electron microscopy. Fertil Steril 24: 746
3. Coppleson M, Reid B (1967) Preclinical carcinoma of the cervix uteri, 1st ed. Oxford, Pergamon
4. Coppleson M, Pixley E, Reid B (1971) Colposcopy. A scientific and practical approach to the cervix in health and disease, 1st ed. Springfield Ill, Charles C Thomas
5. Czernobilsky B, Moll R, Franke WW, et al. (1984) Intermediate filaments of normal and neoplastic tissues of the female

genital tract with emphasis on problems of differential tumor diagnosis. Pathol Res Pract 179: 31
6. Fand SB (1973) The histochemistry of human cervical epithelium. In: Blandau RJ, Moghissi KS (eds). The biology of the cervix. Chicago, University of Chicago Press, pp 103–124.
7. Feldman D, Romney SL, Edgcomb J, Valentine T (1984) Ultrastructure of normal, metaplastic and abnormal human uterine cervix: Use of montages to study the topographical relationship of epithelial cells. Am J Obstet Gynecol 150: 573
8. Ferenczy A, Richart RM (1974) Female reproductive system. Dynamics of scan and transmission electron microscopy, 1st ed. New York, John Wiley & Sons
9. Fetissof F, Berger G, Dubois MP, et al. Endocrine cells in the female genital tract. Histopathology 9: 133
10. Fluhman CF (1961) The cervix uteri and its diseases, 1st ed. Philadelphia, W.B. Saunders
11. Foraker AG, Marino G (1961) Glycogen-synthesizing enzymes in the uterine cervix. Obstet Gynecol 17: 311
12. Foraker AG, Wingo WJ (1956) Protein-bound sulfhydryl and disulfide group in squamous carcinoma of the uterine cervix. Am J Obstet Gynecol 71: 1182
13. Fox H, Kazzaz B, Langley FA (1964) Argyrophil and argentaffin cells in the female genital tract and in ovarian mucinous cysts. J Pathol Bacteriol 88: 479
14. Friedrich ER (1973) The normal morphology and ultrastructure of the cervix. In: Blandau RJ, Moghissi KS (eds). The biology of the cervix. Chicago, University of Chicago Press, pp 79–102
15. Gould RR, Barter RA, Papadimitriou JM (1979) An ultrastructural, cytodynamical and autoradiographic study of the mucous membrane of the human cervical canal with reference to subcolumnar cells. Am J Pathol 95: 1
16. Johnson LD (1973) Dysplasia and carcinoma in-situ in pregnancy. In: Norris HJ, Hertig AT, Abell MR (eds). The uterus. Internatl. Acad. Path. Monogr. Baltimore, Williams & Wilkins, pp 382–412
17. Kolstad P. Stafl A (1977) Atlas of colposcopy, 2nd ed. Baltimore, University Park Press
18. Koss LG (1979) Diagnostic cytology and its histopathologic bases, 3rd ed. Philadelphia, J.B. Lippincott
19. Krantz KE (1973) The anatomy of the human cervix, gross and microscopic. In: Blandau RJ, Moghissi K (eds). The biology of the cervix. Chicago, University of Chicago Press, pp 57–69.
20. Meyer R (1941) The basis of the histological diagnosis of carcinoma with special reference to carcinoma of the cervix and similar lesions. Surg Gynecol Obstet 73: 14
21. Moll R, Levy R, Czernobilsky B, Hohlweg-Majert P, et al. (1983) Cytokeratins of normal eptihelia and some neoplasms of the female genital tract. Lab Invest 49: 599
22. Naftolin F, Stubblefield PG (eds) (1980) Dilatation of the uterine cervix. Connective tissue biology and clinical management. New York, Raven Press
23. Odeblad E (1968). The functional structure of human cervical mucus. Acta Obstet Gynecol Scand 47 [Suppl 1]: 57
24. Reiffenstuhl G (1964). The lymphatics of the female genital organs, 1st ed. Philadelphia, J.B. Lippincott
25. Richart RM (1973) Cervical intraepithelial neoplasia. In: Sommers SC (ed). Pathology annual. New York, Appleton-Century-Crofts, pp 301–328
26. Robboy SJ, Taguchi O, Cunha R (1982) Normal development of the human female reproductive tract and alterations resulting from experimental exposure to diethylstilbesterol. Hum Pathol 13: 190
27. Warhol MJ, Antonioli DA, Pinkus GS, et al. Immunoperoxidase staining for involucrin: A potential diagnostic aid in cervicovaginal pathology. Hum Pathol 13: 1095

6

Benign Diseases of the Cervix

Alex Ferenczy, M.D., and Barbara Winkler, M.D.

Inflammatory Diseases

Cervicitis can be divided into noninfectious and infectious etiologies. Whatever the etiology, the tissue response of the cervix to injury is limited and reflects the basic mechanisms of inflammation and repair. Two types of morphologic changes, however, that are often encountered in association with a variety of inflammatory diseases deserve specific attention. These are atypia of repair and hyperkeratosis and parakeratosis.

Atypia of Repair

In cases of severe, acute or long-standing chronic inflammation or infection and with epithelial injury of any kind—true erosion, biopsy, or conization—the squamous and endocervical epithelia undergo reactive changes characterized by epithelial disorganization and nuclear atypia (Figs. 6.1 and 6.2a,b,c). These changes are often confused, histologically[65] and cytologically,[53] with intraepithelial neoplasia. In reactive atypia, the cytoplasmic membrane is better defined, the nuclei are uniform in shape and size, and the chromatin is aggregated in prominent chromocenters. The epithelium is often studded with migrating inflammatory cells. Mitotic figures are normal and are confined to the proliferating basal and parabasal cell populations. Characteristically, the cells in the upper half of the epithelium are not abnormal, and maturation occurs in an orderly fashion. In the endocervical columnar cells, the reparative morphologic alterations include nuclear enlargement and hyperchromasia, cytoplasmic eosinophilia, and loss of mucinous droplets (Fig. 6.2). Although this type of glandular epithelium appears highly atypical, the changes are focal, alternating with normal mucinous columnar cells, and are confined to areas with massive inflammation or mucosal injury. In addition, the deep cytoplasmic eosinophilia (which is presumably caused by an increase

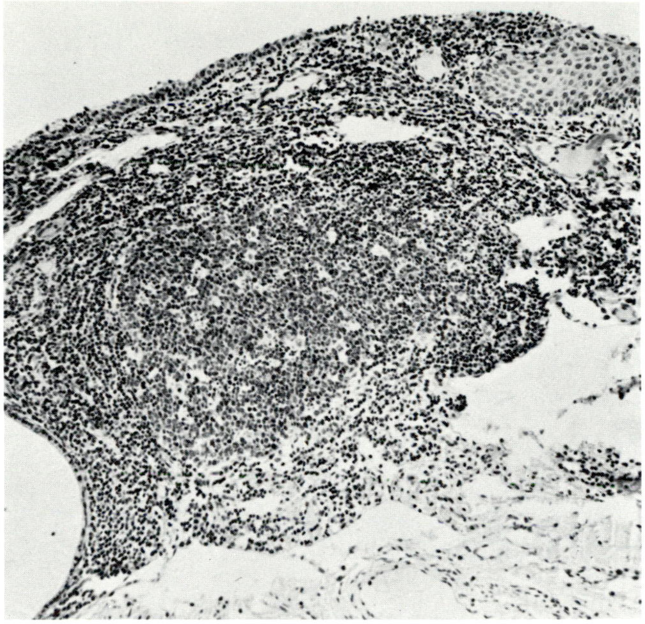

FIG. 6.1. A subepithelial lymphoid follicle with a prominent germinal center. When lymphoid follicles are numerous, the condition is referred to as *follicular cervicitis*.

in ribosomes and mitochondria) and the absence of abnormal mitoses are features that distinguish the inflammatory lesions from an in situ adenocarcinoma of the endocervix. The atypical cellular changes accompany the increased DNA and RNA synthesis that occurs during the repair of the damaged or inflamed epithelium.

Hyperkeratosis and Parakeratosis

Cervical hyperkeratosis or parakeratosis usually involves portio vaginalis and clinically appears as a whitish or greasy plaque (leukoplakia). The origins of focal hyperkeratosis are varied, but they are generally associated with local or circumscribed chronic irritation. When cervical hyperkeratosis is diffuse, the portio is covered by a thickened, white, and wrinkled epithelial membrane. Most patients with diffuse hyperkeratosis have prolapsed uteri. Microscopically, the whitish plaque corresponds to the presence of a thick keratin layer, which is referred to as *hyperkeratosis* (Fig. 6.3). When pyknotic nuclei are found within the keratin layer, the term *parakeratosis* is used (Fig. 6.4). The epithelium is often acanthotic with a well-developed granular layer, prominent intercellular bridges, and elongated rete pegs. Characteristically, the epithelial cells contain sparse glycogen, but cytologic atypicality is absent. There is neither morphologic nor clinical evidence that either hyperkeratosis or parakeratosis represents precursor lesions to cervical neoplasia. However, it should be emphasized that hyperkeratosis or parakeratosis may occasionally be features of cervical intraepithelial neoplasia or invasive carcinoma, and, consequently, all clinical white plaques on the portio vaginalis or vaginal epithelium should be biopsied.

This is particularly important in colposcopic evaluation because the keratotic surface epithelium is opaque and obscures accurate colposcopic definition of abnormal vascular patterns. The reactive nature of hyperkeratosis and parakeratosis is evidenced by a consistent association with epithelial hyperplasia and chronic inflammation. The etiologic and histogenetic mechanisms of cervical hyperkeratosis are poorly understood.

Noninfectious Cervicitis

Noninfectious cervicitis is, for the most part, chemical or mechanical in nature, and the inflammatory response is nonspecific. Common causes include chemical irritation secondary to use of deodorants or douching and local trauma produced by foreign bodies, including tampons, diaphragms, pessaries, and intrauterine contraceptive devices. Surgical instrumentation and therapeutic intervention are common iatrogenic causes of cervical tissue injury and inflammation. Acute cervicitis is characterized by stromal edema, vascular congestion, and neutrophilic infiltration of the stroma and epithelium. Clinically, the cervix appears swollen, erythematous, and friable, and there may be an associated purulent endocervical discharge. Prolonged or severe acute inflammation eventually leads to degenerative changes in the epithelial surface, loss of endocervical secretory activity, and ulceration.

In chronic cervicitis, round cells, including lymphocytes, plasma cells, and histiocytes, predominate in the inflammatory infiltrate and are associated with varying amounts of granulation tissue and stromal fibrosis. On gross and colposcopic examination, the cervical mucosa is hyperemic because of an increased number of terminal vessels and may contain true epithelial erosions (ulcerations) or lacerations. The cervical stroma contains a normal, physiologic population of inflammatory cells, and the diagnosis of chronic cervicitis should be reserved for cases where there is definite clinical and histologic evidence of a significant chronic inflammatory process. Otherwise a histologic diagnosis based on the presence of a few scattered lymphocytes has no clinical significance and is meaningless. Occasionally, lymphoid follicles with germinal centers are found beneath the epithelium (see Fig. 6.1). In a certain proportion of patients with extensive proliferation of lymphoid follicles, *Chlamydia trachomatis* is isolated from cervical secretions.[42] In other instances, a florid lymphoid inflammatory reaction may produce lymphoma-like lesions, raising the question of lymphoma.[95]

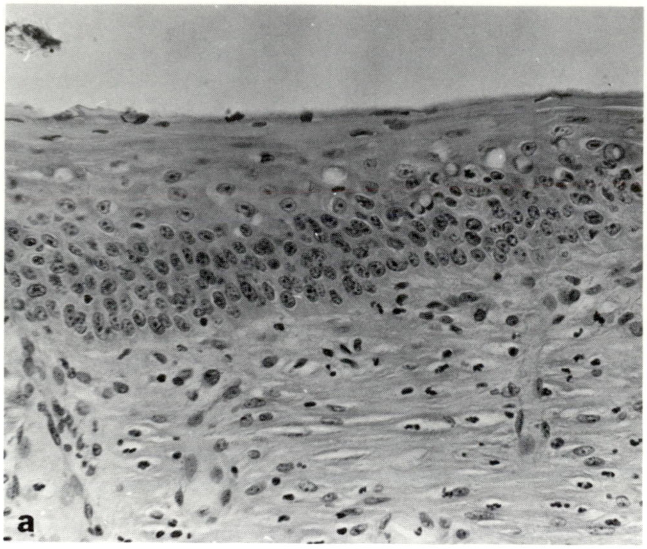

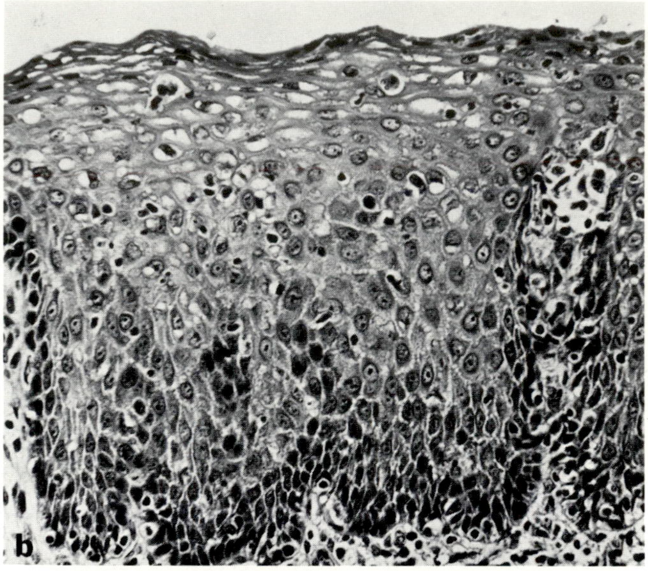

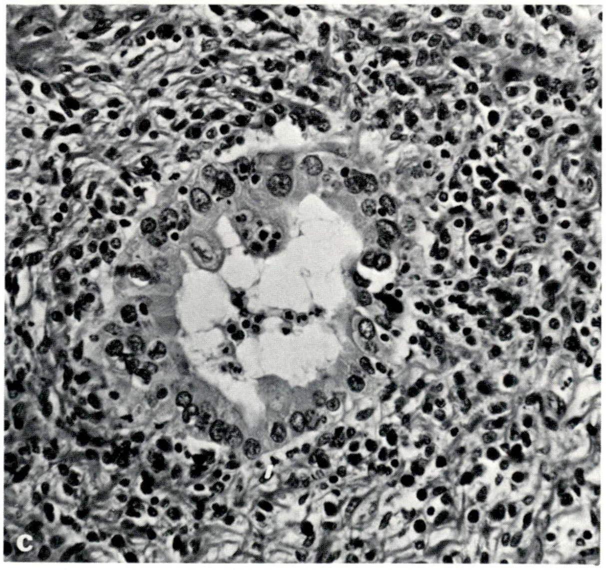

FIG. 6.2. Atypia of repair. *a*. Basal cell hyperplasia involving the lower one third of the squamous epithelium of the cervix. The nuclei contain prominent chromocenters but lack nuclear abnormalities associated with neoplasia. The epithelial cells above the enlarged basal zone display normal maturation. These alterations are often associated with mucosal denudation caused by either trauma or severe inflammation. *b*. Trichomonal cervicitis. The epithelium exhibits intercellular edema, elongation of rete pegs, and poor glycogenization. The lower half is occupied by parabasal-type cells with prominent nucleoli and intercellular bridges. Both the epithelium and the stromal papillae are infiltrated by acute inflammatory cells. *c*. Trichomonal cervicitis. Endocervical epithelium with nuclear enlargement, mitosis, microabscesses, and inconspicuous intracellular mucus. Note the diffuse distribution of nuclear chromatin, the cytoplasmic eosinophilia, and the absence of abnormal mitoses, features distinguishing endocervical atypia of inflammation from in situ adenocarcinoma of the cervix.

Infectious Cervicitis

Table 6.1 summarizes some of the important or pathologically significant etiologic organisms of infectious cervicitis. It is apparent from this listing that infectious cervicitis is of major epidemiologic importance because of its epidemic proportion and because of its central role in the pathogenesis of sexually transmitted diseases[45,94] (Fig. 6.5).

Bacterial Cervicitis

Bacterial infection of the cervix is the most common cause of infectious cervicitis and is associated with a nonspecific inflammatory response. Susceptibility of the cervix to bacterial infection is dependent on a number of interacting factors, primarily the virulence of the organism, epithelial integrity, and vaginal pH. Many cases of bacterial cervicitis are due to opportunistic infection by endogenous vaginal bacteria when epithelial atrophy, trauma, ulceration, alterations in vaginal pH, local obstruction, or stasis predisposes to infection. Infection by pathogenic, sexually transmitted organisms, such as *Chlamydia* or *Neisseria gonorrhoeae*, requires no predisposing factors and is primarily dependent on exposure and size of inoculum.[45,94] The columnar epithelium of the endocervix is much more susceptible to bacterial infection than is the surrounding squamous epithelium, and endocervicitis is characteristic. Consequently, patients with a large columnar ectropion, as is seen in young women or during pregnancy, are at higher risk for bacterial infection and acute endocervicitis.[44,45,93]

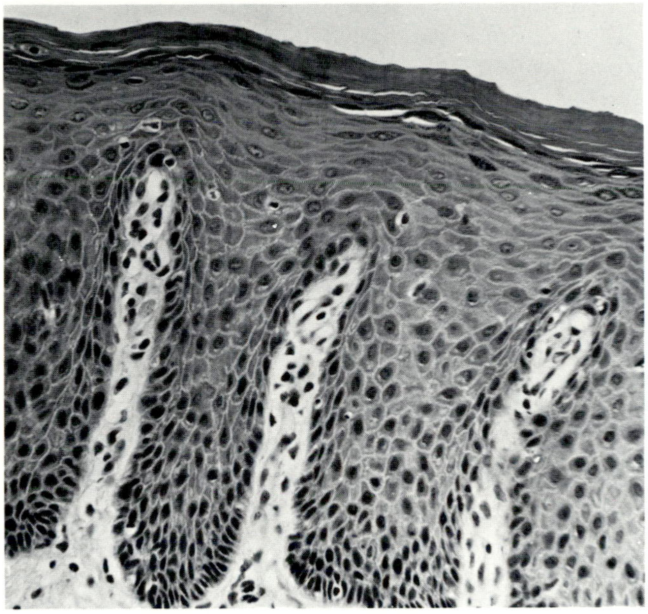

FIG. 6.3. Hyperkeratosis. A prominent keratin layer covers the epithelium of the portio.

TABLE 6.1. Etiologic organisms in infectious cervicitis.

Bacteria
Polymicrobial, endogenous vaginal aerobes and anaerobes
Chlamydia trachomatis
Neisseria gonorrhoeae
Mycoplasma hominis
Group B *Streptococcus*
Ureaplasma ureolyticum
Gardnerella vaginalis
Actinomyces israelii
Mycobacterium tuberculosis
Treponema pallidum
Viruses
Human papillomavirus
Herpes simplex virus
Cytomegalovirus
Fungi
Candida
Aspergillus
Protozoa and parasites
Trichomonas vaginalis
Ameba
Schistosomes

Bacterial infection of the cervix is infrequent in older postmenopausal women and is unusual before menarche. Sexually transmitted virulent bacteria, however, such as *N. gonorrhoeae* and *Chlamydia*, are occasionally reported in children and may affect the atrophic vaginal epithelium as well as the cervix, producing cervicovaginitis. Chronic infection is enhanced by local stasis, obstruction, and bacterial sequestration in the endocervical crypts. Asymptomatic, latent infection is common.

Clinically, bacterial cervicitis is of paramount importance because of its association with ascending infection to the endometrium, fallopian tubes, and pelvic peritoneum as well as vertical transmission to the fetus and neonate. In our current understanding of the pathogenesis of pelvic inflammatory disease, infectious cervicitis is the initial event; it is also the primary infectious focus in related syndromes, such as postpartum and postabortal endometritis. Spontaneous abortion, premature delivery, chorioamnionitis, stillbirth, and neonatal pneumonia

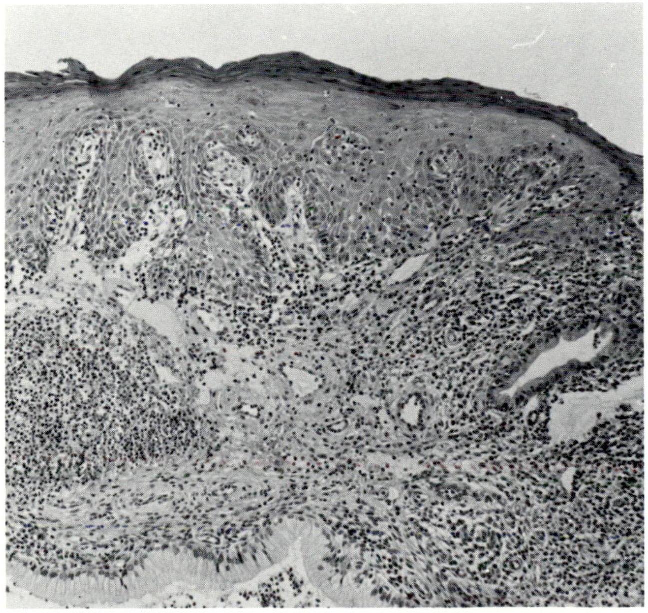

FIG. 6.4. Parakeratosis. Within the keratin layer are pyknotic nuclei. The epithelium and the subjacent stroma are infiltrated by chronic inflammatory cells.

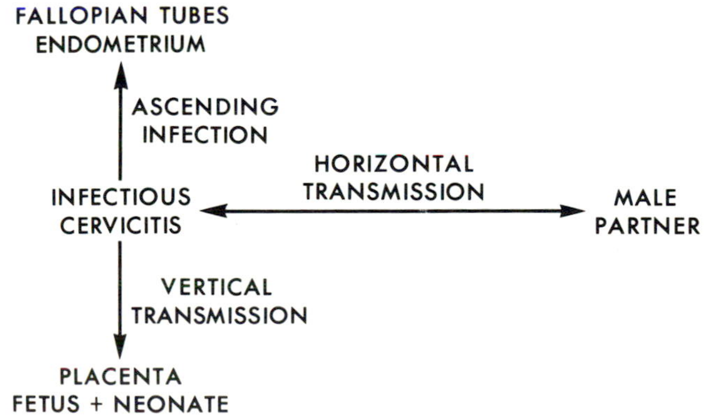

FIG. 6.5. The pivotal role of infectious cervicitis in the pathogenesis and propagation of sexually transmitted diseases. (Adapted by permission of Winkler and Richart, Ref. 94.)

and septicemia have been directly related to concurrent bacterial infection of the cervix.[38,43,45,62,89,94]

Chlamydia Trachomatis. Recent epidemiologic data indicate that *Chlamydia trachomatis* infection (CT) is the most common sexually transmitted disease in the Western world, with a prevalence far exceeding that of gonorrhea.[15,71,80,88] Chlamydial cervicitis will, therefore, be considered as a model for bacterial infectious cervicitis in general. Chlamydial cervicitis has been associated with semispecific morphologic findings, including epithelial inclusions and follicular cervicitis, and is of interest from a pathologic standpoint as well. The chlamydia organisms preferentially infect glandular epithelia, and, hence, vaginal infection is extremely rare.[72] The prevalence of CT cervicitis ranges from 1 to 3% of randomly screened women to up to 40% of women at clinics treating sexually transmitted disease. In pregnant women and young women under 20 years of age, isolation rates for CT from cervices of asymptomatic patients are as high as 10–22%.[61,73,80,88,93] Symptomatic women with acute mucopurulent cervicitis, defined by the presence of a visible, yellow-green, endocervical exudate or by the presence of ≥10 neutrophils per 100× field in a smear of endocervical mucus, have culture-positive CT infection in 58% of cases.[12] Generalized lower genital tract infection is common, often involving the urethra (so-called urethral syndrome) and the rectum.[45,47] The high risk of exposure of these patients to multiple sexually transmitted diseases is highlighted by the frequent finding of other concurrent bacterial infections, principally gonorrhea, as well as cervicitis of viral etiology.[45,51,80,88]

Inflammatory and reactive colposcopic patterns in women with CT cervicitis include hypertrophic ectopy, atypical transformation zone epithelium that may be confused with low-grade cervical intraepithelial neoplasia.[42,60,61] The association between CT infection and follicular cervicitis has been confirmed histologically, and CT is now presumed to be a major cause of this condition.[25,42,60,61,93] CT cervicitis has also been associated with a dense, severe inflammatory exudate and reactive squamous and endocervical atypia.[25,51,78] Cytoplasmic inclusions in endocervical columnar or metaplastic cells, representing aggregates of chlamydia organisms at different stages of development, may be identified in some cases and confirmed immunohistochemically with immunofluorescent or immunoperoxidase methods[25,52] (Fig. 6.6). Although cytoplasmic epithelial inclusions are identifiable in a small number of cervical Papanicolaou smears and biopsies, this finding is too insensitive and nonspecific to be of use diagnostically.[37,51,52,64,78,93]

CT cervicitis is most accurately diagnosed by culture,[72] immunofluorescence, or immunoperoxidase technique using monoclonal antibodies to CT. Since endometritis and salpingitis (see Chapter 10, Benign Diseases of Endometrium, and Chapter 14, Diseases of Fallopian Tube) complicate CT cervicitis in approximately 40% and 11% of cases, respectively, and are often subclinical,[38,62,80,88,89] the patient with CT cervicitis and her sexual partner(s) should be treated. Postinfectious sequelae include pelvic inflammatory disease, tubal infer-

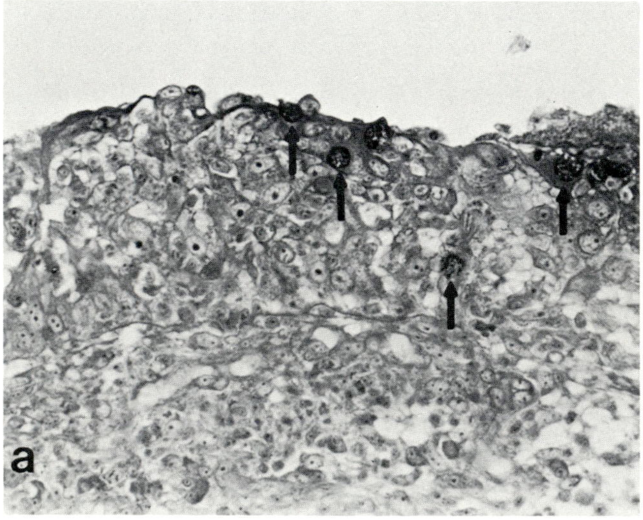

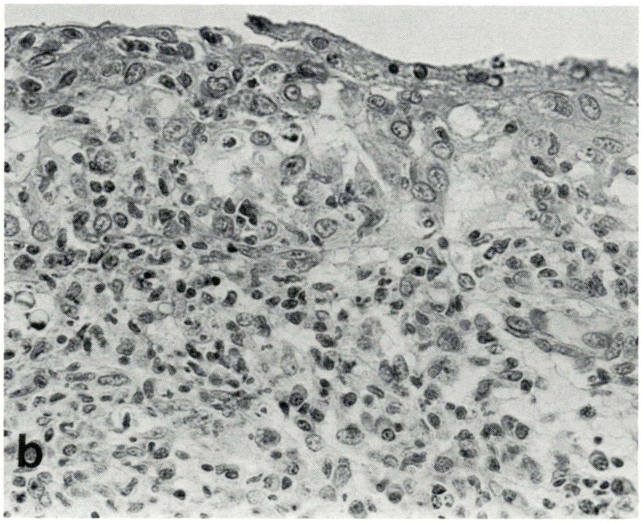

FIG. 6.6.*a*. Immunoperoxidase staining for chlamydial antigens. Several rounded cytoplasmic inclusions are seen. Note the particular character of the inclusions. *b*. The epithelium and stroma are infiltrated by acute and chronic inflammatory cells, partially obscuring the epithelial–stromal junction. The metaplastic epithelium displays reactive atypia. Scattered cytoplasmic vacuoles are present, but the finding is not specific for the definitive diagnosis of chlamydia infection. (Courtesy of C. P. Crum, M.D., New York.)

tility, and neonatal pneumonia. Symptomatic infection in the male is more commonly manifested as acute urethritis,[12,43,62,82,88,89] but the infection may be asymptomatic.

Actinomycosis. Actinomycosis infection of the female genital organs, including the cervix,[11,34,66] is caused by *Actinomycoes israelii* and results from surgical instrumentation, clinical abortion, intrauterine contraceptive devices (see Chapter 10, Benign Diseases of Endometrium, and Chapter 14, Diseases of Fallopian Tube), and direct extension from parametrial and appendiceal lesions or from the anus. More than 300 cases of genital actinomycosis are reported in the literature.[11,66] The diagnosis is made by demonstrating the organism (classified between true bacteria and complete fungi) in the center of large abscesses, occasionally with granuloma formation. The lesions appear yellow and granular to the naked eye, hence the term *sulfur granules*. They are composed of branching, gram-positive filaments with peripheral palisading clubs. Chronic infection of the cervix by *Actinomyces* may produce significant fibrosis and scarring.[11,94]

Tuberculosis. Tuberculosis of the cervix[27,74] is almost invariably secondary to tuberculous salpingitis and endometritis and is typically[27] associated with pulmonary tuberculosis (see Chapter 10, Benign Diseases of Endometrium and Chapter 14, Diseases of Fallopian Tube). The incidence of cervical tuberculosis in a population with genital tuberculosis varies between 2 and 60%, with an incidence rate of 5% in the United States.[74] Macroscopically, the cervix may appear normal or inflamed or may resemble its appearance in invasive carcinoma. Histologically, tuberculous infection of the cervix is recognized by the presence of multiple granulomas or tubercles characterized by central caseous necrosis, epithelioid histiocytes, and multinucleated Langhan's giant cells. The periphery of the tubercle is made of a heavy lymphoplasmocytic infiltrate (Fig. 6.7). Tuberculous cervicitis may often appear as a noncaseating, granulomatous lesion, and caseating, nontuberculous granulomas[31] (lymphogranuloma venereum and sarcoidosis) may be encountered in the cervix. Therefore, the unequivocal diagnosis requires demonstration of acid-fast *Mycobacterium tuberculosis*, a straight, rod-shaped bacillus, by Ziehl-Neelsen-stained sections, by culture, or by animal inoculation of cervical tissue. Because culture or inoculation yields far better results than staining of tissue sections, unfixed biopsy material should be obtained for microbiologic testing whenever tuberculosis is suspected. The most common granulomatous lesions to be distinguished from tuberculous cervicitis include foreign body giant cell granulomas to sutures, crystals, or cotton, lymphogranuloma venereum, schistosomiasis, and sarcoidosis. Cervical granuloma may occasionally develop postoperatively as a reaction to local tissue necrosis.[31]

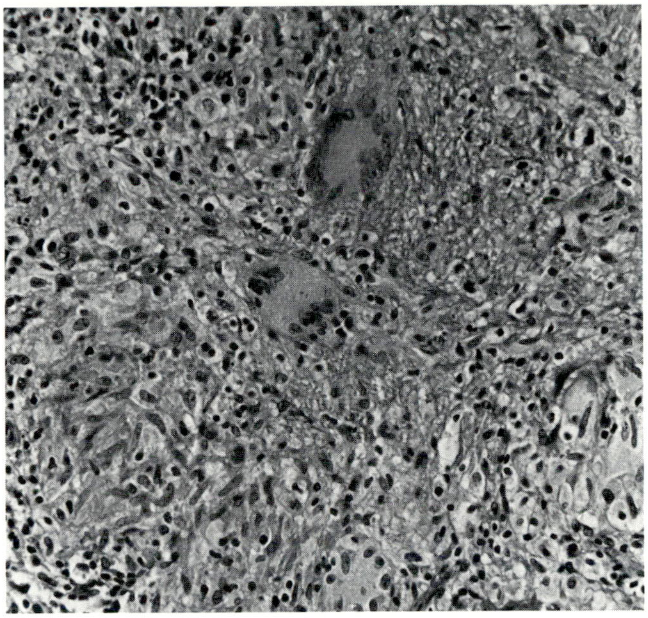

FIG. 6.7. Tuberculous cervicitis. Typical granuloma with palisading epithelioid cells, multinucleated Langhan's giant cells, and central caseous necrosis. Acid-fast stain for *Mycobacterium tuberculosis* was positive.

Other Granulomatous Infections. Certain venereally transmitted diseases commonly encountered in the vulva may also involve the cervix (see Chapter 3, Diseases of Vulva). These include syphilis, either as the primary chancre, secondary mucous patches, or tertiary gumma,[23,27,84] lymphogranuloma venereum,[27] granuloma inguinale,[7,27] and chancroid.[34] All these conditions may resemble carcinoma clinically. In addition to characteristic morphologic features, specific bacteriologic and immunologic techniques are available for identifying each of these diseases.

Viral Cervicitis

In contrast to bacterial infections of the cervix, the prevalent agents of viral cervicitis—human papillomavirus (HPV) and herpes simplex virus (HSV)—have a predilection for the squamous epithelium and produce characteristic morphologic changes. Cytomegalovirus, although often isolated from cervical secretions, is not typically associated with cervicitis, and its role in cervical infection is poorly understood.[45] Human papillomavirus infection of the cervix is discussed in detail in Chapter 7, Cervical Intraepithelial Neoplasia.

Herpesvirus Infection. Although the precise incidence of cervical HSV infection (herpes genitalis) is not known, it is far greater than generally recognized.[5,6] This is because a large number of patients experience mild symptoms or no symptoms at all. It has been shown, however, that 9% of patients seen in private gynecologic practice and 22% of those seen in hospital outpatient gynecologic clinics have positive serology for HSV type 2 (HSV-2) infection.[5,6] The Centers for Disease Control estimated 295,000 patient visits for consultation for genital herpes infections in the United States during the year 1981.[16] Genital herpesvirus infections are caused chiefly by HSV-2 and occasionally by HSV-1.[56]

Herpes simplex viruses types 1 and 2 have several common features, including architecture, size, envelope, mode of multiplication, and double-stranded DNA genetic content. However, HSV-1 is chiefly found in the oropharyngeal region (herpes buccalis) and has different biologic and epidemiologic properties from those of HSV-2 virus.[56] HSV-2 has been identified as a DNA-containing virus, and ultrastructurally,[87] the virions measure 150 nm (1 nm = 10^{-9}m) in diameter. They are surrounded by a hexogonal protein capsid of about 100 nm in diameter. The capsid, in turn, is enveloped by an inner glycoprotein-rich and an outer lipid-rich membrane of about 150–200 nm (Fig. 6.8). Viral particles are thought to replicate within the host cell nuclei, where they synthesize viral proteins necessary for replication of viral DNA.[87]

HSV-2 is acquired through sexual contact, and most female patients are teenagers or are unmarried. Primary herpetic infections produce symptoms within 3–7 days after exposure. When the vulva is involved symptoms include severe vulvar pain, tenderness, painful urination, and profuse watery vaginal discharge.[21,22,49] The symptoms of recurrent herpes genitalis are comparatively less severe than those experienced during the primary infection. The disease is characterized by the development of multiple, painful vesicles involving the vulva, perineum, vagina, and cervix that rapidly evolve into shallow, painful ulcerations.[40] Occasionally, the ulceronecrotic process is so extensive that a fungating, necrotic mass appears on the cervical portio, which can be mistaken for carcinoma.[81] Shedding of herpesvirus from asymptomatic, clinically inapparent cervical lesions occurs in 4–10% of infected women and serves as a hidden reservoir for propagation of infection.[4]

Herpesvirus infection may be diagnosed by cervical cultures, neutralizing antibodies serology,[5,6] and Papanicolaou smears. In the Papanicolaou smear, large multinucleated cells with the characteristic intranuclear ground-glass viral inclusions are observed. Occasionally, during the vesicular phase, a biopsy may reveal the presence of suprabasal intraepidermal vesicles filled with serum, degenerated epidermal cells, and multinucleated giant cells, some containing eosinophilic, intranuclear inclusions surrounded by a clear halo (Fig. 6.9). Diagnostic yield by isolation and cytology is most efficient within 2–3 days after the onset of symptoms.[40]

Herpes genitalis has two important clinical implications. First, it may result in spontaneous abortion, fetal morbidity, and fetal mortality.[21] Second, there may be an association between HSV infections of the female genital tract and the genesis of cervical carcinoma[32] (see Chapter 7, Cervical Intraepithelial Neoplasia).

Herpes-Like Lesions. Vesicular and bullous lesions of the cervical squamous mucous membrane, other than

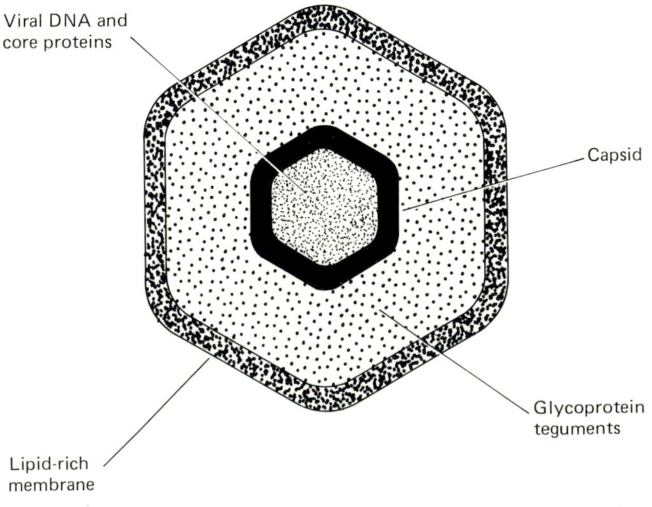

Fig. 6.8. Drawing of a virion of herpes simplex virus type 2.

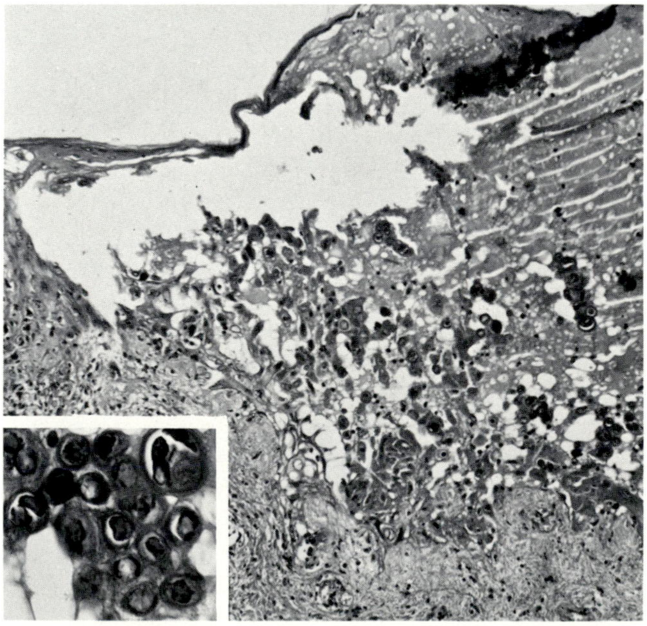

Fig. 6.9. Suprabasal herpetic vesicle in squamous epithelium of the portio. *Inset:* High-power view of acantholytic intravesicular epithelial cells with ground-glass intranuclear viral inclusions.

herpetic cervicitis, have been reported.[10] Pemphigus vulgaris of the cervix[48] is a rather common finding in women with generalized disease. Microscopically, there are multiple intraepithelial bullae in a suprabasal location containing the characteristic acantholytic Tzanck cells.

Isolated arteritis of the cervix, histologically identical with but clinically unrelated to polyarteritis nodosa, may rarely be encountered.[24] The etiology of this condition is unknown. It may be asymptomatic or may be associated with bleeding and may clinically resemble cancer.

Fungal Cervicitis

Cervical fungal infection by *Candida albicans* usually occurs as part of a generalized lower genital tract infection involving the vagina and vulva. Alkalinization of vaginal pH, antibiotic therapy, and poorly controlled diabetes mellitus all favor fungal overgrowth.[94] Typically, *Candida* infection is associated with a viscous vaginal discharge containing white flakes, often accompanied by vulvar pruritus. *Aspergillus* infection of the cervix is uncommonly reported and is prevalent only in the immunosuppressed host.[94]

Protozoal and Parasitic Cervicitis

Cervical infestation by *Trichomonas vaginalis* is quite frequent and most often associated with concurrent trichomonal vaginitis. A foamy, yellow-green vaginal discharge is typically described. Acute trichomonal cervicitis may provoke an intense inflammatory response, with prominent reparative atypia in exfoliated squamous and endocervical cells, with corresponding gross and colposcopic abnormalities[53] (see Fig. 6.2). Diagnosis is usually made by a wet mount or by identification of the organism on Papanicolaou smear (see Chapter 4, Diseases of Vagina and Chapter 25, Cytology).

Rare instances of parasitic infestations, such as echinococcosis or hydatid cysts[54] and ulceronecrotic amebiasis[20] (Fig. 6.10), have been encountered in the cervix. In contrast, schistosomiasis (bilharziasis) of the cervix,[9,30,76] generally caused by *Schistosoma haematobium* and occasionally by *Schistosoma mansoni*, is very common in Africa (Egypt), South America, Puerto Rico, and several Asian countries. A large number of cases of cervical schistosomiasis are associated with urinary schistosomiasis and sterility. The latter condition is presumably related to increased *Schistosoma*-stimulated antispermatozoal antibodies.[30] Microscopically, noncaseating granulomas (pseudotubercles) with ova surrounded by multinucleated giant cells are seen (Fig. 6.11), and the ova are often calcified. *S. mansoni* has a long lateral spine, whereas *S. haematobium* has a short spine extending from one of its poles. Cervical schistosomiasis may be associated with extensive pseudoepitheliomatous hyperplasia of the cervical squamous epithelium, masquerading both clinically and histologically as carcinoma. Chronic, untreated infection has been implicated in the genesis of cervical carcinoma in populations where schistosomiasis is prevalent.[76]

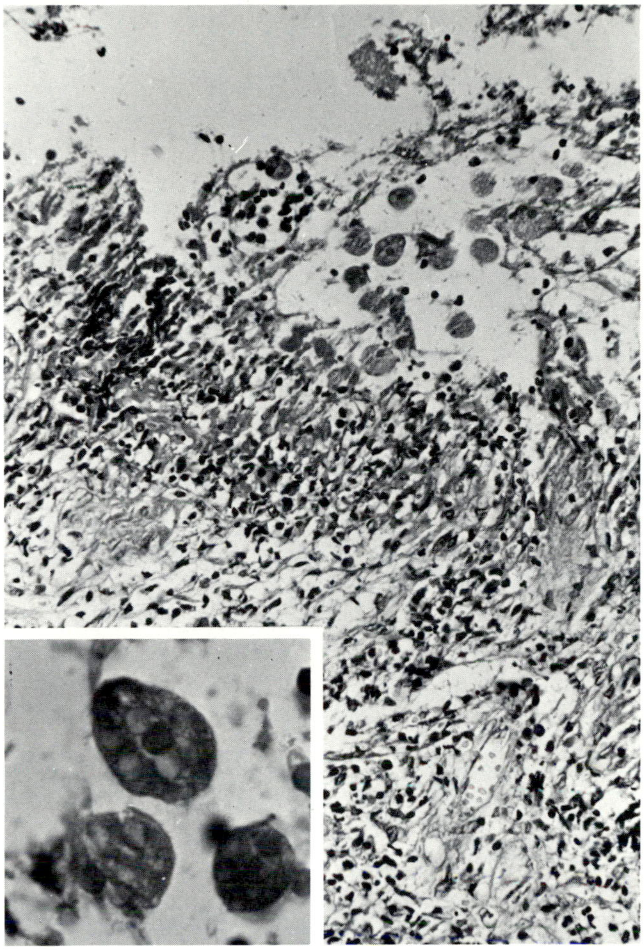

Fig. 6.10. Ulceronecrotic amebiasis of cervix with numerous amebae in the superficial exudate. *Inset:* Detail of *Entamoeba histolytica* with vacuolated cytoplasm.

Cervicovaginitis Emphysematosa

This unusual disease is characterized by multiple, blue-gray, subepithelial cysts of the portio vaginalis and vagina.[36,90] The cause of this condition is unknown, but it is often associated with trichomoniasis.[36,90] Gas-forming bacteria have never been identified. The cysts are dilated connective tissue spaces without lining epithelium that contain air and carbon dioxide.[36] Some of the cysts are surrounded by multinucleated foreign body giant cells, and often the subepithelial veins and lymphatics are dilated. The disappearance of the disease after eradication of trichomoniasis and the experimental production of gas by *T. vaginalis* in subcutaneous tissue of guinea pigs[57] suggest an etiologic relationship.

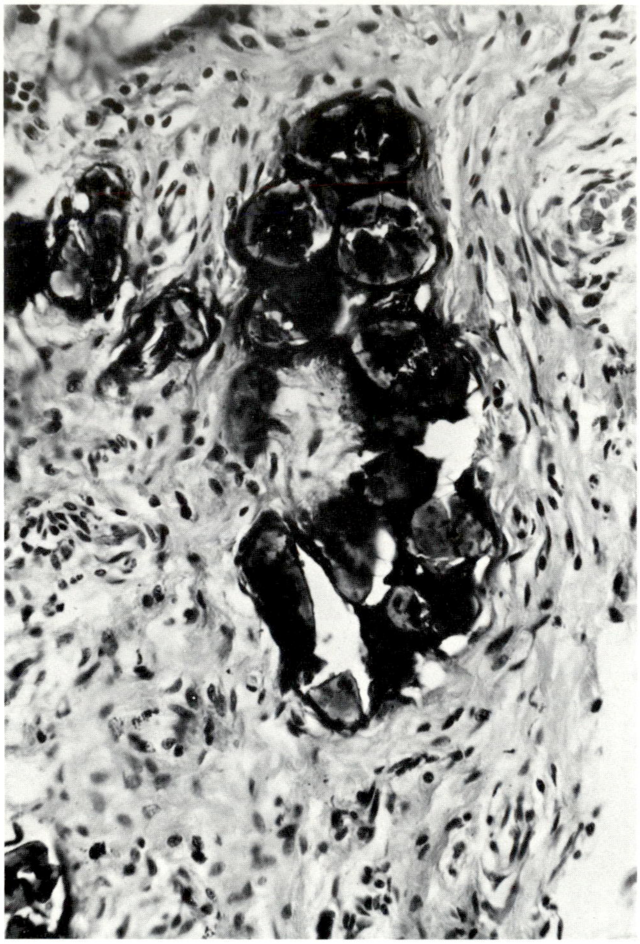

FIG. 6.11. Cervical schistosomiasis. Note calcified *Schistosoma haematobium* ova.

Pseudotumors

Endocervical Polyps

Endocervical polyps[1,27,34] constitute the most common new growths of the uterine cervix. Cervical polyps are focal, hyperplastic protrusions of endocervical folds, including the epithelium and substantia propria, rather than true neoplasms. The stimulus for the polypoid outgrowths is at present unknown. Cervical polyps are most often found during the fourth to sixth decades and in multigravidas.[1] They may be a cause of profuse leukorrhea or abnormal bleeding.[1] These symptoms are caused by hypersecretion of mucus by severely inflamed endocervical epithelium and ulceration of the surface epithelium, respectively. Clinically, cervical polyps are rounded or elongated structures with a smooth or lobulated surface that is often reddened because of increased vascularity. Most polyps occur singly and measure from a few millimeters to 2–3 cm. In rare instances they may

TABLE 6.2. Differential diagnosis of polypoid lesions of the cervix—macroscopy.

Polyp	Condyloma acuminatum
Microglandular endocervical hyperplasia	Papillary adenofibroma
Leiomyoma	Squamous cell carcinoma
Adenomyoma	Adenocarcinoma
Fibroadenoma	Sarcoma, primary or secondary
Squamous papilloma	

TABLE 6.3. Histologic patterns of cervical polyps.

Endocervical mucosal type (cervical mucous polyp)	Inflammatory type (polypoid granulation tissue)
Fibrous type	
Vascular type	Pseudodecidual type
Mixed endocervical–endometrial type	Pseudosarcomatous type

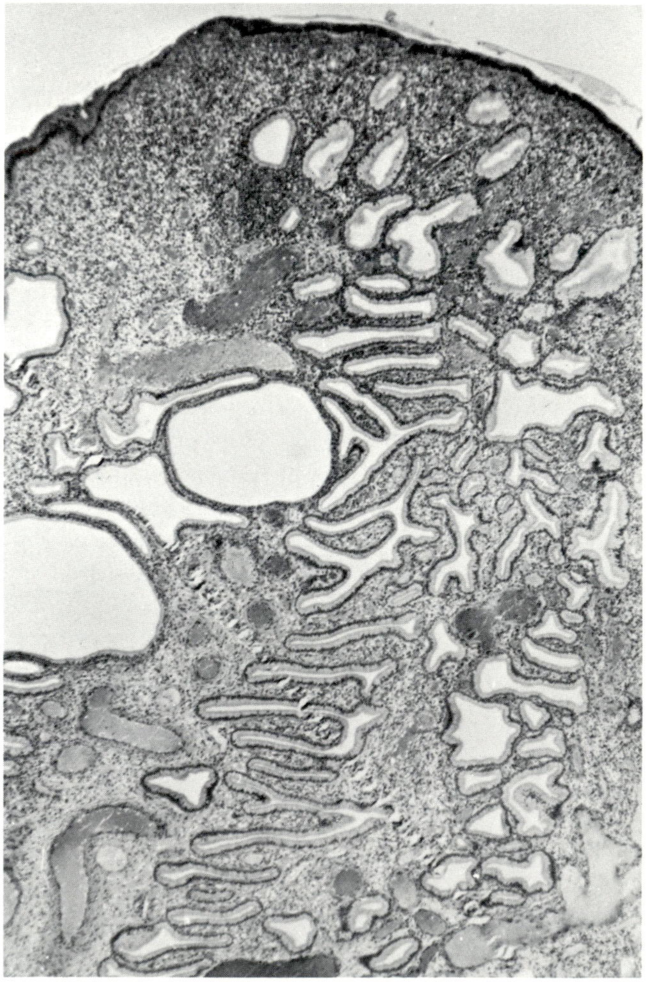

FIG. 6.12. Tip of endocervical mucous polyp.

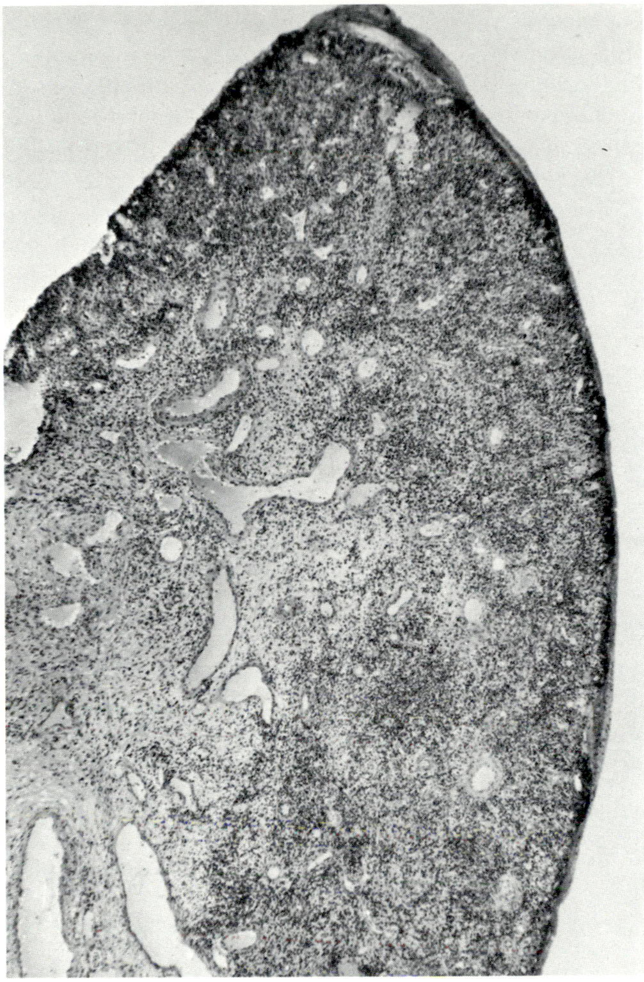

FIG. 6.13. Endocervical polyp with extensive inflammation resembling polypoid granulation tissue. This type of lesion often leads to bleeding.

reach gigantic dimensions, protruding beyond the introitus and resembling carcinoma.[55] Various cervical lesions with a polypoid gross appearance are presented in Table 6.2. Microscopically, cervical polyps display a variety of structural patterns that vary according to the preponderance of one or another tissue component normally found in all cervical polyps (Table 6.3). The most common type is the endocervical mucosal polyp. It is composed of mucinous epithelium that lines crypts, with or without cystic or adenomatous glandular changes (Fig. 6.12). Occasionally, they may be mainly fibrous, representing an overgrowth of the connective tissue stroma of the portio. This type of lesion is referred to as *cervical fibrous polyp*. When vascular structures predominate, the lesion is called a *vascular polyp*. Squamous metaplasia involving the surface or glandular epithelium of polyps is frequently observed. These changes are not difficult to differentiate from carcinoma arising in a polyp. The supporting connective tissue of polyps is generally loose, with centrally placed feeding vessels, and is almost always infiltrated by a chronic inflammatory exudate. Occasionally, such infiltration may be so extensive as to be the principal tissue constituent of the polyp. In these cases, polypoid granulation tissue devoid of surface epithelium is observed (Fig. 6.13). Polyps originating in the isthmus often have an admixture of endocervical- and endometrial-type epithelial components and are referred to as *mixed polyps* (Fig. 6.14).

During gestation, cervical polyps may contain focal stromal decidual changes. Rarely, massive decidualization of endocervical stroma produces a polypoid protrusion from the endocervix, the so-called *true decidual polyp* (Fig. 6.15). In addition to decidua-like cytoplasmic changes, focal areas of bizarre stromal cell reaction with irregular, hyperchromatic nuclei resembling radiation fibroblasts are seen that may simulate the subepithelial

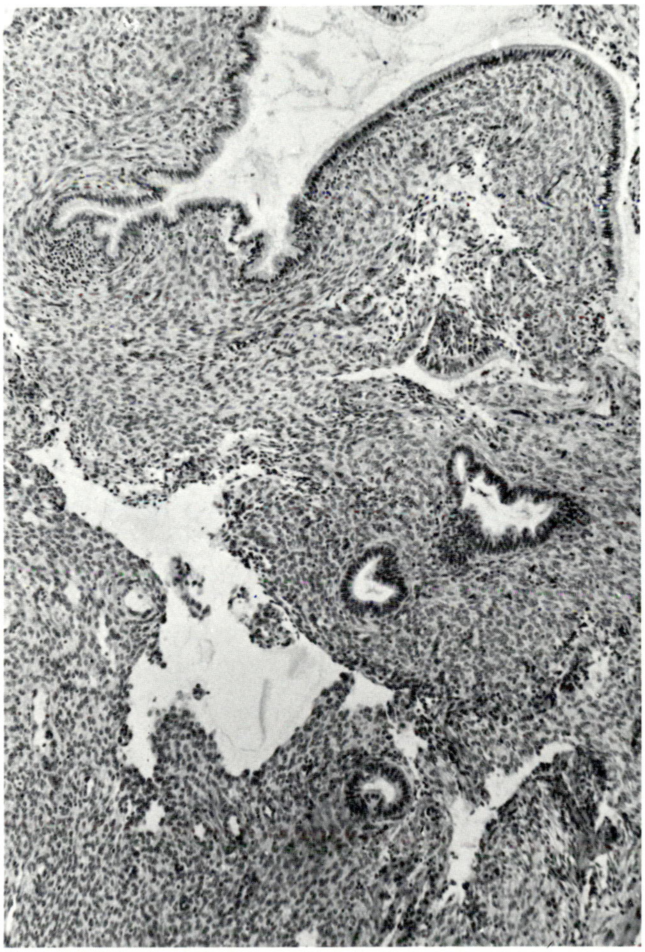

FIG. 6.14. Mixed endocervical–endometrial polyp of uterine isthmus origin. Note dense endometrial stroma with endometrial glands admixed with mucinous endocervical epithelium (*top*).

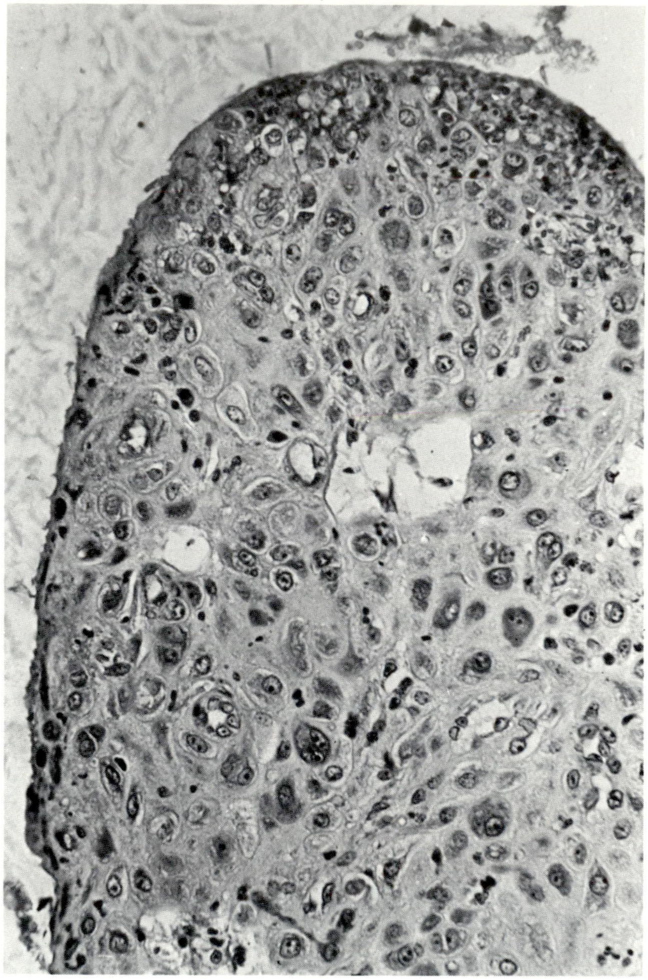

FIG. 6.15. True decidual polyp of cervix in pregnancy. Note typical decidual cells.

cambium layer seen in sarcoma botryoides[28,29] (Fig. 6.16). Similar morphologic alterations are encountered in pseudosarcomatous botryoid polyps of the cervix[29] and vagina,[59] as well as in the subepithelial myxoid stromal zone, which is often seen running from the endocervix to the vulva in adult women.[18,28] All these conditions are benign, most likely representing a peculiar form of stromal cell hyperplasia. Carcinoma, either in situ or invasive (adeno- or squamous), arising in cervical polyps is extremely rare, with an incidence of 0.2–0.4%.[1] Endocervical polyps with adenocarcinomatous changes (Fig. 6.17) must be differentiated from polypoid adenocarcinoma of the endocervix and from endocervical polyps that are secondarily involved by adjacent adenocarcinoma. The most useful criterion for differentiating between the two conditions is to determine whether or not the base of the pedicle of the polyp is involved by carcinoma. The base of a polyp that harbors primary malignancy is free of disease, and the carcinoma usually has a focal distribution within an otherwise benign polyp. In a polypoid carcinoma, the entire mass is malignant, including its base and neighboring areas. A focus of carcinoma in a cervical polyp without involvement of its base but associated with similar carcinoma in the adjacent regions should be regarded as a secondary rather than a primary focus. Adenocarcinoma confined to a polyp has an excellent prognosis.[3]

Microglandular Endocervical Hyperplasia

Clinically, this benign condition most often resembles a cervical polyp measuring 1–2 cm in size. Some patients complain of postcoital bleeding or spotting. Microglandular endocervical hyperplasia (MEH) occurs in most instances in women with a history of oral contraceptive use or in pregnant or postpartum patients.[14,58,91] It is, therefore, considered that MEH is a reflection of proges-

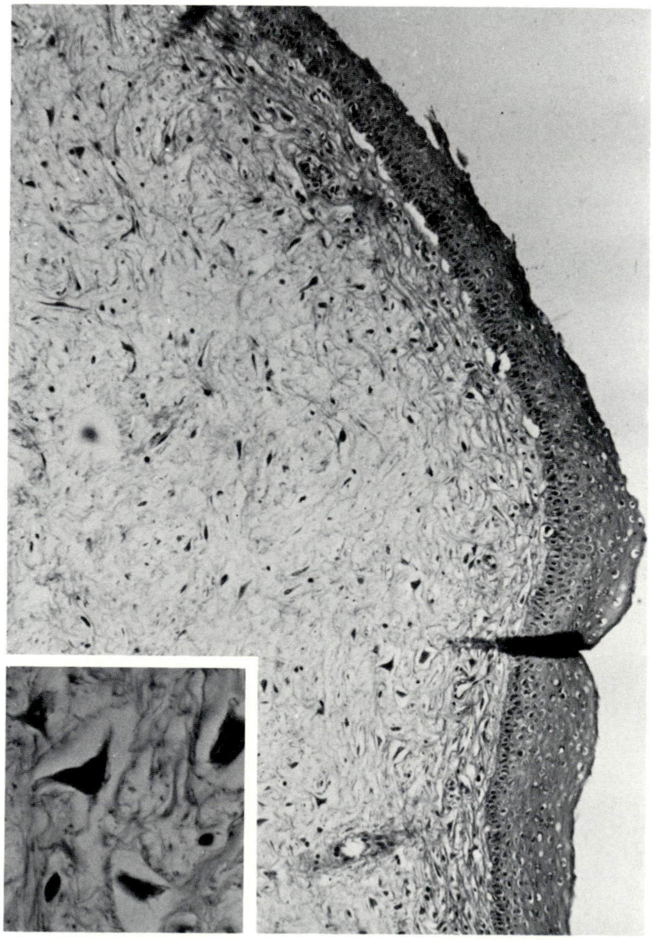

FIG. 6.16. Pseudosarcomatous botryoid polyp of cervix. Spindle-shaped and stellate fibroblasts are embedded in a loose myxoid stroma simulating sarcoma botryoides. Note absence of subepithelial cambium layer. *Inset:* High magnification of stellate atypical fibroblasts.

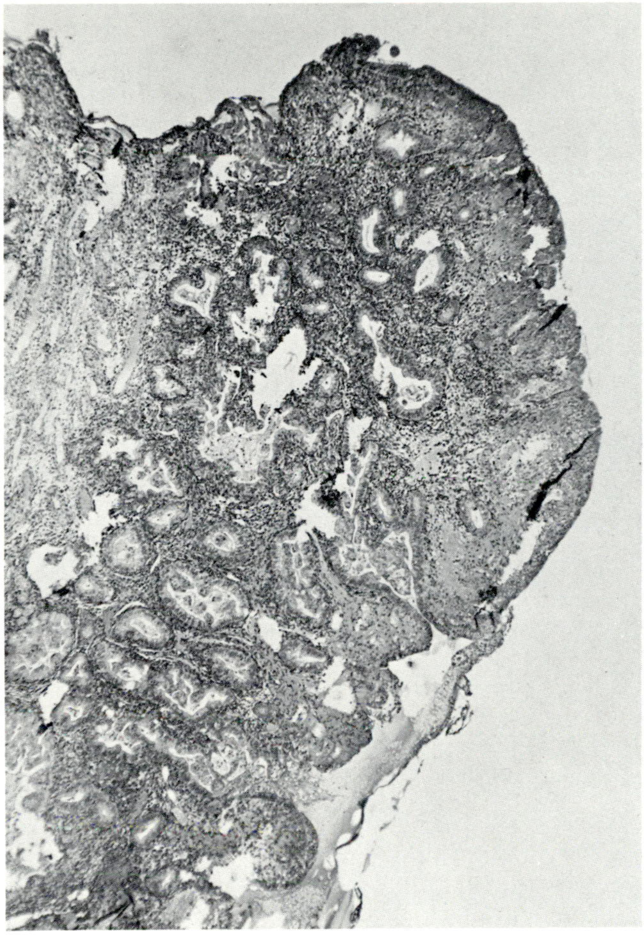

FIG. 6.17. Adenocarcinoma in situ within endocervical polyp. The neoplastic growth is confined to the superficial area of the polyp.

tagenic stimulation.[58] Persistence of the condition for long periods of time after discontinuation of pills or termination of pregnancy suggests that increased hormone levels are needed for inducing but not for maintaining the lesion.[58] Several cases have been reported in which there was no associated hormonal history. Other authors have described the sporadic occurrence of MEH in patients with hyperestrogenism or exogenous estrogen therapy.[85,91]

Histologically, MEH may be single or distributed in multiple foci. It may involve the surface and/or deeper portions of endocervical clefts. Two histologic types of MEH are recognized. The most common form, termed *microglandular hyperplasia*, consists of tightly packed, varying-sized glandular or tubular units lined by flattened to cuboidal cells with eosinophilic granular cytoplasm containing small quantities of mucin (Fig. 6.18). The nuclei are uniform, with occasional pleomorphism and hyperchromasia. Associated squamous metaplasia and subcolumnar reserve cell hyperplasia are seen in a large number of cases. The second form was described by Taylor et al.[83] under the term *atypical endocervical hyperplasia*. This type of florid microglandular proliferation can be mistaken for adenocarcinoma, in particular, clear cell adenocarcinoma.[69] In these lesions the glandular elements are arranged in a reticulated or solid pattern with areas of nuclear hyperchromasia and pleomorphism, features that may cause concern about whether the lesion is malignant (Fig. 6.19). However, the benign nature of the lesion is supported by lack of stromal invasion, scant mitotic activity, and the consistently irregular nuclear morphology as compared to the inconsistently irregular nuclear pattern of endocervical adenocarcinoma. More importantly, unlike clear cell carcinoma, MEH lacks intracellular glycogen. Other evidence in favor of the benign nature of atypical microglandular hyperplasia is that no patients are yet reported to have developed malignancies subsequent to the diagnosis.

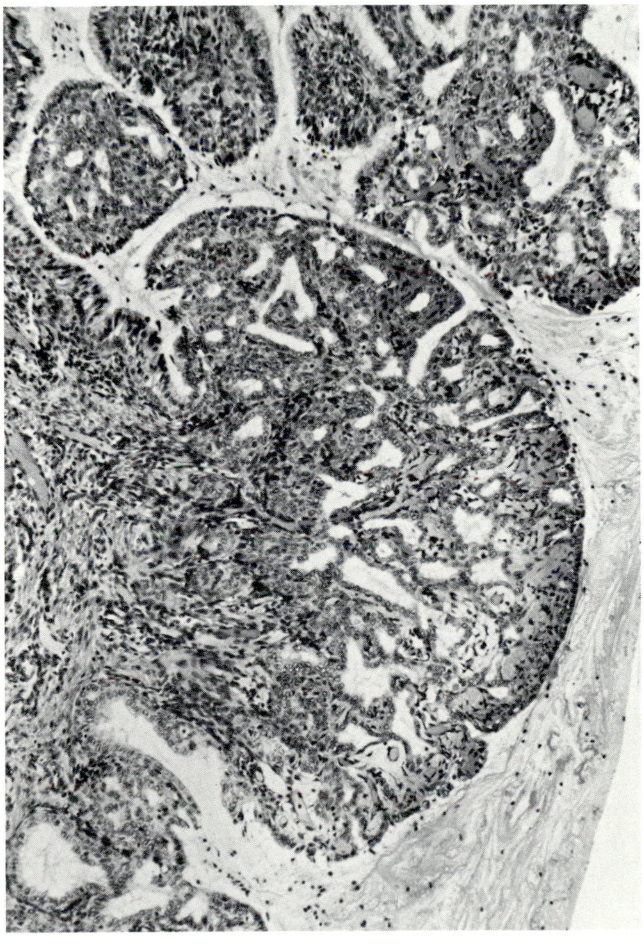

FIG. 6.18. Polypoid microglandular hyperplasia associated with oral contraceptives. Adenomatous pattern with cuboidal lining cells and focal squamous metaplasia.

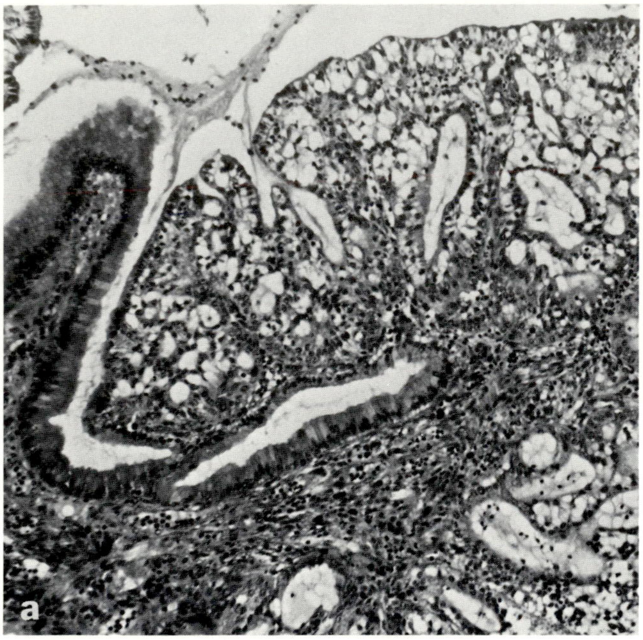

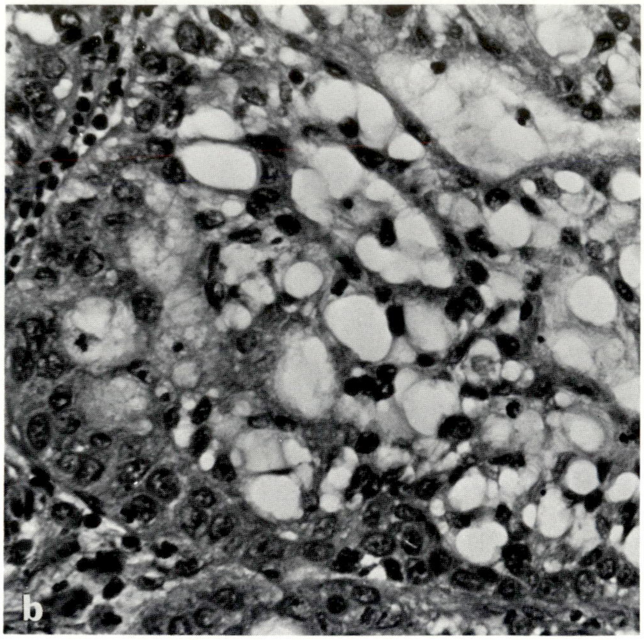

FIG. 6.19.*a*. Polypoid atypical microglandular hyperplasia associated with oral contraceptives. The hyperplastic cells contrast sharply with adjacent normal endocervical picket cells. *b*. High magnification illustrating the reticulated pattern of atypical microglandular hyperplasia. Note extensive vacuolization, which is caused by cystic dilatation of intercellular spaces. There is a paucity of intracellular mucin.

Epithelial Inclusion Cysts

These are solitary, unilocular cystic structures measuring 1–2 cm in diameter and lined by nonkeratinizing squamous epithelium.[34] They are found beneath the native portio epithelium and are believed to result from misplaced portio epithelium after surgical or obstetric trauma rather than from squamous metaplasia of a dilated endocervical gland.

Benign Neoplasms

Leiomyomas

Cervical leiomyomas represent about 8% of all uterine myomas.[33] They usually occur singly and produce unilateral enlargement of the cervical portio. At times the lesion may protrude from the canal, resembling an endocervical polyp, and in pregnancy may produce dystocia. Cervical leiomyomas are similar grossly, microscopically, and ultrastructurally to those observed in the myometrium; bizarre histologic patterns, including nuclear palisading, hyalinization, and giant nuclei, may be encountered (Fig. 6.20). A variant of cervical, as well as myometrial, leiomyomas is the so-called vascular leiomyoma. In these lesions, the muscular growth is associated with an abundance of varying-sized, thick-walled, hyalinized blood vessels. Histologic continuity between the smooth muscle fibers and the muscular wall of blood vessels is often demonstrated, suggesting that the latter represents the source of the neoplastic growth.

Hemangiomas and Other Rare Neoplasms

Hemangiomas are rarely found in the cervix[41] and may be of capillary or cavernous type. A single instance of cervical lymphangioma was reported by Stout[82] and several cases of lipoma of the cervix are on record.[68] Neoplasms of neurogenic derivation arising in the cervix are extremely rare and include neurofibroma[13] and ganglioneuroma.[33] Benign blue nevi of the endocervix, indistinguishable from those arising in the dermis, are seen occasionally.[26,63] They are composed of melanin-containing fusiform cells with dendritic cytoplasmic processes, located in the stroma of the endocervix.

Papillary Adenofibroma

In 1971, Abell[2] described three polypoid lesions of endocervical origin that contained branching clefts and papillary excrescences lined by mucinous epithelium with foci of squamous metaplasia (Fig. 6.21). The epithelium was supported by a compact, cellular, fibrous tissue composed of spindle-shaped and stellate fibroblasts, with an occasional storiform pattern. The stroma was devoid

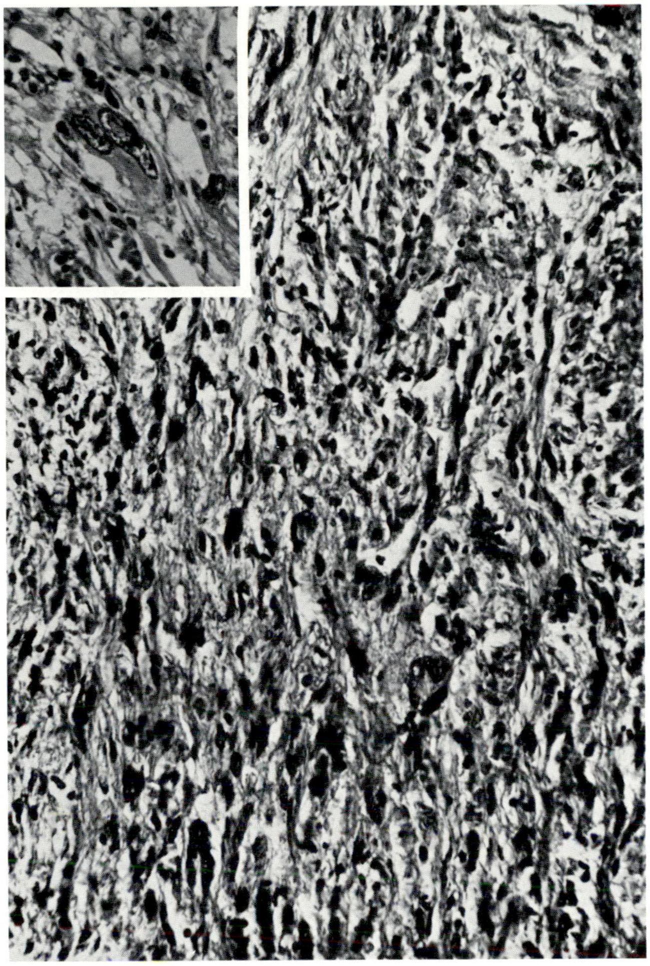

Fig. 6.20. Cellular (atypical) leiomyoma of the cervix in a pregnant woman with atypical giant cells and pleomorphism but no mitotic figures. Such neoplasms should not be interpreted as sarcoma. *Inset:* Detail of atypical neoplastic smooth muscle cells. (Courtesy of Dr. B. Bigelow, New York.)

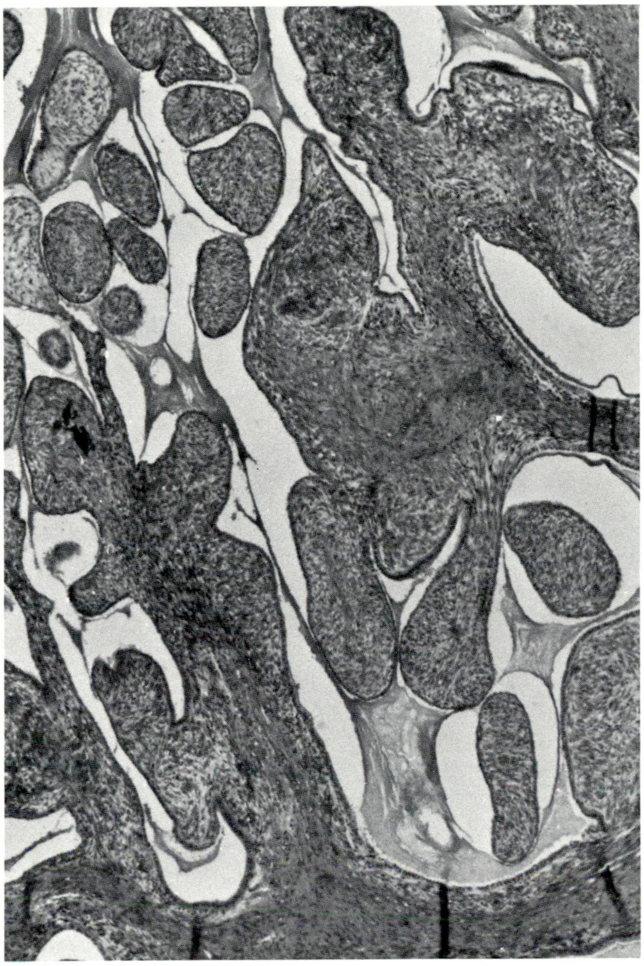

Fig. 6.21. Papillary adenofibroma of the endocervix. Fibroepithelial papillae project into cystic spaces. The endocervical lining epithelium produces abundant mucin.

of smooth muscle fibers and mitoses were rare. Because of their resemblance to adenofibroma of the ovary, the term *papillary adenofibroma of the cervix* was suggested.[2] The lesions are regarded as true benign neoplasms. Similar papillary growths have since been reported in the endometrium[39,86] and fallopian tube. Although a focus of adenocarcinoma has been found[86] in one case of papillary adenofibroma of the endometrium, to date all the patients are alive and well. Papillary adenofibroma of the female reproductive tract, including the cervix, occurs exclusively in perimenopausal and postmenopausal women.

The hypercellular stromal component of papillary adenofibroma may resemble cervical stromal sarcoma. The latter is usually not papillary and the nuclei are pleomorphic and mitoses are frequent. Papillary adenofibroma must also be distinguished from its malignant counterpart, the so-called müllerian adenosarcoma.[19] In this lesion, there is increased mitotic activity in the stromal elements (see Chapter 13, Mesenchymal Tumors of Uterus).

Adenomyoma and Fibroadenoma

These neoplasms are rare and are composed of an admixture of fibroconnective tissue and smooth muscle elements intermingling with mucinous endocervical epithelium.[39] Depending on the predominance of the fibrous or muscular tissue component, they are classified as fibroadenoma or adenomyoma.

Mesonephric Papilloma of Children

Rare instances of benign, papillary growths of the cervix in children have been described.[46,50,77] They are composed of complex papillary projections lined by flat cubiodal epithelium with cores of loose fibrovascular tissue. Cytologic atypia and mitoses are absent. The lesions are thought to be of mesonephric duct origin, although they have not been encountered in association with mesonephric remnants.

Endometriosis

The term *endometriosis* refers to lesions that are composed of ectopic endometrial glands and stroma (see Chapter 17, Endometriosis). Endometriosis of the cervix is not as uncommon as originally believed[67] and may occur on the portio or in the endocervical canal.[35,67] Most areas of endometriosis of the exocervix appear as one or more, small, blue or red nodules, measuring a few millimeters in diameter. Occasionally, however, the lesion may be larger or cystic and may produce abnormal vaginal bleeding. Histologically, the glands and stroma are identical with the endometrium. The glands as well as the stroma usually have a proliferative pattern (Fig. 6.22) but may contain extravasated red blood cells or respond to hormonal stimuli with differentiation into secretory glands and pseudodecidua. A case of adenocarcinoma arising within cervical endometriosis has been reported.[17]

During pregnancy, the ectopic glands occasionally exhibit gestational Arias–Stella reaction (Fig. 6.23). The development of cervical endometriosis may be explained by Samson's implantation theory.[67] According to this theory, endometrial tissue is implanted into the cervical mucosa or submucosa following postmenstrual cauterization[67] or during delivery.

Mesonephric Remnants

The vestigial elements of the distal ends of the mesonephric ducts are found in about 1% of cervices. They consist of small tubules or cysts[75] and are located deep in the lateral cervical wall. Characteristically, the tubules are arranged in small clusters or have an orderly distribution reminiscent of the ampullary portion of the fetal mesonephric duct. The tubules are lined by a nonciliated,

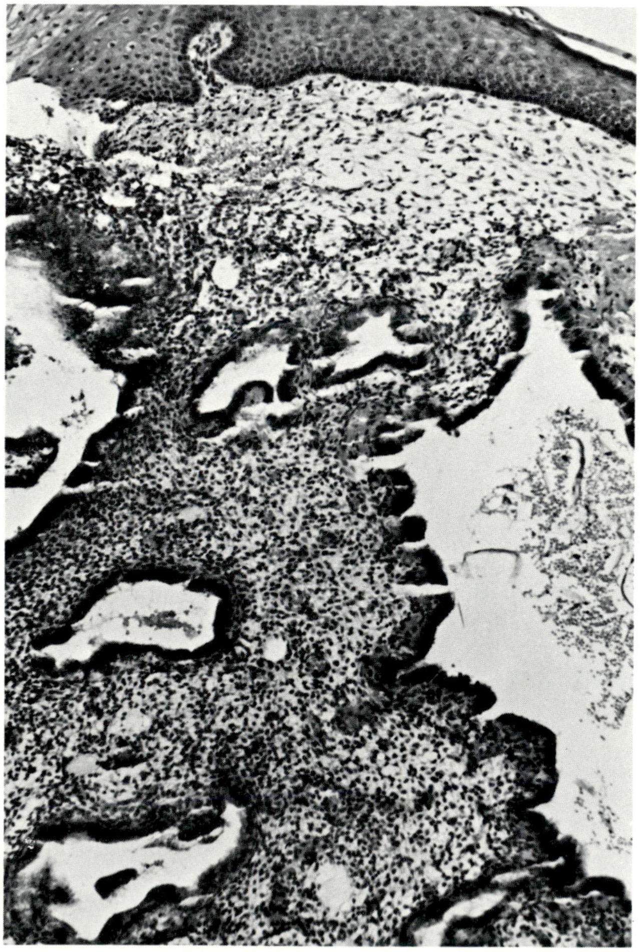

FIG. 6.22. Endometriosis containing typical endometrial glands and stroma subjacent to the squamous portio epithelium. (Courtesy of Dr. A. Blaustein, New York.)

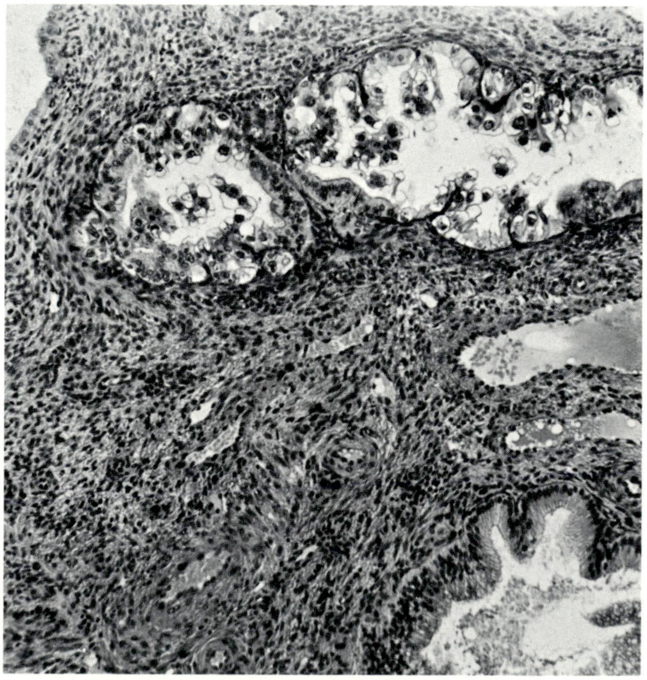

FIG. 6.23. Arias–Stella reaction in the gestational endocervix. Such cellular changes should not be confused with clear cell adenocarcinoma of the cervix.

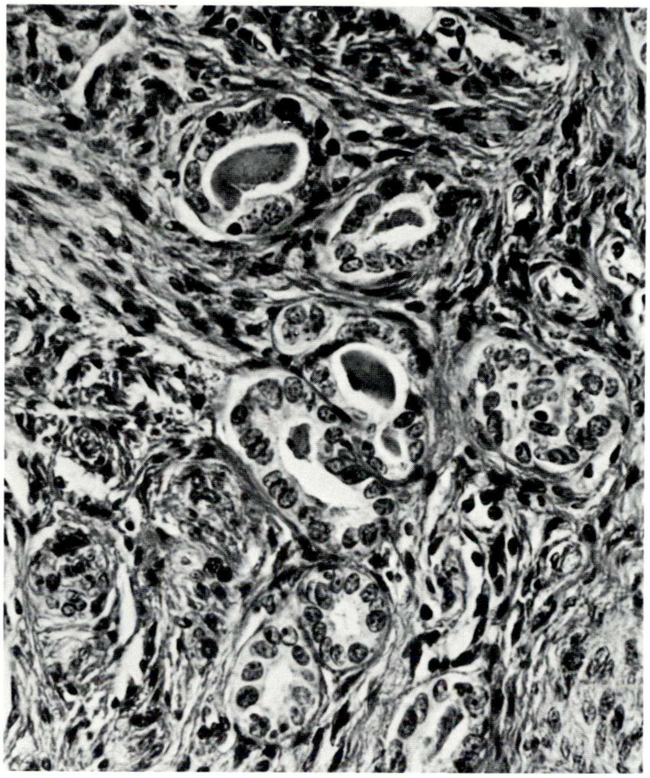

FIG. 6.24. Mesonephric tubules with pink, homogeneous intraluminal secretions.

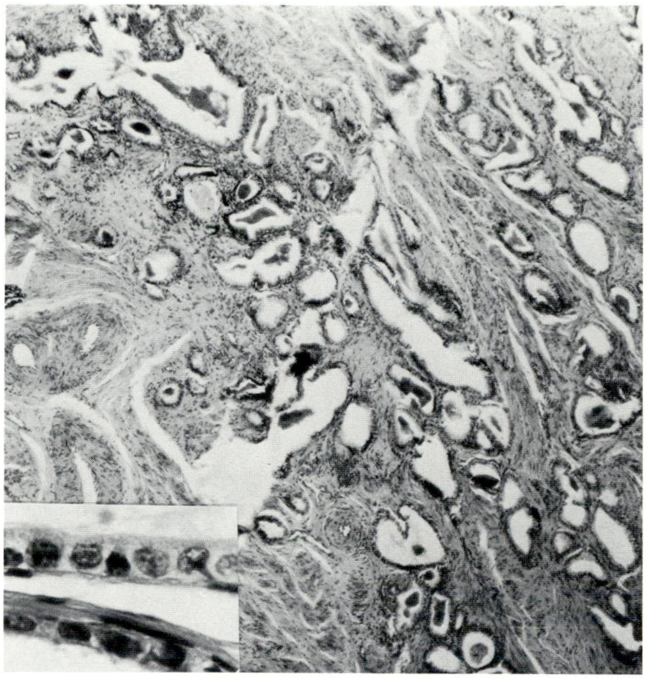

FIG. 6.25. Florid mesonephric hyperplasia. Extensive mesonephric tubular–ductal proliferation in the deeper portion of the cervix, resembling an invasive adenocarcinoma. Unlike the latter, the former lacks papillary growth pattern, periglandular edema, and complex architectural alterations. *Inset:* At magnification of duct lining, cuboidal cells are devoid of atypia. (Reprinted by permission of Ayroud et al., Ref. 8.)

low columnar or cuboidal epithelium.[75] The lining cells contain no glycogen or mucin, features that distinguish them from the endocervical epithelium. The tubular lumen, however, is often filled with pink, homogeneous, PAS-positive secretions (Fig. 6.24). Mesonephric remnants may rarely appear as a florid, tubuloglandular proliferation with transmural involvement of the cervix (Fig. 6.25), masquerading as a minimal deviation adenocarcinoma of the endocervix (see Chapter 8, Cervical Carcinoma). Florid mesonephric hyperplasia is a benign condition and is distinguished from carcinoma by lack of complex glandular configuration, mitosis, intracellular mucin, and periglandular stromal edema. Also, CEA is absent in florid mesonephric hyperplasia, and normal mesonephric remnants are usually admixed with their larger, often cystic counterparts.[8]

Heterologous Tissue

Glia

There are 15 recorded cases of neuroglial tissue in the cervix or the endometrium (see Chapter 10, Benign Diseases of Endometrium).[79] Although the term *glioma* is used for this condition, the high degree of differentiation of the glial tissue, the absence of mitoses, and the absence of recurrence are against its being neoplastic (Fig. 6.26). The lesion should not be confused with a pure heterologous sarcoma or a teratoma. The neural tissue is believed to represent either implantation of fetal cerebral glia at the time of instrumentation of the gravid uterus[79] or heterotopic maldevelopment during embryogenesis. When the cervix is involved, the lesion usually appears as a polyp that bleeds readily.

Skin

Among the pathologic curiosities of the cervix are reports of true epidermidization of the cervical mucosa. In these instances sebaceous glands,[92] hair, and sweat glands are found. The presence of these ectodermal structures, which are normally appendages of the epidermis, on a mucous membrane of mesodermal derivation is difficult to explain. It is conceivable, however, that stratified squamous epithelium under certain circumstances, such as long-standing chronic inflammation, can form the appendages of its epidermal analogue.

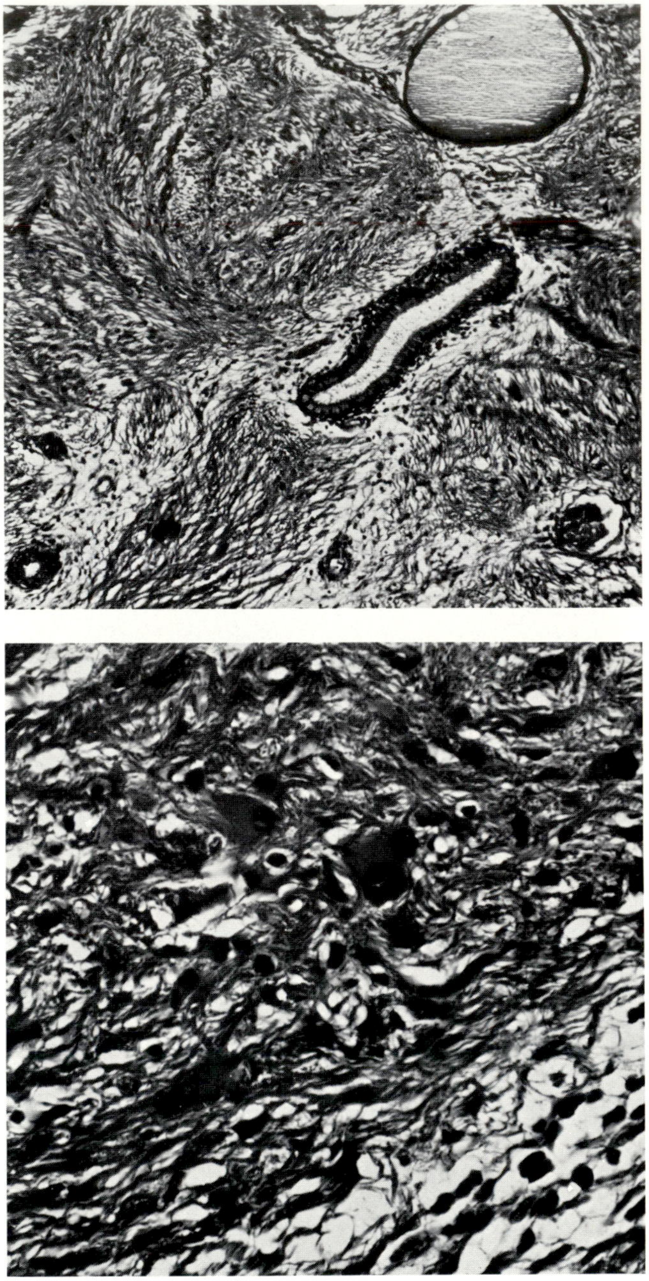

FIG. 6.26. Glioma of the endocervix. *Top:* Bundles of well-differentiated neuroglial tissue intermingle with normal endocervical epithelium. *Bottom:* Higher magnification view. (Courtesy of Dr. Y. Boivin, Montreal.)

Cartilage

Four cases of heterotopic mature cartilage in the cervix are on record.[70] The finding of these structures alone has no clinical significance. They should not be confused with a malignant mixed mesodermal tumor.

References

1. Aaro LA, Jacobson LJ, Soule EH (1963) Endocervical polyps. Obstet Gynecol 21: 659
2. Abell MR (1971) Papillary adenofibroma of the uterine cervix. Am J Obstet Gynecol 110: 990
3. Abell MR, Gosling JRG (1962) Gland cell carcinoma (adenocarcinoma) of the uterine cervix. Am J Obstet Gynecol 83: 729
4. Adam E, Kaufman RH, Mirkovic RR, Melnick JL (1979) Persistence of virus shedding in asymptomatic women after recovery from herpes genitalis. Obst Gynecol 54: 171
5. Adam E, Kaufman RH, Melnick JL, et al. (1973) Seroepidemiologic studies of herpesvirus type 2 and carcinoma of the cervix. III. Am J Epidemiol 96: 427
6. Adam E, Kaufman RH, Melnick JL, et al. (1973) Seroepidemiologic studies of herpesvirus type 2 and carcinoma of the cervix. IV. Dysplasia and carcinoma in situ. Am J Epidemiol 98: 77
7. Adams JQ, Packer H (1955) Granuloma inguinale of the cervix. South Med J 48: 27
8. Ayroud Y, Gelfand MM, Ferenczy A (1985) Florid mesonephric hyperplasia of the cervix: A report of a case with review of the literature. Int J Gynecol Pathol 4: 245
9. Berry A (1966) A cytopathological and histopathological study of bilharziasis of the female genital tract. J Pathol Bacteriol 9: 325
10. Burd LI, Esterly JR (1971) Vesicular lesions of the uterine cervix. Am J Obstet Gynecol 110: 887
11. Burkman RT, Damewood MT (1985) Actinomyces and the intrauterine contraceptive device. In: Zatuchni, GI, Goldsmith A, Sciarra J. (eds). Intrauterine contraception. Advances and future prospects. New York, Harper & Row, pp 427–437
12. Burnham RC, Paavonen J, Stevens CE, et al. (1984) Mucopurulent cervicitis: The ignored counterpart of urethritis in the male. N Engl J Med 311: 1
13. Busby JG (1952) Neurofibromatosis of the cervix. Am J Obstet Gynecol 63: 674
14. Candy J, Abell MR (1968) Progestogen-induced adenomatous hyperplasia of the uterine cervix. JAMA 203: 323
15. Centers for Disease Control. Morbidity and Mortality Weekly Report. (1982) Sexually transmitted diseases treatment guidelines 31: 355
16. Centers for Disease Control (1983) Morbidity Mortality Weekly Report 32: 306
17. Chang SH, Maddox WA (1971) Adenocarcinoma arising within cervical endometriosis and invading the adjacent vagina. Am J Obstet Gynecol 110: 1015
18. Clement PB (1985) Multinucleated stromal giant cells of the uterine cervix. Arch Pathol Lab Med 109: 200
19. Clement PB, Scully RE (1974) Müllerian adenocarcoma of the uterus. Cancer 34: 1138
20. Cohen C (1973) Three cases of amoebiasis of the cervix uteri. J Obstet Gynecol Br Commonw 80: 476
21. Corey L (1984) Genital herpes. In: Holmes KK, Mardh PA, Sparling PF, Wiesner PJ (eds). Sexually transmitted diseases. New York, McGraw-Hill Book Company, pp 449–474

22. Corey L, Holmes KK (1983) Genital herpes simplex virus infection: Current concepts in diagnosis, treatment and prevention. Ann Intern Med 98: 973
23. Crossen RJ (1930) A case of gumma of cervix. Am J Obstet Gynecol 19: 708
24. Crow J, McWhinney N (1979) Isolated arteritis of the cervix uteri. Br J Obstet Gynecol 86: 393
25. Crum CP, Mitao M, Winkler B, et al. (1984) Localizing chlamydial injection in cervical biopsies with the immunoperoxidase technique. Int J Gynecol Pathol 3: 191
26. De Molnar AMD, Guralnick M, Ferenczy A (1978) Blue nevus of the endocervix: Report of two cases and ultrastructure. Gynecol Oncol 6: 373
27. Dougherty CM, Moore WR, Cotten N (1962) Histologic diagnosis and clinical significance of benign lesions of the nonpregnant cervix. Ann NY Acad Sci 97: 683
28. Elliott GB, Elliott JDA (1973) Superficial stromal reactions of lower genital tract. Arch Pathol 95: 100
29. Elliott GB, Reynolds HA, Fidler HK (1967) Pseudosarcoma botryoides of cervix and vagina in pregnancy. J Obstet Gynecol Br Commonw 74: 728
30. El-Mahgoub S (1972) Antispermatozoal antibodies in infertile women with cervicovaginal schistosomiasis. Am J Obstet Gynecol 112: 781
31. Evans CS, Goldman RL, Klein HZ, Kohout ND (1984) Necrobiotic granulomas of the uterine cervix. A probable postoperative reaction. Am J Surg Pathol 8: 841
32. Fenoglio CM, Galloway DA, Crum CO, et al. (1981) Herpes simplex virus and cervical neoplasia. In: Fenoglio CM, Wolff M (eds). Progress in surgical pathology. New York, Masson, Vol 4, pp 45–82
33. Fingerland A, Sikl H (1938) Ganglioneuroma of cervix uteri. J Pathol Bacterol 47: 631
34. Fluhman CF (1961) The cervix uteri and its diseases, 1st ed. Philadelphia, W.B. Saunders
35. Gardner HL (1966) Cervical and vaginal endometriosis. Clin Obstet Gynecol 9: 358
36. Gardner HL, Fernet P (1964) Etiology of vaginitis emphysematosa. Am J Obstet Gynecol 88: 680
37. Giampaolo C, Murphy J, Benes S, McCormack WM (1983) How sensitive is the Papanicolaou smear in the diagnosis of infections with *Chlamydia trachomatis?* Am J Clin Pathol 80: 844
38. Gjonnaess H, Dalaker K, Anestad G, et al. (1982) Pelvic inflammatory disease: Etiologic studies with emphasis on chlamydial infection. Obstet Gynecol 59: 550
39. Grimalt M, Argueles M, Ferenczy A (1975) Papillary cystadenofibroma of endometrium. A histochemical and ultrastructural study. Cancer 36: 137
40. Gurman ME, MacCalman J, Kern ER, et al. (1981) The course of untreated recurrent genital herpes simplex infection in 27 women. N Engl J Med 304: 759
41. Gusdon JT (1965) Hemangioma of the cervix. Am J Obstet Gynecol 91: 204
42. Hare MJ, Toone E, Taylor-Robinson D, et al. (1981) Follicular cervicitis—Colposcopic appearances and association with *Chlamydia trachomatis*. Br J Obstet Gynecol 88: 174
43. Harrison HR, Alexander ER (1984) *Chlamydia trachomatis* infections of the infant. In: Holmes KK, Mardh PA, Sparling PF, Weisner PJ (eds). Sexually transmitted diseases. New York, McGraw-Hill Book Co., pp 270–80
44. Hobson D, Karayiannis P, Byng RE, et al. (1980) Quantitative aspects of chlamydial injection of the cervix. Br J Vener Dis 56: 56
45. Holmes KK (1984) Lower genital tract infections in women: Cystitis/urethritis, vulvovaginitis and cervicitis. In: Holmes KK, Mardh PA, Sparling PF, Weisner PJ (eds). Sexually transmitted diseases. New York, McGraw-Hill Book Co, pp 557–589
46. Janovski MS, Kasdon EJ (1963) Benign mesonephric papillary and polypoid tumors of the cervix in childhood. J Pediatr 63: 211
47. Jones RB, Rabinovitch RA, Katz BP, et al. (1985) *Chlamydia trachomatis* in the pharynx and rectum of heterosexual patients at risk for genital infection. Ann Intern Med 102: 757
48. Kaufman RH, Watts JM, Gardner HL (1969) Pemphigus vulgaris genital involvement. Obstet Gynecol 33: 264
49. Kaufman RH, Gardner HL, Rawls WE, et al. (1973) Clinical features of herpes genitalis. Cancer Res 33: 1446
50. Kistner RW, Hertig AT (1955) Papillomas of the uterine cervix—Their malignant potentiality. Obstet Gynecol 6: 147
51. Kiviat NB, Paavonen JA, Brockway J, et al. (1985) Cytologic manifestations of cervical and vaginal infections. I. Epithelial and inflammatory cellular changes. JAMA 253: 989
52. Kiviat NB, Peterson M, Kinney-Thomas E, et al. (1985) Cytologic manifestations of cervical and vaginal infections. II. Confirmation of *Chlamydia trachomatis* infection by direct immunofluorescence using monoclonal antibodies. JAMA 253: 997
53. Koss LG, Wolinska WH (1959) *Trichomonas vaginalis* cervicitis and its relationship to cervical cancer: A histocytological study. Cancer 12: 1171
54. Langley GF (1943) Primary echinococcal cyst of the uterus. Br J Surg 30: 278
55. Lippert LJ, Richart RM, Ferenczy A (1974) Giant benign endocervical polyp: Report of a case. Am J Obstet Gynecol 118: 1140
56. Nahmias AJ, Roizman B (1973) Infection with herpes simplex viruses 1 and 2. N Engl J Med 289: 667, 719, 781
57. Newton WL, Reardon LV, DeLeva AM (1960) A comparative study of the subcutaneous inoculation of germ-free and conventional guinea pigs with two strains *Trichomonas vaginalis*. Am J Trop Med Hyg 9: 56
58. Nicolas TM, Fidler HK (1971) Microglandular hyperplasia in cervical cone biopsies taken for suspicious and positive cytology. Am J Clin Pathol 56: 424
59. Norris HJ, Taylor HB (1966) Polyps of the vagina: A benign lesion resembling sarcoma botryoides. Cancer 19: 226
60. Paavonen JA, Vesterinen E, Meyer B, Saksela E (1982) Colposcopic and histological findings in cervical chlamydial infection. Obstetrics 59: 712
61. Paavonen JA, Brunham R, Kiviatt N, et al. (1982) Cervicitis—Etiologic, clinical and histopathologic findings. In:

Mardh PA, Holmes KK, Oriel JD, et al. (eds). Chlamydial infections. New York, Elsevier, pp 141–146
62. Paavonen JA, Kiviat N, Brunham RC, et al. (1985) Prevalence and manifestations of endometritis among women with cervicitis. Am J Obstet Gynecol 152: 280
63. Patel DS, Bhagavan BS (1985) Blue nevus of the uterine cervix. Hum Pathol 16: 79
64. Purola E, Paavonen JA (1982) Routine cytology as a diagnostic aid in chlamydial cervicitis. Scand J Infect Dis B345: 55
65. Richart RM (1973) Cervical intraepithelial neoplasia. In: Sommers SC (ed). Pathology annual. New York, Appleton-Century-Crofts, pp 301–328
66. Richter GA, Pratt JH, Nicolas DR, Coulam CV (1972) Actinomycosis of the female genital organs. Minn Med 55: 1003
67. Ridley JH (1968) The histogenesis of endometriosis. A review of facts and fancies. Obstet Gynecol Surv 23: 1
68. Rilke F, Cantaboni A (1964) Lipomas of the uterus. Presentation of 2 cases and review of the recent literature. Ann Obstet Gynecol 86: 645
69. Robboy SJ, Welch WR (1977) Microglandular hyperplasia in vaginal adenosis associated with oral contraceptives and prenatal diethylstilbestrol exposure. Obstet Gynecol 49: 430
70. Roth E, Taylor HB (1966) Heterotopic cartilage in the uterus. Obstet Gynecol 27: 838
71. Schacter J (1978) Chlamydial infections. N Engl J Med 298: 428, 490, 540
72. Schacter J (1984) Biology of *Chlamydia trachomatis*. In: Holmes KK, Mandh PA, Sparling PF, Weisner PJ (eds). Sexually transmitted diseases. New York, McGraw-Hill Book Co., pp 243–257
73. Schacter J, Stoner E, Moncada J (1983) Screening for chlamydial infections in women attending family planning clinics. West J Med 138: 375
74. Schaefer C (1970) Tuberculosis of female genital tract. Clin Obstet Gynecol 13: 965
75. Scherrick JC, Vega JG (1962) Congenital intramural cysts of the uterus. Obstet Gynecol 19: 486
76. Schwartz DA (1984) Carcinoma of the uterine cervix and schistosomiasis in West Africa (Review of the literature). Gynecol Oncol 19: 365
77. Selzer F, Nelson HM (1962) Benign papilloma (polypoid tumor of the cervix uteri in children: Report of two cases. Am J Obstet Gynecol 84: 165
78. Shafer MA, Chen KL, Kromhout LK, et al. (1985) Chlamydial endocervical infections and cytologic findings in sexually active female adolescents. Am J Obstet Gynecol 151: 767
79. Slavutin L (1979) Uterine gliosis and ossification. Am J Diagn Gynecol Obstet 1: 351
80. Stamm WE, Holmes KK (1984) *Chlamydia trachomatis* infections of the adult. In: Holmes KK, Mandh PA, Sparling PF, Weisner PJ (eds). Sexually transmitted diseases. New York, McGraw-Hill Book Co., pp 258–269
81. Stein BJ, Siciliano A (1966) Necrotizing herpes simplex viral infection of the cervix during pregnancy: Mimic of squamous cell carcinoma. Am J Obstet Gynecol 94: 249
82. Stout AP (1943) Hemangioendothelioma: A tumor of blood vessels featuring vascular endothelial cells. Ann Surg 118: 445
83. Taylor HB, Irey NS, Norris HJ (1967) Atypical endocervical hyperplasia in women taking oral contraceptives. JAMA 202: 637
84. Tchertkoff V, Ober WB (1966) Primary chancre of the cervix uteri. NY State J Med 66: 1921
85. Tsukada Y, Piver MS, Barlow JT (1977) Microglandular hyperplasia of the endocervix following long-term estrogen treatment. Am J Obstet Gynecol 127: 888
86. Vellios F, Ng ABP, Reagan JW (1973) Papillary adenofibroma of the uterus. A benign mesodermal mixed tumor of müllerian origin. Am J Clin Pathol 60: 543
87. Wagner ED (1974) The replication of herpesvirus. Am Sci 62: 584
88. Westrom L, Mardh PA (1972) Genital chlamydial infections in the female. In: Mardh PA, Holmes KK, Oriel JD, et al. (eds). Chlamydial infections. New York, Elsevier, pp 121–141
89. Westrom L, Mardh PA (1984) Salpingitis. In: Holmes KK, Mardh PA, Sparling PF, Weisner PJ (eds). Sexually transmitted diseases. New York, McGraw-Hill Book Co., pp 615–632
90. Wilbanks GD, Carter B (1963) Vaginitis emphysematosa. Obst Gynecol 22: 301
91. Wilkinson E, Dufour DR (1976) Pathogenesis of microglandular hyperplasia of the cervix uteri. Obstet Gynecol 47: 189
92. Willis RA (1962) The borderland of embryology and pathology, 2nd ed. Washington D.C., Butterworth
93. Winkler B, Crum CP (1986) *Chlamydia trachomatis* infection of the female genital tract: Pathogenetic and clinicopathologic considerations. In: Sommers SC, Fechner RE, Rosen PP (eds). Pathology annual. E. Norwalk, CT, Appleton-Century-Crofts
94. Winkler B, Richart RN (1985) Cervical/uterine pathologic considerations in pelvic infection. In: Zatuchni GI, Goldsmith A, Sciarra JJ (eds). Intrauterine contraception: Advances and future prospects. New York, Harper & Row, pp 438–449
95. Young RH, Harris NL, Scully RE (1985) Lymphoma-like lesions of the lower female genital tract: A report of 16 cases. Int J Gynecol Pathol 4: 289

7

Cervical Intraepithelial Neoplasia and Condyloma

Alex Ferenczy, M.D., and Barbara Winkler, M.D.

Terminology and Definitions

The nomenclature and classification of intraepithelial squamous lesions of the cervix have a controversial history,[17] now further complicated by the introduction of new terminology for the classification of cervical human papillomavirus (HPV) infection.[39] The classic terminology separates noninvasive cervical lesions into two groups: dysplasia and carcinoma in situ (CIS), implying a biologic distinction between these two entities that can be reproducibly distinguished histologically.[21,151] In the cytologic nomenclature using this system, dysplasia is considered a benign to possibly malignant squamous epithelial atypia, whereas CIS is designated as positive for malignant cells. In 1961, at the First International Congress on Exfoliative Cytology, the Committee on Histological Terminology for Lesions of the Uterus Cervix defined CIS as follows[231]: "Only those cases should be classified as CIS which, in the absence of invasion, show a surface lining epithelium in which, throughout its whole thickness, no differentiation takes place. The process may involve the lining of the cervical glands." It is recognized that the cells of uppermost layers may show some slight flattening. The very rare case of an otherwise characteristic CIS that shows a greater degree of differentiation belongs to the exceptions for which no classification can provide. Dysplasia of the cervix was defined as[231]: ". . . all other (than CIS) disturbances of differentiation of the squamous epithelial lining of surface and glands. . . . They may be characterized as of high or low degree, terms which are preferable to suspicious and non-suspicious, as the proposed terms describe the histological appearance and do not express an opinion." The narrow and arbitrary definition of CIS and the broad, all encompassing definition of dysplasia led to diagnostic uncertainties and to a classification based solely on histology, divorced from clinical and therapeutic considerations.[21,102,173]

Because of management problems with the classification of dysplasia and CIS and the inability to reproducibly distinguish severe dysplasia from CIS, investigators turned to biologic definitions of cervical cancer precursors based on the behavior of these lesions. Studies demonstrated that the cellular changes of dysplasia and CIS were qualitatively similar and remained constant throughout the histologic spectrum. Both dysplasia and CIS could be defined as monoclonal proliferations of abnormal squamous epithelial cells with an aneuploid nuclear DNA content.[65,66] Quantitative differences in the extent of maturation and variable rates of cell cycle turnover were evidence of differing degrees of differentiation but were of limited value in clinical management.[179] From these studies, a unified concept of a single disease process was developed and termed *cervical intraepithelial neoplasia* (CIN).[8] CIN defines a spectrum of histologic changes that share a common etiology, biology, and natural history.[173] The use of the diagnostic term *CIN* implies that there is a malignant precursor lesion present, that is, a lesion that, if left untreated, has a significant, albeit individually unknown, risk of developing into invasive carcinoma at some time in the future.[65,66,173] As a corollary, it is presumed that when the histologic changes of CIN are diagnosed and the lesion is treated adequately, the development of invasive cancer can be prevented. Use of the CIN system deemphasizes lesion grade and provides a rationale approach[17,18,173] to patient management based on cytologic and histologic correlation and colposcopic determination of lesion size and distribution.[174,216]

In recent years, there has been a virtual explosion of information about genital HPV as a sexually transmitted pathogen of major epidemiologic importance and as a possible oncogenic virus in the pathogenesis of CIN and invasive squamous carcinoma. Unfortunately, the identification of HPV in cervical condyloma as well as CIN and invasive carcinoma has further complicated cervical nomenclature and classification.[13,39,62] Synonymous terms, such as flat condyloma, condyloma planum, subclinical papillomavirus infection, koilocytotic atypia, condylomatous atypia, and warty atypia, proliferate in the literature, clouding the basic issues.[62] The so-called transition lesions and atypical condylomas add further to this confusion. Based on the management protocols outlined later in this chapter, these names take on less importance because the clinical approach to them is the same.

Clinicians and pathologists must bear in mind that HPV infections of the cervix, whatever their association with invasive carcinoma, represent sexually transmitted diseases of epidemic proportions that must be controlled by effective treatment of infected individuals and their sexual partners. In addition, there is mounting concern that increased diagnostic use of the terms *condyloma* and *koilocytosis* will lead to inadequate treatment and surveillance of precursor lesions, with a recrudesence of cervical cancer mortality in the future.[96] A 1983 publication addresses these issues and concludes that[96]:

> The presence of the virus-associated (morphologic) component may be mentioned as a part of the microscopic diagnosis but should not modify the clinical approach to these lesions. Women bearing the virus-associated lesions should receive the same clinical and colposcopic evaluation, treatment and follow-up as usually administered to women with conventional forms of CIN, until more data on the natural history of these lesions are obtained.

This chapter reviews and summarizes the clinicopathologic and molecular studies of HPV infections of the cervix and CIN in relation to routine pathologic practice and management.

Epidemiology and Etiology

Both cervical condyloma and CIN are diseases of young women, with a large population impact and risk factors characteristic of a sexually transmitted disease. More than 65% of patients with genital warts are aged 15–29 years, the highest risk group being in the 20–24-year range in both males and females.[29,132] The incidence of HPV infection of the genitalia as manifested clincially by visible condylomata acuminata has increased more than sixfold in the last two decades alone, and, in 1983, the Centers for Disease Control in Atlanta estimated an annual incidence of 2 million persons with the disease.[29] The prevalence of HPV infection continues to increase, with between 60 and 85% of the sexual partners of HPV-infected individuals developing genital condylomas; the incubation period averages 2–3 months.[147] Cytologic evidence of cervical HPV infection is detectable in as many as 3% of women under the age of 30.[29,130] Moreover, HPV DNA was recently found in as many as 10% of cytologically normal smears,[119,225] implying an enormous pool for propagation of the infection.

Although there have been significant declines in the incidence and mortality of invasive cervical carcinoma, both carcinoma and its precursors remain a major health problem.[47] The 1984 cancer statistics for the United States projected over 45,000 new cases of CIN grade 3 and 16,000 new cases of invasive cervical carcinoma annually, with an estimated annual mortality rate of 7000.[196] With the decline of invasive cervical carcinoma, there has been an increase in the incidence of CIN, reflecting not only a relative increase because of screening detection at the preinvasive stage but also a true increase in the incidence of premalignant lesions of the cervix.[242] The annual reported incidence of CIN is currently two to four times the annual incidence of invasive cervical carcinoma.[47] The mean age of patients with CIN 3 is 35 years, 15 years younger than that of patients with invasive disease.[37] The age incidence peaks at 34 years and decreases rapidly thereafter; the risk continues to decrease with advancing age.[37] Although accurate figures are not available, the average incidence rates of CIN 1 and 2 appear higher than that of CIN 3, and the peak incidence occurs several years earlier.[206,207]

The clinical scope and epidemiology of CIN have undergone dramatic changes in the past decade. The age-specific incidence curve for CIN is decreasing, as both the incidence and prevalence of CIN rise steadily, particularly in teenagers and women under 30.[12,188] The incidence of CIN in teenagers and young adults was 18.8/1000 for ages 15–19 years.[188] When specifically focusing on CIN 3, a rate of 2.6/1000 was projected for the teenage population in 1981 compared to an incidence of 0.1/1000 in the 15–19-year-old age group in the late 1960s, indicating a highly significant rise.[37,188] Similarly, studies of Jewish Israeli women have indicated a substantial increase in the incidence of CIN and invasive cervical cancer in this population,[7,209] historically at low risk for the development of cervical malignancy.[84,215] The incidence of cervical cancer in all ages of Israeli-born Jewish women rose from 2.7/100,000 in 1960–1966 to 4.6/100,000 in 1972–1976.[7,209] These epidemiologic changes have been attributed to changes in sexual behavior patterns and corroborate previous epidemiologic data suggesting a direct causal relationship between sexual activity and the pathogenesis of cervical neoplasia.[51] The results of extensive epidemiologic studies focus on two independent variables, early sexual activity and multiple sexual partners, as the principal risk factors for the development of CIN.[104,162,189,223,224] Early sexual activity during active development of the cervical transformation zone (see discussion of management of CIN) appears to be an essential prerequisite and probably plays a pivotal role in susceptibility to carcinogens.[189] There are, in addition, a large number of covariables[162] that are believed to be secondarily related to the incidence of cervical carcinoma because they are a common feature of the population that has early, multiple sexual contacts[31,51,162] (Table 7.1). Similarly, certain venereally transmitted diseases, such as syphilis, gonorrhea, chlamydial infection, and *Trichomonas* vaginitis, that are reported in association with cervical neoplasia seem to characterize the sexual history of the population at risk rather than playing an etiologic role themselves.[30,82,222,224]

The concept of CIN as a sexually transmitted disease is further substantiated by the epidemiologic characterization of the high-risk male (Table 7.2). These studies document the relevance of the male partner's sexual history in determining a woman's risk for the development of CIN and cervical carcinoma and support the idea of transmissible neoplasia.*

* References 9, 27, 79, 97, 98, 121, 123, 158, 184, 197, 199, 205, 215.

Table 7.1. Epidemiologic risk factors for CIN.

Sexual activity
Independent variables
Early sexual activity (especially less than 16 years of age)
Multiple sexual partners
High-risk male sexual partner
Smoking
Dependent variables
Multiple pregnancies
Early age of first pregnancy
Early age of first marriage
Unstable marital history
Low socioeconomic status
Sexually transmitted diseases
Independent of sexual activity
Human papillomavirus
Dependent on sexual activity
Herpes simplex virus
Chlamydia
Gonorrhea
Syphilis
Trichomonas
Immunosuppression

Table 7.2. Epidemiologic characterization of the high-risk male sexual partner.

History of genital carcinoma (especially penile carcinoma)
History of sexually transmitted disease (especially penile or urethral condylomas)
History of CIN or cervical carcinoma in first wife
Low socioeconomic status
Multiple sexual partners

Human Papillomaviruses

Because CIN has all the characteristics of a sexually transmitted disease, investigations have focused on the identification of a venereally transmitted carcinogen that acts preferentially on the immature transformation zone.[52] Most recently, attention has focused on HPVs as primary etiologic agents in a multifactorial pathogenesis of CIN and cervical carcinoma (Fig. 7.1). This association is substantiated by a large number of epidemiologic, clinicopathologic, and molecular studies.*

HPV is a heterogeneous group of double-stranded DNA viruses that cause a variety of proliferative squamous lesions of the skin and mucous membranes in the conjunctiva, oral cavity, larynx, tracheobronchial tree, esophagus, bladder, anus, and genital tract of both sexes.[73,89,102,246] Although little is known about their mechanisms of action in humans, the HPVs appear to

* References 38, 73–77, 108–112, 239, 246–248.

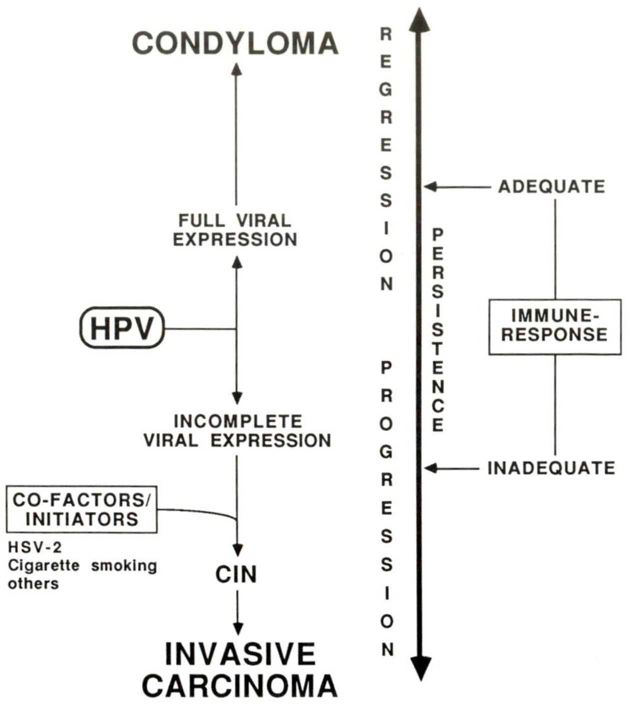

FIG. 7.1. Multifactorial pathogenesis of cervical condyloma and neoplasia. Full viral expression leads to productive infection of cervical squamous cells and is characterized by proliferation (early viral gene effect), maturation, viral replication (late viral gene effect), and the formation of ordinary condylomas. HPV 6/11 are found in most ordinary condylomas. Incomplete viral expression leads to cell proliferation without maturation (late genes are nonfunctional) in which viral integration into host cell chromosomes is enhanced. Clones of cells are produced in which viral DNA can be amplified (promotional effect of HPV) and be transformed to intraepithelial/invasive neoplastic disease by carcinogenic initiators. HPV 16/18 are found in the majority of cervical neoplasias. Regression, persistence, and progression to neoplasia are probably influenced by the immunocompetence of the host. (Adapted by permission of Zur Hausen, Ref. 246.)

be fastidious in their growth requirements. They are remarkably site specific and replicate only in the nucleus of mature, terminally differentiated keratinocytes of the upper intermediate and superficial layers of the squamous epithelia.[80,113] Their study has been hampered by the inability to grow papillomavirus in culture and by the variability of copy number (viral content in infected cells) and viral replication in in vitro and in vivo systems.[73,159,213] Over 40 distinct types of HPV have now been characterized, and their clinical and morphologic expressions form characteristic groupings[80,81,89] (Table 7.3). In addition, specific HPV types have been associated with clinically benign disease, whereas others have been linked to malignant neoplasms.[49,148,248]

Certain HPVs may act synergistically with other

TABLE 7.3. The human papillomaviruses.

Type	Associated lesion
1	Plantar and palmar warts
2	Common warts
3	Juvenile flat warts
4	Plantar and common warts
5	EV[a]
6	Genital condyloma, laryngeal papilloma, GTN[b]
7	Butcher's wart
8, 9	EV
10	Juvenile flat wart, EV
11	Genital condyloma, laryngeal papilloma, GTN
12	EV
13	Oral focal epithelial hyperplasia (Heck's disease)
14, 15	EV
16	GTN, Bowenoid papulosis, genital condyloma
17	EV
18	GTN, genital condyloma
19–25	EV
26–29	Immunosuppressed host, EV
30	Immunosuppressed host, laryngeal carcinoma
31	GTN
32	Oral focal epithelial hyperplasia (Heck's disease)
33	GTN, Bowenoid papulosis
34	Premalignant squamous lesions of skin (actinic keratosis, Bowen's disease)
35	GTN
36	EV, premalignant squamous lesions of skin (actinic keratosis, Bowen's disease, keratoacanthoma)
37	Malignant melanoma[c]

[a] EV, epidermodysplasia verruciformis.
[b] GTN, genital tract neoplasia (including intraepithelial neoplasia and squamous cell carcinoma).
[c] One case reported.

carcinogens.[73] For example, malignant transformation of papillomavirus-induced skin warts in the domestic rabbit and the alimentary tract in cattle is greatly enhanced by the topical application of methylcholanthrene and the feeding of radiomimetic bracken fern, respectively.[72,146] In humans with erythrodysplasia verruciformis, pityriasis-like skin lesions containing HPV 5 and 8 that are exposed to sunlight (ultraviolet radiation) often (35%) undergo malignant transformation.[120,148] These observations provide analogous models for the oncogenic potential of HPVs in the cervical epithelium. Certain HPVs, furthermore, have been shown to be capable of transforming cultured cell lines in vitro with subsequent tumorigenicity in nude mice.[73,107]

The initial clinicopathologic studies correlating HPV infection and CIN stem largely from the 1977 description of Meisels et al. of the pathologic features of flat condyloma of the cervix.[129] Since that time, it has become apparent that up to 80% of lesions previously classified as CIN 1 (very mild to mild dysplasia) are actually flat condylomas.[130,153,211] Experimental evidence for HPV as the infectious agent responsible for flat condylomas includes the ultrastructural identification of intranuclear viral particles and the immunohistochemical localization of papillomavirus group-specific antigens in the koilocytes of these lesions.[57,109,110,131] Furthermore, Kreider et al.[107] have demonstrated the koilocytotic, morphologic transformation by HPV (derived from condylomata acuminata) of normal human cervix grafted beneath the renal capsule of nude mice. This experiment fulfills Koch's postulates for a direct causal relationship between HPV and flat condylomas. It also lays the groundwork for an in vivo transformation assay for HPV and a system with which to study the interactions of HPV with other possible cofactors in the genesis of cervical carcinoma.

The clinicopathologic and epidemiologic evidence for an association between condyloma and CIN is manifold. Coexistent condylomatous features are seen in 25–50% of high-grade CIN lesions and intermixed condylomatous features in up to 73% of cases studied.[13,130,153,159,211] The presence of HPV in association with CIN affects the morphologic appearance of these lesions and possibly the course of CIN. Several investigations have reported that patients with concomitant condyloma and CIN are younger than patients with CIN alone and that their lesions progress at a faster rate.[42,124,130]

A previously unsuspected reservoir of HPV infection in males has recently been detected (see Table 7.2). The high incidence of male HPV infection was previously not fully appreciated because the lesions are small and subtle and are best visualized under magnification. These flat or papular lesions of the penile shaft and distal urethra may serve as a hidden source of HPV infection and can be identified by colposcopic examination in 60–80% of the male partners of women with lower genital tract neoplasia (Fig. 7.2).[11,21,26,117,155] In homosexual males, the frequency of anal condylomas has risen steadily and is associated with a 20–50 times higher risk of the development of anal squamous cell carcinoma than in heterosexual males.[44,114,238]

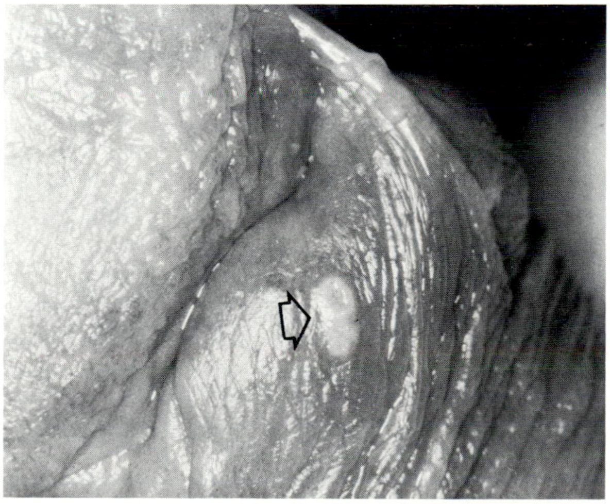

FIG. 7.2. Condyloma of the penis. Two small papules (*arrow*) are seen on the inner surface of the prepuce.

The most substantive evidence for a relationship between HPV and cervical carcinogenesis comes from molecular hybridization studies referred to as *Southern blot hybridization*. This technique detects HPV DNA in cytologic or tissue specimens by incubating radiolabeled ^{32}P-HPV DNA (produced by cloning HPV in *Escherichia coli*) with HPV DNA extracted from nuclear DNA of infected cells. The presence of HPV DNA has been documented in a variety of cervical lesions, including condyloma, squamous intraepithelial neoplasia, verrucous carcinoma, and squamous cell carcinoma.* HPV DNA has been detected by the hybridization technique in over 90% of flat condylomas and CIN, 100% of the verrucous carcinomas studied and 89% of cervical carcinoma.[73] Furthermore, HPV DNA has been isolated in tissues from metastatic cervical carcinoma[112] and in tumor cell lines established from cervical carcinoma.[73,115,150,244,245] Southern blot hybridization not only detects HPV DNA but also can distinguish between different HPV types. Certain HPV types appear to infect specifically the lower genital tract (see Table 7.3). These have differing oncogenic potentials in the cervix. HPV 6 and 11 are most often found in typical, benign condylomas, whereas HPV 16, 18, 31, 32, 36 and other, as yet uncharacterized HPVs are identified in CIN and invasive carcinoma.[40,41,74–80,125,144]

The physical state of papillomaviral DNA may greatly influence the natural history of HPV infections, particularly with regard to cervical carcinogenesis (see Fig. 7.1). When HPVs are found in the nucleus as free extrachromosomal circular episomes, productive infection develops. This is characterized by cell maturation (differentiation) and eventually cell death and is not believed to be related to carcinogenesis. Such a viral stage is particularly frequent with HPV 6/11, although other HPV types may also demonstrate full viral expression. On the other hand, when HPVs are not fully expressed, cell differentiation and cell death do not occur, and carcinogenic activity may thus be enhanced. HPV 16 and 18 often lack full viral expression and, in addition, may be found integrated into the host cell (neoplastic) DNA.[49,73,115] HPVs are promoters rather than initiators of cancer. Their promotional activity lies in producing clones of cells in which viral DNA amplification by carcinogenic initiators may occur. Amplification of *c-myc* and *c-ha-ras* oncogenes has been demonstrated in HPV DNA-containing invasive cervical cancers, as has homology between early regions of the HPV genome and certain cellular oncogenes.[244]

* References 73–77, 125, 144, 247, 248.

HPV 18 genes from early regions are present in transformed cells, and they are suspected of playing an important role in the promotion and possibly the maintenance of cancer cell growth.[150,244]

Mixed low-risk HPV 6–11 and high-risk HPV 16–18 were found in about one-third of lesions in the same patient as well as within a single lesion from the same patient.[191] Whether or not carcinoma can evolve from benign condyloma or arises only de novo in established intraepithelial neoplasia associated with a specific HPV type or types is also not clear at present. The available data suggest that those HPVs that can integrate into host cell DNA, such as HPV 16 and 18 (and possibly 31, 33, and 35), are the most likely to promote events that in concert with cocarcinogens (initiators) eventually lead to the development of cervical carcinoma. New HPV types associated with genital infection are currently being cloned and characterized.

In addition to HPV, other sexually transmitted organisms have been implicated in the pathogenesis of cervical neoplasia, include herpes simplex, *Chlamydia trachomatis, Neisseria gonorrhoeae, Gardnerella vaginalis, Mycoplasma hominis, trichomonas vaginalis*, and cytomegalovirus. In a case-control study of the prevalence of these pathogens in women with CIN, only HPV was found to be present more frequently in patients than in controls when analyzed independently of sexual activity.[82] In view of the high prevalence and multiplicity of sexually transmitted diseases in these patients, an interaction between other forms of infectious cervicitis and HPV is a possibility. Acute infectious cervicitis, especially that caused by chlamydia, has been associated with reparative cytologic atypias as well as with an abnormal transformation zone in young women.[30,31,85,136,149,190] Infectious cervicitis, particularly that seen in adolescents and young women, may contribute substantially to repair and remodeling of the transformation zone, stimulating squamous epithelialization and metaplasia, and may have an important indirect role in the susceptibility of the cervix to HPV infection and the development of CIN in this age group.

Herpes Simplex Virus Type 2

Herpes simplex virus type 2 (HSV-2) previously received considerable attention in relation to the etiology of CIN, with studies linking HSV-2 to CIN and cervical carcinoma biologically and epidemiologically.[53,97,138] Herpesvirus antigens have been detected by immunofluorescence in exfoliated cervical squamous carcinoma cells,[186] and the virus has been identified sporadically at the ultrastructural level in cervical carcinoma cells grown in tissue culture (Fig. 7.3). In contrast, whole viral particles consistent with HSV-2 virions have not been visualized in genital tract carcinoma. Herpesvirus has been demonstrated to transform cultured cell lines and produce malignant tumors when injected into newborn hamsters and nude mice.[70,91,127] Aurelian[3] demonstrated the presence of a tumor-specific antigen, AG-4, in cervical cancers and showed that AG-4 is an HSV-related structural polypeptide located on the cell surface. In situ hybridization studies have shown that cervical biopsies containing CIN, when probed with fragments of radiolabeled DNA from HSV-2, hybridized with the corresponding viral RNA within the cells in the absence of active infection.[71,126] HSV-2 genomic sequences are neither consistently retained nor exposed in experimental models, with the result that no particular transcriptional product could be assigned to maintenance of the transformed state.[70]

Retrospective seroepidemiologic studies have shown that patients with invasive and noninvasive cancers of the cervix have a higher frequency of neutralizing antibodies against HSV-2 than have controls matched for race, age, and socioeconomic status.[135,138] Patients with antibodies to HSV-2 are 7 and 10 times more likely to develop invasive cervical carcinoma and CIN than are women without antibodies to the virus.[139] In contrast to the retrospective studies, a recent, prospective serologic study of over 10,000 women in Prague, Czechoslovakia, with a follow-up of at least 4 years, found no difference in the prevalence of HSV-2 antibody between patients with CIN and invasive carcinoma and matched controls.[224] Moreover, no differences were observed in the prevalence of HSV-2 antibody titers between patients having disease at entry and those developing disease during the study.[223]

Despite the lack of convincing data associating HSV-2 with cervical neoplasia, several hypotheses have been proposed for a possible etiologic mechanism for HSV as a cofactor with HPV in the genesis of cervical cancer.[70,127,246] A hit-and-run mechanism for HSV has been hypothesized by Galloway and McDougall,[70] postulating that HSV may cause transformation without continued viral presence or expression by activating cellular oncogenes, mediating gene amplification, or acting as a mutagen. Zur Hausen has suggested that HSV may act synergistically as an initiator or promotor in HPV-stimulated epithelium, providing for more efficient cellular transformation.[246] Evidence for coexisting viral footprints of both HSV and HPV in the same tumors has been provided by serologic and in situ hybridization studies (Fig. 7.4).[53,127] Furthermore, HPV DNA integration into host cell DNA is facilitated in cells that have previously been infected with HSV.[23]

Other Etiologic Factors

Besides infectious agents, other etiologic cofactors, including iatrogenic and environmental carcinogens and

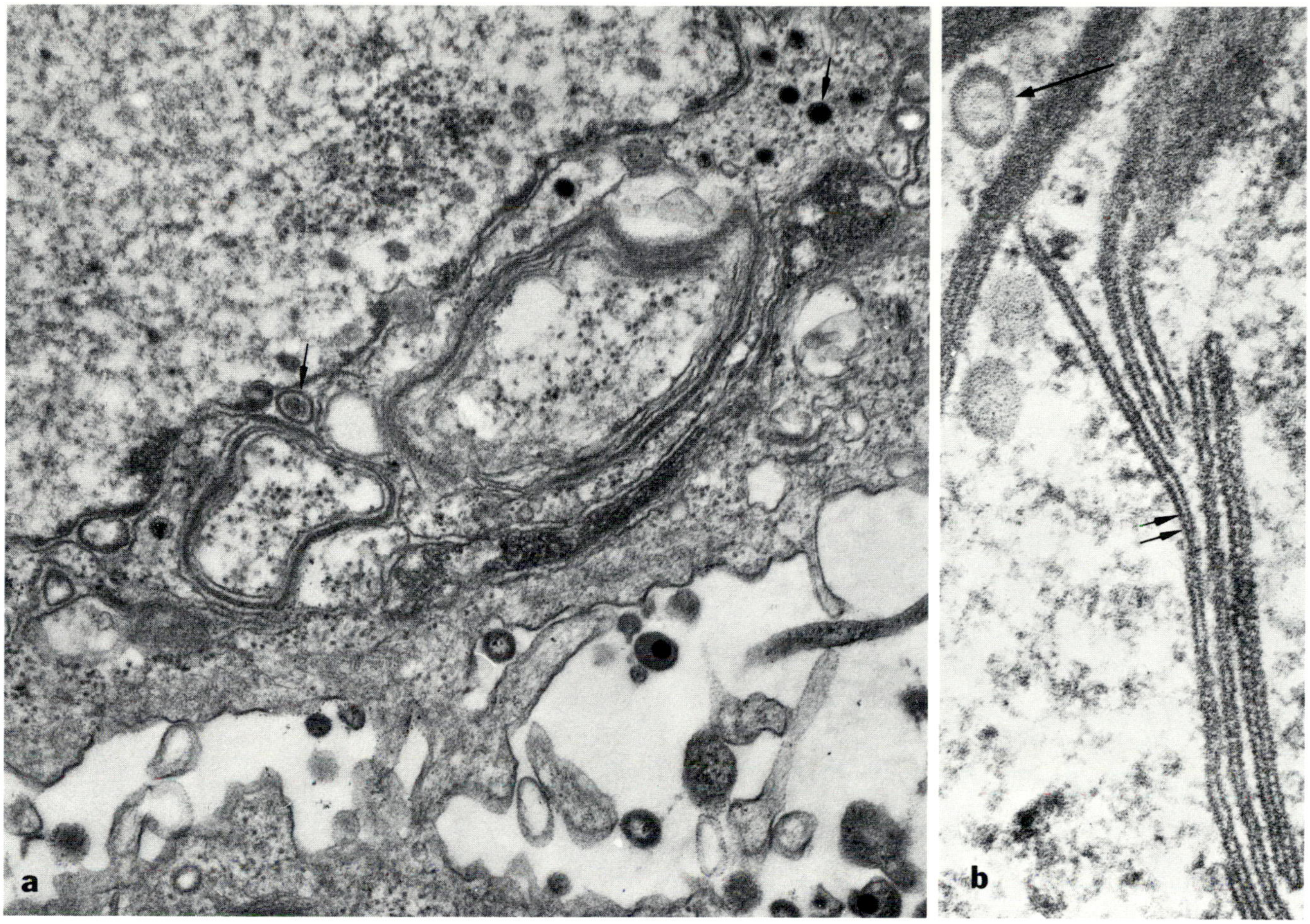

FIG. 7.3. Electron micrographs of two areas from HEp-2 cells infected with HSV-2 isolated from cervical carcinoma cells in vitro. *a*. Most of the infected HEp-2 cells have an obviously productive infection and contain viral components in all stages of maturation (*arrows*). ×27,000. *b*. A smaller number of cells contain intranuclear arrays of capsomeres (*double arrow*) and empty viral capsids (*long arrow*). In these cells complete virion formation is not observed. (Courtesy of L. Aurelian, Johns Hopkins University, Laboratory of Animal Medicine, Baltimore.)

nutritional influences, have been studied. Barrier methods of contraception, particularly condoms and diaphragms, appear to decrease the risk of cervical neoplasia.[164,243] Oral contraceptive (OCP) users have been reported in several studies to have an increased incidence of CIN and cervical carcinoma.[134,221,233,234] Other studies have suggested that OCP use, although not directly implicated in the development of CIN, may influence its natural history by accelerating lesion progression.[54,134,221] Other investigators have been unable to substantiate any causal relationship between OCPs and CIN.[33,180,210,221] Correlations between prenatal diethylstilbestrol (DES) exposure and cervicovaginal intraepithelial neoplasia have been similarly conflicting.[180–185] Despite early observations to the contrary,[182] a recent study by the Diethylstilbestrol Adenosis (DESAD) Project of 3980 DES-exposed women in the United States described a two- to fourfold increased incidence rate of CIN in DES progeny over matched controls.[181] The DESAD project data has to be interpreted with caution. Indeed, immature squamous metaplasia in the DES offspring is often confused with CIN even by expert pathologists. Also, condyloma, which was not recognized or recorded in the DESAD project, might have been included in the CIN group. Such diagnostic pitfalls might have contributed to the relatively high CIN incidence in the DES offspring.

Epidemiologic studies have suggested that cigarette smoking[19,32,33,217,223,224] may be associated, independently of sexual activity, with an increased risk of CIN and that the risk may be duration and dose dependent in women who smoke more than a half pack of cigarettes per day. It is possible, although not proven, that carcinogens in cigarette smoke may act in concert with cervical carcinoma promoters, such as certain HPVs, leading to the development of cervical neoplasia. Nutritional and

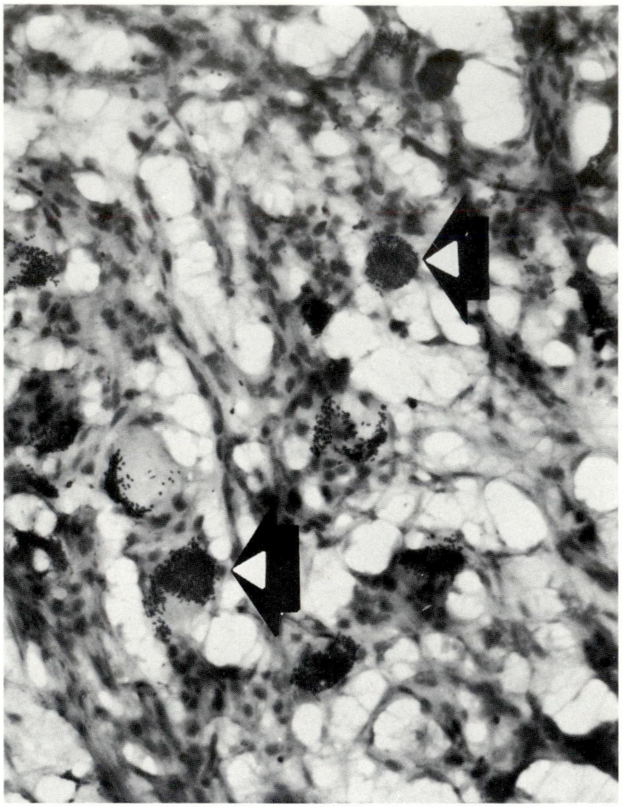

Fig. 7.4. Historadioautograph of frozen-section sensory ganglion demonstrating the hybridization reaction product to HSV-2 DNA using the in situ hybridization technique. Radioautographic grains are present over the Nissl substance in the ganglion cells (*arrow*). These correspond to the presence of herpes-specific message in the messenger RNA. (Courtesy of Drs. Denise A. Galloway and James McDougall, Seattle, and Cecilia M. Fenoglio, Albuquerque.)

dietary factors have also been investigated as covariables in the development of cervical carcinoma. Deficiencies of vitamins A and C in women with CIN have been documented and speculated to interact in the metaplastic epithelium of the transformation zone.[78,183,228] Folate deficiency has been implicated in the genesis of cervical cytologic abnormalities[24] and is a documented cause of cytomegaly in the squamous and columnar epithelia[220,231,232,240] (see Chapter 25, Cytology).

Our understanding of carcinogenesis is now based on the interaction of initiators and promotors, with neoplastic transformation the result of a series of multiple, synergistic, events.[187,246] The host immune system plays an important role in this multifactorial process. Immune suppression provides a background for the development of neoplasia by predisposing to infection by oncogenic viruses and by allowing neoplastic proliferations to escape immune surveillance and other host regulatory mechanisms.[154] With respect to cervical carcinogenesis, there is evidence for an interaction with the immune system. HPV infection is increased in frequency in immunosuppressed individuals, and the acquired condylomas tend to be larger in size, multicentric, and refractory to treatment. Progression of condyloma to intraepithelial neoplasia and invasive carcinoma occurs with greater frequency in the immunosuppressed patient.[119,194,195] Vulvovaginal neoplasia, CIN, and cervical carcinoma are more common in patients on immunosuppressive therapy. It has been proposed that the cytostatic and cytotoxic effects of therapeutic agents, such as azathioprine, corticosteroids, and alkylating agents, potentiate the effects of the already compromised immune regulation. In renal transplant patients, there is a 14-fold increase in the frequency of lower genital tract neoplasia, with carcinoma of the cervix comprising 8% of de novo cancers in organ homograft recipients.[240]

Clinical Features and Natural History

The contrasting clinical features of cervical condyloma and CIN are summarized in Table 7.4.

Cervical Condyloma

Up to 90% of cervical condylomas occur as grossly inapparent flat condylomas (planum), requiring the application of acetic acid and colposcopic magnification for their delineation.[132,134] Typical flat condylomas are slightly raised, sharply circumscribed, irregular plaques with an undulating granular or spiked surface (Fig. 7.5). After application of 5% acetic acid (vinegar) to their surface, they appear white, and the degree of whiteness depends largely on the thickness of associated surface hyperkeratosis. Flat condylomas are commonly multifocal and may involve the mature squamous epithelium of the native cervical portio as well as the immature squamous epithelium of the transformation zone, including metaplastic squamous epithelium replacing endocervical glands. Extension into the endocervical canal may occur. Diffuse

Table 7.4. Contrasting clinical features of cervical condyloma and CIN.

	Condyloma	CIN
Mean age at diagnosis	Early 20s	Late 20s
Cervical portio	+	−
Transformation zone	+	+
Multifocal	+	−
Regression	±	−
Persistence	±	+
Progression	Very low risk	High risk

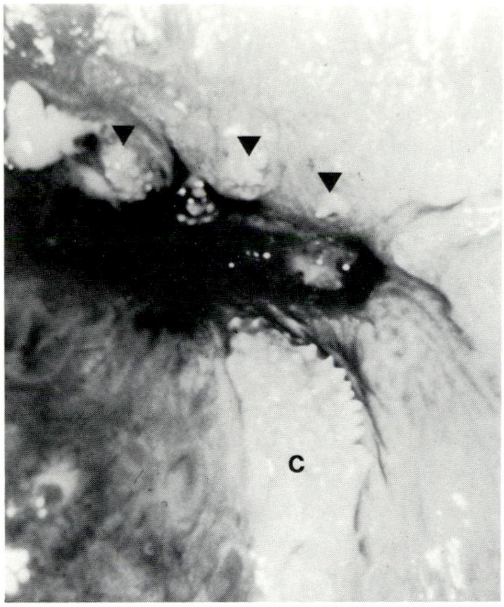

FIG. 7.5. Multifocal spiked condylomas of the cervix. The predominant lesion (C) is located on the posterior lip. Note the surface spikes and satellite lesions (*arrows*) on the anterior lip. (Courtesy of Christopher P. Crum, M.D., New York.)

infection of the lower anogenital tract epithelium by HPV may produce multicentric disease (Fig. 7.6). When florid condylomas of the vulva are identified, internal vaginal or cervical lesions are detectable in greater than 70% of patients.[185] Condylomata acuminata, with their exophytic, papillary growth pattern, are characteristic of the cornified epithelium of the perineum and vulva and are unusual in the nonkeratinizied squamous epithelium of the vagina and cervix (Fig. 7.7). Other configurations of cervical HPV infection include myriads of minute, maculopapular, flat condylomas involving the vagina and cervix.

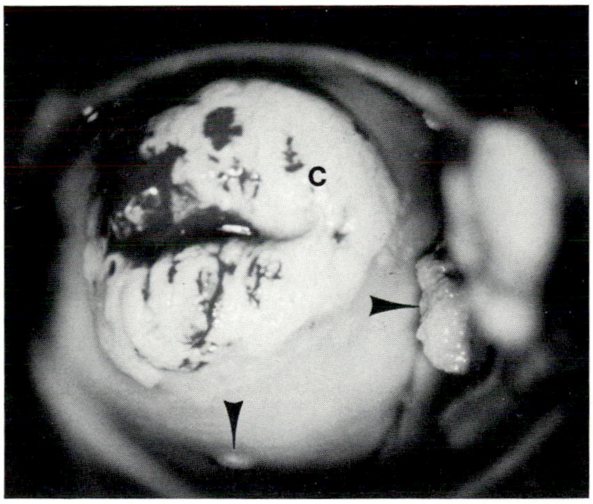

FIG. 7.6. Multicentric condylomas of the cervix and vagina. The cervical condyloma (C) is a four-quadrant white lesion with a thick, opaque, roughened surface. The endocervical limit of the lesion cannot be seen. The darker areas represent bleeding secondary to friability. Coexisting vaginal condylomas can be seen on the right and posteriorly (*arrows*). (Courtesy of Burton Krumholz, M.D., New York.)

The natural history of HPV 6/11-containing cervical condyloma is one of spontaneous regression, good response to conservative therapy, unpredictable recurrence, and often persistence if untreated. Lesion regression or apparent cure following biopsy occurs in 20–65% of patients, whereas there is persistence in 35–80%.[66,129–133,212,239] Latent, nonproductive HPV infection, as indicated by the finding of HPV DNA in normal-appearing genital skin adjacent to clinical anogenital disease, appears to influence subsequent recurrences.[59] Detectable HPV DNA in cervical smears from cytologically disease-free women[119,227] may presage the subsequent development of cervical lesions and indicates latency in the colposcopically normal cervix.[73] Progression of cervical condyloma to CIN and microinvasive carcinoma has been observed in some 10%[212] of patients in a follow-up period of 2–3 years.[132] However, information about whether these condylomas were exclusively diploid or polyploid lesions or whether some had aneuploid DNA content was not given. Since CIN 1 with koilocytosis had similar progression rates (11%),[212] it is likely that the progression rates reported for "ordinary condyloma" include also many well-differentiated aneuploid lesions.

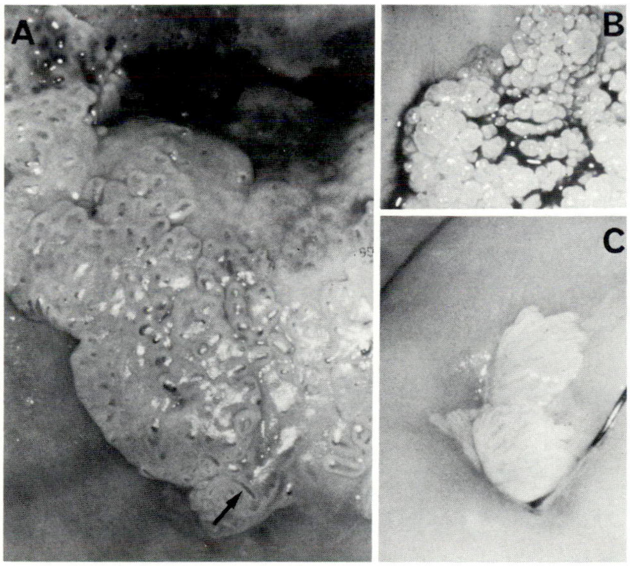

FIG. 7.7. Papillary condylomata acuminata of the cervix and vagina. *A*. Colposcopy of extensive confluent lesion with flattened papillae showing vascular loops (*arrow*). *B*. Vaginal lesion with multinodular surface. *C*. Two papillary lesions protruding from the external os. An IUD string is seen (*right*). (Courtesy of Burton Krumholz, M.D., New York.)

Long-term prospective studies of the progression rates of carefully ascertained cases of cervical condylomas with nuclear polyploidy and their natural history in a statistically significant number of affected women are necessary.

The natural history of genital condylomas may be modified by host factors, notably immunosuppression and steroid hormone levels.[119,154] Recurrence of condyloma during early and midtrimester pregnancy is reported commonly, with the lesions increasing in size and multifocality until term. After delivery, spontaneous regression of the condylomas is the rule. There is increasing concern about genital HPV infection during pregnancy because of the possibility of vertical transmission of infection to the fetus and neonate. There are anecdotal reports of infants born with genital condylomas or developing them in the immediate postnatal period.[132] Of even greater concern is the risk of development of laryngeal papillomatosis because of the morbidity and mortality associated with this disease. Although correlated with similar genital HPV types and linked causally to infection in the mother, the factors requisite for the development of laryngeal papillomatosis are not fully understood, and clinically apparent disease occurs in only a relatively small number of children at risk for exposure.[143,191a] Intrauterine infection of the fetus is also possible.[191a]

Cervical Intraepithelial Neoplasia

Colpomicroscopic studies[169] have shown that CIN occurs on the anterior lip of the cervix twice as commonly as on the posterior lip and is rarely seen at the lateral cervical angles. The distribution of CIN is similar to the distribution of both the everted endocervical epithelium and the transformation zone during the postpartum period.[236] CIN may expand horizontally and involve the entire transformation zone, but it stops abruptly at the junction with the native portio epithelium.[169,172] The area of the transformation zone, therefore, predetermines the distribution and extent of CIN on the exposed portion of the cervix.[20,171] The mechanism by which CIN is able to extend into normal squamous epithelium and into the columnar epithelium of the endocervix is a matter of contention. Some believe that CIN spreads by transformation of cells from normal to neoplastic in a vertical direction.[34,35,92,157] Others have suggested, on the basis of colpomicroscopy,[169] tissue culture studies,[168] and light and electron microscopy,[56] that CIN spreads horizontally along the basement membrane by mechanically lifting the adjacent normal squamous and endocervical columnar cells (Fig. 7.8). Ultrastructural observations[193] of the junction of CIN and the endocervical epithelium have failed to demonstrate subcylindrical reserve cells or metaplastic squamous cells at the interface of these lesions and normal tissues, suggesting that the expansion is not through transformation of metaplastic cells. The mechanical expansion of CIN is not confined to the endocervix, as it may extend along the entire endocervical canal to involve rarely the endometrial cavity.[45,58] The size and endocervical distribution of CIN tend to vary directly with increasing severity of grade, CIN 3 lesions usually having the largest surface area and more frequent involvement of the endocervical canal.

Opinions vary whether the origin is multicellular or unicellular. The proponents of the multicellular theory[22,34,35,92] suggest that CIN arises in a predetermined field or fields in transformation zone epithelium containing an abnormal cell population. This primary lesion, originating from either metaplastic epithelium[35,157] or subcylindrical cells of the endocervix,[92,157] eventually progresses in a vertical fashion by tranforming the adjacent normal epithelium into neoplastic epithelium or by coalescence of multiple predetermined neoplastic fields, producing a larger lesion. This theory of the multicellular origin of CIN and its vertical proliferation is based primarily on histologic[92] and colposcopic observations.[34,35] The unicellular theory proposes that CIN begins in a single cell or at most in an extremely circumscribed group of cells. Support for the unicentric single-cell origin theory has been offered by direct colpomicroscopic[170] and histologic[152] observations, as well as by cytogenetic chromosomal preparations[201] and glucose-6-phosphate dehydrogenase (G-6-PD) X-linked chromosome marker studies.[198] Using colpomicroscopy, Richart and Lerch[176] showed that 95% of early CIN lesions were confined to a single focus. Although they were not able to trace these lesions back to a single-cell origin, some of them were as small as 10 cells in diameter. Multifocal lesions or coalescence of multiple lesions was only rarely observed.

Colpomicroscopic follow-up of patients with minute CIN lesions has shown that the lesions expand centrifugally by mechanically displacing and eventually replacing the adjacent benign squamous or endocervical epithelium. Histologically, CIN lesions were demonstrated to be unifocal and confluent in nearly 95% of serially step-sectioned conization specimens.[152] In direct chromosomal preparations,[201] dysplasia, CIS, and microinvasive carcinoma were shown to contain the same neoplastic clone, which presumably was derived from a single cell. The evidence consisted of finding similar abnormal modal number and marker chromosomes in dysplasia and CIS as well as in microinvasive carcinoma.

The electrophoretic variants of the X-linked enzyme G-6-PD have been applied to determine the unicellular versus multicellular origin of cervical neoplasia. The results with CIN lesions were in most cases consistent with a single-cell origin, again suggesting that the initial tumorigenic event affects one cell rather than a large number of cells simultaneously.[198] At present, there is no unanimous opinion on the cellular origin of CIN.

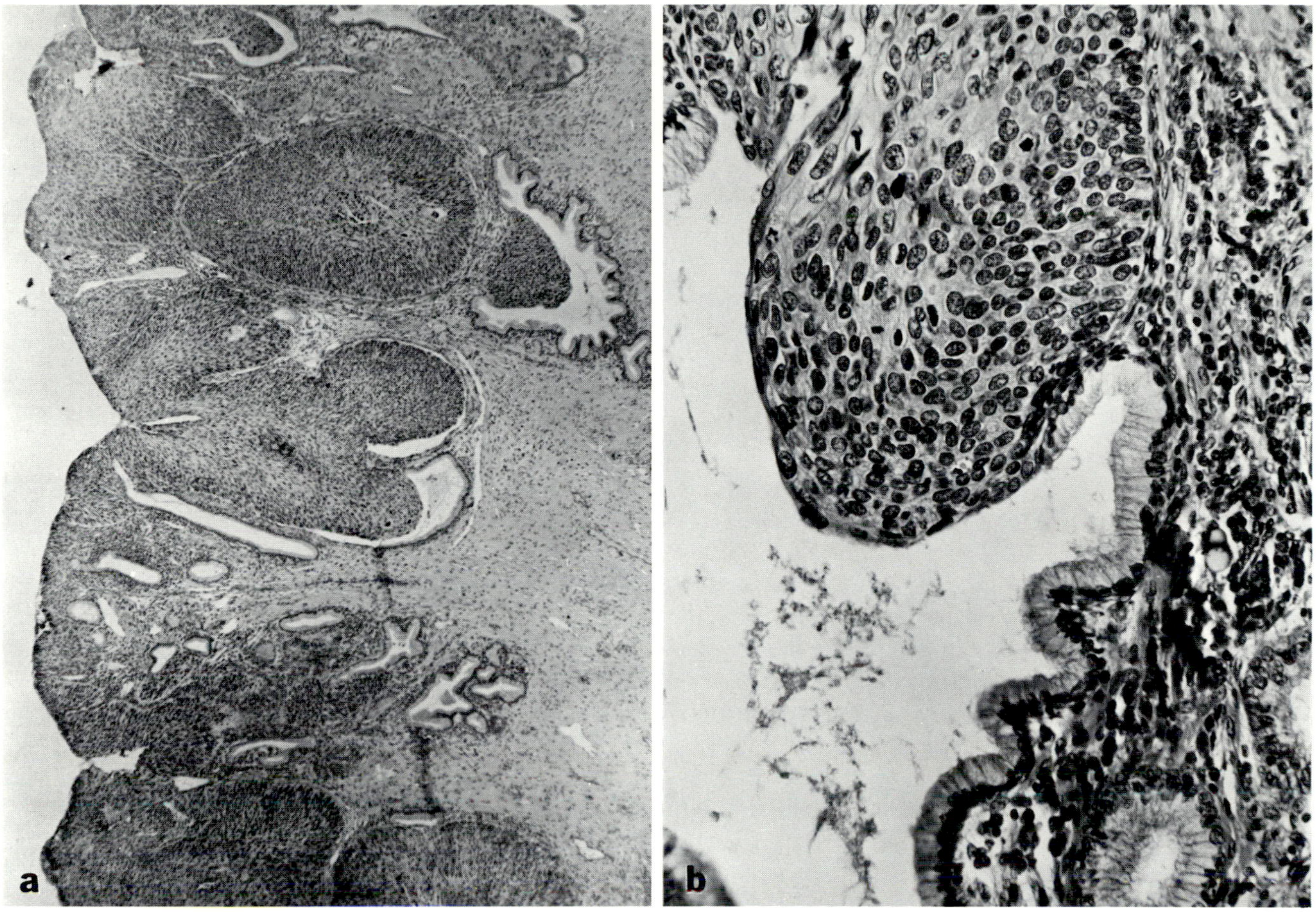

FIG. 7.8. Endocervical gland involvement by CIN. *a*. Masses of neoplastic cells grow into and distend endocervical clefts. Note the smooth margins of ingrowing neoplastic epithelium retaining the normal configuration of endocervical mucosa. *b*. The neoplastic cells grow between the endocervical epithelium and its basal lamina.

Three cellular sites of origin have been proposed: basal cells of the squamous epithelium of the portio, basal cells of the transformation zone epithelium, and subcylindrical reserve cells of the endocervix.[92] Colposcopic, colpomicroscopic, and histologic observations have shown that virtually all CIN begins at the squamocolumnar junction of the transformation zone, with one edge of the lesion bordering the endocervical columnar epithelium.[170] The line of demarcation between the squamous epitheium of the native portio or transformation zone and CIN is sharp and perpendicular to the surface. Early, well-differentiated, preinvasive disease is usually found in the squamous epithelium at the squamocolumnar junction and is seldom seen in the endocervix. In general, the exposed portion of CIN is well differentiated and of the CIN 1 type, whereas the endocervical involvement is less well differentiated and of the CIN 3 type. From these observations it is now proposed that most CIN arises in the basal cells of the transformation zone epithelium, which is formed by the coalescence of squamous metaplastic epithelium with native squamous epithelium. In the metaplastic squamous epithelium, the cell of origin is the subcylindrical reserve cell of the everted endocervix, whereas in the native portio epithelium, the cell of origin is the basal cell of the native squamous epithelium.

The natural history of CIN has been studied extensively.* Large-scale studies with follow-up using cytology and colpomicroscopy alone, without biopsy altering the natural course of the disease, are the most useful.[63,90,171,214] A study of women with CIN ascertained initially by two or three consecutive abnormal smears, followed only by cytology and colpomicroscopy for 9 years, demonstrated that about 50% of women with CIN 1 progressed to CIN 3.[10,175] In the remaining cases, the lesions either developed to CIN 2 or remained persistent at the same grade (28%).[9,175] Although spontaneous regressions did occur, they were confined to patients with "very mild dysplasia" (CIN 1), and their number

* References 58, 60, 61, 93, 99, 102, 165, 208.

was negligible (6%) when compared to the progression rates. The absence of progression in some women and the spontaneous regression in others can now be accounted for by the reclassification of at least some of these lesions as flat condylomas. Follow-up examinations showed that the rate of progression increased and the transit time became shorter with increasing severity of CIN. Therefore, the probability that an untreated, low-grade CIN will progress to CIN 3 is directly dependent on the grade of the lesion. These observations also suggest that lesions develop progressively from a better to a lesser differentiated state. The median transit time to CIN 3 was approximately 6 months to 3 years for CIN 1, 2 years for CIN 2, and 4 years for all the CIN 1–2 lesions taken together.[9,175]

Other rates of regression, persistence, and progression have been reported in a number of large-scale investigations, but this may reflect differences in diagnostic criteria and study design. For example, studies in which punch biopsy and endocervical curettage are used to establish the diagnosis may remove (treat) the lesion. Their use, therefore, may interfere with long-term analysis by increasing the frequency of spontaneous regression and decreasing the frequency of progression.[139,171] Nasiell et al. focused on long-term follow-up of CIN 2 lesions. In the subgroup of patients followed without biopsy, CIN 2 spontaneously regressed in 28% of patients. However, progression occurred in 50% in an average follow-up time of 51 months.[139] These studies emphasize a substantial risk for persistence and progression in lesions classified as low-grade CIN.[105,212] Statistical results are more conclusive in regard to lesions defined as CIN 3.[10,128] In a prospective analysis, CIN 3 progressed to invasive carcinoma in 29% of patients followed from 1 to 20 years, and the rate of progression increased directly with the length of follow-up, peaking at 34.6% in patients followed for 14 years.[60,61,93,99,102] In another study, 71% of women with CIN 3 developed invasive carcinoma during a minimum follow-up period of 12 years.[106] Other long-term retrospective studies have demonstrated progression of CIN 3 to invasive cancer in 60–70% of cases.[15,106]

The prospective follow-up data are in agreement with epidemiologic investigations of patients with CIN 1–2 and CIN 3. The prevalence of CIN 1–2 proportionally decreases with age.[21,93,207] New lesions arise in the form of CIN 1 instead of CIN 3, as determined by calculations of the incidence rate,[93,207] and there is a 1000–2000 times higher annual incidence of CIN 3 in women with CIN 1–2 compared than in those with normal cytologic findings.[214] In animals, cervical lesions also develop through progressive stages of CIN 1 to CIN 3 and invasive carcinoma.[187]

It must be emphasized that these observations apply only to the aggregate (a large group of women) and provide no objective means to predict the potential of regression or persistence of CIN or its progression to a more severe form of CIN or to invasion in the individual patient.[9,102] Since it is impossible to predict which patients will progress to invasion with a given CIN at a given time, a CIN lesion once detected, regardless of degree of morphologic severity, should be treated immediately to prevent the development of invasive carcinoma.

Pathologic Features

Condyloma

The contrasting histologic features of cervical condyloma and CIN are summarized in Table 7.5. The most characteristic cytopathic effects of HPV infection are perinuclear cytoplasmic vacuolization or koilocytosis, the presence of superficial or intermediate squamous epithelial cells with anisocytosis, and nuclear pyknosis or hyperchromaticity (Fig. 7.9). Koilocytes were described in cervical smears associated with dysplasia and carcinoma by Koss and Durfee in 1956.[103] Koilocytosis is derived from the Greek word *koilos,* meaning *hollow* or *empty.* It was not until the studies by Meisels et al.[130] and Purola and Savia,[153] however, that koilocytes were recognized as a cytohistologic manifestation of HPV infection. Cytologically, koilocytes are enlarged intermediate or superficial cells with an irregular cytoplasmic border, a distinct perinuclear zone of cytoplasmic clearing, and a surrounding, peripheral zone of dense cytoplasm (Fig. 7.9). The nuclear changes of koilocytes are variable but most often are degenerative in nature. They are characterized by pyknosis, chromatin margination, and fragmentation. Nuclear enlargement, giant nuclei, and binucleation or multinucleation are common in koilocytotic lesions and may produce an increase in nuclear/cytoplasmic ratio that cannot be distinguished readily from CIN 1. Although koilocytosis is a relatively specific cytopathic effect of HPV, it may occur as a reflection of atrophy-related vacuolar degeneration (in postmenopausal

Table 7.5. Contrasting histologic features of cervical condyloma and CIN.

	Condyloma	CIN
Koilocytosis	+	±
Abnormal mitotic figures	−	+
Basal polarity	+	−
Basal crowding and disorganization	−	+
Chromatin clumping	−	+
Anisonucleosis	+	+
Multinucleation	+	+

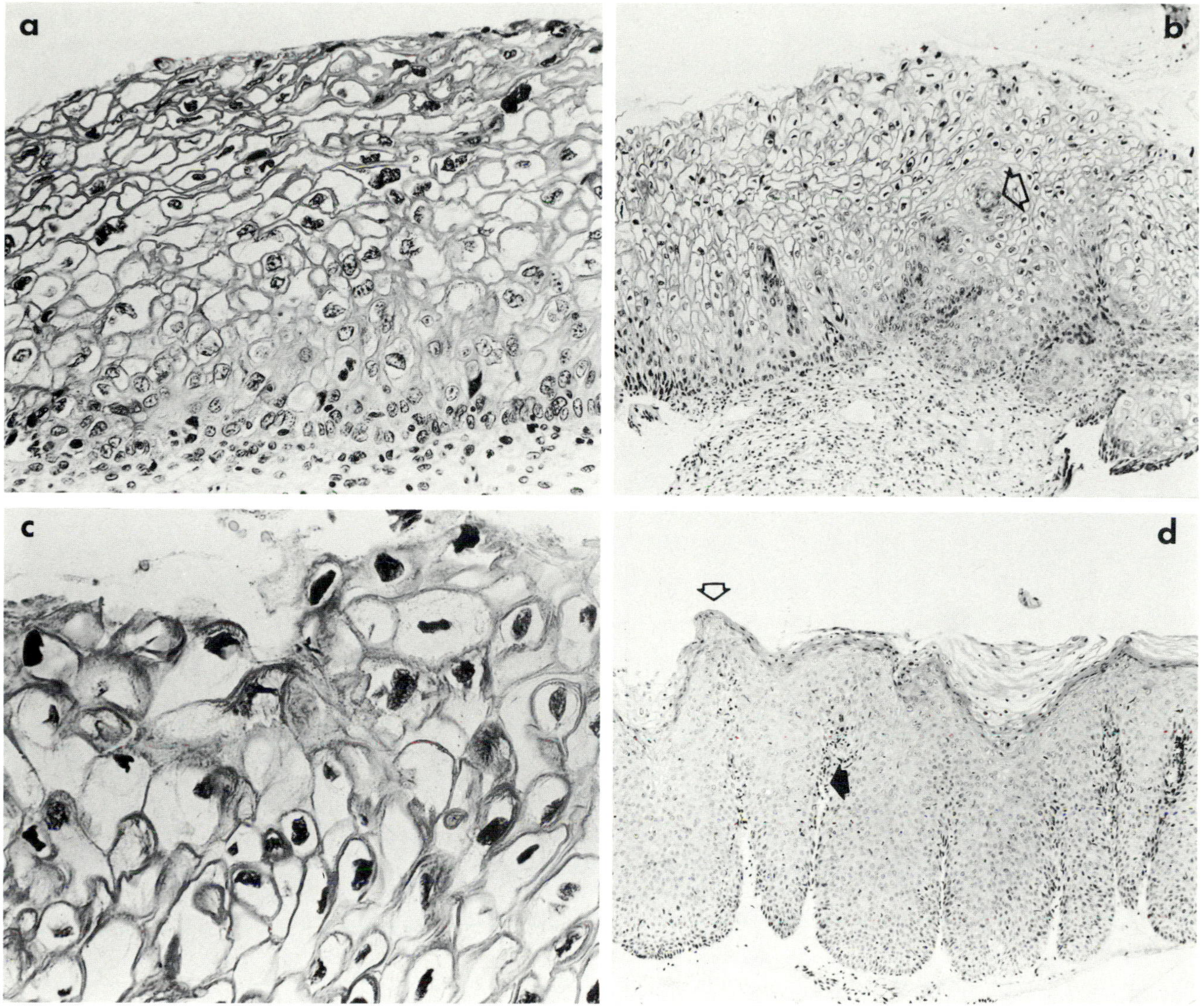

FIG. 7.9. Condylomas of cervix. *a*. Flat condyloma. Thickened epithelium with irregular cytoplasmic cavitation (ballooning), enlarged, occasionally binucleated, degenerated nuclei in the upper strata of the epithelium, and thickened cytoplasmic membranes. These changes are referred to as koilocytosis. *b*. Flat condyloma. Slightly tangential sectioned epithelium with stromal papillae (*arrow*). Note intact, well-defined basal cell layer in *a* and *b*. *c*. Higher magnification of koilocytotic cells with cytoplasmic ballooning, degenerated, hyperchromatic nuclei, and thickened cytoplasmic membranes. The intracellular vacuoles are devoid of glycogen. *d*. Spiked condyloma. The club-shaped rete pegs are prominent, as are the stromal papillae (*dark arrow*) extending to the surface. Koilocytotic atypia is reduced and is limited to the surface. The latter contains parakeratosis and spikes (*light arrow*) corresponding to spikes seen colposcopically (see Fig. 7.5).

women) or in non-HPV-related infections, such as trichomoniasis, *G. vaginalis*, and candidiasis. Therefore, koilocytosis should be considered as a marker of HPV infection only when present in concert with the architectural and epithelial abnormalities associated with HPV.

These architectural findings are less specific than are the cytologic changes but correlate with the patterns seen macroscopically and colposcopically (see Figs. 7.5 and 7.6). Epithelial hyperplasia, characterized primarily by acanthosis and papillomatosis, is almost always present but varies in degree and configuration (Fig. 7.9a,b,d). The most common pattern is that of the flat condyloma (planum) with moderate epithelial thickening and an undulating, slightly raised surface. Pointed tufts of superficial epithelium containing fibrovascular cores may produce surface spikes typical of the spiked condyloma (Figs. 7.5 and 7.9a). When gland involvement and acanthosis predominate, the pattern appears endophytic, resem-

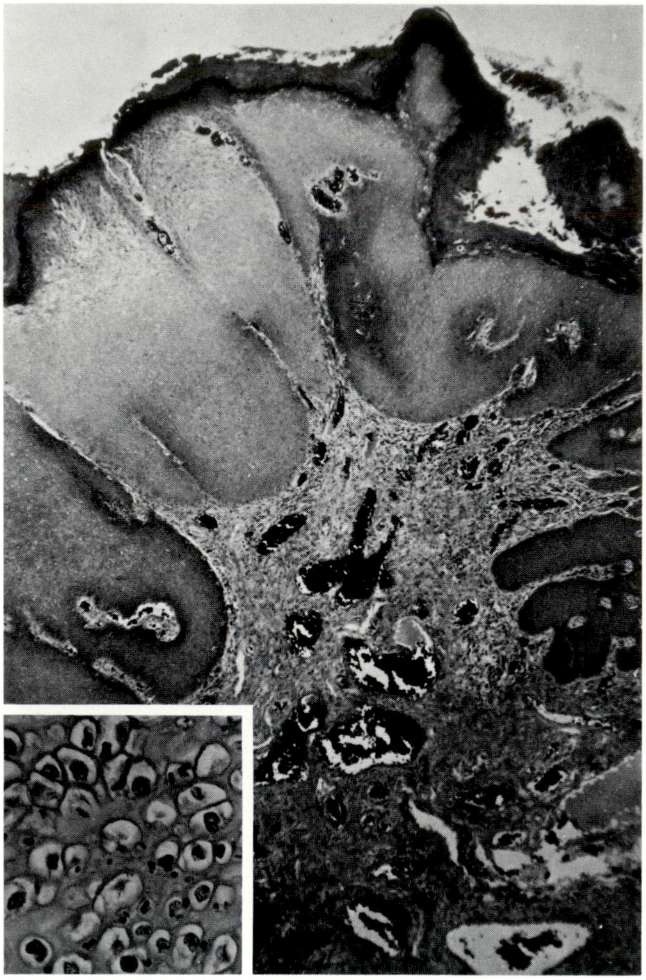
a

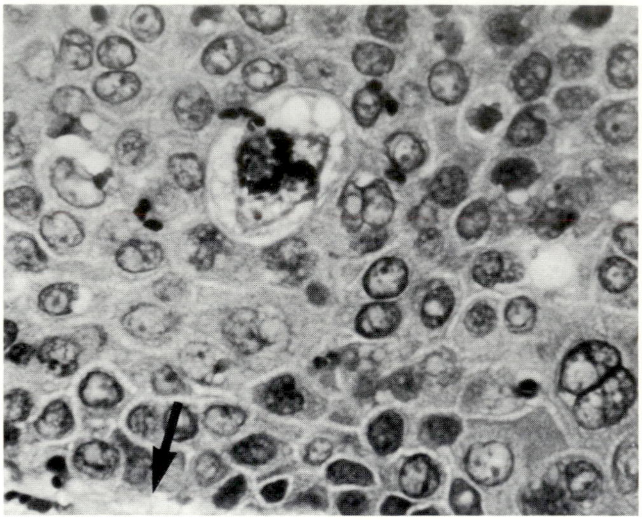
b

FIG. 7.10.*a*. A condyloma acuminatum involving endocervical glands. Acanthotic rete pegs converge toward the vascular base and are separated from each other by stromal papillae. Note the surface hyperkeratosis. *Inset:* High power view of vacuolated koilocytotic cells with atypical nuclei in the upper strata. *b*. Tripolar mitotic figure in a cell undergoing vacuolar cytoplasmic degeneration. The surrounding cells in the parabasal cell layer display little pleomorphism and have uniform nuclear chromatin and occasionally double or multiple nuclei. Such changes are associated with productive HPV infections, that is, ordinary condyloma. Hybridization in this case showed HPV 6. *Arrow* points to basal cell-stromal junction.

bling the configuration of inverted papilloma of the nasal cavity (Fig. 7.10). HPV may also affect the immature metaplastic epithelium of the transformation zone, producing cytologic atypia with only minimal or focal koilocytosis (Fig. 7.11). Papillary condylomas, identical to condylomata acuminata of the vulva, occur on the mucous membrane of the cervix but are unusual. Proliferation of basal or parabasal cells in condylomas of the cervix is minimal, and basal polarity and organization are, for the most part, retained. The well-structured organization and bland cytology of the basal portion of the epithelium often contrasts sharply with the prominent cytologic and architectural abnormalities of the superficial and intermediate layers, with their ballooning koilocytes.

Abnormal keratinization is a prominent, albeit nonspecific, feature of HPV infection. It is manifested by varying amounts of dyskeratosis (individual cell keratinization) and surface hyperkeratosis and parakeratosis (Figs. 7.9a and 7.10). Hypergranulosis may or may not be present and may be marked. Mitotic figures in cervical condyloma are generally confined to the lower portion of the epithelium.[64,239,241] They are usually normal in configuration. Exceptions to the rule are tripolar and dispersed metaphases (Fig. 7.10b). Although these are abnormal in their configuration, they are seen in benign virus infections and regenerative processes unrelated to neoplasia.[14] As a result, they should not be confused with other forms of abnormal mitotic figures typically seen in CIN (see Fig. 7.30).

Ultrastructural studies of the koilocytotic cells of cervical condyloma have confirmed the presence of intranuclear HPV virions. Viral particles can be detected in 30–60% of flat cervical condylomas.[28,55,131] The virions are typically arranged in crystalline arrays, sometimes in association with filaments, and distributed throughout all or part of the nucleoplasm (Fig. 7.12). Other ultrastructural alterations of the koilocytotic cells parallel the light microscopic findings[131,144] and are not dependent on the presence of viral particles. Chromatin clumping and reduction of nuclear size characteristic of karyopyknosis are often demonstrable and are consistent with irreversible cell injury and productive viral infection. Nuclear irregularity, enlargement, binucleation, and polylobulation are also common. The peripheral cyto-

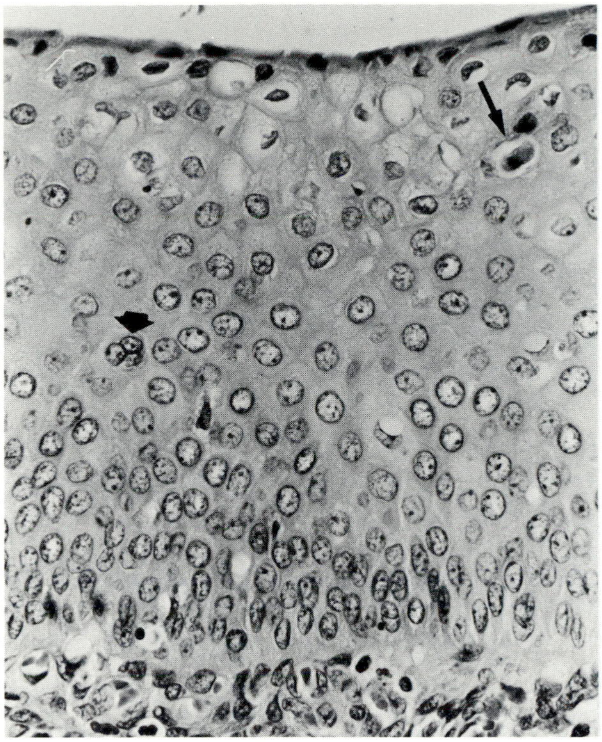

FIG. 7.11. Immature squamous metaplasia with koilocytosis. This cervical lesion is composed of immature squamous metaplastic cells occupying the lower two-thirds of the epithelium. There are a few superficial koilocytes, dyskeratocytes (*long arrow*), trinucleated cells (*short arrow*), and a fine parakeratotic layer.

plasm contains aggregates of tonofilaments that are increased in thickness and irregularly distributed. The perinuclear clear zone is poor in cellular organelles, containing only scattered ribosomes and sparse glycogen particles (Fig. 7.12).

Cervical Intraepithelial Neoplasia

In contrast to condylomas, in CIN, basal polarity is lost and accompanied by a crowded, overlapping basal growth pattern and generalized cellular disorientation (Table 7.5). Cytologic abnormalities that are characteristic of CIN include hyperchromaticity, abnormal chromatin distribution, nuclear pleomorphism, and increased nuclear: cytoplasmic ratio. The nuclear borders are irregular, and the chromatin is coarse, granular (salt and pepper), or filamentous throughout the nuclear mass. The abnormal chromatin patterns are the most important factors in the histologic identification of CIN and serve to distinguish it from lesions that mimic intraepithelial neoplasia. Increased frequency of mitotic activity at all epithelial levels and the presence of morphologically abnormal mitotic figures are typical of CIN and are important diagnostic criteria (Fig. 7.13).[65–67,239,241] Nuclear alterations consistent with neoplasia are found in CIN at all levels of the epithelium regardless of the degree of cytoplasmic maturation.

CIN 1, 2, and 3 may demonstrate koilocytosis, the degree of which is proportional to the number of mature, neoplastic cells in which HPV can replicate and produce visible cytopathic changes. However, the presence of koilocytosis should not be construed as diagnostic of condyloma when associated with nuclear changes of neoplasia. Rather, diagnostic terms, such as CIN 1, 2, or 3, noting that koilocytosis is present should be used. The terms *atypical condyloma* or *transitional lesions* are confusing and, based on their morphology, their HPV 16 or 18 content, and their biologic behavior, represent very well differentiated CIN 1 with koilocytosis.

Grading of intraepithelial neoplasia is classically based on the proportion of the epithelium occupied by basaloid, undifferentiated cells, reflecting a progressive loss of epithelial maturation and decreasing glycogenization with increasing lesion severity (Fig. 7.14). The spectrum of epithelial alterations that comprises CIN can, therefore, be semiquantitatively classified into three categories: CIN grade 1—neoplastic, basaloid cells occupying the lower third of the epithelium (Fig. 7.15), CIN grade 2–basaloid cells occupying the lower third to two-thirds of the epithelium (Fig. 7.16), and CIN grade 3–basaloid cells occupying two-thirds to full thickness of the epithelium (Figs. 7.17 and 7.18). Although grading is useful as a diagnostic reference for statistical analysis and for teaching purposes, it has little if any clinical or therapeutic relevance (see section on management of CIN).

Ultrastructurally,[193] both the nuclear and cytoplasmic alterations of CIN are consistent with a progressive lack of normal differentiation (Figs. 7.19 and 7.20). There is a decrease in glycogen, tonofilaments, desmosomes, and specialized junctional units or nexuses (see Chapter 8, Cervical Carcinoma) with increasing histologic dedifferentiation. These alterations are correlated with a progressive decrease in cellular adhesions, basal pseudopodia, and cell contact inhibition demonstrated by time-lapse cinematography in cells grown in vitro.[176,179,218] The surface ultrastructure of cervical cancer precursors also differs from the normal architecture.[59] The most outstanding feature is the absence of surface microridges and the presence of abundant microvilli (Fig. 7.21).

CIN 3 lesions are classified by some investigators into three main cytologic subtypes[151,156]: small cell anaplastic, large cell keratinizing, and large cell nonkeratinizing CIN. The small cell variety is usually found within the external os or endocervical canal and is composed of small, undifferentiated, malignant cells of the basal cell type (Fig. 7.18). The large cell keratinizing lesion originates on the exposed portion of the cervix and displays prominent intercellular bridges, macronucleoli, and ex-

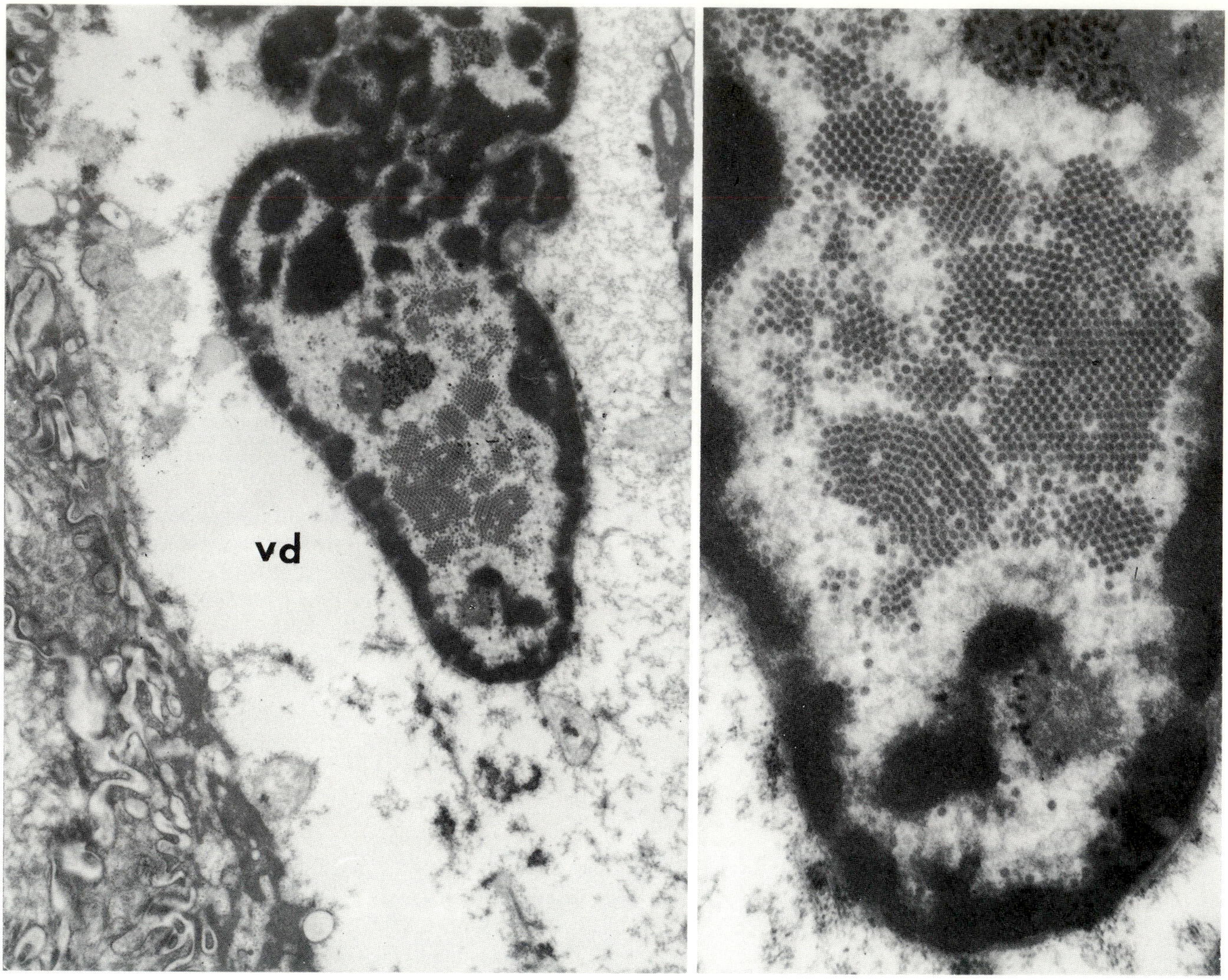

FIG. 7.12. Electron microscopy of human papillomavirus (HPV) particles. *a*. Note intranuclear aggregates of HPV in a koilocytotic, superficial cell of the flat condyloma shown in Fig. 7.9*a*. The marginated nuclear chromatin is agglutinated, and the cytoplasmic substance displays vacuolar degeneration (vd). The latter corresponds to koilocytotic ballooning on light microscopy. *b*. Closer view of HPV particles confined in the nuclear substance.

tensive surface keratinization (Fig. 7.22). Surface keratinization correlates clinically with the presence of a white patch, and, therefore, all lesions with a white surface must be biopsied to rule out the presence of an underlying intraepithelial carcinoma. Large cell nonkeratinizing lesions are by far the most frequent of all intraepithelial carcinomas of the cervix and are found within the cervical transformation zone. The epithelium is composed of undifferentiated cells the size of normal parabasal cells. Individual cell keratinization may be encountered (Fig. 7.23). Because accurate studies concerning the invasive potential of each of these subtypes are lacking, it is felt that prediction of the likelihood of progression to invasive carcinoma should not be based on the above subclassification.

Parallel to the epithelial abnormalities observed in CIN, the subepithelial vascular network undergoes profound alterations, as determined by histochemical vascular preparations and colposcopic observations.[202] These presumably develop to provide an adequate supply of oxygen and nutrients that are necessary for neoplastic growth. The flat capillary network, which is found beneath the normal cervical epithelium, becomes tortuous and compressed vertically by the neoplastic epithelium, with extension close to the surface (Fig. 7.24), producing a colposcopic pattern of punctation (Fig. 7.25a). Further proliferation and interconnection of proliferating masses of neoplastic tissue result in compression of the vascular network into basket-like structures around the neoplastic epithelium, producing a colposcopic mosaic (Fig. 7.25b).

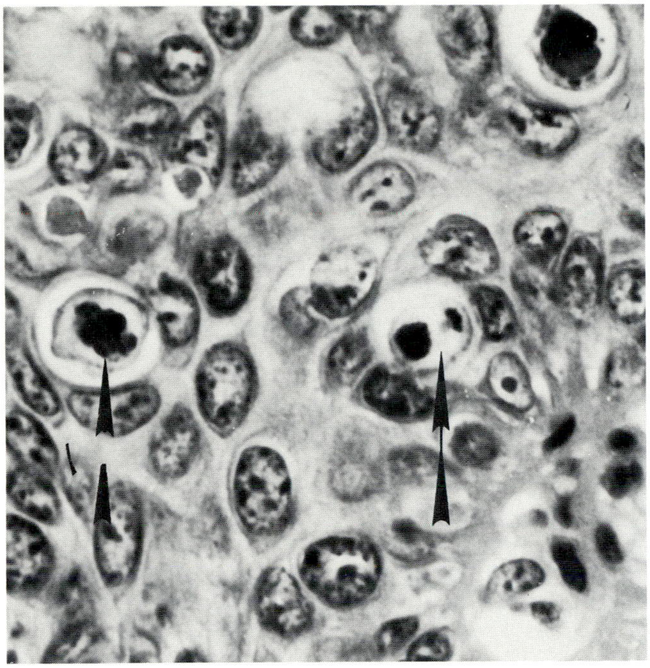

Fig. 7.13. Cervical intraepithelial neoplasia. Abnormal chromatin patterns with coarse granular chromatin, chromatin clumping, and margination are evident. Scattered abnormal mitotic figures (*arrows*) are present.

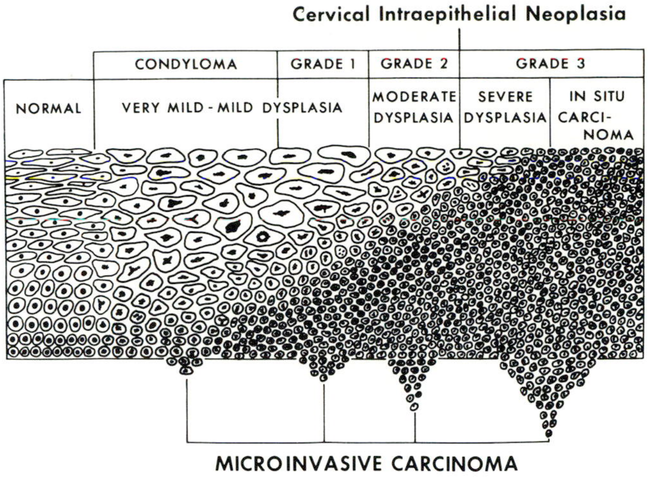

Fig. 7.14. Schematic representation of cervical cancer precursors. Grade 1, 2, and 3 CIN correspond to the traditional very mild–mild, moderate, and severe dysplasia to CIS, respectively. They are characterized by a progressive increase in the number of undifferentiated, malignant cells with nuclear aneuploidy and a decrease in superficial cell differentiation of koilocytotic cells paralleling the increase in severity of CIN. Lesions traditionally referred to as very mild dysplasia and a certain proportion of mild dysplasia or grade 1 CIN are today best referred to as condylomas. These lesions contain normal to reactive basal and parabasal cells with nuclear diploidy to polyploidy and numerous koilocytes in the upper two-third layers of the epithelium. A certain proportion of condylomatous lesions contain abnormal cells in the lower one-third layer of the epithelium with nuclear polyploidy to aneuploidy. These lesions represent the most differentiated form of CIN. This scheme also illustrates that microinvasion, although significantly more frequently associated with a grade 3 lesion, may also develop directly from any given stage of untreated CIN and even condyloma. The risk of developing microinvasion from different stages of CIN is arbitrarily represented and is not necessarily proportional to that illustrated in this scheme.

Because of severe compression, some of the capillaries eventually disappear, resulting in an increase in the intercapillary distance. Although frequently less prominent, similar vascular changes may be seen with flat condyloma of the cervix and cannot be differentiated from low-grade CIN.[133,161] In early invasive carcinoma, a system of new capillaries is generated from capillaries of punctation or mosaic structures and is observed to run parallel to and beneath the surface of neoplastic epithelium (Fig. 7.24c); this is the so-called horizontal capillary network. These vascular changes and variation in the intercapillary distance are the most important diagnostic colposcopic criteria and serve to distinguish noninvasive from invasive cervical squamous carcinoma.

Differential Diagnosis

Intraepithelial abnormalities of the cervix are a spectrum of histologic changes with differing etiologies and clinical outcomes. The benign end of this spectrum is composed of a variety of lesions that are usually reactive or infectious in nature. Nonspecific epithelial hyperplasia, cervicitis, and reparative atypia (Fig. 7.26) may produce lesions that mimic condylomas. They often contain degenerative cytoplasmic vacuolization, which may be confused with koilocytosis. Differentiation from condyloma can be made by noting the absence of the ballooning cytoskeletal irregularities, generalized anisocytosis, nuclear pyknosis, and epithelial and architectural abnormalities that comprise the constellation of findings associated with HPV infection. Immature squamous lesions of the cervix, including squamous metaplasia with or without koilocytosis and atrophy, should be differentiated from CIN 3 (Fig. 7.27). Although these lesions lack the normal maturation process, they are devoid of the nuclear chromatin abnormalities, abnormal mitotic figures, cytonuclear pleomorphism, and epithelial disorganization that are seen in intraepithelial neoplasia (Fig. 7.26). A careful clinical history, cytologic and colposcopic correlation, and cytologic and culture examination of the cervix for infectious organisms other than HPV may elucidate the etiology.

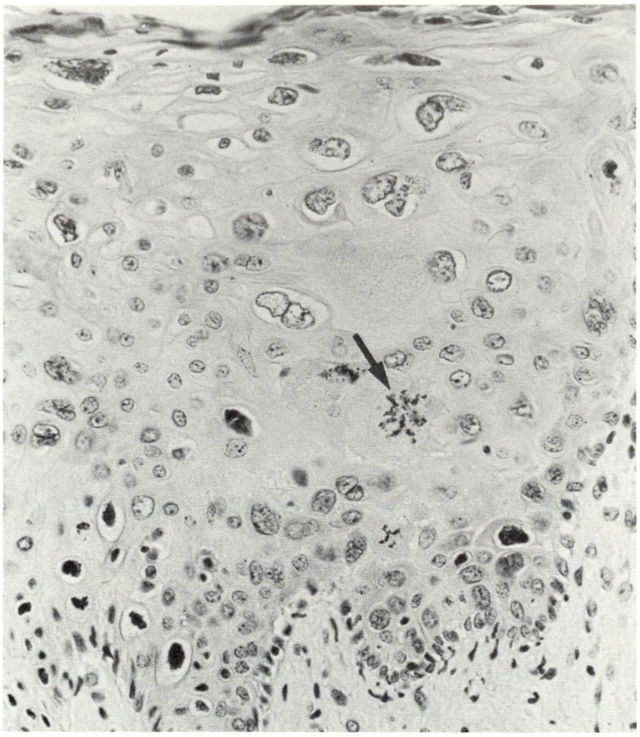

FIG. 7.15. Grade 1 CIN with koilocytosis (mild dysplasia). Well-differentiated lesion in which the upper two-thirds of the epithelium is occupied by single and multinucleated koilocytes. Despite cytoplasmic maturation, the neoplastic nature of the cells is evidenced by the coarse chromatin pattern of pleomorphic nuclei and abnormal mitotic figures (*arrow*). The basal cell layer is not as well defined as in ordinary condyloma.

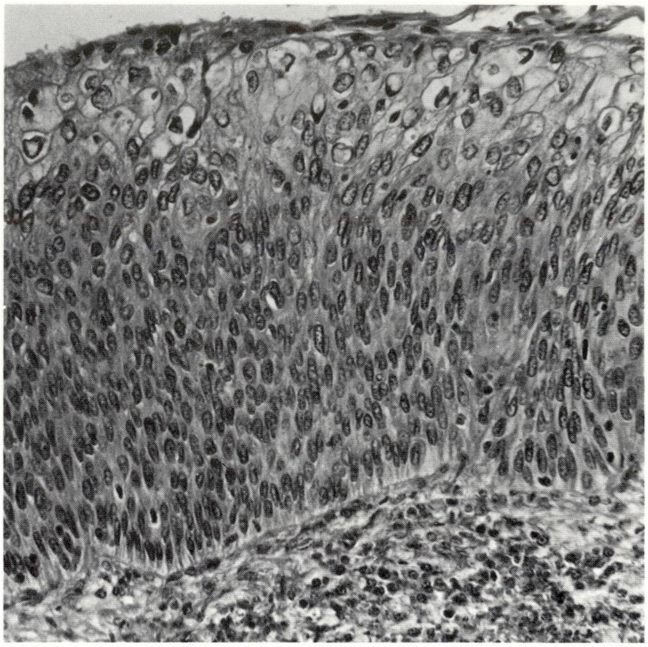

FIG. 7.17. Grade 3 CIN with koilocytosis (severe dysplasia). Undifferentiated basal-type cells involve approximately two-thirds of the full thickness of the epithelium. Koilocytes are limited to the upper one-third of the neoplastic epithelium.

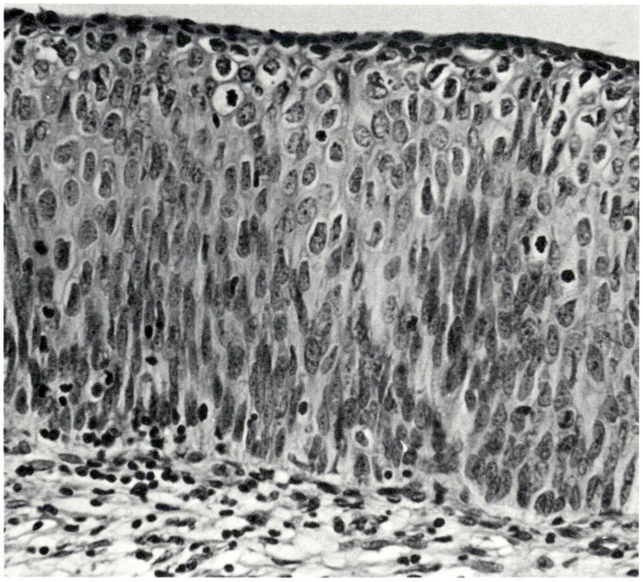

FIG. 7.16. Grade 2 CIN with koilocytosis (moderate dysplasia). Undifferentiated neoplastic cells replace 50–70% of the epithelium. The nucleus/cytoplasm ratio is in favor of the nucleus, and the cytoplasmic membranes and the basal layer are indistinct. A few koilocytes are seen in the superficial strata.

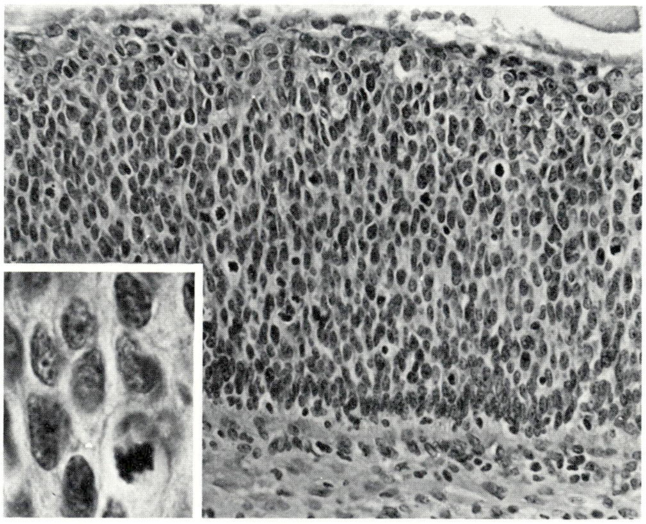

FIG. 7.18. Grade 3 CIN (carcinoma in situ). The full thickness of the epithelium is composed of small, undifferentiated neoplastic cells. This is the classic small cell carcinoma in situ. Note numerous mitotic figures, loss of cellular maturation and organization, and lack of koilocytes. *Inset:* Aggregated nuclear chromatin and mitosis. Characteristically, cell membranes are ill defined.

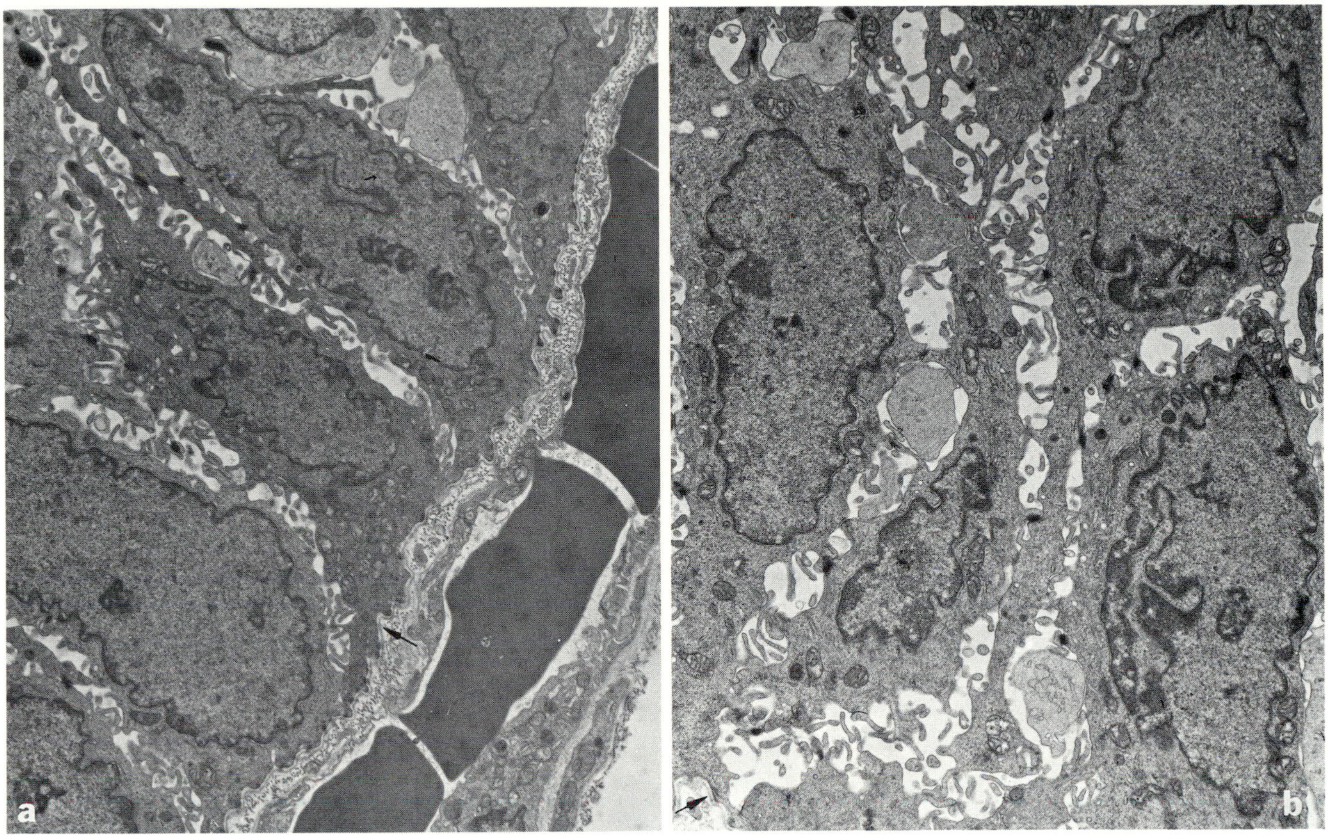

FIG. 7.19. Electron microscopic appearance of the basal cells in (*a*) grade 1 CIN and (*b*) grade 3 CIN. The cells contain identical ultrastructural features, including nuclear pleomorphism, convoluted nuclear membranes, and spare desmosomal attachments. The *arrows* indicate the basal lamina. A subepithelial capillary with red blood cells is seen in (*a*). *a*. ×3973. *b*. ×5160.

Immunohistochemistry

Immunohistochemistry affords pathologists a highly specific and sensitive technique with which to study changes in antigenic expression in tissue sections. Antibodies generated against various cellular proteins and infectious microorganisms have been used to elucidate the biochemical alterations that accompany cervical infections and intraepithelial neoplasia.

The papillomaviruses share a group-specific antigen, probably related to an internal capsid protein, that can be detected by immunoperoxidase staining. The staining localizes the capsid protein specifically to the nuclei of superficial cells, most often koilocytes, and correlates well with the presence of intranuclear virions by electron microscopy[28,57,109,131] (Fig. 7.28). Positive staining requires productive infection as well as terminal squamous differentiation and varies directly with the degree of koilocytosis.[57,108] Even in overt, ordinary condyloma, antigenic expression can be demonstrated in only 50% of cases studied, and staining is often focal or patchy.[83,109–111] Occasional positive staining can be demonstrated in squamous metaplasia with koilocytosis.[43] In a review of over 300 cases, HPV antigens were demonstrated by immunoperoxidase in only 29% of CIN 1, 16% of CIN 2, and 3% of CIN 3.[109] Because of either periodic expression of viral proteins or the sensitivity of immunohistochemical staining of HPV antigens only 50% of overt condylomas show positive staining. Since positive staining may occur in condylomas and in CIN lesions, this technique is impractical for differential diagnosis. If positive, however, it is the only method, besides electron microscopy, that indicates that infectious virus is present.

Biochemical markers for epithelial differentiation have been applied to the study of cervical abnormalities.[1,118] Complex, high molecular weight keratins characteristic of terminal squamous differentiation[68] can be demonstrated in condylomas and low-grade CIN, although their distribution is abnormal. In contrast, they are absent in high-grade CIN, which may contain simple, low molecular weight keratins not normally expressed in squamous epithelium.[118,122,137] Involucrin expression, a marker of suprabasal differentation unrelated to keratini-

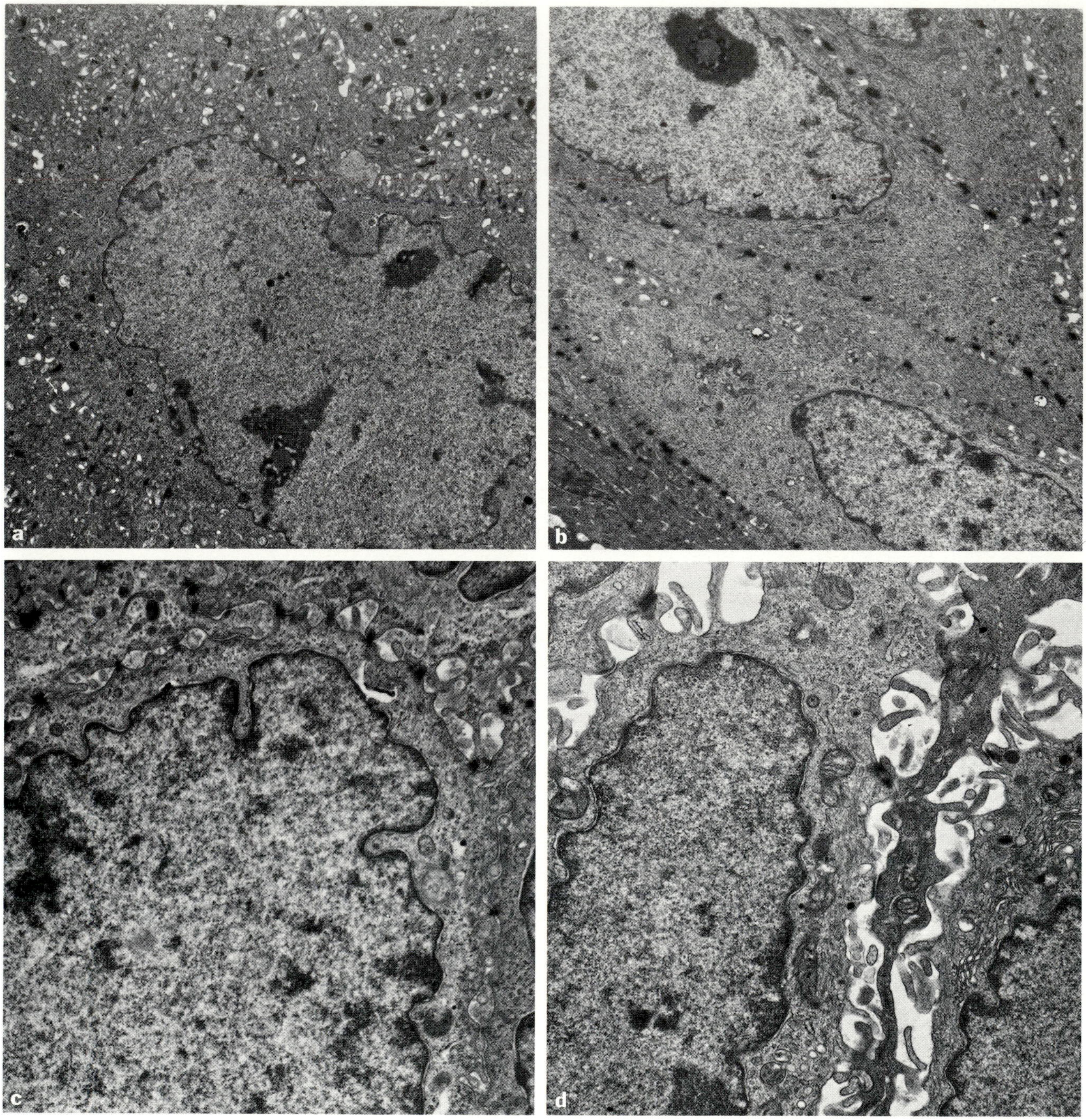

FIG. 7.20. Electron micrographs of neoplastic cells from the middle third of the epithelium in (*a*) grade 1 CIN, (*b*) grade 2 CIN, and (*c* and *d*) two cases of grade 3 CIN. The common features include increased nucleus:cytoplasm ratio, irregular nuclear contour, prominent nucleoli, and abundant free and bound ribosomes. Note the gradual decrease in the number of desmosomes, tonofilaments, and glycogen particles from (*a*) to (*d*). *a*. ×5000. *b*. ×5000. *c*. ×10,200. *d*. ×10,200.

zation, can be detected in condyloma (Fig. 7.29) and low-grade CIN but is absent from immature, high-grade CIN.[163,226] Concurrent positive staining for both involucrin and HPV antigens varies inversely with the degree of epithelial atypia and maturational abnormality, with both antigens expressed in 39% of CIN 1 and 2.[227] Because the expression of involucrin and high-molecular-weight keratins is maturation dependent, there is a substantial overlap in staining between condyloma and low-grade CIN, and they cannot be used as a specific diagnostic tool to discriminate these lesions. The absence of staining in physiologically normal, immature metaplastic

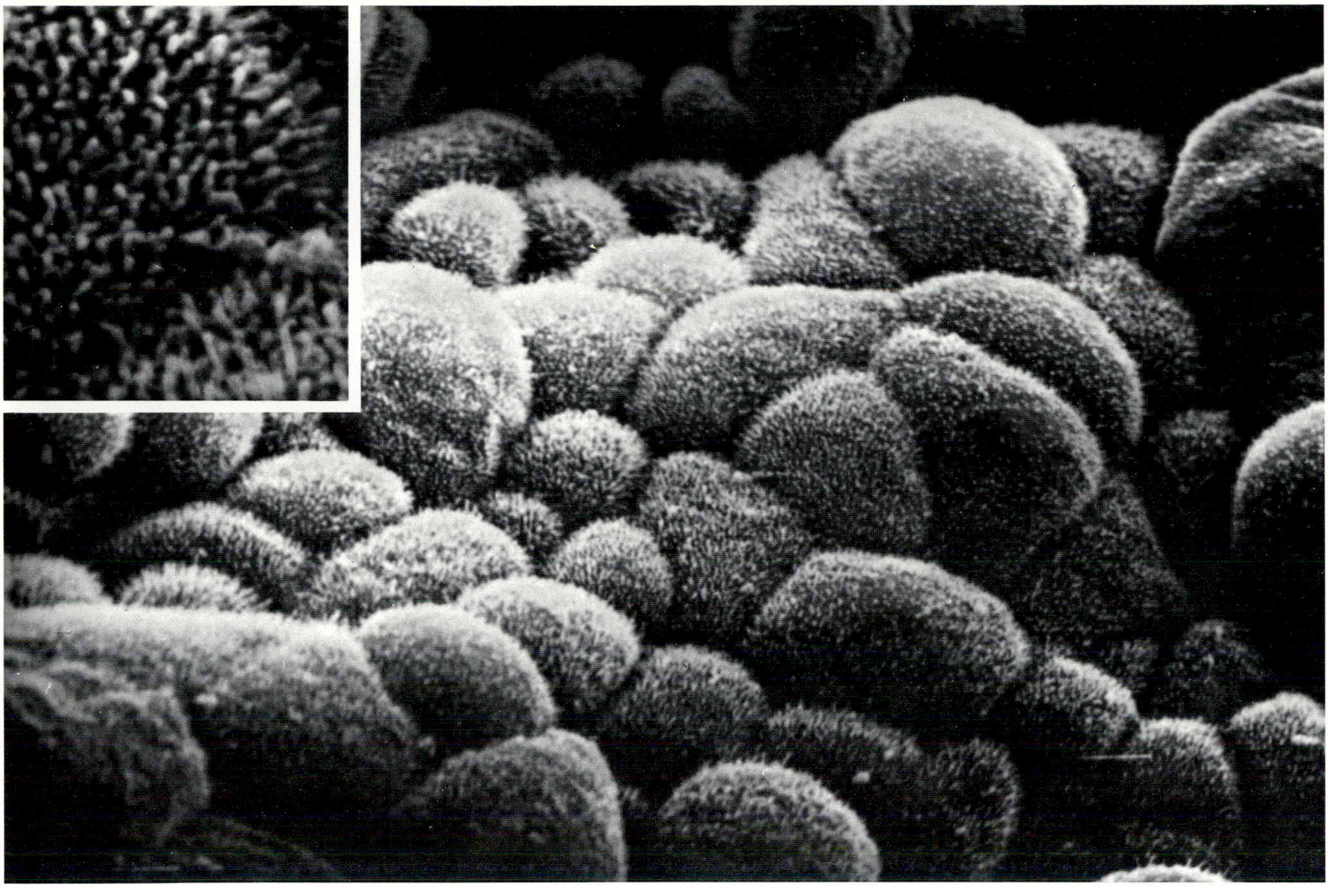

FIG. 7.21. Scanning electron microscopy of the surface of grade 3 CIN. Note cellular disorganization, pleomorphism, and bulging microvillous surface membranes and lack of intercellular terminal bars. ×2280. *Inset:* Higher magnification of tightly packed surface microvilli. ×9120.

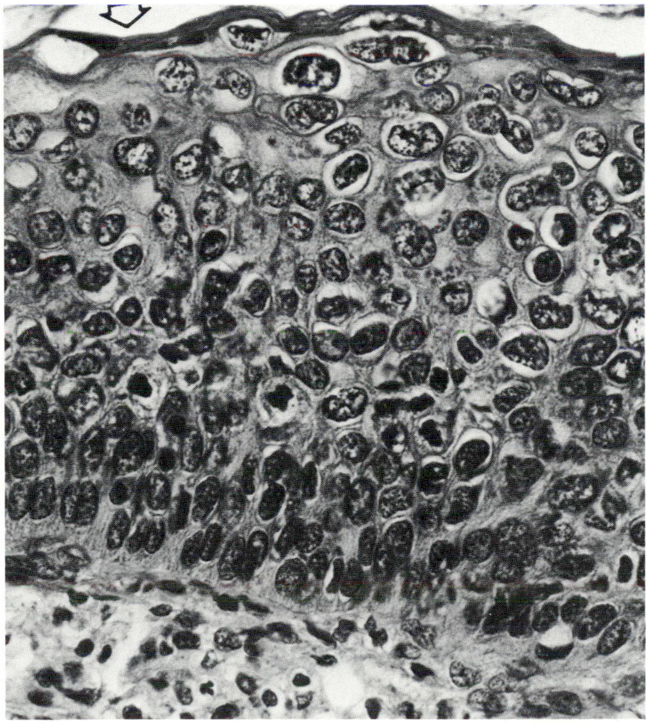

FIG. 7.22. Large cell keratinizing CIN 3. Note cellular prominence, well-defined cytoplasmic membranes, occasional koilocytes, and fine surface keratinization (*arrow*).

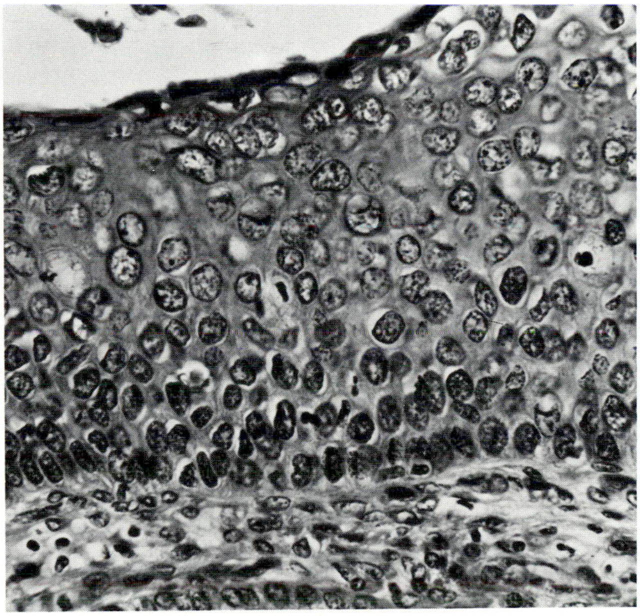

FIG. 7.23. Large cell nonkeratinizing CIN 3. The neoplastic cells have hyperchromatic nuclei with clumping of chromatin. There is a high degree of cellular disorderliness, and cytoplasmic membranes are indistinct.

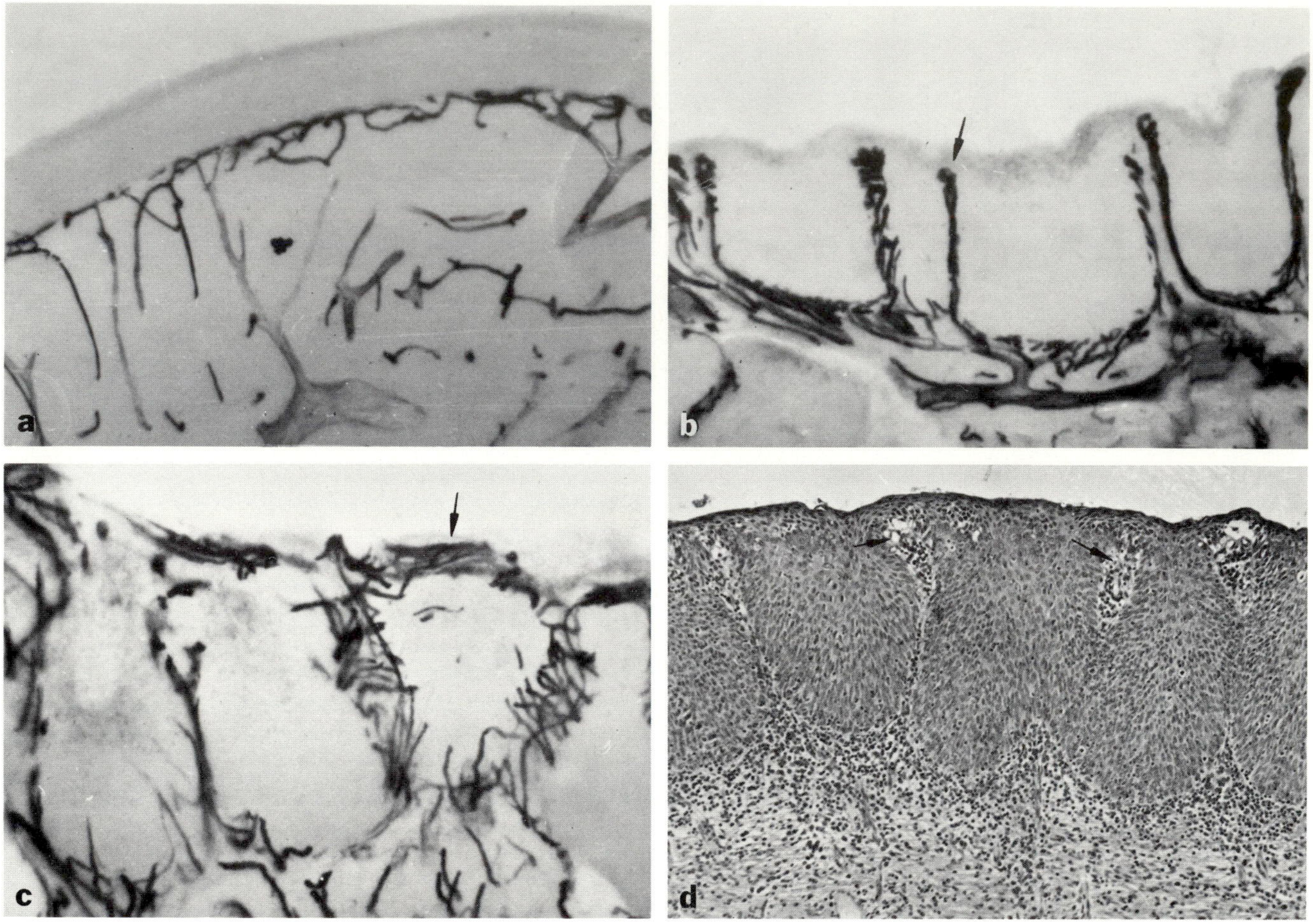

FIG. 7.24. Histochemical preparations of the terminal vascular network of the cervix. *a*. Flat capillary network beneath normal squamous epithelium. *b*. Abnormal vascular growth (*arrow*) in advanced CIN, producing colposcopic mosaic pattern. *c*. Abnormal horizontal vascular pattern (*arrow*) in early invasive carcinoma of cervix. *d*. Histology of CIN 3, in which the vascular stromal papillae are compressed vertically by masses of neoplastic cells, with extension near the surface (*arrows*) producing a colposcopic pattern of punctation. (Courtesy of Dr. A. Stafl, Milwaukee.)

or atrophic epithelium further diminishes the diagnostic usefulness of involucrin.

Epithelial membrane antigen (EMA), a marker of columar and transitional epithelia, is expressed in CIN and in squamous carcinoma but is absent from normal squamous epithelium.[6,219] Similarly, carcinoembryonic antigen (CEA) can be detected in CIN and squamous cell carcinoma but is absent from normal squamous epithelium.[25,86] Positivity of EMA and CEA in immature metaplasia limits their diagnostic usefulness, however.[6,25,86] Newly synthesized heterologous and monoclonal antisera to CIN and cervical carcinoma are potentially useful and are currently being studied.

Ploidy Level Analysis

One of the more successful techniques for the evaluation of cervical epithelial lesions has been nuclear DNA content analysis. Initial studies of CIN by chromosomal karyotyping showed that these lesions, at all maturational levels, had aneuploid patterns similar to those in invasive cervical carcinoma.[100] The techniques of Feulgen microspectrophotometry and computerized image analysis have expanded on these early studies, providing clinicopathologic evidence for the definition of aneuploid CIN lesions as cervical cancer precursors.[66,237] Lesion ploidy level, as estimated from the distributional histogram of nuclear DNA content, has been shown to be a fairly accurate predictor of biologic behavior of cervical epithelial abnormalities.[65,66,69] In a prospective study by Fu et al.,[67] it was found that 100% of lesions that progressed were aneuploid, as were 95% of lesions that persisted. Diploid or polyploid lesions, on the other hand, regressed in 91% of patients and persisted in only 9%. In a retrospective analysis,[66] of 40 lesions that clinically regressed, 85% were diploid or polyploid and 15% were aneuploid. Of 65 lesions that persisted for 1 year or longer, 92% had an aneuploid histogram, whereas only 8% had a

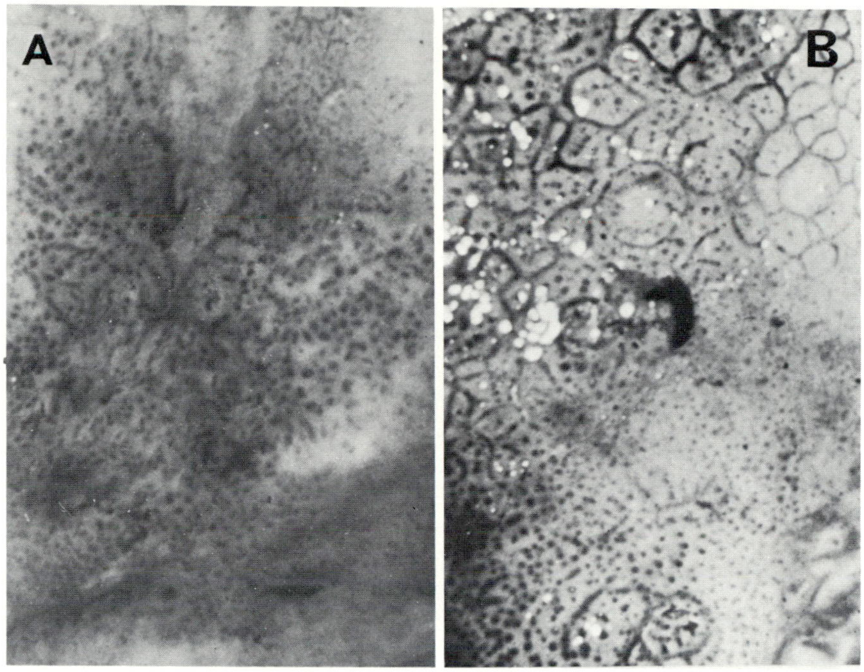

FIG. 7.25. Cervical intraepithelial neoplasia. *A*. Colposcopic pattern of punctation. Note variation in size of punctate vessels and intercapillary distance. *B*. Colposcopic pattern of mosaic. The epithelium is compartmentalized into irregular baskets and is associated with a coarse punctation pattern.

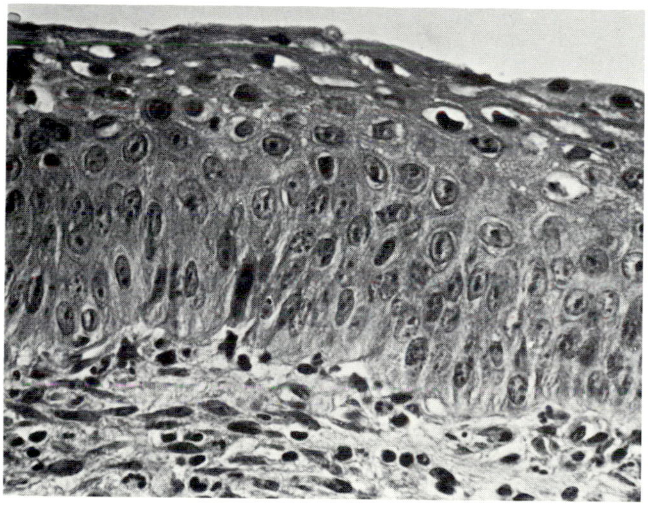

FIG. 7.26. Atypia of repair. Note disorganization in normal maturation. Atypical basal cells occupy the lower half of the epithelium, simulating CIN 2 lesion with koilocytosis. Unlike CIN, however, the basal cells in atypia of repair have a regular nuclear outline, prominent nucleoli, and distinct cell membranes. Additionally, cells in the upper half of the epithelium are not koilocytotic but contain degenerative perinuclear elliptoid-shaped halos.

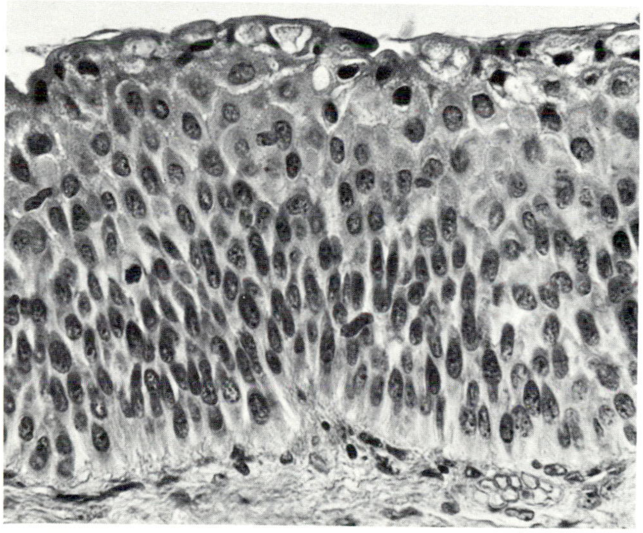

FIG. 7.27. Immature squamous metaplastic epithelium of the transformation zone. The newly formed cells proliferate beneath the mucinous endocervical cells. These may be confused with koilocytes; however, their vacuolar features are due to mucinous–vacuolar degeneration secondary to their separation from the basal lamina rather than papillomavirus infection. Note hyperplasia of basal cells, with occasional mitotic divisions and attempt at cytoplasmic maturation in the upper half of the epithelium. The cells in the upper strata of the epithelium are regularly orientated, with uniformly disposed nuclear chromatin and cellular borders. Intercellular bridges are well defined.

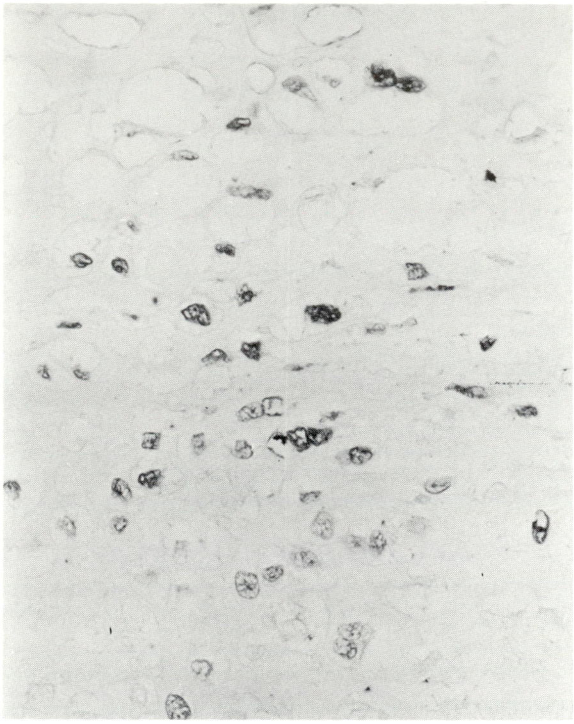

FIG. 7.28. Cervical condyloma stained with immunoperoxidase technique using antibody to HPV DNA extracted from plantar wart. Note positive reaction in darkly staining nuclei of koilocytes.

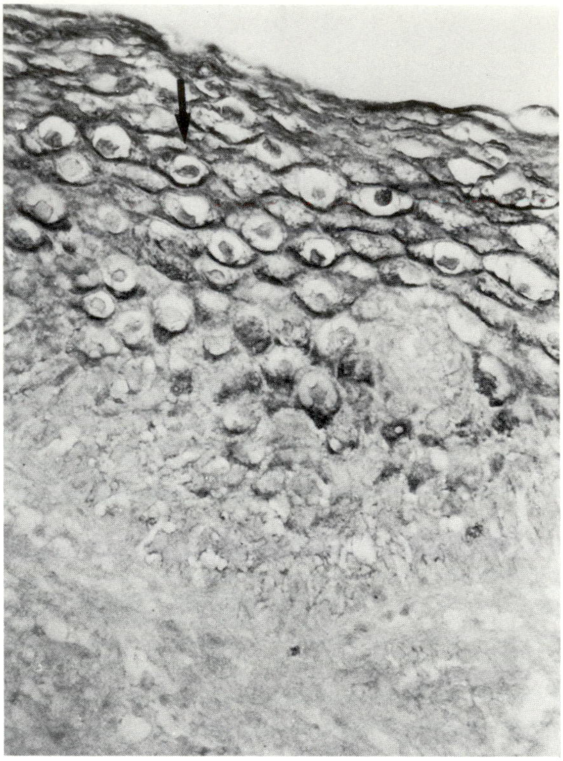

FIG. 7.29. Cervical condyloma stained with anti-involucrin. Arrow points to peripheral staining pattern. (Courtesy of Michael J. Warhol, M.D., Boston.)

diploid or polyploid pattern. Of 8 lesions that progressed to invasive carcinoma, 100% were aneuploid on the original biopsy specimens. Application of these techniques to koilocytotic lesions of the cervix has yielded results that corroborate ploidy level as a useful clinical marker. The vast majority of ordinary condylomas have a diploid or polyploid DNA pattern.[51,67,69,160,192] In contrast, CIN lesions, regardless of their grade and extent of koilocytosis, are generally aneuploid.[51,67,160] Further correlative studies between histologic features and ploidy histograms have defined the presence of morphologically abnormal mitotic figures (AMF) to be one of the most reliable histologic criteria for lesional aneuploidy (Fig. 7.30). This is also true for lesions with extensive koilocytosis of the very well differentiated CIN 1 type.[67,69,241] For example, a lesion with extensive koilocytosis but with a few to several aneuploid type nuclei and abnormal mitotic figures (other than tripolars or dispersed metaphases) is considered to be CIN 1 rather than an ordinary condyloma.

Analysis of ploidy distribution can also be used to identify nonneoplastic atypias of the cervix other than HPV infection and to differentiate them from CIN. These include the reparative atypias, immature squamous metaplasia associated with inflammation, infectious cervicitis, and atrophy. All these conditions have polyploid DNA patterns.

Feulgen microspectrophotometry has not been used as a routine diagnostic tool because it is so labor intensive, time consuming, and expensive. Advances in computerized image analysis have allowed for more rapid, less laborious analyses. They may provide a mechanism for routine diagnostic testing of lesion nuclear DNA content as equipment costs decrease and processing is streamlined.

Molecular Hybridization for Human Papillomavirus Typing

Recent studies have suggested that the genital HPV types have differing oncogenic potentials and that specific types may serve as markers for neoplasia.[39,73–77,125] Crum et al.[40] analyzed 23 koilocytotic lesions of the cervix for HPV 6/11, 16, and 18 by molecular hybridization. HPV 16 was identified in 7 of 10 CIN (with koilocytosis) with abnormal mitotic figures and in only 1 of 13 ordinary condylomas.[40] Similarly, HPV 16 was identified in 29 of 31 CIN lesions and in 0 of 22 ordinary condylomas, whereas HPV types 6/11 were detected in 10 of 22

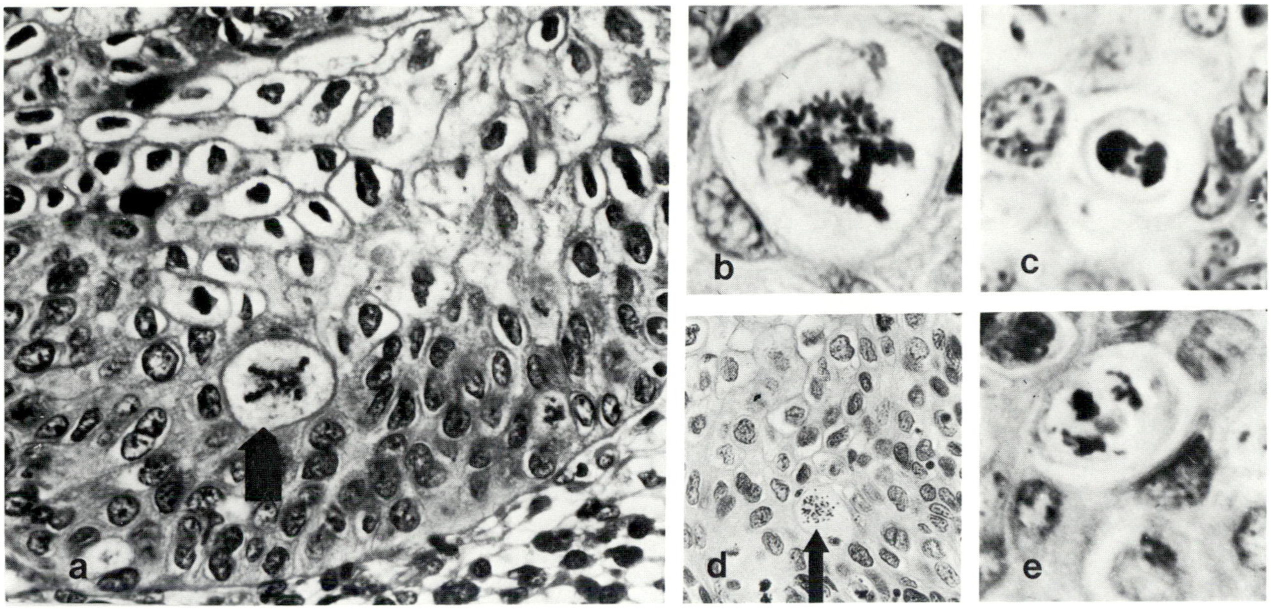

FIG. 7.30. Morphologic variability of abnormal mitotic figures in aneuploid CIN lesions. *a*. Quadripolar mitotic figure (*arrow*) in a lesion with extensive koilocytosis. *b*. Bizarre mitotic figure with Y shape and numerous poorly organized chromosomes. *c*. Two group metaphase. *d*. Dispersed mitotic figure (*arrow*) with finely distributed chromosomes. *e*. Three group metaphase.

ordinary condylomas.[41] Wagner et al.[225] analyzed 47 cervical lesions and found that 68% of CIN 3 were positive for a mixture of HPV 16 and 18, whereas only 18% of CIN 3 reacted with HPV 6 or 11. These preliminary studies suggest that HPV 16 and, to a lesser extent, HPV 18 may be more closely associated with CIN and may serve as a marker for patients at high risk for malignant progression. HPV 6/11, on the other hand, are most closely associated with ordinary condylomas, which in turn carry a low carcinoma risk potential.

The biologic behavior of mixed HPV-type infections and the significance of HPV types other than 6, 11, 16, and 18 have yet to be studied. At present, molecular hybridization is too time consuming and expensive to be used as a diagnostic tool. Prospective follow-up studies demonstrating the behavior of lesions with different HPV types must be performed. More rapid methods of DNA analysis, such as in situ dot hybridization, may have potential for future routine testing.[38,73,225]

Management of Cervical Intraepithelial Neoplasia

Current management of cervical epithelial abnormalities, including cervical condyloma and CIN, depends on a combination of cytology, colposcopy, and directed biopsy as outlined in Fig. 7.31.[141,142,174] This management protocol provides a logical approach to therapy based on lesion size and distribution regardless of lesion grade. In most instances, treatment is conservative and individualized because leison grade is not a major consideration; the need for therapeutic cervical conization is greatly reduced, as are its attendant complications of bleeding and infection. The primary objectives for the clinician are (1) to rule out invasive cancer, (2) to determine the extent and distribution of noninvasive lesions, and (3) to eradicate the lesion by the easiest, most reliable, and most cost-effective method available, preserving reproductive capacity when possible. These considerations in the therapeutic management of cervical condyloma and CIN are examined in the following sections.

Detection and Diagnosis

Cytology

The cytology of the cervix is described in detail in Chapter 25, Cytology, but certain aspects about cell collection techniques deserve special mention in this chapter. The major goal of cervical cytology is to achieve a high detection rate and a high degree of diagnostic predictability. When these criteria are met, cytology can be used as an important tool in the clinical management of patients with CIN. Previous experience[178] has shown that the most accurate sampling technique combines the use of an aspirator for recovering a specimen from the external

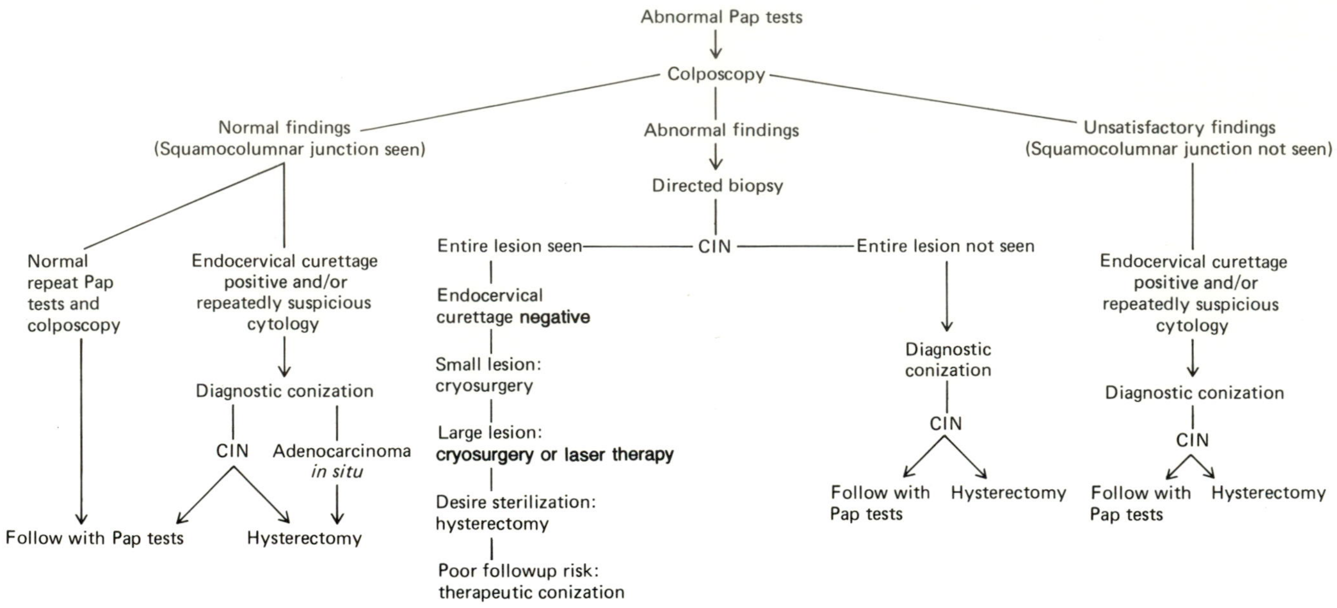

FIG. 7.31. Diagnostic evaluation, treatment, and follow-up of patients with abnormal cytology.

os and a wooden spatula for obtaining a sample from the exposed portion of the cervix (Fig. 7.32). It should be emphasized that a large (25 ml) rubber bulb must be used to provide adequate suction force and that the pipette must have a narrowed tip. The tip of the aspirator is placed at the os, the canal contents are aspirated, and the material obtained is put on a glass slide. By placing the tip of the pipette against the glass slide at a 45° angle and then pressing on the rubber bulb one or more times until the sample is fully recovered. In cases of severe cervical stenosis or dry cervical os, a saline-moistened cotton-tipped applicator can be used instead of a cytopipette. Os aspiration is immediately followed by circumferential scraping of the exposed portion of the cervix with a wooden spatula. The specimen obtained is then gently mixed with the aspiration sample, and the two are evenly smeared on the same glass slide and fixed immediately. When a combination of aspiration and scraping is employed and two or more specimens are obtained over a period of time, the diagnostic accuracy of cytology can reach 98%.[178] When cellular samplings are performed by os aspiration or cervical scraping alone, the diagnostic accuracy is reduced to 93% and 85%, respectively.[178] Cytologic reporting should include a narrative description using diagnostic terminology that corresponds to histologic classification (Table 7.6).[145,174]

Colposcopy

Within the last two decades, colposcopy has been accepted as a complementary technique to exfoliative cytology in the detection of cervical disease and is the current standard of practice in the evaluation of abnormal cytology.[140,174] The colposcope in and of itself is not a diagnostic instrument and must be supplemented by cytology and biopsy to achieve reproducible results. Colposcopy, furthermore, is not a practical screening method for cervical pathology because it is time consuming and expensive, requiring a skilled, experienced clinician for successful performance. However, when colposcopy and cytology are combined to evaluate an abnormal smear, their diagnostic accuracy approaches 100%.[36,203] Physicians without colposcopic training or without access to a skilled pathology laboratory should refer patients for colposcopic consultation. In locales where colposcopic consultation is unavailable, cervical conization remains the preferred management choice.

The colposcope (Fig. 7.33) is a stereoscopic binocular magnifying instrument that provides a three-dimensional image of the tissue surfaces of the vulva, vagina, and cervix. Morphologic modifications of the epithelium that accompany condyloma and intraepithelial neoplasia can, therefore, be visualized and magnified from 4 to 40 times. Application of a 4–5% solution of acetic acid to the surfaces awaiting examination serves to remove mucus and dehydrate cells. In areas with abnormal surface keratinization, epithelial hyperplasia, or nuclear crowding, the abnormal, desiccated mucosa has decreased transparency and appears white (Fig. 7.34). This acetic acid application, or Hinselman test,[88] is essential to the colposcopic procedure. Colposcopic examination of the cervix is limited to the portio and outer third of the endocervical

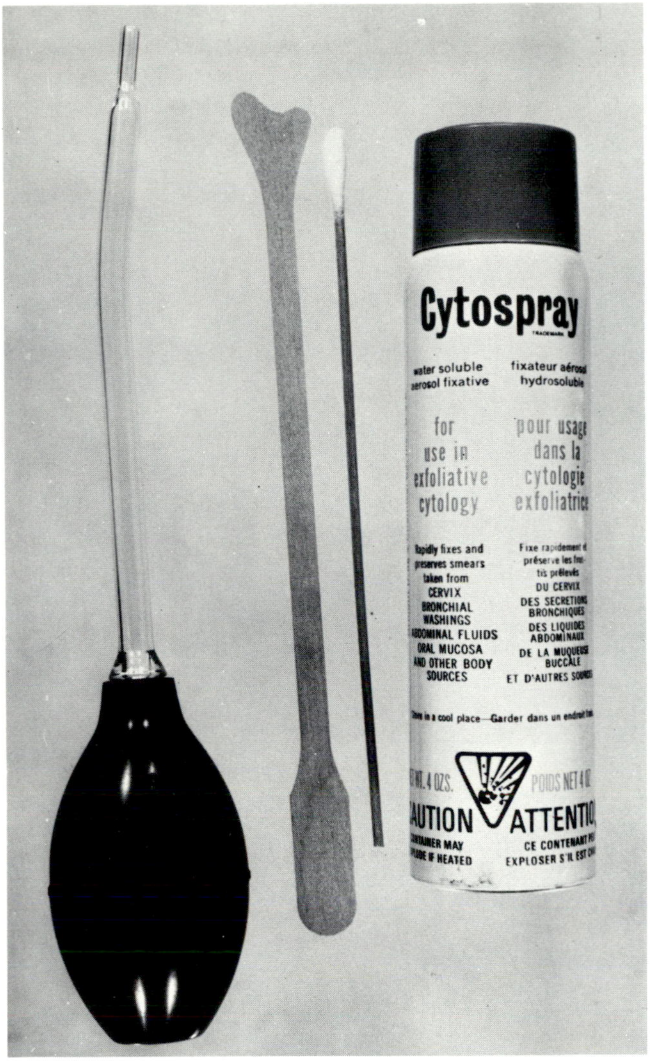

FIG. 7.32. Equipment for exfoliative cervical cytology: endocervical cytopipette, wooden spatula, cotton-tipped applicator, and cytospray fixative.

TABLE 7.6. Nomenclature for histologic reporting of cervical biopsy and endocervical curettings.

Cervical biopsy
  No significant pathologic alterations[a]
  Condyloma
  Cervical intraepithelial neoplasia (CIN) with or without koilocytosis, grade 1, 2, 3
  Microinvasive carcinoma
  Invasive carcinoma
Endocervical curettings
  Fragments of negative endocervix
  Strips of neoplastic squamous epithelium
  Strips of condylomatous epithelium

[a] Includes immature squamous metaplasia, atrophy and repair atypia.

canal and is inadequate for the evaluation of endocervical neoplasms. Pattern recognition in colposcopic diagnosis is based on the evaluation of the surface contour, color tone (degree of opacity), and clarity of demarcation of lesions. Visualization of the subepithelial capillary system allows for additional evaluation of vascular patterns and intercapillary distance.[36,101,203] The most widely used descriptive terminologies for reporting normal and abnormal colposcopic findings are presented in Tables 7.7 through 7.11. Table 7.12 correlates the tissue basis for colposcopic findings. Because of the high resolution capability of the colposcope, the distribution and extent of cervical lesions can be determined accurately and abnormal areas can be selected for directed biopsy.

Staining Tests

Examination of the cervix with the naked eye generally reveals no significant differences between the cervix with CIN and one without a lesion. When a weak aqueous iodine solution is applied to the exposed portion of a normal cervix, the entire mucous membrane stains a deep mahogany brown (iodine-positive or Schiller dark areas) caused by the presence of intracellular glycogen. Areas of clinically normal appearing squamous epithelium that fail to stain (iodine-negative or Schiller light areas) may be composed of neoplastic or metaplastic epithelium, devoid of glycogen (Fig. 7.35). This Schiller test or iodine test is widely used as a tool to aid in the delineation of suspicious areas for biopsy. There are several drawbacks, however, in the application of the Schiller test. These are that not all areas of the cervix that fail to take the iodine represent foci of neoplasia, since columnar epithelium, inflammatory regions, and metaplastic regions also fail to stain with iodine, and a certain number of cases of cervical neoplasia remain iodine positive. Indeed, Richart[167] found that 18% of patients with advanced CIN were iodine positive and 72% were iodine negative. In patients with lower grade CIN lesions, the iodine test failed nearly half the time. In addition, the test failed to detect the actual distribution of CIN in a high proportion of patients. In view of the relatively high false-negative rate of the Schiller test, its use must be combined with considerable clinical experience focusing on the delineation of the limits of the transformation zone because the limits of CIN will be within the limits of that zone. Toluidine blue dye has also been used as a clinical staining procedure, staining dark blue in regions of high nuclear concentration.[166] Although the test yields a comparatively lower false-negative rate than the Schiller test, it suffers from many of the pitfalls of the Schiller test. Other staining tests that have been suggested but have not proved to be of substantial value include acridine orange fluorescence and tetracycline fluorescence.[235]

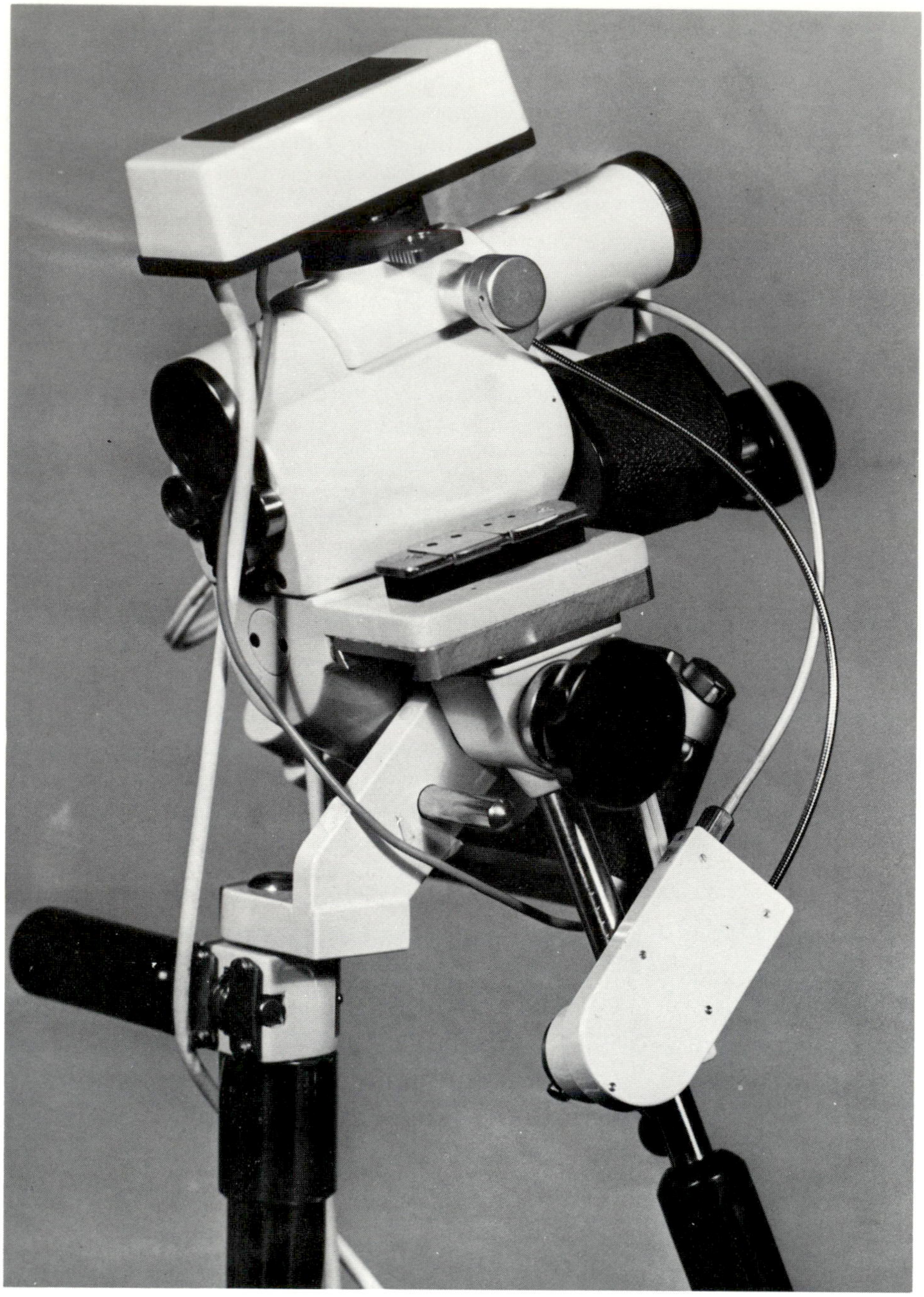

FIG. 7.33. Photograph of a colposcope with a camera attachment for colpophotographs. The basic principle of colposcopy is high-magnification examination of tissue surfaces with bright illumination.

Punch Biopsy

Areas with the most pronounced colposcopic abnormality are delineated and representatively sampled by punch biopsy using a small instrument, such as the square-jawed Kevorkian biopsy punch (Fig. 7.36) (see Chapter 27, Gross Description and Processing of Gynecologic Tissue). Diagnostic histologic terms that are useful to the clinician for the treatment of patients are shown in Table 7.6.

Endocervical Curettage

Endocervical curettage (ECC) is performed to evaluate lesion distribution and morphology within the endocervical canal and to exclude the presence of invasive carcinoma. Endocervical curettage contributes greatly to the diagnostic accuracy of colposcopic evaluation, particularly in patients in whom no exocervical lesion can be visualized or in whom the squamocolumnar junction resides within the endocervical canal.[48,87] Endocervical cu-

TABLE 7.7. Colposcopic terminology.

Normal colposcopic findings
1. Original squamous epithelium
2. Columnar epithelium
3. Normal transformation zone

Abnormal colposcopic findings
1. Abnormal transformation zone
   a. White epithelium
   b. Punctation
   c. Mosaic
   d. Hyperkeratosis
   e. Abnormal blood vessels
2. Suspect invasive cancer

Unsatisfactory colposcopy

Miscellaneous colposcopic findings
1. Vaginocervicitis
2. True erosion
3. Atrophic epithelium
4. Condyloma, papilloma, polyp

rettage should be performed in all patients before outpatient management. It helps also in the post treatment follow-up to evaluate the presence of persistent or recurrent disease.[87] The endocervical curettage specimen consists of endocervical tissue fragments, blood, mucus, and when positive, strips of neoplastic epithelium (Fig. 7.37).

TABLE 7.8. Normal colposcopic findings.

1. Original (native) squamous epithelium
   A smooth, pink membrane that has originally been established on the cervix and vagina. There is no evidence of columnar epithelium, such as mucus-secreting epithelium, gland openings, or nabothian cysts, within or underneath native squamous epithelium.
2. Columnar epithelium
   Mucus-producing and extends between the endometrium cranially and the squamous epithelium caudally. The columnar epithelium has irregular surface with long stromal papillae and deep clefts. After application of acetic acid, it has a typical grape-like appearance. Columnar epithelium may be present in the endocervix, on the portio, or even in the vagina.
3. Transformation zone
   The area between the original squamous epithelium and columnar epithelium in which squamous epithelium in varying degrees of maturation is identified. The squamous epithelium, unlike its native counterpart, is acquired in the process of reepithelialization of previously everted endocervical columnar epithelium. Components of a normal transformation zone may be islands of columnar epithelium surrounded by squamous epithelium, gland openings, and nabothian cysts. In normal transformation zones, there are no colposcopic findings suggestive of CIN.

TABLE 7.9. Abnormal colposcopic findings.

1. Atypical transformation zone
   A transformation zone in which there are colposcopic findings suggestive of condyloma or cervical neoplasia
   a. White epithelium
      A focal area that is seen only after application of acetic acid. The white epithelium is a transient phenomenon that is seen in areas of increased nuclear density.
   b. Punctation
      A focal area in which the capillaries have a stippled pattern.
   c. Mosaic
      A focal area in which the epithelium has been compartmentalized into a mosaic pattern by blood vessels containing stromal papillae.
   d. Hyperkeratosis or parakeratosis
      Appears as elevated whitened plaque seen before the application of acetic acid.
   e. Abnormal blood vessels
      Irregular vessels with abrupt courses appearing as commas, corkscrew capillaries, or spaghetti-like forms.

TABLE 7.10. Miscellaneous colposcopic findings.

1. Vaginocervicitis
   Diffuse, regular punctation.
2. True erosion
   An area denuded of epithelium, usually by trauma.
3. Atrophic epithelium
   An estrogen-deprived squamous epithelium in which the vascular pattern is more readily identified due to the relative thinness of the overlying squamous epithelium.
4. Condyloma, papilloma, polyps
   Exophytic or flat lesions that may be inside or outside the transformation zone. Although papillary or spiked condylomas may be identified colposcopically, flat condylomas cannot be distinguished from CIN 1.

TABLE 7.11. Colposcopic grading (Coppleson).

The atypical transformation zone may be graded in relationship to the quality of the surface appearance. The quality depends on the following:
1. A flat or irregular surface contour
2. A regular or irregular punctation or mosaic pattern
3. Fine or coarse blood vessels
4. The whiteness of epithelium

There are three grades of atypical transformation zone:

Grade 1	Flat epithelium with a regular pattern and fine caliber vessels
Grade 2	Flat, whiter epithelium usually with an irregular pattern and/or coarse caliber vessels
Grade 3	White epithelium with an irregular pattern, coarse caliber and coiled vessels, and an irregular surface contour

TABLE 7.12. Correlation between colposcopy and histology.

Colposcopic terminology	Colposcopic appearance	Histologic correlates
Original squamous epithelium	Smooth, pink with indefinitely outlined vessels; no change after acetic acid application	Squamous epithelium
Columnar epithelium	Grapelike mucosa after acetic acid application	Columnar epithelium
Transformation zone	Tongues of squamous epithelium with gland openings and/or nabothian cysts	Immature to mature squamous stratified epithelium
White epithelium	White, sharp-bordered lesion visible only after acetic acid application; vessels are not visible	From flat condyloma to CIN (grade 1 to grade 3)
Punctation	Sharp-bordered lesion with red stippling; epithelium whiter after acetic acid application	From flat condyloma to CIN (grade 1 to grade 3)
Mosaic	Sharp-bordered lesion with mosaic pattern; epithelium white after acetic acid application	From flat condyloma to CIN (grade 1 to grade 3)
Hyperkeratosis	White patch with rough surface visible before acetic acid application	Usually hyperkeratosis or parakeratosis, sometimes condyloma or CIN
Atypical vessels	Horizontal vessels running parallel with surface; constricted and dilated vessels with atypical branching	From CIN grade 3 to invasive carcinoma

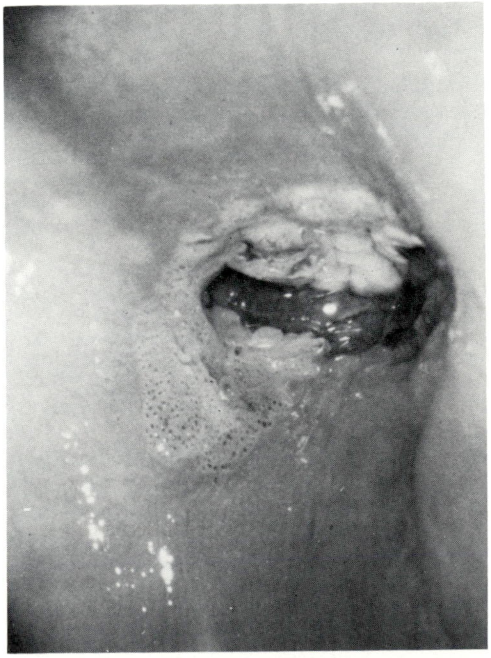

FIG. 7.34. The epithelium around the external cervical os is white with punctation pattern (*lower left*) after the application of 5% acetic acid. The sharply demarcated lesion was CIN 2 with koilocytosis on biopsy.

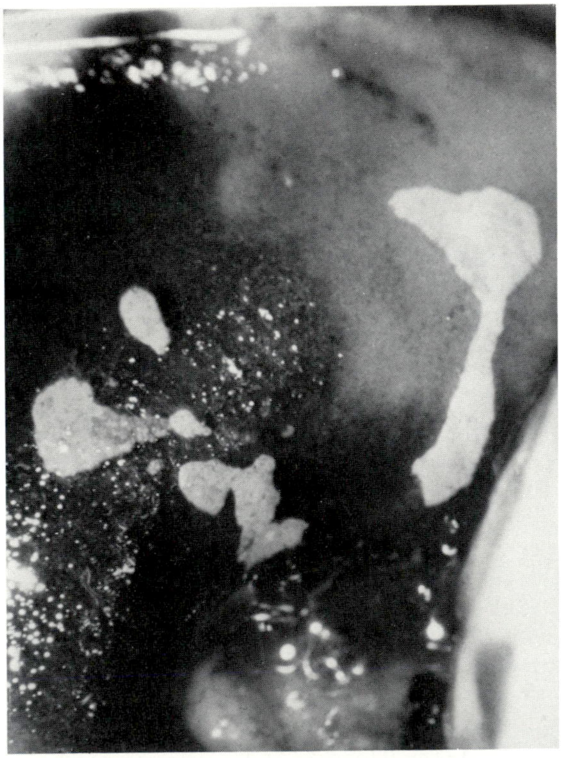

FIG. 7.35. Iodine (Schiller) staining of the cervix. Iodine-negative areas, which appear white in this photograph, are sharply circumscribed, flat lesions contrasting with the surrounding glycogen containing mahogany brown epithelium. (Courtesy of Christopher P. Crum, M.D., New York.)

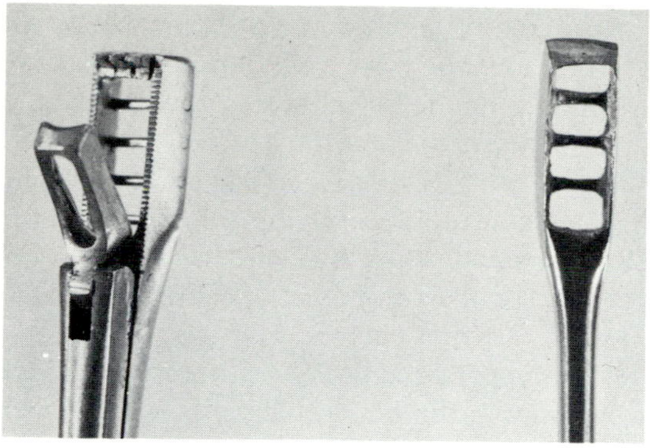

Fig. 7.36. Kevorkian cervical biopsy punch and endocervical curette. *Left:* The rectangular jawed biopsy punch has shallow penetration into the cervical stroma, resulting in little discomfort for the patient, and the tissue removed has straight edges, facilitating orientation. The curette is rectangular with sharp edges.

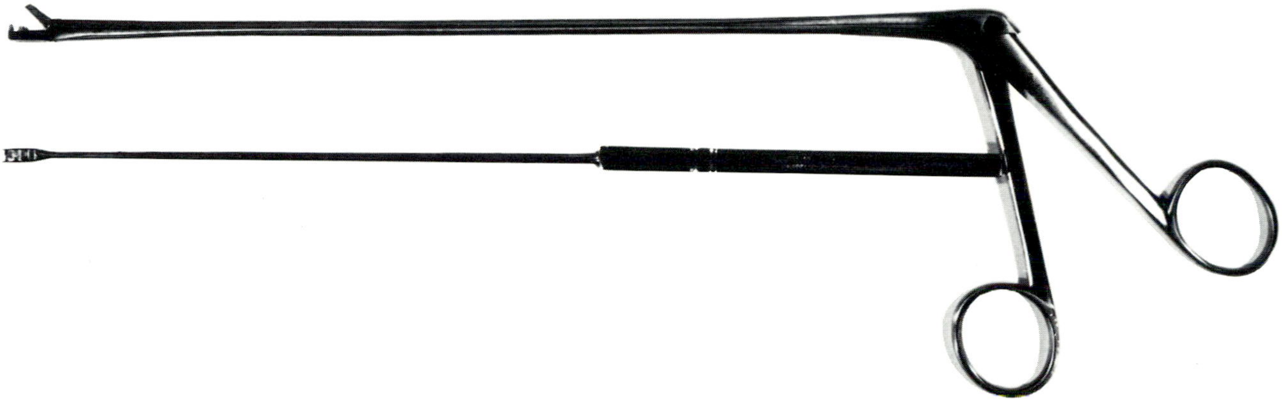

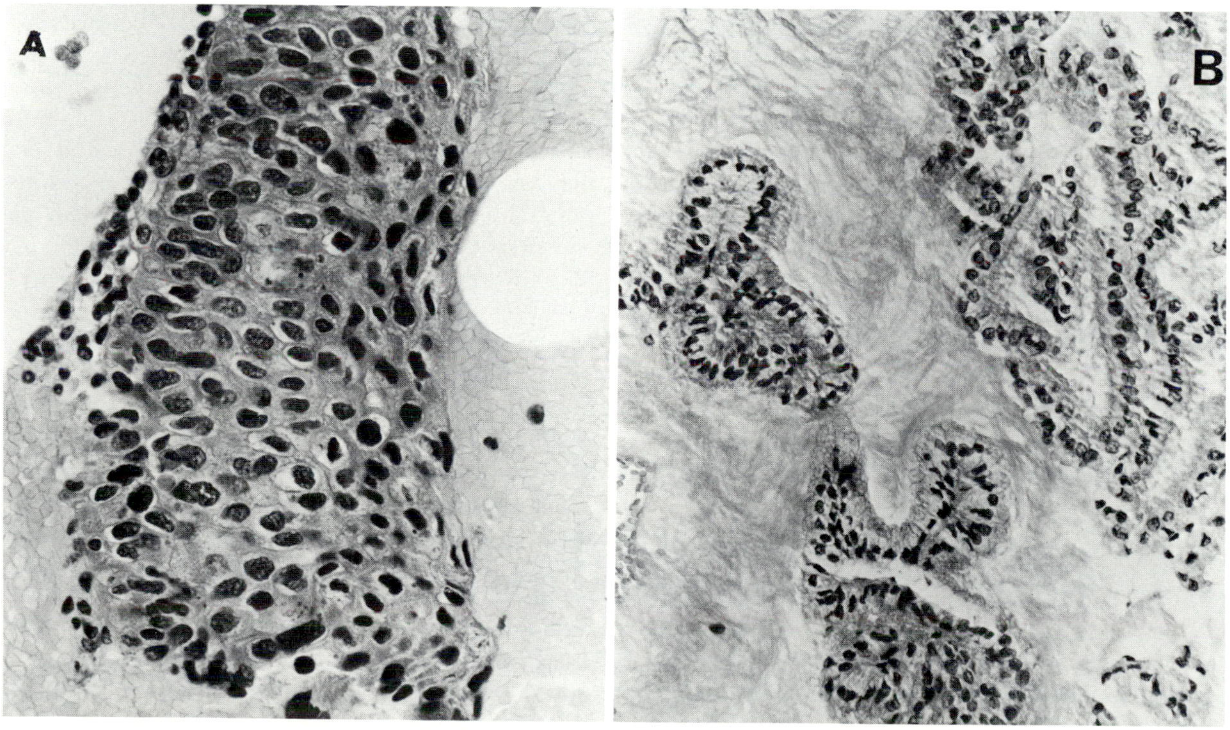

Fig. 7.37. Endocervical curettings. *A*. Positive endocervical curettings with a strip of neoplastic squamous epithelium. The latter lacks orientation and underlying stroma. As a result, grading cannot be performed, and the possibility of an associated (underlying) lesion cannot be ruled out. *B*. Negative endocervical curettings with fragments of endocervical epithelium.

In most instances, the neoplastic epithelium lacks underlying stroma and orientation is therefore not possible. As a result, the pathologist can neither rule out underlying invasion nor grade appropriately the neoplastic process. Even in cases where the neoplastic epithelium is well oriented, grading of CIN has no relevance to the management of the patient. Whether the patient has CIN 1, 2, or 3 or still condylomatous epithelium in the ECC, she must receive a diagnostic conization to rule out associated invasive disease. If the cone contains only noninvasive lesion, it may be considered therapeutic as well. Consequently, the most appropriate term indicating to the clinician to proceed with a diagnostic cone is *strips of neoplastic or condylomatous squamous epithelium* (see Table 7.6). If the clinician bases management on grades and considers CIN 1 a clinically unimportant lesion, a CIN 1 diagnosis in an ECC may not necessarily lead to a diagnostic conization. Instead, the patient may either be followed or treated on an outpatient basis and may run the risk of developing invasive disease in the endocervical canal. When an ECC contains *only a few fragments of neoplastic epithelium,* it is preferable to reexamine the patient with the colposcope than to proceed directly with conization. In many such cases, the ECC has inadvertently been contaminated by CIN with limited extension to the endocervical canal, and its limits are fully visible. A second, carefully performed ECC usually yields no neoplastic tissue and the patient may be managed on a conservative, outpatient basis. In order to avoid the loss of tiny tissue fragments during processing, the clinician should collect and concentrate the sample, including mucus and blood, on a small square of lens paper and immediately place it in the fixative. By this method, even the smallest tissue fragments can be recovered easily in the laboratory, embedded, and sectioned in entirety.

Treatment

Following colposcopic examination patients are placed into three major management triage groups: (1) patients with normal colposcopic findings, (2) patients with abnormal colposcopic findings, and (3) patients with unsatisfactory colposcopic findings (see Table 7.7).

Patients with Normal Colposcopy Findings

In this group the squamocolumnar junction is fully visible, and there is no colposcopic evidence of cervical, vaginal, or vulvar lesions (see Table 7.8). When there is no evidence of disease on repeat smears, colposcopy, and endocervical curettage, the patient should be followed cytologically every 3–4 months for 1 year and, if smears remain negative, yearly thereafter. Review of the original abnormal smear should be done to determine the nature of the referral abnormality. Patients with reactive atypia may benefit from a workup for infectious cervicitis, including endocervical cultures. A diagnostic conization is indicated in women with abnormal colposcopic findings when (1) the endocervical curettage contains strips of neoplastic or condylomatous epithelium and (2) cytology remains positive and is unexplained by cervical–vaginal–vulvar colposcopy or the penile status of the patient's sexual partner. (Invasive squamous cell carcinoma of the penis has occasionally been detected by cervical cytology in the female sexual partner.)

Patients with Abnormal Colposcopy Findings

If there is no cytologic, histologic, or colposcopic evidence of invasion and the lesion is confined to the exocervix with a negative endocervical curettage (see Table 7.9), the patient may be managed effectively with local ablative therapy on an outpatient basis. This may be electrocauterization,[216] cryosurgery,[16,95,216] or carbon dioxide laser therapy.[4,55,204] The patients are followed with triannual cytology for the first year to rule out persistent disease and annually thereafter to detect recurrent disease.

Cryosurgery is one of the most frequently used techniques for lesions limited to the portio. The failure or residual rate (5–10%) and the long-term recurrence rate (1 of 1000 women per year develops a new CIN following successful cryotherapy) in experienced hands do not exceed that of therapeutic conization.[95,216] Cure rates are not affected by the grade of the lesion treated, with only lesion size and quality of freeze proving to be prognostic variables of statistical significance.[2,55] Furthermore, complications and costs of cryosurgery are negligible compared to those of conization. Cryosurgery is preferable to electrocautery because it is less painful and does not interfere with fertility.[177,230] Cryoinjury to cervical tissue is caused by freezing tissue below −22°C with a cryoprobe applied to the cervix. Intracellular and extracellular crystallization leads to dehydration of cells. This results in high electrolyte concentrations that produce biochemical injury associated with lysosomal enzyme release and cell destruction. The only significant endpoint for successful cryosurgical management of CIN is that the margins of the iceball extend 5 mm and preferably 10 mm beyond the limits of the lesion. Postcryotherapy cervical epithelium quickly sloughs, and healing is generally completed within approximately 12 weeks.

The carbon dioxide (CO_2) laser (the term *laser* is an abbreviation for *l*ight *a*mplification by *s*timulated *e*mission of *r*adiation) is the newest treatment modality for noninvasive neoplasms of the cervix, vagina and vulva. Unlike conventional light, which is emitted in all directions and has a low energy, laser light is composed of parallel beams of uniform wave lengths (10.6 μm). As a result, the laser beam can be directed onto a small spot, where it produces a very high-energy density. In the CO_2 laser, a mixture of CO_2, nitrogen, and helium is excited by an electrical discharge, and the excited CO_2 molecules give off photons of light energy in the infrared (invisible) part of the spectrum. The light energy is amplified, focused, and directed by a luminous spot of the target beam. Energy output ranges from 1 to 100 W. The laser beam energy is absorbed by the intracellular and extracellular water in tissues, and tissue temperatures rise instantaneously above 100°C. The tissue fluids boil and expand, and the exploded cells are evaporated. As a result, CO_2 laser treatment produces considerably less necrosis than cryosurgery. Evaporation of tissues permits more rapid healing without scarring and less vaginal discharge than is associated with cryosurgery.[204] The failure and recurrence rates of laser treatment of cervical lesions are similar to those of cryosurgery.[4,204,216] The expensive equipment cost is its major disadvantage when compared to cryotherapy.[5,216] Extensive cervical lesions and associated vaginal or vulvar lesions can be more easily and appropriately treated by laser surgery than by cryotherapy.[55]

If the patient has colposcopic evidence of an exocervical lesion that extends into the endocervical canal and the limits of the lesion cannot be visualized with the colposcope, a diagnostic conization should always be performed. If the disease in the conization specimen is not invasive, the patient may be followed cytologically every 3–4 months for the first year and once a year thereafter, so long as the smears remain negative.

Patients with Unsatisfactory Colposcopy

These are patients in whom the squamocolumnar junction is not fully visible and in whom one cannot exclude colposcopically the possibility of a lesion higher in the endocervical canal. In these patients, a diagnostic conization is indicated. If the diagnostic cone obtained from patients with either normal or unsatisfactory colposcopic findings contains CIN, the patients may be followed with repeated Papanicolaou smears, colposcopy, and endocervical curettage. In patients with a histologic diagnosis of invasive carcinoma, the treatment will depend on the stage of the disease, including hysterectomy, radical surgery, radiotherapy, and chemotherapy (see Chapter 8, Cervical Carcinoma).

Cervical Conization

Indications for diagnostic cervical conization are summarized in Table 7.13. Using the management protocol previously described, the use of diagnostic conization can be avoided in 95% of nonpregnant and 99% of pregnant patients.[46,203] In the absence of evidence of invasive carcinoma, the selection of cervical conization should be carefully considered in light of lesion size and distribution and should not be a knee-jerk reaction to a diagnosis of CIN 3 or carcinoma in situ.[16] Bleeding is the main complication of cone biopsy, occurring in approximately 10% of all conization procedures.[93,94] Large cones, greater than 2 cm in height or 4 ml in volume, can be significantly correlated with subsequent spontaneous midtrimester abortion and premature labor.[116] In small cones, cervical stenosis secondary to postoperative scarring may be an additional complication.[116] Vaginal or abdominal hysterectomy with a 5% complication rate has no biologic rationale in the management of CIN. Hysterectomy is the treatment of choice, however, when the patient with CIN has associated endomyometrial pathology, is at high risk for pelvic inflammatory disease, and wants no pregnancies, or CIN extends to the endometrium. The last phenomenon is an extremely rare event, however.[45,58] Even patients with margin involvement on a conization specimen can be managed conservatively and need no hysterectomy as long as invasive cancer is not a differential consideration.[200] Postconization healing frequently dislodges small foci of residual neoplasia and results in effective cure. The incidence of residual neoplasia in hysterectomy specimens subsequent to conization is less than 10%.[200] Postconization follow-up with cytology and endocervical curettage serves as a reliable means to identify recurrent or residual neoplasia and reduces the need for immediate hysterectomy. Recurrence rates in patients treated by cervical conization range from 5 to 7%.[15]

A cervical conization specimen represents a conically shaped section of cervix performed for both diagnostic and therapeutic purposes. The cone size varies according to lesion distribution and corresponding operative plan: a shallow conization for a predominantly exocervical lesion or a deep cone for a predominantly endocervical lesion. The apex and base of the sample represent the endocervical and exocervical margins, respectively. The technique for processing the specimen is discussed in

TABLE 7.13. Indications for diagnostic cervical conization.

Normal colposcopy,[a] persistent abnormal cytology or positive endocervical curettage
Abnormal cytology, squamocolumnar junction not visualized
Limits of lesion not visualized
Microinvasive carcinoma on biopsy or colposcopy suspicious of invasive carcinoma
Adenocarcinoma in situ on biopsy or endocervical curettage
Lack of correlation among cytologic, colposcopic, and histologic findings[b]

[a] Including the vagina, vulva, and urethra.
[b] Includes condyloma/CIN and invasive carcinoma, i.e., condyloma on cytology and histology, invasion on colposcopy or invasion by cytology, CIN on histology and colposcopy.

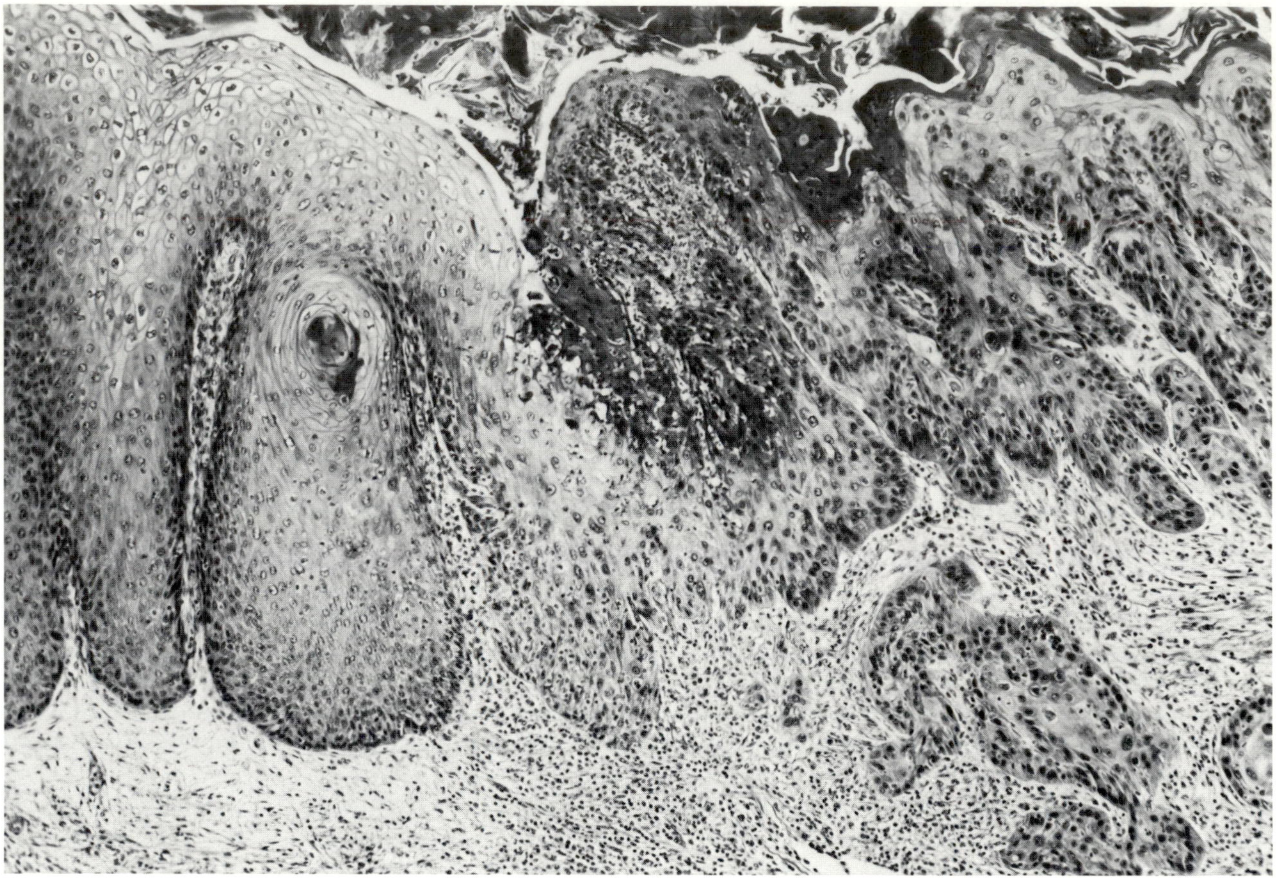

FIG. 7.38. Invasive carcinoma arising in a cervical condyloma. The epithelium on the left is a typical condyloma with bland cytology and minimal pleomorphism and was the only portion of this lesion visible on the exocervix. On the right, an invasive carcinoma arising within the condyloma is present. [Reprinted by permission of Baggish (ed.), Ref. 239]

Chapter 27, Gross Description and Processing of Gynecologic Tissue.

Management of Cervical Condyloma

The rationale underlying the removal of cervical condyloma is twofold: (1) to prevent the spread of a highly infectious sexually transmitted disease and (2) to diminish the risk (presumably low) of progression to CIN and invasive cancer. Management protocols for cervical condyloma are similar to those outlined for CIN. Cure rates for cryosurgical and laser treatment of cervical condylomas appear to be comparable to those for CIN. They are enhanced by treating penile lesions in the male partner simultaneously. The use of barrier methods of contraception may be effective to prevent reinfection.[164,243] In women with condylomatous endocervical involvement, cervical conization is indicated, as with CIN, to rule out associated invasive carcinoma (Fig. 7.38).

References

1. Antonio DA, Fu YS, Warhol M, et al. (1983) Multifactorial approach to the detection of cervical squamous cell dysplasia. Lab Invest 48: 4A
2. Arof HM, Gerbie MV, Smeltzer J (1984) Cryosurgical treatment of cervical intraepithelial neoplasia: Four-year experience. Am J Obstet Gynecol 150: 865
3. Aurelian L (1976) Sexually transmitted cancers? The case for genital herpes. J Am Vener Dis Assoc 2: 10
4. Baggish MS (1980) High-power density carbon dioxide laser therapy for early cervical neoplasia. Am J Obstet Gynecol 136: 117
5. Baggish MS (1981) Complications associated with carbon dioxide laser surgery in gynecology. Am J Obstet Gynecol 139: 568
6. Bamford PN, Ormerod MG, Sloane JP, Warburton MJ (1983) An immunohistochemical study of the distribution of epithelial antigens in the uterine cervix. Obstet Gynecol 61: 603
7. Baram A, Schacter A (1982) Cervical carcinoma: Disease of the future for Jewish women. Lancet 1: 747

8. Barron BA, Richart RM (1968) A statistical model of the natural history of cervical carcinoma based on a prospective study of 557 cases. J Natl Cancer Inst 41: 1343
9. Barron BA, Richart RM (1970) A statistical model of the natural history of cervical carcinoma. II. Estimates of the transition time from dysplasia to carcinoma in situ. J Natl Cancer Inst 45: 1025
10. Barron BA, Cahill MC, Richart RM (1978) A statistical model of the natural history of cervical neoplastic disease: The duration of carcinoma in situ. Gynecol Oncol 6: 196
11. Benedictis TJ, Marmar JL, Praiss DE (1977) Intraurethral condylomata acuminata management and review of the literature. J Urol 118: 767
12. Berkowitz RS, Ehrmann RL, Lavizzo-Mourey R, Knapp RC (1979) Invasive cervical carcinoma in young women. Gynecol Oncol 8: 311
13. Binder MA, Cates GW, Emson HE, et al. (1985) The changing concepts of condyloma. A retrospective study of colposcopically directed cervical biopsies. Am J Obstet Gynecol 151: 213
14. Boon ME, Fox CH (1981) Simultaneous condyloma acuminatum and dysplasia of the uterine cervix. Acta Cytol 25: 393
15. Boyes DA, Fidler HK, Lock DR (1963) The significance of in situ carcinoma of the uterine cervix. In : Proceedings of the First International Congress of Exfoliative Cytology. Philadelphia, J.B. Lippincott
16. Bryson SCP, Lenehan, P, Lickrish GM (1985) The treatment of grade 3 cervical intraepithelial neoplasia with cryosurgery: An 11-year experience. Am J Obstet Gynecol 151: 201
17. Buckley CH, Butler EB, Fox H (1982) Cervical intraepithelial neoplasia. J Clin Pathol 35: 1
18. Buckley CH, Butler EB, Fox H (1983) Cervical intraepithelial neoplasia. Lancet 1: 1389
19. Buckley JD, Doll R, Harris RWC, et al. (1981) Case control study of the husbands of women with dysplasia or carcinoma of the cervix uteri. Lancet 2: 1010
20. Bullough WS, Laurence EB (1967) Epigenetic mitotic control. In: Tier H, Rytomaa T (eds). Control of Cellular Growth in Adult Organisms. New York, Academic Press, pp 28–40
21. Burghart E (1973) Early histological diagnosis of cervical cancer, 1st ed. Philadelphia, W.B. Saunders Co.
22. Burghart E, Ostor AG (1983) Site and origin of squamous cervical cancer: A histomorphologic study. Obstet Gynecol 62: 117
23. Burnett TS, Gallimore PH (1982) Personal communication, Cold Spring Harbor, N.Y.
24. Butterworth CE, Hatch KD, Gore H, et al. (1982) Improvement in cervical dysplasia associated with folic acid therapy in users of oral contraceptives. Am J Clin Nutr 35: 73
25. Bychkov V, Rothman M, Bardawil WA (1983) Immunocytochemical localization of carcinoembryonic antigen (CEA), alpha-fetoprotein (AFP) and human chorionic gonadotropin (HCG) in cervical neoplasia. Am J Clin Pathol 79: 414
26. Campion MJ, Singer A, Clarkson PK, McCance DJ (1985) Increased risk of cervical neoplasia in consorts of men with penile condylomata acuminata. Lancet 1: 943
27. Cartwright RA, Sinson JD (1981) Carcinoma of penis and cervix. Lancet 1: 97
28. Casas-Cordero M, Morin C, Roy M, et al. (1981) Origin of the koilocyte in condylomata of the human cervix. Ultrastructural study. Acta Cytol 25: 383
29. Centers for Disease Control (1983) Morbidity, Mortality Weekly Report 32: 306
30. Cevenini R, Costa S, Rumpanesi F, et al. (1981) Cytological and histopathological abnormalities of the cervix in genital *Chlamydia trachomatis* infections. Br J Vener Dis 57: 334
31. Christopherson WM, Parker JE (1960) A study of the relative frequency of carcinoma of the cervix in the Negro. Cancer 13: 711
32. Clarke EA, Morgan RW, Newman AM (1982) Smoking as a risk factor in cancer of the cervix: Additional evidence from a case control study. Am J Epidemiol 115: 59
33. Clarke EA, Hatcher J, McKeowyn-Eyssen GE, Lickrish GM (1985) Cervical dysplasia: Association with sexual behavior, smoking and oral contraceptive use? Am J Obstet Gynecol 151: 612
34. Coppleson M (1970) The origin and nature of premalignant lesions of the cervix uteri. Int J Gynecol Obstet 8: 539
35. Coppleson M, Reid B (1967) Preclinical carcinoma of the cervix uteri, 1st ed. Oxford, Pergamon Press
36. Coppleson M, Pixley E, Reid B (1971) Colposcopy. A scientific and practical approach to the cervix in health and disease, 1st ed. Springfield, Ill., Charles C Thomas
37. Cramer DW, Cutler SJ (1974) Incidence and histopathology of malignancies of the female genital organs in the United States. Am J Obstet Gynecol 118: 443
38. Croissant O, Bonneaud G, Orth G (1972) Detection of the vegetative viral DNA replication in papillomavirus-induced tumors by in situ molecular hybridization. Cr Acad Sci Paris 274: 614
39. Crum CP, Levine RU (1984) Human papillomavirus infection and cervical neoplasia: New perspectives. Int J Gynecol Pathol 3: 376
40. Crum CP, Ikenberg H, Richart RM, Gissman L (1984) Human papillomavirus type 16 and early cervical neoplasia. N Engl J Med 310: 880
41. Crum CP, Mitao M, Levine RU, Silverstein SJ (1985) Cervical papillomaviruses segregate within morphologically distinct precancerous lesions. J Virol 54: 675
42. Crum CP, Egawa K, Barron B, et al. (1983) Human papillomavirus infection (condyloma) of the cervix and cervical intraepithelial neoplasia: A histological and statistical analysis. Gynecol Oncol 15: 88
43. Crum CP, Egawa K, Fu YS, et al. (1983) Atypical immature metaplasia (AIM): A subset of human papillomavirus infection of the cervix. Cancer 51: 2214
44. Daling JR, Weiss ND, Klopfenstein LL, et al. (1982) Correlates of homosexual behavior and the incidence of anal cancer. JAMA 247: 1988
45. Daniele E, Perino A, Catinella E (1985) Superficial endometrial involvement by cervical intraepithelial neoplasia detected by intrauterine cytology. Acta Cytol 29: 411

46. De Petrillo AD, Townsend DE, Morrow CP, et al. (1975) Colposcopic evaluation of the abnormal Papanicolaou test in pregnancy. Am J Obstet Gynecol 121: 441
47. De Vesa SS (1984) Descriptive epidemiology of cancer of the uterine cervix. Obstet Gynecol 63: 605
48. Drescher CW, Peters WA, Roberts JA (1983) Contribution of endocervical curettage in evaluating abnormal cervical cytology. Obstet Gynecol 62: 343
49. Durst M, Kleinheinz MH, Gissmann L (1985) The physical state of human papillomavirus type 16 DNA in benign and malignant genital tumors. J Gen Virol: 66: 1515
50. Durst M, Gissman L, Ikenberg H, Zur Hausen H (1983) A papillomavirus DNA from a cervical carcinoma and its prevalence in cancer biopsy samples from different geographical regions. Proc Natl Acad Sci USA 80: 3812
51. Evans AS, Monaghan JM (1983) Nuclear DNA content of normal, neoplastic and "wart affected" cervical biopsies. Analyt Quant Cytol 5: 111
52. Fenoglio CM, Ferenczy A (1982) Etiologic factors in cervical neoplasia. Semin Oncol 9: 349
53. Fenoglio CM, Galloway DA, Crum CP, et al. (1981) Herpes simplex virus and cervical neoplasia. In: Fenoglio CM, Wolff M (eds). Progress in Surgical Pathology. New York, Masson, Vol. 4, pp 45–82
54. Ferenczy A (1978) Steroid contraception and cervical and ovarian neoplasia. In: Sciarra JJ, Zatuchni GI, Speidel J (eds). Risks, Benefits and Controversies in Fertility Control. Hagerstown, Maryland, Harper & Row, pp 194–210
55. Ferenczy A (1985) Comparison of cryo- and carbon dioxide laser therapy for cervical intraepithelial neoplasia. Obstet Gynecol 66: 793
56. Ferenczy A, Richart RM (1974) Female reproductive system. Dynamics of Scan and Transmission Electron Microscopy, 1st ed. New York, John Wiley & Sons
57. Ferenczy A, Braun L, Shah KV (1981) Human papillomavirus (HPV) in condylomatous lesions of cervix. Am J Surg Pathol 5: 661
58. Ferenczy A, Richart RM, Okagaki T (1971) Endometrial involvement by cervical carcinoma in situ. Am J Obstet Gynecol 110: 590
59. Ferenczy A, Mitao M, Nagai N, et al. (1985) Latent papillomavirus and recurring genital warts. N Engl J Med 313: 784
60. Fidler HK, Boyes DA, Worth AJ (1968) Cervical cancer detection in British Columbia. J Obstet Gynecol Br Commonw 75: 392
61. Fidler HK, Boyes DA, Nichols TM, Worth AJ (1970) Cervical cytology in the control of cancer of the cervix. Mod Med Can 25: 9
62. Fletcher S (1983) Histopathology of papillomavirus infection of the cervix uteri: The history, toxonomy, nomenclature and reporting of koilocytotic dysplasias. J Clin Pathol 36: 616
63. Fox CH (1967) Biologic behavior of dysplasia and carcinoma in situ. Am J Obstet Gynecol 99: 960
64. Friedell GH, Hertig AT, Younge PA (1960) Carcinoma in Situ of the Uterine Cervix, 1st ed. Springfield, Ill. Charles C Thomas, pp 108–109
65. Fu YS, Reagan JW, Richart RM (1981) Definitions of precursors. Gynecol Oncol 12: S220
66. Fu YS, Reagan JW, Richart RM (1983) Precursors of cervical cancer. Cancer Surv 2: 359
67. Fu YS, Braun L, Shah KV, et al. (1983) Histologic, nuclear DNA, and human papillomavirus studies of cervical condyloma. Cancer 52: 1705
68. Fuchs E, Green H (1980) Changes in keratin gene expression during terminal differentiation of the keratinocyte. Cell 19: 1033
69. Fujii T, Crum CP, Winkler B, et al. (1984) Human papillomavirus infection and cervical intraepithelial neoplasia: Histopathology and DNA content. Obstet Gynecol 63: 99
70. Galloway DA, McDougall JK (1985) The oncogenic potential of herpes simplex viruses: Evidence for a "hit-and-run" mechanism. Nature 302: 21
71. Galloway DA, Fenoglio CM, Shevchuk M, McDougall JK (1979) Detection of herpes simplex RNA in human sensory ganglia. Virology 95: 265
72. Garrett WFH, Murphy J, O'Neil BW, Laird HM (1978) Virus-induced papillomas of the alimentary tract of cattle. Int J Cancer 22: 323
73. Gissmam L (1984) Papillomaviruses and their association with cancer in animals and in man. Cancer Surv 3: 162
74. Gissmam L, Zur Hausen H (1980) Partial characterization of viral DNA from human genital warts (condylomata acuminata). Int J Cancer 25: 605
75. Gissmam L, De Villiers EM, Zur Hausen H (1982) Analysis of human genital warts (condylomata acuminata) and other genital tumors for human papillomavirus type 6 DNA. Int J Cancer 29: 143
76. Gissmam L, Boshart M, Durst M, et al. (1984) Presence of human papillomavirus in genital tumors. J Invest Dermatol 83: 265
77. Gissmam L, Wolnik L, Ikenberg H, et al. (1983) Human papillomavirus types 6 and 11 DNA sequences in genital and laryngeal papillomas and in some cervical cancers. Proc Natl Acad Sci USA 80: 560
78. Graham S (1984) Epidemiology of retinoids and cancer. J Natl Cancer Inst 73: 1423
79. Graham S, Priore R, Graham M, et al. (1979) Genital cancer in wives of penile cancer patients. Cancer 44: 1870
80. Gross G, Ikenberg H, Gissmam L, Hagedorn M (1985) Papillomavirus infection of the anogenital region: Correlation between histology, clinical picture and virus type. Proposal of a new nomenclature. J Invest Dermatol 85: 147
81. Gross G, Pfister H, Hagedorn M, Gissmam L (1982) Correlation between human papillomavirus (HPV) type and histology of warts. J Invest Dermatol 78: 160
82. Guijon FB, Paraskevas M, Brunham R (1985) The association of sexually transmitted diseases with cervical intraepithelial neoplasia: A case-control study. Am J Obstet Gynecol 151: 185
83. Gupta JW, Gupta PK, Shah KV, Kelly DP (1982) Distribution of human papillomavirus antigen in cervicovaginal smears and cervical tissues. Int J Gynecol Pathol 2: 160
84. Handley WS (1936) The prevention of cancer. Lancet 1: 987

85. Hare MJ, Taylor-Robinson D, Cooper P (1982) Evidence for an association between *Chlamydia trachomatis* and cervical intraepithelial neoplasia. Br J Obstet Gynecol 89: 489
86. Harlozinska A, Kula J, Stepinska B, et al. (1985) Cervical carcinoma antigen, carcinoembryonic antigen (CEA) and non specific cross-reacting antigen (NCA) in appraisal of uterine cervix smears. Am J Clin Pathol 83: 301
87. Hatch KD, Singleton HM, Orr JW, et al. (1985) Role of endocervical curettage in colposcopy. Obstet Gynecol 65: 403
88. Hinselmann H, Schmitt AW (1954) In: Girardet VW (ed). Die Kolposkopie. Wuppertal-Elberfeld
89. Howley PM (1982) The human papillomaviruses. Arch Pathol Lab Med 106: 429
90. Hulka BS (1968) Cytological and histological outcome following an atypical cervical smear. Am J Obstet Gynecol 101: 190
91. Jariwalla RJ, Aurelian L, Ts'O PDP (1979) Neoplastic transformation of cultured Syrian hamster embryo cells by DNA of herpes simplex virus type 2. J Virol 30: 404
92. Johnson LD (1969) The histopathological approach to early cervical neoplasia. Obstet Gynecol Surv 24: 735
93. Johnson LD, Nickerson RJ, Easterday CL, et al. (1968) Epidemiologic evidence for the spectrum of change from dysplasia through carcinoma in situ to invasive cancer. Cancer 22: 901
94. Jones HW, Butler RE (1980) The treatment of cervical intraepithelial neoplasia by cone biopsy. Am J Obstet Gynecol 137: 882
95. Kaufman RH, Irwin JF (1978) The cryosurgical therapy of cervical intraepithelial neoplasia. III. Continuing follow-up. Am J Obstet Gynecol 131: 381
96. Kaufman R, Koss LG, Kurman RJ, et al. (1983) Caution in interpreting papillomavirus-associated lesions (Letter). Obstet Gynecol 62: 269
97. Kessler II (1974) Perspectives on the epidemiology of cervical cancer with special reference to the herpes virus hypothesis. Cancer Res 34: 1091
98. Kessler II (1977) Venereal factors in human cervical cancer: Evidence from marital clusters. Cancer 39: 1912
99. Kirkland JA (1963) Atypical epithelial changes in the uterine cervix. J Clin Pathol 16: 150
100. Kirkland JA, Stanley MA, Cellier KM (1967) Comparative study of histologic and chromosomal abnormalities in cervical neoplasia. Cancer 20: 1934
101. Kolstad P, Stafl A (1978) Atlas of Colposcopy, 2nd ed. Baltimore, University Park Press
102. Koss LG (1978) Dysplasia. A real concept or a misnomer? Obstet Gynecol 51: 374
103. Koss LG, Durfee GR (1956) Unusual patterns of squamous epithelium of the uterine cervix: Cytologic and pathologic study of koilocytotic atypia. Ann NY Acad Sci USA 63: 1235
104. Koss LG, Phillips A (1974) Summary and recommendations of the workshop on uterine cervical cancer. Cancer 33: 1753
105. Koss LG, Stewart FW, Foote FW, et al. (1963) Some histological aspects of behavior of epidermoid carcinoma in situ and related lesions of the uterine cervix. A long-term prospective study. Cancer 16: 1160
106. Kottmeier H (1961) Evolution et traitement des épithéliomas. Rev Franç Gynécol 56: 821
107. Kreider JW, Howett MK, Wolfe SA, et al. (1985) Morphological transformation in vivo of human uterine cervix with papillomavirus from condylomata acuminata. Nature 317: 641
108. Kurman RJ, Jenson AB, Lancaster WD (1983) Papillomavirus infection of the cervix. II. Relationship to intraepithelial neoplasia based on the presence of specific viral structural proteins. Am J Surg Pathol 7: 39
109. Kurman RJ, Jenson AB, Sinclair CF, Lancaster WD (1984) Detection of human papillomaviruses by immunocytochemistry. In: De Lellis RA (ed). Advances in Immunohistochemistry. Chicago, Year Book Medical Publishers, pp 201–221
110. Kurman RM, Shah KH, Lancaster WD, Jenson AB (1981) Immunoperoxidase localization of papillomavirus antigens in cervical dysplasia and vulvar condylomas. Am J Obstet Gynecol 140: 931
111. Kurman RL, Sanz LE, Jenson AB, et al. (1982) Papillomavirus infection of the cervix. I. Correlation of histology with viral structural antigens and DNA sequences. Int J Gynecol Pathol 1: 17
112. Lancaster WD, Castellano C, Santos C, et al. (1986) Human papillomavirus deoxyribonucleic acid in cervical carcinoma from primary and metastatic sites. Am J Obstet Gynecol 154: 115
113. La Porta RF, Taichma LB (1979) Human papillomaviral DNA replicates as a stable episome in cultured epidermal keratinocytes. Proc Natl Acad Sci USA 179: 3393
114. Lee SH, McGregor DH, Kuziez MN (1981) Malignant transformation of perianal condyloma acuminatum: A case report with review of the literature. Dis Colon Rectum 24: 462
115. Lehn H, Krieg P, Sauer G (1985) Papillomavirus genomes in human cervical tumors: Analysis of their transcriptional activity. Proc Natl Acad Sci USA 82: 5540
116. Leiman G, Harrison N, Rubin A (1980) Pregnancy following conization of the cervix: Complications related to cone size. Am J Obstet Gynecol 136: 14
117. Levine RM, Crum CP, Herman E, et al. (1984) Cervical papillomavirus infection and intraepithelial neoplasia: A study of male sexual partners. Obstet Gynecol 64: 16
118. Loning TH, Kuhler CH, Caselitz J, Stegner HE (1983) Keratin and tissue polypeptide antigen profiles of the cervical mucosa. Int J Gynecol Pathol 2: 105
119. Lorincz AT, Temple GF, Patterson JA, et al. (1986) Correlation of cellular atypia and human papillomavirus DNA sequences in exfoliated cells of the uterine cervix. Obstet Gynecol 68: 508
120. Lutzner MA (1983) The human papillomaviruses. Arch Dermatol 119: 631
121. Macgregor JE, Innes G (1980) Carcinoma of penis and cervix. Lancet 1: 1246
122. Makin CA, Bobrow LG, Bodmer WF (1984) Monoclonal antibody to cytokeratin for use in routine histopathology. J Clin Pathol 37: 975
123. Martinez I (1969) Relationship of squamous cell carcinoma

of the cervix uteri to squamous cell carcinoma of the penis. Cancer 24: 777
124. Mazur MT, Cloud GA (1984) The koilocyte and cervical intraepithelial neoplasia: Time-tread analysis of a recent decade. Am J Obstet Gynecol 150: 354
125. McCance DJ, Walker PG, Dyson JL, et al. (1983) Presence of human papillomavirus DNA sequences in cervical intraepithelial neoplasia. Br Med J 287: 784
126. McDougall JK, Galloway DA, Fenoglio CM (1980) Cervical carcinoma: Detection of herpes simplex virus RNA in cells undergoing neoplastic change. Int J Cancer 25: 1
127. McDougall JK, Nelson JA, Myerson D, et al. (1984) HSV, CMV and HPV in human neoplasia. J Invest Dermatol 83: 725
128. McIndoe WA, McLean MR, Jones RW, Mullins PR (1984) The invasive potential of carcinoma in situ of the cervix. Obstet Gynecol 64: 451
129. Meisels A, Fortin R, Roy M (1977) Condylomatous lesions of the cervix. II. Cytologic, colposcopic and histopathologic study. Acta Cytol 21: 379
130. Meisels A, Morin C, Casas-Cordero M (1982) Human papillomavirus infection of the uterine cervix. Int J Gynecol Pathol 1: 75
131. Meisels A, Morin C, Casas-Corder M (1984) Lesions of the uterine cervix associated with papillomaviruses and their clinical consequences. Adv Clin Cytol 2: 1–31
132. Meisels A, Roy M, Fortier M, et al. (1981) Human papillomavirus (HPV) infections of the cervix: The atypical condyloma. Acta Cytol 25: 7
133. Meisels A, Roy M, Fortier M, Morin C (1979) Condylomatous lesions of the cervix. Morphologic and colposcopic diagnosis. Am J Diagn Gynecol Obstet 1: 109
134. Melamed MR, Flehinger BJ (1973) Early incidence rates of precancerous lesions in women using oral contraceptives. Gynecol Oncol 1: 290
135. Melnick JL, Adam E, Rawls WE (1974) The causative role of herpes virus type 2 in cervical cancer. Cancer 34: 1375
136. Mitao M, Reumann W, Winkler B, et al. (1984) Chlamydial cervicitis and cervical intraepithelial neoplasia: An immunohistochemical analysis. Gynecol Oncol 19: 90
137. Mole R, Levy R, Czernobilsky B, et al. (1983) Cytokeratins of normal epithelia and some neoplasms of the female genital tract. Lab Invest 49: 599
138. Nahmias AJ, Roizman B (1973) Infection with herpes simplex viruses 1 and 2. N Engl J Med 289: 667, 719, 781
139. Nasiell K, Nasiell M, Vaclavinkova V (1983) Behavior of moderate cervical dysplasia during long-term follow-up. Obstet Gynecol 61: 609
140. Navratil E, Burghardt E, Bajardi F, Nash W (1958) Simultaneous colposcopy and cytology used in screening for carcinoma of the cervix. Am J Obstet Gynecol 75: 1292
141. Nelson JH Jr, Hall JE (1970) Detection, diagnostic evaluation and treatment of dysplasia and early carcinoma of the cervix. Cancer J Clinicians 20: 150
142. Nelson JH, Averette HE, Richart RM (1984) Dysplasia, carcinoma in situ and early invasive carcinoma. CA 34: 306
143. Nikolaidis ET, Trost DC, Buchholz CL, Wilkinson EJ (1985) The relationship of histologic and clinical factors in laryngeal papillomatosis. Arch Pathol Lab Med 109: 24
144. Okagaki T, Clark BA, Brooker DC, Williams PP (1978) Koilocytosis in dysplastic and reactive cervical squamous epithelium: An ultrastructural study. Acta Cytol 22: 95
145. Okagaki T, Twiggs LB, Zachow KR, et al. (1983) Identification of human papillomavirus DNA in cervical and vaginal intraepithelial neoplasia with molecularly cloned virus-specific probes. Int J Gynecol Pathol 2: 153
146. Olson C, Gordon DE, Robl MG, Lee KP (1969) Oncogenicity of bovine papillomavirus. Arch Environ Health 19: 827
147. Oriel JD (1971) Natural history of genital warts. BR J Vener Dis 47: 1
148. Orth G, Favre M, Breitburg F, et al. (1980) Epidermodysplasia verruciformis: A model for the role of papillomaviruses in human cancer. In: Essex M, Todaro G, Zur Hausen H (eds). Viruses in Naturally Occurring Cancer. Cold Spring Harbor, N.Y., Cold Spring Harbor Laboratory Press, Vol. A, p 259
149. Paavonen J, Verterinen E, Meyer B, et al. (1979) Genital *Chlamydia trachomatis* infections in patients with cervical atypia. Obstet Gynecol 54: 289
150. Pater MM, Pater A (1985) Human papillomavirus types 16 + 18 sequences in carcinoma cell lines of the cervix. Virology 145: 313
151. Patten SF Jr (1969) Diagnostic Cytology of the Uterine Cervix, 1st ed. Baltimore, Williams & Wilkins
152. Przybora LA, Plutowa A (1959) Histological topography of carcinoma in situ of the cervix uteri. Cancer 12: 263
153. Purola E, Savia E (1977) Cytology of gynecologic condyloma acuminatum. Acta Cytol 21: 26
154. Purtilo DT (1984) Defective immune surveillance in viral carcinogenesis. Lab Invest 51: 373
155. Ray B (1977) Condyloma acuminatum of the scrotum. J Urol 117: 739
156. Reagan JW, Hamonic MJ (1956) The cellular pathology in carcinoma in situ; a cytohistopathological correlation. Cancer 9: 385
157. Reagan JW, Ng ABP, Wentz WB (1969) Concepts of genesis and development in early cervical neoplasia. Obstet Gynecol Surv 24: 860
158. Reid BL, Coppleson M (1978) The natural history of the origin of cervical cancer. In: MacDonald RR (ed). Scientific Basis of Obstetrics and Gynecology. London, Churchill Livingstone, pp 427–468
159. Reid R (1984) Papillomavirus and cervical neoplasia. Modern implications and future prospects. Colposcopy Gynecol Laser Surg 1: 3
160. Reid R, Fu YS, Herschmann BR (1984) Genital warts and cervical cancer. VI. The relationship between aneuploid and polyploid cervical lesions. Am J Obstet Gynecol 150: 189
161. Reid R, Herschmann BR, Crum CP, et al. (1984) Genital warts and cervical cancer. V. The tissue basis of colposcopic change. Am J Obstet Gynecol 149: 293
162. Report of the Task Force of the Department of Health and Welfare of Canada. Cervical Cancer Screening Pro-

grams. The Walton Report (1982). Can Med Assoc J 127: 581
163. Rice RH, Pinkus GS, Warhol MJ, Antonioli DA (1984) Involucrin: Biochemistry and immunohistochemistry. In: DeLellis RA (ed). Advances in Immunohistochemistry. Chicago, Year Book Medical Publishers, pp 111–125
164. Richardson AC, Lyon JB (1981) The effect of condom use on squamous cell cervical intraepithelial neoplasia. Am J Obstet Gynecol 140: 909
165. Richart RM (1963) A radioautographic analysis of cellular proliferation in dysplasia and carcinoma in situ of the uterine cervix. Am J Obstet Gynecol 86: 925
166. Richart RM (1963) A clinical staining test for the in vivo delineation of dysplasia and carcinoma in situ. Am J Obstet Gynecol 86: 703
167. Richart RM (1964) The correlation of Schiller-positive areas on the exposed portion of the cervix with intraepithelial neoplasia. Am J Obstet Gynecol 90: 697
168. Richart RM (1964) The growth characteristics in vitro of normal epithelium, dysplasia and carcinoma in situ of the uterine cervix. Cancer Res 24: 662
169. Richart RM (1965) Colpomicroscopic studies of the distribution of dysplasia and carcinoma in situ on the exposed portion of the human uterine cervix. Cancer 18: 950
170. Richart RM (1966) Colpomicroscopic studies of cervical intraepithelial neoplasia. Cancer 19: 395
171. Richart RM (1966) The influence of diagnostic and therapeutic procedures on the distribution of cervical intraepithelial neoplasia. Cancer 19: 1635
172. Richart RM (1969) A theory of cervical carcinogenesis. Obstet Gynecol Surv 24: 874
173. Richart RM (1973) Cervical intraepithelial neoplasia. In: Sommers SC (ed). Pathology Annual. New York, Appleton-Century-Crofts, pp 301–328
174. Richart RM (1980) The patient with an abnormal Pap smear: Screening techniques and management. N Engl J Med 302: 332
175. Richart RM, Barron BA (1969) A follow-up study of patients with cervical dysplasia. Am J Obstet Gynecol 105: 386
176. Richart RM, Lerch V (1966) Time-lapse cinematographic observations of normal human cervical epithelium, dysplasia and carcinoma in situ. J Natl Cancer Inst 37: 317
177. Richart RM, Sciarra JJ (1968) Treatment of cervical dysplasia by out-patient electrocauterization. Am J Obstet Gynecol 101: 200
178. Richart RM, Vaillant HW (1965) Influence of cell collection technic upon cytologic diagnosis. Cancer 18: 1474
179. Richart RM, Lerch V, Barron BA (1967) A time-lapse cinematographic study in vitro of mitosis in normal human cervical epithelium, dysplasia and carcinoma in situ. J Natl Cancer Inst 39: 571
180. Robboy SJ, Truslow GY, Anton J, Richart RM (1981) Role of hormones, including diethylstilbestrol in the pathogenesis of cervical and vaginal intraepithelial neoplasia. Gynecol Oncol 12: S98
181. Robboy SJ, Noller KL, O'Brien P, et al. (1984) Increased incidence of cervical and vaginal dysplasia in 3,980 diethylstilbestrol-exposed young women. JAMA 252: 2979
182. Robboy SJ, Szyfelbein WM, Goellner JR, et al. (1981) Dysplasia and cytologic findings in 4,589 young women enrolled in diethylstilbesterol-adenosis (DESAD) project. Am J Obstet Gynecol 140: 579
183. Romney SL, Palan PR, Dattagupta C, et al. (1981) Retinoids and the prevention of cervical dysplasias. Am J Obstet Gynecol 141: 890
184. Rotkin ID (1973) A comparison review of key epidemiological studies in cervical cancer related to current searches for transmissible agents. Cancer Res 33: 1353
185. Roy M, Meisels A, Fortier M, et al. (1981) Vaginal condylomata: A human papillomavirus infection. Clin Obstet Gynecol 24: 261
186. Royston I, Aurelian L (1970) Immunofluorescent detection of herpes virus antigens in exfoliated cells from human cervical carcinoma. Proc Natl Acad Sci USA 67: 204
187. Rubio CA, Lagerlof B (1974) Studies on the histogenesis of experimentally induced cervical carcinoma. Acta Pathol Microbiol Scand 82: 153
188. Sadeghi SB, Hsieh EW, Gunn SW (1984) Prevalence of cervical intraepithelial neoplasia in sexually active teenagers and young adults. Am J Obstet Gynecol 148: 726
189. Sebastian JA, Leeb BO, See R (1978) Cancer of the cervix—A sexually transmitted disease. Cytologic screening in a prostitute population. Am J Obstet Gynecol 131: 620
190. Schachter J, Hill EC, King EB (1975) Chlamydial infection in women with cervical dysplasia. Am J Obstet Gynecol 123: 753
191. Schneider PS, Krumholz BA, Topp WC, et al. (1984) Molecular heterogeneity of female genital wart (condylomata acuminata) papillomaviruses. Int J Gynecol Pathol 2: 329
191a. Shah K, Kashima H, Polk BF, et al (1986) Rarity of cesarean delivery in cases of juvenile-onset respiratory papillomatosis. Obstet Gynecol 68:795
192. Shevchuk MM, Richart RM (1982) DNA content of condyloma acuminatum. Cancer 49: 489
193. Shingleton HM, Richart RM, Wiener J, Spiro D (1968) Human cervical intraepithelial neoplasia. Fine structure of dysplasia and carcinoma in situ. Cancer Res 28: 695
194. Shorkri-Tobibzadeh S, Koss LG, Molnar J, Romney S (1981) Association of human papillomavirus with neoplastic processes in the genital tract of four women with impaired immunity. Gynecol Oncol 12: S129
195. Sillman F, Stanek A, Sedlis A, et al. (1984) The relationship between human papillomavirus and lower genital intraepithelial neoplasia in immunosuppressed women. Am J Obstet Gynecol 150: 300
196. Silverberg E (1983) Cancer statistics, 1983. CA 33: 9
197. Singer A, Reid BD, Coppleson M (1976) A hypothesis: The role of a high risk male in the etiology of cervical carcinoma. A correlation of epidemiology and molecular biology. Am J Obstet Gynecol 126: 111
198. Smith JW, Townsend DE, Sparks RS (1971) Genetic variants of glucose-6-phosphate dehydrogenase in the study of carcinoma of the cervix. Cancer 28: 529
199. Smith PG, Kinlen LJ, White GC, et al. (1980) Mortality of wives of men dying with cancer of the penis. Br J Cancer 41: 422
200. Sprang ML, Isaacs JH, Boraca CT (1977) Management

of carcinoma-in-situ of the cervix. Am J Obstet Gynecol 129: 47

201. Spriggs AI, Bowey CE, Cowdell RH (1971) Chromosomes of precancerous lesions of the cervix uteri. Cancer 27: 1239
202. Stafl A, Mattingly RF (1975) Angiogenesis of cervical neoplasia. Am J Obstet Gynecol 121: 845
203. Stafl A, Mattingly RF (1973) Colposcopic diagnosis of cervical neoplasia. Obstet Gynecol 41: 168
204. Stafl A, Wilkinson EJ, Mattingly RF (1977) Laser treatment of cervical and vaginal neoplasia. Am J Obstet Gynecol 128: 14
205. Stein DS (1980) Transmissible venereal neoplasia. Am J Obstet Gynecol 137: 864
206. Stern E (1969) Epidemiology of dysplasia. Obstet Gynecol Surv 24: 711
207. Stern E, Neely PM (1963) Carcinoma and dysplasia of the cervix: A comparison of rates for new and returning populations. Acta Cytol 7: 357
208. Sugimori H, Matsuyama T, Kashimura M, et al. (1979) Histological study of microinvasive carcinoma of the uterine cervix. Gynecol Oncol 7: 153
209. Suprun HZ, Schwartz J, Spira H (1985) Cervical intraepithelial neoplasia and associated condylomatous lesions. A preliminary report on 4,764 women from northern Israel. Acta Cytol 29: 334
210. Swan SH, Brown WL (1981) Oral contraceptive use, sexual activity and cervical carcinoma. Am J Obstet Gynecol 139: 52
211. Syrjanen KJ, Heinonen UM, Kauraniemi T (1981) Cytologic evidence of the association of condylomatous lesions with dysplastic and neoplastic changes in the uterine cervix. Acta Cytol 25: 17
212. Syrjanen KJ, Yayrynen M, Saarikoski S, et al. (1985) Natural history of cervical human papillomavirus (HPV) infections based on prospective follow-up. Br J Obstet Gynaecol 92: 1086
213. Taichman LB, Breitbind F, Croissant O, Orth G (1984) The search for a culture system for papillomaviruses. J Invest Dermatol 83: 25
214. Takeuchi A, McKay DB (1960) The area of the cervix involved by carcinoma in situ and anaplasia (atypical hyperplasia). Obstet Gynecol 15: 134
215. Terris M, Wilson F, Nelson JH Jr (1973) Relation of circumcision to cancer of the cervix. Am J Obstet Gynecol 117: 1056
216. Townsend DE, Richart RM (1983) Cryotherapy and carbon dioxide laser management of cervical intraepithelial neoplasia. A controlled comparison. Obstet Gynecol 61: 75
217. Trevathan E, Layde P, Webster LA, et al. (1983) Cigarette smoking and dysplasia and carcinoma in situ of the uterine cervix. JAMA 250: 499
218. Twiggs LB, Clark BA, Okagaki T (1981) Basal cell pseudopodia in cervical intraepithelial neoplasia; progressive reduction of number with severity: A morphometric quantification. Am J Obstet Gynecol 139: 640
219. Valkova B, Ormerod MG, Moncrieff D, Colemen DV (1984) Epithelial membrane antigen in cells from the uterine cervix: Immunocytochemical staining of cervical smears. J Clin Pathol 37: 984
220. VanNiekerk WA (1962) Cervical cells in megaloblastic anemia of puerperium. Lancet 1: 1277
221. Vessey MP (1984) Exogenous hormones in the aetiology of cancer in women. J Roy Soc Med 77: 542
222. Vessey MP, McPherson K, Lawless M, Yeates D (1983) Neoplasia of the cervix and contraception: A possible adverse effect of the pill. Lancet 2: 930
223. Vonka V, Kanka J, Hirsch I, et al. (1984) Prospective study on the relationship between cervical neoplasia and herpes simplex type 2 virus. II. Herpes simplex type 2 antibody presence in sera taken at enrolment. Int J Cancer 33: 61
224. Vonka V, Kanka J, Jelinek I, et al. (1984) Prospective study on the relationship between cervical neoplasia and herpes simplex type-2 virus. 1. Epidemiological characteristics. Int J Cancer 33: 49
225. Wagner D, Ikenberg H, Boehm N, Gissmam L (1984) Identification of human papillomavirus in cervical swabs by deoxyribonucleic acid in situ hybridization. Obstet Gynecol 64: 767
226. Warhol MJ, Antonioli DA, Pinkus GS, et al. (1982) Immunoperoxidase staining for involucrin: A potential diagnostic aid in cervicovaginal pathology. Hum Pathol 13: 1095
227. Warhol MJ, Pinkus GS, Rice RH, et al. (1984) Papillomavirus infection of the cervix. III. Relationship of the presence of viral structural proteins to the expression of involucrin. Int J Gynecol Pathol 3: 71
228. Wassertheil-Smoller S, Romney SL, Wylie-Rosset J, et al. (1981) Dietary vitamin C and uterine cervical dysplasia. Am J Epidemiol 114: 714
229. Watts SL, Phelps WC, Ostrow RS, et al. (1984) Cellular transformation by human papillomavirus DNA in vitro. Science 225: 634
230. Weed JC, Curry SL, Duncan ID, et al. (1978) Fertility after cryosurgery of the cervix. Obstet Gynecol 52: 245
231. Weid GL (1961) Proceedings of the First International Congress on Exfoliative Cytology, 1st ed. Philadelphia, J. B. Lippincott
232. Whitehead N, Reyner F, Lindenbaum J (1973) Megaloblastic changes in the cervical epithelium: Association of oral contraceptive therapy and reversal with folic acid. JAMA 266: 1421
233. WHO Scientific Group: Neoplasia of the uterine cervix. (1978) In: WHO Scientific Group: Steroid Contraception and the Risk of Neoplasia. (Technical Report Series 619). World Health Organization, Geneva, Switzerland, pp. 26–33
234. WHO collaborative study of neoplasia and steroid contraceptives (1985) Invasive cervical cancer and combined oral contraceptives. Br Med J 290: 961
235. Wilbanks GD, Carter B (1970) Fluorescence of cervical intraepithelial neoplasia induced by tetracycline and acridine orange. Am J Obstet Gynecol 106: 726
236. Wilbanks GD, Richart RM (1967) The peurperal cervix, injuries and healing: A colposcopic study. Am J Obstet Gynecol 97: 1105
237. Wilbanks GD, Terner JY, Richart RM (1967) The DNA

content of cervical intraepithelial neoplasia studies by two-wave length Feulgen cytophotometry. Am J Obstet Gynecol 98: 792
238. William DC (1977) Venereally transmitted anal warts: Medical aspects. Human Sexuality 11: 77
239. Winkler B, Richart RM (1985) The histology of CIN, VIN, and VAIN. In: Baggish MS (ed). Basic and Advanced Laser Surgery in Gynecology. Norwalk, Conn, Appleton-Century-Crofts, pp 131–159
240. Winkler B, Norris HJ, Fenoglio CM (1982) The female genital tract. In: Ridell RH (ed). Pathology of Drug-induced and Toxic Diseases. New York, Churchill Livingstone
241. Winkler B, Crum CP, Fujii T, et al. (1984) Koilocytotic lesions of the cervix: The relationship of mitotic abnormalities to the presence of papillomavirus antigens and nuclear DNA content. Cancer 53: 1081
242. Wolfendale MR, King S, Usherwood M (1983) Abnormal cervical smears: Are we in for an epidemic? Br Med J 287: 525
243. Wright NH, Vessey MP, Kenward B, et al. (1975) Neoplasia and dysplasia of the cervix uteri and contraception: A possible protective effect of the diaphragm. Br J Cancer 38: 2783
244. Yee C, Krishnan-Hewlett I, Baker CC, et al. (1985) Presence and expression of human papillomavirus sequences in human cervical carcinoma cell lines. Am J Pathol 119: 361
245. Zur Hausen H (1977) Human papillomaviruses and their possible role in squamous cell carcinomas. Curr Top Microbiol Immunol 78: 1
246. Zur Hausen H (1982) Human genital cancer: Synergism between two virus infection or synergism between a virus infection and initiating events? Lancet 2: 1370
247. Zur Hausen H, de Villiers EM, Gissmam L (1981) Papillomaviruses and human genital cancer. Gynecol Oncol 12: 124
248. Zur Hausen H, Gissman L, Boshart M, et al. (1984) Presence of human papillomavirus in genital tumors. J Invest Dermatol 83: 26S

8

Carcinoma and Metastatic Tumors of the Cervix

Alex Ferenczy, M.D., and Barbara Winkler, M.D.

Invasive Squamous Carcinoma

Microinvasive Squamous Carcinoma

Terminology and Definitions

The concept of microinvasive carcinoma of the cervix was first introduced in 1947 by Mestwerdt.[125] Microinvasive carcinoma (MICA) is considered a preclinical stage in the progressive spectrum of cervical intraepithelial neoplasia (CIN) and frank clinical invasive carcinoma of the cervix uteri. It is classified as clinical stage Ia according to the 1985 FIGO (International Federation of Gynecologists and Obstetricians) staging of carcinoma of the cervix (Table 8.1). Because the lesion cannot be visualized on gross inspection, the diagnosis is based on histologic examination of cervical tissue.

The definition of MICA has been controversial.[13,20,28,50,94] The main subjects of contention concern measurement of the depth of stromal invasion and the significance of vascular invasion and confluency between invasive tongues of neoplastic epithelium, as related to the frequency of pelvic node metastasis, vaginal recurrence, and death of patients. The maximal permissible depth of stromal invasion reported in the literature varies from 1 mm to 5 mm.[20,50,94] Some characterize microinvasion by the absence of confluency of invasive foci[20] and/or the absence of vascular permeation,[20] whereas for others, lymphatic involvement[36,154] and confluency[154] do not exclude the diagnosis of microinvasive disease. The lack of a uniform definition is reflected in the conflicting reports about the frequency of pelvic node metastasis associated with microinvasion, which varies from 0 to 7%.[13,18] These figures are difficult to interpret, since in most studies no information is given about the methods used to measure the depth of stromal invasion (see below, Microscopic Features). In other series, the depth of stromal penetration is not even stated. Similarly, precise data on the frequency of recurrences and survival rates are not available because of the lack of uniform definitions, follow-up, and different diagnostic and treatment methods used (punch biopsy, cone biopsy, hysterectomy, radical hysterectomy, irradiation) for early invasive lesions.[13] Despite these pitfalls, analysis of the least bi-

TABLE 8.1. 1985 modification of FIGO staging of carcinoma of the cervix uteri.

Stage[a]	Description
0	Preinvasive carcinoma (intraepithelial carcinoma, carcinoma in situ)
I	Carcinoma strictly confined to the cervix (extension to the corpus should be disregarded)
Ia	Preclinical carcinomas of the cervix, that is, those diagnosed only by microscopy.
Ia1	Minimal microscopically evident stromal invasion.
Ia2	Lesions detected microscopically that can be measured. The upper limit of the measurement should not show a depth of invasion of more than 5 mm taken from the base of the epithelium, either surface or glandular, from which it originates, and a second dimension, the horizontal spread, must not exceed 7 mm. Larger lesions should be staged as Ib.
Ib	Lesions of greater dimensions than Stage Ia2 whether seen clinically or not. Preformed space involvement should not alter the staging but should be specifically recorded so as to determine whether it should affect treatment decisions in the future.
IIa	Invasive carcinoma that extends beyond the cervix involving the upper two thirds of the vagina with parametrial infiltration that has not reached either lateral pelvic wall
IIb	Invasive carcinoma that involves the upper two thirds of the vagina with parametrial infiltration that has not reached the pelvic side wall
III	Invasive carcinoma that extends to either lateral pelvic wall and/or the lower third of the vagina and/or hydronephrosis or nonfunction of kidney due to tumor
IV	Invasive carcinoma that involves the mucosa of the urinary bladder and/or rectum or extends beyond the true pelvis

[a] Notes to the Staging:

Stage 0 comprises those cases with full thickness involvement of epithelium with atypical cells but with no signs of invasion into the stroma.

Over the last several decades there has been continued confusion about the stages of preclinical invasive carcinoma of the cervix. Several classification systems which have not been generally satisfactory have been developed. The addition of colposcopy in many countries has caused further confusion as to what is a clinical lesion for obvious reasons. There has also been an increased pressure to put measurements into the definition. As a result of the above, a new definition is proposed in this volume which is as follows:

Stage Ia Carcinoma should include minimal microscopically evident stromal invasion as well as small cancerous tumors of measurable size. Stage Ia should be divided into those lesions with minute foci of invasion visible only microscopically as Stage Ia1, and the macroscopically measurable microcarcinomas as Stage Ia2 in order to gain further knowledge of the clinical behavior of these lesions. The term Ib Occult should be omitted.

The diagnosis of both Stages Ia1 and Ia2 should be based on microscopic examination of removed tissue, preferably a cone, which must include the entire lesion. As noted above, the lower limit of Stage Ia2 should be that it can be measured macroscopically (even if dots need to be placed on the slide prior to measurement) and the upper limit of Ia2 is given by measurement of the two largest dimensions in any given section. The depth of invasion should not be more than 5 mm taken from the base of the epithelium, either surface or glandular, from which it originates. The second dimension, the horizontal spread, must not exceed 7 mm. Vascular space involvement, either venous or lymphatic, should not alter the staging, but should be specifically recorded as it may affect treatment decisions in the future.

Lesions of greater size should be staged as Ib.

As a rule, it is impossible to estimate clinically whether a cancer of the cervix has extended to the corpus or not. Extension to the corpus should therefore be disregarded.

ased reports indicates that lymph node metastases, recurrences, and deaths tend to occur with lesions that invade the stroma more than 3 mm or demonstrate invasion of vascular spaces, including lymphatic, blood, and capillary-like spaces.[13,20,108,158,160] Depth of stromal invasion is of key clinical significance. Pelvic node metastases or recurrences were not observed in 162 women with MICA in whom the depth of stromal penetration did not exceed 1 mm and contained no vascular invasion or confluency.[20] In 397 women who underwent radical hysterectomy and bilateral lymphadenectomy, only 1 had positive lymph nodes (0.2%) with up to 3 mm deep stromal invasion, whereas 8.1% of 98 women with 3.1–5 mm deep lesions had positive nodes. This gives an overall pelvic node metastasis rate of 1.8% (Table 8.2).

Although vascular space invasion (see below, Microscopic Features) and confluency could not be correlated with pelvic node involvement in the previously described reports, in another study[160] one of four 3-mm-deep lesions with vascular invasion had metastasis to pelvic nodes, whereas 37 women with similar deep lesions devoid of vascular invasion were free of node metastasis. Results of studies of vascular invasion in MICA are somewhat conflicting[36] but suggest that vascular involvement increases the risk of pelvic node metastases and vaginal recurrences (Table 8.3).[13,22,72,176] In one series, none

TABLE 8.2. Pelvic node metastasis with early invasive carcinoma according to depth of stromal penetration.

Depth of invasion (mm)[a]	No. of patients	Node metastasis: No. of patients	Node metastasis: (%)
0.1–3.0	397	1	0.2
3.1–5.0	98	8	8.1
TOTAL 0.1–5.0	495	9	1.8

[a] Stromal invasion from 0.1 to 5.0 mm with and without vascular invasion and confluency. [Adapted from (by permission of) Benson and Norris, Ref. 13, Hasumi et al., Ref. 72, and Van Nagell et al., Ref. 176.]

TABLE 8.3. Significance of vascular invasion in early invasive carcinoma[a] (114 cases).

	No. of cases	(%)
Positive pelvic nodes	4	3.5
Vaginal recurrence	8	7.0
Death	6	5.0

[a] Stromal invasion from 0.1 to 5 mm deep. [Adapted (by permission of) from Bohm et al., Ref. 18, Burghart and Holzer, Ref. 25, Hasumi et al., Ref. 72, Leman et al., Ref. 108, Sedlis et al., Ref. 158, Seski et al., Ref. 160, and Van Nagell et al., Ref. 176.]

TABLE 8.4. Residual invasive tumor in postconization hysterectomy specimens according to lateral extent of carcinoma with up to 5 mm stromal invasion.

Lateral extent (mm)	Residual disease (%)
<4	2
<8	27
>8	35

[Adapted from (by permission of) Sedlis et al. (1979) Microinvasive carcinoma of the uterine cervix: A clinico-pathologic study. Am J Obstet Gynecol, 33: 64]

of the 74 women with stromal invasion up to 5 mm had positive pelvic nodes,[158] however, 2 patients with 3-mm-deep invasive disease and extensive vascular invasion developed vaginal recurrences. In another study,[25] the only patient who presumably died of carcinoma with less than 5 mm stromal invasion had vascular involvement, although the 9 other women with vascular involvement had a benign clinical course. In a compilation of seven studies in which vascular invasion was identified in 114 patients, the frequency of positive pelvic lymph nodes was 3.5%, vaginal recurrence 7%, and death from disease 5% (Table 8.3). Furthermore, vascular invasion has also been related to residual MICA in hysterectomy specimens. Based on recent studies, confluency of neoplastic epithelium in MICA was not associated with pelvic node metastases, vaginal recurrence, or cancer death.[13,154,176] A mortality rate of 5% is estimated in women with MICA and was found only with well-established, confluent lesions with 3–5 mm deep stromal penetration; none of 285 women with early, multiple and superficial (less than 3 mm) invasive foci had vaginal recurrences or death due to carcinoma.[111,112]

The data, although incomplete, suggest that lesions with 3 mm or less stromal penetration, measured from the point of origin of invasion and without vascular space involvement, have virtually no potential for metastasis or recurrences. On the other hand, those with vascular invasion may potentially metastasize, although the risk is small, about 3.5%. Consequently, the definition of MICA proposed in 1974 by the Committee on Nomenclature for the Society of Gynecologic Oncologists (SGO) in the U.S.A. seems to be more appropriate than that proposed by the FIGO: *A microinvasive lesion should be defined as one in which neoplastic epithelium invades the stroma in one or more places to a depth of 3 mm or less below the basement membrane of the epithelium and in which lymphatic or blood vascular involvement is not demonstrated.* Accordingly, histologically detected lesions with 3.1–5 mm deep stromal invasion or vascular space invasion but less than 3.1 mm deep stromal invasion represent stage Ib "occult" carcinomas of the cervix (see section, Invasive Squamous Carcinoma, Terminology and Definitions).

In recent years, the morphologic evaluation of the lateral and frontal extent of MICA as well as that of the surgical margins of cone specimens has been emphasized. Burghardt and Holzer[25] have introduced the concept of tumor volume as applied to MICA and have reported no pelvic node metastases with 420 cu mm of cancer or less, with the exception of one in which vascular invasion was noted. However, their method of measuring volume by serially sectioning cone specimens is extremely cumbersome and time-consuming and is unlikely to become a routine laboratory method. Perhaps measuring only the lateral extent of lesions on well-oriented histologic sections together with evaluating the depth of stromal invasion and presence or absence of vascular invasion will prove to be an acceptable alternative to the three-dimensional evaluation of MICA (see section, Invasive Squamous Carcinoma, Terminology and Definitions). The lateral extent of MICA has been correlated with the rate of residual neoplasia in the post-cone hysterectomy specimens.[158] Table 8.4 shows that the greater the lateral diameter of MICA, the greater the risk of finding residual invasive neoplasia in the hysterectomy specimen. In a series of 134 patients, 3 women with tumor widths up to 10 mm died of their disease.[112]

Perhaps one of the most important contributions to the appropriate management of MICA is the emphasis of evaluating surgical lines of conization specimens.[36,108,158,160] In fact, the status of cone margins may well be the most important single parameter in deciding the therapeutic approach to patients with MICA. Indeed, MICA with either intraepithelial or invasive disease on cone margins is often associated with residual neoplasia including the invasive carcinoma in hysterectomy specimens (Table 8.5). In one study,[108] 39% of women with

TABLE 8.5. Frequency of residual neoplasia[a] according to status of cone margins.

Cone margins	Residual disease (%)
Positive	50[b]–78[c]
Negative	0

[a] Intraepithelial or invasive.
[b] From Leman et al., Ref. 108.
[c] From Seski et al., Ref. 160.

positive cone margins had residual invasive disease in the hysterectomy specimens, and on occasion the residual invasion was deeper than the one found in the cone specimens. By contrast, when the margins were free on extensive sampling, no residual neoplasia was found. Moreover, a positive correlation has been found between the rate of postcone residual invasive disease and depth of stromal penetration and vascular invasion in the cone specimens.[158] There was no residual disease with 1 mm deep or less MICA versus a 61% residual invasive neoplasia rate with 3 mm or deeper carcinoma. Vascular invasion was associated with invasive disease in the hysterectomy specimens in up to 80% of the cases versus 20% when no vascular involvement was seen in the cone.

Frequency and Age Distribution

According to various investigators, the frequency of microinvasion in patients with CIN varies from 4%[23] to over 50%.[105] The significant variations reflect wide differences in the definition of MICA and methods of sampling of cervical specimens. A 4% frequency was demonstrated by serial step sections in specimens with CIN by Boyes et al.[23] and is the figure that has gained general acceptance. However, the Boyes et al. series involved lesions with up to 5 mm stromal invasion, and consequently, the frequency of MICA as defined in this chapter is probably less than 4%.

The majority of MICA are found in patients in their early 40s, between two extremes of age, early 20s and 70s.[53]

Clinical Aspects

The majority of patients with microinvasive disease are asymptomatic and are seen for routine pelvic examination. The cervix demonstrates a grossly normal appearance or nonspecific findings, such as chronic cervicitis or true erosion. A definitive diagnosis of microinvasion is made on histologic evaluation of cervical tissue removed by conization or at hysterectomy. Cytopathologists and colposcopists with wide experience are able to predict early stromal invasion with a high degree of accuracy. Ng et al.,[130] on the basis of cellular characteristics, correctly predicted 27 of 31 patients with proved MICA, an accuracy of 87%. According to these authors, the major cytologic features diagnostic of microinvasion are coarse, irregular chromatin distribution, micro- and macronucleoli, background of exudate and cellular debris (tumor diathesis), and syncytial arrangement of neoplastic cells. The colposcopic diagnosis of MICA[12,20,166] is based on abnormal vascular patterns of the cervical epithelium. Characteristically, the epithelium displays a marked degree of whiteness consistent with CIN in which one or more foci contain bizarre surface branching vessels. The recommended approach in diagnosing microinvasion is colposcope-oriented punch biopsy of the area suspicious for microinvasion, followed by conization in order to exclude the possibility of more advanced disease. The cone is completely and serially sampled for microscopic examination, and the pathologist evaluates the surgical margins, depth of stromal invasion, the greatest lateral extent of the lesion, and whether vascular space invasion is present.

Microscopic Features and Ultrastructure

According to the definition of MICA of the cervix, the diagnosis is based on the presence of one or more tongues of malignant cells penetrating through the plane of the basement membrane of the epithelium (Fig. 8.1a). The latter invariably demonstrates intraepithelial neoplasia (CIN) of varying severity, and in most instances the underlying endocervical glands are extensively replaced by the intraepithelial disease. Typically in the microinvasion foci, the cells are better differentiated than those in the associated CIN, with abundant cytoplasm and prominent nucleoli. Occasionally, small foci of keratinization are seen. Because of focal disruption of the basement membrane, the margin of the invading nests is ragged, flanked by intact basement membrane on either side (Fig. 8.1b). This irregular contour is probably the most reliable criterion in the diagnosis of MICA. It is easily distinguished from the smooth and regular contour of masses of neoplastic cells that represent endocervical gland involvement by intraepithelial carcinoma.

At the site of initial stromal invasion, disruption of the basement membrane is confirmed by electron microscopy. The neoplastic cells are seen encroaching directly onto the collagen fibers of the stroma, and their cytoplasmic membrane is markedly convoluted, with numerous microvilli. The factors that initiate a clone or clones of cells to invade the stroma are obscure. Morphologically, invasive squamous cells have fewer cellular attachments and presumably elaborate more lysosomal lytic substances than their intraepithelial counterparts. It is conceivable that these morphophysiologic changes, when acquired in a small group of intraepithelial neoplastic cells, can lead to a decrease in cellular adhesiveness, loss of contact inhibition, and presumably disruption of the basement membrane, thus enabling them to penetrate the underlying connective tissue stroma. Host factors probably also play an important role in containing the neoplastic cells within the basement membrane, as evidenced by the often conspicuous lymphoplasmacytic infiltrates surrounding the tips of invasive epithelial prongs. The local interactions among tumor cells, inflammatory cells, and capillary endothelial cells may play a role in angiogenesis and tumor neovascularization.[54]

The presence of lymphatic or venous involvement by

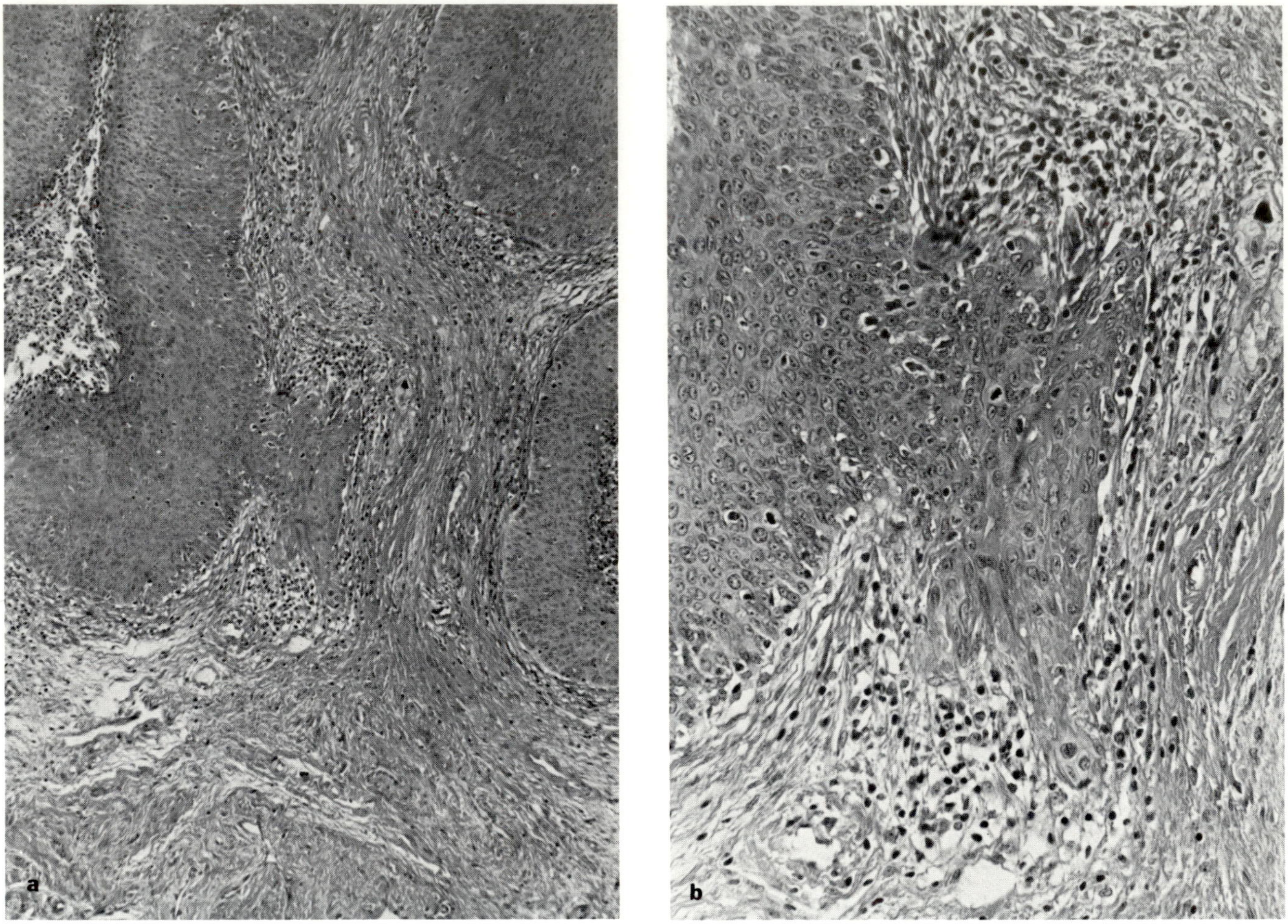

FIG. 8.1. Microinvasive squamous carcinoma of the cervix. *a*. Minute tongue of neoplastic epithelium projecting into the stroma from an area of grade 3 CIN that has replaced a preexisting endocervical cleft. Stromal extension is less than 1 mm in depth. *b*. Higher magnification of the microinvasive focus, which characteristically displays irregular margin and better differentiated neoplastic cells than those above the basal lamina. The stromal epithelial junction of the invasive focus is typically infiltrated by chronic inflammatory cells.

the tumor regardless of the size of the lesion should exclude the disease from the microinvasive category (Fig. 8.2). Identification of early lymphatic and vascular space invasion, particularly in the upper one-third layer of the cervical stroma, may be difficult and is often hampered by technical processing artifacts (Fig. 8.3). More scientific study is required to define the cellular and histologic correlates of vessel invasion and their relationship to routes of metastatic spread.[54] Roche and Norris[154] define lymphatic space invasion as endothelial-lined (capillary-like) spaces containing tumor cells that are contiguous with the stroma. In view of the difficulties in distinguishing small blood vessels and capillaries from small lymphatic channels, the term *vascular space(s)* is used in this chapter.

For consistency in the measurement of the depth of stromal invasion, the following guidelines are recommended. The depth of neoplastic projections should not exceed 3 mm from the initial site of invasion either from the basal lamina of the surface epithelium or from endocervical glands replaced by intraepithelial neoplasia (Fig. 8.4). There are cases, however, in which a direct histologic continuity between invasive foci and CIN cannot be demonstrated even in deeper cuts of the paraffin block. In such instances, it is assumed that invasion originated from the basal cells of the overlying CIN. As a result, depth of invasion is arbitrarily measured from the basal lamina of the surface CIN (Fig. 8.4).

The most accurate method to measure the depth of stromal penetration is with a calibrated slide of ocular microscale,[146,147] although such devices are seldom used in routine practice. A more convenient but perhaps less accurate method of establishing the size of penetrating foci consists of using a microscopic field that corresponds to a diameter of 1 mm. This may be determined by direct microscopic visualization with a transparent metric

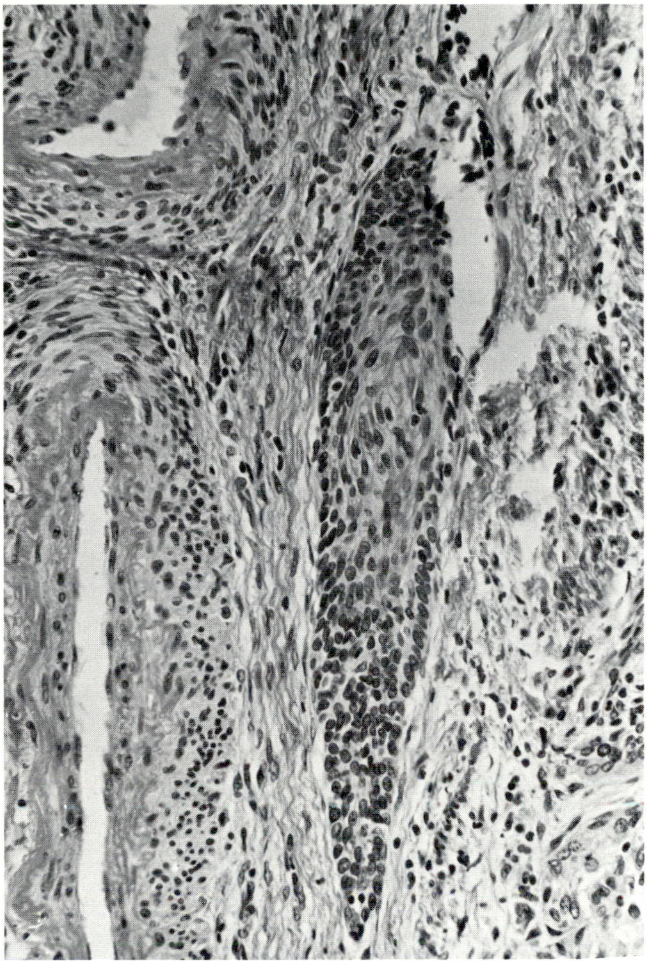

FIG. 8.2. Lymphatic invasion by tumor cells. Neoplastic cells adhere to the endothelial lining of a lymphatic capillary space. Although the lesion contained nonconfluent, less than 2 mm-deep microinvasive sprouts, because of vascular invasion the lesion was interpreted as preclinical, occult invasive carcinoma. Two of 28 pelvic lymph nodes contained metastasis.

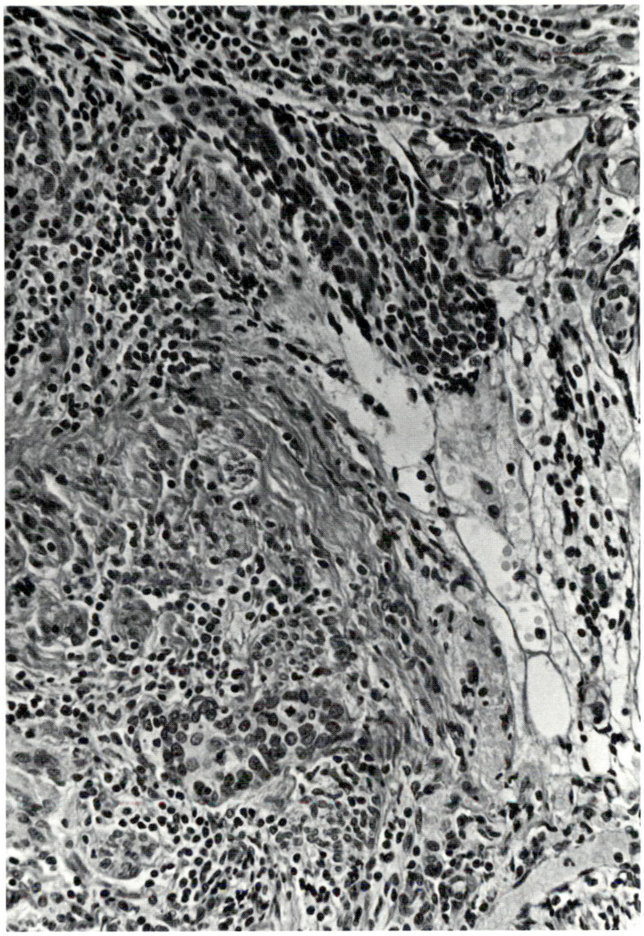

FIG. 8.3. Implanted nests of neoplastic epithelium at the site of previous biopsy site for CIN. Note artifact of shrinkage characterized by irregular outline and absence of endothelial lining of the space surrounding tumor cells. Edema, extravasated red blood cells, and inflammatory exudate indicate response to injury. Such phenomena should not be interpreted as microinvasion of stroma or lymphatic penetration.

ruler. Although variation in microscopic objective and ocular lenses exists, in general a microscopic field of 160× measures a little more than 1 mm in diameter. The depth of penetration also depends on the angle at which sections are prepared, and efforts should be made to secure vertically sectioned tissue samples. The lateral extent of MICA is measured as described for the depth of stromal penetration. Measurements are made between the two points where the neoplastic epithelium (regardless of whether it is microinvasive or CIN) meets the adjacent normal epithelium.

Special attention should be paid to the interpretation of recently biopsied conization specimens. These often harbor individual nests of neoplastic epithelium scattered within the cervical stroma at the site of a previous punch biopsy (Fig. 8.3). Such nests represent clusters of intraepithelial carcinoma that may be disrupted and incorporated into the stroma by the punch biopsy and masquerade as MICA. Therefore, a diagnosis of microinvasion should be carefully evaluated when such a phenomenon is seen at or near a recent biopsy site. CIN or immature squamous metaplasia with extensive gland involvement and pseudoepitheliomatous hyperplasia should also be distinguished from MICA.

Treatment

Many methods of treatment for early invasion are used, ranging from cervical conization to radical hysterectomy with pelvic node dissection and from radium insertion to total pelvic irradiation. The trend appears to be in the direction of more conservative management, with attempts at individualization of treatment based on (1)

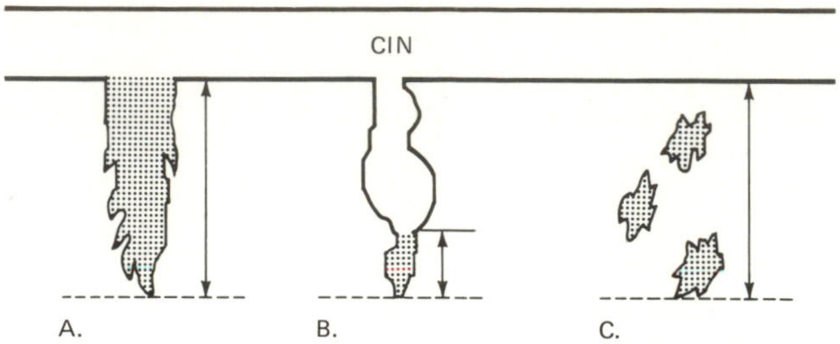

FIG. 8.4. Different stromal depth measurements for different patterns of stromal invasion. *A*. Origin of invasion at surface CIN—depth of stromal invasion is measured from point of origin of invasion downward to the last cell of invasive focus. *B*. Origin of invasion at CIN with gland involvement—depth of stromal invasion is measured from site of origin downward to the last cell of invasive focus. *C*. Origin of invasion not seen—depth of stromal invasion is measured from basal lamina of surface CIN downward to the last cell of invasive focus.

the definition of the lesion, (2) lateral extent, and (3) involvement of cone margins.

The treatment modalities based on the above parameters are outlined in Fig. 8.5. If the cone margins are free of disease, the depth of invasion is less than 3 mm, vascular invasion is absent, and the lateral extent is no greater than 10 mm, a transabdominal hysterectomy is performed. Lesions measuring more than 3 mm but not more than 5 mm in depth or containing vascular invasion and/or with their lateral extent greater than 10 mm regardless of depth of stromal invasion are stage Ib occult carcinoma (see section, Invasive Squamous Carcinoma, Terminology and Definitions) rather than MICA. As a result, for these lesions radical hysterectomy and lymphadenectomy are performed, even though the cone margins are free of tumor. This procedure is preferred in view of the high risk of finding residual disease, including invasion, in the hysterectomy specimens in these patients and to rule out the possibility of associated pelvic node metastasis. Should the margins of the cone be positive, radical hysterectomy and lymphadenectomy are carried out for the same reasons as described above. Some investigators perform a *simple hysterectomy* with lymphadenectomy rather than radical hysterectomy with lymphadenectomy.[111,112] This change in surgical approach may be justified by the observations that early invasive carcinoma with less than 5 mm stromal penetration *does not extend or metastasize to the paracervical regions*.[112] Rather, metastatic disease is confined to the pelvic nodes. This modified surgical technique reduces considerably the risk of ureteral injury. Radiation is limited to those women who clearly represent high operative risks.

If conception is desired and the patient is reliable for close, long-term follow-up and has a 3 mm or less lesion without vascular invasion, free surgical lines, and lateral extension less than 10 mm, the initial cone may be considered sufficient therapy by some investigators[112,169] (Fig. 8.5). These patients, however, must be monitored carefully at 3–6-month intervals by means of cytology, histology, and colposcopy. Regardless of whether the squamocolumnar junction is seen in its entirety, an endocervical curettage should be performed during each visit in these women to make sure that the endocervical canal is free of recurrent or residual disease. It should be pointed out that this management approach is not universally accepted. In fact it may be severely criticized as undertreating MICA. The presently available data indicate that women with MICA, that is, lesions that are limited to a depth of 3 mm, have less than 10 mm lateral extension, are devoid of vascular invasion, and have free surgical lines on serially sectioned cone specimens, have virtually no risk of morbidity or mortality associated with MICA. These data, however, are based on patients treated by hysterectomy.

Invasive Squamous Carcinoma

Terminology and Definitions

Over the last several decades there has been considerable confusion and debate about the terminology and staging of preclinical invasive carcinoma of the cervix (stage Ia). Clinically apparent carcinoma is classified as stage Ib. In 1974 the Society of Gynecologic Oncologists proposed the term "Ib occult" for small invasive carcinomas that could not be detected on gross examination and were

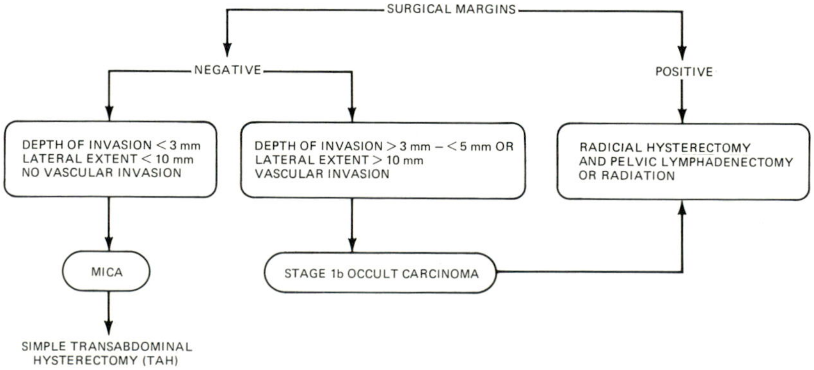

FIG. 8.5. Management modalities of early (microinvasive and stage Ib occult) carcinoma of cervix.

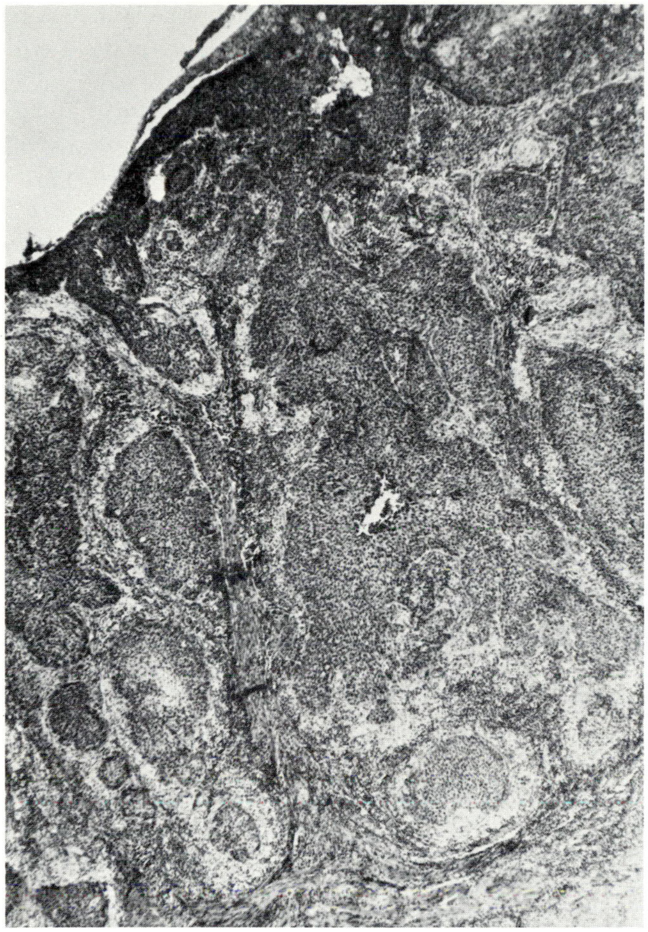

FIG. 8.6. Unifocal, preclinical, occult invasive squamous carcinoma of the cervix. The lesion was not visible to the naked eye. The entire lesion measured 4 mm in diameter and maximum penetration. In contrast to MICA, in this lesion invasive tongues are confluent. Note the extensive inflammatory infiltration at the interface between tumor cells and stroma.

discovered on microscopic examination to have invaded beyond 3 mm in depth and, regardless of size, demonstrated vascular space involvement (Figs. 8.2 and 8.6). This type of lesion is usually unifocal and measures in depth from 3 mm to over 1 cm.[23] The introduction of colposcopy, by permitting enhanced visualization of the cervix, has further complicated the definition of what constitutes a clinical lesion. Also there has been an increased emphasis on making the definition more quantifiable. As a result a modification of the International Federation of Gynecologists and Obstetricians (FIGO) staging system has been recently proposed (Table 8.1). Invasive carcinomas that demonstrate minimal microscopic stromal invasion as well as cancers of measureable size are classified as stage Ia. This category is subdivided into stage Ia1 which includes lesions with minute foci of invasion visible only microscopically and stage Ia2 which includes macroscopically measureable small carcinomas. The diagnosis of stages Ia1 and Ia2 is based on microscopic examination of a cone biopsy specimen that includes the entire lesion. The lower limit of stage Ia2 is that it can be measured macroscopically (even if this measurement is made with a ruler on a microscopic slide). The upper limit of stage Ia2 is a depth of invasion, in any given section, that does not exceed 5 mm from the base of the epithelium, either surface or glandular from which it originates, and a horizontal dimension that does not exceed 7 mm. Vascular space involvement should not alter the staging, but should be specifically recorded since it may affect treatment. Lesions of greater size are classified as stage Ib. In addition, it was recommended that the term "Ib occult" be abandoned although the basis for this recommendation is not clear. In the last 10 years, since the term was introduced, a large number of studies have been published that provide considerable information concerning the behavior and treatment of cervical cancers as defined by this term. In order for these studies to be comprehensible to the reader the term "occult invasive carcinoma" has therefore been retained in this chapter.

Several large series of patients with preclinical malignant cervical neoplasms with more than 3-mm stromal extension demonstrated a close relationship between the extent of stromal extension vascular invasion and lymphatic permeation as well as lymph node involvement and death rate.* Boyes et al.[23] found lymphatic vessel invasion in one third of 218 cases of occult confluent lesions. The mortality rate is 4–7%.[23] Patients who die of disseminated carcinoma in general have lymphatic channel involvement[23,94] and tumors measuring more than 5 mm in greatest extent.[23] In view of these data, the pathologist should specify the extent of the disease and the presence or absence of vascular penetration in order to predict the prognosis of the patient. The better 5-year survival rate (96%)[23] of patients with occult invasive carcinoma as compared to stage Ib frank invasive carcinoma (5-year survival rate, 86%) justifies the former being distinguished from the latter variety.

Incidence and Age Distribution

According to the 1969–1970 Third National Cancer Survey,[34] invasive squamous carcinoma of the uterine cervix represents the most common malignancy in the female reproductive system in American women, both white and black, aged younger than 50. Geographic factors are significant in the incidence of invasive cervical carcinoma, the Southern United States with its low socioeconomic background having the highest rates for both black and white women.[34] The age-adjusted incidence rates

* References 20, 22, 23, 37, 94, 110, 183.

per 100,000 women for invasive cervical cancer fell from 34 in 1947 (Second National Cancer Survey) to 15.3 in 1970, an approximately 58% decrease. This spectacular decline results partly from the increased use of mass cervical cancer screening by cervical cytology, which significantly contributes to the early detection and treatment of invasive cervical cancer precursors.[33,150] The important role of cytology in reducing cervical cancer is also supported by the different incidences reported in screened (4.5 cases per 100,000) and unscreened (29 cases per 100,000) populations, both cohorts exhibiting similar epidemiologic characteristics.[53] The decline of cervical carcinoma accounts for a decrease in all female genital malignancies, which fell from 118 cases per 100,000 women aged 20 and over in 1947 to 88 cases per 100,000 in 1970.[34] Whereas the cervix comprised over 50% of the invasive cancers in the 1947 survey, in 1970 it accounted for less than a third of the cases.[34] A positive correlation between the rate of effective cancer detection programs used in each state of the United States and a decrease in mortality rate can be demonstrated.[33] In areas with mass screening cytologic programs, there has been over 50% reduction in the death rate from cervical carcinoma.[148,150] Despite the success so far achieved in reducing the mortality rate, only half of the United States women aged 20 or over have ever received a Pap test. As a result, cervical malignancy is the fourth most frequent cause of death from cancer (after breast, colon, rectum, and lung) in women 35–54 years old according to the 1980 Cancer statistics from the American Cancer Society.[163] There are 16,000 new cases a year of invasive cervical carcinoma in the United States, and 7000 women died of the disease in 1984. The average age of patients with invasive squamous cell carcinoma is 51.4 years, 15–23 years older than patients with high-grade cervical intraepithelial neoplasia (carcinoma in situ)[34] and 8 years older than patients with microinvasive carcinoma (Fig. 8.7).[150] Cervical cancer occurs, however, at almost any age between 17 and 90 years. In recent years, there has been an increasing frequency of cervical carcinoma in women under 35 years of age, accounting for 24.5% of all invasive lesions of the cervix in one American institution.[16] The epidemiologic characteristics, including socioeconomic status and sexual history, of these patients are similar to those of the older group.[67] Contrary to earlier studies, indicating a less favorable prognosis for young women with invasive cervical neoplasia, recent data[102] showed no significant differences in the histologic differentiation, stage of disease, and survival rates between young women and patients in the perimenopausal and menopausal periods. Patients aged 70 years and older have the lowest risk of developing invasive squamous cell carcinoma, as only 4.5% of all invasive cervical cancers are observed in this age group.[1]

Pathogenesis

A considerable body of evidence has been accumulated in the past decade suggesting that invasive squamous cell carcinoma develops from CIN.[168] Patients with invasive disease have similar epidemiologic characteristics to those with preinvasive precursor lesions (see Chapter 7, Cervical Intraepithelial Neoplasia). The majority of women with invasive cancer of the cervix classically are from lower socioeconomic groups, have begun heterosexual activity early in life, marry early, are multiparous, and have many sexual partners. Most of these are covariables and are related to sexual intercourse. Also, significantly more women (8 times as many as expected) with

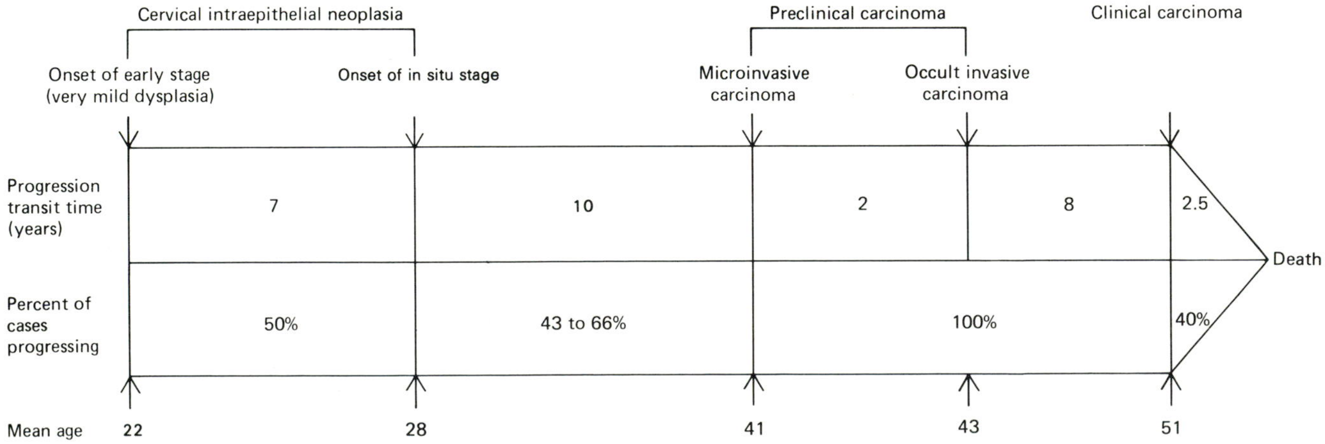

FIG. 8.7. Diagram of the progression, transit time, and proportion of cases of CIN progressing to invasive squamous carcinoma estimated according to the mean age of the patients. [Adapted from Fidler et al. (1970) Mod Med Can 25: 9.]

cervical cancer are observed among spouses of men with cancer of the penis.[66] There is increasing evidence for an association between human papillomavirus (HPV) infection and cervical carcinoma. HPV DNA has been detected in 89% of cervical squamous cell carcinomas[62] and tumor cell lines established from cervical carcinoma.[187] In patients with metastatic cervical carcinoma, HPV DNA can also be identified in lymph node metastases, with viral DNA hybridization patterns matching those of the primary cervical site.[103] A detailed review of the postulated role of HPV in the pathogenesis of cervical carcinoma is presented in Chapter 7, Cervical Intraepithelial Neoplasia.

The usual, but by no means the only, pathogenetic sequence of events of cervical carcinoma is mild to moderate to severe dysplasia to carcinoma in situ, microinvasive carcinoma, preclinical occult invasive carcinoma, and frank clinical invasive carcinoma.[32,53] The mean progression transit time of low-grade CIN (very mild dysplasia) to high-grade CIN (carcinoma in situ) as determined by cytology and colpomicroscopy is approximately 7 years.[152] Based on estimates of the age-specific incidence and prevalence rates of CIS, Barron et al.[11] found that the duration of CIS in the aggregate is a variable that has a distribution with upper limits of 10 years and lower limits of 3 years. Earlier studies[31] suggested an inverse relationship between the incident age and the duration of CIS (i.e., the younger the patient at the time of discovery of newly established CIS, the longer its duration, and vice versa). The Barron et al. study found that the natural history of CIS is independent of the age of the patient at the time of diagnosis.[11] It has been estimated that only 43–66% of untreated intraepithelial lesions eventually progress to MICA.[53] The estimated average duration of preclinical microinvasive disease to occult invasive carcinoma is 2 years and that of occult carcinoma to overt clinical carcinoma is about 8–9 years[150] (Fig. 8.7).

Clinical Aspects

Nearly all patients (99%) with clinically visible invasive carcinoma of the cervix complain of abnormal vaginal bleeding. The most significant and common feature is bleeding following intercourse or douching. Intermittent spotting, serosanguineous discharge, and frank hemorrhage are also frequently encountered. Ten to twenty percent of patients complain of bloody malodorous discharge and pain, often radiating to the sacral region. Weakness, pallor, weight loss, edema of the lower extremities, rectal pain, and hematuria are symptoms and signs of either locally advanced or metastatic disease.

Means for accurate detection and diagnosis of frank invasive carcinoma include cytology, colposcopy, and colposcope-directed punch biopsy. Although the high degree of diagnostic accuracy of cytology (95% of cases)[148] and colposcopy[20,167] (Fig. 7.15d) is no longer questioned, a tissue diagnosis is required for definitive histologic confirmation. Thorough rectovaginal examination, intravenous pyelography (IVP), cystoscopy, proctosigmoidoscopy, and skeletal survey are required to assess the clinical stage of the disease.

Gross Features

The appearance of invasive cervical carcinoma on gross inspection depends on the extent of involvement. The early lesions may produce focal induration, shallow ulcerations, or a slightly elevated granular area that bleeds readily on touch. Approximately 98% of early carcinomas are localized within the transformation zone, with variable degrees of encroachment onto the neighboring native portio. The more advanced growths have two major types of gross appearance: endophytic and exophytic. Endophytic carcinomas are either ulceroinvasive or noduloinvasive (Fig. 8.8), whereas the exophytic variety

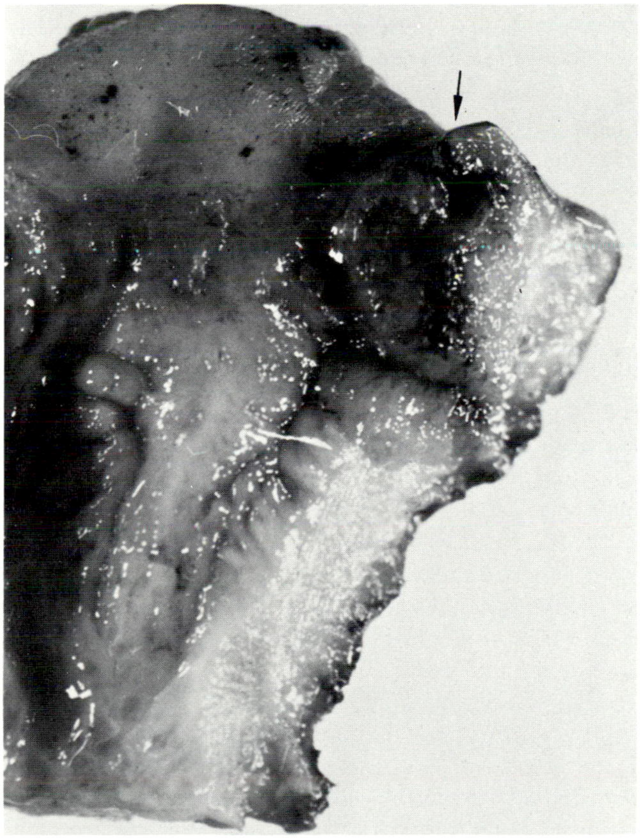

FIG. 8.8. Noduloinvasive squamous carcinoma of the cervix. Note the circumscribed margin of the tumor elevating the squamous portio epithelium (*arrow*), which is devoid of ulceration.

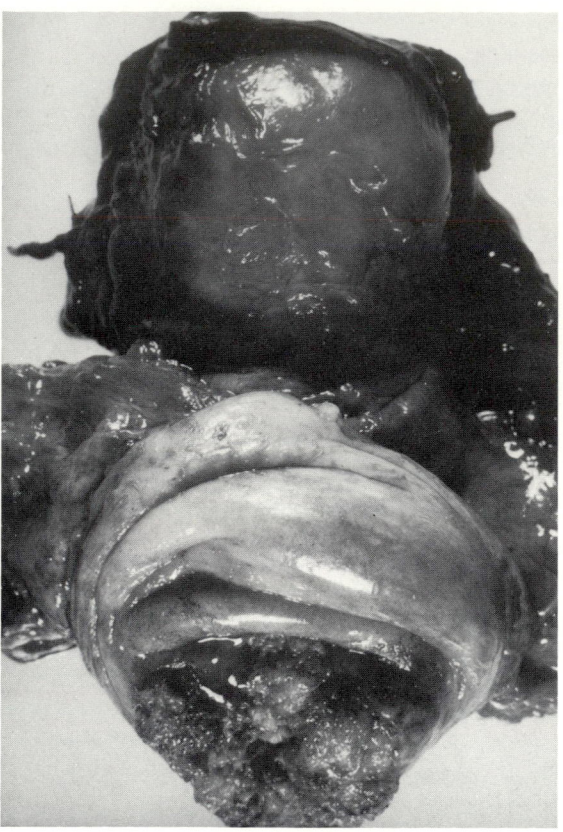

Fig. 8.9. Polypoid, invasive squamous carcinoma of the cervix. A bulky friable mass projects from the external os. (Courtesy of Dr. B.K. Chun, Washington, D.C.)

Table 8.6. Histologic classification of invasive carcinomas of the uterine cervix.

Squamous carcinoma
Microinvasive carcinoma
Occult carcinoma
Clinical invasive carcinoma
Adenocarcinoma
Typical endocervical adenocarcinoma
Endometrioid adenocarcinoma
Clear cell adenocarcinoma (tubulocystic and papillary)
Papillary mucinous adenocarcinoma
Papillary serous adenocarcinoma
Mucinous (colloid) intestinal adenocarcinoma
Medullary adenocarcinoma
Specific variants of adenocarcinoma
Adenoma malignum (minimal deviation adenocarcinoma, very well differentiated adenocarcinoma)
Adenoid cystic carcinoma
Mesonephric carcinoma
Mixed epithelial carcinoma
Adenosquamous carcinoma
Glassy cell carcinoma
Mucoepidermoid carcinoma
Dual primary carcinoma
Neuroendocrine carcinoma
Carcinoid
Small cell carcinoma

may be polypoid (Fig. 8.9) or papillary (verrucous carcinoma).

Microscopic Features

The majority (94%) of malignant epithelial neoplasms of the cervix used to be classified microscopically as squamous (epidermoid) carcinomas. However, a recent analysis of large series of cervical cancers[1,149] revealed that when rigid histologic criteria are used in the histologic classification of cervical carcinomas, only 75–77% are of the squamous type. The remainder, 23–25%, include various types of adenocarcinomas, adenosquamous carcinoma, and undifferentiated carcinoma (Table 8.6). In general, invasive squamous carcinomas are characterized by anastomosing tongues or solid masses of neoplastic epithelium infiltrating the fibrous stroma of the cervix (Fig. 8.10). Characteristically, the contour of the infiltrating nests and clusters is irregular and ragged.

Several attempts have been made to classify cervical squamous carcinomas according to the predominant cell type or degree of differentiation. Reagan and Ng[149] proposed classifying them into large-cell keratinizing, large-cell nonkeratinizing, and small-cell nonkeratinizing carcinomas. In their experience the best 5-year survival rate was associated with large-cell nonkeratinizing carcinomas (68.3%), followed by the large-cell keratinizing type (41.7%), whereas small-cell carcinomas had a 20% 5-year survival rate. Others, however, found no significant difference in prognosis between the different histologic types of cervical squamous tumors.[65] To date, the most accepted and widely used histologic classification is based on the degree of differentiation. The lesions are divided into well-differentiated (grade 1), moderately differentiated (grade 2), and poorly differentiated (grade 3) carcinomas. Most squamous carcinomas are moderately differentiated (grade 2), followed by poorly differentiated (grade 3) and well-differentiated lesions (grade 1).

In the well-differentiated type, the most striking feature is the abundance of keratin formation, which is deposited as concentric whorls (keratin pearls) in the centers of neoplastic epithelial nests (Fig. 8.11). The cells appear mature, with voluminous, eosinophilic cytoplasm. Individual cell keratinization (dyskeratosis) is recognized by intense cytoplasmic eosinophilia. Occasionally, the cells assume a clear appearance, which is caused by the accumulation of intracytoplasmic glycogen (Fig. 8.12). The cells are tightly packed together and produce well-developed intercellular bridges. The nuclei are large, irregular, and hyperchromatic, with numerous

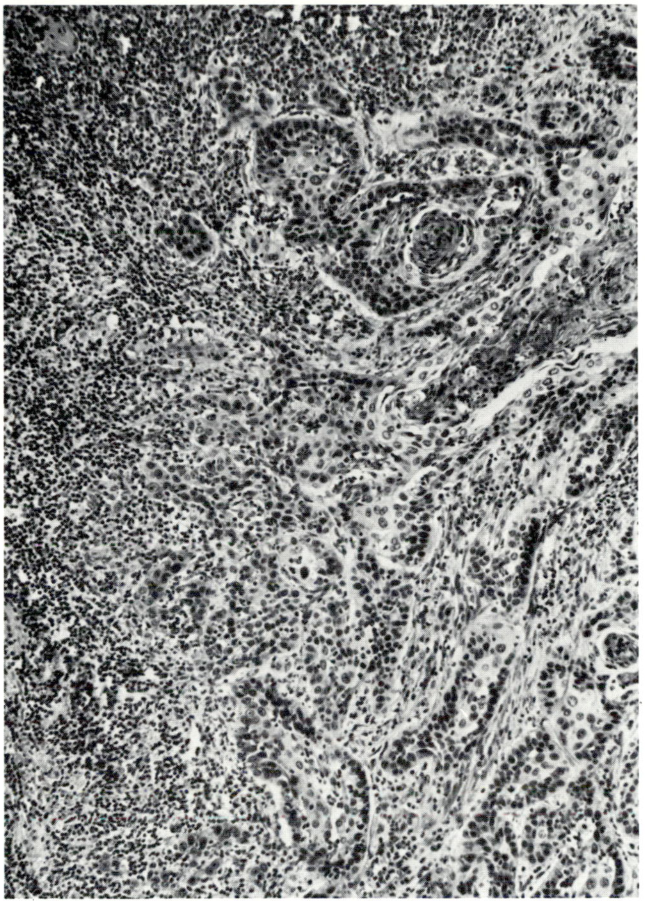

FIG. 8.10. Invasive squamous carcinoma of the cervix. Note the irregular contour of infiltrative nests. There is evidence of neoplastic cell degeneration and conspicuous inflammatory exudate at the epithelial–stromal junction.

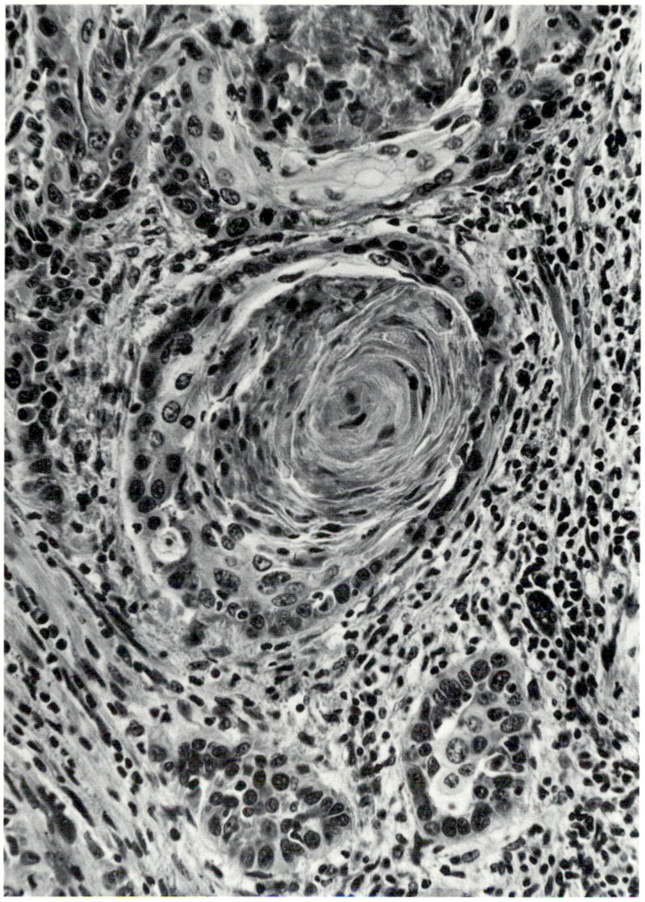

FIG. 8.11. Well-differentiated (grade 1) invasive squamous carcinoma of the cervix. Keratin pearl formation is evident.

chromocenters. Mitotic divisions are present, with maximum concentration at the periphery of the advancing epithelial nests. The stroma is often infiltrated by chronic inflammatory cells, and, occasionally, a foreign body giant cell reaction is observed (Fig. 8.13).

In moderately differentiated carcinomas, the neoplastic cells are more pleomorphic than in grade 1 lesions, are characterized by large irregular nuclei, and have a less abundant cytoplasmic matrix. The cellular borders, as well as intercellular bridges, appear indistinct. Keratin pearl formation is virtually nonexistent, but individual cell keratinization is seen in the center of nests of tumor cells. Mitotic figures are more numerous than in the better differentiated lesions (Fig. 8.14).

Poorly differentiated squamous carcinomas are generally composed of cells with hyperchromatic oval nuclei and scant indistinct cytoplasm, resembling the malignant basal cells of grade 3 intraepithelial neoplasia or CIS (Fig. 8.15). Search for squamous differentiation reveals rare foci of abortive dyskeratosis. Mitoses and areas of necrosis are abundant. Poorly differentiated lesions are occasionally composed of large, pleomorphic cells with giant, bizarre nuclei and abnormal mitotic figures. In rare instances, the neoplastic cells assume a spindle-shaped configuration resembling a sarcoma (Fig. 8.16). In these instances, reticulum stain demonstrates the epithelial nature of the spindle-shaped growth (fibrils encircle nests of cells rather than individual cells), and in most instances histologic continuity between the spindle-shaped neoplastic cells and the usual squamous epithelial cells can be demonstrated (Fig. 8.17).

Differential Diagnosis

Histologically, the lesions most commonly confused with invasive squamous cell carcinomas are squamous metaplasia with extensive endocervical gland involvement, gestational decidual reaction with degenerative features, condylomata acuminata, and pseudoepitheliomatous hyperplasia associated with chronic granulomatous diseases, such as lymphogranuloma venereum and granuloma inguinale. Careful evaluation of the cytonuclear appearance of these lesions, however, reveals their be-

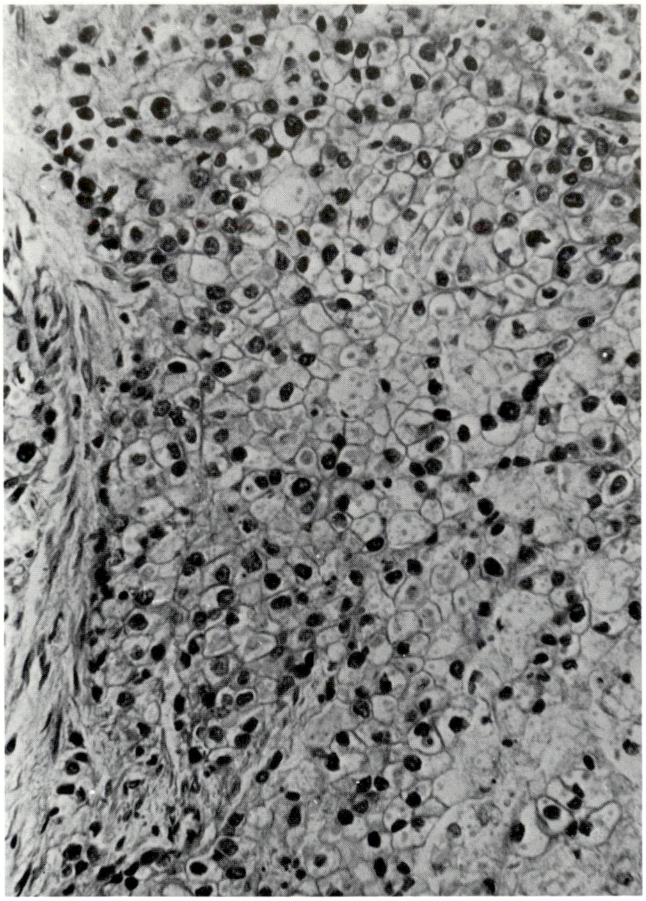

FIG. 8.12. Invasive squamous carcinoma of the cervix with clear cell features. The cells are rich in glycogen, which results in their flocculent, clear cytoplasmic appearance. The cellular borders are well defined.

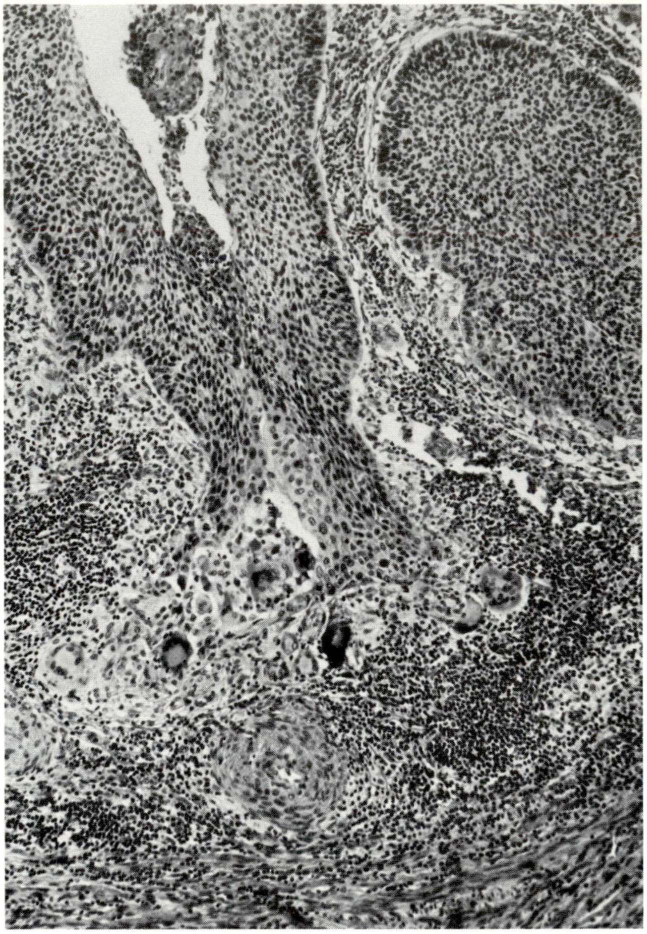

FIG. 8.13. Moderately differentiated (grade 2) squamous carcinoma of the cervix. Note foreign body giant cell reaction to infiltrating tumor cells.

nign nature. Verrucous carcinoma (Figs. 8.18 and 8.19) may also be mistaken for ordinary squamous carcinoma.

Immunohistochemistry

Because of the rapid strides made in antibody technology, a number of immunohistochemical analyses have been applied to the study of cervical carcinoma. Studies of intermediate filaments of cervical carcinoma show a pattern paralleling that of histologic differentiation.[38,128] Poorly differentiated, nonkeratinizing, and undifferentiated carcinomas contain a complex variety of keratins differing in pattern and number from those of normal tissue. Differentiated, keratinizing cervical carcinomas have a less complex pattern of keratin intermediate filaments and contain polypeptides characteristic of terminal differentiation. The heterogeneous intermediate filament patterns expressed in cervical carcinoma indicate that some sets of keratin polypeptides are conserved during malignant transformation whereas others reflect a selection of a minor cell type or clone during carcinogenesis or even de novo expression.[128] Involucrin, a marker for squamous differentiation distinct from keratin, can also be identified in differentiated areas of squamous carcinoma in 93% of patients, indicating conservation of this protein during transformation.[156] After further studies are completed, it is likely that differentiation markers and intermediate filaments may prove useful in better understanding the pathogenesis of cervical carcinoma and as tools in differential diagnosis.[38,156]

Monoclonal antibodies, derived from cervical carcinomas, are being developed and tested. The most promising studies have been those with a tumor-associated antigen, TA-4,[91,118,175] found to be an as yet uncharacterized glycoprotein of 48,000 molecular weight. Elevations of serum TA-4 have been observed in women with cervical carcinoma and can be used to monitor the effects of therapy and detect tumor recurrence.[91,118] In tissue sections, TA-4 is localized in differentiated and keratinized cells

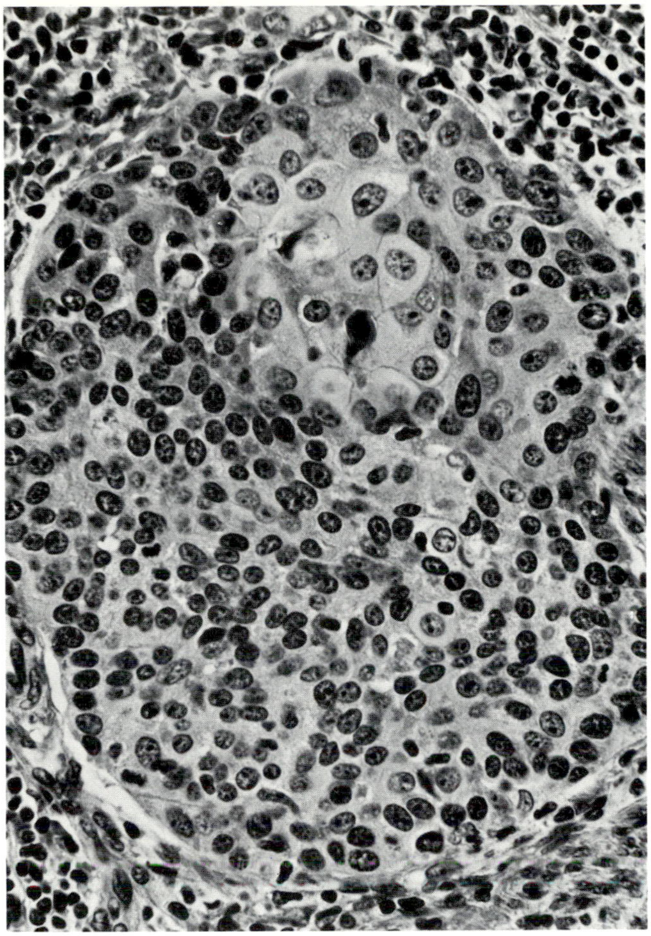

FIG. 8.14. Moderately differentiated (grade 2) squamous carcinoma of the cervix. Note attempt at keratinization.

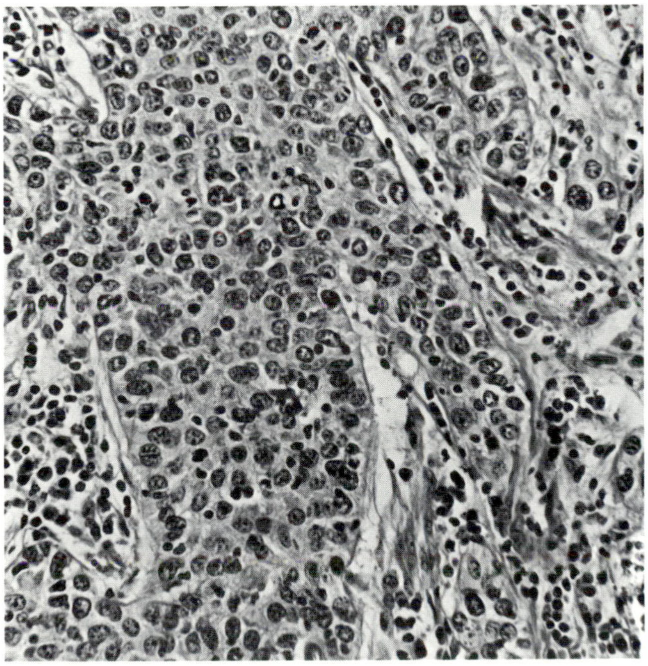

FIG. 8.15. Poorly differentiated (grade 3) squamous carcinoma. Note anisonucleosis, scant cytoplasm, and indistinct cell membranes.

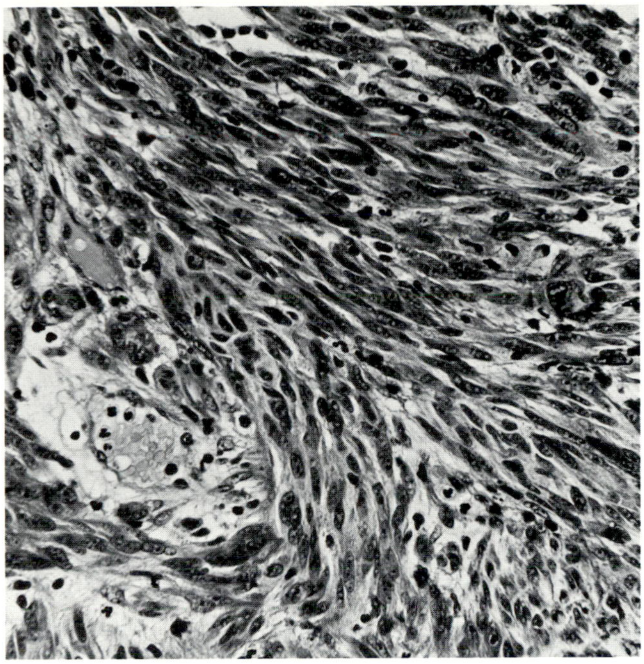

FIG. 8.16. Invasive squamous carcinoma with spindle-shape features. Note fusiform configuration of cells, resembling a sarcoma. This area was continuous, with moderately differentiated squamous carcinoma.

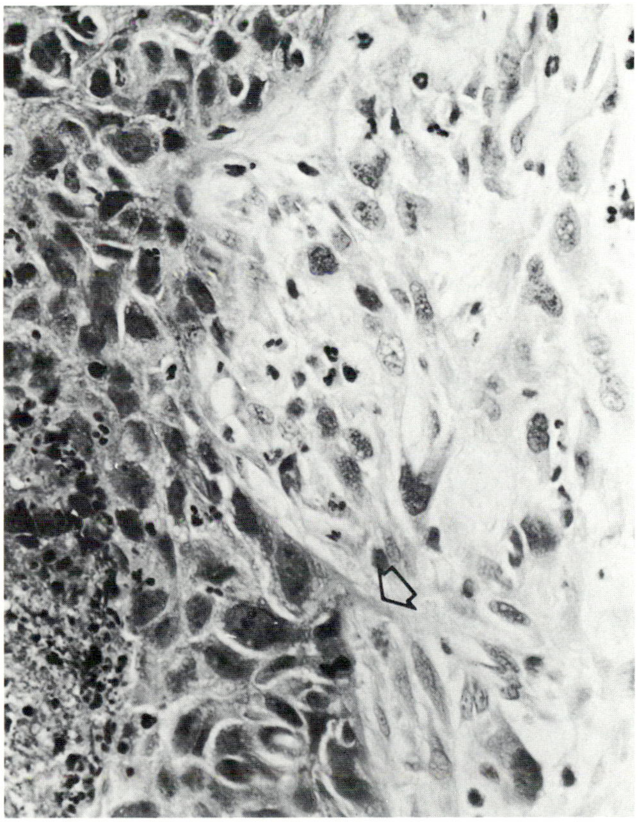

FIG. 8.17. Squamous carcinoma with pseudosarcomatous stromal features. The neoplastic cells in the stroma masquerade as malignant mesenchymal cells. They are squamous cells with spindle-shape. Note continuity between sarcoma-like cells and neoplastic squamous epithelium (*arrow*).

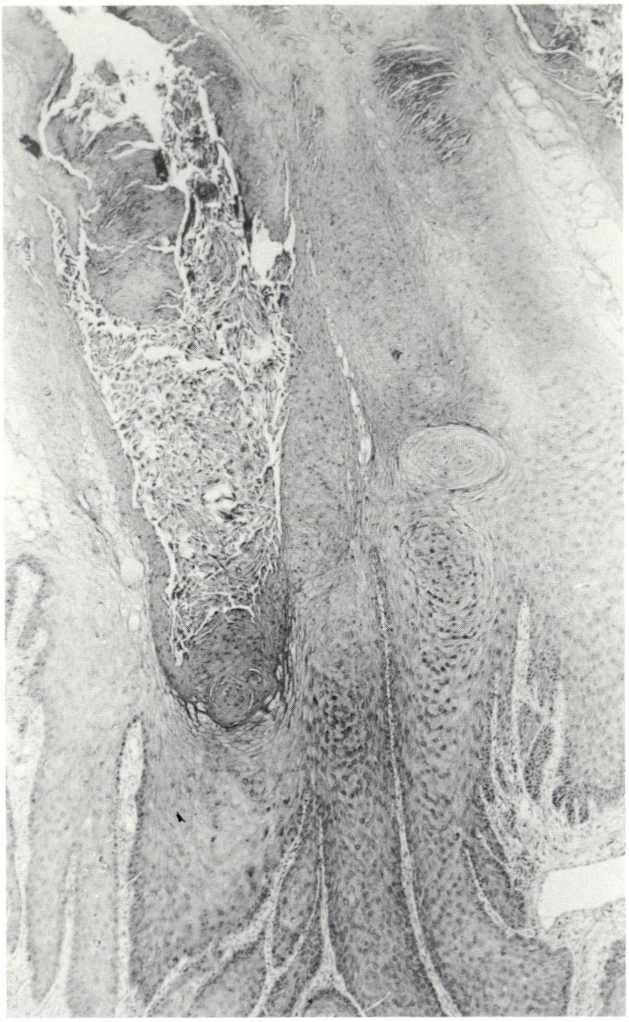

FIG. 8.18. Verrucous carcinoma of the cervix. Note frond-like papillae with extensive surface keratinization. The circumscribed, cone-shaped edges of neoplastic fronds expand into the underlying stroma. There are no stromal papillae in the upper strata of the neoplastic process.

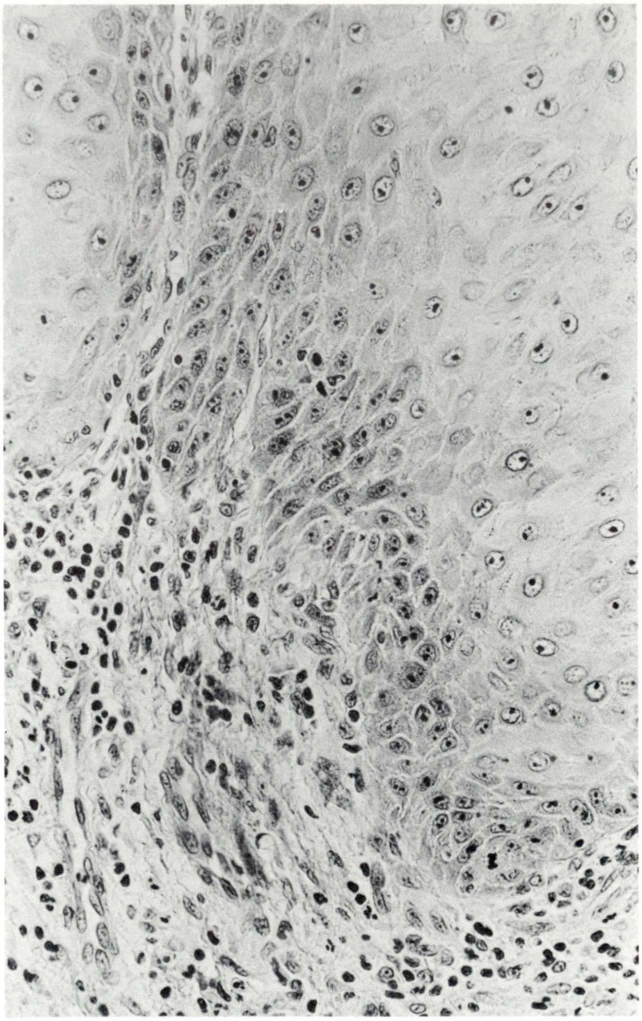

FIG. 8.19. Verrucous carcinoma of the cervix. High-power view illustrating the regular contour of advancing epithelial fronds. Note lack of significant nuclear atypia.

in normal cervical squamous epithelium and malignant tumors. Antigen expression in carcinomas is linked to differentiation and cannot be identified in small cell undifferentiated tumors.[118] The efficacy of TA-4 and other new cervical carcinoma monoclonal antibodies is at present unknown.

Ultrastructure

The ultrastructural hallmarks of neoplastic cells of squamous origin include intracytoplasmic bundles of tonofilaments, desmosome–tonofilament complexes, and finger-like intercellular microvilli.[51] These alterations are readily identified in well- and moderately differentiated neoplasms.[51] The tonofilaments may be aggregated and form large globular masses, resulting in intense cytologic eosinophilia of neoplastic cells that are engaged in individual cell keratinization (Fig. 8.20). In the lesser differentiated lesions, tonofilaments and desmosomal plates are reduced and poorly developed. Loss of desmosomal attachments and separation of desmosomal–tonofilament complexes lead to loss of cellular cohesion. Another characteristic feature of squamous carcinoma cells is the profound decrease in gap–junction nexuses compared to normal cervical squamous epithelium.[123] The nexus consists of closely packed, hexagonal tubules forming an open-channel system between adjacent cells. The system facilitates the passage of electrolytes and proteins from one cell to another without traversing the intercellular space. It has been suggested that nexuses play a role in cell contact inhibition and in the formation of low-resistance electrical coupling sites between normal

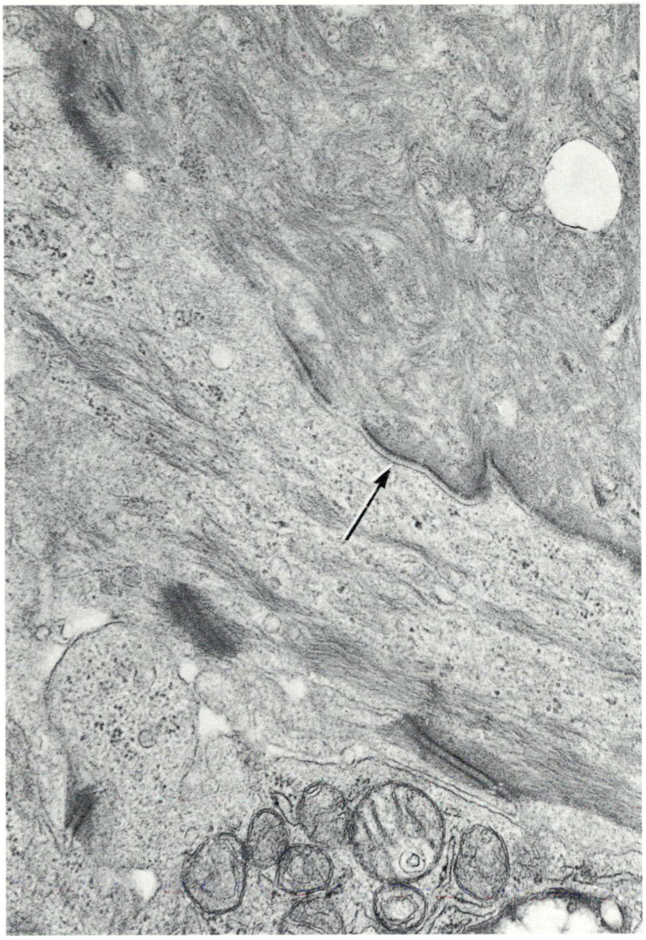

FIG. 8.20. Well-differentiated invasive squamous carcinoma of the cervix. Electron microscopic appearance of individual cell keratinization (dyskeratosis). Lobular masses of tonofilaments are responsible for intense eosinophilia on light microscopy. Aggregation of tonofilament is caused by separation and retraction of desmosomal tonofilament attachments (*arrow*). The intercellular space (I) contains interdigitating microvilli. ×7438.

cells.[123] A deficiency of nexuses in invasive cervical carcinoma may therefore be responsible for the reduced cellular adhesiveness, cell contact inhibition, and altered electrical coupling that have been observed in malignant neoplastic cells[123] and perhaps the invasive character of malignant neoplasms. A well-developed basement membrane is produced by the invading neoplastic cells, although it often appears fragmented.

Modes of Spread

Squamous carcinoma of the cervix spreads principally by direct local invasion to the adjacent tissues and by lymphatics and less commonly through blood vessels. Initially, the tumor grows by direct continuity along tissue spaces of least resistance, the perineural and perivascular tissues, into the paracervical and parametrial areas and into the cardinal and uterosacral ligaments. Ultimately, lateral spread may reach the bony pelvis and so encompass and obstruct one or both ureters. Direct extension may also involve the uterine cavity and vagina, with extension into the urinary bladder and rectum resulting in vesicovaginal and rectovaginal fistulas.

The spread of cervical cancer via lymphatics occurs relatively early in the course of the disease and is found in 25–50% of patients with stage Ib and II carcinomas.[27,92] The preferential course of dissemination is via the paracervical, hypogastric, and external iliac lymph nodes[132,143] and then extension to lateral sacral, common iliac, paraaortic, and inguinal nodes. Isolated invasion of the sacral, external iliac, and hypogastric nodes is occasionally observed. Distant lymph node metastases above the diaphragm including the supraclavicular lymph nodes are uncommon[44] and are a feature of widespread disease. In these cases, cancer cells are transported from the paraaortic nodes into the mediastinum and then into the thoracic duct.

Hematogenous dissemination is the least common metastatic pathway of cervical carcinoma, although nearly 50% of surgically removed specimens may contain histologic evidence of blood vessel invasion.[60] Blood-borne metastases are generally seen in stage IV lesions or when the local growth has previously been irradiated. They are produced in the lung, liver, bone, heart, skin, and brain.

Behavior and Treatment

The three basic modalities in the treatment of invasive carcinoma of the cervix are radiation, surgery, and a combination of radiation and surgery. At present, radical hysterectomy with pelvic lymphadenectomy is considered the most appropriate therapeutic approach for occult invasive carcinoma of the cervix. In selected early stage Ib and II cases, radical hysterectomy and bilateral pelvic lymphadenectomy or intracavitary radiation followed by radical surgery may be carried out. Results of radical surgery and radiation therapy are essentially similar. Because metastatic lymph node involvement remains one of the most important prognostic factors, the use of preoperative lymphography has been recommended in recent years as an aid during the dissection and excision of the pelvic lymphatic system.[96] Accurate staging may be facilitated by the use of percutaneous fine needle aspiration biopsy.[21,60]

The preferred treatment for most stage II and III patients is combined external and intracavitary radiotherapy. Modern techniques of radiotherapy use a variety of intracavitary radium applicators and low-intensity needles. External megavoltage with cobalt-60 is required for adequate radiation of the pelvis. The total cancericidal dose of both radium and x-rays to control squamous carcinoma of the cervix is in the order of 6000–7000 rads. The frequency of serious morbidity and mortality from irradiation is 30% and 2.4%, respectively.[177] The most common complications in decreasing frequency are: proctitis, vault necrosis, hemorrhagic cystitis, peritonitis resulting from obstruction, perforation, and necrosis of the bowel, vesicovaginal fistula, and profuse hemorrhage. The frequency of major complications associated with radical surgery is about 3% and includes bladder atony, thrombophlebitis, cuff abscesses, and hematoma. The operative death rate is 0.6%.[139] Chemotherapy, using methotrexate and 5-fluorouracil, is employed in carcinomas with widespread distribution or recurrent neoplasms, but the results are disappointing. Immunotherapy with DNA from patient's tumor plus Freund's adjuvant and autogenous vaccine made from patient's tumor has been attempted without significant success.[66]

Stage is the most important prognostic factor in cervical carcinoma (Table 8.7). Within a particular stage, however, other factors have been evaluated for their prognostic significance, including depth of invasion,[78] size or bulk of lymph node metastases,[80] and parametrial extension.[79] Large primary tumors, lymph node metastases, and parametrial extension are indicators of tumor burden and are poor prognostic variables within comparable stages.[78–80]

The general 5-year survival for adequately treated patients of all stages is 60%. Local recurrences of invasive disease are principally located in the vaginal vault, pelvis, bladder, and rectum and occur in about 15% of patients. Typically, the majority of recurrences appear within 2 years after initial therapy. Persistent disease, recurrent disease, and metastasis are best detected by a combination of physical examination, chest x-ray, and IVP. Suspicious masses can be sampled percutaneously by fine needle aspiration to confirm the clinical and radiologic findings.[21,161] The 5-year survival rate after treatment of recurrent disease by means of irradiation or exenteration is 20–35%.[69] The actuarial 5-year salvage rates according to the FIGO clinical stages are: stage I, 85–90%; stage II, 70–75%; stage III, 30–35%; stage IV, 10%.[92] In general, the survival rates are reduced to 30–50%, even in the early stages (Ib), when metastatic lymph nodes are discovered compared to those patients without node involvement.[92] Metastatic node involvement occurs in 8–25% of stage I, 21–38% of stage II, and 32–46% of stage III lesions.[92,132]

Elevated levels of plasma carcinoembryonic antigen (CEA), a tumor-associated antigen, were reported in 50% of patients with invasive squamous carcinoma of the cervix and 84% of the patients with recurrent carcinoma.[46] Carcinoembryonic antigen determinations may be used as an aid in the early detection of recurrent disease or metastasis. A tumor-specific complement-fixing antibody, induced by HSV-2 (AG-4), has been detected in 91% of untreated invasive carcinomas, 68% of in situ lesions, and 5% of control patients studied.[8] The latter test may be of considerable prognostic value in evaluating the clinical course as well as the therapeutic response of patients with cervical neoplasia. Tumor-associated antigen TA-4, a monoclonal antibody developed from cervical carcinoma, has also been shown to be of value in monitoring selected patients with cervical carcinoma.

TABLE 8.7. Distribution of carcinomas (squamous and adenocarcinomas) of the uterine cervix by clinical stage.

	Stage			
Series	I	II	III	IV
Campos[26] (311 patients)	27%	34%	27%	2%
Abell[1] (3694 patients)[a]	30%	35%	23%	6.5%
TOTAL	33.5%	34.5%	30%	4.2%

[a] In Abell's series, the clinical stage was not available in 5.5% of patients.

Other factors that influence prognosis are the gross characteristics of invasive cervical carcinomas; polypoid lesions are less aggressive than noduloinvasive or ulceroinvasive cancers. In general, histologic grading has no direct influence on survival within any stage.[66] Although well-differentiated neoplasms progress slower than poorly differentiated lesions, the latter have a better response to ionizing irradiation therapy than the former, and so the overall end results are similar for carcinomas of different grades.[1] However, neoplasms with marked lymphoplasmocytic and foreign body giant cell granulomatous stromal infiltration (Fig. 8.13) appear to have a more favorable course than those without significant stromal inflammatory reaction.[1]

Ureteral compression caused by both ureteral wall compression and periureteral lymphatic obstruction by the tumor leads to hydroureter, hydronephrosis, hydronephrotic renal atrophy, pyelonephritis, and loss of renal function. Obstruction of both ureters results in uremia and is the leading cause of death, being found in about 40–50% of patients dying with cervical carcinoma.[165] Peritonitis caused by obstruction and perforation of large or small bowel, respiratory failure associated with pulmonary metastasis, or massive edema are the other major causes of death. Hemorrhage, cardiac failure, massive venous thrombosis, pulmonary embolism, and complications of radiation therapy represent the less common causes of death.

Carcinoma of the Cervical Stump

Invasive carcinoma of either the squamous or glandular type may develop in the cervical stump that remains following subtotal hysterectomy in 0.2–3% of patients.[184] According to various series, patients with cervical stump cancer represent 0.5–10% of all cancers of the cervix uteri. In a study of 173 women with carcinoma of the cervical stump, Wolff et al.[184] divided their patients into those in whom the neoplasm was found within 2 years of the subtotal hysterectomy and those in whom the lesion appeared more than 2 years after the operation. The 5-year survival of patients of the first subgroup was found to be worse (30%) than either those of the second subgroup (49%) or those with cancer of the cervix in general. The prognosis for patients of the second subgroup was comparable to that for patients with cancer of the cervix in general. Similarly, metastatic disease developed more frequently (17%) in the first subgroup than in the second group of patients. On the basis of these observations, the authors[184] postulated that cervical stump cancers occurring within the first 2 years following surgery represent "left behind" or residual malignancy, whereas those discovered after 2 years are "new" cancers arising de novo from the cervical stump. The existence of two such distinct groups of patients, however, remains speculative as no morphologic data were available either on the subtotal hysterectomy specimens or on the cervix before or after removal of the fundus. Since carcinoma may arise in the cervical stump, subtotal hysterectomy should not be performed except under unusual circumstances dictated at the time of surgery.

Carcinoma in Pregnancy

Invasive carcinoma of the cervix is uncommon during gestation, occurring approximately once in 3500 pregnancies in a high-risk population for cervical cancer.[48] In the general population, the frequency is about 1 in 6000 pregnancies or less. Routine cervical cytology should be part of the initial prenatal examination. The treatment of pregnant patients with invasive cervical cancer depends on the clinical stage of the disease. Patients with stage Ia MICA (with less than 3 mm stromal invasion and no vascular invasion) are allowed to progress to term under careful and frequent colposcopic examinations and then treated either by vaginal hysterectomy after vaginal delivery or by cesarean section hysterectomy.[43] Stages Ib or more are immediately treated without regard to the fetus. Exceptions are made, however, during the last trimester when treatment may be delayed to carry the infant to viability. The management of stage Ib and some IIa lesions is radical hysterectomy and bilateral pelvic lymphadenectomy[53] or combined radiation therapy.[35] Irradiation is the therapeutic choice for patients with more advanced disease, those with medical contraindications, or those who refuse radical surgery. External radiation usually causes abortion in about 6 weeks, and intracavitary radium is applied to the cervix to complete therapy. Pregnancy or young age per se does not influence the prognosis of cancer of the cervix.[16,48]

Verrucous Carcinoma

Verrucous carcinoma is a rare variant of well-differentiated squamous cell carcinoma. In the female genital tract, the most commonly involved region is the vulva, but well-documented cases have been described in the cervix.* Clinically, the lesion is a slow-growing but potentially lethal and locally invasive verrucous neoplasm. Five of eight patients with verrucous carcinoma of the cervix died of tumor shortly after the diagnosis.[113] In the past, this distinctive tumor has often been reported under the term *giant condyloma acuminatum of Buschke and Lowenstein*.[61,113,140,141] Histologically, the neoplasm is composed of well-differentiated squamous cells arranged in frond-like papillae (Fig. 8.18) with or without surface keratinization. The epithelium lacks significant cytologic atypia, although in some cases numerous mitoses may be found in the lower layers. The edges of the invading tongues are broad and expansile without infiltrating ragged edges (Fig. 8.19). There is a conspicuous inflammatory reaction at the epithelial stromal junction. Verrucous carcinoma has been strongly associated with HPV 6 infection.[3,107,135]

Verrucous carcinoma should be distinguished from well-differentiated squamous carcinoma with a keratinized papillary surface and from condylomata acuminata.[140,141] Verrucous carcinoma lacks the small infiltrating clusters of anaplastic cells and central fibroconnective tissue cores in the epithelial papillae that are seen in warty squamous carcinoma and condylomata, respectively.[101] Verrucous carcinoma in the absence of deep stromal invasion or metastasis may be difficult to distinguish histologically from well-differentiated squamous carcinoma or large condylomata acuminata of the cervix.[90,113] As a result, the correct diagnosis is not apparent until local recurrence after surgical removal occurs. Typically, these tumors recur locally but do not metastasize unless they are inadequately radiated, in which case accelerated growth and metastasis may occur.[3,27,90] The

* References 42, 49, 81, 90, 101, 113, 141.

most appropriate therapy is wide local excision. Regional lymph nodes are rarely involved, and distant metastases are exceedingly rare.[113]

Adenocarcinoma

Adenocarcinoma In Situ

The criteria for the diagnosis of adenocarcinoma in situ (ACIS) of the endocervix are controversial and, for the most part, ill defined. The lesions of ACIS may be focal or superficial and, consequently, are often underdiagnosed. In contrast, the more extensive, multicentric lesions are difficult to distinguish from early invasive adenocarcinoma. In ACIS the general characteristics of the endocervical epithelium are retained, and the dominant abnormalities are cytologic, including nuclear enlargement, nuclear hyperchromaticity, mitotic activity, and the presence of abnormal mitotic figures. There is an increase in architectural irregularity and complexity, consisting of papillary infolding, outpouching, and focal cribriform pattern. Nuclear stratification may also be seen (Figs. 8.21 and 8.22). Ostör et al.[136] cite the following characteristics to classify ACIS and to distinguish it from early invasive adenocarcinoma: (1) limitation of lesion to the glandular field (no extension past the normal endocervical crypts—3–5 mm depth), (2) admixture of neoplastic and normal glands, and (3) absence of stromal response, including edema and inflammatory cell infiltrate. The diagnosis of ACIS should be made only on adequate conization or hysterectomy specimens and may only be suspected in punch biopsy samples. The clinical and biologic significance of less severe endocervical lesions variably termed *atypical hyperplasia* or *dysplasia of the columnar endocervix* has not been well studied, and a spectrum of premalignant endocervical changes cannot, as yet, be documented.[6,171]

Although the morphologic and clinical characteristics of microinvasive squamous carcinoma are now well defined, those of its endocervical glandular counterpart are not. The main difficulty in defining microinvasive adenocarcinoma of the endocervix stems from the difficulty in recognizing microinvasion. Unlike squamous disease, in which invasion occurs by breakthrough of single cells or tongues of cells with ragged contours, many adenocarcinomas invade by entire glands without an associated stromal response. As a result, it is impossible to assess with certainty whether the glands are truly invasive, the precise depth of invasion, and where the origin of invasion is. Although lesions with less than 5-mm depth of penetration behaved in a benign fashion in one series,[146] we have seen cases in consultation in which the deepest gland was uninvolved, yet the disease recurred and gave rise to metastasis. Until endocervical microinvasion is clearly defined, there are two clinically meaningful lesions: adenocarcinoma in situ and invasive (early and advanced) carcinoma.

Invasive Adenocarcinoma

Incidence and Age Distribution

The frequency of primary adenocarcinoma has been variously assessed as 5–8% of all epithelial malignancies of the cervix, with a range from 0.42 to 11.7%.[1,40,56] In recent years the average frequency has doubled,[1,148] and rates as high as 34% are reported in certain series.[40] Whether the increase is absolute or related to improved cytologic detection and decreasing numbers of squamous carcinomas[34,53,148] has not been clearly established. Adenocarcinoma in situ often coexists (up to 43% in some series)[115] with CIN. Since the latter has increased in recent years it is possible that the increase in adenocarcinomas is proportional to the increase in squamous lesions. The mean age of patients with invasive adenocarcinoma is 56 years, 5 years older than those with squamous carcinoma.[34] Reports of endocervical adenocarcinoma in premenopausal women under the age of 50 suggest that the age incidence may be decreasing.[39]

Pathogenesis

At present, there is little definitive information on the etiology and pathogenesis of endocervical adenocarcinoma. Unlike squamous carcinoma of the cervix, endocervical adenocarcinoma has not been clearly associated with venereal etiologic factors. Indeed, Menczner et al.[124] found a comparatively higher incidence of adenocarcinoma in ethnic groups such as Israeli women who had a low risk for squamous carcinoma. The not uncommon finding of coexistent squamous carcinoma and adenocarcinoma in situ in the same cervix suggests certain epidemiologic similarities in these two lesions. Epidemiologic risk factors for adenocarcinoma of the cervix are being investigated. Numerous studies have suggested a causal relationship between progestin administration, particularly oral contraceptive use, and the genesis of endocervical adenocarcinoma, but the number of cases have been too small for meaningful statistical analysis.[39] Of interest is the report of cervical adenocarcinoma in 2/12 rhesus monkeys treated with medroxyprogesterone acetate for 10 years.[39] Other studies have found no correlation between oral contraceptive use and the development of endocervical adenocarcinoma. Controlled prospective studies correlating the type of oral contraceptive or gestagen used, dosage, and duration of use with endocervical glandular changes must be undertaken to substantiate a relationship between oral contraceptives and progestins and endocervical adenocarcinoma. A generalized predisposition to the development of adenocarcinoma, possibly a field effect or genetic predisposition, is suggested by the finding of dual primary endocervical and ovarian adenocarcinomas in some women.[87] A genetic predisposition to endocervical adenocarcinoma is documented in women with Peutz–Jeghers syndrome, in whom minimal deviation adenocarcinoma of the cervix occurs more frequently than in the general population.[121,189] Recent studies report the finding of HPV 16 and 18 DNA in some cases of endocervical adenocarcinoma and adenosquamous carcinoma, but too few cases have been analyzed to determine whether or not this association is more than coincidental.[62,103,188]

The cell of origin of endocervical adenocarcinoma is thought to be the pluripotential subcolumnar reserve cell of the columnar endocervical epithelium. Although its natural history and histologic definition have not been well established, ACIS is regarded as the immediate precursor to invasive endocervical adenocarcinoma. Adenocarcinoma in situ occurs 5–20 years earlier than invasive adenocarcinoma[19,146] and can be identified with and without coexistent invasive disease in surgical specimens.[180] In one retrospective clinicopathologic analysis, ACIS was found at the margin of 43% of invasive adenocarcinomas.[2]

Clinical Aspects

The presenting symptom is abnormal vaginal bleeding in about 75% of patients. The disease is confined to the cervix (stage I) or the parametrium or vagina (stage II) in 80% of women at the time of discovery.[1,41,56,73,77]

The diagnostic accuracy of cytopathology in the detection of cervical adenocarcinoma varies according to the cytologic experience of the pathologist and the techniques used for material sampling. When the sampling technique includes aspiration of the endocervical canal with an endocervical pipette, the diagnostic accuracy can reach 95%. The definitive diagnosis of invasive adenocarcinoma[149] is achieved by microscopic examination of punch biopsies or conization biopsy.

Gross Features

On gross examination, 50% of the patients have a fungating, polypoid, or papillary mass, whereas nearly 15% have no gross lesion as the carcinoma is located within the canal or deep within the endocervical clefts. The internal location of endocervical adenocarcinomas makes their early detection and colposcopic definition very difficult.

Microscopic Features and Ultrastructure

Histologically, there are many variations in both the cell types and growth patterns.[1] The diagnosis is not always obvious, particularly in lesions that are very well differentiated or undifferentiated. In assessing whether the malignancy is of primary endocervical origin or metastatic in the cervix, the pathologist should evaluate the following morphologic features: (1) neoplastic growth pattern, (2) coexistent in situ changes, (3) cell type and (4) histochemical characteristics. Transition between in situ and invasive carcinoma[146] provides the strongest evidence for a primary origin and is found in certain series in up to 43% of the cases.[1] Pure adenocarcinomas arising within the endocervix are subclassified by the predominant architectural growth pattern, epithelial arrangement, and cytologic characteristics (Table 8.6). Conventional endocervical adenocarcinomas are of the endocervical columnar cell type and contain intracellular mucin. Foci of well-differentiated neoplastic glands may closely resemble those of the normal columnar endocervix. The majority are well to moderately differentiated[1] and arranged in a complex, racemose, glandular pattern reproducing the cleft–tunnel configuration of the normal

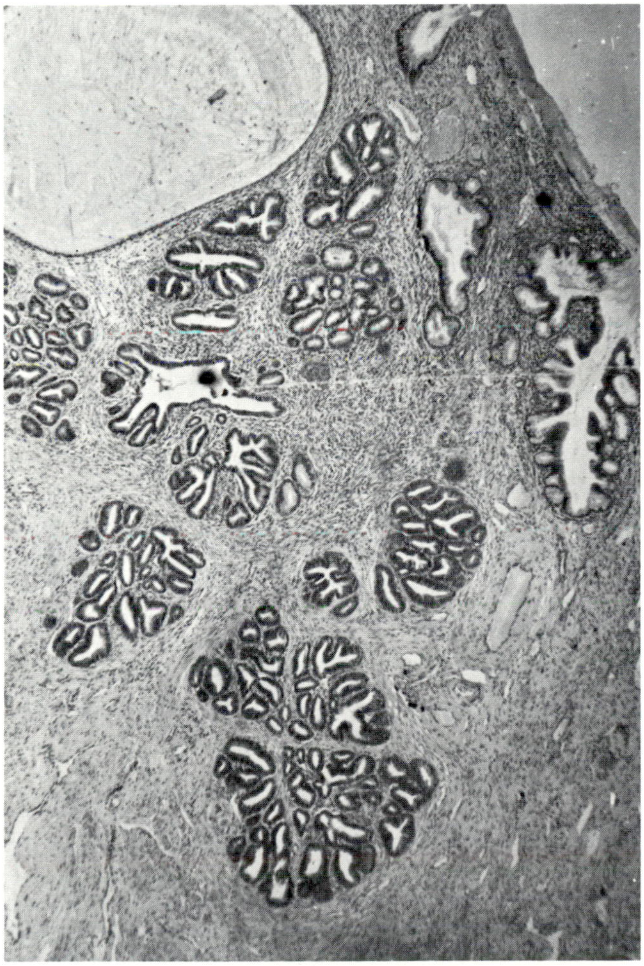

FIG. 8.21. In situ adenocarcinoma of the cervix. The neoplastic glands contrast with normal endocervical epithelium in their arrangement and staining characteristics.

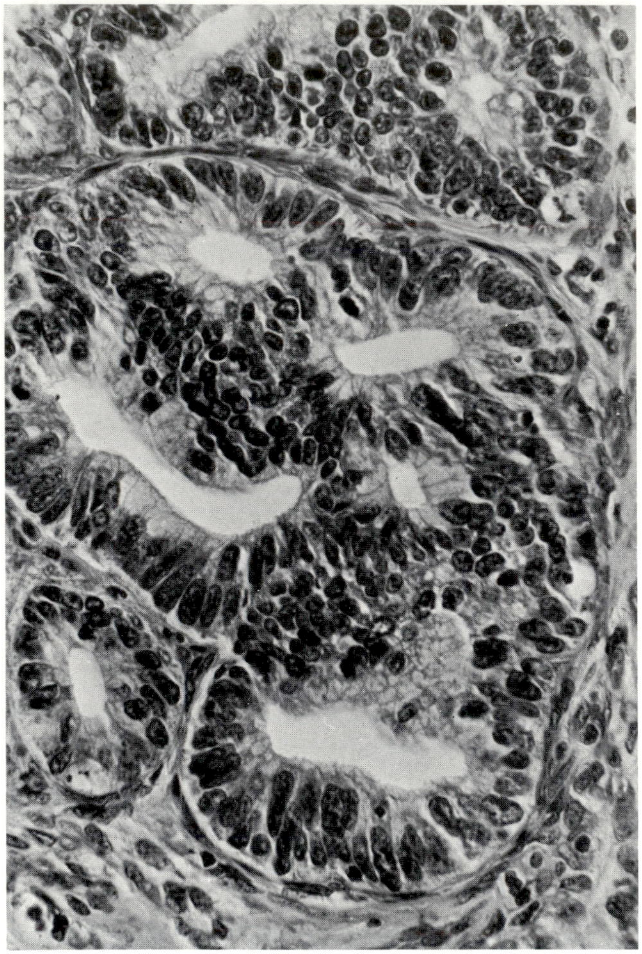

Fig. 8.22. In situ adenocarcinoma of the endocervix. Note the nuclear enlargement and pseudostratification with coarse chromatin, mitoses, and reduced intracytoplasmic mucin.

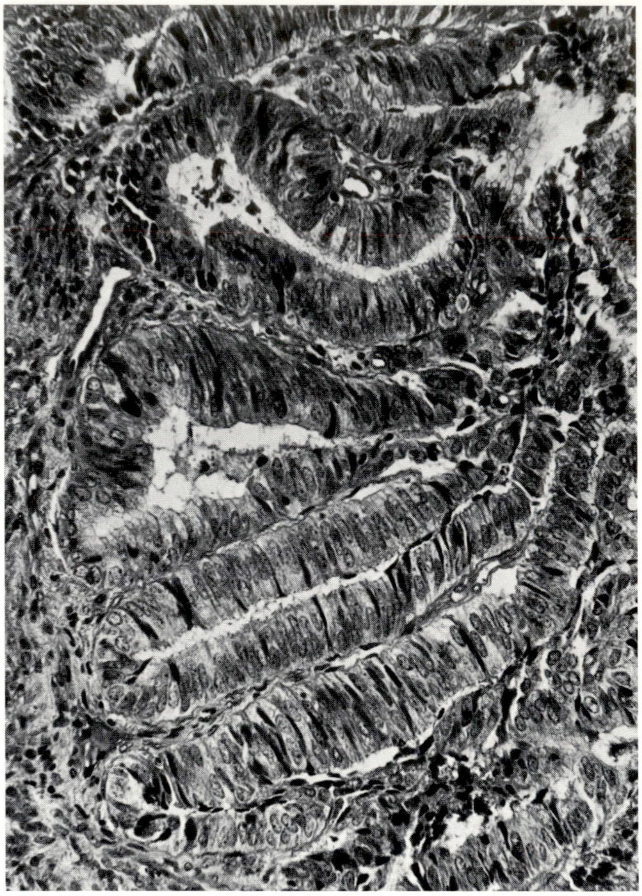

Fig. 8.23. Moderately differentiated invasive adenocarcinoma of the cervix.

endocervical mucosa. Other less common subtypes of endocervical adenocarcinoma recapitulate the varied morphology of the müllerian epithelium and may be of endometrioid, papillary serous, or clear cell type. Some tumors contain goblet cells and are termed *mucinous intestinal (colloid) adenocarcinoma.* In general, these histologic subtypes can be correlated with the clinical course and survival rates.[56,77]

Adenocarcinoma of the endocervical columnar cell type represents the most common variety of cervical glandular malignancies. Histologically, it varies from well-differentiated carcinoma[29,146,180] to poorly differentiated adenocarcinoma without an easily recognizable glandular pattern. The most common type is moderately differentiated, with interbranching glands and variable amount of intracytoplasmic mucin (Figs. 8.23 and 8.24). Transmission electron microscopy (Fig. 8.25) confirms the light microscopic and histochemical observations (Fig. 8.26) of a gradual decrease and an eventual loss of mucin production in increasingly dedifferentiated adenocarcinoma of the cervix.[51] The less frequent histologic varieties of pure adenocarcinoma of the endocervix are müllerian–metaplastic in type[106] and include papillary mucinous and serous carcinomas, both of which arise from the surface epithelium of the endocervix, the latter resembling papillary serous carcinoma of the ovary including psammoma bodies (Fig. 8.27), mucinous (colloid) carcinoma with conspicuous mucin production (Fig. 8.28), identical with adenocarcinoma of the large bowel with occasional argentaffin and Paneth cells,[1] and endometroid carcinoma with or without foci of squamous metaplasia, in all respects similar to endometrial adenocarcinoma. Endometrioid-type adenocarcinoma of the endocervix is probably more common than is usually recognized,[56,131,171] occurring in 4/55 pure adenocarcinomas of the cervix in one series.[56] Such lesions may be impossible to differentiate histologically from endometrial adenocarcinoma. On occasion, endocervical adenocarcinoma incites a stromal fibroplastic or lymphocytic response to produce a scirrhous-type carcinoma or med-

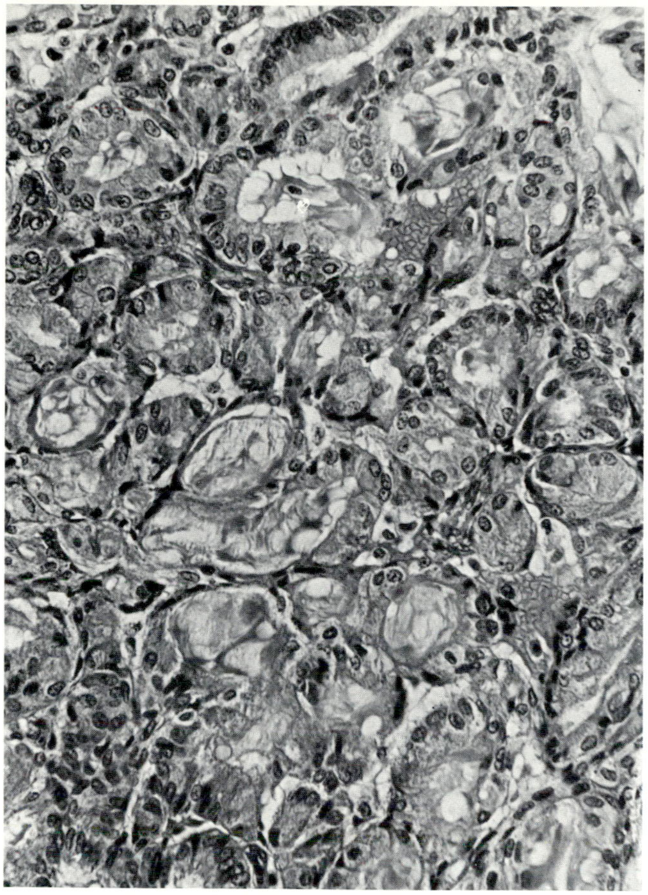

FIG. 8.24. Moderately differentiated invasive adenocarcinoma of the cervix. Note the conspicuous mucin production and finely granular pale cytoplasm of the neoplastic cells.

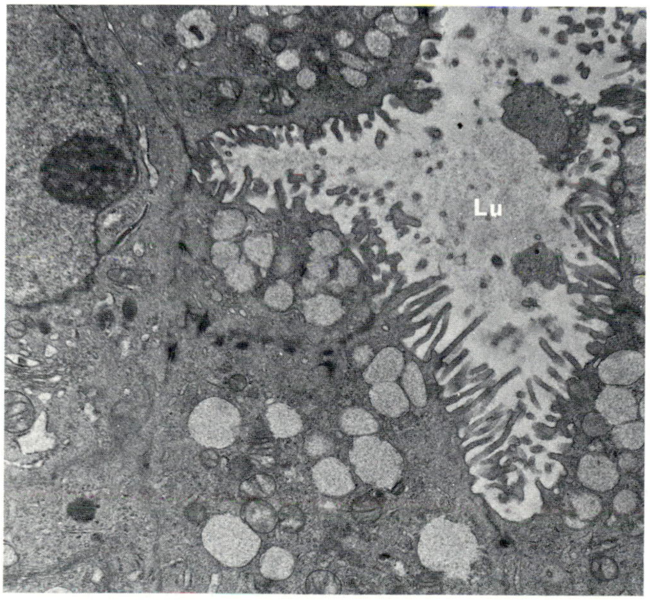

FIG. 8.25. Electron micrograph of neoplastic endocervical gland cells with apical, mucin-containing secretory granules. Mucinogenesis is reduced in neoplastic as compared to normal endocervical epithelium. Lu, lumen. ×6810.

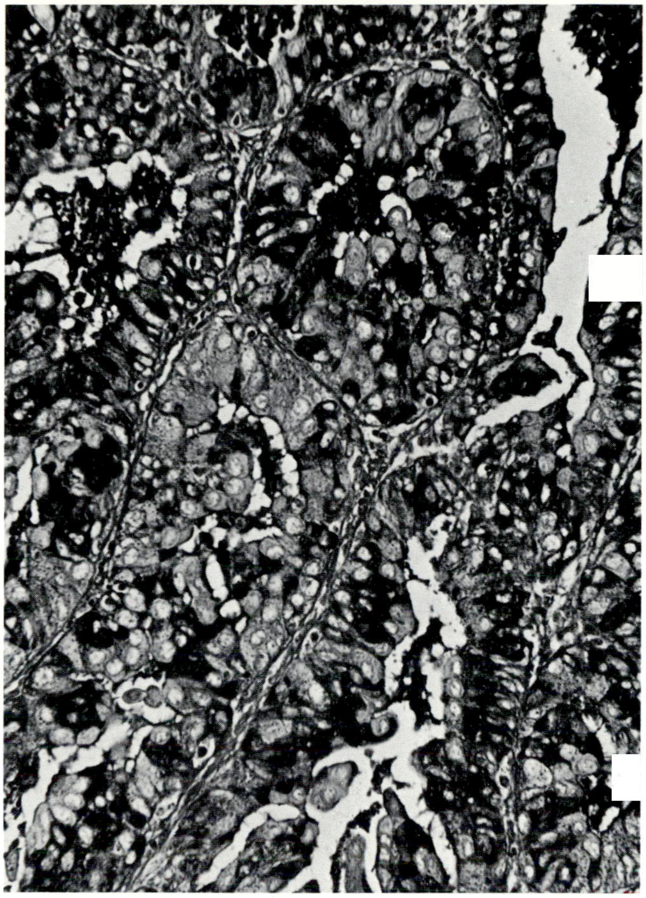

FIG. 8.26. Moderately differentiated adenocarcinoma of the cervix. The endocervical origin of the lesion is confirmed by the finding of abundant intracytoplasmic acid mucin in neoplastic gland cells. Alcian blue.

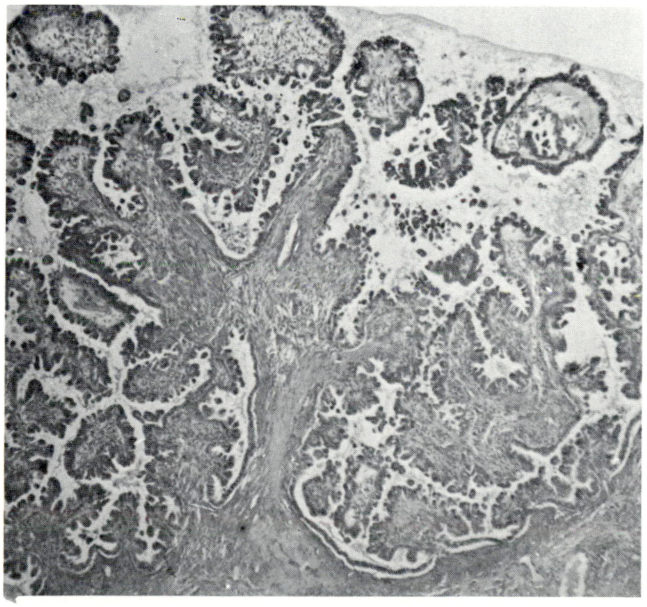

FIG. 8.27. Papillary adenocarcinoma of the cervix. Note the branching papillae lined by atypical epithelium and supported by connective tissue stroma resembling papillary serous carcinoma of the ovary.

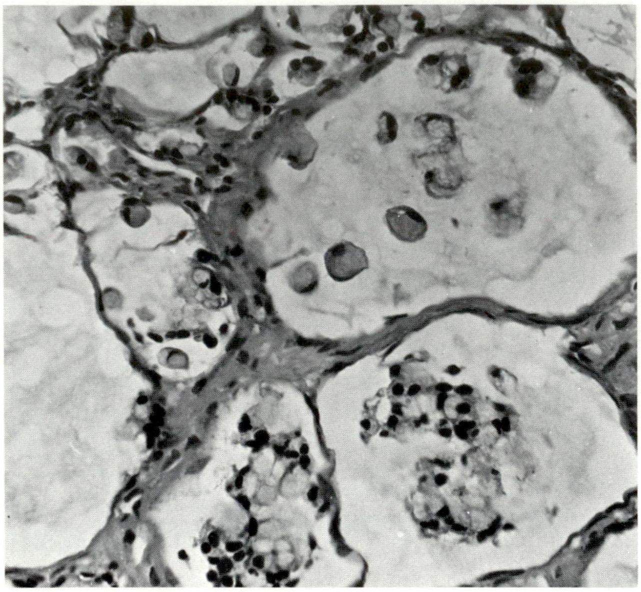

FIG. 8.28. Mucinous, colloid carcinoma of the cervix. Note the malignant signet-ring cells in lakes of extracellular mucin.

ullary-type carcinoma resembling those seen in the female mammary gland. Clear cell adenocarcinoma may also occur in the cervix. Clear cell endocervical adenocarcinoma is of particular interest, since more than 380 cases (60% in the vagina and 40% in the cervix) have

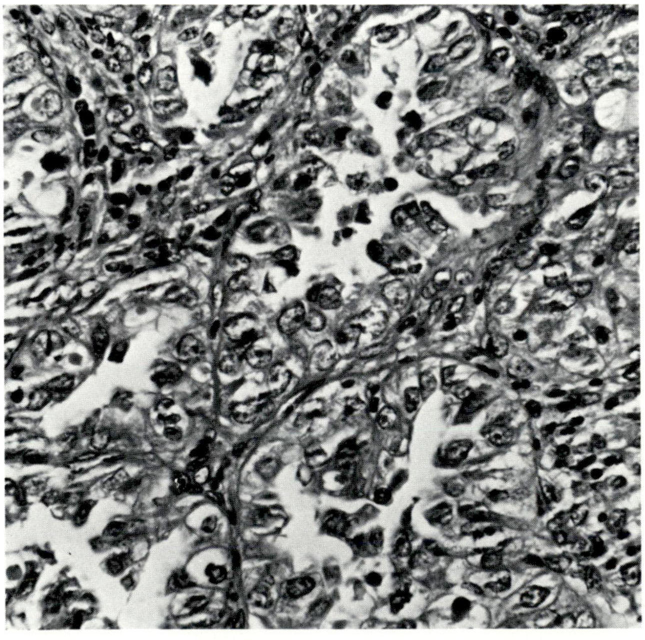

FIG. 8.29. Clear cell carcinoma of the cervix in a young woman with a history of prenatal exposure to diethylstilbestrol. Clear cells and hobnail cells are present.

been reported in young women with a history of prenatal exposure to diethylstilbestol (DES)[74,153] (see Chapter 4, Diseases of Vagina). In the cervix, as in the vagina, the lesion presumably arises from tuboendometrial type gland cells within the endocervical mucosa and is arranged in glands, tubules, cysts, and solid nests (Fig. 8.29). The tubulocystic variety has a comparatively better prognosis than its solid or papillary counterpart.[74] The neoplastic cells have abundant clear cytoplasm and hyperchromatic pleomorphic nuclei, which often are in an apical position resulting in a hobnail cytonuclear pattern. Ultrastructurally (Fig. 8.30) there is abundant intracytoplasmic PAS-positive diastase-labile glycogen, which is thought to be responsible for the clear cytoplasmic appearance of the neoplastic cells. The presently available morphologic[74,145] and experimental[55] data favor a müllerian rather than a mesonephric[70] origin for clear cell adenocarcinomas of the cervix and vagina. Consequently, the term *mesonephric carcinoma* should not be used for clear cell adenocarcinoma of the female genital tract and should be distinguished from rare carcinomas of true mesonephric origin (see below, Mesonephric Carcinoma).[71,86,155]

Differential Diagnosis

Unfortunately, histochemistry, including the Alcian blue stain, has little if any value in differentiating between adenocarcinoma of the cervix (Fig. 8.26) and metastatic adenocarcinoma of endometrial origin. Although more endocervical lesions than endometrial carcinomas stain (rather strongly) positive with Alcian blue, there is sufficient overlap[38] between the two lesions to consider histochemistry of no diagnostic value. The same is true for CEA, secretory component, fat globule membrane antigens, and keratin.[76,178]

Occasionally, mucinous adenocarcinoma of the endocervical type may arise in the endometrium. In such cases, the location of the tumor indicates the appropriate diagnosis. Another condition likely to be confused with invasive adenocarcinoma, especially clear cell carcinoma of the cervix, is atypical microglandular hyperplasia of the endocervical epithelium (see Chapter 6, Benign Lesions of Cervix). Similarly, endocervical epithelial atypia associated with trauma or severe inflammation (see Fig. 6.2c) should be distinguished from in situ adenocarcinoma. The Arias–Stella reaction (see Chapter 9, Uterine Corpus) occurs on occasion in endocervical epithelium with intrauterine or ectopic pregnancy and may be mistaken for clear cell adenocarcinoma. Arias–Stella cells are distinctive by their cytonucleomegaly; they contain no mitoses, and their clear cytoplasmic appearance is not caused by glycogen but by increased cytoplasmic matrix in which the organelles are dispersed.

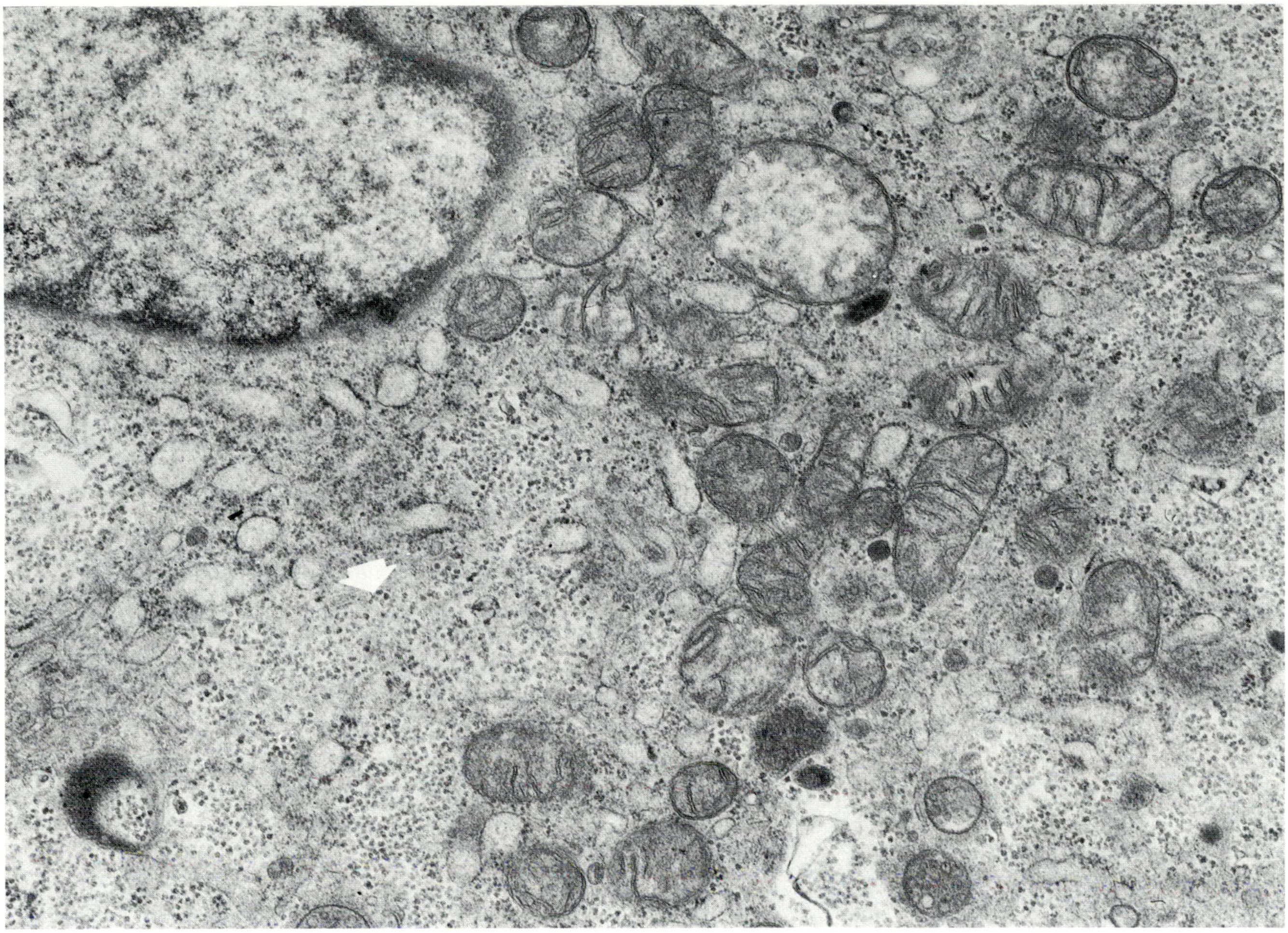

FIG. 8.30. Electron microscopy of Fig. 8.29. The clear cytoplasmic appearance of neoplastic gland cells is caused by the massive accumulation of glycogen granules (*arrow*). ×18,250.

Modes of Spread and Prognosis

Endocervical adenocarcinoma follows similar pathways of progression, including lymphatic metastasis, to that of squamous carcinoma. However, local extension[1] as well as lymph node metastases[15,97,132] occur comparatively earlier in adeno- than squamous carcinoma. As a result, the overall 5-year survival rates are lower for adenocarcinoma (48%–56%)[56] than for squamous carcinoma patients (68%)[1] and recurrences are a common feature (25%).[1,56]

Behavior and Treatment

Poor prognostic factors include tumor size greater than 4 cm, uterine enlargement, and high grade.[15,97] Ploidy level (nuclear DNA content) can be correlated with histologic grade and appears to have prognostic significance.[7,58] Low ploidy level, with stem cell modal values less than triploid, are associated with well differentiated adenocarcinoma, whereas poorly differentiated adenocarcinomas have high ploidy, greater than triploid. In one study women with hypotriploid tumors had a significantly higher survival rate (45–55%) than women with hypertriploid tumors (10–18%).[58]

Determinations of serum CEA may be of value in the follow-up and management of women with cervical adenocarcinoma. A high initial CEA titer (over 15 μg/liter) has been associated with poor prognosis.[95] Papillary clear cell adenocarcinoma[95] and endometrioid carcinoma[52] are associated with the best survival rates.

The two most widely used therapeutic modalities for stages I and II adenocarcinoma are radiation alone and radiation followed by simple hysterectomy.[84,144] Although not generally agreed on, the latter approach seems to yield better results: 80% 5-year survival compared to 66% 5-year survival rate with radiation alone.[84,144] For patients with ACIS, hysterectomy is considered to be the treatment of choice.

Specific Variants of Adenocarcinoma

Adenoma Malignum

An uncommon variant of endocervical columnar type adenocarcinoma of the cervix is adenoma malignum or minimal deviation adenocarcinoma (MDA).[85,88,122,164] This lesion is regarded as an extremely well differentiated adenocarcinoma, with minimal deviation from the normal endocervical columnar epithelium (Fig. 8.31). The cytoplasm remains tall columnar with abundant mucin, and nuclear atypia is inconspicuous or focal. The lesion may exhibit a similar branching arrangement to that of the normal endocervical glands, although bizarre angular outpouchings are often seen. When the pathologist is confronted with such a well-differentiated growth, it is difficult to recognize it as a neoplastic process.[85,88,126,164] The most reliable criteria to assess the malignant nature of MDA are the presence of occasional mitoses in gland cells and the presence of endocervical glands past the usual depth of 5 mm (Fig. 8.32). MDA often involves more than two-thirds of the thickness of the cervical stroma and should be regarded as invasive because the normal endocervical crypts and tunnels do not extend beyond that level. Although earlier reports suggested an extremely poor prognosis for women with MDA, recent experience shows similar survival rates to those with well-differentiated ordinary adenocarcinoma.[164] The discrepancy in observations is apparently due to the fact that the earlier cases did not receive appropriate therapy for cervical cancer. Accurate diagnosis of MDA requires an adequate conization specimen or hysterectomy specimen and cannot be made on a punch biopsy. MDA of the cervix has been strongly associated with Peutz-Jeghers syndrome,[121,189] developing in 4/27 women with this condition in one series.[189] Close clinical surveillance of women with Peutz-Jeghers syndrome is recommended, including careful endocervical cytologic examination and periodic endocervical curettage.

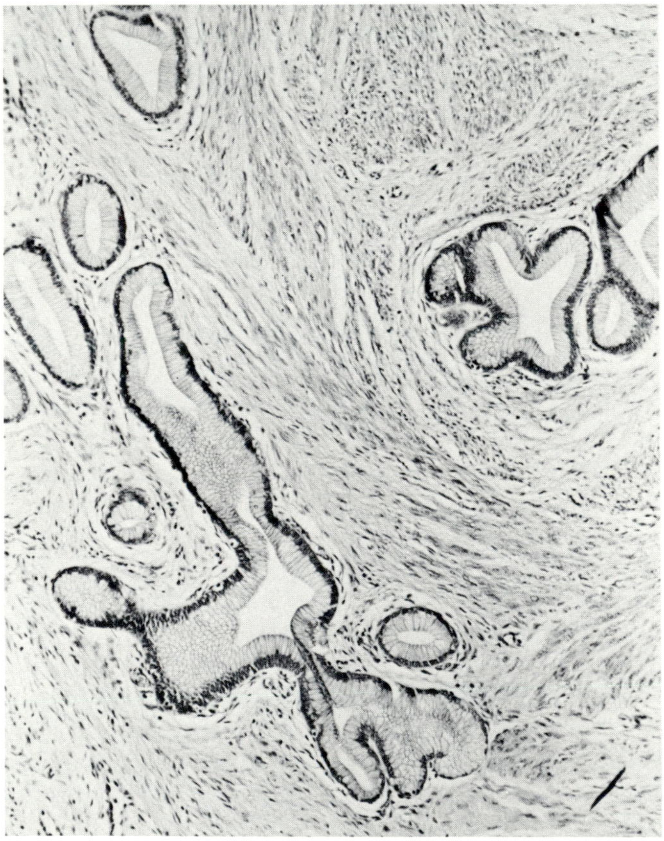

FIG. 8.31. Adenoma malignum or minimal deviation adenocarcinoma representing extremely well differentiated adenocarcinoma of the cervix. Note complex glandular branching pattern and close resemblance of lining cells to normal endocervical epithelium. There is a discrete rim of periglandular stromal edema.

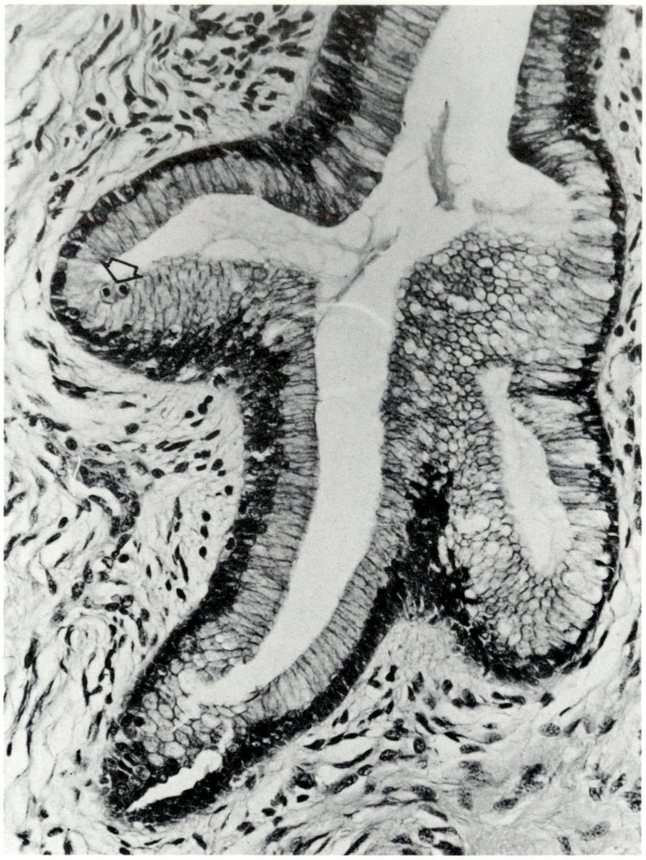

FIG. 8.32. Higher magnification of minimal deviation adenocarcinoma cells with slightly enlarged nuclei in a basal position and occasional mitotic figures (*arrow*). Note periglandular stromal edema.

Adenoid Cystic Carcinoma

Adenoid cystic carcinoma (cylindroma) of the cervix[75,119,127] is characterized by cylindrical hyaline bodies and/or small acini or cysts lying within solid nests or between interanastomosing cords of uniform basaloid tumor cells. In cross section, hyaline cylinders appear round or ovoid, giving the neoplasm a sieve-like appearance (Fig. 8.33). Curiously, the hyaline material at the electron microscopic level was shown to be partly composed of coalesced masses of basal lamina produced by the epithelial tumor cells[99,119] and partly of fine precollagen and collagen fibers of fibroblastic origin. Inconspicuous glandular lumina are sometimes filled with amorphous material, representing partly digested cellular debris. Adenoid cystic carcinoma may be associated with squamous and adenocarcinoma as well as carcinosarcoma of the cervix.[1] The lesion is most often seen in patients between the sixth and seventh decades and behaves more aggressively than most cervical adenocarcinomas.[75] Adenoid cystic carcinoma should be differentiated from adenoid basal carcinoma.[45] In adenoid basal carcinoma, the epithelial nests are morphea-like, smaller, with only rare cystic pseudoglands. Hyalin is absent. Pure adenoid basal carcinomas have an indolent growth pattern and can be managed conservatively by simple hysterectomy.[10,45]

Mesonephric Carcinoma

In contrast to the superficial location of cervical clear cell adenocarcinomas, true mesonephric adenocarcinomas are found deep in the lateral wall of the cervix, in a site corresponding to the location of mesonephric duct remnants. Histologic transitions between mesonephric duct remains and carcinomas have rarely been demonstrated;[71,86,155] the cells of mesonephric adenocarcinoma are not clear and have negligible amount of intracytoplasmic glycogen (Fig. 8.34). Mesonephric carcinoma should also be distinguished from florid mesonephric hyperplasia (see Chapter 6, Benign Lesions of Cervix).

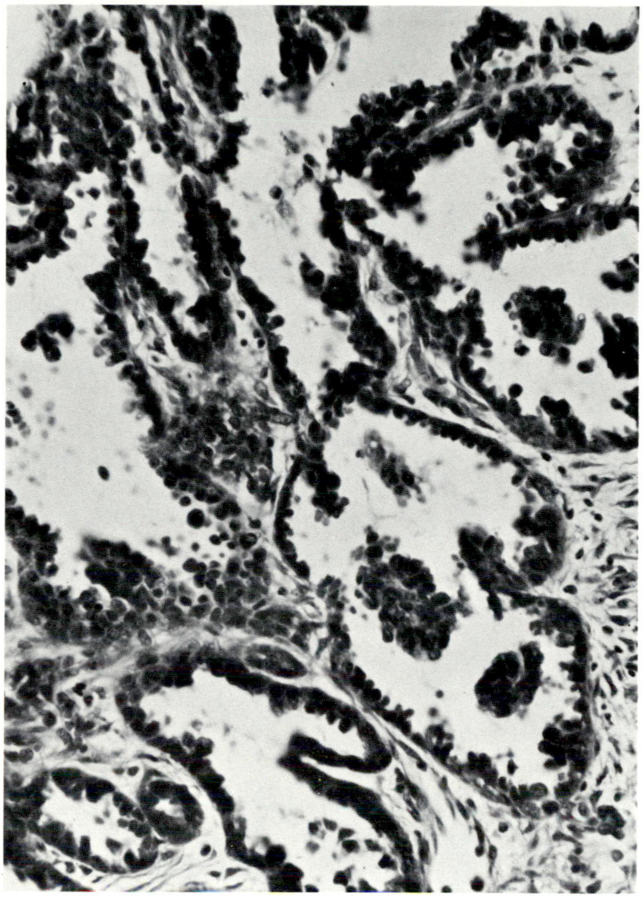

FIG. 8.34. Mesonephric carcinoma of the cervix. The neoplastic cells demonstrate a hobnail pattern. The cytoplasm is not clear and contains an inconspicuous amount of glycogen. The lesion was continuous with mesonephric remnants in the cervix. (Courtesy of Dr. A. Blaustein, New York.)

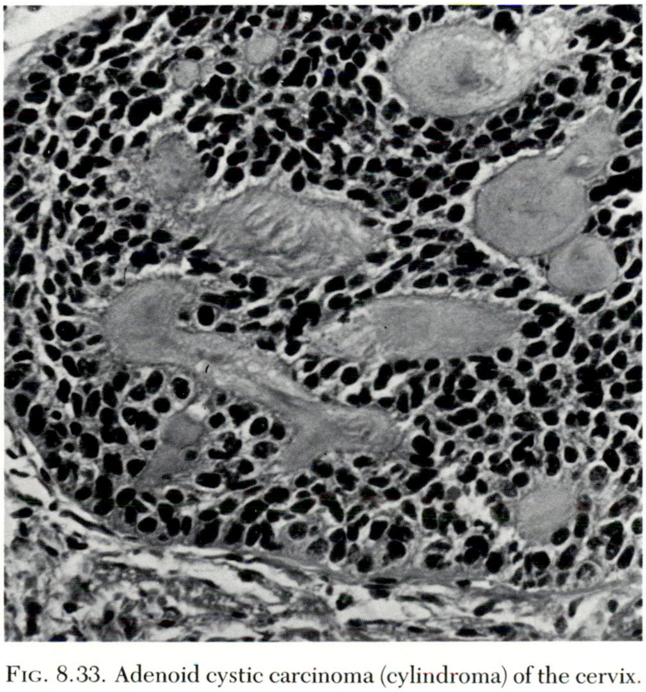

FIG. 8.33. Adenoid cystic carcinoma (cylindroma) of the cervix. Within solid nests of basaloid tumor cells are cylindrical hyaline bodies.

Mixed Epithelial Carcinoma

Adenosquamous Carcinoma

Lesions with mixed patterns of epithelial differentiation are believed to arise from the subcolumnar reserve cells of the endocervical mucous membrane.[1] Adenosquamous carcinomas[47,162,182,185] contain an admixture of histologi-

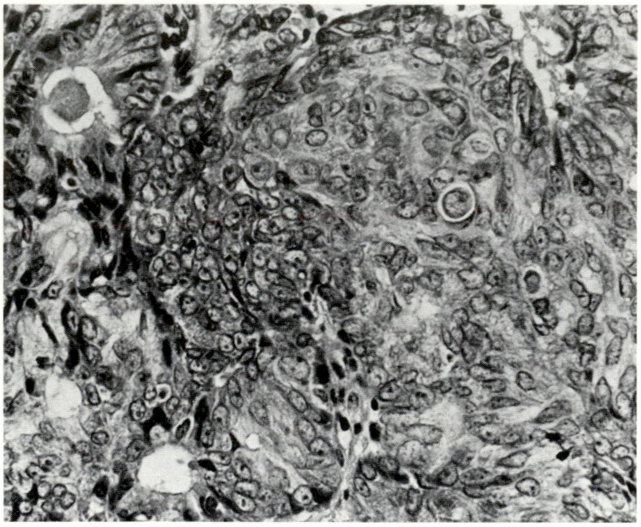

Fig. 8.35. Adenosquamous carcinoma of the cervix.

cally malignant squamous and glandular cells (Fig. 8.35). Carcinomas with a mixed epithelial pattern are being recognized with increased frequency with the aid of ultrastructural and immunohistochemical studies.[151] They constitute approximately 10% of all cervical carcinomas[1] and apparently have a less favorable prognosis than pure squamous cell carcinomas of comparable clinical stage.[59,182]

Glassy Cell Carcinoma

A poorly differentiated form of adenosquamous carcinoma has been referred to as glassy cell carcinoma.[63] This type of lesion comprises 1.2% of cervical cancers and has an extremely aggressive clinical course, with a poor response to radiation and surgery.[59,110,159] Because of its poor prognosis, glassy cell carcinoma should be distinguished from large cell nonkeratinizing squamous carcinoma with which it may be confused. Unlike glassy cell carcinoma, the latter is relatively radiosensitive.

The following are the major morphologic alterations present in glassy cell carcinomas: (1) large cells with finely granular ground glass-type cytoplasm, hence the name *glassy cell*, (2) distinct cell membranes, and (3) prominent nuclei and nucleoli (Fig. 8.36).[133,151,185] In addition, the cells lack intercellular bridges and dyskeratotic cells, and intracellular glycogen is inconspicuous. The stroma is characteristically heavily infiltrated by a lymphoplasmacytic and eosinophilic inflammatory exudate. Occasionally, areas of keratin pearl and abortive lumen formations are seen together with signet-ring cells and intracellular mucin. The overlying surface squamous epithelium may be normal or may contain CIN of the ordinary squamous cell type or glassy cell carcinoma in

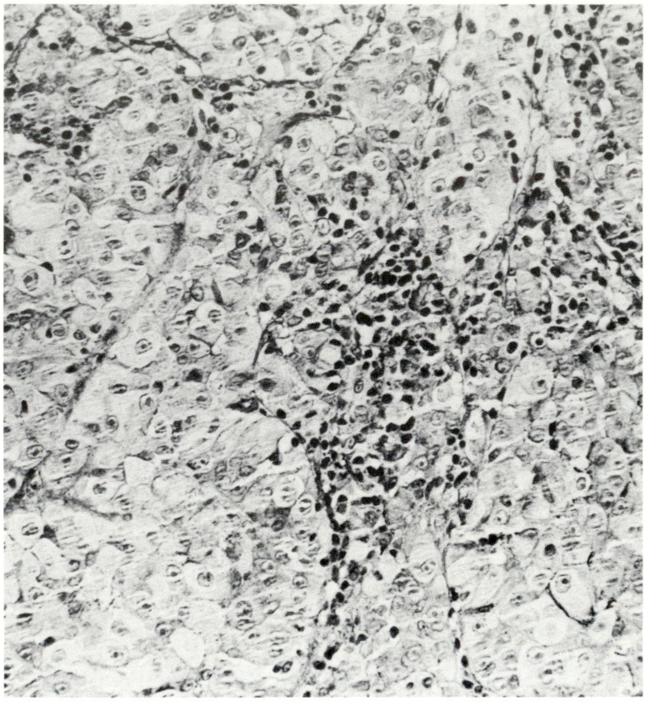

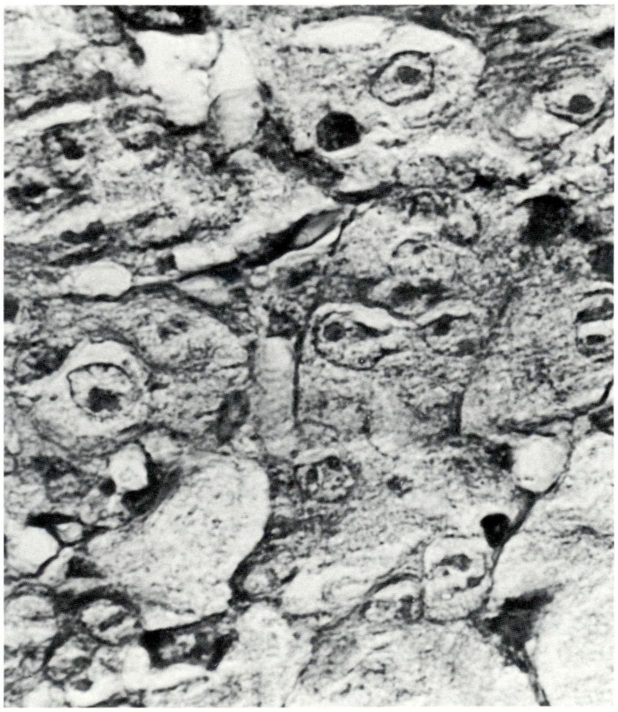

Fig. 8.36. Glassy cell carcinoma. *Top:* Lobules made of compact neoplastic cells. There is no apparent squamous or glandular differentiation. The stroma contains an abundant chronic inflammatory exudate. *Bottom:* Detailed view of granular glassy cytoplasm, well-defined cytoplasmic membranes and prominent nucleoli.

situ type. Ultrastructurally, the adenosquamous nature of glassy cell carcinoma is evidenced by rare abortive glandular lumina formations together with well-developed tonofilament–desmosonal complexes, interdigitating microvilli, and cytoplasmic microfilaments.[151]

Mucoepidermoid Carcinoma

Mucoepidermoid carcinomas[47,138] consist preponderantly of malignant squamous cells disposed in sheets, clumps, and ribbons in which are scattered mucin-secreting cells (Fig. 8.37). The mucin from these cells is extruded into the intercellular spaces or fibrous stroma, where it may collect in small or large lakes. The mucinous cellular elements most often are of the goblet or signet-ring cell type and contain mucinocarminophilic, PAS-positive, diastase-resistant mucopolysaccharides. They presumably develop from neoplastic squamous cells or cells intermediate between squamous and mucinous cells. Mucoepidermoid carcinoma is separated from the squamous cell carcinoma group because the distribution of this lesion in other parts of the body is chiefly confined to glandular tissues, such as the salivary glands, and because subcolumnar reserve cells of the endocervix are capable of differentiating into both squamous and glandular cell lines. The prognosis of mucoepidermoid carcinoma of the cervix is extremely poor.

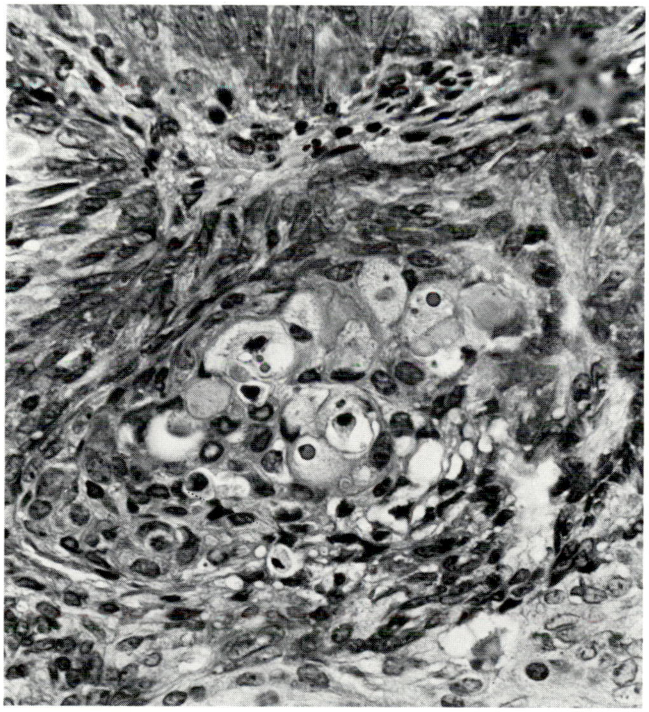

FIG. 8.37. Mucoepidermoid carcinoma of the cervix. Note the pale, mucin-containing cells within masses of neoplastic squamous cells.

Dual Primary Carcinoma

Examples of synchronous adenocarcinoma and squamous cell carcinoma occurring independently in the cervix have been reported.[51,184] They may be either invasive or in situ. In the invasive form, one carcinoma often invades the other, resulting in a collision tumor. Although such lesions closely resemble adenosquamous carcinomas, the different neoplastic components remain histologically distinct, separated from each other by narrow stroma or their respective basal lamina. Because direct transition from one cell type into another, as occurs in adenosquamous carcinoma, is not seen, these tumors are best considered separate primary carcinomas.

Neuroendocrine Carcinomas

Carcinoid

Neuroendocrine carcinomas of the cervix are believed to arise from either the subcolumnar reserve cells of the endocervix or from endocervical neuroendocrine cells. Neuroendocrine cells can be identified histochemically in the normal endocervix.[9,52,57] Carcinoid tumors of the cervix,[45,129,170] in particular, are considered to originate from argyrophil cells of the endocervical epithelium and are a part of tumors of the APUD (amine precursor uptake and decarboxylation) cell system. Cervical carcinoids are malignant, with local and distant metastasis, but to date none of the cases reported has been associated with the carcinoid syndrome. Microscopically, they vary from well to poorly differentiated tumors. The former grow in solid sheets, and trabeculae and glandular lumina are found scattered throughout the tumor (Fig. 8.38). The neoplastic cells have round to oval, spindle-shaped nuclei and finely granular cytoplasm. Tumors with foci of squamous differentiation and crystal violet and Congo red-positive amyloid stroma are occasionally seen. Mitoses may be numerous, and the vessels are often invaded (Fig. 8.38, right).

Small Cell Carcinoma

The poorly differentiated variety resembles small cell carcinoma of the lung without (oat cell type) and with a spindle-shaped growth pattern (Fig. 8.39, left).[68] In these lesions, Grimelius staining (Fig. 8.39, right) or electron microscopy can be carried out to demonstrate the presence of argyrophilic neurosecretory gran-

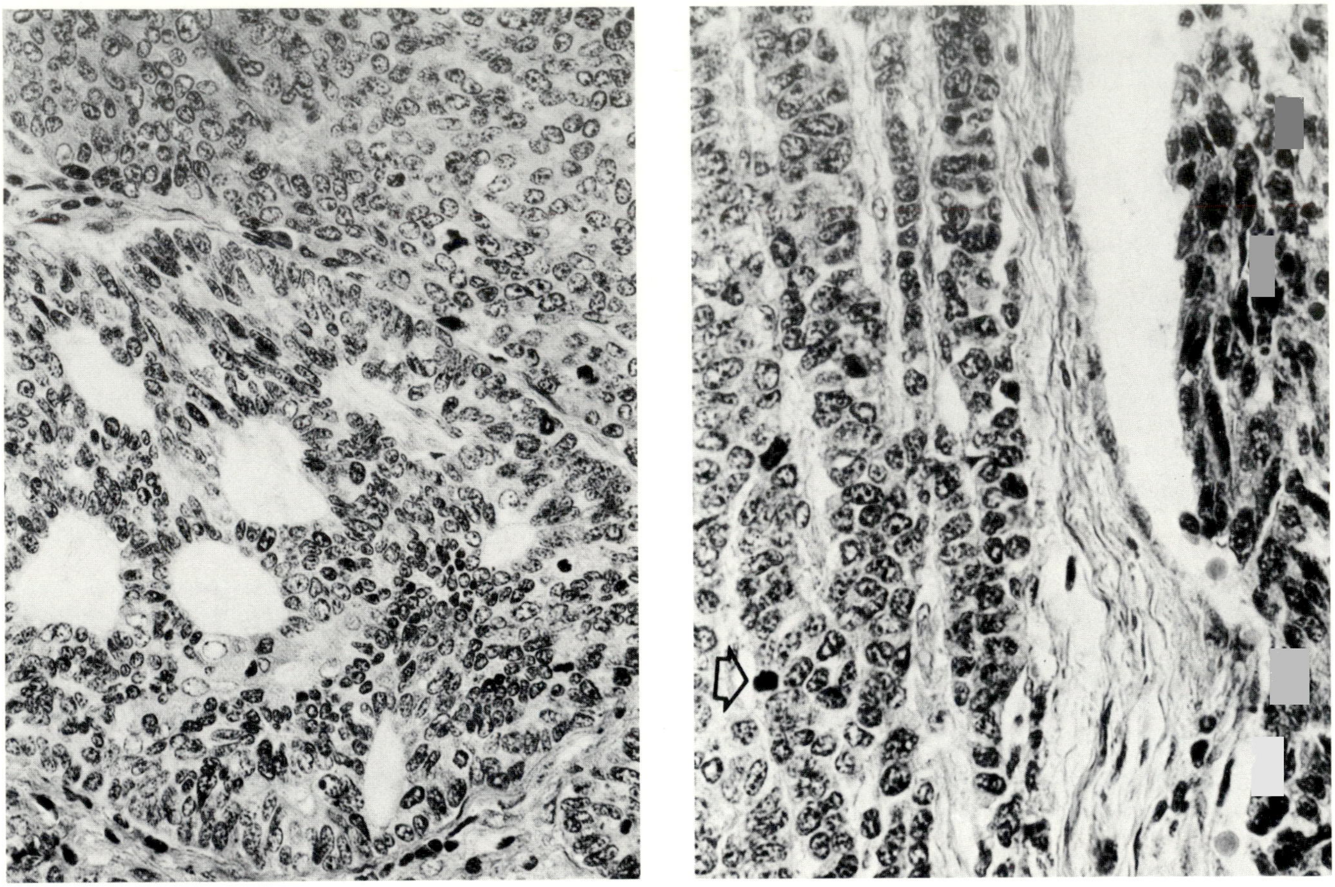

Fig. 8.38. Carcinoid of cervix. *Left:* Acini with spindle-shaped cells forming solid masses. Such a picture may be confused with adenocarcinoma or adenosquamous carcinoma. *Right:* Trabecular pattern with numerous mitoses (*arrow*) and vascular invasion. The cytoplasmic membrane is indistinct and the nuclear chromatin is coarse. (Courtesy of Dr. Walter Schurch, Montreal.)

ules.[82,129,170,174,186] (Fig. 8.40a, b). These poorly differentiated small (oat) cell carcinomas have been associated with ectopic ACTH,[17,82] insulin,[93] and gastrin production.[157,186] The prognosis for poorly differentiated small (oat) cell carcinoma of the cervix is comparatively worse than that of its well-differentiated carcinoid counterpart[4,5] and also worse than that of stage-comparable, poorly differentiated small cell squamous carcinomas.[23,68]

The well-differentiated carcinoid variant should be distinguished from adenocarcinoma, adenosquamous carcinoma, and squamous carcinoma, whereas the poorly differentiated form should be differentiated from nonendocrine, poorly differentiated small cell carcinoma (Fig. 8.41). The latter lacks histochemical, immunohistochemical, and electron microscopic evidence of neuroendocrine differentiation.[58] Besides the rather characteristic histology and cytology of cervical carcinoids, histochemical or ultrastructural demonstration of neurosecretory, argyrophilic granules is diagnostic of neuroendocrine tumors of the cervix.

Rare Tumors

Primary malignant melanoma is among the least common of the malignancies that arise in the cervix. Nine patients have been reported in the literature.[83] All the patients in whom follow-up was available died with widespread metastases from 6 months to 14 years after diagnosis. In most instances, the lesion is pigmented and dark brown. The diagnosis of primary melanoma of the cervix uteri is based on the histologic demonstration of junctional changes in the cervical squamous epithelium and the absence of similar lesions elsewhere in the body (Fig. 8.42). Morphologically, it is identical to melanoma arising in the skin and extragenital mucous membranes; it frequently contains intracytoplasmic melanin pigment granules.

The pathogenesis of malignant melanoma of the cervix is unclear, although its origin may be ascribed to the melanin-containing cells of the schwannian sheath of the normal cervix.[30]

Primary choriocarcinoma in the cervix, is rare and

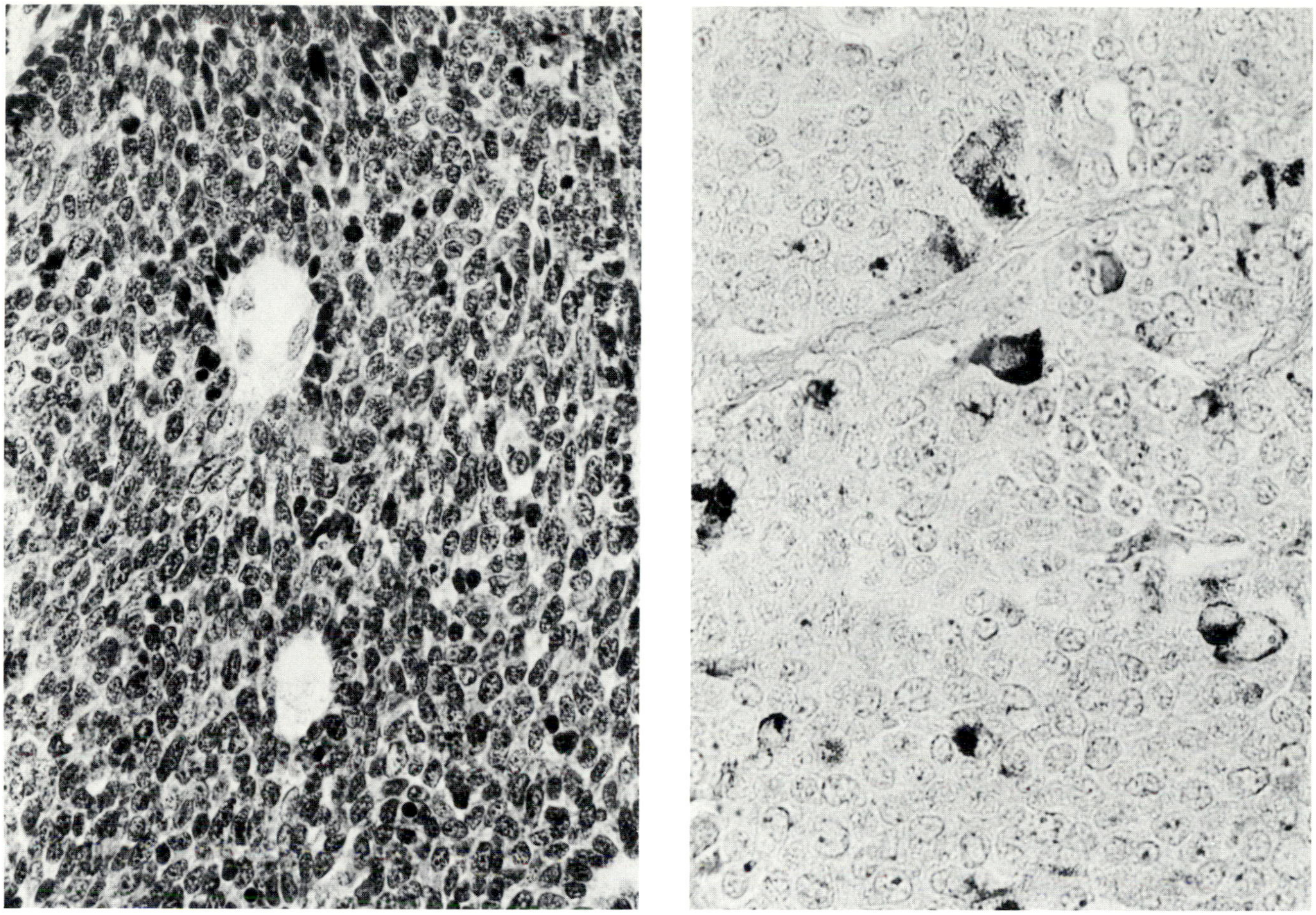

FIG. 8.39. Carcinoid tumor. *Left:* Masses of poorly differentiated small cells (oat cell) with rare acini. *Right.* Grimelius-positive intracytoplasmic argyrophilic granules in scattered neoplastic cells. (Courtesy of Dr. Walter Schurch, Montreal.)

presumably results from a preexisting cervical pregnancy or displaced intrauterine molar tissue. Nearly 50 such cases are recorded in the literature.[172] The gross and microscopic appearance, as well as the clinical course, are identical with those found in the uterine corpus.

Metastatic Tumors

Direct extension from local pelvic tumor is the most common source of cervical involvement by secondary carcinoma, often originating in the endometrium, rectum, or bladder. Intrapelvic and intragenital, lymphatic or vascular metastases to the cervix[24] occur less often but are associated with ovarian carcinoma, endometrial adenocarcinoma, and uncommonly with transitional cell carcinoma of the bladder.[98,109] Another lesion that has a relatively high rate of cervical metastasis is choriocarcinoma. Sarcomas of the uterine corpus may also involve the cervix. Metastases to the cervix from distant primary foci are rare,[24] the most common sites being the gastrointestinal tract (colon and stomach),[109,190] the ovary,[109] and the female mammary gland[98,179] (Fig. 8.43). Instances of metastatic carcinoma of the kidney, gallbladder, pancreas, lung, thyroid,[109,173] and malignant melanoma have also been described.* On occasion, metastases may occur primarily as cervical involvement and pose a differential diagnostic problem. Unusual gross morphology or histologic patterns, e.g., signet-ring cell carcinoma or clear cell carcinoma, may provide a clue to the possibility of origin in a distant primary site. Leukemic infiltration of the cervix, especially of the granulocytic type, is a rather common occurrence at autopsy in women with leukemia.[114] Secondary lymphomatous involvement of the cervix is reported in 6% of women dying with generalized disease.[104]

---

* References 24, 98, 120, 173, 179, 190.

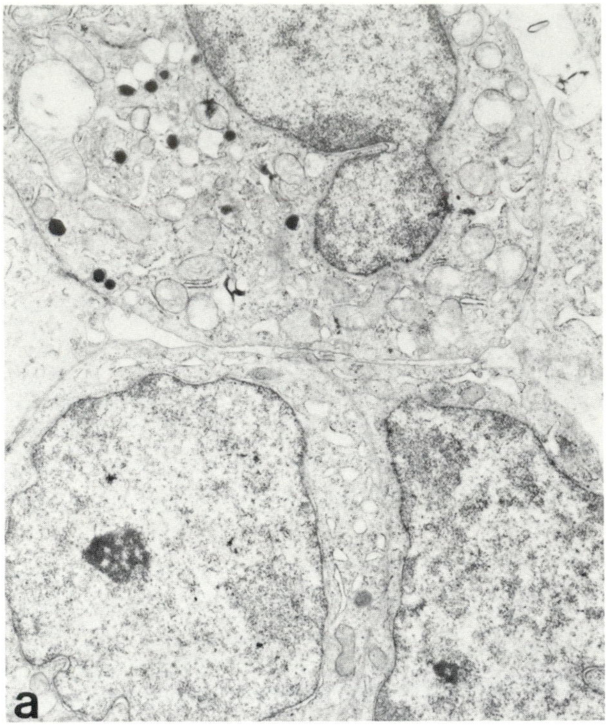

FIG. 8.40. Carcinoid tumor. *a*. Electron microscopy of intracytoplasmic uniform sized, membrane-bound neurosecretory granules with homogenous, electron-dense content. The cells are rich in organelles and are attached by small desmosomes and have irregular nuclear membranes ×7000.

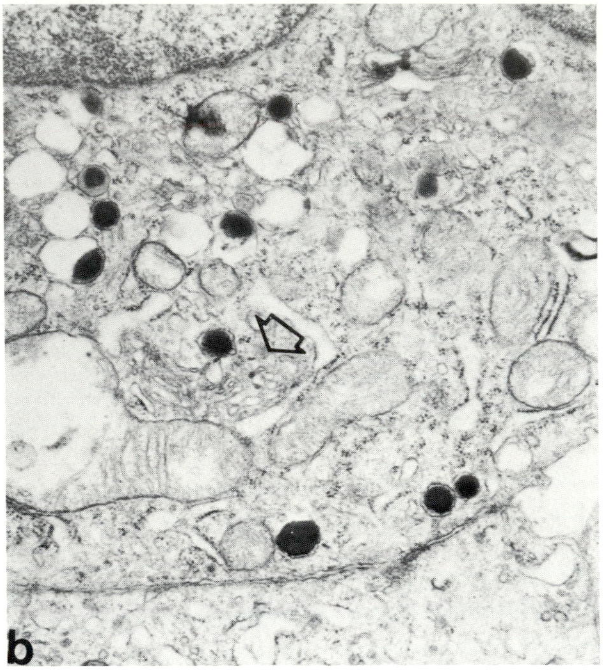

FIG. 8.40.*b*. Higher magnification of membrane-bound argyrophilic, neurosecretory granules near the Golgi (*arrow*), typical of carcinoid tumor cells ×15,000. (Courtesy of Dr. Walter Schurch, Montreal.)

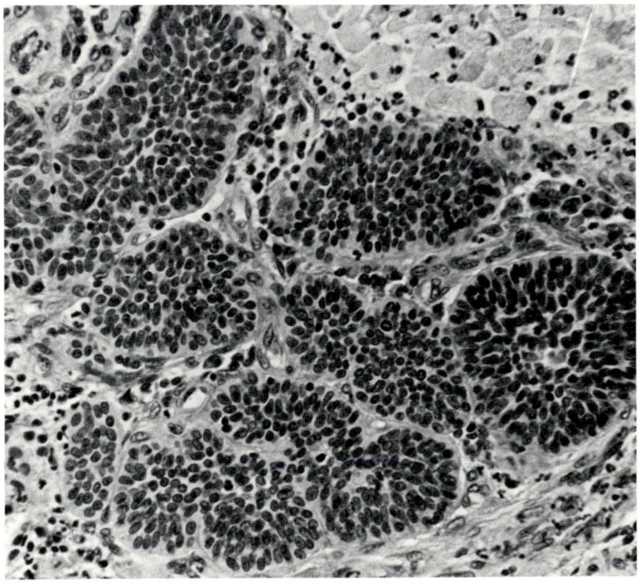

FIG. 8.41. Undifferentiated nonendocrine, small cell carcinoma of the cervix. The cells have small, hyperchromatic nuclei and scant, indistinct cytoplasm, resembling subcolumnar reserve cells. Note the lobular configuration of the tumor, reminiscent of endocervical glandular units.

Effects of Radiation

In general, electromagnetic irradiation in the form of either x-rays or γ-rays produces cellular injury that affects especially the nucleus.[14] Characteristic cytologic changes are observed in the nucleus during different phases of mitotic division, such as chromosome breaks (scission), bridge formation between chromosomes at anaphase, and chromosomal fragmentation. Cells in mitosis, late G_1, and early DNA-synthesis phases are the most sensitive to ionizing radiation.

The morphologic effects of radiation on the cervix are well described by Kraus.[100] The normal cervical squamous cells, immediately after intracavitary radiation for cervical carcinoma, demonstrate cytoplasmic swelling and vacuolization. The nuclei are enlarged and contain one or two prominent nucleoli. The intercellular spaces are dilated (spongiosis) because of the accumulation of intercellular edema, with concomitant loss of desmosomal attachments. The underlying supportive connective tissue is necrotic and contains numerous inflammatory cells. By the sixth postirradiation week there is severe atrophy of the squamous epithelium, and nuclear enlargement associated with a decrease in mucin content is seen in the endocervical epithelial cells. The cervical fibrous

Fig. 8.42. Primary malignant melanoma of the cervix. Note junctional changes in squamous epithelium and spindle-shaped configuration of neoplastic cells. Fontana stain was strongly positive for melanin.

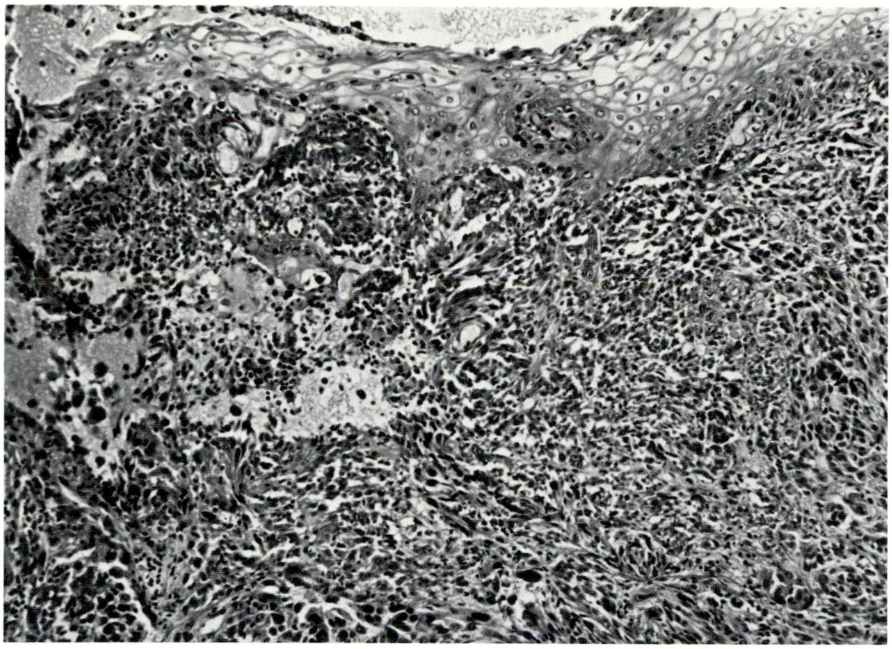

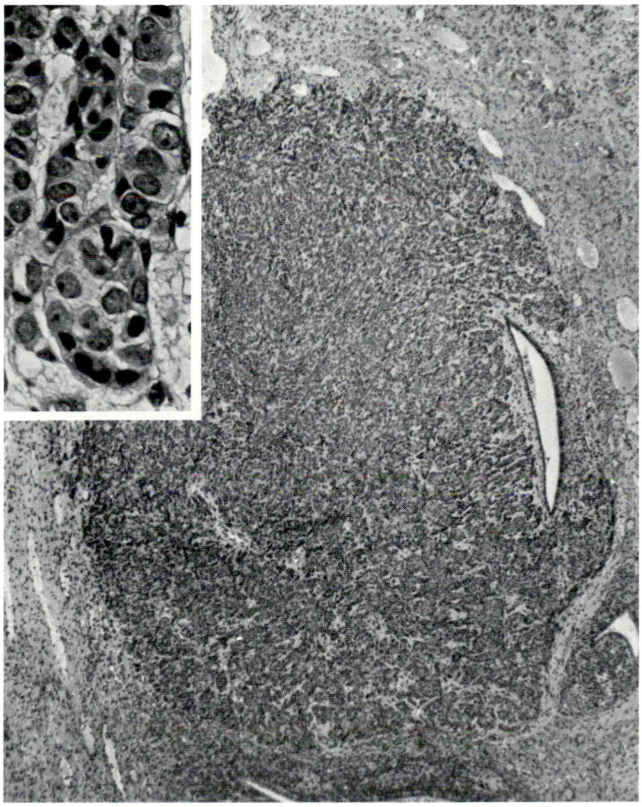

Fig. 8.43. Metastatic breast carcinoma in the cervix. *Inset:* Cellular detail of neoplastic cells arranged in typical narrow cords.

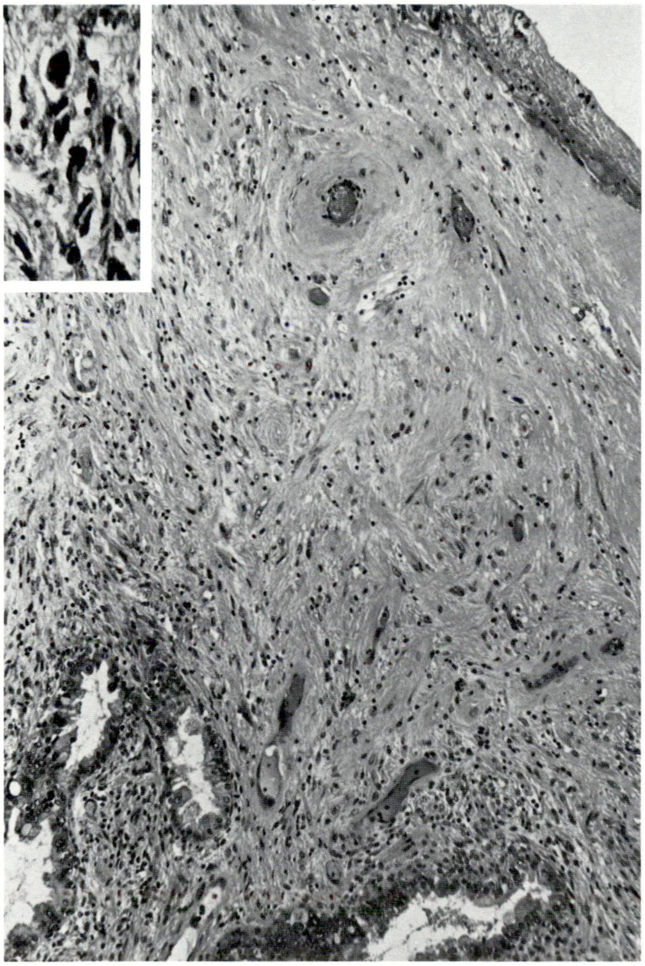

Fig. 8.44. Cervix 6 weeks after intracavitary radiation. Note the amorphous, hyalinized appearance of stroma, decreased mucin in endocervical epithelium, fibroblasts with atypical nuclei, and hyalin obliteration of vessels. *Inset:* Atypical giant fibroblasts are a characteristic feature of radiated connective tissue.

stroma is obscured by chronic inflammatory cells and macrophages and contains foci of partly necrotic, partly hyalinized collagen tissue with a few scattered atypical fibroblasts. These have abundant fibrillar cytoplasm and voluminous dark nuclei with several enlarged nucleoli (Fig. 8.44). Characteristically, the small arteries near the surface are obliterated by hyaline tissue, whereas others have intimal thickening (Fig. 8.44). The endothelial cells lining the capillaries are often enlarged, with hyperchromatic nuclei. In the following years, radiation changes are recognized by extensive hyalinization of the cervical fibrous tissue, which results in severe contraction. Most vessels are transformed into circular fibrohyaline masses surrounded by fragmented, wrinkled elastic fibers. Giant atypical fibroblasts with bizarre nuclear architecture can be found even 10 years after radiation. The squamous mucous membrane of the cervix remains atrophic with minimal intracytoplasmic glycogen.

Radiation of invasive squamous cell carcinoma of the cervix produces a decrease in tumor size and eventual regression.[116] Although tumor regression is generally faster in neoplasms of small size and in those confined to the cervix (stage I) than in larger advanced stage lesions, 90% of 493 patients with all stages had no gross tumor 12 weeks after termination of combined external radiation (^{60}Co, 5000 R) and intracavitary radium (4000 R) therapy. The rapidity of tumor regression is apparently unrelated to histologic patterns and degree of differentiation. Morphologic changes in cervical squamous carcinoma cells that are considered evidence of response to ionizing radiation are cellular differentiation with keratinization, cell degeneration with cytoplasmic vacuolization, pyknosis, and nucleomegaly[64] with polyploid DNA content. Nuclear polyploidy, i.e., generation of multiple double sets of DNA, is the result of arrest of mitotic activity caused by radiation. Radiation-induced changes

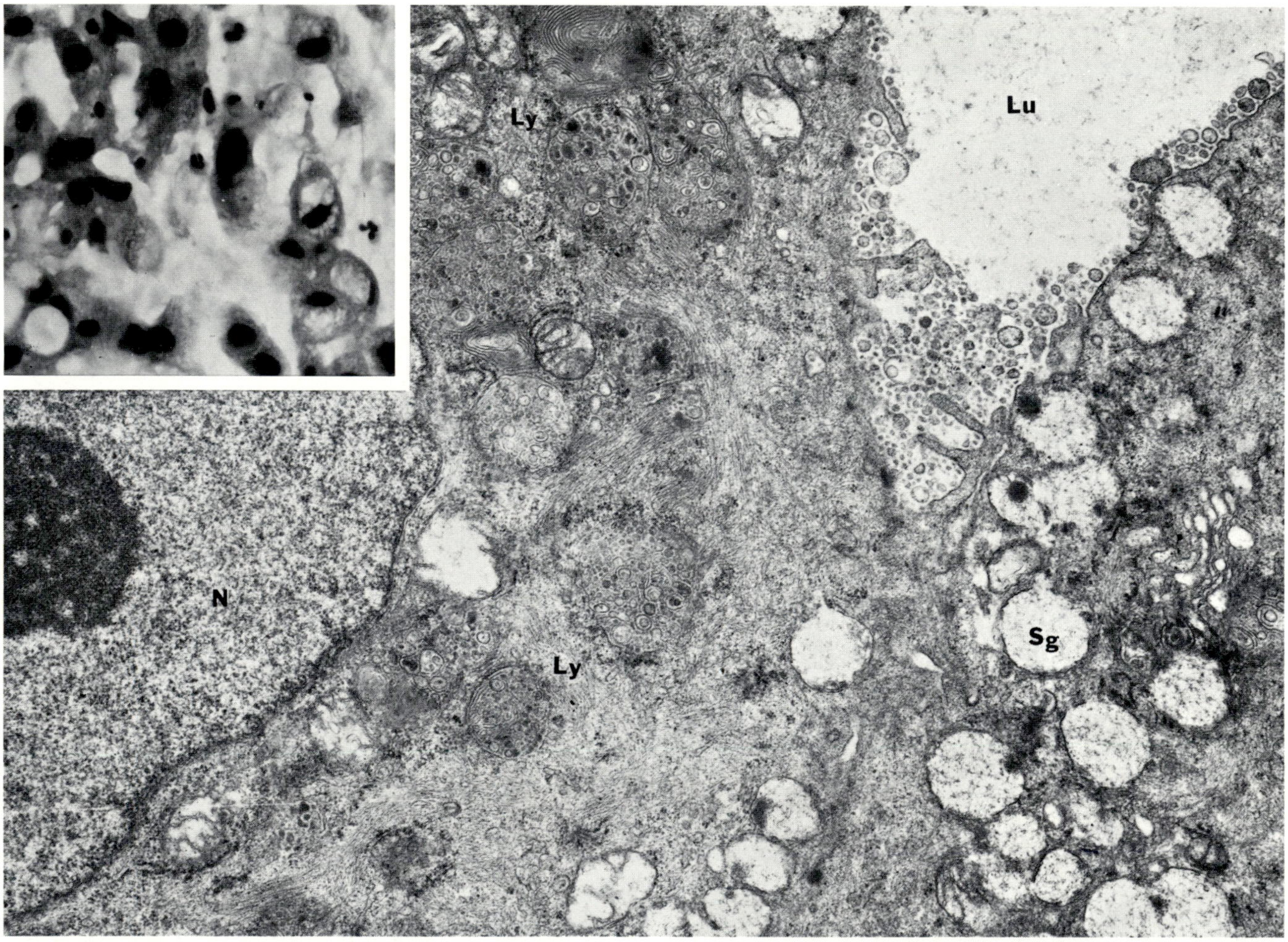

FIG. 8.45. Ultrastructural appearance of invasive adenocarcinoma of the cervix 6 weeks postirradiation. The cells are rich in membrane-bound autophagosomes (Ly), in which are incorporated cytoplasmic vesicles and membranes. The number of secretory granules (Sg) is considerably reduced as compared to normal or moderately differentiated neoplastic endocervical cells without radiation effect. N, nucleus; Lu, glandular lumen. ×19,435. *Inset:* Histologic appearance of heavily irradiated adenocarcinoma of the cervix. Note shrunken pyknotic nuclei, vacuolization, and inconspicuous intracytoplasmic mucin.

in adenocarcinoma of the cervix include nuclear shrinkage and pyknosis, cytoplasmic vacuolization, decrease in mucin synthesis, and a striking abundance of intracytoplasmic cytophagosomes (Fig. 8.45).

The frequency of a squamous carcinoma of the cervix or vagina or adenocarcinoma of the endometrium after irradiation for antecedent cervical malignancy or benign gynecological diseases is not greater than in the general population.[137] Only 1% of 1297 patients treated with radiation for invasive carcinoma of the cervix subsequently developed independent vaginal carcinomas.[89] It is not certain whether the second vaginal malignancy is initiated by radiation or represents a delayed multicentric development in the lower female genital tract. Morphologic alterations of the squamous epithelium of the uterine cervix and vagina of women who have been successfully treated with irradiation for cervical carcinoma occur in approximately 23% of cases.[181] The condition, termed *postirradiation dysplasia*[142] (PRD), is thought to be specifically induced by ionizing radiation and to be pathogenetically unrelated to spontaneously occurring CIN. The abnormal epithelial cells, both in smears and in histologic sections, have large nuclei and a variable degree of cytoplasmic differentiation. Histologically, the lesion resembles early CIN (mild dysplasia) (Fig. 8.46). The clinical significance of PRD, according to Wentz and Reagan,[181] lies in the positive correlation between the early appearance of PRD and the subsequent recurrence of cervical carcinoma. Indeed, if PRD is detected within 3 years of irradiation for carcinoma of the cervix, the likelihood of recurrence is considerably increased, and there is only a 34% 5-year survival rate. In contrast, if PRD occurs after 3 years, a 100% 5-year survival rate is observed, and in many instances the abnormal changes revert to normal without therapy. Attempts were made with the aid of microspectrophotometry to separate PRD with nuclear diploidy (normal DNA content) and polyploidy (multiple normal DNA content) from those with aneuploidy (abnormal DNA content, interclass values).[134] Patients with PRD of the aneuploid type, in which the nuclei contain all the characteristic changes of malignancy, had significantly higher recurrence and death rates than those with nuclear diploidy or polyploidy. In view of these observations, careful evaluation of the cytonuclear changes of PRD is recommended because it may provide useful information for the early detection and treatment of recurrences and contribute to the improvement in patient survival.

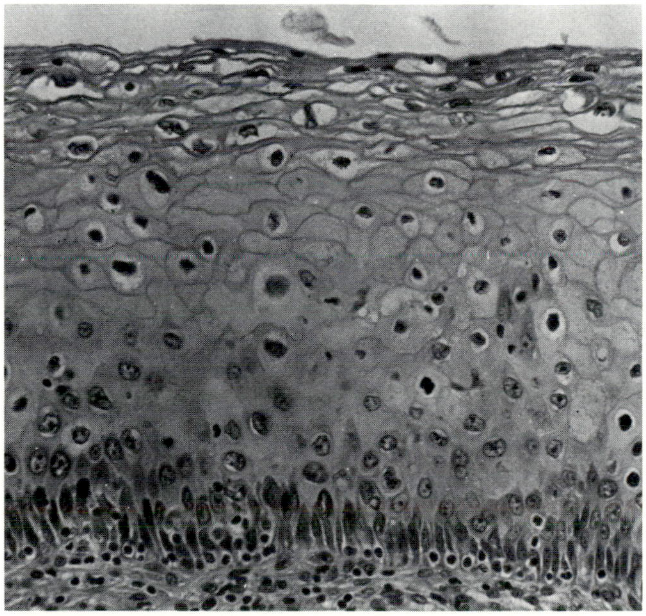

Fig. 8.46. Postirradiation dysplasia of the cervix observed 26 months after irradiation of invasive squamous carcinoma of the cervix.

References

1. Abell MR (1973) Invasive carcinomas of uterine cervix. In The Uterus, Norris HJ, Hertig AT, Abell MR (eds.) Internatl. Acad. Path. Monogr. Baltimore, Williams & Wilkins Co., pp 413–456
2. Abell MR, Gosling JRG (1962) Gland cell carcinoma (adenocarcinoma) of the uterine cervix. Am J Obstet Gynecol 83: 729
3. Abramson AL, Brandsma J, Steinberg B, Winkler B (1985) Verrucous carcinoma of the larynx, possible human papillomavirus etiology. Arch Otolaryngol 111: 709
4. Albores-Saavedra J, Rodriguez-Martinez HA, Larraza-Hernandez O (1979) Carcinoid tumors of the cervix. Pathol Annu 14: 273
5. Albores-Saavedra J, Larraza O, Poucell S, Rodriguez-Martinez HA (1976) Carcinoid of the uterine cervix. Additional observation on a new tumor entity. Cancer 38: 2328
6. Alva J, Lauchlan SC (1975) The histogenesis of mixed cervical carcinomas. The concept of endocervical columnar cell-dysplasia. Am J Clin Pathol 64: 20
7. Atkin NB (1976) Prognostic significance of ploidy level in human tumors. I. Carcinomas of the uterus. J Natl Cancer Inst 56: 909
8. Aurelian L, Schumann B, Marcus RL, Davis HJ (1973) Antibody to HSV-2-induced tumor specific antigens in serums from patients with cervical carcinoma. Science 181: 161
9. Azzopardi JG, Hou LT (1965) Intestinal metaplasia with argentaffin cells in cervical adenocarcinoma. J Pathol Bacteriol 90: 686
10. Baggish M, Woodruff JD (1971) Adenoid basal lesions of the cervix. Obstet Gynecol 37: 807
11. Barron BA, Cahill MC, Richart RM (1978) A statistical model of the natural history of cervical neoplastic disease: The duration of carcinoma in situ. Gynecol Oncol 6: 196
12. Benedet JL, Anderson GH, Boyes DA (1985) Colposcopic accuracy in the diagnosis of microinvasive and occult invasive carcinoma of the cervix. Obstet Gynecol 65: 557

13. Benson WL, Norris HJ (1977) A critical review of the frequency of lymph node metastasis and death from microinvasive carcinoma of the cervix. Obstet Gynecol 49: 632
14. Berdjis CC (1971) Pathology of Irradiation, 1st ed. Baltimore, Williams & Wilkins Co.
15. Berek JS, Hacker NF, Fu YS, Sokale JR, Leuchter RC, Lagasse LD (1985) Adenocarcinoma of the uterine cervix: Histologic variables associated with lymph node metastases and survival. Obstet Gynecol 65: 46
16. Berkowitz RS, Ehrmann RL, Lavizzo-Mourey R, Knapp RC (1979) Invasive cervical carcinoma in young women. Gynecol Oncol 8: 311
17. Berthelot P, Benhamon JP, Fauvert R (1961) Hypercorticisme et cancer de l'utérus. Nouv Presse Med 69: 1899
18. Bohm JW, Krupp PJ, Lee FYL, Batson HWK (1976) Lymph node metastasis in microinvasive epidermoid cancer of the cervix. Obstet Gynecol 48: 65
19. Boon MA, Baak JPA, Kurver PJH, Overdiep SH, Verdonk GW (1981) Adenocarcinoma in situ of the cervix. An underdiagnosed lesion. Cancer 48: 768
20. Boronow RC, Averette HE, Nelson JH Jr., Richart RM, Townsend DE (1975) Defining cervical microinvasive carcinoma. Contemp Obstet Gynecol 5: 121
21. Bottles K, Winkler B, Lacey C, Stern J, Braga CA, Miller T Fine needle aspiration biopsy in the management of cervical carcinoma following primary therapy. Gynecol Oncol (In press)
22. Boyce JG, Fruchter RG, Nicastri AD, et al. (1984) Vascular invasion in stage I carcinoma of the cervix. Cancer 53: 1175
23. Boyes DA, Worth AJ, Fidler HK (1970) The results of treatment of 4389 cases of preclinical squamous carcinoma. J Obstet Gynaecol Br Commonw 77: 769
24. Brady LW, O'Neill EA, Farber SH (1977) Unusual sites of metastasis. Semin Oncol 4: 59
25. Burghart E, Holzer E (1977) Diagnosis and treatment of microinvasive carcinoma of the uterine cervix. Obstet Gynecol 49: 641
26. Campos JL (1971) Mortality trends in carcinoma of the cervix uteri. J Chronic Dis 24: 701
27. Cherry CP, Glucksmann A (1955) Lymphatic embolism and lymph node metastasis in cancers of vulva and of uterine cervix. Cancer 8: 564
28. Christopherson WM, Parker JE (1964) Microinvasive carcinoma of the uterine cervix: A clinical–pathological study. Cancer 17: 1123
29. Christopherson WM, Nealon N, Gray LA, Sr (1979) Noninvasive precursor lesions of adenocarcinoma and mixed adenosquamous carcinoma of the cervix uteri. Cancer 44: 975
30. Cid JM (1959) La pigmentation mélanique de l'endocervix. Un argument viscéral "neurogénique." Ann Anat Pathol 4: 617
31. Coppleson LW, Brown B (1975) Observations on a model of the biology of carcinoma of the cervix. Am J Obstet Gynecol 122: 127
32. Coppleson M (1970) The origin and nature of premalignant lesions of the cervix uteri. Int J Gynecol Obstet 8: 539
33. Cramer DW (1974) The role of cervical cytology in the declining morbidity and mortality of cervical cancer. Cancer 34: 2018
34. Cramer DW, Cutler SJ (1974) Incidence and histopathology of malignancies of the female genital organs in the United States. Am J Obstet Gynecol 118: 443
35. Creasman WT, Rutledge F, Fletcher GH (1970) Carcinoma of the cervix associated with pregnancy. Obstet Gynecol 36: 495
36. Creasman WT, Fetter BF, Clarke-Pearson DL, Kaufman L, Parker RT (1985) Managment of stage IA carcinoma of the cervix. Am J Obstet Gynecol 153: 164
37. Crissman JD, Makuch R, Budhraja M (1985) Histopathologic grading of squamous cell carcinoma of the uterine cervix: An evaluation of 70 Stage 1b patients. Cancer 55: 1590
38. Czernobilsky B, Moll R, Franke WW, Dallenbach-Hellweg G, Hohlweg-Majert P (1984) Intermediate filaments of normal and neoplastic tissues of the female genital tract with emphasis on problems of differential diagnosis. Pathol Res Pract 179: 31
39. Dallenbach-Hellweg G (1984) On the origin and histological structure of adenocarcinoma of the endocervix in women under 50 years of age. Pathol Res Pract 179: 38
40. Davis JR, Moon LB (1975) Increased incidence of adenocarcinoma of uterine cervix. Obstet Gynecol 45: 79
41. Deligdisch L, Escay-Martinez E, Cohen CJ (1984) Endocervical carcinoma: A study of 23 patients with clinicopathologic correlation. Gynecol Oncol 18: 326
42. Demian SDE, Bushkin FL, Echevarria RA (1973) Perineural invasion and anaplastic transformation of verrucous carcinoma. Cancer 32: 395
43. De Petrillo AD, Townsend DE, Morrow CP, Lickrish GM, Di Saia PJ, Roy M (1975) Colposcopic evaluation of the abnormal Papanicoleou test in pregnancy. Am J Obstet Gynecol 121: 441
44. Diddle AW (1972) Carcinoma of the cervix uteri with metastases to the neck. Cancer 29: 453
45. Dinh TV, Woodruff JD (1985) Adenoid cystic and adenoid basal carcinomas of the cervix. Obstet Gynecol 65: 705
46. Di Saia PJ, Haverbeck BJ, Dyce BJ, Morrow CP (1975) Carcinoembryonic antigen in patients with gynecologic malignancies. Am J Obstet Gynecol 121: 159
47. Dougherty CM, Cotten N (1964) Mixed squamous-cell and adenocarcinoma of the cervix: Combined, adenosquamous and mucoepidermoid types. Cancer 17: 1132
48. Dudan RC, Yon JL, Ford JH, Averette HE (1973) Carcinoma of the cervix and pregnancy. Gynecol Oncol 1: 283
49. Faaborg LL, Smith ML, Newland JR (1979) Case report: Uterine cervical and vaginal verrucous squamous cell carcinoma. Gynecol Oncol 8: 104
50. Fennell RH, Jr (1978) Microinvasive carcinoma of the uterine cervix. Obstet Gynecol Surv 33: 406
51. Fereczy A, Richart RM (1974) Female Reproductive System. Dynamics of Scan and Transmission Electron Microscopy, 1st ed. New York, John Wiley & Sons
52. Fetissof F, Berger G, Dubois MP, Arbeille-Brassart B, Lansac J, Sam-Giao M, Jobard P (1985) Endocrine cells in the female genital tract. Histopathology 9: 133
53. Fidler HK, Boyes DA, Worth AJ (1968) Cervical cancer

detection in British Columbia. J Obstet Gynecol Br Commonw 75: 392
54. Forsberg JG (1983) Estrogen, vaginal cancer and vaginal development. Am J Obstet Gynecol 113: 83
55. Fox H, Kazzaz B, Langley FA (1964) Argyrophil and argentaffin cells in the female genital tract and in ovarian mucinous cysts. J Pathol Bacteriol 88: 479
56. Fu YS, Reagan JW, Fu AS, Janiga KE (1982) Adenocarcinoma and mixed carcinoma of the uterine cervix. II. Prognostic value of nuclear DNA analysis. Cancer 49: 2571
57. Fu YS, Reagan JW, Hsiu JG, Storaasli JP, Wentz WB (1982) Adenocarcinoma and mixed carcinoma of the uterine cervix. I. A clinicopathologic study. Cancer 49: 2560
58. Fujii S, Konishi I, Ferenczy A, Imai K, Okamura H, Mori T (1986) Small cell undifferentiated carcinoma of the uterine cervix. Ultrastruct Pathol 10: 337
59. Gallup DG, Harper RH, Stock RJ (1985) Poor prognosis in patients with adenosquamous cell carcinoma of the cervix. Obstet Gynecol 65: 416
60. Gardner HL, Parsons L (1962) Blood vessel invasion in cancer of the cervix. Cancer 15: 1269
61. Gilbert EF, Palladino A (1966) Squamous papillomas of the uterine cervix: Review of the literature and report of a giant papillary carcinoma. Am J Clin Pathol 46: 115
62. Gissman L (1984) Papillomaviruses and their association with cancer in animals and in man. Cancer Surv 3: 161
63. Glucksmann A, Cherry CP (1956) Incidence, histology and response to radiation of mixed carcinomas (adenoacanthomas) of the uterine cervix. Cancer 9: 971
64. Glucksmann A, Spear FG (1945) The qualitative and quantitative histological examination of biopsy material from patients treated by radiation for carcinoma of the cervix uteri. Br J Radiol 18: 313
65. Goellner JR (1976) Carcinoma of the cervix. Clinicopathologic correlation of 196 cases. Am J Clin Pathol 66: 775
66. Graham J, Graham R, Hirabayaski K (1968) Recurrent cancer of the cervix uteri. Surg Gynecol Obstet 126: 799
67. Graham S, Priore R, Graham M, Browne R, Burnett W, West D (1979) Genital cancer in wives of penile cancer patients. Cancer 44: 1870
68. Groben P, Reddick R, Askin F (1985) The pathologic spectrum of small cell carcinoma of the cervix. Int J Gynecol Pathol 4: 42
69. Halpin TF, Frick HC, Munnell EW (1972) Critical points of failure in the therapy of cancer of the cervix: A reappraisal. Am J Obstet Gynecol 114: 755
70. Hameed K (1968) Clear cell "mesonephric" carcinoma of uterine cervix. Obstet Gynecol 32: 564
71. Hart WR, Norris HJ (1972) Cervix adenocarcinoma of mesonephric type. Cancer 29: 106
72. Hasumi K, Sakamoto A, Sugano H (1980) Microinvasive carcinoma of the uterine cervix. Cancer 45: 928
73. Hepler TK, Dockerty MB, Randall LM (1952) Primary adenocarcinoma of cervix. Am J Obstet Gynecol 63: 800
74. Herbst AL, Cole P, Norusis MJ, Welch WR, Scully RE (1979) Epidemiologic aspects and factors related to survival in 384 Registry cases of clear cell adenocarcinoma of the vagina and cervix. Am J Obstet Gynecol 135: 876
75. Hoskins WJ, Averette HE, Ng ABP, Yon JL (1979) Adenoid cystic carcinoma of the cervix uteri: Report of six cases and review of the literature. Gynecol Oncol 7: 371
76. Hurlimann J, Gloor E (1984) Adenocarcinoma in situ and invasive adenocarcinoma of the uterine cervix. An immunohistologic study with antibodies specific for several epithelial markers. Cancer 54: 103
77. Hurt WG, Silverberg SG, Frable WJ, Belgrad R, Crooks LD (1977) Adenocarcinoma of the cervix: Histopathologic and clinical features. Am J Obstet Gynecol 129: 304
78. Inoue T (1984) Prognostic significance of the depth of invasion relating to nodal metastases, parametrial extension and cell types. Cancer 54: 3035
79. Inoue T, Okumura M (1984) Prognostic significance of parametrial extension in patients with cervical carcinoma stages Ib, IIa and IIb. Cancer 54: 1714
80. Inoue T, Chihara T, Morita K (1984) The prognostic significance of the size of the largest nodes in metastatic carcinoma from the uterine cervix. Gynecol Oncol 19: 187
81. Jennings RH, Barclay DL (1972) Verrucous carcinoma of the cervix. Cancer 30: 430
82. Jones HW, Plymate S, Gluck FB, Miles PA, Greene JF (1976) Small cell nonkeratinizing carcinoma of the cervix associated with ACTH production. Cancer 38: 1629
83. Jones WH, Droegemueller W, Makowski ELA (1971) A primary melanocarcinoma of the cervix. Obstet Gynecol 111: 959
84. Kagan AR, Nussbaum H, Chan P. Ziel HK (1973) Adenocarcinoma of the uterine cervix. Am J Obstet Gynecol 117: 464
85. Kaku T, Enjoji M (1983) Extremely well differentiated adenocarcinoma ("adenoma malignum") of the cervix. Int J Gynecol Pathol 2: 28
86. Kaminski PF, Maier RC (1983) Clear cell adenocarcinoma of the cervix unrelated to diethylstilbestrol exposure. Obstet Gynecol 62: 720
87. Kaminski PF, Norris HJ (1984) Coexistence of ovarian neoplasms and endocervical adenocarcinoma. Obstet Gynecol 64: 553
88. Kaminski PF, Norris HJ (1983) Minimal deviation carcinoma (adenoma malignum) of the cervix. Int J Gynecol Pathol 2: 141
89. Kanbour AI, Klionsky B, Murphy AI (1974) Carcinoma of the vagina following cervical cancer. Cancer 34: 1838
90. Kashimura M, Tsukamoto N, Matsukama K, Matsuyama T, Sugimore H, Taki I (1984) Verrucous carcinoma of the uterine cervix: Report of a case with follow-up of 6½ years. Gynecol Oncol 19: 204
91. Kato H, Morioka H, Aramaki S, Tamai K, Torigou T (1983) Prognostic significance of tumor antigen TA-4 in squamous cell carcinoma of the uterine cervix. Am J Obstet Gynecol 145: 350
92. Ketcham AS, Hoye RC, Taylor PT, Deckers PJ, Thomas LB, Chretien PB (1971) Radical hysterectomy and pelvic lymphadenectomy for carcinoma of the uterine cervix. Cancer 28: 1271
93. Kiang DT, Bauer GE, Kennedy BT (1973) Immunoassayable insulin in carcinoma of the cervix associated with hypoglycemia. Cancer 31: 801

94. Kirk ME (1974) Carcinoma of the cervix, stage Ia. Human Pathol 5: 253
95. Kjorstad KE, Orjasaeter H (1984) The prognostic significance of carcinoembryonic antigen determinations in patients with adenocarcinoma of the cervix. Gynecol Oncol 19: 284
96. Kolbenstvedt A, Kolstad P (1974) Pelvic lymph node dissection under preoperative lymphographic control. Gynecol Oncol 2: 39
97. Korhonen MD (1984) Adenocarcinoma of the uterine cervix. Prognosis and prognostic significance of histology. Cancer 53: 1760
98. Korhonen M, Stenback F (1984) Adenocarcinoma metastatic to the uterine cervix. Gynecol Obstet Invest 17: 57
99. Koss LG, Brannan CD, Ashikari R (1970) Histologic and ultrastructural features of adenoid cystic carcinoma of the breast. Cancer 26: 1271
100. Kraus FT (1973) Irradiation changes in the uterus. In The Uterus, Norris HJ, Hertig AT, Abell MR (eds.) Internal. Acad. Pathol. Monograph. Baltimore, Williams & Wilkins Co., pp 457–488.
101. Kraus FT, Perez-Mesa C (1966) Verrucous carcinoma. Cancer 19: 26
102. Kyriakos M, Kempson RL, Perez CA (1971) Carcinoma of the cervix in young women. Obstet Gynecol 38: 930
103. Lancaster WD, Castellano C, Santos C, Delgado G, Kurman RJ, Jenson AB (1986) Human papillomavirus deoxyribonucleic acid in cervical carcinoma from primary and metastatic sites. Am J Obstet Gynecol 154: 115
104. Lathrop JC (1967) Views and reviews: Malignant pelvic lymphomas. Obstet Gynecol 30: 137
105. Latour JPA (1961) Results in the management of preclinical carcinoma of the cervix. Am J Obstet Gynecol 81: 511
106. Lauchlan SC (1984) Metaplasias and neoplasias of müllerian epithelium. Histopathology 8: 543
107. Lehn H, Ernst TM, Sauer G (1984) Transcription of episomal papillomavirus DNA in human condylomata acuminata and Buschke-Lowenstein tumors. J Gen Virol 65: 2003
108. Leman MH, Benson WL, Kurman RJ, Park RC (1976) Microinvasive carcinoma of the cervix. Obstet Gynecol 48: 571
109. Lemoine NR, Hall PA (1986) Epithelial tumors metastatic to the uterine cervix. A study of 33 cases and review of the literature. Cancer 57: 2238
110. Littman P, Clement PB, Henriksen B, Wang CC, Robboy SJ, Taft PD, Ulfelder H, Scully RE (1976) Glassy cell carcinoma of the cervix. Cancer 37: 2238
111. Lohe KJ (1978) Early squamous cell carcinoma of the uterine cervix. I. Definition and histology. Gynecol Oncol 6: 10
112. Lohe KJ (1978) Early squamous cell carcinoma of the uterine cervix. III. Frequency of lymph node metastases. Gynecol Oncol 6: 51
113. Lucas WE, Benirschke K, Lebherz TB (1974) Verrucous carcinoma of the female genital tract. Am J Obstet Gynecol 119: 435
114. Lucia SP, Mills H, Lowenhaupt E, Hunt ML (1952) Visceral involvement in primary neoplastic diseases of the reticuloendothelial system. Cancer 5: 1193
115. Maier RC, Norris HJ (1980) Coexistence of cervical intraepithelial neoplasia with primary adenocarcinoma of the endocervix. Obstet Gynecol 56: 361
116. Marcial VA, Bosch A (1970) Radiation-induced tumor regression in carcinoma of the uterine cervix. Prognostic significance. Am J Roentgenol 108: 113
117. Martzloff KH (1923) Carcinoma of the cervix uteri: A pathological and clinical study with particular reference to the relative malignancy of the neoplastic process as indicated by the predominant cell of cancer cell. Bull Johns Hopkins Hosp 34: 141, 184
118. Maruo T, Shibata K, Kimura A, Hoshina M, Mochizuki M (1985) Tumor-associated antigen, TA-4, in the monitoring of the effects of therapy for squamous cell carcinoma of the cervix. Cancer 56: 302
119. Mazur MT, Battifora HA (1982) Adenoid cystic carcinoma of the uterine cervix: Ultrastructure, immunofluorescence and criteria for diagnosis. Am J Clin Pathol 77: 494
120. Mazur MT, Hsueh S, Gersell DJ (1984) Metastases to the female genital tract, analysis of 325 cases. Cancer 53: 1978
121. McGowan L, Young RH, Scully RE (1980) Peutz-Jeghers syndrome with "adenoma malignum" of the cervix. A report of two cases. Gynecol Oncol 10: 125
122. McKelvey JL, Goodlin RR (1963) Adenoma malignum of the cervix: A cancer of deceptively innocent histologic pattern. Cancer 16: 549
123. McNutt NS, Weinstein RS (1969) Carcinoma of the cervix. Deficiency of nexus intercellular junctions. Science 165: 597
124. Menczner J, Modan B, Oelsner G, Sharon Z, Steintiz R, Sampson S (1978) Adenocarcinoma of the uterine cervix in Jewish women. A distinct epidemiologic entity. Cancer 41: 2464
125. Mestwerdt G (1947) Probeexzision und kolposkopie in des fruhdiagnose des portiokarcinoms. Zentr Gynak 4: 326
126. Michael H, Grawe L, Kraus FT (1984) Minimal deviation endocervical adenocarcinoma: Clinical and histologic features, immunohistochemical staining for carcinoembryonic antigen and differentiation from confusing benign lesions. Int J Gynaecol Pathol 3: 261
127. Miles PA, Norris HJ (1971) Adenoid cystic carcinoma of the cervix: An analysis of 12 cases. Obstet Gynecol 38: 103
128. Moll R, Levy R, Czernobilsky B, Hohlweg-Majert P, Dallenbach-Hellweg G, Franke WW (1983) Cytokeratins of normal epithelial and some neoplasms of the female genital tract. Lab Invest 49: 599
129. Mullins JD, Hilliard GD (1981) Cervical carcinoid ("argyrophil cell" carcinoma) associated with an endocervical adenocarcinoma: A light and ultrastructural study. Cancer 47: 785
130. Ng ABP, Reagan JW, Lindner EA (1972) The cellular manifestations of microinvasive squamous cell carcinoma of the uterine cervix. Acta Cytol 16: 5

131. Noda K, Kimura K, Ikeda M, Teshima K (1983) Studies on the histogenesis of cervical adenocarcinoma. Int J Gynecol Pathol 1: 336
132. Nogales F, Bottela-Llusia J (1965) The frequency of invasion of the lymph nodes in cancer of the uteri cervix: A study of the degree of extension in relation to the histological type of tumor. Am J Obstet Gynecol 93: 91
133. Nunez C, Abdul-Karim FW, Somrak TM (1985) Glassy cell carcinoma of the uterine cervix. Acta Cytol 29: 303
134. Okagaki T, Meyer AA, Sciarra JJ (1974) Prognosis of irradiated carcinoma of cervix uteria and nuclear DNA in cytologic post-irradiation dysplasia. Cancer 33: 647
135. Okagaki T, Clark BA, Zachow KR, et al. (1984) Presence of human papillomavirus in verrucous carcinoma (Ackerman) of the vagina. Arch Pathol Lab Med 108: 567
136. Ostör AG, Pagano R, Davoren RAM, Fortune DW, Chanen W, Rome R (1984) Adenocarcinoma in situ of the cervix. Int J Gynaecol Pathol 3: 179
137. Palmer JP, Spratt DW (1956) Pelvic carcinoma following irradiation for benign gynecological diseases. Am J Obstet Gynecol 72: 497
138. Papadia S (1962) Mucinous patterns in epidermoid carcinomas. Gynecologia 153: 337
139. Park RC, Patow WE, Rogers RE, Zimmerman EA (1973) Treatment of stage I carcinoma of the cervix. Obstet Gynecol 41: 117
140. Patridge EE, Murad T, Shingleton HM, Austin JM, Hatch KD (1980) Verrucous lesions of the female genitalia. I. Giant condylomata. Am J Obstet Gynecol 137: 412
141. Patridge EE, Murad T, Shingleton HM, Austin JM, Hatch KD (1980) Verrucous lesions of the female genitalia. II. Verrucous carcinoma. Am J Obstet Gynecol 137: 419
142. Patten SF Jr., Reagan JW, Obenauf M, Ballard L (1963) Post-irradiation dysplasia of uterine cervix and vagina. An analytical study of cells. Cancer 16: 173
143. Pilleron JP, Durand JC, Hamelin JP (1974) Location of lymph node invasion in cancer of the uterine cervix: Study of 140 cases treated at the Curie Foundation. Am J Obstet Gynecol 119: 453
144. Prempree T, Amornmarn R, Wizenberg MJ (1985) A therapeutic approach to primary adenocarcinoma of the cervix. Cancer 56: 1264
145. Puri S, Fenoglio CM, Richrat RM, Townsend DE (1977) Clear cell carcinoma of cervix and vagina in progeny of women who received diethylstilbestrol: Three cases with scanning and transmission electron microscopy. Am J Obstet Gynecol 128: 550
146. Qizilbash A-H (1975) In situ and microinvasive adenocarcinoma of the uterine cervix. A clinical, cytologic and histologic study of 14 cases. Am J Clin Pathol 64: 155
147. Rampone JF, Klem W, Kolstad P (1973) Combined treatment of stage Ib carcinoma of the cervix. Obstet Gynecol 41: 163
148. Reagan JW (1974) Cellular pathology and uterine cancer. Am J Clin Pathol 62: 150
149. Reagan JW, Ng ABP (1973) The cellular manifestations of uterine carcinogeneis. In The Uterus, Norris NJ, Hertig AT, Abell MR (eds.) Internatl. Acad. Path. Monogr. Baltimore, Williams & Wilkins Co., pp 320–347.
150. Report of the Task Force of the Department of National Health and Welfare of Canada. Cervical cancer screening programs. The Walton Report. Cana Med Assoc J 144: 2
151. Richard L, Guralnick M, Ferenczy A (1981) Ultrastructure of glassy cell carcinoma of cervix. Diagn Gynecol Obstet 3: 31
152. Richart RM, Barron BA (1969) A follow-up study of patients with cervical dysplasia. Am J Obstet Gynecol 105: 386
153. Robboy SJ, Herbst AL, Scully RE (1974) Clear-cell adenocarcinoma of the vagina and cervix in young females: Analysis of 37 tumors that persisted or recurred after primary therapy. Cancer 34: 606
154. Roche WD, Norris HJ (1975) Microinvasive carcinoma of the cervix. The significance of lymphatic invasion and confluent patterns of stromal growth. Cancer 36: 180
155. Rosen Y, Dolan TE (1975) Carcinoma of the cervix with cylindromatous features believed to arise in mesonephric duct. Cancer 36: 1739
156. Sassoon AF, Said JW, Nash G, Shintaku IP, Banks-Schlegel S (1985) Involucrin in intraepithelial and invasive squamous cell carcinomas of the cervix: An immunohistochemical study. Human Pathol 16: 467
157. Scully RE, Aguirre P, De Lellis RA (1984) Argyrophilia, serotonin and peptide hormones in the female genital tract and its tumors. Int J Gynaecol Pathol 3: 51
158. Sedlis A, Sall S, Tsukada Y, Park R, Mangan C, Shingleton H, Blessing JA (1979) Microinvasive carcinoma of the uterine cervix: A clinical-pathologic study. Am J Obstet Gynecol 133: 64
159. Seltzer V, Sall S, Castadot MJ, Muradian-Davidian M, Sedlis A (1979) Glassy cell cervical carcinoma. Gynecol Oncol 8: 141
160. Seski JC, Abell MR, Morley GW (1977) Microinvasive squamous carcinoma of the cervix. Definition, histologic analysis, late results of treatment. Obstet Gynecol 50: 410
161. Sevin BU, Nadji M, Greening SE, Ng ABP, Nordqvist SRB, Girtanner, Averette HE (1980) Fine needle aspiration cytology in gynecologic oncology: Early detection of occult persistent or recurrent cancer after radiation therapy. Gynecol Oncol 9: 351
162. Sidhu GS, Koss LG, Barber HRK (1970) Relation of histologic factors to the response of stage I epidermoid carcinoma of the cervix to surgical treatment: Analysis of 115 patients. Obstet Gynecol 35: 329
163. Silverberg E (1985) Cancer statistics. Cancer J Clin 30: 23
164. Silverberg SG, Hurt WG (1975) Minimal deviation adenocarcinoma ("adenoma malignum") of the cervix: A reappraisal. Am J Obstet Gynecol 121: 971
165. Sotto LSJ, Graham JB, Pickren JW (1960) Post-mortem findings in cancer of the cervix. Am J Obstet Gynecol 80: 791
166. Stafl A, Mattingly RF (1975) Angiogenesis of cervical neoplasia. Am J Obstet Gynecol 121: 845
167. Stafl A, Friedrich EG Jr., Mattingly RF (1973) Detection

of cervical neoplasia. Reducing the risk of error. Clin Obstet Gynecol 16: 238
168. Stern E (1969) Epidemiology of dysplasia. Obstet Gynecol Surv 24: 711
169. Taki I, Sugimori H, Matsuyama T, Kashimura Y, Yoshino T (1979) Treatment of microinvasive carcinoma. Obstet Gynecol Surv 34: 839
170. Tateishi R, Wada A, Hayakawa K, Hongo J, Ishii S, Terakawa N (1975) Argyrophil cell carcinomas (apudomas) of the uterine cervix. Virchows Arch Pathol Anat Histol 366: 257
171. Teshima S, Shimosato Y, Kishi K, Kasamatsu T, Ohmi K, Uei Y (1985) Early stage adenocarcinoma of the uterine cervix. Cancer 56: 167
172. Tsukamoto N, Nakamura M, Kashimura M, Saito (1980) Primary cervical choriocarcinoma. Gynecol Oncol 9: 99
173. Twombley GH, Di Palma S (1951) Growth and spread of cancer of cervix uteri. Am J Roentgenol 65: 691
174. Ueda G, Yamasaki M, Inoue M, Tanaka Y, Hiramatsu K, Inoue Y, Abe Y (1984) Immunohistochemical demonstration of peptide hormones in cervical adenocarcinomas with argyrophil cells. Int J Gynaecol Pathol 2: 373
175. Ueda G, Inoue Y, Yamasaki M, Inoue M, Tanaka Y, Hiramatsu K, Saito J, Nishino T, Abe Y (1984) Immunohistochemical demonstration of tumor antigen TA-4 in gynecologic tumors. Int J Gynaecol Pathol 3: 291
176. Van Nagell JR, Greenwell N, Powell DF, Donaldson ES, Hanson MS, Gay EC (1983) Microinvasive carcinoma of the cervix. Am J Obstet Gynecol 145: 981
177. Villasanta U (1972) Complications of radiotherapy for carcinoma of the uterine cervix. Am J Obstet Gynecol 114: 717
178. Wahlstrom T, Lindgren J, Korhonen M, Seggala M (1979) Distinction between endocervical and endometrial adenocarcinoma with immunoperoxidase staining of carcinoembryonic antigen in routine histological tissue specimens. Lancet 2: 1159
179. Way S (1980) Carcinoma metastatic to the cervix. Gynecol Oncol 9: 298
180. Weisbort IM, Stabinsky C, Davis AM (1972) Adenocarcinoma in situ of the uterine cervix. Cancer 29: 1179
181. Wentz WB, Reagan JW (1970) Clinical significance of post-irradiation dysplasia of the uterine cervix. Am J Obstet Gynecol 106: 812
182. Wheeless CR, Graham R, Graham JB (1970) Prognosis and treatment of adenoepidermoid carcinoma of the cervix. Obstet Gynecol 35: 928
183. White CD, Morley GW, Kumar NB (1984) The prognostic significance of tumor emboli in lymphatics or vascular spaces of the cervical stroma in stage Ib squamous cell carcinoma of the cervix. Am J Obstet Gynecol 149: 342
184. Wolff JP, Lacour J, Chassagne D, Berend M (1972) Cancer of the cervical stump. Obstet Gynecol 39: 10
185. Yajima A, Fukuda M, Noda K (1984) Histopathological findings concerning the morphogenesis of mixed carcinoma of the uterine cervix. Gynecol Oncol 18: 157
186. Yamaski M, Tateishi R, Hongo J, Ozaki Y, Inoue M, Ueda G (1984) Argyrophil small cell carcinomas of the uterine cervix. Int J Gynecol Pathol 3: 146
187. Yee C, Krishnan-Hewlett I, Baker CC, Schlegel R, Howley PM (1985) Presence and expression of human papillomavirus sequences in human cervical carcinoma cell lines. Am J Pathol 119: 361
188. Yoshikawa H, Matsukara T, Yamamoto E, Kawana T, Mizuno M, Yoshiike K (1985) Occurrence of human papillomavirus types 16 and 18 DNA in cervical carcinomas from Japan: Age of patients and histological type of carcinoma. Jpn J Cancer Res 76: 667
189. Young RH, Welch WR, Dickersin R, Scully RE (1982) Ovarian sex cord tumor with annular tubules. Review of 74 cases including 27 with Peutz-Jeghers syndrome and four with adenoma malignum of the cervix. Cancer 50: 1384
190. Zhang YC, Zhang PF, Wei YH (1983) Metastatic carcinoma of the cervix uteri from the gastrointestinal tract. Gynecol Oncol 15: 287

9

Anatomy and Histology of the Uterine Corpus

Alex Ferenczy, M.D.

Elizabeth Ramsey's review of the history of anatomic studies of the human uterus is among the best available in the English literature, and the interested student is referred to her chapter in *Biology of the Uterus.*[65] Briefly, the first comprehensive description of the external anatomy of the human uterus was made by the Greek physician Soranus of Ephesus in the second century A.D. Until the Renaissance in Europe, several misconceptions prevailed about the function and internal anatomy of the uterus. For example, it was believed that the cervix had a spongy consistency similar to that of the lungs and served the function of respiration. Others suggested that the uterus was analogous to the scrotum and migrated into the abdominal cavity. The theory of a multicompartmentalized uterus with seven chambers was held for centuries, as was the concept that the uterine arteries convey menstrual blood to the mammary glands, where it is converted into milk during pregnancy. The anatomy of the uterus became better known when dissection of cadavers became a part of medical practice—Leonardo da Vinci in the 15th century and Vesalius in the 16th century demonstrated that the human uterus had a single cavity lined by decidua and supported by muscular layers. In the 18th century, William Hunter described the gestational uterus including the placenta and the uteroplacental vascular system. Development of histology and microscopy led to an explosive growth of knowledge of the uterus, with detailed descriptions of the embryology by Müller in the 19th century and hormone-mediated cyclic endometrial changes by Hitschmann and Adler and later by Robert Schroeder in the early 20th century.

Developmental Anatomy

Embryologically, the endometrium and myometrium are of mesodermal origin, and both structures are formed secondary to fusion of the müllerian ducts between the eighth and ninth postovulatory weeks.[59] Until the 20th week of gestation, the endometrium is composed of a single layer of columnar epithelium supported by a thick layer of fibroblastic stroma. By the 20th gestational week, the surface epithelium invaginates into the underlying stroma, forming glandular structures that extend toward

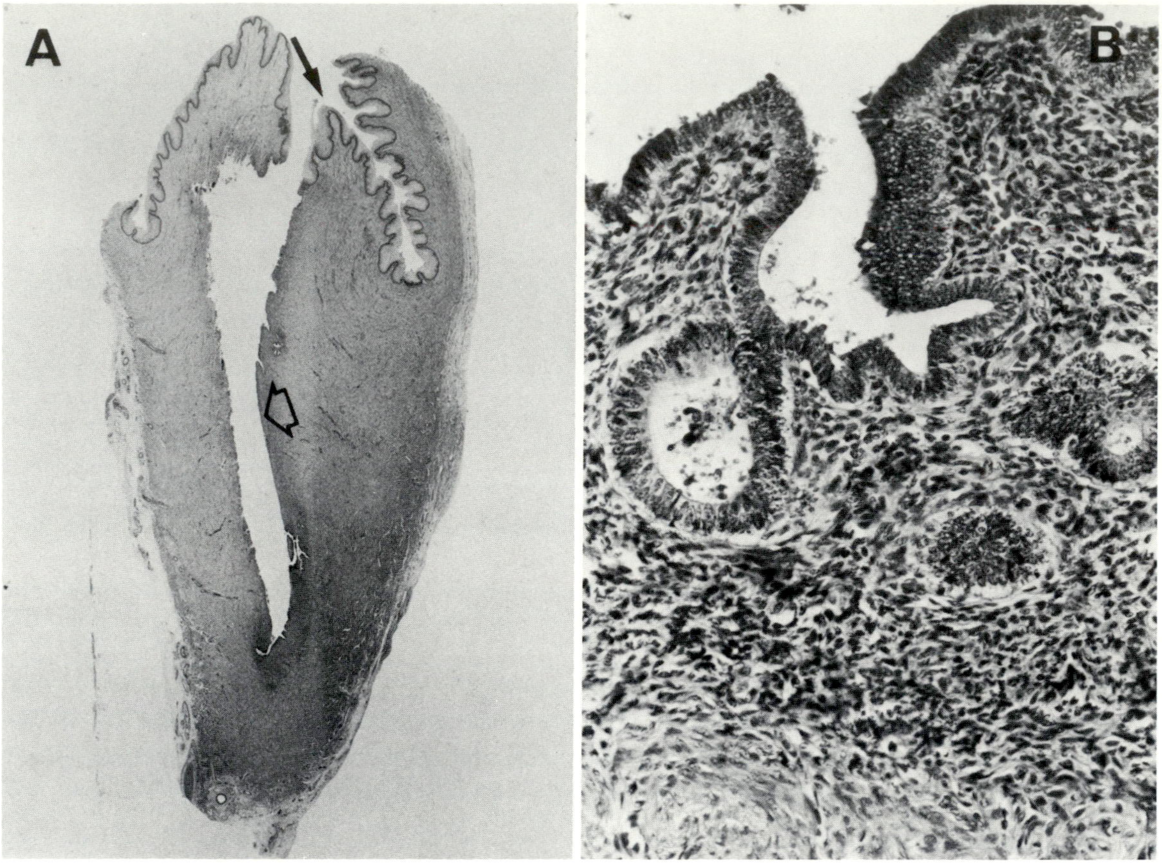

FIG. 9.1. Neonatal uterus. *A*. Whole mount section of a 4-day old baby's uterus. The cervix (*narrow and open arrows*) is the dominant part of the uterus. *B*. The endometrium is thin and has few glands, and the lining epithelium is of the inactive type. The stroma is dense and compact, resembling the basalis layer of the endometrium during the postpubertal period.

the underlying myometrium. At birth the uterus measures about 4 cm in length, much of which is made up of the cervix (Fig. 9.1A). The endometrial surface and glands are lined by a low columnar to cuboidal epithelium, which in general is devoid of either proliferative or secretory changes; it resembles the inactive endometrium in menopausal or in castrated premenopausal women (Fig. 9.1B). The endometrial mucosa measures less than 0.5 mm in thickness.

During the prepubertal period, the endometrial mucosa remains inactive, and the cervix comprises the predominant portion of the uterus. In the reproductive years, the size and weight of a normal uterus vary according to parity. In nulliparous women, it measures 8 cm in length, 5 cm in width at the fundus level, and 2.5 cm in thickness and weighs between 40 and 100 g. Multigravid uteri (four deliveries or more) measure about 10–12 cm × 5–7 cm × 2.5–3.5 cm and weigh up to 250 g.[46] The corpus uterus is divided into fundus, corpus, and isthmus regions. The uterus is located between the rectum (posteriorly) and urinary bladder (anteriorly); it is supported by the round and utero-ovarian ligaments and is covered by the pelvic peritoneum. The endometrium during the reproductive period undergoes cyclic morphologic changes. These are particularly evident in the upper two-thirds of the mucosa, the so-called functionalis layer. Morphologic alterations are minimal in the lower one-third of the basalis layer. In postmenopausal life, the endometrium recapitulates the neonatal–fetal period, being thin with relatively few glands and lined by cuboidal epithelium that is devoid of proliferative or secretory activity (see section on inactive and atrophic endometrium). Endometrial stromal fibroblasts are relatively more abundant, however, in the neonatal period than in advanced postmenopausal atrophy.

Vascular Anatomy

The blood supply of the uterus is provided by the left and right uterine arteries, which originate from the hypogastric arteries.[66] At the isthmus, the uterine arteries

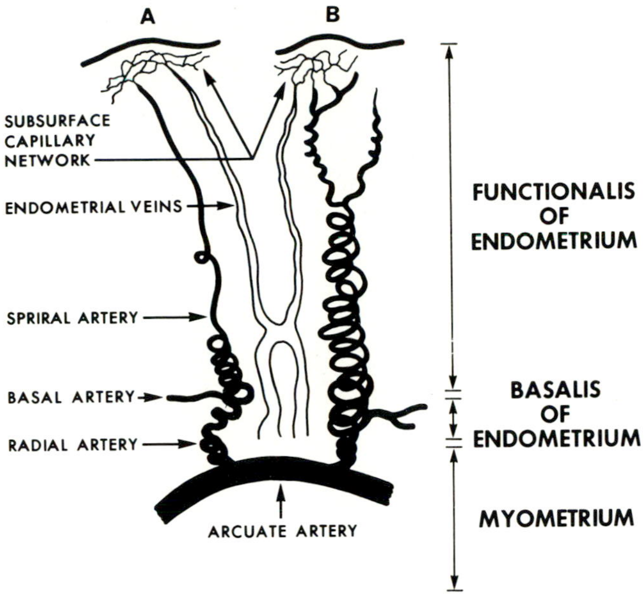

FIG. 9.2. Endometrial vessels. The coiled endometrial spiral arteries originate from the myometrial arcuate arteries and have connections with the subsurface capillary network, which in turn is drained by dilated veins. Arborization and coiling of spiral arteries are amplified in the postovulatory period (*B*) compared to the preovulatory phase (*A*) of the menstrual cycle.

divide, and the ascending branches anastomose with the ovarian arteries, whereas the descending branches anastomose with the vaginal arteries. The endometrial mucosa has an abundant vascular supply originating from the radial arteries of the subjacent myometrium (Fig. 9.2). These penetrate the endometrium at regular intervals and give rise to the basal arteries. These in turn divide into horizontal and vertical branches, the former providing the blood supply to the basal layer of the endometrium and the latter to the overlying functionalis layer. The endometrial vessels in the functionalis layer are referred to as *spiral arterioles* (Fig. 9.2). Their development and arborization near the surface and their connections with the subsurface epithelial precapillary system, as well as extreme coiling during the menstrual cycle (Figs. 9.2 and 9.3), are influenced by the ovarian steroid hormones and, presumably, prostaglandins. The latter are likely also to influence contraction of the endometrial basal and myometrial radial arteries.[6,14,51,60]

Histologically the feature differentiating the endometrial and myometrial arteries is the absence of subendothelial elastica in the endometrial arteries except for the basal portion[60] and its presence in the myometrial arteries (Fig. 9.4). The specific morphologic constitution of endomyometrial arteries is related to the control of endometrial bleeding (see section on steroid hormone and receptor interactions in the normal endometrial cy-

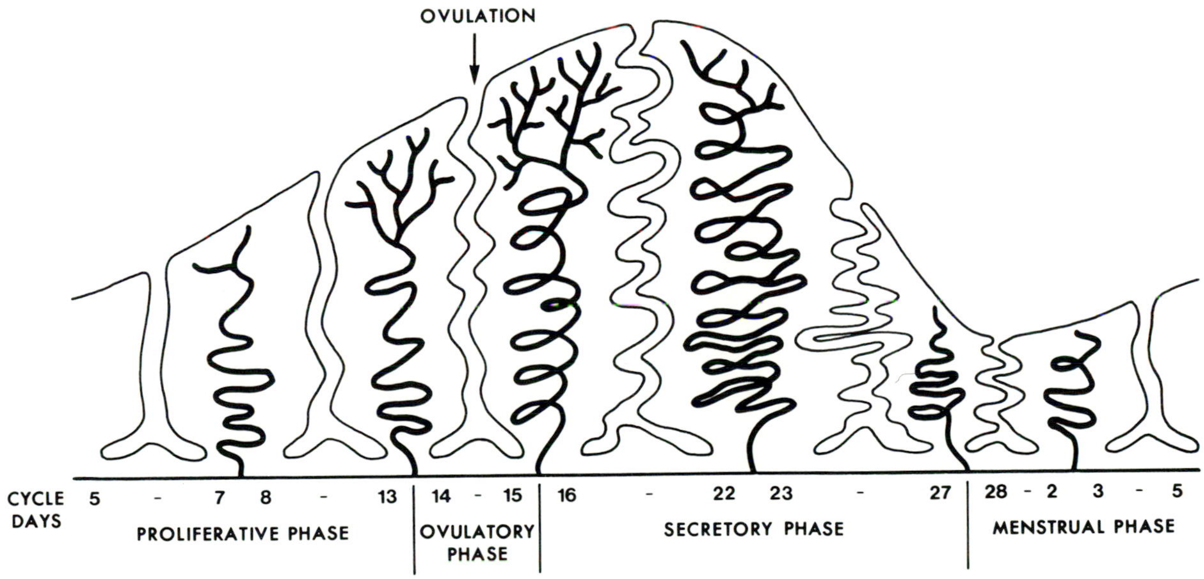

FIG. 9.3. Diagrammatic representation of endometrial vascular alterations during the menstrual cycle. There is a gradual increase in the arborization and coiling of spiral arteries during the preovulatory–ovulatory and postovulatory periods up to cycle days 23–25. The spiral arterial growth parallels the gradual increase in length and coiling of endometrial glands (hollow tubules). During the late secretory phase and menstrual period, collapse of the vascular and glandular systems predominates, whereas both the vessels and glands remain essentially unchanged in the lower one-third of the basal layer throughout the menstrual cycle.

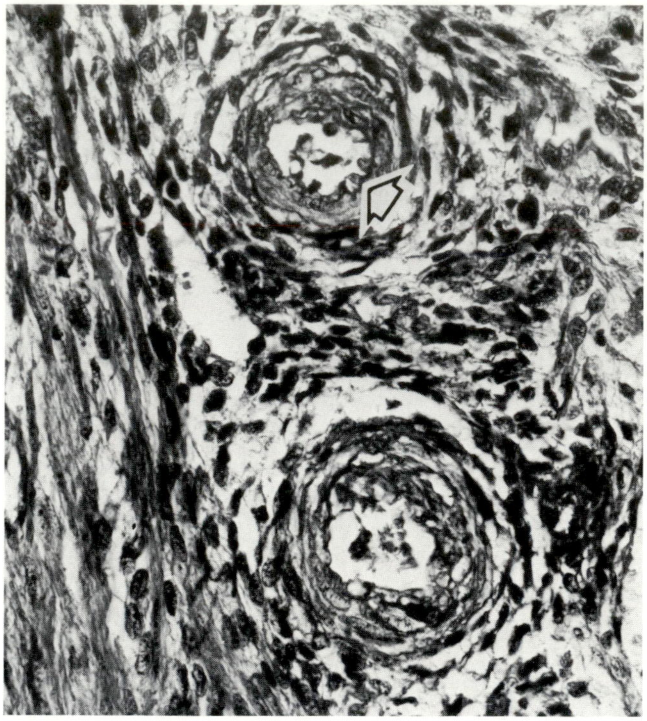

FIG. 9.4. Basal endometrial and myometrial arcuate arteries. Both arterial systems contain fine Weigert stain-positive elastic membranes (*arrow*) that presumably contribute to vascular constriction and ischemic necrosis during periods of menstruation. Elastica is absent in arteries of the endometrial functionalis.

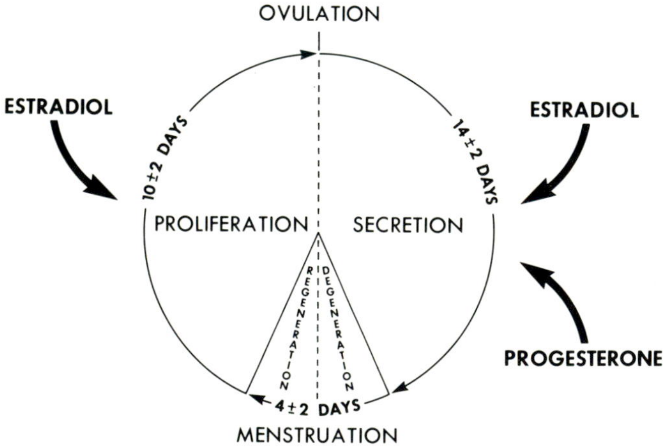

FIG. 9.5. Schematic representation of steroid hormone–morphologic interactions during the endometrial cycle. Estradiol promotes endometrial proliferation, whereas after ovulation, progesterone converts estradiol-primed endometrium into secretory tissue. Postovulatory estradiol amplifies the progesterone effect, and after withdrawal of both estradiol and progesterone, the endometrial mucosa degenerates and regenerates within the period of menstruation. (Reprinted by permission of Ferenczy and Guralnick, Ref. 24.)

cle). Veins and lymphatics are closely associated with the endometrial arteries and glands, respectively. Uterine lymphatics drain from subserosal uterine plexuses to the pelvic and periaortic lymph nodes.[61] The lymphatic drainage has important clinical implications with regard to management of patients with carcinoma of the endometrium (see Chapter 12, Endometrial Carcinoma).

Steroid Hormone and Receptor Interactions in the Endometrial Cycle

The endometrial cycle in women follows a precisely scheduled series of morphologic and physiologic events characterized by proliferation, secretory differentation, degeneration, and regeneration of the uterine lining (Fig. 9.5). These alterations are controlled by cyclically released ovarian estradiol (E_2) and progesterone (P). As a result, the endometrium is a highly sensitive indicator of the hypothalamopituitary–ovarian axis and serves to determine whether the infertile patient has ovulatory cycles.[57] Steroid hormone control of endometrial, epithelial, stromal, and presumably endothelial cells is mediated by estrogen receptors (E_2R) and progesterone (PgR) receptors. These steroid receptors are specific proteins concentrated in the nuclei of endometrial cells and have high affinity to bind E_2 and P, respectively.[40] Because they are sex steroid hormone (ligand) specific, a particular receptor may display high affinity for a closely related class of hormones, and the same class may compete for available binding sites. For example, E_2R effectively binds not only E_2 but also estrone (E_1), as well as synthetic estrogens, such as diethylstilbestrol (DES). E_2R and PgR concentrations are routinely determined by the dextran-coated charcoal binding assay. This technique uses homogenates prepared from fresh-frozen (−70°C) tissues. The quantity of E_2R and PgR is measured by their respective binding capacity to tritiated E_2 and synthetic progestagens R-5020/ORG-2058 with liquid scintillation counting spectrophotometer and is expressed in femtomoles (fmol/mg cytoplasmic protein or nuclear DNA). The clinical utility of the steroid receptor determination lies in the appropriate selection of patients with endometrial carcinoma, hyperplasias, or breast carcinoma for suppressive endocrine therapy (see Chapter 12, Endometrial Carcinoma). Neoplastic target tissues containing 10 fmol/mg protein E_2R and 50 fmol PgR or more generally respond to suppressive hormonal therapy.

The concentrations of E_2R and PgR in the normal endometrium vary during the normal menstrual cycle according to fluctuating plasma levels of E_2 and P. The highest values of E_2R (400 fmol/mg protein) and PgR

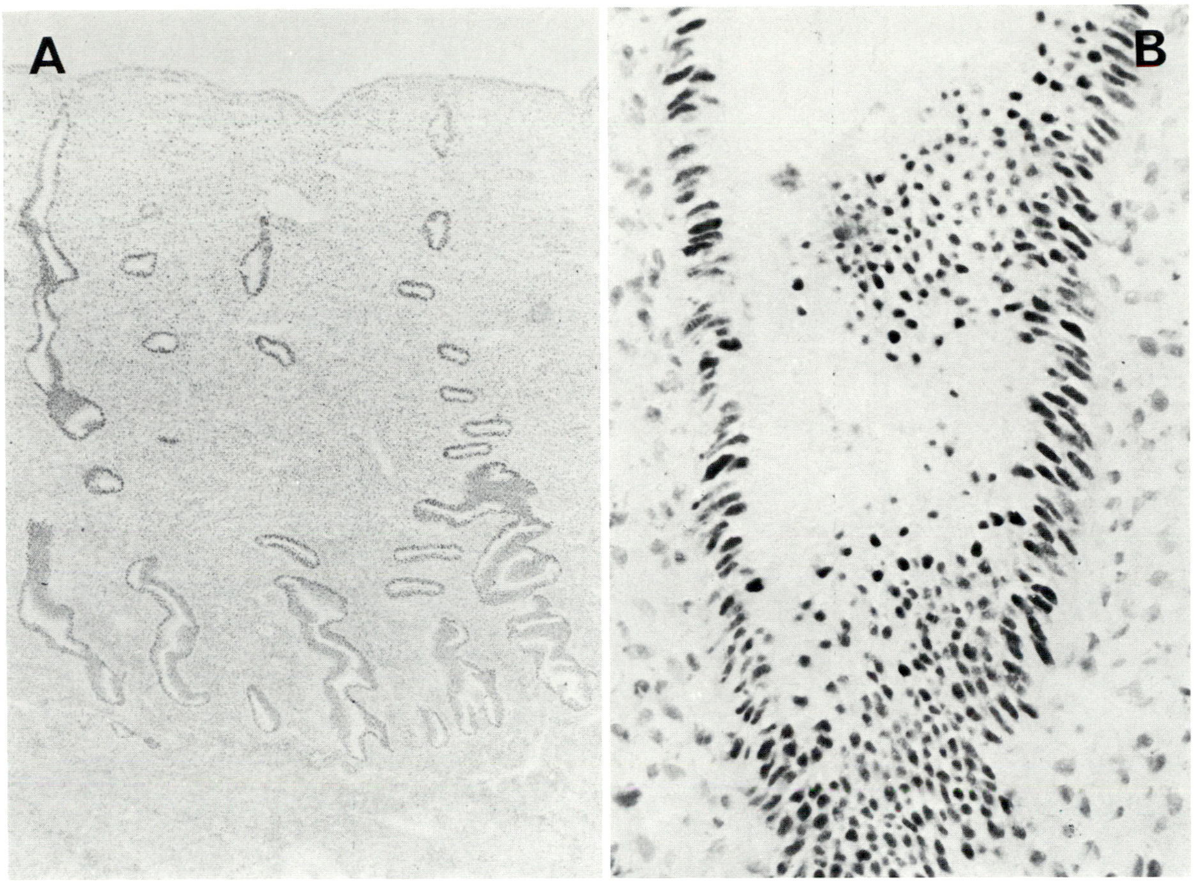

FIG. 9.6. Immunohistochemical localization of estrogen receptor (estrophilin). *A*. Estrogen receptors are present in midproliferative phase endometrium, as indicated by the dark (gray to black) diaminobenzidine reaction product within cell nuclei. *B*. Receptors are localized to epithelial and stromal cell nuclei, although the intensity of specific staining is stronger in most epithelial cell nuclei than in most stromal cell nuclei. (Reprinted by permission of Press et al., Ref. 62.)

(1000 fmol/mg protein) concentrations occur during the midproliferative phase (8th–10th day of the cycle)[7,34,74] and correspond to rising plasma levels of E_2 during the preovulatory and early postovulatory secretory phases of the cycle. E_2 promotes the synthesis of both E_2R and PgR,[40] whereas P inhibits the synthesis of E_2R. Recently developed monoclonal antibodies to E_2R (estrophilin) derived from MCF-7 human breast cancer cell lines permit[33] the precise intracellular localization of E_2R by means of immunohistochemistry in frozen tissue sections.[43,62] Most of E_2R is localized in the nuclei[62] rather than the cytoplasm[7,31,32] of endometrial epithelial and stromal cells (Fig. 9.6). Endothelial cells fail to stain with antiestrophilin antibody.[62] Malignant breast tissue also has intranuclear E_2R.[43] The concept of the mechanisms of sex steroid hormone–receptor action in target cells[7,32] is illustrated in Fig. 9.7 and includes the following major steps[38]: (1) circulating and unbound (from sex hormone-binding globulin) steroid hormone molecules are taken up from the cytoplasmic membrane presumably by cytoplasmic receptors, (2) the hormone molecules enter the nucleus, which contains most (90–95%) of the cellular receptors, (3) the intranuclear hormone molecules induce conversion of the inactive (nonfunctional) 4S form of receptor to active (functional) 5S form of receptor, (4) the hormonally activated 5S receptor binds to acceptor genes in the nucleus and influences gene expression by stimulating RNA polymerase and thus messager RNA (mRNA) transcription, and (5) the newly formed mRNA is transported to the cytoplasm, where it is translated into proteins, including anabolic and catabolic enzymes as well as new receptors (receptor replenishment). According to this concept, the most significant effect of sex hormones is intranuclear activation of receptors that in turn initiate a sequence of events that lead to alterations in physiologic functions of target cells.

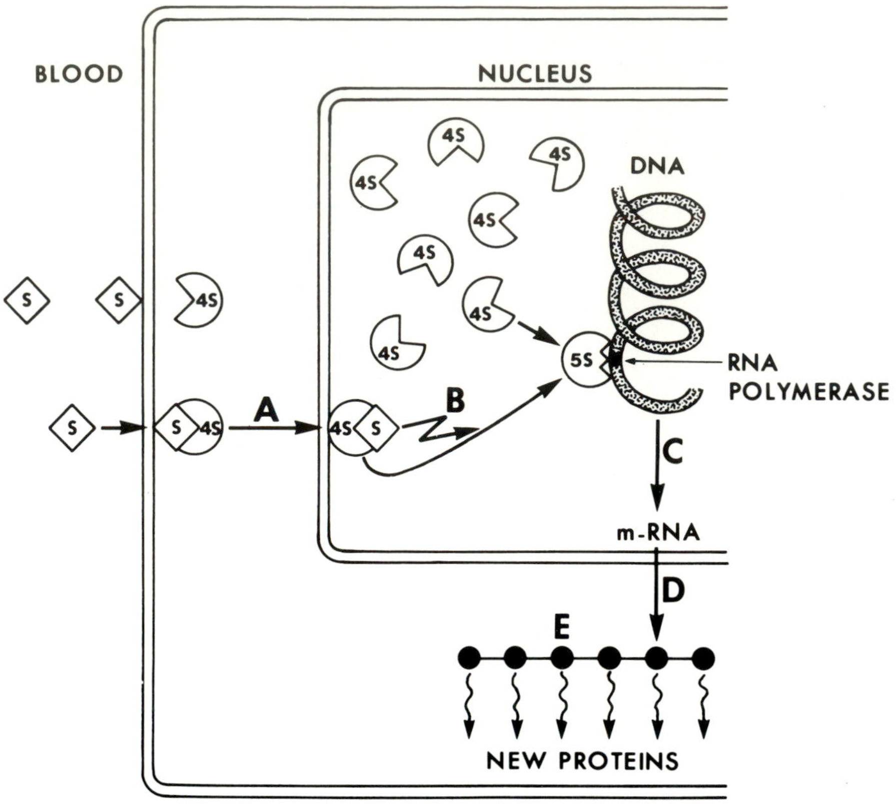

FIG. 9.7. Schematic representation of sex steroid hormone–receptor interaction in target cells. Circulating, free hormone molecule(s) following their passage through cell membranes are bound to cytoplasmic 4S receptors; the hormone–receptor complex is transported (*A*) to and in the nucleus, where the biologically active 5S steroid receptor complex is formed (*B*) from either the inactive 4S cytoplasmic steroid–receptor complex or by interaction of the 4S nuclear receptor with the steroid dissociated from 4S cytoplasmic receptor. The 5S receptor stimulates RNA polymerase and transcription (*C*) of messenger RNA; mRNA is transported (*D*) to cytoplasm, where it is translated (*E*) into new proteins related to physiologic cell functions. Most cellular receptors are intranuclear and are in equilibrium with small amounts of cytoplasmic receptors.

Morphology and Physiology of the Normal Endometrium

Precise knowledge and understanding of the endocrinologic morphology of the endometrium throughout the cycle is important not only for appropriately dating the endometrium but also for distinguishing pathologic or physiologic alterations from normal physiologic events. The major morphologic features that occur in the endometrium throughout the cycle are shown in Fig. 9.8. To avoid bias, the pathologist should read the clinical information, including the date of the last menstrual period, after evaluating the histologic section. The first day of bleeding is considered day 1 of the cycle (Fig. 9.8).[56,57] During the proliferative phase, daily morphologic alterations are not sufficiently obvious to permit accurate dating. Also, since proliferation precedes the ovulatory period, dating proliferative endometrium gives the clinician no relevant information indicating whether or not ovulation has occurred. On the other hand, the daily changes in the endometrium during the postovulatory period are sufficiently distinct to permit accurate evaluation of the endometrial cycle.[16,35]

Proliferative Phase

The preovulatory endometrium is characterized by proliferation of gland cells, stromal fibroblasts, and vascular endothelial cells,[23] leading to an increase in the volume of the uterine mucosa. Synthesis of nuclear DNA is increased[18] (Fig. 9.9A), and mitoses are numerous (Fig. 9.9B). As a result, the straight glands in the early proliferative phase (Fig. 9.9C) become progressively more voluminous and tortuous (Fig. 9.10) during the mid and late phases of proliferation. The changes are under the influence of E_2, which stimulates the DNA-promoter enzyme, thymidilate synthetase.[23,26] The endometrium demonstrates zonal variations in its response to hormonal

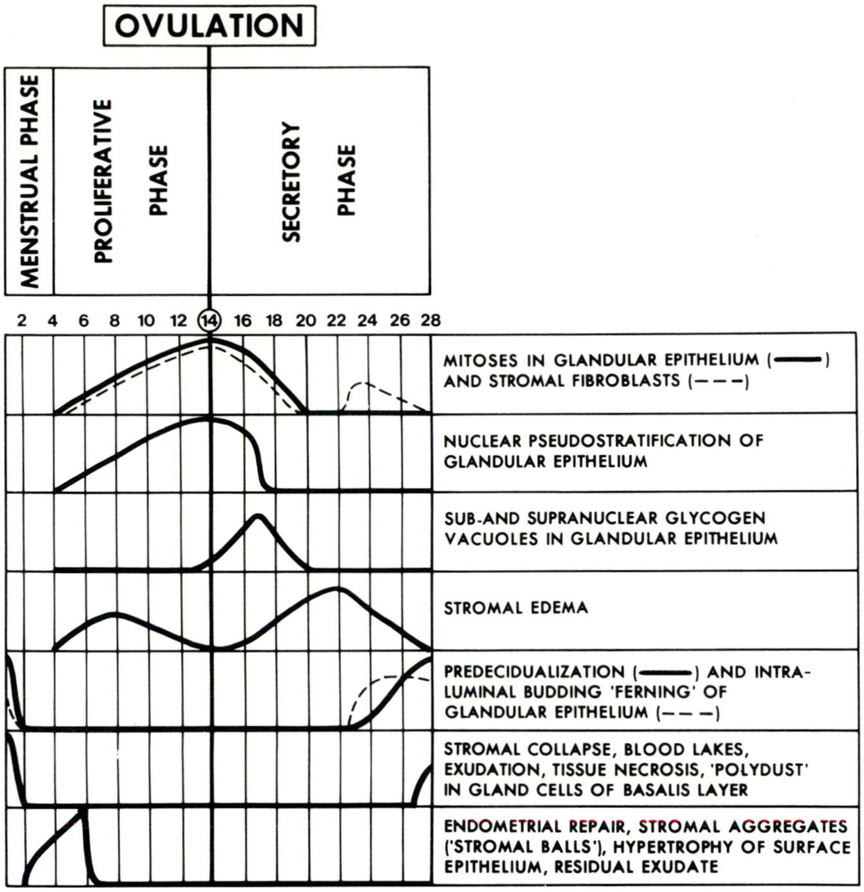

FIG. 9.8. The major morphologic characteristics of the endometrium during the menstrual cycle. (Adapted by permission of Noyes et al., Ref. 57.)

stimuli. For example, DNA synthesis is more intense in the upper two-thirds of the functionalis of the fundus and corpus than in the lower third, the isthmic and cornual regions and the basalis layer.[26] The geographic variation in the sensitivity of the endometrium to hormonal stimulation correlates with different biologic functions. The upper functional layer serves as the implantation site, providing an appropriate metabolic and physical environment for the implanted blastocyst. The lower functionalis provides the integrity of the endometrial mucosa. The maximum number of endometrial cells engaged in DNA synthesis is seen between cycle days 8 and 10 (Fig. 9.11) and corresponds to maximal mitotic activity, peak plasma E_2 levels, and maximum concentration of E_2R. The decline in the E_2-promoted DNA activity by days 11–14 (Fig. 9.11) when P levels are low is possibly related to endometrial refractoriness to relative hyperstimulation of the preovulatory endometrium by E_2. Indeed, DNA synthesis in rat uteri decreases rather than increases after 2 days of continuous estrogen administration.[31] In this system, nucleic acid synthesis is inhibited in the absence of low levels of P and is not due to loss of E_2R but rather to the presence of a chalone-like inhibitor of DNA synthesis. Although uterine chalone has not been biochemically demonstrated, chalones are known to be potent DNA inhibitors in other tissue systems, particularly in the skin,[52] and thus the uterine chalone hypothesis seems plausible.

In addition to growth promotion, E_2 stimulates the formation of ultrastructural organelles in gland cells and stromal fibroblasts as well as the vascular endothelium.[26] These include free and bound ribosomes, ATP-rich mitochondria, and Golgi and primary lysosomes (Fig. 9.12A). These structures provide a protein matrix, energy, and synthesis and storage of enzymes, respectively. Endometrial enzymes, such as the Golgi-related lactate dehydrogenase, hexokinase, pyruvate kinase, and glucose-6-phosphatase (the last is especially abundant in the granular endoplasmic reticulum),[25] are all involved in carbohydrate metabolism during the postovulatory phase of the menstrual cycle. Acid phosphatase and presumably B-glucuronidase confined within membrane-bound pri-

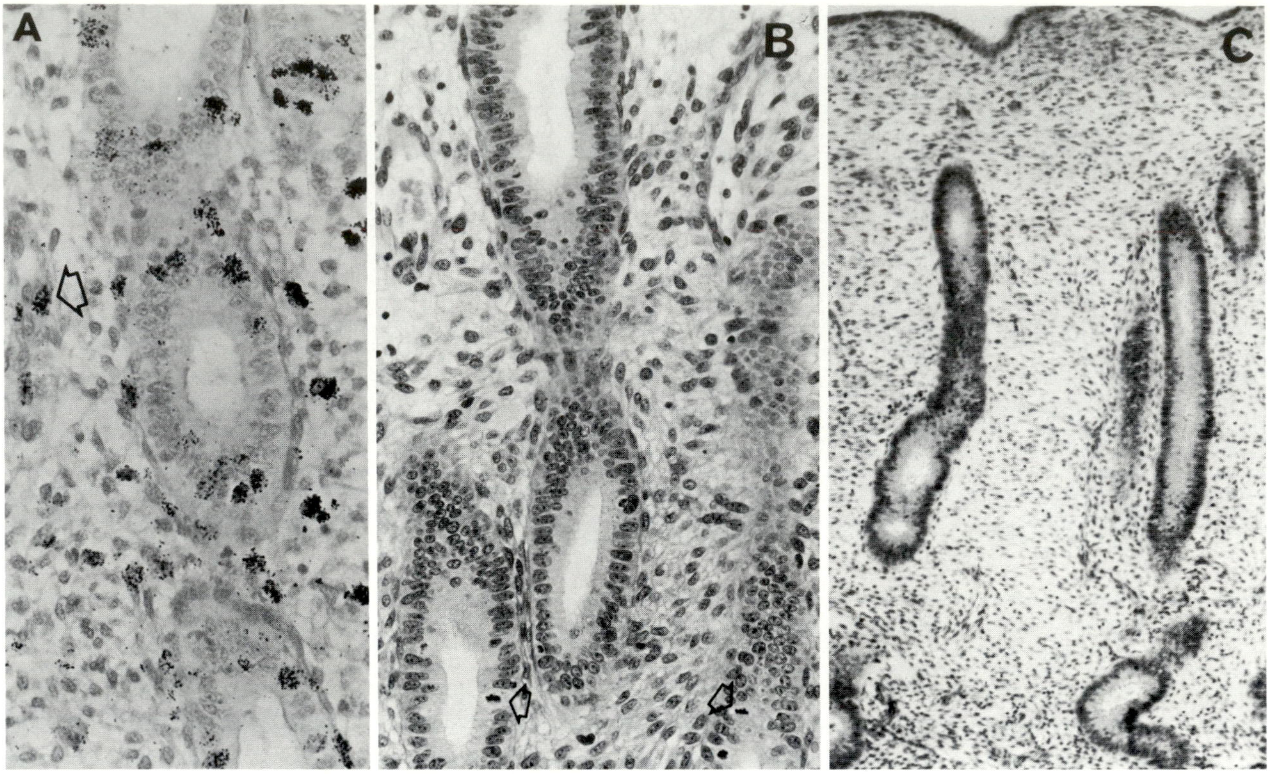

FIG. 9.9. Proliferative endometrium. *A*. Historadioautography of proliferative endometrium, cycle day 12. Radiothymidine granules are heavily incorporated into the nuclei of endometrial gland cells, stromal fibroblasts, and capillary endothelium (*arrow*). *B*. Routine histologic staining of proliferative glands lined by columnar cells with pseudostratified, pencil-shaped nuclei. Mitoses (*arrows*) are seen. (Reprinted by permission of Ferenczy and Guralnick, Ref. 24.) *C*. Cycle day 8. Straight glands with narrow lumens oriented perpendicular to the surface. The stroma is edematous and well vascularized.

mary lysosomes derived from the Golgi complex contribute to endometrial destruction during the menstrual period.[34,36] According to animal experimental studies,[72] sex steroid molecules may be transported from the cytoplasm into the nucleus by endometrial lysosomes that migrate into the nucleus. Other endometrial enzymes with obscure functional significance are alkaline phosphatase[79] and peroxidase. The former is produced by epithelial and endothelial cells and stromal elements in the human, whereas the latter is found in the stroma of the rodent uterus.

Characteristically, the proliferative epithelial cells are rich in intracytoplasmic intermediate filaments that serve as a supportive skeleton to maintain their integrity (Fig. 9.12B). Also, the surface and gland cells acquire numerous cilia and microvilli (Fig. 9.13A). Ciliary shafts have a strong forward and slow recovery ciliary beat pattern, and cilia are particularly numerous around gland openings (Fig. 9.13B).[19,20,22] These findings are consistent with their role in facilitating mobilization and distribution of endometrial secretions during the progestational phase of the menstrual cycle.[27] Surface microvilli are extensions of the cytoplasmic substance and serve to increase the overall cell surface. This situation enhances excretory, secretory, and adsorptive functions of gland cells.

Lymphoid aggregates resembling follicles (Fig. 9.14A) may be seen in the endometrial stroma, particularly during the proliferative phase of the cycle. Although they stain for IgA, IgM, or IgG, they are unlikely to play a significant role, if any, in the local secretory immune system. Indeed, endometrial epithelial cells synthesize negligible amounts of immunoproteins,[67] and IgG-containing plasma cells are absent in normal endometria. The observations are consistent with the sterile nature of normal endometrium.

Secretory Phase

Postovulation Days 1–3

Following ovulation, under the influence of P, the E_2-primed endometrium undergoes rapid secretory differentiation.[26,56,57] The morphologic alterations that

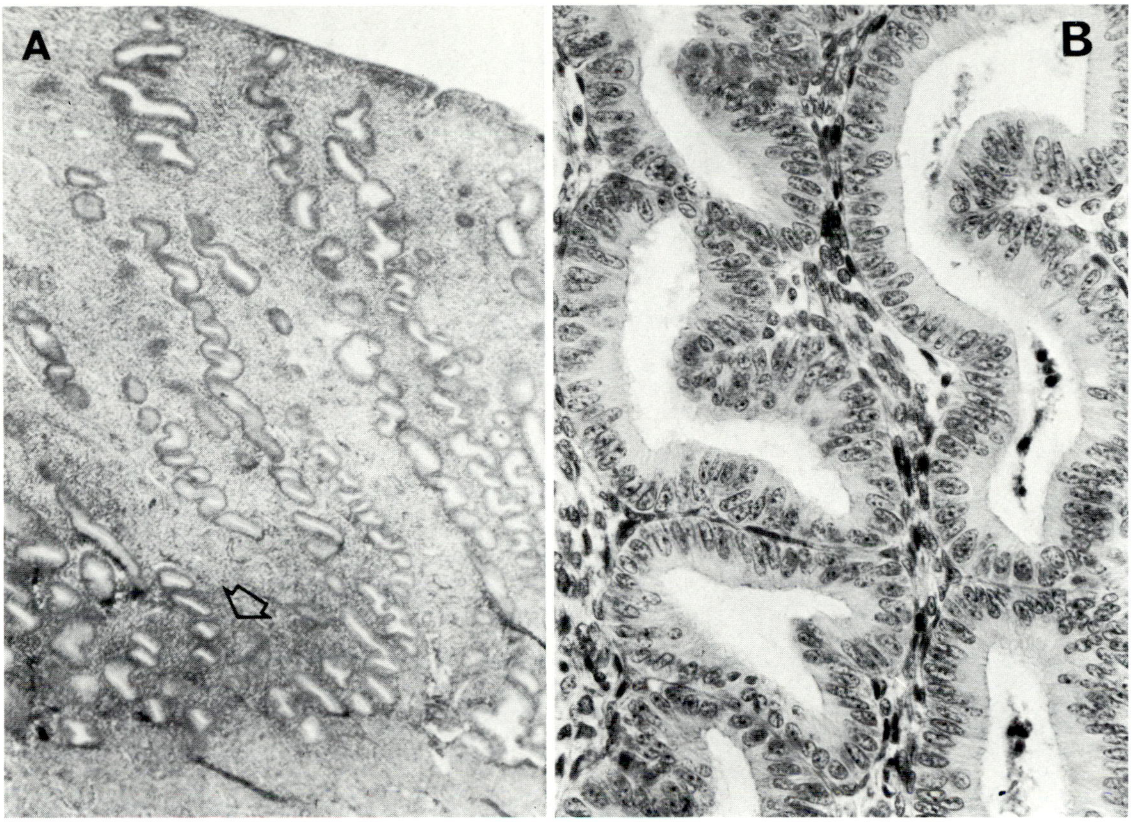

FIG. 9.10. Proliferative endometrium, cycle day 12. *A*. Rows of voluminous, tortuous glands arranged at regular intervals characterize the preovulatory endometrium. The somewhat edematous stroma of the functionalis layer contrasts with the dense, compact stroma of the lower basalis layer (*arrow*). *B*. The glands have an S-shaped configuration, are closely apposed, and the lining cells have pseudostratified nuclei.

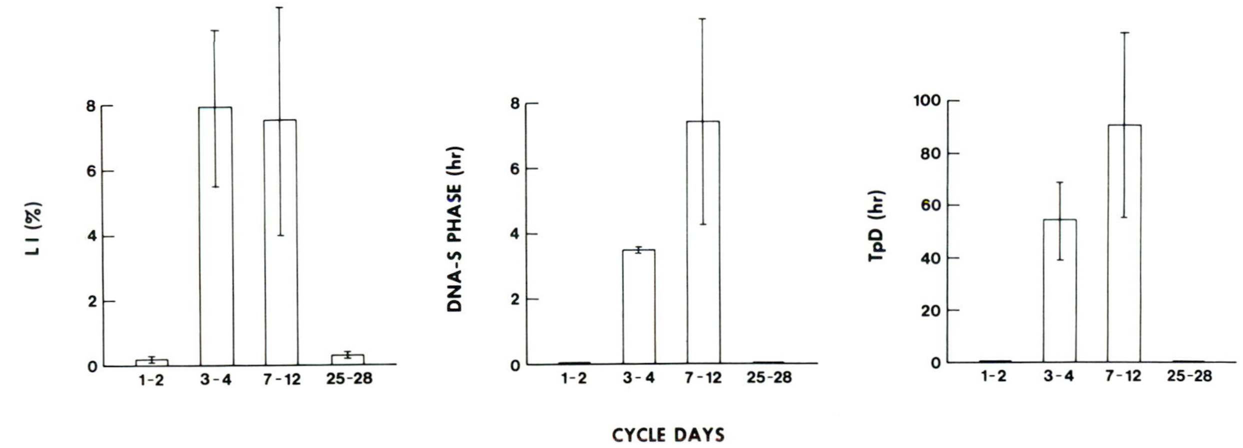

FIG. 9.11. Kinetic characteristics of the endometrium during the menstrual cycle according to in vitro historadioautography using the double-labeling technique with ^{3}H-thymidine. Labeling index (LI), DNA synthesis phase (DNA-S phase), and potential doubling time (TpD) are negligible during the premenstrual and early menstrual periods. Note the sudden increase in LI and shortening of the DNA-S phase and tissue turnover time during the regenerative period on cycle days 3–4. The postregenerative period (cycle day 5 on) is characterized by prolongation of both the DNA-S phase and tissue turnover time. (Reprinted by permission of Ferenczy, Ref. 22.)

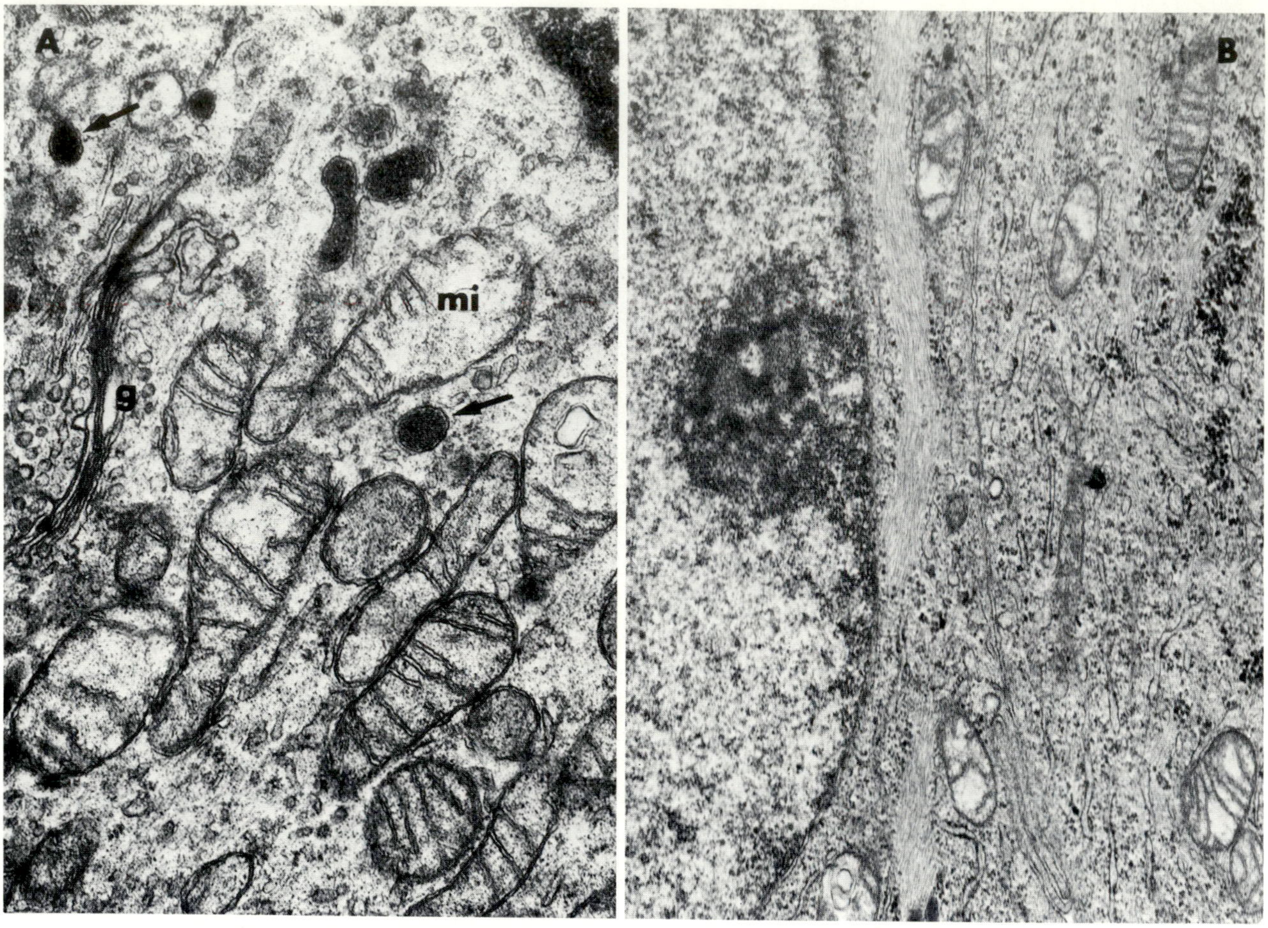

FIG. 9.12. Proliferative endometrium, cycle day 10. *A*. Gland cells have well-developed intracytoplasmic mitochondria (mi). The Golgi complex (g) has periogolgian vesicles from which originate membrane-bound, hydrolytic enzyme-containing electron-dense primary lysosomes (*arrows*). Free and bound ribosomes provide for basic proteins. ×32,000. *B*. Bundles of intermediate filaments serve as a cytoskeleton to tall, late proliferative endometrial gland cells. ×9000. (Reprinted by permission of Ferenczy and Guralnick, Ref. 24.)

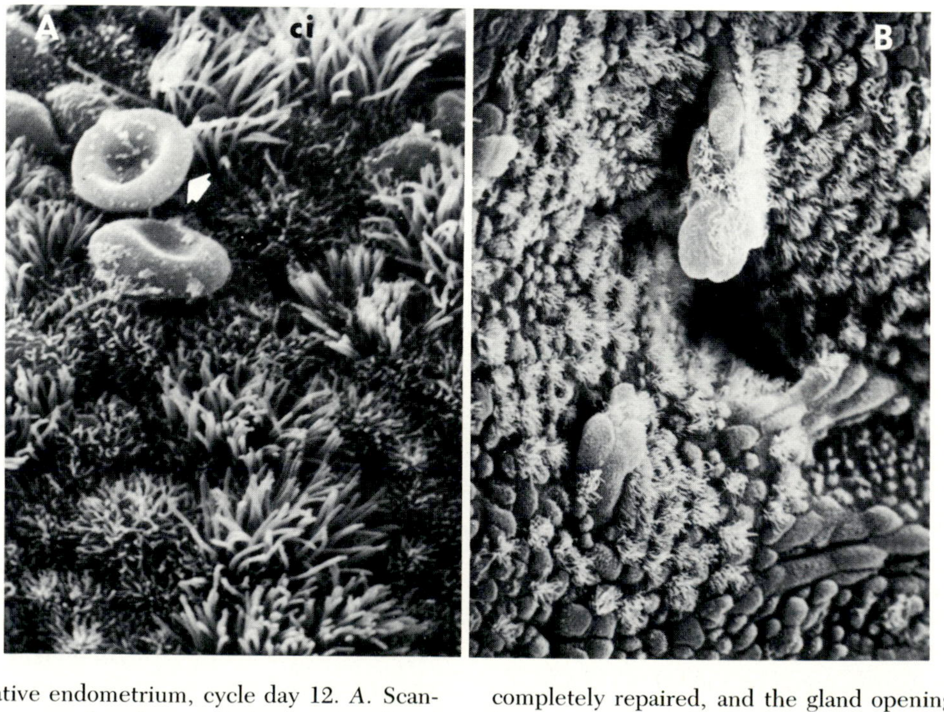

FIG. 9.13. Proliferative endometrium, cycle day 12. *A*. Scanning electron microscopy of surface epithelium with ciliated cells (ci) and microvillous cells. Red blood cells 7 μm in size (*arrow*) are seen. ×3000. *B*. On cycle days 5–6 the surface is completely repaired, and the gland openings are surrounded by ciliated cells. ×1000. (Reprinted by permission of Ferenczy and Guralnick, Ref. 24.)

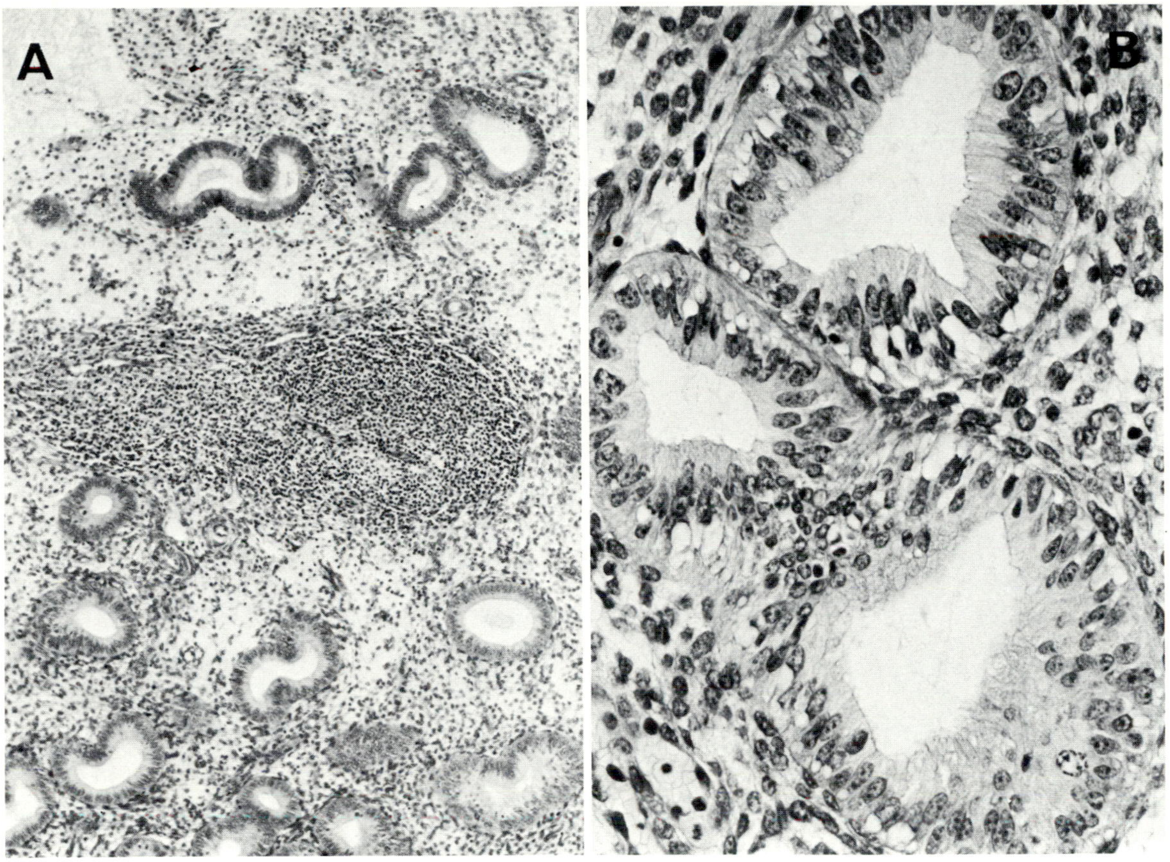

FIG. 9.14. Proliferative endometrium. *A*. Aggregates of mature lymphocytes forming lymphoid follicle-like structures in the basalis layer of the endometrium. *B*. Day 16 endometrium. Gland cells with small, abortive, subnuclear glycogen vacuoles. Many gland cells are devoid of vacuoles, and nuclear pseudostratification is maintained. The overall histology is that of glands of the late proliferative rather than the postovulatory phase. Similar changes may be seen in anovulatory endometrium.

are used to date the endometrium are shown in Table 9.1. During cycle days 14 and 15 (postovulation day, POD, 1), the morphology of the endometrium is not significantly different from that seen in the late proliferative phase of the menstrual cycle. On the 16th day (POD 2) of the cycle, small cylindrical vacuoles appear in the base of the gland cells in the functional layer. Otherwise, the epithelium is indistinguishable from that of the late proliferative phase; the gland cells remain tall and the nuclei pseudostratified (Fig. 9.14B). Similar changes may be produced by estrogens alone in the absence of ovulation. As a result, incomplete or abortive subnuclear vacuolization is not considered specific to ovulation. The first reliable histologic alterations that are considered specific to ovulation are seen on the 17th day (POD 3) of the cycle.[24,56,57] These include well-developed subnuclear glycogen vacuoles in gland lining cells and palisading of gland cell nuclei. Both phenomena involve every cell in a given gland (Fig. 9.15A, B).

Ultrastructurally[25,26,80] and histochemically,[79] the vacuoles correspond to pools of glycogen granules (Fig. 9.16A). Accumulation of glycogen and its synthesis are unique phenomena of the endometrium in that this occurs in the absence of excessive glycogen intake or exer-

Table 9.1. Morphologic evidence of ovulation.

Morphology	Cycle days
Nucleolar channel system[a] in gland cells	15–25
Subnuclear vacuolization with nuclear palisading of gland cells	17–18
Stromal edema with ferning of glandular epithelium	22–23
Perivascular and stromal predecidualization	23–28
Diffuse predecidual and glandular necrosis, inflammation, and vascular thrombosis	1–2
Inflammatory exudate, aggregates of stromal cells (stromal balls) with or without hypertrophic surface epithelial cells, diffuse	2–4

[a] At transmission electron microscopic level.

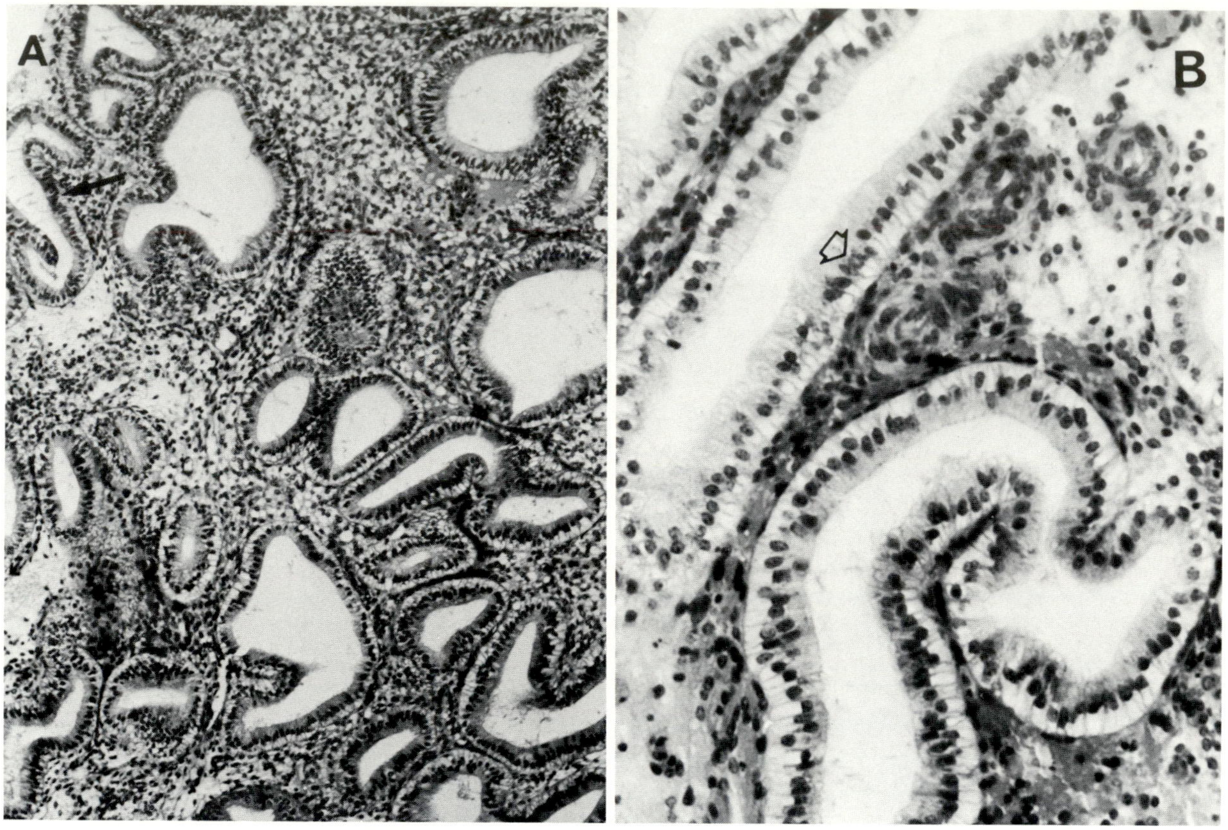

FIG. 9.15. Postovulatory, secretory endometrium. *A*. Many glands on cycle day 17 (POD 3) have S-shaped configurations (*arrow*), conspicuous subnuclear vacuolization, and nuclear palisading. The stroma is relatively edematous. *B*. Detailed view of the 17th day secretory endometrium. Each gland cell has a well-developed subnuclear vacuole. As a result, the nuclei are pushed up to the center of the cells producing nuclear palisading (*arrow*). These are the fist morphologic features in the menstrual cycle that are indicative of ovulation.

cise. Mitochondrial gigantism, with increased numbers of cristae (Fig. 9.16B), occurs in response to the increased demand for energy for glycogen metabolism.[80] The intracellular glycogen is broken down by enzymes of oxidative phosphorylation into glycoproteins and synthesized via the Golgi complex in the supranuclear region.

At the ultrastructural level, ovulation is manifested by the appearance of giant mitochondria and the so-called nucleolar channel system (NCS) formed by the helical infolding of the nuclear membranes into the nuclear or nucleolar substance[55] in gland cells (Table 9.1, Fig. 9.17A, B). NCS is seen as early as the 15th day of the cycle, but its significance is not known. These structures are unique to women and are seen only during the postovulatory phase.[25,80] However, NCS may be produced both in vivo and in vitro by progesterone or its synthetic variants.[63]

Postovulation Days 4–6

On cycle day 18 (POD 4) supranuclear vacuolization is established (Fig. 9.18A), and between days 19 and 20 (POD 5 and 6), the glycoprotein-rich and mucopolysaccharide-rich supranuclear cytoplasmic products are expelled into the glandular lumen by apocrine-type secretion.[24,25,80] This is characterized by protrusion and eventual detachment of the apical portion of cells (Fig. 9.18B). Uterine secretory fluids also contain plasma transudates derived from circulating blood in the endometrial mucosa. The peak of intraglandular secretions coincides with the time of implantation of the free blastocyst, on cycle day 21 (POD 7) if fertilization takes place.

DNA synthesis and cell divisions in gland cells cease (Fig. 9.11 and 9.18B) concomitantly with the initiation of apocrine secretory activity by day 19.[26] Mitosis is further inhibited by the rising levels of postovulatory P. Progesterone antagonizes the action of E_2 by interfering with either the recycling or replenishment or both of cytoplasmic E_2R[12] and through the action of the P-specific enzyme 17β-hydroxydehydrogenase (E_2DH).[34] E_2DH converts the potent uterotropic E_2 into relatively weak E_1, which rapidly leaves the cell without significantly stimulating the nuclei of target cells. As a result, an increase in E_2DH lowers the intracellular concentration

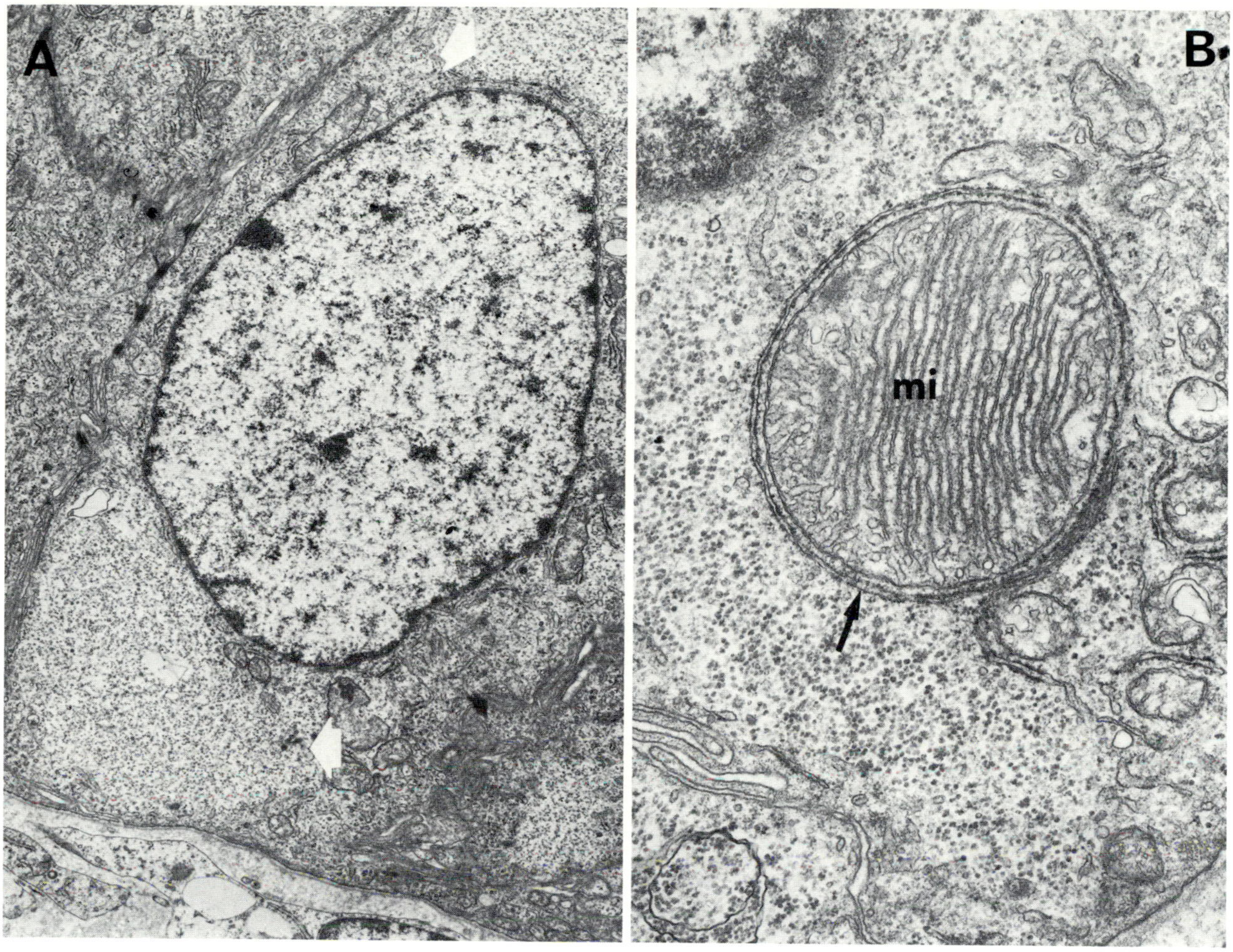

FIG. 9.16. Postovulatory, secretory endometrium, cycle day 18. *A*. Ultrastructure of gland cells with abundant sub- and supranuclear glycogen granules (*arrows*). ×11,000. *B*. Detailed view of glycogen–giant mitochondria (mi)–granular endoplasmic reticulum (*arrow*) complex. Their close ultrastructural relationship is geared for glycoprotein synthesis. ×23,000. (Reprinted by permission of Ferenczy and Guralnick, Ref. 24.)

of E_2 and its receptors. Progesterone prevents the epithelial cells from entering the premitotic (G_1 and S) phases of the cell cycle.[81]

Postovulation Days 7–10

From day 20 on, the changes in the stroma rather than the glands are evaluated in dating the endometrium (see Table 9.1). These changes are edema (days 20–23), coiling of spiral arterioles (days 22–25), and predecidualization of the stroma (days 23–28). These alterations are mediated by prostaglandin F_2 (PGF_2) and PGE_2.[48] Experimentally, PG synthesis is stimulated by estrogens in primed secretory endometrium. Inhibitors of PG biosynthesis, such as indomethacin and mefenamic acid (Motrin, Ponstan), as well as P, reduce the levels of PG. The elevated concentrations of midluteal phase E_2 on cycle day 22 (POD 8) increase the synthesis of the enzyme, cyclooxygenase, responsible for PG production.[2] PGE_2 in turn promotes capillary permeability,[22,41] leading to maximal stromal edema on day 22 (POD 10) (Fig. 9.19A). PGE_2 presumably also promotes vascular endothelial mitotic activity, perivascular concentrations of filaments (Fig. 9.19B), and mitoses that are first seen in the postovulatory endometrium on day 22 of the cycle (Fig. 9.19C). Endothelial proliferation leads to coiling of the arterial system of the endometrium (Fig. 9.20A), a phenomenon that produces vascular clusters in the upper functionalis layer, seen on histologic sections (Fig. 9.20B).

Vascular permeability and edema of the stroma are essential prerequisites for the predecidual transformation (Fig. 9.20B) of uncommitted stromal fibroblasts.[64,68] The roles of endometrial histamine,[13] bradykinin, and

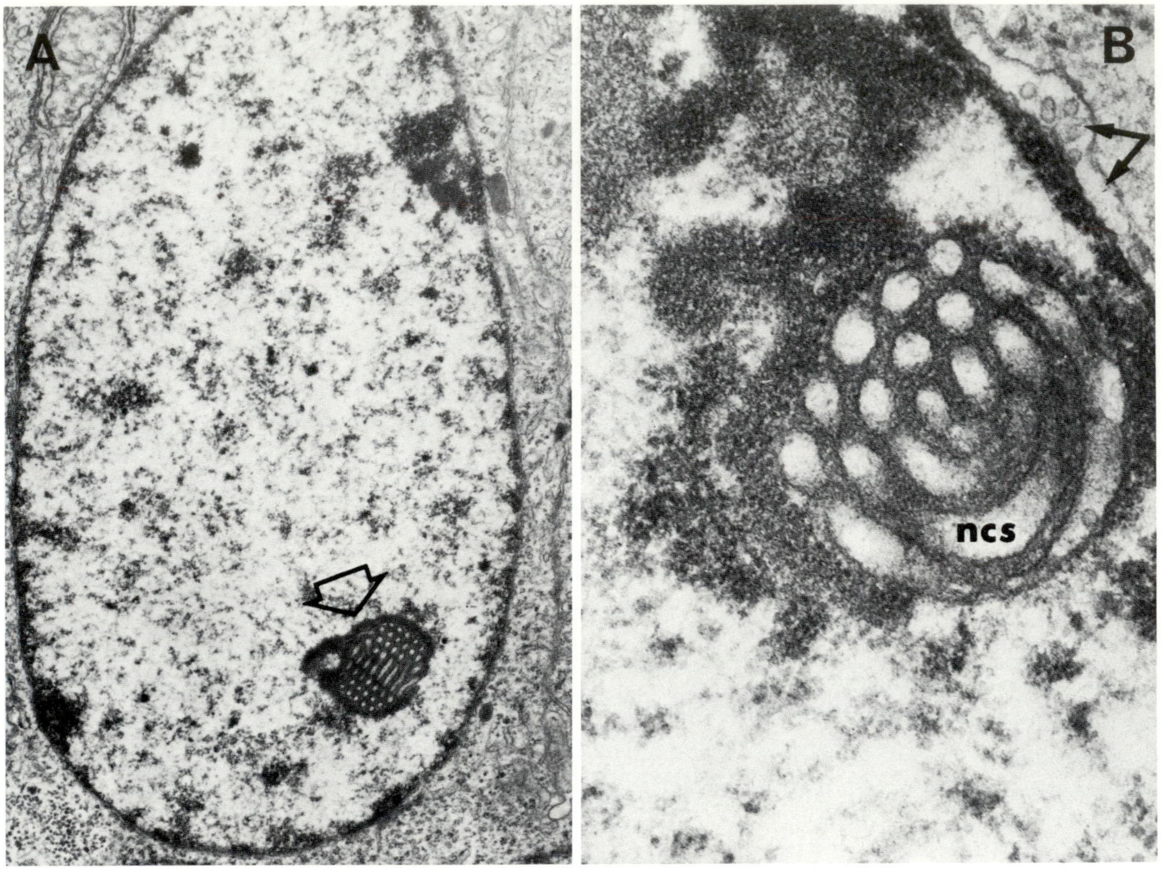

FIG. 9.17. Postovulatory secretory endometrium, cycle day 17 (POD 3). *A*. Gland cell with a nucleolar channel system (*arrow*), subnuclear glycogen, and giant mitochondria enveloped by parallel membranes of glandular endoplasmic reticulum. These ultrastructural features are typical of postovulatory endometrium. ×8000. *B*. Detailed view of nucleolar channel system made of hollow, membrane-bound tubules embedded in dark granular nucleolonema. Vesicular structures seen in ncs are also seen between the inner and outer nuclear membrane (*arrows*). ×60,000.

serotonin[75] in these biologic events are not completely understood. In experimental animal systems, release of histamine from mast cells and the subsequent edematous response occur within a few hours of E_2 stimulation.[39] Endometrial cell membranes and blastocyst membranes in the rabbit and rat, respectively, have receptors for histamine.[39] It is also possible that histamine is synthesized by the implanted blastocyst itself as well as the endometrium, and it may facilitate the implantation process. In the human endometrium, however, mast cells are rare, and antihistamines do not prevent stromal edema, whereas indomethacin does.[13] These observations suggest that histamine may act on the endometrium indirectly by the production of PG.[39] Endometrial vascular proliferation at the implantation site is related to the blastocyst rather than to histamine or PGE_2. The blastocyst has a unique biologic property that is shared only with tumor cells producing the so-called angiogenesis factor, a substance capable of inducing growth of new capillaries.[30]

Stromal predecidualization (not pseudodecidualization; the prefix *pre* refers to decidual transformation of stromal cells before their further decidual development during pregnancy) begins by day 22–23 (POD 8–9) (see Table 9.1) around spiral arterioles and capillaries of the functional layer (Fig. 9.20B). Coinciding with the beginning of the predecidual reaction on cycle day 23, the glands form intraluminal epithelial projections, so-called ferning (see Table 9.1; Fig. 9.21A). Perivascular predecidualization is more obvious on day 24 (POD 10) and is characterized by the conversion of uncommitted spindle-shaped fibroblasts into plump epithelial-like cells with enlarged nuclei and increased cytoplasm. Ultrastructurally, the cells lack the typical features of epithelial cells, such as bundles of intermediate tonofilaments, glandular lumens, or desmosomal connections. On the other hand,

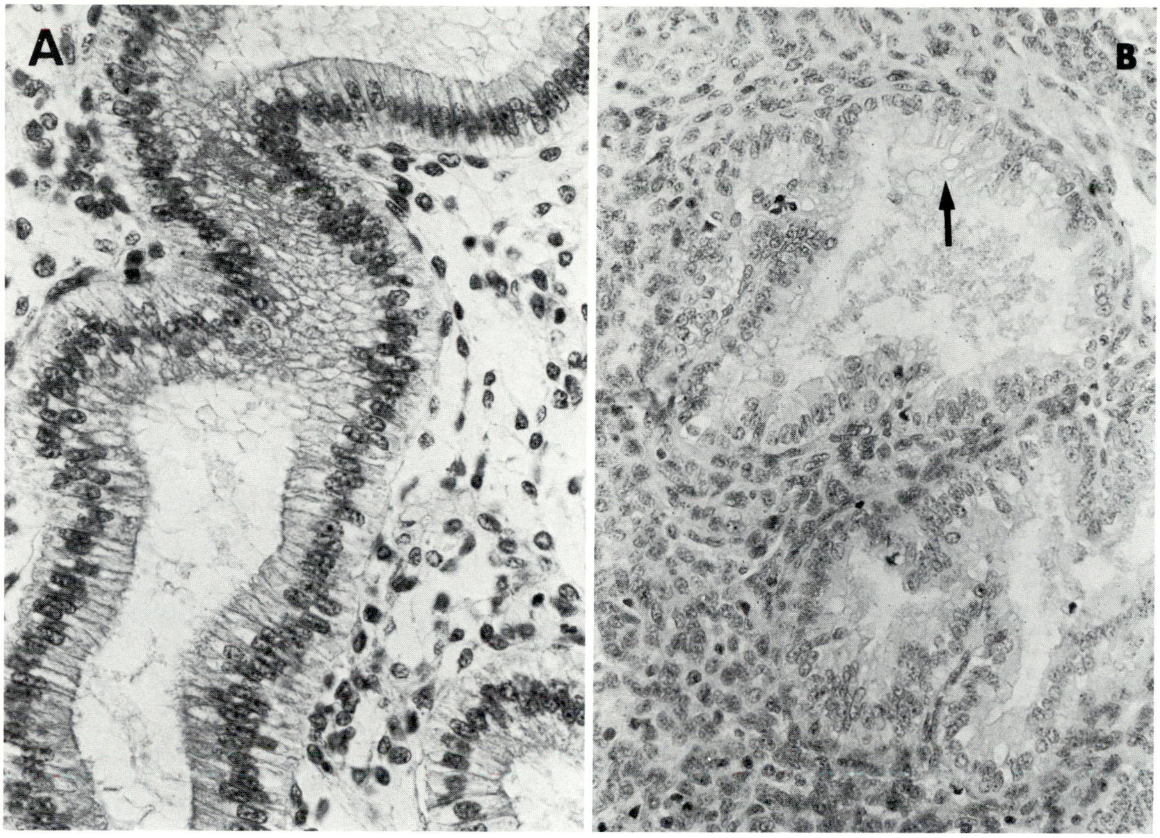

FIG. 9.18. Postovulatory secretory endometrium, cycle day 18 (POD 4). *A*. Endometrial gland cells have well-developed sub- and supranuclear vacuoles, and nuclear palisading is evident. Many cells contain finely granular cytoplasmic substance, and intraluminal vacuolated secretory products are abundant. *B*. Historadioautograph of secretory endometrium. Lack of uptake of radiothymidine by gland cells coincides with conspicuous apocrine secretory activity (*arrow*) and accumulation of intraluminal secretory products.

they have intercellular gap-junction nexuses (Fig. 9.21C). The latter are composed of hexagonal microtubules forming an open-channel system between adjacent cells that facilitates passage of electrolytes and molecules and plays a role in cell contact inhibition.[24,47,80] Histochemically, the predecidual cells contain glycogen and PAS-positive mucosubstances. Predecidual cells represent precursor forms of gestational decidual cells (decidus vera). Since they develop after implantation, they are not involved in the implantation process per se. The cells have several metabolic functions related either to pregnancy or, if conception has not occurred, to menstrual breakdown of the endometrium. For example, the decidual cells have phagocytotic properties (Fig. 9.21B, C) and digest extracellular collagen matrix.[24,47] Decidual phagocytosis may facilitate the development of the decidual reaction by removing collagen from the endometrial stroma. The latter may represent a mechanical obstacle to proliferating and expanding predecidual cells. If conception does not occur, predecidual cells, by removing collagen, may contribute to menstrual breakdown of the endometrial stroma (Fig. 9.21B, C).

Postovulation Days 11–13

Predecidual transformation of stromal fibroblasts under the surface epithelium is achieved by day 25 (POD 11), producing the compacta layer (Fig. 9.22). On days 26 and 27 (POD 12 and 13), the upper two-thirds of the functionalis becomes predecidualized, and the glands demonstrate coiling and ferning (Fig. 9.23A). The endometrial stroma during 26 and 27 is infiltrated by extravasated polymorphonuclear leukocytes and the so-called metrial cells or granulocytes. Their number is greater on day 27 than on day 26. Metrial granulocytes have a granular eosinophilic cytoplasm resembling eosinophils, except that they have a single, kidney-shaped nucleus

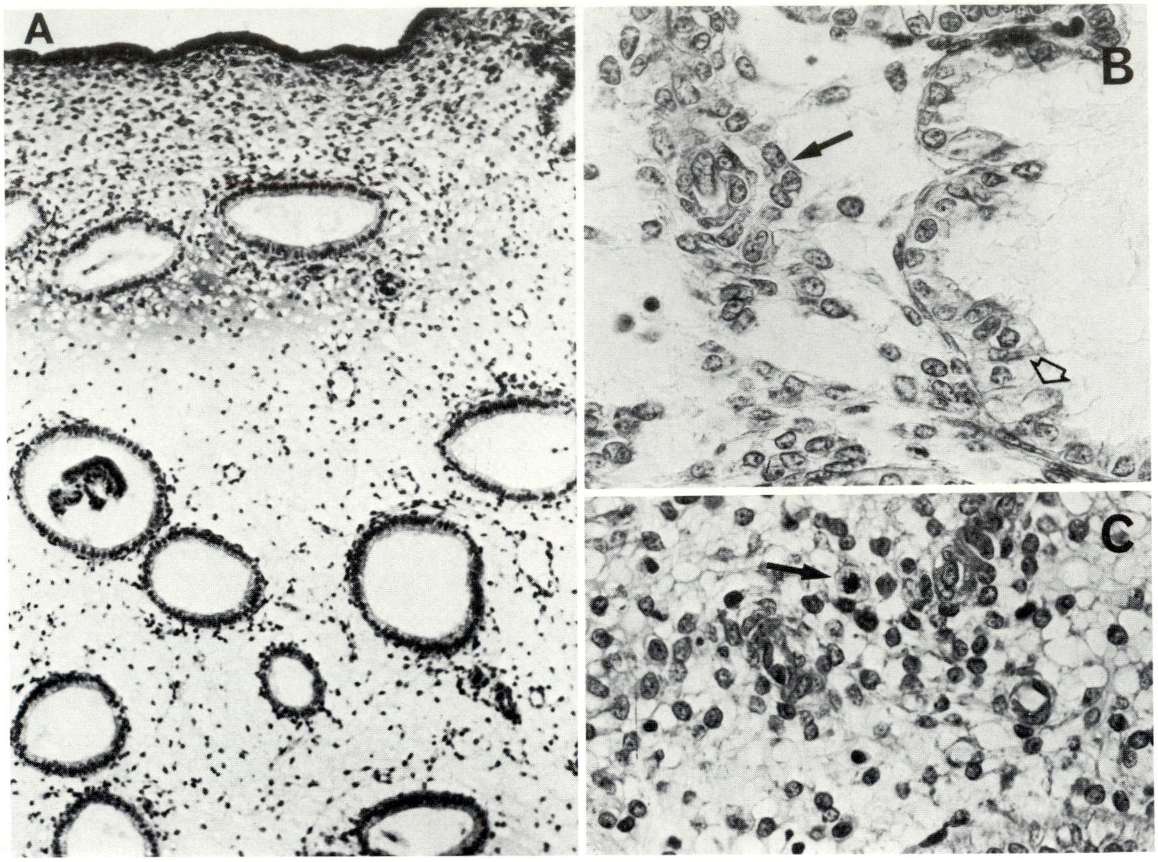

FIG. 9.19. Postovulatory, secretory endometrium, cycle day 22 (POD 8). *A*. There is marked stromal edema producing a naked glands–stromal cells pattern. The glands have somewhat dilated lumens with secretions, and the lining epithelium is low, columnar, and devoid of intraluminal projections. *B*. Detailed view of perivascular thickening due to hypertrophy of perivascular stromal cells (*arrow*). The gland cells are low columnar to cuboidal and have apical apocrine secretory protuberances (*open arrow*). *C*. Mitoses (*arrow*) in perivascular stromal cells reappear on late 22nd–early 23rd day of the menstrual cycle.

(Fig. 9.23B, C). Immunohistochemical studies[15] show relaxin-containing secretory granules in these cells. Gestational decidua has also been shown to produce relaxin.[9] During labor, relaxin, a polypeptide hormone (disulfide homologue of insulin), activates the collagenolytic system (collagen peptidase), causing weakening, rupture, and eventually detachment of fetal membranes, as well as contributing to cervical dilation.[28] Because metrial granulocytes are numerous during implantation (20–22 days) and before menstruation (days 27–28), it is conceivable, although not proven, that relaxin may similarly affect the endometrial stroma, facilitating implantation and, if conception does not occur, breakdown of menstrual stroma.[16] Degenerated nuclear debris of acute and chronic inflammatory cell origin is often seen to be phagocytosed by intact gland cells of the lower spongiosa and basalis layers on cycle days 28, 1, and 2 (Fig. 9.24B).

Menstrual Phase

A normal menstrual period lasts 4 days ± 1 day. During this time, the endometrial mucosa rapidly degenerates, and 50% of the menstrual detritus is expelled in the first 24 hours of menses. Tissue shedding is followed by regeneration. The upper two-thirds of the endometrium on cycle days 28–2 contains fissures and degenerative predecidual cells admixed with epithelial glandular cells as well as acute and chronic (lymphoid) inflammatory cells (Figs. 9.25 and 9.26).

Ultrastructural enzyme tracing studies[36,80] of the upper two-thirds of late secretory endometrium show that it gradually involutes, degenerates, and undergoes necrosis (Fig. 9.26C). The mechanisms by which degeneration occurs are shown in Fig. 9.27. During endometrial proliferation, E_2 stimulates the development of Golgi-derived, primary lysosomes in the epithelial, stromal, and en-

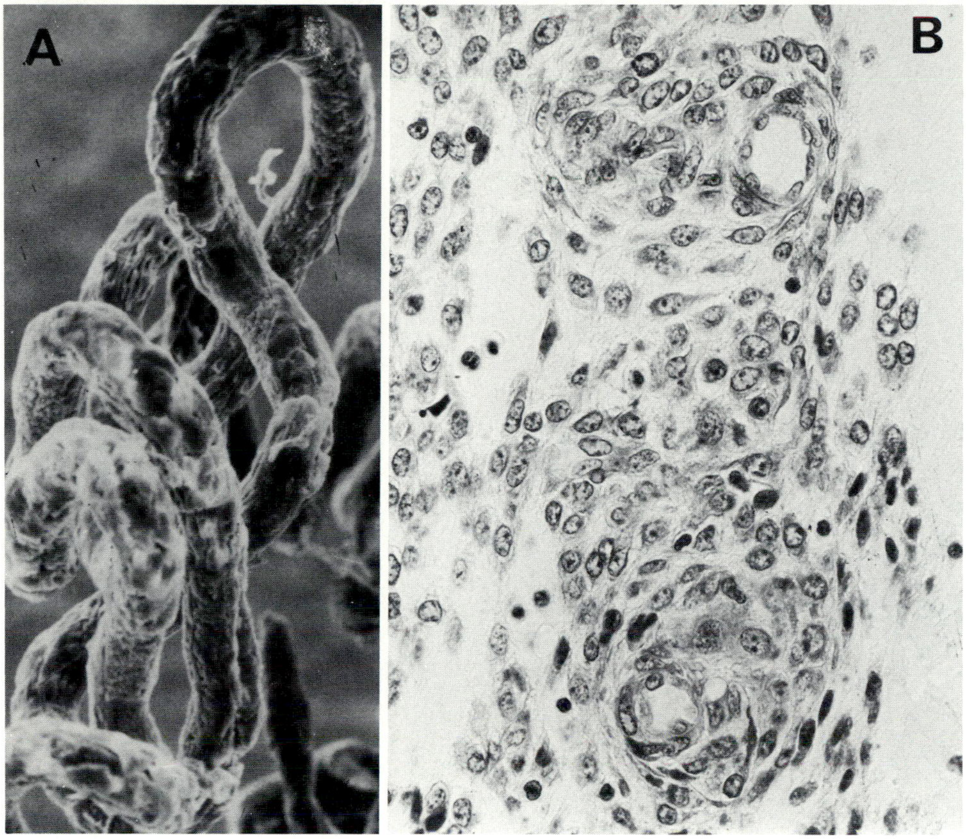

FIG. 9.20. Postovulatory, secretory endometrium, cycle day 23 (POD 9). *A*. Vascular preparation of spiral arteries seen with scanning electron microscopy. *B*. Predecidual thickening around spiral arteries can better be appreciated on cycle day 23. This is due to enlargement and rounding of the cytoplasm and nuclei of perivascular stromal cells. (Reprinted by permission of Ferenczy and Guralnick, Ref. 24.)

dothelial cells of the functional layer of the endometrium.[22,36] These contain highly potent proteolytic enzymes. During the first half of the postovulatory period, lytic enzymes, including acid phosphatase, are confined to membrane-bound lysosomes by the action of P that stabilizes lysosomal membranes.[77] Coinciding with the fall of E_2 and P by day 25, the integrity of lysosomal membrane is no longer maintained. As a result, lysosomal enzymes are released intracellularly as well as into the intercellular space. Acid hydrolases digest the cytoplasmic elements, intercellular desmosomes, and ultimately the entire cellular system.[36] Lysosomal autodigestion destroys the glandular and stromal cells and also the vascular endothelium. Vascular luminal surface membrane injury promotes platelet deposits.[11,71] These alterations presumably are mediated by prostaglandin–thromboxane, and the final results are manifest by multiple minute foci of ischemic tissue necrosis.[11,60] In addition, acute swelling of the endothelial cells of endometrial arterioles contributes to obliteration of the vascular lumen.[36] Paralleling these events, PGE_2 and particularly PGF_2 significantly increase in the late secretory endometrium and reach maximum concentrations during the menstrual period.[48] It has been speculated that the high levels of PGF_2 may also release acid hydrolases from lysosomes and, during menstruation, stimulate the onset of ischemic necrosis via vasoconstriction of myometrial and basal arteries. Expulsion of degenerated endometrium is enhanced by PGF_2-mediated myometrial contractions.[48] The menstrual fluid is composed of autolyzed tissue admixed with a heavy polymorphonuclear exudate, red blood cells, and proteolytic enzymes.[8] One of the latter is blood protease plasmin, a potent fibrinolytic agent that prevents clotting of menstrual blood and facilitates expulsion of the degenerated functionalis. The fibrinolytic activity of the endometrium, which characteristically disappears during the implantation period (cycle day 21), may play a role in preventing this process from occurring during the menstrual period. Plasminogen activators, which convert plasminogen into plasmin, are

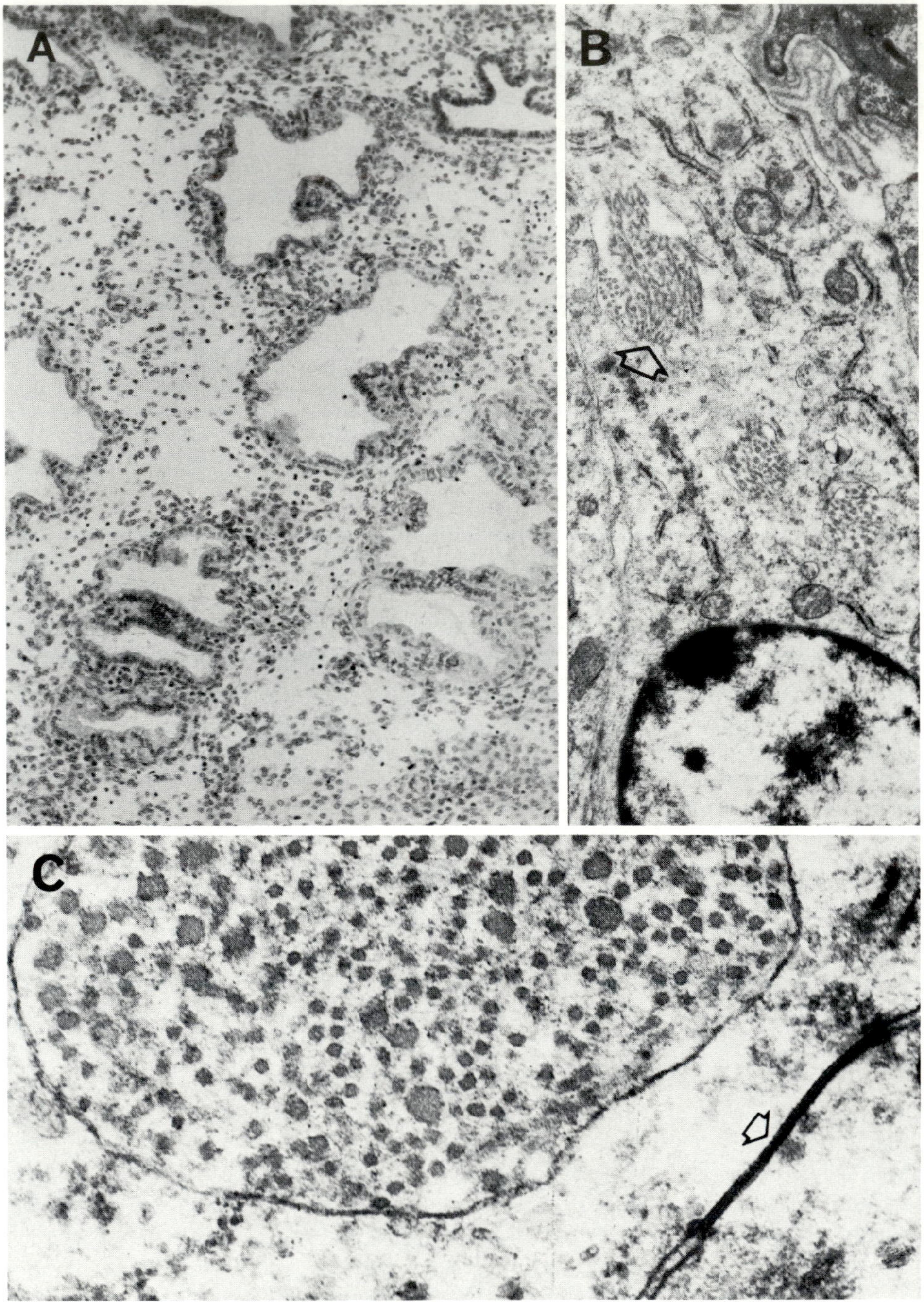

FIG. 9.21. Postovulatory, secretory endometrium, cycle day 23 (POD 9). *A*. In addition to predecidual vascular cuffing, intraluminal epithelial projections (glandular ferning) and stromal edema are typical features of cycle day 23. *B*. Predecidual stroma cells with membrane-bound heterocytophagolysosomes (*arrow*) containing extracellular collagen fibers. ×7000. *C*. Higher magnification of heterocytophagolysosome with cross-sectioned, partially digested, extracellular collagen fibers. A tight junctional nexus (*arrow*) is seen in between predecidual cells. ×10,000. (Reprinted by permission of Ferenczy and Guralnick, Ref. 24.)

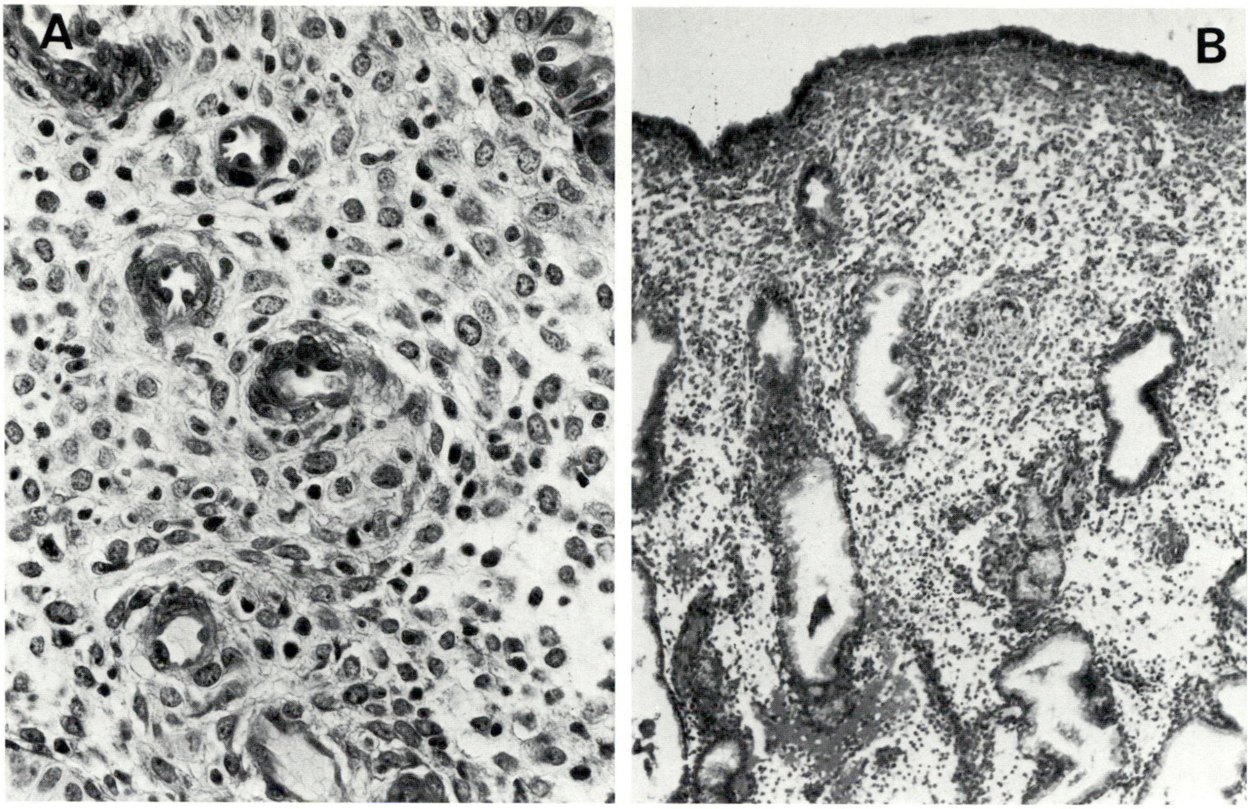

FIG. 9.22. Postovulatory, secretory endometrium, cycle days 24 and 25. *A*. On cycle day 24 (POD 10), predecidual transformation of perivascular stromal cells is evident. Note the well-defined cytoplasmic membranes and round nuclei of predecidual cells resembling epithelial cells. *B*. On cycle day 25 (POD 11), predecidualization of fibroblasts beneath the surface epithelium produces a band-like cellular plate, the so-called compacta layer.

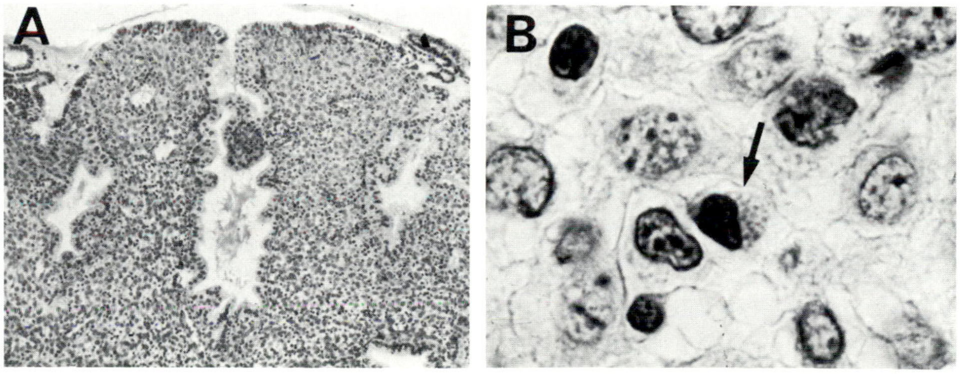

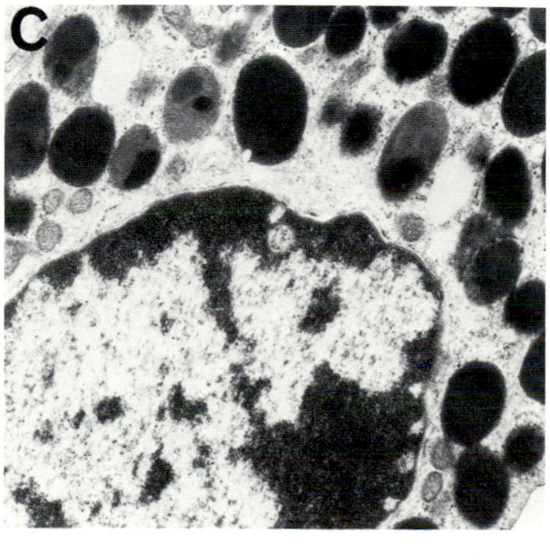

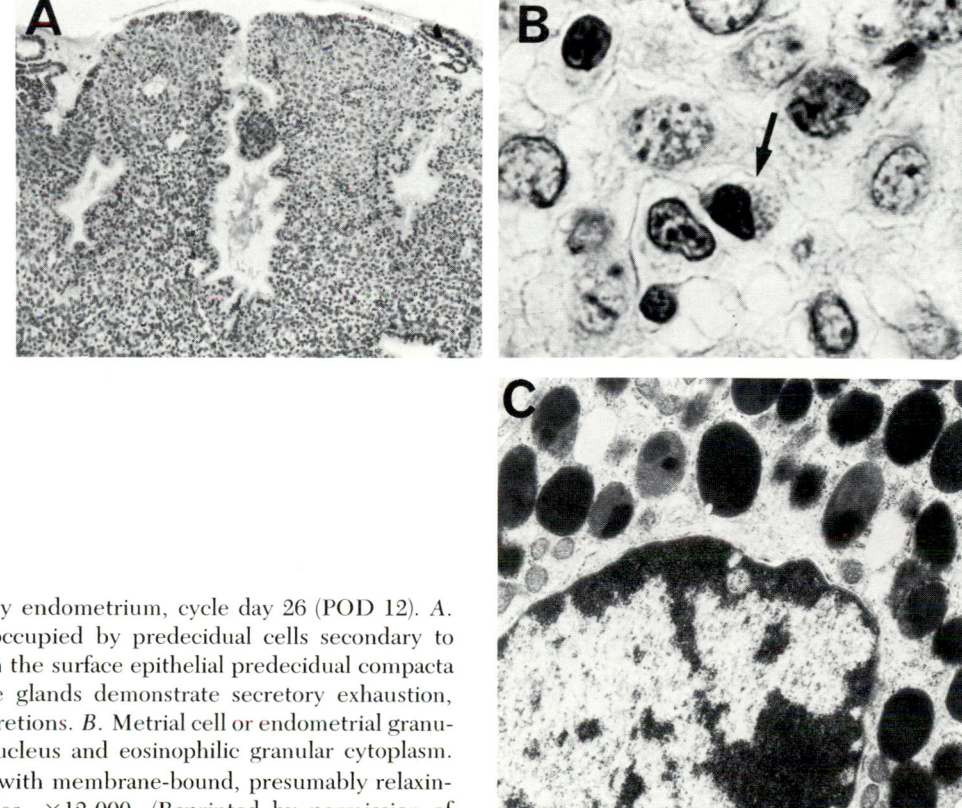

FIG. 9.23. Postovulatory, secretory endometrium, cycle day 26 (POD 12). *A*. The entire functionalis layer is occupied by predecidual cells secondary to expansion and confluency between the surface epithelial predecidual compacta and perivascular predecidua. The glands demonstrate secretory exhaustion, with inspissated intraglandular secretions. *B*. Metrial cell or endometrial granulocyte (*arrow*) with a unilobed nucleus and eosinophilic granular cytoplasm. *C*. Ultrastructure of a metrial cell with membrane-bound, presumably relaxin-containing, electron-dense granules. ×12,000. (Reprinted by permission of Ferenczy and Guralnick, Ref. 24.)

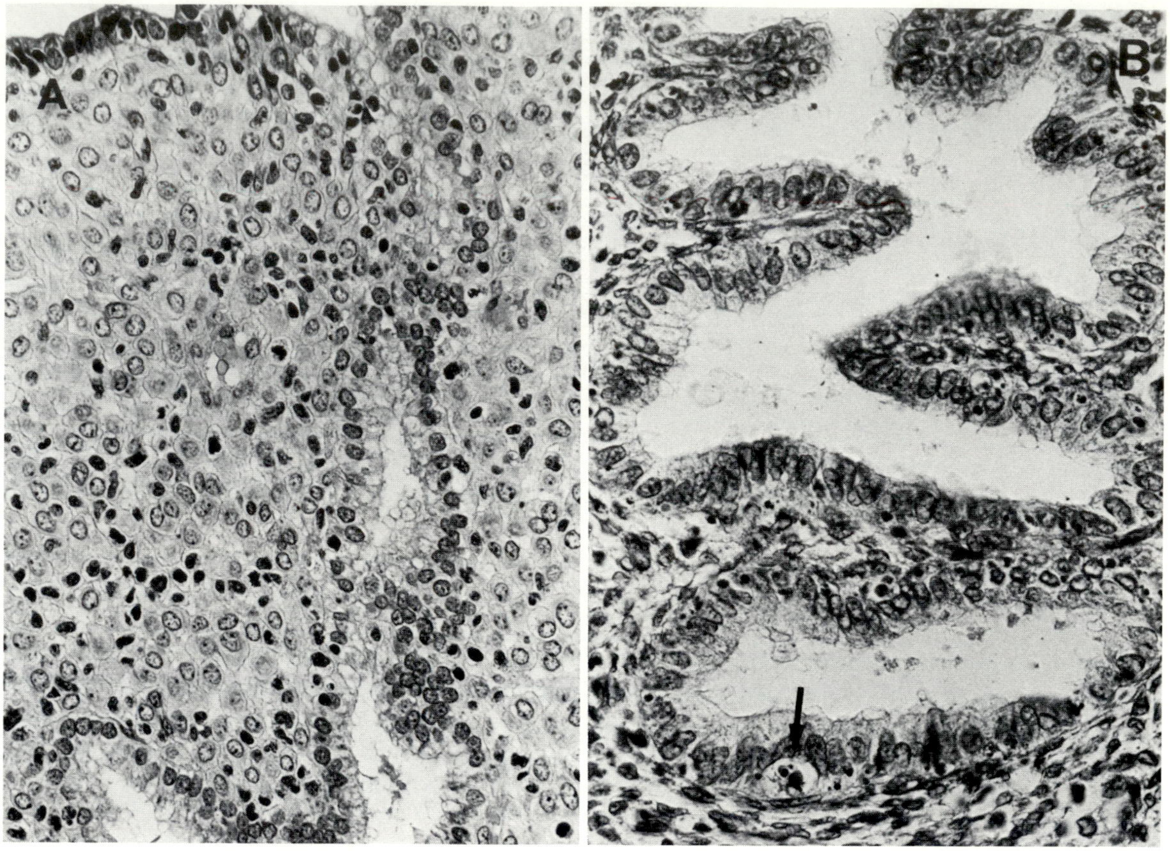

FIG. 9.24. Postovulatory secretory endometrium, cycle day 27 (POD 13). *A*. The predecidua is scattered with inflammatory cells; they are more conspicuous on cycle day 27 than day 26. *B*. Polydust (*arrow*) in gland cells and the stroma is a typical feature of impending (cycle day 28) or ongoing (cycle days 1 and 2) menstrual degeneration. Polydusts represent nuclear debris of inflammatory cell origin that has been phagocytosed by gland cells of the lower functionalis and basal layers.

found in and released from degenerated endometrial vascular endothelium.[44,60]

Menstrual bleeding is controlled by vasoconstriction of the ruptured basal arteries in the denuded basal layer and radial and arcuate arteries in the myometrium.[60] Rapid denudation of the basal layer reduces menstrual blood loss considerably. The arteries of the functionalis layer lack elastin[60] and consequently cannot contract. In addition, they are shed with the functionalis and fail, therefore, to contribute to uterine hemostasis.

On days 2–4, the functionalis becomes gradually detached from the underlying basalis.[19–22,56,57,60] Detachment starts from the fundus and slowly extends toward the isthmus, as observed by hysteroscopy.[50] The cleaved mucosa rolls on itself until it is detached from the basalis and is shed from the endometrial cavity. Shedding is most prominent during the first 2 days of the menstrual period, and endometrial biopsy or curettage yields abundant tissue. On the other hand, the next 2 days are dominated by proliferation of the residual basal gland epithelium in areas of complete denudation,[19–22] and the material obtained for histology during these days is generally scant. Reepithelialization occurs by extension of the residual glandular epithelium over the denuded surface (Fig. 9.28A). Essentially similar phenomena are observed in the spontaneously menstruating monkey and in the rabbit[21] in which the endometrium has been artificially denuded. The peripheral regions of the endometrial cavity, such as the isthmus and peritubal ostium, both of which remain intact during the menstrual period,[19,20] also contribute to resurfacing the epithelium. These converging epithelial proliferations interanastomose, leading to a new surface epithelium by cycle day 5 (Fig. 9.28B). Bleeding ceases when the surface has been completely reepithelialized (see Fig. 9.13B).

Epithelial cell migration followed by replication characterizes the biodynamics of endometrial surface repair.[22] The first-generation, resurfacing epithelial cells are flattened (Fig. 9.29) and have abundant surface microvilli, intracellular intermediate filaments, microtubules, and

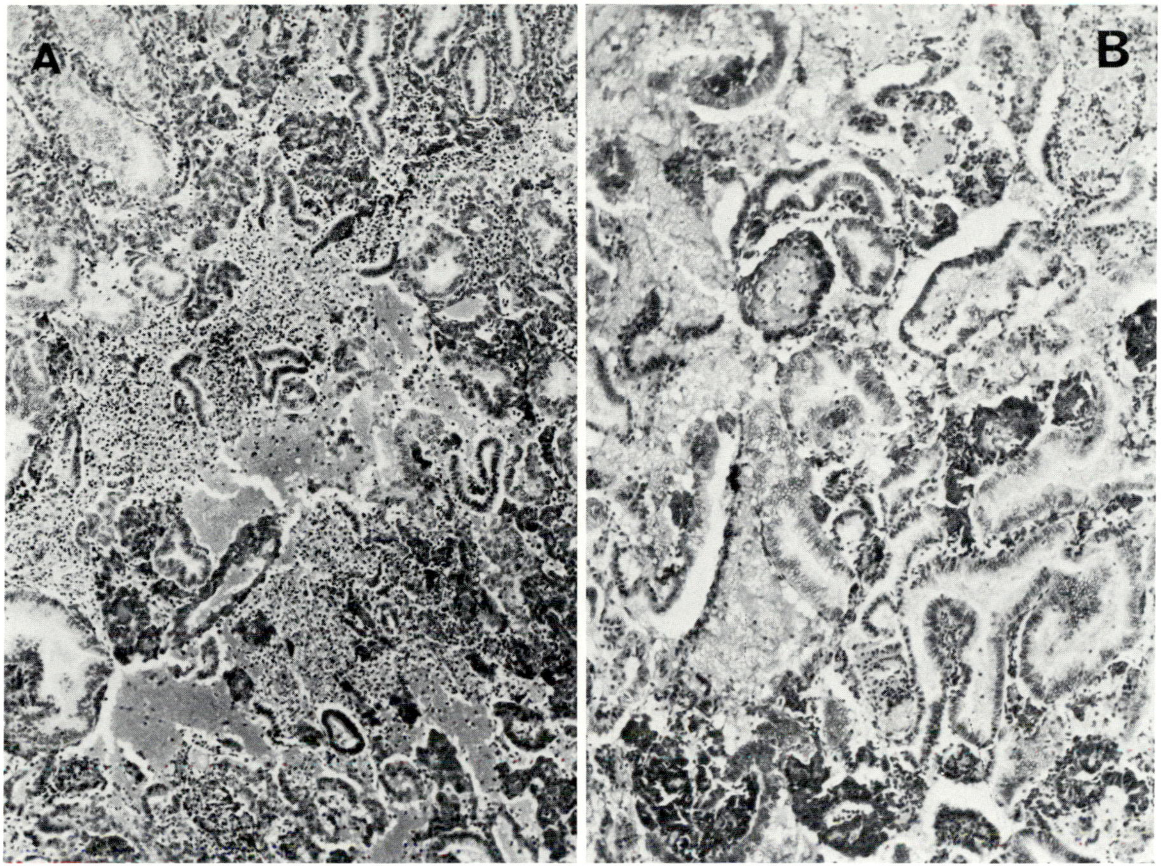

FIG. 9.25. Menstrual endometrium, degenerative phase. *A*. On cycle days 1–2, the endometrium contains collapsed stroma, ruptured glands with secretory exhaustion, degenerated predecidua, and inflammatory cells. *B*. Menstrual endometrium in a 42-year-old woman. The glands are larger and less exhausted than in *A;* however, degeneration is diffuse, a feature typical of estrogen–progestogen withdrawal type of bleeding endometrium.

pseudopodial projections. These alterations reflect ameboid motility promoted by cyclic adenosine monophosphate and by the interaction of actin-containing filaments with myosin-containing plasma membranes. Nuclear and nucleolar enlargement (Fig. 9.30C) in regenerative cells also promotes cellular motility by providing increased DNA and RNA, respectively. Following the initial epithelial spread, mitosis and migration operate simultaneously until a confluent surface layer has been regenerated on cycle day 5. The sudden increase in DNA synthesis and the shortened DNA synthesis phase of regenerative cells provide for accelerated tissue turnover (see Fig. 9.11). The cellular migration and the rapid wound healing capability observed in the human endometrium together with the kinetic and ultrastructural data do not support the view that new endometrium is regenerated directly from persistent, secretory spongiosa[29] or stromal fibroblasts.[5] The latter are believed to contribute to endometrial epithelial repair[21] indirectly, presumably by their positive influence on growth factors[69] and by providing cellular support to the newly resurfacing surface epithelial cells. The latter event is recognized by aggregates of stromal cells beneath resurfacing epithelial cells. These so-called stromal balls (Fig. 9.30A, B) are typical features of endometrial stromal breakdown following uterine bleeding associated with tissue regeneration (see Fig. 9.8). The deep blue staining characteristic of aggregated stromal cells with H&E stain is due to their prominent nuclei and scant cytoplasm. The stromal aggregates are not pathonomonic of postovulatory menstrual regeneration, since they are also seen in endometrium after anovulation, estrogen or progestogen breakthrough bleeding, or withdrawal of exogenous estrogen and progestogens.

Postmenstrual endometrium repair is not induced by E_2. During cycle days 3 and 4, despite increased DNA synthesis, circulating estrogens and receptors for E_2 and P are low, unchanged from the premenstrual values.[22] In experimental endometrial regeneration in the rabbit, similar proliferative and morphologic patterns are ob-

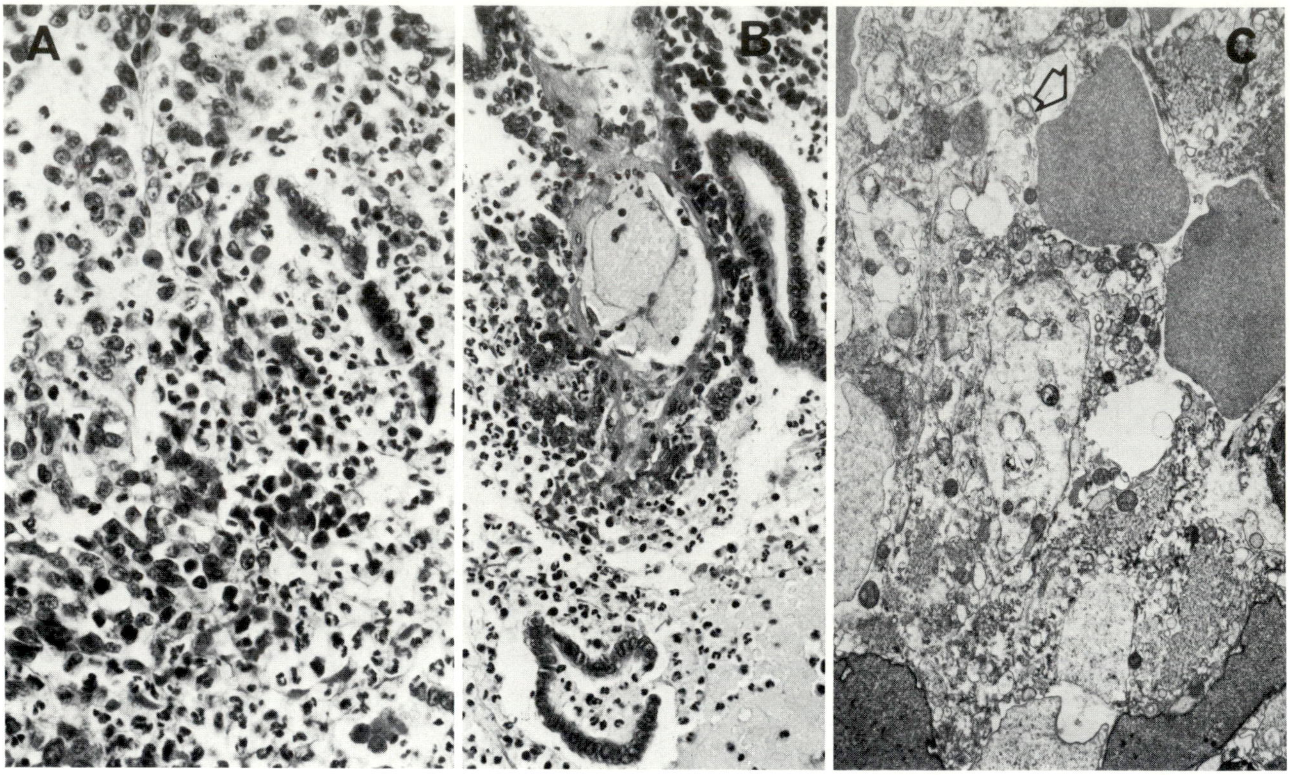

FIG. 9.26. Menstrual endometrium, degenerative phase. *A*. Ruptured, collapsed, exhausted glands and degenerative stromal cells intermingling with acute inflammatory cells, edema, and red blood cells. *B*. Ruptured endometrial vessel with fibrinoid deposit surrounded by degenerated predecidua and polymorphs. *C*. Ultrastructurally, there is severe cytologic, organellar, and nuclear degeneration, consistent with irreversible cell injury. Red blood cells (*arrow*) are seen. (Reprinted by permission of Ferenczy and Guralnick, Ref. 24.)

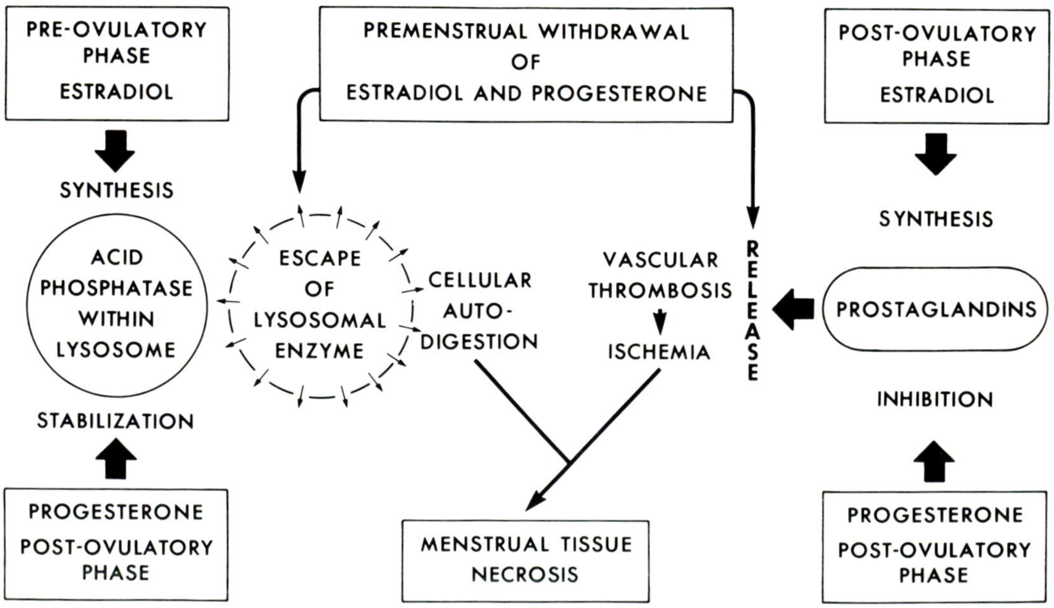

FIG. 9.27. Schematic representation of the morphobiochemical events that lead to the menstrual breakdown of the endometrium. The *large arrows* indicate the stimulatory effects of ovarian hormones. (Reprinted by permission of Ferenczy (1981) Contemp Obstet Gynecol 18: 115.)

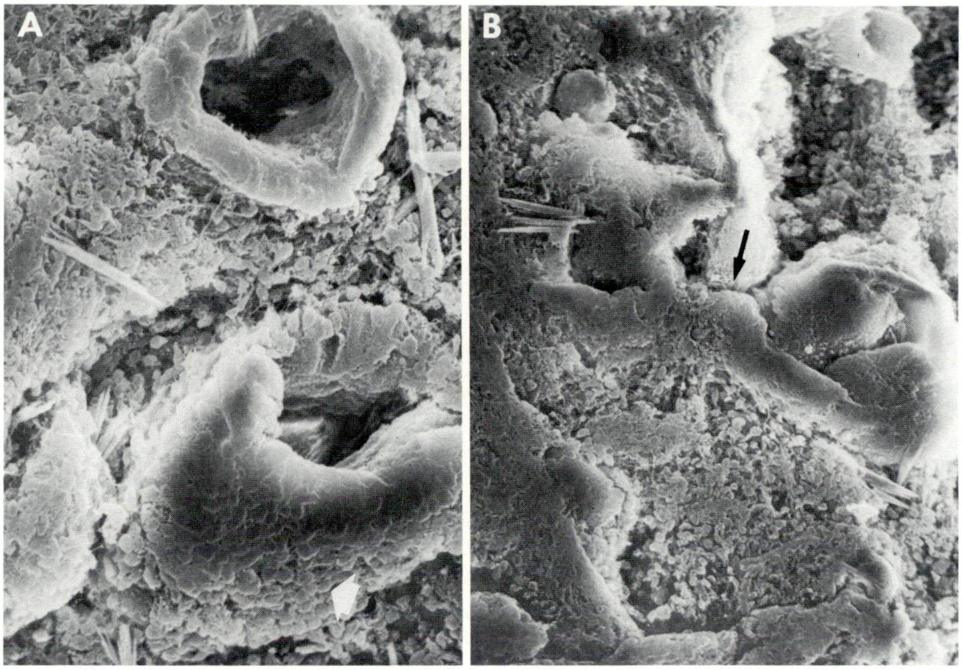

FIG. 9.28. Menstrual endometrium, reparative phase. *A*. Scanning electron microscopy of regenerative endometrium. On cycle day 3, gland stumps of residual basal glands have epithelial extensions (*arrow*) onto denuded stroma. *B*. Cycle day 4 is dominated by anastomoses of epithelial membranes (*arrow*) from adjacent basal gland opening. (Reprinted by permission of Ferenczy, Ref. 23.)

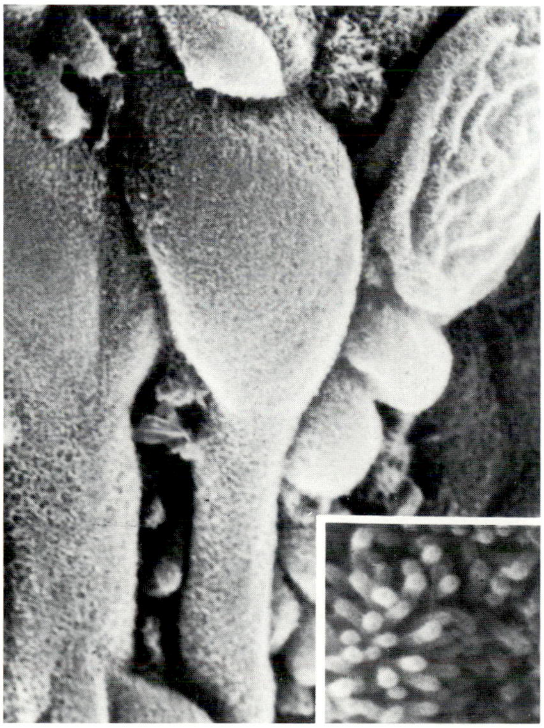

FIG. 9.29. Menstrual endometrium, regenerative phase. On cycle days 3 and 4, the newly formed epithelial cells have flattened cytoplasm and prominent pseudopodial projections. ×24,000. *Inset:* Higher magnification of hair-like surface microvilli. ×50,000. (Reprinted by permission of Ferenczy, Ref. 22.)

served, regardless of whether the animals are ovariectomized or have intact ovaries.[21] On cycle days 7–12, however, there is a marked increase in DNA synthesis (see Fig. 9.11) and mitotic activity in all cell components of the regenerated human endometrium. This coincides with an increase in plasma estrogens and E_2R–PgR concentrations and a slight decrease in serum pituitary hormones. These alterations reflect target cell sensitivity and response to preovulatory E_2.

Morphology of Gestational Endometrium

Glandular Epithelium

If pregnancy occurs, the secretory phase endometrium undergoes further morphophysiologic development and achieves its raison d'être, that is, to provide an appropriate environment for the conceptus. Between days 22 and 28, the endometrium displays hypertrophic and hypersecretory features that many refer to as "gestational hyperplasia.[37] The endometrium is characterized by (1) glandular ferning with epithelial and intraluminal se-

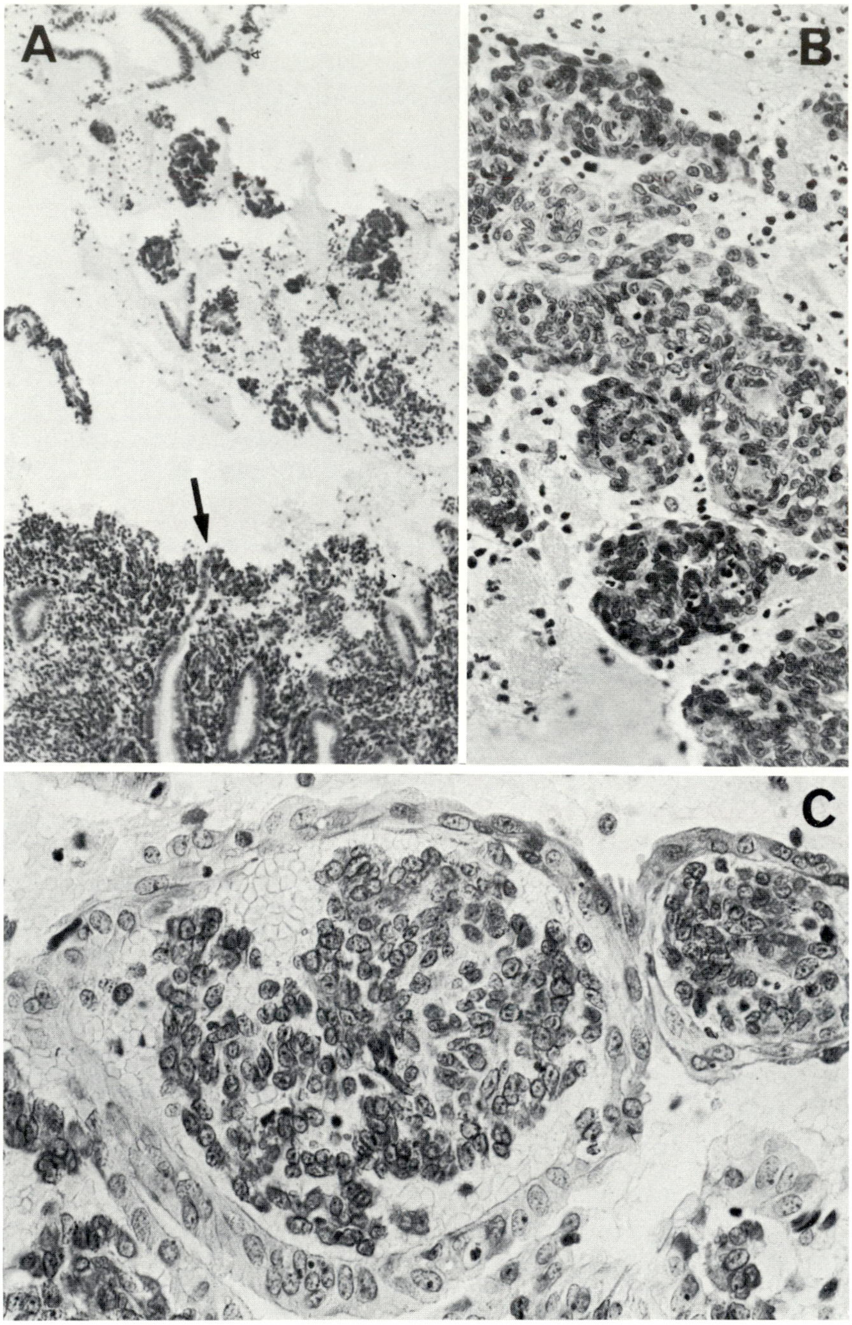

FIG. 9.30. Menstrual endometrium, regenerative phase. *A*. After expulsion of the functionalis layer, the basalis appears denuded (*arrow*) and is cleaved from the upper residual degenerated endometrial mucosa. The latter is made of stromal aggregates, ruptured glands, and inflammatory cells. *B*. Aggregates of residual stromal fibroblasts (stromal balls) are typical of late degenerative–early regenerative phase endometrium. *C*. Endometrial stromal fibroblasts forming the stromal balls are surrounded by resurfacing regenerative epithelial cells, which typically have flattened cytoplasm, enlarged nuclei and nucleoli consistent with repair, and nuclear polyploidy.

cretions, (2) stromal edema and vascular congestion, and (3) transmucosal predecidual reaction devoid of inflammatory exudate. The changes are similar to but quantitatively exaggerated from nongestational 22–26-day secretory endometrium. In the latter, each of the above alterations is prominent on a given day of the secretory phase, whereas during early pregnancy, they occur simultaneously. However, gestational hyperplasia is not diagnostic of early pregnancy unless a 9–13 POD ovum is seen implanted in the endometrium or an elevated serum hCG is detected.[4,35] The presence of fibrinoid with syncytial giant cells representing the placental site is diagnostic. Indeed, morphologic modification similar to gestational hyperplasia may also be found in association with double (twin) corpora lutea[37] and persistent corpus luteum cyst.[35] The only pathognomonic feature of intrauterine pregnancy is chorionic tissue, embryonic tissue, or a fibrinoid layer with placental site syncytial giant cells (Fig. 9.31).

The gestational endometrium becomes distinctive by

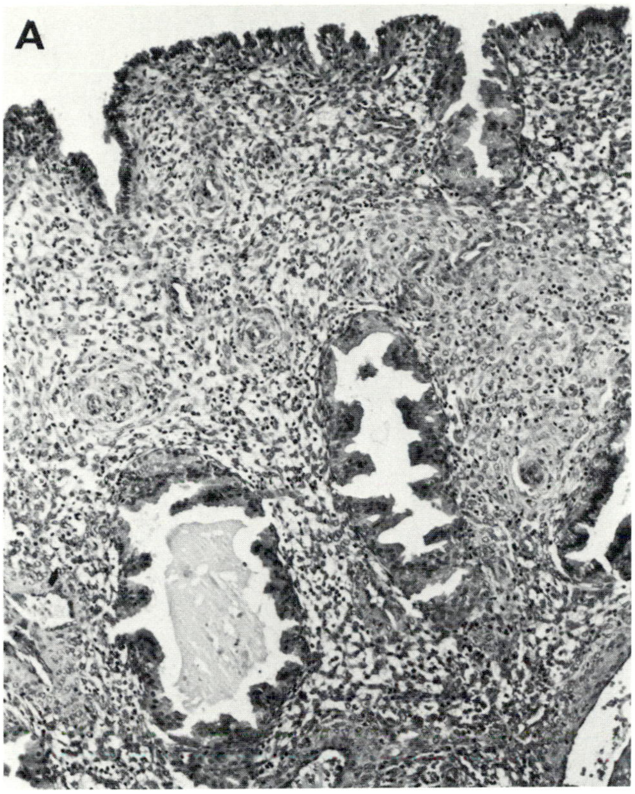

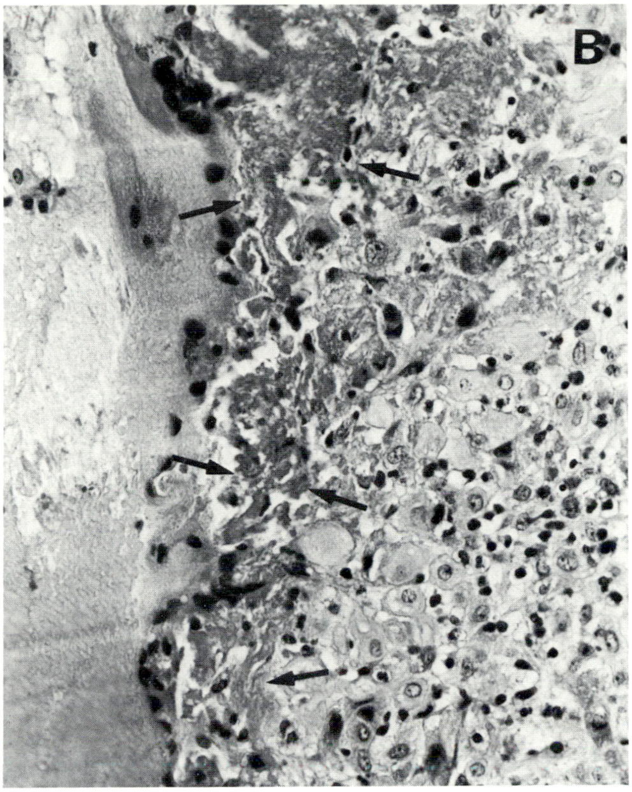

FIG. 9.31. Gestational endometrium. *A*. Voluminous secretory glands with numerous, prominent intraluminal epithelial projections and secretions are associated with dense predecidua (*right*), stromal edema (*left*), and a well-developed arterial system. When these changes are seen in the upper one-third of the spongiosa layer, they are suggestive but not diagnostic of early gestation. *B*. Fibrinoid (Nitabuch's) layer (*arrows*), with placental site multinucleated syncytial cells on one side (*left*) and gestational decidua vera cells on the other side (*right*), is pathognomonic of intrauterine pregnancy.

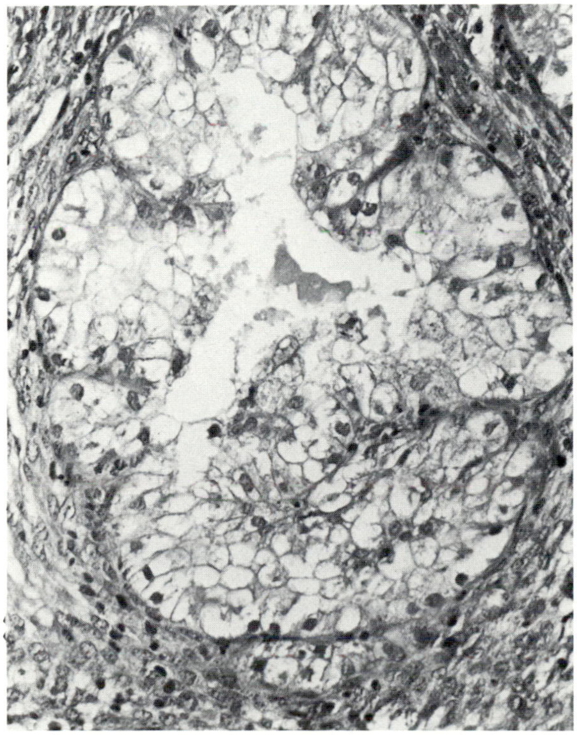

FIG. 9.32. Hypersecretory gland with thickened, hypertrophic, pseudostratified cells with clear cytoplasm and blunt-ended epithelial projections into the lumen. The nuclei are round, and unlike those in the Arias–Stella reaction, are small. Both the glandular and cellular alterations are suggestive but not pathognomonic of early pregnancy.

the fourth week of gestation. Many gestational glands display intraluminal epithelial projections (ferning), and often they are lined with large cells with clear or eosinophilic cytoplasm and varying sized nuclei (Fig. 9.32). Exaggeration of these cytonuclear alterations produces the so-called Arias-Stella reaction (ASR),[3] characterized by voluminous cells with large hyperchromatic nuclei and irregular nuclear membranes. The cytoplasm is often clear and vacuolated. ASR, when extensive, may be confused with clear cell carcinoma by the uninitiated. Unlike clear cell carcinoma, ASR is typically focal, and the adjacent endometrium shows normal gestational changes, that is, a prominent decidual reaction. In addition, in the malignant clear cells, the nucleocytoplasmic (N/C) ratio is in favor of the nuclei, whereas ASR cells have normal N/C ratios, both the cytoplasm and nucleus being enlarged (cytonucleomegaly) (Fig. 9.33). Nuclear enlargement in ASR is a consequence of nuclear polyploidy, which presumably occurs by endomitosis and subsequent fusion of divided nuclei.[76] This is in contrast with the near diploid or aneuploid nuclear DNA content of endometrial carcinoma. ASR is a hormonally related gland cell hypertrophy associated with intra- or extrauterine pregnancy or trophoblastic disease.[70] The hormones involved are presumably chorionic gonadotropin, estrogen, and progesterone. ASR may also be seen in the glandular epithelium of the cervix, the fallopian tube, endometriosis, or vaginal adenosis.[70] In spontaneous abortion or later gestation, ASR demonstrates nuclear aberrations consistent with degenerative features, including agglutinated nuclear DNA, cytoplasmic vacuolization, and apical nuclear position (hobnail cells) (Fig. 9.33). These observations suggest that ASR in endometrial gland cells results from hyperstimulation induced by high levels of gestational hormones. These changes regress and disappear after withdrawal of hormonal stimulation.

Another distinctive feature in endometrial gland cells associated with intrauterine pregnancy and trophoblastic disease is nuclear vacuolization, so-called optically clear nuclei (Fig. 9.34), resembling the ground-glass appear-

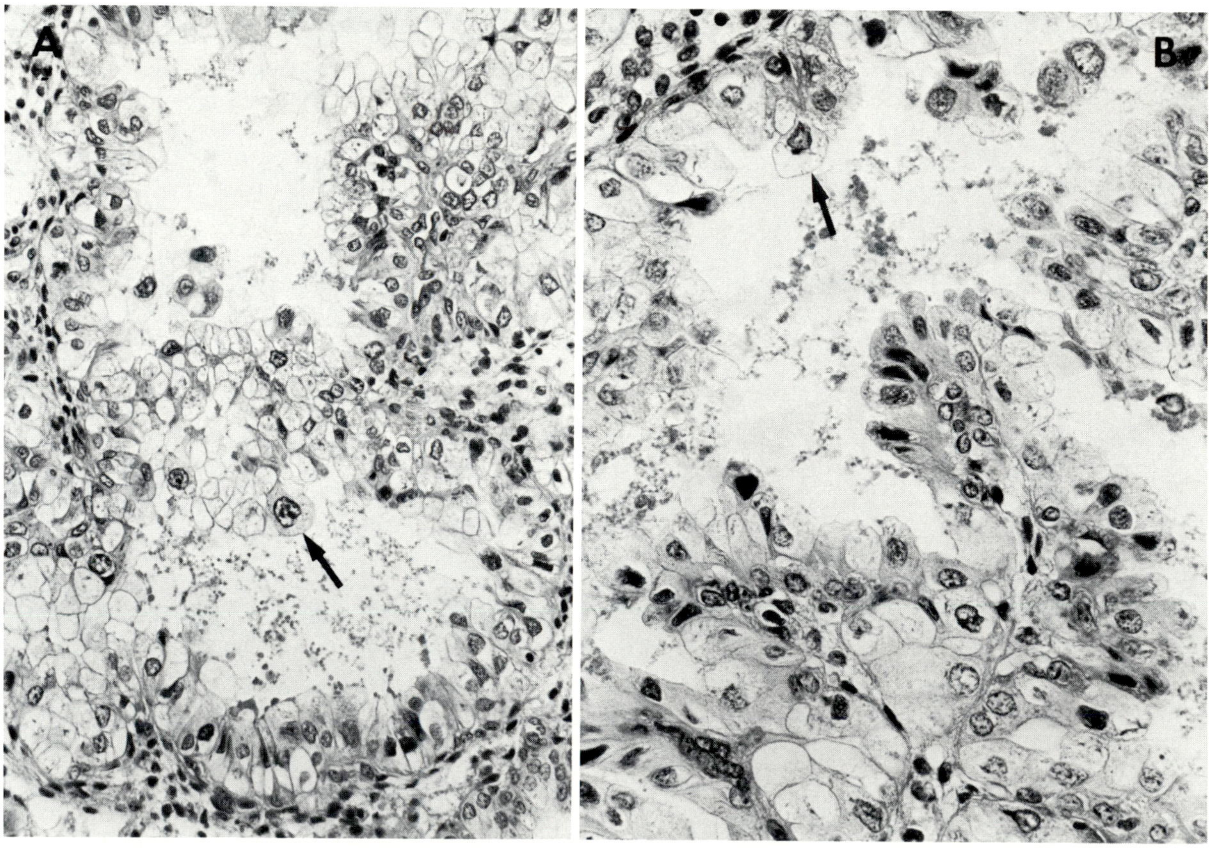

FIG. 9.33. Gestational endometrium with Arias-Stella reaction (ASR). *A*. Voluminous gland in which some of the lining cells demonstrate ASR (*arrow*), characterized by cytonucleomegaly, hyperchromatic nuclei, and enlarged nucleoli. Note the well-preserved, finely granular cytoplasmic substance and nuclear chromatin of ASR cells. These are seen in the early developmental phase of ASR. *B*. ASR cells with shrunken, degenerated nuclei and vacuolated cytoplasm (*arrow*). This is the degenerative phase of ASR and is seen in missed abortions.

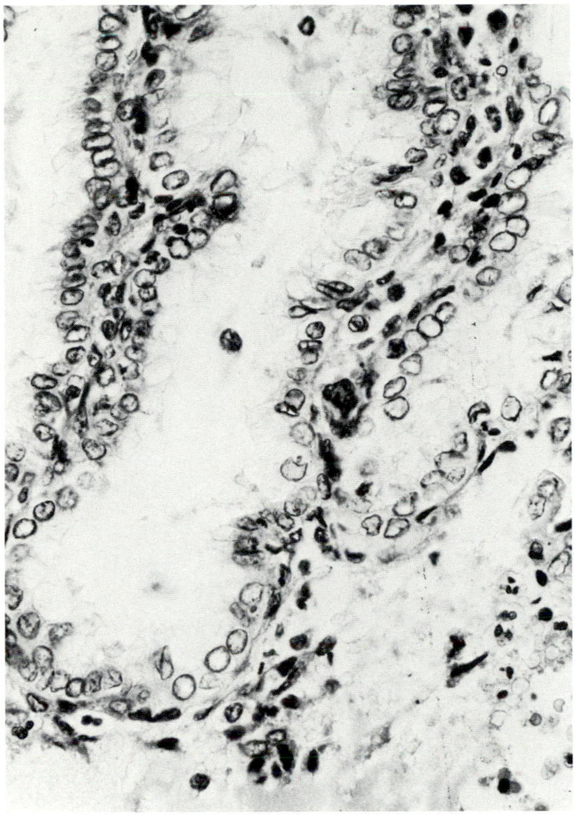

FIG. 9.34. Gestational endometrium. Intranuclear clearing resembling the ground-glass appearance of nuclei with herpes simplex virus inclusions. In gestational endometrial gland cells, however, the nuclei contain thread-like filaments rather than viral particles.

ance of herpes virus inclusions.[53] Ultrastructurally, however, nuclear clearing corresponds to strands of 70–80 A thick filaments. This in turn may correspond to a filamentous presentation of nuclear chromatin, secondary to gestational hormonal hyperstimulation.

Stroma

The predecidual cells are transformed into larger epithelioid decidual cells termed *decidua vera*. They are particularly prominent in the upper one-third of the endometrium and produce the compacta layer. Ultrastructurally, gestational decidual cells contain comparatively more organelles, including intermediate filaments, cigar-shaped mitochondria, and granular endoplasmic reticulum, than their predecidual nongestational counterparts.[25,47,80] Whereas predecidual cells are interconnected by tight junctional nexuses, the gestational variant has nexuses between cytoplasmic filipodial projections (Fig. 9.35). The gestational decidual reaction is not pathognomonic of intrauterine pregnancy in general, since similar changes may be seen in ectopic pregnancy or as a result of exogenous progestational therapy.

Near the implantation site, cells resembling decidual cells often contain significant nuclear atypia to mimic malignancy. However, immunohistochemistry localizes human placental lactogen in these cells, indicating that they are intermediate-type trophoblasts rather than decidual cells (see Chapter 23, Diseases of Placenta and Chapter 24, Gestational Trophoblastic Disease).[45] This is also true for the so-called placental site reaction, which is produced by trophoblastic cells infiltrating the decidua near the implantation site. In both instances, the atypical cytologic features are often those of degeneration with agglutinated nuclear DNA and are focal, and the neighboring endometrium contains gestational decidual cells and glandular secretory features. Occasionally, however, cytologic atypia seems to be a reflection of active trophoblastic cells that extend into the decidua. The decidual cells have phagocytic properties (see Fig. 21B, C) and digest the extracellular collagen matrix.[24,47] Decidual phagocytosis may facilitate the development of the decidual reaction by removing collagen from the endometrial stroma, which may represent a mechanical obstacle to proliferating and expanding decidual cells.

Another important function of decidual cells is related to the maintenance of the fetal allograft (fetus).[42] Indeed, it is likely that decidual cells control the invasive nature of the normal trophoblast. Lack of a decidual reaction in the endometrium as occurs in the isthmus or in the fallopian tubal mucosa is accompanied by deep myometrial implantation of the placenta (placenta accreta) and invasion of the myosalpinx, respectively. An abdominal pregnancy may be viable because the subcoelomic mesenchymal cells of the pelvic and abdominal peritoneum are capable of decidual transformation.[58] The factors that control decidual transformation in different sites are unknown, however, immunologic mechanisms may be involved.[9] The immunologic role of decidua is suggested by its suppression of the antibody response of spleen cultures to DNP–polylysine, as well as its suppression of the mixed lymphocyte reaction and proliferative response of lymphocytes to allogeneic graft cells and to T cell mitogens.[42] Furthermore, recent studies have traced the origin of decidual cells in the bone marrow.[42] Decidual cells have been found to have surface antigens ($H\text{-}2K^k$ and $H\text{-}2K^b$) similar to splenic lymphocytes and macrophages admixed with decidual cells.[42] The human nongestational and, particularly, gestational decidua also has been reported to have endocrinologic functions,[9] which apparently synthesize and release prolactin (PRL) that is immunologically identical to pituitary PRL. However, immunocytochemistry has not convincingly demonstrated PRL in decidual cells. Also, decidual cells lack ultrastructural similarity to pituitary cells and are devoid of secretory granules.[25] Decidual cells are also suspected

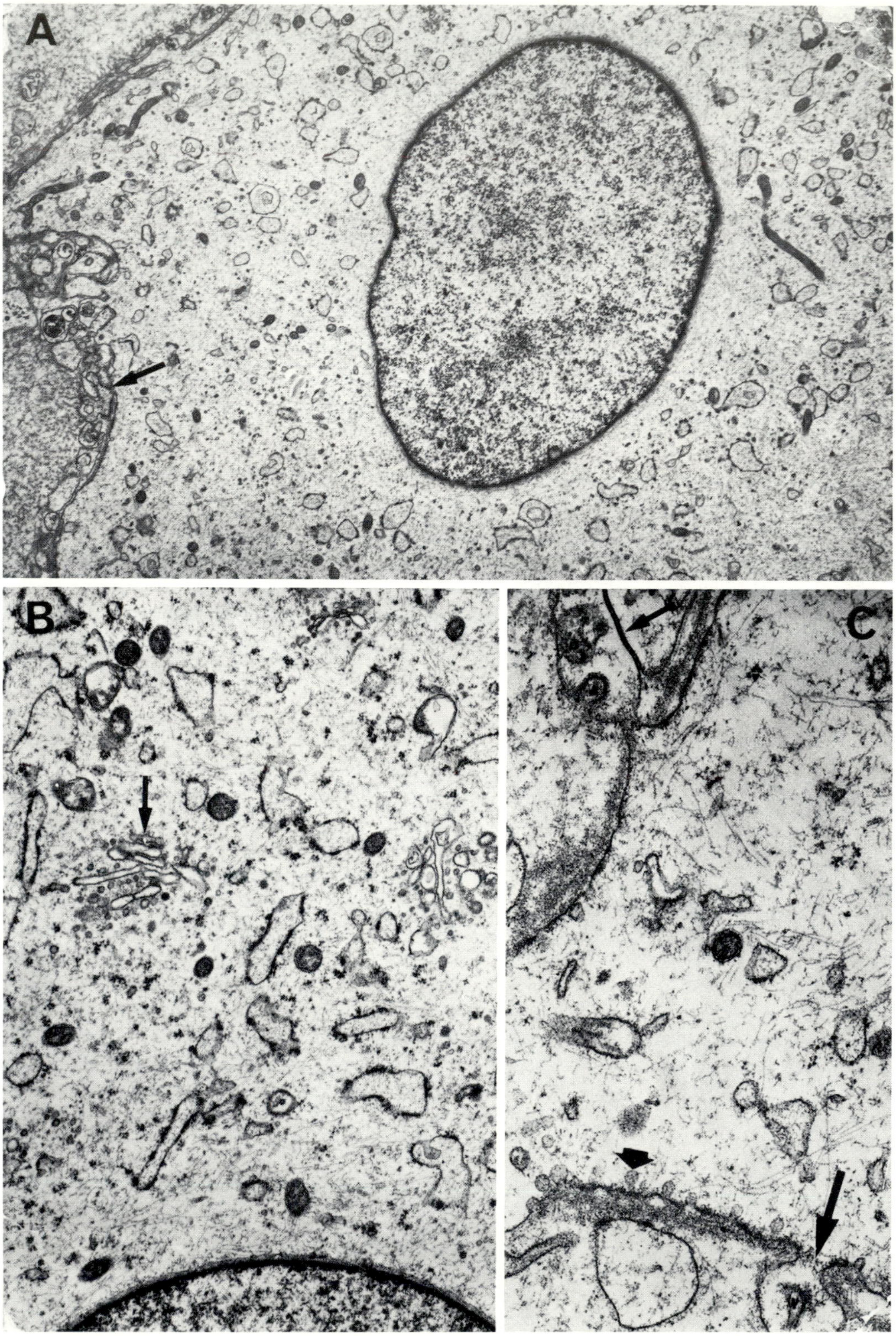

Fig. 9.35. Ultrastructure of 10-week-old gestational decidual cells. *A*. The prominent cytoplasm is centered by a round nucleus and contains scattered organelles. The cytoplasmic membrane contains club-shaped filopodial processes (*arrow*) projecting into the extracellular space. ×6000. *B*. Detail of organelles including the Golgi complex (*arrow*), intermingling with intermediate filaments. ×12,000. *C*. The cytoplasmic membrane contains micropinocytic vesicles (*short arrow*) and club-shaped cytoplasmic processes (*long arrow*). A tight junctional nexus (*fine arrow*) connects to cytoplasmic projections. ×22,000.

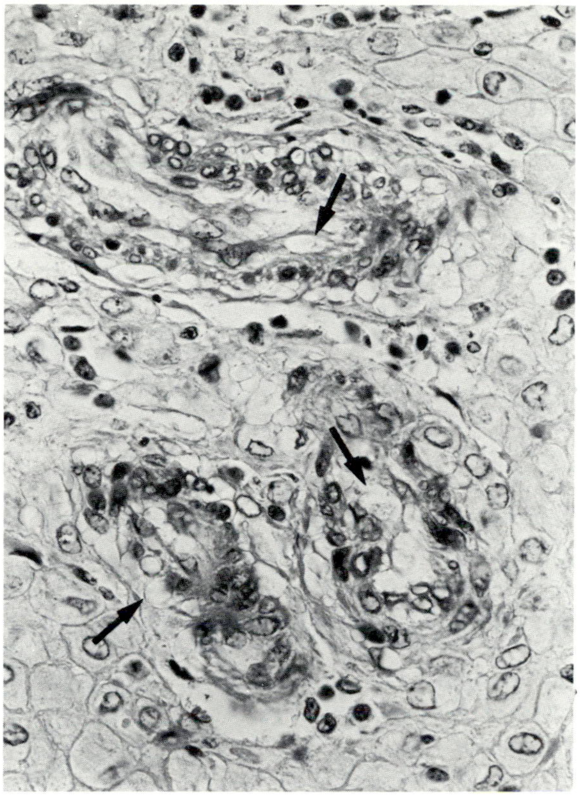

FIG. 9.36. Gestational endometrium. Atherosis of endometrial vessels with foamy vacuolization (*arrows*) of endothelial cells.

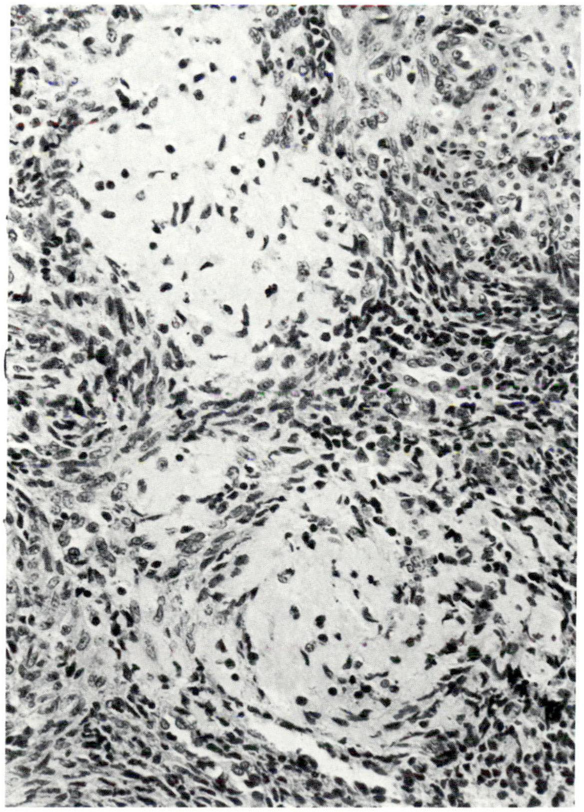

FIG. 9.37. Fibrohyaline nodules scattered with fibroblasts. These structures represent obliterated endometrial arteries at previous placental site. This patient delivered her baby 8 weeks before curettings for postpartum bleeding.

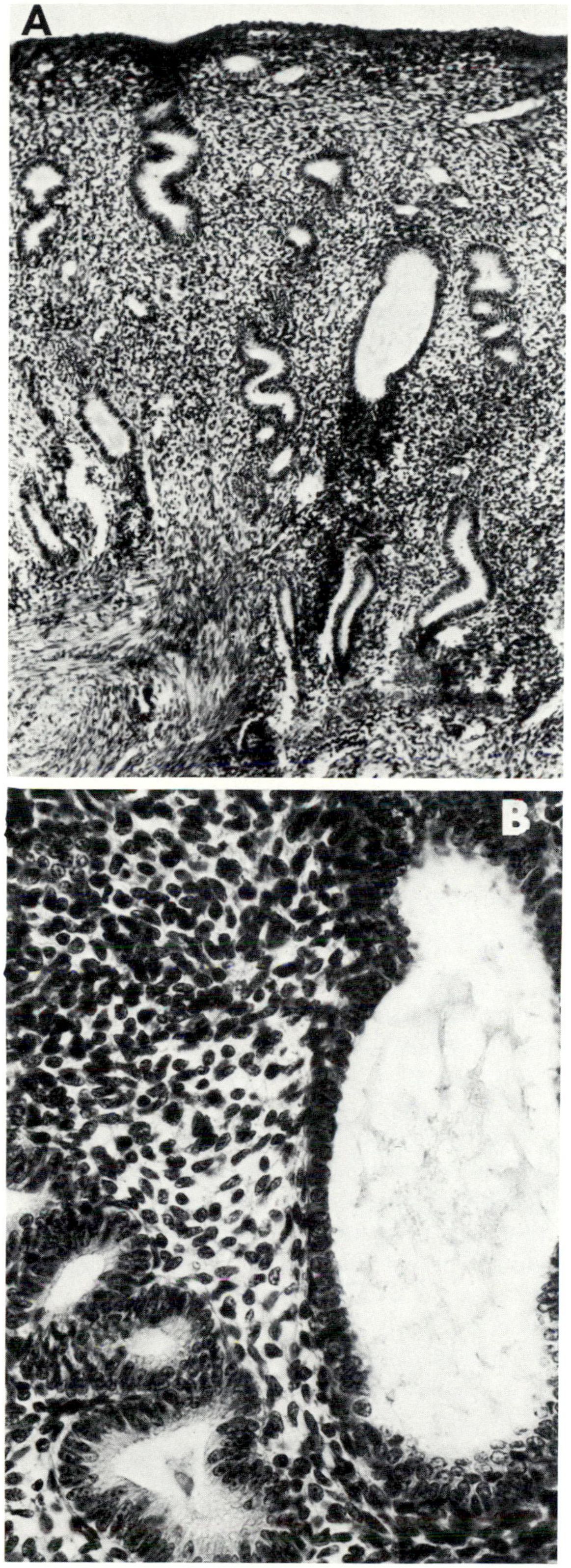

FIG. 9.38. Inactive endometrium. *A*. The endometrial stroma is uniformly dense without clear-cut separation between the upper functionalis and the lower basalis layers. The glandular architecture is similar to that of midproliferative phase endometrium; however, there are fewer glands, and some of them are oriented parallel to the surface. *B*. Inactive glandular epithelium has pseudostratified nuclei devoid of mitoses, and the surrounding stroma is dense and cellular, resembling the stroma of the basalis layer of cyclic endometrium.

of synthesizing PGF_2 from archidonic acid released from intracellular stores of phospholipids.[28] Phospholipase A_2 that releases arachidonic acid is found in intracytoplasmic lysosomes. Release of PGF_2 from gestational decidual cells may play a role in the initiation of labor.[1]

Spiral arteries are larger and their walls are thicker than those found in nongestational secretory endometrium. Some of them display acute atherosis, with concentric intimal proliferation of myofibroblasts and foamy cells (Fig. 9.36). These alterations apparently occur in response to trophoblastic invasion of endometrial vessels; they are focal and are more frequent in primigravidas.[73] They are not associated with preeclampsia, eclampsia, diabetes, or hypertension.[49] Following delivery, the endometrial vessels near the implantation site undergo thrombosis and later hyalinization, as does the surrounding decidua. These alterations produce fibrohyaline nodules typical of recent to remote (several years) intrauterine pregnancy (Fig. 9.37). When the placental site becomes acutely or chronically inflamed, the partially hyalinized and thrombosed vessels cannot contract, which leads to postpartum bleeding of the subinvoluting uterus.

Morphology of Inactive and Atrophic Endometrium

An endometrium that is as thick as early to midproliferative phase endometrium but is devoid of morphologic features of either active proliferation or secretion may be considered inactive as far as its response to hormonal stimuli is concerned. The glands and stroma resemble proliferative endometrium, but the glands usually are oriented parallel rather than perpendicular to the surface epithelium. The surface epithelium as well as that lining the glands is columnar to cuboidal and contains pseudostratified nuclei without mitoses, and occasional ciliated cells are seen. The stroma is generally dense throughout, without a clear-cut separation between the basalis and functionalis layer (Fig. 9.38A, B). Such endometrial changes are found in the early postmenopausal years when ovarian hormonal stimuli have decreased to levels not sufficient to induce endometrial proliferation.

There are several morphologic manifestations of atrophic endometrium, but all have in common a thin mucosa that measures about half or less the thickness of a basal layer of cyclic endometrium (less than 0.5 mm). Typically, in the curettings, the entire atrophic endometrial mucosa, including its basalis layer, can be seen within a microscopic field of ×250. There is a further decrease in the number and volume, respectively, of glands and stroma and most commonly the glands are oriented parallel to the surface (Fig. 9.39A, B). The lining epithelium of both the surface and glands is low and cuboidal and devoid of cilia, although cilia may be quite frequent in surface epithelial cells. The stroma is often collagenized and resembles the stroma of the isthmus or lower uterine segment in premenopausal women. Endometrial vascular alterations are seldom seen in women with atrophic endometrium, including those with abnormal uterine bleeding. In fact, in more than 50% of patients, no pathology is found in the uterus.[10,54] The most frequent morphologic changes that can be related to clinical bleeding are (1) arteriosclerosis of the myometrial arteries, including the arcuate and radial arteries, with medial hypertrophy and calcification and narrowing of the lumen, and (2) rupture of dilated and engorged endometrial veins secondary to uterine prolapse or compression by dilated atrophic endometrial cysts.[10,54] The former condition when associated with cardiovascular collapse may lead to hemorrhagic necrosis of the endometrial mucosa, producing apoplexia uteri.[17] At other times, coexistent chronic endometritis, submucous leiomyomata, or endometrial polyps may be the organic causes of uterine bleeding.

Often, atrophic endometrium has cystically dilated glands. Whether these represent the atrophic variants of cystically dilated glands that are seen in the lower functionalis in virtually all women aged 35 years and over[40] is not clear. However, the condition is often referred to as *cystic atrophy* (Fig. 9.40A). Cystically dilated glands are also seen in cystic glandular hyperplasia with retrogressive atrophy. In this case the endometrial mucosa retains the thickness of an otherwise active hyperplasia, but the glandular epithelium is atrophic and the stroma is collagenized (Fig. 9.38B). On occasion, both the surface and glandular epithelium is composed of tall columnar to cuboidal cells, including ciliated cells resembling those seen in hyperplasia. Unlike true hyperplasia, this form of atrophy lacks mitotic figures, the mucosa is thin, and the stroma is relatively rich in collagen fibers (Fig. 9.41A). It is possible that the changes reflect estrogenic response of otherwise atrophic endometrial epithelium that has been under either endogenous or exogenous estrogenic stimulation. The morphologic changes, furthermore, appear to be confined to the epithelial cells without stromal cell participation. In extreme atrophy, there is endometrial stromal fibrosis, and only the surface epithelium and rare glands remain lined by low cuboidal cells (Fig. 9.41B). In such cases, the isthmic ostium (internal os), as well as the external cervical os, may be completely stenotic, resulting in pyometra. In response to long-standing irritation by the chronic inflammatory exudate, the surface epithelium may undergo squamous metaplasia, which in extreme cases lines the entire endometrial cavity, resulting in the condition, referred to as *icthyosis psoriasis uteri.*

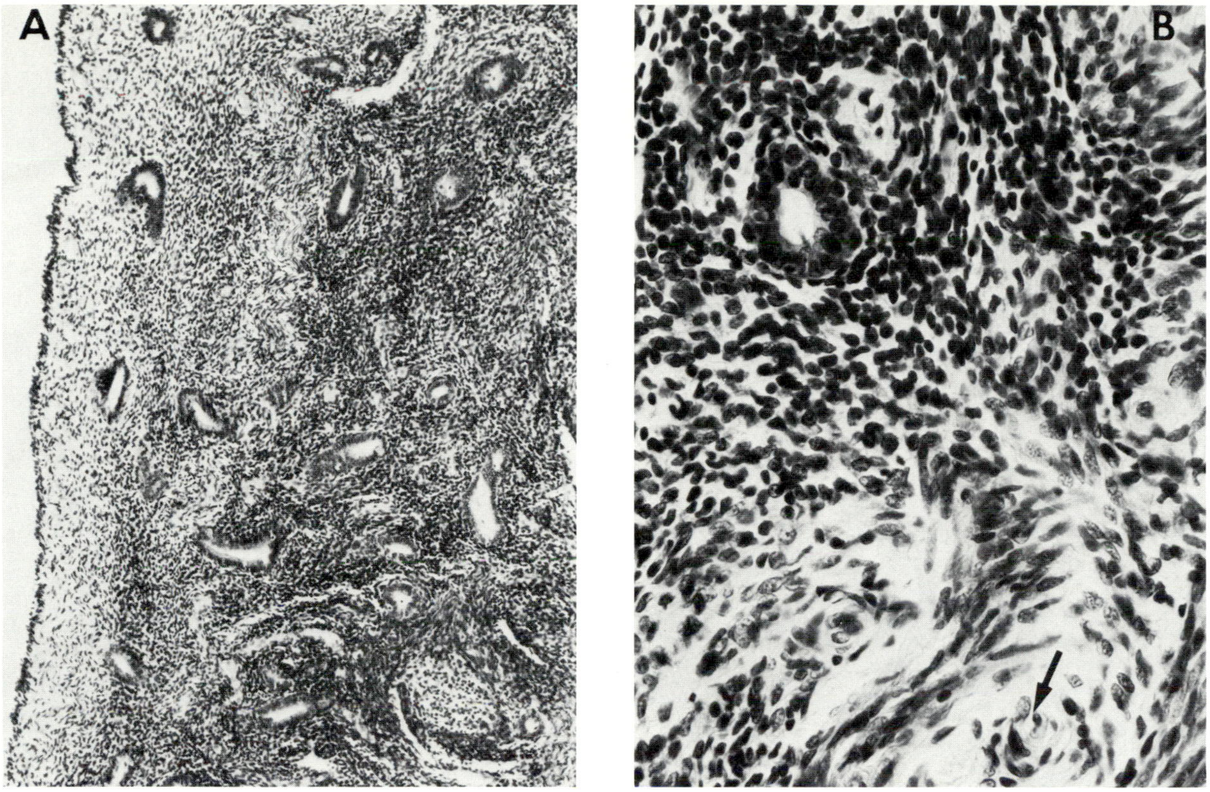

FIG. 9.39. Atrophic endometrium. *A*. The endometrial mucosa is thin, made of dense fibrocellular stroma and a few small glands with narrow lumens. *B*. Detailed view of endometrial arteries in basalis layer. There is severe obliterative endarteritis with minute lumens (*arrow*). The gland in the upper left is the size of a capillary, has a narrow lumen, and is lined by low cuboidal cells.

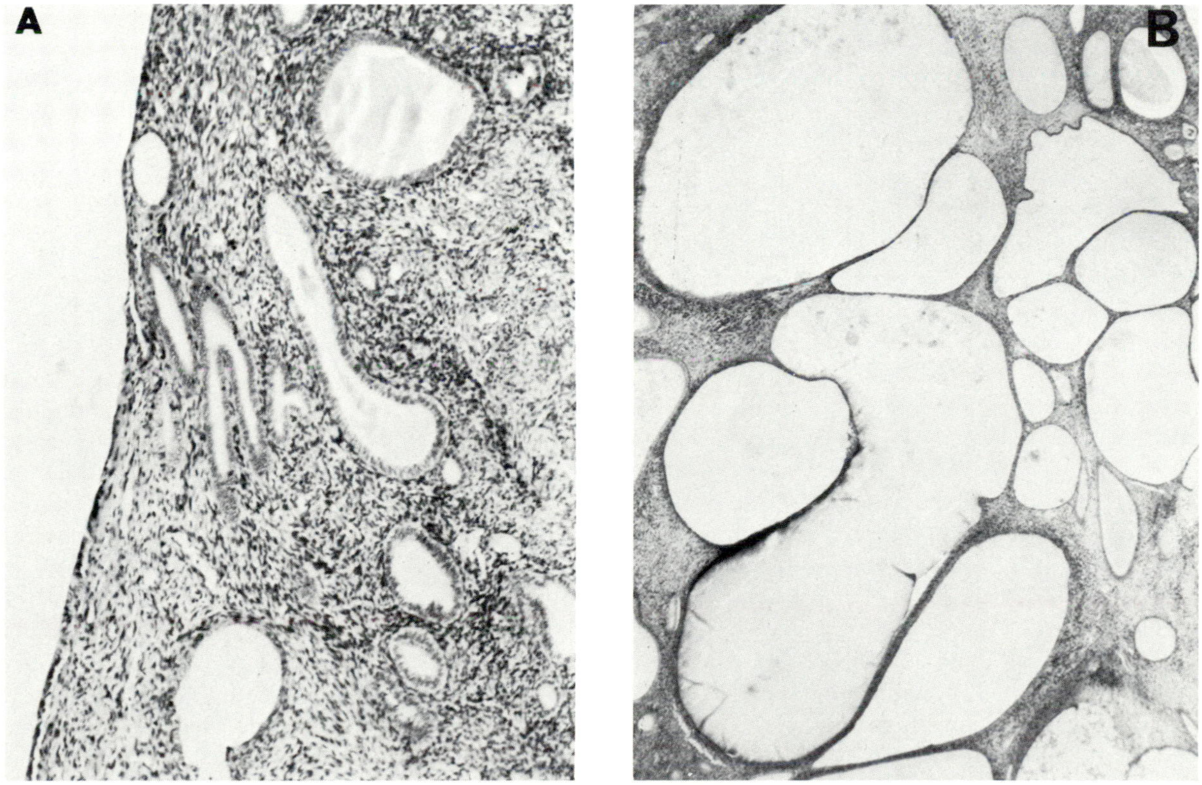

FIG. 9.40. Atrophic endometrium. *A*. Several cystically dilated glands, particularly at the endomyometrial junction, are often seen in otherwise atrophic endometrium. Their significance, if any, is unknown, but they are not considered to reflect previous hyperplasia. *B*. Cystic glandular hyperplasia with retrogressive atrophic glandular and stromal features is characterized by a relatively tall endometrial mucosa in which there are multiple cystic spaces lined by atrophic epithelium and surrounded by dense fibrous stroma.

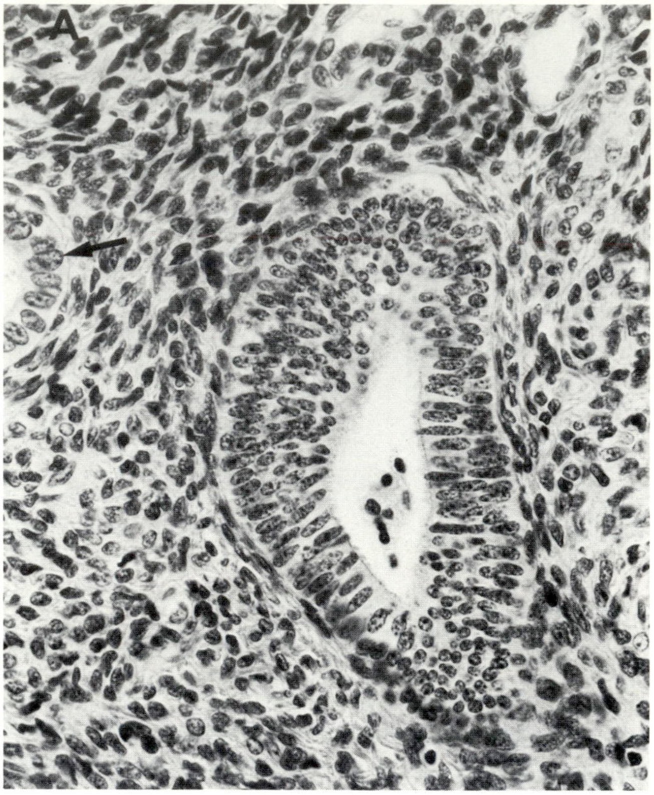

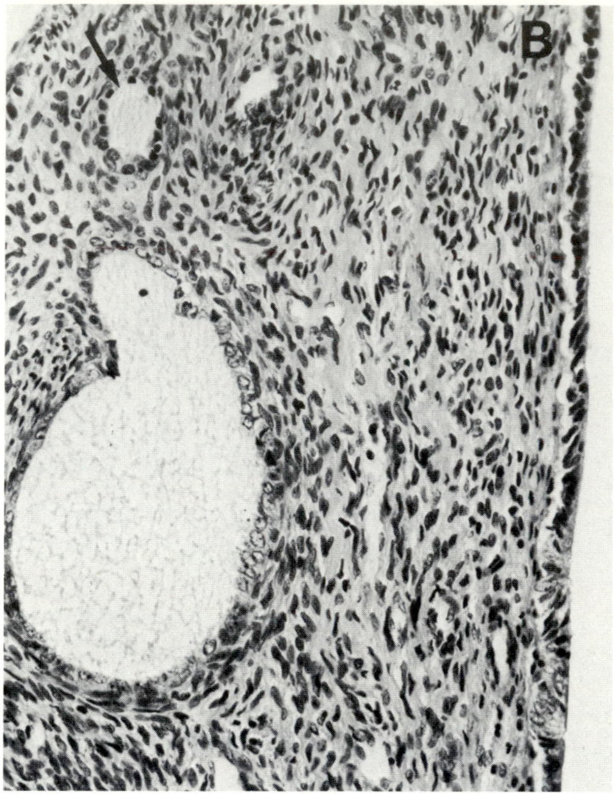

FIG. 9.41. Atrophic endometrium. *A*. The gland lining cells are tall columnar with pencil-shaped pseudostratified nuclei and cilia resembling those found in endometrial hyperplasia. However, the endometrium is thin, and the stroma is dense fibrocellular with many glands lined by atrophic epithelium (*arrow*). *B*. On the other end of the spectrum, in severe glandulostromal atrophy, both the surface- and gland-lining epithelium is low cuboidal, and the stroma is collagenous. Some of the glands resemble capillaries (*arrow*).

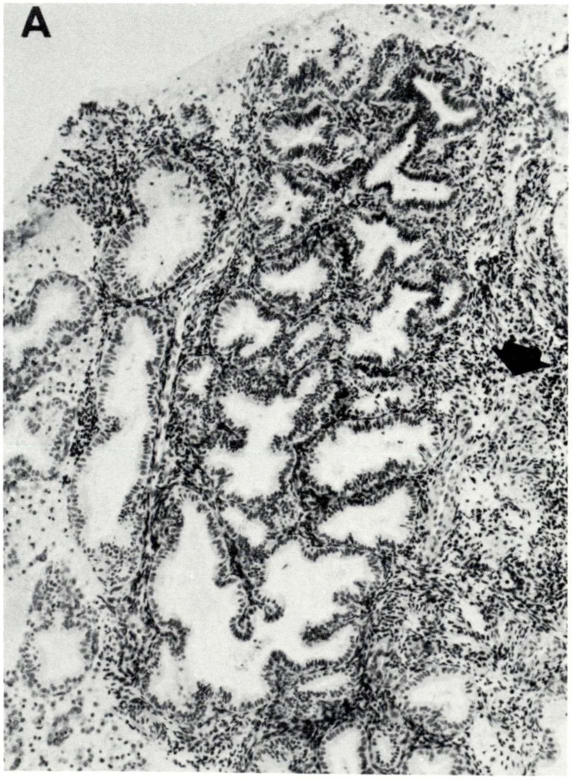

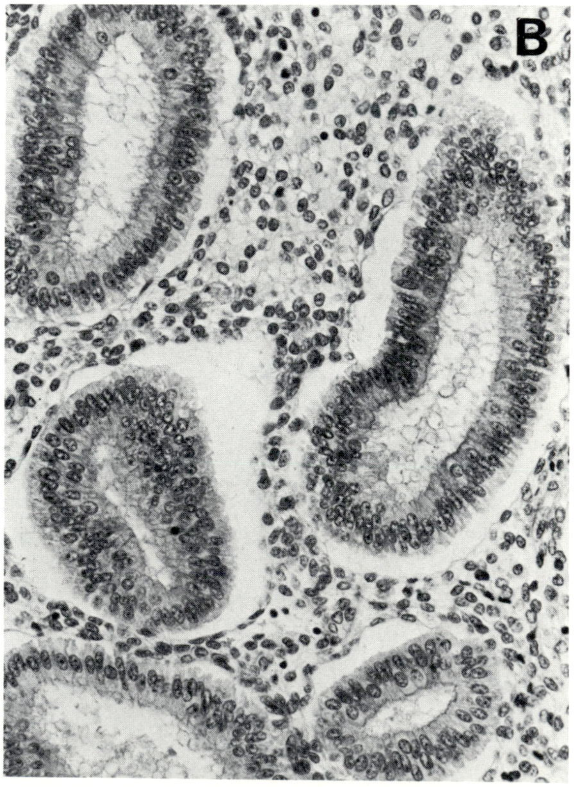

FIG. 9.42. Basalis endometrium. *A*. Clusters of tortuous glands in a back-to-back position masquerading as hyperplasia. The glandular aggregate is focal and flanked by clusters of basal arteries (*right*) (*arrow*) and degenerative spongiosa (*left*). Note the absence of surface epithelium. *B*. Delayed fixation artifact of endometrial specimens results in separation of glands from the supportive stroma, producing periglandular spaces. Such endometrium is difficult to date accurately.

Technical Consideration and Pitfalls in Interpretation of Biopsies

Accurate morphologic interpretation is achieved when either the biopsy sample or the curetting is taken from the body or fundus region and fixed immediately in either Bouin's solution or 10% buffered formalin. Bouin's solution is preferred because it preserves cytologic characteristics, whereas formalin is a tissue fixative that yields comparatively poor cytologic details. If Bouin's solution is used, the jaw of the curette should not be immersed in the fixative, since Bouin's solution contains highly corrosive glacial acetic acid, which quickly blunts the cutting edge of the curette. Instead, the specimen should be removed from the curette with forceps, placed on a lens paper, and immersed in the fixative. The specimen adheres to the lens paper, thereby minimizing the possibility that the tissue may be lost during processing (see Chapter 27, Gross Description and Processing).

Morphologic interpretion, including dating of the endometrium, is based on the assessment of the functionalis of the endometrium, which is identified by its covering surface epithelium (see Figs. 9.22B and 9.23A). An endometrial specimen devoid of surface epithelium may lead to an inaccurate diagnosis because, in many instances, such endometrium represents the basalis layer, which does not respond to cyclic hormonal stimuli, the specimen cannot be dated. In addition, since it often contains voluminous glands and compact stroma, with clusters of basal arteries (Fig. 9.42A), it may be confused with an endometrial polyp or hyperplasia. The endometrium in hysterectomy specimens often contains autolytic artifacts, which are due to the high proteolytic enzyme content of the endometrium.[8,44] This high enzyme content quickly produces autolytic changes if the specimen is not fixed immediately after removal of the uterus. The major morphologic autolytic artifacts include gland and stromal cell retractions (Fig. 9.42B). The best time to confirm ovulation is on cycle day 22 (POD 8) or later. Some investigators, including myself, advocate endometrial sampling at the onset of uterine bleeding.[4,23] By obtaining samples at the time of early uterine bleeding, the pathologist is able to determine whether the bleeding is caused by breakdown of postovulatory, secretory endometrium, focal necrosis of the endometrium associated with anovulation or other pathologic states, or exogenous sex steroid hormone administration. In addition, since with a few exceptions (inadequate luteal phase), the secretory phase of the cycle is constant in length (14 days ± 2 days), the time of ovulation can be estimated if the endometrium is of the normal menstrual type. During the period of bleeding, both the external os and the lower uterine segment are dilated, facilitating introduction of a curette into the endometrial cavity, thereby minimizing the discomfort associated with the endometrial biopsy. When the pathologist is confronted often with the morphology of menstrual endometrium, his diagnostic expertise of this condition is considerably improved. This, in turn, prevents the confusion of menstrual endometrium with endometrial carcinoma. Such a mistake is seen somewhat frequently in routine pathology practice.[23,78] Secretory endometrium may be relatively more difficult to date precisely than menstrual endometrium. Indeed, secretory endometrium often demonstrates subtle changes and combinations of morphologic patterns that may result in errors of ±4–5 days. This can be improved to ±2 days, however, by basing the date on the endometrial alterations that represent the most advanced phase of the menstrual cycle. For example, an endometrial biopsy may show changes consistent with the 16th, 17th, and 18th days of the cycle; the diagnosis should be based on the most advanced date and, therefore, reported as 18th day secretory endometrium instead of averaging cycle days and reporting 17th day secretory endometrium.

References

1. Abel MH (1979) Production of prostaglandins by the human uterus: Are they involved in menstruation? Res Clin Forum 1: 33
2. Abel MH, Baird DT (1980) The effect of 17β-estradiol and progesterone on prostaglandin production by human endometrium maintained in organ culture. Endocrinology 106: 1599
3. Arias-Stella J (1972) Atypical endometrial changes produced by chorionic tissue. Hum Pathol 3: 450
4. Arronet GH, Berquist GA, Parekh MC, Latour JPA, Marshall KG (1973) Evaluation of endometrial biopsy in the cycle of conception. Int J Fertil 18: 220
5. Baggish MS, Pauerstein CJ, Woodruff JD (1967) Role of stroma in regeneration of endometrial epithelium. Am J Obstet Gynecol 99: 453
6. Bartelemez GW (1957) The form and the functions of the uterine blood vessels in the rhesus monkey. Contrib Embryol Carnegie Inst Wash 36: 153
7. Bayard F, Damilano S, Robel P, Beaulieu EE (1978) Cytoplasmic and nuclear estradiol and progesterone receptors in human endometrium. J Clin Endocrinol Metab 46: 635
8. Beller FK, Schewppe KW (1979) Review on the biology of menstrual blood. In: Beller FK, Schaumacher GFB (eds), The biology of the fluids of the female genital tract. Amsterdam, New York, Elsevier-North Holland Press, pp 231–245
9. Bigazzi M (1983) Specific endocrine function of human decidua. Semin Reprod Endocrinol 1: 343
10. Choo YC, Mak KC, Hsu C, Wong TS, Ma HK (1985) Postmenopausal uterine bleeding of nononcogenic cause. Obstet Gynecol 66: 225
11. Christiaens GCML, Sixma JJ, Haspels AA (1980) Morphology of haemostasis in menstrual endometrium. Br J Obstet Gynecol 87: 425

12. Clark JH, Hseuh AJW, Peck EJ Jr (1977) Regulation of estrogen receptor replenishment by progesterone. Ann NY Acad Sci 286: 161
13. Clark KE, Farley DB, Van Orden DE, Brody MJ (1977) Estrogen-induced uterine hyperemia and edema persist during histamine receptor blockade. Proc Soc Exp Biol Med 156: 411
14. Czekanowski R (1975) Investigations into spontaneous contractile activity of isolated human uterine arteries in vitro. Am J Obstet Gynecol 121: 718
15. Dallenbach FD, Dallenbach G (1964) Immunohistologische untersuchungen zur lokalisation des relaxins in menschlichen placenta und decidua. Virchows Arch [Pathol Anat] 337: 301
16. Dallenbach-Hellweg G (1975) Histopathology of the endometrium, 2nd ed. New York, Springer-Verlag
17. Daly JJ, Balogh K Jr (1968) Hemorrhagic reaction of the senile endometrium ("apoplexia uteri"). Relation to superficial hemorrhagic necrosis of the bowel. N Engl J Med 278: 709
18. Epivanova OI (1971) Effects of hormones on the cell cycle. In: Baserga R (ed) The cell cycle and cancer. New York, Dekker, pp 145–190
19. Ferenczy A (1976) Studies on the cytodynamics of human endometrial regeneration: I. Scanning electron microscopy. Am J Obstet Gynecol 124: 64
20. Ferenczy A (1976) Studies on the cytodynamics of human endometrial regeneration: II. Transmission electron microscopy and histochemistry. Am J Obstet Gynecol 124: 582
21. Ferenczy A (1977) Studies on the cytodynamics of experimental endometrial regeneration in the rabbit: Historadioautography and ultrastructure. Am J Obstet Gynecol 128: 536
22. Ferenczy A (1980) Regeneration of the human endometrium. In: Fenoglio CM, Wolff M (eds) Progress in surgical pathology. New York, Masson Publishing USA Inc., Vol 1, pp 157–173
23. Ferenczy A (1981) The endometrial cycle. In: Sciarra JJ (ed) Gynecology and obstetrics. New York, Harper & Row, Vol 5, pp 1–14
24. Ferenczy A, Guralnick M (1983) Endometrial microstructure: Structure-function relationships throughout the menstrual cycle. Semin Reprod Endocrinol 1: 205
25. Ferenczy A, Richart RM (1974) Female reproductive system: Dynamics of scan and transmission electron microscopy. New York, John Wiley & Sons
26. Ferenczy A, Bertrand G, Gelfand MM (1979) Proliferation kinetics of human endometrium during the normal menstrual cycle. Am J Obstet Gynecol 133: 859
27. Ferenczy A, Richart RM, Agate FJ Jr, Purkerson ML, Dempsey EW (1972) Scanning electron microscopy of the endometrial surface. Fertil Steril 23: 515
28. Fitzpatrick RL, Liggins GC (1980) Effects of prostaglandins on the cervix of pregnant women and sheep. In: Naftolin F, Stubblefield PF (eds) Dilatation of the uterine cervix. New York, Raven Press, pp 287–300
29. Flowers CE Jr, Wilborn WH (1978) New observations on the physiology of menstruation. Obstet Gynecol 51: 16–24
30. Folkman J (1976) The vascularization of tumors. Sci Am 234: 58
31. Gorski J, Stornshak F, Harris J, Wertz N (1977) Hormone regulation of growth: Stimulatory and inhibitory influences of estrogens on DNA synthesis. J Toxicol Environ Health 3: 271
32. Gorski J, Toft D, Shyamala G, Smith D, Motides A (1968) Hormone receptors: Studies on the interaction of estrogen with the uterus. Recent Prog Horm Res 24: 45
33. Greene GL, Nolan C, Engner JP, Jensen EW (1980) Monoclonal antibodies to human estrogen receptors. Proc Natl Acad Sci USA 77: 5115
34. Gurpide E, Tseng L, Gusberg SB (1977) Estrogen metabolism in normal and neoplastic endometrium. Am J Obstet Gynecol 129: 809
35. Hendrickson MR, Kempson RL (1980) Surgical pathology of the uterine corpus. In: Bennington JL (ed) Major problems in pathology. Philadelphia W.B. Saunders, Vol 12
36. Henzl MR, Smith RE, Boost G, Tyler ET (1972) Lysosomal concept of menstrual bleeding in humans. J Clin Endocrinol Metab 34: 860
37. Hertig AT (1964) Gestational hyperplasia of endometrium. A morphologic correlation of ova, endometrium and corpora lutea during pregnancy. Lab Invest 13: 1153
38. Jensen EV (1984) Intracellular localization of estrogen receptors: Implications for interaction mechanism (Editorial). Lab Invest 51: 487
39. Johnson DC, Dey SK (1980) Role of histamine in implantation: Dexamethasone inhibits estradiol-induced implantation in the rat. Biol Reprod 22: 1136
40. Katzenellenbogen BS (1980) Dynamics of steroid hormone receptor action. Annu Rev Physiol 42: 17
41. Kennedy TG (1980) Prostaglandins and the endometrial vascular permeability changes preceding blastocyst implantation and decidualization. Prog Reprod Biol 7: 234
42. Kerns M, Lala PK (1983) Life history of decidual cells: A review. Am J Reprod Immunol 3: 78
43. King W, Greene GL (1984) Monoclonal antibodies localize estrogen receptor in the nuclei of target cells. Nature 307: 745
44. Kok P (1979) Separation of plasminogen activators from human plasma and a comparison with activators from human uterine tissue and urine. Thromb Haemost 4: 734
45. Kurman RJ, Young RH, Norris HJ, Main CS, Lawrence WD, Scully RE (1984) Immunocytochemical localization of placental lactogen and chorionic gonadotropin in the normal placenta and trophoblastic tumors, with emphasis on intermediate trophoblast and the placental site trophoblastic tumor. Int J Gynecol Pathol 3: 101
46. Langlois PL (1970) The size of the normal uterus. J Reprod Med 4: 220
47. Lawn AM, Wilson EW, Finn CA (1971) The ultrastructure of human decidual and predecidual cells. J Reprod Fertil 26: 85
48. Levitt MJ, Tobon H, Josimovich JB (1975) Prostaglandin content of human endometrium. Fertil Steril 26: 296
49. Lichtig C, Deutch M, Barnes J (1984) Vascular changes of endometrium in early pregnancy. Am J Clin Pathol 81: 702

50. Lindeman HJ (1979) Hysteroscopic data during menstruation. In: Beller FK, Schaumacher GFB (eds) The biology of the fluids of the female genital tract. Amsterdam, New York, Elsevier-North Holland Press, pp 225–229
51. Markee JE (1940) Menstruation in intraocular endometrial transplants in the rhesus monkey. Contrib Embryol Carnegie Inst Wash 28: 219
52. Marks I (1976) The epidermal chalones. In: Houck JC (ed) Chalones. Amsterdam, North Holland Publishing Co., pp 173–227
53. Mazur MT, Hendrickson MR, Kempson RL (1983) Optically clear nuclei. An alteration of endometrial epithelium in the presence of trophoblast. Am J Surg Pathol 7: 415
54. Meyer WC, Malkasian GD, Dockerty MB, Decker DG (1971) Postmenopausal bleeding from atrophic endometrium. Obstet Gynecol 38: 731
55. More IAR, Armstrong EM, McSeveney D, Chatfield WR (1974) The morphogenesis and fate of the nucleolar channel system in the human endometrial glandular cells. J Ultrastruct Res 47: 74
56. Noyes RW (1973) Normal phases of the endometrium. In: Norris HJ, Hertig AT, Abell MR (eds) The uterus. Baltimore, Williams & Wilkins Co., pp 110–135
57. Noyes RW, Hertig AT, Rock J (1950) Dating the endometrial biopsy. Fertil Steril 1: 3
58. Ober WB (1979) Carcinosarcoma of the ovary. Case report, review of literature and comment on the subcoelomic mesenchyme. Am J Diag Gynecol Obstet 1: 73
59. O'Rahilly R (1977) Prenatal human development. In: Wynn RM (ed) Biology of the uterus. New York, Plenum Press, pp 35–57
60. Orcel L, Smadj A, Roland J, Minh HN (1973) Nouvelle hypothèse sur le méchanisme intime de la menstruation. Rev Fr Gynecol 68: 477
61. Plenzl AA, Friedman EA (1971) Lymphatic system of the female genitalia. The morphologic basis of oncologic diagnosis and therapy. Philadelphia, W.B. Saunders Co.
62. Press MF, Goebl-Novsek M, King WJ, Herbst AL, Greene GL (1984) Immunohistochemical assessment of estrogen receptor distribution in the human endometrium throughout the menstrual cycle. Lab Invest 51: 495
63. Pryse Davies J, Ryder TA, Mackenzie ML (1979) In vivo production of the nucleolar channel system in postmenopausal endometrium. Cell Tissue Res 203: 493
64. Psychoyos A (1973) Endocrine control of egg implantation. In: Greep RO, Astwood EB, Geiger SR (eds) Handbook of physiology. Washington, American Physiol Soc, Vol 11, pp 187–215
65. Ramsey EM History. In: Wynn RM (ed) Biology of the uterus. New York, Plenum Press, pp 1–34
66. Ramsey EM (1977) Vascular anatomy. In: Wynn RM (ed) Biology of the uterus. New York, Plenum Press, pp 59–76
67. Rebello R, Green FHY, Fox H (1975) A study of the secretory immune system of the female genital tract. Br J Obstet Gynaecol 82: 812
68. Sananes N, Baulieu EE, Le Goascogne C (1976) Prostaglandin(s) as inductive factor of decidualization in the rat uterus. Mol Cell Endocrinol 6: 153
69. Shyamala G, Ferenczy A (1984) Mammary fat pad may be a potential site for initiation of estrogen action in normal mouse mammary glands. Endocrinology 115: 1078
70. Silverberg SG, Arias-Stella J (1972) Phenomenon in spontaneous and therapeutic abortion. Am J Obstet Gynecol 112: 777
71. Srivastava, KC (1978) Prostaglandins and platelet function. S Afri J Sci 74: 290
72. Szego CM (1972) Lysosomal membrane stabilization and antiestrogen action in specific hormonal target cells. Gynecol Invest 3: 63
73. Taylor PV, Hancock KW (1975) Antigenicity of trophoblast and possible antigen-marking effects during pregnancy. Immunology 28: 973
74. Tseng L (1979) Physiologic changes in binding and metabolism of estradiol and progesterone in human endometrium during the menstrual cycle. Obstet Gynecol Annu 8: 1
75. Van Orden DE, Clancey CJ, Farley DB (1981) Uterine serotonin and receptor blockage during estrogen-induced uterine hyperemia. Proc Soc Exp Biol Med 167: 469
76. Wagner D, Richart RM (1968) Polyploidy in the human endometrium with the Arias-Stella reaction. Arch Pathol 85: 475
77. Weissman G (1964) Labilization and stabilization of lysosomes. Fed Proc 23: 1038
78. Winkler B, Alvarez S, Richart RM, Crum CP (1984) Pitfalls in the diagnosis of endometrial neoplasia. Obstet Gynecol 64: 185
79. Wood JC, Williams EA, Barley VL, Cowdell RH (1969) The activity of hydrolytic enzymes in the human endometrium during the menstrual cycle. J Obstet Gynaecol Br Commonw 76: 724
80. Wynn RM (1977) Histology and ultrastructure of the human endometrium. In: Wynn RM (ed) Biology of the uterus. New York, Plenum Press, pp 341–376
81. Zhinkin LD, Samoshkina NA (1967) DNA synthesis and cell proliferation during formation of deciduomata in mice. J Embryol Exp Morphol 17: 598

10

Benign Diseases of the Endometrium

Robert J. Kurman, M.D., and Michael T. Mazur, M.D.

A wide variety of benign diseases, from rare infections to commonplace polyps, occurs in the endometrium. Furthermore, since the uterus is a target organ for hormonal stimulation, morphologic changes involving the endometrium may reflect disorders in the hypothalamic–pituitary–ovarian axis. The histologic changes are typically manifested by abnormal uterine bleeding, and an endometrial biopsy or curettage is commonly performed to control excessive bleeding or, more often, to determine its cause. The endometrial biopsy also continues to be an important and integral part of the infertility work-up. This chapter considers various benign conditions involving the uterus, with emphasis on the interpretation of endometrial biopsies and curettings. Congenital abnormalities of the uterus are also discussed.

Congenital Abnormalities

Congenital abnormalities of the uterus are uncommon.[10] Many of these abnormalities are due to the effects of exogenous hormones, such as diethylstilbestrol (DES),[74]

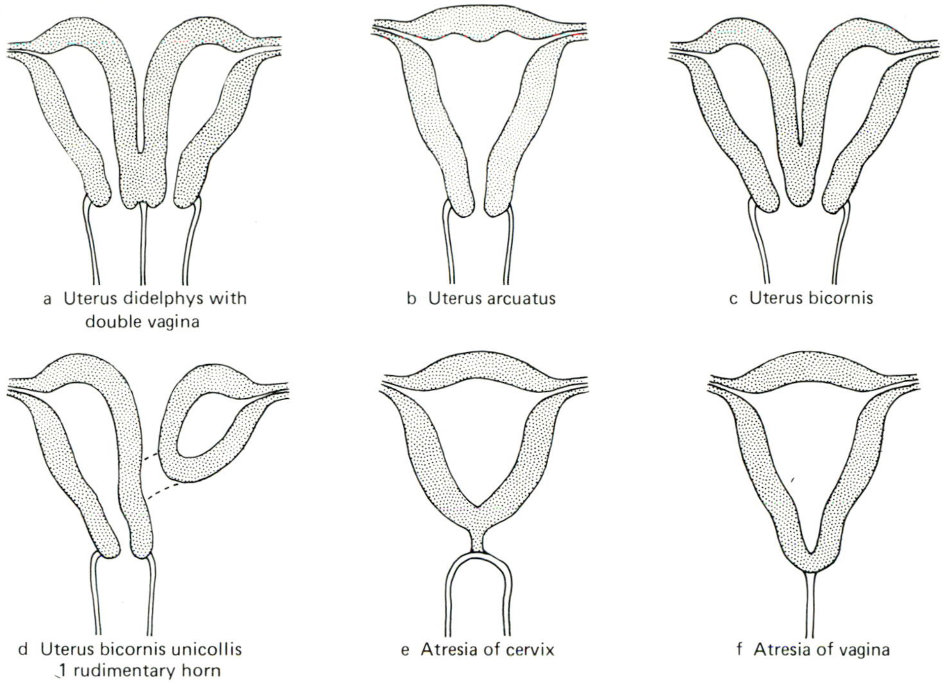

FIG. 10.1. Schematic representation of the main congenital abnormalities of the uterus and vagina caused by persistence of the uterine septum or obliteration of the lumen of the uterine canal. (From Sadler TW: Langman's Medical Embryology, Fifth edition. 1985, Williams & Wilkins Company. Reproduced by permission.)

in utero or endogenous hormones associated with abnormal gonads, and chromosomal defects. The latter group of congenital disorders is described in Chapter 2, Abnormal Sexual Development, and the upper and lower genital tract structural abnormalities associated with in utero DES exposure are discussed in Chapter 4, Diseases of Vagina. Another group of müllerian duct abnormalities occurs in genotypically normal females with normal gonads. These developmental aberrations, such as defects in the fusion of the müllerian ducts, are due to faulty morphogenesis and are similar to those occurring in other organ systems of the embryo. Little is known of their precise etiology. Some may result from abnormal hormonal stimulation, and others may be of genetic origin. These disorders may be quite complex and are frequently associated with malformations in the urinary system and the distal gastrointestinal tract (see Chapter 1, Embryology). For practical purposes, these müllerian duct abnormalities can be divided into two categories: (1) abnormalities of fusion and (2) abnormalities due to atresia (Fig. 10.1).

Fusion Defects of the Müllerian Ducts

Normally, the upper one-third of the vagina and the uterus are formed by fusion of the paired müllerian ducts. Following fusion, the intervening wall degenerates, forming the endometrial cavity and upper vaginal canal. Two types of abnormalities can occur depending on whether fusion or subsequent degeneration is the pathologic process. Nonfusion of the müllerian ducts gives rise to the *uterus bicornis* (Fig. 10.1c). Persistence of the fused ducts with failure of degeneration results in the development of a septum. If the defect is minor and confined to the fundus, the uterus is referred to as *arcuatus* (Fig. 10.1b). If the septum persists throughout the full length of the uterus and upper vagina, a *uterus didelphys* with a partially double vagina results (Fig. 10.1a). These congenital anomalies may cause infertility or spontaneous abortion and therefore require surgical correction.[48,166]

Atresia of the Müllerian Ducts and Vagina

Atresia can be partial or complete, but a wide range of intermediate degrees of atresia may be encountered. The etiology of this condition is obscure, although a genetic cause is sometimes apparent since siblings may be affected. The pattern of inheritance may be autosomal recessive[92,177] or dominant.[36]

If just one of the müllerian ducts is involved, only the fimbriae and a small muscular mass at the pelvic side wall will form. Occasionally, a rudimentary structure remains as an appendage attached to the unaffected side, giving rise to what is referred to as *uterus bicornis unicollis with a rudimentary horn* (Fig. 10.1d) With bilateral atresia, the upper genital tract may consist of bilateral noncanalized strands of muscular tissue located on the lateral pelvic walls. In severe defects, there is müllerian and vaginal aplasia. This abnormality, referred to as the *Rokitansky-Kuster-Hauser syndrome*, is frequently associated with urinary tract anomalies, such as a pelvic kidney or absence of a kidney. Vertebral and other skeletal abnormalities may also occur, suggesting a severe generalized morphogenetic abnormality involving several organ systems simultaneously.

Patients with these conditions are endocrinologically normal and have complete gonadal development. If the anomaly results in obstruction of the vagina with functional endometrial tissue present, hydrocolpos may be present at birth, or adolescents may present with primary amenorrhea. If only one müllerial duct is affected, giving rise to a rudimentary horn of a uterus bicornis unicollis, a young woman may have regular menstrual cycles associated with a pelvic mass and cyclic pelvic pain. A number of multiple malformation syndromes have been associated with müllerian or vaginal agenesis, such as the Winter syndrome, characterized by vaginal agenesis, renal agenesis, and middle ear anomalies.[176] This condition is inherited in an autosomal recessive manner.

Treatment of patients with complete vaginal atresia requires surgery to create a neovagina. If the anomaly is isolated *vaginal atresia* (Fig. 10.1f), as most commonly occurs, the patient will usually be fertile if a normal uterus and fallopian tubes are present.

Inflammation

Endometritis is divided into acute and chronic forms, depending on the type of inflammatory infiltrate. Chronic endometritis is further subdivided into specific types, depending on whether specific morphologic changes or an etiologic agent can be recognized.

Acute Endometritis

Pathology. The presence of necrosis, hemorrhage, and a polymorphonuclear leukocytic (PML) infiltrate is a normal physiologic event occurring in menstrual endometrium and shedding decidua following pregnancy. Consequently, the histologic diagnosis of acute endometritis is based on finding focal aggregates of PMLs in the stroma, that is, forming microabscesses or disrupting and filling gland lumens (Fig. 10.2). Even during the late phase of menstruation, cells having the appearance of neutrophils are found in great abundance in the stroma, but few are present within gland lumens. Some cells with lobated nuclei have been termed *stromal granulocytes*.[28] These cells closely resemble PMLs and eosinophils, having dark, lobate nuclei and intracytoplasmic eosinophilic granules. Electron microscopic and immunohistochemical studies have shown that the cytoplasmic granules in these cells, unlike leukocytes and eosinophils, contain relaxin, which may play a role in the dissolution of the endometrial stroma at the time of menses. This has led some observers[28] to propose that the endometrial stromal cell differentiates along two lines, one terminating in the formation of a decidual cell and the other in the formation of a granulocyte (see Chapter 9, Uterine Corpus).

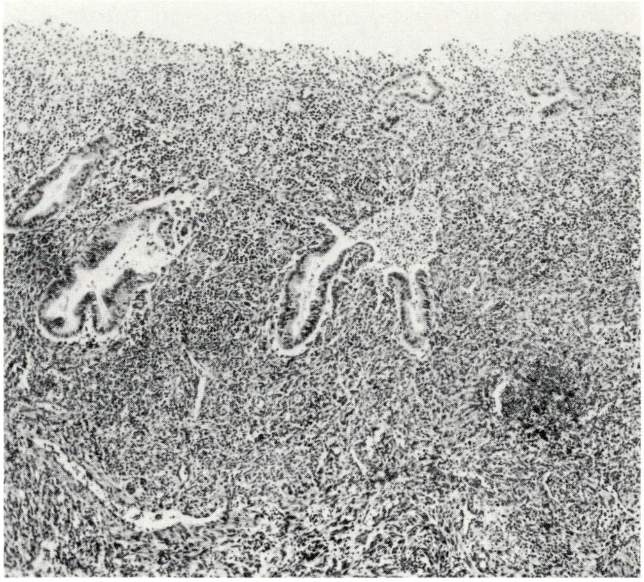

FIG. 10.2. Acute endometritis. A profuse infiltrate of polymorphonucelar leukocytes disrupts and fills gland lumens. Microabscess is shown on the *right*.

Clinical Aspects. The cervix acts as a barrier to the entry of microorganisms into the endometrial cavity. Except for rare forms of endometritis established by hematogenous implantation or descending infection from the fallopian tubes (e.g., tuberculosis), most types of endometritis result from ascending infection through the cervix. The usually impervious cervical barrier is compromised during menses, abortion, parturition, and instrumentation (e.g., curettage, insertion of an intrauterine device, cervical conization). In such instances, bacteria, some of which comprise the normal vagina flora, gain access to the endometrial cavity but usually without colonizing or producing infection.

Clinically significant acute endometritis is usually associated with pregnancy or abortion. The complex clinical aspects of postpartum and postabortal endometritis are beyond the scope of this presentation and are detailed elsewhere.[82,100] Most acute endometritis is caused by hemolytic *Streptococcus*, anaerobic *Streptococcus*, *Sta-*

phylococcus, *Neisseria gonorrhoeae*, and *Clostridium welchii*. The inflammatory reaction is nonspecific, and these organisms can only be identified by culture. The diagnosis of acute endometritis is made on clinical grounds; curettage in such instances is performed to remove devitalized and necrotic tissue that serves as a nidus of infection.

Chronic Endometritis—Nonspecific

Pathology. Lymphocytes that are not arranged in distinct aggregates occur in normal endometrium.[126] Moreover, granulation tissue seldom develops in the endometrium despite marked chronic inflammation. The diagnosis of chronic endometritis, therefore, rests on the identification of plasma cells (Fig. 10.3).[15,17,35,138] Plasma cells may be scant and difficult to identify in some instances. They should not be confused with stromal cells that have a dense, eccentrically placed nucleus and pale-staining cytoplasm. Close scrutiny for the clockface nucleus of the plasma cell should resolve equivocal cases. Immunohistochemical stains for immunoglobulins may also be helpful. The inflammatory infiltrate in chronic endometritis is composed of variable numbers of lymphocytes, plasma cells, and macrophages. The heterogeneous nature of the infiltrate is a useful feature in distinguishing chronic endometritis from the rare examples of lymphoma that may involve the endometrium[56] (see Chapter 13, Mesenchymal Tumors of Uterus).

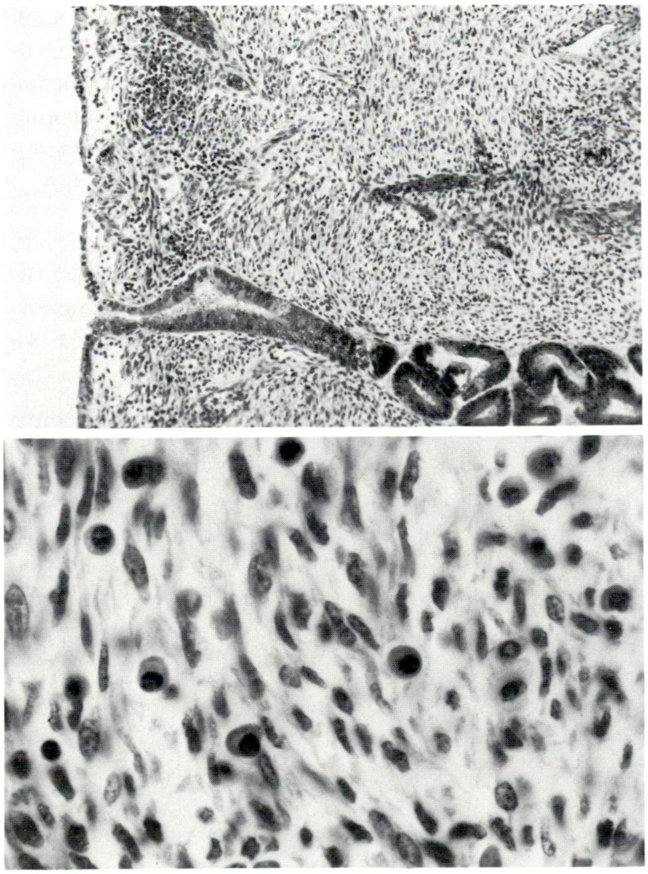

FIG. 10.3. *Top*. Chronic endometritis characterized by aggregates of lymphocytes and plasma cells. *Bottom*. Plasma cells with eccentrically placed nuclei and clockface chromatin pattern.

Under low magnification, two important clues alert the pathologist to look carefully for plasma cells. First, with chronic inflammation, the endometrium is difficult to date.[113] Frequently, this is manifested by either a wide variation in the maturation of the glands or a dyssynchrony between the glands and the stroma. Some glands are inactive, and it may be difficult to decide whether they are proliferative or secretory. Second, the stromal cells undergo a characteristic spindle cell alteration. The nuclei become enlarged, oval, or spindle-shaped and tend to palisade around glands in a pinwheel arrangement (Fig. 10.4). Occasionally, regenerative activity is more pronounced, and the glandular cells become stratified, with enlarged rounded nuclei and prominent nucleoli. Squamous metaplasia may be found in association with chronic endometritis.

Clinical Aspects. Chronic endometritis has been observed in 3–10% of women undergoing an endometrial biopsy for irregular bleeding.[49,138] Patients may have menometrorrhagia, mucopurulent cervical discharge, uterine tenderness, or an elevated erythrocyte sedimen-

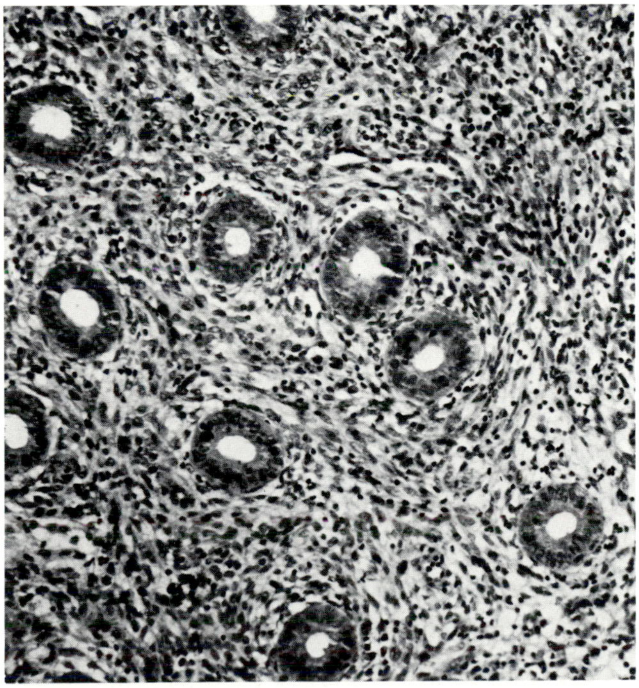

FIG. 10.4. Chronic endometritis. Note the spindle-shaped stromal cells surrounding glands in a pinwheel arrangement.

tation rate and/or white blood cell count, but some women are asymptomatic. Chronic endometritis has been associated with an abortion in 41%, with salpingitis in 25%, with an intrauterine device (IUD) in 14%, and with a recent pregnancy in 12%.[17] It also occurs in association with necrotic tissue, such as an infarcted polyp or carcinoma, or in association with cervical stenosis secondary to radiation or cryosurgery.

The histologic diagnosis of chronic endometritis in an asymptomatic patient who has not been recently pregnant, has had an abortion, or is using an IUD should be followed by an endocervical culture for gonococci and *Chlamydia*. In a study of women with mucopurulent cervicitis, attending a sexually transmitted disease clinic, 40% were found to have chronic endometritis.[125] *Chlamydia trachomatis* and/or *N. gonorrhoeae* was isolated from the cervix but not from the endometrium in 58%.

A major problem in the diagnosis of *Chlamydia* infection has been the requirement of a mammalian cell culture system. In the future, an immunofluorescence stain using monoclonal antibodies on cervical smears may aid in its detection.[157] Nonetheless, *Chlamydia* has been identified in the endometrium by culture[124] as well as by immunocytochemical techniques on paraffin-embedded tissue.[175] In immunocytochemical analysis, *Chlamydia* was found in only 4% of 90 endometrial biopsies showing chronic endometritis; this percentage rose to 57% in biopsies of patients with severe chronic endometritis and superimposed acute inflammation. Besides the inflammatory reaction, positive cases were associated with stromal necrosis and reparative cytologic atypia in the glandular and surface epithelium. Chlamydial inclusions were difficult to identify, being obscured by the inflammatory infiltrate (see Fig. 6.6). *Chlamydia* does not usually produce severe pain and fever and, consequently, may be responsible for most cases of tubal damage associated with infertility in which there is no apparent history of pelvic inflammatory disease. Because of the difficulty in identifying *Chlamydia*, it may be prudent to treat asymptomatic women with negative cultures for 2 weeks with oral antibiotics, such as tetracycline.

Chronic Endometritis—Specific Types

Mycoplasma

Pathology. *Mycoplasma* infection of the endometrium has been associated with infertility and fetal wastage.[155,161,162] Three species of *Mycoplasma*, *Mycoplasma hominis*, *Mycoplasma fermentans*, and *Ureaplasma urealyticum*, have been demonstrated in the lower female genital tract.[19,42,43,121,161] Although some studies have associated *M. hominis* with reproductive failure, *U. urealyticum* has been most strongly associated with infertility and reproductive failure.[19,43,154]

Significant endometrial infection with *U. urealyticum* should cause an identifiable inflammatory response. Horne et al. have identified a lesion termed *subacute focal inflammation* (SFI), associated with *U. urealyticum*.[61] The lesion is characterized by focal collections of lymphocytes; plasma cells and PMLs are rarely seen. The lymphoid aggregates may be small and few in number, making their detection, at times, difficult. They are mostly easily identified from the 20th to the 23rd (POD 6–9) days of the cycle, when there is maximal stromal edema. The lesions are usually without germinal centers and tend to be localized just beneath the surface endometrium, adjacent to glands, or around spiral arterioles.

Clinical Aspects. Genital mycoplasmas are generally transmitted by sexual contact but the organisms have been cultured from prepubertal girls and women who have denied sexual contact. Other modes of transmission, such as autoinfection from the anal canal, may therefore occur.[66a] Although *Mycoplasma* species, especially *U. urealyticum*, appear to have a role in some cases of unexplained infertility, the relationship of this organism to endometrial infection is controversial.[19,20,50] Data regarding both the culture of the organism from the endometrium and the association of positive cultures with an inflammatory endometrial response have been conflicting.[19,20,50,61] The differences in isolation rate in infertile women may be due to cervical contamination, since mycoplasmas more frequently colonize the lower genital tract.[161] Cervicovaginal isolation of *U. urealyticum* was associated with male factor infertility in one study,[20] suggesting that the organism may be a more significant pathogen in males, where it can interfere with spermatogenesis and reduce spermatozoa motility[20] rather than affecting the endometrium.

The effect of ureaplasmas on infertility also may be indirect in women. For example, in a recent study of 262 patients, it was reported that 87% of women with SFI had pelvic adhesions evident at laparoscopy compared to only 11% who did not have SFI ($P = 0.0001$).[16] It has been postulated that ureaplasmas, if they cause the lesions, may be responsible for producing adhesions or may place the patient at risk for developing more severe adhesions (see Interpretation of the Endometrial Biopsy).

Tuberculosis

Pathology. The endometrium is affected in one-half to three-quarters of patients with genital tuberculosis.[111] Endometrial involvement occurs from seeding by organisms draining from the fallopian tubes directly. Infection in the fallopian tubes is acquired by hematogenous or, rarely, lymphatic spread from a primary focus in the lung or gastrointestinal tract.[56]

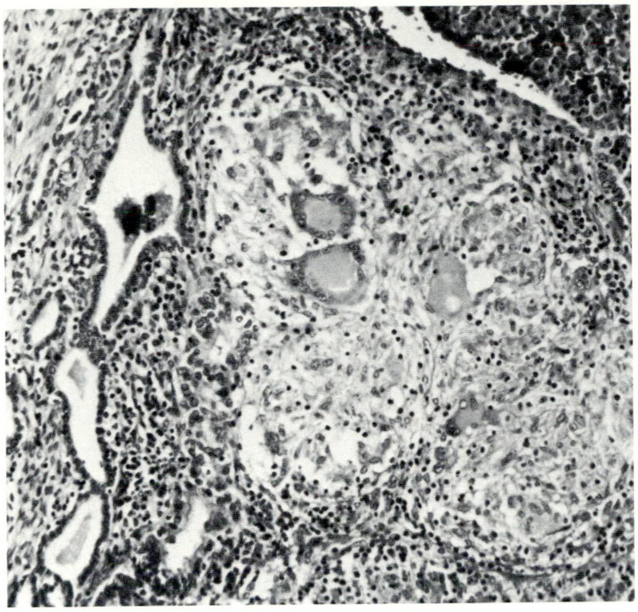

FIG. 10.5. Tuberculous endometritis with multiple granulomas containing Langhan's giant cells.

The extent of the inflammatory involvement in tuberculous endometritis varies from a focal process with very few granulomas to a diffuse process with ulceration of the mucosa and extensive caseous necrosis. The typical granulomatous inflammation with Langhan's giant cells (Fig. 10.5) is not always present. The process may be manifested only by a nonspecific endometritis with focal or diffuse infiltrates of plasma cells and lymphocytes.[28] Frequently, destruction of glands occurs, with the inflammatory infiltrate filling gland lumens, as in nonspecific endometritis. The inflammation is usually confined to the superficial and intermediate portion of the endometrium, with transmural involvement occurring only in very severe infections.[111] A reactive proliferative epithelial response with cellular stratification, mild nuclear atypia, and squamous metaplasia may occur. This atypical proliferation should not be confused with a neoplastic process.

Clinical Aspects. Tuberculous endometritis is a manifestation of a systemic disease; its frequency parallels that of pulmonary tuberculosis in the population. Rare in the United States, Germany, and eastern Europe, tuberculous endometritis is more common in England, Spain, and India.[14,66,104,111,156] It is generally found in women during their reproductive years, but it also occurs in postmenopausal women. Sometimes, genital tuberculosis is discovered during the course of an investigation for infertility. The diagnosis of tuberculous endometritis in this setting terminates the work-up, as such patients are nearly always sterile. Following appropriate antimicrobial therapy, the tubercles become hyalinized, but the inflammatory infiltrate may persist for years. In the rare instances of subsequent fertility, implantation is likely to occur in the fallopian tube. Intrauterine pregnancy may terminate in fatal miliary tuberculosis. In addition to infertility, other clinical manifestations of genital tuberculosis may include a pelvic mass or lower abdominal pain. Often the diagnosis of tuberculous endometritis is not made until the time of hysterectomy, when caseating granulomas are found in the fallopian tubes.

Histologic diagnosis of tuberculosis is difficult because the tubercles are often focal and take up to 2 weeks to develop, and the functionalis, where the tubercles usually occur, is shed every 4 weeks.[111] Thus, if tuberculosis is suspected, a curettage, rather than an endometrial biopsy, should be performed during the late secretory or menstrual phase of the cycle. Specific diagnosis requires culture or identification of acid-fast organisms, because other microorganisms may be associated with granulomatous inflammation. Acid-fast bacilli are rarely demonstrated, even when cultures are positive.[111]

Sarcoidosis

A few cases of sarcoid have had endometrial involvement in association with systemic sarcoidosis.[58,159] In contrast to tuberculosis, the granulomas in sarcoidosis are noncaseating, and acid-fast bacilli are not identified. Since these features may also be absent in tuberculous endometritis, every effort should be made to distinguish sarcoidosis from tuberculosis in view of the different prognosis and approach to treatment.

Fungal Infections

Blastomycosis (*Blastomyces dermatitidis*)[38] and coccidioidomycosis (*Coccidioides immitis*)[54,140] may produce granulomatous endometritis as part of a disseminated infection. The Gomori silver-methenamine stain and periodic acid-Schiff (PAS) reactions are helpful in distinguishing these infections from tuberculosis. There have been case reports of mycotic infection consistent with Candida[135] and cryptococcosis (*Cryptococcus glabratus*)[129] in the endometrium.

Viral Infections

Herpes virus (HSV),[132a,142] cytomegalovirus (CMV)[31,90,169] and human papillomavirus (HPV)[165a] are the only viruses known to infect the endometrium. HSV and CMV may be a source of neonatal infection, and CMV has been considered responsible for spontaneous abortion. In herpes infection, the glandular cells show nuclear enlargement, with round eosinophilic inclusions surrounded by a halo. There is associated necrosis in the stroma.[142] In CMV infection, the epithelial cells have

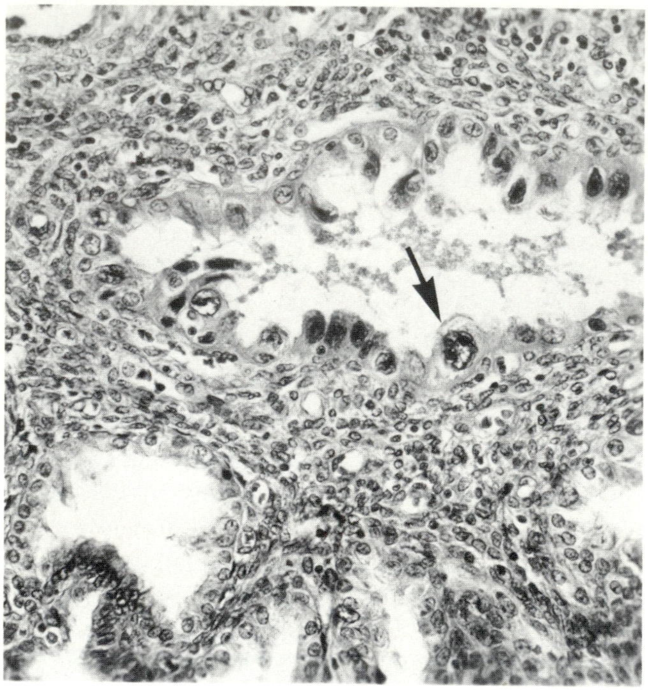

FIG. 10.6. Endometritis caused by infection with cytomegalovirus. Glandular cells are markedly enlarged and contain large, round basophilic inclusions (*arrow*).

a ground-glass appearance, are markedly enlarged, and contain large, round basophilic inclusions (Fig. 10.6). The Arias–Stella reaction (see Chapter 9, Uterine Corpus) that can occur in pregnancy and gestational trophoblastic disease may be confused with CMV because of the marked nuclear enlargement. In contrast to the Arias–Stella reaction, endometritis due to CMV has a plasma cell infiltrate and nuclear inclusions and lacks the associated features of gestational endometrium, such as decidua. Diffuse condylomatous involvement of the endometrium occurring secondary to cervical infection with HPV has been reported.[165a] The histologic features are the same as those observed in the cervix (see Chapter 7, Cervical Intraepithelial Neoplasia).

Parasitic Infections

Schistosoma,[11,103,174] *Enterobius vermicularis*,[141] and *Echinococcus granulosus*[167] are rare causes of endometritis in the United States, but schistosomiasis is endemic in Central America, Africa, the Middle East, and the Far East. Patients usually present with amenorrhea and infertility. The infection may be mild or severe and is characterized by granulomatous inflammation with lymphocytes, plasma cells, eosinophils, and histiocytes closely simulating a tubercle. The endometrial surface may ulcerate and be replaced by granulation tissue. Diagnosis is made by identifying the ova in tissue sections or in smears of vaginal secretions.

Toxoplasmosis (*Toxoplasma gondii*)[132,153] produces a nonspecific inflammation of the endometrium. The microorganism can be identified by immunofluorescence. Fragmentary data implicate this organism in the endometrium as a cause of congenital toxoplasmosis and habitual abortion.

Granulomatous Foreign Body Infections

Rarely, talc or other foreign substance may elicit a foreign body reaction in the endometrium.[28] Talc may be introduced into the endometrial cavity by instruments contaminated with talcum powder or by gloves during a pelvic examination. Patients may be asymptomatic or may have menorrhagia. Microscopically, the exent of the granulomatous inflammatory reaction depends on the quantity of the talc inoculated. The infiltrate is characterized by histiocytes and foreign body multinucleated giant cells surrounding the talc crystals, along with lymphocytes and plasma cells. The crystals appear as refractile, birefringent, needle-like, or fan-shaped splinters in polarizing light.

Miscellaneous Infections

Two rare forms of endometritis of probable bacterial origin that produce specific morphologic changes are pneumopolycystic endometritis[127] and malakoplakia.[131,164] The former is characterized by the presence of multiple thin-walled cysts and vesicles lined by flattened cells. Multinucleated giant cells are occasionally present. A similar condition can be seen in the vagina (see Chapter 4, Diseases of Vagina). The disease in the vagina is thought to result from infection by *Haemophilus vaginalis* or *Trichomonas*, but the precise origin of this condition in the endometrium is not known.

Malakoplakia is an unusual type of chronic inflammation most often involving the urinary bladder and only rarely affecting the genital tract. Of the 17 reported cases of genital malakoplakia, 4 have involved the endometrium.[23,99,131,164] On gross examination, the lesion is firm and indurated and may simulate a malignant tumor. Microscopically, malakoplakia is characterized by a monomorphic population of histiocytes containing eosinophilic or clear cytoplasm (Von Hansemann cells) and may, therefore, simulate a xanthogranulomatous inflammation or clear cell carcinoma.

The diagnosis of malakoplakia is made by the identification of intracellular and extracellular calcified spherules (Michaelis–Gutman bodies). *Escherichia coli* has been cultured from these lesions. It is thought that a defect in the phagocytic function of monocyte–macrophages leads to persistence of bacteria, which calcify to form Michaelis–Gutman bodies. Patients with malakoplakia involving the genital tract range in age from 29 to 84 years (mean 62), and the majority experience vaginal bleeding. Treatment consists of a course of antibiotics and surgical excision.

Functional Disorders

The endometrium is a sensitive bioassay for estrogen and progesterone. During the reproductive years, the endometrium in response to physiologic changes in estrogen and progesterone levels proliferates, differentiates, and sheds in a cyclical, generally predictable fashion. In ovulatory cycles, the luteal phase is 14 days in length, whereas the follicular phase is variable and may range from 10 to 20 days, yielding a wide range of cycle lengths among normal, ovulating women. Abnormalities along the hypothalamic–pituitary–ovarian axis may result in a derangement of follicular maturation, ovulation, or corpus luteum development, with subsequent abnormal hormone secretion. These alterations in the normal hormonal patterns are manifested by abnormal uterine bleeding, infertility, or both.

Dysfunctional Uterine Bleeding

This term is used for bleeding not attributable to underlying organic pathologic conditions.* Dysfunctional uterine bleeding is, therefore, synonymous with abnormal uterine bleeding resulting from derangements in the magnitude or duration of estrogen and progesterone effects on the endometrium.[51] Many uterine lesions can produce bleeding, and these should be excluded before making the diagnosis of dysfunctional uterine bleeding. Conditions that can cause abnormal bleeding include endometrial polyps, adenomyosis, leiomyomas, endometritis, atrophy, IUDs, oral contraceptive use, abortion, ectopic pregnancy, hyperplasia, malignant tumors, and gestational trophoblastic disease.

Estrogen withdrawal as a result of anovulatory cycles is the most common cause of dysfunctional uterine bleeding, but early decline of the corpus luteum or inadequate luteal function (luteal phase defect) is another cause. Failure of the corpus luteum to regress at the appropriate time can produce irregular shedding, a rare cause of dysfunctional uterine bleeding.

Estrogen Withdrawal Bleeding and Anovulation

Anovulatory cycles occur when there is development of one of more follicles in the ovary with estradiol synthesis by granulosa and theca cells. The estradiol promotes endometrial proliferation, however, there is no ovulation and subsequent progesterone production by a corpus luteum. Consequently, the endometrium grows without the stromal and glandular differentiation of the secretory phase. The follicles may persist and continue to produce estradiol, or they may regress, ending the estrogen production. When estrogen levels decline, the endometrium can no longer be maintained, and bleeding ensues. Bleeding in this situation is variable in amount and erratic in its pattern.

Dysfunctional uterine bleeding as a result of anovulatory cycles can occur at any time during the reproductive years, but it occurs characteristically at menarche and at menopause.[112] Nearly 60% of all cycles in the first year after menarche are anovulatory. For the vast majority of these women, ovulatory cycles ensue, but some women never establish normal cycles.[150] Women in this latter group have infrequent, irregular periods, occasionally marked by extremely heavy bleeding, which may require hospitalization. Typically, these women are also obese, infertile, and hirsute and are considered to have polycystic ovarian disease (Stein–Leventhal syndrome) (see Chapter 16, Nonneoplastic Lesions of Ovary). Many women in the reproductive age group with anovuluatory cycles, however, do not manifest these classic clinical features. Most of the cycles in a patient with polycystic ovarian disease are anovulatory, but as many as 25% of the cycles may be ovulatory, as documented by the presence of a corpus luteum.

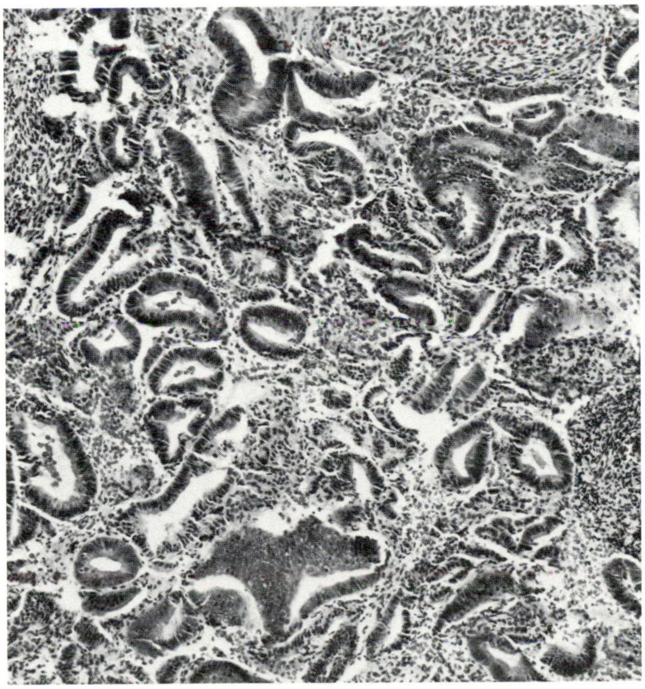

Fig. 10.7. The endometrium associated with estrogen withdrawal bleeding is characterized by fragmented proliferative glands, stromal necrosis, and hemorrhage. Compare with Fig. 10.10.

* References 2, 3, 9, 65, 72, 112, 130, 143, 148.

Pathology. The endometrium associated with anovulatory cycles reflects the effect of estrogen stimulation without subsequent progesterone stimulation from an intervening luteal phase. Typically, the glands are proliferative, but the degree of proliferation depends mainly on the duration of unopposed estrogenic stimulation. Over a period of months to years a variety of metaplasias, hyperplasia, and carcinoma can be produced (see Chapter 11, Endometrial Hyperplasia and Metaplasia, and Chapter 12, Endometrial Carcinoma).

An endometrial sample obtained during the bleeding phase is characterized by extensive tissue fragmentation that is readily apparent under low magnification (Fig. 10.7). As the ground substance undergoes dissolution, stromal cells condense and form compact nests of cells with hyperchromatic nuclei and little or no cytoplasm (Fig. 10.8). The normal architecture collapses. Isolated, fragmented glands lie in haphazard disarray without surounding stroma. Because of the profound degree of stromal necrosis and collapse, endometrial glands become artifactually crowded (Figs. 10.7 and 10.9). It is important not to confuse this appearance with the true glandular crowding of hyperplasia and carcinoma. Stromal breakdown also occurs in menstrual endometrium, but the glandular secretion and the predecidual reaction distinguish menstrual endometrium (Fig. 10.10) from the endometrial breakdown associated with estrogen withdrawal. Under higher magnification, the glandular epithelium displays no nuclear atypia (Fig. 10.11). Nuclear debris from necrotic cells is frequently phagocytized by glandular cells and appears as dark granules within the cytoplasm (Figs. 10.8 and 10.11). Scant focal subnuclear vacuolization may be seen (Fig. 10.11), but the extensive vacuolization characteristic of the early secretory phase does not occur.

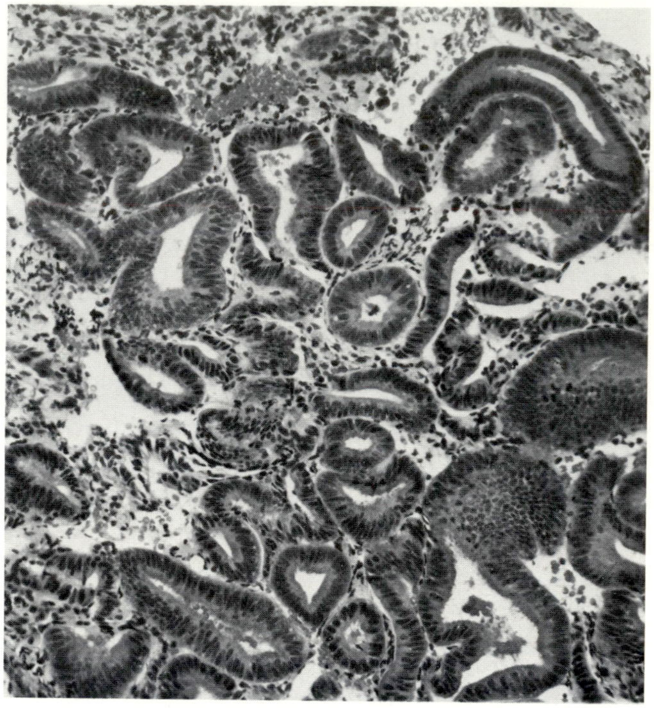

FIG. 10.9. Pseudoglandular crowding in the endometrium associated with estrogen withdrawal bleeding. The glands have fallen together and become crowded as a result of the dissolution of the intervening stroma. This should not be confused with crowding as a result of hyperplasia.

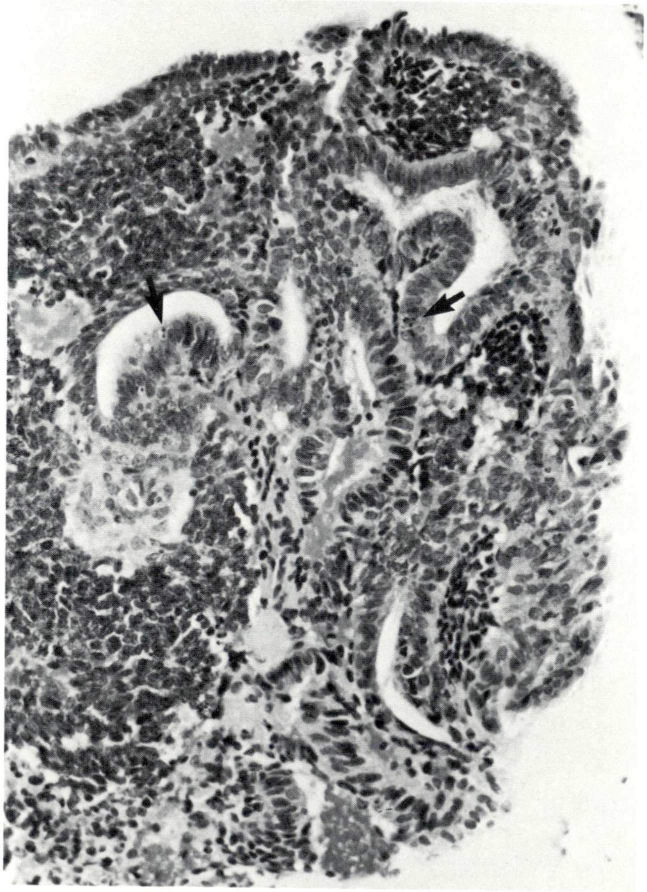

FIG. 10.8. Higher power of estrogen withdrawal bleeding, showing stromal collapse and condensation. Cellular necrosis is evidenced by nuclear debris (*arrows* within endometrial glandular epithelial cells).

In addition to the stromal and glandular changes, there are profound vascular alterations characterized by inhibition of spiral arterioles and an increase in thin-walled venules, many of which are ectatic. Typically, these blood vessels contain prominent fibrin thrombi (Fig. 10.12), a feature seldom encountered in normal menstrual endometrium.

When this pattern of collapse and bleeding is seen in proliferative endometrium, the diagnosis of *estrogen withdrawal endometrial breakdown* is made. This histologic pattern reflects endometrial breakdown due to falling estrogen levels. The endometrium was primed by

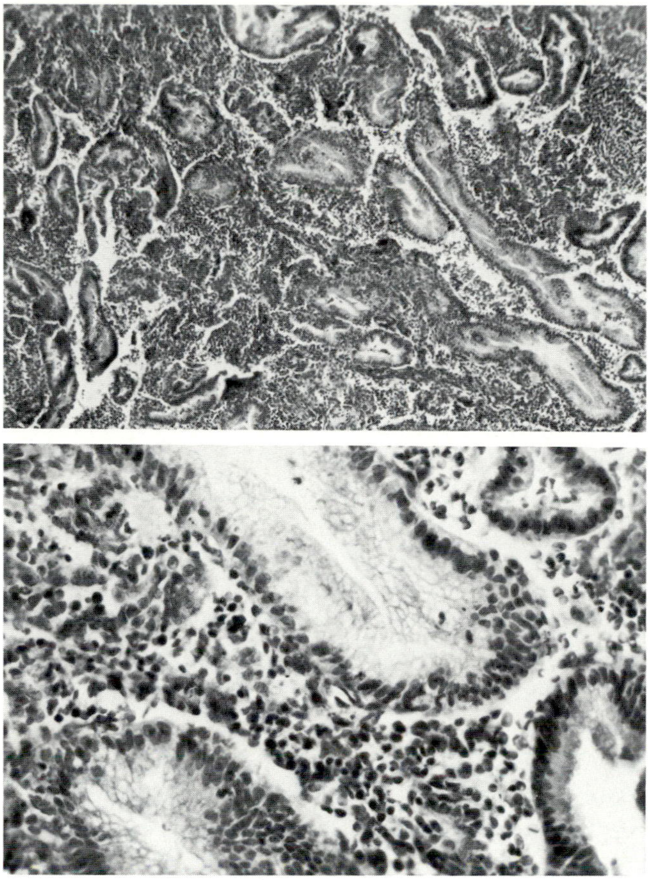

FIG. 10.10. *Top:* Menstrual endometrium showing diffuse hemorrhage, necrosis, and stromal breakdown. *Bottom:* Numerous glands containing vacuolated cytoplasm.

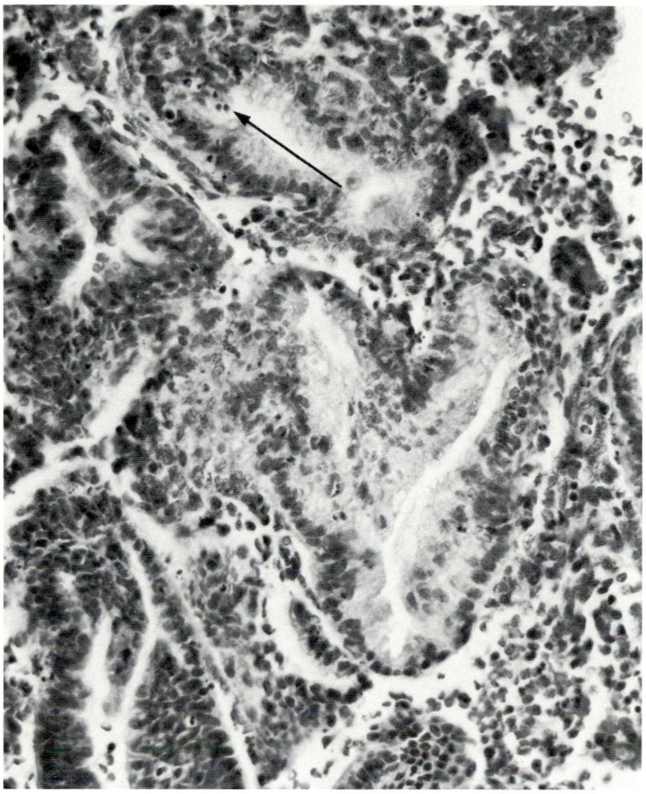

FIG. 10.11. Endometrial glands in association with estrogen withdrawal bleeding may contain nuclear debris (*arrow*) and show focal cytoplasmic vacuolation. This should not be interpreted as menstrual endometrium. Gland at lower *left* is clearly proliferative.

estrogen without adequate progesterone stimulation, and the bleeding is due to a relative lack of estrogen. The microscopic appearance is not specific and may reflect estrogen withdrawal associated with an anovulatory cycle, replacement estrogen therapy alone, or cyclic therapy with progesterone if the progesterone dose is inadequate to produce secretory differentiation.

Clinical Aspects. The bleeding during a normal menstrual cycle is a consequence of rhythmic vasospasm and relaxation of the spiral arterioles, resulting in a complete, yet self-limited sloughing of the functionalis layer (see Chapter 9, Uterine Corpus).[85,134] In anovulatory cycles, spiral arterioles fail to develop adequately, and the dilated, thin-walled venules undergo thrombosis. Stromal necrosis involving random portions of the endometrium results in incomplete shedding. Consequently, the bleeding pattern is asynchronous and highly variable in duration. Histologic examination of endometrial tissue removed at the time of bleeding may be scanty or abundant, depending on the duration and amount of bleeding that preceded the curettage.

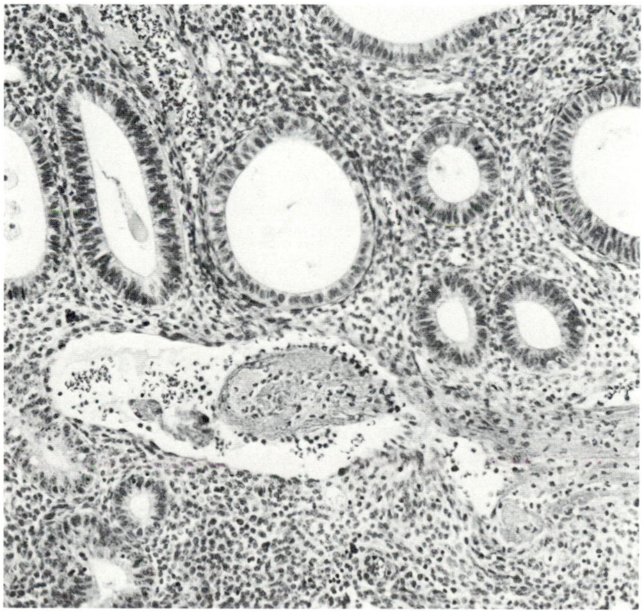

FIG. 10.12. Anovulatory cycles may be associated with mild endometrial hyperplasia. Bleeding is caused, in part, by disruption of thin-walled ectatic capillaries, many containing fibrin thrombi.

Treatment depends on the age of the patient. An acute bleeding episode in a women under the age of 35 years is best treated the first time with oral progestin–estrogen combination birth control pills.[151] The progestin stabilizes the uterine vasculature, differentiates the glands and stroma, and results in a complete shedding of the endometrium when therapy is discontinued, usually after 5–7 days. Bleeding may be heavy but is self-limited. In women over the age of 35 years and in young women whose bleeding is not controlled with hormones, an endometrial biopsy is necessary to rule out organic pathology. In young women with recurrent anovulatory cycles who are not immediately desirous of childbearing, a week's course of oral medoxyprogesterone acetate (Provera) every 2 months will prevent excessive endometrial buildup and should give controlled withdrawal bleeding. If bleeding occurs in an anovulatory patient who is infertile, induction of ovulation with clomiphene will result in ovulatory cycles and a normal menstrual pattern of bleeding.

Inadequate Luteal Phase

Inadequate luteal phase, also referred to as luteal phase defect (LPD), is generally thought to result from inadequate progesterone secretion by the corpus luteum. Recent studies suggest that LPD may also be the result of an end-organ receptor defect, in view of the finding of a reduced number of endometrial progesterone receptor binding sites in some patients with LPD.[79,152] As a result, menses occurs 6–9 days after the luteinizing hormone (LH) surge.[68,69,102] This disorder is primarily of concern in the evaluation of infertility. It may also be a factor in abnormal uterine bleeding.

The pathogenesis of this abnormality is complex and not completely understood. In many cases, LPD develops when the corpus luteum either fails to develop adequately or regresses prematurely. It is postulated that a poorly formed corpus luteum may be due to decreased FSH levels during the follicular phase or to lowered FSH and LH peaks at midcycle, resulting in deficient luteinization of the granulosa cells.[151] Elevated prolactin levels may also lead to LPD by suppressing progesterone release by the granulosa cells. Any of these processes could result in a reduction of the total amount of progesterone secreted by the corpus luteum.

Pathology. The pathologic features of LPD are not completely defined, mainly because there is no consensus on the exact criteria for the diagnosis. Characteristically, the endometrium in LPD has a normal secretory appearance but shows a lag of greater than 2 days from the expected day of the cycle, according to the basal body temperature graph and the onset of menses after biopsy (e.g., a day 22 pattern on day 26).[102,149] In normally cycling women, endometrial dating is, at best, an approximation, with variation from one microscopic field to another and between observers. Reproducibility of endometrial dating is within 2 days of the expected date in about 80% of cases.[114]

Depending on the relative amounts of hormones being secreted, the secretory patterns can become abnormal.[46] Precise dating is not possible in some instances. Terms, such as glandular–stromal dissociation, dyssynchrony, or irregular maturation, are applied to these patterns. In general, the glands and stroma are discordant in their development.[29] Glands may show secretory changes but lack the complex tortuosity expected. The stroma may remain nonreactive, without edema or predecidua formation, although the glands demonstrate secretory exhaustion.

The pathologic changes in secretory endometrium attributable to abnormal hormone relationships have not been well studied by careful clinicopathologic correlations of hormone levels, receptor status, and endometrial history. Consequently, although abnormally developed secretory phase endometrium may reflect LPD, the pathologic changes are not diagnostic.

Clinical Aspects. LPD is an uncommon cause of infertility, being found in only 3–5% of infertile women in most studies.[171] The significance and even the existence of the condition remains controversial because there is a lack of controlled studies evaluating its role in infertility. Luteal phase defect has also been suggested as a factor in early habitual spontaneous abortions and in abnormal uterine bleeding.[62]

To be significant, LPD must be demonstrated in at least two consecutive cycles because sporadic LPD occurs in normal women.[70] The endometrial biopsy is believed to be one of the best methods of establishing the diagnosis,[4,30,170] but basal body temperature graphs showing a temperature rise that is sustained for less than 10 days and low serum progesterone levels are valuable adjuncts.[26,30,136,151]

Various forms of treatment have been used. If LPD is thought to be due to low FSH and LH levels, clomiphene citrate or human menopausal gonadotropin is used to cause an elevation of FSH.[34,151] Progesterone replacement, in the form of daily progesterone vaginal suppositories following the midcycle temperature rise, is another type of treatment, since there is a deficiency of progesterone in LPD.[69,149,172] Alternatively, human chorionic gonadotropin (hCG) is administered to stimulate the corpus luteum to produce progesterone.[151] Bromocriptine, which inhibits prolactin secretion, is used in patients with LPD due to hyperprolactinemia.[32]

Irregular Shedding

Irregular shedding is characterized by prolonged, heavy bleeding at the time of menses, sometimes lasting longer

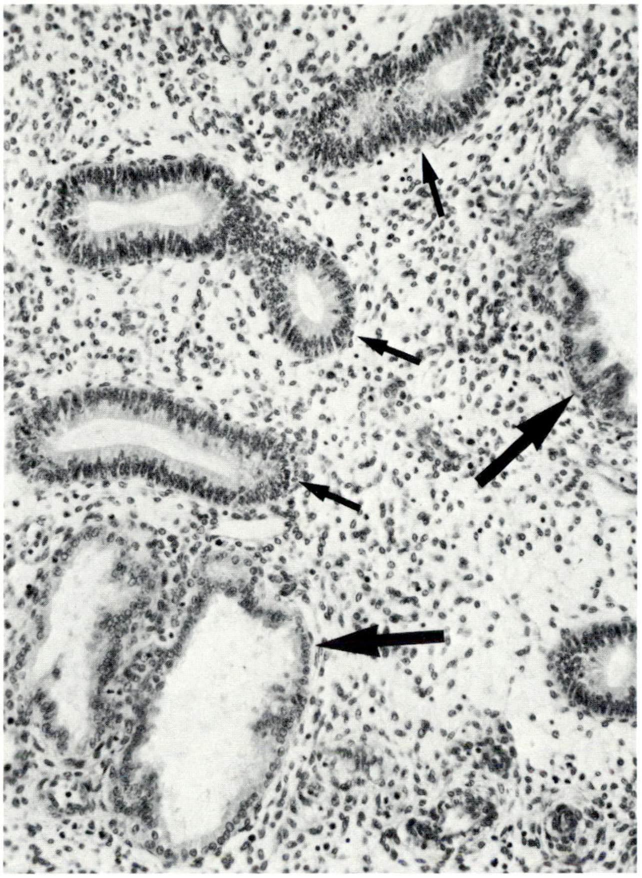

FIG. 10.13. Irregular shedding. Glands showing secretory exhaustion (*large arrows*) lie immediately adjacent to proliferative glands (*small arrows*) in an edematous, secretory-type, stroma.

than 2 weeks.[93,147] The continued bleeding appears to be caused by persistent corpus luteum function and continued secretion of progesterone, as irregular shedding can be produced by injecting small doses of progesterone during the menstrual phase of the cycle.[60]

Pathology. This entity is diagnosed on curettings obtained at least 5 days after the onset of bleeding and is characterized by a mixture of secretory and proliferative patterns (Fig. 10.13). There is a diverse array of endometrial fragments containing irregular star-shaped secretory glands admixed with early proliferative glands.[28] The stroma around these glands is dense and compact, with many stromal granulocytes. In areas containing secretory-type glands, the stroma is edematous and the stromal cells may be converted into predecidual cells (Fig. 10.14). Fibrin thrombi may be present, as in anovulatory cycles, but unlike irregular shedding, which demonstrates secretory and proliferative changes, anovulatory cycles demonstrate proliferative glands only. Luteal phase defect, in contrast, shows only secretory changes.

Clinical Aspects. This condition develops during the reproductive years, especially between the ages of 24 and 50 years.[91,163] Irregular shedding may occur at every menstrual period or only once, such as after a persistent corpus luteum cyst. Irregular shedding is a rare cause of abnormal bleeding. Other endometrial disorders, including abortions, polyps, and chronic endometritis, may produce bleeding patterns that mimic irregular shedding. These other lesions should be ruled out before making the diagnosis of irregular shedding.

The Endometrial Biopsy in Infertility

Infertility, defined as the inability to conceive over a period of at least 12 months, affects approximately 10% of American couples. In this section we consider uterine factors in infertility and consequently present a small aspect of a very complex problem. For example, male factors, which account for about 40% of infertility problems, are not considered here. In women, infertility may be the result of a variety of pathologic processes involving all levels of the female genital tract. For a discussion of the pathologic factors of infertility involving

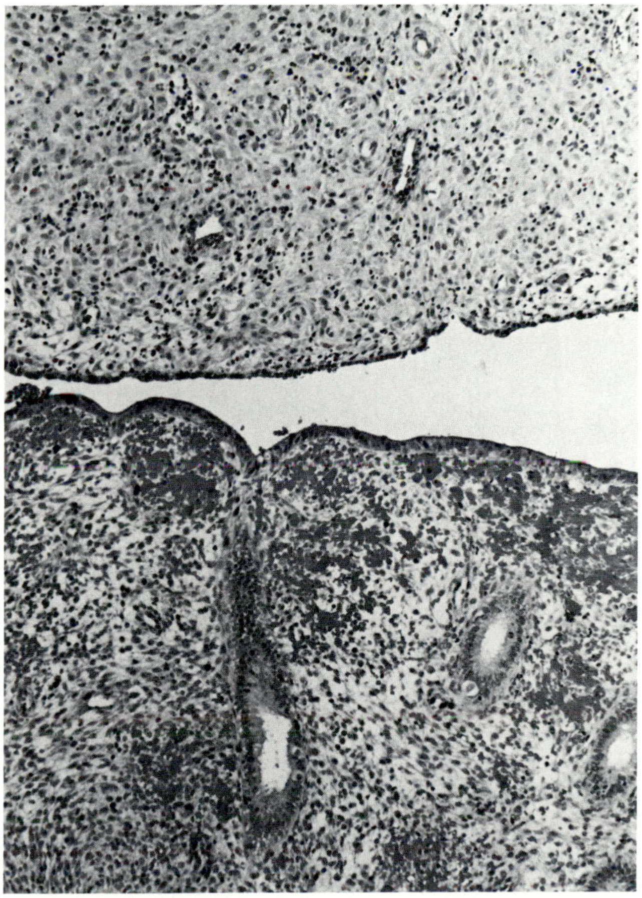

FIG. 10.14. Irregular shedding, with a secretory pattern showing a predecidual reaction (*top*) and a proliferative pattern (*bottom*).

the cervix, fallopian tubes, and ovary the reader is directed to Chapter 6, Benign Diseases of Cervix, Chapter 14, Diseases of Fallopian Tube, Chapter 16, Nonneoplastic Lesions of Ovary, and Chapter 17, Endometriosis, respectively. Uterine factors in infertility either are due to organic disorders, such as the presence of adhesions or leiomyomas, or reflect functional disorders due to gonadal disturbances, such as anovulation or LPD.[29] In addition, the presence of intrinsic organic disease, such as endometritis, can serve as an indicator of what is primarily an extrinsic process, that is, pelvic inflammatory disease involving the fallopian tubes and ovaries. An endometrial biopsy is, therefore, an important component of an evaluation of infertility.

Organic Disorders

Organic causes of infertility include chronic inflammation, leiomyomas, congenital uterine anomalies, and intrauterine adhesions.[27,166] Except for chronic endometritis, the diagnosis of the organic conditions can only be inferred by the biopsy findings. For example, thin, atrophic-appearing endometrium overlying a submucous leiomyoma cannot be reliably distinguished from atrophic endometrium reflecting premature ovarian failure, resistant ovary syndrome, or abnormalities at the hypothalamic–pituitary level with abnormal gonadotropin secretion.

Although inflammation of the endometrium creates an environment that is unfavorable to implantation, the diagnosis of endometritis on a biopsy specimen also is an indicator of the presence of pelvic inflammatory disease. In a study comparing endometrial biopsy, clinical examination, and laparoscopy in the diagnosis of acute pelvic inflammatory disease, Paavonen et al.[123] found that the presence of chronic endometritis in the endometrial biopsy correlated with the presence of acute salpingitis at laparoscopy in 89% of patients, compared to only a 67% correlation between bimanual examination and laparoscopy. These findings, in conjunction with the high correlation of mucopurulent cervicitis and endometritis with salpingitis, suggest that chronic endometritis represents an intermediate stage of pelvic inflammatory disease between cervicitis and salpingitis. In a similar study correlating the presence of subacute focal inflammation in endometrial biopsies (see section on mycoplasma) and laparoscopic findings, Burke et al.[16] found a highly statistically significant correlation between subacute focal inflammation and the presence of pelvic adhesions and tubal occlusion. The sensitivity of the endometrial biopsy in that study was 87%. Furthermore, significant pelvic adhesions can be found at laparoscopy despite normal hysterosalpingography,[84] thereby emphasizing the value of the endometrial biopsy as a predictor of pelvic inflammatory disease.

Since chronic endometritis is found in the absence of salpingitis[123] and half of women with tubal infertility do not have a history of pelvic inflammatory disease,[101] it is conceivable that early endometritis can cause infertility. Thus, the endometrial biopsy can serve as a method for directing specific therapy or as an indicator of the need for laparoscopic examination.

Functional Disorders

The endometrial biopsy should be obtained in the luteal phase of the cycle to determine if ovulation has occurred and, if it has, to correlate the development of the secretory endometrium with the expected day of the cycle according to the basal body temperature graph.[29,170] Usually, the biopsy is performed 2–3 days before the expected first day of menses, although some investigators advocate a biopsy at the midsecretory phase, the time of blastocyst implantation. Relevant clinical information that should accompany the biopsy specimen includes the age of the patient, the date of the biopsy, the last menstrual period, and any hormonal medication.

An endometrial biopsy usually consists of one or more

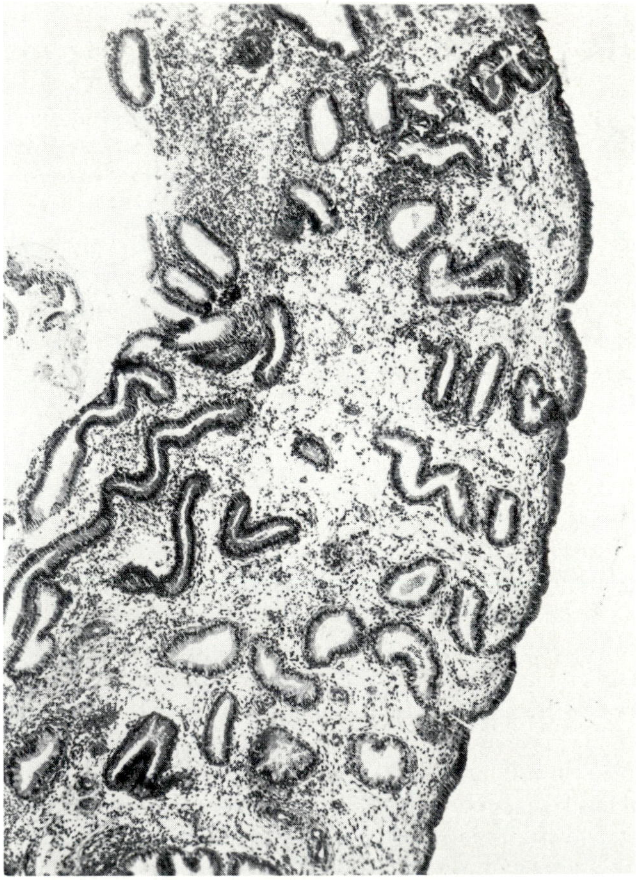

Fig. 10.15. An endometrial biopsy for dating must contain surface endometrium in order to be accurately dated.

strips of endometrium that are haphazardly oriented. For dating, endometrium from the functionalis must be evaluated, since fragments of basalis endometrium and the lower uterine segment do not respond to hormonal stimulation. The functionalis is best identified by finding surface epithelium (Fig. 10.15). Endometrium in which the stroma is fibrous represents tissue from the lower uterine segment and is inadequate for dating. The specific features of functional disorders that are associated with infertility, such as anovulation and LPD, have been described previously.

Benign Tumors

Endometrial Polyps

Endometrial polyps are common. They originate as focal hyperplasias of the basalis and develop into benign, localized overgrowths of endometrial tissue covered by epithelium and containing a variable amount of glands, stroma, and blood vessels.

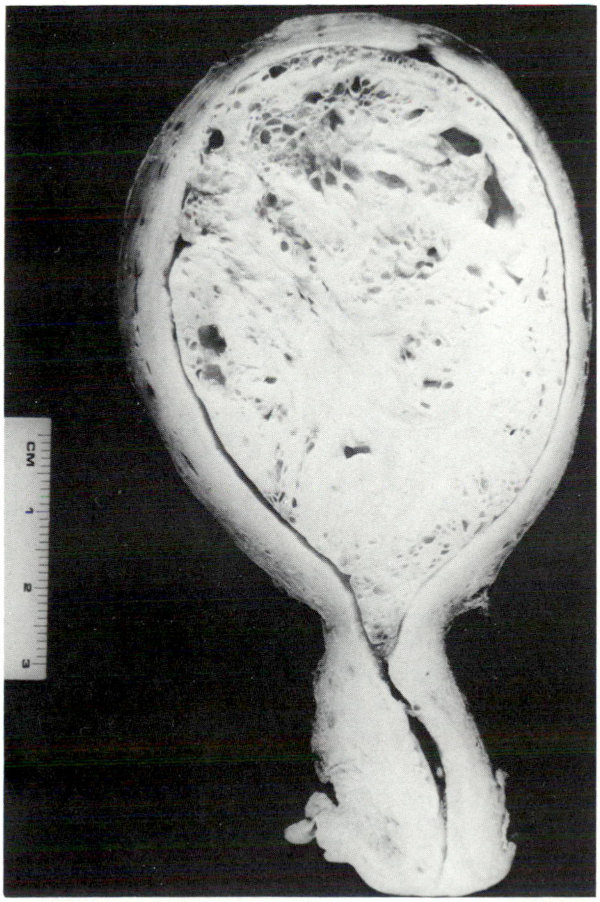

Fig. 10.16. Endometrial polyp entirely filling and distending the endometrial cavity.

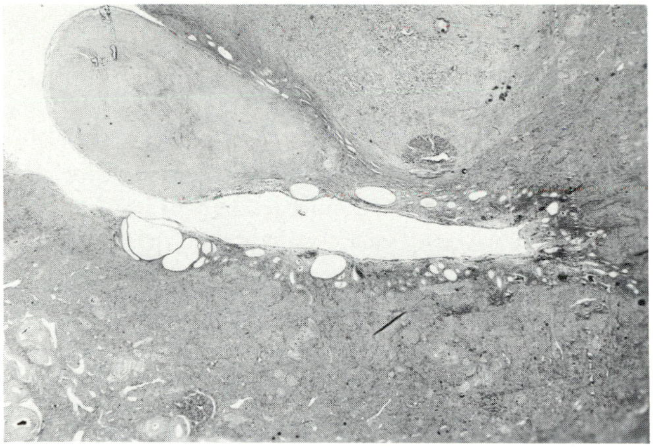

Fig. 10.17. Pedunculated endometrial polyp composed almost entirely of fibrous tissue.

Pathology. Polyps may be broad based and sessile, pedunculated, or attached to the endometrium by a slender stalk. Furthermore, they vary in size from 1.0 mm to a mass that fills and expands the entire endometrial cavity (Fig. 10.16). Large polyps may extend down the endocervical canal and through the cervix, being visible on physical examination. The surface is tan and glistening, but occasionally the tip or the entire polyp is hemorrhagic due to irritation or infarction. Polyps are generally solitary, but about 20% are multiple. These growths may originate anywhere in the uterine cavity, but most occur in the fundus, usually the cornual region. Polyps sometimes arise in the lower uterine segment. Upper endocervical polyps and mixed endometrial–endocervical polyps contain glandular epithelium from both components.

Characteristically, a varying proportion of the glands of a polyp are out of synchrony with the endometrium. The glands usually show some degree of irregularity in outline. In addition, fibrous tissue (Fig. 10.17) and sometimes smooth muscle are observed. A polyp with significant amounts of smooth muscle is referred to as an *adenomyomatous polyp*. Hyperplasia (Fig. 10.18) and, occasionally, even a focal area of well-differentiated carcinoma (Fig. 10.19) occur.[78] Rare examples of carcinosarcomas confined to an otherwise benign polyp have also been reported.[73] Secretory changes in the glandular epithelium of a polyp are seldom encountered. Rarely, these are seen focally in women with secretory endometrium. Various types of metaplasia, most often squamous metaplasia (Fig. 10.20), of the epithelium may also occur. The endometrial stroma surrounding the glands resembles the stroma of proliferative endometrium. A decidual reaction in the stroma, rarely described in polyps when patients have received progestins, is even less common in women with normal cycles.[56] The blood vessels lying at the base of a polyp are usually thick walled but are

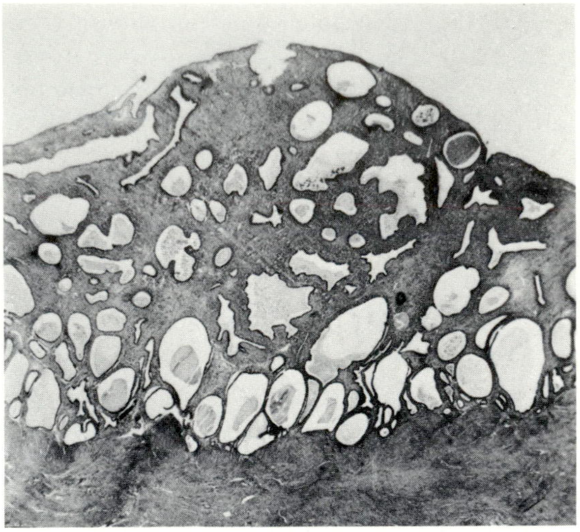

FIG. 10.18. Broad-based endometrial polyp showing hyperplastic glands.

sometimes abundant and dilated, simulating a hemangioma.

Because of their morphologic diversity, polyps have defied subclassification to any great extent. Most polyps can be placed into one of three broad groups: hyperplastic, atrophic, or functional.

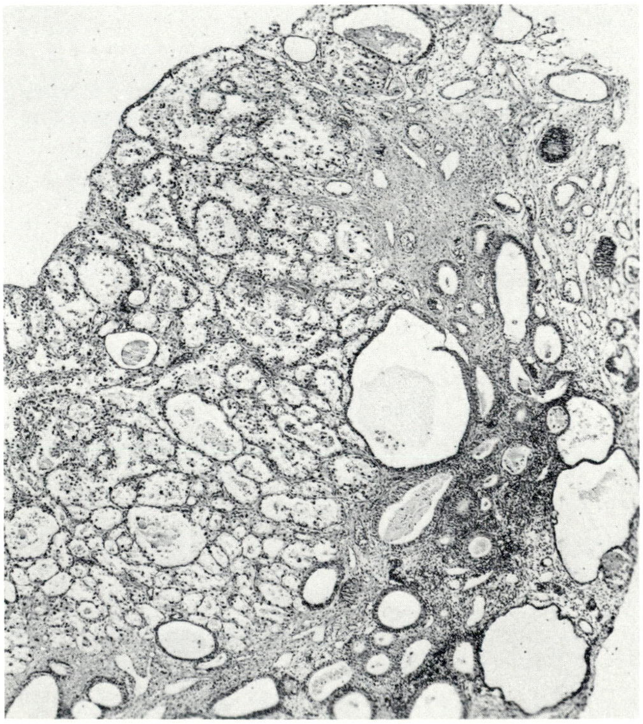

FIG. 10.19. Microscopic clear cell carcinoma confined to the tip of an endometrial polyp. (Reprinted by permission of Kurman and Scully, Ref. 78.)

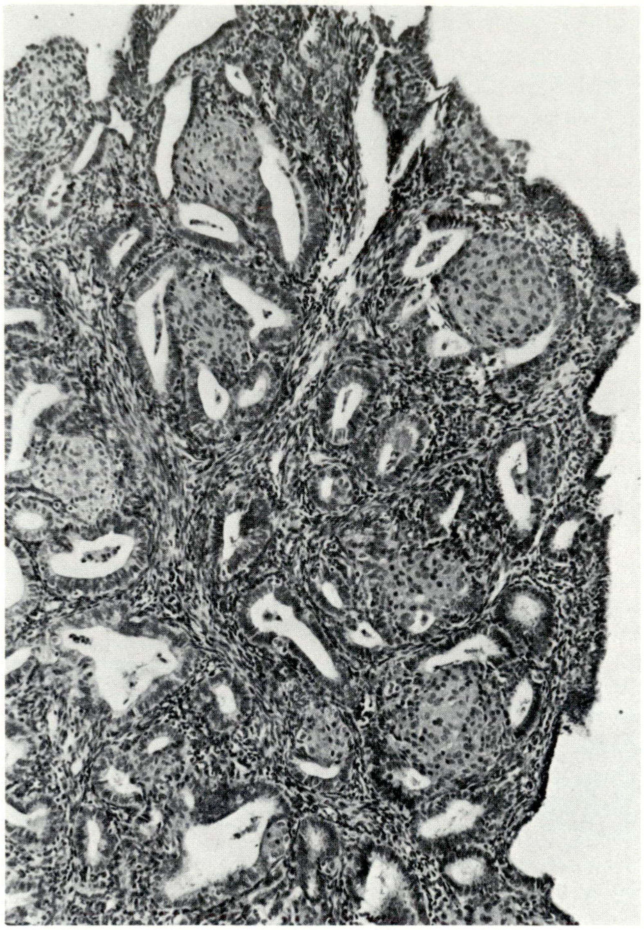

FIG. 10.20. A benign hyperplastic polyp shows irregular glands and squamous metaplasia.

In hyperplastic polyps, the glands resemble those encountered in diffuse hyperplasia of the endometrium, showing active growth and irregular shapes and sizes (Fig. 10.17). This is a frequent form of polyp, since these tumors are derived from the basalis, which is sensitive to estrogens but much less so to progesterone. Consequently, the varying degrees of proliferative and hyperplastic changes occurring in these polyps results from estrogen stimulation during successive menstrual cycles. Hyperplastic polyps are distinguished from hyperplasias, since they are only focal, pedunculated abnormalities in otherwise normal endometrium, whereas hyperplasias are diffuse.

Atrophic polyps show atrophic glandular epithelium that is low columnar to cuboidal. The glands tend to be enlarged and cystically dilated. This form of polyp is typically found in the postmenopausal patient and probably represents regressive changes in a hyperplastic or functional polyp.

Functional polyps are the least frequent. These polyps show glandular changes resembling those of the surrounding endometrium, since they respond to hormones of the menstrual cycle.

Polyps may be difficult to recognize in curettage specimens. Ideally, they should appear as polypoid-shaped fragments of tissue, with epithelium on three sides. This criterion is difficult to fulfill in many cases, however, because of fragmentation of the specimen or sampling of only a portion of the lesion. In addition, normal endometrium has an irregular surface that may appear polypoid with surface epithelium on three sides when sectioned tangentially; therefore, a polypoid configuration in itself is rarely a suitable diagnostic feature. Other clues to the recognition of a polyp include irregular glands that do not resemble those of surrounding endometrium, dense or fibrous stroma, and thick-walled vessels. These features should be seen in fragments of tissue with surface epithelium attached, since glands, stroma, and vessels of the basalis can resemble those seen in polyps.

The differential diagnosis of polyps includes hyperplasias, polypoid adenocarcinomas, adenofibromas, and adenosarcomas. Hyperplasias are most likely to cause difficulty in the differential diagnosis, since these abnormalities have polypoid growth when they are florid. In contrast to benign polyps, however, hyperplasias are diffuse abnormalities; when encountered in curettings, all, or most of, the tissue should show hyperplastic changes—in contrast to the focal change found in polyps. Adenocarcinomas with polypoid growth will retain diagnostic features of malignancy. Adenosarcoma is distinguished from a benign polyp by the distinctive characteristics of the stroma. The stromal cells demonstrate increased mitotic activity and cytologic atypia and tend to be closely applied to the glands (see Chapter 13, Mesenchymal Tumors of Uterus).

Clinical Aspects. Polyps are most commonly encountered in women between 40 and 50 years of age. Rare before menarche, polpys occur relatively frequently after the menopause. The most common clinical presentation is abnormal bleeding. During the reproductive years, intermenstrual bleeding or menometrorrhagia is the usual presenting symptom. For some patients, polyps may be the cause of infertility.[41] A polyp should always be considered if abnormal bleeding persists after curettage because a polyp on a delicate, pliable stalk may be easily missed by the curette. In postmenopausal women, endometrial carcinoma should always be considered when a patient has vaginal bleeding, although endometrial polyps are a more common cause.

The occurrence of carcinoma in benign polyps has been reported to be no more than 0.5%. However, polyps have been found in 12–34% of uteri with endometrial carcinoma.[128,139] A long-term prospective study[6] of patients with endometrial polyps reported that endometrial carcinoma ultimately developed in 3.5% of the patients, but nearly one half of the women in whom carcinoma developed had been treated earlier with intracavitary radium. From these data, it appears that women with polyps may be at greater risk for carcinoma than is anticipated for women of the same age. The increased risk stems from the general proliferative trend of endometria harboring polyps. There is no evidence to suggest that polyps have a greater propensity for developing carcinoma than has the adjacent endometrium.

For perimenopausal or postmenopausal women in whom atypical hyperplasia or carcinoma is present in a polyp, hysterectomy is indicated. For lesser degrees of hyperplasia in a polyp, the only treatment needed is polypectomy and curettage. In young women, if the atypical hyperplasia or carcinoma is confined to the polyp, that is, the adjacent endometrium is uninvolved, and the gynecologist is confident that the entire endometrial cavity has been curetted (if hysteroscopy was performed following the curettage), polypectomy is probably curative.

Atypical Polypoid Adenomyoma

Pathology. The atypical polypoid adenomyoma (APA) grossly resembles an endometrial polyp (Fig. 10.21) and often involves the lower uterine segment. Microscopically, the APA is composed of irregularly shaped hyperplastic glands that are haphazardly arranged within smooth muscle[88,184] (Fig. 10.22). Squamous metaplasia is very common within the glands, complicating the gland patterns. The glandular cells display nuclear atypia, loss of polarity, and cytoplasmic eosinophilia (Fig. 10.23).

The lesion may be difficult to identify in curettings and must be distinguished from hyperplasias, infiltrating carcinomas, and mixed müllerian tumors. The focal na-

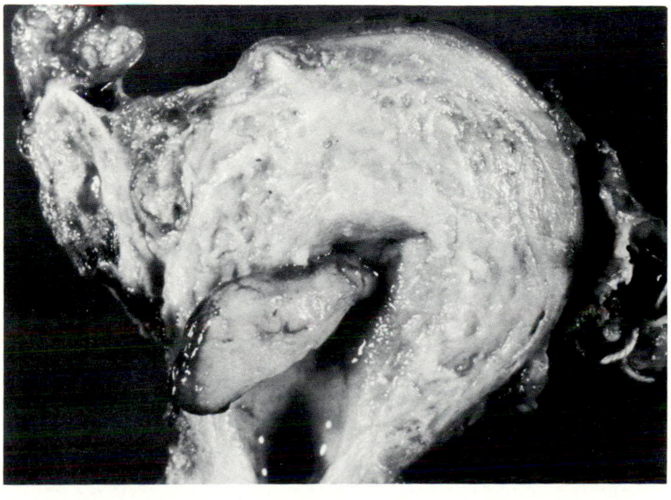

Fig. 10.21. Atypical polypoid adenomyoma occurs as a discrete pedunculated polypoid mass within the uterine cavity.

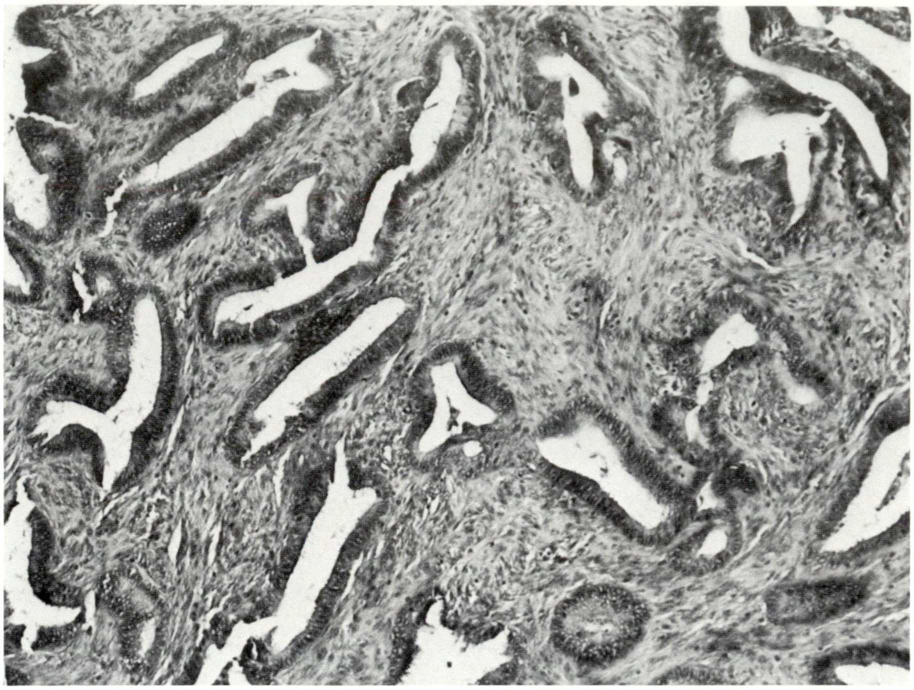

FIG. 10.22. Large and atypical glands in the smooth muscle of an atypical polypoid adenomyoma. (Reprinted by permission of Mazur, Ref. 88.)

ture of the APA and the presence of smooth muscle around the glands distinguish this lesion from atypical hyperplasia (see Chapter 11, Endometrial Hyperplasia and Metaplasia). Infiltrating adenocarcinoma is associated with a reactive fibrous stroma, in contrast to the smooth muscle that surround glands in APA (see Chapter 12, Endometrial Carcinoma). Furthermore, carcinomas usually show more marked atypia and frequently cribriform bridging that contrasts with the milder degree of atypia of APA. Both adenocarcinomas and APA (Fig. 10.23) can show bland squamous differentiation in glands, and this feature is not helpful in separating these entities.

In rare instances, it may not be possible to distinguish an APA from a well-differentiated carcinoma, and a hysterectomy will be necessary. The smooth muscle of APA may show focal mitotic activity, but this is generally less than two mitoses per 10 high-power fields, in contrast to higher rates in sarcomatous patterns. The uniformity of the smooth muscle cells and the lack of high mitotic activity are important features that separate APA from mixed müllerian tumors (see Chapter 13, Mesenchymal Tumors of Uterus).

Clinical Aspects. The APA occurs in the reproductive years and the perimenopausal period, although rare cases have been seen in postmenopausal women. The lesion, like other polyps, usually occurs with abnormal uterine bleeding. Despite the atypical cytologic features of APA, this lesion does not show aggressive behavior. Follow-up has shown that a curettage may be curative in premenopausal women who wish to preserve their fertility, and pregnancy has followed curetting of the lesion.[88,184]

Teratoma

Primary benign teratomas of the uterus are extremely rare,[80,86,160] and immature teratomas are even more unusual.[56] These must not be confused with the more common types of metaplasia, inherent in the uterus, and implantation of fetal tissues. Nearly 20 teratomas have been reported, but most of those in the older literature are of dubious authenticity. Nicholson[109] concluded in 1956 that only four cases were acceptable, and since then three additional cases have been reported. Microscopically, the appearance of the uterine tumor is similar to that of its ovarian counterpart. The neoplasm is lined by squamous epithelium and contains respiratory epithelium, adipose tissue, and sebaceous glands (Fig. 10.24).[86] A remnant of an embryo should be excluded, and placental and decidual tissue in the surrounding endometrium should be absent.

Brenner Tumor

One tumor with the histologic features of a Brenner tumor located in the myometrium immediately beneath the uterine serosa has been reported.[5] The lesion was

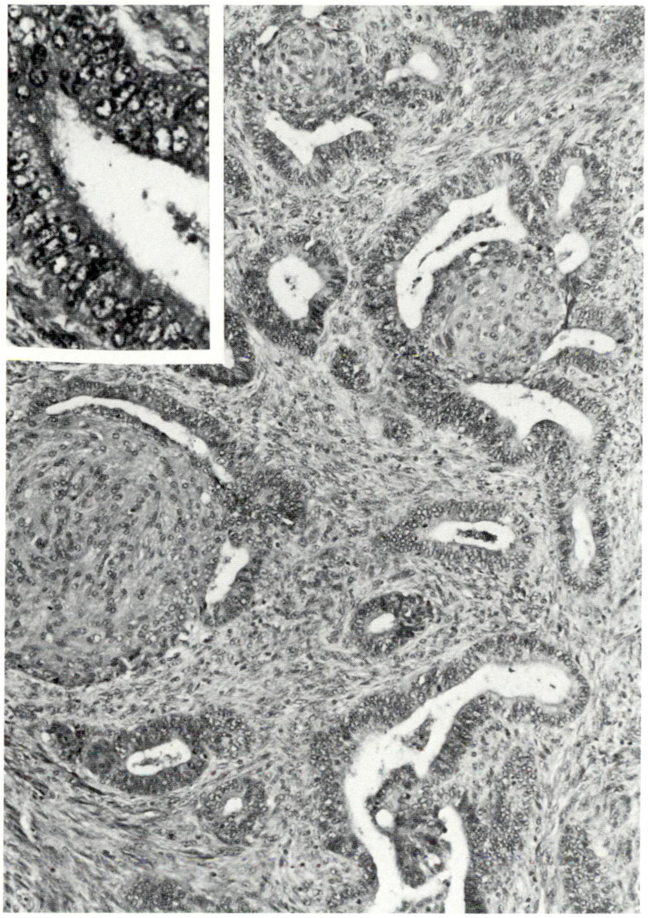

FIG. 10.23. Atypical polypoid adenomyoma with irregular glands containing foci of squamous metaplasia haphazardly arranged and surrounded by smooth muscle. *Inset:* Cytologic atypia is characterized by enlarged nuclei with prominent nucleoli.

described as arising from a metaplasia of peritoneal epithelium within the uterus, and not as an endometrial growth. Other examples of ectopic Brenner tumor have been paracervical.

Heterologous Tissue

Heterologous tissues are defined as those not native to the endometrium. There have been reports of benign heterologous bone,[24,44,63,107] cartilage,[1,107,137] smooth muscle,[13] and glial tissue.[107,110,133,185] The two theories advanced to account for their presence are (1) metaplastic transformation of the endometrial stromal cell and (2) implantation of fetal tissue after abortion and instrumentation, with the fetal tissue persisting and growing as a homograft. Before making the diagnosis of benign heterologous tissue, the pathologist should determine if the

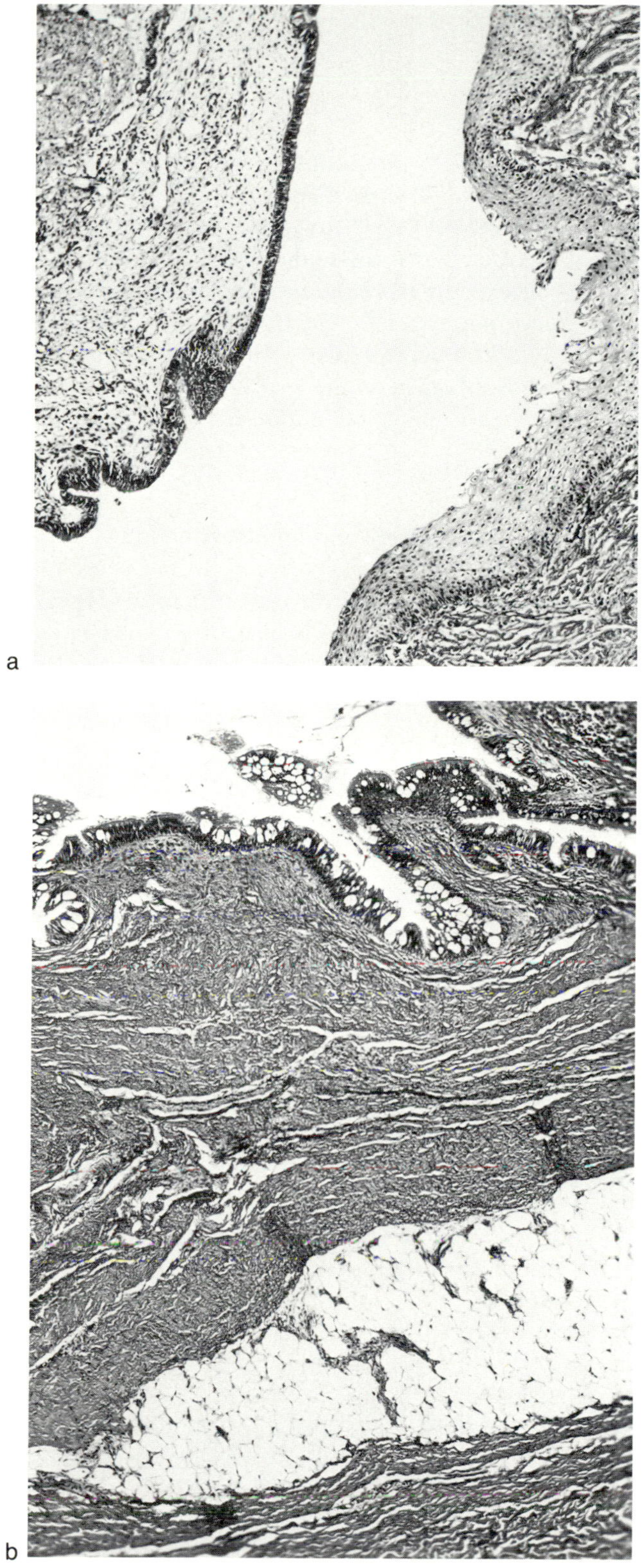

FIG. 10.24. *a.* Mature teratoma of the uterus containing squamous and glandular epithelium. *b.* Respiratory epithelium and adipose tissue present elsewhere in this mature uterine teratoma.

element is benign or malignant, the latter being a component of a malignant mixed mesodermal tumor.

Bone

Heterotopic bone in the endometrium is characteristically found in women with a history of repeated abortions and endometritis.[24,44,63,107] In rare instances, the bone represents a metaplastic phenomenon of the endometrial stroma, triggered by the inflammatory reaction. In most cases, the strong association with prior pregnancy, the immaturity of the heterologous element, and the rarity of osseous metaplasia in other types of endometritis indicate that it represents implantation from fetal parts.

Cartilage

Heterotopic cartilage in the endometrium (Fig. 10.25) is frequently associated with a history of prior abortion and is, therefore, caused by implantation of fetal tissue.[107] In a few patients, there is no history of pregnancy, and furthermore, in the series reported by Roth and Taylor,[137] the age of the patients ranged to 52 years. Microscopically, the cartilage was mature, and a transition from endometrial stromal cells to chondrocytes was found in some, suggesting that a metaplastic phenomenon also occurs.

Smooth Muscle

Smooth muscle is heterologous only in relation to the endometrium, as it is obviously a normal component in the myometrium. Occasionally, fascicles and even nodules of benign smooth muscle occur within the endometrium. Some develop without continuity to the underlying myometrium. It is likely that they develop as a metaplastic process from endometrial stromal cells, as the two have a common anlage.[13]

Glia

Twenty-five examples of mature glial tissue in the endometrium have been reported.[110,133,185] Microscopically, these occur as multiple foci of mature glial tissue, with an absence of mitotic activity (Fig. 10.26). These foci are often surrounded by a lymphocytic and plasma cell infiltrate, as in a graft rejection. Most have a history of instrumented termination of pregnancy. This history, together with the unlikely occurrence of endometrial tissue undergoing metaplasia exclusively into glial tissue or monophytic differentiation of germ cells, supports the theory that the presence of glial tissue in the endometrium is a result of fetal implantation. Rarely, the glial tissue may be a true neoplasm, which is then referred to as a *glioma of the uterus*. In the one case reported, the follow-up was uneventful.[183]

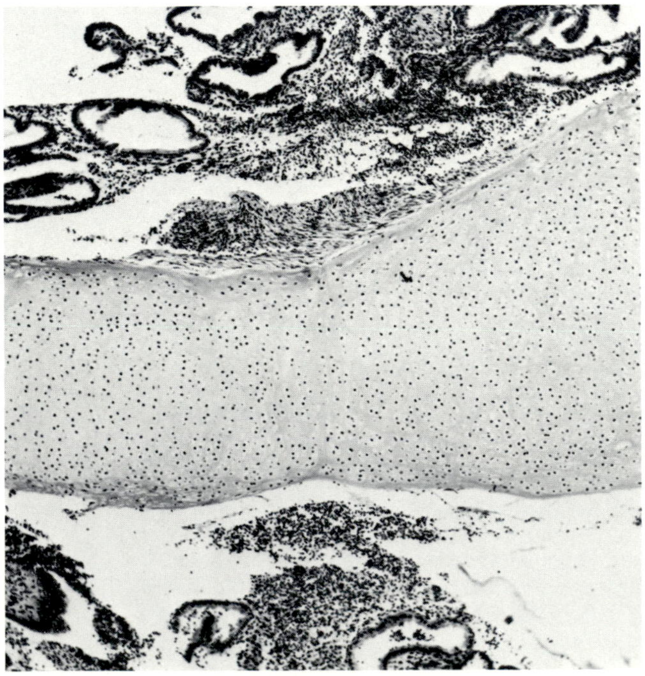

Fig. 10.25. Heterotopic cartilage in the endometrium.

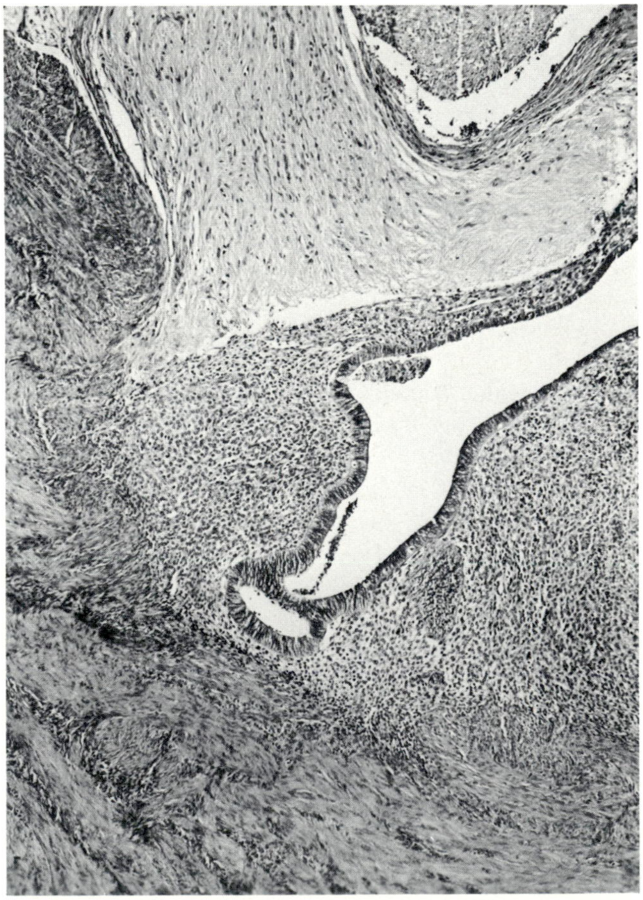

Fig. 10.26. Mature glial implant (*top*) in endometrium.

Effects of Drugs on the Endometrium

Estrogens

Estrogens can stimulate the endometrium even in low concentrations. The duration of exposure rather than the dose of estrogen appears to be more important in the pathologic effect on the endometrium. It has been shown in rabbits that estrogen given over a prolonged period induces endometrial carcinoma,[96] whereas high doses given to monkeys result in atrophy.[55] In humans, prolonged administration of estrogens may result in varying degrees of hyperplasia[117] and, in a small percentage of patients, in low-grade carcinoma. These are discussed in greater detail in Chapter 11, Endometrial Hyperplasia and Metaplasia, and Chapter 12, Endometrial Carcinoma.

In addition to their proliferative effects, estrogens have other specific morphologic effects on the endometrium, for example, various types of epithelial differentiation, such as the formation of cilia (tubal metaplasia), and cytoplasmic eosinophilia[56] (see Chapter 11, Endometrial Hyperplasia and Metaplasia). These effects may involve the surface of the endometrium or the glandular epithelium.

Contraceptive Steroids (Progestin–Estrogen Agents)

Contraceptive steroids differ chemically from and are metabolized differently than natural hormones and should, consequently, be regarded as inducing a pharmacologic and not a physiologic state. The naturally occurring estrogens are inactivated when administered orally, but by the addition of an ethinyl group at the 17 position, the resulting agent 17-alpha-ethinylestradiol is orally active. This compound and the 3-methyl ether of ethinylestradiol, mestranol, are used as the estrogenic components of the oral contraceptives. Mestranol is less potent. Synthetic progestins are either derived from acetylation of the 17-alpha-hydroxyl group of 17-hydroxyprogesterone or by removal of a 19 carbon from the androgen ethisterone, resulting in the formation of the 19-nortestosterone derivatives. These agents have profound progestational activity; some progestins may be 50 times more potent than natural progesterone. Also, progestational agents are metabolized to estrogenic compounds in the body.[151] The potencies of the various progestins vary considerably, and their biologic effect depends mainly on the potency rather than on the dose of drug administered.

The progestational agent in the combination pill prevents ovulation by inhibiting LH secretion through a negative feedback effect on the hypothalamus. Although the estrogenic agent exerts a similar effect on follicle-stimulating hormone (FSH), its primary function is to stimulate the endometrium, thereby preventing breakthrough bleeding, as well as to potentiate the negative feedback action of the progestational agent, thereby permitting reduction in dose of the progestin. This latter effect is attributed to estrogen's stimulating an increase in the concentration of intracellular progestin receptors.[151]

Pathology. The histologic alterations produced by exogenous estrogen–progestin oral contraceptives on the endometrium are a function of (1) whether the drugs are administered in the combined or sequential regimen, (2) the dose and duration of drug used, (3) the morphologic appearance of the endometrium before the start of therapy, and (4) the time of the cycle when the tissue is obtained for study.[57,115,116]

During the first cycle of the combined regimen in women who had previously been ovulating normally, the proliferative phase is markedly shortened, with an arrest in both the growth and differentiation of the glandular epithelium. The glands remain straight and are lined by a single layer of low, inactive columnar epithelium. Glycogen vacuoles appear prematurely and tend to be randomly distributed (Fig. 10.27). Glandular growth is inhibited, and secretory changes develop slowly, if at all. Stromal edema, which can be striking early in therapy, gives way to a distinct decidual change, and numerous stromal granulocytes appear (Fig. 10.28).

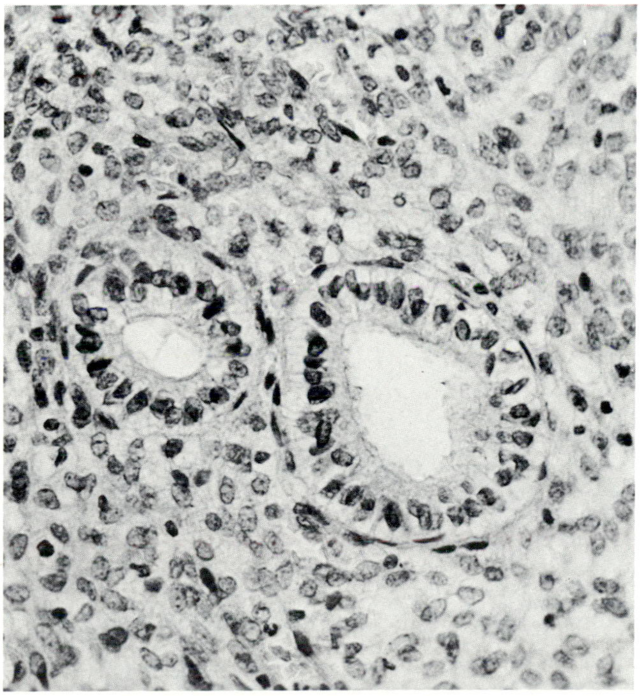

FIG. 10.27. Secretory vacuoles appear prematurely in endometrial glands early during the course of combined oral contraceptive administration.

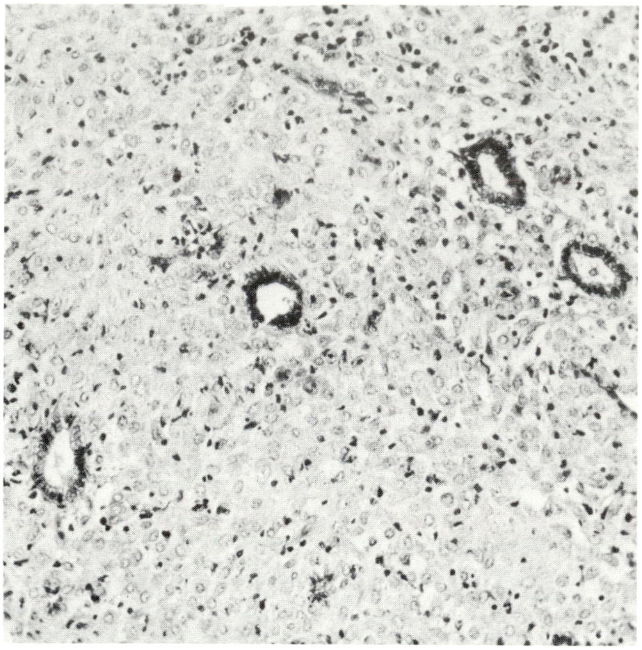

FIG. 10.28. After several cycles of oral contraceptives, the endometrium shows a marked decidual reaction. Glands are small and lined by inactive epithelium.

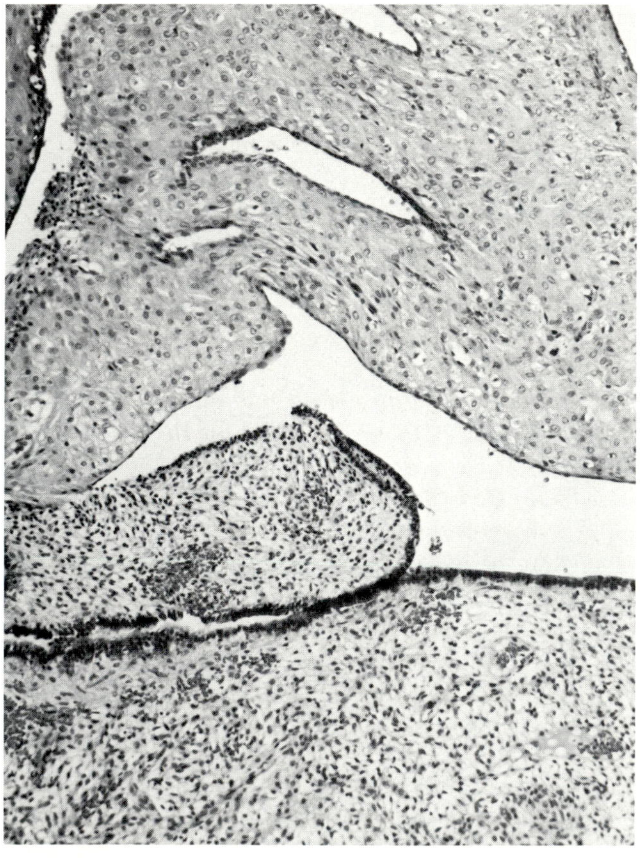

FIG. 10.29. An unusual spindle cell alteration of stromal cells on the *bottom* and the typical decidual change on the *top* in a patient treated with high doses of medroxyprogesterone.

An unusual type of stromal atypia, referred to as *pseudomalignant*[33] or *pseudosarcoma*,[25] has been reported in women receiving high-dose progestational oral contraceptives (Figs. 10.29 and 10.30). Although this lesion is rarely seen now because of the use of low-dose oral contraceptives, the change may be seen in women being treated with progestational agents for endometrial hyperplasia.

After long-term contraceptive use, there is no evidence of secretory activity. The endometrium undergoes atrophy and is composed of sparse, narrow glands.[22] Most glands disappear, and those remaining are composed of flattened epithelial cells, making the glands difficult to distinguish from capillaries. Changes in the endometrial vasculature also occur. Spiral arterioles are inhibited, and thin-walled vascular sinusoids appear. The stroma consists primarily of collagenous fibers, and a decidual reaction may not be evident. This is the usual appearance of the endometrium of women using the low-dose pills.

The ultrastructural features of endometria stimulated

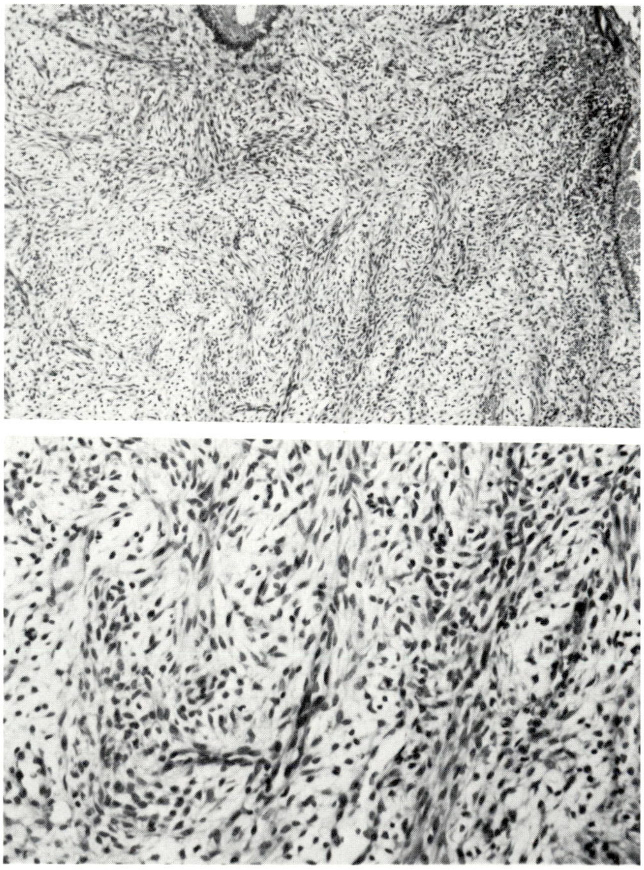

FIG. 10.30. The spindle cell alteration associated with high-dose progestin treatment should not be confused with an endometrial stromal sarcoma. The absence of mitotic activity, as noted in the higher magnification on the *bottom*, distinguishes this lesion from a stromal sarcoma.

by oral contraceptives have been summarized by Cavazos and Lucas.[21] Under the influence of a combined regimen, the estrogen-dependent cell functions are depressed, and an intracellular progresterone-type milieu appears. An increase in ribosomal activity and development of the Golgi apparatus is evident during the early phase of the cycle, but the same activities are depressed during the second half of the cycle. Large mitochondria, intranuclear canaliculi, increased glycogen, and rough endoplasmic reticulum characteristic of the secretory phase appear but are suppressed during the latter half of the cycle and do not achieve the development found during the normal postovulatory phase of the cycle.

Clinical Aspects. In the past, contraceptive steroids were administered in two regimens. (1) In the combined regimen, a synthetic estrogen is combined with a synthetic progestin in a single tablet taken on day 5 of the cycle and continued for 21 days. (2) In the sequential regimen, an estrogen alone is taken for 14–16 days, followed by 5–6 days during which the estrogen and progestin are given in a single tablet, as in the combined regimen. The sequential regimen was introduced with the expectation that it would be better tolerated because it more closely simulated a women's natural endocrine milieu. The sequential pills proved to be less reliable contraceptive agents, as breakthrough ovulations were reported in about 8% of women who used them.[95] They were withdrawn from the market in the United States and Canada in 1976 following reports linking them to endometrial cancer.[76,83,145,146]

Evaluation of the women in whom endometrial carcinoma developed while they were using sequential contraceptives demonstrated that 82% used Oracon.[83,145] Weiss and Sayvetz[168] found that women taking Oracon had a risk of endometrial carcinoma substantially higher than did a control group of women who did not use oral contraceptives. The study also provided evidence that the risk of endometrial carcinoma is reduced in women taking combined oral contraceptives, as would be expected from the suppressive effect of progestin-dominated combined regimens. The carcinogenic effect of Oracon does not appear to be attributable to the unopposed estrogen regimen alone because the other sequential pills were not associated with the development of endometrial carcinoma. The difference is that Oracon used a high dose of the potent estrogen (100 μg ethinylestradiol) and a weak progestin insufficient to mitigate the effect of the estrogen.

Continued use of oral contraceptives, particularly the low-dose preparations (20–35 μg ethinylestradiol), may result in breakthrough bleeding or amenorrhea.[98] Secondary amenorrhea may occur because the low estrogen content of the pill is frequently inadequate to stimulate endometrial growth. Consequently, there is insufficient tissue to produce withdrawal bleeding at the end of a pill cycle. A pill with a slightly higher estrogen content helps in this situation. Prolonged use of oral contraceptives results in the development of thin-walled vascular sinusoids located beneath the endometrial surface, which become ectatic (Fig. 10.31) and undergo thrombosis. The endometrial vessels become disrupted and bleed; the surrounding tissue shrinks but is not actually shed, and this is clinically manifested as breakthrough bleeding. A 7-day course of conjugated estrogens or ethinylestradiol daily will build up the endometrium and result in uniform withdrawal bleeding.[151]

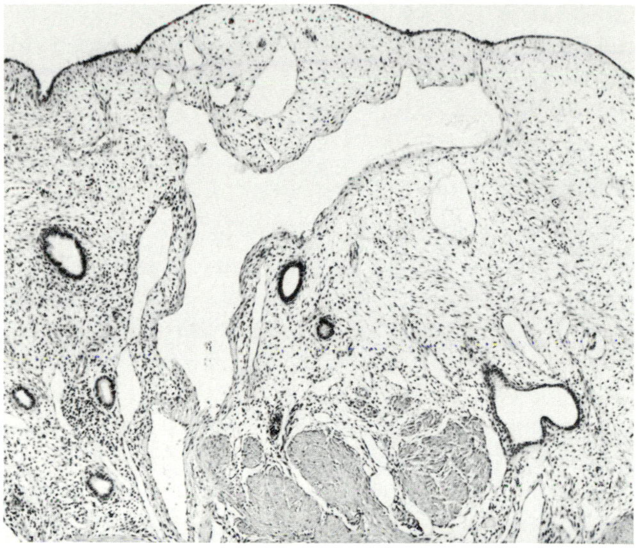

FIG. 10.31. Thin-walled capillaries are frequently present in the endometrium of women taking oral contraceptives.

Progestins

The effects of these drugs alone on the endometrium are the same as those described for the combined oral contraceptives, but atrophy ensues earlier. The same marked decidual reaction and glandular suppression on the endometrium may be induced with intramuscular injection of medroxyprogesterone acetate (Depo-Provera). A similar effect is observed with IUDs impregnated with progesterone, but the effect is confined to the superficial portions of the endometrium.

Clomiphene Citrate

Clomiphene citrate (Clomid) is an orally active nonsteroidal compound structurally similar to DES that binds to estrogen receptors. Clomiphene reduces estrogen receptors in the hypothalamus by inhibition of the process of receptor replacement. Endogenous estrogen levels, therefore, appear to be low, and gonadotropin-releasing hormone is secreted, stimulating pituitary secretion of FSH and LH. When clomiphene is used to induce ovulation, the endometrium reflects the changes of a normal menstrual cycle.[81]

Prostaglandins

Prostaglandin production by the endometrium increases through the secretory phase. Primary dysmenorrhea is thought to be caused by myometrial contractions induced by prostaglandins. This correlates with the association of dysmenorrhea with ovulatory cycles and may explain the beneficial effect of oral contraceptives on primary dysmenorrhea because the resulting atrophic endometrium has lower prostaglandin levels. The mophologic effects of prostaglandins on the endometrium are as yet undetermined.[8]

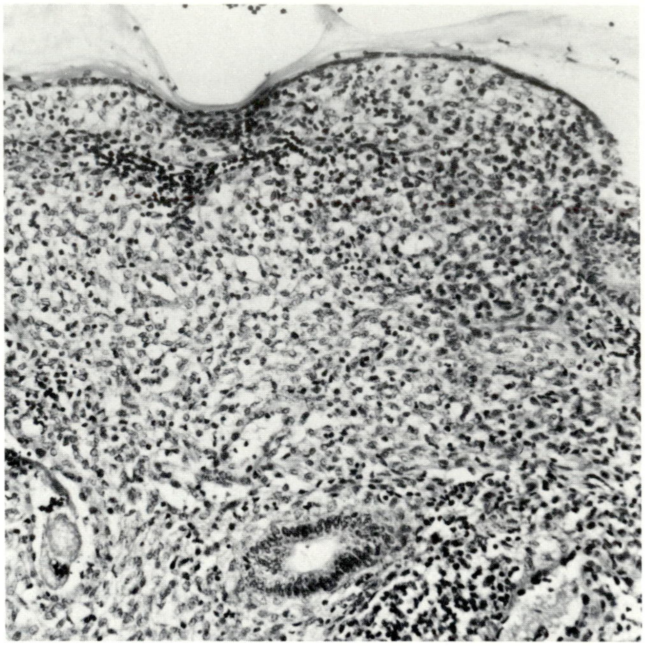

FIG. 10.32. Endometrium in vicinity of intrauterine device showing chronic inflammatory infiltrate.

Miscellaneous Effects on the Endometrium

Intrauterine Devices

A resurgence of interest in IUDs as a method of contraception occurred during the 1960s with the introduction of polyetheylene plastic inert devices. In the mid 1980s, however, as a result of litigation, the copper IUD and several of the plastic devices have been removed from the market.

Pathology. The histologic effects on the endometrium depend on the composition of the IUD. The plastic devices induce a focal acute and chronic inflammatory response (Fig. 10.32) composed of leukocytes, lymphocytes, plasma cells, macrophages, and, rarely, foreign body giant cells.[105,106,118] A significant degree of chronic inflammation is observed in 25–40% of IUD users and may be related to the duration of use.[118] Squamous metaplasia is occasionally present, and a premature predecidual reaction, thought to be related to local trauma from the device, also occurs.[118,180,181] The endometrium immediately beneath the device may show focal fibrosis and pressure atrophy, whereas surrounding regions may be completely unaffected. With copper-bearing devices, inflammatory reactions occur slightly less frequently. Leukocytes are commonly confined to the gland lumens, with exudation on the endometrial surface and sparing of the endometrial stroma. Devices impregnated with progesterone released in a slow, continuous fashion produce a marked, but sharply demarcated, decidual reaction in the endometrium immediately adjacent to the device.[87]

Electron microscopic studies of the effects of the plastic devices reveal giant mitochondria in the glandular epithelial cells during the proliferative phase and premature predecidual changes during the secretory phase.[181,182] An ultrastructural study[45] of endometria in which the copper devices were used shows as increase in the number of mitochondria and lysosomes. The mitochondria show vacuolization of the matrix. Myelin figure formation occurs in 70–80% of the epithelial cells. Specific vascular effects include endometrial degeneration, necrosis, and formation of defects between endometrial cells and adjacent basement membranes.[59] This effect, together with the increase in vessel density,[144] may account for the increased bleeding associated with IUD use.

Clinical Aspects. The mechanism by which the IUD prevents pregnancy is not entirely clear. For the plastic devices, the inflammatory reaction, in conjunction with an asynchronous premature decidual reaction, results in an unfavorable local environment for implantation of the blastocyst. In addition to these effects, copper ions released by the copper-bearing devices may have direct metabolic effects on endometrial cells, inhibiting several enzyme systems.[122] Energy-dispersive x-ray analysis[45] has failed to demonstrate significant amounts of copper in the various organelle studies. However, this may represent a sampling artifact or rapid turnover of the endometrial cells. The mechanism of action for the progesterone-releasing devices is that the induced decidual reaction probably hinders implantation and the local progesterone effect on cervical mucus may render the cervix impermeable to sperm.

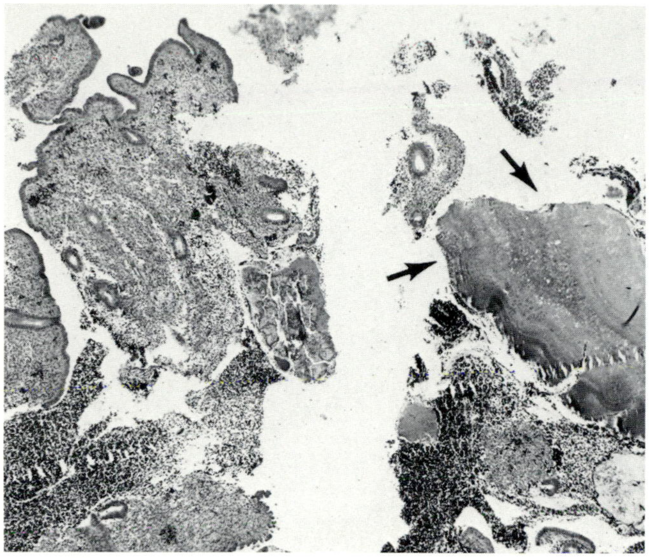

FIG. 10.33. Sulfur granules (*arrows*) can be identified under low magnification in endometrial curettings infected with *Actinomyces*.

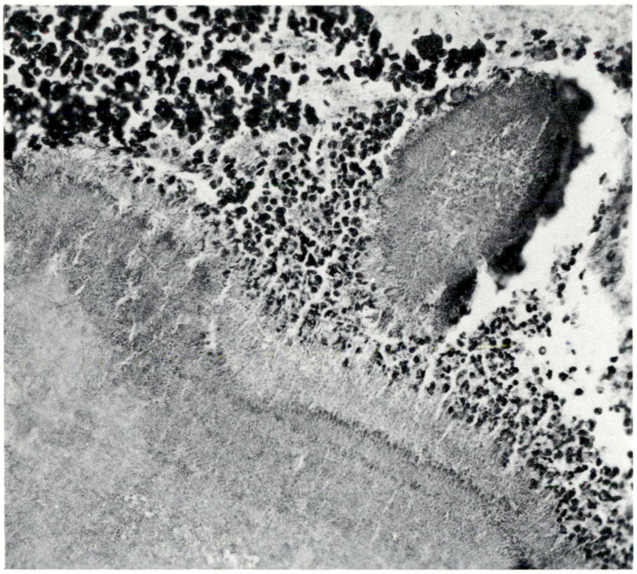

FIG. 10.34. Sulfur granules are composed of a dense central basophilic mass of tangled hyphae surrounded by peripheral radiating filaments.

Early reports during the 1960s suggested that bacteria introduced into the endometrial cavity at the time of insertion were cleared within 24 hours and that endometrial cultures 30 days after insertion were sterile.[97] Several case-controlled studies have subsequently provided strong evidence that among IUD users, pelvic infections are three to nine times more likely to develop than among nonusers.* These infections are often serious and are occassionally fatal.[94] The exact prevalence of IUD-associated pelvic infection is difficult to determine because of many uncontrolled variables. For example, many reports fail to distinguish between the device and promiscuity as relative risk factors. Eshenbach et al.[37] estimated that there are 200,000 cases of IUD-related pelvic inflammatory disease in the United States each year.

IUD-associated pelvic infections are polymicrobial and include aerobic and anaerobic bacteria, *Mycoplasma*, and *Chlamydia*. Pelvic infection in IUD users by *Actinomyces israelii* also occurs.[12,52,53,89] *Actinomyces* is an anaerobic, gram-positive organism classified between true bacteria and complete fungi. The presence of any type of IUD, regardless of its duration of use, predisposes a patient to colonization or infection with *Actinomyces*.[53] The typical sulfur granules, composed of a dense central basophilic mass of tangled hyphae surrounded by peripheral radiating filaments, is characteristic (Figs. 10.33 and 10.34). The organism can be demonstrated in Papanicolaou-stained cervical vaginal smears.[12]

Actinomyces is not normally found in the cervix and vagina but is part of the normal flora of the oral cavity and gastrointestinal tract. It is likely that the organism is introduced into the lower genital tract during coitus. Because this organism does not ordinarily invade mucosal surfaces, the presence of a foreign body, that is, the IUD, associated tissue injury, and decreased oxygenation may promote colonization by *Actinomyces* and other anaerobic organisms. When tubo-ovarian abscesses occur in association with the IUD, they tend to be unilateral, especially when associated with *Actinomyces*. For patients with disease apparently confined to one side, unilateral salpingo-oophorectomy may be sufficient, since it has been shown that in association with an IUD, the opposite adnexa may be completely free of disease.[108,179]

A serious but rare complication of the IUD is perforation through the uterus, with involvement of the omentum and possible bowel obstruction. Bowel obstruction is more likely to occur with copper devices because they are more reactive in the peritoneal cavity than are plastic IUDs. In one study, all seven copper devices that perforated into the abdominal cavity required laporotomy to be removed because of the intense peritoneal reaction, in contrast to noncopper devices, which could be removed during laparoscopy.[120]

Curettage (Asherman's Syndrome)

Hypomenorrhea or amenorrhea and infertility may follow injury to the endometrium (Asherman's syndrome).[7,18,64,67] This condition may develop after a curettage performed during the postpartum or postabortal period, particularly if uterine infection is present. Rarely,

* References 37, 39, 47, 75, 119, 158, 173.

tuberculous endometritis or myomectomy is the predisposing factor. Curettage of the nonpregnant uterus does not appear to have an adverse effect on the endometrium and rarely, if ever, produces secondary amenorrhea. In one large study, it was found that after a curettage, more than 83% of women had their menstrual period on schedule, whereas in 10% it was delayed, and in 7% it was early.[69]

Pathology. Curettings obtained from women with Asherman's syndrome usually contain scant tissue. The uterine synechiae seen at the time of hysteroscopy consist of fibrous tissue or smooth muscle (Fig. 10.35), with no significant inflammation.

Clinical Aspects. The diagnosis is made by hysterography or hysteroscopy, which demonstrates bands of tissue traversing, but rarely obliterating, the endometrial cavity.[40] Many cases of Asherman's syndrome show poor correlation between the diminution of menstrual bleeding and the surface area of the endometrium involved by the adhesions. The lack of correlation appears even more exaggerated when the cervicoisthmic area is involved. In these patients, after penetration of the obliterated endocervical canal at the time of cervical dilatation and hysteroscopy, a normal endometrial cavity without abnormal accumulation of blood is encountered.[165] On the basis of these findings, it has been suggested that a visceral reflex originating in the area of the isthmus may inhibit endometrial proliferation and lead to hypomenorrhea.[165] It has also been postulated that the intrauterine adhesions are a manifestation of a more widespread process in which the endomyometrium is replaced by fibrous tissue.[182]

Treatment of Asherman's syndrome consists of curettage to break the synechiae and placement of an IUD to keep the endometrial surfaces apart.[18] Cyclic estrogen–medroxyprogesterone treatment is administered to induce endometrial proliferation. This form of treatment is curative in most patients, but occasionally intrauterine adhesions reform.[165]

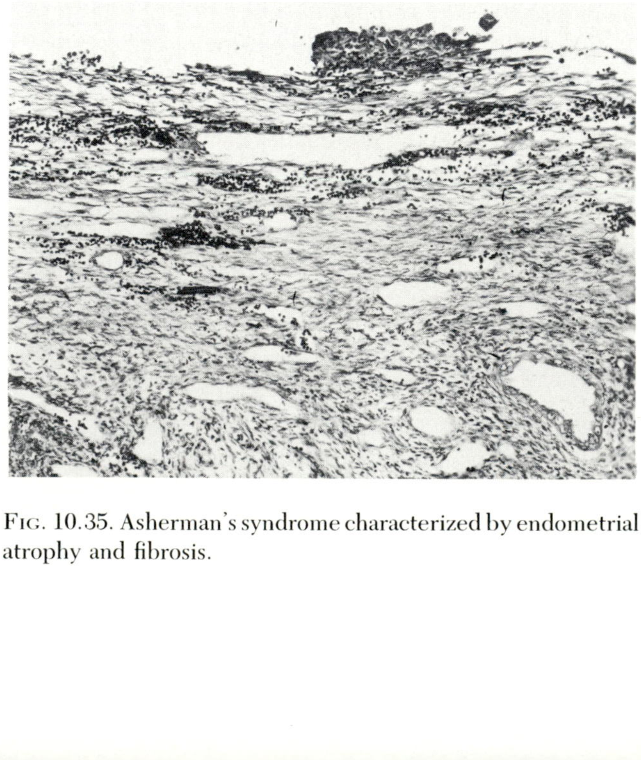

Fig. 10.35. Asherman's syndrome characterized by endometrial atrophy and fibrosis.

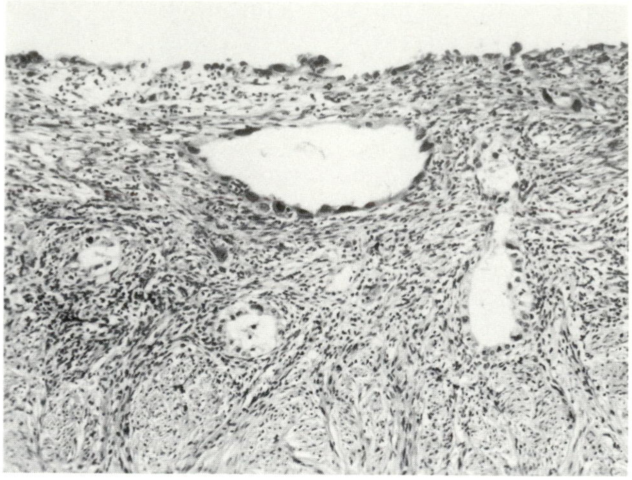

Fig. 10.36. Nuclear atypia in benign gland of irradiated uterus.

Radiation

The morphologic changes induced by radiation are described in Chapter 12, Endometrial Carcinoma. Briefly, the nuclear changes include enlargement, pleomorphism, and hyperchromasia (Fig. 10.36). The cytoplasm of irradiated cells is often granular and vacuolated. A more detailed discussion of radiation-induced endometrial changes is presented by Kraus.[77]

References

1. Aabye R (1955) Cartilage in the endometrium. Acta Obstet Gynecol Scand 34: 105
2. Aksel S, Jones GS (1974) Etiology and treatment of dysfunctional uterine bleeding. Obstet Gynecol 44: 1
3. Altchek, A (1977) Dysfunctional uterine bleeding in adolescence. Clin Obstet Gynecol 20: 633
4. Annos T, Thompson IE, Taymor ML (1980) Luteal phase deficiency and infertility: Difficulties encountered in diagnosis and treatment. Obstet Gynecol 55: 705
5. Arhelger RB, Bocian JJ (1976) Brenner tumor of the uterus. Cancer 38: 1741
6. Armenia CC (1967) Sequential relationship between endometrial polyps and carcinoma of the endometrium. Obstet Gynecol 30: 524
7. Asherman JG (1948) Amenorrhoea traumatica (atretica). J Obstet Gynaecol Br Emp 55: 23
8. Auletta FJ, Caldwell BV, Speroff L (1976) Estrogen-induced luteolysis in the rhesus monkey: Reversal with indomethacin. Prostaglandins 11: 745

9. Beer, AE (1970) Differential diagnosis and clinical analysis of dysfunctional uterine bleeding. Clin Obstet Gynecol 13: 434
10. Benirschke, K (1973) Congenital anomalies of the uterus with emphasis on genetic causes. In: Norris HT, Hertig AT, Abel MR (eds) International Academy of Pathology monograph number 14, The uterus. Baltimore, Williams & Wilkins, pp 68–79
11. Berry A (1966) A cytopathological and histopathological study of bilharziasis of the female genital tract. J Pathol Bacteriol 91: 325
12. Bhagavan BS, Gupta, PK (1978) Genital actinomycosis and intrauterine contraceptive devices. Hum Pathol 9: 567
13. Bird CC, Willis RA (1965) The production of smooth muscle by the endometrial stroma of the adult human uterus. J Pathol Bacteriol 90: 75
14. Botella-Llusia J (1967) Tuberculosis of the endometrium. In: Bertelli A, Houck JC (eds) Proceedings of the 5th World Congress on Fertility and Sterility. Stockholm 1966. Amsterdam, Excerpta Medica, International Congress Series 188, p 514
15. Brudenell JM (1955) Chronic endometritis and plasma cell infiltration of the endometrium. J Obstet Gynaecol Br Emp 62: 269
16. Burke RK, Hertig AT, Miele CA (1985) Prognostic value of subacute focal inflammation of the endometrium, with special reference to pelvic adhesions as observed on laparoscopic examination. An eight-year review. J Reprod Med 30: 646
17. Cadena D, Cavanzo FJ, Leone CL, Taylor HB (1973) Chronic endometritis. A comparative clinicopathologic study. Obstet Gynecol 41: 733
18. Carmichael DE (1970) Asherman's syndrome. Obstet Gynecol 36: 922
19. Cassell GH, Cole BC (1981) Mycoplasmas as agents of human disease. N Engl J Med 304:80
20. Cassell GH, Younger JB, Brown MB, Blackwell RE, Davis JK, Marriott P, Stagno S (1983) Microbiologic study of infertile women at the time of diagnostic laparoscopy. N Engl J Med 308: 502
21. Cavazos F, Lucas FV (1973) Ultrastructure of the endometrium. In: Norris HJ, Hertig AT, Abel MR (ed) International Academy of Pathology monograph number 14, The uterus. Baltimore, Williams & Wilkins, pp 136–174
22. Charles D (1964) Iatrogenic endometrial patterns. J Clin Pathol 17: 205
23. Chen KTK, Hendricks EJ (1985) Malakoplakia of the female genital tract. Obstet Gynecol 65: 84s
24. Courpas AS, Morris JD, Woodruff JD (1964) Osteoid tissue in utero. Report of 3 cases. Obstet Gynecol 24: 636
25. Cruz-Aquino M, Shenker L, Blaustein A (1967) Pseudosarcoma of the endometrium Obstet Gynecol 29: 93
26. Cumming DC, Honore LH, Scott JZ, Williams KP (1985) The late luteal phase in infertile women: Comparison of simultaneous endometrial biopsy and progesterone levels. Fertil Steril 43: 715
27. Czernobilsky B (1978) Endometritis and infertility. Fert Steril 30: 119
28. Dallenbach-Hellweg G (1981) Histopathology of the endometrium, 3rd ed. New York, Heidelberg, Berlin, Springer-Verlag
29. Dallenbach-Hellweg G (1984) The endometrium in infertility. Pathol Res Pract 178: 527
30. Daly DC, Walters CA, Soto-Albors CE, Riddick DH (1983) Endometrial biopsy during treatment of luteal phase defects is predictive of therapeutic outcome. Fertil Steril 40: 305
31. Dehner LP, Askin FB (1975) Cytomegalovirus endometritis. Report of a case associated with spontaneous abortion. Obstet Gynecol 45: 211
32. Del Pozo E, Wyss H, Tolis G, Alcaniz J, Campana A, Naftolin F (1979) Prolactin and deficient luteal function. Obstet Gynecol 53: 282
33. Dockerty MB, Smith, RA, Symmonds RE (1950) Pseudomalignant endometrial changes induced by administration of new synthetic progestins. Proc Mayo Clin 34: 321
34. Downs KA, Gibson M (1983) Basal body temperature graph and the luteal phase defect. Fertil Steril 40: 466
35. Dumoulin JG, Hughesdon PE (1951) Chronic endometritis. J Obstet Gynaecol Br Emp 58: 222
36. Edwards JA, Gale RF (1972) Camptobrachydactyl: A new autosomal dominant trait with two probably homozygotes. Am J Hum Genet 24: 464
37. Eschenbach DA, Harnisch JP, Holmes KK (1977) Pathogenesis of acute pelvic inflammatory disease: Rose of contraception and other risk factors. Am J Obstet Gynecol 128(8): 838
38. Farber ER, Leahy MS, Meadows TR (1968) Endometrial blastomycosis acquired by sexual contact. Obstet Gynecol 32: 195
39. Faulker WL, Ory HW (1976) Intrauterine devices and acute pelvic inflammatory disease. JAMA 235: 1851
40. Foix A, Bruno RO, Davison T, Lema B (1966) The pathology of postcurettage intrauterine adhesions. Am J Obstet Gynecol 96: 1027
41. Foss BA, Horne HW, Hertig AT (1958) The endometrium and sterility. Fertil Steril 9: 193
42. Friberg J, (1978) Genital mycoplasma infections. Am J Obstet Gynecol 132: 573
43. Friberg J (1980) Mycoplasmas and ureaplasmas in infertility and abortion. Fertil Steril 33: 351
44. Ganem KJ, Parsons L, Friedell GH (1982) Endometrial ossification. Am J Obstet Gynecol 83: 1592
45. Gonzalez-Angulo A, Aznar-Ramos R (1976) Ultrastructural studies on the endometrium of women wearing TCu-200 intrauterine devices by means of transmission and scanning electron microscopy and x-ray dispersive analysis. Am J Obstet Gynecol 125: 170
46. Good RG, Moyer DL (1968) Estrogen–progesterone relationships in the development of secretory endometrium. Fertil Steril 19: 37
47. Gray RH (1976) Pelvic inflammatory disease and intrauterine contraceptive devices. Lancet 2: 521
48. Gray SW, Skandalakis JE (1972) Embryology for surgeons: The embryological basis for the treatment of congenital defects. Philadelphia, W.B. Saunders Co., pp 633–664
49. Greenwood SM, Moran JJ (1981) Chronic endometritis: Morphologic and clinical observations. Obstet Gynecol 58: 176

50. Gump DW, Gibson M, Ashikaga T (1984) Lack of association between genital mycoplasmas and infertility. N Engl J Med 310: 937
51. Gurpide E, Tseng L, Gusberg SB (1977) Estrogen metabolism in normal and neoplastic endometrium. Am J Obstet Gynecol 129: 809
52. Hager WD, Majmudar B (1979) Pelvic actinomycosis in women using intrauterine contraceptive devices. Am J Obstet Gynecol 133: 60
53. Hager, WD, Douglas B, Majmudar B, Naib ZM, Williams OJ, Ramsey C, Thomas J (1979) Pelvic colonization with Actinomyces in women using intrauterine contraceptive devices. Am J Obstet Gynecol 135: 680
54. Hart WR, Prins RP, Tsai JC (1976) Isolated coccidioidomycosis of the uterus. Hum Pathol 7: 235
55. Hartman CG, Geschikter GF, Speert H (1941) Effects of continuous estrogen administration in very large doses. Anat Rec [Suppl 2]79: 31
56. Hendrickson MR, Kempson RL (1980) In: Bennington JL (ed) Surgical pathology of the uterine corpus. Philadelphia, London, Toronto, W.B. Saunders Co.
57. Hilliard GD, Norris JH (1979) The pathologic effects of oral contraceptives. In: Lingeman C (ed) Recent results in cancer research. Carcinogenic steroids. New York, Springer-Verlag, Vol 66, pp 49–71
58. Ho KH (1979) Sarcoidosis of the uterus. Hum Pathol 20: 219
59. Hohnman WR, Shaw ST Jr, Macaulay L, Moyer DL (1977) Vascular defects in human endometrium caused by intrauterine contraceptive devices. Contraception 16: 507
60. Holmstrom EG, McLennan CE (1947) Menorrhagia associated with irregular shedding of the endometrium. Am J Obstet Gynecol 53: 727
61. Horne HW Jr, Hertig AT, Knudsin RB (1973) Sub-clinical endometrial inflammation and T-Mycoplasma. Int J Fertil 18:226
62. Horta JLH, Fernandez JG, Soto de Leon B, Cortes Gallegos V (1977) Direct evidence of luteal insufficiency in women with habitual abortion. Obstet Gynecol 49: 705
63. Hsu C (1975) Endometrial ossification. Br J Obstet Gynaecol 82: 836
64. Hunt JE, Wallach EE (1974) Uterine factors in infertility; An overview. Clin Obstet Gynecol 17: 44
65. Israel R, Mishell DR Jr, Labudovich M (1970) Mechanisms of normal and dysfunctional uterine bleeding. Clin Obstet Gynecol 13: 386
66. Israel SL, Roitman, HB, Clancy C (1963) Infrequency of unsuspected endometrial tuberculosis. JAMA 183: 63
66a. Iwasaka T, Wada T, Kidera Y, Sugimori H (1986) Hormonal status and mycoplasma colonization in the female genital tract. Obstet Gynecol 68:263
67. Jewelewicz R, Khalaf S, Neuwirth RS, Vande Wiele RL (1976) Obstetric complications after treatment of intrauterine synechiae (Asherman's syndrome). Obstet Gynecol 47: 701
68. Jones GS (1972) Luteal phase insufficiency. Clin Obstet Gynecol 16:255
69. Jones GS (1975) Luteal phase defects. In: Behrman SJ, Kistner RW (eds) Progress in infertility, 2nd ed. Boston, Little, Brown, pp 299–324
70. Jones GS, Aksel S, Wentz AC (1974) Serum progesterone values in the luteal phase defects. Effects of chorionic gonadotropin. Obstet Gynecol 44: 26
71. Jorgensen V, Enevoldsen B (1964) The occurrence of the first menstruation after curettage. Acta Obstet Gynecol Scand 42 [Suppl 6]: 159
72. Judd HL (1978) Endocrinology of polycystic ovarian disease. Clin Obstet Gynecol 21: 99
73. Kahner S, Ferenczy A, Richart RM (1975) Homologous mixed müllerian tumors (carcinosarcoma) confined to endometrial polyps. Am J Obstet Gynecol 121: 278
74. Kaufman RH, Binder GL, Gray PN, et al. (1977) Upper genital tract changes associated with exposure in utero to diethylstilbestrol. Am J Obstet Gynecol 128: 51
75. Kaufman DW, Shapiro S, Rosenberg L, Monson RR, Miettnen OS, Stolley PD, Slone D (1980) Intrauterine contraceptive device use and pelvic inflammatory disease. Am J Obstet Gynecol 136: 159
76. Kelly HW, Miles PA, Buster JE, Scragg WH (1976) Adenocarcinoma of the endometrium in women taking sequential oral contraceptives. Obstet Gynecol 47: 200
77. Kraus FT (1973) Irradiation changes in the uterus. In: Hertig AT, Norris HJ, Abell MR (eds) International Academy of Pathology monograph number 14, The uterus. Baltimore, Williams & Wilkins, pp 457–488
78. Kurman RJ, Scully RE (1976) Clear cell carcinoma of the endometrium. An analysis of 21 cases. Cancer 37: 872
79. Laatikainen T, Anderson B, Karkkainen J, et al. (1983) Progestin receptor levels in endometria with delayed or incomplete secretory changes. Obstet Gynecol 62: 592
80. Lackner JE, Krohn L (1932) Report of a case of teratoma of the uterus. Am J Obstet Gynecol 25: 735
81. Lamb EJ, Colliflower WW, Williams JW (1972) Endometrial histology and conception rates after clomiphene citrate. Obstet Gynecol 39: 389
82. Ledger WJ (1977) Infection in the female. Philadelphia, Lea & Febiger
83. Lyon FA, Frisch MJ (1976) Endometrial abnormalities occurring in young women on long-term sequential oral contraception. Obstet Gynecol 47: 639
84. Maathius JB, Horbach JGM, Hall EV (1972) A comparison of the results of hysterosalpingography and laporoscopy in the diagnosis of fallopian tube dysfunction. Fertil Steril 23: 428
85. Markee JE (1948) Morphological basis for menstrual bleeding. Bull NY Acad Med 24: 253
86. Martin E, Scholes J, Richart RM, Fenoglio CM (1979) Benign cystic teratoma of the uterus. Am J Obstet Gynecol 135: 429
87. Martinex-Manautou J, Maqueo M, Aznar R, Phariss BB, Zaffaroni A (1975) Endometrial morphology in women exposed to intrauterine systems releasing progesterone. Am J Obstet Gynecol 121: 175
88. Mazur MT (1981) Atypical polypoid adenomyoma of the endometrium. Am J Surg Pathol 5: 473
89. McCormick JF, Scorgie RDF (1977) Unilateral tubo-ovarian actinomycosis in the presence of an intrauterine device. Am J Clin Pathol 68: 622
90. McCracken AW, D'Agostino AN, Brucks AB, Kingsly

WB (1974) Acquired cytomegalovirus infection presenting as viral endometritis. Am J Clin Pathol 61: 556
91. McKelvey JL (1942) Irregular shedding of the endometrium. Lancet 2: 434
92. McKusick VA, Welbalcher RG, Gragg GW (1968) Recessive inheritance of a congenital malformation syndrome. JAMA 204: 113
93. McLennan CE (1952) Current concepts of prolonged or irregular endometrial shedding. Am J Obstet Gynecol 64: 988
94. Mead PB, Beecham JB, Van S Maeck J (1976) Incidence of infections associated with the intrauterine contraceptive device in an isolated community. Am J Obstet Gynecol 125: 79
95. Mears E (1965) Handbook on oral contraception. London, Churchill
96. Meissner WA, Sommers SC, Sherman G (1957) Endometrial hyperplasia, endometrial carcinoma, and endometriosis produced experimentally by estrogen. Cancer 10: 500
97. Mishell DR Jr, Moyer DL (1969) Association of pelvic inflammatory disease with the intrauterine device. Clin Obstet Gynecol 12: 179
98. Moghissi KS (1975) Endometrium and endosalpinx of women treated with microdose progestogens. J Reprod Med 14: 217
99. Molnar JT, Poliak A (1983) Recurrent endometrial malakoplakia. Am J Clin Pathol 80: 762
100. Monif GRR (1974) Infectious diseases in obstetrics and gynecology. New York, Harper & Row
101. Moore DE, Spandoni LR, Foy HH, et al. (1982) Increased frequency of serum antibodies to *Chlamydia trachomatis* in infertility due to distal tubal disease. Lancet 1: 574
102. Moszkowski E, Woodruff JD, Jones GS (1962) The inadequate luteal phase. Am J Obstet Gynecol 83: 363
103. Mouktar M (1966) Functional disorders due to bilharzial infection of the female genital tract. J Obstet Gynecol Br Commonw 73: 307
104. Moyer DL (1975) Endometrial lesions in infertility. In: Behrman SJ, Kistner RW (eds) Progress in infertility, 2nd ed. Boston, Little, Brown, pp 91–115
105. Moyer DL, Mishell DR Jr (1971) Reactions of human endometrium to the intrauterine foreign body. II. Long-term effects on the endometrial histogy and cytology. Am J Obstet Gynecol 111: 66
106. Moyer DL, Mishell DR Jr, Bell J (1970) Reactions of human endometrium to the intrauterine device. I. Correlation of the endometrial histology with the bacterial environment of the uterus following short-term insertion of the IUD. Am J Obstet Gynecol 106: 799
107. Newton CW III, Abell MR (1973) Iatrogenic fetal implants. Obstet Gynecol 40: 686
108. Niebyl JR, Parmley TH, Spence MR, Woodruff JD (1978) Unilateral ovarian abscess associated with the intrauterine device. Obstet Gynecol 52: 165
109. Nicholson GW (1956) Studies of tumour formation: Polypoid teratoma of the uterus. Guy's Hosp Rep 205: 157
110. Niven PAR, Stansfeld AG (1973) "Glioma" of the uterus: A fetal homograft. Am J Obstet Gynecol 115: 434
111. Nogales-Ortiz F, Taranco I, Nogales FF Jr (1979) The pathology of female genital tuberculosis. A 31-year study of 1436 cases. Obstet Gynecol 53: 422
112. Novak E (1933) Recent advances in the physiology of menstruation. Can menstruation occur without ovulation? JAMA 94: 833
113. Noyes RW (1973) Normal phases of the endometrium. In: Norris HJ, Hertig AT, Abell MR (eds) The uterus. Baltimore, William & Wilkins, pp 110–135
114. Noyes RW, Haman JO (1954) Accuracy of endometrial dating. Fertil Steril 4: 504
115. Ober WB (1966) Synthetic progesten-oestrogen preparations and endometrial morphology. J Clin Pathol 19: 138
116. Ober WB (1977) Effects of oral and intrauterine administration of contraceptives on the uterus. Hum Pathol 8: 513
117. Ober WB, Bronstein SB (1967) Endometrial morphology following oral administration of quinestrol. Int J Fertil 23: 210
118. Ober WB, Sobrero AJ, Kurman R, Gold S (1968) Endometrial morphology and polyethylene intrauterine devices. A study of 200 endometrial biopsies. Obstet Gynecol 32: 782
119. Ory HW (1978) A review of the association between intrauterine devices and acute pelvic inflammatory disease. J Reprod Med 20: 200
120. Osborne JL, Bennett MJ (1978) Removal of intraabdominal intrauterine contraceptive devices. Br J Obstet Gynecol 85: 868
121. Osborne NG (1977) The significance of mycoplasma in pelvic infection. J Reprod Med 19: 39
122. Oster G, Salgo MP (1975) The copper intrauterine device and its mode of action. N Engl J Med 293: 432
123. Paavonen J, Aine R, Teisala K, et al. (1985) Comparison of endometrial biopsy and peritoneal fluid cytologic testing with laporoscopy in the diagnosis of acute pelvic inflammatory disease. Am J Obstet Gynecol 151: 645
124. Paavonen J, Aime K, Teisala K, et al. (1985) Chlamydial endometritis. J Clin Pathol 38: 726
125. Paavonen J, Kiviat N, Brunham RC et al. (1985) Prevalence and manifestations of endometritis among women with cervicitis. Am J Obstet Gynecol 152: 280
126. Payan H, Daino J, Kish M (1964) Lymphoid follicles in endometrium. Obstet Gynecol 23: 570
127. Perkins MB (1960) Pneumopolycystic endometritis. Am J Obstet Gynecol 80: 332
128. Peterson WF, Novak ER (1956) Endometrial polyps. Obstet Gynecol 8: 40
129. Plaut A (1950) Human infection with *Cryptococcus glabratus*. Report of case involving uterus and fallopian tube. Am J Clin Pathol 20: 377
130. Povey WG (1970) Abnormal uterine bleeding at puberty and climacteric. Clin Obstet Gynecol 13: 474
131. Rao NB (1969) Malacoplakia of broad ligament, inguinal region and endometrium. Arch Pathol 88: 85
132. Remington JS (1973) Toxoplasmosis. In: Charles D, Finland M (eds) Obstetric and perinatal infections. Philadelphia, Lea & Febiger, pp 27–74
132a. Robb JA, Benirschke K, Barmeyer R (1986) Intrauterine latent herpes simplex virus infection: I. Spontaneous abortion. Hum Pathol 17:1196

133. Roca AN, Guajardo M, Estrada WJ (1980) Glial polyp of the cervix and endometrium. Report of a case and review of the literature. Am J Clin Pathol 73: 718
134. Rock J, Garcia CR, Menkin, MF (1959) A theory of menstruation. Ann NY Acad Sci 75: 831
135. Rodriguez M, Okagaki T, Richart RM (1972) Mycotic en dometritis due to *Candida*. A case report. Obstet Gynecol 39: 292
136. Rosenfeld DL, Chudow S, Bronson RA (1980) Diagnosis of luteal phase inadequacy. Obstet Gynecol 56: 193
137. Roth E, Taylor HB (1966) Heterotopic cartilage in uterus. Obstet Gynecol 27: 838
138. Rotterdam H (1978) Chronic endometritis: A clinicopathologic study, Pathol Annu 13: 209
139. Salm R (1972) The incidence and significance of early carcinomas in endometrial polyps. J Pathol 108: 47
140. Saw, EC, Smale LE, Einstein H, Huntington RW (1975) Female genital coccidioidomycosis. Obstet Gynecol 45: 199
141. Schenken JR, Tamisiea J (1956) *Enterobius vermicularis* (pinworm) infection of the endometrium. Am J Obstet Gynecol 72: 913
142. Schneider V, Behm FG, Mumaw VR (1982) Ascending herpetic endometritis. Obstet Gynecol 59: 259
143. Scommegna A, Dmowski WP (1973) Dysfunctional uterine bleeding. Clin Obstet Gynecol 16: 221
144. Shaw ST, Maucaulay LK, Hohman WR (1979) Vessel density in endometrium of women with and without intrauterine contraceptive devices. A morphometric evaluation. Am J Obstet Gynecol 135: 101
145. Silverberg SG, Makowski EL (1975) Endometrial carcinoma in young women taking oral contraceptive agents. Obstet Gynecol 46: 503
146. Silverberg SG, Makowski EL, Roche WD (1977) Endometrial carcinoma in women under 40 years of age: Comparison of cases in oral contraceptive users and nonusers. Cancer 39: 592
147. Sinykin MB, Goodlin RC, Barr MM (1956) Irregular shedding of the endometrium. Am J Obstet Gynecol 71: 990
148. Sobrino LG, Kase N (1970) Endocrinologic aspects of dysfunctional uterine bleeding. Clin Obstet Gynecol 13: 400
149. Soules MR, Wiebe RH, Aksel S, Hammond CB (1977) The diagnosis and therapy of luteal phase deficiency. Fertil Steril 28: 1033
150. Southam AL, Richart RM (1966) The prognosis for adolescents with menstrual abnormalities. Am J Obstet Gynecol 94: 637
151. Speroff L, Glass RH, Kase NG (1983) Clinical gynecologic endocrinology and infertility, 3rd ed. Baltimore, Williams & Wilkins, pp 467–492
152. Spirtos NJ, Yurewicz EC, Moghisii KS, et al. (1985) Pseudocorpus luteum insufficiency: A study of cytosol progesterone receptors in human endometrium. Obstet Gynecol 65: 535
153. Stray-Pedersen B, Lorentzen-Styr A-M (1977) Uterine toxoplasma infections and repeated abortions. Am J Obstet Gynecol 128: 716
154. Stray-Pedersen B, Bruu A-L, Molne K (1982) Infertility and uterine colonization with *Ureaplasma urealyticum*. Acta Obstet Gynecol Scand 61: 21
155. Stray-Pedersen B, Eng J, Reikvam TM (1978) Uterine T-mycoplasma colonization in reproductive failure. Am J Obstet Gynecol 130: 307
156. Sutherland AM (1958) Tuberculosis of endometrium: A report of 250 cases with results of drug treatment. Obstet Gynecol 11: 527
157. Tam MR, Stamm WE, Handsfield HH, et al. (1984) Culture-independent diagnosis of *Chlamydia trachomatis* using monoclonal antibodies. N Engl J Med 310: 1146
158. Targum SD, Wright NH (1974) Association of the intrauterine device and pelvic inflammatory disease: A retrospective pilot study. Am J Epidemiol 100: 262
159. Taylor AB (1960) Sarcoidosis of the uterus. J Obstet Gynecol Br Emp 67: 32
160. Taylor RN, Welch KL, Sklar DM, et al. (1984) Heterotopic skin in the uterus. A report of an unusual case. J Reprod Med 29: 837
161. Taylor-Robinson D, McCormack WM (1980) The genital mycoplasmas. Part 1. N Engl J Med 302: 1003
162. Taylor-Robinson D, McCormack WM (1980) The genital mycoplasmas. Part 2. N Engl J Med 302: 1063
163. Thiery M (1955) Irregular shedding of the endometrium. Gynaecologia (Basel) 139: 1
164. Thomas W Jr, Sadeghieh B, Fresco R, Rubenstone AI, Stepto RC, Carasso B (1978) Malacoplakia of the endometrium, a probable cause of postmenopausal bleeding. Am J Clin Pathol 69: 637
165. Toaff R, Ballas S (1978) Traumatic hypomenorrhea–amenorrhea (Asherman's syndrome). Fertil Steril 30: 379
165a. Venkataseshan VS, Woo TH (1985) Diffuse viral papillomatosis (condyloma) of the uterine cavity. Int J Gynecol Pathol 4:370
166. Wallach EE (1972) The uterine factor in infertility. Fertil Steril 23: 138
167. Weicker ML, Kaneb GD, Goodale RH (1940) Primary echinococcal cyst of the uterus. N Engl J Med 223: 574
168. Weiss NS, Sayvetz TA (1980) Incidence of endometrial cancer in relation to the use of oral contraceptives. N Engl J Med 302: 551
169. Wenckelbach GFC, Curry B (1976) Cytomegalovirus infection of the female genital tract. Histologic findings in three cases and review of the literature. Arch Pathol Lab Med 100: 1609
170. Wentz AC (1980) Endometrial biopsy in the evaluation of infertility. Fertil Steril 33: 121
171. Wentz AC (1982) Diagnosing luteal phase inadequacy. Fertil Steril 37: 334
172. Wentz AC, Herbert CM, Maxson WS, Garner CH (1984) Outcome of progesterone treatment of luteal phase inadequacy. Fertil Steril 41: 856
173. Westrom L, Bentsson LP, Mordh PA (1976) The risk of pelvic inflammatory disease in women using intrauterine contraceptive devices as compared to nonusers. Lancet 2: 221
174. Williams AO (1967) Pathology of schistosomiasis of the uterine cervix due to *S. haematobium*. Am J Obstet Gynecol 98: 784

175. Winkler B, Reumann W, Mitao M (1984) Chlamydial endometritis. A histological and immunohistochemical analysis. Am J Surg Pathol 8: 771
176. Winter JD, Faiman C, Reyes FI (1978) Normal and abnormal pubertal development. Clin Obstet Gynecol 21: 67
177. Winter JD, Kohn G, Mellinin WJ, et al. (1968) A familial syndrome of renal, genital, and middle ear anomalies. J Pediatr 72: 88
178. Wolfe SA, Mackles A (1960) Malignant lesions arising from benign endometrial polyps. Obstet Gynecol 20: 542
179. Woodruff JD, Pauerstein CJ (1969) The fallopian tube structure: Function, pathology and management. Baltimore, Williams & Wilkins
180. Wynn RM (1967) Intrauterine devices: Effects on ultrastructure of human endometrium. Science 156: 1508
181. Wynn RM (1968) Fine structural effects of intrauterine contraceptives on the human endometrium. Fertil Steril 19: 867
182. Yaffe H, Ron M, Polishuk WZ (1978) Amenorrhea, hypomenorrhea, and uterine fibrosis. Am J Obstet Gynecol 130: 599
183. Young RH, Kleinman GM, Scully RE (1981) Glioma of the uterus. Am J Surg Pathol 5: 695
184. Young RH, Treger T, Scully RE (1986) Atypical polypoid adenomyoma of the uterus. A report of 27 cases. Am J Clin Pathol 86: 139
185. Zettergren L (1973) Glial tissue in the uterus. Am J Pathol 171: 419

11

Endometrial Hyperplasia and Metaplasia

Robert J. Kurman, M.D., and Henry J. Norris, M.D.

Abnormal endometrial proliferations form a morphologic continuum ranging from focal glandular crowding through various degrees of hyperplasia and carcinoma. Classifications have evolved in which degrees of proliferation are separately labeled, although objective criteria are few and only simple hyperplasia and frank carcinoma, at the extreme ends of the spectrum, are consistently identified. Proliferations composed of closely packed complex glands displaying cytologic atypia comprise a gray area in the spectrum and provide the greatest difficulty in interpretation since some carcinomas of the endometrium lack atypia and some hyperplasias show atypia to a marked degree. Terms that have been used to describe lesions in the borderline area include *adenomatous hyperplasia*, *atypical hyperplasia*, and *carcinoma in situ*, but criteria for distinguishing them have been loosely and variably applied by different authors, and follow-up studies that might justify and validate their existence as discrete entities are difficult to interpret meaningfully.[39]

Endometrial proliferations are divided into noninvasive and invasive forms. Invasive lesions comprise all types of endometrial carcinoma and are considered in Chapter 12, Endometrial Carcinoma. Noninvasive lesions are the subject of this chapter and are considered as follows: (1) a brief review of terms and classifications in use, (2) the histopathologic features of hyperplasia and metaplasia, (3) adjunctive techniques in the characterization of hyperplasia, (4) behavior of the various forms of hyperplasia, (5) hyperplasia as a precursor of endometrial carcinoma, and (6) management of patients with endometrial hyperplasia.

Terminology in a Historical Perspective

Cystic Hyperplasia

This is the most common form of hyperplasia. It is characterized by dilated glands of varying sizes lined by tall columnar or cuboidal epithelium, usually showing some degree of mitotic activity and mild stratification. The stratification and columnar shape of the cells distinguish it from cystic (senile) atrophy and the isolated inactive cystic glands occasionally observed in normal proliferative or secretory endometrium, since the latter are lined by a single layer of flattened or low cuboidal epithelium.

Adenomatous Hyperplasia

This term has been applied by different authors to describe widely differing patterns. Gusberg used it to include all categories of endometrial hyperplasia beyond cystic hyperplasia.[19–21] He subdivided adenomatous hyperplasia into mild, moderate, and severe forms. Severe adenomatous hyperplasia corresponds to the pattern others designate as atypical hyperplasia. In contrast, Hertig and Sommers[26] used the term adenomatous hyperplasia to denote a histologic pattern exhibiting glandular projections and budding into the surrounding stroma. Vellios[45] and Buehl et al.[4] used the term in a similar fashion but restricted it to endometria with little or no cytologic atypia.

Atypical Hyperplasia

This term was introduced by Novak and Rutledge[40] to describe proliferative endometria characterized by a greatly increased number of glands, with very little intervening stroma. Although they described the glandular pattern as closely resembling carcinoma and described the presence of moderately large uniform nuclei, they did not mention nuclear atypia. Campbell and Barter[5] used a similar terminology but divided atypical hyperplasia into grades 1, 2, and 3, depending on how closely the lesion resembled carcinoma. They used complexity of the pattern rather than cytologic atypia as the main basis for subdividing atypical hyperplasia. In contrast, Vellios[45] restricted atypical hyperplasia to endometria showing degrees of cellular atypia even in the absence of glandular crowding. This discrepancy in what constitutes atypia persists in the literature in that some authors use the term *atypical hyperplasia* to describe abnormally complex architectural patterns regardless of cytologic atypia, whereas others limit the term to endometria with cytologic atypia regardless of architectural pattern, and some authors require that both be present.[33,47]

Carcinoma In Situ

The term *carcinoma in situ* (CIS) was introduced by Hertig et al.[26,27] to describe a focal lesion with cytologic alterations in which glandular crowding was not usually a prominent feature. The cells were large, with loss of polarity and abundant amphophilic or eosinophilic cytoplasm. The nuclei were pale, with fine granular chromatin and irregular nuclear membranes, but were not hyperchromatic. The glands had some cellular disorientation, disparity in size, and duplication of lumens. Intraglandular tufting was sometimes present. Buehl et al.[4] and Vellios,[45] however, used the term to denote a process at the extreme end of the proliferative continuum, with cytologic and architectural features consistent with carcinoma. Nuclear hyperchromatism and irregular nuclear outlines, clumping of chromatin, enlarged nucleoli, and usually eosinophilic cytoplasm were major features. Architectural changes included intraglandular cribriform arrangements and epithelial bridges. This lesion was distinguished from well-differentiated carcinoma on the basis of crowding. If glands having the characteristics of CIS were crowded together to the point that the likelihood of stromal invasion was high, the lesion was designated invasive carcinoma. Welch and Scully[47] defined CIS as a small lesion involving no more than five or six glands in which cytologic features of carcinoma are present, but in which there is no evidence of invasion. If the change involves more than five or six glands, a diagnosis of invasive carcinoma is made arbitrarily. It is clear that in some instances, invasion is impossible to identify in areas of crowded glands, just as cytologic atypia is not found in every endometrial carcinoma. Many authors do not regard CIS as a replicable diagnosis for these reasons.

Classification

Until recently, the confusion in terminology and uncertainty over the behavior of various forms of hyperplasia have led to misleading diagnoses and inappropriate treatment. A clinically useful classification should be objective and reproducible, categorizing endometrial proliferations according to their behavior. Individualized management based on the natural history of the disease can then be undertaken. The classification proposed by the International Society of Gynecological Pathologists (ISGP) takes into account the inability to recognize some fully transformed malignant cells by any technique that is presently available until invasion of the adjacent tissue occurs. Abnormal endometrial proliferations are, therefore, divided into noninvasive and invasive forms according to the presence or absence of endometrial stromal invasion.[34] This classification may not necessarily distin-

TABLE 11.1. Classification of endometrial hyperplasia.[a]

Simple hyperplasia
Complex hyperplasia (Adenomatous hyperplasia without atypia)
Atypical hyperplasia (Adenomatous hyperplasia with atypia)

[a] International Society of Gynecological Pathologists

guish a benign lesion from a malignant one, but it is the most useful means of separating a biologically inert lesion from one capable of metastasis.[31,34] Although stromal invasion is defined arbitrarily, applying quantifiable measurements makes its recognition less subjective than it was in the past. The criteria for invasion are discussed in Chapter 12, Endometrial Carcinoma.

Noninvasive proliferations are subdivided into two categories, hyperplasia without cytologic atypia and hyperplasia with cytologic atypia (atypical hyperplasia). The rationale for this division is based on the natural history of the disease as shown in a long term follow-up study.[36] It is now known that less than 2% of hyperplasia without cytologic atypia progresses to carcinoma, no matter how architecturally complex, whereas 23% of hyperplasia with cytologic atypia (atypical hyperplasia) progresses to carcinoma. Increasing degrees of glandular complexity and crowding (architectural atypia) also appear to increase the likelihood of progression to carcinoma but not to the extent that cytologic atypia does. The classification proposed by the International Society of Gynecological Pathologists (Table 11.1), therefore, takes into account cytologic abnormalities primarily. Proliferations displaying no evidence of cytologic atypia are classified as either simple or complex hyperplasia depending on the extent of glandular complexity and crowding (architectural abnormalities) whereas those displaying cytologic atypia regardless of the architectural pattern are classified as atypical hyperplasia.

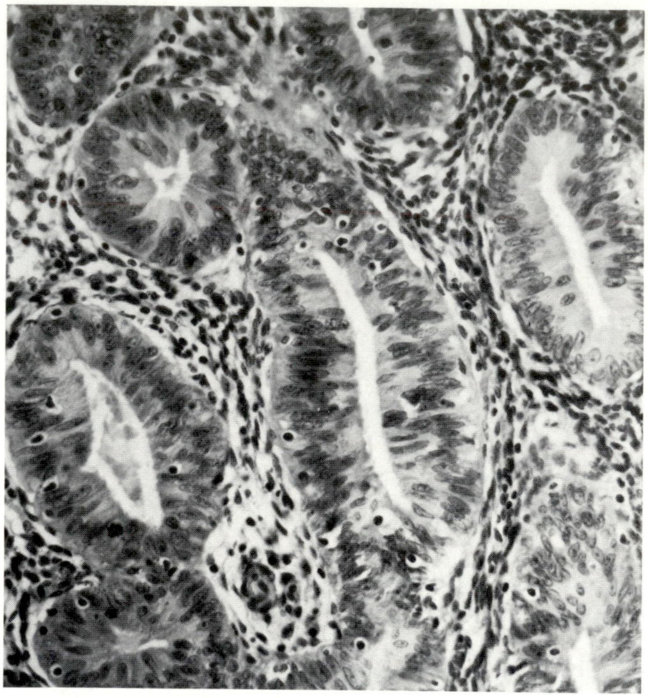

FIG. 11.1. Hyperplastic glands lacking cytologic atypia. The nuclei are cigar-shaped and resemble those in proliferative endometrium.

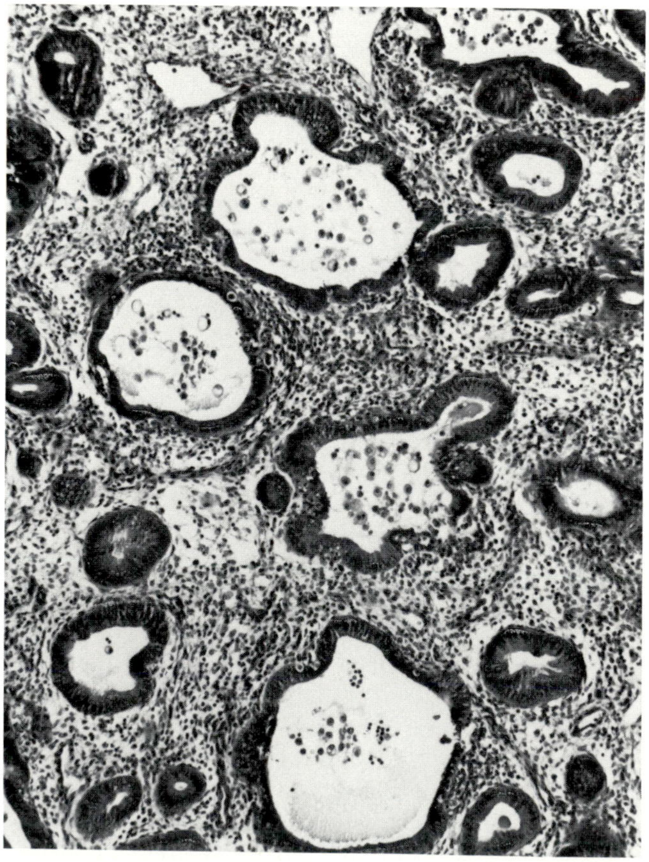

FIG. 11.2. Simple hyperplasia characterized by cystically dilated glands with occasional outpouchings and surrounded by abundant stroma.

Pathology

Gross Appearance

Hyperplastic endometrium is not distinctive grossly. Diffuse thickening is typical, but focal overgrowth may occur and simulate a polyp. The volume of tissue is usually increased, but it may be quite variable and less than obtained during the secretory phase of the normal cycle. The diagnosis of hyperplasia, therefore, depends on the histologic pattern and not on the volume of tissue. A small volume of tissue may reflect inadequate sampling, particularly if the specimen is a biopsy. In hysterectomy specimens, hyperplasia usually presents a velvety, knobby surface of pale, spongy tissue with vague borders.

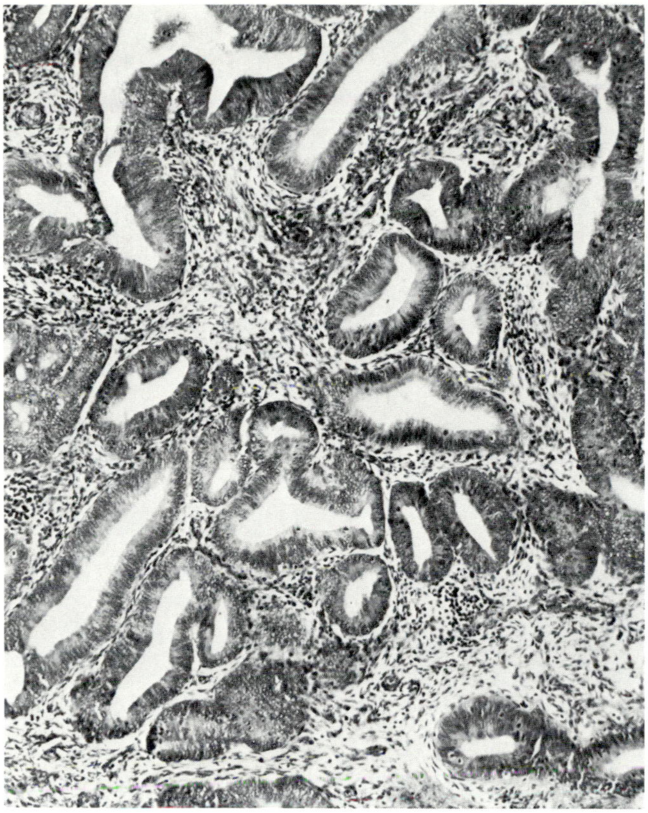

FIG. 11.3. Simple hyperplasia in which there is some crowding but the glands are not back to back. (Reprinted by permission of Kurman et al., Ref. 36.)

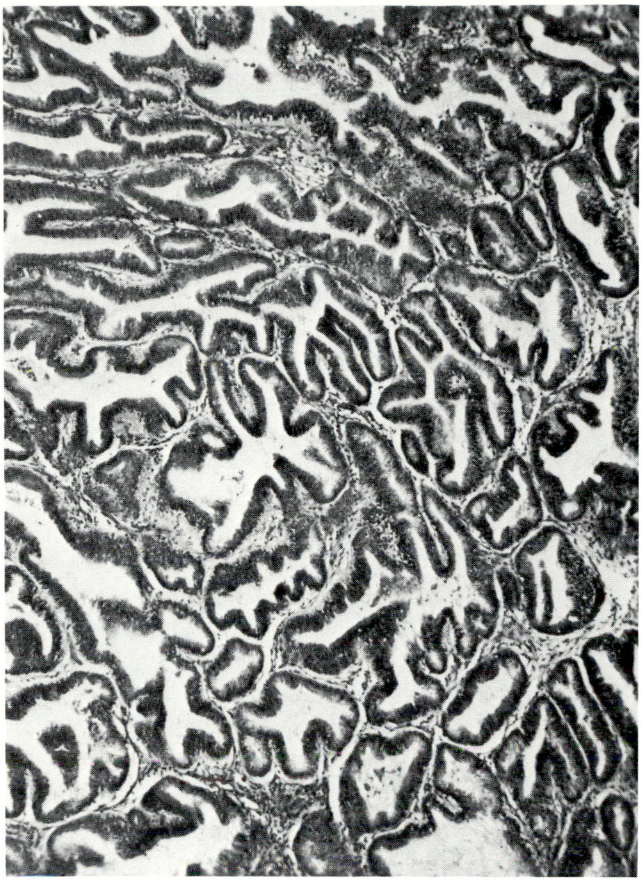

FIG. 11.4. Complex hyperplasia characterized by glands with complex glandular outlines that are markedly crowded. There is no cytologic atypia. (Reprinted by permission of Kurman et al., Ref. 36.)

Microscopic Appearance

Hyperplasia Without Atypia

Microscopically, this type of hyperplasia is characterized by an increase in the number of endometrial glands relative to the stroma. The glands are lined by cells displaying no cytologic atypia. The epithelial cells have oval, basally oriented, bland nuclei that resemble those in normal proliferative glands, although the cell size including nuclei may be slightly enlarged (Fig. 11.1).

Simple Hyperplasia. The glands are cystically dilated, with occasional outpouchings surrounded by an abundant cellular stroma. In other instances, the glands are only minimally dilated but focally crowded. Admixtures of the various patterns frequently occur (Figs. 11.2 and 11.3).

Complex Hyperplasia. These proliferations are composed of highly complex, crowded glands with little intervening stroma (Fig. 11.4).[36] Epithelial stratification and mitotic activity generally parallel the architectural complexity, but sometimes they are discordant. Epithelial stratification can range from two to four layers, but some glands may exhibit little or no stratification. Mitotic activity may range from less than 5 to greater than 10 mitotic figures per 10 high-power fields (HPF), but even in highly complex hyperplasia with marked stratification, mitotic figures may be inconspicuous.

Hyperplasia with Atypia (Atypical Hyperplasia)

Atypical hyperplasia is characterized by an increase in the number of endometrial glands lined by cells displaying cytologic atypia. Enlarged cells that show loss of polarity and an increase in the nuclear/cytoplasmic ratio are considered atypical (Fig. 11.5). Nuclei are enlarged, irregular in size and shape, and have a thickened nuclear membrane, coarse chromatin clumping, and prominent nucleoli. They tend to be round as compared to the oval nuclei of proliferative endometrium and simple and complex hyperplasia. As a result, the nuclei often have a cleared or vesicular appearance despite peripherally clumped chromatin. The glands may be relatively simple and separated by fairly abundant stroma, so-called simple atypical hyperplasia (Fig. 11.6), or have irregular outlines and demonstrate marked structural complexity and back-to-back crowding, so-called complex atypical hyperplasia

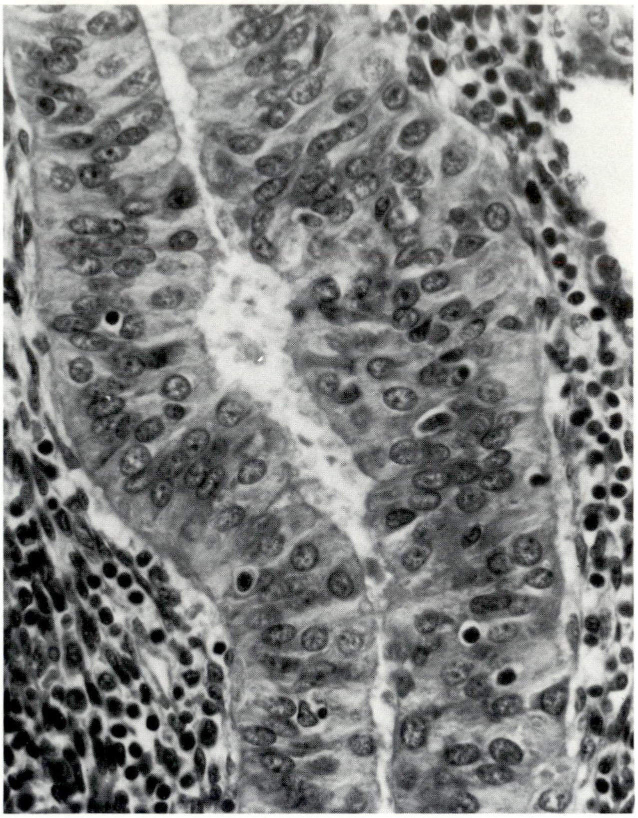

FIG. 11.5. Cells displaying cytologic atypia have nuclei that frequently appear clear or vesicular.

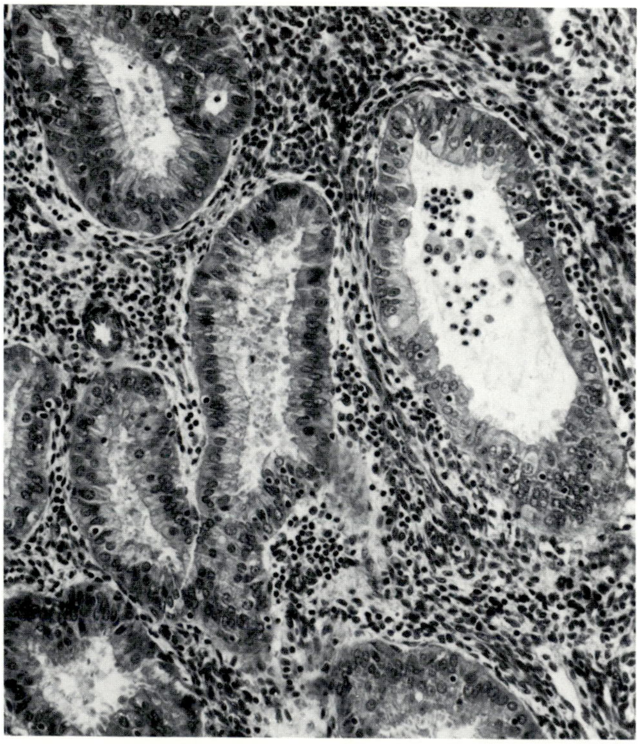

FIG. 11.6. Simple atypical hyperplasia (atypical hyperplasia in the International Society of Gynecological Pathologists Classification), in which glands showing cytologic atypia are separated by fairly abundant endometrial stroma. (Reprinted by permission of Kurman and Norris, Ref. 35.)

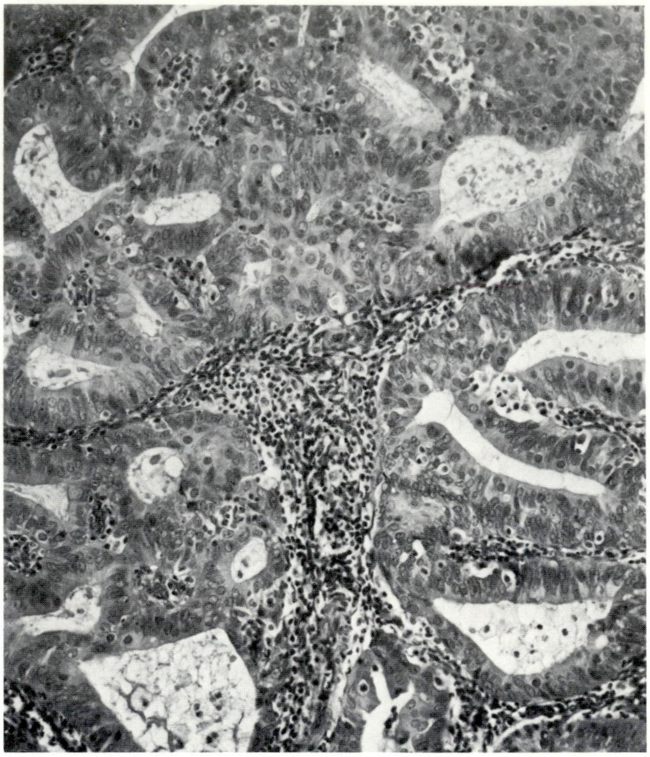

FIG. 11.7. Complex atypical hyperplasia (atypical hyperplasia in the International Society of Gynecological Pathologists Classification), characterized by glands lined by cells showing cytologic atypia with a complex glandular pattern. A focus of squamous metaplasia is present in the *upper right*.

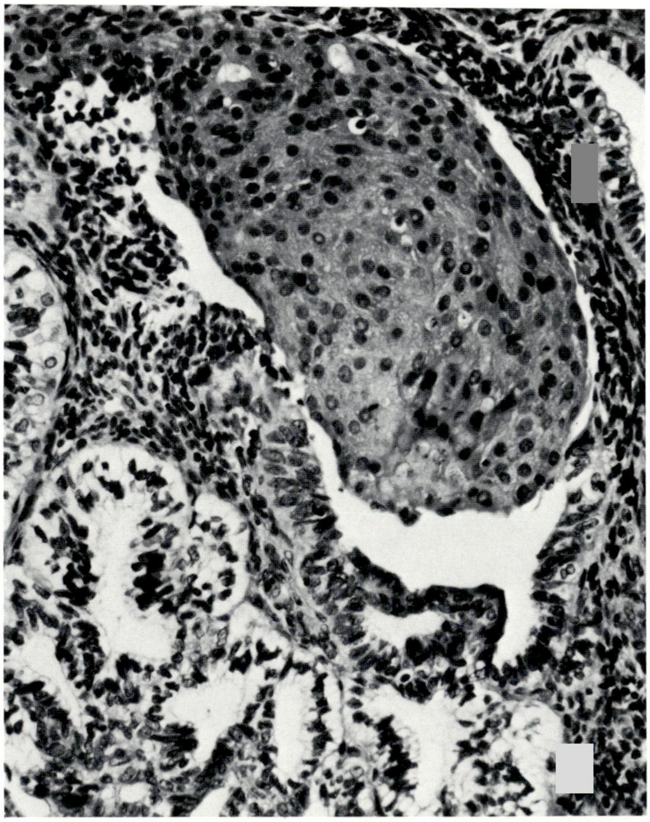

FIG. 11.8. Squamous metaplasia in secretory endometrium.

(Fig. 11.7).[36] As in hyperplasias without atypia, epithelial stratification and mitotic activity are variable. Some atypical hyperplasias may have little stratification, and mitotic activity may be inconspicuous. Cytologic atypia is also variable, but the quantification of atypia is subjective and not very reproducible. Generally, increasing degrees of nuclear atypia, mitotic activity, and stratification of cells in curettings are associated with a higher frequency of carcinoma in the uterus.[34]

Metaplasia

Metaplasia commonly occurs in association with endometrial hyperplasia. It is defined as the replacement of typical endometrial epithelium by another type not found normally in the endometrium. Metaplasia may occur in association with various benign conditions, including polyps, endometritis, trauma, vitamin A deficiency, and hyperplasia, and in carcinoma.[8,17,24,25] The presence of metaplasia in a hyperplasia may produce a dramatic alteration that can be confused microscopically with carcinoma. The various types of metaplasias do not, however, appear to influence the behavior of the underlying process.

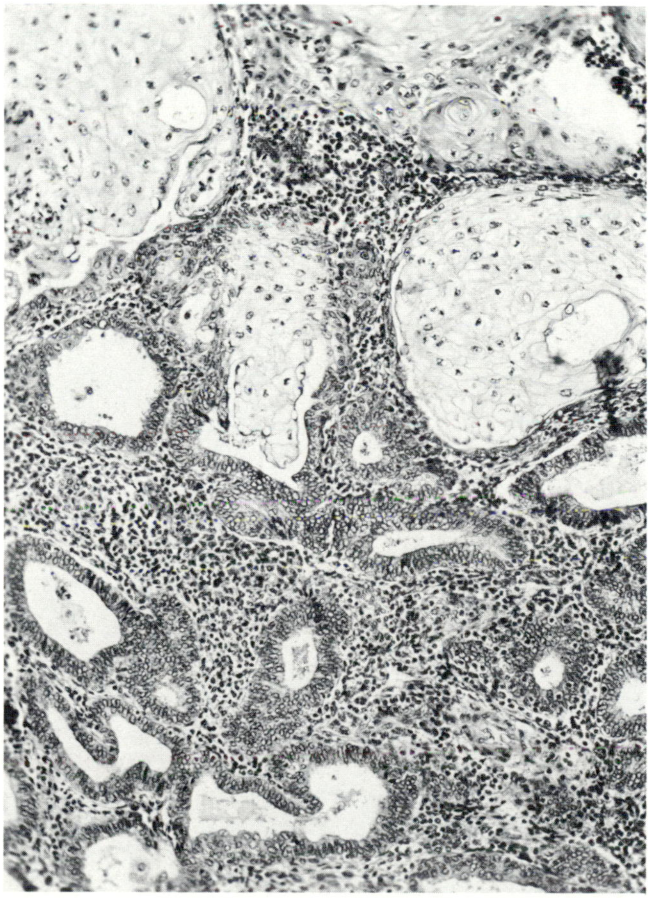

FIG. 11.9. Squamous metaplasia in simple hyperplasia. Both the squamous and the glandular cells lack cytologic atypia.

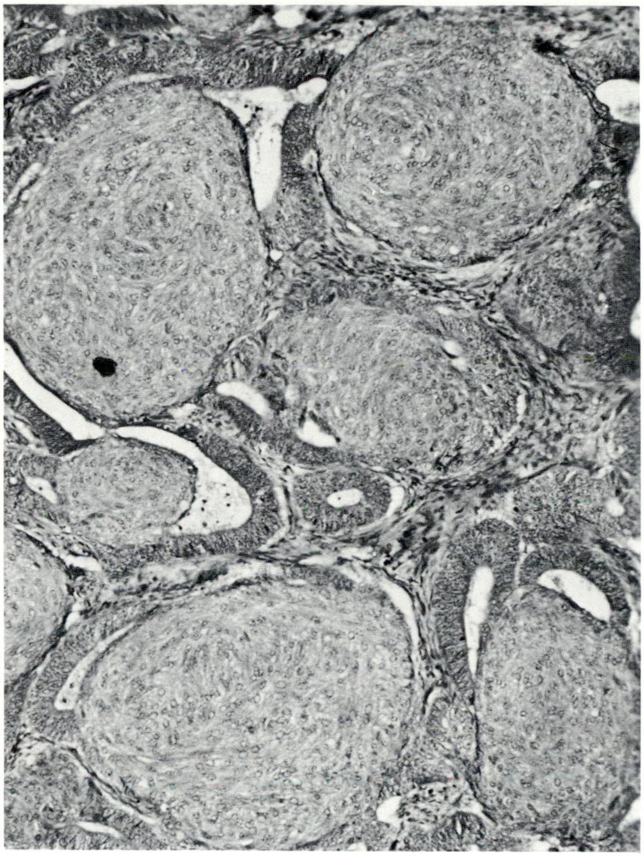

FIG. 11.10. Atypical hyperplasia with squamous metaplasia. The squamous cells have almost entirely obliterated the gland lumens.

Squamous Metaplasia. Squamous differentiation occurs in all forms of hyperplasia as well as in carcinoma. There is a tendency for it to be more common in the more atypical endometrial proliferations. Thus, squamous metaplasia is rare in normally cycling endometrium (Fig. 11.8) but is encountered in approximately 5% of simple and complex hyperplasias (Fig. 11.9) and a quarter of atypical hyperplasias (Fig. 11.10). Adenoacanthosis is another name for hyperplasia with squamous metaplasia.[8]

Metaplastic squamous cells are usually cytologically bland. The degree of nuclear atypia generally parallels that of the glandular cells. Thus, in an atypical hyperplasia with squamous metaplasia, the squamous component will display a comparable or perhaps a lesser degree of nuclear atypia than that observed in the glandular cells. Typically, the squamous cells have a moderate amount of eosinophilic cytoplasm and are surrounded by a well-defined cell membrane. They tend to be rounded or polygonal but may be spindle-shaped, forming a circumscribed nest, so-called squamous morule, within the

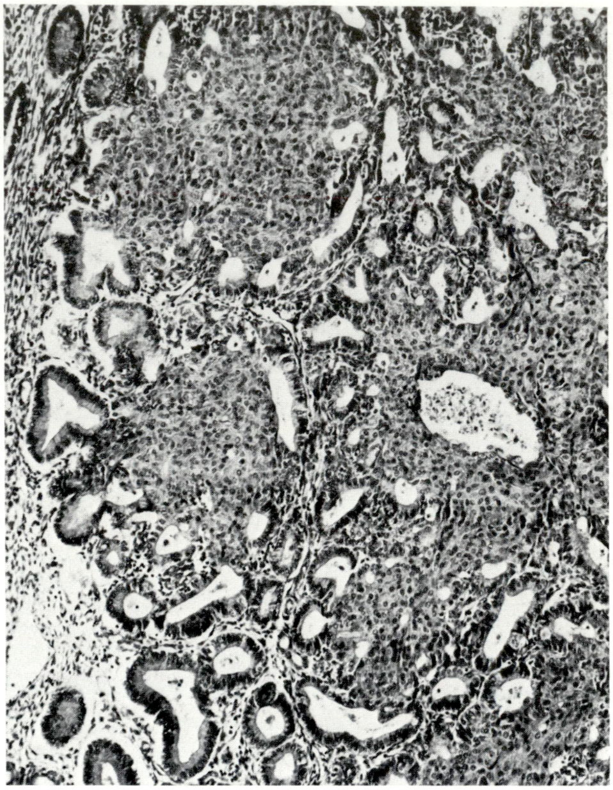

FIG. 11.11. Extensive squamous metaplasia in association with atypical hyperplasia can look ominous.

gland lumen. Morules reflect immature or incomplete squamous differentiation. The cells are smaller, and the cytoplasm is less prominent than in the more completely differentiated squamous metaplasia. Central keratinization and necrosis rarely occur. Eventually, proliferation results in protrusion of the squamous cells into the lumen, leading to replacement of the lumen by nests of squamous cells or coalescence with neighboring glands undergoing the same process. Mitotic activity is rare. Masses of coalescent squamous epithelium that obliterate gland lumens in an atypical hyperplasia make it look ominous (Fig. 11.11), but in the absence of solid replacement of the stroma over 2 sq mm by these masses (stromal invasion) (see Chapter 12, Endometrial Carcinoma), the process is not interpreted as carcinoma.

Ciliated Cell (Tubal) Metaplasia. Proliferative endometrial gland cells with cilia are not usually evident microscopically.[37] Ciliated cells occasionally are observed in senile endometrium or polyps. The presence of a significant number of ciliated glandular cells is generally referred to as *ciliated* or *tubal metaplasia* because the ciliated epithelium bears a close resemblance to the ep-

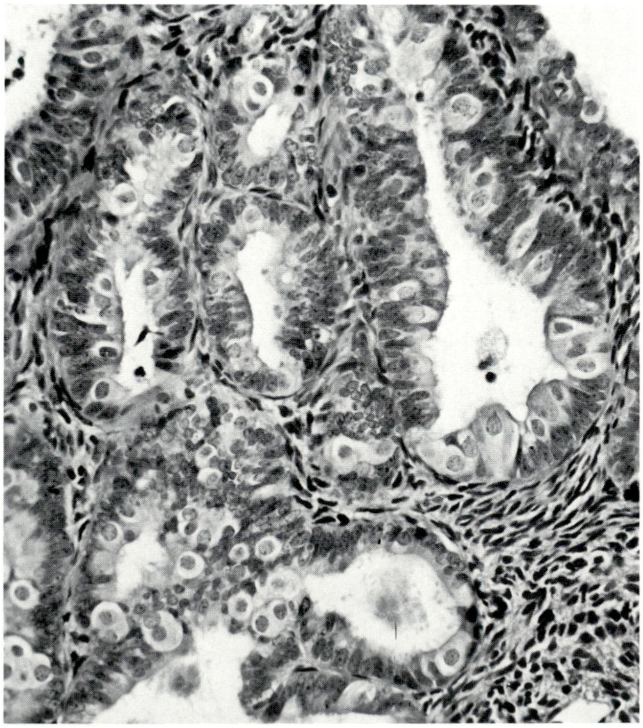

FIG. 11.12. Ciliated (tubal) metaplasia in complex hyperplasia. Numerous ciliated cells with round, bland nuclei and clear cytoplasmic halos are present.

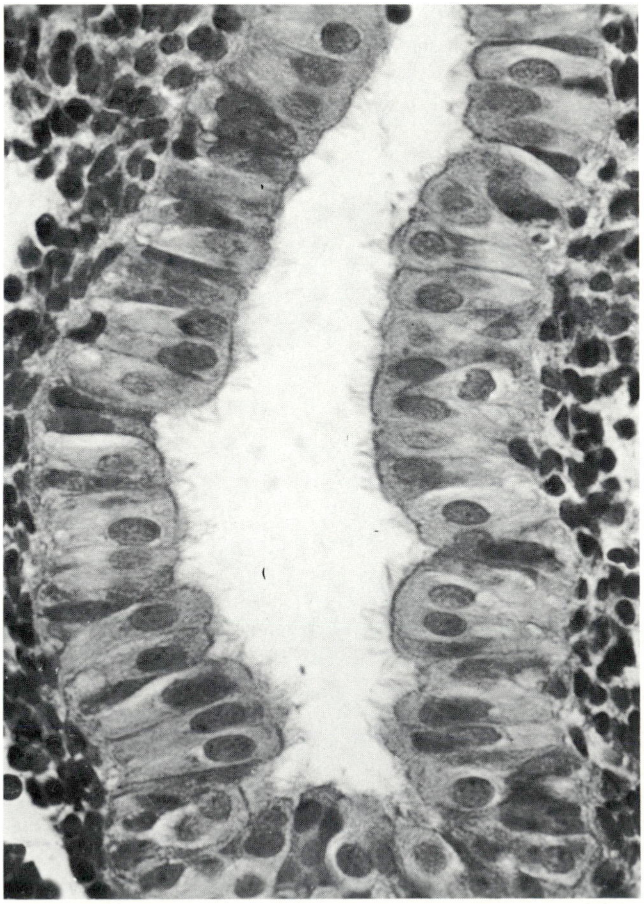

FIG. 11.13. High magnification of ciliated cells along with intercalated (peg) cells closely resembling the epithelium of the fallopian tube.

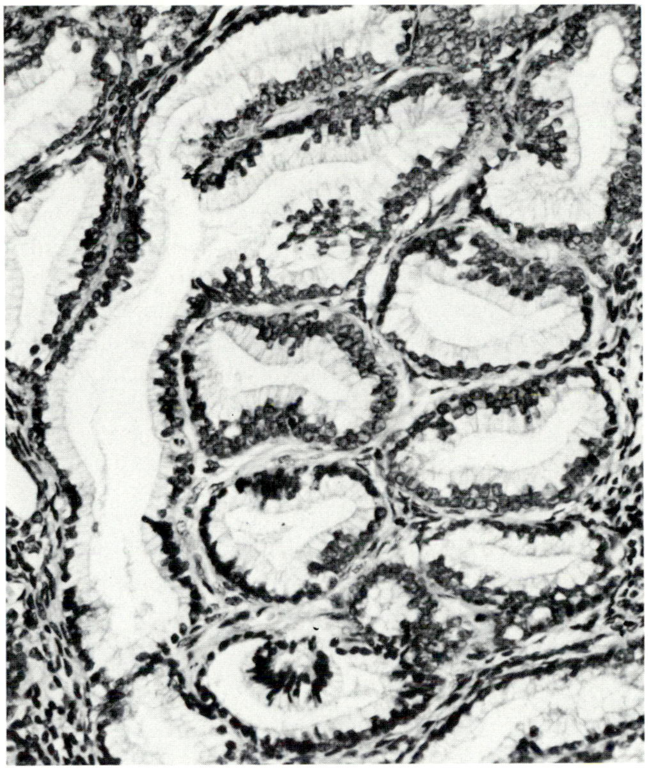

FIG. 11.14. Mucinous metaplasia in complex hyperplasia. The nuclei of the glandular cells are closely applied to the basement membrane. The cytoplasm is intensely positive with mucicarmine stains but contains no stainable glycogen.

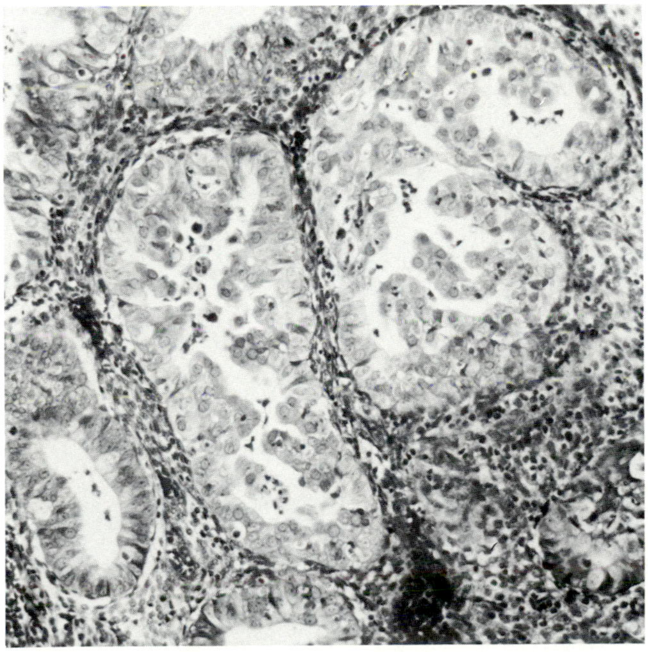

FIG. 11.15. Eosinophilic (pink) cell metaplasia in an atypical hyperplasia. In the past, lesions such as this were called carinoma in situ. The cells lining the glands are large, with eosinophilic cytoplasm and atypical nuclei. Intraglandular tufting is present.

ithelium of the fallopian tube. The ciliated cells are bland and interspersed singly or in small groups among nonciliated cells (Figs. 11.12 and 11.13). Mitotic activity is limited to the adjacent nonciliated cells. Ciliated cell metaplasia is usually found with milder forms of hyperplasia.

Mucinous Metaplasia. This form of metaplasia is characterized by mucinous epithelium resembling that of the endocervix. It is one of the least commonly encountered types of metaplasia. The mucinous epithelium tends to be distributed focally and is composed of tall columnar cells with bland, basally oriented nuclei and clear cytoplasm (Fig. 11.14). Mitotic figures are rare. The cytoplasm is clear on H&E stains because it contains mucin, which is periodic acid-Schiff (PAS) positive and diastase resistant. It stains with mucicarmine, toluidine blue, and Alcian blue. The cytologic, ultrastructural, and histochemical features of metaplastic mucinous epithelium differ from those of normal secretory endometrium by more closely resembling endocervical glandular epithelium.[10]

Other Metaplasias. The most common metaplasia in this category is eosinophilic metaplasia. In eosinophilic metaplasia, inactive or hyperplastic glands may be composed entirely or in part of enlarged glandular cells with abundant eosinophilic cytoplasm. The nuclei are generally round and vesicular and may display a variable degree of atypia. Atypical hyperplasia commonly is composed of eosinophilic cells (Fig. 11.15). On rare occasions, bland cells with clear cytoplasm containing glycogen and hobnail-type nuclei are found in glands or on the surface of the endometrium. These lesions are referred to as *clear cell metaplasia* (Fig. 11.16) and *hobnail metaplasia* (Fig. 11.17), respectively.[24] *Papillary metaplasia* (Fig. 11.18) has processes composed of cytologically bland cells with pyknotic nuclei, usually on the endometrial surface and less frequently in gland lumens.[24,25] Mitotic figures are rare. Some believe that papillary metaplasia is a form of hyperplasia. Typically, the papillary processes lack connective tissue support and are infiltrated with polymorphonuclear leukocytes.

Mixtures of different types of metaplasias are common. It is likely that most of the metaplasias are closely related and represent different morphologic expressions of a particular form of cellular differentiation.[24] For example, both papillary and eosinophilic metaplasia have a squamoid appearance at times and are often associated with squamous metaplasia. Likewise, eosinophilic and tubal metaplasias are closely related, since many of the cells in eosinophilic metaplasia resemble those in tubal metaplasia.

The frequent association of endometrial metaplasia with hyperplasia is probably due to the fact that both are often associated with a hyperestrogenic state. In one study, over 70% of perimenopausal and postmenopausal

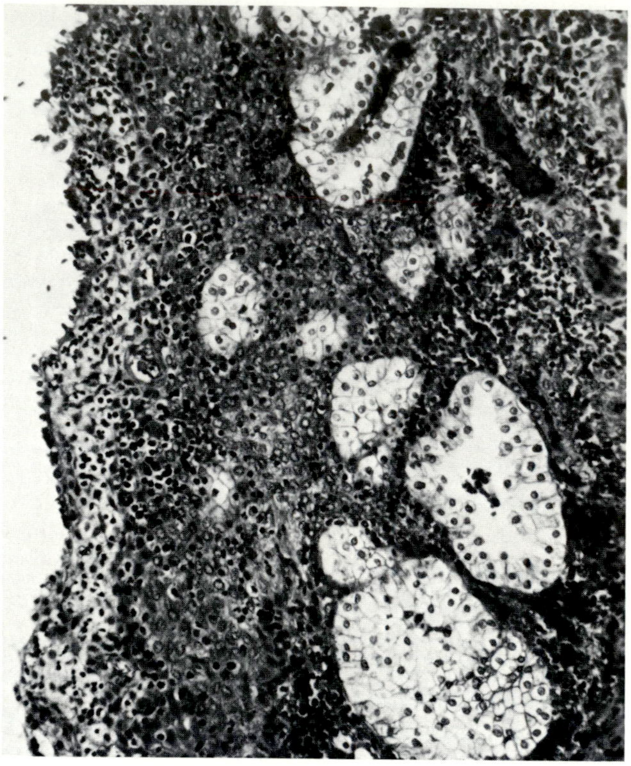

FIG. 11.16. Clear cell metaplasia characterized by glycogen-containing clear cells lining the endometrial glands.

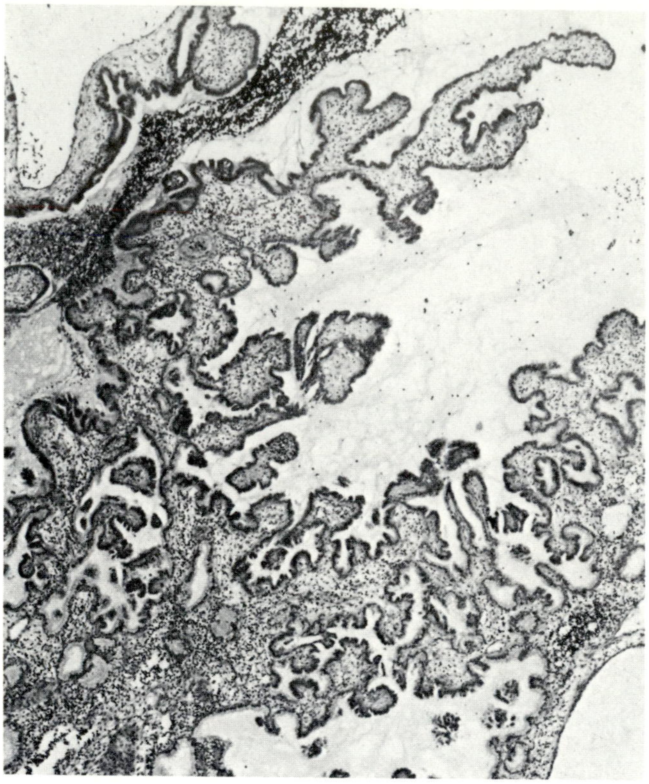

FIG. 11.18. Papillary metaplasia characterized by papillary fronds that are thin, delicate, and lined by cells with bland nuclei.

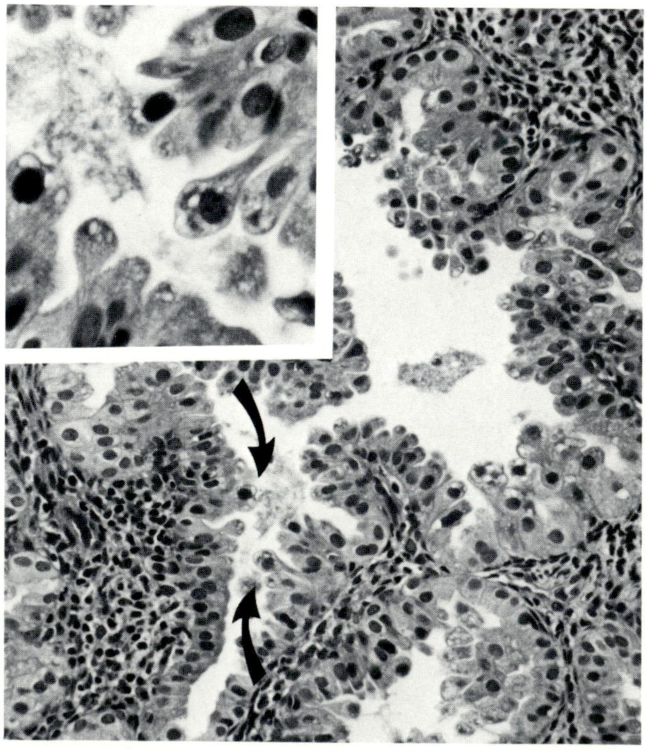

FIG. 11.17. Hobnail cell metaplasia is present in this complex hyperplasia. *Inset:* High magnification of the area designated by *arrows*.

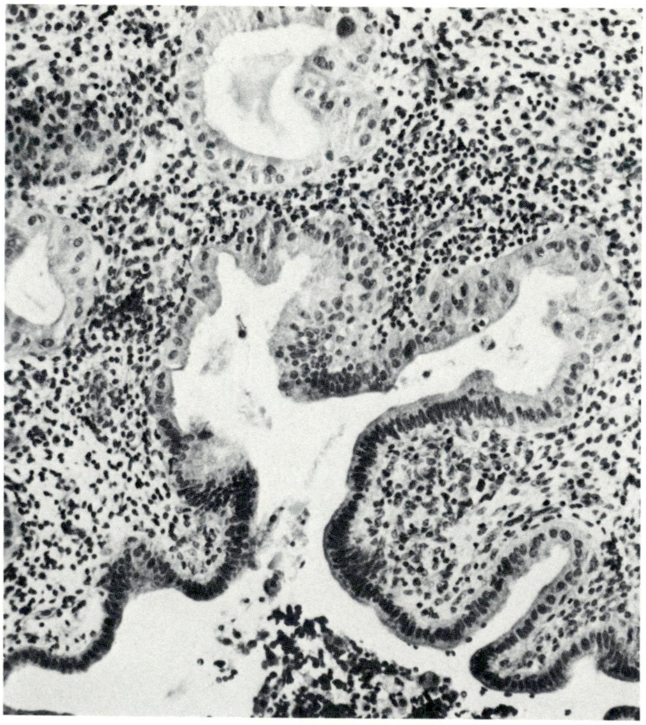

FIG. 11.19. Simple hyperplasia in which hyperplastic glands are surrounded by abundant stroma. Nuclei of stromal cells are plump and spindle-shaped, with indistinct (naked nucleus) cytoplasm.

women with metaplasia had received exogenous estrogen.[24] In addition, the vast majority of young women with metaplasia have clinical manifestations of persistent anovulation and primary infertility, features of polycystic ovarian disease.[3,8,24]

Metaplasia occurring in the absence of hyperplasia or carcinoma is rare except for senile or inactive endometrium, where it is known to have no influence on prognosis. Long-term follow-up studies specifically designed to determine the behavior of endometrial metaplasia have not been performed, and, therefore, its malignant potential is unknown. However, the association of hyperplasia and carcinoma is so frequent that evaluation of a metaplasia alone is rare. Bland metaplasias were not associated with aggressive behavior in a study of 89 patients by Hendrickson and Kempson.[24] In a long-term follow-up study of endometrial hyperplasia,[36] 5 of 11 patients with atypical hyperplasia and associated squamous metaplasia eventually developed carcinoma, indicating that atypical hyperplasia with squamous metaplasia has malignant potential.[36] It is doubtful that the metaplasia has any prognostic significance; the importance of recognizing metaplasia lies in not confusing a benign process with carcinoma.

Stroma

Stromal hyperplasia usually exists with endometrial glandular hyperplasia. In simple hyperplasias, the stromal cells are more densely packed than in proliferative endometrium. The cells retain their spindle shape but are plump, with enlarged nuclei and indistinct cytoplasm (Fig. 11.19). Mitotic activity in endometrial stromal cells is variable but may be increased. Cytologic atypia is rarely observed. In the complex forms of hyperplasia, the stromal cells are spindle shaped and become compressed by the glandular proliferation (Fig. 11.20).

In addition to densely packed stromal cells, clusters of foamy, lipid-laden cells (Fig. 11.21) occur in the stroma of 30% of the simple and complex hyperplasias and in 53% of atypical hyperplasias. These cells also occur in 3–43% of well-differentiated adenocarcinomas.[9,11,22,43] Foam cells have small pyknotic nuclei and abundant foamy cytoplasm that contains lipid droplets but no mu-

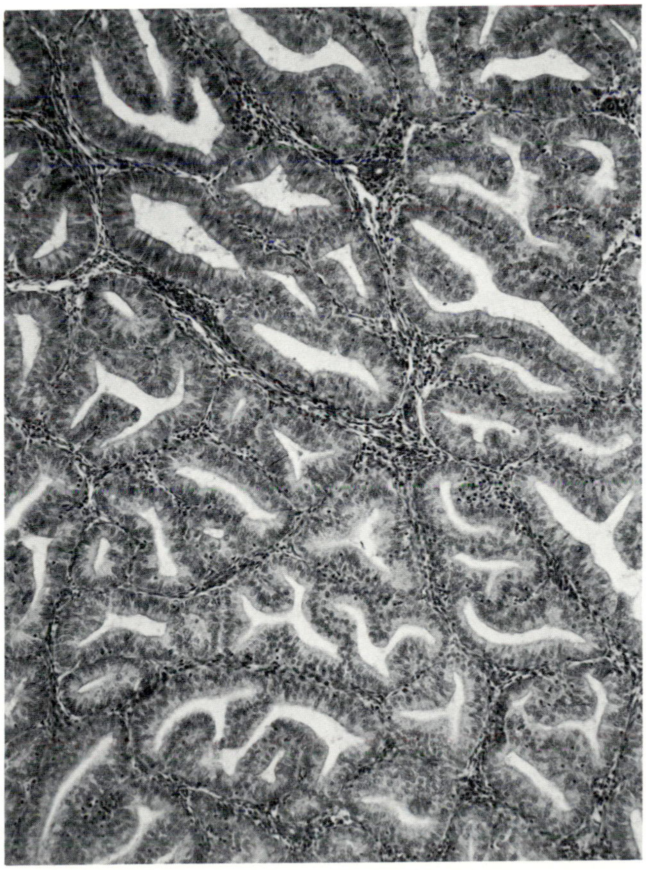

Fig. 11.20. Atypical hyperplasia with marked glandular crowding, resulting in compression of endometrial stroma. The stromal cells are spindle-shaped.

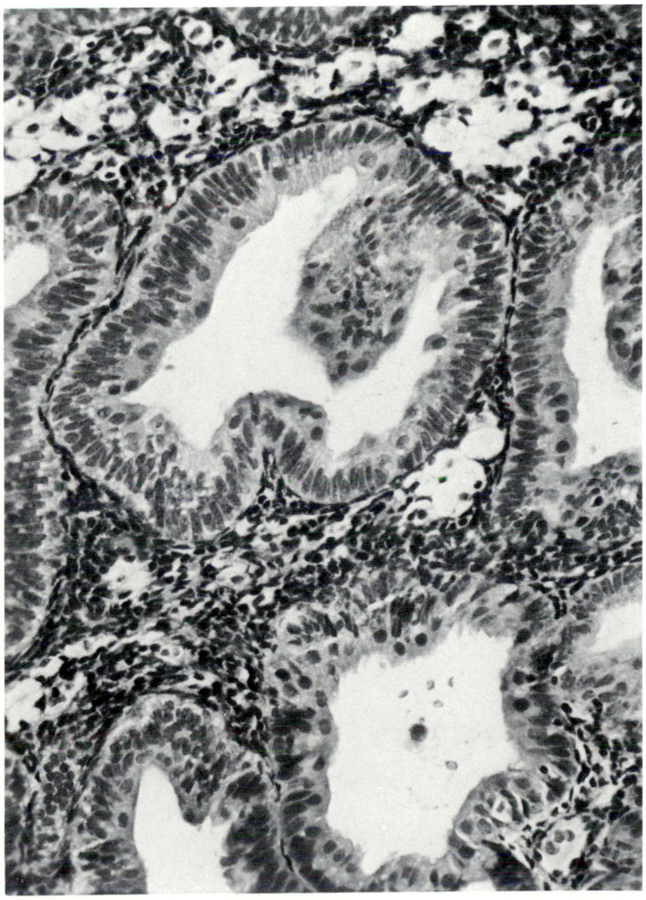

Fig. 11.21. Clusters of foamy, lipid-laden stromal cells in atypical hyperplasia.

cin. Although the foam cells were once considered macrophages, an ultrastructural study has shown that they are altered endometrial stromal cells.[12] Foam cells are rarely observed in nonneoplastic endometria, and their presence in curettings serves to warn of endometrial hyperplasia or carcinoma.

Adjunctive Techniques in the Characterization of Hyperplasia

Electron Microscopy

Scanning and transmission electron microscopic studies[15,16,32,41] reveal that the nonatypical forms of hyperplasia have an increase in the number of estrogen-related organelles in the glandular epithelial cells. These include cilia and microvilli and an increase in free ribosomes, rough endoplasmic recticulum, and complexes of glycogen, Golgi, and mitochondria. Lipid bodies and microfilaments are also increased. These are nonspecific features; ultrastructural analysis does not permit distinction between the cells of the nonatypical hyperplasias (Fig. 11.22) and those of normal proliferative endometrium. In hyperplasia with cytologic atypia, there are corresponding ultrastructural changes. As the lesion approaches carcinoma, estrogen-related features diminish. Cilia and surface microvilli are less frequent, and the mitochondria and rough endoplasmic reticulum are increased and show greater variation. Microfilaments are arranged in a more haphazard fashion than in nonatypical hyperplasia. These bizarre epithelial alterations may closely approach well-differentiated adenocarcinoma but are not as marked (Fig. 11.23). Atypical hyperplasia appears to be comprised of a heterogeneous population of cells, ranging from those that are indistinguishable from normal proliferative endometrium to those that exist in well-differentiated adenocarcinoma. Estrogen-related characteristics are reduced in carcinoma. Unfortunately, electron microscopy, with its limited sample size, does not aid in the distinction between atypical hyperplasia and well-differentiated adenocarcinoma.

Quantitative Microscopy

Quantitative cytomorphology offers a reproducible method to identify degrees of architectural and cytologic atypia,[1,2,7,39] provided that the fixation, embedding, and staining of the samples are uniform and selectivity is controlled. Profiles of glandular form, nuclear size, and nuclear shape can be measured so that one lesion can be compared with another. Degrees of atypia can be

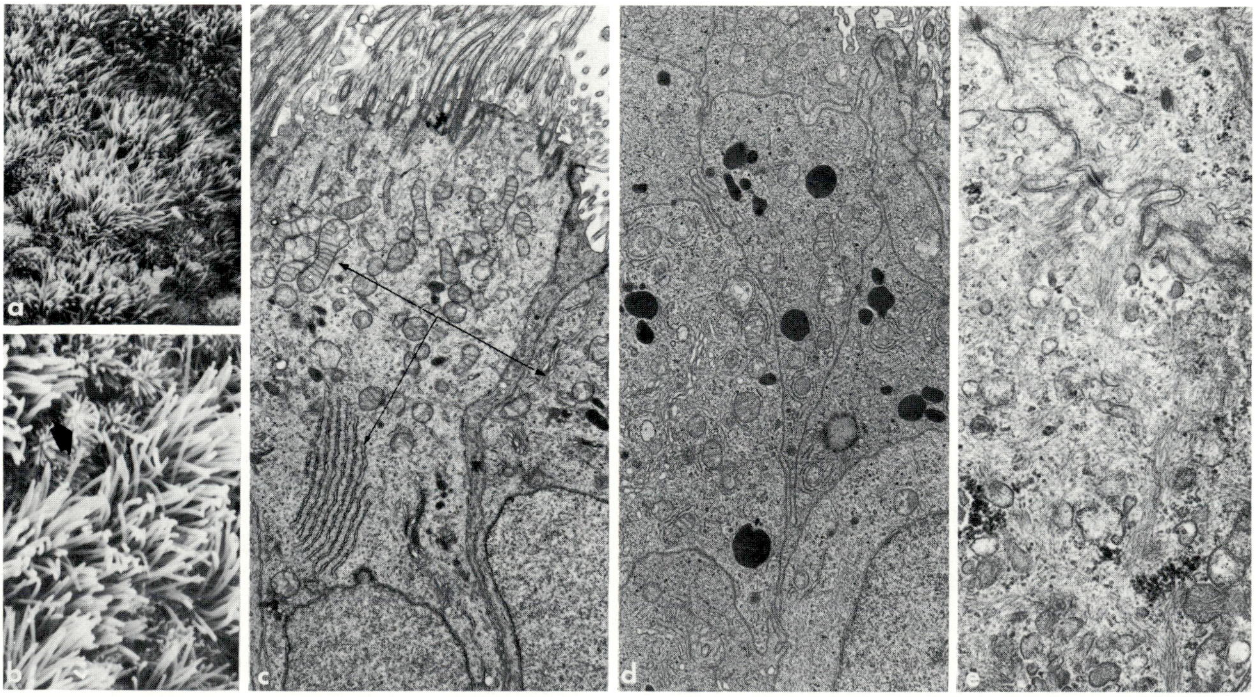

FIG. 11.22. Ultrastructure of hyperplasia without atypia. *a*. Scanning electron microscopy demonstrating abundance of ciliated cells. ×950. *b*. Nonciliated cells are covered by prominent surface microvillus promontories. ×2850. *c*. A well-developed mitochondria–granular endoplasmic reticulum–Golgi complex (*arrow*) in gland-lining cells. ×570. *d*. Abundant electron-dense, membrane-bound lysosomes in gland-lining cells. ×7125. *e*. Glycogen granules intermingling with microfilaments in gland-lining cells. ×45,600. (Adapted and reprinted by permission of Ferenczy, Ref. 16.)

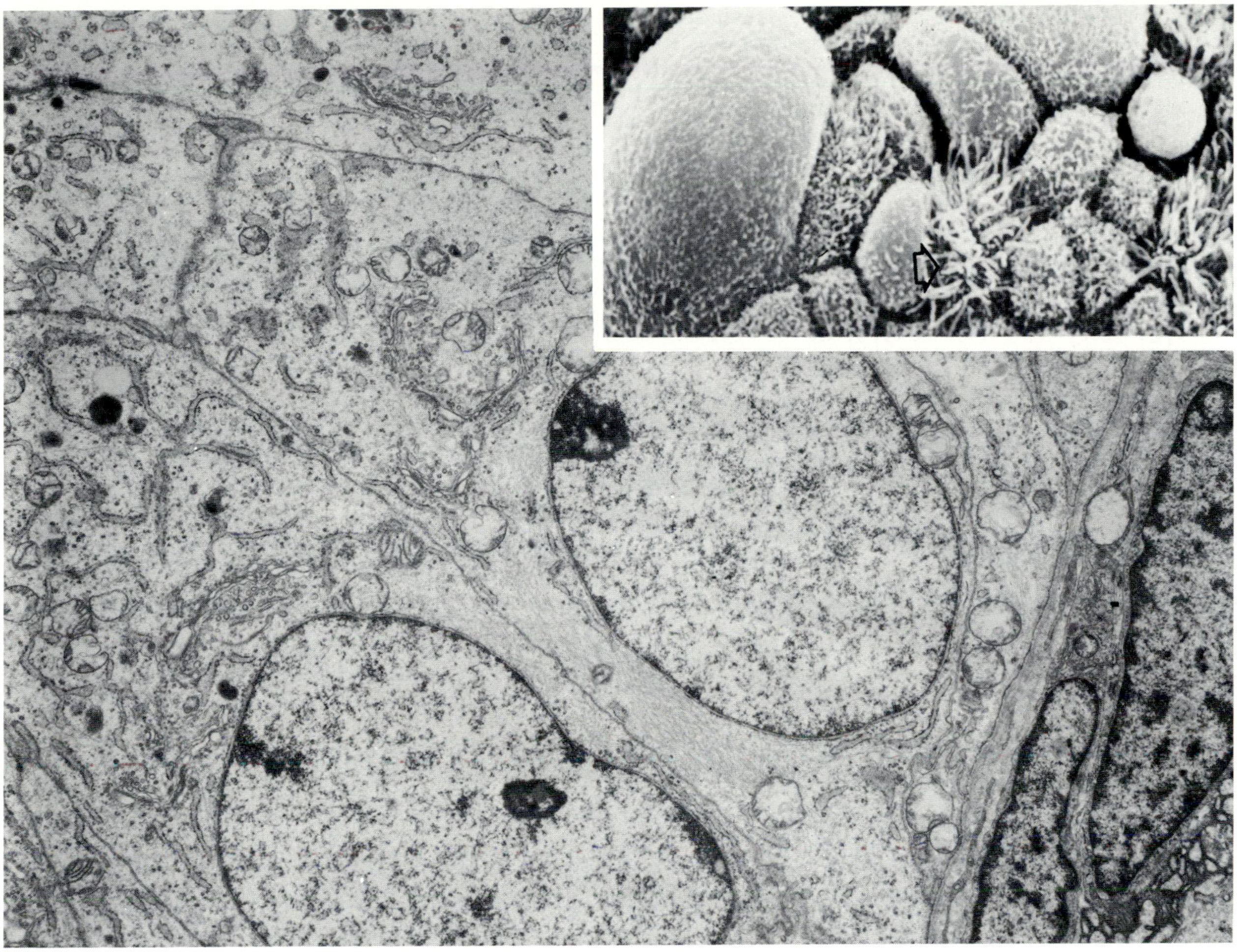

FIG. 11.23. Electron microscopy of atypical hyperplasia. Note the well-developed Golgi and pleomorphic disposition of microfilaments. Free ribosomes are sparse. ×9300. *Inset:* Scanning electron microscopy showing that ciliated cells (*arrow*) are few and nonciliated cells are pleomorphic, with short and sparse microvilli. ×1900. (Reprinted by permission of Ferenczy, Ref. 16.)

further quantitated by measuring nuclear texture, DNA content, and nuclear thickness. These techniques offer the promise of reducing the subjectivity of the diagnosis that currently prevails. One study[1] showed that volume percentage and inner surface density of the glands showed significant differences between atypical hyperplasia and carcinoma. In another study, measurements of nuclear size in curettings of patients with atypical hyperplasia provided a means of predicting with 83% accuracy which atypical hyperplasia in curettings would progress to carcinoma.[7]

DNA Microspectrophotometry and In Vitro Histoautoradiography

Aneuploidy is a feature of malignant cells, with the exception of some carcinomas of endocrine organs.[29,42] Microspectrophotometric studies demonstrate an aneuploid DNA distribution in some atypical hyperplasia,[30,46] although a significant number of well-differentiated endometrial carcinomas may be diploid or peridiploid.[29,30] Thus, some hyperplasias with a potential to progress cannot be identified or predicted from cell measurements or DNA content.

In vitro DNA labeling with [^{3}H]thymidine or [^{14}C]thymidine shows atypical hyperplasia to have a prolonged DNA synthesis (S-1 phase) coupled with a shorter cell doubling time, as in carcinoma.[14,15] In this respect, the extreme forms of atypical hyperplasia are similar to those of invasive carcinoma. These techniques may assist in identifying severe forms of atypical hyperplasia and carcinoma and may be useful in predicting the likelihood of progression.

Immunocytochemistry

Carcinoembryonic antigen (CEA), human chorionic gonadotropin (hCG), lutenizing hormone (LH), alpha-fetoprotein (AFP), and casein have been analyzed in endometrial hyperplasia and carcinoma.[13,23,28] Hustin[28] localized CEA in all atypical hyperplasias and in 60% of carcinomas. Casein was also demonstrated in all grades of hyperplasia,[28] but AFP and LH were not.[23,28] Reports of the localization of hCG have been conflicting, since some investigators have identified hCG in more than a third of atypical hyperplasias[28] and others have been unable to identify it in any of them.[13] The number of cases thus far studied is too small to draw conclusions about the role of immuncytochemistry in distinguishing atypical hyperplasia from carcinoma.

Behavior of Endometrial Hyperplasia

Endometrial proliferations without evidence of invasion constitute a group of heterogeneous lesions of differing biologic potential displaying a continuum of cytologic and architectural alterations. Most sudies[4,6,20,26,38] designed to determine the fate of untreated hyperplasia fail to consider the cytologic and architectural abnormalities separately.[47] Some reports are further confounded by including irradiated patients, thereby altering the natural history of the study condition.

Recently, 170 patients with all grades of endometrial hyperplasia in curettings were followed (mean 13.4 years) without a hysterectomy being performed for at least 1 year.[36] None of the women had been irradiated. Various histologic features were evaluated, and cytologic and architectural abnormalities were analyzed independently in an effort to delineate the histologic features associated with an increased risk of progression to carcinoma. Those without cytologic atypia (see section on microscopic pathology) were designated *hyperplasia*, and those with cytologic atypia were designated *atypical hyperplasia*. *Hyperplasia* thus defined is equivalent to what is termed *simple and complex hyperplasia* in the classification proposed by the International Society of Gynecological Pathologists. A third of the patients with both types of hyperplasia (nonatypical and atypical) were asymptomatic after the diagnostic curettage and required no further treatment. Only 2 (2%) of 122 patients with hyperplasia lacking cytologic atypia progressed to carcinoma, whereas 11 (23%) of the 48 women with atypical hyperplasia progressed to carcinoma ($p = 0.001$). The 2 cases of hyperplasia that progressed underwent an alteration to atypical hyperplasia before developing into carcinoma. Clearly, cytologic atypia is the most useful feature in identifying a lesion that might progress to carcinoma.

Subdivision of hyperplasia by the degree of glandular complexity and crowding can be made (see section on microscopic pathology). A proliferative lesion displaying no evidence of cytologic atypia and not having back-to-back glands or intraluminal papillary processes is a simple hyperplasia, whereas one with back-to-back glands and intraluminal papillary processes is a complex hyperplasia. A simple hyperplasia with cytologic atypia is a simple atypical hyperplasia, and one accompanied by a complex glandular pattern is a complex atypical hyperplasia. Progression to carcinoma occurs in only 1% of patients with simple hyperplasia and in 3% of patients with complex hyperplasia. In contrast, 8% of patients with simple atypical hyperplasia and 29% of patients with complex atypical hyperplasia will progress to carcinoma (Table 11.2). The presence of glandular complexity and crowding superimposed on atypia, therefore, appears to place the patient at greater risk than does cytologic atypia alone. The differences among the four subgroups, however, are not statistically significant.

Endometrial Hyperplasia as a Precursor of Endometrial Carcinoma

The carcinomas that develop in patients with simple, complex, and atypical hyperplasia are relatively innocuous.[20,36] The mean duration of progression of hyperplasia without atypia to carcinoma is nearly 10 years, and it takes a mean of 4 years to progress from atypical hyperplasia to clinically evident carcinoma.[36]

It has been shown that 17–25% of women with atypical

TABLE 11.2. Follow-up comparing cytologic and architectural abnormalities in 170 patients.[a]

Type of hyperplasia	No. of patients	Regressed		Persisted		Progressed to carcinoma	
		No.	(%)	No.	(%)	No.	(%)
Simple	93	74	(80)	18	(19)	1	(1)
Complex	29	23	(80)	5	(17)	1	(3)
Simple atypical	13	9	(69)	3	(23)	1	(8)
Complex atypical	35	20	(57)	5	(14)	10	(29)

[a] Adapted with permission of Kurman et al., Ref. 36.

hyperplasia in curettings will have a well-differentiated carcinoma in the uterus if a hysterectomy is performed within 1 month of the curettage.[31,34,44] Yet with long-term follow-up, only 11–23% of women with atypical hyperplasia develop carcinoma if a hysterectomy is not done.[20,36] Thus, the lesion designated *well-differentiated carcinoma* usually remains stable for a long period of time. Several reasons may account for the relatively low rate of progression to carcinoma in untreated patients with atypical hyperplasia. First, there is a general tendency for the highest grade of atypical hyperplasia to be selected for hysterectomy, leaving the lesser degree of atypia for conservative management. Second, atypical hyperplasia may not be the precursor of all forms of endometrial cancer but only of a type that is slow-growing and not always progressive. The different forms of endometrial carcinoma and how they relate to atypical hyperplasia are discussed in Chapter 12, Endometrial Carcinoma.

Treatment

Management of patients with noninvasive endometrial proliferations is based on consideration of clinical factors in addition to the microscopic findings.[33] A plan for the management of women with abnormal bleeding using the classification of the International Society of Gynecological Pathologists is shown in Figure 11.24.

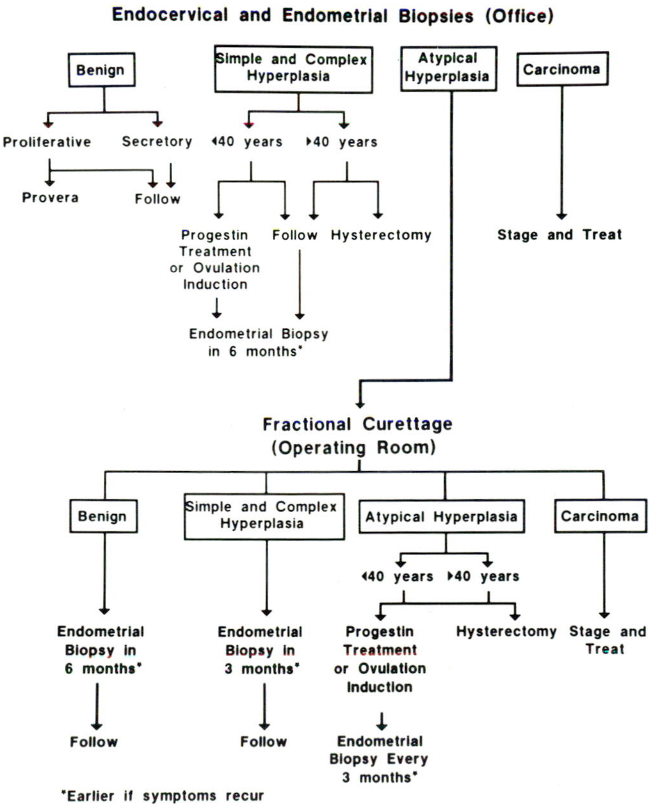

FIG. 11.24. Plan for management of women with abnormal bleeding using the classification of the International Society of Gynecological Pathologists.

Women 40 Years and Younger

Women with simple and complex hyperplasia based on an endometrial biopsy can be treated conservatively, since these lesions have an extremely low risk (1–2%) of progression to carcinoma. Moreover, since the transit time to carcinoma is approximately 10 years and proliferations without cytologic atypia first progress through atypical hyperplasia before becoming carcinoma, close follow-up and periodic endometrial biopsies suffice.[36]

Women with atypical hyperplasia on an endometrial biopsy require a fractional curettage (endocervical and endometrial curettage) in the operating room to make certain that the uterine cavity has been thoroughly sampled. The distinction of atypical hyperplasia from carcinoma is important in young women who want to retain their fertility. The likelihood of residual carcinoma in the uterus after curettage increases with age (Fig. 11.25) and is low in women younger than 40 years of age. Only 2 of 17 patients under age 40 with atypical hyperplasia in curettings had carcinoma in the uterus (Table 11.3), and both neoplasms were well differentiated and confined to the endometrium. In contrast, if well-differentiated carcinoma is present in the curettings as determined by the identification of stromal invasion, more than a third of women younger than age 40 will have residual carcinoma in the uterus. Furthermore, nearly a quarter of the residual tumors are moderately differentiated, and the majority invade the myometrium.[34]

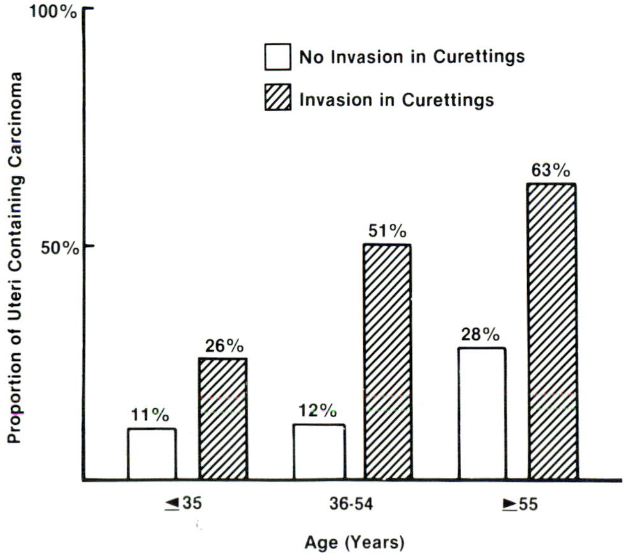

FIG. 11.25. Residual carcinoma in uterus according to age and presence of stromal invasion in curettings of 204 patients. (Adapted by permission of Kurman and Norris, Ref. 35.)

TABLE 11.3. Residual carcinoma in the uterus according to the presence or absence of stromal invasion in 52 women under 40 years of age.[a]

	Curettings	
	No invasion	Invasion
Hysterectomy findings	17	35
Residual carcinoma	2(12%)	13(37%)
Grade 1	2(100%)	10(77%)
Grade 2	0	3(23%)
Endometrium only	2(100%)	3(23%)
Myometrium		
Inner one third	0	9(69%)
Middle one third	0	1(8%)

[a] Adapted from Kurman and Norris, Ref. 34.

Therefore, young women with atypical hyperplasia who wish to retain their fertility can have hormonal treatment, either by suppression with progestins or induction of ovulation, but close follow-up and periodic endometrial biopsies are necessary. A conservative plan of management is justified, since young women with atypical hyperplasia who progress to carcinoma rarely if ever die of their tumor, and nearly a quarter of those less than 40 years of age will have normal deliveries.[6,36] In contrast, women less than 40 years of age with bona fide well-differentiated carcinoma (using the criteria outlined in Chapter 12, Endometrial Carcinoma) require surgical treatment.

Women Older than 40 Years

Most simple and complex hyperplasias in this age group are related to anovulation associated with the menopause and are self-limited. Conservative management, either observation only or treatment with medroxyprogesterone to produce a medical curettage, therefore, is adequate. Repeated episodes of irregular bleeding that is not responsive to hormone treatment may require a hysterectomy. The majority (80%) of these nonatypical hyperplasias regress.

Nearly 60% of atypical hyperplasias also regress, but since the likelihood of residual carcinoma in the uterus after a curettage increases with age (Fig. 11.25), hysterectomy is the treatment of choice for women over 50. For patients in the 40–50-year age range, treatment should be individualized. Regression occurs frequently, and the risk of residual carcinoma is lower than in older women. Therefore, observation or suppression with progestins monitored by repeat endometrial biopsies every 3 months and repeat curettage may suffice. If the lesion persists, a hysterectomy should be performed.

In perimenopausal or menopausal women with either simple, complex, or atypical hyperplasia who are receiving exogenous estrogen, termination of the estrogen usually suffices even for atypical hyperplasia, since these proliferations are iatrogenic and regress after the stimulus for their growth has been removed. Alternatively, cyclic courses of medroxyprogesterone have been advocated in women being treated with estrogen as a means of preventing the development of endometrial hyperplasia and carcinoma. Using a 7–14 day regimen of orally administered 10 mg of medroxyprogesterone to postmenopausal women receiving estrogen, 5 endometrial carcinomas were detected in 5402 woman-years of continuous estrogen therapy.[18] This incidence is not greater than that of untreated postmenopausal women, in whom the expected incidence of endometrial cancer is 1–2 per 1000 woman-years, that is, 5.4–9.8 cases.

References

1. Ausems, WEMA, van der Kamp J-K, Baak, JAP (1985) Nuclear morphometry in the determination of the prognosis of marked atypical endometrial hyperplasia. Int J Gynecol Pathol 4: 180
2. Baak JPA, Kurver PHJ, Diegenbach PC, Delemarre JFM, Brekelmans ECM, Nieuwlaat JE (1981) Discrimination of hyperplasia and carcinoma of the endometrium by quantitative microscopy—A feasibility study. Histopathology 5: 61
3. Blaustein A (1982) Morular metaplasia misdiagnosed as adenoacanthoma in young women with polycystic ovarian disease. Am J Surg Pathol 6: 223
4. Buehl IA, Vellios F, Carter JE, Huber CP (1964) Carcinoma in situ of the endometrium. Am J Clin Pathol 42: 594
5. Campbell PE, Barter RA (1961) The significance of atypical hyperplasia. J Obstet Gynaecol Br Commonw 68: 668
6. Chamlian DL, Taylor HB (1970) Endometrial hyperplasia in young women. Obstet Gynecol 36: 659
7. Colgan TJ, Norris HJ, Foster W, Kurman RJ, Fox CH (1983) Predicting the outcome of endometrial hyperplasia by quantitative analysis of nuclear features using a linear discriminant function. Int J Gynecol Pathol 1: 347
8. Crum CP, Richart RM, Fenoglio CM (1981) Adenoacanthosis of the endometrium. A clinicopathologic study in premenopausal women. Am J Surg Pathol 5: 15
9. Dewagne MP, Silverberg SG (1982) Foam cells in endometrial carcinoma. A clinicopathologic study. Gynecol Oncol 13: 67
10. Demopoulos RI, Greco MA (1983) Mucinous metaplasia of the endometrium: Ultrastructural and histochemical characteristics. Int J Gynecol Pathol 1: 383
11. Fechner RE (1980) Ultrastructure of endometrial stromal foam cells (Letter to Editor). Am J Clin Pathol 73: 731
12. Fechner RE, Bossart MI, Spjut HJ (1979) Ultrastructure of endometrial stromal foam cells. Am J Clin Pathol 72: 628
13. Fenoglio CM, Crum CP, Ferenczy A (1982) Endometrial hyperplasia and carcinoma. Are ultrastructural, biochemical, and immunocytochemical studies useful in distinguishing between them? Pathol Res Pract 174: 257
14. Ferenczy A (1983) Cytodynamics of endometrial hyperpla-

sia and neoplasia. Part II: In vitro DNA histoautoradiography. Hum Pathol 14: 77
15. Ferenczy A (1982) Cytodynamics of endometrial hyperplasia and neoplasia. I. Histology and ultrastructure. In: Fenoglio CM, Wolff M (eds) Progress in surgical pathology. New York Masson Publishing USA, Vol 4, p 95
16. Ferenczy A (1979) Recent advances in endometrial neoplasia. Exp Mol Pathol 31: 226
17. Fluhman CF (1954) Comparative studies of squamous metaplasia of the cervix uteri and endometrium. Am J Obstet Gynecol 68: 1447
18. Greenblatt RB, Gambrell RD Jr, Stoddard LD (1982) The protective role of progesterone in the prevention of endometrial cancer. Pathol Res Pract 174: 297
19. Gusberg SB (1974) Precursors of corpus carcinoma. Estrogens and adenomatous hyperplasia. Am J Obstet Gynecol 54: 905
20. Gusberg SB, Kaplan AL (1963) Precursors of corpus cancer. IV. Adenomatous hyperplasia as stage 0 carcinoma of the endometrium. Am J Obstet Gynecol 87: 661
21. Gusberg SB, Moore DB, Martin F (1954) Precursors of corpus cancer. II. A clinical and pathological study of adenomatous hyperplasia. Am J Obstet Gynecol 68: 1472
22. Harris HR (1958) Foam cells in the stroma of carcinoma of the body of the uterus and uterine cervical polypi. J Clin Pathol 11: 19
23. Hayata T, Fenoglio CM, Crum CP, Richart RM (1981) The simultaneous expression of human chorionic gonadotropin and carcinoembryonic antigen in the female genital tract. Diag Gynecol Obstet 3: 309
24. Hendrickson MR, Kempson RL (1980) Endometrial epithelial metaplasias—Proliferations frequently misdiagnosed as adenocarcinoma: Report of 89 cases and proposed classification. Am J Surg Pathol 4: 525
25. Hendrickson MR, Kempson RL (1980) In: Bennington JL (ed) Surgical pathology of the uterine corpus. Major problems In pathology. Philadelphia, London, Toronto, W.B. Saunders Co.
26. Hertig AT, Sommers SC (1949) Genesis of endometrial carcinoma. I. Study of prior biopsies. Cancer 2: 946
27. Hertig AT, Sommers SC, Bengaloff H (1949) Genesis of endometrial carcinoma. III. Carcinoma in situ. Cancer 2: 964
28. Hustin J (1978) Imunohistochemical demonstration of several tumor markers in neoplastic and preneoplastic states of the uterine mucosa. Gynecol Obstet Invest 9: 3
29. Hustin J (1976) Morphology and DNA content of endometrial cancer nuclei under progestogen treatment. Acta Cytol 20: 556
30. Katayma KP, Jones HW (1967) Chromosomes of atypical (adenomatous) hyperplasia and carcinoma of the endometrium. Am J Obstet Gynecol 97: 978
31. King A, Seraj IM, Wagner RJ (1984) Stromal invasion in endometrial carcinoma. Am J Obstet Gynecol 149: 10
32. Klemi PJ, Gronroos M, Rauramo L, Punnonen R (1980) Ultrastructural features of endometrial atypical adenomatous hyperplasia and adenocarcinomas and the plasma levels of estrogens. Gynecol Oncol 9: 162
33. Kraus FT (1985) High-risk and premalignant lesions of the endometrium. Am J Surg Pathol 9(3) [Suppl]: 31
34. Kurman RJ, Norris HJ (1982) Evaluation of criteria for distinguishing atypical endometrial hyperplasia from well-differentiated carcinoma. Cancer 49: 2547
35. Kurman RJ, Norris HJ (1986) Endometrium. In: Henson D, AlboresSaavedra J (eds) The pathology of incipient neoplasia. Philadelphia, W.B. Saunders Co., p 265
36. Kurman RJ, Kaminski PF, Norris HJ (1985) The behavior of endometrial hyperplasia. A long-term study of "untreated" hyperplasia in 170 patients. Cancer 56: 403
37. Masterson R, Armstrong EM, Moore IAR (1975) The cyclical variation in the percentage of ciliated cells in the normal human endometrium. J Reprod Fertil 42: 537
38. McBride JM (1959) Pre-menopausal cystic hyperplasia and endometrial carcinoma. J Obstet Gynaecol Br Emp 66: 288
39. Norris HJ, Tavassoli FA, Kurman RJ (1983) Endometrial hyperplasia and carcinoma. Diagnostic considerations. Am J Surg Pathol 7: 839
40. Novak E, Rutledge F (1948) Atypical endometrial hyperplasia simulating adenocarcinoma. Am J Obstet Gynecol 55: 46
41. Richart RM, Ferenczy A (1974) Endometrial morphologic response to hormonal environment. Gynecol Oncol 2: 180
42. Richart RM, Ludwig AS (1969) Alterations in chromosomes and DNA content in gynecologic neoplasms. Am J Obstet Gynecol 104: 463
43. Salm R (1962) Macrophages in endometrial lesions. J Pathol Bacteriol 83: 405
44. Tavassoli FA, Kraus FT (1978) Endometrial lesions in uteri resected for atypical endometrial hyperplasia. Am J Clin Pathol 70: 770
45. Vellios F (1974) Endometrial hyperplasia and carcinoma in situ. Gynecol Oncol 2: 152
46. Wagner D, Richart RM, Terner JY (1967) Deoxyribonucleic acid content of presumed precursors of endometrial carcinoma. Cancer 20: 2067
47. Welch WR, Scully RE (1977) Precancerous lesions of the endometrium. Hum Pathol 8: 503

12

Endometrial Carcinoma

Robert J. Kurman, M.D., and Henry J. Norris, M.D.

Etiology

Endometrial carcinoma has become the most common invasive neoplasm of the female genital tract in the United States. In 1984 there were an estimated 39,000 new cases and 2900 deaths from endometrial cancer.[161] A rising incidence has been observed also in Canada and western and eastern Europe.[11,92,182] There is a much lower incidence in Asia, Africa, and South America than in North America.[43] Migration studies of Japanese women who have a low incidence of endometrial cancer in Japan show an increase in the rates of endometrial carcinoma in first and second generations born in California.[66] These findings have been attributed to the high content of animal fat in the Western diet,[64] but this does not explain the dramatic rise in the incidence of endometrial carcinoma in the United States and Europe.

There is a strong association between replacement estrogen therapy and the development of endometrial cancer.* This is partly reflected in the parallel rise and fall in the incidence of endometrial cancer and estrogen sales in the United States.[183] The decline in rates of endometrial cancer since 1975 is confined to women in their 50s, whereas a slight, continuous rise in endometrial cancer rates is observed for women over 60. This difference suggests that there may be two different forms of endometrial cancer: a low-grade neoplasm that is estrogen-related and occurs in younger, perimenopausal

* References 60, 62, 116, 121, 167, 192.

TABLE 12.1. Endometrial carcinoma: two types.

	Type I	Type II
Unopposed estrogen	Present	Absent
Menopausal status	Pre- and perimenopausal	Postmenopausal
Hyperplasia	Present	Absent
Race	White	Black
Grade	Low	High
Myometrial invasion	Minimal	Deep
Specific subtypes	Adenoacanthoma	Adenosquamous
	Secretory	Serous
	Ciliated	Clear cell
Behavior	Stable	Progressive

women and a second, more virulent form, unrelated to estrogenic stimulation, that occurs in older postmenopausal women.[17,168] Several lines of epidemiologic and clinicopathologic evidence support the hypothesis that there are two pathogenetic forms of endometrial carcinoma, which for purposes of this discussion are designated type I (estrogen related) and type II (nonestrogen related) (Table 12.1). Robboy and Bradley[143] showed that the carcinomas in estrogen users are better differentiated than are those in nonestrogen users. Also, only 4 (12%) of 33 of the estrogen users had poorly differentiated adenocarcinoma compared to 30 (37%) of 81 of the nonusers, suggesting that the development of poorly differentiated adenocarcinoma is unrelated to the use of estrogen.

Among nontumor risk factors, the presence of endometrial hyperplasia is the single most important factor in identifying patients with a favorable prognosis. The presence of hyperplasia correlates with low tumor grade and lack of myometrial invasion.[13,60] In contrast, high-grade tumors are more often associated with an atrophic endometrium.[17] Atypical hyperplasia in curettings is associated with well-differentiated carcinoma in the uterus in 17–25% of women if a hysterectomy is performed within 1 month.[100,172] In contrast, 11–23% of women with atypical hyperplasia in curettings develop low grade carcinoma if they do not undergo a hysterectomy but are followed.[65,103] These findings suggest that endometrial hyperplasia is a precursor of type I but not necessarily type II endometrial carcinoma.

Unfavorable endometrial carcinoma subtypes, such as serous carcinoma, adenosquamous carcinoma, and clear cell carcinoma, may be unrelated to estrogen use also because they occur at an older age (mean of 66 years) than the usual endometrial carcinoma (mean age of 59 years) and are rarely associated with hyperplasia.[41] Race also appears to be related to the two different forms of endometrial cancer. In the United States, a higher frequency of the favorable types of carcinoma occur in white women than in black women.[33] In Miyagi Prefecture, Japan, the risk factors associated with type I endometrial cancers, such as obesity and estrogen use, are considerably lower than in the United States. There, adenosquamous carcinoma represents 41% of all endometrial carcinomas whereas in two different series in the United States, adenosquamous carcinoma represented only 18–23% of endometrial cancers.[165]

Of the constitutional factors associated with endometrial carcinoma, such as obesity, hypertension, diabetes mellitus, and nulliparity, obesity has received the greatest attention. The effect of obesity is related to the enhanced conversion of androstenedione to estrone from aromatization of androstenedione to estrogen in fat cells.[18,112,113,133,155] Nonetheless, slender women, ovulating women, and women who are pregnant may also develop endometrial carcinoma.[142] These women represent a subgroup of patients whose endocrine–metabolic profiles are not significantly different from those of control subjects, suggesting that their tumors are not associated with an obvious endocrine or metabolic disorder[113] or that their neoplasms are estrogen-related but arise in progesterone refractory endometrium.[142] These endometrial carcinomas are frequently occult and not associated with vaginal bleeding.

Several studies have shown a high incidence of both endometrial carcinoma and breast cancer among sisters, mothers, and aunts of individuals with endometrial carcinoma,[115,127,185] suggesting a genetic predisposition. In a review of endometrial carcinoma in Israel, 3% of the patients had breast carcinoma that preceded the diagnosis of the uterine neoplasm.[154] In one study, adenosquamous carcinoma of the endometrium, in particular, tended to coexist with breast carcinoma.[16]

Other known carcinogens, such as radiation and smoking, appear to have no role in the etiology of endometrial cancer. Cigarette smoking was found to decrease the risk of endometrial carcinoma in postmenopausal women, including those receiving exogenous estrogens.[54,106] It is postulated that the reduction in endometrial carcinoma associated with smoking may be due to the enhanced clearance of estrogen resulting from the induction of hepatic microsomal enzymes by cigarette smoking.[34] In several large series, from 5–7% of patients with endometrial carcinoma had received prior radiation, but this experience does not appear to differ significantly from that of control patients.[146]

Clinical and Pathologic Features

Gross Appearance

The gross appearance of the various types of endometrial carcinoma is not distinctive. The endometrial surface is shaggy, glistening, and tan and may be focally hemorrhagic. Necrosis is usually not evident macroscopically in well-differentiated carcinomas but may be seen in poorly differentiated tumors, sometimes in association with ulcerated or firm areas. Myometrial invasion by carcinoma may result in enlargement of the uterus, but a small, atrophic uterus may harbor carcinoma diffusely invading the myometrium. Myometrial invasion appears as well-demarcated, firm, gray-white tissue with linear extensions beneath and exophytic mass or as multiple, white nodules with yellow areas of necrosis within the uterine wall.

Microscopic Appearance and Clinicopathologic Correlation

Endometrial Stromal Invasion as a Criterion of Malignancy

Most endometrial carcinomas are readily identified, but it may be difficult to distinguish well-differentiated carcinoma from atypical hyperplasia.[21] A diagnosis of well-differentiated carcinoma is established easily when there is myometrial invasion, but this is usually not apparent in curettings. The two conditions can be separated if arbitrary criteria are used to reduce the subjectivity of the appraisal. The stroma interacts with invasive carcinoma,[80,81,109] and the morphologic changes it undergoes can serve as a means of identifying carcinoma. The stromal and epithelial alterations associated with invasive carcinoma are referred to collectively as *endometrial stromal invasion*. There are four useful criteria, any of which identifies stromal invasion: (1) an irregular infiltration of glands associated with an altered fibroblastic stroma (desmoplastic response); (2) a confluent glandular pattern in which individual glands, uninterrupted by stroma, merge and create a cribriform pattern; (3) an extensive papillary pattern; and (4) replacement of the stroma by masses of squamous epithelium. A process manifesting the features of invasion must be sufficiently extensive to involve half (2.1 mm) of a low-power field 4.2 mm in diameter, or it will not have value in predicting the presence of a biologically significant carcinoma in the uterus.[100] The four signs of invasion are amplified below:

1. Infiltration of endometrial stroma by neoplastic glands frequently induces a desmoplastic or fibrous stromal

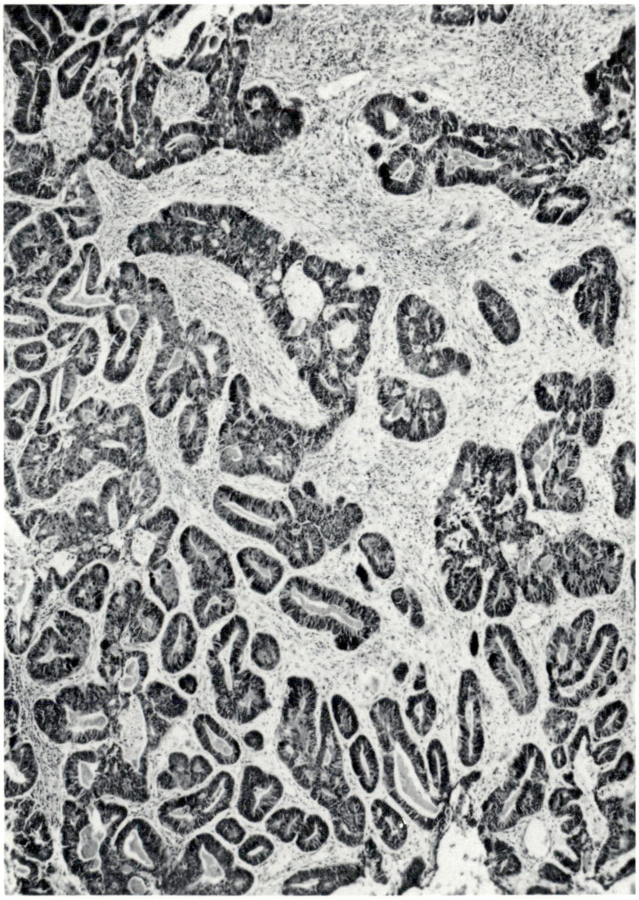

FIG. 12.1. Well-differentiated carcinoma. A desmoplastic stromal response results in a haphazard glandular pattern.

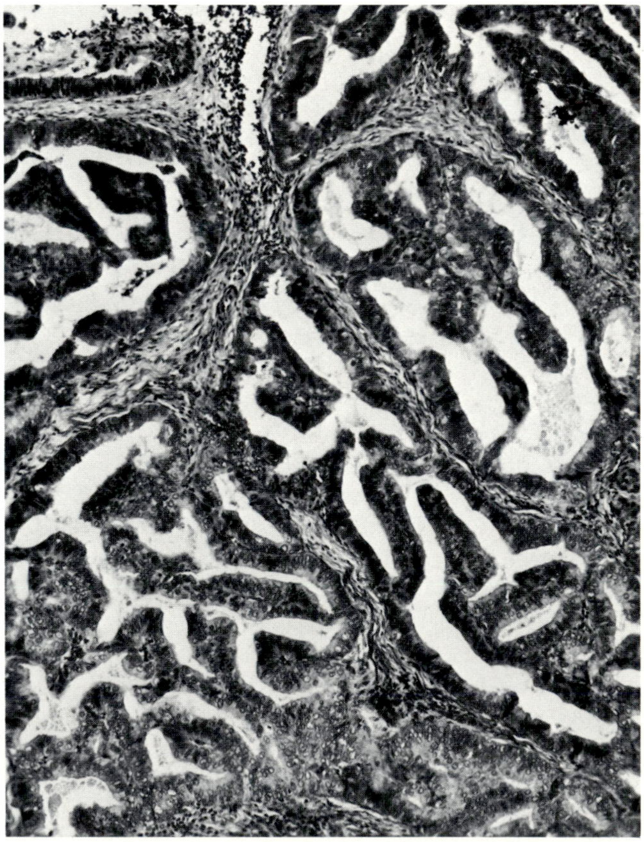

FIG. 12.2. Well-differentiated carcinoma. The altered desmoplastic stroma contains parallel fibroblasts that produce collagen and have an eosinophilic wavy appearance. Compare with Fig. 12.3.

response. The altered stroma of invasion contains parallel, densely arranged fibroblasts with more fibrosis than normal endometrial stroma, disrupting the usual glandular pattern (Fig. 12.1). The stromal cells are more spindle-shaped than are the stromal cells of proliferative endometrium, and their nuclei are more elongated. Collagen compresses the stromal cells so that they have an eosinophilic and wavy appearance (Fig. 12.2) compared to the basophilic naked-nucleus appearance of stromal cells found in proliferative endometrium and hyperplasia (Fig. 12.3). In some curettings, fragments of fibrous, relatively aglandular polyps or stroma from the lower segment of the uterus may be similar and obscure a diagnosis of carcinoma. Atypical adenomyomatous polyps (see Chapter 10, Benign Diseases of Endometrium) contain areas that are difficult to distinguish from invasion (Fig. 12.4).[119] When a polyp is suspected or fragments of lower segment are in the curettings, other features than the altered stroma must be used to support the diagnosis of adenocarcinoma.

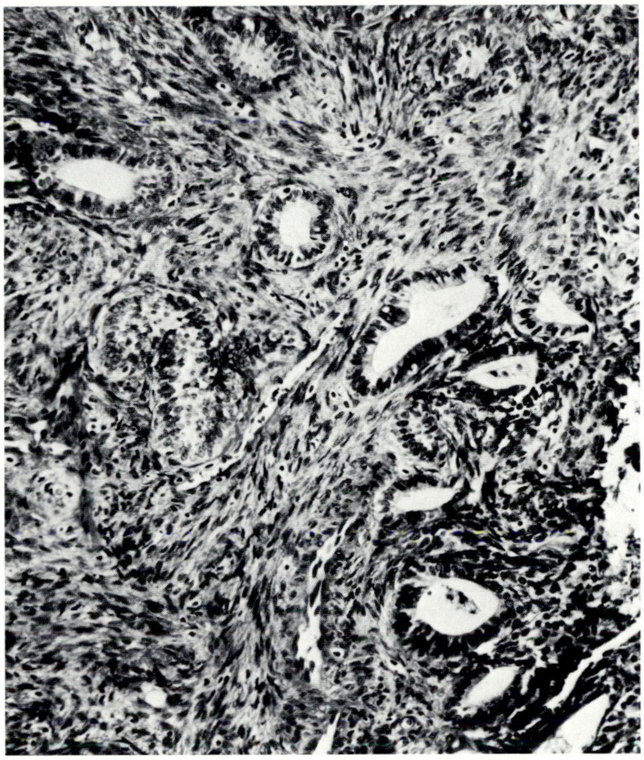

Fig. 12.4. Atypical adenomyomatous polyp. The stroma is composed of smooth muscle and myofibroblasts in bundles and fascicles simulating the desmoplastic response of invasive carcinoma. The glands show minimal atypia and complexity.

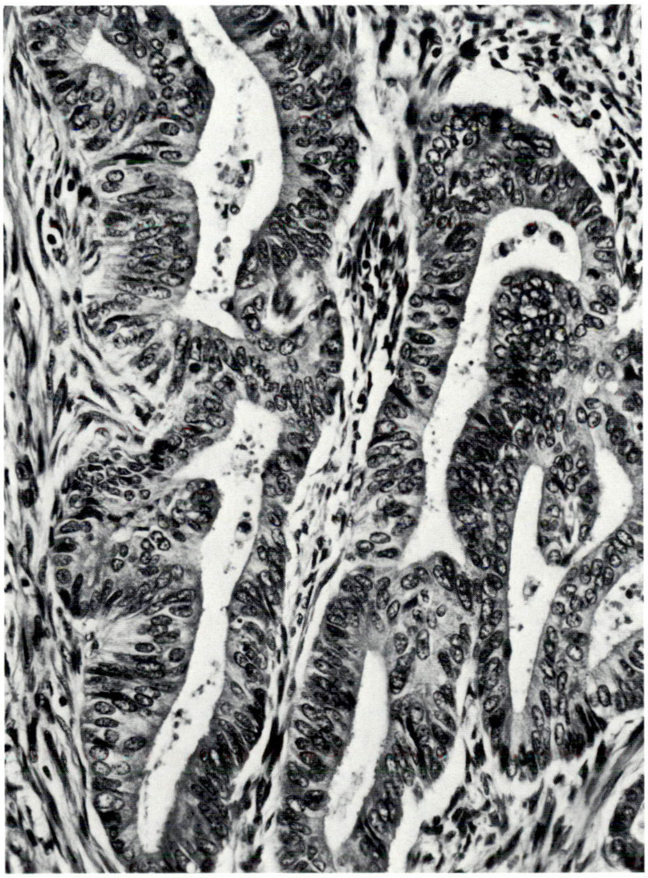

Fig. 12.3. Atypical hyperplasia. The endometrial stromal cells have a basophilic naked-nucleus appearance similar to that found in proliferative endometrium and hyperplasia. The cells are, however, more compact.

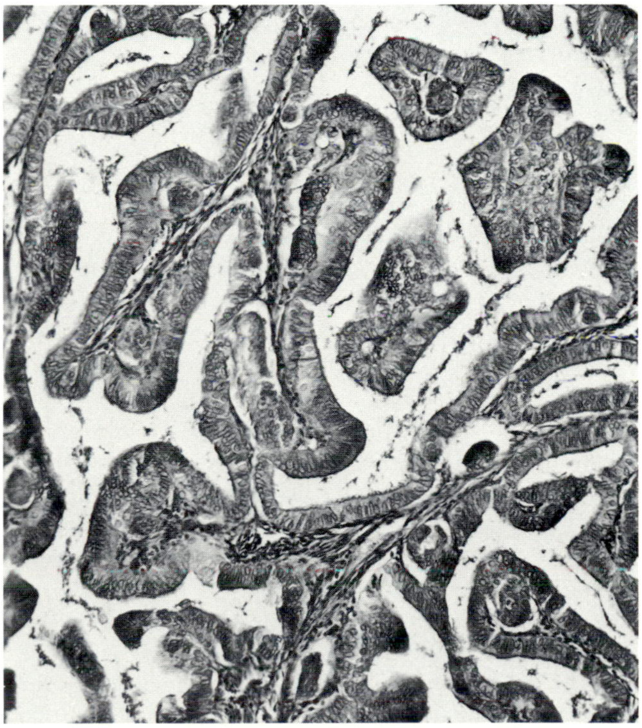

Fig. 12.5. Well-differentiated carcinoma. Stromal invasion is manifested by a confluent glandular pattern in which glandular epithelium interconnects one gland with another.

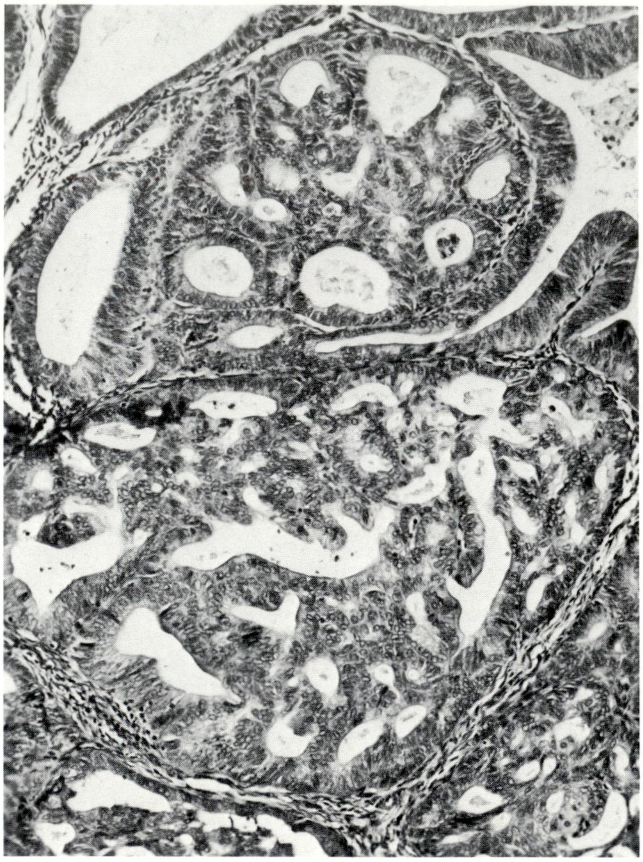

FIG. 12.6. Well-differentiated carcinoma. A confluent glandular pattern of stromal invasion in a cribriform arrangement. (Reprinted by permission of Kurman and Norris, Ref. 100.) Compare to Fig. 12.7.

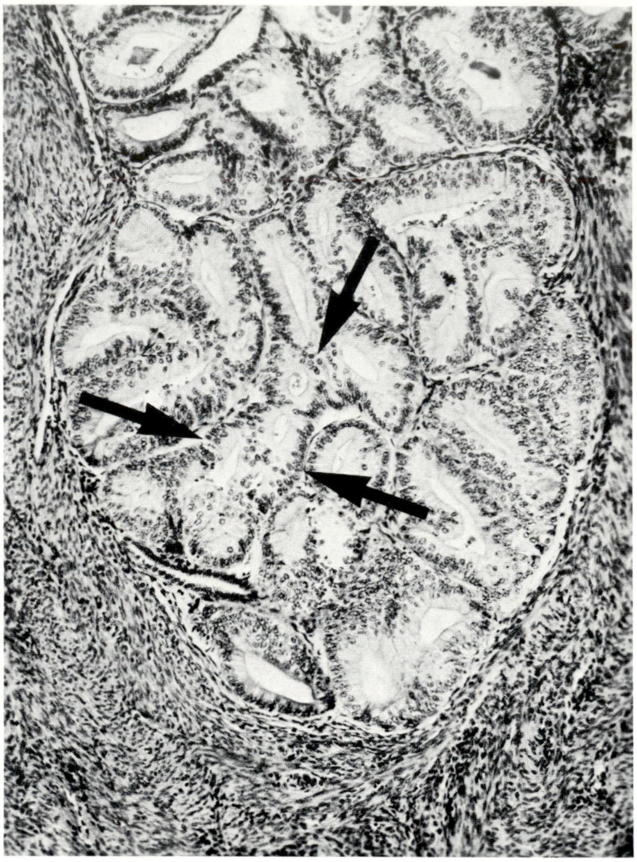

FIG. 12.7. Atypical hyperplasia showing a focal cribriform area (*arrows*). The cribriform area, however, occupies less than a half a low-power field and, consequently, does not qualify as invasion.

2. Confluent glandular aggregates reflect invasion when half a low-power field is occupied without intervening stroma (Fig. 12.5). Some proliferations are cribriform, resulting from proliferation and bridging of epithelium (Fig. 12.6). Hyperplasia may display a cribriform pattern in focal areas, but it does not occupy half a low-power field without intervening stroma (Fig. 12.7).
3. Complex papillary patterns represent stromal invasion if multiple, branching, fibrous processes lined by epithelium involve at least half a low-power field (Fig. 12.8).
4. A proliferation of squamous cells that fills, expands, and coalesces glands to form solid sheets of cells replacing the stroma represents invasion if it occupies at least half a low-power field (Fig. 12.9). The squamous cells (morules and squamous metaplasia) show little or no cytologic atypia.

Increasing degrees of nuclear atypia, mitotic activity, necrosis, and stratification of cells in curettings are associated with a higher frequency of carcinoma in the uterus but are of limited value because even a mild degree of these changes is associated with carcinoma in nearly one-third of cases.[100] Even with mild atypia, low mitotic activity, and lesser degrees of stratification in curettings, when the uterus is removed, 20% of residual carcinomas are moderately or poorly differentiated, and 10% deeply invade the myometrium.[100] These features in curettings, although useful, are not sufficiently accurate to predict whether a biologically significant lesion is present in the uterus. In addition, assessing varying degrees of nuclear atypia in this borderline group of lesions is subjective and not easily reproduced. In contrast, when stromal invasion is absent in curettings, carcinoma is found in the uterus in only 17% of cases, and all the carcinomas are well-differentiated and either confined to the endometrium or only superficially invasive (Table 12.2). If stromal invasion is present in curettings, residual carcinoma is found in the uterus in half; more than one-third of the carcinomas are moderately or poorly differen-

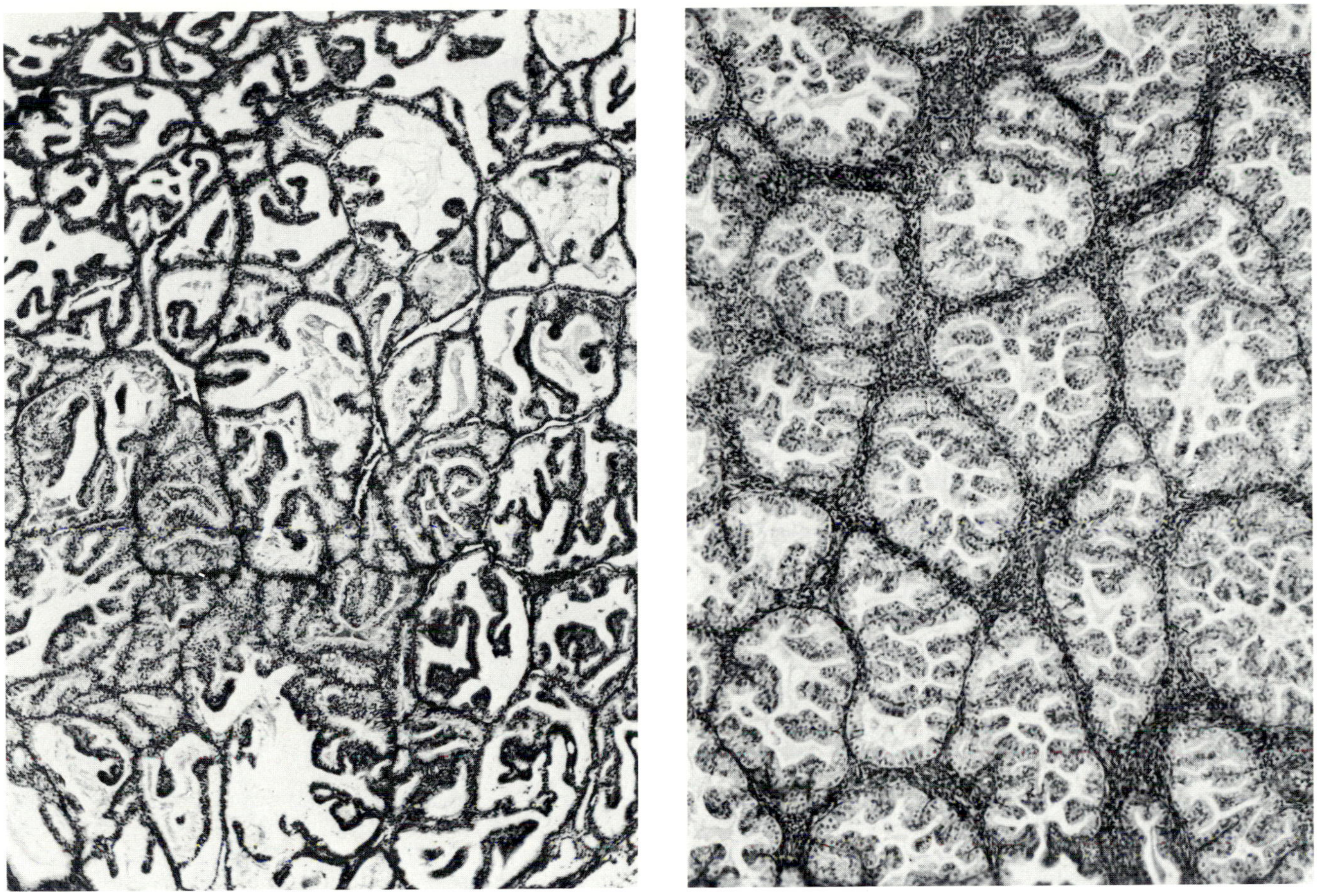

FIG. 12.8. *Left:* Well-differentiated carcinoma with a complex papillary pattern extensive enough to indicate stromal invasion. *Right:* Atypical hyperplasia in which papillary tufts are lying within individual gland lumens. Stroma surrounds each individual gland.

tiated, and a fourth of them invade deeply into the myometrium (Table 12.3). A small proportion (7%) of patients will have extrauterine metastases at hysterectomy, and half with metastasis will die of tumor.[100] Thus, the absence of stromal invasion provides the basis for distinguishing atypical hyperplasia from a biologically significant, well-differentiated carcinoma.[90,100] The identification of stromal invasion in curettings has two advantages: (1) it is semiquantifiable and, therefore, less subjective than other criteria, and (2) it delineates a biologically significant lesion—one having a much greater likelihood of metastasis than one in which invasion is absent.

Experimental studies of neoplasms from the breast, colon, pancreas, and lung lend support to the division of endometrial proliferations into noninvasive and invasive forms based on the histologic alterations observed in the endometrial stroma. These studies demonstrate profound molecular and structural alterations in the stroma adjacent to invasive as compared to noninvasive tumors.[80,109,158] Invasive tumors can induce a conversion of stromal fibroblasts into myofibroblasts, which elaborate extracellular matrix components, such as type V collagen and proteoglycans,[10,81] that are detected in increased amounts in desmoplasia and are readily observed by light microscopy using the criteria for stromal invasion as outlined.

Histopathologic Classification

A classification of endometrial carcinoma proposed by the International Society of Gynecological Pathologists is shown in Table 12.4. The relationship of the behavior to the type of carcinoma is shown in Table 12.5.

TYPICAL ENDOMETRIAL (ENDOMETRIOID) CARCINOMA

This is the common form of endometrial carcinoma, accounting for over three-fourths of all cases. The tumors in this category do not contain significant areas of squa-

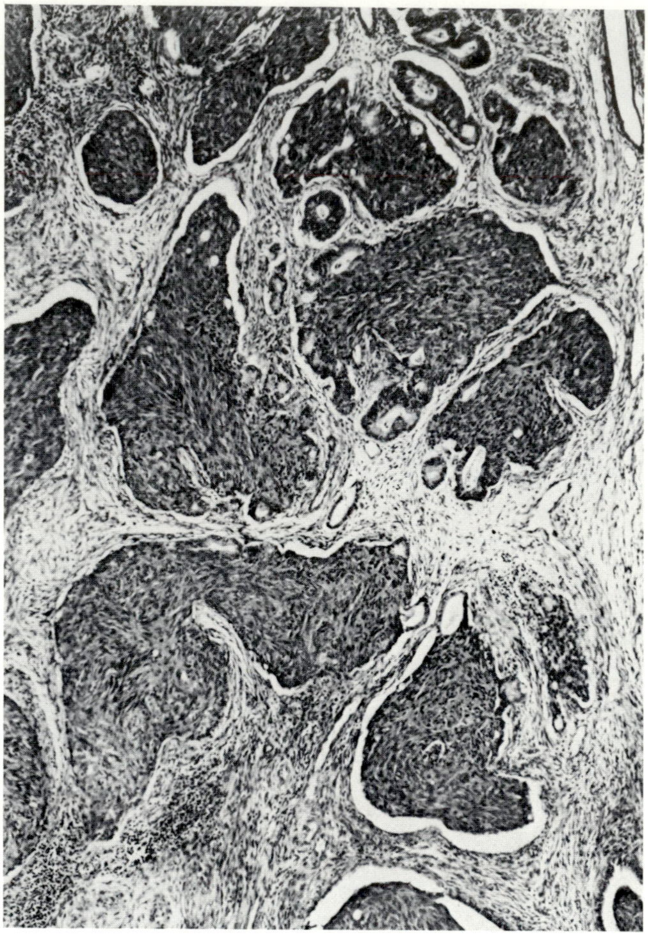

FIG. 12.9. Well-differentiated carcinoma in which stromal invasion is manifested by a proliferation of squamous cells expanding out of gland lumens into the surrounding stroma. The stroma shows an early desmoplastic reaction.

TABLE 12.2. Hysterectomy findings when stromal invasion is absent in curettings (89 patients).[a]

Finding	No.	(%)
Residual carcinoma	15	(17)
Grade		
Well differentiated	15	(100)[b]
Moderately differentiated	0	
Poorly differentiated	0	
Myometrial invasion		
None	8	(53)[b]
Inner one third	7	(47)[b]
1 mm or less	5	
2–4 mm	2	

[a] Adapted by permission of Kurman and Norris, Ref. 100.
[b] The percentages refer to the proportion of carcinomas in the hysterectomy specimen.

TABLE 12.3. Hysterectomy findings when stromal invasion is present in curettings (115 patients).[a]

Finding	No.	(%)
Residual carcinoma	58	(50)
Grade 1	38	(66)[b]
Grade 2	14	(24)[b]
Grade 3	6	(10)[b]
Myometrial invasion	42	(72)
Depth of invasion		
Inner one third	28	(48)[b]
Middle and outer thirds	14	(24)[b]

[a] Adapted by permission of Kurman and Norris, Ref. 100.
[b] The percentages refer to the proportion of carcinomas in the hysterectomy specimen.

TABLE 12.4. Classification of endometrial carcinoma.[a]

Endometrioid adenocarcinoma
- Papillary
- Secretory
- Ciliated cell
- Adenocarcinoma with squamous differentiation
  - Adenocarcinoma with squamous metaplasia (adenoacanthoma)
  - Adenosquamous carcinoma

Mucinous carcinoma
Serous carcinoma
Clear cell carcinoma
Squamous carcinoma
Undifferentiated carcinoma
Mixed types of carcinoma
Miscellaneous carcinomas
Metastatic carcinoma

[a] International Society of Gynecological Pathologists.

TABLE 12.5. Survival at 5 years for stage I endometrial cancer according to subtype.[a]

Subtype	Alive (%)	DOD[b] (%)
Adenocarcinoma with squamous metaplasia[c]	88	6
Adenocarcinoma, NSF[d]	80	6
Papillary serous	70	21
Adenosquamous	53	33
Clear cell	44	51

[a] Adapted and reprinted by permission of Christopherson et al., Ref. 31.
[b] Dead of disease.
[c] Adenoacanthoma.
[d] No specific features; includes secretory carcinoma.

mous, serous, mucinous, or clear cell differentiation. The carcinomas range from well-differentiated to poorly differentiated carcinomas. The latter would be regarded as undifferentiated carcinomas except for rare foci showing glandular differentiation.

The existence of papillary patterns within endometrial carcinoma has been recognized since the turn of the century.[39] Subsequently, sporadic reports drew attention to the presence of psammoma bodies in primary papillary endometrial carcinomas,[50,69,88,104,105,111] focusing on the similarity with a metastasis from the ovary. A serous form of papillary endometrial carcinoma is a highly malignant subtype.[30,73] Papillary processes, however, also occur in endometrioid carcinoma and clear cell carcinoma. Christopherson et al.[30] included papillary carcinoma containing clear cells in the category of clear cell carcinoma, but papillary tumors displaying endometrioid and serous patterns were included together in the category of papillary adenocarcinoma. In contrast, Hendrickson et al.[73] regarded papillary carcinomas with an endometrioid pattern as "villoglandular-type papillary carcinoma" and those with the serous pattern as "uterine papillary serous carcinoma." Included in the latter category were clear cell carcinomas with a papillary pattern. Because different definitions were used to categorize papillary endometrial neoplasms in these two studies, their findings are not directly comparable, but both found papillary serous carcinoma distinctive and highly malignant. Papillary carcinomas composed predominantly of clear cells should be included in the clear cell category, in keeping with clear cell carcinoma occurring elsewhere in the female genital tract.[28,102] Papillary carcinomas composed of delicate fibrovascular processes lined by low-grade columnar epithelial cells are a variant of typical endometrioid carcinoma with a good prognosis[26] and should be designated as *papillary carcinoma.* Papillary carcinomas with broad fibrovascular processes lined by atypical cells containing high-grade nuclei that resemble serous carcinomas of the ovary should be designated *serous carcinoma.* These tumors have a poor prognosis.

Clinical Aspects. Patients with typical endometrial carcinoma range in age from the teens to the eighth decade, with a mean of 59 years. More than three quarters are obese. Nearly half of women under the age of 40 are nulliparous, and lowered parity is characteristic.[135,137,189] In contrast to the consistent reports of obesity and low parity in women with endometrial carcinoma, an association with diabetes mellitus and abnormal glucose tolerance tests is not clear.[137,189] Overt diabetes has been reported in under 2% to over 40%[57,145] and abnormal glucose tolerance tests from 10% to 65%.[45,145,189]

Microscopic Appearance. Typical endometrial adenocarcinoma is usually well differentiated, and its microscopic features and distinction from atypical hyperplasia have been described (see section on endometrial stromal invasion as a criterion of malignancy). The microscopic appearance of higher-grade carcinoma depends on the extent of architectural and nuclear alterations associated with increasing grade (see section on pathologic risk factors).

Behavior. Typical adenocarcinoma of the endometrium spreads by lymphatic dissemination, direct extension to contiguous organs, transperitoneal and transtubal seeding, and hematogenous spread.[12] Lymphatic metastasis is three times as common as hematogenous spread,[22] but involvement of the lungs without metastasis to mediastinal lymph nodes suggests that hematogenous spread may occur early in the course of disease.

Endometrial carcinoma tends to spread to the pelvic nodes before involving para-aortic lymph nodes. In a surgical staging study of stage I carcinoma in which selective pelvic and para-aortic lymphadenectomy was performed, 6.8% had pelvic lymph node metastasis and 2.5% had para-aortic lymph node metastasis.[20] Pelvic lymph nodes were accurate predictors of para-aortic involvement. When pelvic lymph nodes were negative, the risk of para-aortic lymph node metastasis was low, whereas if pelvic nodes were positive, the para-aortic lymph nodes were involved in two thirds of the patients.[20]

The interval for recurrence after initial treatment depends on the histologic grade of the tumor and the clinical stage.[150] For grade 1 tumors, the mean time to recurrence

TABLE 12.6. Sites of metastasis from endometrial carcinoma at autopsy.

Organ site	Relative frequency (%)
Lung	41
Peritoneum and omentum	39
Ovary	34
Liver	29
Bowel	29
Vagina	25
Bladder	23
Vertebra	20
Spleen	14
Adrenal	14
Ureter	8
Brain or skull	5
Vulva	4
Breast	4
Hand	
Femur	Rare
Tibia	Rare
Pubic bone	Rare
Skin	Rare

From Hendrickson E (1975), The lymphatic dissemination in endometrial carcinoma. A study of 188 necropsies. Am J Obstet Gynecol 123: 570. Reprinted by permission.

TABLE 12.7. Sites of lymph node metastasis from endometrial carcinoma at autopsy.

Lymph nodes	Relative frequency (%)
Para-aortic	64
Hypogastric	61
External iliac	48
Common iliac	40
Obturator	37
Sacral	22
Mediastinal	18
Inguinal	16
Supraclavicular	12

From Hendrickson E (1975), The lymphatic dissemination in endometrial carcinoma. A study of 188 necropsies. Am J Obstet Gynecol 123: 570. Reprinted by permission.

is 38 months, for grade 2 tumors, it is 21 months, and for grade 3 tumors, it is 14 months.[191] Nearly 80% of failures occur within 3 years, but recurrence can appear as late as 5 years after treatment. One-half of treatment failures occur in the pelvis and one-half at distant sites, but of the patients who die, the majority do so from effects of distant metastasis rather than local recurrence.[12,150] The relative frequency of metastasis to various organs and lymph node groups is shown in Tables 12.6 and 12.7.

The 10-year actuarial survival by nuclear grade for stage I typical adenocarcinoma was 97% for grade 1, 88% for grade 2, and 71% for grade 3.[31] In a related study by the same investigators,[33] the 5-year actuarial survival for all grades of typical carcinoma in stage I was 100% if tumor was confined to the endometrium, 97% when there was invasion of the inner third of the myometrium, 86% for middle-third myometrial invasion, and 83% for outer-third invasion.

Papillary Carcinoma. This is a variant of typical endometrial carcinoma that displays a papillary pattern in which the papillary fronds are composed of a delicate fibrovascular core covered by cells with bland nuclei.[26,73]

Clinical Aspects. There is only limited published experience with tumors of this type, and consequently the clinical profile of these patients is sketchy. The mean age is similar to that of women with typical endometrial carcinoma (61 years). All patients reported thus far are white. In all other respects, women with these tumors are similar to patients with typical endometrial carcinoma.

Microscopic Appearance. The papillary fronds that characterize this tumor are thin, delicate, and covered by stratified columnar epithelial cells with oval nuclei that generally display grade 1 or 2 atypia (Figs. 12.10 and 12.11). Although grade 3 nuclei may occur, marked nuclear atypia and pleomorphism are more often features of (papillary) serous carcinoma. Mitotic activity is variable, and abnormal mitotic figures are rare.[26,73] Myometrial invasion is superficial.

Behavior. These carcinomas generally reflect a low-grade tumor that rarely invades deeply or involves the cervix and, consequently, has an excellent prognosis. Typically, these tumors are at an early stage at the time of diagnosis. Treatment is the same as for typical endometrial carcinoma of comparable stage, grade, and depth of invasion.

Secretory Carcinoma. This is a variant of typical endometrial carcinoma in which the majority of cells exhibit subnuclear or supranuclear cytoplasmic vacuoles resembling early secretory endometrium. A rare pattern, it represents 1–2% of endometrial carcinomas.[49,75,102,175]

Clinical Aspects. All patients thus far reported are white. The age range is from 35 to 78 years, with a mean age of 58. A majority are postmenopausal and experience abnormal bleeding. In all other respects, including the association of obesity, hypertension, diabetes mellitus, and exogenous estrogen administration, patients with secretory carcinoma are similar to women with typical endometrial carcinoma.

Microscopic Appearance. Carcinomas with a secretory pattern display a well-differentiated glandular pattern

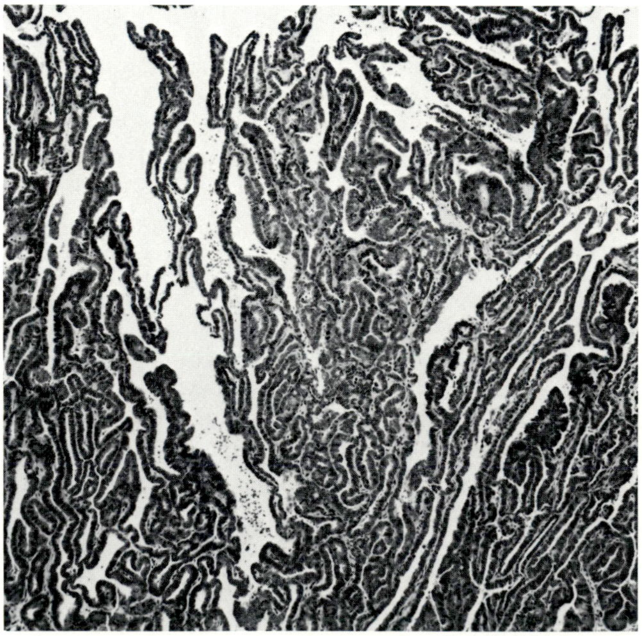

FIG. 12.10. Well-differentiated papillary endometrial carcinoma composed of papillary fronds with delicate fibrovascular cores covered by stratified columnar epithelium.

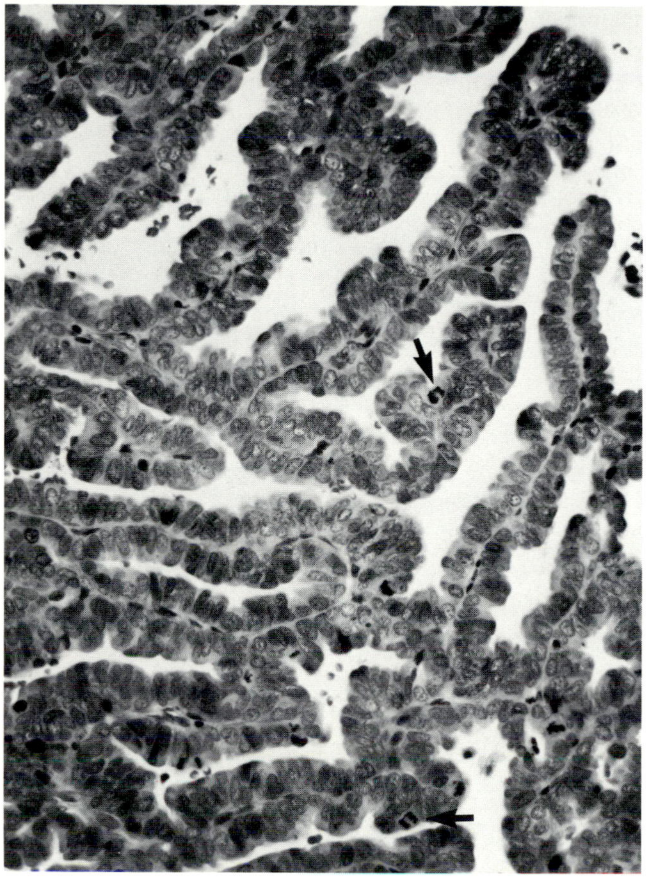

FIG. 12.11. Higher magnification of a papillary endometrial carcinoma with delicate fibrovascular cores and low-grade nuclei. Mitotic activity is present (*arrows*).

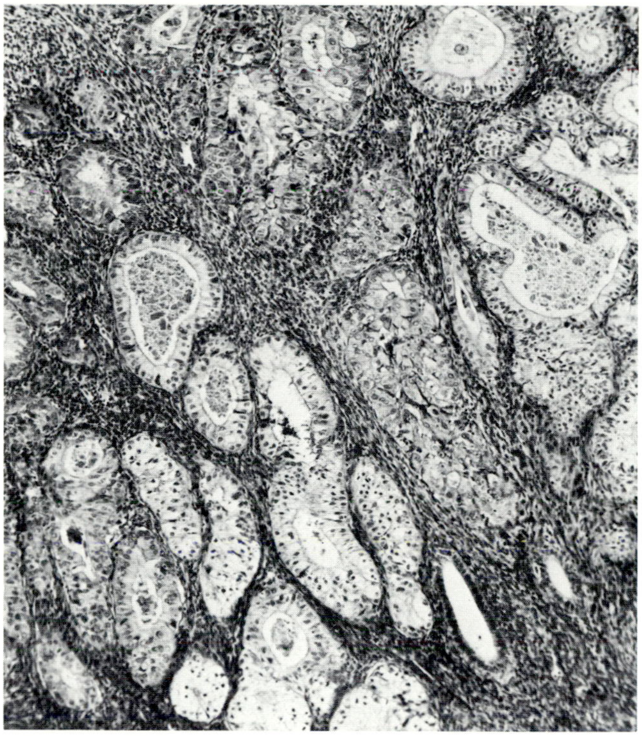

FIG. 12.12. Secretory carcinoma is typically low grade, composed of crowded glands lined by relatively unstratified cells with bland nuclei. The subnuclear or supranuclear vacuolization resembles secretory endometrium 4–6 days after ovulation.

and are composed of columnar cells, often unstratified, with subnuclear or supranuclear vacuolization closely resembling 17–20-day secretory endometrium (Fig. 12.12). Usually the nuclei are grade 1. The secretory pattern may be focal or diffuse, and it is frequently admixed with typical endometrial adenocarcinoma.[49,75,102]

It is important to distinguish secretory carcinoma from clear cell carcinoma in view of the excellent prognosis of the former and unfavorable prognosis of the latter. Although both tumors are composed of cells with clear, glycogen-rich cytoplasm, the histologic features are distinctive. Clear cell carcinoma has pleomorphic cells with high-grade nuclei in solid, papillary, tubular, or cystic patterns, whereas secretory carcinoma has little nuclear atypia; it forms a well-differentiated glandular pattern and has more uniform subnuclear or supranuclear vacuolization. The distinction of secretory carcinoma from atypical hyperplasia with secretory effect is more difficult and is based on the presence of stromal invasion in the carcinoma.

Behavior. The endometrium adjacent to secretory carcinoma in young women typically shows a secretory pattern that is more advanced than 17 days, and a corpus luteum is found in the majority of patients when a hysterectomy and bilateral salpingo-oophorectomy are performed.[102] Nonetheless, a relationship to progesterone stimulation is not always demonstrable, and most of the women are postmenopausal. The secretory activity in the tumor may be transient, since it has been observed in curettings but not in the later hysterectomy specimen.[30] Secretory carcinoma may occur spontaneously in postmenopausal women without exogenous or abnormal levels of progesterone, and the secretory pattern has also been observed in an adenocarcinoma of the stomach in a male.[102]

Treatment is the same as that for typical endometrial carcinoma of the same stage and grade. Since secretory carcinoma is usually low grade, the 5-year survival is 87%. Death from recurrent disease occurs rarely.[30]

Ciliated Carcinoma. This is a rare form of differentiation in typical endometrial carcinoma.[72,144,166] Ciliated carcinoma has an association with exogenous estrogen treatment; 4 of 10 patients in one study[72] had received estrogen, and in another study, ciliated cells were found in 37% of carcinomas in estrogen users compared to 12% of nonusers ($p < 0.005$).[143] Estrogen induces cilia formation in the normal endometrium. Despite the prevalence of estrogen use, ciliated carcinoma is an extremely rare

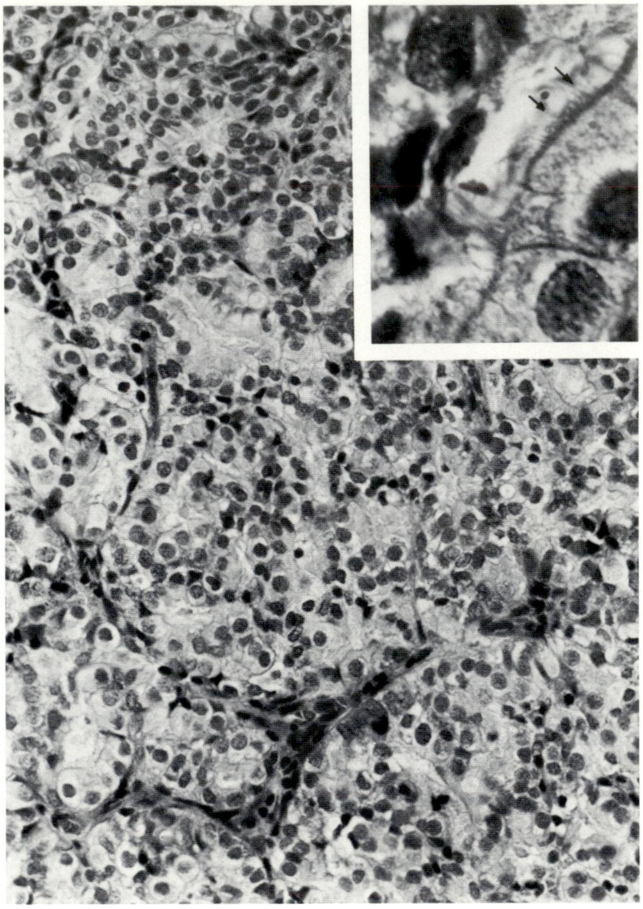

FIG. 12.13. Ciliated cell carcinoma composed of well-differentiated glands. *Inset:* Cell with minimal cytologic atypia showing cilia (*arrows*) on luminal surface. The tumor invaded two thirds into the myometrium. (Courtesy of M. R. Hendrickson, M.D.)

carcinoma, and most endometrial proliferations in which cilia are observed represent hyperplasias associated with eosinophilic or tubal metaplasia.

Clinical Aspects. Patients range in age from 42 to 79 years. All of the women reported by Hendrickson and Kempson[72] were postmenopausal and had bleeding.

Microscopic Appearance. The tumors are well to moderately differentiated and often display a cribriform pattern. The gland lumens in the cribriform areas are lined by cells with prominent eosinophilic cytoplasm and cilia (Fig. 12.13). The nuclei of ciliated cells generally have an irregular nuclear membrane and display coarse nuclear chromatin with prominent nucleoli.[72] In the majority of cases, ciliated carcinoma is admixed with typical nonciliated carcinoma and even areas of mucinous carcinoma.

Behavior. Although some ciliated carcinomas are moderately differentiated and invade to the middle third of the myometrium, none of the patients has developed recurrence or died of disease. Thus, the presence of cilia in a bona fide carcinoma identifies a low-grade neoplasm.

Adenocarcinoma with Squamous Differentiation

Most endometrial adenocarcinomas contain squamous differentiation, but the amount of squamous epithelium can vary widely. In a well-sampled neoplasm, the squamous element should constitute at least 10% of a tumor to qualify as an adenocarcinoma with squamous differentiation.

In the past, an adenocarcinoma containing squamous elements often was designated an adenoacanthoma. Originally it was thought to be rare and low grade,[134] but when less stringent quantitative criteria were applied, the frequency rose to as high as 44% of the endometrial carcinomas.[25] Adenocarcinomas with squamous elements can be divided into those with benign-appearing squamous differentiation (adenoacanthoma or adenocarcinoma with squamous metaplasia) and those with malignant-appearing squamous epithelium (adenosquamous carcinoma).[129,131] These neoplasms differ markedly in their behavior; the 5-year survival for adenosquamous carcinoma is 19–40% compared to about 70–80% for adenocarcinoma with squamous metaplasia.[2,85,143,149,164] Thus, adenocarcinoma with squamous metaplasia is a relatively well differentiated carcinoma with an excellent prognosis, whereas adenosquamous carcinoma is a poorly differentiated carcinoma with an unfavorable outlook. Because the term *adenoacanthoma* has not been uniformly applied, use of the term *adenocarcinoma with squamous metaplasia* (ASM) more clearly defines a carcinoma with benign-appearing squamous epithelium.

To a large extent, the difference in behavior between ASM and adenosquamous carcinoma reflects the difference in grade of the glandular as well as the squamous component.[164] Silverberg et al.[164] found that the 5-year actuarial survival of 35% for adenosquamous carcinoma was similar to the 40% survival for poorly differentiated typical adenocarcinoma. A similar relationship was suggested for ASM and typical well-differentiated adenocarcinoma, although the 5-year survival was higher for ASM (83% versus 61%). Other studies[33,85,143,149] have also shown a more favorable survival for ASM as compared to well-differentiated adenocarcinoma, but the difference is not significant. Adenocarcinoma with squamous metaplasia and adenosquamous carcinoma are terms used to describe low and high grades of carcinoma with squamous differentiation. Since grade is one of the most important pathologic prognostic factors, these terms identify tumors with a favorable and unfavorable prognosis, respectively. An alternative terminology that we prefer is adenocarcinoma with squamous differentiation graded

1, 2, or 3. Often the squamous component in these neoplasms displays some cytologic atypia, and it is difficult to decide whether it is benign-appearing or sufficiently atypical to qualify as malignant. By using the term *adenocarcinoma with squamous differentiation*, the distinction is not necessary. The tumor is graded on the basis of the glandular component as well, moderately, or poorly differentiated (grade 1, 2, or 3, respectively) using a nuclear grading system (see section on pathologic risk factors). Almost invariably the grades of the glandular and the squamous components correspond closely.

An early report stated that the frequency of adenosquamous carcinoma had increased to a point where it represented nearly a third of all endometrial carcinomas in a 5-year period ending in 1971. More recent studies,[2,143] however, show that the relative frequency of this tumor has remained relatively constant over the last 30 years, representing 7% of endometrial carcinoma.

Adenocarcinoma with Squamous Metaplasia (Adenoacanthoma). Adenocarcinoma with squamous metaplasia is characterized by a mixture of adenocarcinoma and squamous epithelium arising in the glands. By definition, the squamous epithelium is cytologically benign, and usually the glandular component is well-differentiated, both from an architectural (FIGO) and nuclear grade standpoint.

Clinical Aspects. There are no differences in the clinical features of ASM and typical adenocarcinoma. Thus, there are no differences in the frequency of obesity, hypertension, diabetes, and nulliparity among the large series in which this has been analyzed.[33,85,149] Most studies, however, have consistently shown that women with ASM are slightly younger than women with typical adenocarcinoma (median age of 58 years) and are more often premenopausal, but this may be a reflection of the younger age. Typically, there is a higher proportion of estrogen users among patients with ASM.[143,166] In one study,[143] half of the patients had used extrogen compared to a quarter of patients with other types of endometrial carcinoma.

Microscopic Appearance. The tumor is composed of glandular and squamous elements but generally the glandular component predominates; the nests of squamous epithelium are confined to gland lumens (Fig. 12.14). The squamous epithelium resembles metaplastic squamous cells of the cervical transformation zone. Frequently, a prominent oval-to-spindle cell appearance, referred to as morules, is observed.[46] Intracellular bridges can be identified within the squamous epithelium, and keratin formation is common. The nuclei of the squamous cells are bland, uniform, and lack prominent nucleoli. Mitotic figures are rare.

The most frequent differential diagnosis is with atypical hyperplasia showing squamous metaplasia. To distinguish the two, the criteria for identifying endometrial stromal invasion should be employed. At times, ASM may be confused with a high-grade carcinoma because the masses of squamous epithelium are misconstrued as a solid proliferation of neoplastic cells. The nuclear grade is high in poorly differentiated carcinoma, however. Occasionally, squamous morules may be confused with granulomas, but the presence of foreign body giant cells and an inflammatory infiltrate helps identify the latter.

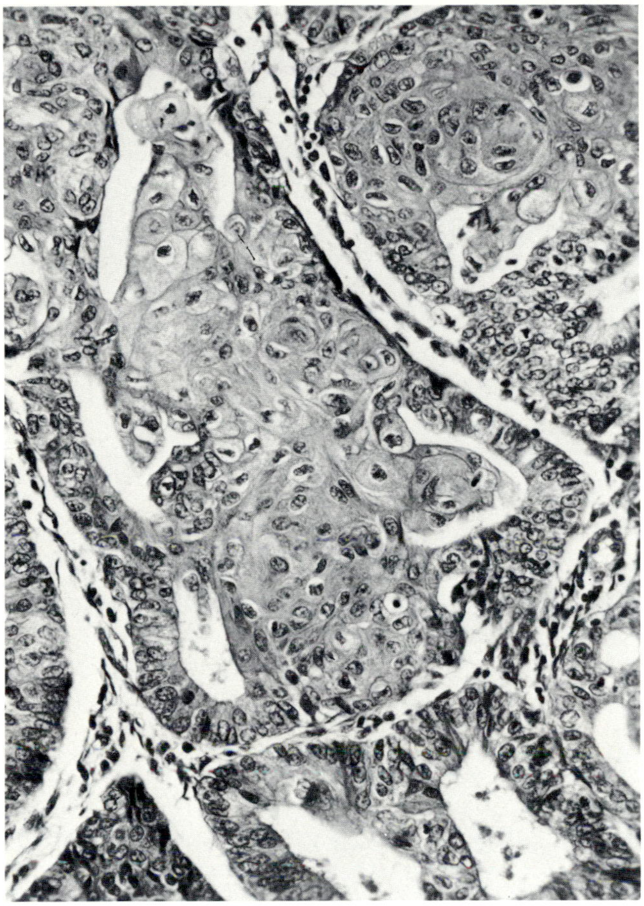

FIG. 12.14. Well-differentiated adenocarcinoma with squamous metaplasia. Both the glandular and squamous elements are grade 1.

Behavior. Although not statistically significant, some studies show that ASM has the same or slightly better prognosis than typical adenocarcinoma,[110,128,164] even when stratified according to grade and stage.[33] With stage I, grade 1, disease there are few deaths with either type of tumor for patients younger than 50 years of age.[33] The good prognosis may reflect the younger age of the patients or the biology of the tumor, since the benign-appearing squamous epithelium indicates that the carcinoma has partially differentiated into mature tissue. One of the rare examples of spontaneous regression of endometrial carcinoma was a patient with widespread metastatic ASM.[14]

Adenosquamous Carcinoma. Adenosquamous carcinoma is defined as an adenocarcinoma in which at least 10% of the tumor contains malignant squamous epithelium.

Clinical Aspects. The clinical features of women with adenosquamous carcinoma are similar to those of women with ASM and typical adenocarcinoma except the patients are older (median age 65). In the largest series,[2] 37% of the patients were nulliparous, 15% had diabetes mellitus, half were obese, and half were hypertensive. Over 90% experienced abnormal bleeding.

Microscopic Appearance. Cytologically malignant squamous epithelium is the diagnostic feature. Unlike ASM, the squamous element in adenosquamous carcinoma is cytologically malignant and is not confined to gland lumens but often extends out from the glands (Figs. 12.15 and 12.16). It may not be in direct continuity with the

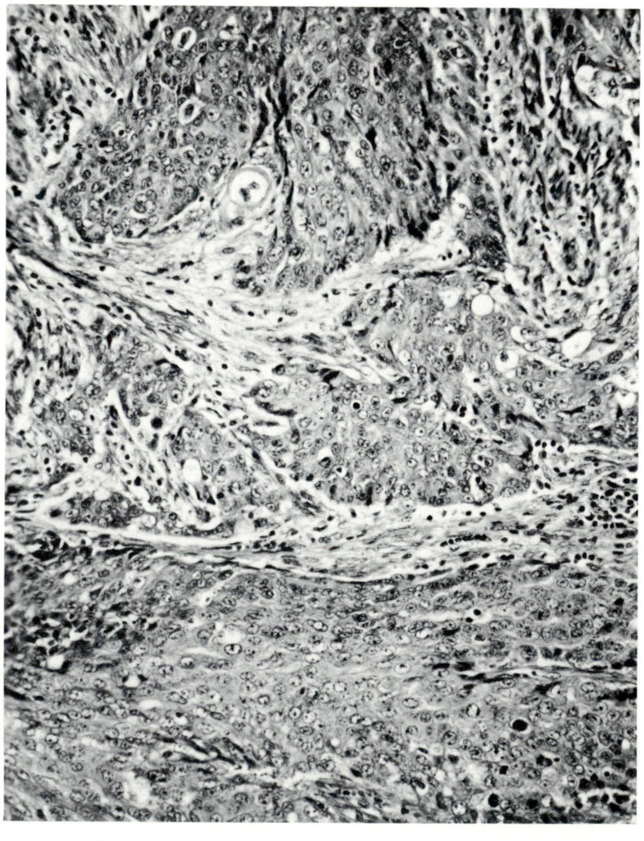

FIG. 12.15. Adenosquamous carcinoma. Sheets of cytologically malignant squamous cells in a poorly differentiated adenocarcinoma with squamous differentiation.

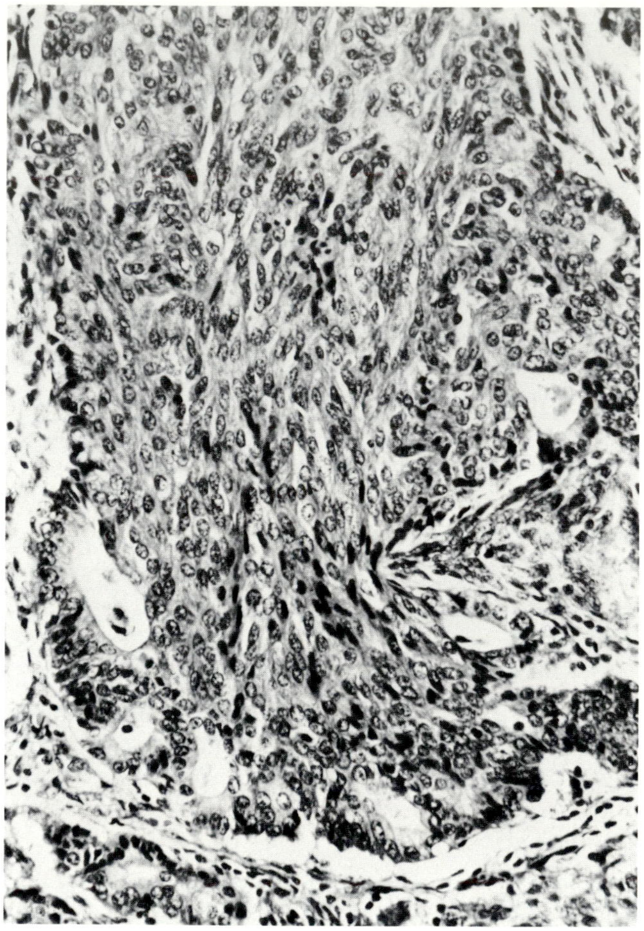

FIG. 12.16. Adenosquamous carcinoma in which the squamous cells show a prominent spindle cell arrangement. This spindle cell pattern should not be confused with sarcoma.

glandular epithelium, appearing in isolated nests within the myometrium or in vascular spaces. Keratinization and pearl formation occur to varying degrees. Generally, the glandular component predominates, but masses of undifferentiated cells that may represent poorly differentiated glandular or squamous cells lie between glands. This undifferentiated epithelium should be considered glandular unless intercellular bridges are demonstrated or the cells have prominent eosinophilic cytoplasm, well-defined cytoplasmic borders, and a sheet-like proliferation without evidence of gland formation.

Both the glandular and squamous components display grade 2 or 3 nuclear atypia, an increased nuclear cytoplasmic ratio, and increased mitotic activity. The glandular architecture usually is moderately or poorly differentiated.

The major problem in differential diagnosis in curettings is distinguishing adenosquamous carcinoma of the endometrium from adenosquamous carcinoma arising in the endocervix. In the cervix, the squamous component usually predominates, whereas in the endometrium, the glandular component predominates. A profusion of cell types, especially mucinous or signet-ring cells, is more characteristic of an endocervical neoplasm.

Behavior. Patients with adenosquamous carcinoma have a lower 5-year survival than do those with typical adenocarcinoma, with a mean of 70% for typical adenocarcinoma and 40% for adenosquamous carcinoma.[2,85,128,149,164] The difference in survival is a result of the cytologic grade of both components, not just the squamous component. It is doubtful that adenosquamous carcinoma displays behavioral characteristics that differ from a typical adenocarcinoma of similar grade. Patients with adenosquamous carcinoma have a high frequency of deep myometrial invasion, vascular space involvement, and pelvic and para-aortic lymph node metastasis.[162] Metastasis occurs widely throughout the pelvis and abdomen, involving bowel, mesentery, liver, kidney, spleen, and lymph nodes. Distant metastasis may involve the lungs, heart, skin, and bones.[2] Nearly two-thirds of metastases contain both glandular and squamous elements, but pure adenocarcinoma or squamous carcinoma is encountered in 20% and 8%, respectively.[131]

Mucinous Carcinoma

This uncommon type of endometrial carcinoma has the same appearance as mucinous carcinoma in the ovary and endocervix.[152,174] It occurs as a focal component of otherwise typical adenocarcinoma in up to 42% of endometrial carcinomas[32] but represents the dominant cellular population in only 9%.[148] To qualify as a mucinous carcinoma, more than one half of the cell population of the tumor must contain PAS-positive, diastase-resistant intracytoplasmic mucin.

Clinical Aspects. Judging from the small number of cases available, the clinical features of patients with mucinous carcinoma of the endometrium do not differ from those with typical endometrial carcinoma.

Microscopic Appearance. Pure mucinous tumors are rare. Curiously, mucinous differentiation is often associated with squamous differentiation, but the most frequent architectural pattern is glandular, often in a papillary configuration. Cribriform areas are unusual; cystically dilated glands filled with mucin and papillary fronds surrounded by extracellular lakes of mucin, containing neutrophils, are typical. The epithelial cells lining the glands and papillary processes tend to be uniform columnar cells with minimal stratification (Fig. 12.17). Nuclear atypia is mild to moderate, and mitotic activity is not prominent.

The presence of intracytoplasmic mucin can be identified on H & E stains by its distinctive granular, foamy or bubbly appearance and can be confirmed by PAS, mucicarmine, or Alcian blue stains. The intracytoplasmic mucin is variable in both the number and distribution of mucinous cells in the tumor and in the location of the mucin within individual cells. Mucin may be diffusely present in the cytoplasm, confined to the apical area, or may show a combination of both patterns.

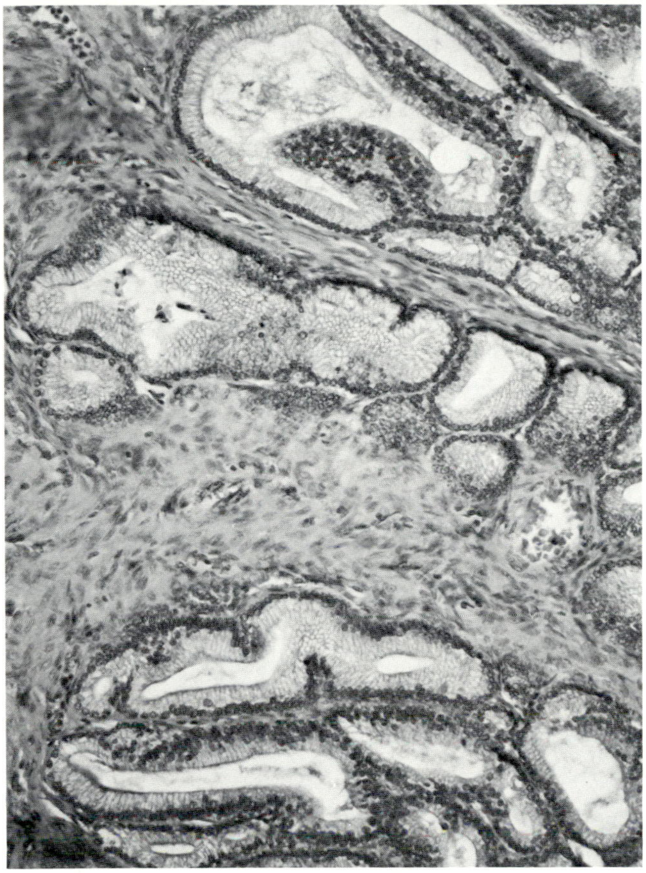

Fig. 12.17. Mucinous carcinoma characterized by glands with uniform columnar cells having basally oriented nuclei and minimal atypia. The tumor is invading the myometrium.

Since the endocervical epithelium merges with the endometrium in the lower uterine segement, it is not surprising that the distinction of primary endocervical from endometrial mucinous carcinoma in curettings can be difficult. There is no distinction by histochemical staining pattern.[40] Immunohistochemically, CEA is more common in endocervical than in endometrial mucinous carcinomas, but significant overlap occurs, rendering this technique of limited value in the differential diagnosis.[181] The presence of an associated endometrial hyperplasia suggests an endometrial primary neoplasia. Conversely, the presence of cervical intraepithelial neoplasia favors an endocervical primary site.

The distinction of mucinous carcinoma of the endometrium from clear cell or secretory carcinoma is made on the basis of morphology and PAS and mucin stains. The cells in secretory carcinoma are clear (not granular or foamy) because of the presence of glycogen, which is PAS-positive and is removed by diastase treatment. Mucin in these tumors is focal at most.

Behavior. Mucinous tumors tend to be low grade and behave as ordinary endometrial carcinomas.[148] Thus, the presence of intracytoplasmic mucin in an endometrial carcinoma does not appear to have prognostic significance but serves to point out that a mucinous carcinoma identified in curettings does not necessarily indicate that the tumor is a primary endocervical neoplasm.

Serous Carcinoma

Clinical Aspects. Patients with serous carcinoma, in contrast to women with typical endometrial carcinoma, are older (mean age of 66 years versus 59), are less likely to have received estrogens (21% versus 53%), and are more likely to have an abnormal cervical cytology (23% versus 5%). In other respects, they appear similar.

Microscopic Appearance. Serous carcinoma is characterized by a complex papillary architecture resembling serous carcinoma of the ovary (Fig. 12.18). The papillary fronds are usually densely fibrotic and covered by stratified epithelial cells, many with a hobnail appearance, forming smaller papillary tufts (Fig. 12.19). The cells are serous or mesothelial in character. There may be considerable cytologic variability throughout the tumor as the cells tend to show marked cytologic atypia manifested by nuclear pleomorphism, hyperchromasia, and macronucleoli. Multinucleated cells, giant nuclei, and bizarre forms occur in half the patients. Psammoma bodies are encountered in a third.

It may be difficult to distinguish serous carcinoma from a clear cell carcinoma that displays a prominent papillary pattern. The presence of associated areas containing clear cells with a solid or tubulocystic pattern is characteristic of clear cell carcinoma. If the two tumor types are admixed, the diagnosis is based on the predominant component.

Behavior. Serous carcinoma has a propensity for myometrial and lymphatic invasion (Fig. 12.20). The hysterectomy specimen often discloses tumor in lymphatics

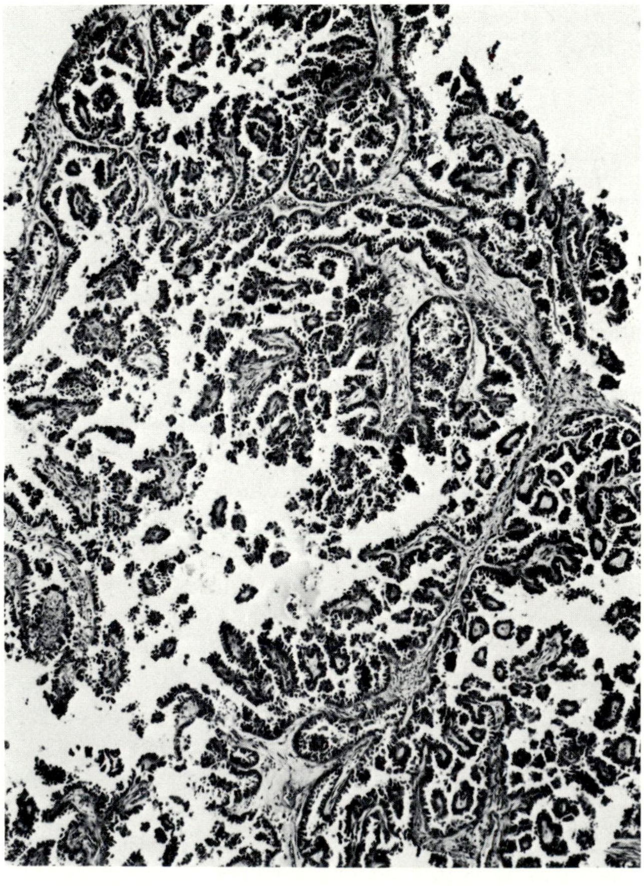

Fig. 12.18. Serous carcinoma characterized by a complex papillary architecture resembling serous carcinoma of the ovary.

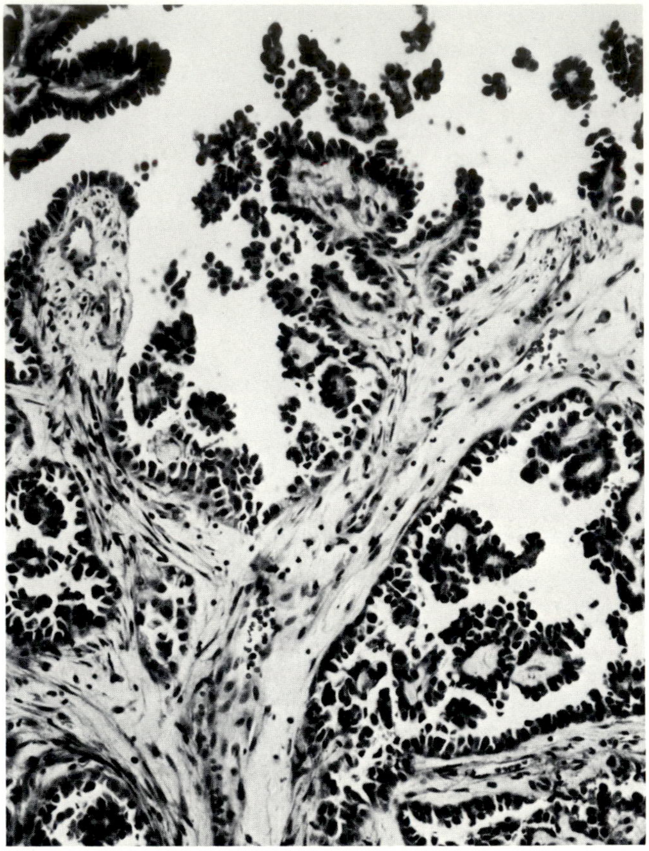

Fig. 12.19. Higher magnification of a serous carcinoma. Dense fibrotic fibrovascular cores are covered by papillary tufts, with cells often having a hobnail appearance. The nuclei are characteristically grade 2–3.

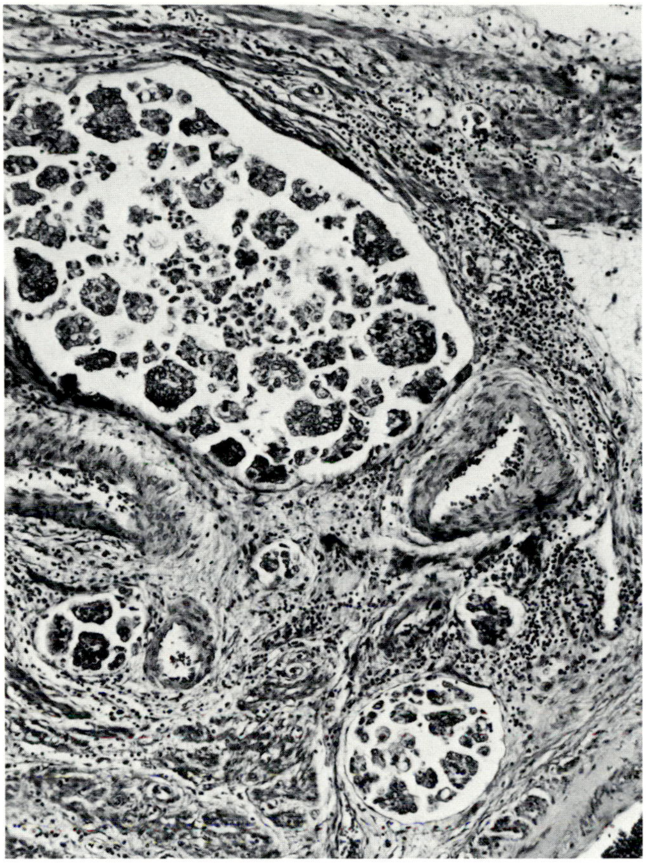

FIG. 12.20. Serous carcinoma often permeates lymphatics within the myometrium far removed from the tumor mass. The papillary serous architecture is retained in the metastasis.

within the broad ligament and ovarian hilus as well as in the lumen of the fallopian tube and cervix. Like ovarian serous carcinoma, uterine serous carcinoma spreads early and involves peritoneal surfaces in the pelvis and abdomen. This may be a manifestation of multifocal disease arising synchronously or asynchronously in the endometrium and the secondary müllerian system (see Chapter 17, Endometriosis) rather than a metastasis from a primary uterine tumor. In patients with high-stage disease, it may be impossible to distinguish a primary serous carcinoma of the ovary from one arising in the uterus. A large amount of myometrial and lymphatic spread with minor endometrial involvement favors the ovary as the primary site. Whether primary in the ovary or endometrium, the prognosis is equally unfavorable. With both sites involved, treatment is usually that employed for ovarian cancer.

In a series of 256 stage I endometrial carcinomas at Stanford University Hospital, serous carcinoma accounted for half of all relapses from endometrial carcinoma.[73] In view of the poor prognosis and the tendency of serous carcinoma to spread throughout the abdominal cavity (like ovarian cancer), patients with pathologic stage I disease exhibiting myometrial invasion probably should receive adjuvant chemotherapy or pelvic and upper abdominal irradiation. In women who do not have myometrial invasion, no further treatment is recommended, since none of these patients have had recurrent tumor.

Clear Cell Carcinoma

Clear cell carcinoma is a distinctive type of endometrial carcinoma similar to those that occur in the ovary, vagina, and cervix. In young women, clear cell carcinoma of the vagina and cervix is associated with in utero diethylstilbestrol exposure, but in the endometrium it occurs in older women without a history of exogenous hormone use. Previously, clear cell carcinoma was regarded as mesonephric in origin because of its resemblance to renal carcinoma, but the occurrence of clear cell carcinoma in the endometrium, a müllerian derivative, is evidence of its müllerian origin.[102]

Clinical Aspects. As with the other subtypes of endometrial carcinoma with an unfavorable prognosis, such as serous and adenosquamous carcinoma, women with clear cell carcinoma are older than women with typical carcinoma (mean age 67 versus 59 years). They also have a higher likelihood of abnormal cytology (58% versus 5%) and a lower frequency of some of the associated constitutional symptoms, such as obesity and diabetes mellitus.[28]

Microscopic Appearance. Clear cell carcinoma may exhibit solid, papillary, tubular, and cystic patterns. The solid pattern is composed of masses of clear cells intermixed with eosinophilic cells, whereas papillary, tubular, and cystic patterns are composed predominantly of hobnail-shaped cells with interspersed clear and eosinophilic cells. Cystic spaces are frequently lined by flattened cells. Psammoma bodies can be found in association with papillary areas within the tumor.[102]

The cells are typically large, with clear or lightly stained eosinophilic cytoplasm (Fig. 12.21). The clear cytoplasm is due largely to the presence of glycogen, demonstrated with a PAS stain and diastase digestion. Cells that have discharged their glycogen and lost most of their cytoplasm are characterized by a naked nucleus, the hobnail cells. Nuclear atypia is generally marked, manifested by pleomorphic, often large, multiple nuclei with prominent nucleoli. Mitotic activity is high, and abnormal mitoses are readily seen. The nuclear grade is generally high.[28,147,163] PAS-positive, diastase-resistant intracellular and extracellular hyaline bodies, similar to those in endodermal sinus tumors, can be found in nearly two-thirds of clear cell carcinomas and serve as a useful identifying feature.[28] The differential diagnosis is be-

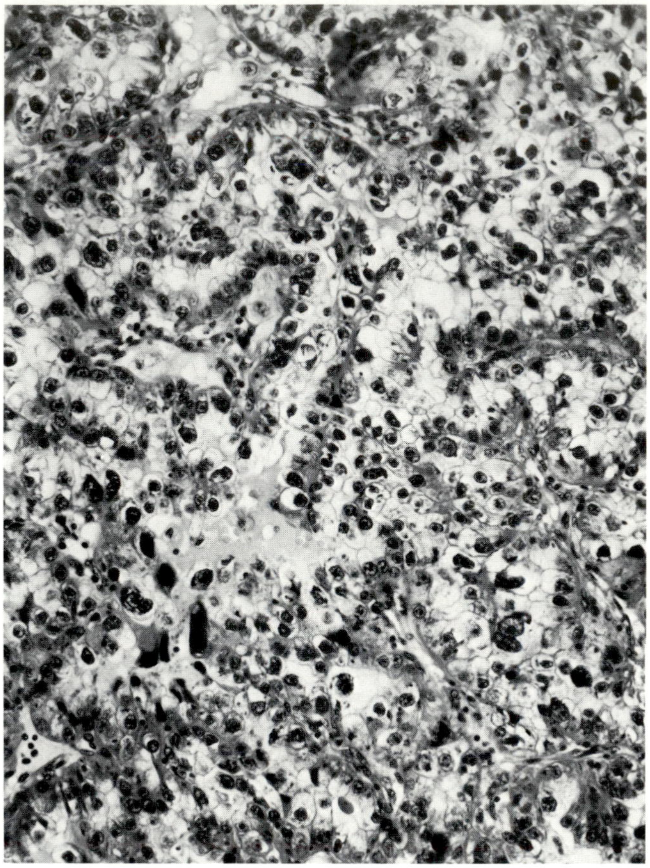

FIG. 12.21. Clear cell carcinoma composed of sheets of large cells with clear cytoplasm and marked nuclear atypia.

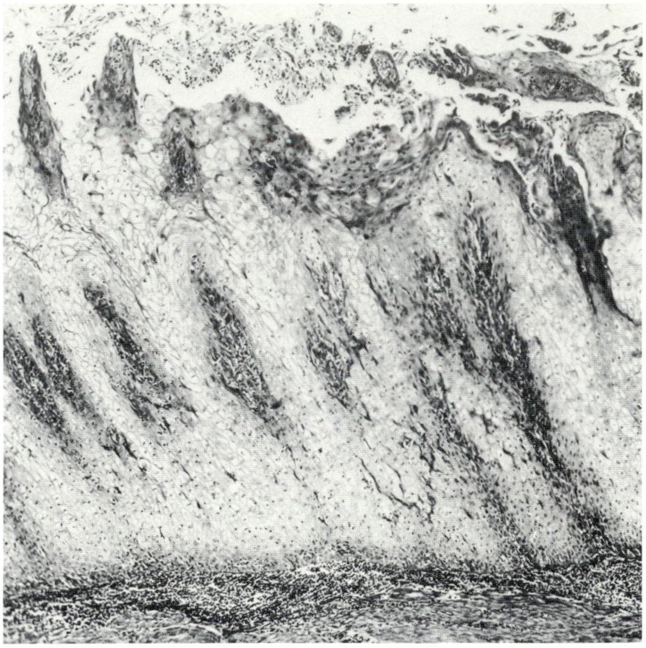

FIG. 12.22. Squamous carcinoma of the endometrium in which there is complete replacement of the surface by squamous carcinoma.

tween serous carcinoma and secretory carcinoma, both of which were discussed previously.

Behavior. Clear cell carcinoma has a tendency to be high grade, deeply invasive, and present in an advanced stage. None of the patients with tumor beyond stage I survived for 5 years in the series reported by Christopherson et al.[28] Even in stage I, the 5-year survival is only 44%. The mean length of survival for those who fail treatment is 19 months.

Squamous Carcinoma

Squamous carcinoma develops in the endometrium, but it is extremely rare (Fig. 12.22). There is a strong association with cervical stenosis, pyometria, and chronic inflammation. The tumor may arise from icthyosis uteri, a condition in which the endometrium is replaced by keratinized squamous epithelium. In the past, this condition was considered a sequela of the use of steam as treatment for endometritis. With the abandonment of this procedure, icthyosis uteri has become quite rare.

There have been 25 cases of squamous carcinoma in the endometrium reported in association with squamous carcinoma in situ of the cervix.[87] Rare examples in which carcinoma in situ of the cervix involves the endometrium, fallopian tube, and surface of the ovary also have been reported.[87] Some of these may have arisen in the endometrium, but in order to justifiably identify primary squamous carcinoma of the endometrium, three criteria must be met: (1) adenocarcinoma is not present in the endometrium; (2) the squamous carcinoma in the endometrium does not have any connection with the squamous epithelium of the cervix; and (3) squamous carcinoma is not present in the cervix.[53] By these criteria, only 21 cases of primary squamous carcinoma of the endometrium have been reported.[122]

Undifferentiated Carcinoma

Tumors that fail to show evidence of either glandular or squamous differentiation are regarded as undifferentiated carcinomas. Some of these are small cell carcinomas (Fig. 12.23). These may show neuroendocine differentiation. Tumors in which the neoplastic cells demonstrate argyrophilia with the Grimelius stain have been termed *argyrophil cell adenocarcinoma*[178] (see section in Immunocytochemistry). Rare neoplasms may contain multinucleated giant cells resembling osteoclastic giant cells (Fig. 12.24) or syncytiotrophoblast. PAS and mucicarmine stains are helpful in identifying glandular differentiation and immunocytochemical localization of hCG for demonstrating trophoblastic differentiation. Rarely, primary choriocarcinoma of the endometrium may develop in a postmenopausal woman (Figs. 12.25 and 12.26), repre-

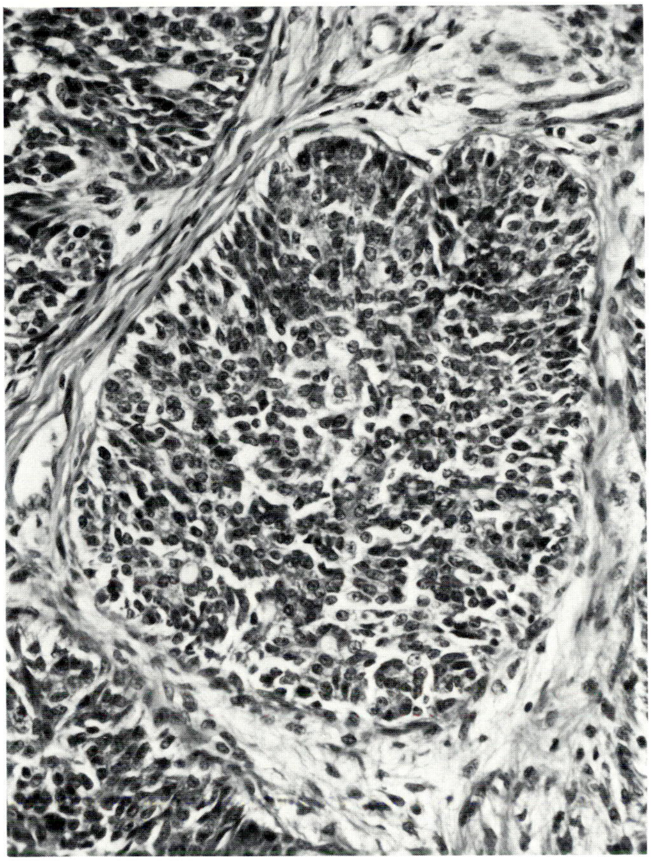

FIG. 12.23. An undifferentiated small cell carcinoma of the endometrium composed of a relatively uniform population of cells with small round to oval nuclei and scant cytoplasm.

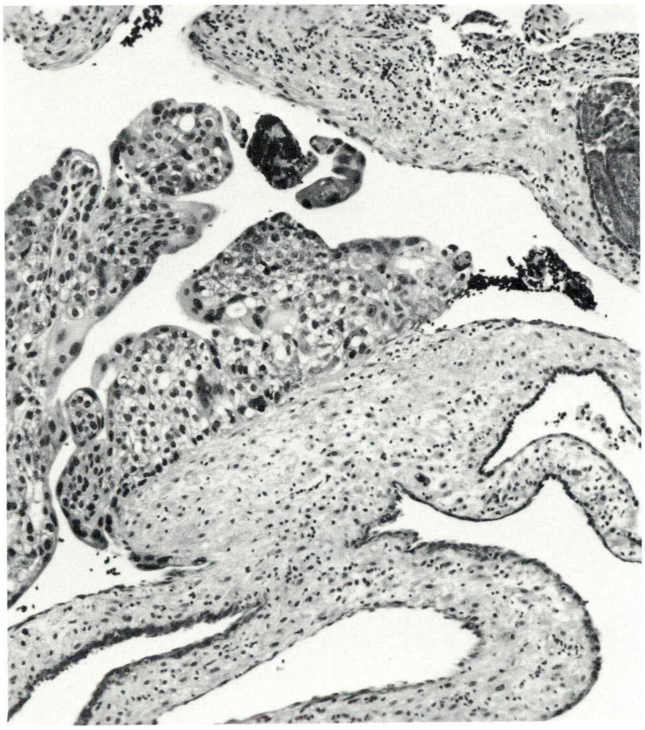

FIG. 12.25. Primary choriocarcinoma of the endometrium in a 64-year-old woman. Neoplasm closely associated with poorly differentiated adenocarcinoma showing squamous differentiation. The endometrial stroma has undergone a decidual reaction.

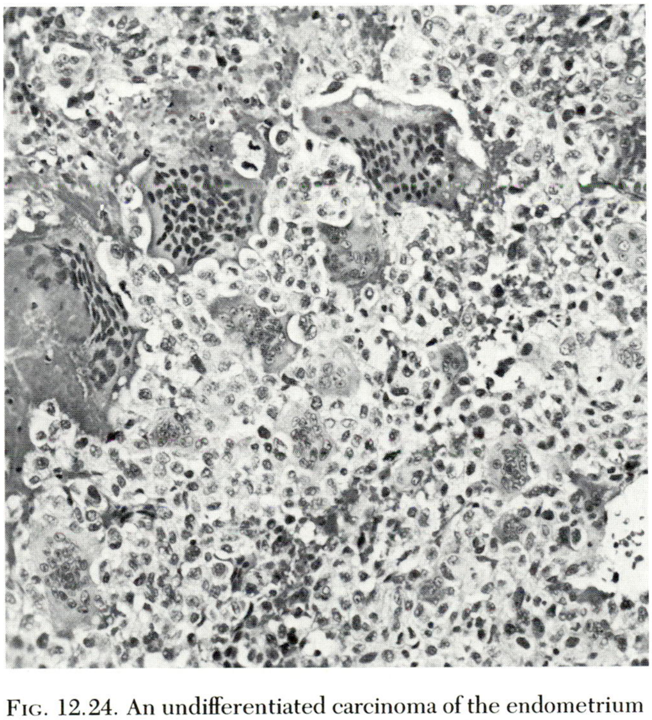

FIG. 12.24. An undifferentiated carcinoma of the endometrium containing multinucleated giant cells resembling osteoclastic giant cells.

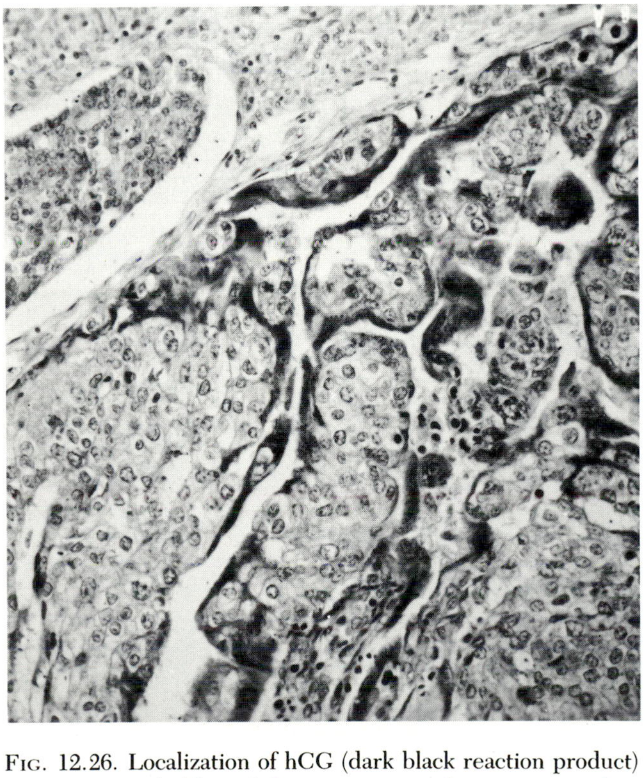

FIG. 12.26. Localization of hCG (dark black reaction product) in syncytiotrophoblast of choriocarcinoma. Immunoperoxidase with hematoxylin.

senting a form of differentiation of a carcinoma derived from somatic cells and not a germ cell or trophoblastic neoplasm.

Mixed Types of Carcinoma

An endometrial carcinoma may show combinations of two or more of the pure types. The tumor should be classified according to the dominant component, since there are no studies delineating the behavior of mixed tumors.

Nonspecific Carcinomas Including Glassy Cell Carcinoma

A number of rare examples of unusual neoplasms arising in the endometrium have been reported, but the data consist largely of case reports precluding a detailed clinicopathologic analysis. One of these, glassy cell carcinoma, is regarded as a variant of a mixed adenosquamous carcinoma and occurs in the endometrium.[29] First described in the cervix, glassy cell carcinoma is a poorly differentiated neoplasm with little or no glandular or squamous differentiation and is composed of masses and nests of characteristic polygonal cells separated by a fibrous stroma that often contains an abundance of inflammatory cells. The cells have well-defined borders and granular eosinophilic or amphophilic cytoplasm, giving a ground-glass appearance. The nuclei are enlarged and round, with centrally placed, prominent, eosinophilic nucleoli (Fig. 12.27). Mitotic activity, including the presence of abnormal mitotic figures, is high. The behavior, based on a small series of cases, is highly aggressive.

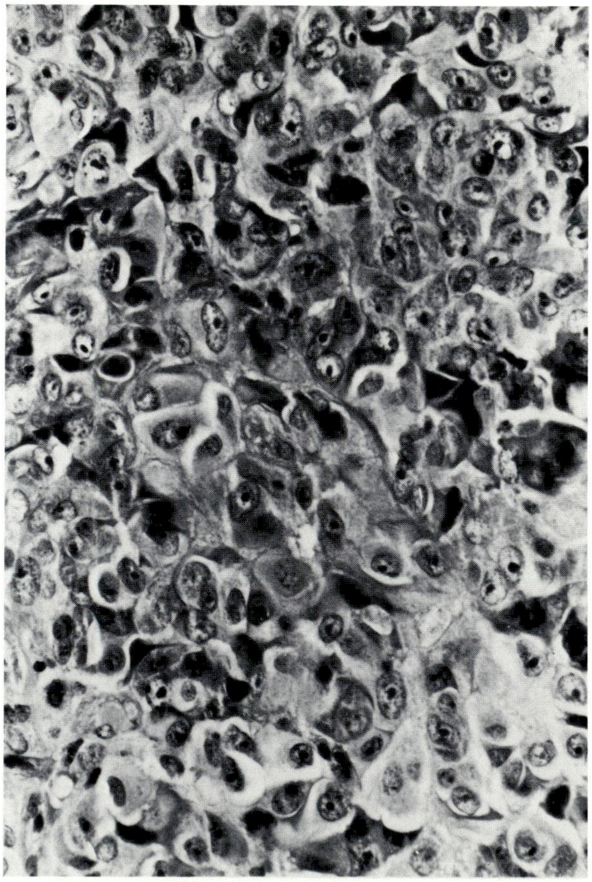

Fig. 12.27. Glassy cell carcinoma composed of masses and nests of polygonal cells with well-defined borders, granular cytoplasm, and enlarged nuclei with prominent nucleoli. (Courtesy of W.M. Christopherson, M.D.)

Tumors Metastatic to the Endometrium

Ovary. Simultaneous cancers involving the endometrium and the ovary may represent (1) metastasis from the endometrium to the ovary, (2) metastasis from the ovary to the endometrium, or (3) independent primary tumors (see Chapter 22, Metastatic Ovarian Tumors). The distinction is important because the prognosis and treatment differ. Scully et al.[157] suggested that when the endometrial carcinoma is small and minimally invasive, the two neoplasms are independent. Eifel et al.[48] found that if the two carcinomas have an endometrioid pattern, the prognosis is good, and therefore the two neoplasms are probably independent. When serous or clear cell carcinoma is found, the prognosis is poor, and a primary tumor with metastasis is likely. The primary neoplasm is identified by its larger size or more advanced stage. Ulbright and Roth[179] classified tumors as primary in the endometrium with metastasis to the ovaries when there is multinodular ovarian involvement or at least two of the following criteria are met: (1) small (< 5 cm) ovaries, (2) bilateral ovarian involvement, (3) deep myometrial invasion, (4) vascular invasion, or (5) fallopian tube involvement. When these criteria are used, there is a significant difference in the frequency of distant metastasis in the group classified as metastatic versus the group classified as an independent primary. Metastasis from the endometrium to the ovary occurs more often than the reverse. About a third of the cases are independent tumors involving both sites simultaneously. Independent tumors display either well-differentiated endometrioid or nonendometrioid patterns, whereas grade 3 endometrial carcinoma, adenosquamous carcinoma, and malignant mixed mesodermal tumors are generally metastatic when detected.

Extragenital Sites. When an extragenital tumor metastasizes to the uterus it usually is a manifestation of obvious dissemination.[98] The mean age of patients is 60 years, and they have abnormal bleeding. The diagnosis in curettings may, on rare occasion, be the first clue of an occult primary tumor usually from the breast, stomach, or

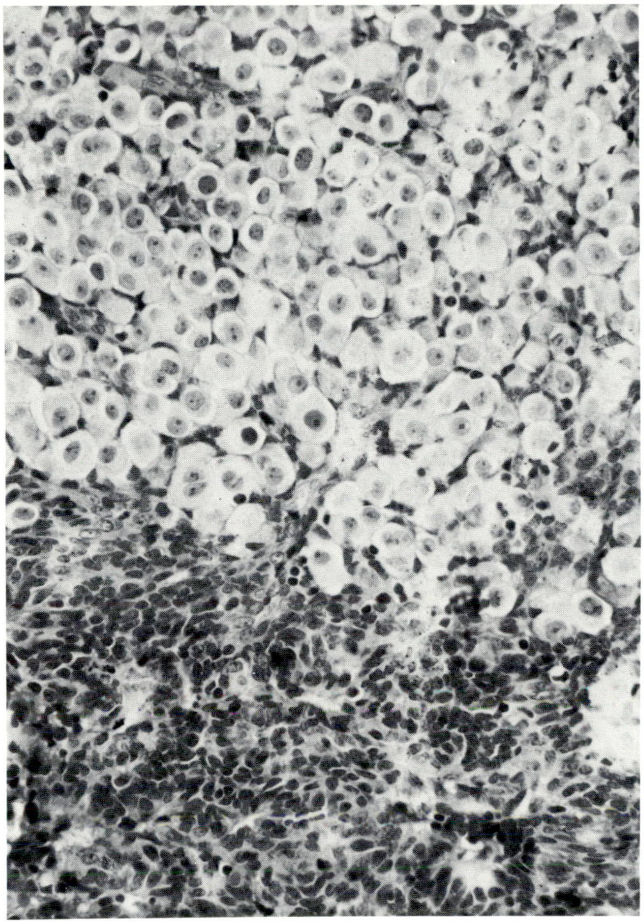

Fig. 12.28. Metastatic breast carcinoma in the endometrium. Metastatic carcinoma should not be mistaken for primary, undifferentiated carcinoma of the endometrium.

ovary.[99] Metastatic breast cancer is the most frequent extragenital tumor that metastasizes to the uterus (47%), followed by stomach (29%), melanoma (5%), colon (3%), pancreas (3%), and kidney (3%). In addition, rare examples of metastasis from the gallbladder, appendix, pleura, liver, lung, urinary bladder, and thyroid have been reported.[99]

Metastatic neoplasms to the endometrium frequently infiltrate the endometrium diffusely, sparing the glands (Fig. 12.28). Most neoplasms metastatic to the endometrium are poorly differentiated and lack squamous metaplasia, unlike primary endometrial carcinoma. The myometrium can contain metastatic nodules as well. Mean survival after metastasis to the uterus is 20 months.

Ultrastructure

Electron microscopy can be employed as an aid in the differential diagnosis of an undifferentiated endometrial carcinoma.

Typical Endometrial (Endometrioid) Carcinoma

The neoplastic cells have striking structural variability, paralleling the observations made using light microscopy.* Ultrastructurally, endometrioid carcinoma is composed of a heterogenous population of cells. There are four distinct cell types and two different nuclear forms that differ from normal endometrium. The four cell types are (1) a large round cell containing a large nucleus and scant cytoplasm with a highly variable content of organelles; (2) an irregularly shaped, elongated cell frequently containing cytoplasmic projections; (3) a clear cell with a paucity of organelles; and (4) a dark cell with dense cytoplasmic contents and pyknotic nucleus.

One form of nucleus in endometrial carcinoma is a large, rounded nucleus with a relatively smooth margin. The other has an elongated nucleus with numerous deep irregular clefts, producing a lobulated appearance. The nucleolus of these cells is large, but a nucleolar channel system has not been identified.

The cell membrane of adenocarcinoma cells typically has small sparse microvilli, but occasionally long microvilli are present (Fig. 12.29). The lateral cell membrane is more irregular than in normal cells and tends to undergo dehiscence, leading to the formation of intracellular spaces. The basal cell membrane is also irregular and discontinuous due to the presence of complex cytoplasmic projections irregularly extending into the stroma. There is marked variation in the development of rough endoplasmic reticulum and considerable variation in ribosomal content. Autophagosomes and giant lysosomes are prominent in some cells. Cells may have dense cytoplasm due to the presence of abundant ribosomes, whereas some have clear cytoplasm due to almost complete absence of ribosomes. The variability in organelle content, size, and shape exceeds that of endometrial hyperplasia. The Golgi apparatus of endometrial carcinoma cells tends to be poorly developed, and there is scant smooth endoplasmic reticulum as well. Mitochondria show considerable variation in size, shape, and number, and glycogen and lipid are increased. Microtubules and microfibrils are rare, and annulate lamellae are absent.

Adenocarcinoma with Squamous Metaplasia (Adenoacanthoma)

The squamous component of adenoacanthoma resembles squamous metaplasia in normal endometrium and other epithelia. Although keratohyaline granules, specific for squamous cells, are scanty and membrane-coated granules are not evident, frank keratinization may be ob-

* References 1, 8, 23, 51, 56, 58, 132, 173, 188.

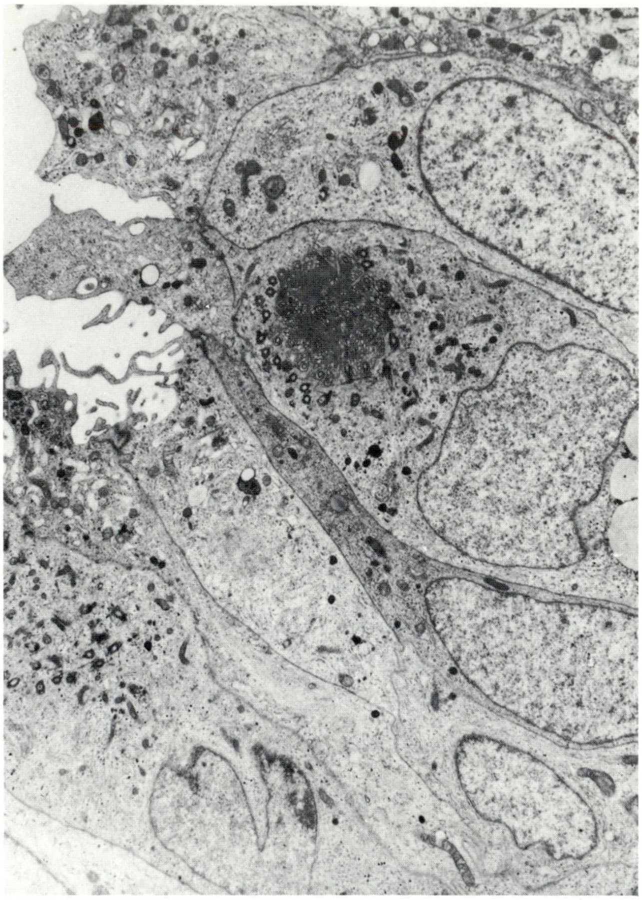

FIG. 12.29. Electronmicrograph of adenocarcinoma showing ciliated cells with considerable pleomorphism. Microvilli are prominent. ×2900. (Reprinted by permission of Cavazos and Lucas, Ref. 23.)

served. The basal lamina surrounding the squamous cells is, for the most part, complete and usually reduplicated.[59]

ADENOSQUAMOUS CARCINOMA

The squamous and glandular elements can be clearly distinguished. The squamous cells may contain keratohyaline granules, have abundant tonofilaments and tonofibrils, and are joined by numerous desmosomal junctions. Golgi apparatus is scant. In contrast, the glandular cells show luminal formation and have numerous microvilli, and there is a paucity of tonofilaments. They contain abundant Golgi apparatus and vacuoles in the cytoplasm. Cells intermediate between glandular and squamous cells can be seen in clusters extending into gland lumens, suggesting that the two types of cells differentiate from the same stem cell.[56]

SEROUS CARCINOMA

In a study comparing the ultrastructural features of serous carcinoma, typical endometrial carcinoma, and clear cell carcinoma, Sato et al.[153] found similarities among all three types of neoplasms, particularly between serous carcinoma and clear cell carcinoma. Numerous secretory granules, large nuclei, prominent nucleoli, and a paucity of microfilaments are features that differ from the typical endometrial carcinoma and more closely resemble serous carcinoma of the ovary. The nuclear findings are a reflection of the poorly differentiated nature of serous carcinoma in contrast to the better-differentiated endometrial carcinoma.

CLEAR CELL CARCINOMA

The clear cells contain abundant glycogen, parallel stacks of granular endoplasmic reticulum, numerous free ribosomes, and small, uniform, rounded mitochrondria. Supranuclear Golgi complex and microvesicles are present in some of the cells. Nuclei are irregularly shaped and show shallow indentations. The hobnail-type cells have an abundant supranuclear cytoplasmic matrix and a prominent bulging nucleus.[147,163]

Quantitative Microscopy

There have been only a few studies of endometrial carcinoma by Feulgen cytomorphometry. About 30% of endometrial carcinomas are euploid. One study reported that tumors with near diploid DNA distribution are better differentiated and have a more favorable prognosis than those with high ploidy levels.[6] The 8-year survival for women with diploid tumors is nearly 80%, compared to 18% for those with aneuploid tumors.[124] Ploidy is as good as or a better predictor of survival than either histologic grade or stage.

Immunocytochemistry

Immunocytochemical investigations of endometrial carcinoma have been used primarily for research to correlate biochemical features of the neoplastic cells with morphologic patterns of cytodifferentiation. The availability of specific and standardized antibodies against various cellular proteins, particularly intermediate filaments, permits greater use of the technique in diagnostic pathology. Monoclonal antibodies to estrogen receptor protein detect estrogen receptor protein in the nuclei of the majority of epithelial and stromal cells in normal proliferative endometrium, but the antibodies react only on frozen tissue, limiting their utility in diagnostic surgical pathology.[138,139]

CEA has been described in both endometrial carcinoma and endocervical carcinoma.* A higher proportion of endocervical carcinomas than endometrial carcinomas

* References 79, 123, 148, 169, 180, 181.

contain CEA. At present, it does not appear that localization of CEA is useful in the differential diagnosis of endometrial and endocervical carcinoma. CEA and related oncofetal proteins, such as alpha-fetoprotein (AFP) and hCG, are serum tumor markers that can be monitored. CEA has been detected in the serum of approximately 30%[93,160,180] of patients with endometrial carcinoma, but there is no consistent relationship between the histologic grade of the tumor by tissue localization and the stage of disease by serum measurement. All patients with persistent serum elevations of CEA develop recurrence, but many patients with widespread disease have normal levels of CEA.

Elevated serum levels of AFP and beta-hCG occur in 50% and 21%, respectively, of patients with endometrial carcinoma,[44] but Hustin,[79] using immunocytochemical methods, was unable to detect either marker in tissue sections of endometrial hyperplasia or carcinoma. At present, these tumor markers are of doubtful value in the diagnosis and management of patients with endometrial neoplasia.

Immunocytochemical studies reveal peptide hormones and other gastrointestinal hormones in 26–68% of endometrial carcinomas.[9,156,178] These tumors can also be identified by the Grimelius stain or the presence of dense core granules by electron microscopy and the term *argyrophil cell adenocarcinoma* has been proposed.[178] Only a small proportion of the argyrophilic cells resemble the hormone-containing cells of the gastrointestinal tract, but it is these cells that stain for serotonin and, less frequently, somatostatin, ACTH, and calcitonin.[9,156] None of the carcinomas with argyrophilic cells or hormone immunoreactivity have exhibited clinical evidence of hormone activity. Bannatyne et al.[9] observed argyrophilia in 8% of normal endometria. Endometrial carcinomas with neuroendocrine granules do not assume a specific glandular pattern or resemble carcinoids and do not behave differently from ordinary endometrial carcinoma of the same stage and grade.[177,178]

Clinical and Pathologic Risk Factors

Clinical Risk Factors

Age

Although younger patients tend to have better differentiated, less advanced disease and a better prognosis as a consequence, age may be an independent prognostic factor. In a study from the National Cancer Institute's Surveillance, Epidemiology, and End Results (SEER) Program, stage and age were found to be the major prognostic indicators, followed by race, average family income, and highest education received.[170] In a clinicopathologic analysis of 989 women with endometrial carcinoma from the Louisville Uterine Cancer Registry, the percentage of women dead of disease at 5 and 10 years, respectively, was 0 and 1% for women under the age of 50 compared to 5% and 7% for women over 50 (p = 0.001). There were few patients with grade 3 tumors, but all of the women younger than 50 years of age survived compared with only 57% of women over 50 years.[31]

Race

The 5- and 10-year survival rates for black women are significantly lower than for white women. Black women have a higher proportion of high-grade, high-stage tumors and also seek medical attention at a more advanced age compared to white women (median age of 62 years versus 58). In the Louisville Uterine Cancer Registry, 92% of white women had stage I disease compared to 76% of black women, and 58% of white women had grade 1 tumors compared to 39% of black women. Even after correcting for stage and grade, a difference in survival rate persisted.[31] Similar findings were reported in the SEER analysis.[170]

Stage

The stage describes the extent of disease at the time of diagnosis. It is important in determining prognosis and treatment as well as in providing a standardized method of reporting data among different investigators. The staging system adopted by the International Federation of Gynecology and Obstetrics (FIGO) classifies endometrial carcinoma stage I if it is confined to the corpus, stage II if it involves the corpus and cervix, stage III if carcinoma is outside the uterus but confined to the pelvis, and stage IV if carcinoma is either outside the true pelvis or involves the mucosa of the bladder or rectum. The clinical stage is determined preoperatively. More extensive disease discovered after hysterectomy does not alter the clinical stage but is referred to as the surgical, pathologic, or surgical–pathologic stage. It has been shown that the inaccuracy of clinical staging when compared to the surgical–pathologic stage may be as high as 51%.[35] Patients are more often understaged.

Clinical Staging. Approximately 80% of women with endometrial carcinoma are clinically stage I. In the Louisville Uterine Cancer Registry study, 5- and 10-year survival rates of patients with stage I disease were 81% and 65%, respectively, for stage II, 41% and 33%, for stage III, 42% and 25%, and for stage IV, only 9% and 0.[33] Extrauterine spread is one of the most important clinical prognostic variables.[42] When tumor is confined to the uterus, 93% of patients will remain free of disease, but if disease extends beyond the uterus, only 57% of the patients will be free of disease in a follow-up interval ranging from 3 to 6 years.

Pathologic Staging. The mortality rate increases with increasing stage even when there is only microscopic disease. A fractional curettage is, therefore, performed before hysterectomy in order to identify microscopic involvement of the cervix, which, in the absence of tumor elsewhere, alters the stage from I to II. The increased mortality for stage II disease is related to an increased frequency of lymph node metastasis and the presence of higher grade, more deeply invasive tumors in stage II patients.[15] A definitive diagnosis of cervical involvement requires the presence of endometrial carcinoma cells attached or within endocervical tissue (Fig. 12.30). Unattached, free-floating tumor in endocervical curettings is probably not significant. In one study, it was associated with stage II disease in 23% of cases,[186] but in another study, the survival was similar to that of patients with stage I disease,[86] suggesting that unattached tumor in endocervical curettings is a contaminant and can be disregarded.

Pathologic staging after hysterectomy is also important in the determination of occult stage II and stage III disease. Patients with microscopic stage III disease, even after complete surgical eradication of tumor and additional radiotherapy, have a 50% recurrence rate. Disseminated disease is often present at the time of hysterectomy, since 50% of patients with clinical stage I disease who have adnexal involvement discovered at surgery also have pelvic lymph node metastasis.[20] A quarter of these patients die with distant metastasis, usually to the lung, brain, and bone.[3]

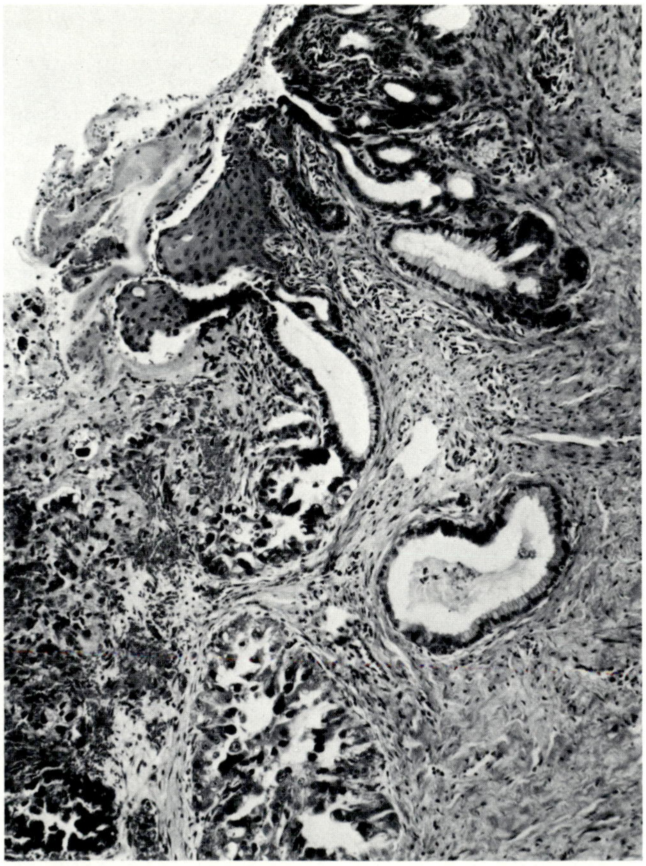

FIG. 12.30. Clear cell carcinoma of the endometrium invading the endocervix. Neoplastic glands are present in the stroma adjacent to endocervical glands.

Estrogen and Progesterone Receptors

The presence of estrogen and progesterone receptors by dextran-coated charcoal or sucrose gradient analysis is of prognostic value in women with breast cancer. Similar studies have been performed for endometrial carcinoma, but much of the data has been inconclusive. The early studies were compromised by the limited number of cases analyzed and the wide variety of methodologies and experimental conditions used for the assays. Monoclonal antibodies against estrogen receptor demonstrate the receptor only in the nucleus.[138] Thus, it appears that the native estrophilin in target cells identified in the cytosol fraction of tissue homogenates actually resides in the nucleus. Since the receptor in this location is loosely bound, it is readily extractable into the homogenization medium when the cells are disrupted. As a result, the following scheme has been proposed for estrogen–receptor interaction: (1) The majority of native receptor is in the nucleus in equilibrium with a small amount in the cytoplasm; (2) the cytoplasmic receptor takes up the hormone into the target cell because of its high binding capacity compared to serum transport proteins; (3) the inactive receptor is activated in the nucleus, where it binds tightly to the chromatin, removing it from solution and resulting in the transport of additional occupied receptor into the nucleus for activation[83] (see Chapter 9, Uterine Corpus).

Measurable amounts of estrogen receptor are present in 67–100% of endometrial carcinomas.[67,82,108,126] Generally, there is a correlation between the degree of differentiation, the prognosis, and the presence of estrogen and progesterone receptors.[36,47,118,120] When the effects of conventional histopathologic risk factors are controlled, estrogen and progesterone receptor status, individually and combined, appear to be independent risk factors for predicting survival.[38] Estrogen and progesterone receptors are both positive in 70% of grade 1, 55% of grade 2, and 41% of grade 3 carcinomas. Conversely, both receptors are negative in 10% of grade 1, 18% of grade 2, and 33% of grade 3 neoplasms. Discordance between estrogen or progesterone receptor status occurs in nearly a quarter of the tumors irrespective of grade. Because estrogen induces progesterone receptors,[24,63,77] it has been postulated that the response to hormonal manipulation may be more accurately predicted by measuring progesterone receptor alone.[36,47]

Pathologic Risk Factors

In addition to the histologic type, the grade, depth of myometrial invasion, and presence or absence of vascular invasion should be included in the surgical pathology report because they are prognostic determinants that play an important role in guiding treatment.[33]

Grade

Numerous studies have confirmed the value of grading.[7,27,55,117,128,130] The 5-year survival rate for patients with grade 1 tumors is 81%, with grade 2 tumors 74%, and with grade 3 tumors 50%.[84] The depth of myometrial invasion and the frequency of lymph node metastasis are also related to tumor grade. Only 12% of patients with grade 1 tumors have deep myometrial invasion, whereas 46% of those with grade 3 tumors have deep myometrial invasion.[27] Patients in the latter group have only a 30% 5-year survival. Metastasis to lymph nodes occurs in 5% of patients with well-differentiated tumors but in 26% of those with poorly differentiated carcinoma.[107]

There are two methods of grading. One is based on architectural criteria (FIGO), and one is a nuclear grade. A well-differentiated adenocarcinoma has a prominent and easily recognizable glandular pattern (Fig. 12.31), whereas a poorly differentiated adenocarcinoma is characterized by solid masses of cells in which gland formation is barely evident (Fig. 12.32). Moderately differentiated adenocarcinoma (Fig. 12.33) has histologic characteristics midway between the well-differentiated and poorly differentiated forms. For tumors displaying widely disparate grades, the architectural (FIGO) grade is grade 1 if less than 10% grows in a solid pattern, grade 2 if the tumor is composed mostly of glands but 10–50% of the tumor grows in solid sheets, and grade 3 if more than 50% is solid.

Nuclear grading may be slightly better than histologic grading in predicting outcome, especially for nuclear

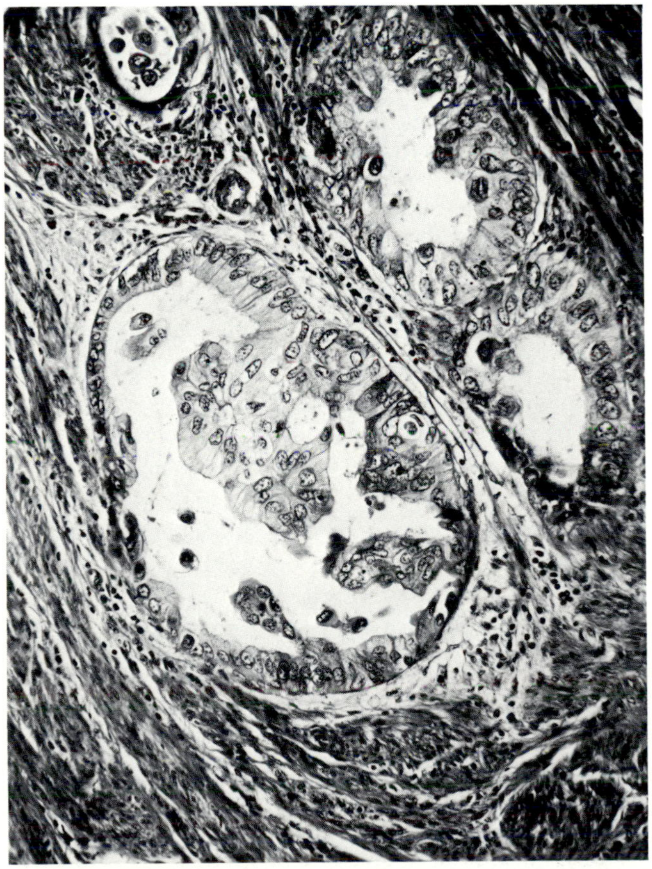

FIG. 12.31. Well-differentiated adenocarcinoma characterized by well-defined glands invading the myometrium. (Reprinted by permission of Kurman and Norris, Ref. 101.)

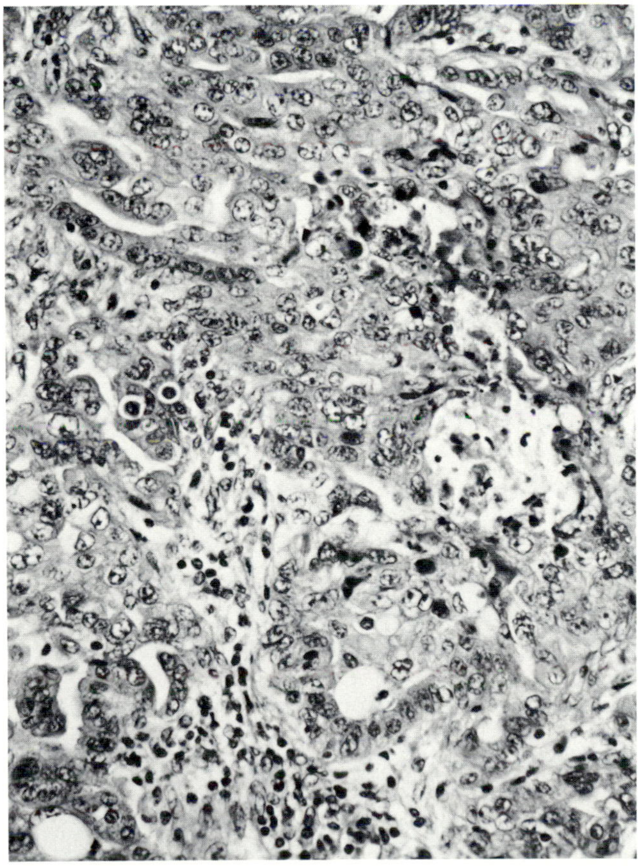

FIG. 12.32. Poorly differentiated adenocarcinoma. Only rare gland lumens are present in an otherwise solid proliferation of epithelium.

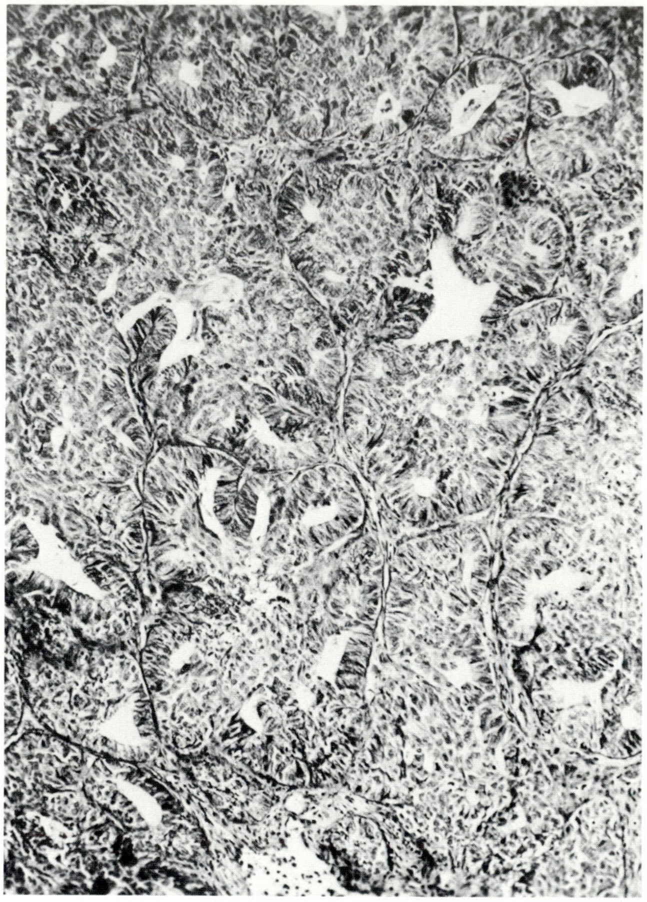

FIG. 12.33. Moderately differentiated adenocarcinoma, showing more solid proliferation of epithelium than in well-differentiated carcinoma, but numerous gland lumens are still present.

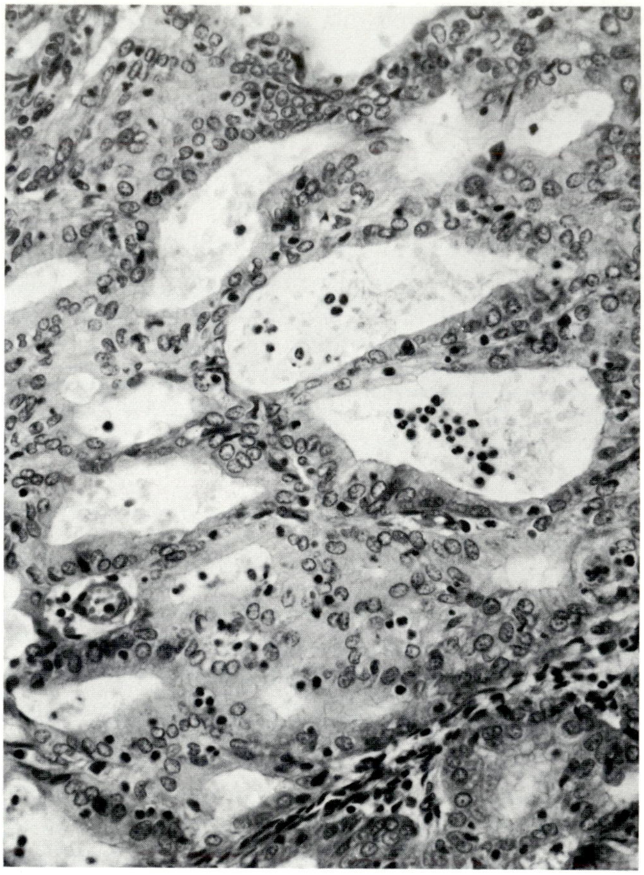

FIG. 12.34. Adenocarcinoma of the endometrium with grade 1 nuclear atypia. The cells have oval nuclei and evenly dispersed chromatin.

grade 3 lesions.[33] The 5-year survival rate ranges from 84% for nuclear grade 1 to 52% for grade 3. An advantage of the nuclear grading system is that it more reliably identifies the tumors with poor prognosis, that is, clear cell and serous carcinomas, which typically have grade 3 nuclei. Since these tumors may display a prominent papillary pattern, they are undergraded using an architectural grade in which papillary tumors are considered well differentiated. Cells with oval nuclei and evenly dispersed chromatin are considered grade 1 (Fig. 12.34). Cells with markedly enlarged, pleomorphic nuclei displaying irregular coarse chromatin and prominent, eosinophilic nucleoli are considered grade 3 (Fig. 12.35). Those falling between grades 1 and 3 are designated grade 2 (Fig. 12.36). Mitotic activity is an independent histologic variable but is generally increased, as are abnormal mitotic figures, with increasing degrees of nuclear atypia.

Occasionally, a neoplasm may exhibit wide variation in differentiation within different parts of the tumor. Well-differentiated glandular components may coexist in adjacent fields with solid sheets of cells. The nuclear grade of the cells in the glandular and solid components usually is similar, supporting nuclear as opposed to histologic grading. Less commonly, the nuclear grade within different parts of the tumor also may differ. In this instance the nuclear grade is assigned according to the least differentiated area. The heterogeneity in differentiation that a tumor may exhibit accounts, in part, for the differences in grade that can be observed between the endometrial curettings and the hysterectomy specimen. A discordance as high as 30% has been reported.[35,100,136]

Myometrial Invasion

Myometrial invasion, independent of tumor grade, is also important in predicting prognosis. The 5-year survival rate for patients with tumor either limited to the endometrium or showing only superficial myometrial invasion is 80%, in contrast to those with deep myometrial invasion, in whom the 5-year survival rate is 60%.[84] The frequency of lymph node metastasis is also related to the depth of myometrial invasion. In clinical stage I

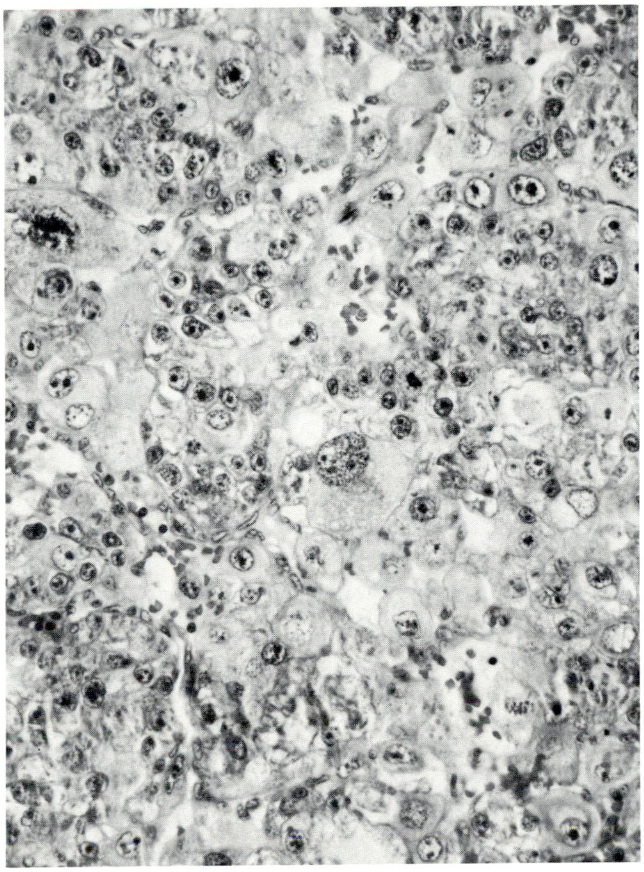

FIG. 12.35. Adenocarcinoma of the endometrium nuclear grade 3. The cells are markedly enlarged, with pleomorphic nuclei displaying irregular coarse chromatin and prominent nucleoli.

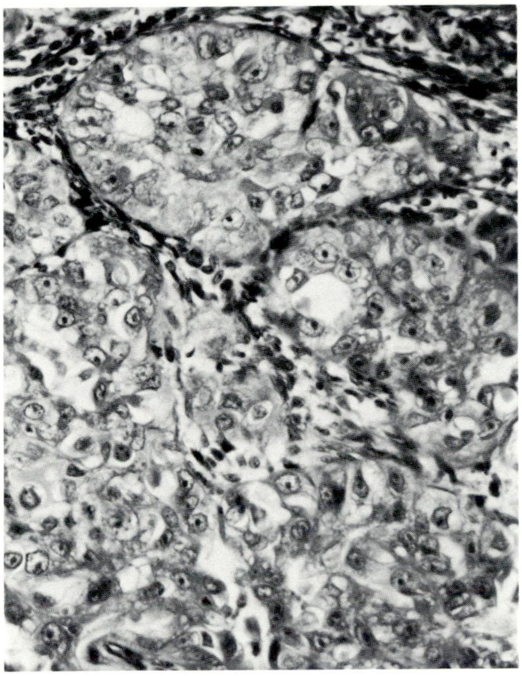

FIG. 12.36. Adenocarcinoma of the endometrium nuclear grade 2. The cells are enlarged, but pleomorphism is not as marked as in grade 3 nuclei. Prominent nucleoli are present, but the degree of chromatin clumping is not as marked as in nuclear grade 3.

endometrial carcinoma, inner third myometrial invasion was associated with lymph node metastasis in 5% of cases, middle third invasion with metastasis in 23%, and outer third invasion with 33%. Stage I well-differentiated carcinoma must invade halfway through the myometrium before there is a risk of metastasis. When grade and myometrial invasion are analyzed together, grade 1 tumors invading the inner third of the myometrium are not associated with pelvic node metastasis, but with outer third invasion, pelvic node metastasis is 25%. A similar trend occurs with higher-grade tumors.

Depth of myometrial invasion is expressed in percentage by dividing the uterine wall into thirds and determining and the maximum depth of invasion. Tumor in vascular spaces beyond the deepest point of invasion should not be used for this measurement. An alternate method for assessing depth of invasion is to measure the uninvolved myometrium, in millimeters, from the serosa to the point of maximum tumor invasion.[114] This approach has the advantage of a more accurate measurement, since the uterine serosa is readily identified in contrast to the boundary of the endomyometrium, and a measurement in millimeters may be more easily reproducible.

In patients with concomitant adenomyosis, it may be difficult to distinguish myometrial invasion from extension of the carcinoma into adenomyosis. The distinction, however, is important because the presence of carcinoma in adenomyosis deeper than the maximum depth of true tumor invasion does not worsen the prognosis.[68,74] The diagnosis of carcinoma extending into adenomyosis depends on the demonstration of endometrial stroma. Tumor involving adenomyosis frequently has a smooth, rounded outline in contrast to the more irregular margin of invasive carcinoma.

Vascular Invasion

The presence of vascular invasion should be specified, since it is a useful predictor of recurrence. In a retrospective study of 379 patients with recurrent endometrial carcinoma,[4] vascular invasion was found in 54%. Usually, vascular invasion is associated with high-grade tumors and deep myometrial invasion. A study of stage I endometrial carcinoma, however, revealed a significant correlation between vascular invasion and tumor recurrence independent of differentiation and depth of myometrial invasion.[70] Also, the interval from treatment to recurrence is shorter in patients with vascular invasion.[4]

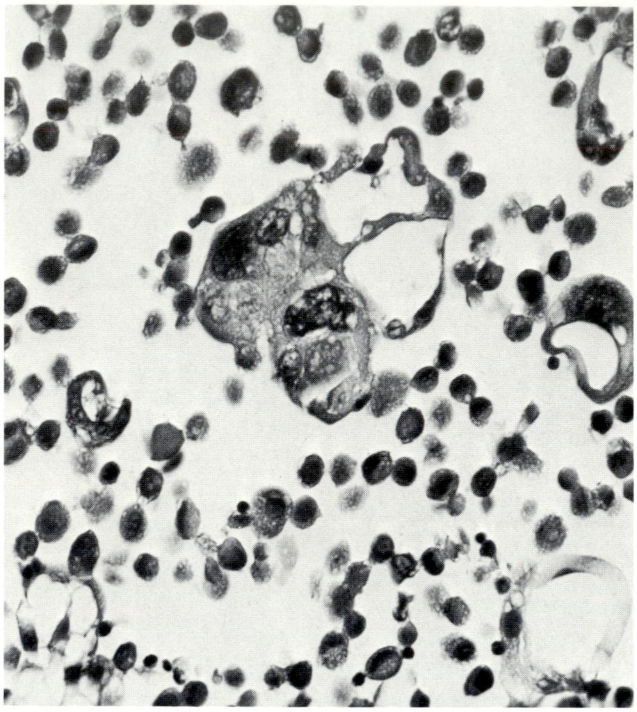

FIG. 12.37. Endometrial carcinoma cells in the peritoneal fluid.

Peritoneal Cytology

The status of peritoneal cytology as an independent risk factor is not clear. Of 167 patients with clinical stage I disease, 38% with positive cytology had recurrences, compared to 10% with negative cytology.[37] Of women with positive cytology and no disease beyond the uterus at the time of hysterectomy, 46% eventually died of carcinoma. Not all studies agree, however. In an analysis of 93 patients with clinical stage I disease by Yazigi et al.,[190] there was no difference in survival among patients with either positive or negative cytology. Both groups had a recurrence rate of approximately 10%.

Since patients with malignant cells in the peritoneal washings (Fig. 12.37) may receive additional treatment, it is important that the pathologist be conservative in the interpretation of pelvic washings. Reactive mesothelial cells may form clusters and have enlarged, atypical nuclei. If there is doubt about the nature of cells in the peritoneal fluid, comparison with the histologic appearance of the tumor in the hysterectomy specimen will resolve the problem.

Treatment

Stage I

Nearly three fourths of patients with endometrial cancer have clinical stage I disease when initially treated. Although several studies describe survival of over 90% with total abdominal hysterectomy and bilateral salpingo-oophorectomy, a survey by the International Federation of Gynecology and Obstetrics in 1979 indicated a 5-year survival rate of approximately 75%.[96] Although hysterectomy or hysterectomy combined with intracavitary radium or whole pelvis external beam therapy are the primary therapeutic modalities, the mode of treatment administered by a particular gynecologist or radiotherapist varies widely, and a difference in survival rate, if any, is minor for stage I carcinoma.*

Judging from a well-designed prospective clinicopathologic study,[42] of patients with grade 1 carcinoma, only 2% have lymph node metastasis, 4% have deep myometrial invasion, and only 4% develop recurrence. Total abdominal hysterectomy and bilateral salpingo-oophorectomy, therefore, are adequate treatment. For the few patients with high-risk prognostic factors, such as deep myometrial invasion, postoperative pelvic radiation is generally recommended.

Of patients with grade 2 carcinomas, 11% have lymph node metastasis, 15% have deep myometrial invasion, and 15% develop recurrence.[42] Total abdominal hysterectomy and bilateral salpingo-oophorectomy with radiotherapy for the pelvic lymph nodes are standard treatment for grade 2 carcinoma with myometrial invasion. The benefit of external radiation, however, is not completely clear, since of the grade 2 tumors confined to the uterus that recur, half recur at distant sites.[42]

Of patients with grade 3 tumors, 27% have lymph node metastasis, 39% have deep myometrial invasion, and 42% develop recurrence.[42] Therefore, initial treatment should include pelvic and para-aortic lymphadenectomy to assess the extent ot disease and guide postoperative radiation. The value of external radiation can be questioned in these instances, since the majority of recurrences are distant, even in patients with grade 3 tumors confined to the inner third of the myometrium. Although external radiation may provide local control, a successful form of chemotherapy or hormonal therapy is needed for distant metastasis.

Stages II–IV

Patients with endometrial carcinoma involving the cervix have stage II disease. These women require adjuvant radiotherapy because these carcinomas mimic the spread of primary cervical cancer and may metastasize even if well differentiated and only superficially invasive. The frequency of pelvic lymph node metastasis rises from 10% for stage I to 36% for stage II tumors.[125]

Patients with spread outside the uterus but confined

* References 19, 76, 84, 89, 95, 125, 151.

to the pelvis have stage III disease. Only 3% of women with endometrial carcinoma are initially diagnosed as clinical stage III, and 5% of women thought to have stage I disease clinically have occult involvement of the adnexal areas (pathologic stage III) at the time surgery.[3] The 5-year actuarial survival rate for pathologic stage III (subclinical) disease is 40%, compared to 16% for clinical stage III disease. Despite treatment by surgery and radiotherapy, 50% recur. Half of these patients die with distant metastasis, although local control is also a major problem. Adjuvant treatment with a progestational drug does not appear to improve the prognosis.

About 4% of patients with endometrial carcinoma have stage IV disease; the actuarial 5-year survival rate is 10%.[5] Spread to the lungs occurs in 36% of patients, followed by multiple other sites, including lymph nodes and the urinary bladder. Radiation is of value for control of local disease, and progestational agents are beneficial, especially for alleviation of symptoms and for treatment of pulmonary metastasis. A remission of all visible lesions (complete response) occurs in 31% of women treated with a progestational agent. The response rate for grade 1 and 2 carcinoma is 83% compared to 14% for grade 3 neoplasms.[5]

Histologic Effects of Treatment

Radiation

There are characteristic histologic changes in both the neoplastic and nonneoplastic tissues after intracavitary radiation.[97,184] These changes, however, are nonspecific and variable, since neoplastic cells may show only minor alterations from their preirradiated state or may show profound morphologic changes. Similarly, nonneoplastic endometrial or endocervical glands may be only minimally affected or show nuclear and cytoplasmic changes indistinguishable from carcinoma cells. It may be difficult to distinguish tumor invading the myometrium from adenomyosis in an irradiated uterus or to distinguish invasion of the endocervix by endometrial carcinoma from radiation-induced atypia of benign endocervical glands.

Because the cytologic changes in both neoplastic and nonneoplastic tissue can be similar, identification of carcinoma largely depends on the recognition of histologic patterns and signs of invasion. Irradiated carcinoma generally retains a haphazard glandular pattern (Fig. 12.38), but nonirradiated, nonneoplastic glands tend to maintain their normal architectural arrangement despite radiation effects in the endometrial stroma and myometrium.

The difference in radiosensitivity of tumor cells and benign cells is due largely to the increased mitotic activity of the neoplastic cells because it is in mitosis and the S-phase of the cell cycle that a cell is most susceptible

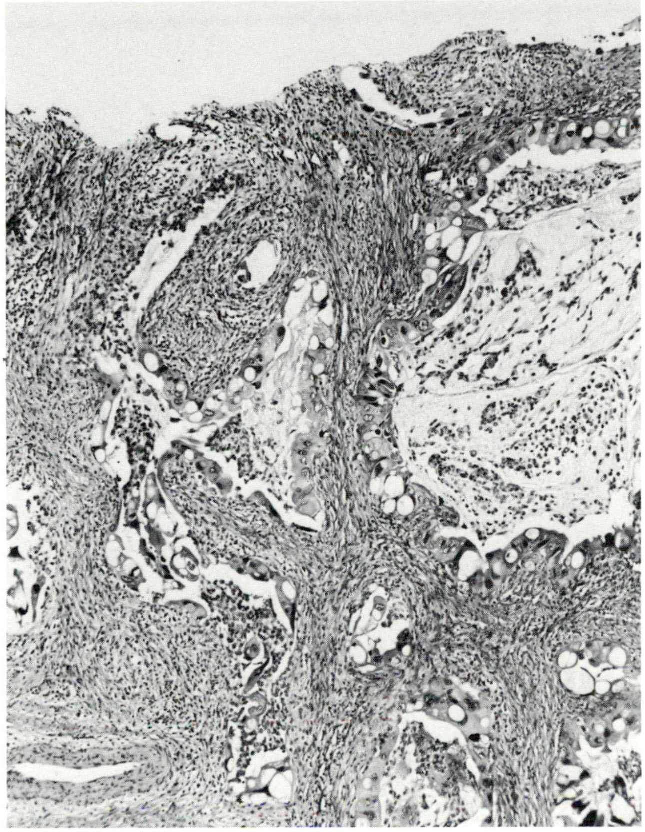

FIG. 12.38. Endometrial carcinoma with radiation-induced cellular alterations. Note the haphazard glandular pattern of carcinoma.

to radiation injury.[176] Also, nonneoplastic cells have a better reparative capacity than do neoplastic cells.[176] In view of the variable morphologic response to radiation, it is often difficult to determine whether irradiated tumor cells are viable or not. It has been shown in animals that some irradiated tumor cells that are morphologically unaltered may nevertheless be unable to proliferate when transplanted.[171] This suggests that these cells are no longer viable despite the absence of morphologically recognizable radiation-induced changes. Nonetheless, on a practical basis, if tumor cells are evident after irradiation, it should be assumed that some retain the capacity to persist however abnormal they appear.

When radiation effect is evident, nuclei tend to be enlarged, highly pleomorphic, and hyperchromatic, with coarsely clumped chromatin. The cytoplasm is often granular and swollen. Vacuolation can be present in both the nucleus and the cytoplasm (Fig. 12.39). The nuclear changes are due to replication of DNA without cell division. Cytoplasmic vacuolation results from dilatation of various organelles and possibly lysis due to damaged lysosomal membranes.[97] In some instances, radiation may enhance cellular differentiation. Occasionally,

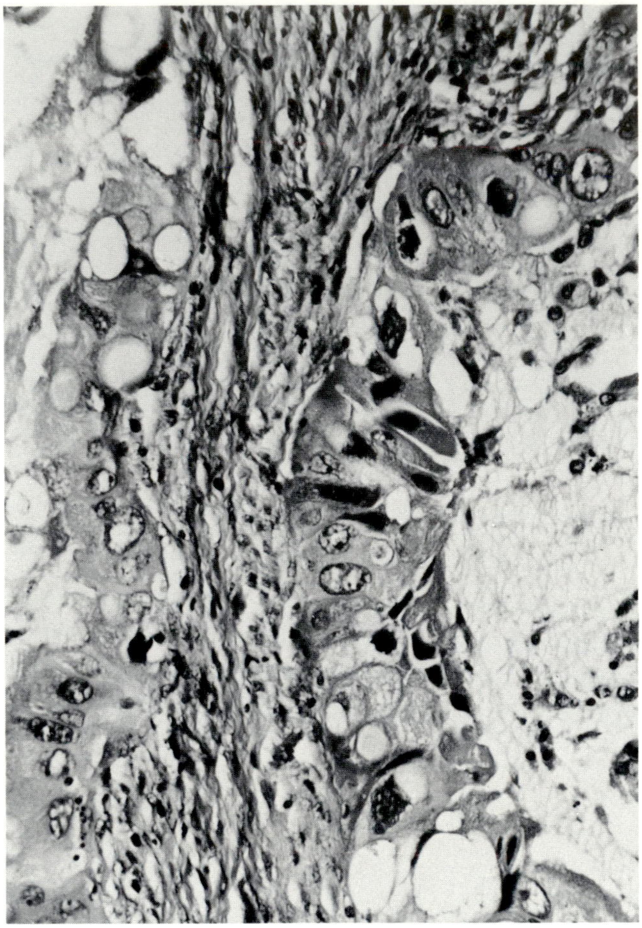

Fig. 12.39. Marked vacuolation, nuclear hyperchromasia, and pleomorphism evident within endometrial carcinoma cells after radiation treatment.

poorly differentiated carcinomas without squamous differentiation in the curettings may have nests of squamous epithelium in the resected uterus after radiation.

Radiation changes in the endometrial stroma and myometrium are greatest in the vicinity of the radiation source. The stromal cells are first converted to giant fibroblasts. The stroma undergoes progressive hyalinization, resulting in a collagenous scar. Elastic tissue is often fragmented and frayed, and blood vessels are thickened and sclerotic.[97] Occasionally, changes similar to those found in atherosclerosis may be present in the intima of blood vessels.[91] Foam cells occur in the intima, and myometrial cells may appear granular and swollen, especially in areas close to the radium source. Longstanding radiation effects are characterized by scarring, atrophy, and sclerosis of vessels. The endometrium is thin and easily traumatized, and small blood vessels in the stroma are thin-walled and ectatic. Some blood vessels form plaques of lipid-filled clear cells (lipid cells) in the media, diagnostic of late effects of radiation.

Progestins

Pharmacologic doses of progestins, such as medroxyprogesterone acetate or megestrol acetate, can produce an objective remission in approximately 30% of endometrial carcinomas.[94,140] Most poorly differentiated adenocarcinomas and some well-differentiated adenocarcinomas, however, fail to show the progestin-induced changes.[52] This lack of response generally reflects a paucity of progesterone receptors.[47,140,187] It appears that carcinomas are composed of a heterogeneous population of cells, some of which contain steroid receptors and are responsive to hormones and some that lack steroid receptors and are unresponsive. Regression also is related to the dose and the duration of progestin treatment; high initial doses must be given, and treatment must be continued for at least 3 months.

Progestin-induced changes include secretory differentiation of glandular cells, mitotic arrest, decrease in estrogen-related cellular changes, such as ciliogenesis, tissue necrosis, and conversion of spindle-shaped stromal cells to decidual cells[78,141,159] (Fig. 12.40). The earliest evi-

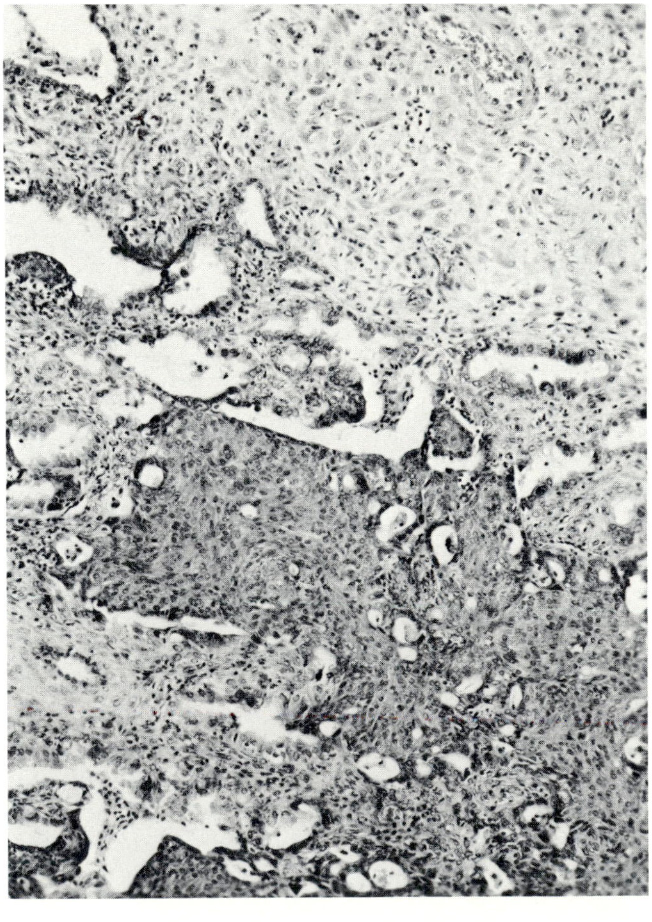

Fig. 12.40. Marked decidual reaction (*upper portion of field*) present in stroma of endometrial carcinoma after 1 month of high-dose progestin treatment.

dence of the progestin effect is subnuclear vacuolization, observed within 2–3 days of treatment. The vacuoles are a manifestation of glycoprotein synthesis, which is followed by an apocrine-type secretion in which the apical portion of the cytoplasm of the cell is discharged into the gland lumen, with reduction in the size of the cell. Concomitantly, there is a marked decrease in mitotic activity and RNA synthesis, as measured by scintillation radioautographs. Lysosomal autodigestion of cells is also stimulated by progestins.[141]

References

1. Aikawa M, Ab P (1973) Mixed (adenosquamous) carcinoma of the endometrium. Electron microscopic observations. Cancer 31: 385
2. Alberhasky RC, Connelly PJ, Christopherson WM (1982) Carcinoma of the endometrium. IV. Mixed adenosquamous carcinoma. A clinical–pathological study of 68 cases with long-term follow-up. Am J Clin Pathol 77: 655
3. Alders JG, Abeler V, Kolstad P (1984) Clinical (stage III) as compared to subclinical intrapelvic extrauterine tumor spread in endometrial carcinoma: A clinical and histopathological study of 175 patients. Gynecol Oncol 17: 64
4. Alders JG, Abeler V, Kolstad P (1982) Recurrent carcinoma of the endometrium: A clinical and pathological study of 379 patients. Gynecol Oncol 17: 85
5. Alders JG, Abeler V, Kolstad P (1982) Stage IV endometrial carcinoma: A clinical and pathological study of 83 patients. Gynecol Oncol 17: 75
6. Atkin NB (1976) Prognostic significance of ploidy level in human tumors. I. Carcinoma of the uterus. J Natl Cancer Inst 56: 909
7. Austin JH, MacMahon B (1969) Indicators of prognosis in carcinoma of the corpus uteri. Surg Gynecol Obstet 128: 1247
8. Aycock NR, Jollie WP, Dunn LJ (1979) An ultrastructural comparison of human endometrial adenocarcinoma with normal postmenopausal endometrium. Obstet Gynecol 53: 565
9. Bannatyne P, Russell P, Wills EJ (1983) Argyrophilia and endometrial carcinoma. Int J Gynecol Pathol 2: 235
10. Barsky SH, Rao CN, Grotendorst GR, Liotta LA (1982) Increased content of type V collagen in desmoplasia of human breast carcinoma. Am J Pathol 108: 276
11. Bean HA, Bryant AJS, Carmichael JA, et al. (1978) Carcinoma of the endometrium in Saskatchewan: 1966 to 1971. Gynecol Oncol 6: 503
12. Beck RP, Latour, JPA (1963) Necropsy reports on 36 cases of endometrial carcinoma. Am J Obstet Gynecol 85: 307
13. Beckner ME, Mori T, Silverberg SG (1985) Endometrial carcinoma: Nontumor factors in prognosis. Int J Gynecol Pathol 4: 131
14. Beller U, Beckman M, Twombly GH (1984) Spontaneous regression of advanced endometrial carcinoma. Gynecol Oncol 17: 381
15. Bigelow B, Vekshtein V, Demopoulis RI (1983) Endometrial carcinoma, stage II: Route and extent of spread to the cervix. Obstet Gynecol 62: 363
16. Blaustein A, Bigelow B, Demopoulis RI (1978) Association of carcinoma of the breast with adenosquamous carcinoma of the endometrium. Cancer 42: 326
17. Bokhman JV (1983) Two pathogenetic types of endometrial carcinoma. Gynecol Oncol 15: 10
18. Bolt HM, Gobel P (1976) Formation of estrogens from androgens by human subcutaneous adipose tissue in vitro. Horm Metab Res 4: 312
19. Boronow RC (1976) Endometrial cancer: Not a benign disease. Obstet Gynecol 47: 630
20. Boronow RC, Morrow CP, Creasman WT, DiSaia PJ, Silverberg SG, Miller A, Blessing JA (1984) Surgical staging in endometrial cancer: Clinical–pathologic findings of a prospective study. Obstet Gynecol 63: 825
21. Buehl IA, Vellios F, Carter JE, Huber CP (1964) Carcinoma in situ of the endometrium. Am J Clin Pathol 42: 594
22. Bunker M (1959) The terminal findings in endometrial carcinoma. Am J Obstet Gynecol 77: 530
23. Cavazos F, Lucas FV (1973) Ultrastructure of the endometrium. In: Norris HJ, Hertig AT, Abel MR (eds) The uterus. Baltimore, Williams & Wilkins Co., p 136
24. Chan L, O'Malley BW (1976) Mechanism of action of the sex steroid hormones. N Engl J Med 294: 1322
25. Charles D (1967) Endometrial adenoacanthoma. A clinicopathologic study of 55 cases. Cancer 18: 737
26. Chen J, Trost DC, Wilkinson EG (1985) Endometrial papillary adenocarcinomas: Two clinicopathologic types. Int J Gynecol Pathol 4: 279
27. Cheon HK (1969) Prognosis of endometrial carcinoma. Obstet Gynecol 34: 680
28. Christopherson WM, Alberhasky RC, Connelly PJ (1982) Carcinoma of the endometrium: I. A clinicopathologic study of clear-cell carcinoma and secretory carcinoma. Cancer 49: 1511
29. Christopherson WM, Alberhasky RC, Connelly PJ (1982) Glassy cell carcinoma of the endometrium. Hum Pathol 13: 421
30. Christopherson WM, Alberhasky RC, Connelly PJ (1982) Carcinoma of the endometrium. II. Papillary adenocarcinoma: A clinical pathological study of 46 cases. Am J Clin Pathol 77: 534
31. Christopherson WM, Connelly PJ, Alberhasky RC (1983) Carcinoma of the endometrium. V. An analysis of prognosticators in patients with favorable subtypes and stage I disease. Cancer 51: 1705
32. Cohen C, Shulman G, Budgeon LR (1982) Endocervical and endometrial adenocarcinoma. An immunoperoxidase and histochemical study. A J Surg Pathol 6: 151
33. Connelly PJ, Alberhasky RC, Christopherson WM (1982) Carcinoma of the endometrium. III. Analysis of 865 cases of adenocarcinoma and adenoacanthoma. Obstet Gynecol 59: 569
34. Conney AH (1967) Pharmacological implications of microsomal enzyme induction. Pharmacol Rev 19: 317
35. Cowles TA, Magrina JF, Masterson BJ, et al. (1985) Comparison of clinical and surgical staging in patients with endometrial carcinoma. Obstet Gynecol 66: 413

36. Creasman WT, McCarty KS Sr, Barton TK, McCarty KS Jr (1980) Clinical correlates of estrogen and progesterone-binding proteins in human endometrial adenocarcinoma. Obstet Gynecol 55: 363
37. Creasman WT, DiSaia PJ, Blessing J, et al. (1981) Prognostic significance of peritoneal cytology in patients with endometrial cancer and preliminary data concerning therapy with intraperitoneal radiopharmaceuticals. Am J Obstet Gynecol 141: 921
38. Creasman WT, Soper JT, McCarty KS Jr, McCarty KS Sr, Hinshaw W, Clarke-Pearson DL (1985) Influence of cytoplasmic steroid receptor content on prognosis of early stage endometrial carcinoma. Am J Obstet Gynecol 151: 922
39. Cullen TS (1900) Cancer of the uterus: Its pathology, symptomatology, diagnosis and treatment. New York, D. Appleton, p 374
40. Czernobilsky B, Katz Z, Lancet M, Galton E (1980) Endocervical-type epithelium in endometrial carcinoma. A report of 10 cases with emphasis on histochemical methods for differential diagnosis. Am J Surg Pathol 4: 481
41. Deligdisch L, Cohen CJ (1985) Histologic correlates and virulence implications of endometrial carcinoma associated with adenomatous hyperplasia. Cancer 56: 1452
42. DiSaia PJ, Creasman WT, Boronow MD, Blessing JA (1985) Risk factors and recurrent patterns in stage I endometrial cancer. Am J Obstet Gynecol 151: 1009
43. Doll R, Muir C, Waterhouse J (1970) Cancer incidence in five continents. International Union Against Cancer. Berlin, Springer-Verlag, Vol 2
44. Donaldson ES, van Nagell JR Jr, Pursell S, Gay EC, Mecker WR, Kashmiri R, Van de Voorde J (1980) Multiple biochemical markers in patients with gynecologic malignancies. Cancer 45: 948
45. Dunn LJ, Merchant JA, Bradbury JT, Stone DB (1968) Glucose tolerance and endometrial cancer: A controlled study. Arch Intern Med 121: 246
46. Dutra F (1959) Intraglandular morules of the endometrium. Am J Clin Pathol 31: 60
47. Ehrlich CE, Young PCM, Cleary RE (1981) Cytoplasmic progesterone receptors in normal, hyperplastic, and carcinomatous endometrium: Therapeutic implications. Am J Obstet Gynecol 141: 539
48. Eifel P, Hendrickson M, Ross J, et al. (1982) Simultaneous presentation of carcinoma involving the ovary and uterine corpus. Cancer 50: 163
49. Elton NW (1942) Morphologic variations in adenocarcinoma of the fundus of the uterus, with reference to secretory activity and clinical interpretations. Am J Clin Pathol 12: 32
50. Factor SM (1974) Papillary adenocarcinoma of the endometrium with psammoma bodies. Arch Pathol 98: 201
51. Fasske E, Morgenroth K, Theman H, Verhagen A (1965) Vegleichende elektronmikroskopishe untersuchungen von proliferationsphase glandular cystischer hyperplasie und adenocarcinom der schleimhaut des corpus uteri. Arch Gynaekol 200: 473
52. Ferenczy A (1980) Morphological effects of exogenous gestagens on abnormal human endometrium. In: Dallenbach-Hellweg G (ed) Functional morphologic changes in female sex organs induced by exogenous hormones. Berlin, Heidelberg, New York, Springer-Verlag, p 101
53. Fluhmann CF (1928) Squamous epithelium in the endometrium in benign and malignant conditions. Surg Gynecol Obstet 47: 309
54. Franks AL, Kendrick JS, Tyler CW Jr (1987) Postmenopausal smoking, estrogen replacement therapy and the risk of endometrial cancer. Am J Obstet Gynecol 156: 20
55. Frick HC, Munnell EW, Richart RM, Berger AP, Lawry MF (1973) Carcinoma of the endometrium. Am J Obstet Gynecol 115: 663
56. Fu YS, Parks PJ, Reagen JW, Wentz WB, Storaasli JP (1979) The ultrastructure and factors relating to survival of endometrial cancers. Am J Diag Gynecol Obstet 1: 55
57. Glicksman AS, Rawson RW (1956) Diabetes and altered carbohydrate metabolism in patients with cancer. Cancer 9: 1127
58. Gompel C (1971) Ultrastructure of endometrial carcinoma: Review of 14 cases. Cancer 28: 745
59. Gould VE, Sommers SC, Terzakis JA (1976) Squamous differentiation and basal lamina deposition in endometrial adenoacanthoma. Am J Pathol 84: 25
60. Gray LA, Christopherson WM, Hoover RN (1977) Estrogens and endometrial carcinoma. Obstet Gynecol 49: 385
61. Gray LA, Robertson RW, Christopherson WM (1971) Atypical endometrial changes associated with carcinoma. Gynecol Oncol 2: 93
62. Greenwald P, Caputo TA, Wolfgang PE (1977) Endometrial cancer after menopausal use of estrogens. Obstet Gynecol 50: 239
63. Gurpide E, Tseng L, Gusberg SB (1977) Estrogen metabolism in normal and neoplastic endometrium. Am J Obstet Gynecol 129: 809
64. Gusberg SB (1980) Current concepts in cancer. The changing nature of endometrial cancer. N Engl J Med 302: 729
65. Gusberg SB, Kaplan AL (1963) Precursors of corpus cancer. IV. Adenomatous hyperplasia as stage 0 carcinoma of the endometrium. Am J Obstet Gynecol 87: 662
66. Haenszel W, Kurihara M (1968) Studies of Japanese migrants. I. Mortality from cancer and other diseases among Japanese in the United States. J Natl Cancer Inst 40: 43
67. Hahnel R, Martin JD, Masters AM, Ratajczak T, Twaddle E (1979) Estrogen receptors and blood hormone levels in endometrial carcinoma. Gynecol Oncol 8: 209
68. Hall JB, Young RH, Nelson JH (1984) The prognostic significance of adenomyosis in endometrial carcinoma. Gynecol Oncol 17: 32
69. Hameed K, Morgan DA (1972) Papillary adenocarcinoma of endometrium with psammoma bodies: Histology and fine structure. Cancer 29: 1326
70. Hanson MB, van Nagell JR Jr, Powell DE, Donaldson ES, Gallion H, Merhige M, Pavlik EJ (1985) The prognostic significance of lymph–vascular space invasion in stage I endometrial cancer. Cancer 55: 1753
71. Hendrickson E (1975) The lymphatic dissemination in endometrial carcinoma. A study of 188 necropsies. Am J Obstet Gynecol 123: 570

72. Hendrickson MR, Kempson RL (1983) Ciliated carcinoma—A variant of endometrial adenocarcinoma: A report of 10 cases. Int J Gynecol Pathol 2: 1
73. Hendrickson M, Ross J, Eifel P, Martinez A, Kempson R (1982) Uterine papillary serous carcinoma. A highly malignant form of endometrial adenocarcinoma. Am J Surg Pathol 6: 93
74. Hernandez E, Woodruff JD (1980) Endometrial adenocarcinoma arising in adenomyosis. Am J Obstet Gynecol 138: 827
75. Hertig AT, Gore H (1960) Atlas of tumor pathology, Section IX—Fascicle 33. Tumors of the female sex organs. Part 2 with supplement. Tumors of the vulva, vagina, and uterus. Washington, D.C., Armed Forces Institute of Pathology, pp 177–258
76. Homesley HD, Boronow RC, Lewis JL Jr (1976) Treatment of adenocarcinoma of the endometrium at Memorial-James Ewing Hospital, 1949–1965. Obstet Gynecol 47: 100
77. Horowitz KB, McGuire WL (1978) Estrogen control of progesterone receptor in human breast cancer. Correlation with nuclear processing of estrogen receptor. J Biol Chem 253: 2223
78. Hustin J (1973) Hormonal therapy on endometrial cancer: Effects of large doses given by parenteral or intracavity routes. In: Brush MG, Taylor RW, Williams DC (eds) Symposium on endometrial cancer. London, Cassell Ltd, p 246
79. Hustin J (1978) Immunohistochemical demonstration of several tumour markers in neoplastic and preneoplastic states of the uterine mucosa. Gynecol Obstet Invest 9: 3
80. Iozzo RV (1984) Proteoglycans and neoplastic–mesenchymal cell interactions. Hum Pathol 15: 2
81. Iozzo RV, Bolender RP, Wight TN (1982) Proteoglycan changes in the intercellular matrix of human colon carcinoma: An integrated biochemical and stereologic analysis. Lab Invest 47: 124
82. Janne O, Kauppila A, Kontula K, Syrjala P, Vihko R (1979) Female sex steroid receptors in normal, hyperplastic and carcinomatous endometrium. The relationship to serum steroid hormones and gonadotropins and changes during medroxyprogesterone acetate administration. Int J Cancer 24: 545
83. Jenson EF (1984) Intracellular localization of estrogen receptors: Implications for interaction mechanisms. Lab Invest 51: 487
84. Jones HW III (1975) Treatment of adenocarcinoma of the endometrium. Obstet Gynecol Surv 30: 147
85. Julian CG, Daikoku NH, Gillespie A (1977) Adenoepidermoid and adenosquamous carcinoma of the uterus. A clinicopathologic study of 118 cases. Am J Obstet Gynecol 128: 106
86. Kadar RD, Kohorn EI, LiVolsi VA, Kapp DS (1982) Histologic variants of cervical involvement by endometrial carcinoma. Obstet Gynecol 59: 85
87. Kanbour AI, Stock RJ (1978) Squamous cell carcinoma in situ of the endometrium and fallopian tube as superficial extension of invasive cervical carcinoma. Cancer 42: 570
88. Karpas CM, Bridge MR (1963) Endometrial carcinoma with psammomatous bodies. Am J Obstet Gynecol 87: 935
89. Keller D, Kempson RL, Levine G, McLennan C (1974) Management of the patient with early endometrial carcinoma. Cancer 33: 1108
90. King A, Seraj IM, Wagner RJ (1984) Stromal invasion in endometrial carcinoma. Am J Obstet Gynecol 149: 10
91. Kirkpatrick JB (1967) Pathogenesis of foam cell lesions in irradiated arteries. Am J Pathol 50: 291
92. Kjellgren O (1977) Epidemiology and pathophysiology of corpus carcinoma. Acta Obstet Gynecol Scand [Suppl] 65: 77
93. Kjorstad KE, Orjaseter H (1977) Studies on carcinoembryonic antigen levels in patients with adenocarcinoma of the uterus. Cancer 40: 2953
94. Kohorn EI (1976) Gestagens and endometrial carcinoma. Gynecol Oncol 4: 398
95. Koller O (1964) Results of treatment of adenocarcinoma of the uterine body. Natl Cancer Inst Monogr 15: 99
96. Kottmeier HL (ed) (1979) Annual report on the results of treatment in gynecologic cancer. Stockholm, Sweden, International Federation of Gynecology and Obstetrics, Vol 17
97. Kraus FT (1973) Irradiation changes in the uterus. In: Norris HJ, Hertig AT, Abell MR (eds) The uterus. Baltimore, William & Wilkins Co., p 457
98. Kumar A, Schneider V (1983) Metastases to the uterus from extrapelvic primary tumors. Int J Gynecol Pathol 2: 134
99. Kumar NB, Hart WR (1982) Metastases to the uterine corpus from extragenital cancers. A clinicopathologic study of 63 cases. Cancer 50: 2163
100. Kurman RJ, Norris HJ (1982) Evaluation of criteria for distinguishing atypical endometrial hyperplasia from well-differentiated carcinoma. Cancer 49: 2547.
101. Kurman RJ, Norris HJ (1986) Precursors of endometrial cancer. In: Henson DE, Albores, Savedra JA (eds) Pathology of incipient neoplasia. Philadelphia, W.B. Saunders Co.
102. Kurman RJ, Scully RE (1976) Clear cell carcinoma of the endometrium. An analysis of 21 cases. Cancer 37: 872
103. Kurman RJ, Kaminski PF, Norris HJ (1985) The behavior of endometrial hyperplasia. A long-term study of "untreated" hyperplasia in 170 patients. Cancer 56: 403
104. Lauchlan SC (1968) Conceptual unity of the müllerian tumor group. Cancer 22: 601
105. Lauchlan SC (1981) Tubal (serous) carcinoma of the endometrium. Arch Pathol 105: 615
106. Lesko SM, Rosenberg L, Kaufman DW, et al. (1985) Cigarette smoking and the risk of endometrial cancer. N Engl J Med 313: 593
107. Lewis BV, Stallworthy JA, Cowdell R (1970) Adenocarcinoma of the body of the uterus. J Obstet Gynaecol Br Commonw 77: 343
108. Lindahl B, Alm P, Ferno M, Norgren A, Trope C (1984) Plasma steroid hormones, cytosol receptors, and thymidine incorporation rate in endometrial carcinoma. Am J Obstet Gynecol 149: 607

109. Liotta LA, Rao CN, Barsky SH (1983) Tumor invasion and the extracellular matrix. Lab Invest 49: 636
110. Liu CT (1972) A study of endometrial adenocarcinoma with emphasis on morphologically variant types. Am J Clin Pathol 57: 562
111. LiVolsi VA (1977) Adenocarcinoma of the endometrium with psammoma bodies. Obstet Gynecol 50: 725
112. Longscope C, Pratt JH, Schneider SH, Fineberg SE (1978) Aromatization of androgens by muscle and adipose tissue in vivo. J Clin Endocrinol Metabl 46: 146
113. Lucas WE, Yen SSC (1979) A study of endocrine and metabolic variables in postmenopausal women with endometrial carcinoma. Am J Obstet Gynecol 134: 180
114. Lutz MH, Underwood PB Jr, Kreutner A Jr, et al. (1978) Endometrial carcinoma: A method of classification of therapeutic and prognostic significance. Gynecol Oncol 6: 83
115. Lynch HT, Krush AH, Larsen AL (1967) Heredity and endometrial carcinoma. South Med J 60: 231
116. Mack TM, Pike MC, Henderson BE, Pfeffer RI, Gerkins VR, Arthur M, Brown SE (1976) Estrogens and endometrial cancer in a retirement community. N Engl J Med 294: 1262
117. Mahle A (1923) The morphological histology of adenocarcinoma of the body of the uterus in relation to longevity. Surg Gynecol Obstet 36: 385
118. Martin JD, Hahnel R, McCartney AJ, Woodings TL (1983) The effect of estrogen receptor status on survival in patients with endometrial cancer. Am J Obstet Gynecol 147: 322
119. Mazur MT (1981) Atypical polypoid adenomyomas of the endometrium. Am J Surg Pathol 5: 473
120. McCarty KS Jr, Barton TK, Fetter BF, Creasman WT, McCarty KS Sr (1979) Correlation of estrogen and progesterone receptors with histologic differentiation in endometrial adenocarcinoma. Am J Pathol 96: 171
121. McDonald TW, Annegers JF, O'Fallon WM, Dockerty MB, Malkasian GD, Kurland LT (1977) Exogenous estrogen and endometrial carcinoma: Case-control and incidence study. Am J Obstet Gynecol 127: 572
122. Melin JR, Wanner L, Schulz DM, Cassel EE (1979) Primary squamous cell carcinoma of the endometrium. Obstet Gynecol 53: 115
123. Michael H, Grawe L, Kraus FT (1984) Minimal deviation endocervical adenocarcinoma: Clinical and histologic features, immunohistochemical staining for carcinoembryonic antigen, and differentiation from confusing benign lesions. Int J Gynecol Pathol 3: 261
124. Moberger B, Forsslun AG, Moberger G (1984) The prognostic significance of DNA measurements in endometrial carcinoma Cytometry 5: 430
125. Morrow CP, DiSaia PJ, Townsend DE (1973) Current management of endometrial carcinoma. Obstet Gynecol 42: 399
126. Muechler EK, Flickinger GL, Mangan CE, Mikhail G (1975) Estradiol binding by human endometrial tissue. Gynecol Oncol 3: 244
127. Musubuchi K, Nemoto H (1972) Epidemiologic studies on uterine cancer at Cancer Institute Hospital, Tokyo, Japan. Cancer 30: 268
128. Nahhas WA, Lund CJ, Rudolph JH (1971) Carcinoma of the corpus uteri: A 10-year review of 225 patients. Obstet Gynecol 38: 564
129. Ng ABP (1968) Mixed carcinoma of the endometrium. Am J Obstet Gynecol 102: 506
130. Ng ABP, Reagan JW (1970) Incidence and prognosis of endometrial carcinoma by histologic grade and extent. Obstet Gynecol 35: 437
131. Ng ABP, Reagan JW, Storaasli JP, Wentz WB (1973) Mixed adenosquamous carcinoma of the endometrium. Am J Clin Pathol 59: 765
132. Nilsson O (1962) Electron microscopy of human endometrial carcinoma. Cancer Res 22: 491
133. Nimrod A, Ryan KJ (1975) Aromatization of androgens by human abdominal and breast fat tissue. J Clin Endocrinol Metab 40: 367
134. Novak ER, Nalley WB (1957) Uterine adenoacanthoma. Obstet Gynecol 9: 396
135. Peterson EP (1968) Endometrial carcinoma in young women. A clinical profile. Obstet Gynecol 31: 702
136. Piver MS, Lele S, Barlow J, et al. (1982) Paraaortic lymph node evaluation in stage I endometrial cancer. Obstet Gynecol 59: 97
137. Prem KA, Mensheha NM, McKelvey JL (1965) Operative treatment in adenocarcinoma of the endometrium in obese women. Am J Obstet Gynecol 92: 16
138. Press MF, Nousek-Goebel N, Greene, GL (1985) Immunoelectron microscopic localization of estrogen receptor with monoclonal estrophilin antibodies. J Histochem Cytochem 33: 915
139. Press MF, Nousek-Goebel N, King WJ, Herbst AL, Greene GL (1984) Immunohistochemical assessment of estrogen receptor distribution in the human endometrium throughout the menstrual cycle. Lab Invest 51: 495
140. Reifenstein EC Jr (1974) The treatment of advanced endometrial cancer with hydroxyprogesterone caproate. Gynecol Oncol 2: 377
141. Richart RM, Ferenczy A (1974) Endometrial morphologic response to hormonal environment. Gynecol Oncol 2: 180
142. Risberg B, Grotoft O, Westholm B (1983) Origin of carcinoma in secretory endometrium—A study using a whole organ sectioning technique. Gynecol Oncol 15: 32
143. Robboy SJ, Bradley R (1979) Changing trends and prognostic features in endometrial cancer associated with exogenous estrogen therapy. Obstet Gynecol 54: 269
144. Robboy SJ, Miller AW III, Kurman RJ (1982) The pathologic features and behavior of endometrial carcinoma associated with exogenous estrogen administration. Pathol Res Pract 174: 237
145. Roberts DWT (1961) Carcinoma of the body of the uterus at Chelsea Hospital for Women, 1943–1953. J Obstet Gynaecol Br Commonw 68: 132
146. Rodriguez J, Hart WR (1982) Endometrial cancers occurring 10 or more years after pelvic irradiation for carcinoma. Int J Gynecol Pathol 1: 135
147. Rorat E, Ferenczy A, Richart RM (1974) The ultrastructure of clear cell adenocarcinoma of endometrium. Cancer 33: 880
148. Ross J, Eifel PH, Cox RS, Kempson RL, Hendrickson MR (1983) Primary mucinous adenocarcinoma of the en-

dometrium. A clinicopathologic and histochemical study. Am J Surg Pathol 7: 715
149. Salazar OM, DePapp EW, Bonfiglio TA, Feldstein MK, Rubin P, Rudolph JH (1977) Adenosquamous carcinoma of the endometrium. An entity with an inherently poor prognosis? Cancer 40: 119
150. Salazar OM, Feldstein ML, DePapp EW, et al. (1977) Endometrial carcinoma: Analysis of failures with special emphasis on the use of initial preoperative external pelvic radiation. Int J Radiat Oncol Biol Phys 2: 1101
151. Salazar OM, Feldstein ML, DePapp EW, et al. (1978) The management of clinical stage I endometrial carcinoma. Cancer 41: 1016
152. Salm R (1962) Mucin production of normal and abnormal endometrium. Arch Pathol 73: 30
153. Sato N, Mori T, Orenstein JM, Silverberg SG (1984) Ultrastructure of papillary serous carcinoma of the endometrium. Int J Gynecol Pathol 2: 337
154. Schenker JG (1980) Adenocarcinoma of the endometrium in Israel, 1960–1968. Cancer 46: 2752
155. Schenker JG, Weinstein D, Okon E (1979) Estradiol and testosterone levels in the peripheral and ovarian circulations in patients with endometrial cancer. Cancer 44: 1809
156. Scully RE, Aguirre P, DeLellis RA (1984) Argyrophilia, serotonin, and peptide hormones in the female genital tract and its tumors. Int J Gynecol Pathol 3: 51
157. Scully RE, Richardson G, Barlow JF (1966) The development of malignancy in endometriosis. Clin Obstet Gynecol 9: 384
158. Seemayer TA, Schurch W, Lagace R, Tremblay G (1979) Myofibroblasts in the stroma of invasive and metastatic carcinoma. Am J Surg Pathol 3: 525
159. Sekiya S, Takeda B, Kikuchi Y, Sakaguchi S, Takamizawa H (1977) Morphologic and enzyme–cytochemical changes in uterine adenocarcinoma cells of a rat by direct application of progesterone in vitro. Gynecol Oncol 5: 5
160. Seppala M, Pihko H, Ruoslahti E (1975) Carcinoembryonic antigen and alpha-fetoprotein in malignant tumors of the female genital tract. Cancer 35: 1377
161. Silverberg E (1984) Cancer Statistics. 34: 7
162. Silverberg SG (1981) Significance of squamous elements in carcinoma of the endometrium: A review. Prog Surg Pathol 4: 115
163. Silverberg SG, De Giorgi LS (1973) Clear cell carcinoma of the endometrium: Clinical, pathologic, and ultrastructural findings. Cancer 31: 1127
164. Silverberg SG, Bolin MG, De Giorgi LS (1972) Adenoacanthoma and mixed adenosquamous carcinoma of the endometrium: A clinicopathologic study. Cancer 30: 1307
165. Silverberg SG, Sasano N, Yajima A (1982) Endometrial carcinoma in Miyagi Prefecture, Japan: Histopathologic analysis of a cancer-based series and comparison with cases in American women. Cancer 49: 1504
166. Silverberg SG, Mullen D, Faraci JA, Makowski EL, Miller A, Finch JL, Sutherland JV (1980) Endometrial carcinoma: Clinical–pathologic comparison of cases in postmenopausal women receiving and not receiving estrogens. Cancer 45: 3018
167. Smith DC, Prentice R, Thompson DJ, Hermann WL (1975) Association of exogenous estrogen and endometrial carcinoma. N Engl J Med 293: 1164
168. Smith M, McCartney AJ (1985) Occult, high-risk endometrial cancer. Gynecol Oncol 22: 154
169. Speers WC, Picaso LG, Silverberg SG (1983) Immunohistochemical localization of carcinoembryonic antigen in microglandular hyperplasia and adenocarcinoma of the endocervix. Am J Clin Pathol 79: 105
170. Steinhorn SC, Myers MH, Hankey BF, Pelham VF (1986) Factors associated with survival differences between black and white women with cancer of the uterine corpus. Am J Epidemiol 124: 85
171. Suit HD, Gallagher HS (1964) Intact tumor cells in irradiated tissue. Arch Pathol 78: 648
172. Tavassoli F, Kraus FT (1978) Endometrial lesions in uteri resected for atypical endometrial hyperplasia. Am J Clin Pathol 70: 770
173. Thrasher TV, Richart RM (1972) An ultrastructural comparison of endometrial adenocarcinoma and normal endometrium. Cancer 29: 1713
174. Tiltman AJ (1980) Mucinous carcinoma of the endometrium. Obstet Gynecol 55: 244
175. Tobon H, Watkins GJ (1985) Secretory adenocarcinoma of the endometrium. Int J Gynecol Pathol 4: 328
176. Tubiana M (1971) The kinetics of tumour cell proliferation and radiotherapy. Br J Radiol 44: 325
177. Ueda G, Yamasaki M, Inoue M, Kurachi K (1979) A clinicopathologic study of endometrial carcinomas with argyrophil cells. Gynecol Oncol 7: 223
178. Ueda G, Sato Y, Yamasaki M, et al. (1978) Argyrophil cell adenocarcinoma of the endometrium. Gynecol Oncol 6: 467
179. Ulbright TM, Roth LM (1985) Metastatic and independent cancers of the endometrium and ovary: A clinicopathologic study of 34 cases. Hum Pathol 16: 28
180. van Nagell JR Jr, Donaldson ES, Wood EG, Sharkey RM, Goldenberg DM (1977) The prognostic significance of carcinoembryonic antigen in the plasma and tumors of patients with endometrial adenocarcinoma. Am J Obstet Gynecol 128: 308
181. Wahlstrom T, Korhonen M, Lindgren J, Markku S (1979) Distinction between endocervical and endometrial adenocarcinoma with immunoperoxidase staining of carcinoembryonic antigen in routine histologic tissue sections. Lancet 2: 1159
182. Walker AM, Jick H (1979) Cancer of the corpus uteri: Increasing incidence in the United States. Am J Epidemiol 110: 47
183. Walker AM, Jick H (1980) Declining rates of endometrial cancer. Obstet Gynecol 56: 733
184. Warren S (1961) The pathology of ionizing radiation. Springfield, Ill., Charles C Thomas
185. Way S (1954) The aetiology of carcinoma of the body of the uterus. J Obstet Gynaecol Br Empire 61: 46
186. Weiner J, Bigelow B, Demopoulis RI (1980) The value of endocervical sampling in the staging of endometrial carcinoma. Diag Gynecol Obstet 2: 265
187. Wentz WB (1964) Effect of a progestational agent on endometrial hyperplasia and endometrial cancer. Obstet Gynecol 24: 370

188. Wessel W (1965) Endometrials adenocarcinome verschiedener differenzierungsgrade und ihr stroma in elektronenmikroskopishen bild. Z Krebsforsch 66: 421
189. Wynder EL, Escher GC, Mantel N (1966) An epidemiological investigation of cancer of the endometrium. Cancer 19: 489
190. Yazigi R, Piver MS, Blumenson L (1983) Malignant peritoneal cytology as a prognostic indicator in stage I endometrial cancer. Obstet Gynecol 62: 359
191. Yoonessi M, Anderson DG, Morley GW (1979) Endometrial carcinoma: Causes of death and sites of treatment failure. Cancer 43: 1944
192. Ziel HK, Finkle WD (1975) Increased risk of endometrial carcinoma among users of conjugated estrogens. N Engl J Med 293: 1167

13

Mesenchymal Tumors of the Uterus

Charles Zaloudek, M.D., and Henry J. Norris, M.D.

This chapter deals with neoplasms of the uterus in which there is mesenchymal differentiation. Purely mesenchymal tumors, such as those derived from smooth muscle and endometrial stroma, are considered, as are benign and malignant neoplasms in which there are mixtures of epithelium and connective tissue.

The capacity of neoplasms arising in the uterus to form heterologous mesenchymal elements is a reflection of the potentiality of the uterine primordium, which is formed from an anlage of coelomic lining cells and subjacent mesenchymal cells.[59,110] Within the mesodermal primordium that is to become the uterus, the distinction between müllerian duct epithelium and mesenchyme is lost.[16] The müllerian duct epithelial cells seem to form part of the mesenchyme accompanying the duct before the formation of the uterus (see Chapter 1, Embryology).[59] A distinction between the precursors of the endometrium and myometrium is not possible, and neoplasms that subsequently arise in the uterus may express the bipotentiality of their ancestry by forming a mixture of epithelial and mesodermal components, as in the biphasic adenofibroma, adenosarcoma, and mixed müllerian tumor.

Mesenchymal tumors of the uterus, other than leiomyomas, are uncommon.[139] Sarcomas, for example, constitute only 3% of uterine malignancies.[24] A simplified classification of uterine sarcomas is suitable for daily practice (Table 13.1), but a more complex one is needed to embrace all types (Table 13.2).[68,110,124]

Proper pathologic study of a mesenchymal tumor of the uterus is predicated upon careful gross examination and prompt, thorough fixation. If indicated, fresh tissue

TABLE 13.1. Classification and relative frequency of uterine sarcomas.[a]

Type	% of uterine sarcomas
Mixed müllerian tumor (homologous or heterologous)	30
Leiomyosarcoma	27
Endometrial stromal sarcoma (including low-grade forms)	26
Adenosarcoma	8
Unclassified sarcoma	6
Miscellaneous sarcomas	3

[a] The frequency estimate is based on sarcomas in the Armed Forces Institute of Pathology files.

should be appropriately fixed or frozen for immunocytochemistry and fixed in glutaraldehyde for electron microscopy. Large tumors should be sectioned to ensure adequate penetration of the fixative. After fixation, the tumor should be thoroughly examined, and one block of tissue should be taken for each centimeter of tumor diameter, except from grossly typical leiomyomas.[183] Even the latter may have to be examined extensively if the microscopic appearance is unusual. In addition to the histologic diagnosis three major goals of the pathologic examination are to determine the type of tumor margin (expansile or infiltrating), to evaluate the depth of myometrial invasion, and to determine whether the tumor involves the serosa or extends beyond the uterus. Tissue samples should be taken with these requirements in mind.

TABLE 13.2. Detailed classification of uterine sarcomas.

- Pure sarcomas
  - Pure homologous
    - Leiomyosarcoma
    - Low-grade endometrial stromal sarcoma
    - High-grade endometrial stromal sarcoma
    - Angiosarcoma
  - Pure heterologous
    - Rhabdomyosarcoma (including sarcoma botryoides)
    - Chondrosarcoma
    - Osteosarcoma
- Mixed sarcomas (homologous or heterologous)
- Mixed müllerian tumors
  - Müllerian adenosarcoma (homologous or heterologous)
  - Malignant mixed müllerian tumors (homologous or heterologous)
- Sarcoma unclassified
- Malignant lymphoma

Modified by permission of Hendrickson and Kempson, Ref. 68.

Smooth Muscle Tumors

Leiomyoma

Leiomyomas, which occur in 20–30% of women older than 30 years of age, are the most common uterine neoplasms. Usually found in middle-aged women, some leiomyomas apparently regress after menopause, as they are less frequent in older women. Leiomyomas are rare in women younger than 18 years; the youngest patient on record was 13 years old.[177] Leiomyomas are more common in black women than in white women. Evaluation of a glucose-6-phosphate dehydrogenase marker in leiomyomas of the uterus suggests that they are a proliferation of a single clone of smooth muscle cells. Some leiomyomas increase in size while women are taking estrogen, and leiomyomas decrease in size in women treated with luteinizing hormone-releasing hormone agonists.[94] The concentration of cytosol estrogen and progesterone receptors is similar in leiomyomas and the adjacent myometrium.[123,129,148,150,175] Immunocytochemical studies using monoclonal antibodies to estrogen receptors reveal that the receptors are in the nucleus,[127] however, and when total cellular (cytosol plus nuclear) receptor levels are measured, there appears to be more estrogen receptor in leiomyomas than in myometrium.[150] The ratio of estrogen to progesterone receptors is significantly higher in leiomyomas than in normal myometrium, suggesting that the relative concentrations of these receptors may influence the growth of leiomyomas.[150] Progestins,[20,56,99] progesterone,[73] clomiphene,[48] and pregnancy have been associated in a few instances with a rapid increase in size and hemorrhagic degeneration of leiomyomas.

Clinical Aspects. The clinical presentation depends on the size, location, and number of tumors. Leiomyomas characteristically cause a wide variety of signs and symptoms, the most common of which are pain, a sensation of pressure, and abnormal uterine bleeding. Even small leiomyomas, when submucosal, can cause bleeding, which is due to compression of the overlying endometrium and compromise of its vascular supply. In some instances, infertility is attributed to the presence of leiomyomas.[7]

Large tumors are detected during pelvic examination because they produce uterine enlargement or an irregular uterine contour. Some leiomyomas are pedunculated and protrude through the cervical os. Subserosal pedunculated leiomyomas may undergo torsion, infarction, and separation from the uterus. Secondary infection of myomas can be responsible for fever, leukocytosis, elevated sedimentation rates, and even septicemia. Among the complications of pregnancy ascribed to leiomyomas are abortion, disseminated intravascular coagulation, hemo-

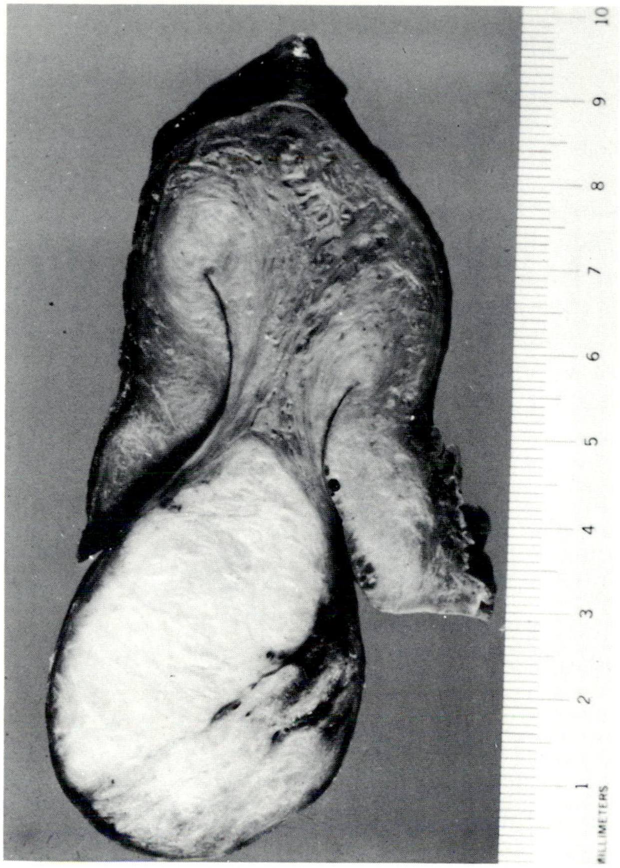

FIG. 13.1. Prolapsed submucosal leiomyoma. (Courtesy of Dr. David Taylor, Rotorua, New Zealand.)

peritoneum, premature rupture of membranes, dystocia, inversion of the uterus, and postpartum hemorrhage.[102] Unusual clinical syndromes associated with leiomyomas include ascites, ascites with hydrothorax,[174] and polycythemia secondary to erythropoietin production by the leiomyoma.[169]

Gross Pathology. Despite the variety in the histologic subtypes of leiomyomas, all are grossly similar. Multiple leiomyomas are present in two-thirds of the women with these neoplasms. Leiomyomas are spherical and firm, and they bulge above the surrounding myometrium. The cut surfaces are white to tan in color, with a whorled trabecular pattern. Leiomyomas can be located anywhere in the myometrium. *Submucosal* leiomyomas compress the overlying endometrium. As they enlarge, they may bulge into the endometrial cavity. Rare examples become pedunculated and prolapse through the cervix (Fig. 13.1). *Intramural* leiomyomas are the most common. *Subserosal* leiomyomas can become pedunculated, and, in the event of torsion with necrosis of the pedicle, the leiomyoma can lose its connection with the uterus and, in some instances, become attached to other pelvic structures (parasitic leiomyoma).

The appearance of a leiomyoma is often altered by degenerative changes. Submucosal leiomyomas frequently become hemorrhagic and ulcerated. Hemorrhage and necrosis occur in large leiomyomas, particularly in women who are pregnant or who are undergoing high-dose progestin therapy.[56] Dark red areas represent hemorrhage, and sharply demarcated yellow areas reflect necrosis. The damaged smooth muscle is eventually replaced by firm, white or translucent, collagenous tissue. Cystic degeneration also occurs (Fig. 13.2), but palpable calcified areas are infrequent.

Microscopic Pathology. Leiomyomas consist of whorled, anastomosing fascicles of uniform, fusiform, smooth mus-

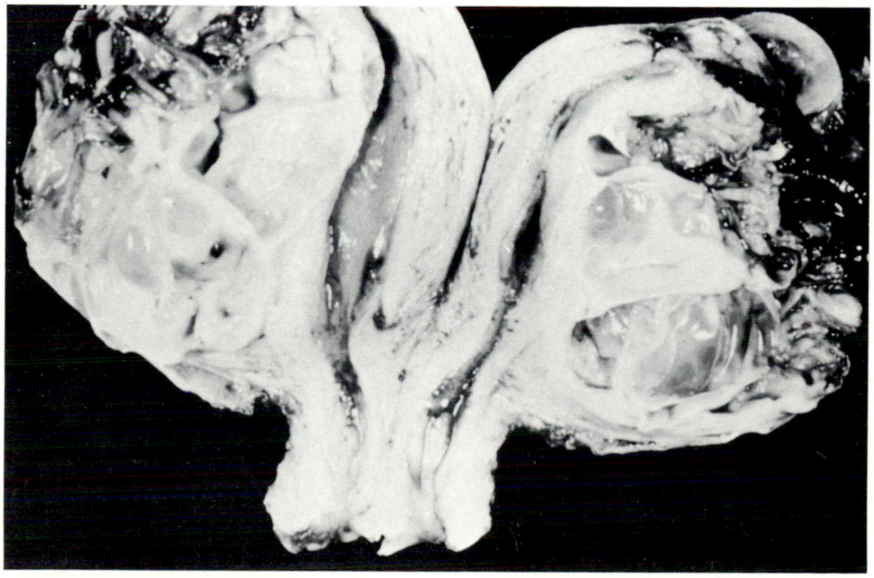

FIG. 13.2. Cystic subserosal leiomyoma.

cle cells. The spindle-shaped cells have indistinct borders and abundant fibrillar, eosinophilic cytoplasm. The nuclei are elongated, with blunt or tapered ends, and have finely dispersed chromatin and small nucleoli. Mitotic figures are rare. Most leiomyomas are more cellular than the surrounding myometrium. Those that are not can be identified by their nodular circumscription and by the disorderly arrangement of the smooth muscle fascicles within the tumor, out of phase with the surrounding myometrium.

Degenerative changes are commonly observed in leiomyomas.[119] Hyaline fibrosis is present in more than 60% of them and edema in about one-half. Significant areas of hemorrhage, which tend to be zonal and sharply demarcated, are observed in about 10% of leiomyomas, and cystic degeneration and microcalcification each occur in about 4%. Hemorrhage, edema, myxoid change, hypercellular foci, and muscle hypertrophy occur in leiomyomas in women who are pregnant or are taking progestins.[102,119] Progestational agents are associated with a slight increase in mitotic activity,[161] but not to the level observed in a leiomyosarcoma.[41,161]

Ultrastructure. Leiomyomas are characterized by the presence of a folded nucleus, an abundance of cytoplasmic myofilaments, dense bodies among the filaments and dense plaques on the cytoplasmic aspect of the cell membrane, prominent pinocytotic vesicles, a well-defined basal lamina, and a prominent extracellular collagenous matrix (Fig. 13.3).[46,51] The cells within leiomyomas differ from those of the normal myometrium by virtue of their increased nuclear size, more numerous mitochondria, and increased amounts of free ribosomes.[46]

Treatment and Prognosis. Many leiomyomas are asymptomatic, and not all require treatment. Only those that are symptomatic, enlarge rapidly, or pose diagnostic problems are removed. In some instances, leiomyomas can be excised (myomectomy), but if they are large or multiple, a hysterectomy may be required.

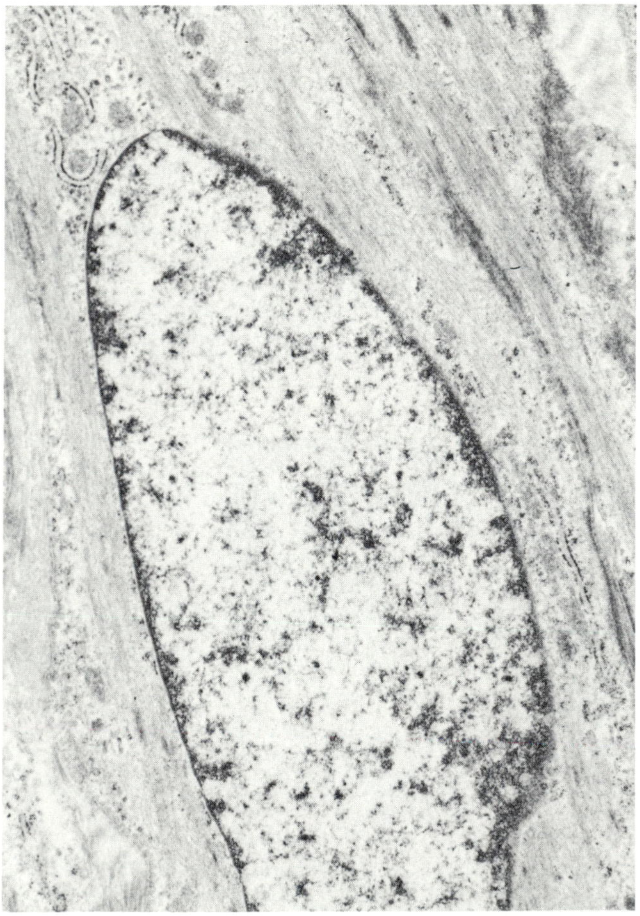

FIG. 13.3. Ultrastructure of smooth muscle cell from a typical leiomyoma showing myofibrils in cytoplasm and pinocytotic vesicles (*top*) on the plasma membrane. ×8000. (Courtesy of Dr. George Hilliard, San Antonio, Texas.)

Specific Subtypes of Leiomyoma

Several specific subtypes of leiomyoma must be distinguished from leiomyosarcoma. These are cellular leiomyomas, atypical leiomyomas (leiomyomas with atypical nuclei), and epithelioid leiomyomas.

Cellular Leiomyoma

These are composed of densely cellular fascicles of smooth muscle with little intervening collagen. Their extreme cellularity may suggest a leiomyosarcoma, but cellular leiomyomas have fewer mitotic figures (fewer than 5/10 HPF), and usually there is little or no cytologic atypia.* Cellular leiomyomas composed of small cells with scanty cytoplasm can be confused with endometrial stromal tumors. Features that help distinguish a cellular leiomyoma from a stromal tumor are the fusiform shape of the nuclei, the spindled shape of the cells, the reticulin pattern, and the lack of a prominent vascular bed in a cellular leiomyoma. Reticulin fibers tend to parallel the fascicles of cells in a leiomyoma, but the reticulin network surrounds individual tumor cells in an endometrial stromal tumor.

Palisades of nuclei reminiscent of those seen in the Verocay bodies of a neurilemoma are present in some cellular leiomyomas. Electron microscopic evaluation has shown that the cells in these, as in ordinary leiomyomas, contain myofilaments, pinocytotic vesicles, and other ultrastructural features of smooth muscle cells.[51]

* References 9, 21, 24, 80, 95, 135, 155, 170.

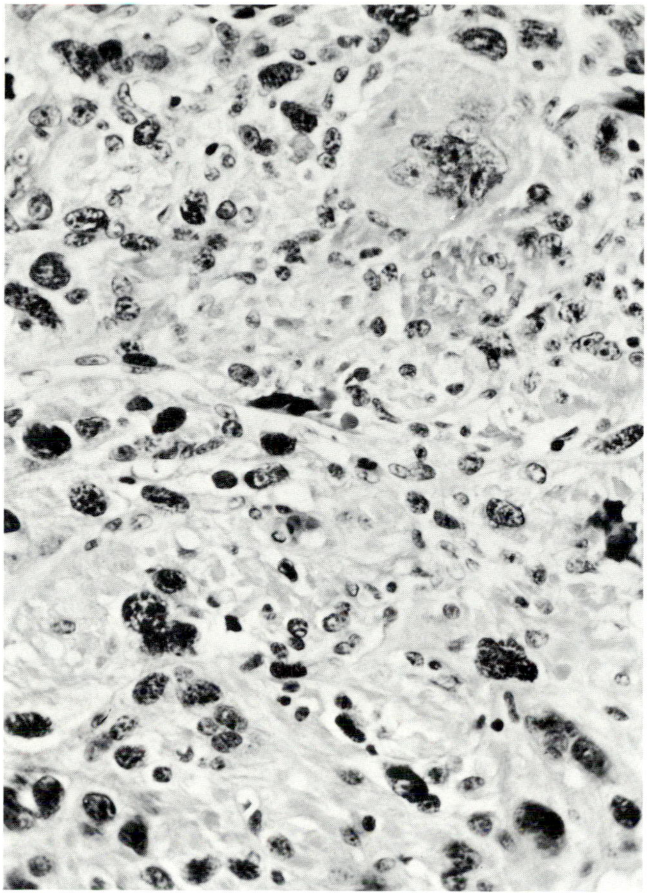

Fig. 13.4. Atypical or symplastic leiomyoma.

Atypical Leiomyoma

Leiomyomas that contain atypical cells are designated as atypical leiomyomas. The atypical cells may be distributed throughout the leiomyoma, or they may be clustered. They have enlarged hyperchromatic nuclei with prominent chromatin clumping and, often, smudging (Fig. 13.4). Large intranuclear inclusions of cytoplasm are often present. Multinucleated tumor giant cells can be numerous and prompt the names *bizzare* or *symplastic leiomyoma*.[68]

It may be difficult to distinguish an atypical leiomyoma from a leiomyosarcoma. The main distinguishing feature is that there are fewer than 5 mitotic figures/10 HPF in an atypical leiomyoma (Table 13.3).* Mitotic figures, when present, are most numerous in cellular areas adjacent to clusters of atypical cells. Sarcomas seldom arise in preexisting leiomyomas. Few convincing examples have been reported, since the diagnosis in most cases has been based only on the presence of focal cellular atypia within a circumscribed leiomyoma. Atypia, by itself, has not proven to be a reliable criterion for malignancy in smooth muscle tumors of the uterus, since it occurs in clinically benign leiomyomas, some of which have been excised from women taking progestins.[41,126] Moreover, leiomyosarcomas can be highly variable in their composition and may contain areas that appear benign. Many sections may be required to identify diagnostic areas in which there is high mitotic activity and atypia of the cells.

Epithelioid Leiomyoma

This category includes leiomyoblastoma,[91] clear cell leiomyoma,[132] and plexiform leiomyoma.[57,87] These neoplasms have the same histologic appearance in the uterus as in other sites in the body.

Clinically, the median age of patients with an epithelioid leiomyoma is 48 years. Race and parity do not deviate from the normal population. The major symptoms are abnormal bleeding, abdominal or pelvic pain, and abdominal enlargement.[87] The median duration of symptoms is 2 months.

Grossly, epithelioid leiomyomas do not differ from other leiomyomas. They are yellow or gray (Fig. 13.5) and may contain visible areas of hemorrhage and necrosis. They tend to be softer than the usual leiomyoma. Most are solitary, and they can occur in any part of the uterus. The median diameter is about 7 cm.

Microscopically, the cells are round or polygonal rather

---

* References 9, 21, 24, 65, 80, 95, 135, 155, 170.

Table 13.3. Histologic criteria for the diagnosis of uterine smooth muscle tumors.

Mitotic figures/ 10 HPF	Cytologic atypia	Diagnosis
0–4	−	Cellular leiomyoma
0–4	+	Atypical leiomyoma
5–9	−	Uncertain malignant potential
5–9	+	Leiomyosarcoma
10 or more	+ or −	Leiomyosarcoma

Reprinted by permission of Zaloudek and Norris, Ref. 183.

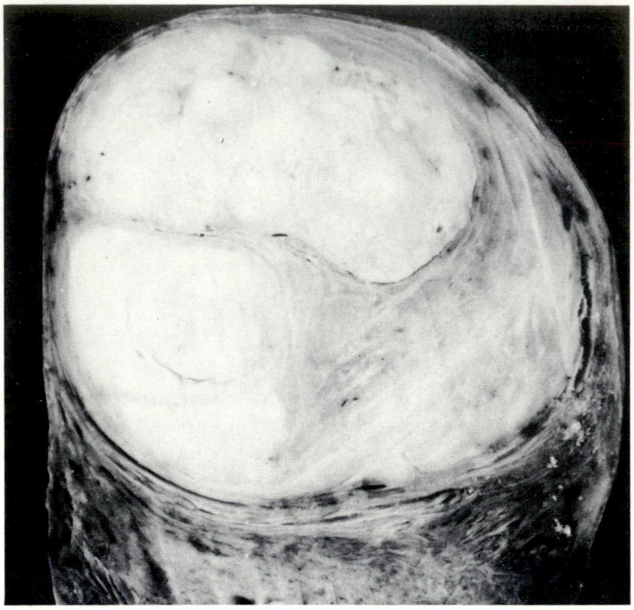

FIG. 13.5. Epithelioid leiomyoma. Cut surface of dense, circumscribed nodule.

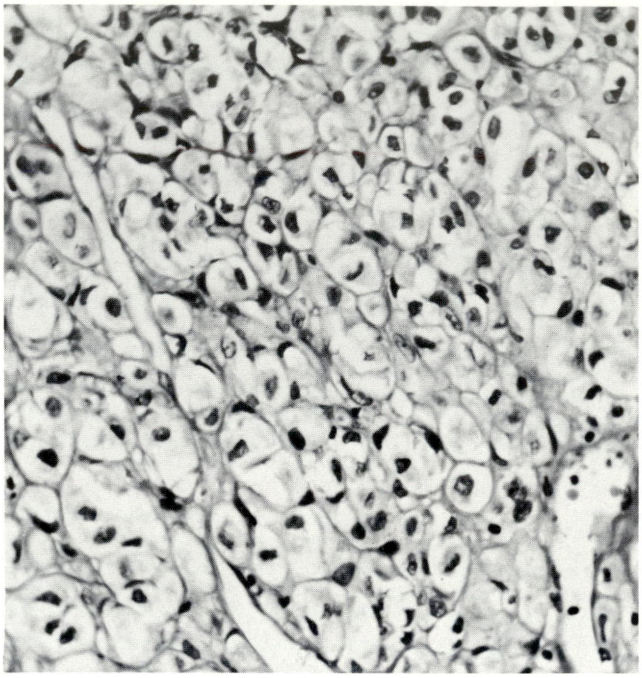

FIG. 13.7. Epithelioid leiomyoma, clear cell type. (Reprinted by permission from Kurman and Norris, Ref. 87.)

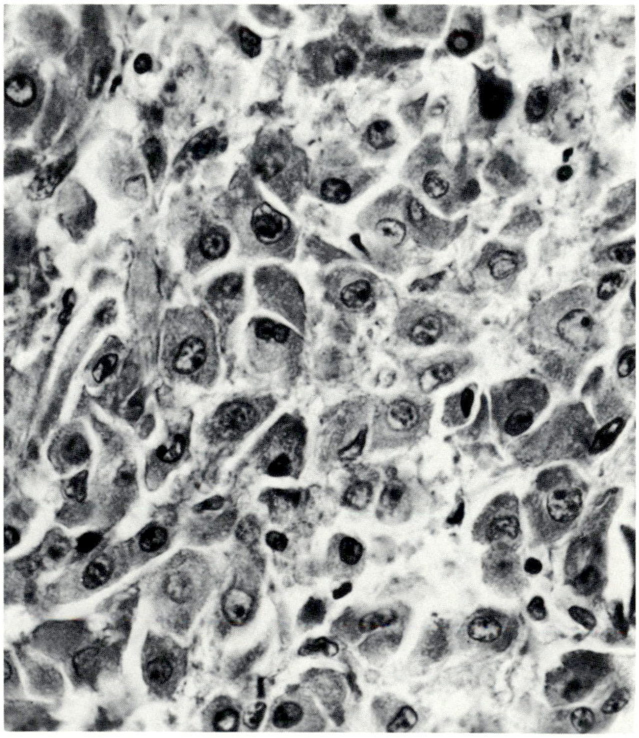

FIG. 13.6. Epithelioid leiomyoma, leiomyoblastoma type. Cellular tumor with little cohesion between cells. (Reprinted by permission of Kurman and Norris, Ref. 87.)

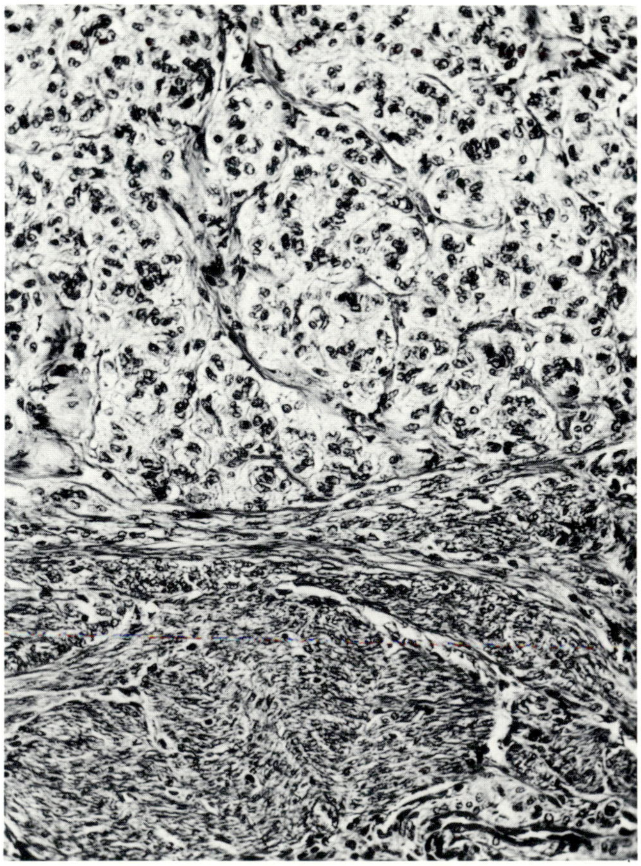

FIG. 13.8. Epithelioid leiomyoma, plexiform type, composed of cells in nested and cord-like configurations.

than spindle-shaped, and they are usually arranged in clusters or cords. The nuclei are round, relatively large, and centrally positioned. There are three basic types of epithelioid leiomyoma: leiomyoblastoma, clear cell leiomyoma, and plexiform leiomyoma. Neoplasms composed of round cells with eosinophilic cytoplasm (Fig. 13.6) are leiomyoblastomas. In clear cell leiomyomas (Fig. 13.7), the cells are polygonal and have abundant clear cytoplasm and well-defined cell membranes. The cells contain a large amount of glycogen, but lipid is minimal and mucin is absent. The nucleus may be displaced to the periphery of the cell, resulting in a signet-ring appearance. Plexiform leiomyomas (Fig. 13.8) are composed of cords or nests of round cells with scanty to moderate amounts of cytoplasm. Small plexiform leiomyomas that are detected only on microscopic examination are referred to as *plexiform tumorlets*.[75] These were formerly thought to be angiomas or endometrial stromal tumors, but ultrastructural examination has revealed the presence of myofilaments (Fig. 13.9) and other features of smooth muscle cells.[75,109] Plexiform tumorlets are usually solitary and submucosal, but they can occur anywhere in the myometrium and even in the endometrium, and multiple tumorlets have been described in a few patients.[75] All reported plexiform leiomyomas have been benign. Mixtures of the various patterns are common, providing the basis for designating the various types as *epithelioid leiomyoma*.

The behavior of epithelioid leiomyomas of the uterus, like that of similar tumors elsewhere in the body, is difficult to predict. Small tumors in which there is neither cytologic atypia nor significant mitotic activity can be safely regarded as benign.[87] Circumscribed margins, extensive hyalinization, and clear cells are histologic features associated with a benign course. Neoplasms with 5 or more mitotic figures/10 HPF metastasize with sufficient frequency that all should be regarded as epithelioid leiomyosarcomas. Epithelioid smooth muscle tumors displaying two or more of the following features have uncertain malignant potential: large size (greater than 6 cm), moderate mitotic activity (2–4 mitotic figures/10 HPF), moderate-to-severe cytologic atypia, and necrosis.[87] Most malignant and borderline epithelioid smooth muscle tumors are of the leiomyoblastoma type.

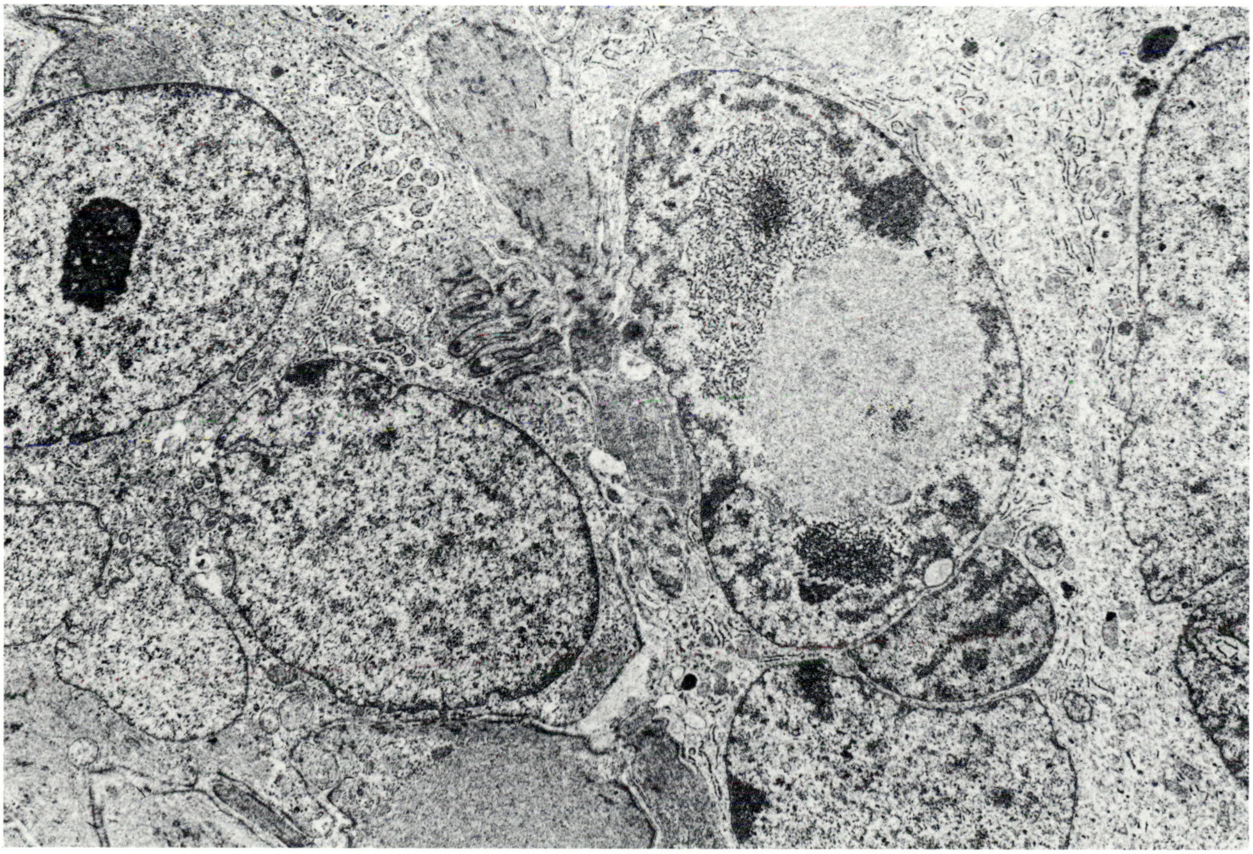

FIG. 13.9. Plexiform leiomyoma with inclusions of fibrillar cytoplasm within the nucleus. ×5790. (Courtesy of F.A. Tavassoli, Washington D.C.)

Other Types of Leiomyoma and Related Entities

Myxoid Leiomyoma

Myxoid leiomyomas are soft and translucent. Microscopically, there is abundant amorphous myxoid substance between the smooth muscle cells. The margins of a myxoid leiomyoma are circumscribed, and neither cytologic atypia nor mitotic figures are present. Large myxoid leiomyomas and those in which an infiltrating margin, cytologic atypia, or mitotic activity are observed microscopically should be regarded with suspicion. Some myxoid smooth muscle tumors exhibiting these features have proven to be leiomyosarcomas, even though they do not meet standard criteria for that diagnosis (see section on leiomyosarcoma).

Vascular Leiomyoma

A vascular leiomyoma contains dense proliferations of large caliber, thick-walled vessels. The distinction between a vascular leiomyoma and a hemangioma may be difficult. Hemangiomas are very rare in the uterus, and they tend to be of the cavernous type, composed of dilated capillary spaces.

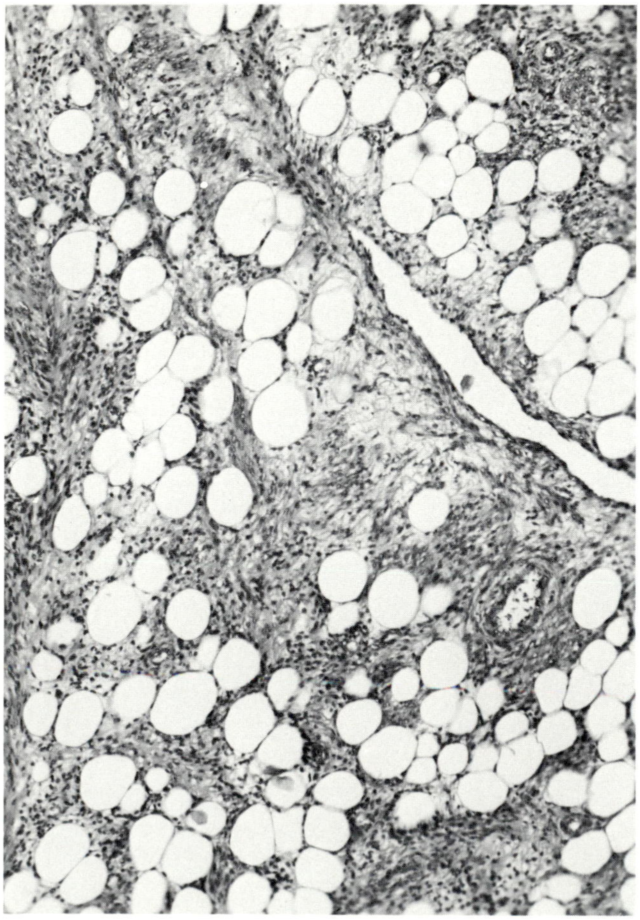

FIG. 13.10. Myolipoma with intermixture of fat cells, smooth muscle, and collagen.

Lipoleiomyoma

Leiomyomas containing significant amounts of fat are called *lipoleiomyomas* or *myolipomas* (Fig. 13.10).[70,71,171] Myolipomas occur in all locations, including the cervix. Some have been reported as being hamartomas. The fat generally occurs in circumscribed areas within a leiomyoma, but it may be present diffusely. Pure lipomas are extremely rare in the uterus.[33,125,171] Smooth muscle tumors containing heterologous elements, such as fat, should be given a descriptive name and should not be reported as a mixed mesodermal tumor.[32] That designation is reserved for tumors containing both epithelium and stroma.

Leiomyoma with Tubules

Very rarely, leiomyomas contain tubular structures.[98] The tubules share some features with epithelial cells in that desmosomes with tonofilaments and a basal lamina are present, a reflection of epithelial differentiation by mesenchymal tissue. At times, mesothelial differentiation also occurs, and in rare instances the light and electron microscopic features of a leiomyoma with tubules merge with those of an adenomatoid mesothelioma.

Diffuse Leiomyomatosis and Myometrial Hypertrophy

Diffuse leiomyomatosis is a peculiar, symmetrical, global enlargement of the uterus (Fig. 13.11), resulting from diffuse nodular myometrial hypertrophy.[90] Only a few cases have been described. With diffuse leiomyomatosis, the uterus is diffusely and symmetrically enlarged, weighing up to 1000 g. The myometrium may be 5–6 cm in thickness and crowded with nodules with ill-defined oulines.[90] Microscopically, there is little or no circumscription to the nodules, and the distinction between the adjoining myometrium and the nodules is obscure. Collagen and vessels do not appear to be increased. The microscopic picture is one of a diffuse nodularity of the myometrium rather than multiple leiomyomas.

In myometrial hypertrophy, the uterus is symmetrically enlarged and free of any discrete pathologic condition. It is abnormal only in size.[92] Weights up to 700 g occur. The cause of the enlargement has been ascribed to chronic myometritis, hyperplasia and/or hypertrophy of muscle fibers, chronic subinvolution, diffuse fibrosis, and fibrosclerosis, but none of these except hyperplasia and hypertrophy of existing muscle fibers explains the diffuse enlargement.[92]

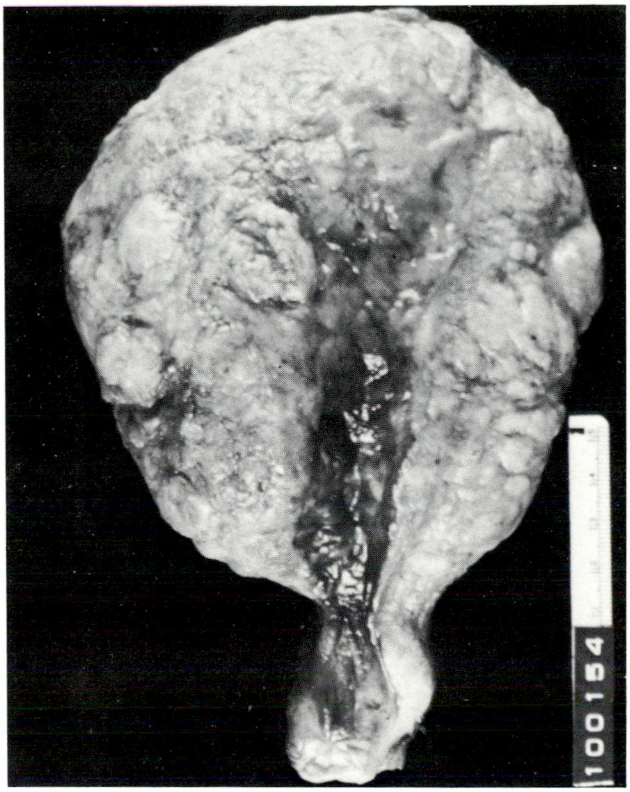

FIG. 13.11. Diffuse leiomyomatosis. The uterus was markedly enlarged, weighing 945 g, but discrete leiomyomas were not evident. [Reprinted with permission from The American College of Obstetricians and Gynecologists. (Obstetrics and Gynecology, [Suppl] 53: 825, 1979.)]

Uterine weight increases with increasing parity and with age, up to 49 years.[88] After menopause, the mean weight of the uterus declines. A very small normal uterus can occur in a postmenopausal woman; a 45 g uterus has been described in a 55-year-old mother of 13 children.[92] Nulliparous black women have larger uteri than do nulliparous white women of the same age.[88] The weight beyond which the uterus is abnormally large, indicative of myometrial hypertrophy, is 130 g for the nulliparous uterus, 210 g for parity 1–3, and 250 g for parity of 4 and above.[88]

Intravenous Leiomyomatosis

Intravenous leiomyomatosis is a very rare smooth muscle tumor characterized by grossly visible nodular masses of histologically benign smooth muscle cells growing within venous channels.

The median age of patients with intravenous leiomyomatosis is 45 years; few patients are younger than 40 years.[104] There is no racial predisposition or history of infertility or decreased parity. Abnormal bleeding and pelvic discomfort are the main symptoms, and most patients have a pelvic mass.

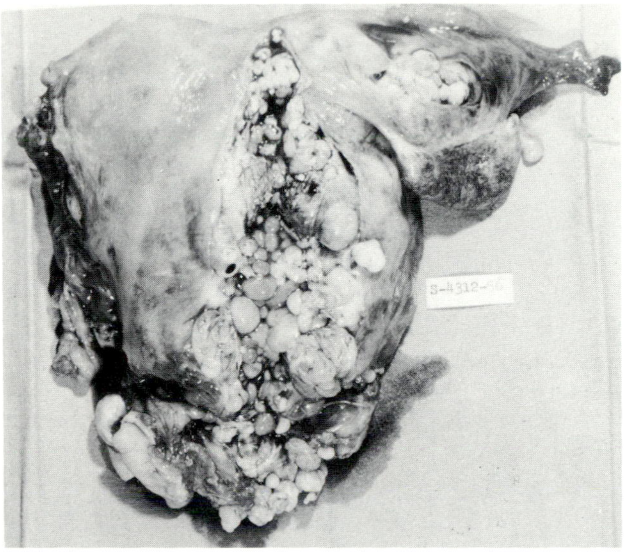

FIG. 13.12. Intravenous leiomyomatosis replacing most of the uterus and extending to both broad ligaments and the uterine and vaginal veins. (Reprinted by permission of Norris and Parmley, Ref. 104.)

Grossly, intravenous leiomyomatosis is a coiled or nodular growth in the myometrium with convoluted, worm-like extensions into the uterine veins within the broad ligament or into other pelvic veins (Fig. 13.12). Extension to the vena cava occurs in more than 10% of patients. The worm-like masses vary from soft and spongy to rubbery and firm, and their color is pinkish white or gray. The tumor is so uncommon that it is often not recognized on gross examination.

Microscopically, the tumor is present in multiple venous channels lined by endothelium. Growth does not occur in arteries. The histologic appearance is highly variable, even within the same tumor. Although the cellular composition of some intravenous leiomyomatosis is similar to a leiomyoma, most examples are fibrous or hyalinized to the degree that smooth muscle cells may be difficult to identify (Fig. 13.13). Clear cells and epithelioid transformation are present in some examples. Vascularity may be so prominent that the intravascular growth resembles an angiofibroma. Nuclear atypia and mitotic activity are usually absent.[104]

Vascular invasion within a leiomyoma does not warrant a diagnosis of intravenous leiomyomatosis if it is a microscopic finding and does not extend beyond the leiomyoma. Microscopic vascular invasion within a leiomyoma has not been shown to have any clinical significance. Grossly visible intravascular growth with extension beyond the leiomyoma in which it may have originated is required for a diagnosis of intravenous leiomyomatosis.

Norris and Parmley concluded, on the basis of their

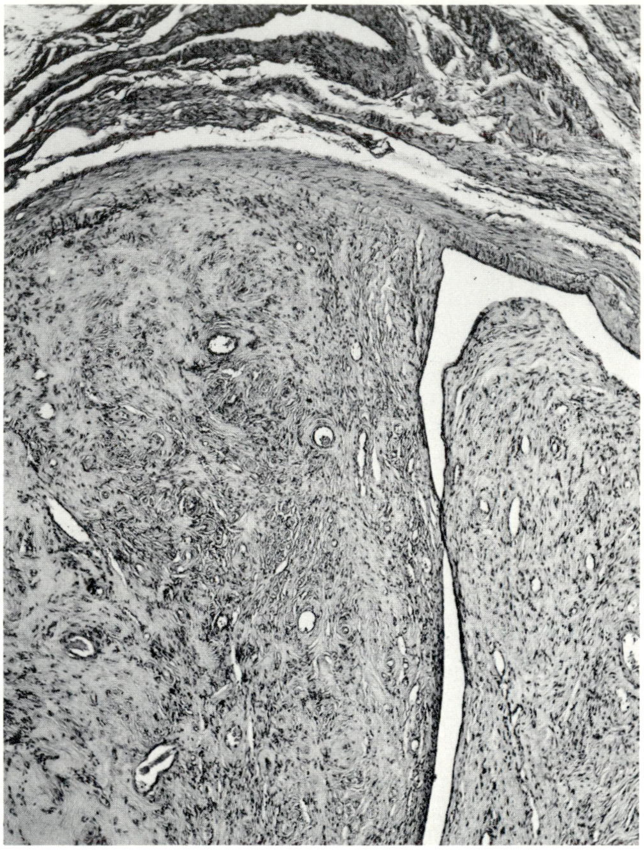

FIG. 13.13. Intravenous leiomyomatosis. Nearly all tumor was within the vascular spaces. (Reprinted by permission of Norris and Parmley, Ref. 104.)

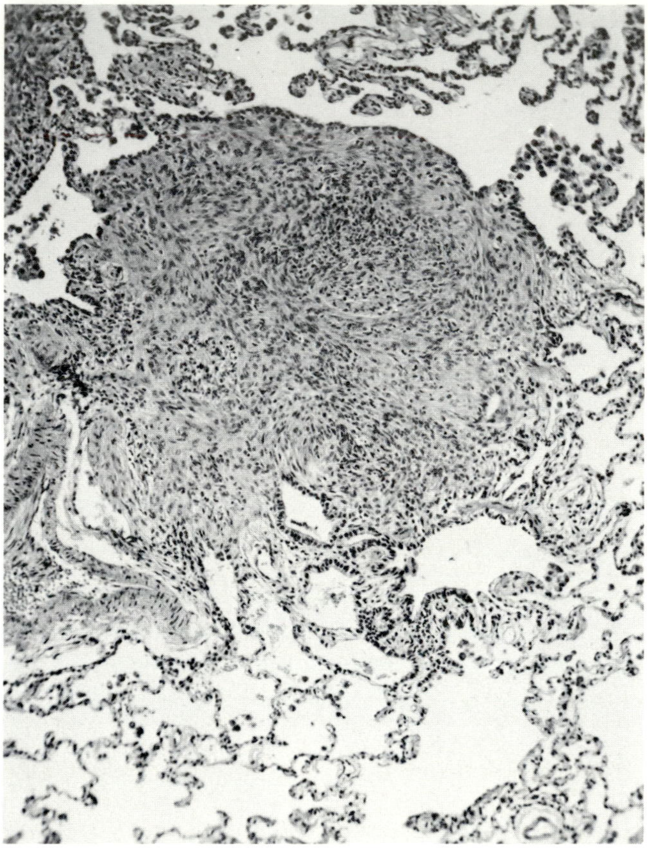

FIG. 13.14. Leiomyoma metastatic to lung was the initial diagnosis until the uterus, removed years earlier, was reexamined and showed intravenous leiomyomatosis.

study of 14 cases,[104] that some cases of intravenous leiomyomatosis originate in vascular smooth muscle, whereas other cases represent extensive vascular invasion by a leiomyoma.[63,158] When intravenous leiomyomatosis results from vascular invasion by a leiomyoma, the bulk of the tumor tends to be extravascular, and sites of origin from a vein wall are not found. In cases developing from venous smooth muscle, the tumor is predominantly or entirely intravascular, and there are many sites of attachment to the vein walls.

Total abdominal hysterectomy and bilateral salpingo-oophorectomy together with excision of any extrauterine extension is indicated. The prognosis of intravenous leiomyomatosis is favorable, even in patients in whom the tumor is incompletely excised. Pelvic recurrences are infrequent and usually amenable to surgical excision. Residual pelvic tumor may remain stable for 5 years or longer, but progression has been described, particularly in women who did not undergo bilateral salpingo-oophorectomy.[38] Excision of lung metastases (Fig. 13.14) and removal of plugs of tumor from the vena cava and right atrium have resulted in long-term survivals.[104,159,162]

Benign Metastasizing Leiomyoma

Only about a dozen cases of benign metastasizing leiomyoma have been reported, and most do not stand up under critical scrutiny. Most reports of benign metastasizing leiomyoma have failed to establish that the primary neoplasms were adequately studied. In some cases, the primary tumors were not examined histologically by the reporting author, and in others, the mitotic counts were not recorded for either the primary tumor or the alleged metastasis. It is possible that smooth muscle cells within cellular leiomyomas or intravenous leiomyomatosis gain access to vascular channels at the time of surgery and are transported to the lungs, where they may become implanted and grow as multiple intrapulmonary nodules of smooth muscle (Fig. 13.14). Other reported implantation sites are in the broad ligament or near the iliac veins. Virtually all patients have been operated on before developing metastases, and some women were treated

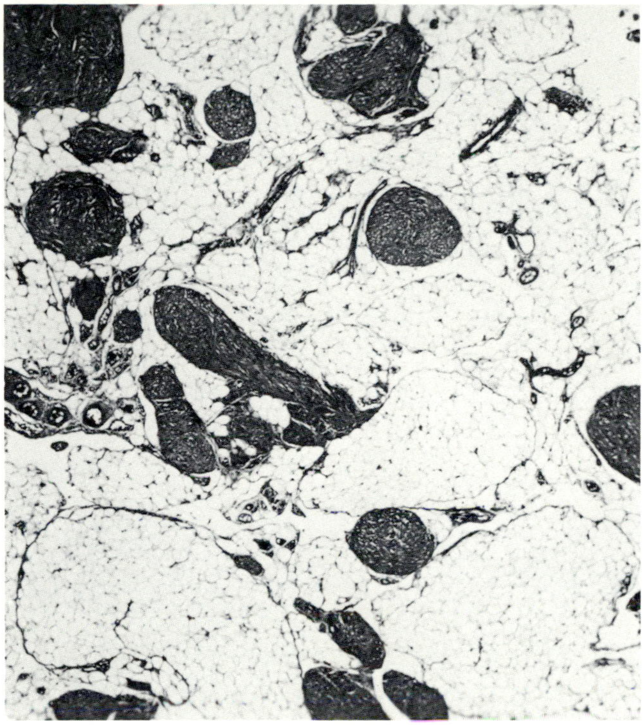

FIG. 13.15. Disseminated peritoneal leiomyomatosis in omentum.

initially by myomectomy or supracervical hysterectomy or had repeated curettage, raising the possibility that tumor spread was enhanced by incomplete surgery.[3] Most cases of benign metastasizing leiomyoma are instances of metastasis from a previously unrecognized low-grade leiomyosarcoma, usually of the uterus. Progression of the metastases frequently takes place over many years.[178]

Disseminated Peritoneal Leiomyomatosis

Disseminated peritoneal leiomyomatosis is a rare condition characterized by the presence of multiple myofibroblastic nodules on the peritoneal surface of the pelvic and abdominal cavities in women of reproductive age.* This condition is discussed in connection with leiomyomas of the uterus because it must be distinguished from metastatic leiomyosarcoma.

Most cases are associated with pregnancy, an estrinizing granulosa tumor, or oral contraceptive use.[54,78,153] Disseminated peritoneal leiomyomatosis is usually discovered as an incidental finding at the time of cesarean section. At surgery, disseminated peritoneal leiomyomatosis appears as multiple, small, granular nodules on the peritoneal surfaces of the uterus and adnexal structures and on the surfaces of the intestines and omentum (Fig. 13.15). Randomly distributed on the peritoneum, few of the nodules exceed 1 cm in diameter. This contrasts with benign metastasizing leiomyoma and metastatic leiomyosarcoma, in which the nodules are fewer in number but larger in size.

Microscopically, the nodules are composed of collagen, decidual cells, fibroblasts or myofibroblasts, and smooth muscle cells (Fig. 13.16). The spindle cell component usually dominates in the proliferation, raising the possibility that disseminated peritoneal leiomyomatosis may be confused with a metastatic sarcoma. The clinical setting is different, however, and mitotic figures are generally infrequent, and nuclear atypia and pleomorphism are minimal or absent. Electron microscopic observations have confirmed that most nodules are composed of smooth muscle and decidual cells, but some are mixtures of decidua and fibroblasts or myofibroblasts.[69,121,153,176] In one instance, endometrial glands were present along with decidual cells and smooth muscle,[78] reflecting the metaplastic potential of the peritoneal mesothelium and the myofibroblasts of adjacent stroma to undergo differentiation or metaplasia to endometrial stromal cells and

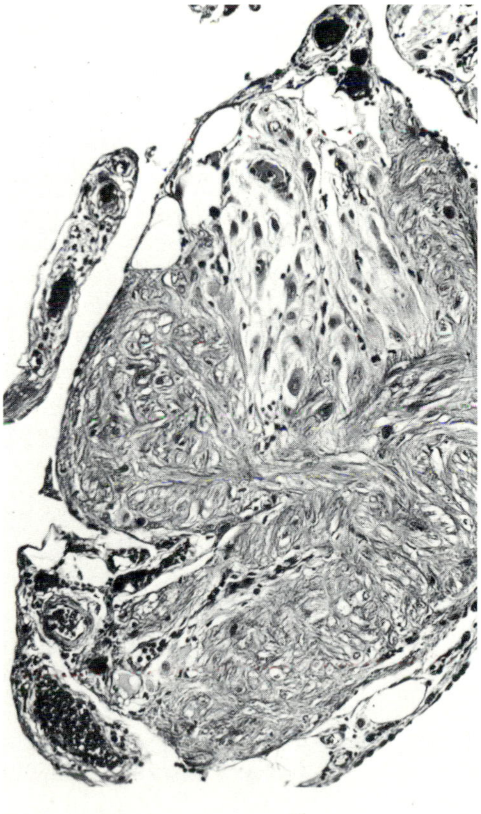

FIG. 13.16. Disseminated peritoneal leiomyomatosis. Decidual cells (*top*) are interspersed with collagen and smooth muscle (*bottom*). (Reprinted by permission of Norris and Parmley, Ref. 104.)

*References 6, 69, 103, 121, 153, 172.

TABLE 13.4. Comparison of the gross pathology of leiomyoma and leiomyosarcoma.

Leiomyoma	Leiomyosarcoma
Usually multiple	Often solitary (½–⅔)
Variable size, usually 3–5 cm	Large, often more than 10 cm
Firm, whorled cut surface	Soft, fleshy cut surface
White	Yellow or tan
Hemorrhage and necrosis infrequent	Hemorrhage and necrosis frequent

glands, decidua, smooth muscle, fibroblasts, and collagen. Disseminated peritoneal leiomyomatosis regresses after delivery, so radical attempts at excision are unnecessary.[153]

Leiomyosarcoma

Leiomyosarcoma represents about 1.3% of uterine malignancies and about one-quarter of uterine sarcomas. Approximately 1 of every 800 smooth muscle tumors of the uterus is a leiomyosarcoma. If the level of mitotic activity is the primary criterion for diagnosis, the incidence rate is about 0.67 per 100,000 women 20 years of age or older.[24]

Clinical Aspects. The mean age of patients with leiomyosarcoma is approximately 52 years, nearly a decade older than the mean age of patients with leiomyomas.* Leiomyosarcoma is perhaps slightly more frequent in black than in white patients, but there is no consistent racial predisposition. The incidence is not related to gravidity or parity. Clinically, a rapid increase in the size of a uterine tumor after menopause arouses the suspicion of sarcoma.[49] The signs and symptoms that occur in women with leiomyomas are also produced by leiomyosarcomas. Vaginal bleeding, lower abdominal pain, and a pelvic or abdominal mass are the usual symptoms and signs. Unlike other uterine sarcomas, there is seldom a history of prior radiation.

Gross Pathology. Most leiomyosarcomas are intramural. A higher proportion involve the cervix than is the case with leiomyomas.[155] Half to two thirds are solitary masses within the uterus.[21,24,155] They have an average size of 9 cm and are soft or fleshy and gray-yellow or pink, with poorly defined margins. Areas of necrosis and hemorrhage occur in three-quarters of them. Leiomyosarcomas tend to be larger and softer than leiomyomas, and they have a more irregular margin, more hemorrhage, and more necrosis (Table 13.4).[21,24,155]

Microscopic Pathology. Leiomyosarcomas are composed of fascicles of spindle cells with abundant eosinophilic cytoplasm (Fig. 13.17). Longitudinal cytoplasmic fibrils, best appreciated with a trichrome stain, are frequently present. The nuclei are fusiform, usually with rounded ends, and tend to be hyperchromatic, with coarse chromatin and prominent nucleoli. Cellular pleomorphism is marked in poorly differentiated neoplasms. Multinucleated tumor cells are common, occurring in half of leiomyosarcomas, and giant cells resembling osteoclasts have been described in a few neoplasms.[31] Vascular invasion occurs in 10–22% of leiomyosarcomas. Leiomyosarcomas infiltrate the myometrium, but infiltration may be difficult to identify, and it also occurs in some leiomyomas, albeit usually not to the degree seen in leiomyosarcoma.[142] Metastasis can occur from a sarcoma with a circumscribed margin.

Mitotic activity is the main criterion for the diagnosis of leiomyosarcoma (Tables 13.3 and 13.5).* In addition the degree of cellular atypia, the presence of abnormal mitotic figures, the extent of necrosis and the presence

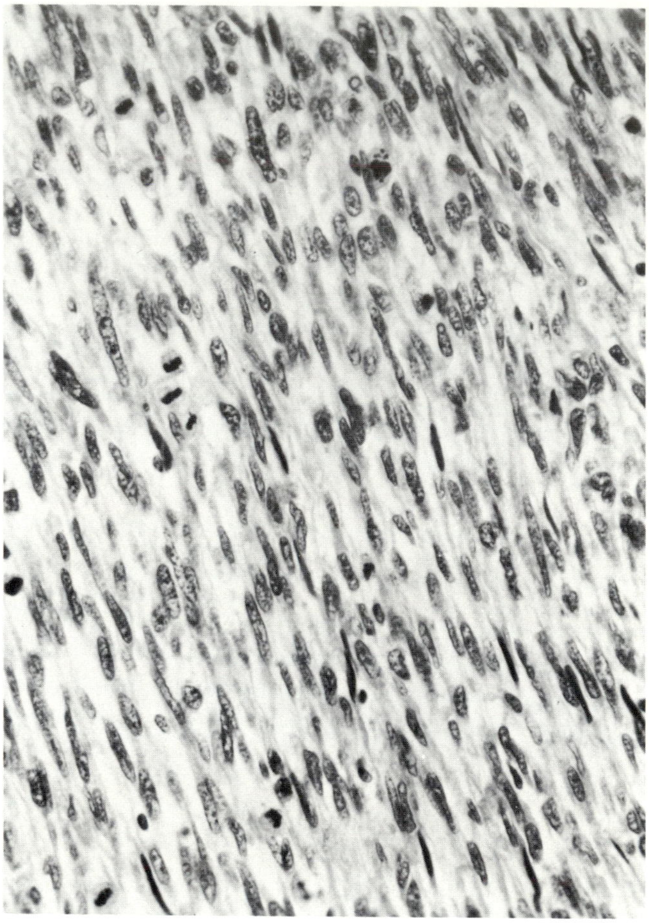

FIG. 13.17. Leiomyosarcoma. Cells are small and uniform. Only increased mitotic activity indicates the metastatic potential of this tumor.

* References 9, 24, 65, 95, 135, 155, 170.

* References 1, 9, 21, 24, 65, 80, 95, 135, 155, 170.

of myometrial or vascular invasion must also be considered. Cellular neoplasms with 10 or more mitotic figures/10 HPF are designated as leiomyosarcomas regardless of the degree of atypia that is present. High mitotic activity is usually associated with marked atypia. Moderate to marked cytologic atypia and a mitotic rate in excess of 10 mitotic figures/10 HPF are found in 75% of leiomyosarcomas. Neoplasms with 5–9 mitotic figures/10 HPF and moderate-to-marked cellular atypia are regarded as leiomyosarcomas, but the behavior of cellular smooth muscle tumors with this degree of mitotic activity and minimal atypia is uncertain. The latter are designated as *smooth muscle tumors of uncertain malignant potential.* Normocellular and hypocellular smooth muscle tumors with 5–9 mitotic figures/10 HPF are very rare. These have not been demonstrated to have metastatic potential and are designated as *leiomyomas with increased mitotic figures* by some. Fortunately, few smooth muscle tumors have mitotic activity in this range.

Rare smooth muscle tumors in which there are fewer than 5 mitotic figures/10 HPF prove to be leiomyosarcomas, and features other than mitotic counts must be employed when evaluating these. Myxoid smooth muscle tumors are in this category.[22,82] Myxoid leiomyosarcomas are large, gelatinous neoplasms that usually appear circumscribed on gross examination. Microscopically, the smooth muscle cells are widely separated by myxoid ground substance (Fig. 13.18). The low cellularity partly accounts for the presence of only a few mitotic figures/10 HPF in most myxoid leiomyosarcomas. Other microscopic features may be helpful in identifying a myxoid leiomyosarcoma since most of them exhibit microscopic infiltration of the surrounding myometrium, and some invade blood vessels. Despite the low mitotic counts, myxoid leiomyosarcomas have the same unfavorable prognosis as have other types of leiomyosarcoma.[82] Even if features diagnostic of leiomyosarcoma are not observed, myxoid smooth muscle tumors should be regarded with suspicion, and all but small, histologically bland, entirely circumscribed examples should be considered smooth muscle tumors of uncertain malignant potential.

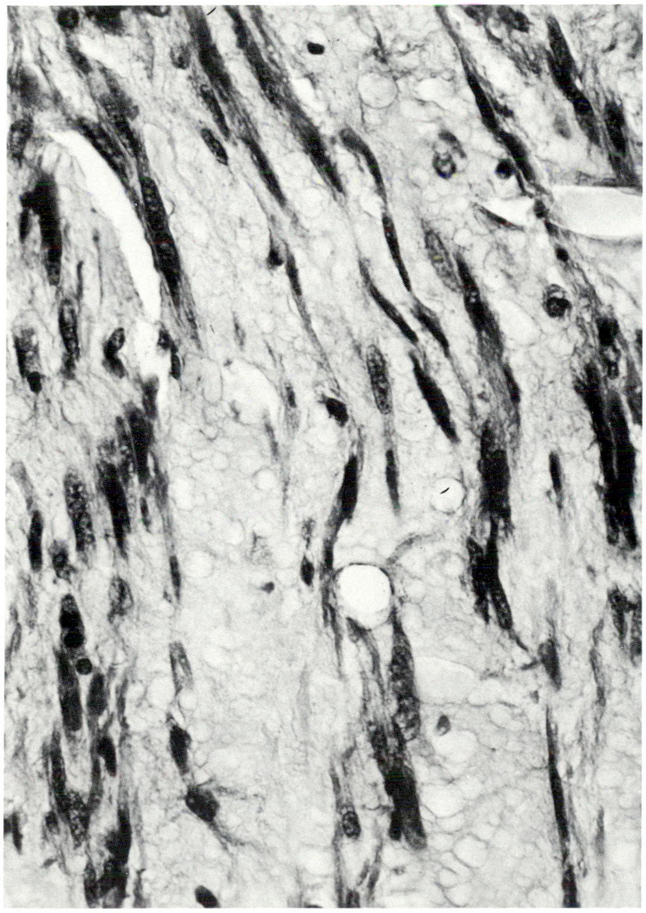

FIG. 13.18. Myxoid ground substance within a smooth muscle tumor. Some myxoid smooth muscle tumors with this degree of atypia and few mitotic figures metastasize.

As previously discussed, epithelioid smooth muscle tumors have unpredictable clinical behavior, and some epithelioid leiomyosarcomas have fewer than 5 mitotic figures/10 HPF. In particular, if there is necrosis, loss of cell cohesion, moderate atypia, and a size larger than 6 cm, the neoplasm is probably malignant.[87]

Finally, an occasional conventional smooth muscle tumor with a low mitotic count proves to be a leiomyosarcoma. Unless the tumor is invasive or contains abnormal mitotic figures or areas of necrosis, there are no grounds for suspecting that it is a leiomyosarcoma until it manifests its true nature by metastasizing. Doubtless, the pulmonary metastases from some benign metastasizing leiomyomas originate from neoplasms in this category.

Ultrastructure. Undifferentiated and myoblastic tumor cells and intermediate forms are present in leiomyosarcomas.[19,46] The myoblastic cells have cytoplasmic features that are incompletely developed and often disorganized. Bundles of thin myofilaments are usually limited to areas along the plasma membranes or parallel to the nuclei. The bundles contain dense bodies and occasionally terminate in marginal plaques. Pinocytotic vesicles are present at the plasma membrane. Intercellular junctions are of the nexus or zonula adherens type; desmosomes are not present. Leiomyosarcomas differ from leiomyomas in that they have greater nuclear pleomorphism, fewer and more disordered myofilaments, free ribosomes, and abundant mitochondria. Leiomyosarcomas also tend to have a less abundant extracellular collagenous stromal matrix. The fine structure of leiomyomas is more like that of normal myometrium.

Treatment and Prognosis. The variation in reported survival rates for leiomyosarcoma is largely a result of the

TABLE 13.5. Relationship between mitotic activity and death from uterine smooth muscle tumors.

Reference	<5 Mitotic figures/ 10 HPF	DOD/AWR[a,b]	≥5 Mitotic figures/ 10 HPF	DOD/AWR
Taylor and Norris[155]	24	0	39	31
Kempson and Bari[80]	10	0	19	14
Silverberg[142]	12	1	22	12
Christopherson et al.[24]	48	0	32	30
Saksela et al.[135]	22	0	28	17
Hart and Billman[65]	13	0	15	15
Burns et al.[21]	64	5	18	11
van Dinh and Woodruff[165]	9	1	21	8
Marchese et al.[95]	6	0	10	7
Barter et al.[9]	9	1	21	19
Wheelock et al.[170]	10	0	19	17
TOTALS	227	8(4%)	244	181(74%)

[a] Some patients were lost to follow-up in most series.
[b] AWR, patient alive with recurrent tumor; DOD, patient dead of tumor.

different criteria used for diagnosis. Survival rates in series selected by the diagnostic criteria previously cited are about 20% (Table 13.5). When stage I and II tumors are considered, the survival rate is 40–50%.[95,113,168] Some investigators have found tumor grade, based on cellularity, pleomorphism, and cytologic atypia, to be a useful prognostic feature,[135] whereas others have found no correlation between tumor grade and clinical behavior.[9,65]

Leiomyosarcomas are treated surgically, usually with hysterectomy and bilateral salpingo-oophorectomy. Extrauterine tumor should be excised to increase the efficacy of postoperative therapy. Most patients with leiomyosarcomas are menopausal or postmenopausal, and ovarian conservation is seldom necessary. Combined therapy (radiation and hysterectomy), used in some centers,[146] has not resulted in an improved survival in any series of leiomyosarcoma diagnosed by objective criteria.[168] Consequently, radiation therapy is of unproved benefit and seldom is used in the initial treatment of leiomyosarcoma, although it is often added as palliation of advanced disease. In view of the poor results obtained by surgery and radiation, adjuvant chemotherapy has been advocated, but currently available regimens have failed to improve the prognosis.[9,60,113]

Recurrent or metastatic leiomyosarcoma is difficult to treat, since neither radiotherapy nor chemotherapy is effective.[61,62,114] Resection of solitary metastatic deposits is possible occasionally.[87]

Endometrial Stromal Tumors

Endometrial stromal tumors occur in two basic forms—a benign endometrial stromal nodule, which is a circumscribed, expansile neoplasm that does not infiltrate the myometrium, and endometrial stromal sarcoma, which infiltrates the myometrium and has metastatic potential.[68,106,183] Endometrial stromal sarcomas also occur in two forms: a relatively high-grade sarcoma and a low-grade neoplasm that is slow to metastasize. In older reports, the low-grade form was designated as *endolymphatic stromal myosis*.[86] The malignant potential and microscopic features of the various types of endometrial stromal tumors are shown in Table 13.6. Variants of endometrial stromal tumors also occur; these include combined smooth muscle–stromal tumors[151] and uterine tumors with a histologic appearance somewhat similar to an ovarian sex cord–stromal tumor.[28] A few endome-

TABLE 13.6. Histologic characteristics of the three main types of endometrial stromal tumors.

Tumor	Malignant potential	Cytologic atypia	Mitoses/10 HPF
Stromal nodule	None	Mild to moderate	Usually 0–3
Low-grade stromal sarcoma	Low to intermediate	Mild to moderate	Less than 10, usually 1–3
High-grade stromal sarcoma	High	Moderate to marked	10 or more

Reprinted by permission of Zaloudek and Norris, Ref. 183.

trial stromal tumors arise outside the uterus from endometriosis.[14,118]

Endometrial Stromal Nodule

Endometrial stromal nodules are rare. They represent about one fourth of endometrial stromal tumors.

Clinical Aspects. Patients with endometrial stromal nodules range in age from 23 to 75 years, with a median age of 47 years.[152] Three-quarters are of reproductive age. There is no unusual racial predisposition. Abnormal bleeding and menorrhagia are the main symptoms, with bleeding occasionally severe enough to cause anemia.[44,106] Pelvic and abdominal discomfort (or pain) are frequent complaints. The duration of symptoms averages 2.2 months.[152] More than 10% of patients are asymptomatic, their tumors being found incidentally in hysterectomy specimens.

Gross Pathology. Endometrial stromal nodules are fleshy and yellow or tan. They have a rounded contour (Fig. 13.19) and bulge above the surrounding myometrium. The size ranges from 0.8 to 15 cm, with a median diameter of 4 cm. Cysts, ranging in size from 0.5 to 5 cm in diameter, are occasionally present, but necrosis and hemorrhage are infrequent. In one study, 11 of 60 nodules were polypoid, protruding into the uterine cavity.[152] About 5% of stromal nodules are multiple.

Slightly more than one-half of endometrial stromal nodules are located entirely within the myometrium in

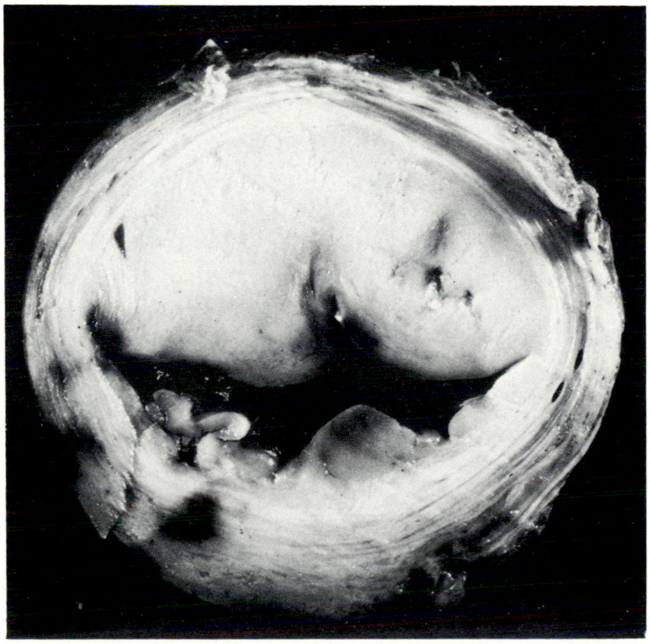

FIG. 13.19. Endometrial stromal nodule with cystic change, showing homogeneous appearance of cut surface. (Reprinted by permission of Zaloudek and Norris, Ref. 183.)

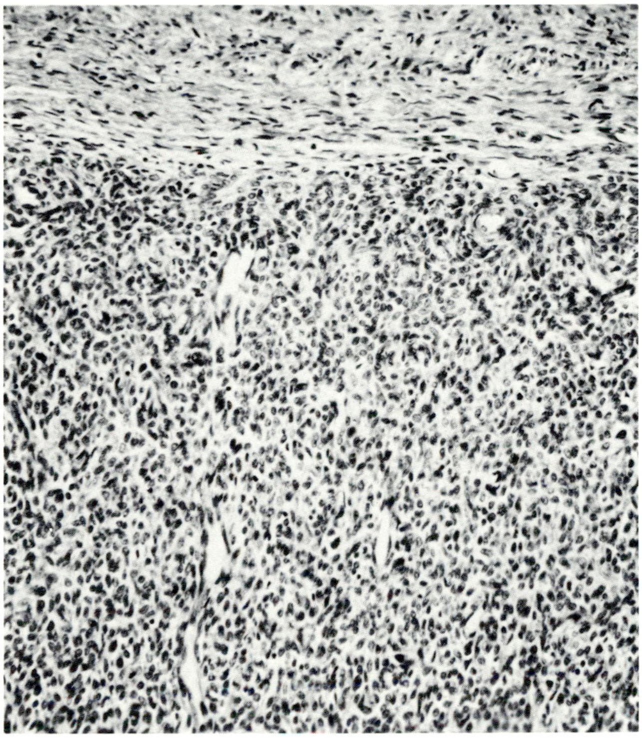

FIG. 13.20. Endometrial stromal nodule. Note the circumscribed, expansile margin that characterizes a stromal nodule. (Reprinted by permission of Tavassoli and Norris, Ref. 152.)

an intramural or subserosal location, with no apparent connection to the endometrium. Endometrial stromal nodules seldom involve the cervix. Subserosal stromal nodules rarely become pedunculated, but their external surface may adhere to the round ligament or omentum.[152]

Microscopic Pathology. Endometrial stromal nodules are composed of cells identical to or closely resembling normal endometrial stromal cells. The tumors have an expansile, noninfiltrative margin that compresses the adjacent endometrium and myometrium (Fig. 13.20).[44,106,152] The neoplastic cells are uniform in size, shape, and staining qualities, and there is minimal cytologic atypia. Decidual change is rare. Mitotic activity ranges from none to 15 mitotic figures/10 HPF in the most active areas of the nodule. It is usually very low (fewer than 3 mitotic figures/10 HPF), and in about one-half of cases, mitotic figures are not seen in 50 consecutive HPF. Only 5–10% of stromal nodules have more than 5 mitotic figures/10 HPF. The behavior of nodules with high mitotic activity is uncertain because only a few have been identified; none are known to have been clinically malignant, however.

A reticulin network encircles individual cells within endometrial stromal nodules. Epithelial configurations, such as cords or trabeculae of tumor cells or gland-like structures, are occasionally present (Fig. 13.21). Small

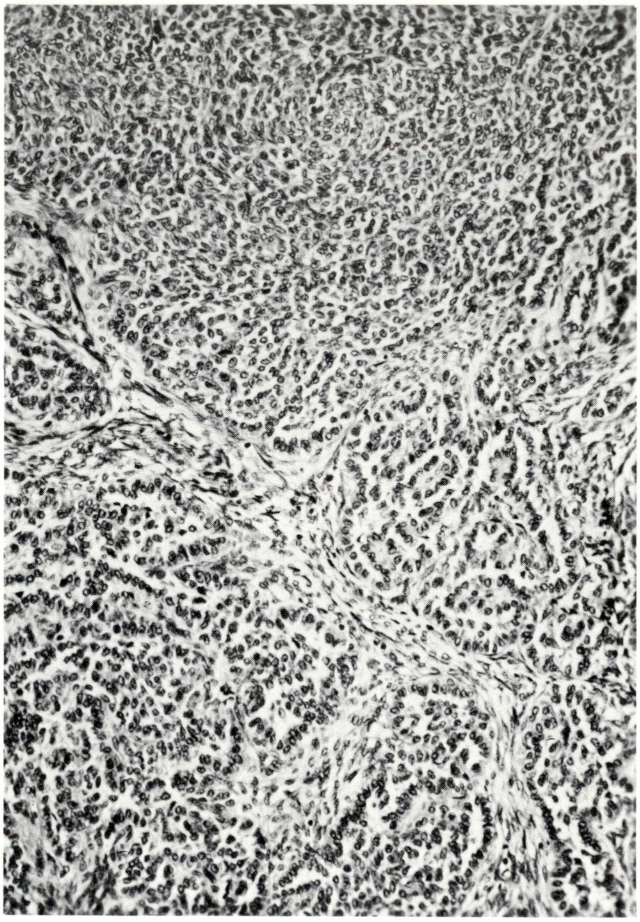

FIG. 13.21. Endometrial stromal nodule. Typical pattern on *top*, cord-like or tubular pattern on *bottom*. (Reprinted by permission of Tavassoli and Norris, Ref. 152.)

areas of necrosis, small cysts, foam cells, and occasional calcium deposits also occur. Focal areas of hyalinized collagen having a starburst pattern are present in some neoplasms, and there are minor areas of smooth muscle cell differentiation in about 10% of them.[152]

Treatment and Prognosis. Hysterectomy is the appropriate therapy for most stromal nodules because the periphery of the nodule must be evaluated to be certain that the tumor is completely circumscribed, with no infiltration of the myometrium. Hysterectomy may not be necessary for smaller nodules that can be completely excised. Regardless of the extent of surgery, none of the patients in the three largest series developed recurrences despite the presence of frequent mitotic figures or minor irregularities of the peripheral margin in a few neoplasms.[44,152,156]

Endometrial Stromal Sarcoma

Endometrial stromal sarcomas infiltrate the myometrium. There are two forms: low-grade stromal sarcoma (LGSS) and high-grade stromal sarcoma (HGSS).[68,106,183] The frequency of endometrial stromal sarcoma is difficult to estimate, because LGSS has been excluded from some reports and included in others. The term *stromatosis*[67,156] has been a major source of confusion because it has been used to identify a benign tumor by some and a malignant tumor by others. Even benign stromal nodules have been included erroneously within some reports of endometrial stromal sarcoma. In the Armed Forces Institute of Pathology (AFIP) files, stromal sarcomas constitute 26% of uterine sarcomas. Two thirds are low grade and one third are high grade. Both forms are included in the following discussion.

Clinical Aspects. The mean age of patients with endometrial stromal sarcoma ranges from 42 to 53 years.* More than one-half of the patients are premenopausal, and stromal sarcoma even occurs in young women and girls.[35,44,80,106] Endometrial stromal sarcoma occurs in younger patients than does malignant mixed mesodermal tumor or endometrial carcinoma. There is no association with endometrial carcinoma risk factors, but a few patients have a history of prior pelvic irradiation.[1,106]

The main symptoms are abnormal vaginal bleeding, cyclic menorrhagia that gradually becomes more severe, and abdominal pain. Enlargement of the uterus, with an irregular contour, is common, and bulky polypoid tumors protrude from the cervical os in a few patients. The usual clinical impression is that the patient has a uterine leiomyoma that is producing an unusual degree of bleeding. A few patients have abdominal metastases; these may pose diagnostic problems if they appear before the patient develops uterine bleeding or enlargement before the true nature of her disease is recognized.

Abnormal cells may be detected in cervical and vaginal smears from patients with HGSS, but cells shed from a stromal nodule or a LGSS are usually not sufficiently atypical to be accurately distinguished from benign endometrial stromal cells.[13,96,100]

A diagnosis of high-grade endometrial stromal sarcoma can be established by pathologic study of curettings. It may be impossible to arrive at a diagnosis before hysterectomy, however, if the neoplasm is entirely intramural or if the periphery of a LGSS is not present in the curettings. At the time of operation, endometrial stromal sarcoma may resemble intravenous leiomyomatosis or a leiomyoma that has extended into the broad ligament. Frozen section examination permits distinction between these entities.

Gross Pathology. Endometrial involvement by LGSS usually takes the form of a smooth-surfaced polypoid growth. Three patterns of intramural growth have been described. First, the myometrium may be diffusely thick-

* References 39, 44, 67, 72, 80, 85, 106, 122, 135, 156, 180.

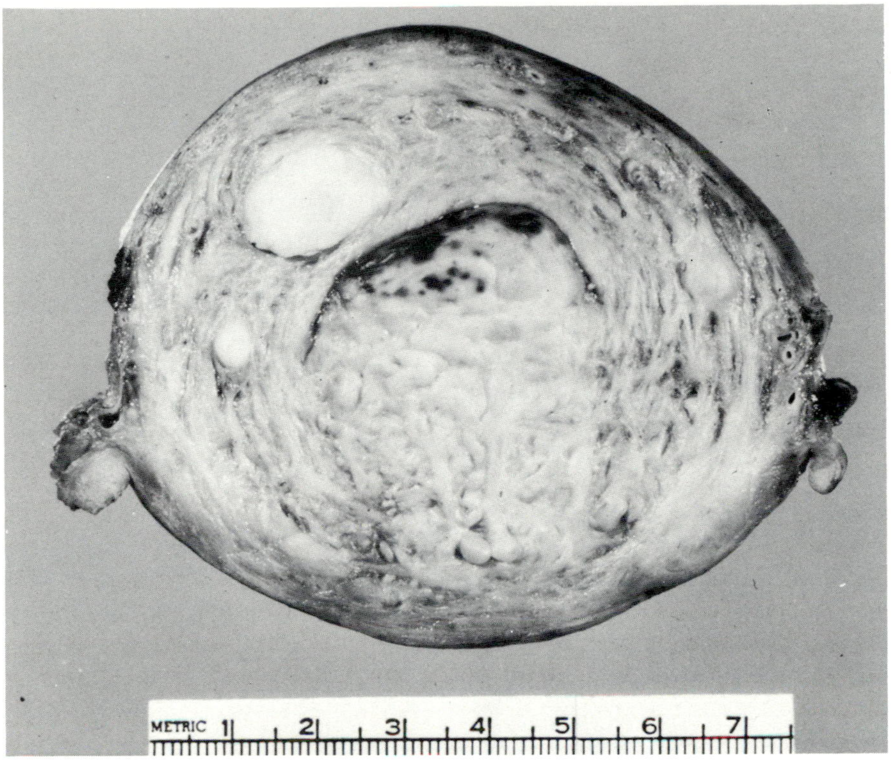

FIG. 13.22. Low-grade endometrial stromal sarcoma (endolymphatic stromal myosis). Extensions of tumor (*lower field*) bulge above the cut surface and obliterate the endometrial cavity. Compare with the leiomyomas in the left half of the myometrium. (Reprinted by permission of Norris and Taylor, Ref. 106.)

ened by infiltration, but a clearly defined tumor is not evident. Second, a nodular tumor with peripheral bosselations may be present. These differ from leiomyomas in that their cut surfaces are tan or yellow-orange and soft, unlike the white, whorled, firm surface of a leiomyoma. The third, and most common, appearance of LGSS is that of a poorly demarcated mass with pink, tan, or yellow cords and nodules permeating the myometrium (Fig. 13.22). LGSS tends to be smaller than HGSS, and its margins are ill-defined and difficult to measure.

High-grade endometrial stromal sarcomas are soft, fleshy, polypoid tumors that bulge into, and often fill, the endometrial cavity.[44,106,180] Multiple, soft, white-to-tan, polypoid masses with focal hemorrhage and necrosis invade the underlying myometrium on a broad front. Both LGSS and HGSS may grow beyond the uterus as infiltrating masses of tan or white tumor that can be palpated as firm, worm-like cords. Pink or tan strands of tumor protrude from the cut surface of the infiltrated tissues and can sometimes be pulled from tissue spaces and vessels.

Microscopic Pathology. Endometrial stromal sarcomas are composed of cells resembling the stromal cells of proliferating endometrium. The cells in a LGSS show little variation and, like those in stromal nodules, have round or ovoid nuclei with dispersed chromatin and small, inconspicuous nucleoli. The cytoplasm is amphophilic, and the cell border is ill defined. The uniformity of the cells imparts a monotonous appearance to LGSS. As many as 9 mitotic figures/10 HPF can be present in a LGSS, but there are fewer than 3 mitotic figures/10 HPF in the most active areas of most of them.[44,67,80,106]

Low-grade stromal sarcoma invades the myometrium and may extensively permeate it (Fig. 13.23). Invasion of lymphatic and vascular channels is a characteristic of LGSS (Fig. 13.24), and it provides the basis for the former designation of this neoplasm as *endolymphatic stromal myosis*.

A prominent vascular pattern is frequently present in LGSS and is the reason that some of these neoplasms have been mistaken for hemangiopericytomas. All types of blood vessels are present, but capillaries and arterioles are prominent.[39,44,67,106] Reticulin fibers surround individual cells or small groups of cells, resulting in a basket-weave pattern.[67,72] The hyalinization, foam cells,[42] and necrosis that are observed within stromal nodules tend to occur more frequently in LGSS. Areas of infarctive necrosis also occur. Decidual change in a stromal tumor is an uncommon response to endogenous progesterone,

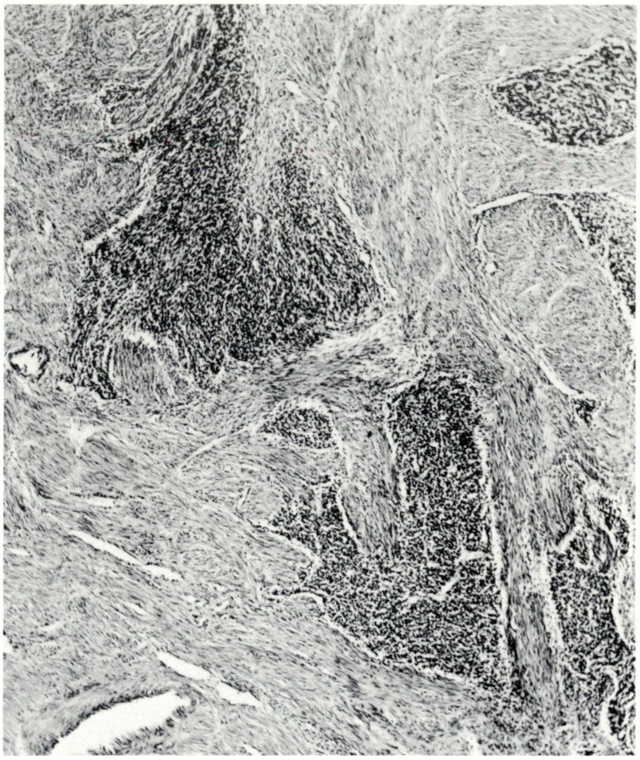

FIG. 13.23. Low-grade stromal sarcoma infiltrating the myometrium in a characteristic pattern. (Reprinted by permission of Norris and Taylor, Ref. 106.)

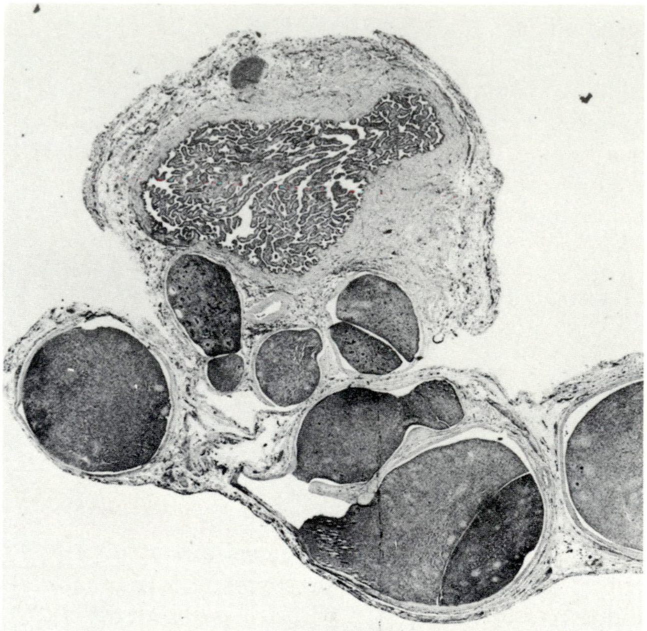

FIG. 13.24. Low-grade endometrial stromal sarcoma growing in the lymphatics of the mesosalpinx and mesovarium.

and it is also infrequent in women receiving exogenous progestogens.

Areas of epithelial differentiation are present in about one quarter of endometrial stromal tumors of all types.[44,106,152] Highly varied in appearance, epithelial differentiation can be manifested as trabecular cords, mesothelial-like structures, endometrial-type glands, or as glands lines by clear cells (see section on endometrial stromal variants).*

High-grade endometrial stromal sarcomas are composed of cells that are usually considerably more atypical than those in LGSS and benign stromal tumors. The degree of atypia is variable, however, and HGSS are distinguished from LGSS most reliably by their increased mitotic activity (Fig. 13.25). HGSS has 10 or more mitotic figures/10 HPF,[44,80,106] and there are typically 20 or more mitotic figures/10 HPF in the most active areas. HGSS often infiltrates the myometrium destructively, with necrosis, rather than with the myometrial permeation characteristic of LGSS. The reticulin meshwork is less uniform in HGSS, and it may be poorly developed or absent in areas of rapid growth.

We reserve the designation *endometrial stromal sarcoma* for a neoplasm that consists exclusively of cells

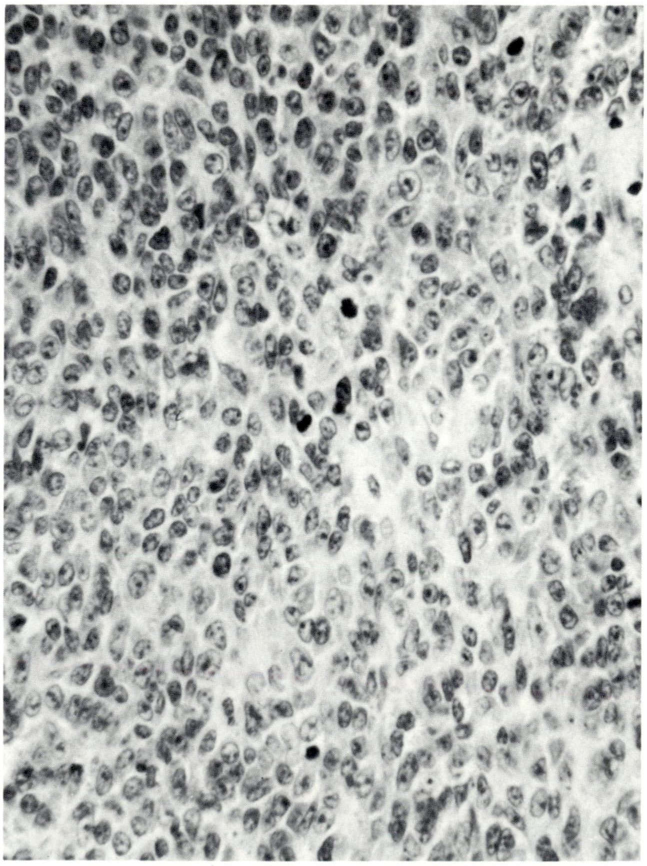

FIG. 13.25. High-grade endometrial stromal sarcoma with frequent mitotic figures.

* References 39, 44, 98, 106, 152, 156.

resembling endometrial stromal cells. A variety of sarcomas that do not qualify for this designation arise in the endometrium. Most are pure or mixed sarcomas that resemble the mesenchymal component of a mixed müllerian tumor. These should be separately classified, since grouping them with pure HGSS, as has been done in some studies,[39] obscures the behavior and response to treatment of both types of neoplasms.

Ultrastructure. The ultrastructural characteristics of the cells in a LGSS are similar to those of stromal cells in early to midproliferative phase endometrium and in stromal nodules.[5,84] The tumor cells (Fig. 13.26) are irregular or spindle shaped, with round or oval nuclei. The cytoplasm is scanty and usually has sparsely distributed organelles. Mitochondria, rough endoplasmic reticulum, free ribosomes, microfilaments, and Golgi vesicles are present, but they are less common than in smooth muscle cells. Some cells are partly surrounded by a basal lamina, and desmosomes are sparse. The ultrastructural similarity to fibroblasts suggests that stromal cells may be specialized or altered fibroblasts. The pleomorphism and cytologic atypia seen in HGSS by light microscopy is also observed at the ultrastructural level.[5] The cytoplasmic content is similar to that of LGSS, except that microfilaments are less prominent.

Treatment and Prognosis. The type and extent of tumor and the type of operation performed determine the risk of recurrence. Recurrence of LGSS is most likely when the tumor has invaded the uterine serosa or into the peritoneum, parametrium, or adnexae.[39,44,85,106] Extensions of tumor into the adnexal area are not always visible at operation, and recurrences have followed preservation of the adnexal structures.

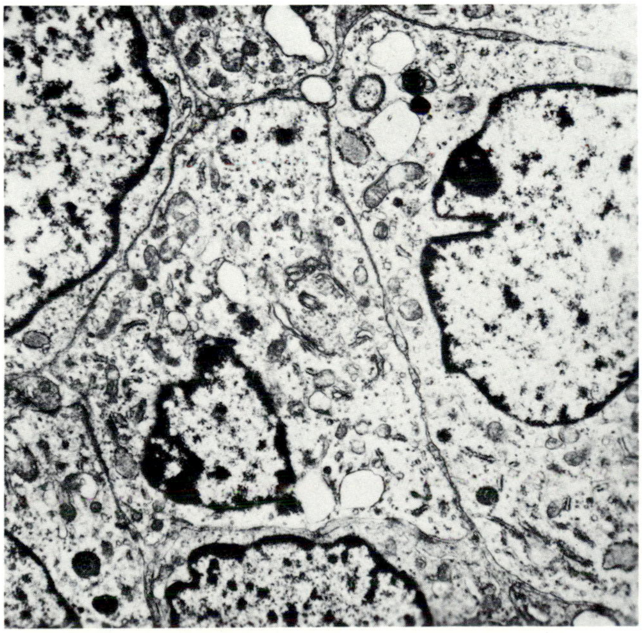

FIG. 13.26. Endometrial stromal sarcoma (low grade). Nuclei are rounded, the chromatin is dispersed, and the cytoplasm contains a few organelles and fibrils. ×8000.

Low-grade stromal sarcomas are usually slow growing, and recurrences, which develop in about 50% of patients, are commonly detected many years (as many as 26 years) after initial treatment.[85] Recurrences are usually in the pelvis and tend to involve the ureter, bladder, vagina, or bowel.[39,72,85,122] Metastases beyond the pelvis are often distributed over the peritoneal surfaces or omentum. Pulmonary metastases develop in 9–43% of the patients with recurrences.[67,72,85,106,122] Histologically, the recurrences are low grade and resemble the primary neoplasms. The median time from diagnosis of LGSS to death is about 11 years.

Complete or partial resolution of recurrent or metastatic LGSS has been documented after treatment with progestational agents,[8,53,89,122,156,163] as has tumor regression after oophorectomy. In one large series, 6 of 13 patients with recurrent LGSS had complete or partial remissions with hormonal therapy, and an additional 6 patients had stable disease.[122] These findings, together with reports by others of similar responses to progestin therapy, have led to the recommendation that women with LGSS should be treated by total abdominal hysterectomy and bilateral salpingo-oophorectomy followed by long-term progestin therapy,[122,156] with the hope that the hormonal therapy might reduce the 50% relapse rate observed historically in patients with LGSS. Steroid hormone receptor assays on tumor tissue have been performed in a few patients with LGSS, and it appears that a woman whose tumor contains high levels of progesterone receptors will have at least an initial response to progestin therapy.[8,53,89,163] The significance of the estrogen receptor level is less certain. Estrogen and progesterone receptor analysis should be performed on all LGSS. Alternative therapy must be considered for women whose neoplasms do not contain significant amounts of progesterone receptors and for those whose neoplasms progress while they are receiving progestins.

Kerby recommended that women with LGSS receive postoperative pelvic radiation.[81] The effectiveness of postoperative radiation is illustrated in several reports in which women treated with radiation did not develop pelvic recurrences as often as expected, even though some had residual tumor after surgery.[122] Patients who are treated with pelvic radiation may still develop distant recurrences. In view of this and the success achieved with progestin therapy, the role of adjuvant radiotherapy for LGSS is limited to patients with recurrent LGSS who are not responsive to progestin therapy. Responses to cytotoxic chemotherapy have been reported in a few instances, but, in general, chemotherapy has proven ineffective in patients with LGSS.[122]

High-grade endometrial stromal sarcomas are characterized by rapid progression. Recurrences are common and are usually evident within 2 years of the initial treatment.* The most common site of recurrence is in the pelvis, particularly in patients who do not receive preoperative or postoperative radiation therapy. Isolated pelvic recurrences are uncommon, as most patients with pelvic metastases also have metastases in the abdomen or lungs. Surgery combined with preoperative or postoperative pelvic radiation offers the best prospect of control of HGSS. Pelvic recurrences are fewer, and survival is better in patients with low-stage disease treated with combined therapy.[138,168,170] Recurrence outside the radiation field is the most common reason for treatment failure in patients who have received combined therapy. Adjuvant chemotherapy has been suggested as a possible means to control such metastases, but an effective drug regimen is not yet available.[60,113] Progestational agents have generally not been effective for HGSS,[180] but one patient with a low estrogen receptor level and an elevated progesterone receptor level remained stable for over a year on progestin therapy.[147] Measurement of estrogen and progesterone receptors may provide guidance as to which patients are likely to respond to hormonal therapy.

The results of treatment of HGSS vary widely, with 5-year survivals ranging from 0 to 62%.† The variation in results is attributable to differences in diagnostic criteria and the inclusion of benign stromal nodules in some series. The most favorable results indicate a 5-year survival of 50–62% for patients with stage I and II sarcomas.[106,113,168]

Endometrial Stromal Variants

There are two neoplasms that contain endometrial stroma that are different from the usual stromal tumors. One has been termed *uterine neoplasm resembling an ovarian sex cord tumor*,[28] and the other is a combined smooth muscle–stromal tumor, designated by some as a *stromomyoma*.[151]

The uterine neoplasm resembling an ovarian sex cord tumor contains variable amounts of typical endometrial stromal cells. Most neoplasms in this category are readily recognized endometrial stromal tumors with epithelial differentiation in the form of trabeculae, nests, and cords (Figs. 13.27, 13.28, and 13.29). In a neoplasm studied ultrastructurally, the stromal cells resembled proliferative endometrial stroma and the cells in stromal neoplasms. The epithelial clusters lacked lumens, and the cells did not have microvilli, but they were joined by occasional desmosomes and contained perinuclear intermediate filaments, features suggestive of differentiation toward endometrial glandular structures (Fig. 13.30).[98] When plexiform and tubular structures dominate the morphologic pattern and endometrial stroma is inconspicuous, the resemblance to other endometrial stromal tumors may be obscure.

Patients having uterine stromal tumors with a sex cord pattern are generally of reproductive age, although a few are perimenopausal or postmenopausal.[28] The neoplasms produce abnormal bleeding and uterine enlargement. Although few cases have been reported, the behavior of the tumor, like that of pure endometrial stomal tumors, is probably dependent on the cytologic characteristics and the type of margin (i.e., circumscribed versus infiltrating).[28,44,152]

Microscopically, in the combined smooth muscle–stromal tumor or stromomyoma, there may be discrete areas

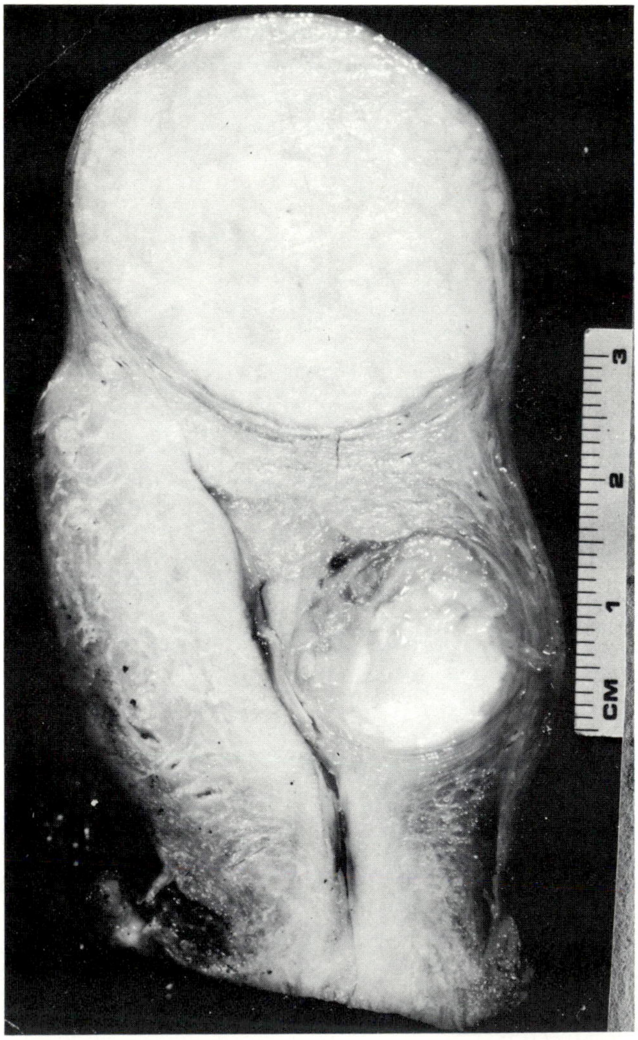

FIG. 13.27. Endometrial stromal variant resembling a sex cord–stromal tumor (small nodule at *right*). The large nodule in the fundus is a leiomyoma.

* References 80, 95, 106, 120, 138, 139, 170, 180.
† References 1, 80, 95, 106, 120, 139, 170, 180.

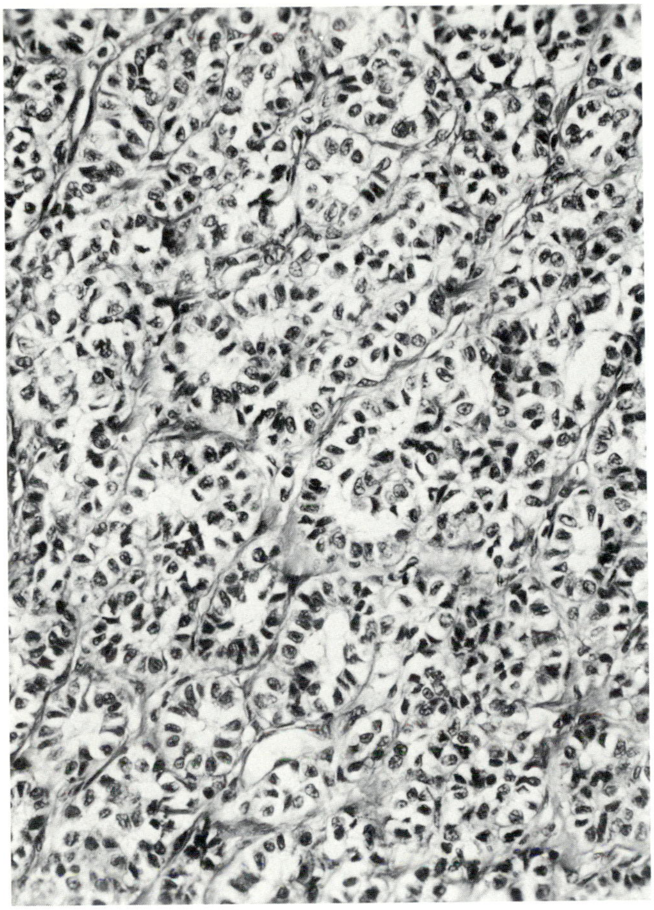

FIG. 13.28. Endometrial stromal tumor variant with a tubular pattern.

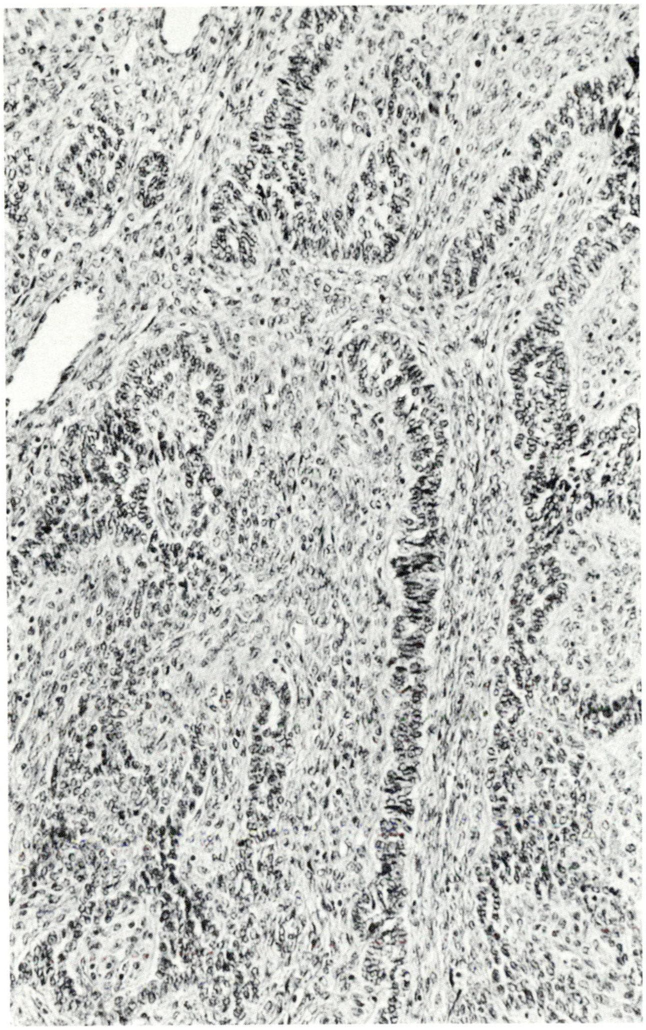

FIG. 13.29. Stromal tumor containing organoid cords that resemble gonadal stroma to some investigators. (Reprinted by permission of Mazur and Kraus, Ref. 98.)

of smooth muscle and endometrial stroma, but nearly all neoplasms have areas in which the cells have characteristics intermediate between muscle and stroma. Ultrastructurally, differentiation to endometrial stroma and smooth muscle is confirmed.[98,151] Bird and Willis thought that the smooth muscle differentiated from stromal cells,[16] a view supported by Hart and Yoonessi[67] and embryologically by Gruenwald.[59] Combined smooth muscle–stromal tumors are more common than realized. In the past, most were designated as leiomyomas or as endometrial stromal sarcomas. Malignant behavior in a combined smooth muscle–stromal tumor has not been reported, but metastasis could occur from a neoplasm that is dominated by endometrial stroma and that has an infiltrating margin.

Mixed Mesodermal Tumors

Mixed mesodermal tumors contain both epithelium and mesenchymal elements as active participants in the neoplastic process. This group of tumors includes adenofibroma, adenosarcoma, and mixed müllerian tumor (MMT) (Table 13.7). There is a gradation of malignant potential in both the epithelium and the stroma ranging from adenofibroma at the benign end of the spectrum, through adenosarcoma, to the highly malignant mixed müllerian tumor. Adenofibroma and adenosarcoma both have a benign glandular component. The stroma is benign in an adenofibroma, whereas an adenosarcoma has a sarcomatous mesenchymal component.[116,182] Both stroma and epithelium are malignant in an MMT. The capacity to form neoplasms with both epithelial and connective tissue differentiation is a result of the embryologic heritage of the epithelium and stroma of the endometrium.

Mixed müllerian tumors are classified as homologous or heterologous, depending on the mesenchymal ele-

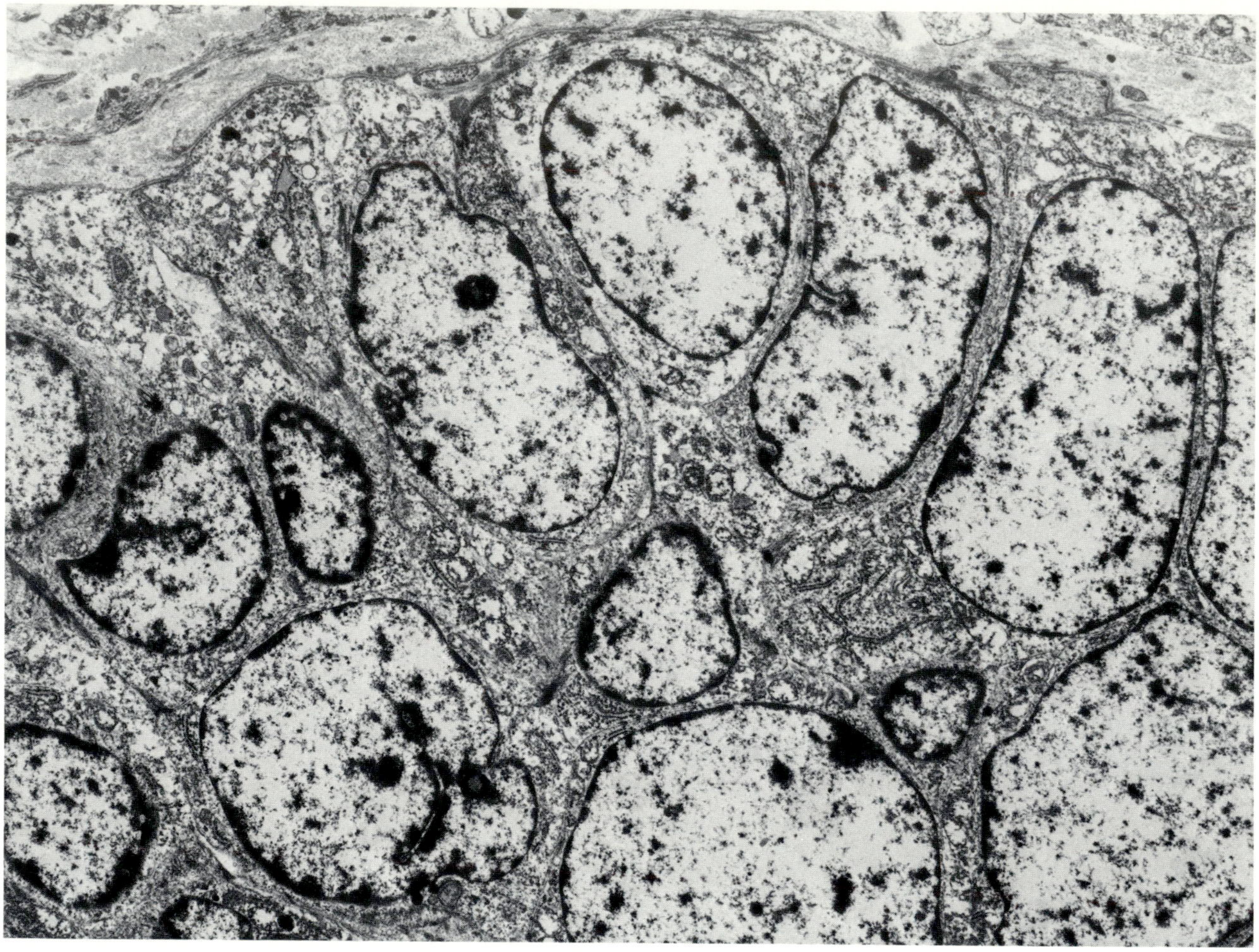

FIG. 13.30. Same tumor as shown in Figure 13.29. An electron microscopic view of epithelial-like cells within one of the cords. A true lumen is absent. Tonofilaments are present in cell to *lower right*. (Reprinted by permission of Mazur and Kraus, Ref. 98.)

ments present.[68,80,110] Homologous tumors, which are also called *carcinosarcomas*, contain mesenchymal cell types that are normally found in the uterus, such as endometrial stromal cells, smooth muscle cells, and fibroblasts. Heterologous tumors, frequently referred to as *malignant mixed mesodermal tumors*, exhibit types of mesenchymal differentiation that are not normally observed in the uterus. Heterologous elements include striated muscle, cartilage, osteoid, and fat.

Adenofibroma and Adenosarcoma

Orginally described in the cervix[2] and endometrium,[110,167] adenofibroma and adenosarcoma have been

TABLE 13.7. Classification of mixed mesodermal tumors.

Tumor	Malignant potential	Epithelial component	Mesenchymal component
Adenofibroma	None	Benign	Benign, homologous
Adenosarcoma	Low to intermediate	Benign	Homologous or heterologous sarcoma
Mixed müllerian tumor			
Homologous	High	Carcinoma	Homologous sarcoma
Heterologous	High	Carcinoma	Heterologous sarcoma

variously designated as adenofibroma, papillary adenofibroma, adenomyomatosis,[144] benign müllerian tumor, müllerian adenosarcoma,[27] and benign and low-grade variants of mixed müllerian tumor.[116] Initially, it was not appreciated that the cellular stroma in some neoplasms diagnosed as adenofibromas had characteristics of malignancy. Not until Clement and Scully described adenosarcoma did it become apparent that adenofibroma and adenosarcoma were closely related but different neoplasms.[27] The distinction between the two is based on the criteria of Zaloudek and Norris.[182]

Adenofibroma and adenosarcoma also occur in extrauterine pelvic locations, such as the fallopian tube, ovary, and paraovarian tissues. Extrauterine adenosarcomas occur in younger women and appear to be more aggressive than their uterine counterparts.[76]

Adenofibroma

Clinical Aspects. Women with adenofibromas generally are elderly; most are either perimenopausal or postmenopausal. The median age is 68 years,[182] but patients have ranged in age from 19 years to more than 80 years.[2,58,116,167,182] There is no known racial predilection, nor does adenofibroma share the epidemiologic features of endometrial carcinoma.[182] Abnormal vaginal bleeding is the most frequent complaint. Less common findings include abdominal pain, abdominal enlargement, or a polypoid tumor projecting from the cervix. Some patients give a history of prior removal of polyps.

Gross Pathology. Adenofibromas are polypoid neoplasms with lobular or papillary surfaces; curettings generally contain large polypoid tissue fragments. They may arise in the cornual region, the fundus, the lower uterine segment, or the cervix. When discovered, their size ranges from 2 to 10 cm, with a median diameter of 7 cm. Large adenofibromas may fill the endometrial cavity, enlarging the uterus. Soft, rubbery to firm, tan or brown with focal hemorrhage, about one-half of the neoplasms contain small cysts that impart a spongy or mucoid appearance to the cut surface.

Microscopic Pathology. Adenofibromas are composed of histologically bland epithelium and mesenchyme. They originate in the endometrium and do not invade the underlying myometrium (Fig. 13.31). Broad papillary fronds covered with epithelium project from the surface and into cystic spaces within the neoplasm. Cysts and cleft-like spaces are lined by columnar or cuboidal epithelial cells of endometrial type. Multiple types of epithelium may occur within the same neoplasm, and the epithelium is often hyperplastic and stratified.

The mesenchymal component is usually fibroblastic (Fig. 13.32), but endometrial stromal cells or mixtures of stromal cells and fibroblasts occur in some neo-

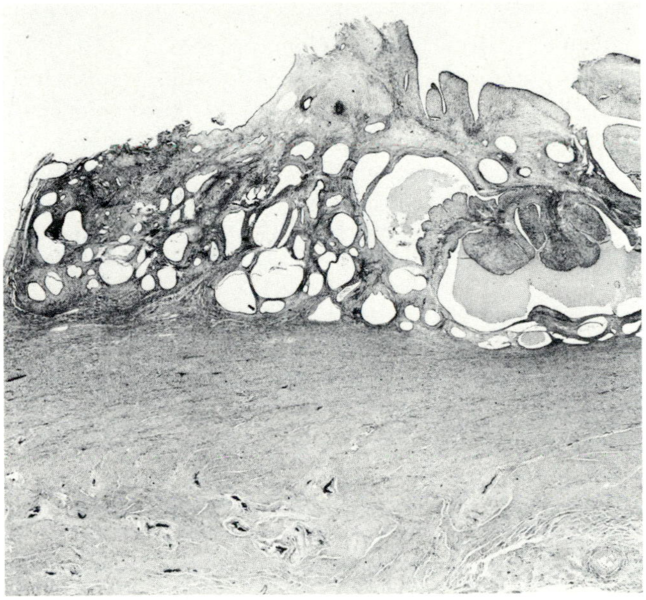

FIG. 13.31. Adenofibroma. Like all adenofibromas, it does not invade the myometrium. (Reprinted by permission of Zaloudek and Norris, Ref. 182.)

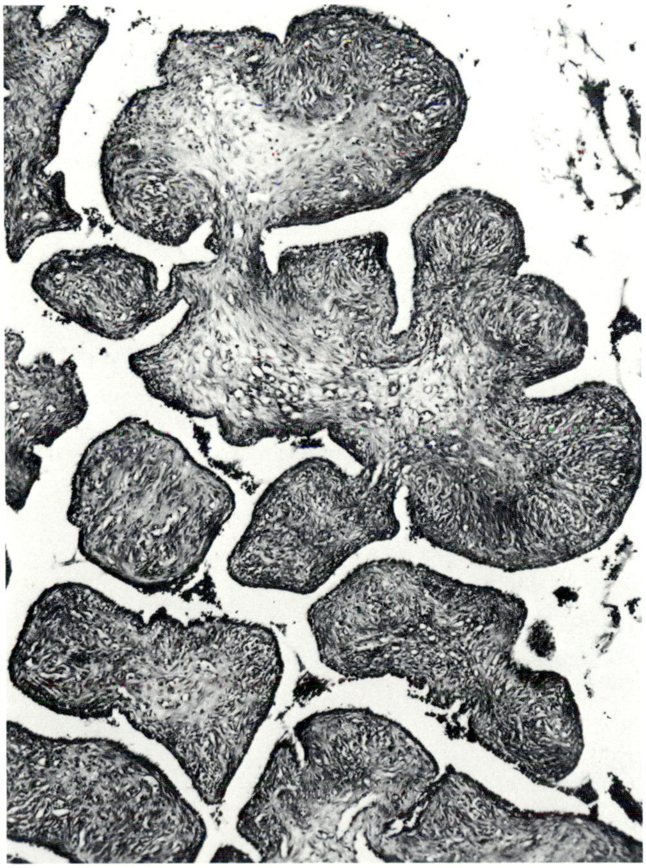

FIG. 13.32. Adenofibroma. Papillae projecting into cystic spaces, showing hypocellular, collagenous stroma. (Reprinted by permission of Zaloudek and Norris, Ref. 182.)

plasms.[58,116,167,182] The fibrotic stroma is more cellular and uniform than in polyps. Characteristically, the stroma is more cellular adjacent to the epithelium. Atypia within the stromal cells is generally absent or mild, and markedly atypical mesenchymal cells are seldom present. Mitotic figures are most numerous in the cellular periglandular stroma, but mitoses are usually few in number, and there are invariably less than 4 mitotic figures/10 HPF.[182]

Treatment and Prognosis. Hysterectomy is the preferred treatment for an adenofibroma because the neoplasm may recur if it is incompletely curetted.[116,182] Hysterectomy ensures complete excision, and it also permits the thorough sampling needed to exclude an adenosarcoma.

Adenosarcoma

Clinical Aspects. Adenosarcomas occur in patients of all ages. The median age is about 57 years, with a range of 14 to 79 years.* There is no association with obesity or hypertension, nor is there any association with prior pelvic radiation. In one study, 3 of 25 women were diabetic.[182] Some patients have a history of prior removal of polyps.

The most common presenting symptom is abnormal vaginal bleeding. Vaginal discharge, pain, nonspecific urinary symptoms, a palpable pelvic mass, and tumor protruding from the vagina are the most common signs and symptoms.[15,27,116,182]

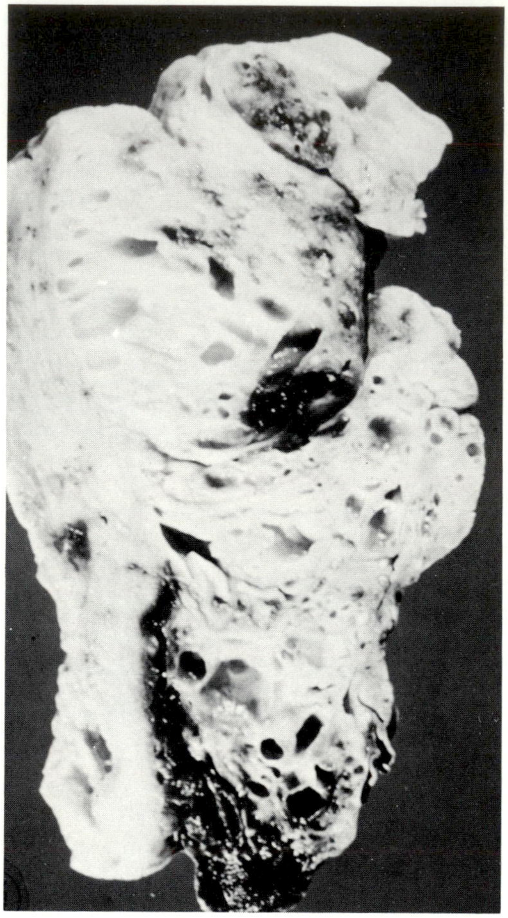

FIG. 13.33. Adenosarcoma in bisected uterus. A polypoid, cystic, partially infarcted mass fills the endometrial cavity and invades the myometrium.

Gross Pathology. On gross examination, a sessile, polypoid neoplasm arises from the cervix or fills the endometrial cavity and enlarges the uterus (Fig. 13.33). A solitary polypoid growth is most characteristic, but multiple papillary and polypoid masses also occur. Adenosarcomas can be soft or firm and are tan, brown, or gray. Visible hemorrhage and areas of necrosis occur in about one-quarter. About one fifth of adenosarcomas have visible cysts filled with mucoid material. Adenosarcomas differ from adenofibromas in that they tend to be larger and softer and have more hemorrhage and necrosis.

Microscopic Pathology. Papillary fronds project from the surface or into cysts (Fig. 13.34). Tubular glands or cleft-like spaces lined by epithelium are dispersed throughout. The most common type of epithelium resembles inactive or proliferative endometrial glands, but the epithelium may be hyperplastic and slightly atypical. Mucinous epithelium and squamous epithelium also occur. Both glands and stroma are present in the invasive component of adenosarcomas, identifying the epithelium as an actively proliferating part of the neoplasm.[15,182]

The mesenchymal component of an adenosarcoma is generally a fibrous sarcoma or a sarcoma composed of small cells differentiated toward endometrial stroma. The stroma is characteristically hypercellular beneath the surface epithelium and around glands and cysts. Mesenchymal cells are mildly atypical in about one-third of these neoplasms, moderately atypical in one-third, and severely atypical in one-third.[182] By definition, 4 or more mitotic figures/10 HPF are found in adenosarcomas. Ostor and Fortune reported two adenosarcomas without mitotic figures that metastasized,[116] but these may not have been adequately sampled for microscopic study. Ten of the 25 adenosarcomas in one study contained bland areas histologically indistinguishable from an adenofibroma, and only thorough examination identified the sarcomatous component.[182] Heterologous mesenchymal components, particularly cartilage, striated muscle, and fat (Fig. 13.35) occur in about one quarter of adenosarcomas.[131,182]

Ultrastructure. Electron microscopic studies support the impression that two distinct components are present.[15,79,112,131] A distinct basal lamina separates the

* References 15, 27, 47, 52, 79, 112, 131, 182.

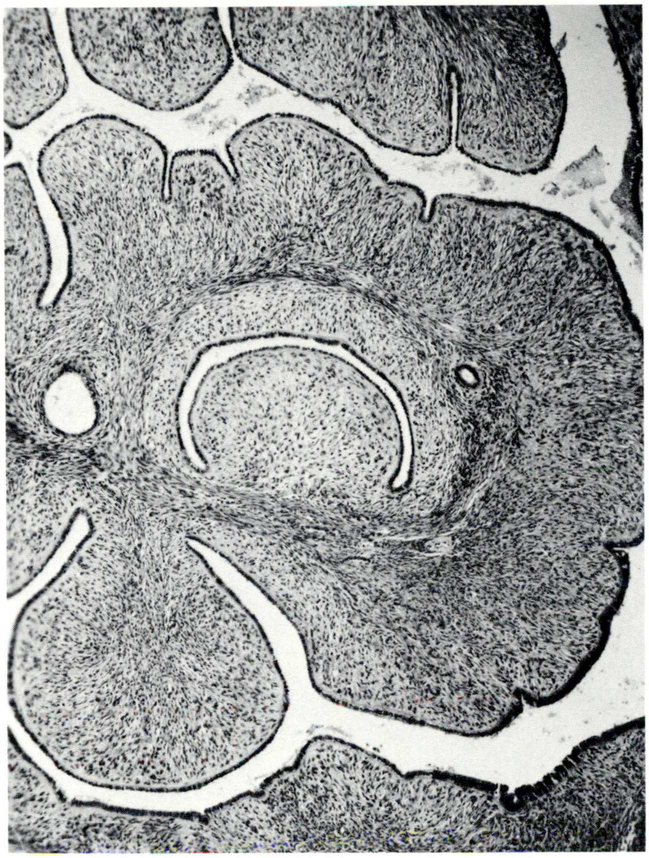

FIG. 13.34. Adenosarcoma. The dense stromal cellularity contrasts with adenofibroma (compare with Fig. 13.32).

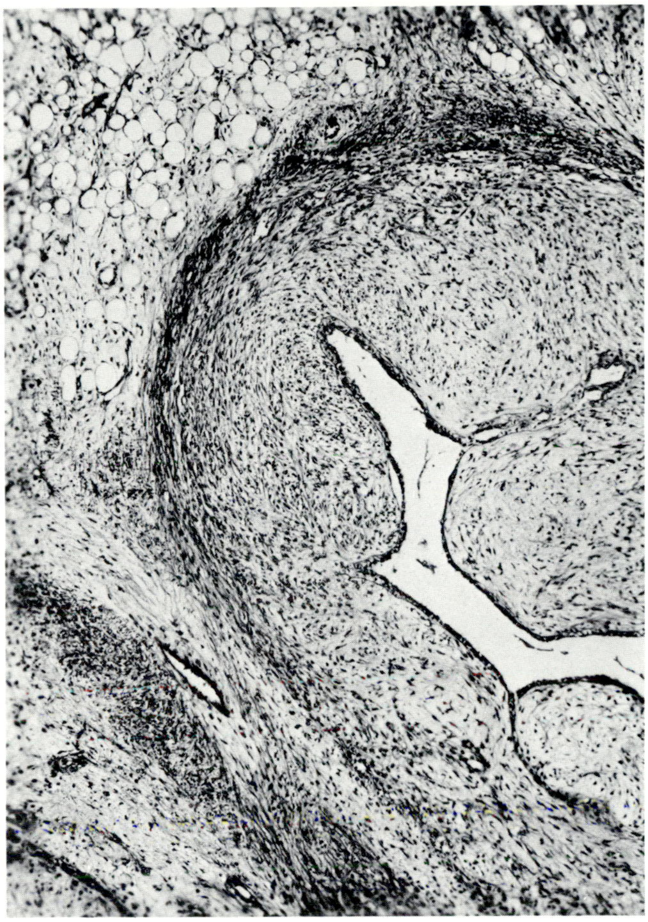

FIG. 13.35. Adenosarcoma containing fat in *upper left* of field. Smooth muscle, cartilage, and striated muscle also occur in adenosarcomas.

stromal cells from the epithelium. The epithelium has typical müllerian characteristics, including cilia, microvilli, and basal orientation of the nuclei (Fig. 13.36). The mesenchymal cells are often similar to preovulatory stromal cells as well as to the cells in endometrial stromal sarcoma, but in some areas the mesenchymal cells have ultrastructural features of fibroblasts or nonspecific mesenchymal cells.[15,79,112,131]

Treatment and Prognosis. The usual treatment is hysterectomy with bilateral salpingo-oophorectomy. Women with superficial adenosarcomas probably do not require radiation therapy, but those with tumors invading more than halfway through the myometrium have a high likelihood of recurrence[182] and might benefit from the type of combined therapy given to women with malignant mixed müllerian tumors. The efficacy of vaginal radium treatment has not been tested, but the frequency of isolated vaginal recurrence is sufficiently high to recommend such therapy.[27,182] The effectiveness of chemotherapy has not been studied.

The results obtained in two teenage girls treated with wide local excision of cervical adenosarcomas[182] suggest that conservative methods of treatment are reasonable in special situations. Gloor reported an adenosarcoma originating in the cervix that was eradicated by local excision and radium application.[52]

Adenosarcoma is not as aggressive as malignant mixed müllerian tumor. Forty percent of adenosarcomas recur or metastasize.[27,182] Common sites of metastasis are in the pelvis or vagina (60%), but in a smaller proportion of patients, metastases develop outside the pelvis. The histologic appearance of recurrent and metastatic adenosarcoma is similar to that of the primary tumor except that epithelium is often absent. Some vaginal and pelvic recurrences have contained an epithelial component.[27,182] In these, the stroma around the epithelium is often hypercellular. About one-half of recurrent tumors manifest greater cellular atypia and mitotic activity than do the primary neoplasms. Heterologous elements, if present originally, may appear in the metastasis. Long-term clinical observation is needed because the median interval between treatment and recurrence is 5 years, and of the 24% of women who die of tumor, the median time to death is 7 years.[182]

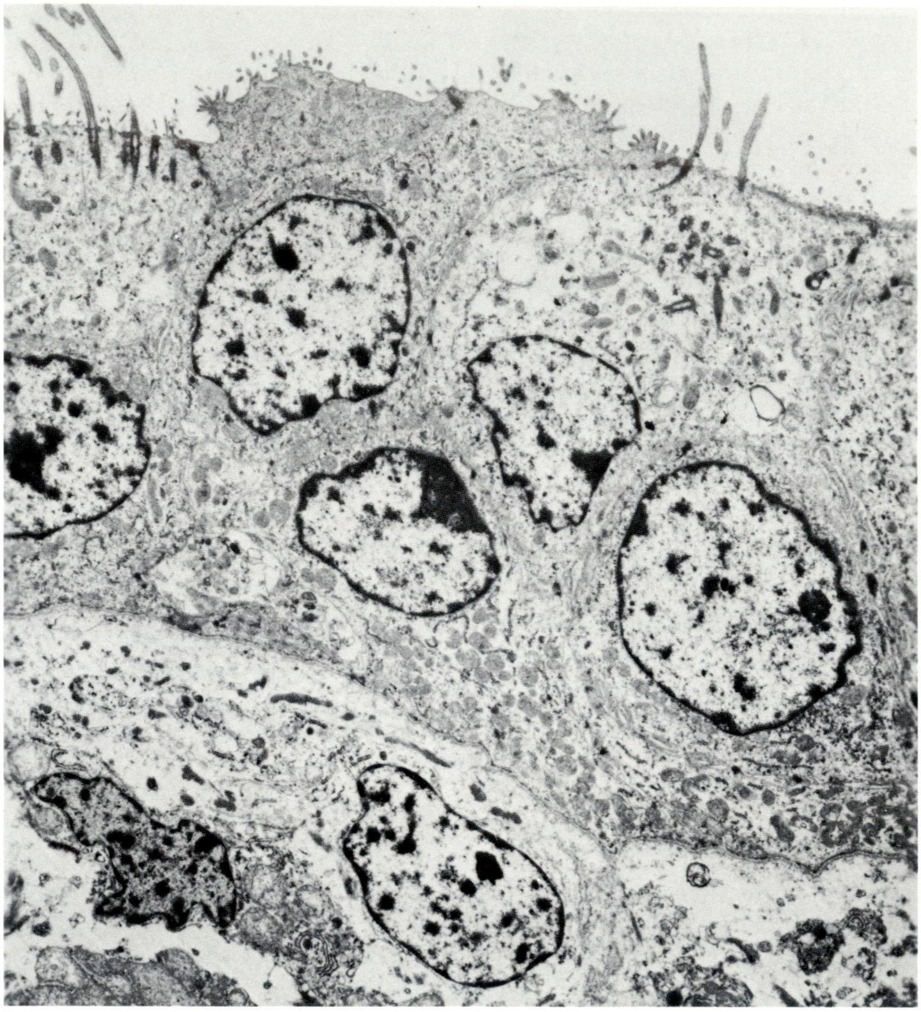

FIG. 13.36. Adenosarcoma. Epithelial cells have microvilli and cilia. Epithelial and stromal cells are separated by a discrete basal lamina. ×4000. (Courtesy of F.A. Tavassoli, Washington, D.C.)

Mixed Müllerian Tumor

The mixed müllerian tumor is the most common uterine sarcoma.[95,137,170] It is nonetheless rare, constituting less than 1.5% of malignant tumors of the uterus.[24] It is increasing in relative frequency, and it is more common than leiomyosarcoma when stringent criteria are used for the diagnosis of the latter neoplasm.

Clinical Aspects. Most patients with MMT are postmenopausal, with a median age of about 65 years.* The most common symptom is postmenopausal bleeding. Lower abdominal pain, abdominal distention, and a palpable abdominal mass are also frequent presenting complaints. An enlarged irregular uterus and tumor protruding through the cervical os are common findings.[93] Extrauterine spread occurs early, and many patients complain of symptoms caused by gastrointestinal or urinary tract involvement. Few patients are asymptomatic at the time of diagnosis.

Infertility, hypertension, obesity, and diabetes occur in patients with MMT,[93,137,173] but their association with MMT is not as clear as it is with endometrial carcinoma. No association between MMT and these risk factors was found in one study.[10] A disproportionate number of uterine tumors developing after pelvic radiation are MMT.[43,105,120,141,157] Norris and Taylor, for example, found 17 postradiation sarcomas in a review of 136 malignant mesenchymal tumors of the uterus, and 13 of the 17 were carcinosarcomas or mixed mesodermal tumors.[105] The median latent period between pelvic irradiation and the discovery of the sarcoma was 16 years. The MMTs that occur in patients who have had pelvic radiation tend to develop at a younger age than those that occur in women who have not been radiated.[105,166]

* References 10, 25, 80, 93, 107, 108, 120, 141, 149, 173.

The proportion of patients with a history of radiation is smaller in recent reports on MMT.

Curettage can be an effective means of establishing a diagnosis,[10,25,93,141] but in some cases the histologic findings may be misleading. Curettings may consist only of fragments of carcinoma or sarcoma, and the biphasic nature of the neoplasm may not become apparent until the entire tumor is studied. Identification of heterologous elements may require extensive sampling.

Cytologic studies have not played a significant role in the diagnosis of MMT.[96] Most patients have symptoms requiring curettage, and cytologic evaluation is performed as part of the initial diagnostic evaluation rather than to detect tumors in asymptomatic patients. Malignant cells may be identified, but they often cannot be specifically classified as epithelial or mesenchymal.[93,96,141] In a few instances, malignant mesenchymal cells, such as rhabdomyoblasts, have been identified.[10,96] Malignant mesenchymal cells in a Pap smear suggest a diagnosis of MMT, as other sarcomas are less common and are rarely evident cytologically.

Gross Pathology. MMTs are polypoid neoplasms that usually fill the endometrial cavity (Fig. 13.37). Many are of sufficient size to protrude through the external os. Some MMTs arise in the cervix, where they grow as polypoid neoplasms similar to those found in the endometrium.[4] MMTs generally have soft tan cut surfaces, with areas of hemorrhage and necrosis. Gritty or hard areas may reflect the presence of bone or cartilage. Cartilaginous areas often have a translucent appearance. Myometrial invasion may be evident.

Microscopic Pathology. A MMT is composed of an intimate admixture of malignant epithelium and sarcomatous stroma, with the latter usually predominating (Fig. 13.38). The epithelial component is typically an adenocarcinoma of the endometrioid type, but clear cell, mucinous, and serous adenocarcinomas also occur in MMT.[80,93,107,108] In 5% of MMT, the epithelial component is a squamous carcinoma. Squamous carcinoma is relatively more common in MMT arising in the cervix than in those of the corpus.[4]

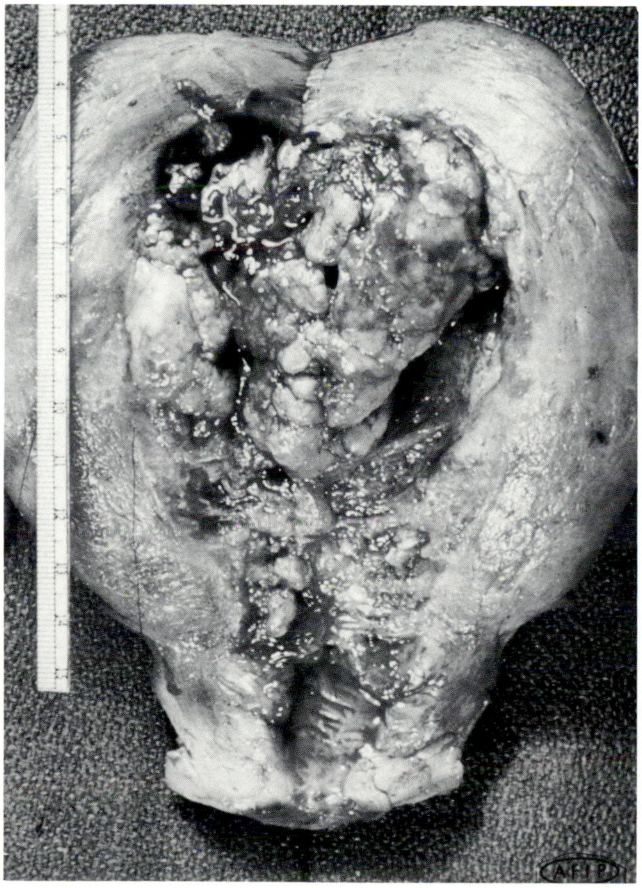

FIG. 13.37. Mixed müllerian tumor of endometrium, showing extension into myometrium and cervix. [Reprinted with permission from The American College of Obstetricians and Gynecologists. (Obstetrics and Gynecology, 28: 57, 1966.)]

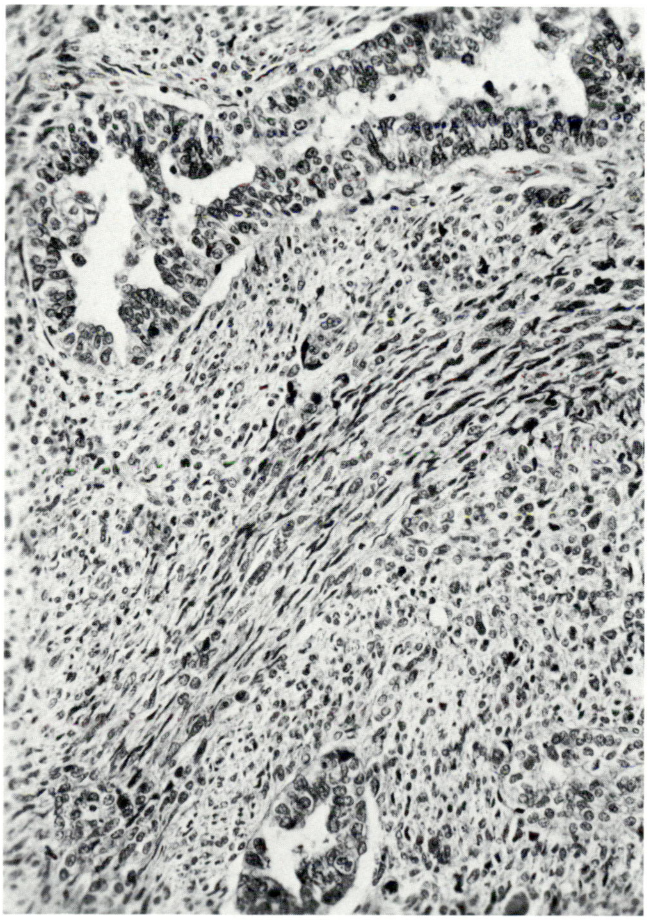

FIG. 13.38. Homologous mixed müllerian tumor (carcinosarcoma).

The most common homologous mesenchymal components are fibrosarcoma and endometrial stromal sarcoma (Fig. 13.38). Leiomyosarcoma is less frequent. Mixtures of fibrosarcoma, leiomyosarcoma, and stromal sarcoma also occur. Heterologous components tend to be found in association with areas of undifferentiated sarcoma or stromal sarcoma. Rhabdomyosarcoma is the most common heterologous element. Rhabdomyoblasts, usually occurring in clusters and associated with undifferentiated sarcoma cells, can be identified with certainty by routine light microscopy when cytoplasmic cross-striations are identified; these are best seen in lightly stained H & E sections. Round cells with atypical nuclei and variable amounts of granular or fibrillar acidophilic cytoplasm are often found in association with striated rhabdomyoblasts, and most pathologists regard them as sufficiently characteristic to permit diagnosis. Immunocytochemical stains for desmin and myoglobin are useful in the identification of rhabdomyoblasts.

Bocker and Stegner[17] traced the development of rhabdomyoblasts from undifferentiated stromal cells using the electron microscope. Partially differentiated rhabdomyoblasts contain conspicuous but nonspecific 100-A filaments in their cytoplasm. Myofilaments are more numerous and better organized in more differentiated rhabdomyoblasts in which well-defined sarcomeric organization and Z bands are present. Cross-striations can be identified at the light microscopic level only in the most differentiated cells.

Cartilage is the second most common heterologous element in heterologous MMT (Fig. 13.39). Silverberg found evidence that the chondroid cells differentiate from stromal cells.[143] Less common heterologous elements include osteoid and fat.

Pure and mixed heterologous endometrial sarcomas occur very rarely. They differ from mixed mesodermal tumors by the absence of an epithelial component. Most are rhabdomyosarcomas,[66,120,140,164] but chondrosarcomas,[26,83,164] osteosarcomas,[30] and tumors containing mixtures of heterologous elements have also been reported. Histologically benign heterotopic cartilage is occasionally found in the uterus.[130] It should not be mistaken for a heterologous endometrial sarcoma or mixed mesodermal tumor.

The histogenesis of mixed mesodermal tumors has been a source of controversy since they were first described. Many of the older theories of histogenesis, summarized by Ober,[110] have been discarded in favor of the concept that these tumors develop by neoplastic transformation of the least differentiated cells in the endometrium (primitive stromal cells).[18] The müllerian epithelium and mesenchyme share a common embryologic background, so neoplastic stromal cells have the potential to differentiate into the rich variety of cell types found in the tumors in this group.

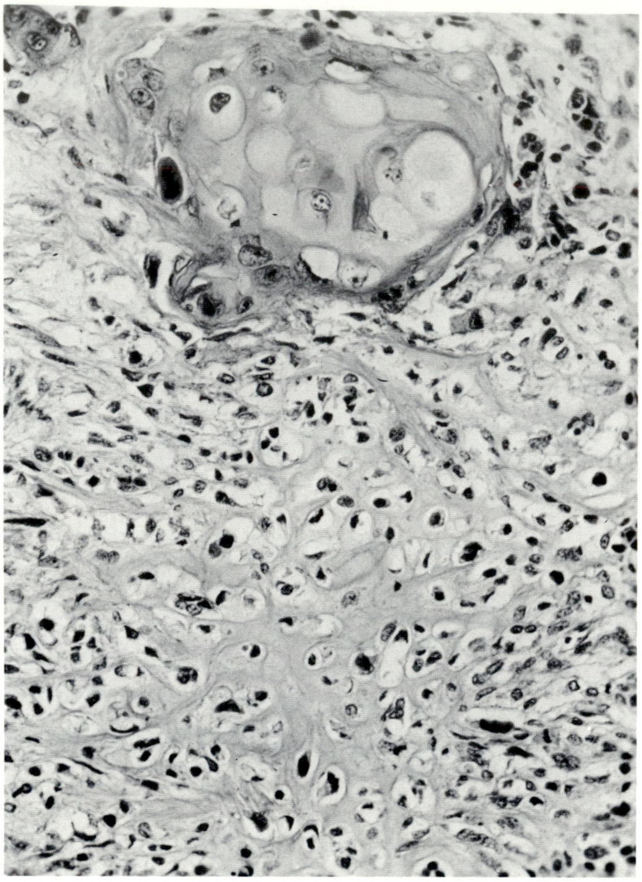

FIG. 13.39. Heterologous mixed müllerian tumor with cartilage (*center*) and squamous epithelium (*top*). [Reprinted with permission from The American College of Obstetricians and Gynecologists. (Obstetrics and Gynecology, 28: 57, 1966.)]

Poorly differentiated pleomorphic carcinomas are often misdiagnosed as carcinosarcomas. A malignant mesenchymal component must be present to establish the diagnosis of MMT and avoid that error. A reticulum stain may be of value, as reticulin fibers tend to surround individual cells or small groups of cells in the sarcomatous component of an MMT, whereas larger groups of cells are typically delineated by reticulin fibers in poorly differentiated carcinomas. Immunocytochemical studies (i.e., keratins, vimentin, desmin, and myoglobin) are capable of resolving this problem, and electron microscopic studies of the tumor may help establish differentiation toward sarcoma or epithelium.

Treatment and Prognosis. Methods of treatment for carcinosarcoma and mixed mesodermal tumor have varied, as have the end results. Five-year survival ranges from 20 to 40%.* The most significant prognostic factor is the extent of tumor when treated and, in those tumors confined to the uterus, the depth of myometrial invasion. Survival is nil when tumor has extended beyond the

* References 93, 95, 120, 135, 141, 149, 170.

uterus (stages III and IV).[117,137,138] Clinical staging underestimates the extent of disease in a significant proportion of patients with MMT. A surgical–pathologic staging system is a more accurate predictor of prognosis.[93,120,149] The relatively large proportion of cases (30–50%) in advanced stages at the time of diagnosis reflects the aggressive nature of the tumor.[10,25,107,108,117] Even those confined to the uterus have a poor 5-year survival rate in comparison to endometrial carcinoma of similar stage. Pathologists must record the depth of myometrial invasion, which is important not only in predicting the ultimate prognosis but also in determining the need for treatment of pelvic and para-aortic lymph nodes.[95] Pelvic lymph node metastases occur in one-third of patients with MMT invading more than halfway through the myometrium.[34,120] A superficial tumor is not a guarantee of survival, however, since many patients with such tumors experience recurrences.[80,141] Some MMTs have developed in an endometrial polyp, and all patients with such tumors have survived.[11,74] There is no difference in survival between patients with homologous and those with heterologous tumors,[†] and it is doubtful whether any morphologic feature of these tumors except the depth of myometrial invasion has prognostic value. About a third of MMTs contain estrogen or progesterone receptors, but the presence of receptors does not correlate with clinical behavior.[147] Too few patients have had hormonal therapy to know whether it has any effect.

Total abdominal hysterectomy and bilateral salpingo-oophorectomy should be performed for stage I and II MMTs. Most oncologists advocate a combined surgical and radiotherapeutic approach for treatment of patients with localized tumors.[50,117,137,168] Patients who are treated only with surgery have a higher frequency of recurrence in the pelvis than do patients who receive combined therapy.[*] In view of the likelihood of pelvic lymph node metastasis in patients with deep invasion of the myometrium by stage I tumors, external radiation should be administered to those patients as well. The pelvis was formerly the most frequent site of metastasis, but in recent studies of women who have been treated with pelvic radiation in addition to surgery, the lungs are the most frequent metastatic site, followed by the abdominal cavity and lymph nodes.[149] The histologic appearance of metastatic MMT is variable; epithelial and mesenchymal components are both present in about a third of metastases, a third are pure carcinoma, and a third are pure sarcoma.[25,107,108]

The prognosis is so poor for patients with stage III and IV tumors that, in some institutions, they are not subjected to extensive surgical procedures. Instead, they are treated with intracavitary and external irradiation, followed by chemotherapy.[117] Occasional patients are cured with this regimen, but survival rates are low.[138] Most patients fail with distant metastases or because of local growth.

The poor survival of patients treated with surgery and radiotherapy, despite control of disease in the pelvis, indicates that occult metastases are present at the time of operation in many patients, even those whose neoplasms are clinically stage I or II. The results in several series suggested the possibility of improved survival in patients with low-stage disease treated with systemic chemotherapy in conjunction with surgery and radiation.[10,95,120] Unfortunately, two prospective trials have failed to demonstrate improved survival in patients who received adjuvant chemotherapy.[60,113] No effective chemotherapy is available for advanced or recurrent MMT.[61,62,114]

Miscellaneous Mesenchymal Conditions

Adenomyosis and Adenomyoma

Adenomyosis is a common condition characterized pathologically by the presence of endometrial glands and stroma within the myometrium. Occurring mainly in perimenopausal women, it is detected in 15–20% of uteri.[160] The usual symptoms are abnormal bleeding and dysmenorrhea. The uterus is enlarged, and as adenomyosis is usually most extensive in the posterior wall, the latter is thickened. The cut surface of the myometrium is trabeculated and contains hemorrhagic foci, but a distinct tumor nodule is not present. Microscopically, there are endometrial glands and stroma within the myometrium (Fig. 13.40). The lower border of the endometrium is irregular and dips into the superficial myometrium. In order to avoid misclassifying a normal histologic finding as adenomyosis, some pathologists make the diagnosis only when the distance between the lower border of the endometrium and the adenomyosis exceeds one half of a low power field (about 2.5 mm). Adenomyosis exhibits a varied functional response to ovarian hormones. Proliferative glands and stroma are generally observed in the first half of the menstrual cycle. Adenomyosis may not respond to physiologic levels of progesterone, and secretory changes are frequently absent or incomplete during the second half of the cycle.

An adenomyoma is a circumscribed, nodular aggregate of smooth muscle, endometrial glands, and, usually, endometrial stroma. It may be located within the myometrium, or it may involve or originate in the endometrium and grow as a polyp. About 2% of endometrial polyps are adenomyomas. A rare variant of the adenomyoma, the atypical polypoid adenomyoma, appears as an endometrial polyp in premenopausal women (see Chapter

† References 10, 25, 93, 113, 120, 134, 141, 149, 170, 173.
* References 50, 117, 138, 149, 168, 170.

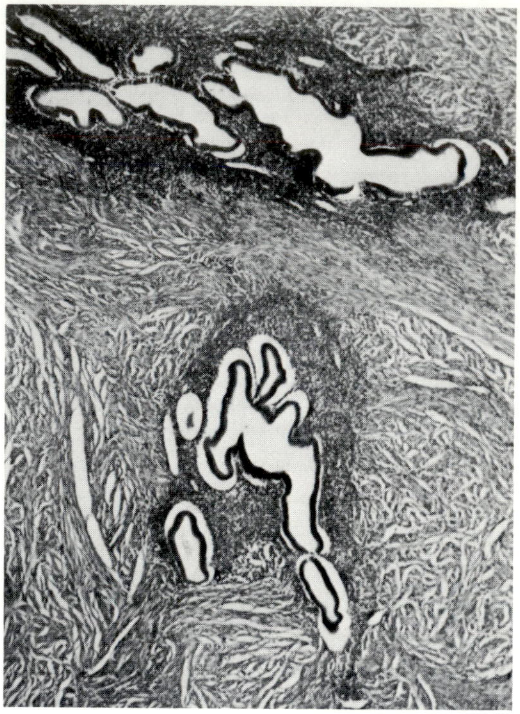

FIG. 13.40. Adenomyosis, showing endometrial glands and stroma within the myometrium.

9, Benign Diseases of the Uterine Corpus).[97] When detected in endometrial curettings, its atypical features may prompt a diagnosis of carcinoma. The atypical polypoid adenomyoma is composed of atypical endometrial glands surrounded by smooth muscle; endometrial stroma is not identified at the light microscopic level. The glands are irregular and hyperplastic and are lined by cells with enlarged, hyperchromatic nuclei and prominent nucleoli. Squamous metaplasia is invariably present. The smooth muscle stroma is benign. All reported examples have followed a benign clinical evolution, but there was residual adenomyoma in the endometrium of two of three patients treated by hysterectomy.[97] Careful follow-up is required if the patient is treated by curettage rather than hysterectomy.

Adenomatoid Mesothelioma

In 1945, Golden and Ash proposed the term *adenomatoid tumor* for a distinctive neoplasm of the genital tract previously described under a variety of terms (lymphangiocystic fibroma, lymphangioma, adenomatoid tumor, adenofibroma, adenoma, and mesothelioma).[55] The term adenomatoid tumor has been gradually supplanted by the name *adenomatoid mesothelioma* as histochemical and ultrastructural evidence relating these neoplasms to mesothelium has accumulated.

Clinical Aspects. Adenomatoid mesotheliomas are usually incidental findings in a uterus removed for other causes. About 1% of uteri contain an adenomatoid tumor, but no specific symptoms are attributable to them.[160] Less than 10% are multiple. The tumors are independent of any other pelvic condition. Women with adenomatoid tumors are usually of reproductive age, with a median age of 42 years.[181] There is no known racial predilection or evidence of impairment of fertility.

Gross and Microscopic Pathology. Adenomatoid mesotheliomas typically measure 0.5–1 cm in diameter and are gray, round, and rubbery, with ill-defined margins. Usually subserosal and located near the cornu, they often resemble leiomyomas or adenomyomas.[179] Small, uniform cystic spaces may be visible. One-half of the reported cases have occurred in the uterus, with most of the others found in the fallopian tube.[160,181] The uterine adnexal ligaments, ovary, and omentum are less common sites.

Microscopically, adenomatoid mesotheliomas consist of spaces lined by flat or cuboidal cells surrounded by a stroma rich in collagen, elastic tissue, and smooth muscle. The smooth muscle fibers may be so prominent that the lesion appears at first glance to be a leiomyoma. Spaces lined by flattened cells resemble lymphatic vessels, reflecting the capacity of mesothelium to resemble endothelium. The cuboidal cells within the lesion are often arranged in cords and tubules. Abundant cytoplasm, round eccentric nuclei, and vacuolation of the cytoplasm may be prominent. The cells may have the appearance of signet cells, producing confusion with metastatic signet-ring cell carcinoma. Nuclear atypia, however, is absent or minimal, and mitotic figures are usually very infrequent. Adenomatoid mesotheliomas may resemble angiomas, but the spaces lack blood. Adenomatoid mesotheliomas of the uterus have a similar appearance to those occurring in the ovary and broad ligament (see Chapter 21, Nonspecific Ovarian Tumors).

Histochemically, the cystic spaces in the tumor contain hyaluronic acid.[181] Mucicarmine stains are negative. Immunocytochemical studies reveal that the tumor cells contain cytokeratin, and electron microscopy displays cells with basal nuclei, dilated intercellular spaces, microvilli, and bundles of cytoplasmic filaments, all characteristics of mesothelial cells.*

Hemangioma and Angiosarcoma

The most common vascular tumor of the uterus is the capillary hemangioma of the cervix. Diffuse ramifying hemangiomas of the corpus occur (Figs. 13.41 and 13.42) but are very rare. Some hemangiomas, identified in cu-

* References 12, 29, 45, 101, 133, 136, 154, 179.

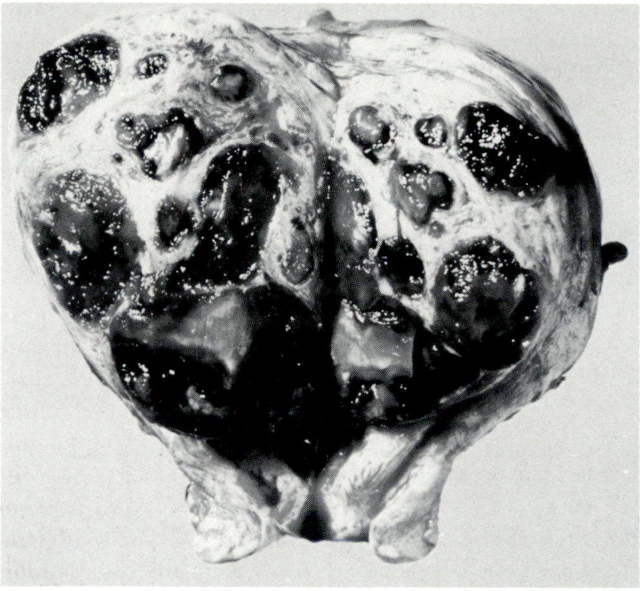

FIG. 13.41. Hemangioma of uterus. Abnormal vessels may extend beyond the uterus.

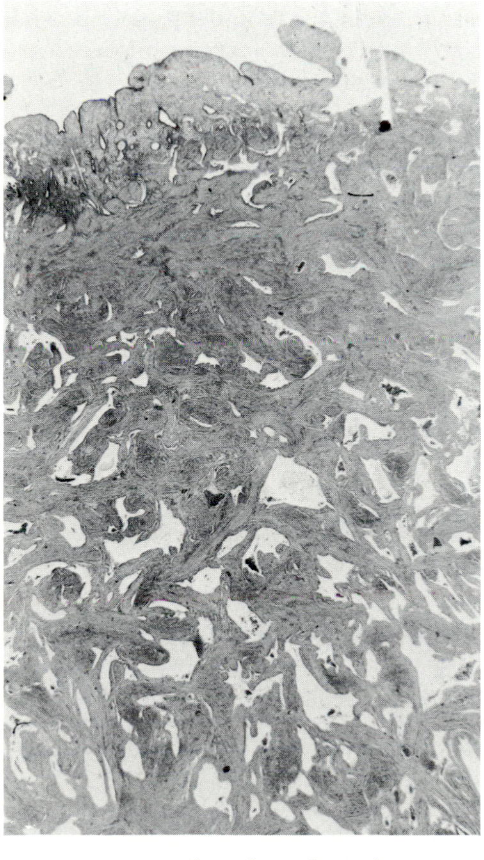

FIG. 13.42. Angioma extending throughout the myometrium.

rettings by markedly dilated capillary and sinusoidal spaces, may extend through the myometrium and into the broad ligament. In these cases, curettage may lead to bleeding that is difficult to control except by a hysterectomy, which may also be associated with marked blood loss. Rarely, a malignant vascular tumor occurs in the uterus.[36,115] Composed of anastomosing vascular channels lined by atypical endothelial cells, angiosarcomas infiltrate the myometrium. Solid growth patterns occur in poorly differentiated angiosarcomas. These neoplasms have a similar appearance to those in the ovary (see Chapter 21, Nonspecific Ovarian Tumors).

Hemangiopericytoma

The entity most often reported as hemangiopericytoma of the uterus is a misidentified endometrial stromal tumor. Few neoplasms reported as examples of hemangiopericytoma of the uterus have closely resembled the hemangiopericytoma of the soft tissues and retroperitoneum.[37] Nonetheless, there is no theoretical reason why a hemangiopericytoma should not occur in the uterus, and the case reported by Silverberg et al.[145] qualifies on histologic and ultrastructural grounds.

The difference between a bona fide hemangiopericytoma and endometrial stromal sarcoma needs emphasis. In hemangiopericytoma, round and ovoid cells are enmeshed in reticulin. The vascular spaces have more irregularity in the caliber of the lumen, and there is a more variable thickness of the vessel wall. The numerous gaping sinusoidal vascular channels and the staghorn configuration of the vascular spaces observed in hemangiopericytoma are not found in endometrial stromal tumors. In hemangiopericytoma, the cells are more spindle shaped and fibroblastic, and there is more intervening collagen than in a typical endometrial stromal tumor. Hemangiopericytomas, unlike endometrial stromal tumors, may show extensive myxoid change. The ultrastructural appearance of the cells of a hemangiopericytoma differs only slightly from that of the cells in an endometrial stromal tumor, both being relatively simple, primitive-appearing cells with few specific ultrastructural characteristics. Pericytes within a hemangiopericytoma tend to be more elongated and contain more cytoplasmic fibrils, and unlike stromal cells, pericytes have a well-defined basal lamina and pinocytotic vesicles on the cell surface away from the endothelium.

Pseudotumor of the Uterus

In the female genital tract, postoperative spindle cell nodules occur most frequently in the vagina,[128] but very rare examples arise in the cervix. The nodules are detected 1–3 months after surgery, grow rapidly, and attain a size of up to 4 cm. Microscopically, they are composed of fascicles of plump spindle cells separated by an edematous stroma containing small blood vessels, chronic inflammatory cells, and small foci of hemorrhage. The nuclei are pale, but numerous mitotic figures are present, which raises the question of leiomyosarcoma. Electron microscopy reveals that the proliferating cells are active fibroblasts, and none of the reported examples has recurred despite inadequate treatment for a sarcoma.[128] Correct diagnosis depends on knowledge of the clinical history and recognition of the characteristic histology, including, notably, the absence of significant nuclear atypia or atypical mitotic figures.

Lymphoma

Lymphoma rarely occurs with uterine involvement as the initial sign or symptom, but when it does, the cervix is the presenting site three times more often than is the endometrium.[23,64] Lymphomas occur predominantly in women aged 20 years or older. The major complaints are an abdominal or pelvic mass, abnormal vaginal bleeding, vaginal discharge, and pelvic discomfort.[23,64] Lymphomas involving the uterus are staged by gynecologic staging criteria and also by a lymphoma-staging classification. The lymphoma is usually a diffuse large cell (histiocytic) or a follicular small, cleaved (poorly differentiated) lymphocytic type.[64] Hodgkin's disease virtually never involves the uterus. The prognosis of lymphoma presenting in the uterus is more favorable than that of lymphoma presenting in the ovary. An 89% survival rate was reported in patients with localized (Ann Arbor stage IE) lymphoma of the uterus and vagina.[64] In women with lymphoma and intact reproductive organs at necropsy, the cervix is involved in 6% and the uterine corpus is involved in 10% of cases. Leukemic infiltrates occur in the uterus in 41% of necropsied women with leukemia and retained reproductive organs, but uterine involvement as an initial manifestation of leukemia is more rare than lymphoma at that site.[23,77]

References

1. Aaro LA, Symmonds RE, Dockerty MB (1966) Sarcoma of the uterus. A clinical and pathologic study of 177 cases. Am J Obstet Gynecol 94: 101
2. Abell MR (1971) Papillary adenofibroma of the uterine cervix. Am J Obstet Gynecol 110: 990
3. Abell MR, Littler ER (1975) Benign metastasizing uterine leiomyoma: Multiple lymph nodal metastases. Cancer 36: 2206
4. Abell MR, Ramirez JA (1973) Sarcomas and carcinosarcomas of the uterine cervix. Cancer 31: 1176
5. Akhtar M, Kim PY, Young I (1975) Ultrastructure of endometrial stromal sarcoma. Cancer 35: 406
6. Aterman K, Fraser GM, Lea RH (1977) Disseminated peritoneal leiomyomatosis. Virchows Arch [Pathol Anat] 374: 13
7. Babaknia A, Rock JA, Jones HW Jr (1978) Pregnancy success following abdominal myomectomy for infertility. Fertil Steril 30: 644
8. Baker VV, Walton LA, Fowler WC Jr, Currie JL, et al. (1984) Steroid receptors in endolymphatic stromal myosis. Obstet Gynecol 63: 72s
9. Barter JF, Smith EB, Szpak CA, Hinshaw W, et al. (1984) Leiomyosarcoma of the uterus: Clinicopathologic study of 21 cases. Gynecol Oncol 21: 220
10. Barwick KW, LiVolsi VA (1979) Malignant mixed müllerian tumors of the uterus. A clinicopathologic assessment of 34 cases. Am J Surg Pathol 3: 125
11. Barwick KW, LiVolsi VA (1979) Heterologous mixed müllerian tumor confined to an endometrial polyp. Obstet Gynecol 53: 512
12. Barwick KW, Madri JA (1982) An immunohistochemical study of adenomatoid tumors utilizing keratin and factor VIII antibodies: Evidence for a mesothelial origin. Lab Invest 47: 276
13. Becker SN, Wong JY (1981) Detection of endometrial stromal sarcoma in cervicovaginal smears: Report of three cases. Acta Cytol 25: 272
14. Berkowitz RS, Ehrmann RL, Knapp RC (1978) Endometrial stromal sarcoma arising from vaginal endometriosis. Obstet Gynecol [Suppl] 51: 34s
15. Bibro MC, LiVolsi VA, Schwartz PE (1979) Adenosarcoma of the uterus: Ultrastructural observations. Am J Clin Pathol 71: 112
16. Bird CC, Willis RA (1965) The production of smooth muscle by the endometrial stroma of the adult human uterus. J Pathol Bacteriol 90: 75
17. Bocker W, Stegner HE (1975) Mixed müllerian tumors of the uterus. Ultrastructural studies on the differentiation of rhabdomyoblasts. Virchows Arch [Pathol Anat] 365: 337
18. Bocker W, Stegner HE (1975) A light and electron microscopic study of endometrial sarcomas of the uterus. Virchows Arch [Pathol Anat] 368: 141
19. Bocker W, Strecker H (1975) Electron microscopy of uterine leiomyosarcomas. Virchows Arch [Pathol Anat] 367: 59
20. Briscoe CC (1964) Acute hemorrhagic degeneration of a leiomyoma following norethindrone acetate. Report of a case. Obstet Gynecol 23: 279
21. Burns B, Curry HR, Bell MEA (1979) Morphologic features of prognostic significance in uterine smooth muscle tumors: A review of eighty-four cases. Am J Obstet Gynecol 135: 109
22. Chen KTK (1984) Myxoid leiomyosarcoma of the uterus. Int J Gynecol Pathol 3: 389
23. Chorlton I, Karnei RF Jr, King FA, Norris HJ (1974) Primary malignant reticuloendothelial disease involving the vagina, cervix and corpus uteri. Obstet Gynecol 44: 735
24. Christopherson WM, Williamson EO, Gray LA (1972) Leiomyosarcoma of the uterus. Cancer 29: 1512
25. Chuang JT, VanVelden DJJ, Graham JB (1970) Carcinosar-

coma and mixed mesodermal tumor of the uterine corpus. Review of 49 cases. Obstet Gynecol 35: 769
26. Clement PB (1978) Chondrosarcoma of the uterus: Report of a case and a review of the literature. Hum Pathol 9: 726
27. Clement PB, Scully RE (1974) Müllerian adenosarcoma of the uterus. A clinicopathologic analysis of ten cases of a distinctive type of müllerian mixed tumor. Cancer 34: 1138
28. Clement PB, Scully RE (1976) Uterine tumors resembling ovarian sex-cord tumors. A clinicopathologic analysis of fourteen cases. Am J Clin Pathol 66: 512
29. Craig JR, Hart WR (1979) Extragenital adenomatoid tumor. Evidence for the mesothelial theory of origin. Cancer 43: 1678
30. Crum CP, Rogers BH, Andersen W (1980) Osteosarcoma of the uterus: Case report and review of the literature. Gynecol Oncol 9: 256
31. Darby AJ, Papadaki L, Beilby JOW (1975) An unusual leiomyosarcoma of the uterus containing osteoclast-like giant cells. Cancer 36: 495
32. Demopoulos RI, Denarvaez F, Kaji V (1973) Benign mixed mesodermal tumors of the uterus. A histogenetic study. Am J Clin Pathol 60: 377
33. Dharkar DD, Kraft JR, Gangadharam D (1981) Uterine lipomas. Arch Pathol Lab Med 105: 43
34. DiSaia PJ, Morrow CP, Boronow R, Creasman W, et al. (1978) Endometrial sarcoma: Lymphatic spread pattern. Am J Obstet Gynecol 130: 104
35. Doolan JJ Jr (1969) Endometrial sarcoma in a 14-year old girl. Am J Obstet Gynecol 103: 909
36. Ehrmann RL, Griffiths CT (1979) Malignant hemangioendothelioma of the uterus. Gynecol Oncol 8: 376
37. Enzinger FM, Smith BH (1976) Hemangiopericytoma. An analysis of 106 cases. Hum Pathol 7: 61
38. Evans AT III, Symmonds RE, Gaffey TA (1981) Recurrent pelvic intravenous leiomyomatosis. Obstet Gynecol 57: 260
39. Evans HL (1982) Endometrial sarcoma and poorly differentiated endometrial sarcoma. Cancer 50: 2170
40. Farrer-Brown G, Beilby JOW, Rowles PM (1970) Microvasculature of the uterus. An injection method of study. Obstet Gynecol 35: 21
41. Fechner RE (1968) Atypical leiomyomas and synthetic progestin therapy. Am J Clin Pathol 49: 697
42. Fechner RE, Bossart MI, Spjut HJ (1979) Ultrastructure of endometrial stromal foam cells. Am J Clin Pathol 72: 628
43. Fehr PE, Prem KA (1974) Malignancy of the uterine corpus following irradiation therapy for squamous cell carcinoma of the cervix. Am J Obstet Gynecol 119: 685
44. Fekete PS, Vellios F (1984) The clinical and histologic spectrum of endometrial stromal neoplasms: A report of 41 cases. Int J Gynecol Pathol 3: 198
45. Ferenczy A, Fenoglio J, Richart RM (1972) Observations on benign mesothelioma of the genital tract (adenomatoid tumor). A comparative ultrastructural study. Cancer 30: 244
46. Ferenczy A, Richart RM, Okagaki T (1971) A comparative ultrastructural study of leiomyosarcoma, cellular leiomyoma, and leiomyoma of the uterus. Cancer 28: 1004
47. Fox H, Harilal KR, Youell A (1979) Müllerian adenosarcoma of the uterine body: A report of nine cases. Histopathology 3: 167
48. Frankel T, Benjamin F (1973) Rapid enlargement of a uterine fibroid after clomiphene therapy. J Obstet Gynaecol Br Commonw 80: 764
49. Gallop DG, Cordray DR (1979) Leiomyosarcoma of the uterus: Case reports and a review. Obstet Gynecol Surv 34: 300
50. Gilbert HA, Kagan AR, Lagasse L, Jacobs MR, et al. (1975) The value of radiation therapy in uterine sarcoma. Obstet Gynecol 45: 84
51. Gisser SD, Young I (1977) Neurilemoma-like uterine myomas: An ultrastructural reaffirmation of their non-Schwannian nature. Am J Obstet Gynecol 129: 389
52. Gloor E (1979) Müllerian adenosarcoma of the uterus. Clinicopathologic study of five cases. Am J Surg Pathol 3: 203
53. Gloor E, Schnyder P, Cikes M, Hofstetter J, et al. (1982) Endolymphatic stromal myosis: Surgical and hormonal treatment of extensive abdominal recurrence 20 years after hysterectomy. Cancer 50: 1888
54. Goldberg MF, Hurt WG, Frable WJ (1977) Leiomyomatosis peritonealis disseminata. Report of a case and review of the literature. Obstet Gynecol [Suppl] 49: 46s
55. Golden A, Ash JE (1945) Adenomatoid tumors of the genital tract. Am J Pathol 21: 63
56. Goldzieher JW, Maqueo M, Ricaud L, Aguilar JA, et al. (1966) Induction of degenerative changes in uterine myomas by high-dosage progestin therapy. Am J Obstet Gynecol 96: 1078
57. Goodhue WW, Susin M, Kramer EE (1974) Smooth muscle origin of uterine plexiform tumors. Arch Pathol 97: 263
58. Grimalt M, Arguelles M, Ferenczy A (1975) Papillary cystadenofibroma of endometrium: A histochemical and ultrastructural study. Cancer 36: 137
59. Gruenwald P (1943) Developmental basis of regenerative and pathological growth in the uterus. Arch Pathol 35: 53
60. Hannigan EV, Freedman RS, Rutledge FN (1983) Adjuvant chemotherapy in early uterine sarcoma. Gynecol Oncol 15: 56
61. Hannigan EV, Freedman RS, Elder KW, Rutledge FN (1983) Treatment of advanced uterine sarcoma with vincristine, actinomycin D, and cyclophosphamide. Gynecol Oncol 15: 224
62. Hannigan EV, Freedman RS, Elder KW, Rutledge FN (1983) Treatment of advanced uterine sarcoma with adriamycin. Gynecol Oncol 16: 101
63. Harper RS, Scully RE (1961) Intravenous leiomyomatosis of the uterus. A report of four cases. Obstet Gynecol 18: 519
64. Harris NL, Scully RE (1984) Malignant lymphoma and granulocytic sarcoma of the uterus and vagina: A clinicopathologic analysis of 27 cases. Cancer 53: 2530
65. Hart WR, Billman JK Jr (1978) A reassessment of uterine

neoplasms originally diagnosed as leiomyosarcomas. Cancer 41: 1902
66. Hart WR, Craig JR (1978) Rhabdomyosarcomas of the uterus. Am J Clin Pathol 70: 217
67. Hart WR, Yoonessi M (1977) Endometrial stromatosis of the uterus. Obstet Gynecol 49: 393
68. Hendrickson MR, Kempson RL (1980) Surgical pathology of the uterine corpus. Philadelphia, WB Saunders
69. Herr JC, Platz CE, Heidger PM, Curet LB (1979) Smooth muscle within ovarian decidual nodules: A link to leiomyomatosis peritonealis disseminata? Obstet Gynecol 53: 451
70. Honore LH (1978) Uterine fibrolipoleiomyoma: Report of a case with discussion of histogenesis. Am J Obstet Gynecol 132: 635
71. Jacobs DS, Cohen H, Johnson JS (1965) Lipoleiomyomas of the uterus. Am J Clin Pathol 44: 45
72. Jensen PA, Dockerty MB, Symmonds RE, Wilson RB (1966) Endometrioid sarcoma ("stromal endometriosis"). Report of 15 cases including 5 with metastases. Am J Obstet Gynecol 95: 79
73. John AH, Martin R (1971) Growth of leiomyomata with estrogen–progestogen therapy. J Reprod Med 6: 56
74. Kahner S, Ferenczy A, Richart RM (1975) Homologous mixed müllerian tumors (carcinosarcoma) confined to endometrial polyps. Am J Obstet Gynecol 121: 278
75. Kaminski PF, Tavassoli FA (1984) Plexiform tumorlet: A clinical and pathologic study of 15 cases with ultrastructural observations. Int J Gynecol Pathol 3: 124
76. Kao GF, Norris HJ (1978) Benign and low-grade variants of mixed mesodermal tumor (adenosarcoma) of the ovary and adnexal region. Cancer 42: 1314
77. Kapadia SB, Krause JR, Kanbour AI, Hartsock RJ (1978) Granulocytic sarcoma of the uterus. Cancer 41: 687
78. Kaplan C, Benirschke K, Johnson KC (1980) Leiomyomatosis peritonealis disseminata with endometrium. Obstet Gynecol 55: 119
79. Katzenstein AA, Askin FB, Feldman PS (1977) Müllerian adenosarcoma of the uterus. An ultrastructural study of four cases. Cancer 40: 2233
80. Kempson RL, Bari W (1970) Uterine sarcomas. Classification, diagnosis, and prognosis. Hum Pathol 1: 331
81. Kerby IJ (1975) Stromal endometriosis. Clin Radiol 26: 99
82. King ME, Dickersin GR, Scully RE (1982) Myxoid leiomyosarcoma of the uterus: A report of six cases. Am J Surg Pathol 6: 589
83. Kofinas AD, Suarez J, Calame RJ, Chipeco Z (1984) Chondrosarcoma of the uterus. Gynecol Oncol 19: 231
84. Komorowski RA, Garancis JC, Clowry LJ Jr (1970) Fine structure of endometrial stromal sarcoma. Cancer 26: 1042
85. Koss LG, Spiro RH, Brunschwig A (1965) Endometrial stromal sarcoma. Surg Gynecol Obstet 121: 531
86. Krieger PD, Gusberg SB (1973) Endolymphatic stomal myosis—A grade I endometrial sarcoma. Gynecol Oncol 1: 299
87. Kurman RJ, Norris HJ (1976) Mesenchymal tumors of the uterus. VI. Epithelioid smooth muscle tumors including leiomyoblastoma and clear-cell leiomyoma. A clinical and pathologic analysis of 26 cases. Cancer 37: 1853.
88. Langlois PL (1970) The size of the normal uterus. J Reprod Med 4: 220
89. Lantta M, Kahanpaa K, Karkkainen J, Lehtovirta P, et al. (1984) Estradiol and progesterone receptors in two cases of endometrial stromal sarcoma. Gynecol Oncol 18: 233
90. Lapan B, Soloman L (1979) Diffuse leiomyomatosis of the uterus precluding myomectomy. Obstet Gynecol [Suppl] 53: 825
91. Lavin P, Hajdu SI, Foote FW Jr (1972) Gastric and extragastric leiomyoblastomas. Clinicopathologic study of 44 cases. Cancer 29: 305
92. Lewis PL, Lee ABH, Easler RE (1962) Myometrial hypertrophy. A clinical pathologic study and review of the literature. Am J Obstet Gynecol 84: 1032
93. Macasaet MA, Waxman M, Fruchter RG, Boyce J, et al. (1985) Prognostic factors in malignant mesodermal (Müllerian) mixed tumors of the uterus. Gynecol Oncol 20: 32
94. Maheux R, Guilloteau C, Lemay A, Bastide A, et al. (1985) Luteinizing hormone-releasing hormone agonist and uterine leiomyoma: a pilot study. Am J Obstet Gynecol 152: 1034
95. Marchese MJ, Liskow AS, Crum CP, McCaffrey RM, et al. (1984) Uterine sarcomas: A clinicopathologic study, 1965–1981. Gynecol Oncol 18: 299
96. Massoni EA, Hajdu SI (1984) Cytology of primary and metastatic uterine sarcomas. Acta Cytol 28: 93
97. Mazur MT (1981) Atypical polypoid adenomyomas of the endometrium. Am J Surg Pathol 5: 473
98. Mazur MT, Kraus FT (1980) Histogenesis of morphologic variations in tumors of the uterine wall. Am J Surg Pathol 4: 59
99. Mixson WT, Hammond DO (1961) Response of fibromyomas to a progestin. Am J Obstet Gynecol 82: 754
100. Morimoto N, Ozawa M, Kato Y, Kuramoto H (1982) Diagnostic value of mitotic activity in endometrial stromal sarcoma: Report of two cases. Acta Cytol 26: 695
101. Mucientes F, Govindarajan S, Burotto S (1985) Immunoperoxidase study on adenomatoid tumor of the epididymis using anti-mesothelial cell serum. Cancer 55: 363
102. Muram D, Gillieson M, Walters JH (1980) Myomas of the uterus in pregnancy: Ultrasonographic follow-up. Am J Obstet Gynecol 138: 16
103. Nogales FF Jr, Matilla A, Carrascal E (1978) Leiomyomatosis peritonealis disseminata. An ultrastructural study. Am J Clin Pathol 69: 452
104. Norris HJ, Parmley T (1975) Mesenchymal tumors of the uterus. V. Intravenous leiomyomatosis. A clinical and pathologic study of 14 cases. Cancer 36: 2164
105. Norris HJ, Taylor HB (1965) Postirradiation sarcomas of the uterus. Obstet Gynecol 26: 689
106. Norris HJ, Taylor HB (1966) Mesenchymal tumors of the uterus. I. A clinical and pathological study of 53 endometrial stromal tumors. Cancer 19: 755
107. Norris HJ, Taylor HB (1966) Mesenchymal tumors of the uterus. III. A clinical and pathologic study of 31 carcinosarcomas. Cancer 19: 1459
108. Norris HJ, Roth E, Taylor HB (1966) Mesenchymal tumors

of the uterus. II. A clinical and pathologic study of 31 mixed mesodermal tumors. Obstet Gynecol 28: 57
109. Nunez-Alonso C, Battifora HA (1979) Plexiform tumors of the uterus: Ultrastructural study. Cancer 44: 1707
110. Ober WB (1959) Uterine sarcomas: Histogenesis and taxonomy. Ann NY Acad Sci 75: 568
111. Oda Y, Nakanishi I, Tateiwa T (1984) Intramural müllerian adenosarcoma of the uterus with adenomyosis. Arch Pathol Lab Med 108: 798
112. Okagaki T, Brooker DC, Adcock LL, Prem KH (1979) Müllerian adenosarcoma of the uterus with rapid progression: An ultrastructural study. Gynecol Oncol 7: 361
113. Omura GA, Blessing JA, Major F, Lifshitz S, et al. (1985) A randomized clinical trial of adjuvant Adriamycin in uterine sarcomas: A Gynecologic Oncology Group study. J Clin Oncol 3: 1240
114. Omura GA, Major FJ, Blessing JA, Sedlacek TV, et al. (1983) A randomized study of Adriamycin with and without dimethyl triazenoimidazole carboxamide in advanced uterine sarcomas. Cancer 52: 626
115. Ongkasuwan C, Taylor JE, Tang C-K, Prempree T (1982) Angiosarcomas of the uterus and ovary: Clinicopathologic report. Cancer 49: 1469
116. Ostor AG, Fortune DW (1980) Benign and low-grade variants of mixed müllerian tumour of the uterus. Histopathology 4: 369
117. Perez CA, Askin F, Baglan RJ, Kao MS, et al. (1979) Effects of irradiation on mixed müllerian tumors of the uterus. Cancer 43: 1274
118. Persaud V, Anderson MF (1977) Endometrial stromal sarcoma of the broad ligament arising in an area of endometriosis in a paramesonephric cyst. Case report. Br J Obstet Gynaecol 84: 149
119. Persaud V, Arjoon PD (1970) Uterine leiomyoma. Incidence of degenerative change and a correlation of associated symptoms. Obstet Gynecol 35: 432
120. Peters WA III, Kumar NB, Fleming WP, Morley GW (1984) Prognostic features of sarcomas and mixed tumors of the endometrium. Obstet Gynecol 63: 550
121. Pieslor PC, Orenstein JM, Hogan DL, Breslow A (1979) Ultrastructure of myofibroblasts and decidualized cells in leiomyomatosis peritonealis disseminata. Am J Clin Pathol 72: 875
122. Piver MS, Rutledge FN, Copeland L, Webster K, et al (1984) Uterine endolymphatic stromal myosis: A collaborative study. Obstet Gynecol 64: 173
123. Pollow K, Geilfub J, Boquoi E, Pollow B (1978) Estrogen and progesterone binding proteins in normal human myometrium and leiomyoma tissue. J Clin Chem Clin Biochem 16: 503
124. Poulsen HE, Taylor CW (1978) Histological typing of female genital tract tumors. In: International Histological Classification of Tumours. Geneva, World Health Organization, Vol 13
125. Pounder DJ (1982) Fatty tumours of the uterus. J Clin Pathol 35: 1380
126. Prakash S, Scully RE (1964) Sarcoma-like pseudopregnancy changes in uterine leiomyomas: Report of a case resulting from prolonged norethindrone therapy. Obstet Gynecol 24: 106
127. Press MF, Nousek-Goebl N, King WJ, Herbst AL, et al. (1984) Immunohistochemical assessment of estrogen receptor distribution in the human endometrium throughout the menstrual cycle. Lab Invest 51: 495
128. Proppe KH, Scully RE, Rosai J (1984) Postoperative spindle cell nodules of genitourinary tract resembling sarcomas. A report of eight cases. Am J Surg Pathol 8: 101
129. Puukka MJ, Kontula KK, Kauppila AJI, Janne OA, et al. (1979) Estrogen receptor in human myoma tissue. Mol Cell Endocrinol 6: 35
130. Roth E, Taylor HB (1966) Heterotopic cartilage in the uterus. Obstet Gynecol 27: 838
131. Roth LM, Pride GL, Sharma HM (1976) Müllerian adenosarcoma of the uterine cervix with heterologous elements. A light and electron microscopic study. Cancer 37: 1725
132. Rywlin AM, Recher L, Benson J (1964) Clear cell leiomyoma of the uterus. Report of two cases of a previously undescribed entity. Cancer 17: 100
133. Said JW, Nash G, Lee M (1982) Immunoperoxidase localization of keratin proteins, carcinoembryonic antigen, and Factor VIII in adenomatoid tumors: Evidence for a mesothelial derivation. Hum Pathol 13: 1106
134. Sakamoto A, Sugano H (1976) Mixed mesodermal tumor of the uterine body: Relationship between histology and survival. Gann 67: 263
135. Saksela E, Lampinen V, Procope BJ (1974) Malignant mesenchymal tumors of the uterine corpus. Am J Obstet Gynecol 120: 452
136. Salazar H, Kanbour A, Burgess F (1972) Ultrastructure and observations on the histogenesis of mesotheliomas "adenomatoid tumors" of the female genital tract. Cancer 29: 141
137. Salazar OM, Bonfiglio TA, Patten SF, Keller BE, et al. (1978) Uterine sarcomas. Natural history, treatment and prognosis. Cancer 42: 1152
138. Salazar OM, Bonfiglio TA, Patten SF, Keller BE, et al. (1978) Uterine sarcomas. Analysis of failures with special emphasis on the use of adjuvant radiation therapy. Cancer 42: 1161
139. Schwartz Z, Dgani R, Lancet M, Kessler I (1985) Uterine sarcoma in Israel: A study of 104 cases. Gynecol Oncol 20: 354
140. Siegel GP, Taylor LL, Nelson KG, Reddick RL, et al. (1983) Characterization of a pure heterologous sarcoma of the uterus: Rhabdomyosarcoma of the corpus. Int J Gynecol Pathol 2: 303
141. Shaw RW, Lynch PF, Wade-Evans T (1983) Müllerian mixed tumour of the uterine corpus: A clinical histopathological review of 28 patients. Br J Obstet Gynaecol 90: 562
142. Silverberg SG (1971) Leiomyosarcoma of the uterus. A clinicopathologic study. Obstet Gynecol 38: 613
143. Silverberg SG (1971) Malignant mixed mesodermal tumor of the uterus: An ultrastructural study. Am J Obstet Gynecol 110: 702
144. Silverberg SG (1975) Adenomyomatosis of endometrium and endocervix—A hamartoma? Am J Clin Pathol 64: 192
145. Silverberg SG, Willson MA, Board JA (1971) Hemangio-

pericytoma of the uterus: An ultrastructural study. Am J Obstet Gynecol 110: 397
146. Smith JP, Rutledge F, Delclos L, Sutow W (1975) Combined irradiation and chemotherapy for sarcomas of the pelvis in females. Am J Roentgenol 123: 571
147. Soper JT, McCarty KS Jr, Hinshaw W, Creasman WT, et al. (1984) Cytoplasmic estrogen and progesterone receptor content of uterine sarcomas. Am J Obstet Gynecol 150: 342
148. Soules MR, McCarty KS Jr (1982) Leiomyomas: Steroid receptor content. Variation within normal menstrual cycles. Am J Obstet Gynecol 143: 6
149. Spanos WJ Jr, Wharton JT, Gomez L, Fletcher GH, et al. (1984) Malignant mixed müllerian tumors of the uterus. Cancer 53: 311
150. Tamaya T, Fujimoto J, Okada H (1985) Comparison of cellular levels of steroid receptors in uterine leiomyoma and myometrium. Acta Obstet Gynecol Scand 64: 307
151. Tang C, Toker C, Ances IG (1979) Stromomyoma of the uterus. Cancer 43: 308
152. Tavassoli FA, Norris HJ (1981) Mesenchymal tumors of the uterus. VII. A clinicopathological study of 60 endometrial stromal nodules. Histopathology 5: 1
153. Tavassoli FA, Norris HJ (1982) Peritoneal leiomyomatosis (leiomyomatosis peritonealis disseminata): A clinicopathologic study of 20 cases with ultrastructural observations. Int J Gynecol Pathol 1: 59
154. Taxy JB, Battifora H, Oyasu R (1974) Adenomatoid tumors: A light microscopic, histochemical, and ultrastructural study. Cancer 34: 306
155. Taylor HB, Norris HJ (1966) Mesenchymal tumors of the uterus. IV. Diagnosis and prognosis of leiomyosarcomas. Arch Pathol 82: 40
156. Thatcher SS, Woodruff JD (1982) Uterine stromatosis: A report of 33 cases. Obstet Gynecol 59: 428
157. Thomas WO Jr, Harris HH, Enden JA (1969) Postirradiation malignant neoplasms of the uterine fundus. Am J Obstet Gynecol 104: 209
158. Thompson JW III, Symmonds RE, Dockerty MB (1962) Benign uterine leiomyoma with vascular involvement. Report of three cases. Am J Obstet Gynecol 84: 182
159. Tierney WM, Ehrlich CE, Bailey JC, King RD, et al. (1980) Intravenous leiomyomatosis of the uterus with extension into the heart. Am J Med 69: 471
160. Tiltman AJ (1980) Adenomatoid tumours of the uterus. Histopathology 4: 437
161. Tiltman AJ (1985) The effect of progestins on the mitotic activity of uterine fibromyomas. Int J Gynecol Pathol 4: 89
162. Timmis AD, Smallpiece R, Davies AC, McCarthur AM, et al. (1980) Intracardiac spread of intravenous leiomyomatosis with successful surgical exploration. N Engl J Med 303: 1043
163. Tsukamoto N, Kamura T, Matsukuma K, Imachi M, et al. (1985) Endolymphatic stromal myosis: A case with positive estrogen and progesterone receptors and good response to progestins. Gynecol Oncol 20: 120
164. Vakiani M, Mawad J, Talerman A (1982) Heterologous sarcomas of the uterus. Int J Gynecol Pathol 2: 211
165. van Dinh T, Woodruff JD (1982) Leiomyosarcoma of the uterus. Am J Obstet Gynecol 144: 817
166. Varela-Duran J, Nochomovitz LE, Prem KA, Dehner LP (1980) Postirradiation mixed müllerian tumors of the uterus: A comparative clinicopathologic study. Cancer 45: 1625
167. Vellios F, Ng ABP, Reagan JW (1973) Papillary adenofibroma of the uterus: A benign mesodermal mixed tumor of müllerian origin. Am J Clin Pathol 60: 543
168. Vongtama V, Karlen JR, Piver SM, Tsukada Y, et al. (1976) Treatment, results and prognostic factors in stage I and II sarcomas of the corpus uteri. Am J Roetgenol 126: 139
169. Weiss DB, Aldor A, Aboulafia Y (1975) Erythrocytosis due to erythropoietin-producing uterine fibromyoma. Am J Obstet Gynecol 122: 358
170. Wheelock JB, Krebs H-B, Schneider V, Goplerud DR (1985) Uterine sarcoma: Analysis of prognostic variables in 71 cases. Am J Obstet Gynecol 151: 1016
171. Willen R, Gad A, Willen H (1978) Lipomatous lesions of the uterus. Virchows Arch [Pathol Anat] 377: 351
172. Williams LJ Jr, Pavlick FJ (1980) Leiomyomatosis peritonealis disseminata. Two case reports and a review of the medical literature. Cancer 45: 1726
173. Williamson EO, Christopherson WM (1972) Malignant mixed müllerian tumors of the uterus. Cancer 29: 585
174. Williamson JG, Patel D, Menzies DN (1972) Leiomyomata of the uterus associated with ascites and hydrothorax. J Obstet Gynaecol Br Commonw 79: 273
175. Wilson EA, Yang F, Rees ED (1980) Estradiol and progesterone binding in uterine leiomyomata and in normal uterine tissues. Obstet Gynecol 55: 20
176. Winn KJ, Woodruff JD, Parmley TH (1976) Electron microscopic studies: Leiomyomatosis peritonealis disseminata. Obstet Gynecol 48: 225
177. Wisot AL, Neimand KM, Rosenthal AH (1969) Symptomatic myoma in a 13-year-old girl. Am J Obstet Gynecol 105: 639
178. Wolff M, Kaye G, Silva F (1979) Pulmonary metastases (with admixed epithelial elements) from smooth muscle neoplasms. Am J Surg Pathol 3: 325
179. Wood C, Bouchelle WH (1978) Benign mesothelioma simulating a uterine leiomyoma. Am J Obstet Gynecol 132: 225
180. Yoonessi M, Hart WR (1977) Endometrial stromal sarcomas. Cancer 40: 898
181. Youngs LA, Taylor HB (1967) Adenomatoid tumors of the uterus and fallopian tube. Am J Clin Pathol 48: 537
182. Zaloudek CJ, Norris HJ (1981) Adenofibroma and adenosarcoma of the uterus. A clinicopathologic study of 35 cases. Cancer 48: 354
183. Zaloudek CJ, Norris HJ (1981) Mesenchymal tumors of the uterus. In: Fenoglio CM, Wolff M (eds), Progress in surgical pathology. New York, Masson, Vol III, pp 1–35, Masson Publishing USA, Inc., 1981

14

Diseases of the Fallopian Tube

James E. Wheeler, M.D.

The function of the fallopian tube, transport of sperm and ovum, may be seriously compromised or entirely destroyed by inflammatory processes or tubal pregnancy. Tumors may interfere with normal function or, if malignant, may lead to death. The etiology and pathophysiology of many tubal diseases are imperfectly understood at present. Progress can take place only with a thorough knowledge of normal anatomy, histology, and physiology.

Anatomy

The normal fallopian tube extends from the area of its corresponding ovary anteriorly and medially to its terminus in the posterosuperior aspect of the uterine fundus. In an adult during the reproductive years, its length is usually between 9 and 11 cm. The tube at the ovarian end opens to the peritoneal cavity and is composed of about 25 irregular finger-like extensions of the tube, the fimbriae. The fimbriae attach to the expanded end of the tube, the infundibulum, which is about 1 cm long and 1 cm in diameter distally. The infundibulum lies within a few mm of the superolateral or tubal end of the ovary. It narrows gradually to about 4 mm in diameter and merges medially with the ampullary portion of the tube, which extends about 6 cm, passing anteriorly as it loops around the ovary. At a point characterized by relative thickening of the muscular wall, the isthmic portion begins and extends some 2 cm to the uterus. Within the myometrium, the tube extends as a 1 cm long intramural segment until it joins the extension of the endometrial cavity at the uterotubal junction.[136]

Throughout its extrauterine course, the tube lies in a peritoneal fold along the superior margin of the broad ligament, the mesosalpinx. The arterial blood supply has a dual origin. A tubal branch of the uterine artery passes in the mesosalpinx laterally from the cornu of the uterus to anastomose with tubal branches of the ovarian artery. Venous drainage parallels the arterial supply via anastomosing tubal branches of uterine and ovarian veins, also located in the mesosalpinx. Tubal lymphatics pass laterally, accompanying the ovarian vessels. Thence, on the right side, lymph drains into nodes in the area of the right renal vein and the inferior vena cava, whereas on the left side, lymph drains into nodes lying between the left ovarian vein and the left renal vein. Lymph also drains into presacral and common iliac nodes. It is apparent that lymphatic spread of tubal malignancy may reach extrapelvic sites in its dissemination.[173]

The nerve supply of the tube is both sympathetic and parasympathetic. Sympathetic fibers from T_{10} through L_2 synapse in the celiac, aortic, renal, inferior mesenteric, cervicovaginal, and possibly presacral plexuses. Postsynaptic fibers pass into the myosalpinx, where they provide adrenergic innervation to the smooth muscle. The fact that isthmic and ampullary tubal muscle is innervated via presacral and ovarian plexuses, respectively, provides a possible neural explanation for differential myosalpingeal activity and formation of a physiologic sphincter. Sensory pain fibers pass along with the sympathetic nerves to the spinal cord at the level of T_{10}–T_{12}. Parasympathetic fibers from the vagus nerve supply the extrauterine tube via postganglionic fibers from the ovarian plexus, whereas the intramural portion is innervated via S_{2-4} parasympathetic fibers synapsing in the pelvic plexuses.[44]

Histology

A mucosal membrane, a wall of smooth muscle, and a serosal coat make up the three histologic layers of the tube. The serosa is lined by flattened mesothelial cells. Beneath the mesothelium lies a small amount of connective tissue containing a few collagen fibers and blood vessels. The tubal muscularis generally has two layers: an outer longitudinal layer and an inner circular layer. At the uterine end, beginning in the intramural tube and extending laterally about 2 cm, there is, in addition, an inner longitudinal layer. The outer longitudinal layer is easily overlooked, as it is composed of inconspicuous bundles of smooth muscle interspersed with loose connective tissue containing numerous small blood vessels. The circular layer forms the major muscle mass of the tube. Its thickness varies, being about 0.5 mm in the isthmus and only about 0.1 mm in the ampulla.

The mucosal layer lies directly on the muscularis. It

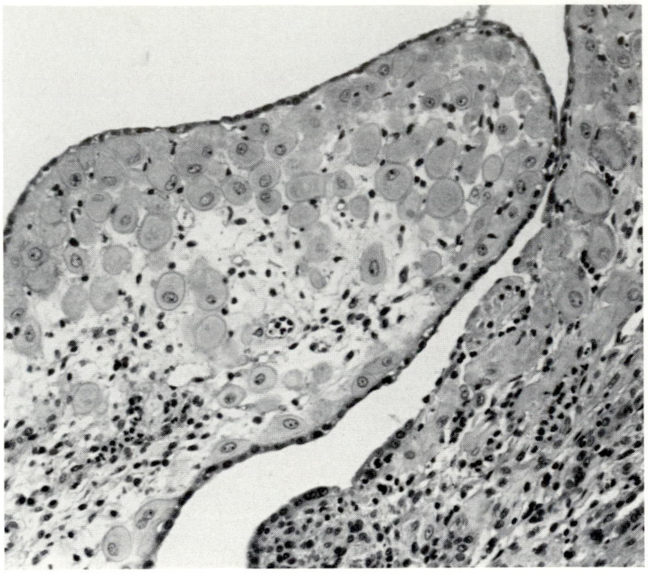

FIG. 14.1. Decidual reaction in tubal mucosa. The endosalpingeal folds are expanded by oval decidualized stromal cells characterized by well defined cytoplasmic membranes.

consists of a luminal epithelial lining and a scanty underlying lamina propria containing vessels and spindly or angular cells. Although these stromal cells seem sparse, they are the cells that lead to focally recognizable decidua in 5–12% of pregnancies (Fig. 14.1).[101,218] The mucosa increases significantly in its gross structural complexity as the lumen enlarges from uterine to ovarian end. The interstitial and intramural portions each contain about five or six blunt plicae, or folds. In the isthmus, the plicae increase in height to more nearly occupy the larger lumen. A dozen or more plicae, some with secondary folds, are present. In the ampulla, the plicae are frond-like and delicate, and both secondary and tertiary branches may be appreciated. The infundibular plical pattern is similar.

The epithelial layer of the mucosa is composed of at least three histologic cell types: ciliated, secretory, and intercalary.[165] About 20–30% of the cells contain prominent cilia,[63] and about 55–65% are secretory (Fig. 14.2). Although investigators[72] have found the ciliated cells in humans to be apparently randomly and equally distributed throughout the isthmic, ampullary, and fimbriated portions, others[160] have found ciliated cells numerous and preferentially located at the apical portions of the plicae, especially in the fimbriae and ampulla. Ciliated cells in the isthmus are less frequent[61] and occur in short strands. Ciliated cells are even scantier in the intramural tubal segment.

The ciliated cell itself is columnar and approximately 20–30 μm long.[73] Electron microscopic study reveals typical ciliary basal bodies and rootlets.[73] The nucleus is oval to round, about 8–10 μm in greatest extent, and

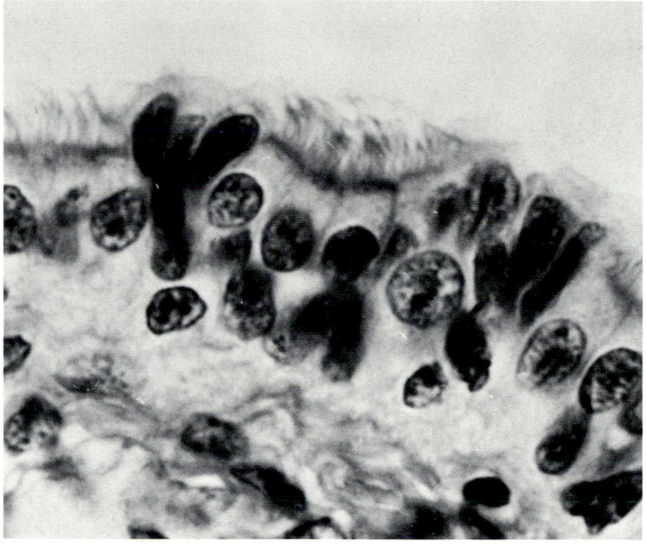

FIG. 14.2. Tubal epithelium. Ciliated cells are numerous. Secretory cells with columnar, somewhat compressed nuclei protrude above the level of the ciliated cells. Note vacuolated apical cytoplasm of secretory cells.

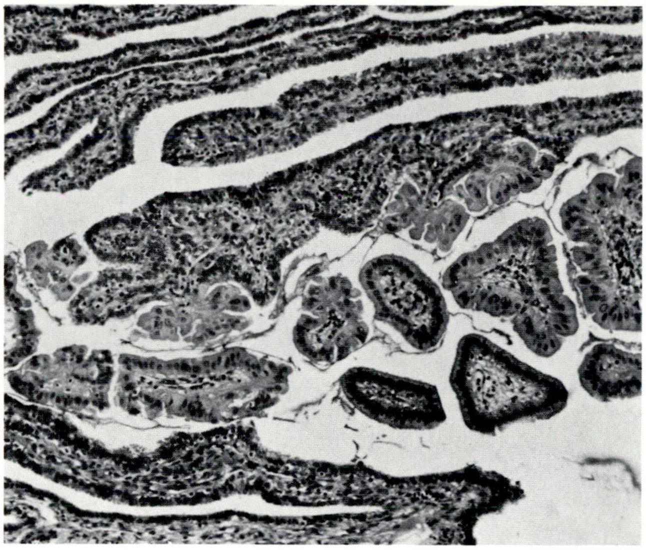

FIG. 14.3. Benign oncocytic (pink cell) metaplasia. Cells with prominent eosinophilic cytoplasm form papillary projections or line modestly distorted plicae. Scattered lymphocytes are present in plicae.

may lie parallel or perpendicular to the long axis of the cell. The chromatin pattern is moderately granular. A distinct but small nucleolus is present.

The secretory cell is also columnar, approximately the same height as the ciliated cell but often narrower (Fig. 14.2). Its nucleus is ovoid and perpendicular to the long axis of the cell. The chromatin pattern may be somewhat denser than that of the ciliated cell, but its nucleolus is similar.

The intercalary, or peg cell is a columnar cell that appears to be occupied mainly by a thin, dark-staining nucleus. It is likely a morphologic variant of the secretory cell.[154]

In addition to the three epithelial types described, a basally located cell with a rounded nucleus and dark-staining chromatin is present. Although this cell has been postulated to be a reserve cell and precursor of the other cell types,[164] electron microscopic evidence indicates that most, if not all, of these cells are actually lymphocytes.[155]

The tubal epithelium may undergo metaplastic changes without apparent reason. The metaplastic cells may be squamous or may be columnar and mucin secreting, resembling endocervical epithelium.[164,233] Mucinous metaplasia may be associated with the Peutz-Jeghers syndrome.[74] Oncocytic metaplasia with marked cytoplasmic eosinophilia on routine H & E staining may occur. When associated with chronic salpingitis and papillary changes (Fig. 14.3), it is occasionally interpreted as a benign neoplasm.[180] Studies delineating the usual extent of epithelial variability demonstrate that focal nuclear crowding and tufting are frequent and normal (Fig. 14.4), but mitoses occur infrequently.

Psammoma bodies are an occasional finding in chronic salpingitis but may be seen in otherwise normal appearing epithelium (Fig. 14.5). A unique case with accumulation of lipofuscin in macrophages in the lamina propria has been reported as *pigmentosis tubae*.[103]

The wolffian or mesonephic duct develops in close proximity to the fallopian tube, and remnants from it normally persist throughout adult life. These remnants consist of 10–15 mesonephric tubules lying in the mesovarium. The tubules are lined by low columnar or cuboi-

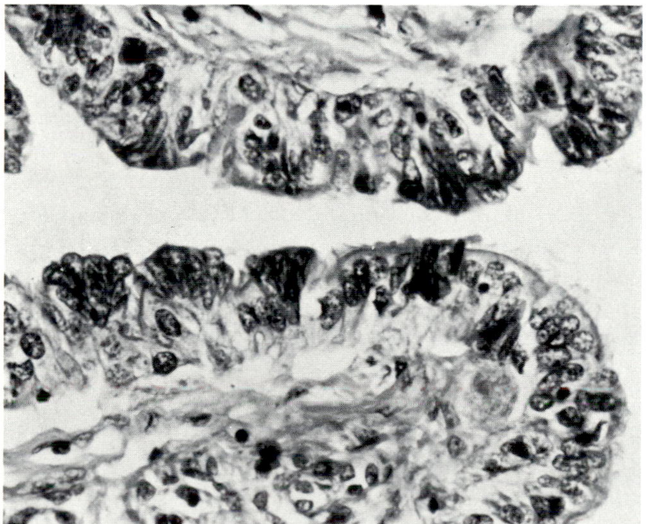

FIG. 14.4. Tubal epithelium. Crowding of nuclei and tufting of epithelial cells is a normal variant.

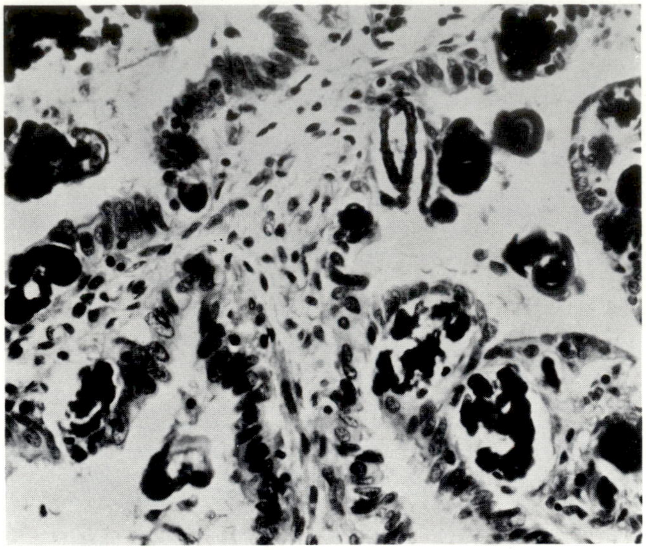

FIG. 14.5. Psammoma bodies in tubal epithelium. These calcific bodies may be found in chronic salpingitis or in relatively normal epithelium containing only rare lymphocytes.

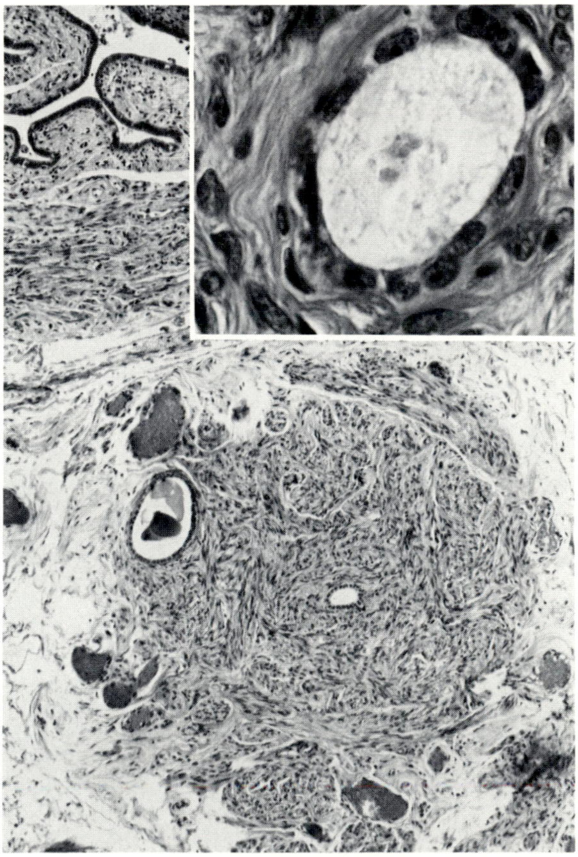

FIG. 14.6. Mesonephric duct remnants. These embryologic rests are commonly found on routine cross-sections. Note tubal lumen and muscle in *upper left corner*. The nodule of mesonephric remnants (*center*) is composed of simple tubules surrounded by an irregular smooth muscle mass. *Inset:* The tubules are lined by low cuboidal to low columnar cells.

dal epithelium containing ciliated and nonciliated cells. There is only a thin, if any, muscular coat.[20] The tubules connect with the mesonephric duct, which runs parallel to the fallopian tube in the mesosalpinx. The duct is lined by non-ciliated cuboidal or columnar cells surrounded by a relatively thick layer of first longitudinal and then circular smooth muscle. It is commonly seen on routine histologic cross-sections of tube lying outside the circular muscularis (Fig. 14.6).

Physiology with Morphologic Correlation

The morphologic characteristics of the tubal epithelium change during life. Ciliated cells appear during early fetal development[159] and persist until the postmenopausal years. At this time, as circulating estrogen levels drop, the cilia are gradually lost.[83] Estrogen therapy in postmenopausal women, however, restores both the cilia and the ability to transport particulate matter.[83,222] The demonstration of a specific estradiol receptor in the human tube[76] suggests that there is a direct action of estrogen on ciliogenesis.

The characteristics of the tubal epithelium change during the course of the menstrual cycle.[154] Early in the cycle, the cells are low, and the secretory cells appear relatively inactive. As the time of ovulation approaches, probably under the influence of an increasing amount of estrogen, the secretory cells become columnar and actually project beyond the ciliated cells (Fig. 14.2). A discharge of PAS-positive material, probably glycogen, into the tubal lumen has been demonstrated.[79] Changes in cilial maturity and repeated ciliation and deciliation of a minor degree have been documented during the menstrual cycle.[61,221] Other cyclic changes in tubal physiology have been reviewed recently.[113]

The cilia play a dominant role in tubal function at the time of ovulation. The cilia beat in synchronized waves in the direction of the uterus.[82] During the course of ovum pickup, there appears to be a realignment of fimbriae in their relationship to the ovary itself. A distinct fimbria, the fimbria ovarica, runs from the tubal ostium to one pole of the ovary. It is thought that, at the time of ovulation, the muscle of the fimbria ovarica contracts, pulling the tube in the direction of the rupturing follicle. At the same time, some muscular elements in the paraovarian tissue contract, pulling the ovary toward the tubal ostium. This realignment of fimbriae over the rupturing follicle has been observed in several laboratory species, but for technical reasons, it has not yet been satisfactorily evaluated in the human. Once the ovum is released from its follicle, surrounded by an entourage of sticky cumulus cells, it is transported along the surface of the fimbriated end of the fallopian tube by the action of the cilia. The ovum is retained within the tube for approximately 3 days,[45] after which it is delivered into the uterus. In Kartagener's syndrome, where cilia are structurally defective and immobile, fertility, although impaired, is preserved. This raises the likelihood that muscular contraction is more important than previously considered. The effect of adrenergic innervation[161] or prostaglandins[42,134] on muscle function and ova transport, is not yet well defined.

Spermatozoa are transported upward through the uterus into the fallopian tube. The mechanisms by which they traverse the uterotubal junction and tubal isthmus in the face of a ciliary beat in a downward direction is still not understood. It is known, however, that spermatozoa can reach the tube within minutes after they are placed in the vagina in the human.[190] It is likely that the fertilizing spermatozoan is already present in the fallopian tube at the time the ovum arrives there.

The environment provided within the tubal lumen is of special importance in reproductive function. The fallopian tube does provide a temporary milieu for spermatozoa, the ovum, and finally the fertilized, cleaving zygote during its initial development. The secretory cells certainly must play a role in the provision of suitable conditions for the processes that occur within the tubal lumen. Contents of the tubal fluid have been studied extensively in the rhesus monkey, but only limited observations have been carried out in the human.[49,135] The salient components of oviductal fluid include metabolic substrates, the most important of which are lactate, pyruvate, and bicarbonate, which appears in tubal fluid as a result of carbonic anhydrase in the tubal epithelium, and electrolytes, including calcium.[144] Tubal fluid also contains trypsin inhibitors, which may influence the fertilization process, and a genital tract isoamylase.[192]

The bicarbonate ion is in part responsible for dispersion of cells that surround the ovum. On reaching the level of the zona pellucida (a protein–mucopolysaccharide layer immediately surrounding the egg), the spermatozoan is able to penetrate by virtue of the presence of a trypsin-like enzyme in its head. Trypsin inhibitors appear in high concentration both before and after ovulation, but for a matter of hours after ovulation, they are at their lowest level of concentration.[197] Some investigators have speculated that trypsin inhibitors control the fertilization process so that aged ova that are in the fallopian tube in the presence of a high concentration of inhibitors are not fertilized. Be that as it may, the 3-day residence in the fallopian tube apparently serves a useful function in several experimental mammals. When zygotes are removed prematurely from the tube and placed in the uterus, implantation is less likely.

Most of the work on tubal physiology has focused on its role in reproduction, and only scanty information is available on the tubal immune system and its role in infection. The immunoglobulin IgG is present in tubal fluid, but immunofluorescent studies show that the only significant tissue immunoglobulin is the secretory component of IgA. It is localized to the apical cytoplasm of the epithelial cells.[172]

Congenital Anomalies

Structural congenital anomalies of the fallopian tube are rare and may be simulated by inflammatory processes or torsion. Tubes associated with uterine abnormalities such as a rudimentary uterine horn or bicornuate uterus may be hypoplastic or partially atretic.[70,122] Bilateral absence of the ampullary muscularis has been reported.[219]

Infertility patients who were exposed in utero to diethylstibestrol (DES), may have shortened, sacculated and convoluted fallopian tubes despite normal salpingograms. The fimbria are described as constricted and the os as pinpoint.[51] No detailed pathologic studies are available. A mouse model of DES exposure produces tubal changes more reminiscent of salpingitis isthmica nodosa.[151]

Apparent congenital absence of a segment of the tube has been reported,[191] as has tubal duplication[50] and accessory tubes.[14] Tubes may be absent in phenotypic females in rare cases.[232]

Torsion, Prolapse, and Intussusception

Among the various anatomic displacements of the tube, torsion is the most common. The usual predisposing factor is cystic enlargement of the ipsilateral ovary. A benign ovarian cyst or tumor is present in 65–80% of patients, and a malignant ovarian tumor is present in 5–15%.[54,131] Paraovarian cysts are also associated with torsion. Tubal enlargement secondary to hydrosalpinx or pyosalpinx[131] or previous gynecologic surgery, especially sterilization,[12] are additional causes, but torsion may occur in the absence of apparent adnexal disease.

The typical patient is in the reproductive years, occasionally pregnant,[112] and complains of the sudden onset of lower abdominal pain. At operation, the adnexa on one side is twisted, usually once or twice. Venous outflow is compromised early, and the resulting congestion may lead to arterial compression. The adnexa is often swollen and edematous, with hemorrhagic infarction and gangrene. If surgical intervention is prompt, the tube may be preserved. Undiagnosed torsion in an infant or adult may result in resorption and total disappearance of the infarcted adnexa or in calcification of the necrotic tissue.[13,32]

Tubal prolapse into the vagina may rarely occur as a complication of hysterectomy, usually vaginal[66,183] (see

Chapter 4, Diseases of Vagina). Clinically this is characterized by vaginal discharge, beginning a few days to several years after vaginal hysterectomy. On examination, an excresence is seen in the vaginal vault, suggestive of granulation tissue or carcinoma. Fimbriae may be apparent grossly. Severe acute and chronic inflammation is present microscopically, and pseudogland formation by the tubal epithelium may mimic adenocarcinoma.[183]

Intussusception of the tube has been reported once.[3] A paraovarian cyst was engulfed by the end of the tube and pulled the fimbriated end into the ampulla. Simple eversion and cystectomy permitted tubal salvage.

Endometriosis and Endosalpingiosis

Endometrial-type tissue may involve the tubal lumen, wall, or serosa. Heterotopic endometrium may entirely replace normal tubal epithelium, with luminal occlusion.[126]

Endosalpingiosis, is the ectopic location of tubal-type epithelium involving peritoneal surfaces. Both endometriosis and endosalpingiosis are discussed in detail in Chapter 17, Endometriosis.

Salpingitis

Salpingitis may be divided into three major types: acute, chronic, and granulomatous.

Acute Salpingitis

Acute salpingitis is a purulent inflammatory process usually secondary to the passage of bacteria from the uterine cavity into the tubal lumen. It is not clear if organisms may be carried upward by sperm or trichomonads as vectors or whether some form of passive transport is in effect.[121] Although *Neisseria gonorrhoeae* has been considered the most common causative organism, meticulous bacteriologic studies indicate that the etiology is polymicrobial and that *Chlamydia trachomatis* and anaerobic bacteria, especially *Bacteroides* species and peptostreptococci, are frequently present, as well as such aerobes as *Escherichia coli*.[36,205,209,216,217] The presence in some of these women of serum antibodies against gonococcal pili, however, suggests that gonococci may initiate the process, only to be supplanted by anaerobes.

Elegant in vitro studies by Ward and others[146,225] have clarified the likely initial steps in gonococcal infection, and the molecular mechanisms involved have been reviewed recently.[25] *N. gonorrhoeae* perfused through the lumen of cultured whole tubes attach only to nonciliated cells. Within 3 hours, microvilli from the cells appear to embrace the gonococci and adhere to them. The bacteria then penetrate both the cells and intercellular junctions, with cell lysis and sloughing. Adjacent ciliated cells are also destroyed but are not invaded directly. Following cell lysis, the bacteria penetrate the subepithelial connective tissue. In vivo, this process is considerably modified by the host response. A brisk diapedesis of granulocytes occurs from capillaries into the mucosa and lumen, and there is vascular engorgement and edema of all tubal layers (Fig. 14.7). In severe cases, transudation of plasma proteins results in a fibrinous exudate on the serosal surface. As the lumen fills with granulocytes and cellular debris and as the tube distends, pus may be seen dripping from the fimbriated end in patients undergoing laparoscopy. The serosa reddens because of vascular dilatation, and the tube attains the classic appearance of a pus tube. The cell necrosis, distention of the tube, and focal peritonitis give rise to fever and abdominal and pelvic pain. The gonococcus gains access to the tube most readily at the time of menstruation. This corresponds to the typical clinical presentation in which the onset of acute pain occurs a few days after menses. The onset of nongonococcal, nonchlamydial acute salpingitis is not, however, clearly related to the recent onset of menses.[206] Over the course of time, repeated invasions will result in recurrent symptoms as well as the anatomic changes of chronic salpingitis, discussed below. Acute salpingitis after tubal ligation is rare.[169]

Although *N. gonorrhoeae* spreads via the epithelial surface and thus causes mucosal changes, other bacteria

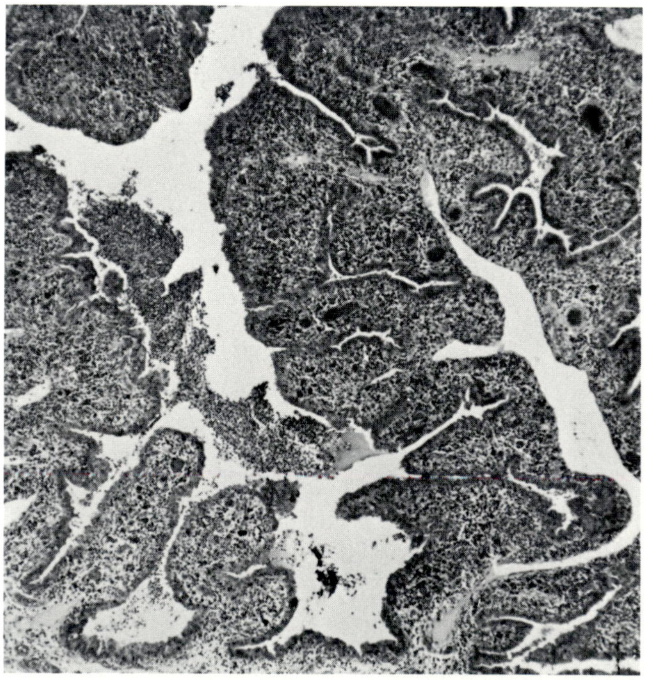

FIG. 14.7. Acute and chronic salpingitis. Plicae are broadened and blunted. Numerous granulocytes, lymphocytes, and plasma cells are present in the mucosa; many granulocytes are present in the lumen.

present in the uterus, such as streptococci, tend to spread into the tube by vascular or lymphatic channels. This results in acute inflammation of the tubal wall, with relative sparing of the mucosa.

The frequency of acute salpingitis is increased at least threefold in women using intrauterine contraceptive devices (see Chapter 10, Benign Diseases of Endometrium.[228] The reason for this is unknown, and nulliparous patients are disproportionately at risk. Acute salpingitis is also increased in frequency in women with multiple sexual partners.

Mycoplasmas have been reported in both acute salpingitis and tuboovarian abscess.[21] Laparoscopically obtained pretreatment cultures from grossly infected tubes occasionally reveal *Mycoplasma hominis*.[141,142] Tubes examined histologically have shown a moderate infiltration with chronic inflammatory cells, some neutrophils, and focal epithelial ulceration.[21] Recent studies suggest that *M. hominis* is not an important cause of salpingitis or infertility.[93,133] *Ureaplasma urealyticum* may also be responsible for acute salpingitis.[207]

C. trachomatis is frequently cultured from the cervix, uterus, and tube in women with acute salpingitis,[124,140] but the histologic changes are not well characterized (see Chapter 6, Benign Lesions of Cervix). Experimentally, there is deciliation of ciliated cells and epithelial cell degeneration;[162] inclusions may be found in both tubal epithelial cell types.[170] Tubal damage may be inferred by subsequent infertility in patients with circulating antichlamydial antibody.[28] The frequency of tubal damage is similar to that caused by the gonococcus.[204] Salpingitis due to chlamydia does not appear to occur with the same degree of pelvic pain as infections with *N. gonorrhoeae* and, in fact, may be clinically silent. There is a close association with chronic endometritis, and, therefore, patients with a diagnosis of chronic endometritis should be carefully evaluated for asymptomatic salpingitis (see Chapter 10, Benign Diseases of Endometrium). Coxsackie viruses B5 and ECHO 6 have been recovered from tubes with acute salpingitis, but no histologic data are available.[142]

An asymptomatic form of acute salpingitis is seen in tubes removed during postpartum ligation. Beginning about 5 hours after delivery and present up to 7–10 days later, a small or moderate number of acute or mixed acute and chronic inflammatory cells are found in the mucosa or lumen of 10% or more of specimens.[101,178] Attempts to culture aerobic or anaerobic bacteria[178,196] have been almost uniformly unsuccessful. The process may be regarded as secondary to the trauma of delivery or intrauterine tissue necrosis.

Chronic Salpingitis

When acute salpingitis resolves through agent–host interaction, residual disease may be found in the fallopian tube. With acute inflammation, the mucosal plicae, secondary to surface fibrin deposition, adhere to one another (Fig. 14.8). Healing and organization then lead to perma-

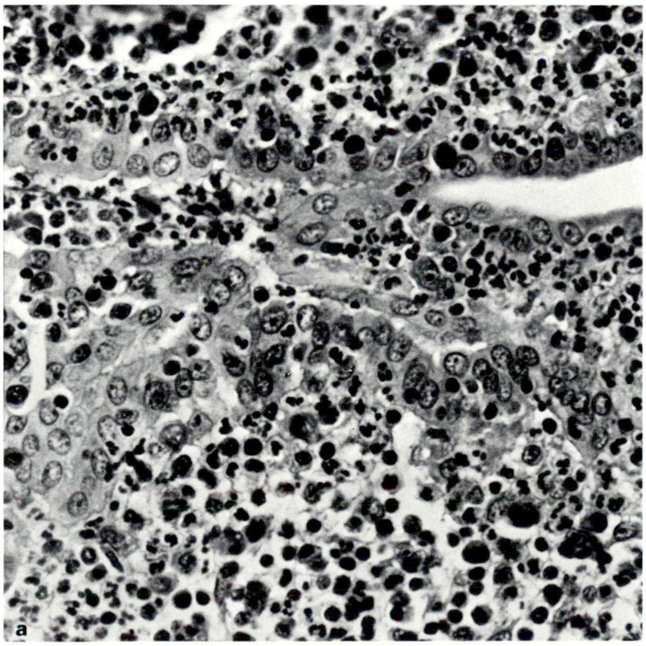

FIG. 14.8 *a*. Acute and chronic salpingitis. Mucosal folds are distended with polymorphonuclear leukocytes, histiocytes, lymphocytes and plasma cells. Fibrin strands lie in lumen at left. Note approximation of plicae and suggestion of early adhesion at center.

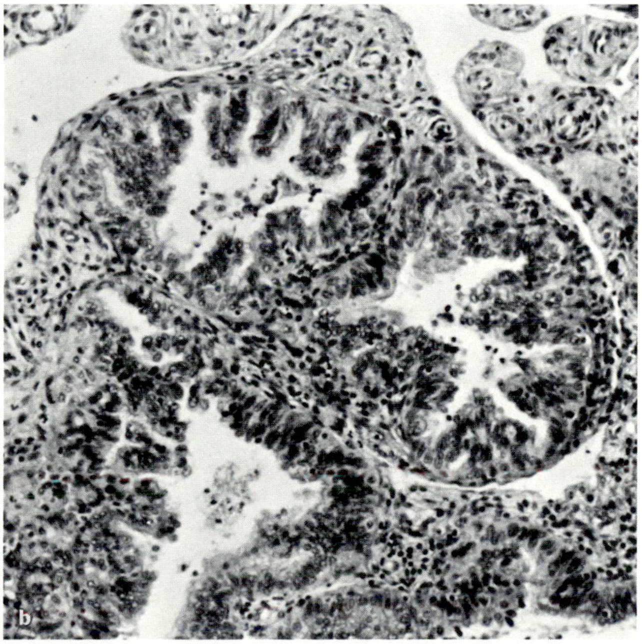

FIG. 14.8.*b*. Chronic salpingitis. Papillary ingrowth of reactive epithelial cells is prominent, but mitoses are absent. A few lymphocytes may be seen in the stroma. This should not be confused with carcinoma.

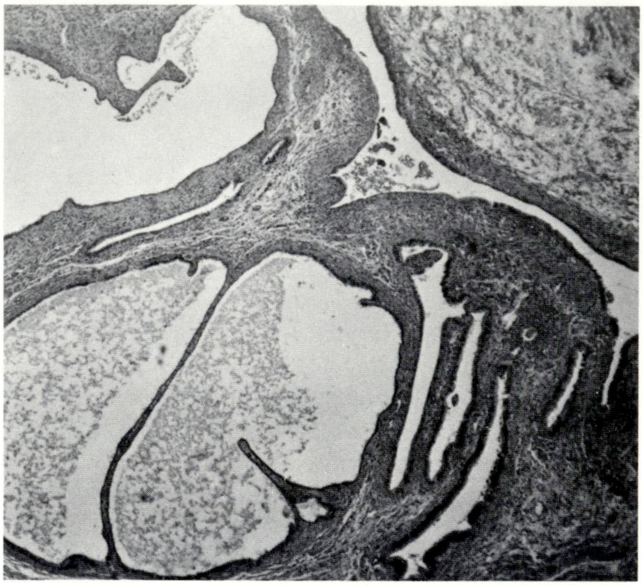

FIG. 14.9. Salpingitis follicularis, showing agglutination of plicae with formation of dilated gland-like spaces between them.

nent bridging between folds. In the classic case, this results in a follicular salpingitis (Fig. 14.9). Plicae may retain much of their size and shape, but plasma cells, lymphocytes, or both are still present in the mucosa. Often the height of the folds appears lowered, or their intricate pattern, so prominent in the ampulla and infundibulum, is subtly altered. Fibrinous adhesions between the serosa and surrounding peritoneal surfaces may organize into thin fibrous adhesions that, unless routinely sought, are easily overlooked. Peritoneal inflammation may be widespread, and thin, violin-string adhesions may form between liver and diaphragm. Agglutination of acutely inflamed fimbriae may be focal or massive. If it is severe enough, the bases of the fimbriae may coalesce in the center, with the fimbriae radiating outward like a daisy, or the tips of the fimbriae may adhere, blocking the lumen and causing a blunted end, the clubbed tube (Fig. 14.10). The proximity of the ovary to the fimbriae allows multiple tuboovarian adhesions to form, with occlusion of the tubal ostium. The ovary itself may then become more directly involved, and a tuboovarian abscess may result (Fig. 14.11).[214] If the fimbriae close before the ovary is seriously involved, the inflamed, dilated tube forms a pyosalpinx full of acute and chronic inflammatory cells. As the inflammation subsides, the acute and most of the chronic inflammatory cells gradually disappear, and the patient is left with either a severely scarred tube or a hydrosalpinx.

Both aerobic and anaerobic cultures of any tuboovarian abscess should be obtained in the operating room or laboratory. Prior treatment with antibiotics may possibly eliminate culturable organisms, but with careful technique, anaerobes are isolated in 63–100% of cases.[127] *E. coli*, *Bacteriodes fragilis*, *Bacterioides* species, *Peptostreptococcus*, *Peptococcus*, and aerobic streptococci are the most commonly found organisms; typically, infection is polymicrobial.[128]

Fungi, including *Blastomyces dermatitidis*, are only rarely cultured from tuboovarian abscesses[149] and may be secondary to hematogenous spread. Tubal coccidioidomycosis may also be found secondary to disseminated

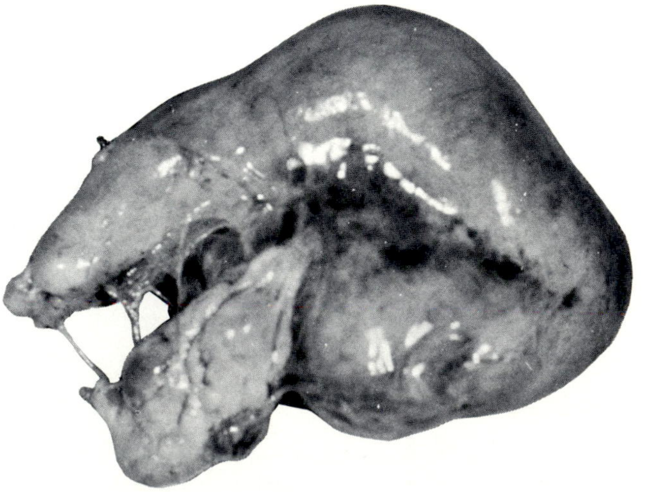

FIG. 14.10. Chronic salpingitis. Multiple, thin, fibrous adherences are present between tube and ovary and between ampulla and infundibulum. Distal portion of tube has clubbed appearance because of obliteration of tubal ostium.

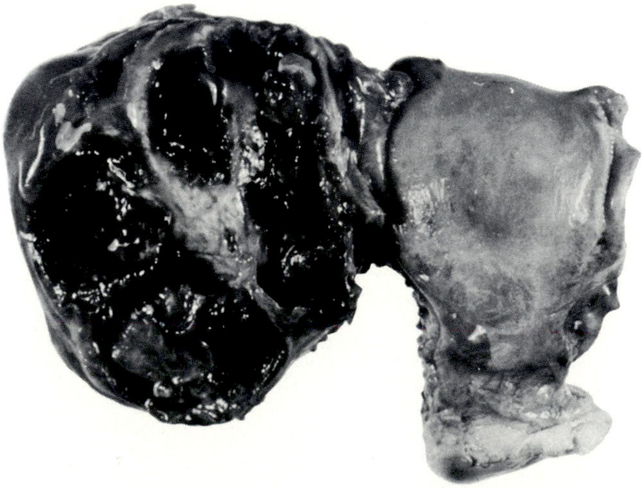

FIG. 14.11. Tuboovarian abscess. Posterior view shows bisected tuboovarian abscess involving entire left adnexa. Tube and ovary have been largely destroyed and replaced by a multiloculated mass containing foul-smelling pus.

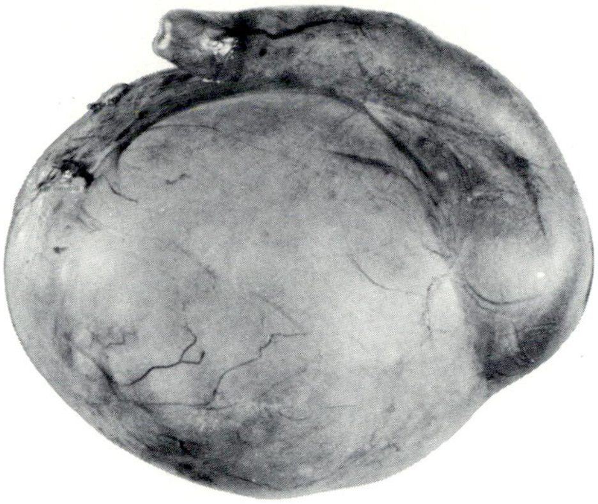

FIG. 14.12. Hydrosalpinx, showing tube, especially in its ampullary portion, dilated with total obliteration of ostium. Wall is fibrous and translucent.

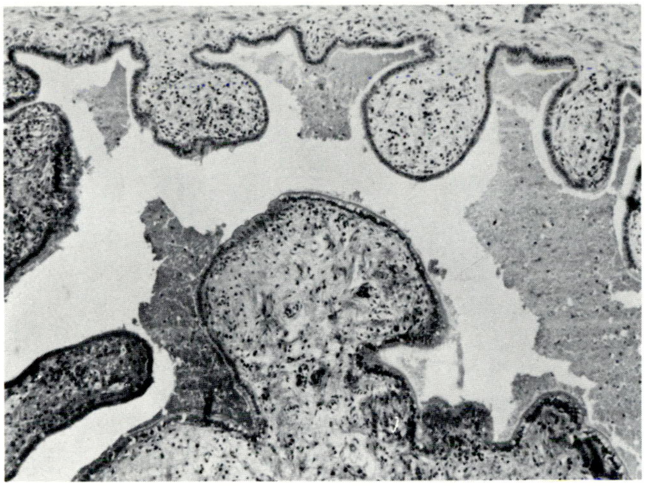

FIG. 14.14. Chronic salpingitis. Transitional stage between chronic salpingitis and hydrosalpinx. Marked blunting of plicae and only a scanty residual lymphocytic infiltrate are shown.

disease.[30] Malacoplakia only rarely involves the fallopian tube.[33]

Hydrosalpinx is one of the complications of salpingitis. It is characterized by obliteration of the fimbriated end and dilation of the tube, usually the ampullary and infundibular portions. If the ovary is first involved by tuboovarian adhesions, the ovary may be compressed by the dilated tube. The dilated tube may resemble the chemist's retort, and the wall is generally whitish, thin, and translucent, with occasional fibrous adhesions on its surface (Fig. 14.12). The tube usually contains clear serous fluid with an electrolyte composition similar to serum but with a low protein content.[48] Since a luminal communication can usually be demonstrated between dilated and nondilated portions of the tube,[36,46] the etiology of the dilatation is obscure[34,48] but it may result in part from a sphincter-like action of the isthmus. The muscle wall is either thin and atrophic or replaced by collagenous connective tissue. Most of the epithelial lining consists of low cuboidal cells, but an occasional plica may persist, with surprisingly intact columnar epithelium with histologically normal ciliated and secretory cells corresponding morphologically with the menstrual phase (Fig. 14.13). The persistence of healthy-appearing plicae suggests that pressure effects from the luminal fluid may not be responsible for the flattened and absent plicae. Instead, the preceding inflammatory process may have selectively damaged the tubal folds, resulting in uneven scarring and plical disappearance (Fig. 14.14). A few lymphocytes may be found in the wall of the hydrosalpinx but are more commonly absent. Recovery of tubal function, even with expert surgery, is unlikely, and the possibility of tubal torsion with subsequent hemorrhagic infarction remains.[58]

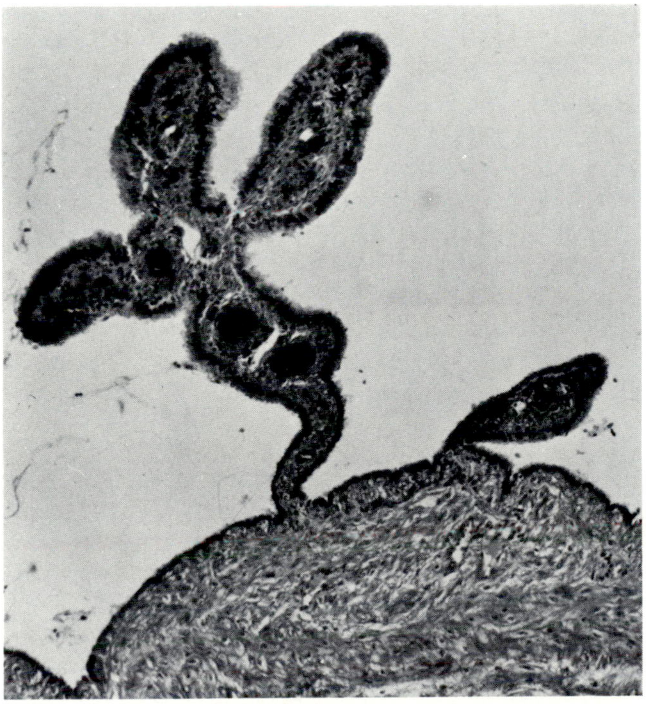

FIG. 14.13. Hydrosalpinx. Although most of the luminal epithelium is cuboidal or flattened, occasional plicae may remain with normal epithelial surface.

Granulomatous Salpingitis

Granulomatous inflammation of the fallopian tube may be provoked by a number of different organisms as well as by a variety of noninfectious processes. The histologic identification of one or more granulomas calls for immediate communication between pathologist and clinician and for attempts to determine the likely etiology.

Tuberculous Salpingitis

Mycobacterium tuberculosis historically has been the predominant etiologic agent of granulomatous salpingitis. The frequency of tuberculous salpingitis in women studied for infertility ranges from about 1% in the United States to more than 10% in India, and 10–20% of women who die from tuberculosis have tubal involvement.[184]

Primary infection of the genitalia, as by coitus with a partner with genitourinary tuberculosis, is extremely rare. Secondary spread, usually from a primary infection, is the normal route of infection. For reasons still unknown, the blood-borne organism preferentially lodges in the tubes rather than the other parts of the female genital tract. The primary pulmonary lesion may not be radiologically evident, but extrapulmonary involvement of the peritoneum, kidneys, or other site may be present. Lymphatic spread from primary intestinal tuberculosis[90] or direct spread from bladder or gastrointestinal tract may occur.

Although the earliest pathologic lesions are microscopic, with advancing disease the tube increases in diameter and may become nodular, mimicking salpingitis isthmica nodosa. In the more common adhesive type of the disease, multiple, dense adhesions may form between the tube and ovary, and the fimbriae and ostium may be obliterated.[94] Frequently, the ostium remains patent, and some investigators, in fact, regard the presence of an identifiable ostium and fimbriae in a grossly diseased tube as characteristic of tuberculous salpingitis.[184] With the exudative type of disease, progressive distention mimics bacterial pyosalpinx. Hematosalpinx or hydrosalpinx may be found late in the disease process. In either form, serosal tubercles may be present.

The earliest microscopic lesions are mucosal, with a typical granulomatous reaction of epithelioid cells and lymphocytes arranged in a nodular configuration. Giant cells are often seen, and central caseation, focal or massive, may be present. Immunosuppressive therapy may modify cellular immunity to a point where granulomas fail to form. With this clinical information, the mere finding of acute and chronic inflammatory cells should lead to consideration of staining for acid-fast organisms. From the mucosa, extension to the muscularis and serosa may occur. As the tubercles enlarge, they may erode through the mucosa and discharge their contents into the tubal lumen (Fig. 14.15). The mucosal inflammatory reaction leads to progressive scarring, with plical distortion and conglutination. Large caseous nodules may form and coalesce, eventually filling the dilated tube. Ectopic calcification may occur in areas of fibrosis. Since tubercles may not be present in a given section, the presence of caseation, fibrosis, or calcification in a tube may be the only histologic finding pointing to the necessity for more thorough study. The presence of severe mucosal atypicality in tuberculous salpingitis and confusion with adenocarcinoma have been stressed by numerous authors, but similar atypia may be found in any chronic salpingitis (see Fig. 14.8b). Complications of tuberculous salpingitis are several. Alteration in function is the rule. Sterility is almost universal because of the common bilaterality of the disease. Rarely, successful pregnancies occur, but ectopic tubal nidation is likely in the event that fertilization is successful.[184]

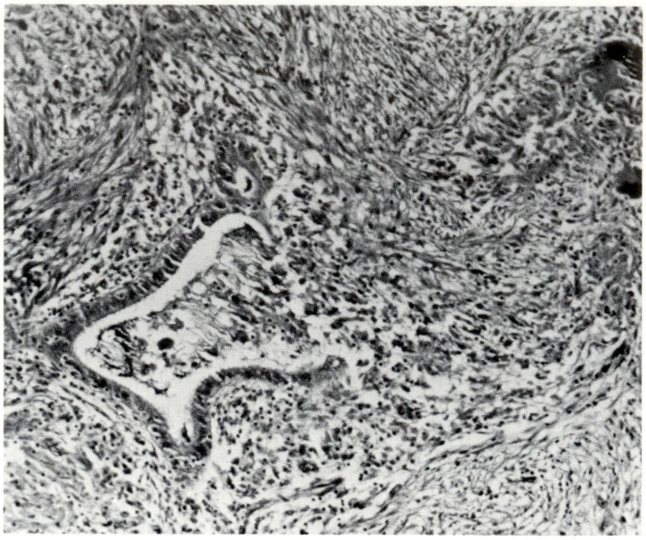

FIG. 14.15. Tuberculous salpingitis, showing two giant cells present in granulomas (*upper right*). There is necrosis and very early caseation in the center of the granulomas. One of the granulomas appears to be rupturing into a pocket of tubal epithelium, illustrating a mechanism whereby *M. tuberculosis* can reach the lumen and then seed the endometrial cavity.

Pelvic pain, sterility, and menstrual irregularities are the most common complaints. Because of repeated seeding of the endometrium from the infected tubes, mycobacterial culture and the histologic finding on curettage of endometrial tubercles are diagnostically useful (see Chapter 10, Benign Diseases of Endometrium). Laparoscopy may cause bowel perforation in cases of extensive pelvic and peritoneal tuberculosis.

Actinomycosis

Actinomycotic infections of the tube may occur, many of them associated with intrauterine contraceptive devices (see Chapter 10, Benign Diseases of Endometrium).[59,203] Recent studies note that actinomycetes are probably part of the indigenous female genital tract flora.[168]

Grossly, a large fibrous mass is present that often includes the ovary. The mass may appear to be a dilated tube or may be more obviously inflammatory, being bound down to pelvic structures with adhesions or fistula formation. Pus is present in the shaggy-walled cavities within the tube. Anaerobic culture is necessary to permit growth of *Actinomyces israelii*. Microscopically, numerous histiocytes, plasma cells, and lymphocytes are present in the abscess walls, and gram-positive, filamentous clumps, sulfur granules, may be recognized in the pus. Complications in unrecognized cases may include dissemination to the liver and lung.

Parasitic Salpingitis

Pinworm. The pinworm, *Enterobius vermicularis*, may migrate up the female genital tract, embed in the tube, and cause an inflammatory reaction. The tube may be involved with the ovary in what appears to be a tuboovarian abscess, or a fibrous nodular area may be present. Acute and chronic inflammatory cells may be found together with eosinophils, Charcot-Leyden crystals, and portions of gravid female worm. Ova may be released into the tissue, where they provoke a granulomatous reaction. The ova may be identified by their size (about 20×50 μm) and ovoid asymmetrical shape,[210] but they may be obscured by calcification of granulomas. The ova may be widely disseminated in the peritoneum in the absence of histologic tubal involvement, and the fibrous granulomas may simulate metastatic carcinoma.[75]

Schistosomiasis. Although tubal bilharziasis is probably one of the commonest causes of granulomatous salpingitis worldwide, it is rare in the United States. In Africa, reported tubal infections occur in as many as 20% of unselected women at autopsy.[80] The ova of *Schistosoma haematobium* are most common, but *Schistosoma mansoni* eggs may be present in some women.[86] If granulomas are present and there is a suspicion of schistosomiasis, sodium hydroxide digestion of the remaining tubal tissue may reveal ova.

Gross findings appear to be related to fibrosis surrounding the ova, producing a nodular or fibrotic tube. Ectopic pregnancy in an infected tube may precipitate its removal, but the granulomas themselves may not always cause sufficient damage to account for abnormal nidation.[16]

Hydatid Disease. Where the condition is common, hydatid disease secondary to *Echinococcus granulosus* infection may involve the female genital tract, including the adnexae.[88]

Sarcoid

Sarcoidosis of the tube is rarely reported[94] and appears to accompany disseminated disease. One patient[119] had gross tubal distention, tuboovarian adhesions, an ovarian abscess, and multiple serosal nodules, but bacterial salpingitis was not excluded as a cause. Histologically, noncaseating granulomas may be seen in the mucosa. Culture, special stains, and clinical information are necessary to exclude other granulomatous diseases.

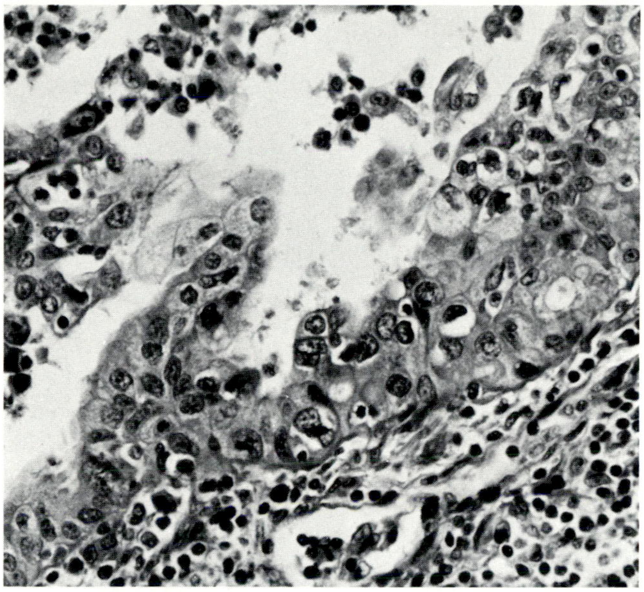

FIG. 14.16. Granulomatous salpingitis secondary to Crohn's disease. Underlying granulomas are not visible here, but severe chronic inflammation is present (*lower right*). Epithelium is piled up and has marked nuclear atypia. This change should not be confused with carcinoma in situ.

Crohn's Disease

Crohn's disease of the ileum, colon, or appendix may secondarily involve the tube and ovary to produce a granulomatous salpingo-oophoritis.[27,231] Noncaseating granulomas may involve the entire thickness of the tubal muscularis as well as the mucosa. The epithelium may react with severe cellular atypia (Fig. 14.16). Fistulas from bowel to tube may also occur (see Chapter 3, Diseases of Vulva).[43]

Foreign Body

Foreign material may be introduced into the tube in the course of gynecologic investigation, especially hysterosalpingography. Lubricant jelly, mineral oil, and starch and talc powder may cause a lipoid or granulomatous salpingitis.[31,65] An intense phagocytic reaction to introduced lipid material causes accumulation of subepithelial foamy histiocytes (Fig. 14.17). If the patient has received a blood substitute containing polyvinylpyrrolidone (PVP), this foreign material may be ingested by macrophages and deposited in many organs, including the tube.[125] The cells formed simulate signet-ring cell carcinoma, with mucicarmine-positive vacuolated cytoplasm. An appropriate history and a negative PAS stain should clarify the benign nature of the lesion. Talc may cause

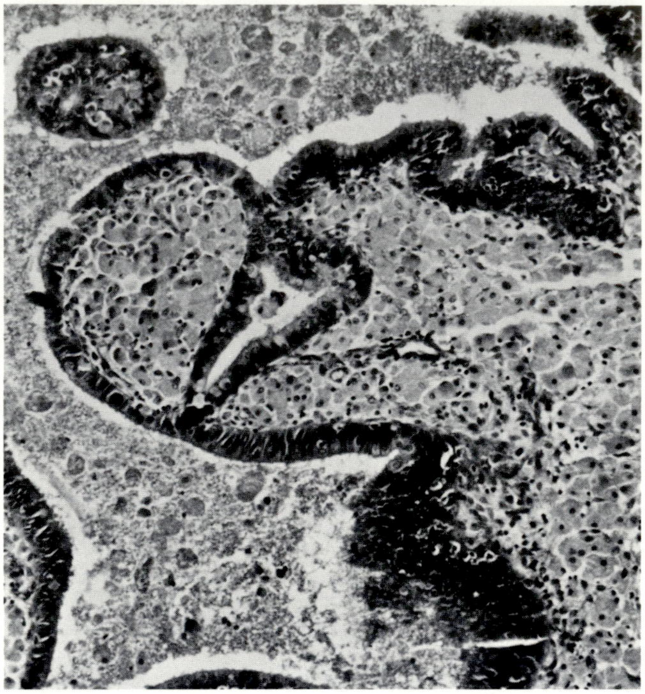

Fig. 14.17. Foreign body reaction in tubal mucosa. Hysterosalpingography or exposure to other foreign material may lead to intense histiocytic reaction, as here, or to formation of foreign body granulomas.

mucosal or serosal granulomas. Examination of all granulomas or foreign body reactions under polarized light is useful in the recognition of these processes. Other disease processes in the tube, such as leprosy[234] or amyloidosis,[40] are so infrequent that they are of little clinical or pathologic significance.

Salpingitis Isthmica Nodosa

This peculiar condition consists of one or more outpouchings or diverticula of tubal epithelium in the isthmic region, often bilateral, and usually accompanied by nodular hyperplasia of the surrounding muscularis.

The etiology is at present unknown. The disease is found in women between the ages of 25 and 60 years, with the average age at diagnosis of about 30 years.[9] Because the lesion is almost unknown before puberty and is not found congenitally, attention has focused on other possible causes, including postinflammatory distortion[186] and an adenomyosis-like process.[9,235] Against the proposed inflammatory etiology is the usual localization of nodularity in the isthmic portion of the tube or immediately adjacent ampulla.[9] Most of the ampulla is uninvolved, unlike the usual picture in inflammatory salpingitis. When salpingitis isthmica nodosa is associated with inflammatory salpingitis, such as pyosalpinx and hydrosalpinx, the inflammatory process is nearly as often contralateral as it is ipsilateral.[9] Although a few lymphocytes are found in the peridiverticular stroma, scarring is usually absent.

Evidence for a noninflammatory adenomyosis-like origin is more convincing. Moderate or large numbers of endometrial-like stromal cells accompany the diverticula in over half the patients.[9] As in uterine adenomyosis, the presence of glands appears to stimulate muscular growth, with subsequent mural thickening. Unilateral tubal involvement is often accompanied by uterine adenomyosis on the same side.[235]

The external gross appearance is of one or more nodular swellings in the isthmus up to 1–2 cm in diameter. The serosa is smooth. On section, the tissue is firm, and careful inspection may disclose some of the dilated diverticula. Microscopically, the diverticula appear on cross-section as dispersed glands of tubal epithelium surrounded by broad bands of muscularis (Fig. 14.18). Diverticula may closely approach the serosal surface but do not normally connect with it. Endometrial-like stromal cells lying beneath the epithelial outpouchings may be abundant, sparse, or absent. If both glands and stroma are really apparent, a diagnosis of tubal endometriosis may well be considered. Because the underlying configuration is diverticular rather than glandular and since the condition is not clearly related to pelvic endometriosis, it seems best to continue using the term *salpingitis isthmica nodosa* until the etiology is better understood.

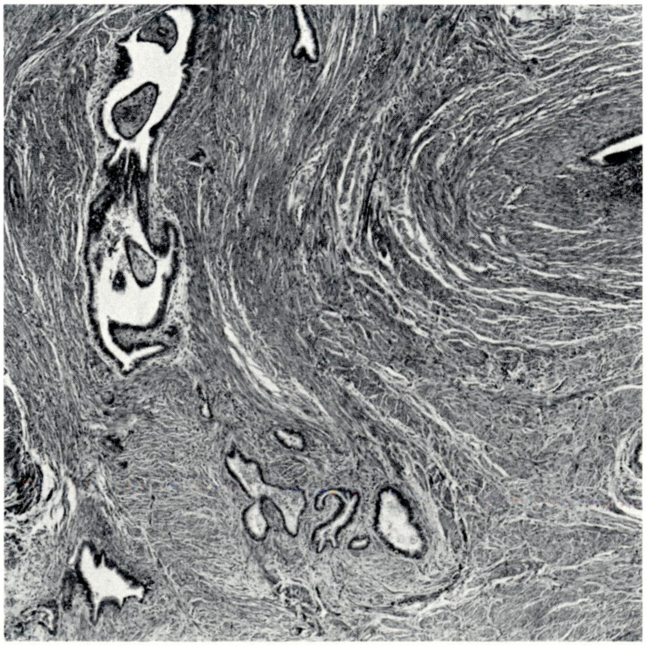

Fig. 14.18. Salpingitis isthmica nodosa. Tubal lumen is visible at *upper right*. Cross-sectioned diverticula are widely separated by broad bands of smooth muscle. A few endometrial-like stromal cells are present (*left center*).

The most serious clinical and pathologic complications of salpingitis isthmica nodosa are infertility and the strong association with ectopic pregnancy.[108,167] Inflammatory tubal disease may be associated with it ipsilaterally or contralaterally. A rare complication that we have seen is rupture of a deep diverticulum through the serosa, with subsequent mild intraabdominal bleeding and pelvic pain.

Ectopic Pregnancy

An ectopic pregnancy occurs when the developing blastocyst implants at a site other than in the endometrium of the fundus or lower uterine segment. Since well over 95% of ectopic pregnancies occur in the fallopian tube, the terms *ectopic pregnancy* and *tubal pregnancy* are nearly synonymous. However, implantation on both tubal fimbriae and ovary, in the abdominal cavity, in the uterine interstitium (intramural pregnancy[147]), in the cervix,[22] or in the retroperitoneum[194] may also occur, in descending order of frequency. Within the tube, most ectopic pregnancies are found in the ampulla (75–80%), with about 10–15% isthmic and 5% at the fimbriae.[22] Right-sided ectopic pregnancies comprise 52–57% of all tubal pregnancies.[18,22,23,115]

Epidemiologic studies note an increasing incidence of ectopic pregnancy.[7,11,106,179,227,229] Currently 1 to 2% of all conceptions are ectopic. Histologic examination of curettings performed for elective termination of pregnancy reveals an absence of villi in 1 of every 100 women, and each has subsequently been shown to have an unsuspected ectopic pregnancy (personal observations). Ectopic pregnancies may be bilateral; in one series[18] the frequency was 2 of 905. Simultaneous ectopic and intrauterine implantations, so-called combined pregnancy, may occur in 1 in 30,000 pregnancies.[230]

Etiology

The mechanisms responsible for ectopic pregnancy are largely unknown, although any disease process that alters the normal tubal anatomy seems to increase the incidence. Whereas delay in entering the uterine cavity may predispose the blastocyst to tubal nidation, experimentally delayed conceptuses in rabbit, guinea pig, and mouse oviducts degenerate and fail to implant.[26] However, ectopic pregnancy is uncommonly reported in nonhuman primates.[129]

A history of previous pelvic inflammatory disease is the single most common antecedent factor in 35–45% of patients,[23,115,229] and the risk of ectopic pregnancy increases seven times after acute salpingitis.[229]

Salpingitis isthmica nodosa,[167] previous pelvic surgery,[23] genital tuberculosis,[95] a history of prenatal DES exposure,[51] and vaginal douching[37] also appear as ectopic risk factors. The risk posed by the use of an intrauterine contraceptive device (IUD) is controversial[97] and may relate to associated salpingitis.[228] Electively induced abortion does not appear to increase the frequency of ectopic pregnancy unless there is postabortal infection.[38] Tubal ectopic pregnancy after tubal sterilization may occur subsequent to tuboperitoneal fistula formation,[199] and repeat ectopic pregnancy on the same or opposite side is common (9%) after one ectopic pregnancy.[98] The increasing use of linear salpingostomy for the removal of an unruptured ectopic pregnancy, especially when only one tube is patent, poses the highest known risk for a repeat ectopic pregnancy (20%) but is tolerated because of the 50–60% chance for intrauterine pregnancy.[52] Ectopic pregnancy after hysterectomy is rare.[238] Abnormalities in the embryo may possibly lead to an increased tendency toward tubal implantation,[29] but subsequent work (C. Oertel and R. Baumiller, Master's thesis) did not confirm this finding.

Clinical Aspects

Although many women with an ectopic pregnancy still appear as emergency patients with tubal rupture and hemorrhagic shock, because of the increasing frequency, clinicians consider any complaint of pelvic pain with or without menstrual irregularity as a possible indication of an ectopic pregnancy. Quantitative, sensitive serum hCG assays and ultrasonography to identify a gestational sac are subsequently performed.[107,176] Early diagnosis and operation result either in salpingostomy with conceptus removal or salpingectomy for an unruptured ectopic pregnancy. Trophoblastic tissue may persist after salpingostomy and conceptus removal. The remaining tissue may retain its viability and form an ectopic-like tubal mass with a persistent hCG titer, requiring reoperation.[174]

Pathologic Features

The unruptured tubal pregnancy is characterized grossly by a somewhat irregular sausage-like dilatation of the tube, with a bluish discoloration due to hematosalpinx (Fig. 14.19). Chorionic villi are usually found in the blood-filled and dilated tubal lumen and, in 75% of cases, appear viable.[152] Nearly two thirds of cases contain a grossly or microscopically identifiable embryo,[152] and multiple pregnancy may occur.[81]

Perhaps because of the limited ability of the endosalpingeal stroma to undergo decidualization, the trophoblast behaves as it does in placenta increta, with penetration deep into the muscularis. Vascular changes in midsized tubal arteries adjacent to ectopic pregnancies are similar to those found in the vessels near uterine implan-

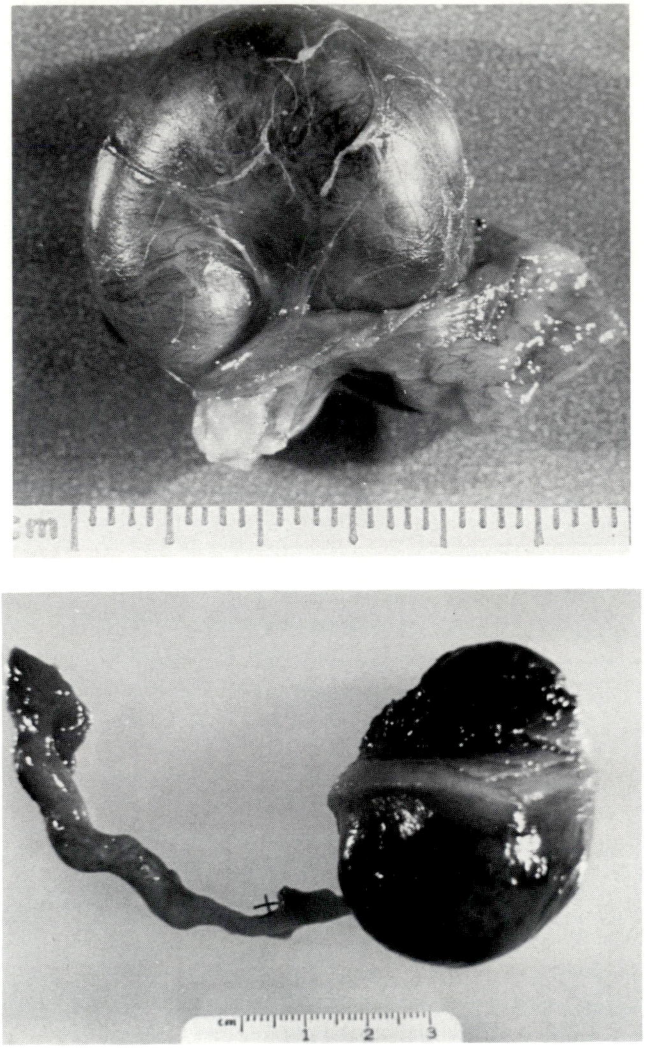

FIG. 14.19. Unruptured ectopic pregnancy. *Top:* Tubal pregnancy. A resected, kinked portion of tube is expanded by the growing pregnancy. Intraluminal blood imparts a bluish discoloration. The thin fibrous peritubal adhesions suggest previous salpingitis. *Bottom:* Cornual pregnancy. The attached tube is normal, but the resected uterine cornu is expanded by the hemorrhagic mass of a nonviable ectopic pregnancy.

tations, with proliferation of the vascular intima and accumulation of foam cells in the intima.[17] Chronic salpingitis is found adjacent to the ectopic pregnancy in nearly half the patients.[152] Ultrastructural studies may demonstrate decreased or absent areas of ciliation in the mucosa adjacent to the ectopic pregnancy.[220] The tubal wall should be examined microscopically for the diverticula of salpingitis isthmica nodosa.

The pathology of extratubal ectopic pregnancy varies according to the site. Cornual or interstitial pregnancies may expand up to about 12 weeks, when rupture may lacerate one of the uterine arteries as well as the entire side of the uterus. Cervical ectopic pregnancy presents much as an incomplete abortion with bleeding. Because of the fibrous cervical tissue underlying placental implantation, control of bleeding may be difficult.[114]

Ovarian pregnancy is clinically similar to tubal pregnancy, including frequent preoperative rupture.[96] More than half of the patients in one series had a history of previous reproductive tract disease or infertility,[91] and 17–25% had an IUD in place.[68,91]

Macroscopic examination typically reveals a hemorrhagic mass replacing the ovary. The pathologic criteria for ovarian pregnancy proposed by Spiegelberg[195] are (1) the tube must be intact and separate from the ovary, (2) the gestational sac must occupy the normal position of the ovary, (3) the gestational sac must be connected to the uterus by the uteroovarian ligament, and (4) ovarian tissue must be demonstrated within the wall of the sac. Pathologic documentation of ovarian tissue within the pregnancy may be difficult or impossible if treatment consists of conservative resection or if the pregnancy has extensively replaced the ovarian tissue.

The endometrial glandular changes described by Arias-Stella (see Chapter 9, Uterine Corpus) may be found in at least 60% of women with ectopic pregnancy. In addition, very similar changes of focal epithelial hyper-

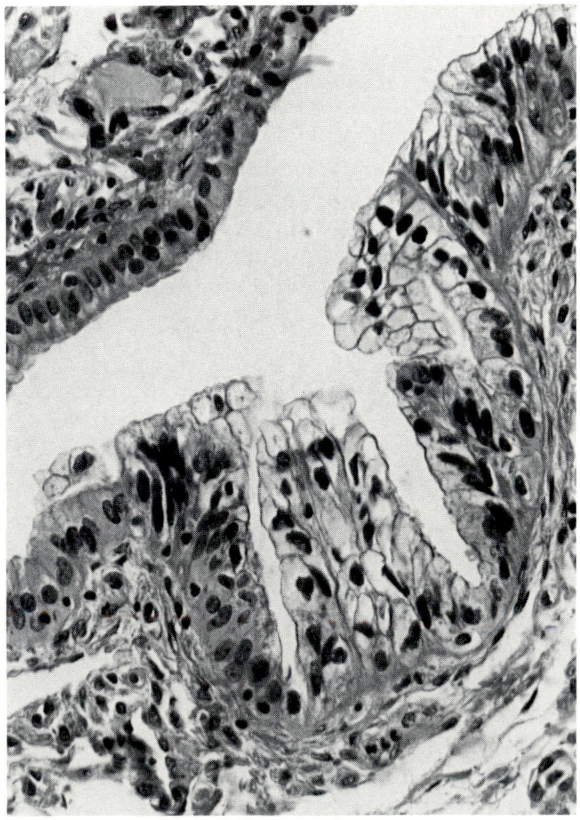

FIG. 14.20. Arias–Stella reaction in tubal epithelium. Note the focally clear epithelial cell cytoplasm, with nuclear enlargement and hyperchromatism.

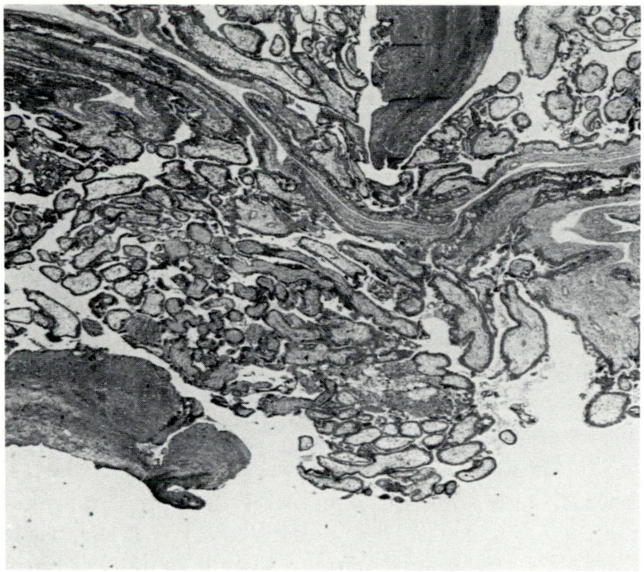

FIG. 14.21. Ruptured tubal pregnancy. Following penetration of the tubal musculature by the trophoblastic cells of the ectopic pregnancy, the muscle wall (*top center and bottom left*) weakens and ruptures, with extrusion of chorionic villi.

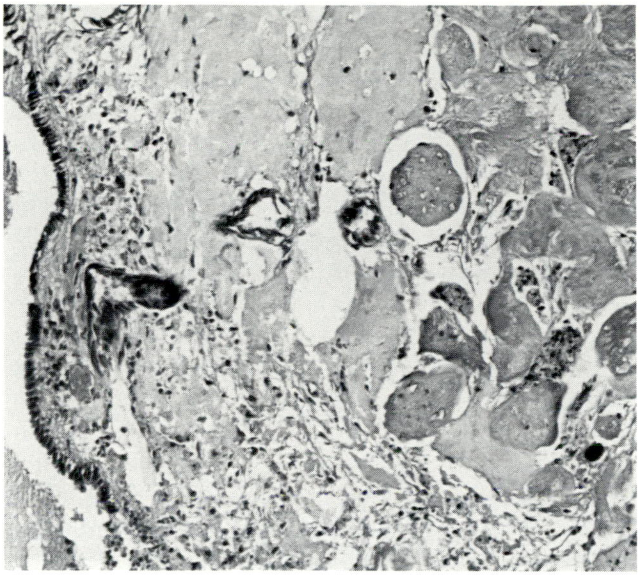

FIG. 14.23. Chronic ectopic pregnancy. Proteinaceous fluid is present in the distorted tubal lumen on the *left*. Fibrotic chorionic villi replacing the normal tubal architecture are present on the *right*. A vew degenerated cells among the ghost villi probably represent residual trophoblast.

plasia, nuclear atypia, and some cytoplasmic vacuolization may be found in about 15% of carefully studied tubes[15] (Fig. 14.20).

Sequelae

The natural history of tubal ectopic pregnancy includes spontaneous expulsion from the fimbriated end—tubal abortion—as well as embryonal death and involution of the conceptus. Typically, however, continued growth of the trophoblast leads to increasing dilatation and weakening of the muscularis, with rupture about the eighth week (Fig. 14.21). Because hemorrhage may be massive, it is a major cause of maternal mortality.[62] A few tubal pregnancies have proceeded to term with fetal viability. Peritoneal irritation and formation of dense intestinal adhesions is likely to occur in these patients.[78]

Some tubal pregnancies form a chronic inflammatory mass that, with involution of trophoblast and reestablishment of the menstrual cycle, may present problems in differential diagnosis. The convoluted, blood-filled tube, often with involved ipsilateral ovary, may simulate tumor[110] or an endometriotic mass (Fig. 14.22). Extensive microscopic sampling of a so-called chronic ectopic pregnancy may be required to demonstrate a few ghost villi (Fig. 14.23).

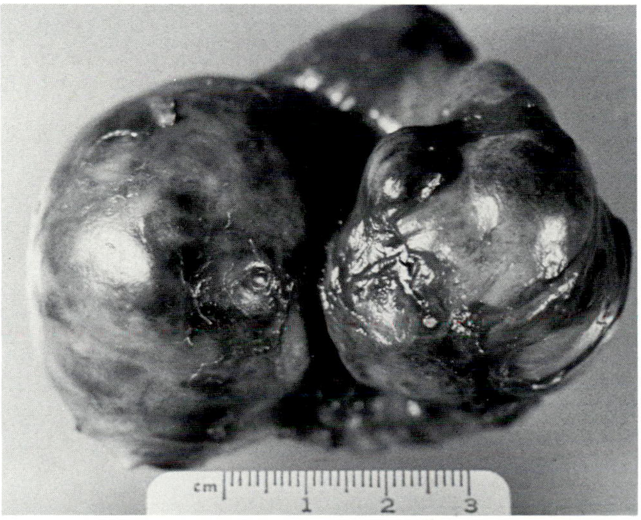

FIG. 14.22. Chronic ectopic pregnancy. This irregularly lobulated mass grossly simulated an ovarian neoplasm.

Infertility

Most of the diseases discussed in this chapter may result in sufficient anatomic distortion to cause infertility. In contrast, purely physiologic tubal dysfunction is not well defined but may be illustrated by the immotile cilia of Kartagener's syndrome that may lead to reduced fertility; only 3 of 12 women in one series succeeded in becoming pregnant.[4]

Peritubal adhesions secondary to endometriosis, prior pelvic inflammatory disease, or appendicitis may interfere with normal tubal motility and ovum pickup. Adhesion lysis may be curative. Multiple fimbrial adhesions secondary to gonococcal or other inflammatory tubal disease may be treated by operative lysis and surgical eversion of tubal mucosa. Obliterative fibrosis, possibly secondary to inflammation within the uterus, may lead to obstruction at the uterotubal junction.[77] Resection of the obstruction and microsurgical anastomosis or tubal reimplantation may result in patency rates of about 80–85% and term pregnancy rates of 50%[150] to nearly 80%.[89] Whereas tubal surgery for infertility has been criticized for lack of convincing evidence of effectiveness,[39] untreated complete bilateral tubal obstruction offers no expectation of spontaneous cure, and surgery offers some hope of pregnancy. Typically, tubal patency rates are approximately double the rates for intrauterine pregnancy, and ectopic pregnancy is an ever-present risk.

Tubal patency is commonly checked by hysterosalpingography,[189] using radiopaque dye or intrauterine dye injection with tubal monitoring via laparoscopy (chromopertubation). More physiologic methods recently reported[201] may, with further experience, prove useful.

Contraception by interference with tubal function involves procedures designed to damage the tube by electrocautery or surgical removal of a segment of the tube or to obstruct it by placement of a clip. Tubal resection should be confirmed by histologic demonstration of a complete cross-section of tubal lumen. In spite of these procedures, spontaneous reanastomosis or fistula formation (Fig. 14.24) may occur in approximately 1% of all patients and may lead to fertilization and ectopic or intrauterine pregnancy.[193] In order to identify the cause of failure of tubal sterilization procedures, careful gross examination of the specimen, occasionally specimen salpingography, longitudinal orientation of the tubal segment in paraffin, and meticulous sectioning techniques may be necessary.[200] Fistula formation at suture and excision sites appears to be the most common cause of failure. Up to 70% of pregnancies after electrocoagulation are ectopic.[211] Other complications of tubal sterilization have been reviewed recently.[35] The success of surgical reanastomosis in reestablishing a patent lumen varies with the extent of the initial procedure and the skill of the surgeon but is reported to be as high as 80%. Only 25–40% of the patients, however, will subsequently become pregnant. The frequency of ectopic pregnancy after reanastomosis is increased.

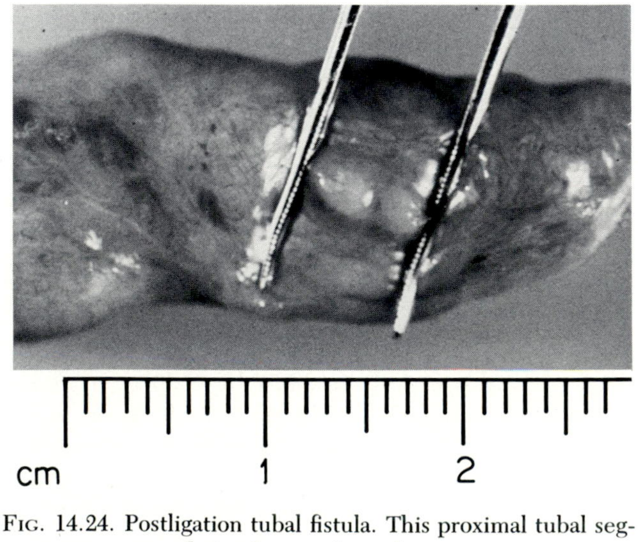

FIG. 14.24. Postligation tubal fistula. This proximal tubal segment was removed simultaneously with an ectopic pregnancy on the opposite side. Slight pressure on the forceps has caused the endosalpingeal mucosa to pout out through a 2–3 mm fistulous opening, with the lumen represented by a small dimple in the *center*.

Benign Neoplasms

Both benign and malignant tumors of the fallopian tube are uncommon. They are frequently mistaken for lesions of chronic salpingitis or pyosalpinx, both preoperatively and during the operative procedure itself. Benign tumors are most often of mesodermal origin and are usually small enough to be incidental findings at laparotomy.

Inclusion Cysts and Walthard Nests

The tubal serosa, by invagination, may give rise to a number of benign inclusion cysts. The simplest is a

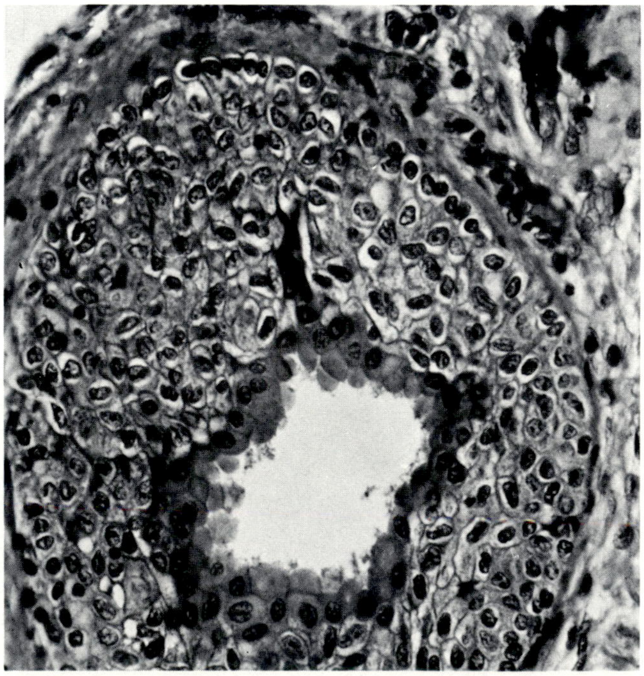

FIG. 14.25. Walthard nest. The most central epithelial cells have undergone columnar metaplasia. Nuclear grooves are visible in many other epithelial cells as dark lines in the long axis of ovoid nuclei. Note the serosal surface at *upper left*.

1–2 mm unilocular cyst lying directly beneath the serosal surface lined by mesothelial cells, a mesothelial inclusion cyst. By a process of metaplasia, these cysts may become filled with polygonal epithelial-like cells to form a Walthard nest. On gross examination, a 1–2 mm yellowish white nodule lies beneath the serosa. The cells of the Walthard nest often fully occupy it. Their nuclei are irregularly ovoid, and a longitudinal nuclear groove gives them a coffee-bean appearance (Fig. 14.25). Columnar metaplasia may occur in the nests and has no known significance. Both mesothelial inclusion cysts and Walthard nests are common incidental findings of no clinical importance.

Epithelial Tumors

Epithelial papillomas or polyps are rare. The only example acquired in our laboratory over the past 40 years was an incidental finding in a 42-year-old woman. It was composed of a delicate, branching stromal stalk lined by a single layer of nonciliated columnar cells with regular nuclei (Fig. 14.26). Whether or not these lesions have malignant potential is unknown. Because papillary proliferations may accompany salpingitis (see Fig. 14.8b), a diagnosis of a papilloma in the presence of inflammation or plical distortion secondary to previous inflammation is probably not warranted.

Mesodermal Tumors

Leiomyoma

Tumors of smooth muscle origin, chiefly leiomyomas, may originate from the tubal muscularis, from smooth muscle of the broad ligament, or from walls of blood

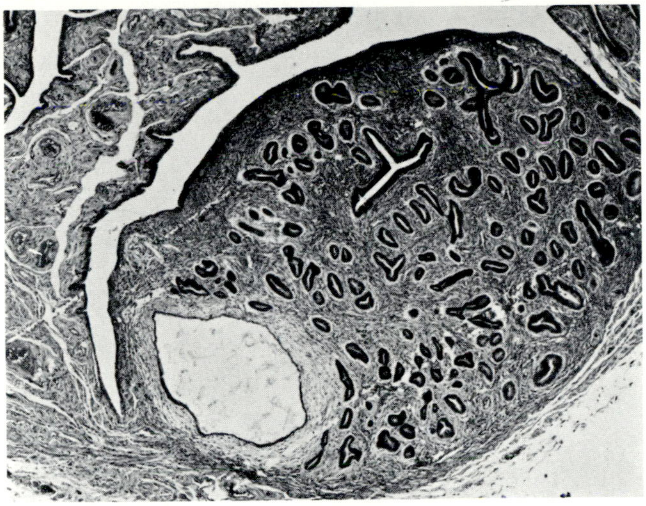

Fig. 14.27. Adenomyoma. A nodule of mixed simple glands and smooth muscle fibers protrudes into the tubal lumen.

vessels in either location. Compared with the frequency of uterine leiomyomas, tubal leiomyomas are quite uncommon.[139,175] Microscopically, they are similar to those found in the uterus, and they can undergo similar degenerative changes. Rarely, benign glands and smooth muscle may be so intimately involved in a tumor that a true adenomyoma is produced (Fig. 14.27).

Adenomatoid Tumor

Adenomatoid tumor (benign mesothelioma) is the most frequent type of benign tubal tumor. Previously reported lymphangiomas[182] probably represent examples of this entity. They are usually only 1–2 cm in diameter, appearing as a nodular swelling beneath the tubal serosa, and

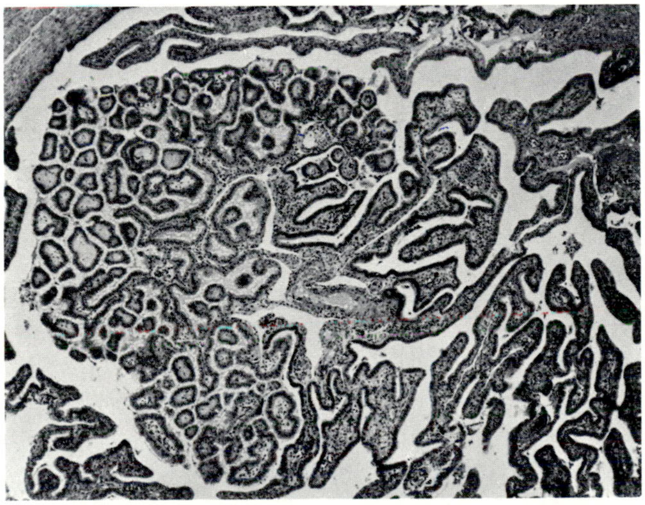

Fig. 14.26. Epithelial papilloma. Single layer of uniform cells lines a delicately branched papillary core.

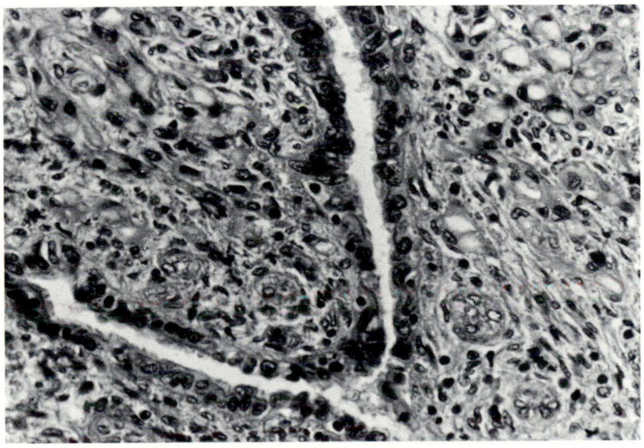

Fig. 14.28. Adenomatoid tumor (benign mesothelioma). Tumor infiltrates mucosal folds in a diffuse manner. Confusion with carcinoma is possible on frozen section. Note the intact epithelium of the tubal lumen.

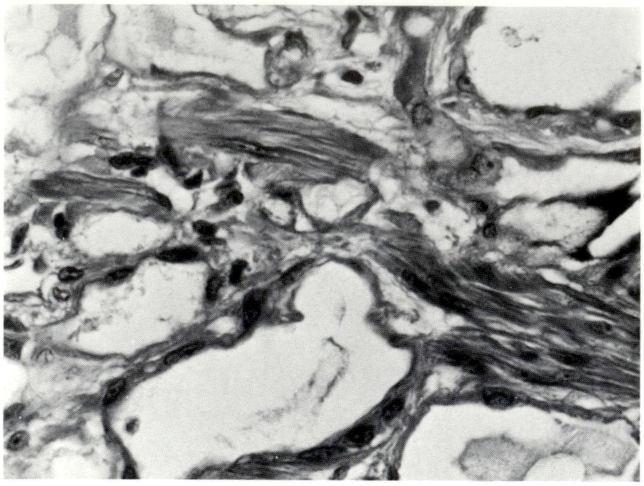

FIG. 14.29. Adenomatoid tumor (benign mesothelioma). Cuboidal or flattened mesothelial cells line dilated slit-like spaces. Penetration between small bundles of smooth muscle is seen here.

are yellow or whitish gray on section. Similar lesions may be found on the uterine surface,[215] in the cul-de-sac,[234] and on the ovary (see Chapter 13, Mesenchymal Tumors of Uterus and Chapter 21, Nonspecific Ovarian Tumors). Their chief importance to the gynecologic pathologist is differentiation from carcinoma on frozen section (Fig. 14.28). Microscopically, multiple, small, slit-like or ovoid spaces are seen lined by a single layer of low cuboidal or flattened endothelial-like cells (Fig. 14.29). Connection with the serosa may be seen on a fortuitous section (Fig. 14.30), but usually the serosa covers the lesion. The tumor may be large enough to displace the tubal lumen eccentrically and may grow into the supporting stroma of the luminal folds in an infiltrating manner (Fig. 14.28). Histochemical studies[213] have shown hyaluronidase-digestible, Alcian blue-positive material in the cells and spaces. No significant glycogen or intracellular mucin is present, as might be found in a tumor of müllerian origin. Electron microscopic[72,213] and immunocytochemical studies support a mesothelial origin for these lesions. Microvilli project from the cell surfaces. Bundles of tonofilaments are present and are occasionally attached to desmosomes. Desmosomes are numerous between cells but are absent along the basal lamina on which the cells lie. These features are not characteristic of endothelial or müllerian epithelium but are seen in benign mesotheliomas[72] as well as in malignant mesotheliomas. Clinically, they are asymptomatic, and rarely, if ever, do they recur after adequate excision.

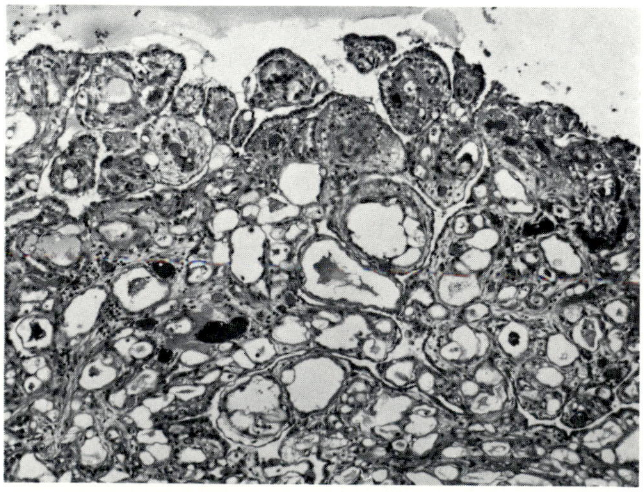

FIG. 14.30. Adenomatoid tumor (benign mesothelioma). Multiple connections with serosal surface are seen at top. Cuboidal or flattened cells line round or slit-like spaces.

Other Mesodermal Tumors

Other benign tumors of mesenchymal origin are rare. Hemangiomas,[64] lipomas,[53] angiomyolipomas,[118] and neural tumors[156,226] have been reported. Their microscopic appearance is identical to that of similar tumors appearing elsewhere in the body. Occasionally, a benign fibroblastic or fatty tumor will contain a focus of cartilage.[8,157]

Benign Teratoma

Tubal teratomas are rare. Clinically, a patient with a tubal teratoma is usually nulliparous and in the fourth decade.[145] Grossly, the tumors are located most frequently in the lumen, often attached by a pedicle to the inner tubal wall. They may, however, be intramural or attached to the serosa. On section, they are more often cystic than solid and may be small (1–2 cm in diameter) or large (10–20 cm in diameter).[145] As in their ovarian counterparts, ectodermal, mesodermal, and endodermal tissues are represented by well-differentiated mature elements. One lesion consisting entirely of mature thyroid tissue was described in the tube of a woman without clinical hyperthyroidism.[104] An isolated nodule of pancreatic tissue has been found beneath the tubal mucosa of one patient.[143] Only a single case of histologically immature tubal teratoma has been described.[208] Although ovarian teratomas appear to originate in abnormally developing ova,[198] only one patient is mentioned in whom ovarian tissue containing ova was found within tubal mucosa.[123]

Malignant Neoplasms

Primary Tumors

Carcinoma in Situ

The great majority of primary malignant lesions of the fallopian tube are adenocarcinomas. Although the typical adenocarcinoma is rarely a diagnostic problem, a good

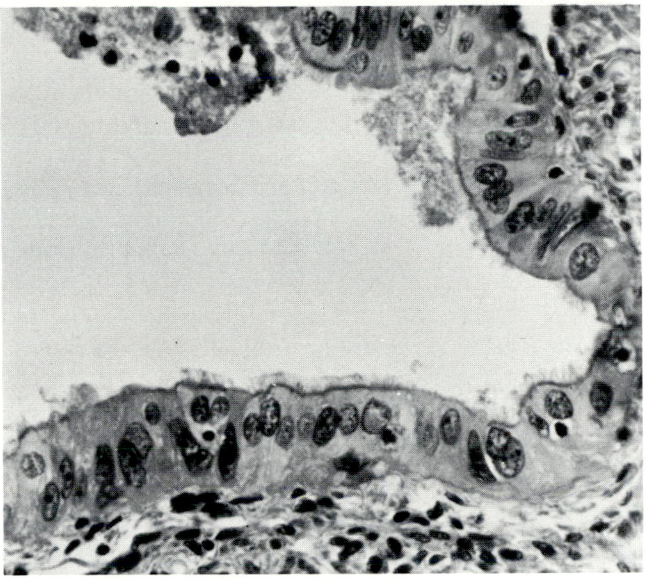

FIG. 14.31. Benign oncocytic (pink cell) metaplasia. Nuclear atypia and cell crowding in absence of papillary formations and mitoses should not be confused with early carcinoma.

deal of confusion has centered on what constitutes the earliest malignant change.[166] Previous authors[164,234] have illustrated cases in which tubal epithelium showed nuclear crowding and atypia and termed it *carcinoma in situ* (CIS). It is now clear that, when carefully studied, similar epithelial changes are present in 18% of routinely accessioned salpingectomy specimens.[148] Frequently, changes are present in only one or two of many sections (see Fig. 14.4). Although the lesions are more common in tubes with salpingitis (see Fig. 14.16), 14% of otherwise normal tubes show changes consisting of nuclear crowding and stratification, loss of polarity, and nuclear atypia. Mitoses are sparse. Papillary formation with bridging reminiscent of some forms of mammary papillomatosis may occur. An oncocytic type of metaplasia with cytoplasmic acidophilia is occasionally present (Figs. 14.3 and 14.31).

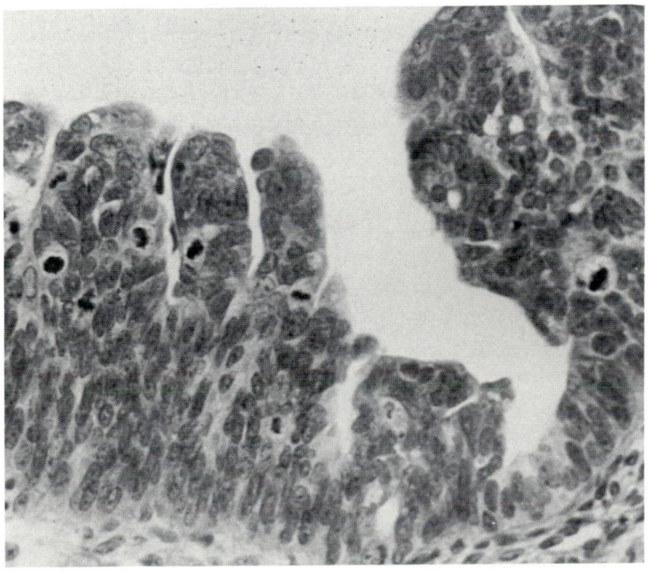

FIG. 14.32. Carcinoma in situ. The epithelial cells have lost their polarity and are growing in papillae without stromal cores. Nuclei are hyperchromatic, large, and irregular, and mitoses are numerous. The basement membrane is intact.

CIS is accurately diagnosed only when papillary formations with mitoses and marked nuclear atypia are present (Fig. 14.32), and one must question whether nonpapillary, noninfiltrative lesions ever represent CIS. As noted previously, papillary formations with atypia are common in various forms of chronic salpingitis. Numerous mitoses or evidence of invasion are lacking, however, in these lesions. Startling epithelial changes that tend to mimic early papillary adenocarcinoma may be produced by accidental exposure of the specimen to heat.[41]

Invasive Adenocarcinoma

Primary adenocarcinoma of the tube is uncommon. A recent study found only 0.2% of primary female genital malignancies to be tubal.[236]

Unfortunately, primary tubal carcinoma is rarely found in the in situ stage. The typical patient is in her fifth or sixth decade and ordinarily has one or more of the classic signs or symptoms of invasive tubal carcinoma: abnormal uterine bleeding, clear or serosanguinous vaginal discharge (hydrops tubae profluens), pelvic pain, or a pelvic mass.[100,188,237] The diagnosis is rarely made before operation, but occasionally positive cytology associated with negative endometrial curettage will indicate the correct location of the malignancy.[10,188]

Grossly, the tube is usually swollen secondary to advanced intraluminal growth. Hydrosalpinx or tuboovarian abscess is ruled out only after the specimen is opened. The lumen is usually filled and dilated by papillary or solid tumor (Fig. 14.33). The fimbriated end is closed in about half the cases.[234]

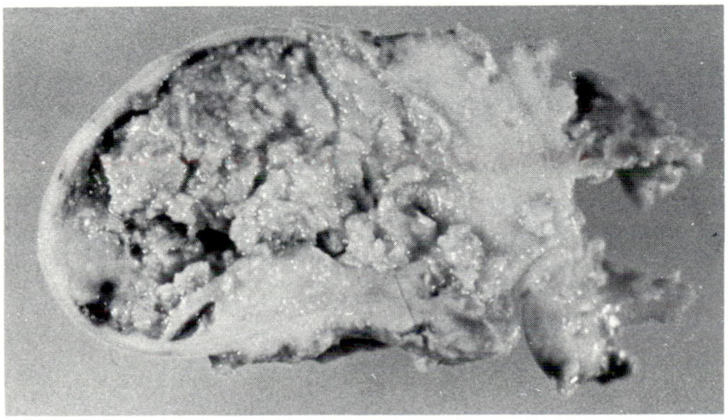

FIG. 14.33. Primary tubal adenocarcinoma. Tube is dilated and filled by papillary and solid tumor, which penetrates the muscularis along the lower margin of the specimen.

Bilateral involvement frequently occurs, but the reason for this is unknown. A common carcinogenic stimulus could cause simultaneous development of tumor in both tubes, or a retrograde lymphatic spread after blockage by advanced tubal carcinoma of one side could lead to metastatic deposits contralaterally. Subsequent growth might then mimic a second primary tumor. The fact that bilateral tubal carcinoma is present in only 7% of stage 0–II lesions but may be seen in as many as 30% of stage III and IV lesions[187] suggests that metastatic spread in advanced lesions is an important cause of bilaterality.

Microscopically, alveolar, papillary, and medullary patterns of tumor growth may be observed, but mixtures are frequent. Disorganized piling up of cells with mitoses, nuclear pleomorphism, and hyperchromaticity is present in virtually all types (Figs. 14.34 and 14.35). Abrupt transitions from normal to neoplastic epithelium may be found. Mucin production is usually inconspicuous but rarely may be prominent.[130] Attempts to grade tumor pattern or degree of nuclear atypia have proved to be of limited prognostic value,[56,100,237] but staging (Table 14.1) is very useful. A number of staging schemes have been proposed based on operative or operative plus pathologic findings.[6,67,187] Once tumor spreads to the serosa, 5-year survival drops to only one patient in six (Table 14.1), and even 5-year survival is not synonymous with cure.[187]

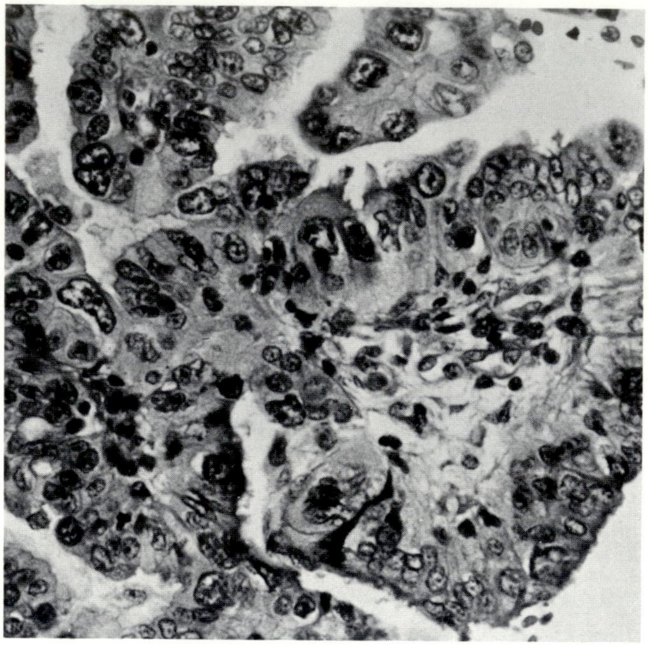

FIG. 14.35. Tubal adenocarcinoma. Papillary projections are lined by piled-up epithelial cells, showing marked nuclear atypia. Mitoses are present in nearby areas.

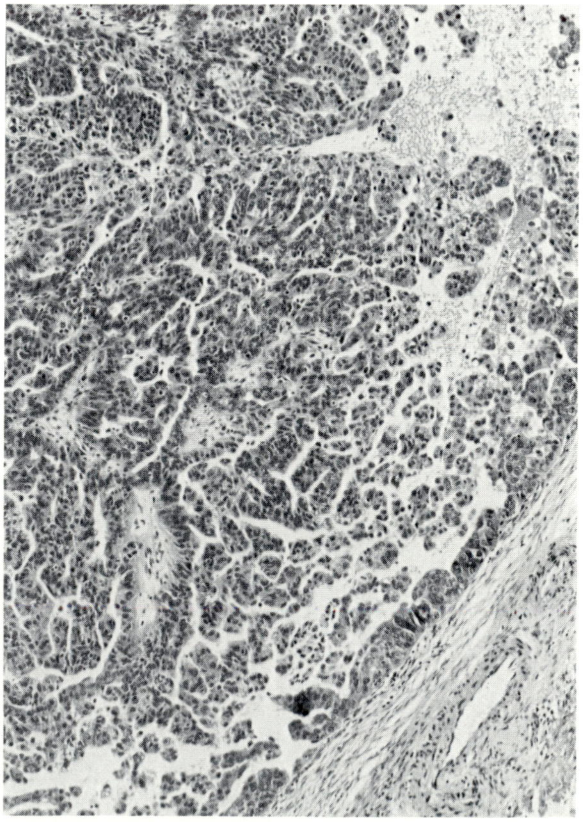

FIG. 14.34. Primary tubal carcinoma. The tubal lumen is dilated by fronds of papillary tumor. Invasion is present in adjacent areas of the wall.

Current treatment by total abdominal hysterectomy and bilateral salpingo-oophorectomy with or without adjuvant radiation or chemotherapy usually fails due to transperitoneal spread.[56] The CA125 antigenic determinant found in ovarian carcinoma is also present in tubal carcinoma[153] and may prove useful in patient follow-up.

TABLE 14.1. Staging and survival in adenocarcinoma of the fallopian tube.

Stage	Definition	Number of patients	Percent 5-year survival without disease
0	Carcinoma in situ	11	82
I	Tumor extends into submucosa or muscularis, not serosa	13	53
II	Tumor extends to serosa	6	16
III	Tumor extends to ovary and/or endometrium	12	8
IV	Tumor extends beyond reproductive organs	34	9

After Schiller and Silverberg, Ref. 187.

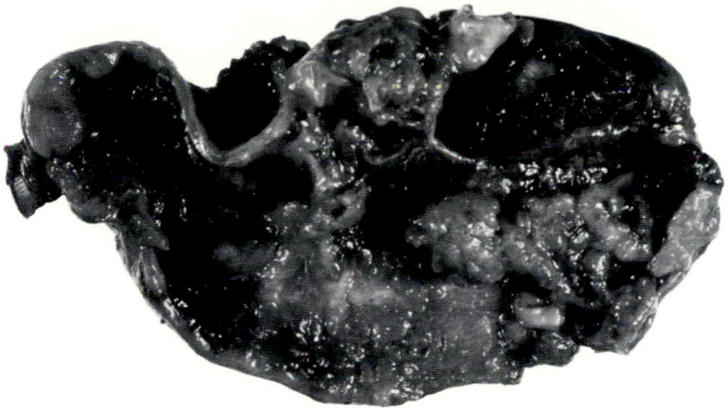

FIG. 14.36. Primary tubal carcinosarcoma. Dilated tube has been opened to illustrate the irregular intraluminal projections and a shaggy, irregular mucosal surface.

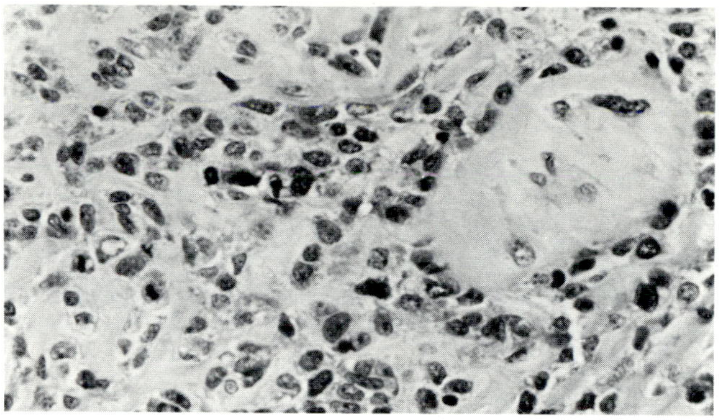

FIG. 14.38. Primary mixed mesodermal tumor of tube. At right is a relatively acellular nodule of osteoid shown lying in a sarcomatous background. Elsewhere, carcinomatous areas are present.

Tubal adenoacanthomas or adenosquamous carcinomas are composed, respectively, of histologic foci of benign-appearing or malignant-appearing squamous epithelium within an adenocarcinoma.[100] Primary squamous,[138] transitional cell,[71] and clear cell[223] carcinomas have been described rarely.

Sarcomas

Sarcomas of the tube are exceedingly uncommon and may be pure or mixed with carcinomatous elements. Pure sarcomas may be histologically classified if sufficient differentiation is present. Leiomyosarcomas[2] are perhaps the most common type and may arise from the tube or broad ligament. Chondrosarcomas have been described.[2,185] Carcinomas mixed with sarcomas containing only elements normally present in the fallopian tubes, such as smooth muscle, are termed *carcinosarcomas* (Figs. 14.36 and 14.37). If heterologous elements not normally found in the tubes, such as cartilage or bone, are present, the tumor is termed *malignant mixed mesodermal tumor* or *heterologous carcinosarcoma* (Fig. 14.38).[99] The number of cases available is too few to prove any prognostic difference between these two groups.

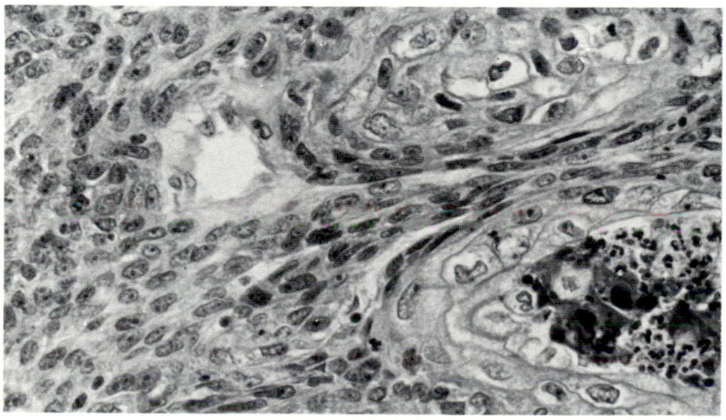

FIG. 14.37. Carcinosarcoma of tube. Two ovoid islands of malignant squamous epithelium (*right*) lie in the stroma of a leiomyosarcoma.

As with tubal carcinomas, patients with sarcomas are frequently postmenopausal. They may have watery or bloody vaginal discharge and abdominal pain and signs of intraperitoneal spread. Life expectancy is usually measured in months, but surgery and chemotherapy may lead to longer remissions.[57,99]

Metastatic Tumors

Metastatic tumors involving the tube are usually secondary to spread from carcinomas of the ovary or endometrium.[233] Peritoneal spread involves the serosal surface, whereas lymphatic metastases from adjacent primary sites may involve the mucosa or muscularis as well. Endolymphatic stromal myosis, originating in the uterus, may extend to involve the tubes and ovaries. Spread takes place by the extension of worm-like tongues of tumor along tubal lymphatics. Blood-borne metastases from breast carcinomas or other extrapelvic tumors may also occur. On occasion, squamous carcinoma of the uterine cervix may spread in an in situ manner to involve the endometrial cavity, tubes, and even the ovarian surface.[171] Primary squamous carcinoma is a rarity.[138]

The presence of a large ovarian primary coupled with tumor in the lumen of the fallopian tube and tumor in the endometrial cavity suggests that the tubal lumen may serve as a conduit for tumor spread. Careful study of the tubes removed at surgery for primary ovarian carcinoma reveals that luminal groups of tumor cells may implant onto endosalpingeal surfaces and simulate CIS or early primary tubal carcinoma (Fig. 14.39). Because of frequent secondary involvement of the tubes, Hu et al.[111] suggested that the following criteria be used

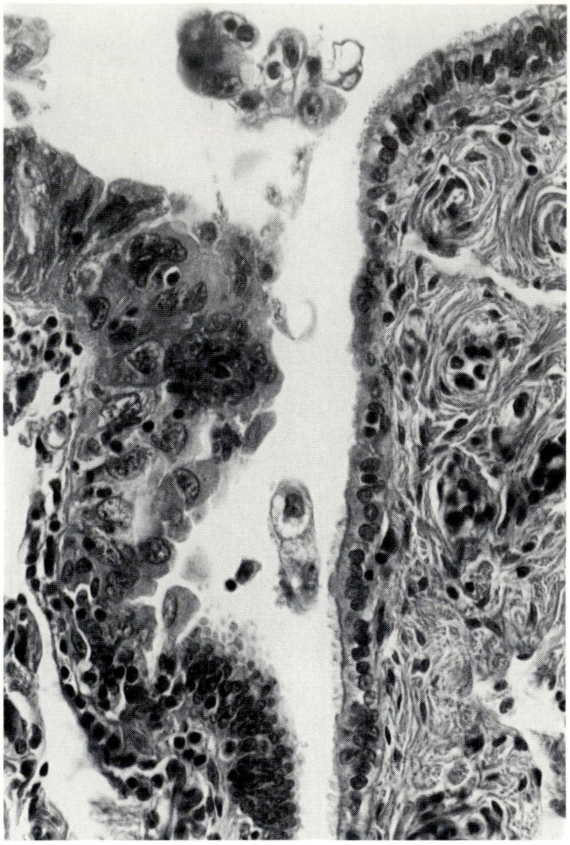

FIG. 14.39. Tubal implantation of ovarian carcinoma. Two clusters of malignant cells from an ipsilateral ovarian carcinoma lie free in the tubal lumen, and on the *left*, carcinoma has implanted and begun to spread over the mucosal surface.

to determine primary tubal carcinoma. Grossly, the main tumor is in the tube; microscopically, chiefly the mucosa is involved and shows a papillary pattern; if the tubal wall is greatly involved, a transition between benign and malignant tubal epithelium should be found. When both tube and ovary are intimately involved by a mass of tumor, the assumption of an ovarian primary tumor may not always be correct.[236]

Lymphoma

Tubal involvement by lymphoma is rare and is almost invariably associated with simultaneous involvement of the ipsilateral ovary.[2] Undifferentiated carcinoma must be ruled out.

Trophoblastic Lesions

Trophoblastic tubal lesions are exceedingly rare. Hydatiform moles usually occur as isolated growths but may be associated with intrauterine pregnancy.[202] Histologically, their appearance is similar to that of an intrauterine molar pregnancy. Clinically, perhaps 1 in 5000 ectopic pregnancies will prove to be a mole.[104] Choriocarcinoma rarely may arise in the tube.[137] Clinically, the patient is believed to have an ectopic pregnancy. At operation, a large and very hemorrhagic, fleshy mass may have largely destroyed the tube. Histologically, the malignant trophoblastic proliferation is similar to that of uterine choriocarcinomas. Response to modern chemotherapy has been gratifying[163] (see Chapter 24, Gestational Trophoblastic Disease).

Paratubal Tumors and Cysts

Adrenal Rests

Adrenal cortical rests, if carefully looked for, may be found in the broad ligament in more than 20% of women. They lie in the ligament "anywhere from its junction with the mesosalpinx to its lateral attachment to the pelvic wall"[69] adjacent to the ovarian vein and just beneath the peritoneum. Grossly, they appear as yellow nodules or disks, but they may be obscured by fat. Medullary tissue is absent, but microscopically all three cortical layers are recognizable. This accessory tissue may hypertrophy secondary to adrenal destruction[116] or may, rarely, give rise to a functional cortical adenoma.[19]

Nests of cells morphologically similar to ovarian hilus cells have been described in the midportion of the tube.[158] In the absence of Reinke crystals, close association with nonmyelinated nerve fibers, or histochemical studies, it is difficult to exclude the possibility of an adrenal rest. Hilus cell nests with Reinke crystals may be seen, however, in fimbrial stroma.[132] These may be the cells responsible for the only case reported of tubal Sertoli-Leydig tumor.[60]

Adnexal Tumor of Probable Wolffian Origin

A small group of distinctive tumors is described as located either within the leaves of the broad ligament or attached to the tube by a pedicle.[117] (These tumors are also described and illustrated in Chapter 21, Nonspecific Ovarian Tumors.) Briefly, patients range in age from 29 to 58 years. Either they have abdominal pain and a palpable mass, or else the tumor is discovered as an incidental finding. The lesions measure from 1.3 to 12 cm in greatest dimension and are lobulated, with gross encapsulation. On section, the consistency may be rubbery or friable, and cysts or calcification may be present.

The microscopic picture varies widely (Fig. 14.40). Solid masses of epithelial cells may be present, or tubular

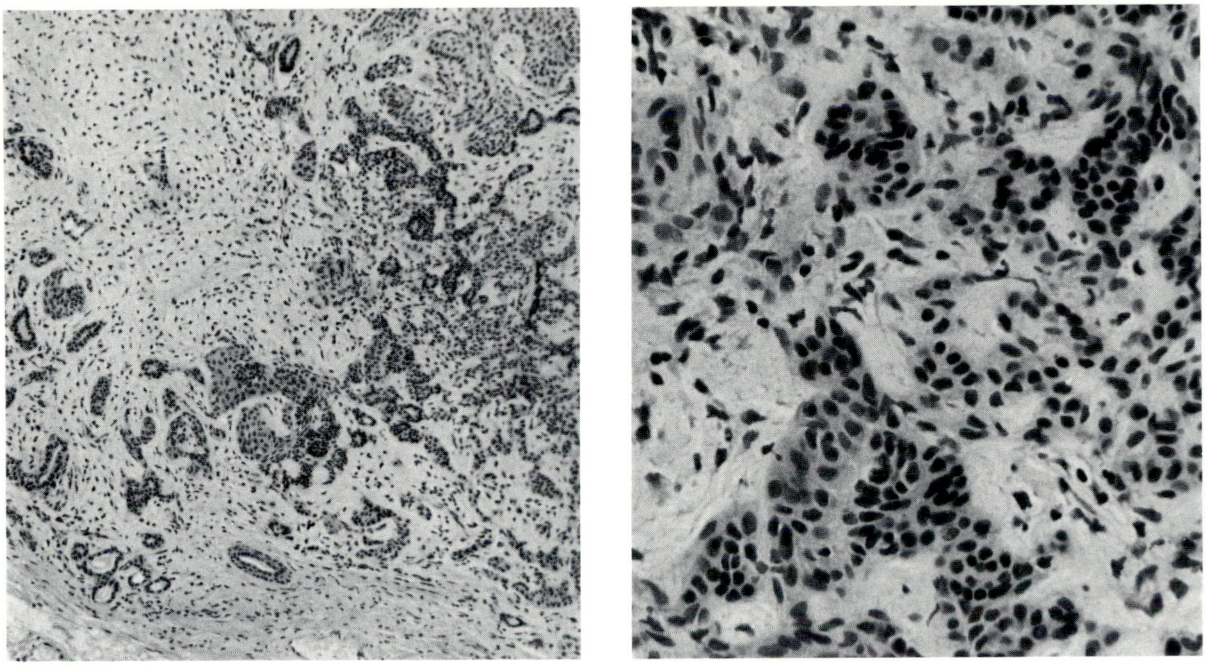

FIG. 14.40. Paratubal wolffian tumor. This was an incidentally found, 4 mm mass. *Left:* The tumor has a nonencapsulated pushing border on the *bottom left*. Irregular cords and trabeculae with abortive tubule formation grow haphazardly in a somewhat cellular spindle cell stroma. *Right:* The nuclei of the abortive tubules and trabeculae are regular and lack mitotic activity. (Courtesy of Dr. V.A. LiVolsi, Philadelphia, PA.)

areas may be found similar to a well-differentiated Sertoli-Leydig tumor of the ovary (Pick's tubular adenoma). A sieve-like pattern reminiscent of benign tubal mesotheliomas may also be seen. Microscopically, the capsule is often breached by tongues of tumor. Ultrastructural analysis has been interpreted as supporting a mesonephric origin.[55,105,117,212] Although most of these tumors behave in a benign fashion, multiple local recurrences[24] and fatal metastases may occur.[1,212]

Other Paraovarian Tumors

Other solid paraovarian tumors are most often leiomyomas. Sarcomas and malignant primary epithelial lesions are rare.[46,85] The rare broad ligament adenocarcinomas reported tend to be in women in the reproductive years and are typically low-grade serous lesions.[177] Overdiagnosis of borderline serous tumors as carcinoma should be avoided.[47] Distinction of a borderline tumor from an invasive serous carcinoma is based on the absence of stromal invasion, using the same criteria that are applied to ovarian serous neoplasms (see Chapter 18, Epithelial Tumors of Ovary). Paraovarian cystadenofibromas are occasional, usually incidental findings.[109] Extraovarian Brenner tumors,[224] mesosalpingeal choriocarcinoma,[120] broad ligament pheochromocytoma,[5] and mesovarial ependymoma[92] are among the rare tumors reported adjacent to tube and ovary.

Paratubal Cysts

Paratubal cysts may arise from mesonephric (wolffian) structures, from paramesonephric (müllerian) structures, or from mesothelial inclusions.[181] Differentiation may be difficult because of compression and atrophy of the lining cells; paramesonephric cysts are lined by epithelium containing numerous ciliated cells. Such cysts may also have papillary infoldings similar to endosalpingeal folds. Mesonephric cysts contain only a few or no ciliated cells and may have a more prominent muscular coat. Ultrastructurally, mesonephric epithelial cells tend to have an inapparent Golgi apparatus, moderate rough endoplasmic reticulum (RER), numerous lysosomes, and minimal glycogen. Paramesonephric epithelial cells tend to have a prominent Golgi apparatus and RER, prominent glycogen, and only rare lysosomes.[54,84]

The hydatid of Morgagni is by far the most common paramesonephric cyst. Grossly, it is found dangling from one of the fimbriae. It is ovoid or round, 2–10 mm in diameter, and contains clear serous fluid surrounded by a thin translucent wall. Microscopically, it is lined by ciliated and nonciliated cells and may have small epithelial-covered plicae projecting into the lumen. The nonciliated cells undergo cyclic changes.[20] A careful study of paraovarian cysts revealed that 86% of those more than 3 cm in diameter were mesothelial, 14% were paramesonephric, and none was mesonephric.[87]

References

1. Abbot RL, Barlogie B, Schmidt WA (1981) Metastasizing malignant juxtaovarian tumor with terminal hypercalcemia: A case report. Cancer 48: 860
2. Abrams J, Kazal HL, Hobbs RE (1958) Primary sarcoma of the fallopian tube. Am J Obstet Gynecol 75: 180
3. Adams BE (1969) Intussusception of a fallopian tube. Am J Surg 118: 591
4. Afzelius BA, Eliasson R (1983) Male and female infertility problems in the immotile-cilia syndrome. Eur J Respir Dis 64 [Suppl 127]: 144
5. Al-Jafari MS, Panton HM, Gradwell E (1985) Phaeochromocytoma of the broad ligament. Case report. Br J Obstet Gynaecol 92: 649
6. American College of Obstetricians and Gynecologists' Committee on Terminology (1972) In: Hughes EC, ed. Obstetric–gynecologic terminology, with section on neonatology and glossary of congenital anomalies. Philadelphia, FA Davis, p 157
7. Aselton PJ, Stergachis A (1984) Increasing incidence of ectopic pregnancy (Letter). JAMA 251: 469
8. Bachmann FF (1961) Ein chondrolipom des Eileiters. Geburts Frauenheilkd 21: 975
9. Benjamin CL, Beaver DC (1951) Pathogenesis of salpingitis isthmica nodosa. Am J Clin Pathol 21: 212
10. Benson PA (1974) Cytologic diagnosis in primary carcinoma of the fallopian tube. Acta Cytol 18:429
11. Beral V (1975) An epidemiological study of recent trends in ectopic pregnancy. Br J Obstet Gynaecol 82: 775
12. Bernardus RE, Van der Slikke JW, Roex AJM, Dijkhuizen GH, Stolk JG (1984) Torsion of the fallopian tube: Some considerations on its etiology. Obstet Gynecol 64: 675
13. Beyth Y, Bar-On E (1984) Tuboovarian autoamputation and infertility. Fertil Steril 42: 932
14. Beyth Y, Kopolovic J (1982) Accessory tubes: A possible contributing factor in infertility. Fertil Steril 38: 382
15. Birch HW, Collins CG (1961) Atypical changes of genital epithelium associated with ectopic pregnancy. Am J Obstet Gynecol 81: 1198
16. Bland KG, Gelfand M (1970) The effects of schistosomiasis on the fallopian tubes in the African female. J Obstet Gynaecol Br Commow 77: 1024
17. Blaustein A, Shenker L (1967) Vascular lesions of the uterine tube in ectopic pregnancy. Obstet Gynecol 30: 551
18. Bobrow ML, Bell HG (1962) Ectopic pregnancy: A 16-year survey of 905 cases. Obstet Gynecol 20: 500
19. Boularan, Cahuzac, Salvador, Genesseau (1945) Macrogenitosomie et gynandrie chez un sujet porteu de deux tumeurs cortico-surrenaliennes incluses dans les ligaments larges. Ann Endocrinol (Paris) 6: 57
20. Bransilver BR, Ferenczy A, Richart RM (1973) Female genital tract remnants. An ultrastructural comparison of hydatid of Morgagni and mesonephric ducts and tubules. Arch Pathol 96: 255
21. Braun P, Besdine R (1971) Tuboovarian abscess with recovery of *T. mycoplasm.* Am J Obstet Gynecol 117: 861
22. Breen JL (1970) A 21-year survey of 654 ectopic pregnancies. Am J Gynecol 106: 1004
23. Brenner PF, Roy S, Mishell DR Jr (1980) Ectopic pregnancy. A study of 300 consecutive surgical treated cases. JAMA 243: 673
24. Brescia RJ, Cardoso de Almeida PC, Fuller AF Jr, Dickersin GR, Robboy SJ (1985) Female adnexal tumor of probable wolffian origin with multiple recurrences over 16 years. Cancer 56: 1456
25. Britigan BE, Cohen MS, Sparling PF (1985) Gonococcal infection: A model of molecular pathogenesis. N Engl J Med 312: 1683
26. Bronson R, Cunnane M (1975) Transfer of uterine implantation blastocysts to the oviduct in mice. Fertil Steril 26: 455
27. Brooks JJ, Wheeler JE (1977) Granulomatous salpingitis secondary to Crohn's disease. Obstet Gynecol 49: 31s
28. Brunham RC, Maclean IW, Binns B, Peeling RW (1985) *Chlamydia trachomatis:* Its role in tubal infertility. J Infect Dis 152: 1275
29. Busch DH, Benirschke K (1974) Cytogenetic studies of ectopic pregnancies. Virchows Arch [Pathol Anat] 16: 319
30. Bylund DJ, Nanfro JJ, Marsh WL (1986) Coccidioidomycosis of the female genital tract. Arch Pathol Lab Med 110: 232
31. Campbell JS, Nigam S, Hurtig A, Sahasrabudhe MR, Marino I (1964) Mineral oil granulomas of the uterus and parametrium and granulomatous salpingitis with Schaumann bodies and oxalate deposits. Fertil Steril 15: 278
32. Case Records of the Massachusetts General Hospital (Case 9–1971) (1971) N Engl J Med 284: 491
33. Chalvardjian A, Picard L, Shaw R, Davey R, Cairns JD (1980) Malacoplakia of the female genital tract. Am J Obstet Gynecol 138: 391
34. Chevallier G, Parent B (1966) L'hydrosalpinx. Etude de 253 cas. Presse Med 74: 2035
35. Chi I-C, Potts M, Wilkens L (1986) Rare events associated with tubal sterilization: An international experience. Obstet Gynecol Surv 41: 7
36. Chow AW, Malkasian KL, Marshall JR, Guze LB (1975) The bacteriology of acute pelvic inflammatory disease. Am J Obstet Gynecol 122: 876
37. Chow W-H, Daling JR, Weiss NS, Moore DE, Soderstrom R (1985) Vaginal douching as a potential risk factor for tubal ectopic pregnancy. Am J Obstet Gynecol 153: 727
38. Chung CS, Smith RG, Steinhoff PG, Mi M-P (1982) Induced abortion and ectopic pregnancy in subsequent pregnancies. Am J Epidemiol 115: 879
39. Collins JA, Wrixon W, Janes LB, Wilson EH (1983) Treatment-independent pregnancy among infertile couples. N Engl J Med 309: 1201

40. Copeland W Jr, Hawley PC, Teteris NJ (1985) Gynecologic amyloidosis. Am J Obstet Gynecol 153: 555
41. Cornog JL, Curie JL, Rubin A (1970) Heat artifact simulating adenocarcinoma of fallopian tube. JAMA 214: 1118
42. Coutinho EM, Maia H Jr, Mattos CER (1975) Contractility of the fallopian tube. Gynecol Invest 6: 146
43. Crohn BB, Yarnis H (1958) Regional ileitis, 2nd ed. New York, Grune & Stratton
44. Crosby EC, Humphrey T, Lauer EW (1962) Correlative anatomy of the nervous system. New York, Macmillan
45. Croxatto HB, Diaz S, Feuntealba B, Croxatto HD, Carrillo D, Fabres C (1972) Studies on the duration of egg transport in the human oviduct. I. The time interval between ovulation and egg recovery from the uterus in normal women. Fertil Steril 23: 447
46. Czernobilsky B, Lancet M (1972) Broad ligament adenocarcinoma of müllerian origin. Obstet Gynecol 40: 238
47. d'Ablaing G, Klatt EC, DiRocco G, Hibbard LT (1983) Broad ligament serous tumor of low malignant potential. Int J Gynecol Pathol 2: 93
48. David A, Garcia C-R, Czernobilsky B (1969) Human hydrosalpinx. Histologic study and chemical composition of fluid. Am J Obstet Gynecol 105: 400
49. David A, Serr DN, Czernobilsky B (1973) Chemical position of human oviduct fluid. Fertil Steril 24: 435
50. Daw E (1973) Duplication of the uterine tube. Obstet Gynecol 42: 137
51. DeCherney AH, Cholst I, Naftolin F (1981) Structure and function of the fallopian tubes following exposure to diethylstilbestrol (DES) during gestation. Fertil Steril 36: 741
52. DeCherney AH, Maheaux R, Naftolin F (1982) Salpingostomy for ectopic pregnancy in the sole patient oviduct: Reproductive outcome. Fertil Steril 37: 619
53. Dede JA, Janovski NA (1963) Lipoma of the uterine tube. Obstet Gynecol 22: 461
54. Demopoulos RI, Bigelow B, Vasa U (1978) Infarcted uterine adnexa: Associated pathology. NY State J Med 78: 2027
55. Demopoulos RI, Sitelman A, Flotte T, Bigelow B (1960) Ultrastructural study of a female adnexal tumor of probable wolffian origin. Cancer 46: 2273
56. Denham JW, Maclennan KA (1984) The management of primary carcinoma of the fallopian tube. Experience of 40 cases. Cancer 53: 166
57. Deppe G, Zbella E, Friberg J, Thomas W (1984) Combination chemotherapy for mixed müllerian tumor of the fallopian tube. Cancer 54: 1517
58. Diamant YZ, Aboulafia Y, Raz S (1972) Torsion of hydrosalpinx. Int Surg 57: 303
59. Dische FE, Burt JM, Davison NJH, Puntambekar S (1974) Tuboovarian actinomycosis associated with intrauterine contraceptive devices. J Obstet Gynaecol Br Commonw 81: 724
60. Dokumov St, Dekov D (1963) A rare case of precocious pseudopuberty due to a Sertoli-Leydig cell tumor originating from the left fallopian tube. J Clin Endocrinol Metab 23: 1262
61. Donnez J, Casanas-Roux F, Caprasse J, Ferin J, Thomas K (1985) Cyclic changes in ciliation, cell height, and mitotic activity in human tubal epithelium during reproductive life. Fertil Steril 43: 554
62. Dorfman SF, Grimes DA, Cates W Jr, Binkin NJ, Kafrissen ME, O'Reilly KR (1984) Ectopic pregnancy mortality, United States, 1979 to 1980: Clinical aspects. Obstet Gynecol 64: 386
63. Dudkiewicz J (1970) Quantitative and qualitative changes of epithelial cells of fallopian tubes in women according to the phase of menstrual cycle. A cytologic study. Acta Cytol 14: 531
64. Ebrahimi T, Okagaki T (1973) Hemangioma of the fallopian tube. Am J Obstet Gynecol 115: 864
65. Elliott GB, Brody H, Elliott KA (1965) Implications of "lipoid" salpingitis. Fertil Steril 16: 541
66. Ellsworth HS, Harris JW, McQuarrie HG, Stone RA, Anderson AE (1973) Prolapse of the fallopian tube following vaginal hysterectomy. JAMA 224: 891
67. Erez S, Kaplan LA, Wall JA (1967) Clinical staging of carcinoma of the uterine tube. Obstet Gynecol 30: 547
68. Evans MI, Angerman NS, Moravec WE, Hajj SN (1979) The intrauterine device and ovarian pregnancy. Fertil Steril 32: 31
69. Falls JL (1955) Accessory adrenal cortex in the broad ligament. Cancer 8: 143
70. Farber M, Mitchell GW Jr (1979) Bicornuate uterus and partial atresia of the fallopian tube. Am J Obstet Gynecol 134: 881
71. Federman Q, Toker C (1973) Primary transitional cell tumor of the uterine adnexa. Am J Obstet Gynecol 115: 863
72. Ferenczy A, Fenoglio J, Richart RM (1972) Observations on benign mesotheliomas of the genital tract (adenomatoid tumor). Cancer 30: 244
73. Ferenczy A, Richart RM (1974) Female reproductive system: Dynamics of scan and transmission electron microscopy. New York, Wiley, pp 212–253
74. Fetissof F, Berger G, Dubois MP, Philippe A, et al. (1985) Female genital tract and Peutz-Jeghers syndrome: An immunohistochemical study. Int J Gynecol Pathol 4: 219
75. Fitzgerald TB, Mainwaring AR, Ahmed A (1974) Pelvic peritoneal oxyuriasis simulating metastatic carcinoma. J Obstet Gynaecol Br Commonw 81: 248
76. Flickinger GL, Meuchler EK, Mikhail G (1974) Estradiol receptor in the human fallopian tube. Fertil Steril 25: 900
77. Fortier KJ, Haney AF (1985) The pathologic spectrum of uterotubal junction obstruction. Obstet Gynecol 65: 93
78. Frachtman KG (1953) Unruptured tubal term pregnancy. Am J Surg 86: 161
79. Fredricsson B (1969) Histochemistry of the oviduct. In: Hafex ESE, Blandau RJ, eds. The mammalian oviduct. Chicago, University of Chicago Press
80. Frost O (1975) Bilharzia of the fallopian tube. S Afr Med J 49: 1201
81. Fujii S, Ban C, Okamura H, Nishimura T (1981) Unilateral tubal quadruplet pregnancy. Am J Obstet Gynecol 141: 840
82. Gaddum-Rosse P, Blandau RJ (1973) In vitro studies on

ciliary activity within the oviducts of the rabbit and pig. Am J Anat 136: 91
83. Gaddum-Rosse P, Rumery RE, Blandau RT, Thiersch JB (1975) Studies on the mucosa of postmenopausal oviducts: Surface appearance, ciliary activity, and the effect of estrogen treatment. Fertil Steril 26: 951
84. Gardner GH, Greene RR, Peckham BM (1948) Normal and cystic structures of broad ligament. Am J Obstet Gynecol 55: 917
85. Gardner GH, Greene RR, Peckham B (1957) Tumors of the broad ligament. Am J Obstet Gynecol 73: 536
86. Gelfand M, Ross MD, Blair DM, Weber MC (1971) Distribution and extent of schistosomiasis in female pelvic organs with special reference to the genital tract, as determined at autopsy. Am J Trop Med Hyg 20: 846
87. Genadry R, Parmley T, Woodruff JD (1977) The origin and clinical behavior of the paraovarian tumor. Am J Obstet Gynecol 129: 843
88. Georgakopoulos PA, Gogas CG, Sariyannis HG (1980) Hydatid disease of the female genitalia. Obstet Gynecol 55: 555
89. Gomel V (1983) An odyssey through the oviduct. Fertil Steril 39: 144
90. Gravaller J, Suranyi S, Berensci G (1956) Neue Gesichtpunkte in der Klinik der Genitaltuberkulos. Zentralbl Gynaekol 78: 496
91. Grimes HG, Nosal RA, Gallagher JC (1983) Ovarian pregnancy: A series of 24 cases. Obstet Gynecol 61: 174
92. Grody WW, Nieberg RK, Bhuta S (1985) Ependymoma-like tumor of the mesovarium. Arch Pathol Lab Med 109: 291
93. Gump DW, Gibson M, Ashikaga T (1984) Lack of association between genital mycoplasm and infertility. N Engl J Med 310: 937
94. Haines M (1958) Tuberculous salpingitis as seen by the pathologist and the surgeon. Am J Obstet Gynecol 75: 472
95. Halbrecht I (1962) Genital tuberculosis. Fertil Steril 13: 371
96. Hallatt JG (1982) Primary ovarian pregnancy: A report of twenty-five cases. Am J Obstet Gynecol 143: 55
97. Hallatt JG (1976) Ectopic pregnancy associated with the intrauterine device: A study of seventy cases. Am J Obstet Gynecol 125: 754
98. Hallatt JG (1975) Repeat ectopic pregnancy: A study of 123 consecutive cases. Am J Obstet Gynecol 122: 520
99. Hanjani P, Petersen RO, Bonnell SA (1980) Malignant mixed müllerian tumor of the fallopian tube. Gynecol Oncol 9: 381
100. Hanton EM, Malkasian GD Jr, Dahlin DC, Pratt JH (1966) Primary carcinoma of the fallopian tube. Am J Obstet Gynecol 94: 832
101. Hellman LM (1949) Morphology of the human fallopian tube in the early puerperium. Am J Obstet Gynecol 57: 154
102. Henriksen E (1955) Struma salpingii. Obstet Gynecol 5: 833
103. Herrera GA, Reimann BEF, Greenberg HL, Miles PA (1983) Pigmentosis tubae, a new entity: Light and electron microscopic study. Obstet Gynecol 61: 80S
104. Hertig AT, Mansell H (1956) Tumors of the female sex organs. Part 1. Hydatiform mole and choriocarcinoma. In: Atlas of tumor pathology, Series 1, Fasc 33, pp 62–63. Washington, DC, Armed Forces Institute of Pathology
105. Hinchey WW, Silva EG, Guarda LA, Ordonez NG, Wharton JT (1983) Paravaginal wolffian duct (mesonephros) adenocarcinoma: A light and electron microscopic study. Am J Clin Pathol 80: 539
106. Hockin JC, Jessamine AG (1984) Trends in ectopic pregnancy in Canada. Can Med Assc J 131: 737
107. Holman JF, Tyrey EL, Hammond CB (1984) A contemporary approach to suspected ectopic pregnancy with use of quantitative and qualitative assays for the beta-subunit of human chorionic gonadotropin and sonography. Am J Obstet Gynecol 150: 151
108. Honore LH (1978) Salpingitis isthmica nodosa in female infertility and ectopic tubal pregnancy. Fertil Steril 29: 164
109. Honore LH, O'Hara KE (1980) Serous papillary neoplasms arising in paramesonephric parovarian cysts. Acta Obstet Gynecol Scand 59: 525
110. Hovadhanakul P, Eachempati U, Cavanagh D (1971) Ureteral observation in chronic ectopic pregnancy. Am J Obstet Gynecol 110: 311
111. Hu CY, Taymor ML, Hertig AT (1950) Primary carcinoma of the fallopian tube. Am J Obstet Gynecol 59: 58
112. Isager-Sally L, Weber T (1985) Torsion of the fallopian tube during pregnancy. Acta Obstet Gynecol Scand 64: 349
113. Jansen RPS (1984) Endocrine response in the fallopian tube. Endocrinol Rev 5: 525
114. Jauchler GW, Baker RL (1970) Cervical pregnancy: Review of the literature and a case report. Obstet Gynecol 35: 870
115. Kallenberger DA, Ronk DA, Jimerson GK (1978) Ectopic pregnancy: A 15 year review of 160 cases. South Med J 71: 758
116. Karakascheff KI (1906) Weitere Beitrage zur pathologischen Anatomie der Nebennieren. Beitr Pathol 39: 373
117. Kariminejad MH, Scully RE (1973) Female adnexal tumor of probable wolffian origin. Cancer 31: 671
118. Katz DA, Thom D, Bogard P, Dermer MS (1984) Angiomyolipoma of the fallopian tube. Am J Obstet Gynecol 148: 341
119. Kay S (1956) Sarcoidosis of the fallopian tubes. J Obstet Gynaecol Br Emp 63: 871
120. Kay S, Schneider V, Litt J (1983) Choriocarcinoma of the mesosalpinx masquerading as congestive heart failure: Ultrastructural observations of the tumor. Int J Gynecol Pathol 2: 72
121. Keith LG, Berger GS, Edelman DA, Newton W, Fullan N, Bailey R, Friberg J (1984) On the causation of pelvic inflammatory disease. Am J Obstet Gynecol 149: 215
122. Knab DR, Blanco LJ (1978) Müllerian duct agenesis with a unilateral functioning segment of the rudimentary uterine horn. Am J Obstet Gynecol 132: 222
123. Kraus FT (1977) Female genitalia. In: Anderson WAD, Kisane JM, eds. Pathology, 7th ed. St. Louis, CV Mosby, p 1726
124. Kristensen GS, Bollerup AC, Lind K, et al. (1985) Infec-

tions with *Neisseria gonorrhoeae* and *Chlamydia trachomatis* in women with acute salpingitis. Genitourin Med 61: 179

125. Kuo T-t, Hsueh S (1984) Mucicarminophilic histiocytosis. A polyvinyl pyrolidone (PVP) storage disease simulating signet-ring cell carcinoma. Am J Surg Pathol 8: 419
126. Kuzela DC, Speers WC (1985) Heterotopic endometrium of the fallopian tube. Fertil Steril 44: 552
127. Landers DV, Sweet RL (1985) Current trends in the diagnosis and treatment of tuboovarian abscess. Am J Obstet Gynecol 151: 1098
128. Landers DV, Sweet RL (1983) Tubo-ovarian abscess: Contemporary approach to management. Rev Infect Dis 5: 876
129. Lapin BA, Yakoleva LA (1963) Comparative physiology in monkeys. Springfield Ill, Charles C Thomas, p 215
130. Lauchlan SC (1984) Metaplasias and neoplasias of müllerian epithelium. Histopathology 8: 543
131. Lee RA, Welch JS (1967) Torsion of the uterine adnexa. Am J Obstet Gynecol 97: 974
132. Lewis JD (1964) Hilus cell hyperplasia of ovaries and tubes. Obstet Gynecol 24: 728
133. Lind K, Kristensen GB, Bollerup AC, et al. (1985) Importance of *Mycoplasma hominis* in acute salpingitis assessed by culture and serological tests. Genitourin Med 61: 185
134. Lindblom B, Hamberger L, Wiqvist N (1978) Differentiated contractile effects of prostaglandins E and F on the isolated circular and longitudinal smooth muscle of the human oviduct. Fertil Steril 30: 553
135. Lippes J, Ender RG, Pragay OA, Bartholomew WR (1972) The collection and analysis of human fallopian tube fluid. Contraception 5: 85
136. Lisa JR, Gioia JD, Rubin IC (1954) Observations on the interstitial portion of the fallopian tube. Surg Gynecol Obstet 99: 159
137. Madden S (1950) Chorionepithelioma of the fallopian tube. J Obstet Gynaecol Br Emp 57: 68
138. Malinak LJ, Miller GV, Armstrong JT (1966) Primary squamous cell carcinoma of the fallopian tube. Am J Obstet Gynecol 95: 1067
139. Mallory T (1935) Case records of the Massachusetts General Hospital. N Engl J Med 213: 1249
140. Mårdh P-A, Ripa T, Svensson L, Weström L (1977) *Chlamydia trachomatis* infection in patients with acute salpingitis. N Engl J Med 296: 1377
141. Mårdh P-A, Weström L (1970) Antibodies to *Mycoplasm hominis* in patients with genital infections and in healthy controls. Br J Vener Dis 46: 390
142. Mårdh P-A, Weström L (1970) Tubal and cervical cultures in acute salpingitis with special reference to *Mycoplasma hominis* and T-strain mycoplasmas. Br J Vener Dis 46: 179
143. Mason TE, Quagliarello JR (1976) Ectopic pregnancies in the fallopian tube. Obstet Gynecol 48: 70s
144. Mastroianni L Jr, Komins J (1975) Capacitation, ovum maturation, fertilization and preimplantation development in the oviduct. Gynecol Invest 6: 226
145. Mazzarella P, Okagaki T, Richart RM (1972) Teratoma of the uterine tube. Obstet Gynecol 39: 381
146. McGee ZA, Stephens DS, Hoffman LH, Schlech WF III, Horn RG (1983) Mechanisms of mucosal invasion by pathogenic *Neisseria*. Rev Infect Dis 5 [Suppl 4]: S708
147. McGowan L (1965) Intramural pregnancy. JAMA 192: 637
148. Moore SW, Enterline HT (1975) Significance of proliferative epithelial lesions of the uterine tube. Obstet Gynecol 45: 385
149. Murray JJ, Clark CA, Lands RH, Heim CR, Burnett LS (1984) Reactivation blastomycosis presenting as a tuboovarian abscess. Obstet Gynecol 64: 828
150. Musich JR, Behrman SJ (1983) Surgical management of tubal obstruction at the uterotubal junction. Fertil Steril 40: 423
151. Newbold RR, Bullock BC, McLachlan JA (1985) Progressive proliferative changes in the oviduct of mice following developmental exposure to diethylstilbestrol. Teratogenesis Carcinogy Mutagen 5: 473
152. Niles JH, Clark JFJ (1969) Pathogenesis of tubal pregnancy. Am J Obstet Gynecol 105: 1230
153. Niloff JM, Klug TL, Schaetzl E, Zurawski VR Jr, Knapp RC, Bast RC Jr (1984) Elevation of serum CA125 in carcinomas of the fallopian tube, endometrium and endocervix. Am J Obstet Gynecol 148: 1057
154. Novak E, Everett HS (1928) Cyclical and other variations in the tubal epithelium. Am J Obstet Gynecol 16: 499
155. Odor DL (1974) The question of "basal" cells in oviductal and endocervical epithelium. Fertil Steril 25: 1047
156. Okagaki T, Richart RM (1970) Neurilemmoma of the fallopian tube. Am J Obstet Gynecol 106: 929
157. Outerbridge GW (1914) Polypoid chondrofibroma of the fallopian tube associated with tubal pregnancy. Am J Obstet NY 70: 173
158. Palomaki JF, Blair OM (1971) Hilus cell rest of the fallopian tube. Obstet Gynecol 37: 60
159. Patek E, Nilsson L (1973) Scanning electron microscopic observations on the ciliogenesis of the infundibulum of the human fetal and adult fallopian tube epithelium. Fertil Steril 24: 819
160. Patek E, Nilsson L, Johannisson E (1972) Scanning electron microscopic study of the human fallopian tube. Report I. The proliferative and secretory stages. Fertil Steril 23: 459
161. Paton DM, Widdicombe JH, Rheaume DE, Johns A (1978) The role of the adrenergic innervation of the oviduct in the regulation of mammalian ovum transport. Pharmacol Rev 29: 67
162. Patton DL (1985) Immunopathology and histopathology of experimental chlamydial salpingitis. Rev Infect Dis 7: 746
163. Patton GW Jr, Goldstein DP (1973) Gestational choriocarcinoma of the tube and ovary. Surg Gynecol Obstet 137: 608
164. Pauerstein CJ (1974) The fallopian tube: A reappraisal. Philadelphia, Lea & Febiger
165. Pauerstein CJ, Woodruff JD (1967) The role of the "indifferent" cell of the tubal epithelium. Am J Obstet Gynecol 98: 121
166. Pauerstein CJ, Woodruff JD (1966) Cellular patterns in proliferative and anaplastic disease of the fallopian tube. Am J Obstet Gynecol 96: 486

167. Persaud V (1970) Etiology of tubal ectopic pregnancy. Radiologic and pathologic studies. Obstet Gynecol 36: 257
168. Persson E, Holmberg K (1984) A longitudinal study of *Actinomyces israelii* in the female genital tract. Acta Obstet Gynecol Scand 63: 207
169. Phillips AJ, D'Ablaing G (1986) Acute salpingitis subsequent to tubal ligation. Obstet Gynecol 67: 55S
170. Phillips DM, Swenson CE, Schachter J (1984) Ultrastructure of *Chlamydia trachomatis* infection of the mouse oviduct. J Ultrastruct Res 88: 244
171. Qizilbash AH, DePetrillo AD (1975) Endometrial and tubal involvement by squamous carcinoma of the cervix. Am J Clin Pathol 64: 668
172. Rebello R, Green FHY, Fox H (1975) A study of the secretory immune system of the female genital tract. Br J Obstet Gynaecol 82: 812
173. Reiffenstuhl G (1964) The lymphatics of the female genital organs. Philadelphia, JB Lippincott
174. Rivlin ME, Meeks GR, Cowan BD, Bates GW (1985) Persistent trophoblastic tissue following salpingostomy for unruptured ectopic pregnancy. Fertil Steril 43: 323
175. Roberts CL, Marshall HK (1961) Fibromyoma of the fallopian tube. Am J Obstet Gynecol 82: 364
176. Romero R, Kadar N, Jeanty P, Copel JA, Chervenak FA, DeCherney A, Hobbins JC (1985) Diagnosis of ectopic pregnancy: Value of the discriminatory human chorionic gonadotropin zone. Obstet Gynecol 66: 357
177. Rojansky N, Ophir E, Sharony A, Spira H, Suprun H (1985) Broad ligament adenocarcinoma—Its origin and clinical behavior. A literature review and report of a case. Obstet Gynecol Surv 40: 665
178. Rubin A, Czernobilsky B (1970) Tubal ligation. A bacteriologic, histologic and clinical study. Obstet Gynecol 36: 199
179. Rubin GL, Peterson HB, Dorfman SF, Layde PM, Maze JM, Ory HW, Cates W Jr (1983) Ectopic pregnancy in the United States, 1970 through 1978. JAMA 249: 1725
180. Saffos RO, Rhatigan RM, Scully RE (1980) Metaplastic papillary tumor of the fallopian tube—A distinctive lesion of pregnancy. Am J Clin Pathol 74: 232
181. Samaha M, Woodruff JD (1985) Paratubal cysts: Frequency, histogenesis, and associated clinical features. Obstet Gynecol 65: 691
182. Sanes S, Warner R (1939) Primary lymphangioma of the fallopian tube. Am J Obstet Gynecol 37: 316
183. Sapan IP, Solberg NS (1973) Prolapse of the uterine tube after abdominal hysterectomy. Obstet Gynecol 42: 26
184. Schaefer G (1970) Tuberculosis of the female genital tract. Clin Obstet Gynecol 13: 965
185. Scheffey LC, Lang WR, Nugent FB (1941) Clinical and pathologic aspects of the uterine tube. Am J Obstet Gynecol 52: 904
186. Schenken JR, Burns EL (1943) A study and classification of nodular lesions of the fallopian tube. Am J Obstet Gynecol 45: 624
187. Schiller HM, Silverberg SC (1971) Staging and prognosis in primary carcinoma of the fallopian tube. Cancer 28: 389
188. Sedlis A (1961) Primary carcinoma of the fallopian tube. Obstet Gynecol Surv 16: 209
189. Seigler AM (1983) Hysterosalpingography. Fertil Steril 40: 139
190. Settlege DSF, Motoshima M, Tredway DR (1973) Sperm transport from the external cervical os to the fallopian tube in women. A time and quantitation study. Fertil Steril 24: 655
191. Silverman AY, Greenberg EI (1983) Absence of segment of the proximal portion of a fallopian tube. Obstet Gynecol 62: 90S
192. Skude G, Mårdh PA, Weström L (1976) Amylases of the genital tract. I. Isoamylases of genital tract tissue homogenates and peritoneal fluid. Am J Obstet Gynecol 126: 652
193. Soderstrom RM (1985) Sterilization failures and their causes. Am J Obstet Gynecol 152: 395
194. Sotus PC (1977) Retroperitoneal ectopic pregnancy: A case report (Letter). JAMA 238: 1363
195. Spiegelberg O (1878) Zur Kasuistik der Ovarialschwanagenschaft. Arch Gynakol 13: 73
196. Spore WW, Moskal PA, Nakamura RM, Mishell OR (1970) Bacteriology of postpartum oviducts and endometrium. Am J Obstet Gynecol 107: 572
197. Stambaugh R, Seitz HM, Mastroianni L Jr (1974) Acrosomal proteinase inhibitors in rhesus monkey (*Macaca mulatta*) oviduct fluid. Fertil Steril 25: 352
198. Stevens LC, Varnum DS (1974) The development of teratomas from pathogenetically activated ovarian mouse eggs. Dev Biol 37: 369
199. Stock RJ, Nelson KJ (1984) Ectopic pregnancy subsequent to sterilization: Histologic evaluation and clinical implications. Fertil Steril 42: 211
200. Stock RJ (1983) Histopathologic changes in fallopian tubes subsequent to sterilization procedures. Int J Gynecol Pathol 2: 13
201. Stone SC, McCalley M, Braunstein P, Egbert R (1985) Radionuclide evaluation of tubal function. Fertil Steril 43: 757
202. Sutherland CG (1953) Tubal mole associated with intrauterine pregnancy. Am J Obstet Gynecol 65: 1164
203. Surur F (1974) Actinomycosis of the female genital tract. NY State J Med 74: 408
204. Svensson L, Mårdh P-A, Weström L (1983) Infertility after acute salpingitis with special reference to *Chlamydia trachomatis*. Fertil Steril 40: 322
205. Sweet RL (1975) Anaerobic infections of the female genital tract. Am J Obstet Gynecol 122: 891
206. Sweet RL, Blankfort-Doyle M, Robbie MO, Schacter J (1986) The occurrence of chlamydial and gonococcal salpingitis during the menstrual cycle. JAMA 255: 2062
207. Sweet RL, Mills J, Hadley KW, Blumenstock E, Schachter J, Robbie MO, Draper DL (1979) Use of laparoscopy to determine the microbiologic etiology of acute salpingitis. Am J Obstet Gynecol 134: 68
208. Sweet RL, Selinger HE, McKay DG (1975) Malignant teratoma of the uterine tube. Obstet Gynecol 45: 553
209. Swenson RM, Michaelson TC, Daly MJ, Spaulding EH (1973) Anaerobic bacterial infections of the female genital tract. Obstet Gynecol 42: 538

210. Symmers W St C (1950) Pathology of oxyuriasis. Arch Pathol 50: 475
211. Tatum HJ, Schmidt FH (1977) Contraceptive and sterilization practices and extrauterine pregnancy: A realistic perspective. Fertil Steril 28: 407
212. Taxy JB, Battifora H (1976) Female adnexal tumor of probable wolffian origin. Cancer 37: 2349
213. Taxy JB, Battifora H, Oyasu R (1974) Adenomatoid tumors: A light microscopic, histochemical, and ultrastructural study. Cancer 34: 306
214. Taylor ES, McMillian JH, Greer BE, Droegemueller W, Thompson HE (1975) The intrauterine device and tubo-ovarian abscess. Am J Obstet 123: 338
215. Teilum G (1971) Special tumors of the ovary and testis. Copenhagen, Munksgard, p 298
216. Thadepalli H, Gorbach SL, Keith L (1973) Anaerobic infections of the female genital tract: Bacteriologic and therapeutic aspects. Am J Obstet Gynecol 117: 1034
217. Thompson C, Allen SD, Stargel MD, Thornsberry C, Benigno BB, Thompson JD, Shulman JA (1980) The microbiology and therapy of acute pelvic inflammatory disease in hospitalized patients. Am J Obstet Gynecol 136: 179
218. Tilden IL, Winstedt R (1943) Decidual reactions in fallopian tubes. Am J Pathol 19: 1043
219. Tulusan AH (1984) Complete absence of the muscular layer of the ampullary part of the fallopian tubes. Arch Gynecol 234: 279
220. Vasquez G, Winston RML, Brosens IA (1983) Tubal mucosa and ectopic pregnancy. Br J Obstet Gynaecol 90: 468
221. Verhege HG, Bareither ML, Jaffe RC, Akbar M (1979) Cyclic changes in ciliation, secretion and cell height of the oviductal epithelium in women. Am J Anat 156: 505
222. Verhege HG, Brenner RM (1975) Estradiol-induced differentiation of the oviductal epithelium in ovariectomized cats. Biol Reprod 13: 104
223. Voet RL, Lifshitz S (1982) Primary clear cell adenocarcinoma of the fallopian tube: Light microscopic and ultrastructural findings. Int J Gynecol Pathol 1: 292
224. Wagner I, Bettendorf U (1980) Extraovarian Brenner tumor. Case report and review. Arch Gynecol 229: 191
225. Ward ME, Watt PJ, Robertson JN (1974) The human fallopian tube: A laboratory model for gonococcal infection. J Infect Dis 129: 650
226. Weber DL, Fazzini E (1970) Ganglioneuroma of the fallopian tube. Acta Neuropathol 16: 173
227. Weinstein L, Morris MB, Dotters D, Christian CD (1983) Ectopic pregnancy—A new surgical epidemic. Obstet Gynecol 61: 698
228. Weström L, Bengtsson LP, Mårdh P-A (1976) The risk of pelvic inflammatory disease in women using intrauterine contraceptive devices as compared to non-users. Lancet 2: 221
229. Westrom L, Bengtsson L PH, Mårdh P-A (1981) Incidence, trends, and risks of ectopic pregnancy in a population of women. Br Med J 282: 15
230. Winer AE, Bergman WD, Fields C (1957) Combined intra- and extrauterine pregnancy. Am J Obstet Gynecol 74: 170
231. Wlodarski FM, Trainer TD (1975) Granulomatous oophoritis and salpingitis associated with Crohn's disease of the appendix. Am J Obstet Gynecol 122: 527
232. Wong S-LR, Lippe BM, Kaplan SA (1971) The XX Turner phenotype with unilateral streak gonad and absent uterus. Am J Dis Child 122: 449
233. Woodruff JD, Julian CG (1969) Multiple malignancy in the upper genital canal. Am J Obstet Gynecol 103: 810
234. Woodruff JD, Pauerstein CJ (1969) The fallopian tube. Baltimore, Williams & Wilkins
235. Wrork DH, Broders AC (1942) Adenomyosis of the fallopian tube. Am J Obstet Gynecol 44: 412
236. Yeung HHY, Bannatyne P, Russell P (1983) Adenocarcinoma of the fallopian tubes: A clinicopathological study of eight cases. Pathology 15: 279
237. Yoonessi M (1979) Carcinoma of the fallopian tube. Obstet Gynecol Surv 34: 257
238. Zolli A, Rocko JM (1982) Ectopic pregnancy months and years after hysterectomy. Arch Surg 117: 962

15

Anatomy and Histology of the Ovary

Philip B. Clement, M.D.

This chapter deals with the normal macroscopic, microscopic, and ultrastructural morphology of the human ovary, and its hormonal function. Since the anatomy and function of the ovary vary considerably at different stages in a woman's life, these aspects will be considered during adulthood, childhood, and after the menopause.

Ovary in Adulthood

Gross Anatomy

The ovaries are paired pelvic organs that lie on either side of the uterus close to the lateral pelvic wall, behind the broad ligament and anterior to the rectum. Each ovary is attached along its anterior margin (or hilus) by a double fold of peritoneum, the mesovarium, to the posterior aspect of the broad ligament. Each ovary is also attached at its medial pole to the ipsilateral uterine cornu by the ovarian (or uteroovarian) ligament and from the superior aspect of its lateral pole to the lateral pelvic wall by the infundibulopelvic (or suspensory) ligament.

Adult ovaries have an ovoid shape, measure approximately 3.0–5 cm by 1.5–3.0 cm by 0.6–1.5 cm, and weigh 5–8 g. Their size and weight, however, vary considerably depending on their content of follicular derivatives. They have a pinkish-white exterior, which in early reproductive life is usually smooth (Fig. 15.1), but with time exhibits increasing numbers of retracted scars and convolutions. Thin-walled, fluid-filled cysts (cystic follicles) and bright yellow structures (corpora lutea) may be partially visible from the external aspect. On cut section, three ill-defined zones are discernible, including an outer cortex, an inner medulla, and the hilus. The stroma of the superficial cortex is typically more fibrotic than elsewhere, and although frequently referred to as the *tunica albuginea*, it lacks the densely collagenous, almost acellular appearance and sharp delineation of this layer in the testis. Follicular structures (cystic follicles, corpora lutea, corpora albicantia) are typically visible in the cortex and medulla (Fig. 15.2).

Blood Vessels

The ovarian artery, a branch of the aorta, courses along the infundibulopelvic ligament and the mesovarial border of the ovary, where it anastomoses with the ovarian

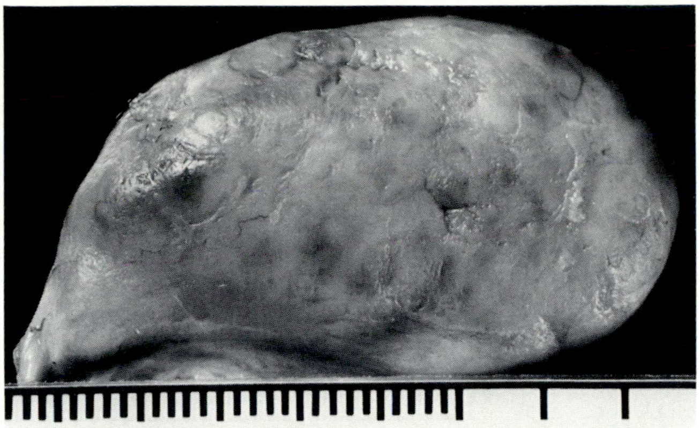

FIG. 15.1. Normal adult ovary from 25-year-old female. Except for occasional fibrous adhesions, the external surface is smooth and white.

branch of the uterine artery. Approximately 10 arterial branches arise from this arcade and penetrate the ovarian hilus and medulla. As they course through the medulla, they exhibit marked coiling and branching.[9,96] These helicine arteries possess, along their length, longitudinal ridges of intimal smooth muscle.[9] At the corticomedullary junction, the medullary arteries and arterioles form a plexus from which smaller, straight cortical arterioles arise and penetrate the cortex in a radial fashion, perpendicular to the ovarian surface. These cortical arterioles branch and anastomose several times, forming sets of interconnected vascular arcades.[96] These arcades give rise to capillaries that form dense networks within the theca layers of the ovarian follicles (Fig. 15.3).

The ovarian veins accompany the arteries. In the medulla they are large and tortuous. The veins join together in the hilus where they form a rich plexus that drains into the ovarian veins,[9,96] that traverse the mesovarium and course along the infundibulopelvic ligament. The left and right ovarian veins drain into the left renal vein and the inferior vena cava, respectively.

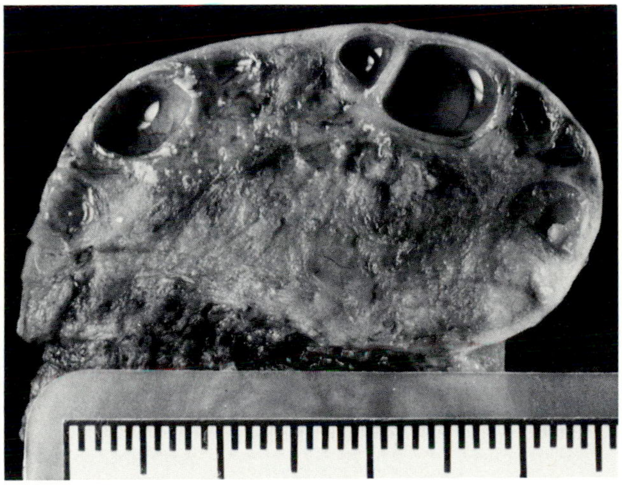

FIG. 15.2. Normal adult ovary (*cut surface*). Occasional cystic follicles are present in the cortex.

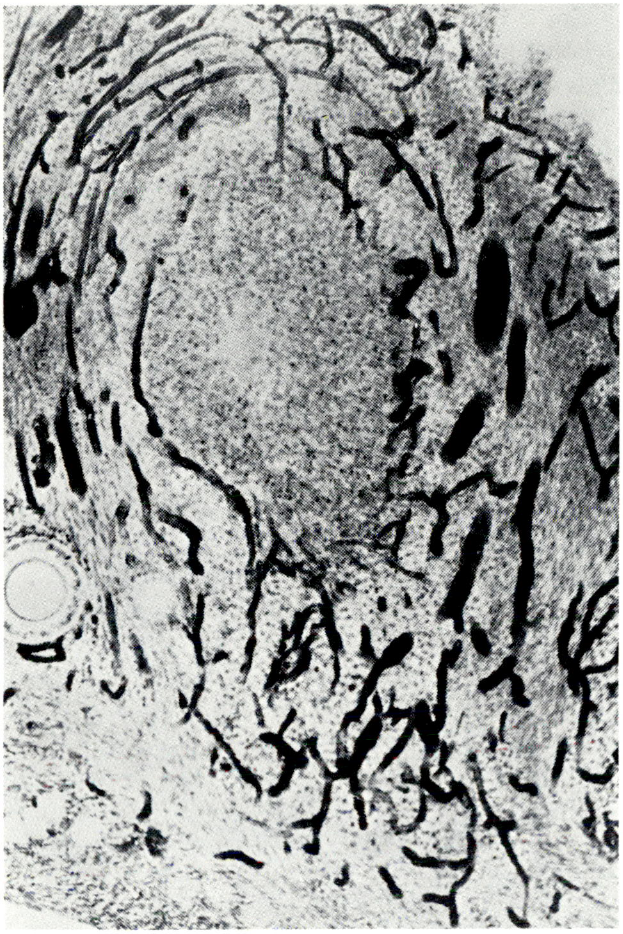

FIG. 15.3. Perifollicular capillary network. Ovarian vessels were injected with colored gelatin before sectioning. [Reprinted by permission of Leeson, Leeson (1970) Histology. Philadelphia, Saunders.]

Lymphatics

The lymphatics of the ovary originate predominantly within the theca layers of the follicles. The granulosa layer of a maturing follicle is devoid of lymphatics in contrast to its counterpart within the corpus luteum, which possesses a rich supply of lymphatics.[90] The lymphatics pass through the ovarian stroma, independent of blood vessels, to drain into larger trunks that form a plexus at the hilus.[90] Within the hilus, the lymphatics and blood vessels converge, with the former coiled around veins in a helicoid fashion.[90] Four to eight efferent channels pass into the mesovarium where they converge to form another plexus (subovarian plexus), which is joined by branches from the fallopian tube and uterine fundus.[90] Leaving the plexus, the drainage trunks diminish in number and size, passing along the free border of the infundibulopelvic ligament enmeshed with the ovarian veins.[90] They then travel with the ovarian vessels, in juxtaposition to the psoas muscle, to drain into the upper para-aortic lymph nodes at the level of the lower pole of the kidney.[28,90,99] The major lymphatic drainage of the ovary is therefore in a cephaloid direction toward the aortic nodes. In some patients, accessory channels exist that bypass the subovarian plexus, passing through the broad ligament to the internal iliac, external iliac, and interaortic lymph nodes or via the round ligament to the iliac and inguinal lymph nodes.[28,90,99]

Nerves

The nerve supply of the ovary arises from a sympathetic plexus that is enmeshed with the ovarian vessels in the infundibulopelvic ligament.[49] Nerve fibers, which are predominantly nonmyelinated, accompany the ovarian artery, entering the ovary at the hilus. Delicate terminal fibers, many surrounding small arteries and arterioles, penetrate the medulla and cortex to terminate as plexi surrounding the follicles.[49,84] Adrenergic nerve fibers and terminals have been shown to be in close contact with smooth muscle cells in the cortical stroma and theca externa. The physiologic significance of ovarian sympathetic innervation is not clear, although it has been suggested that it may play a role in follicular maturation, follicular rupture, or both.[4,49,79] In addition, catecholamines can stimulate progesterone production by the ovarian follicles and androgen production by the ovarian stroma in vitro.[27]

Surface Epithelium

Histology. The ovary is covered by a single, focally pseudostratified layer of modified peritoneal cells that constitute the surface epithelium. The cells vary from flat to cuboidal to columnar, and several types may be seen in different areas of the same ovary (Fig. 15.4). The surface cells are separated from the underlying stroma by a distinct basement membrane. This epithelium is extremely fragile and is almost always denuded in oophorectomy specimens because of handling by the surgeon and pathologist, as well as delayed fixation that results in drying. Preserved epithelium is often confined to areas protected by surface adhesions or lining sulci.[99] Surface epithelium within these crevices may lose connection with the surface, giving rise to surface epithelial inclusion cysts (see Chapter 16, Nonneoplastic Lesions of Ovary).

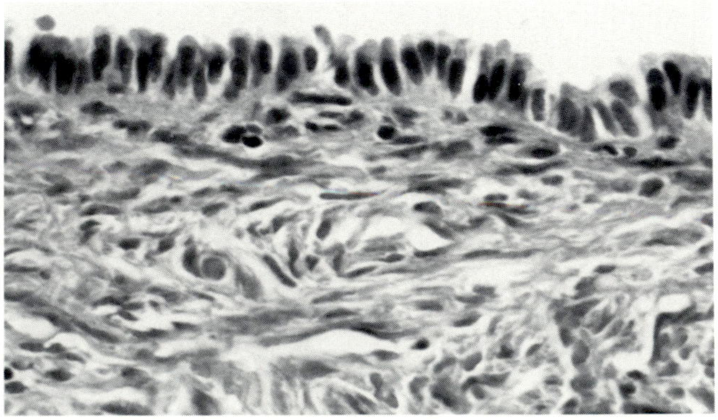

FIG. 15.4. Ovarian surface epithelium composed of a single layer of columnar cells.

Histochemical studies have demonstrated glycogen, as well as acid and neutral mucopolysaccharides, within surface epithelial cells.[8,68] 17-beta-hydroxysteroid dehydrogenase activity, absent in extraovarian mesothelial cells, has also been found in ovarian surface epithelial cells.[8] Immunofluorescent or immunoperoxidase meth-

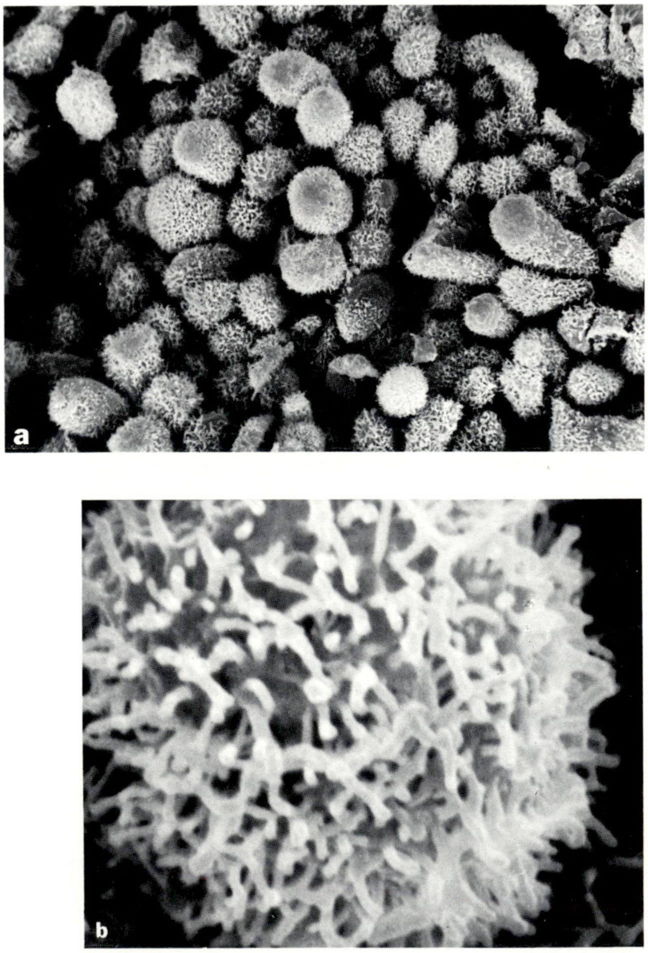

FIG. 15.5. Scanning electron micrograph of ovarian surface epithelium. *a.* Note dome-shaped apices covered by abundant surface microvilli. ×1140. *b.* Branching surface microvilli. ×12,000. (Reprinted by permission of Ferenczy, Richart, Ref. 31. Copyright John Wiley & Sons, Inc., 1974.)

ods have revealed positivity for cytokeratin[22,77] and vimentin[77] but not desmin. Several antigens associated with ovarian tumors of surface epithelial origin have been demonstrated with a variable frequency, including anti-carbohydrate determinant 19–9 (CA 19–9)[16] and MH99,[17] but not carcinoembryonic antigen (CEA)[16] or CA125.[55] The latter antigen, however, is demonstrable within surface epithelial cells lining inclusion cysts and papillary excrescences on the ovarian surface.[55]

Ultrastructure. The ultrastructural appearance of the ovarian surface epithelium is similar to that of the extra-ovarian peritoneum and consistent with functions of active fluid and ion transport, occurring partly through intercellular spaces and partly through surface pinocytosis.[7,31,85] The cell surfaces by scanning and transmission electron microscopy are characterized by dome-shaped apices covered by numerous, often branching, microvilli, occasional single cilia, and pinocytotic vesicles (Figs. 15.5 and 15.6). The cytoplasm contains well-developed organelles, particularly abundant polysomes, free ribosomes, abundant mitochondria, and tonofilaments loosely arranged in bundles. Lipid droplets are sometimes present in the basal cytoplasm. The nuclei have indented nuclear membranes and peripheral nucleoli. Straight or convoluted lateral plasma membranes are reinforced by luminal junctional complexes, scattered desmosomes, and desmosome–tonofilament complexes. The membranes may be widely separated in areas, creating dilated intercellular spaces.[31] There is a well-developed basal lamina that separates the surface epithelial cells from the underlying cortical stroma.

Stroma

Histology. The stroma of the ovarian cortex and medulla is composed of densely cellular whorls of spindle-shaped

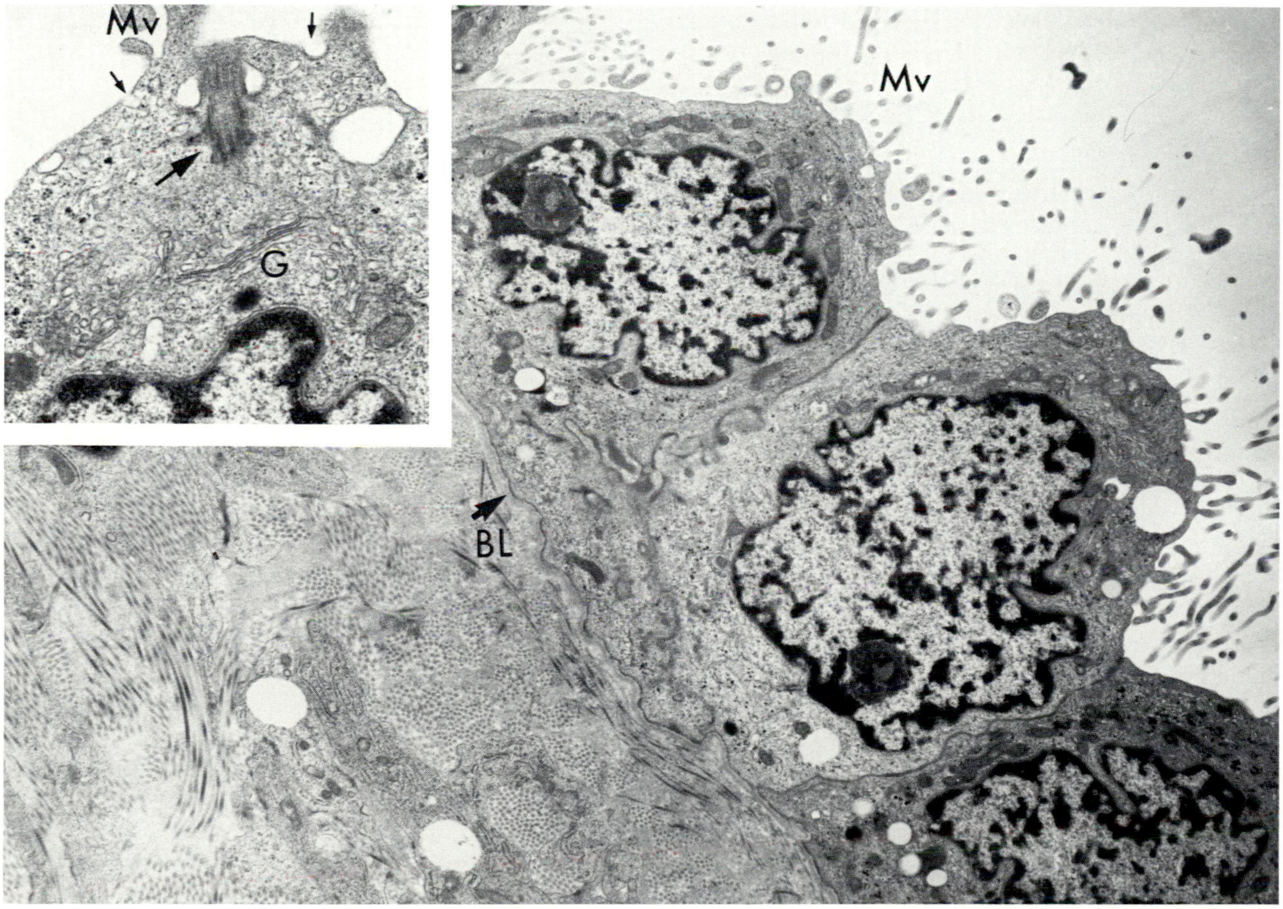

FIG. 15.6. Electron micrograph of ovarian surface epithelium. The cells have numerous microvilli (Mv) and well-developed organelles in a perinuclear location. The nuclei have indented membranes and peripheral nucleoli. The lateral plasma membranes are reinforced by luminal junctional complexes and scattered desmosomes but are occasionally widely separated, producing dilated intercellular spaces. A well-defined basal lamina (BL) separates the cells from the underlying stroma. *Inset:* The surface microvilli are associated with micropinocytotic vesicles (*short arrows*) and occasional single cilia (*long arrow*). G, Golgi. ×6400. Inset ×22,000. (Reprinted by permission of Ferenczy, Richart, Ref. 31.)

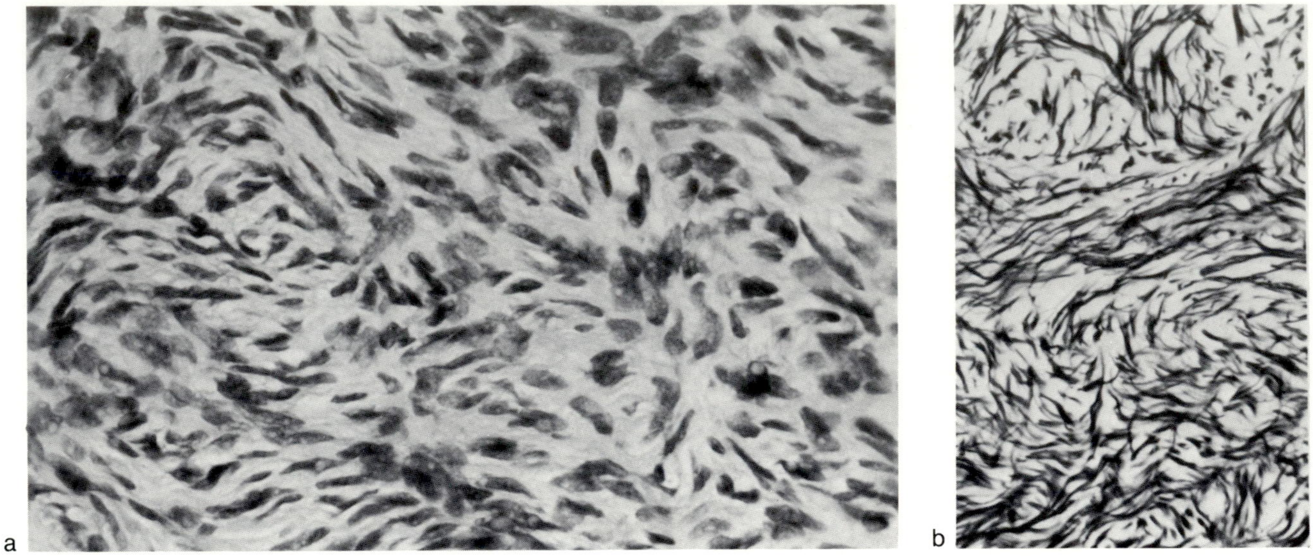

FIG. 15.7. *a*. Ovarian stroma composed of whorls of plump, fibroblastic cells. *b*. Dense pericellular reticulum pattern (reticulin stain).

fibroblastic cells with scant cytoplasm (Fig. 15.7a). Cytoplasmic lipid in the form of fine droplets may be appreciable with special stains, especially in the late reproductive and postmenopausal age groups.[30] The amount of stroma in the cortex and medulla varies considerably from one person to another. In many patients, there is a decrease in stromal volume and stromal cellularity as the menopause is approached (see p. 465). Concurrently, the stromal cell nuclei diminish in size and change from fusiform and vesicular to spindle-shaped and pyknotic. Stromal cells are separated from each other by a dense reticulum network (Fig. 15.7b) and a variable amount of collagen, the latter most abundant in the superficial cortex. The amount of intercellular collagen increases in the late reproductive and postmenopausal age groups.

The fibroblastic ovarian stromal cells differentiate into a variety of other cell types:[99]

(1) Follicular theca interna cells, and at distance from the follicles, luteinized stromal cells. These cells have a similar appearance, characterized by a polygonal shape, abundant eosinophilic to clear cytoplasm containing variable amounts of lipid, a central round nucleus, and a prominent nucleolus. Luteinized stromal cells are found singly or in small nests, most often in the medulla. Their numbers increase during pregnancy and after the menopause, probably secondary to elevated levels of circulating gonadotropins during these periods.[11,30] In one autopsy study, luteinized stromal cells were demonstrated after diligent searching in 13% of women under the age of 55 and in one-third of women over that age. More exhaustive sampling might indicate that luteinized stromal cells may be normal constituents of the ovary, particularly in later life.[11] In this age group, the presence of luteinized cells is not usually associated with clinical evidence of an endocrine disturbance. In some older women, but more often in younger patients, increased degrees of stromal luteinization (stromal hyperthecosis) are frequently associated with androgenic manifestations (see Chapter 16, Nonneoplastic Lesions of Ovary).[11]

(2) Enzymatically active stromal cells (EASC). These cells are characterized by their oxidative and other enzymatic activity.[30,99,101] The frequency of their detection and quantity increase with age, occurring in over 80% of postmenopausal women, typically in the medulla.[101] Some EASC correspond to luteinized stromal cells, but most cannot be distinguished from neighboring, nonreactive stromal cells in routine histologic preparations.[99,101]

(3) Smooth muscle cells.[100] These have been demonstrated in certain pathologic conditions (see Chapter 16), but also within the ovarian stroma in otherwise normal ovaries. Smooth muscle cells have also been identified on ultrastructural examination within the normal theca externa layer of the follicles.[83]

(4) Decidual cells. One of the most consistent changes within the ovary during pregnancy is focal decidual transformation of the ovarian stroma, a finding present in almost every ovary examined at term, and reflecting elevated progesterone levels (see Chapter 16).[5,6,41,48]

(5) Endometrial stromal-type cells (endometrial stromatosis) (see Chapter 16).

(6) Fat cells (see Chapter 16).

(7) Stromal Leydig cells (see Chapter 16).

Rare cells of neuroendocrine or APUD type, which may be of stromal origin, have been demonstrated within the ovarian stroma in fewer than 10% of normal women in one study.[45] Such cells occur in small groups in the corticomedullary stromal junction and exhibit argyrophilia and argentaffinia. Their significance, if any, is unknown.

Ultrastructure. Typical ovarian stromal cells have slender, spindle-shaped nuclei and complex cytoplasmic processes. Their scant cytoplasm is rich in organelles required for collagen synthesis, including free ribosomes and mitochondria.[31] Tropocollagen, concentrated at the periphery of the cytoplasm, is deposited in the extracellular space and eventually converted to collagen (Fig. 15.8a).[31] Rows of micropinocytotic vesicles are found along the plasma membrane and desmosome-like attachments may be found between the cells (Fig. 15.8b). Luteinized stromal cells have abundant cytoplasm containing lipid droplets and organelles required for steroid hormone synthesis, including smooth endoplasmic reticulum, mitochondria with tubular cristae, and Golgi

a
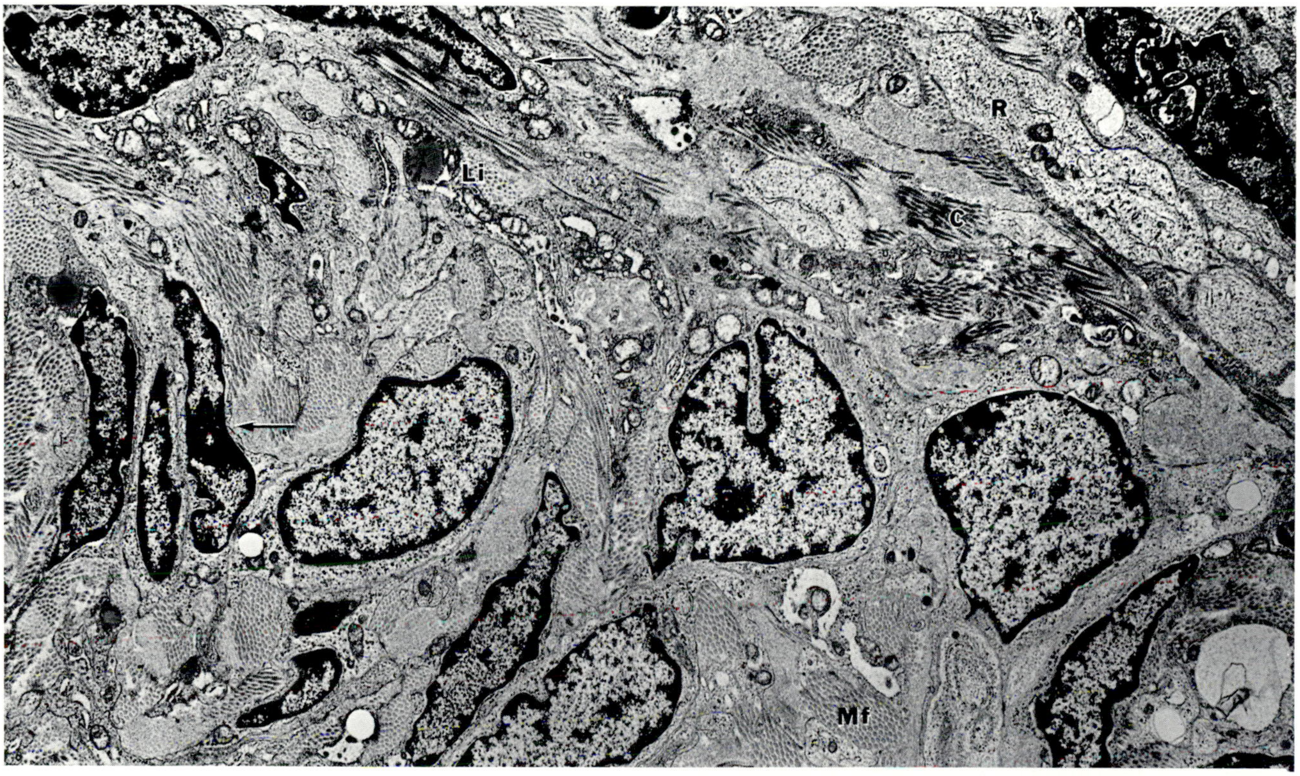

b
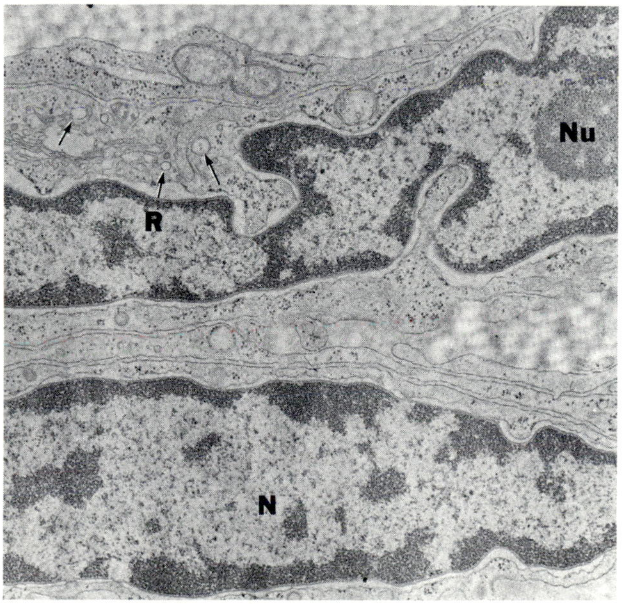

Fig. 15.8. *a.* Electron micrograph of ovarian stromal cells. The cells are fibroblastic in type. C, collagen fibers; Mf, tropocollagen; R, free ribosomes; Li, lipid inclusions; *upper arrow*, perinuclear clustering of mitochondria. ×3000. *b.* Higher power of two stromal cells showing micropinocytotic vesicles (*arrows*). R, ribosomes; N, nucleus; Nu, nucleolus. ×12,000.

complexes.[31,58] Cells with an ultrastructural appearance intermediate in appearance between fibroblastic cells and luteinized cells may also be seen.[31] Electron microscopic examination of the argyrophilic stromal cells reveals electron-dense, membrane-bound, cytoplasmic granules measuring from 300 to 750 nm in diameter.[45]

Hormone Synthesis. Numerous studies have demonstrated the steroidogenic potential and the gonadotropin-responsiveness of the ovarian stroma in both pre- and postmenopausal women.* In vitro incubation of ovarian stromal tissue indicates that its principal steroid product is androstenedione, in addition to smaller quantities of testosterone and dehydroepiandrosterone.[97] In vitro production of these androgens is enhanced by human chorionic gonadotropin and anterior pituitary gonadotropins. To what extent the ovarian stroma contributes to the androgen pool in normal premenopausal women is unknown, but it is likely that it is the source of small amounts of testosterone. With cessation of follicular activity at the time of the menopause, the ovarian stroma becomes, together with the adrenal glands, the major source of androgens (see p. 466).

Primordial Follicles

Histology. Approximately 400,000 primordial follicles are present at the time of birth and decrease progressively until they disappear at the time of the menopause. They are found scattered irregularly in clusters throughout a narrow band in the superficial cortex (Fig. 15.9). Primordial follicles consist of a primary oocyte surrounded by a single layer of flattened, mitotically inactive, granulosa cells resting on a thin basal lamina. Rare primordial (and maturing) follicles may contain multiple oocytes.[35] The oocyte has a diameter of 40–70 μm, a spherical shape, and a regular outline.[3] It is arrested at the dictyate stage of meiotic prophase at the time of birth, entering an interphase period until degeneration of the oocyte or follicular maturation prior to ovulation.[3,31] The interphase period for oocytes that eventually undergo ovulation thus spans a period of about 12 years to several decades. The large (22–24 μm) spherical nucleus of the oocyte has finely granular, uniformly dispersed chromatin and one or more dense, thread-like nucleoli.[3] It is enclosed by a nuclear membrane composed of two leaflets with prominent pores.[44] Rare oocytes may have multiple nuclei.[35] Within the cytoplasm of the oocyte is a paranuclear, eosinophilic, crescent-shaped zone representing a complex of interrelated organelles, so-called Balbiani's vitelline body (Fig. 15.9).[43,44] Within the vitelline body is a dark spot (the centrosome) surrounded by a halo, which in turn is flanked by darker, PAS-positive, granular zones rich in mitochondria.[43,44] Histochemical studies reveal that the oocyte cytoplasm has lost the abundant glycogen and the high alkaline phosphatase activity characteristic of primordial germ cells and oogonia of the embryonic gonad.[99]

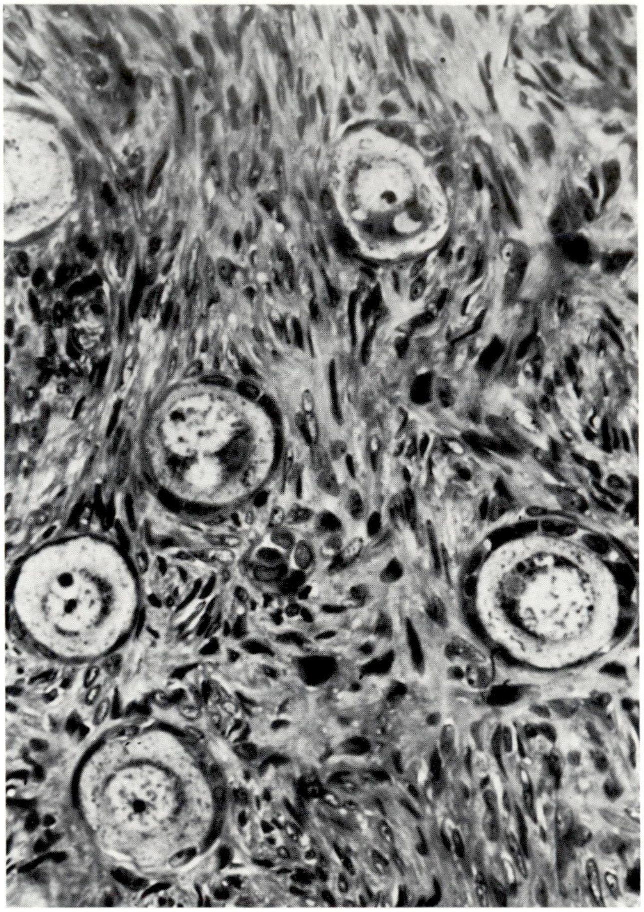

FIG. 15.9. Primordial follicles within ovarian cortex. The primary oocytes are surrounded by a single layer of flattened granulosa cells. Note perinuclear crescentic zones (Balbiani's vitelline body) in the cytoplasm of several of the oocytes. (Reprinted by permission of Baca, Zamboni, Ref. 3.)

Ultrastructure. The granulosa cells of the primodial follicle have sparse organelles, occasional desmosomal attachments with each other, and microvillous projections that attach to the oocyte through tight apposition (Fig. 15.10).[31] Within the oocyte, the juxtanuclear centrosome of Balbiani's vitelline body consists of dense granules, closely packed vesicles, and peripheral dense fibers that form a basket-like structure at the periphery of the centrosome (Figs. 15.11 and 15.12).[43,44] It is surrounded by a zone of smooth endoplasmic reticulum (ER) that represents the halo seen by light microscopy. Surrounding the centrosome and constituting the rest of the vitelline body are a concentration of most of the oocyte's organelles, including multiple Golgi complexes, promi-

* References 15, 26, 39, 53, 54, 65, 67, 71, 74, 108.

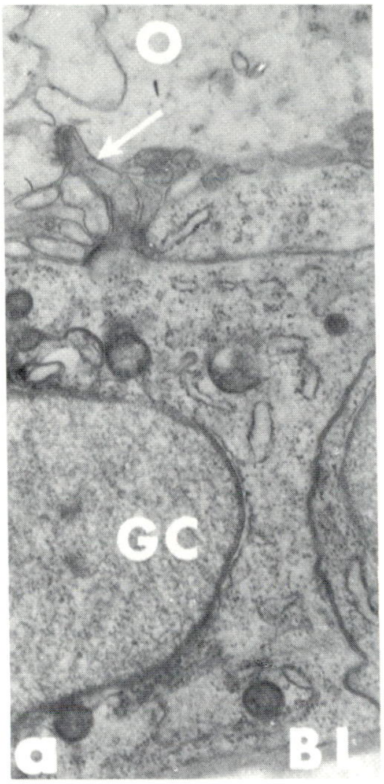

FIG. 15.10. The granulosa cells (GC) of the primordial follicle have microvillous projections that are attached to the oocyte (O) by tight apposition (*arrow*). BL, basal lamina. ×20,000. (Reprinted by permission of Hertig, Ref. 43.)

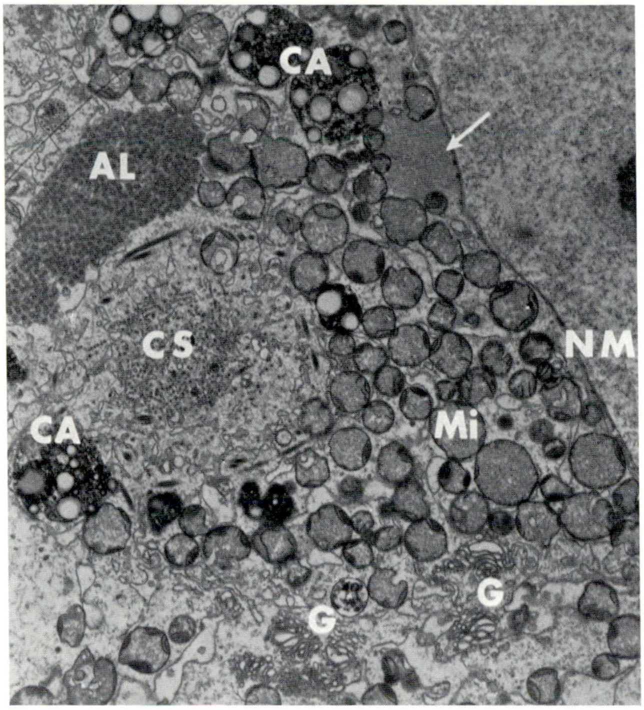

FIG. 15.12. Detailed view of Balbiani's vitelline body. A cluster of closely packed spiral fibrils (*arrow*) is attached to the nuclear envelope (NM). The centrosome (CS) is composed of dense granules, some arranged periodically on fine fibers, and small vesicles, with a peripheral zone of endoplasmic reticulum and dense fibers. Surrounding the centrosome are masses of mitochondria (Mi) and compound aggregates (CA). A stack of annulate lamellae (AL) is seen tangentially. Note the prominent endoplasmic reticulum in close association with multiple Golgi complexes (G) at the periphery of the vitelline body. (Reprinted by permission of Hertig, Ref. 43.)

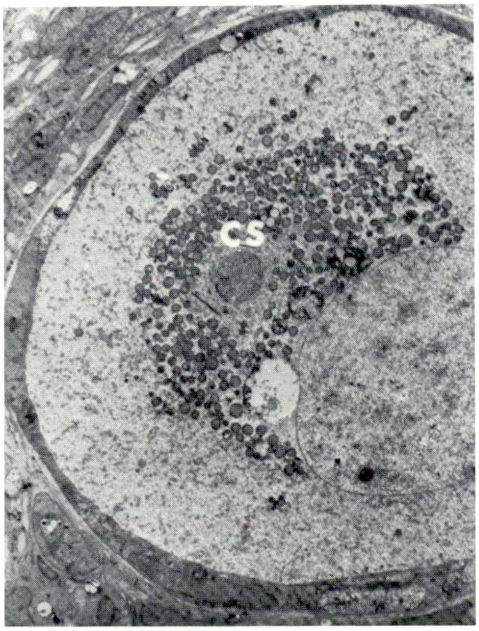

FIG. 15.11. Within a primordial follicle, Balbiani's vitelline body is seen, consisting of a juxtanuclear centrosome (CS) surrounded by a condensation of mitochondria, Golgi, endoplasmic reticulum, and lysosomes. ×2400. (Reprinted by permission of Hertig, Ref. 43.)

nent compound aggregates, numerous mitochondria intimately associated with sparsely granular ER, and annulate lamellae.[43,44] The last structures, which may be attached or immediately adjacent to the nucleus or free within the vitelline body, are constantly present in primary oocytes and other rapidly growing embryonal or neoplastic cells. They are arranged in stacks or concentric arrangements of up to 100 parallel, smooth, paired membranes that delineate greatly flattened cisternal spaces, 30–50 μm wide (Fig. 15.13). At regularly spaced intervals, the paired membranes of each lamellar unit become fused with one another.[3] When the lamellae are sectioned along a tangential plane, the sites of apposition of the membranes are seen as regularly spaced annuli 100 nm in diameter. At their periphery, they are connected to the granular ER.[43] The paired membranes of the annulate lamellae mimic the two leaflets of the nuclear membrane, and it is likely that they are formed by blebbing of its outer leaflet.[3,31,43] Their function is not known with certainty, but it has been suggested that they may have a

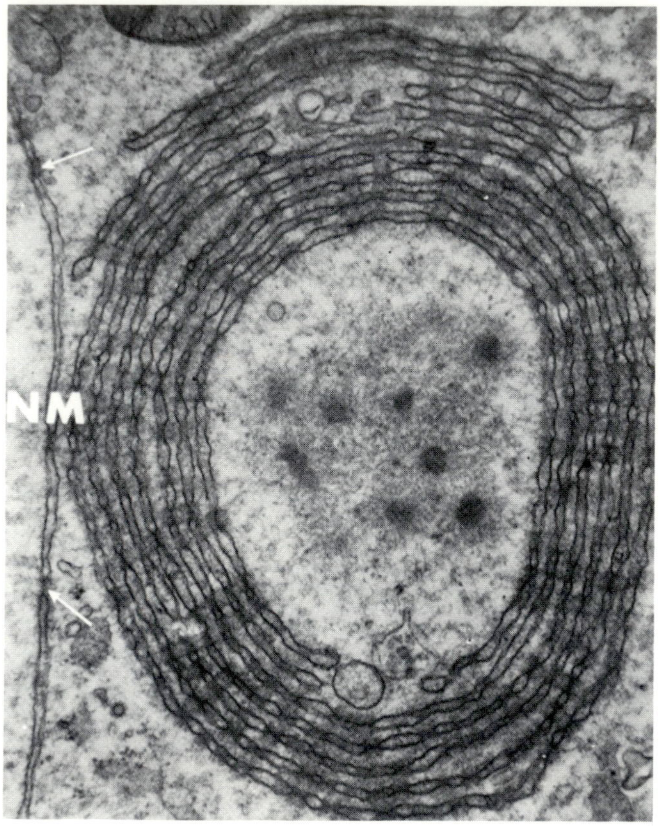

FIG. 15.13. A coiled stack of annulate lamellae from a primordial follicle. NM, nuclear membrane. (Reprinted by permission of Hertig, Ref. 43.)

role in nucleocytoplasmic exchange of substances related to metabolic activity or the transfer of genetic information.[31,43] In some oocytes, Golgi, ER, and mitochondria may also be found outside the vitelline body, closely applied to the entire circumference of the nucleus.[44] Similarly, microtubules present throughout the oocyte cytoplasm are most prevalent around the circumference of the nuclear membrane. Bundles of spiral filaments occasionally abut the nuclear membrane or are seen in the more peripheral cytoplasm (Fig. 15.12).[44] A variety of different vacuoles may also be seen in the peripheral cytoplasm, some containing multiple small vesicles.[44]

Maturing Follicles

Folliculogenesis

Folliculogenesis refers to the continuous process occurring throughout reproductive life whereby cohorts of primordial follicles undergo maturation during each menstrual cycle. Follicular maturation begins during the luteal phase of the preceding cycle and continues through-

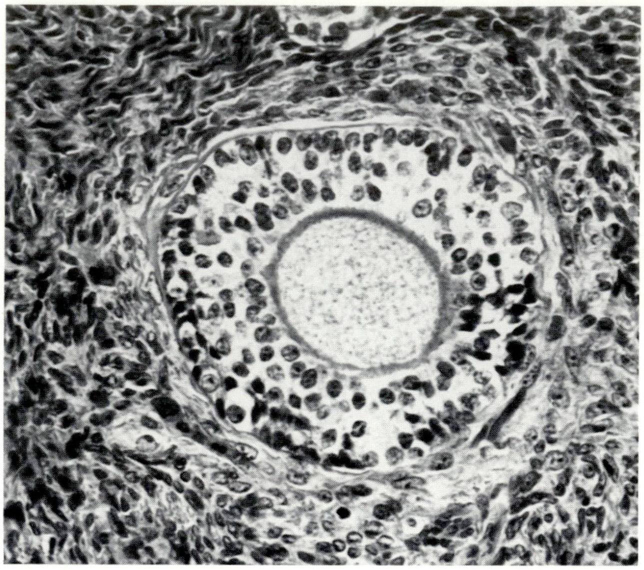

FIG. 15.14. Preantral follicle. Several layers of granulosa cells surround the oocyte. A theca interna layer is not yet apparent.

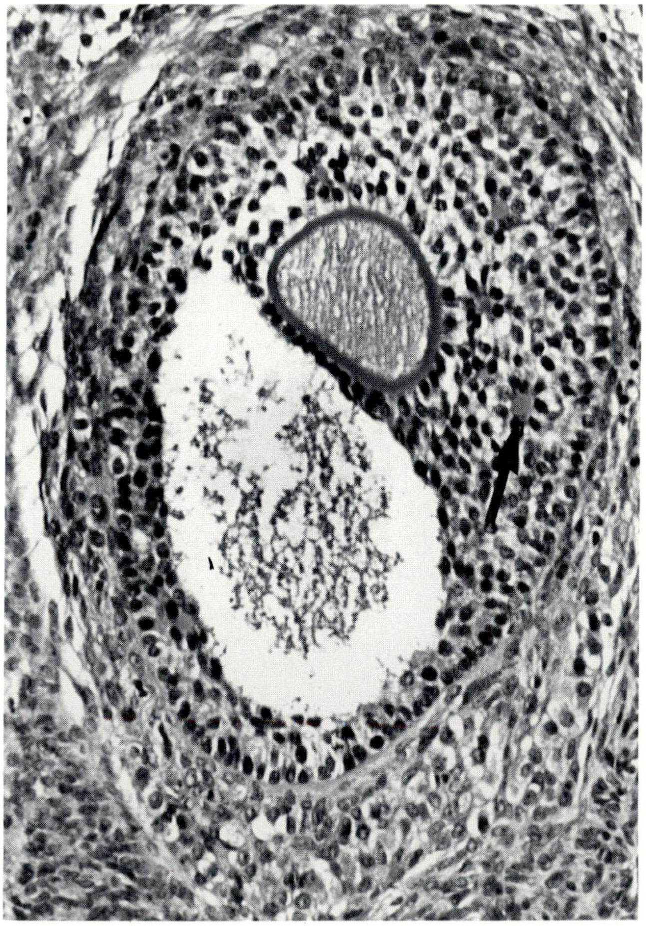

FIG. 15.15. Antral follicle. Note Call–Exner body (*arrow*) within the granulosa layer. A well-developed theca interna layer is now visible.

out the follicular phase. Each month, only one such follicle, the preovulatory follicle, achieves complete maturation, culminating in the release of the oocyte, or ovulation. The other follicles that have begun the maturational process undergo atresia at earlier stages of their development (see p. 457). Folliculogenesis and atresia continue during pregnancy, although the former process does not reach the preovulatory follicle stage.[24,36,66,80]

The first morphological evidence of follicular maturation is the assumption of a cuboidal to columnar shape by the surrounding layer of granulosa cells accompanied by enlargement of the oocyte (primary follicle). Mitotic activity in the granulosa cells results in their stratification, producing three to five concentric layers around the oocyte (secondary or preantral follicle) (Fig. 15.14). Preantral follicles measure from 50 to approximately 400 μm in diameter, and as they increase in size, they migrate into the more vascularized medulla. Simultaneously, the surrounding ovarian stromal cells become specialized into several layers of theca interna cells and an outer, ill-defined layer of theca externa cells. Secretion of mucopolysaccharide-rich fluid by the granulosa cells results in their separation by fluid-filled clefts, which eventually coalesce to form a single large cavity or antrum lined by several layers of granulosa cells (tertiary, antral, or vesicular follicle) (Fig. 15.15). The first evidence of antrum formation occurs in follicles measuring from 200 to 400 μm in diameter, after which there is progressive follicular enlargement due to continued fluid secretion into the antrum. Concurrently, the oocyte reaches its definitive size and assumes an eccentric position at one pole of the follicle. At this site, the granulosa cells proliferate to form the cumulus oophorus. The latter contains the oocyte in its center and protrudes into the antrum (mature or graafian follicle) (Fig. 15.16).

During each cycle, it is likely that only one or two mature follicles continue to grow after reaching a diameter of 4 mm, a size that is attained by the onset of the follicular phase; one of them will become the preovulatory follicle.[73] Late in follicular growth, the oocyte, its surrounding zona pellucida, and a single layer of radially disposed, columnar granulosa cells (the corona radiata) detach from the cumulus oophorus and float in the antral fluid. The preovulatory follicle shortly before ovulation reaches a diameter of 15–25 mm.[4,73] It partially protrudes from the ovarian surface at a point that represents the eventual rupture point, or stigma. Here the overlying surface epithelial cells exhibit progressive flattening, loss of their microvilli, and eventual degeneration and desquamation.[4] The stroma in this area becomes ex-

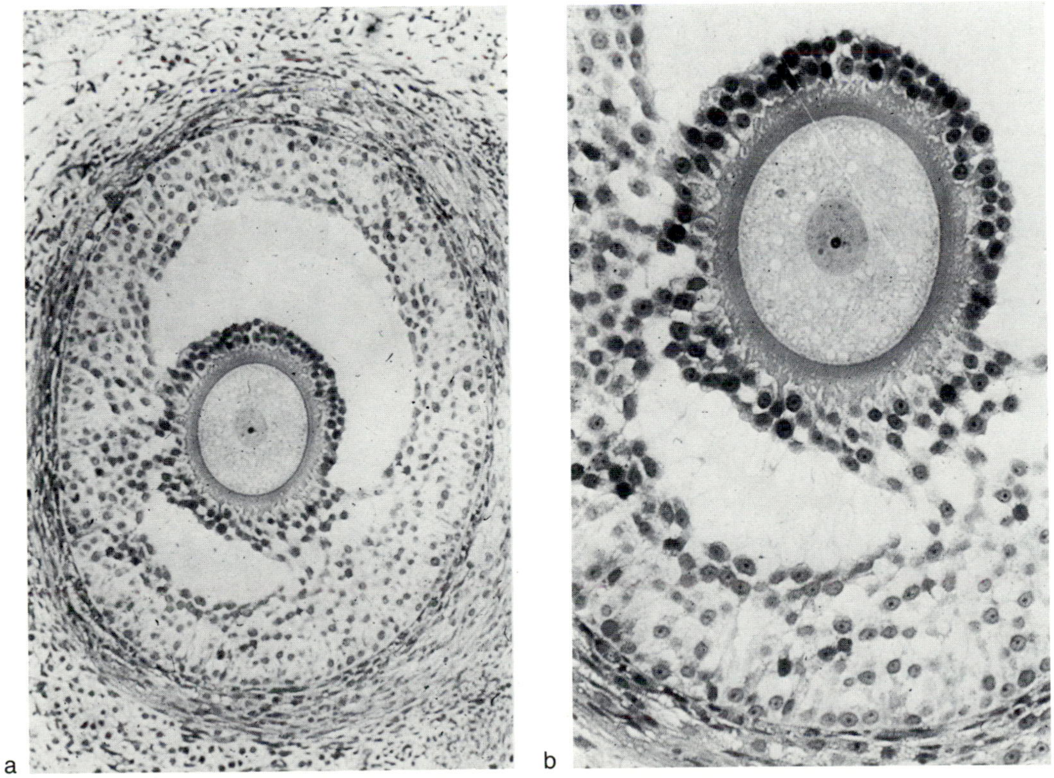

Fig. 15.16. *a*. Graafian follicle with large antrum. *b*. Higher power view. Note the cumulus oophorus containing the oocyte with its surrounding zona pellucida and corona radiata. [Reprinted by permission from Leeson, Leeson (1970) Histology, Philadelphia, Saunders.]

tremely thin, almost avascular, and exhibits degeneration of the stromal cells, fragmentation of collagen fibers, and an accumulation of intercellular fluid.[4] These surface epithelial and stromal changes that immediately precede ovulation may be secondary to local ischemia and release of proteolytic enzymes and prostaglandins into the stroma.[4] The preovulatory follicle then ruptures, possibly secondary to contraction of the perifollicular smooth muscle cells, with liberation of the follicular fluid and oocyte (with its surrounding layers) into the peritoneal cavity. After ovulation, the stigma is occluded by a mass of coagulated follicular fluid, fibrin, blood, granulosa and connective tissue cells. It is eventually converted to scar tissue.[4] The specific components of the maturing follicle will be considered in more detail.

Oocyte and Zona Pellucida

As the oocyte matures and undergoes a threefold increase in its volume, it develops more numerous and better developed organelles (mitochondria, granular endoplasmic reticulum, free ribosomes, Golgi complexes) reflecting increased protein synthesis. The number of annulate lamellae, however, decrease.[3,31] The Golgi complexes at the same time become more dispersed coming to lie in several aggregates under the plasma membrane.[3] The Golgi complexes appear to be the source of dense, membrane-bound, 300–500 nm granules that are diffusely distributed under the plasma membrane (Fig. 15.17).[3] Surface microvilli become prominent and establish a close relationship with the bordering layer of granulosa cells (Fig. 15.17).

When the oocyte of a preantral follicle has reached 80 μm in diameter, light microscopic examination reveals an eosinophilic, PAS-positive, homogeneous, acellular layer, the zona pellucida, encasing the oocyte (Figs. 15.16–15.18). Its formation is usually attributed to the granulosa cells, but the oocyte may also play a role. At the end of its development, the zona pellucida is a 20–25 μm thick membrane consisting of fine filamentous material of medium electron density.[3] It is rich in acid mucopolysaccharides and glycoprotein.[31]

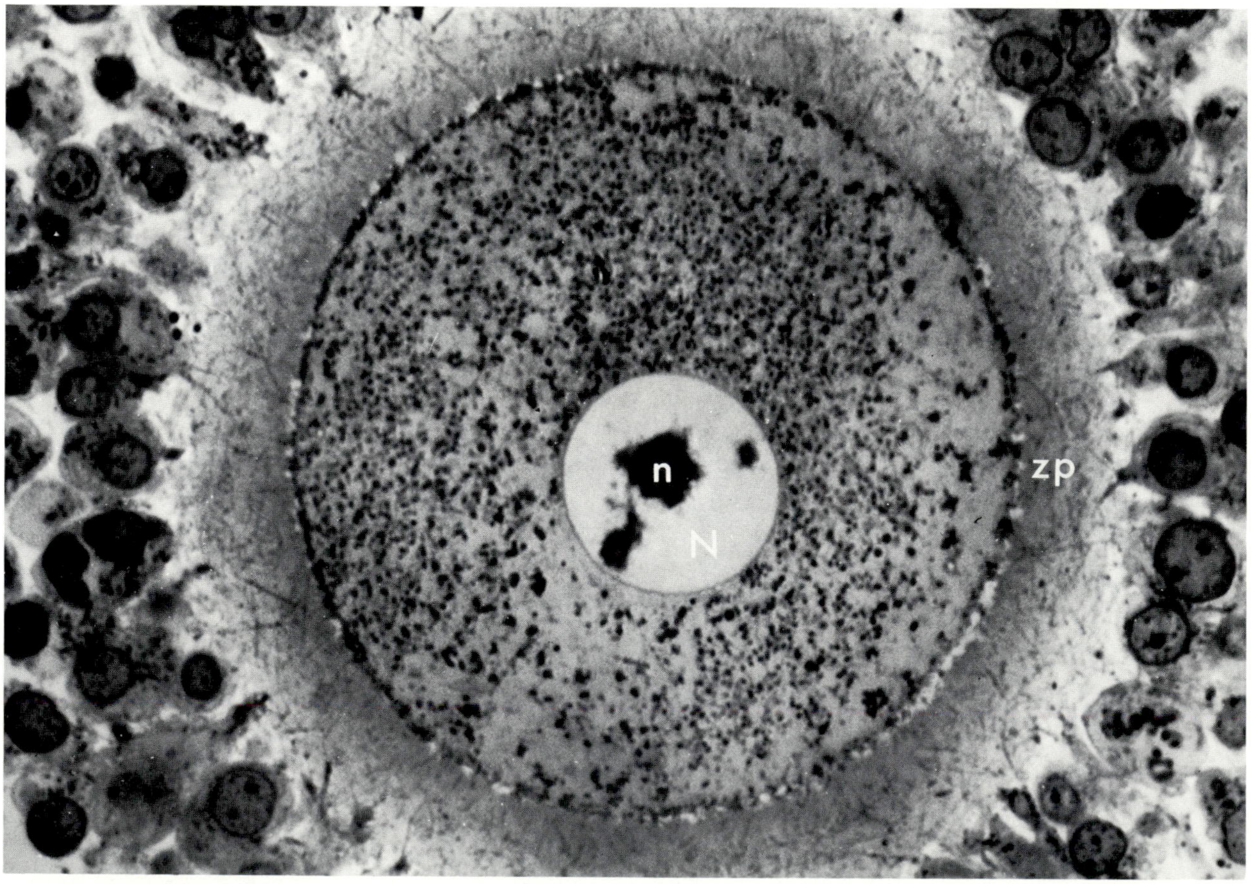

FIG. 15.17. Maturing oocyte. Note the uniform distribution of the organelles and the row of dense granules in the cytoplasm immediately subjacent to the plasma membrane of the oocyte. A continuous zona pellucida (zp) surrounds the oocyte and separates it from the granulosa cells. Numerous cytoplasmic processes of the granulosa cells are visible within the zone pellucida. N, nucleus; n, nucleolus. (Reprinted by permission of Baca, Zamboni, Ref. 3.)

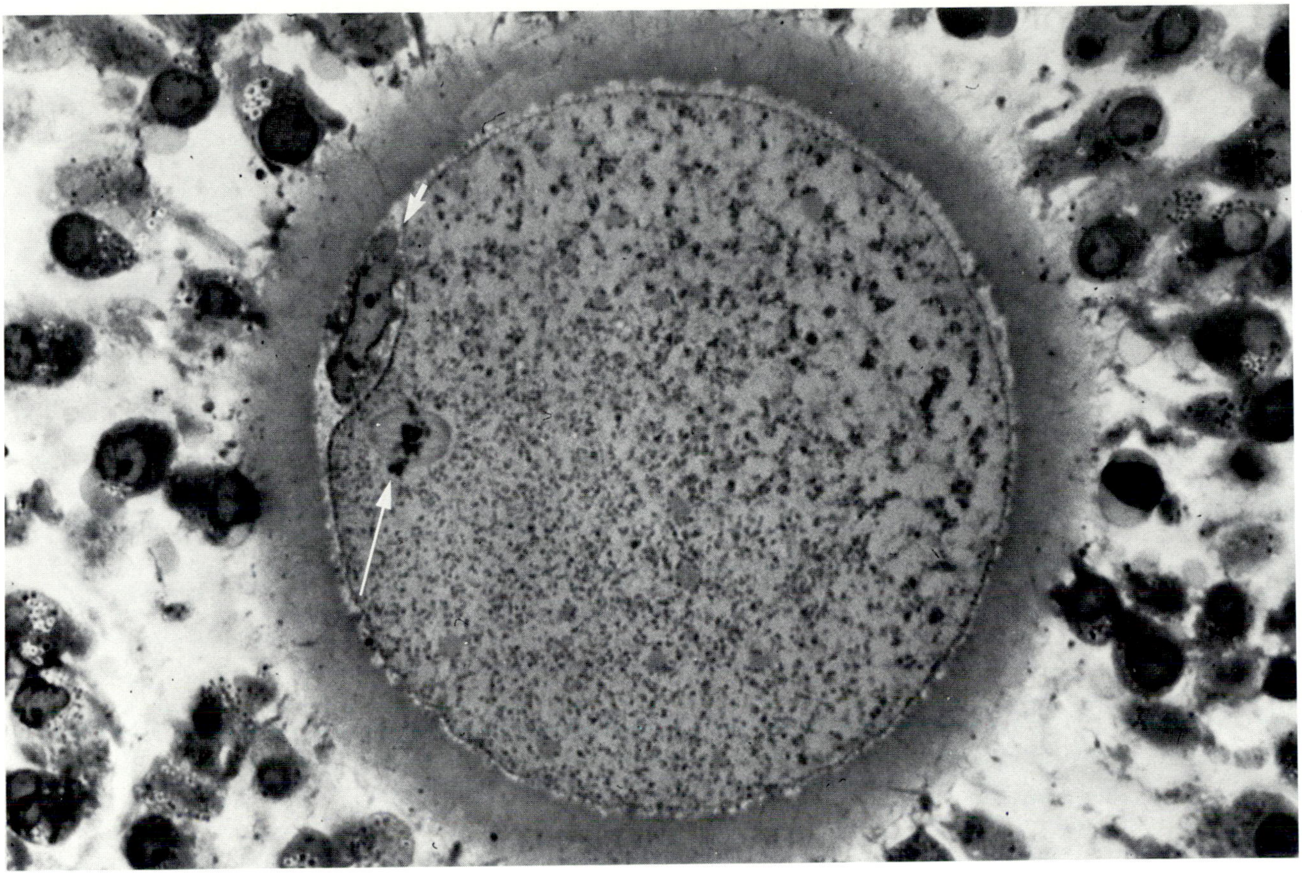

FIG. 15.18. Oocyte shortly after separation of the first polar body. The first polar body (*short arrow*) sits in the perivitelline space. The posttelophasic chromosomes are arranged on the equatorial plate of the meiotic spindle (*long arrow*). (Reprinted by permission of Baca, Zamboni, Ref. 3.)

During the early stages of follicular growth, the oocyte nucleus has a resting appearance similar to that seen in the primordial follicle. Shortly before ovulation, the oocyte within the ovulatory follicle enters telophase of the first meiotic division. This process begins by transformation of the nucleolus into a compact body, followed by chromatin condensation into aggregates that are closely associated with the nucleolus.[3] Chromosomal reduction occurs by migration of one-half the oocyte chromosomes into a portion of the oocyte cytoplasm that separates from the cell as the first polar body. It has an elliptical shape and is contained within a crescentic space (the perivitelline space) between the plasma membrane of the oocyte and the inner aspect of the zona pellucida (Fig. 15.18). It is delimited by a plasma membrane with a few irregular microvilli.[3] The first meiotic division begun in fetal life is now complete, and the oocyte is now designated the secondary oocyte. Immediately after expulsion of the first polar body, the secondary oocyte enters the second meiotic division, arresting at metaphase until fertilization occurs.

Granulosa Layer

Histology. Granulosa cells are almost entirely formed from their embryonic precursors by the time of birth.[99] Those within maturing and graafian follicles are polyhedral cells measuring 5–7 μm in diameter. Cells resting on the basement membrane are often columnar in shape. They have scant, pale, frothy cytoplasm, indistinct cell borders, and small, round to oval, hyperchromatic nuclei that typically lack nuclear grooves (Fig. 15.19a).[114] Cytoplasmic lipid is absent or sparse.[52] Mitotic figures within granulosa cells are usually numerous in maturing follicles, but their numbers decrease in the late stages of follicular growth immediately before ovulation.

The granulosa cells typically surround small cavities, Call-Exner bodies (Fig. 15.15), which have a distinctive appearance, representing one of the most specific features of granulosa cells, both normal and neoplastic. Call-Exner bodies are delimited from the granulosa cells by a basal lamina and contain a deeply eosinophilic, PAS-positive, filamentous material consisting of excess

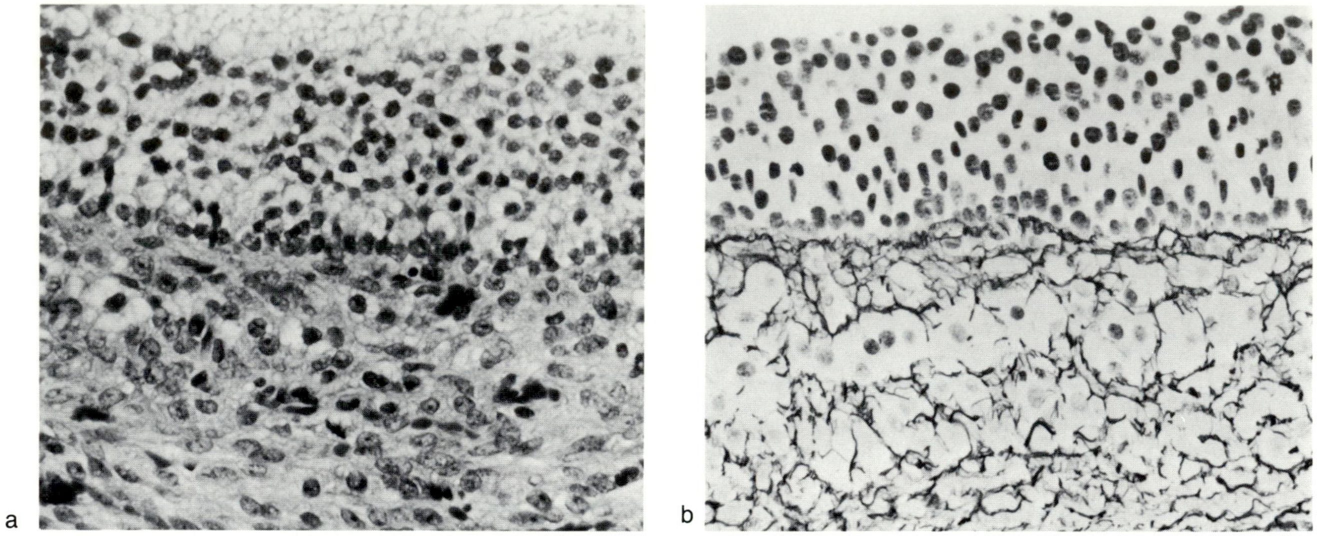

FIG. 15.19. Lining of mature follicle. *a*. The granulosa layer is surrounded by an outer layer of luteinized theca interna cells. *b*. A reticulin stain reveals a reticulum network in the theca interna layer but an absence of reticulin in the granulosa layer.

basal lamina and possible precursors of the pellucid zone.[9,31,99] Unlike the theca layers, the granulosa layer of the maturing and graafian follicles is avascular and devoid of a reticulum framework (Fig. 15.19b).

Ultrastructure. Mitochondria with lamelliform cristae, granular ER, free ribosomes, and Golgi complexes gradually increase in abundance within the granulosa cells of maturing follicles.[9] These ultrastructural features suggest active protein synthesis. Histochemical and ultrastructural features (abundant smooth ER and mitochondria with tubular cristae) indicative of steroid biosynthesis are absent until shortly before ovulation.[23,30,52,76,101] The plasma membranes of the granulosa cells develop specialized membrane contacts in the form of tight junctions that probably facilitate cellular interchange of ions and small-molecular-weight substances.[29,31] The granulosa cells of the corona radiata that border the oocyte possess slender cytoplasmic extensions that traverse the zona pellucida and establish similar junctions with the plasma membrane of the oocyte (Fig. 15.17).[3,31]

Theca Layers

In contrast to granulosa cells, theca cells differentiate continuously from the stromal cells at the periphery of developing follicles, a process beginning during fetal life and ending at the termination of the menopause.[99] The thecal component of the antral follicle is characterized by a well developed theca interna and a less well defined theca externa.

Histology. The theca interna layer is three or four cells in thickness and lies external to that formed by the granulosa cells; the two layers are separated by a basement membrane. Unlike the granulosa cells of the developing and graafian follicles, the theca interna cells typically have a luteinized or partially luteinized appearance, resembling true theca-lutein cells of the corpus luteum. The round to polygonal cells measure 12–20 μm in diameter and have abundant, eosinophilic to clear, vacuolated cytoplasm containing variable amounts of lipid; a central, round, vesicular nucleus typically contains a single, prominent nucleolus (Fig. 15.19a). Luteinization of the theca interna of maturing follicles is particularly prominent during pregnancy. In the larger follicles, many mitoses are present, but they decrease with further follicular maturation. Theca interna cells have the histochemical patterns characteristic of steroid hormone secretion.[23,30,52,99] Occasional darkly eosinophilic, stellate K cells may be seen in the mature graafian follicle within the theca interna, but these cells are more characteristic of the corpus luteum (see p. 453).[114] The theca interna layer of developing follicles contains a rich vascular plexus consisting of dilated capillaries, as well as a dense reticulum network that surrounds each cell (Fig. 15.19b).

The theca externa is an ill-defined layer of variable thickness that surrounds the theca interna and merges imperceptibly with the adjacent ovarian stroma. It is composed of circumferentially arranged collagen bundles, blood and lymphatic vessels, and plump, spindle-shaped stromal cells that lack the histochemical features of steroidogenic cells.[34] The spindle-shaped cells typically exhibit prominent mitotic activity and may be misinterpreted as tumor cells when only the theca externa edge of the follicle is seen on a microscopic section.

Ultrastructure. Ultrastructural examination of theca interna cells reveals the organelles associated with steroidogenesis, similar to those within granulosa-lutein cells (see p. 450). The theca externa cells, some of which exhibit smooth muscle differentiation, lack such organelles.[83]

Hormone Synthesis

As a small antral follicle develops into a preovulatory follicle, a sequence of endocrine events occurs within its antral fluid that differs from most, if not all, other antral follicles in the same ovary.[69,70] Early follicular maturation is under the control of FSH, reflected by the appearance of FSH receptors within the granulosa cells of primary follicles, followed by increasing concentrations of FSH receptors and intrafollicular FSH within the preovulatory follicle.[29,69,70] As the FSH concentration increases, there is a concomitant increase in estradiol receptors within the granulosa cells and estradiol levels within the follicular fluid. The latter reach peak concentrations (10,000 times circulating levels) during the mid to late proliferative phase.[29,69,70] Intrafollicular estradiol likely stimulates, through estradiol receptors, mitotic activity within the granulosa cells and their increased sensitivity to FSH.[29] As the level of circulating estradiol rises, the plasma FSH falls toward basal levels. At this stage the preovulatory follicle has become self-sustaining, continuing to mature under the influence of intrafollicular FSH and estradiol.[71] As the FSH levels fall, the circulating LH levels increase. Whereas circulating estradiol is probably derived from both the granulosa cells and the LH-stimulated theca cells, intrafollicular estradiol is derived almost exclusively from the granulosa cells by both de novo synthesis and by FSH-dependent aromatization of theca-derived androstenedione.[71,72] Aromatase activity is highest in the preovulatory follicle, thereby maintaining a high concentration of estradiol and low levels of androstenedione.[69,70] In contrast, the other follicles are FSH- and aromatase-deficient, with a resultant predominance of intrafollicular androstenedione; these follicles will ultimately undergo atresia (p. 459). Granulosa and theca LH receptors increase gradually throughout follicular development, possibly under the control of FSH, reaching a maximum number just before ovulation.[29,69,70] Simultaneously, the high estrogen levels, through positive feedback, initiate a preovulatory surge of plasma LH.[86,117] Intrafollicular LH leads to a rise in local cyclic AMP, inhibition of mitotic activity in the granulosa cells, resumption of oocyte maturation, luteinization of the granulosa cells, and their production of progesterone and prostaglandins.[32] As a result, there is an increase in intrafollicular progesterone concentration as well as a small but significant preovulatory rise in circulating progesterone.[32,69,70] Shortly before ovulation, the preovulatory follicle contains high concentrations of FSH, LH, and progesterone, but low levels of androstenedione and declining levels of estradiol.[69,70] The rising plasma progesterone levels and the peaking estrogen levels further augment the LH surge, as well as initiating a smaller increase in FSH, triggering ovulation. The latter has been estimated to occur 36–38 hours after the onset of the LH surge, 24–36 hours after the estradiol peak, and 10–12 hours after the LH peak.[32]

Inhibin-F or FSH-suppressing substance, a nonsteroidal polypeptide, has been recently demonstrated in follicular fluid in amounts that correlate with steroid levels.[106] It acts, by negative feedback, to reduce FSH secretion from the hypothalamic-pituitary unit. Inhibin-F is synthesized by the granulosa cells (consistent with their content of rough ER) and is secreted into the follicular fluid and ovarian venous effluent.[32]

Corpus Luteum of Menstruation

Dating the Corpus Luteum. Following ovulation on the 14th day of the typical 28-day menstrual cycle, and in the absence of fertilization, the collapsed ovulatory follicle becomes the corpus luteum of menstruation (CLM). When mature, the latter is a 1.5–2.0 cm, round, yellow structure with festooned contours and a cystic center filled with a gray, focally hemorrhagic coagulum (Figs. 15.20 and 15.21). During the 14 days after ovulation, the CLM undergoes an orderly sequence of histologic changes that allow an approximate estimation of its age. Corner has described these stages in detail, using endometrial histology and menstrual data to establish the age of the CLM.[18,109] A subsequent study correlated the histologic date of the CLM using Corner's criteria with the interval between the LH peak and the biopsy of the CLM.[20] It was determined that the dating of different corpora lutea obtained at the same LH peak-biopsy

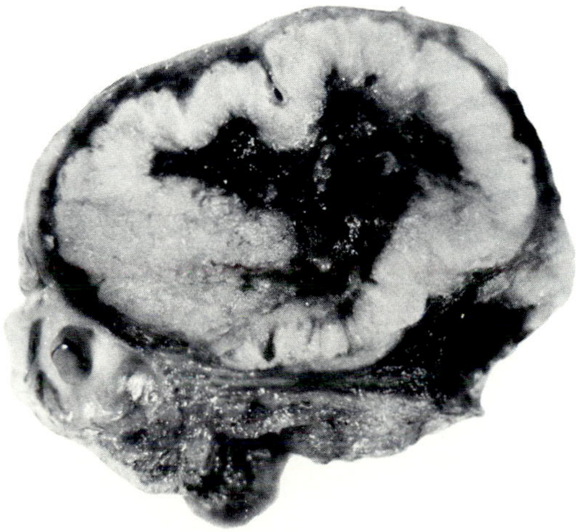

FIG. 15.20. Mature corpus luteum of menstruation. A yellow convoluted border surrounds a central hemorrhagic coagulum.

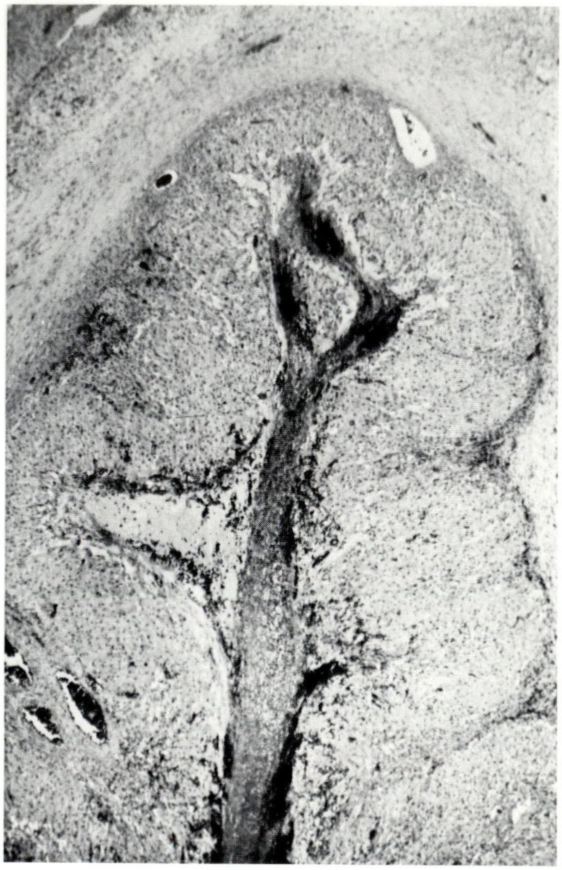

FIG. 15.21. Mature corpus luteum of menstruation. Festooned lining composed of granulosa–lutein cells surrounds central cavity.

interval could differ by as much as 4 days, that stages described by Corner as days 1 and 2 developed within the first 24 hours, and that stages corresponding to his days 4 and 5 each took 2 days to develop. It was concluded that the use of the histology of the CLM for retrospective timing of ovulation is subject to an error of variable magnitude due to unequal duration of each stage and considerable individual variation.

Histology. In contrast to the granulosa cells of the maturing and preovulatory follicles, the luteinized granulosa cells of the mature CLM (granulosa-lutein cells) are large, 30–35 μm, polygonal cells with abundant, pale eosinophilic cytoplasm that may contain numerous small lipid droplets (Fig. 15.22a).[34] The 7–10 μm spherical nucleus contains one or two large nucleoli.[34] The histochemical pattern of these cells varies with the age of the CLM, but generally it is typical of steroid hormone-producing cells.[23,30,115]

The theca interna forms an irregular and often interrupted layer several cells in thickness around the circumference of the CLM as well as ensheathing the vascular septa that extend into its center (Fig. 15.22).[34] When these septa are cut in cross-section, triangular-shaped nests of theca cells appear at intervals throughout the granulosa layer. In all but the earliest stages of the CLM, the theca-lutein cells are approximately half the size of granulosa-lutein cells. They contain a round to oval nucleus with a single prominent nucleolus. Their less abundant, more darkly staining cytoplasm contains lipid droplets that are usually larger than those in granulosa-lutein cells. The nuclear and cytoplasmic density of theca-lutein

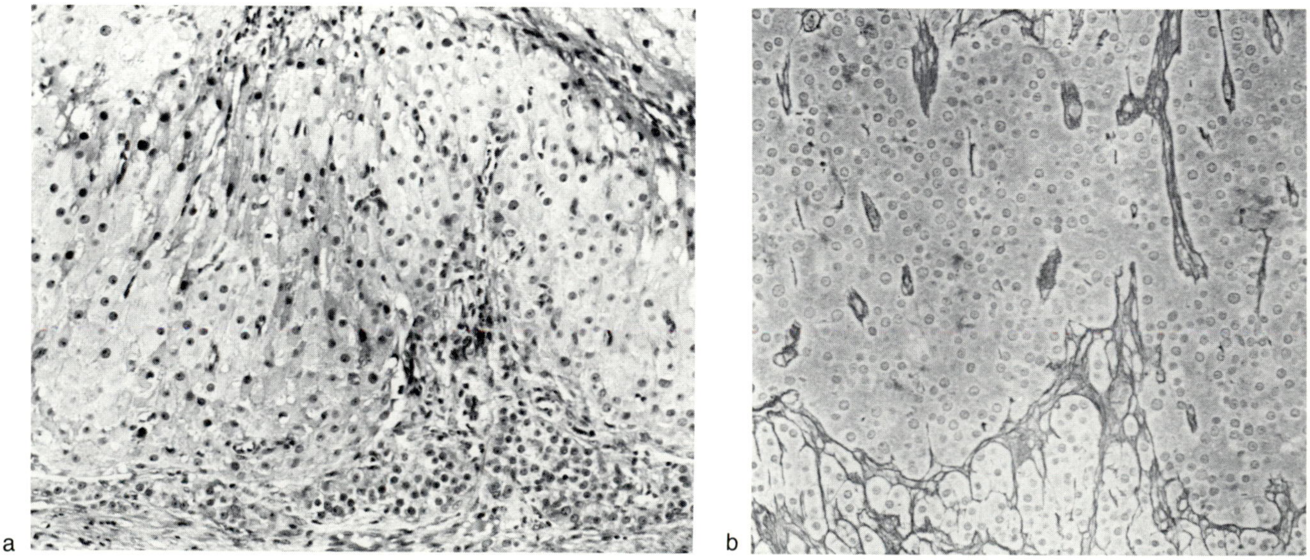

FIG. 15.22. Mature corpus luteum of menstruation. *a.* The lining is composed of a thick layer of large granulosa–lutein cell and an outer, thinner layer of smaller theca–lutein cells. *b.* A reticulin stain shows a dense reticulum network in the theca interna and a beginning reticulum network, predominantly perivascular, within the granulosa–lutein layer.

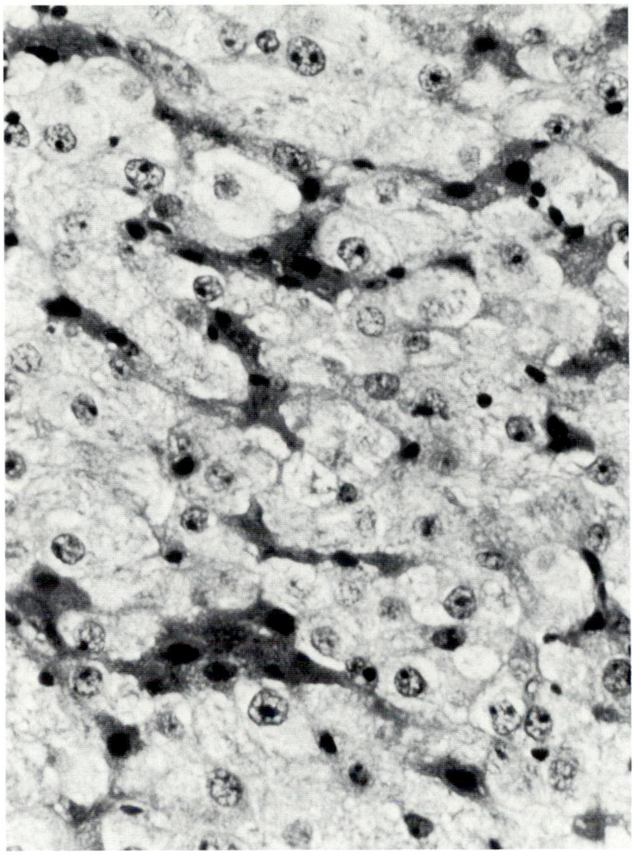

FIG. 15.23. Mature corpus luteum of menstruation. Darkly staining K cells are seen interspersed between granulosa–lutein cells.

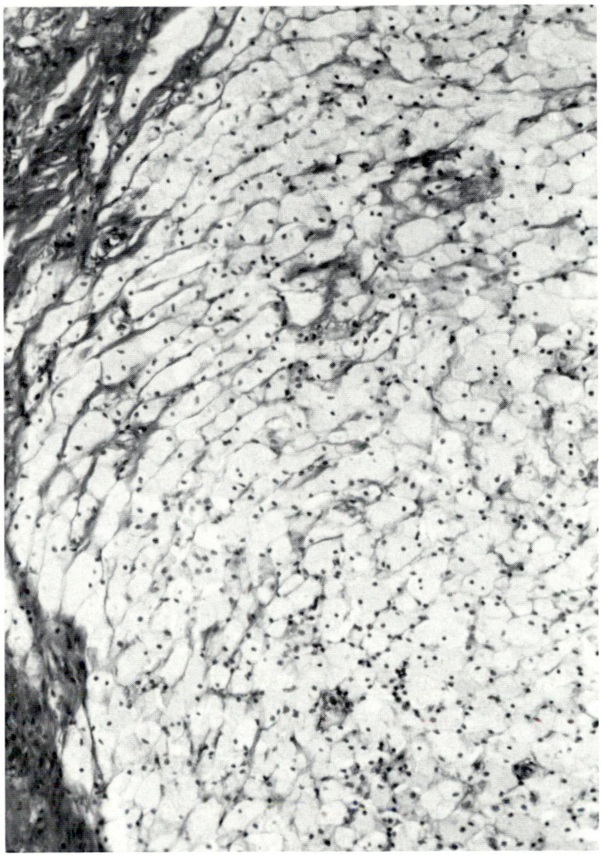

FIG. 15.24. Degenerating corpus luteum of menstruation. Granulosa–lutein cells have pyknotic nuclei and abundant cytoplasmic lipid.

cells is often much more variable than that of the granulosa-lutein cells.

A third type of cell, the so-called K cell which is present in small numbers within the theca interna of the mature follicle, appears in greater numbers within the granulosa layer of the early CLM.[114] K cells persist until menstruation at which time they degenerate. They are characterized by a stellate shape, a deeply eosinophilic cytoplasm and an irregular, hyperchromatic or pyknotic nucleus (Fig. 15.23). The cytoplasm is uniformly sudanophilic due to the presence of phospholipid.[114] K cells lack the histochemical patterns of steroidogenic cells and have been variously considered perivascular macrophages[34] or cells of theca or granulosa origin affected by degenerative changes or altered metabolic activity.[1,80,81,114]

During the maturation of the CLM, capillaries originating from the theca interna layer penetrate the granulosa layer and reach the central cavity. Fibroblasts that accompany the vessels form an increasingly dense reticulum network within the granulosa layer as well as an inner fibrous layer that lines the central cavity (Fig. 15.22b).[68]

In the absence of fertilization, involutional changes begin on the eighth or ninth days following ovulation.[18] The granulosa-lutein cells decrease in size, develop pyknotic nuclei, and accumulate abundant cytoplasmic lipid (Fig. 15.24). There is a decrease in histochemical staining of enzymes associated with steroid biosynthesis and an increase in hydrolytic enzymes.[23] Eventually, the cells undergo dissolution and are phagocytosed.[1] Over a period of several months there is progressive fibrosis and shrinkage of the CLM with conversion to a corpus albicans (p. 457).[68]

Ultrastructure. At the ultrastructural level, luteinization is characterized by a gradually increasing content of steroidogenic organelles, specifically smooth ER and abundant mitochondria with tubular cristae (Fig. 15.25).[1, 19,34,37] The smooth ER exhibits a characteristic regional modification in the form of a folded-membrane complex consisting of highly folded, radiating, tubular cisternae that communicate and interdigitate with adjacent cisternae.[19] Well-developed, dispersed and perinuclear Golgi complexes, free and bound ribosomes, lipid droplets, and lipofuschin pigment are also seen (Fig.

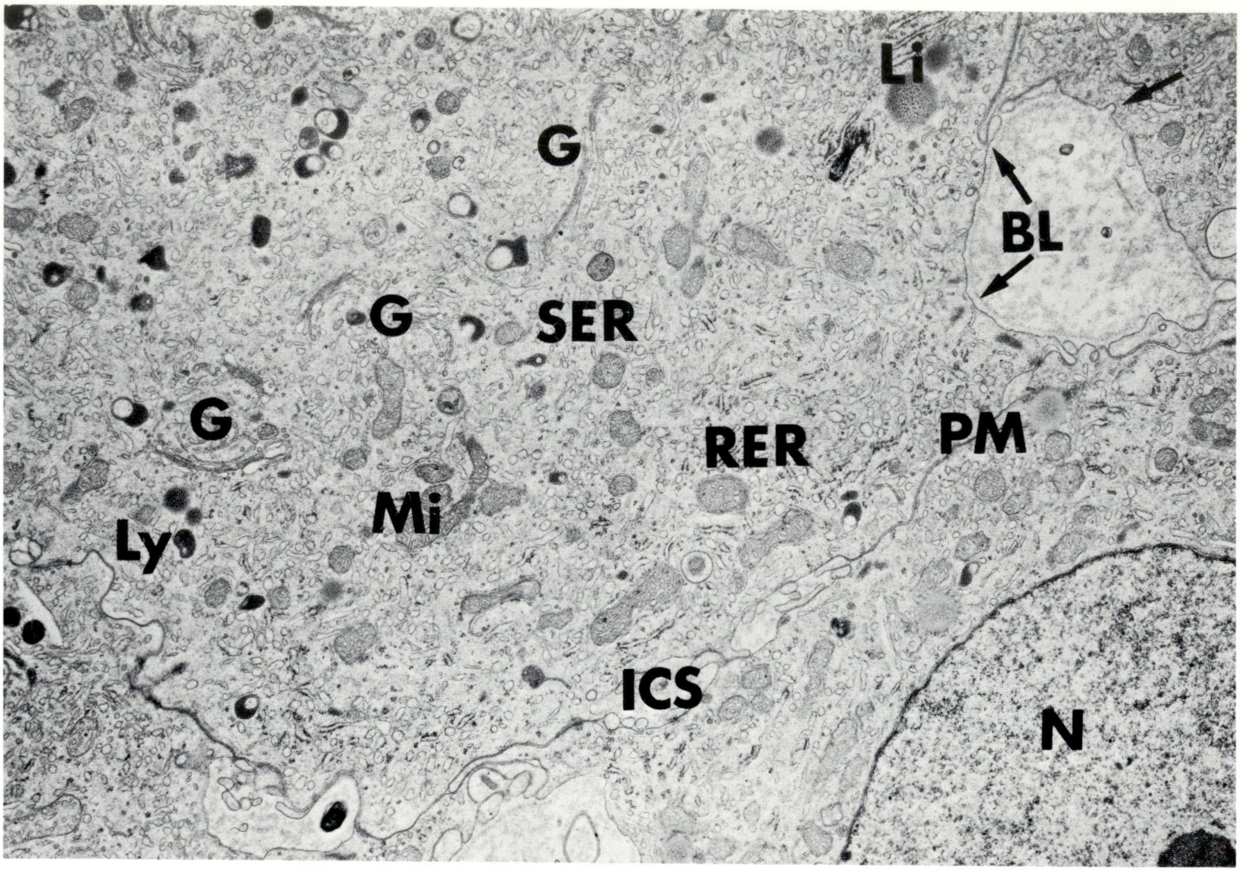

FIG. 15.25. Electron micrograph of granulosa–lutein cell of a mature corpus luteum of menstruation. Note abundant smooth endoplasmic reticulum (SER), mitochondria (Mi), Golgi (G), rough endoplasmic reticulum (RER), lipid droplets (Li), intercellular space (ICS), nucleus (N), lysosomes (Ly), plasma membrane (PM), micropinocytotic vesicle (*arrows*) and basal lamina (BL). (Courtesy of Dr. T. Okagaki. Reprinted by permission of Ferenczy, Richart, Ref. 31. Copyright John Wiley & Sons, Inc., 1974.)

15.25).[1,19,34,37] The cells are separated by a narrow space of variable width, but occasionally the outer leaflets of their plasma membranes become closely apposed and reinforced by desmosomal and pentalaminar tight junctional complexes.[1,19,34] Nearly all the cells have a free surface that borders on a broad pericapillary space from which they are separated by an interrupted basal lamina.[34] Many irregular microvillous cytoplasmic extensions project into these pericapillary, as well as the intercellular, spaces (Fig. 15.25).[1,19,31,34] Occasional interdigitation of these microvilli has been noted between adjacent cells to form intercellular channels.[19] Underlying the microvilli is a narrow zone of cytoplasm filled with a network of filaments that also extend into the microvilli.[34]

Theca-lutein cells are similar ultrastructurally to granulosa lutein cells except for the presence of localized perinuclear Golgi complexes and the absence of folded-membrane complexes, microvilli, and a network of fine filaments.[19,34] The varying degrees of cell density appreciable on histological examination are also seen at the ultrastructural level and may represent an artifact of fixation.[34] The theca externa layer of the CLM does not differ significantly from that of the graafian follicle (see p. 450). K cells have very irregular nuclear membranes, vesicular ER, and pleomorphic mitochondria.[1] They lack ultrastructural evidence of active steroidogenic activity.

The lutein cells of the degenerating CLM exhibit disorganization and fragmentation of the smooth ER, alterations of the mitochondria, and an increase in cytolysosomes.[31] Lipid droplets are increased and irregular in size and show increased osmiophilia.[1]

Hormone Synthesis. The formation and function of the CLM is under the control of LH, reflected by the high content of LH receptors within the granulosa-lutein cells.[32] Although progesterone is the major steroid formed in vivo and in vitro by the CLM, it also synthesizes, both in vitro and in vivo, estrone and estradiol, as well as androgens, mostly androstenedione.[62] In vitro progesterone and estrogen synthesis is stimulated by the addition of both hCG and LH.[98]

After ovulation, LH, FSH, and estradiol levels fall, but the LH concentration is sufficient to maintain the CLM, producing a midluteal peak in progesterone and estradiol concentration. If fertilization does not occur, the increased levels of progesterone and estrogen through negative feedback result in a fall of LH and FSH to basal levels, a reduction in LH and FSH receptors within the CLM, and a marked decline in progesterone and estradiol synthesis after the 22nd day of the cycle.[13,29,32,93] These changes are reflected by morphologic involution of the CLM and the onset of menses. Luteolysis appears to be estrogen-related, possibly secondary to an estrogen-induced reduction in LH receptors or by enhancement of the luteolytic action of prostaglandins synthesized by the CLM.[32] A nonsteroidal LH-receptor-binding-inhibitor, which increases in concentration during the luteal phase, may also play a role.[32]

Corpus Luteum of Pregnancy

Gross Appearance. On gross inspection, the corpus luteum of pregnancy (CLP) is similar to, and may be indistinguishable from, the CLM. However, it usually has a larger size and a color that is more typically bright yellow, compared to the orange-yellow of the late CLM.[42] The larger size, which may account for up to one-half the ovarian volume, is due primarily to the presence of a central cystic cavity filled with fluid or a coagulum composed of fibrin and blood (Fig. 15.26);[81,103,110] the cavity size, however, can be highly variable. When the cavity is large, typically in early pregnancy, the wall of the CLP may lose its convolutions, becoming stretched and thinned to the extent that it may focally consist only of fibrous tissue of the inner fibrous layer.[81] Obliteration of the cavity usually begins by the fifth month and is typically completed by term.[81] The CLP thus gradually decreases in size, and by the last trimester, it is not a conspicuous structure. It may be as small or smaller than the CLM.[81] During the puerperium, the CLP undergoes involution and conversion to a corpus albicans in a fashion similar to that seen with the CLM.[81]

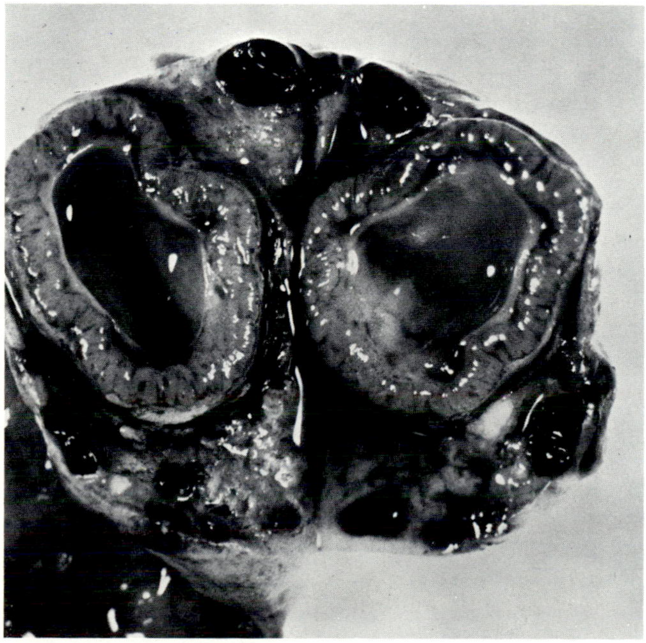

Fig. 15.26. Cystic corpus luteum of pregnancy.

Histology. The CLP, in contrast to the CLM, does not mature in an orderly sequence that allows an estimation of its age. However, early and late stages are recognizable on histologic examination.

Granulosa Layer. The first morphologic evidence within the corpus luteum that conception has occurred is the absence of the regressive changes that normally appear in the CLM on the 9th–12th days. Instead, the granulosa-lutein cells enlarge, reaching their maximum size (50–60 μm) by 8–9 weeks of gestation, and assume a round or polyhedral shape with abundant eosinophilic cytoplasm (Fig. 15.27a). Their round to oval, vesicular nuclei, have one or two prominent nucleoli.[81] They typically have polyploid levels of DNA.[102]

The granulosa cells of the early CLP are characterized by cytoplasmic vacuoles that initially are minute but eventually increase in size to occupy almost the entire cell, often with displacement and flattening of the nucleus (Fig. 15.27a). The vacuoles tend to diminish in number and size as gestation progresses, and typically disappear after the fourth month.[81] Fine, diffusely scattered, cytoplasmic lipid droplets are also commonly seen within the cells, particularly in early CLP. With increasing age of the CLP, the droplets become fewer and larger.[81]

Eosinophilic colloid or hyaline droplets within the granulosa cells of a CLP are almost diagnostic of pregnancy but can be seen very rarely within a CLM.[81] They can be identified as early as 15 days after ovulation.[99] These inclusions initially appear as small, round or irregular, often multiple, droplets but eventually enlarge, possibly by fusion of smaller droplets, into one or several large bodies that may fill the entire cell (Fig. 15.27a). They become more numerous as gestation progresses,[110] although by term their numbers decrease as they undergo calcification, a process that continues into the puerperium (Fig. 15.27b).[81,110] It is likely that these calcified bodies eventually are resorbed, since they are not a feature of corpora albicantia.[81]

K cells, identical to those described within CLM (p. 453), are typically found in the granulosa layer of the early CLP. They are most numerous in the second,

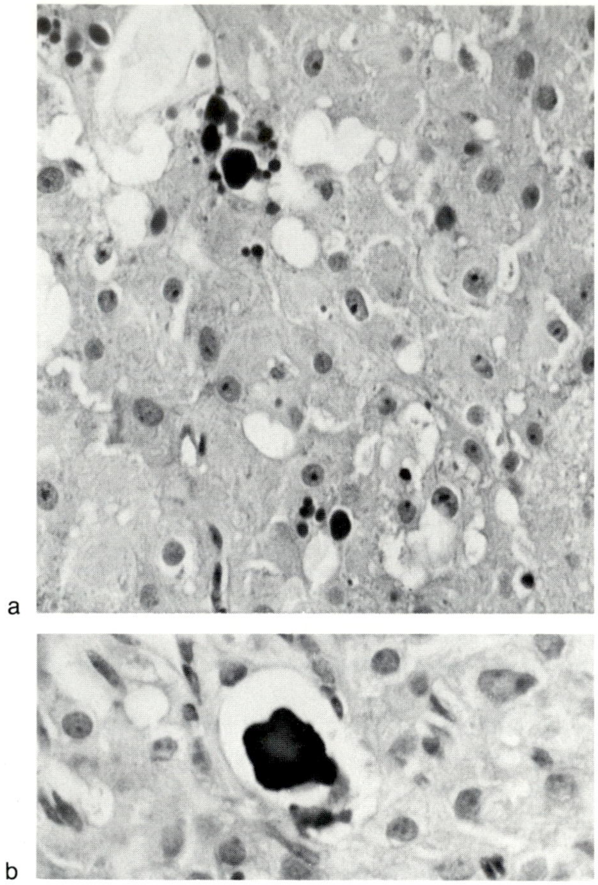

FIG. 15.27. Corpus luteum of pregnancy. *a.* Note granulosa–lutein cells with large irregular vacuoles and numerous, variably sized, darkly staining hyaline bodies. *b.* Focal calcification within a late corpus luteum of pregnancy.

third, and fourth months of gestation after which they are rarely encountered.[80,81,110]

Theca Layer. The theca interna is thickest in the early CLP when it resembles its counterpart in the CLM, surrounding the granulosa-lutein layer and forming triangular-shaped, vascular septa that extend into the latter. In the CLP, the theca cells are polyhedral or round and approximately one-fourth the size of the granulosa-lutein cells. The cytoplasm is more darkly staining and granular than in the latter, and typically nonvacuolated. Their nuclei are central, round, and more hyperchromatic than those of the granulosa cells; one or two prominent nucleoli are usually present.[81] The characteristic colloid inclusions seen within the granulosa cells are absent or very rare within the theca cells.[81] Occasional K cells may be seen in early pregnancy, but in smaller numbers than in the granulosa layer.[110,114] After the fourth month, the theca interna and its septa become much thinner as the theca cells become smaller and fewer in number, with darker, more irregular, oblong to spindle-shaped nuclei, so that they resemble fibroblasts.[110] By term, the theca interna layer has almost completely disappeared.[44,81] The theca externa layer may be more edematous and vascular than that of the CLM[81] or, in other examples, inapparent.[110]

Connective Tissue. As in the mature CLM, the central cystic cavity is typically lined by a layer of fibrous tissue, composed of variable numbers of fibroblasts, collagen and reticulin fibers, and blood vessels.[81] Its thickness is highly variable, not only within the same CLP but also from one CLP to another and from one phase of pregnancy to another.[110] As noted, in some CLP with large cystic cavities, the granulosa layer is focally absent, and its wall is formed entirely by this fibrous layer. As gestation advances, the central cyst or coagulum is eventually obliterated by connective tissue, which may exhibit focal hyalinization and calcification.[80]

Reticulum staining reveals a pattern similar to that of the mature CLM, that is, a dense pattern within the theca interna and inner fibrous layer and a sparser framework within the granulosa layer.[81] In the early CLP, many, often large vessels are present in the theca externa and interna, which give origin to smaller vessels that penetrate the granulosa and inner fibrous layers.[81] In the late CLP, the vessels develop sclerotic walls with luminal narrowing or obliteration.[81,110] The amount of connective tissue around the vessels increases in proportion to the decreasing vascularization and regression of the theca interna layer.[110]

Ultrastructure. The ultrastructural appearance of the CLP is similar to that of the CLM and remains intact throughout pregnancy despite a reduction in its metabolic activity.[2,38,87] The increased cell volume of the granulosa cells in the CLP is reflected by increased smooth ER, which exhibits many folded-membrane complexes. There is also an increase in rough ER, which is localized in stacks and characteristic concentric whorls not usually seen in the CLM.[19,38] Electron-dense, 150–200 nm, membrane-bound granules are closely associated with the cisternae of the rough ER. Mitochondria, including large spherical mitochondria not seen in the CLM, are typically highly variable in their size, shape, and internal structure.[19,38] The colloid or hyaline inclusions consist of homogeneous electron-opaque material that may surround occasional needle-shaped crystals (Fig. 15.28). They typically have no relationship to any organelle, although occasional smaller hyaline bodies are surrounded by rough ER. The vacuoles seen by light microscopy are lined by attenuated microvilli and contain an electron-translucent material.[2] Unlike the CLM, extensive bundles of microfilaments are typically encountered throughout the cytoplasm in most lutein cells and become more prominent as pregnancy progresses.[2,38] Collagen fibrils are encountered more frequently in the

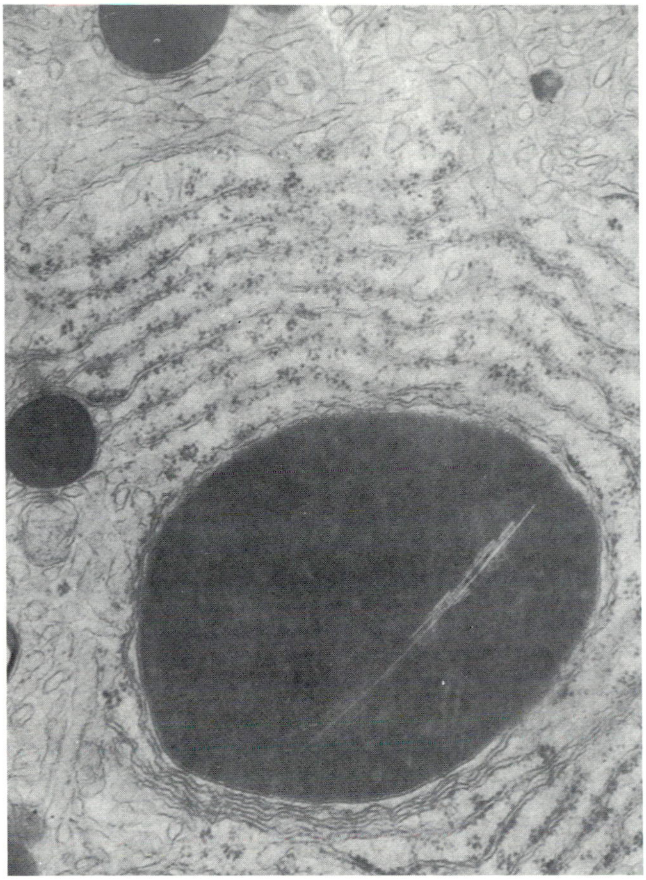

FIG. 15.28. Hyaline bodies within a lutein cell from a corpus luteum of pregnancy consisting of homogeneous, electron-opaque material. Note the needle-shaped cleft within the largest hyaline body. ×22,000. (Reprinted by permission of Adams, Hertig, Ref. 2. Reproduced from *The Journal of Cell Biology*, 1969, 41:716 by copyright permission of The Rockefeller University Press.)

intercellular and perivascular spaces of the term CLP compared to the CLM.[38]

Hormone Synthesis. Following fertilization, chorionic gonadotropin (hCG) of placental origin stimulates progesterone production by the granulosa-lutein cells, with progesterone concentrations within the postovulatory corpus luteum increasing by approximately 600%.[69,70] The estradiol levels drop to 10% of their levels within the preovulatory follicle.[69,70] hCG levels, and as a result, progesterone production by the CLP, begin to decline by the end of the second month of gestation as the production of progesterone is largely assumed by the placenta. However, it has been shown by both in vivo and in vitro studies that the CLP continues to produce progesterone throughout the remainder of gestation, albeit in reduced amounts, a finding consistent with the maintenance of its structural integrity until term.[2,38,62,78,111] It is not known if the progesterone derived from the CLP has a biologic role during this period or is redundant because of the massive progesterone production by the placenta.[63,113] There is a rapid decline in function during the puerperium, reflecting falling hCG levels during this period. The function of the CLP (as determined by plasma progesterone levels) can be maintained during the puerperium by exogenous hCG stimulation.[63] Similarly, in vitro incubation studies of hCG-stimulated tissue removed from puerperal corpora lutea have demonstrated a capacity for progesterone synthesis.[62,63]

Relaxin, a polypeptide hormone, is another substance produced during gestation and the puerperium by the CLP.[112,113] Its concentration in ovarian vein plasma during pregnancy correlates with progesterone levels. The increased amounts of rough ER and the associated membrane-bound granules found in the CLP may represent the sites of relaxin synthesis and storage respectively.[19] The placenta and uterus have also been suggested as additional, but less important, sources for this hormone. Its reported actions include cervical dilatation and softening, inhibition of uterine contractions, and relaxation of the pubic symphysis and other pelvic joints.[112,113]

Corpus Albicans

The regressing CLM is invaded by connective tissue that gradually converts it to a scar, the corpus albicans. The degenerating CLM and the young corpus albicans may contain macrophages laden with ceroid and hemosiderin pigment.[94] The mature corpus albicans is a well-circumscribed structure with convoluted borders composed almost entirely of densely packed collagen fibers with occasional admixed fibroblasts (Fig. 15.29). Most corpora albicantia are eventually resorbed and replaced by ovarian stroma.[51,99] Persistent corpora albicantia are typically found in the medulla of postmenopausal women suggesting that this resorption process may decelerate or terminate prior to the menopause.

Atretic Follicles

Histology. Of the original 400,000 primordial follicles present at birth, approximately 400 mature to the point of ovulation. The remaining 99.9% undergo atresia, a process that begins before birth and continues throughout reproductive life but is most intense immediately after birth, during puberty, and during pregnancy.[14,24,36,66,81] Factors that initiate atresia and determine which follicles will ultimately undergo atresia are unknown. The atretic process varies with the stage of follicular maturation that has been reached.

Atresia of early follicles (primordial and preantral) begins with degeneration of the oocyte, manifested by nuclear changes (chromatin condensation, pyknosis, frag-

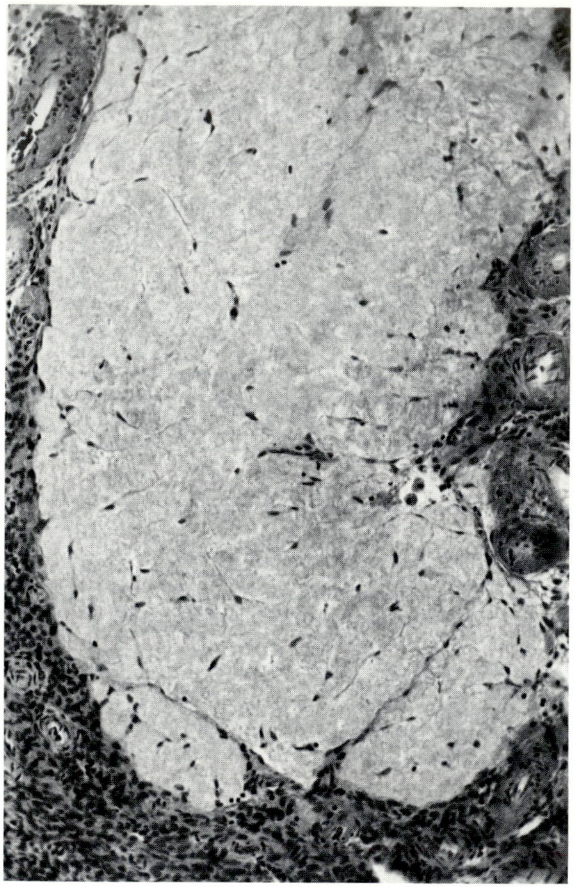

FIG. 15.29. Corpus albicans.

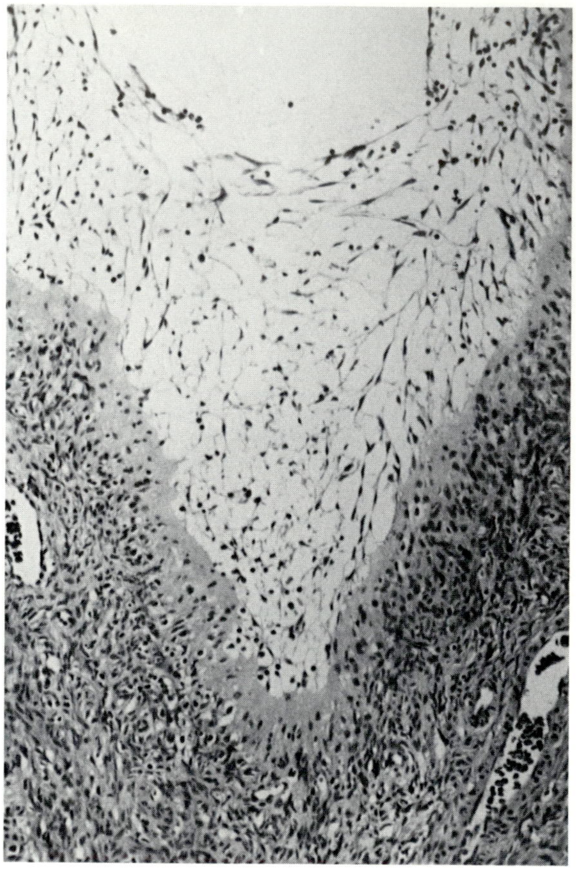

FIG. 15.31. Atretic cystic follicle undergoing obliterative atresia. Loose connective tissue is replacing the central cavity. The wavy basement membrane (glassy membrane) is thickened and hyalinized.

mentation) and cytoplasmic vacuolation. Ultrastructural examination of the degenerating oocyte reveals aggregation of mitochondria, fatty degeneration of the ooplasm, and shrinkage of the zona pellucida.[3] Degeneration of the granulosa cells soon follows, and the follicle disappears without a trace.

In contrast, atresia of follicles that have reached the antral stage of development is more complex and variable but ultimately leads to obliterative atresia and the formation of a scar, the corpus fibrosum.[9] The earliest evidence of this process is mitotic inactivity of the granulosa cells and a decrease in their numbers, manifested by thinning and focal exfoliation of the granulosa layer. Some follicles may persist for an indefinite period of time at this stage as atretic cystic follicles (Fig. 15.30). Ultimately, however, atretic follicles are invaded by vascular connective tissue that eventually fills the central cavity (Fig. 15.31). The oocyte may persist for an indefinite period of time but eventually degenerates.[9] Concurrent with these changes, the basement membrane between the granulosa and theca interna layers becomes transformed into a thick, wavy, eosinophilic, hyalinized band, the so-called "glassy membrane" (Figs. 15.31 and 15.32). The theca interna layer typically persists, often with prominent luteinization, until the late stages of atresia, at which time cords and nests of theca cells become surrounded by proliferating connective tissue (Fig. 15.32). Luteinization of both theca and granulosa layers is particularly striking in atretic follicles during pregnancy.[81] Continued shrinkage and hyalinization produce the corpus fibrosum (or corpus atreticum), a small scar consisting of a wavy strand of hyaline tissue (Fig. 15.33). Like corpora albican-

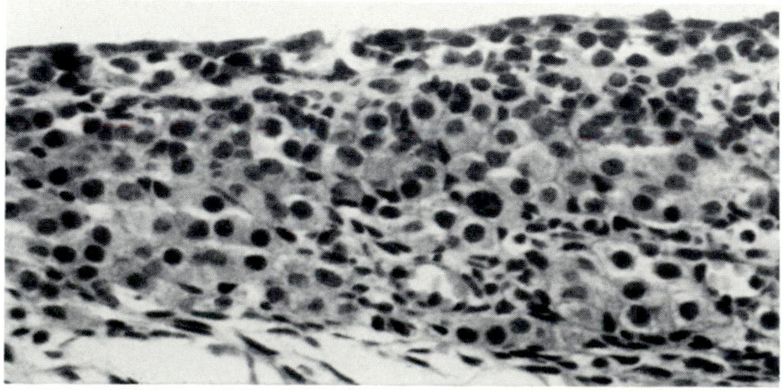

FIG. 15.30. Lining of atretic cystic follicle. The inner layer composed of small granulosa cells is thin and partially exfoliated. The outer, thicker theca interna layer exhibits prominent luteinization.

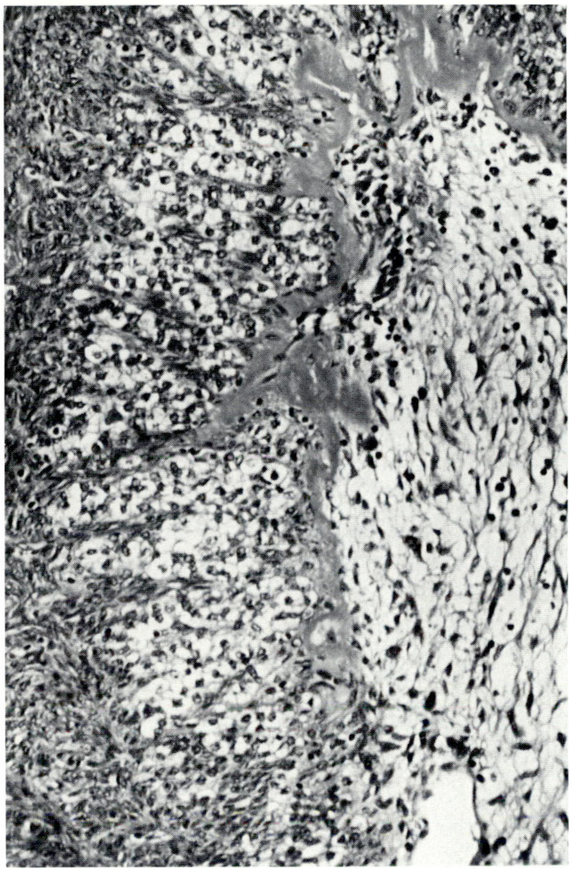

FIG. 15.32. Late stage of obliterative atresia. The thickened basement membrane separates the central fibrous tissue from the prominent luteinized theca interna layer.

tia, most corpora fibrosa are probably resorbed by the ovarian stroma.

Hormone Synthesis. In contrast to preovulatory follicles, the microenvironment of follicles undergoing atresia is predominantly androgenic, with high concentrations of

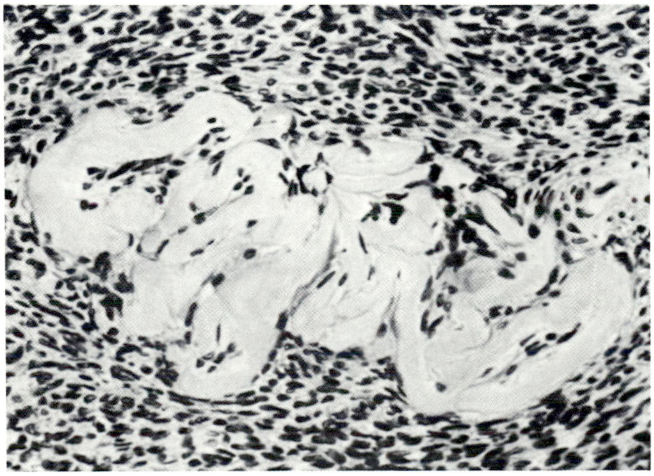

FIG. 15.33. Corpus fibrosum.

intrafollicular androstenedione and low concentrations of FSH and estradiol.[10,69,70,73,82] As noted, these follicles are deficient in granulosa cells, and it has been shown in vitro that residual granulosa cells are incapable of responding to FSH.[73] In addition, oocytes from these follicles are unable to complete the first meiotic division.[73] It is therefore likely that an androgenic intrafollicular milieu is the major factor that halts follicular growth and maturation, ultimately leading to atresia of that follicle.

Hilus Cells

Histology. Ovarian hilus cells, morphologically identical to testicular Leydig cells (with the exception of a female chromatin pattern), are present during fetal life but are not seen during childhood. They reappear at the time of puberty and are demonstrable in virtually all postmenopausal women.[104,105] Their number and location can be highly variable. Their numbers increase during pregnancy and with increasing age after the menopause, as well as with increasing degrees of ovarian stromal proliferation and stromal luteinization.[11] Hilus cell aggregates of variable size and shape are typically found in the ovarian hilus and adjacent mesovarium (Fig. 15.34).

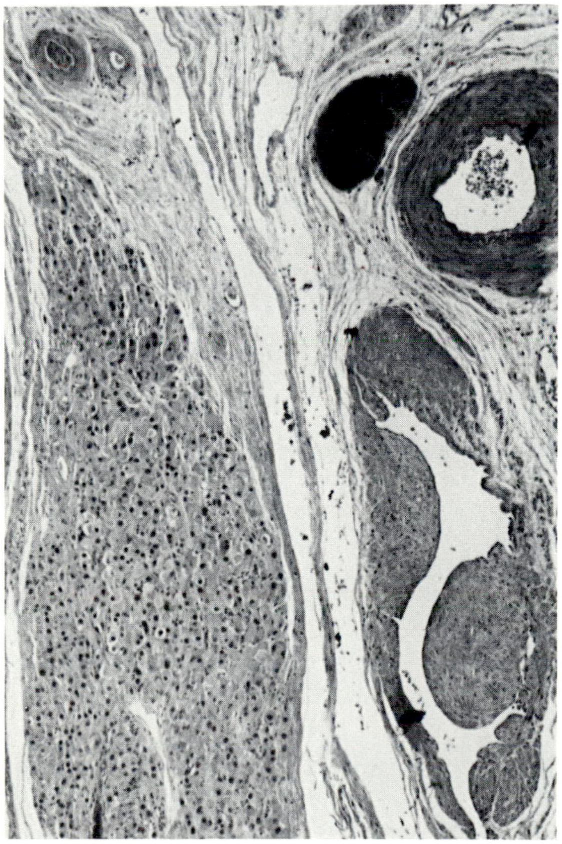

FIG. 15.34. Nest of hilus cells adjacent to large vessels within the ovarian hilus.

They are more numerous in the lateral and medial poles of the hilus and near the junction of the ovarian ligament with the ovary, typically lying close to the junction of the hilus with the medullary stroma.[104] The hilus cells characteristically ensheath nonmedullated nerves; less commonly they are intraneural, separating nerve fibers (Fig. 15.35). Hilus cells and their associated nerves frequently occur in close association with large hilar venous and lymphatic sinusoids and may form nodular protrusions into the lumina of these vessels.[104] Occasionally, hilus cells may surround the rete ovarii.[104] Nests may also be present within the medullary stroma near the hilus, probably representing extensions of the hilus into the medulla and, rarely, as an abnormal finding within the ovarian stroma away from the hilus, i.e., stromal Leydig cells (see Chapter 16, Nonneoplastic Lesions of Ovary). Ectopic hilus cells may also occur in the fallopian tube in a perisalpingeal or endosalpingeal location.[47]

Hilus cells nests are unencapsulated, typically lying within the loose connective tissue of the ovarian hilus, although rarely they may be surrounded by ovarian-type stroma within the hilus.[118] The cells measure 15–25 μm in diameter, are round to oval, less commonly elongate. They have abundant eosinophilic cytoplasm and a spherical vesicular nucleus that contains one or two prominent nucleoli (Fig. 15.36). Rare multinucleated cells may be seen. Those found incidentally in normal postmenopausal women do not exhibit mitotic activity, in contrast to hyperplastic or neoplastic hilus cells. Hilus cells contain crystals of Reinke, which are considered almost specific proteinaceous inclusions, although they are typically unevenly distributed, present in only a minority of cells, and frequently may not be demonstrable.[50] Crystals are homogenous, eosinophilic, nonrefractile, rod-shaped structures, 10–35 μm in length, with blunt, or occasionally tapered, ends (Fig. 15.36, inset). A search for crystals may be facilitated by the use of Masson's trichrome and iron hematoxylin methods, which stain them magenta and black, respectively. They typically lie in a parallel or stacked arrangement within a cell and often are surrounded by a clear halo. Occasionally, they appear to be extending through cell membranes or overlying them. Also present within hilus cells, often in greater numbers than crystals, are spherical or ellipsoidal hyaline structures that have an otherwise identical appearance to crystals and probably represent their precursors. The

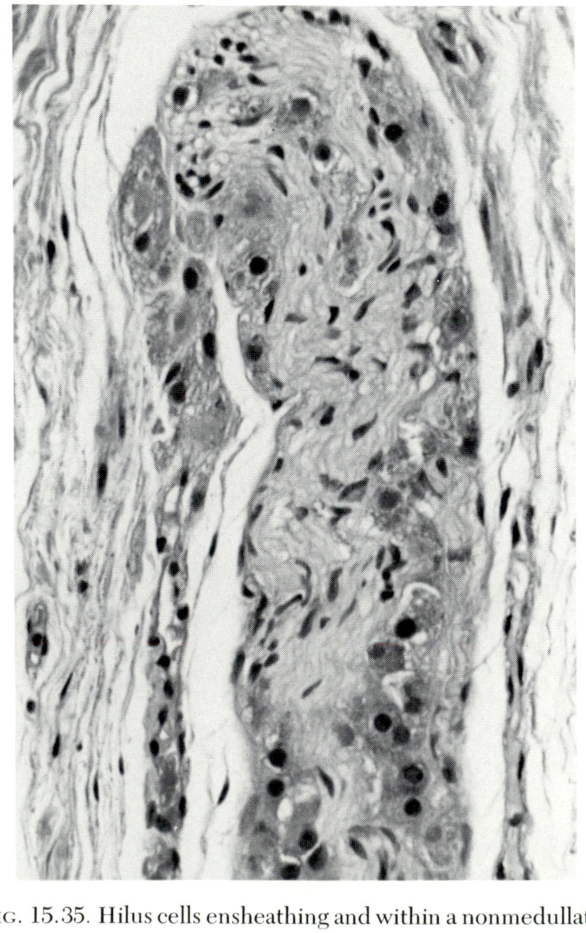

FIG. 15.35. Hilus cells ensheathing and within a nonmedullated nerve.

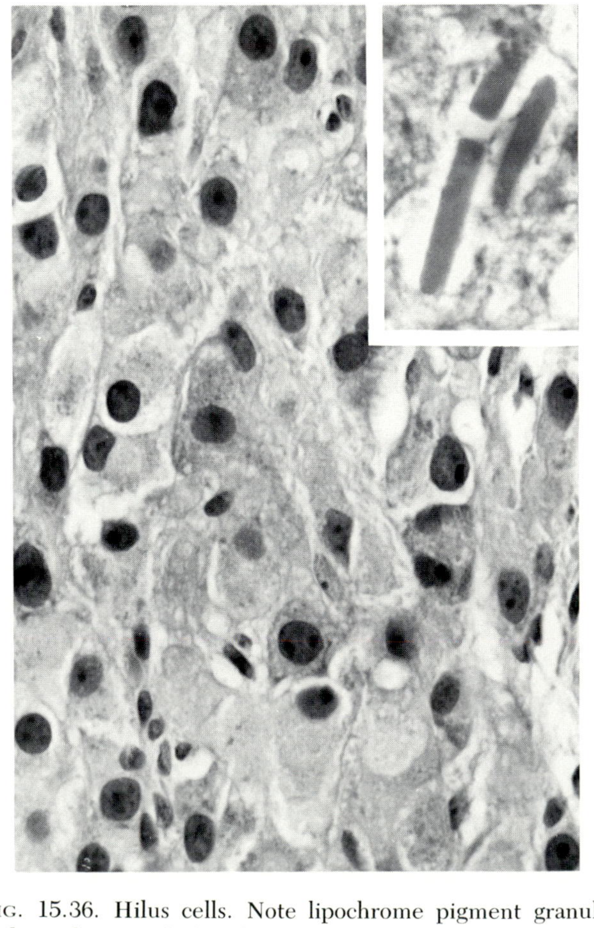

FIG. 15.36. Hilus cells. Note lipochrome pigment granules and Reinke crystals (*inset*).

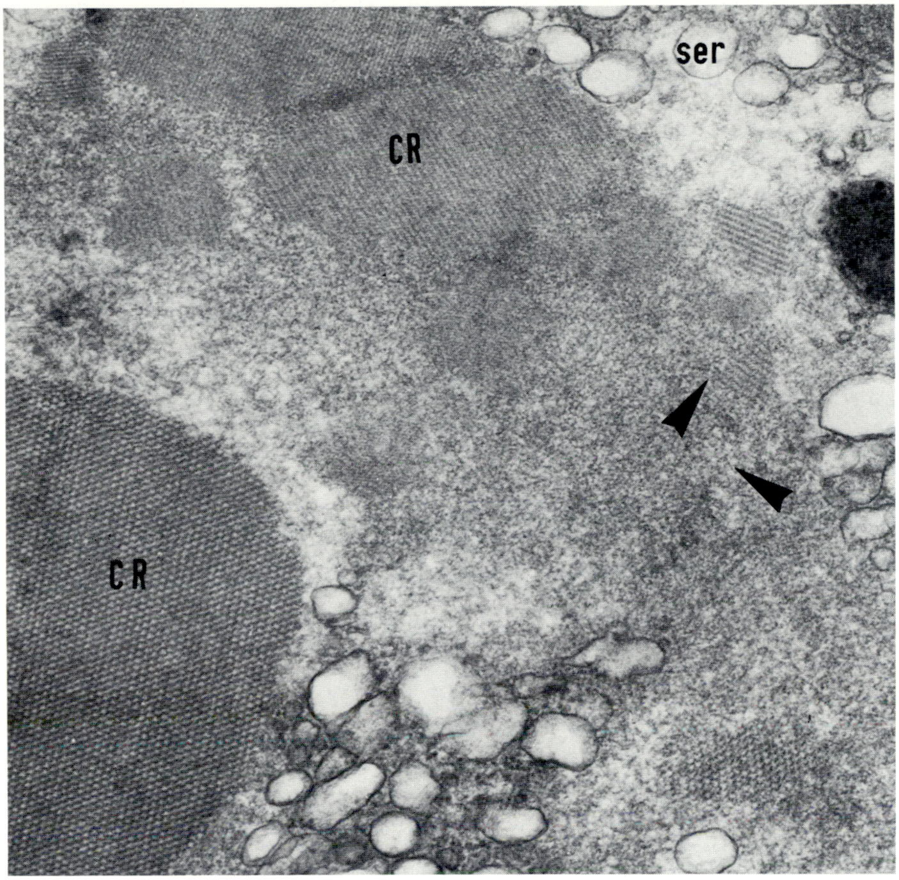

FIG. 15.37. Reinke crystals with hexagonal internal pattern (CR) formed by association of precrystalline units (*arrows*). ser, smooth endoplasmic reticulum. ×25,000. (From Laffargue et al., Ref. 59. Reprinted with permission from W. B. Saunders Co.)

cytoplasm may also contain perinuclear eosinophilic granules, peripheral lipid vacuoles, and golden-brown lipochrome pigment. Delicate collagen fibrils typically surround each cell.

Ultrastructure. Hilus cells have a steroidogenic ultrastructure consisting of prominent smooth ER and mitochondria with tubular cristae, as well as well developed Golgi complexes, large lysosomes, and osmiophilic lipid inclusions.[59] Reinke crystals have a truly crystalline appearance composed of dense parallel hexagonal microtubules with a mean thickness of 12 nm separated by clear spaces 15 nm wide, producing a "woven fabric" appearance (Fig. 15.37).[31,59] The crystals are typically oriented in many directions in the same cell. Crystals are formed by progressive association of precrystalline units each of which is composed of bundles of four or five parallel filaments (Fig. 15.38).[59] Typically found admixed with hilus cells are fibroblasts and cells intermediate in ultrastructural appearance between the two cell types.[59] Hilus cells and intermediate cells have intimate attachments to nerves in the form of simple membranous contacts, invaginations of axon terminals into hilus cells, or surface membrane thickenings resembling a true synapse (Fig. 15.39).[59] These findings suggest that hilus cells most likely originate from hilar fibroblasts, possibly under the inductive influence of hilar nerves.[59,101]

Hormone Synthesis. The light and electron microscopic morphology and enzyme content of hilus cells are those of steroid hormone-producing cells, although to what extent hilus cells contribute to the steroid hormone pool in normal females is unknown.[68,99,101] In vitro incubation studies indicate that the major steroid produced by ovarian hilus cells is androstenedione and that it is produced in amounts higher than that produced from ovarian stroma.[25] Lesser amounts of estradiol and progesterone are also produced in vitro. Steroid synthesis, particularly estradiol, is augmented by the addition of hCG.[25] Hilus cells are also responsive to exogenous and endogenous hCG stimulation in vivo, with an increase in cell size, mitotic activity, and in pregnancy, cell numbers.[105] Hy-

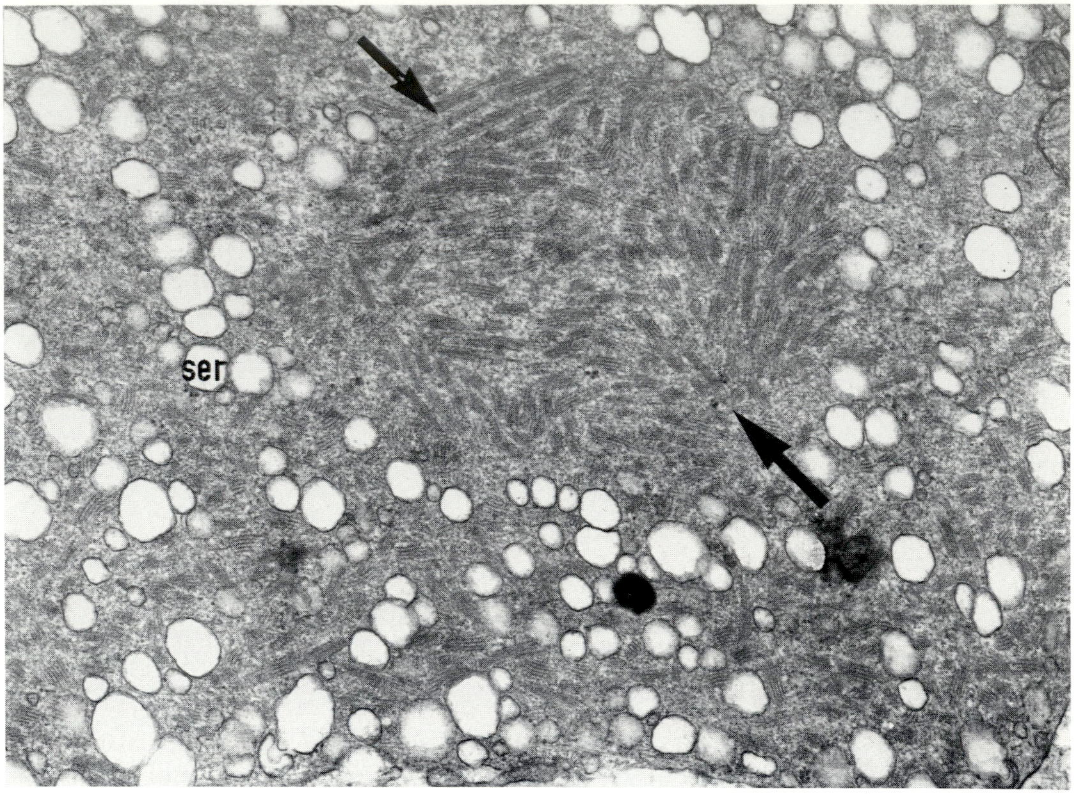

FIG. 15.38. Aggregation of cytoplasmic precystalline inclusions (*between arrows*). ser, smooth endoplasmic reticulum. ×15,700. (From Laffargue et al., Ref. 59. Reprinted with permission from W. B. Saunders Co.)

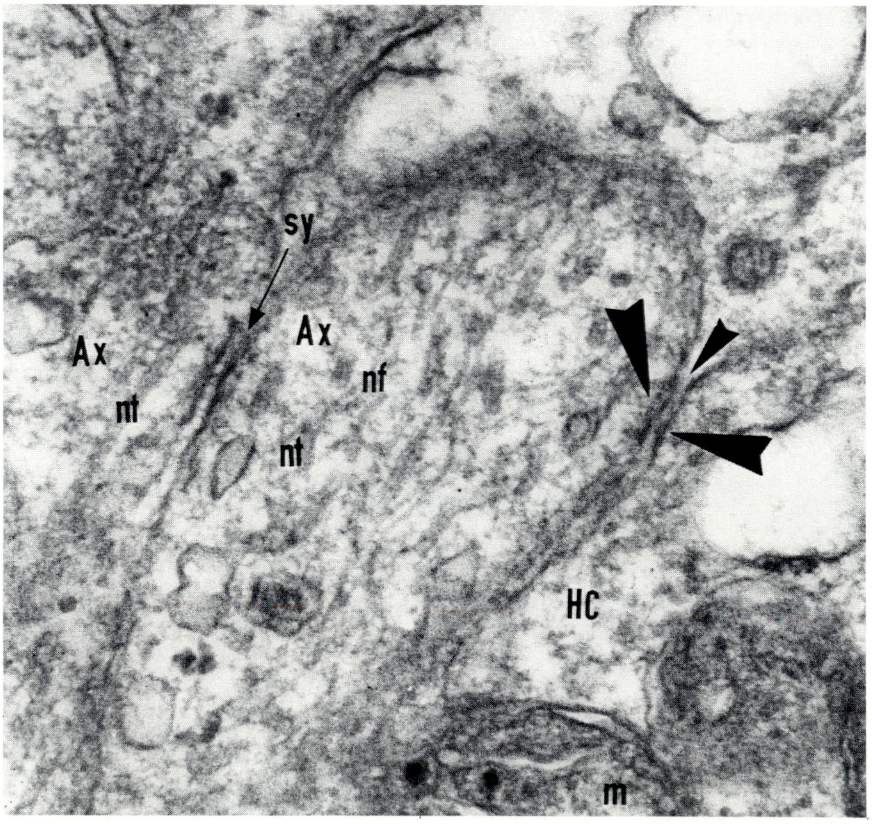

FIG. 15.39. Axon relationships with a hilus cell. Ax, axon terminal; HC, hilus cell; *large arrows*, synaptic membrane-like thickenings; *small arrow*, nonorientated filamentous material; nf, neurofilament; nt, neurotubules; sy, synapse between two axon terminals with parallel intersynaptic filaments; m, mitochondria. ×91,500. (From Laffargue et al., Ref. 59. Reprinted with permission from W. B. Saunders Co.)

perplastic and neoplastic lesions of hilus cells have been associated with virilization secondary to testosterone production by the proliferating cells.

Rete Ovarii

The rete ovarii, the ovarian analogue of the rete testis, is present in the hilus of all ovaries. It consists of a network of irregular clefts, tubules, cysts, and intraluminal papillae, lined by a flat to cuboidal epithelium (Fig. 15.40).[99] Solid cords of similar cells may also be seen. Parts of the rete have a continuous, sharply defined basement membrane.[60] Characteristically, the rete is surrounded by a cuff of spindle-cell stroma morphologically similar to, but discontinuous from, the ovarian stroma. The rete is in juxtaposition to and may communicate with mesonephric tubules within the mesovarium.[33] Small, tumor-like proliferations of the rete have been referred to as *rete adenomas*.[33] Occasional examples of larger tumors (*female adnexal tumor of probable wolffian duct origin*) within the ovary (and broad ligament) may have arisen from the rete or adjacent mesonephric remnants (see Chapter 21, Nonspecific Ovarian Tumors).[56,116] The fine structure of the rete ovarii has not been reported.[12]

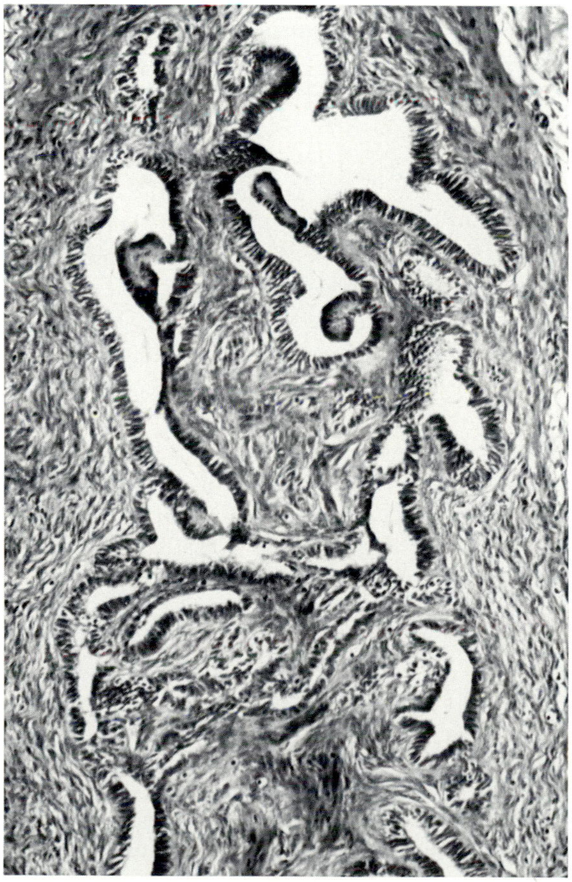

FIG. 15.40. Rete ovarii.

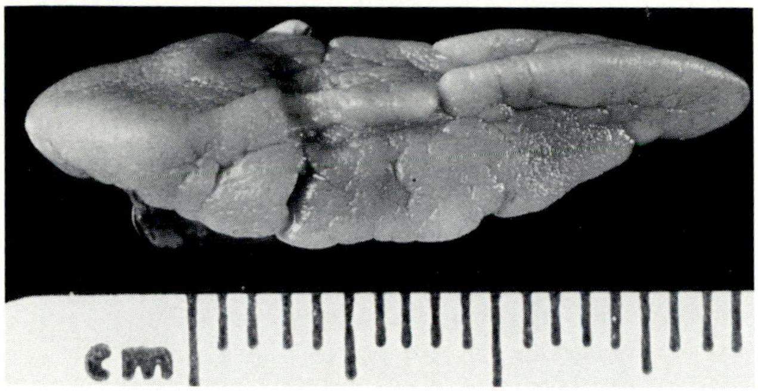

FIG. 15.41. Ovary of newborn.

Ovary in Childhood

Gross Appearance. The ovary in the newborn is a tan, elongated, and flattened structure that lies above the true pelvis. It sometimes has a lobulated appearance with irregular edges (Fig. 15.41).[92] It has approximate dimensions of 1.3 cm by 0.5 cm by 0.3 cm, and weighs less than 0.3 g.[92,99,107] Throughout infancy and childhood, the ovary enlarges, increases in weight 30-fold, and changes in shape, so that by the time of puberty it has reached the size, weight, and shape of the adult ovary (p. 438), and lies within the true pelvis.[92,99,107] Inspection of the external and cut surfaces, particularly during the first few months of life and at puberty, may reveal prominent cystic follicles similar to those seen in polycystic ovary disease (Fig. 15.42).

Histology. At the time of birth, the ovarian cortex is filled with large numbers of closely packed primordial follicles (Figs. 15.43 and 15.44). Some primordial follicles contain two (or rarely a greater number) of oocytes.[107] Follicular maturation and atresia occur prenatally and throughout childhood, becoming more prominent after the age of 6 years.[21,46,75,82,89,107] Deceleration or arrest of folliculogenesis may occur in prepubertal patients with chronic illnesses or Down's syndrome and in those exposed to cytotoxic drugs or radiation, accounting for the conclusion reached in some studies that the normal prepubertal ovary is quiescent.[89] Follicular maturation is

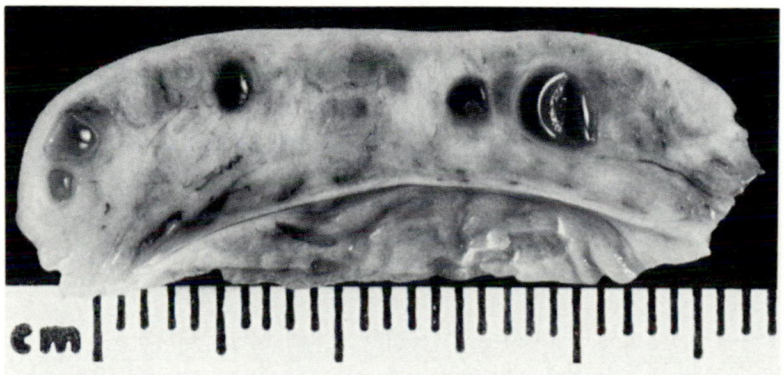

FIG. 15.42. Ovary of 14-year-old girl (*cut surface*). Note multiple cystic follicles within cortex.

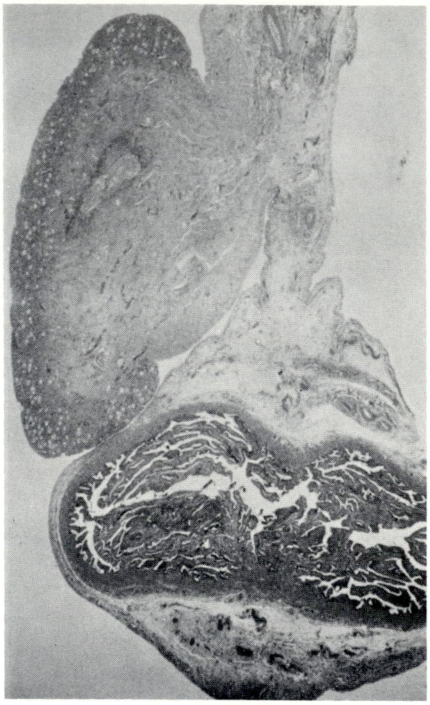

FIG. 15.43. Ovary and fallopian tube of newborn in cross-section. Ovarian cortex is packed with primordial follicles.

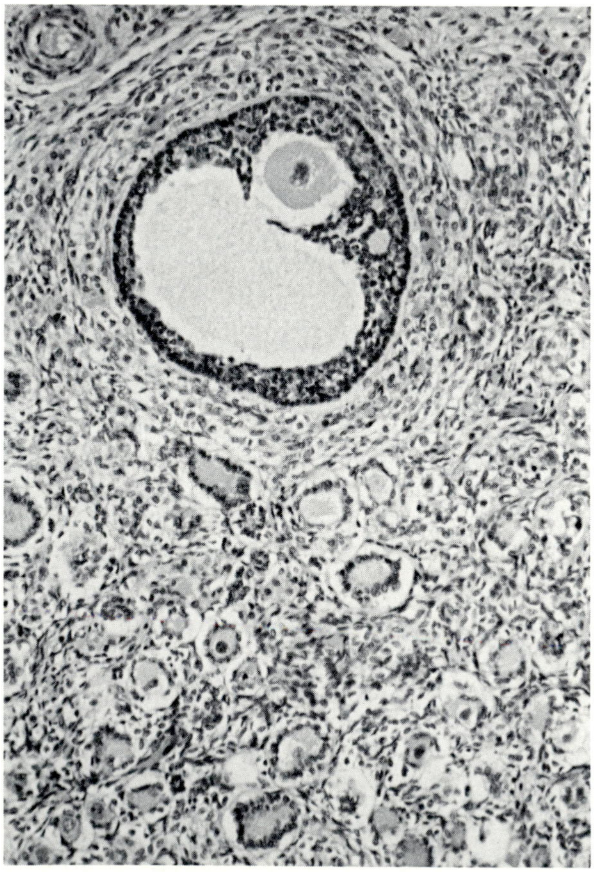

FIG. 15.44. Ovary of newborn. Note closely packed primordial follicles and antral follicle.

identical to that occurring in premenopausal adult subjects, except that it does not proceed beyond antral follicles measuring 5 mm in diameter (Fig. 15.44). Because ovulation does not occur, corpora lutea and corpora albicantia are absent in the prepubertal ovary. All maturing follicles, therefore, undergo atresia in a manner identical to that occurring in adults. Prominent luteinization of the theca interna layer may also be seen in this age group.[57] By puberty, the atretic process has depleted over 90% of the approximately 400,000 primordial follicles that were present at birth. Simultaneous with this depletion, the progressive increase in ovarian size, due primarily to an increase in the amount of ovarian stroma, produces the more sparse distribution of primordial follicles seen in the pubertal and young adult subject.

Adolescent prepubertal ovaries, in addition to prominent cystic follicles with luteinization of the theca interna, may exhibit focal fibrosis of the superficial cortex, further enhancing their resemblance to the ovaries of polycystic ovary disease.[75] This sclerocystic appearance is consistent with the conclusion that such changes are not specific for polycystic ovary disease but are merely a reflection of chronic anovulation (see Chapter 16, Nonneoplastic Lesions of Ovary). As previously noted (p. 459), hilus cells are demonstrable during fetal life but are not seen during infancy and childhood, reappearing at puberty.

Hormone Synthesis. Levels of gonadotropins and sex steroids, largely of placental origin, decline rapidly during the first few days of life. As a result, a rise in FSH and LH levels, paralleled by an elevation in follicle-derived estradiol, begins on the fifth day.[61] All three hormones reach peak levels at 3–4 months of age and then decline to low levels by the age of 2 years due to the increasing sensitivity of the hypothalamic-pituitary unit to negative feedback by estradiol. Low levels of gonadotropins are maintained until 6–8 years of age but are sufficient to maintain the growing ovary and stimulate continuous follicular development and atresia.[61,88] Only minimal quantities of estradiol are produced during this period. The onset of adrenal androgen secretion (adrenarche) at the age of 6 or 7 usually precedes and may promote activation of the hypothalamic gonadostat.[61] As a result, there is a reduction in hypothalamic–pituitary sensitivity to negative feedback by estrogen, and FSH and LH levels progressively increase until menarche. They stimulate the increased production of follicular estrogens that are responsible for the secondary sexual characteristics of puberty.

Ovary in Menopause

Gross Appearance. After the menopause, the ovaries typically shrink to a size approximately one-half of that seen in the reproductive era. Their size varies consider-

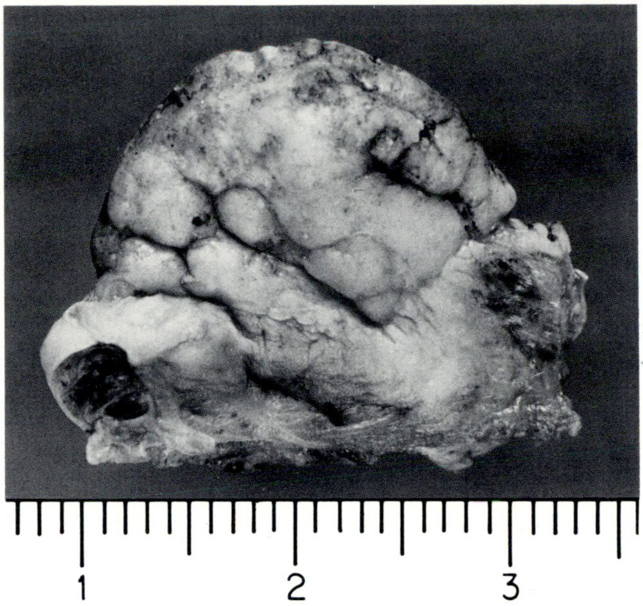

FIG. 15.45. Ovary of postmenopausal woman. Note the markedly irregular cortical surface.

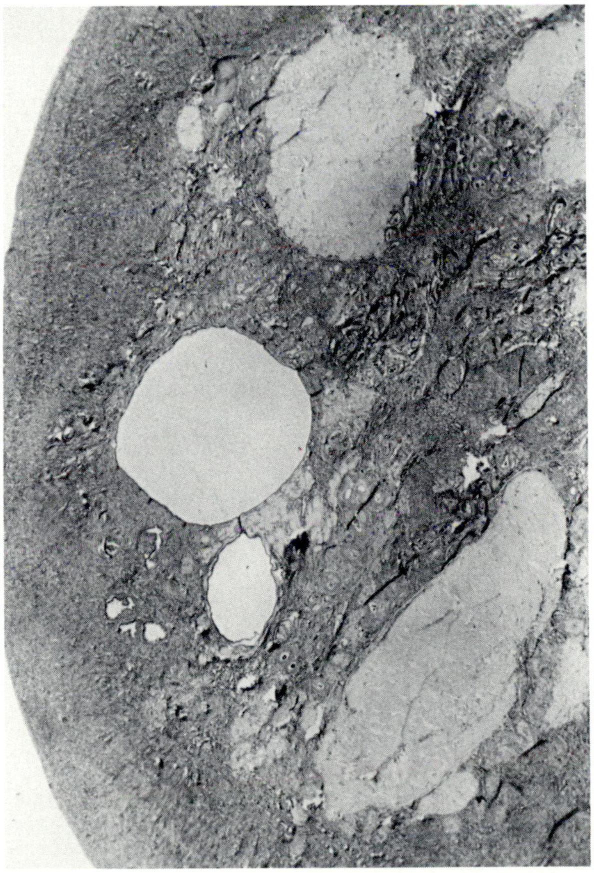

FIG. 15.46. Ovary of postmenopausal woman. Note the thin cortex devoid of follicular structures. Two inclusion cysts are present at the corticomedullary junction. Multiple corpora albicantia occupy the medulla.

ably, however, depending on their content of ovarian stromal cells and the number of unresorbed corpora albicantia.[99] Most postmenopausal ovaries have a shrunken, gyriform, external appearance (Fig. 15.45) whereas some are more smooth and uniform.[99] They have a firm consistency and a predominantly solid, pale cut surface, although occasional inclusion cysts may be discernible within the cortex. Corpora albicantia are typically visible within the medulla.

Histology. The characteristic feature of the postmenopausal ovary is the absence of primordial follicles and, consequently, an absence of maturing follicles, corpora lutea, and atretic follicles. Occasional primordial follicles, however, may persist for several years after cessation of menses, accounting for sporadic ovulation and postmenopausal bleeding in some women. After this period, the only follicle derived structures typically encountered are occasional unresorbed corpora fibrosa and corpora albicantia, the latter typically occupying the medulla (Fig. 15.46).

The ovarian stroma in postmenopausal women exhibits a wide spectrum of appearances.[11] At one extreme there is stromal atrophy manifested by a thin cortex and minimal amounts of medullary stroma (Fig. 15.46). In these subjects, the stroma becomes less cellular due to an increase in intercellular collagen, and its cells exhibit smaller, darker, more inactive appearing nuclei (Fig. 15.47). At the other extreme, there is marked stromal proliferation warranting the designation "stromal hyperplasia" to connote a pathological process (see Chapter 16, Nonneoplastic Lesions of Ovary). Most postmenopausal subjects, however, exhibit varying degrees of nodular or diffuse proliferation of cortical and medullary stromal cells that lie between these two extremes. The normal appearance is therefore difficult if not impossible to define but is probably represented by an indeterminate 80–90% in the middle of this spectrum. Ovarian stromal changes frequently present in postmenopausal women to the extent that they could be considered normal aging phenomena. These include occasional luteinized stromal cells (see p. 442), irregular areas of dense cortical stromal fibrosis,[11] cortical granulomas, spherical, cloud-like, hyaline scars, and surface papillary stromal proliferations (see Chapter 16). Less commonly, focal decidual transformation of the ovarian stroma may be seen in otherwise normal ovaries from postmenopausal subjects (see Chapter 16).

Other common changes within the ovaries of postmenopausal patients include surface epithelial inclusion cysts within the cortex and mild degrees of hilus cell hyperplasia (see Chapter 16). After the menopause, the medullary blood vessels exhibit a greater tortuosity, appearing more numerous and closely packed, and should not be mistaken for a hemangioma. Many of the same

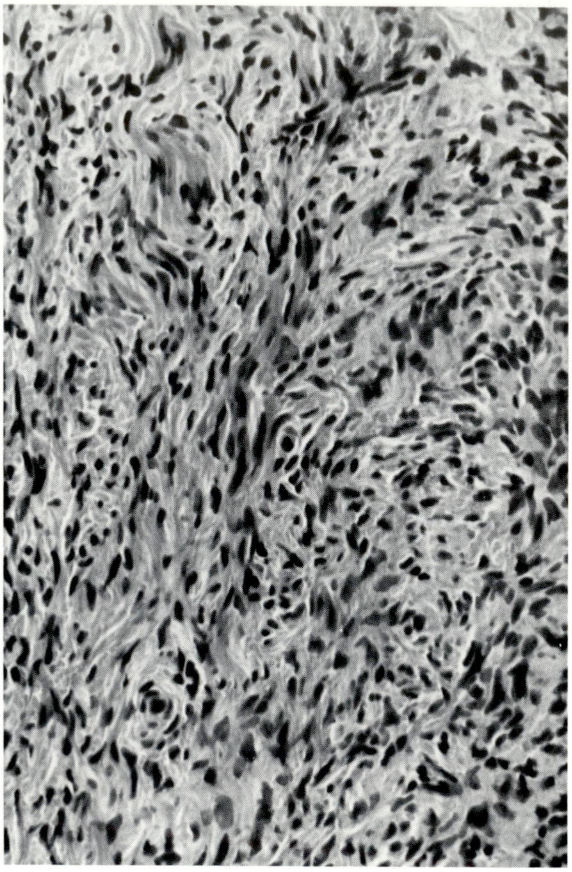

Fig. 15.47. Ovarian stroma in postmenopausal woman. Note the spindle-shaped cells with thin, darkly staining nuclei and abundant intercellular collagen.

vessels and smaller vessels within the cortex have thickened walls and narrowed lumina due to a medial deposition of a hyaline, amyloid-like material.

Hormone Synthesis. The menopause is associated with cessation of follicular activity, including the follicular synthesis of estradiol and other hormones, prompting an increase in secretion of FSH and LH. These hormonal changes are usually associated with the clinical manifestations of estrogen withdrawal. Both in vitro and in vivo studies, however, indicate that the ovarian stroma retains its steroidogenic potential in postmenopausal subjects, continuing to secrete moderate amounts of testosterone and smaller amounts of androstenedione.* In this age group, circulating levels of androstenedione decline by 40–60%, reflecting diminished ovarian secretion. As a result, 80% of the circulating levels of this hormone after the menopause is of adrenal origin.[15,54,65] In contrast, direct ovarian secretion of testosterone is greater in postmenopausal than in premenopausal women, although the mean circulating testosterone levels in premenopausal and postmenopausal women are similar. Androgen production by the ovarian stroma in postmenopausal women can be enhanced by hCG stimulation,[39] consistent with the presence of hCG and LH receptors within the stroma.[93] It is, therefore, likely that continued ovarian androgen production in these women is a result of stimulation by the high circulating levels of endogenous FSH and LH.[15,93]

Despite a cessation of follicular synthesis of estradiol in postmenopausal women, small amounts of this hormone are present in the circulation, probably derived from the adrenal glands, by peripheral conversion of estrone, and from the ovarian stroma itself.[15,65,95] Estrone levels also decrease in the postmenopausal woman, but to a much lesser extent than estradiol, so that estrone becomes the major circulating estrogen.[40,64] Most of the estrone is derived from the peripheral aromatization of androstenedione, which occurs in fat, muscle, liver, kidney, brain, and the adrenals.[15] The daily production rate of estrone by aromatization in postmenopausal women is twice that of premenopausal women and is higher in obese subjects. In some postmenopausal patients, sufficient estrogen may be elaborated by this mechanism to prevent the clinical manifestations of estrogen withdrawal and to play a role in the genesis of endometrial carcinoma.[15] The variations that exist in the ovarian steroid hormone output from one postmenopausal woman to another may correspond to similar variations in the morphologic appearance of the stroma in this age group, although no correlative functional and structural studies have been performed.

Acknowledgement. The author is very grateful to Dr. Robert E. Scully for reviewing parts of the manuscript and offering invaluable constructive criticism.

* References 15, 26, 40, 53, 54, 65, 67, 91, 108.

References

1. Adams EC, Hertig AT (1969) Studies on the human corpus luteum. I. Observations on the ultrastructure of development and regression of the luteal cells during the menstrual cycle. J Cell Biol 41: 696
2. Adams EC, Hertig AT (1969) Studies on the human corpus luteum. II. Observations on the ultrastructure of luteal cells during pregnancy. J Cell Biol 41: 716
3. Baca M, Zamboni L (1967) The fine structure of the human follicular oocyte. J Ultrastruct Res 19: 354
4. Balboni GC (1983) Structural changes: Ovulation and luteal phase. In: The Ovary. Serra GB (ed.) New York, Raven Press
5. Bassis ML (1956) Pseudodeciduosis. Am J Obstet Gynecol 72: 1029
6. Bersch W, Alexy E, Heuser HP, Staemmler HJ (1973) Ectopic decidua formation in the ovary (so-called deciduoma). Virchows Arch [Pathol Anat] 360: 173

7. Blaustein A (1984) Peritoneal mesothelium and ovarian surface epithelial cells—Shared characteristics. Int J Gynecol Pathol 3: 361
8. Blaustein A, Lee H (1979) Surface cells of the ovary and pelvic peritoneum: A histochemical and ultrastructural comparison. Gynecol Oncol 8: 34
9. Bloom W, Fawcett DW (1975) A Textbook of Histology, 10th ed. Philadelphia, Saunders
10. Bomsel-Helmreich O, Gougeon A, Thebault A, Saltarelli D, Milgrom E, Frydman R, Papiernik E (1979) Healthy and atretic human follicles in the preovulatory phase: Differences in evolution of follicular morphology and steroid content of follicular fluid. J Clin Endocrinol Metab 48: 686
11. Boss, JH, Scully RE, Wegner KH, Cohen RB (1965) Structural variations in the adult ovary—Clinical significance. Obstet Gynecol 25: 747
12. Bransilver BR, Ferenczy A, Richart RM (1974) Brenner tumors and Walthard cell nests. Arch Pathol Lab Med 98: 76
13. Centola GM (1983) Structural changes: Follicular development and hormonal requirements. In: The Ovary. Serra GB (ed). New York, Raven Press
14. Centola GM (1983) Structural changes: Atresia. In: The Ovary. Serra GB (ed). New York, Raven Press
15. Chang RJ, Judd HL (1981) The ovary after menopause. Clin Obstet Gynaecol 24: 181
16. Charpin C, Bhan AK, Zurawski VR Jr, Scully RE (1982) Carcinoembryonic antigen (CEA) and carbohydrate determinant 19–9 (CA 19–9) localization in 121 primary and metastatic ovarian tumors: An immunohistochemical study with the use of monoclonal antibodies. Int J Gynecol Pathol 1: 231
17. Cordon-Cardo C, Mattes MJ, Melamed MR, Lewis JL Jr, Old LJ, Lloyd KO (1985) Immunopathologic analysis of a panel of mouse monoclonal antibodies reacting with human ovarian carcinomas and other human tumors. Int J Gynecol Pathol 4: 121–130
18. Corner GW Jr (1956) The histological dating of the human corpus luteum of menstruation. Am J Anat 98: 377–401
19. Crisp TM, Dessouky DA, Denys FR (1970) The fine structure of the human corpus luteum of early pregnancy and during the progestational phase of the menstrual cycle. Am J Anat 127: 37–70
20. Croxatto, H, Ortiz M, Croxatto HB (1980) Correlation between histologic dating of human corpus luteum and the luteinizing hormone peak–biopsy interval. Am J Obstet Gynecol 136: 667–670
21. Curtis EM (1962) Normal ovarian histology in infancy and childhood. Obstet Gynecol 19: 444–454
22. Czernobilsky B, Moll R, Franke WW, Dallenbach-Hellweg G, Hohlweg-Majert P (1984) Intermediate filaments of normal and neoplastic tissues of the female genital tract with emphasis on problems of differential tumor diagnosis. Pathol Res Pract 179: 31–37
23. Deane HW, Lobel BL, Romney SL (1962) Enzymic histochemistry of normal human ovaries of the menstrual cycle, pregnancy, and the early puerperium. Am J Obstet Gynecol 83: 281–294
24. Dekel N, David MP, Yedwab GA, Kraicer PF (1977) Follicular development during late pregnancy. Int J Fertil 22: 24–29
25. Dennefors BL, Janson PO, Hamberger L, Knutsson F (1982) Hilus cells from human postmenopausal ovaries: Gonadotrophin sensitivity, steroid and cyclic AMP production. Acta Obstet Gynecol Scand 61: 413–416
26. Dennefors BL, Janson PO, Knutsson F, Hamberger L (1980) Steroid production and responsiveness to gonadotropin in isolated stromal tissue of human postmenopausal ovaries. Am J Obstet Gynecol 136: 997–1002
27. Dyer CA, Erickson GF (1985) Norepinephrine amplifies human chorionic gonadotropin-stimulated androgen biosynthesis by ovarian theca–interstitial cells. Endocrinology 116: 1645–1652
28. Eichner E, Bove ER (1954) In vivo studies on the lymphatic drainage of the human ovary. Obstet Gynecol 3: 287–297
29. Erickson GF (1978) Normal ovarian function. Clin Obstet Gynecol 21: 31–52
30. Feinberg R, Cohen RB (1965) A comparative histochemical study of the ovarian stromal lipid band, stromal theca cell, and normal ovarian follicular apparatus. Am J Obstet Gynecol 92: 958–969
31. Ferenczy A, Richart RM (1974) Female Reproductive Systems: Dynamics of Scan and Transmission Electron Microscopy. New York, Wiley
32. Futterweit W (1985) In: Polycystic Ovarian Disease. Clinical Perspectives in Obstetrics and Gynecology. Buchsbaum HJ (ed) New York, Springer-Verlag.
33. Gardner GH, Greene RR, Peckham B (1957) Tumors of the broad ligament. Am J Obstet Gynecol 73: 536–555
34. Gillim SW, Christensen AK, McLennan CE (1969) Fine structure of the human menstrual corpus luteum at its stage of maximum secretory activity. Am J Anat 126: 409–428
35. Gougeon A (1981) Frequent occurrence of multiovular follicles and multinuclear oocytes in the adult human ovary. Fertil Steril 35: 417–422
36. Govan ADT (1970) Ovarian follicular activity in late pregnancy. J Endocrinol 48: 235–241
37. Green JA, Maqueo M (1965) Ultrastructure of the human ovary. I. The luteal cell during the menstrual cycle. Am J Obstet Gynecol 92: 946–957
38. Green JA, Garcilazo JA, Maqueo M (1967) Ultrastructure of the human ovary. II. The luteal cell at term. Am J Obstet Gynecol 99: 855–863
39. Greenblatt RB, Colle ML, Mahesh VB (1976) Ovarian and adrenal steroid production in the postmenopausal woman. Obstet Gynecol 47: 383–387
40. Grodin JM, Siiteri PK, MacDonald PC (1973) Source of estrogen production in postmenopausal women. J Clin Endocrinol Metab 36: 207–214
41. Herr JC, Heidger PM Jr, Scott Jr, Anderson JW, Curet LB, Mossman HW (1978) Decidual cells in the human ovary at term. I. Incidence, gross anatomy and ultrastructural features of merocrine secretion. Am J Anat 152:7–28
42. Hertig AT (1964) Gestational hyperplasia of endometrium. A morphologic correlation of ova, endometrium, and cor-

pora lutea during early pregnancy. Lab Invest 13: 1153–1191
43. Hertig AT (1968) The primary human oocyte: Some observations on the fine structure of Balbiani's vitelline body and the origin of the annulate lamellae. Am J Anat 122: 107–138
44. Hertig AT, Adams EC (1967) Studies on the human oocyte and its follicle. I. Ultrastructural and histochemical observations on the primordial follicle stage. J Cell Biol 34: 647–675
45. Hidvegi D, Cibils LA, Sorensen K, Hidvegi I (1982) Ultrastructural and histochemical observations of neuroendorcine granules in nonneoplastic ovaries. Am J Obstet Gynecol 143: 590–594
46. Himelstein-Braw R, Byskov AG, Peters H, Faber M (1976) Follicular atresia in the infant human ovary. J Reprod Fert 46: 55–59
47. Honore LH, O'Hara KE (1979) Ovarian hilus cell heterotopia. Obstet Gynecol 53: 461–464
48. Israel SL, Rubenstone A, Meranze DR (1954) The ovary at term. I. Decidua-like reaction and surface cell proliferation. Obstet Gyncol 3: 399–407
49. Jacobowitz D, Wallach EE (1967) Histochemical and chemical studies of the autonomic innervation of the ovary. Endocrinology 81: 1132–1139
50. Janko AB, Sandberg EC (1970) Histochemical evidence for the protein nature of the Reinke crystalloid. Obstet Gynecol 35: 493–503
51. Joel RV, Foraker AG (1960) Fate of the corpus albicans: A morphologic approach. Am J Obstet Gynecol 80: 314–316
52. Jones GES, Goldberg B, Woodruff JD (1968) Histochemistry as a guide for interpretation of cell function. Am J Obstet Gynecol 100: 76–83
53. Judd HL, Lucas WE, Yen SSC (1974) Effect of oophorectomy on circulating testosterone and androstenedione levels in patients with endometrial carcinoma. Am J Obstet Gynecol 118: 793–798
54. Judd HL, Judd GE, Lucas WE, Yen SSC (1974) Endocrine function of the postmenopausal ovary: Concentration of androgens and estrogens in ovarian and peripheral vein blood. J Clin Endocrinol Metab 39: 1020–1024
55. Kabawat SE, Bast RC Jr, Bhan AK, Welch WR, Knapp RC, Colvin RB (1983) Tissue distribution of coelomic–epithelium-related antigen recognized by the monoclonal antibody OC125. Int J Gynecol Pathol 2: 275–285
56. Kariminejad MH, Scully RE (1973) Female adnexal tumor of probable wolffian origin. A distinctive pathologic entity. Cancer 31: 671–677
57. Kraus FT, Neubecker RD (1962) Luteinization of the ovarian theca in infants and children. Am J Clin Pathol 37: 389–397
58. Laffargue P, Adechy-Benkoel L, Valette C (1968) Ultrastructure du stroma ovarien. Ann Anat Pathol 13: 381–401
59. Laffargue P, Benkoel L, Laffargue F, Casanova P, Chamlian A (1978) Ultrastructural and enzyme histochemical study of ovarian hilar cells in women and their relationships with sympathetic nerves. Hum Pathol 9: 649–659
60. Lamb EJ, Fucilla I, Greene RR (1960) Basement membranes in the female genital tract. Am J Obstet Gynecol 79: 79–85
61. Lee PA (1983) Ovarian function from conception to puberty: Physiology and disorders. In: The Ovary. Serra GB (ed). New York, Raven Press
62. LeMaire WJ, Rice BF, Savard K (1968) Steroid hormone formation in the human ovary: V. Synthesis of progesterone in vitro in corpora lutea during the reproductive cycle. J Clin Endocrinol Metab 28: 1249–1256
63. LeMaire WJ, Conly PW, Moffett A, Spellacy WN, Cleveland WW, Savard K (1971) Function of the human corpus luteum during the puerperium: Its maintenance by exogenous human chorionic gonadotropin. Am J Obstet Gynecol 110: 612–618
64. Longcope C (1971) Metabolic clearance and blood production rates of estrogens in postmenopausal women. Am J Obstet Gynecol 111: 778–781
65. Longcope C, Hunter R, Franz C (1980) Steroid secretion by the postmenopausal ovary. Am J Obstet Gynecol 138: 564–568
66. Maqueo M, Goldzieher JW (1966) Hormone-induced alterations of ovarian morphology. Fertil Steril 17: 676–683
67. Mattingly RF, Huang WY (1969) Steroidogenesis of the menopause and postmenopausal ovary. Am J Obstet Gynecol 103: 679
68. McKay DG, Pinkerton JHM, Hertig AT, Danziger S (1961) The adult human ovary: A histochemical study. Obstet Gynecol 18: 13–39
69. McNatty KP (1978) Follicular determinants of corpus luteum function in the human ovary. In: Ovarian Follicular and Corpus Luteum Function. Advances in Experimental Medicine and Biology. Channing CP, Marsh JM, Sadler WA (eds). New York, Plenum Press, Vol. 112
70. McNatty KP (1978) Cyclic changes in antral fluid hormone concentrations in humans. Clin Endocrinol Metab 7: 577–600
71. McNatty KP, Makris A, DeGrazia C, Osathanondh R, Ryan KJ (1979) The production of progesterone, androgens, and estrogens by granulosa cells, thecal tissue, and stromal tissue from human ovaries in vitro. J Clin Endocrinol Metab 49: 687–699
72. McNatty KP, Makris A, DeGrazia C, Osathanondh R, Ryan KJ (1979) The production of progesterone, androgens, and estrogens by human granulosa cells in vitro and in vivo. J Steroid Biochem 11: 775–799
73. McNatty KP, Smith DM, Makris A, Osathanondh R, Ryan KJ (1979) The microenvironment of the human antral follicle: Interrelationships among the steroid levels in antral fluid, the population of granulosa cells, and the status of the oocyte in vivo and in vitro. J Clin Endocrinol Metab 49: 851–860
74. McNatty KP, Smith DM, Makris A, DeGrazia C, Tulchinsky D, Osathanondh R, Schiff I, Ryan KJ (1980) The intraovarian sites of androgen and estrogen formation in women with normal and hyperandrogenic ovaries as judged by in vitro experiments. J Clin Endocrinol Metab 50: 755–763
75. Merrill JA (1963) The morphology of the prepubertal

ovary: Relationship to the polycystic ovary syndrome. South Med J 56: 225–231

76. Mestwardt W, Muller O, Brandau H (1978) Structural analysis of granulosa cells from human ovaries in correlation with function. In: Ovarian Follicular and Corpus Luteum Function. Advances in Experimental Medicine and Biology. Channing CP. Marsh JM, Sadler WA (eds). New York, Plenum Press, Vol. 112
77. Miettinen M, Lehto V, Virtanen I (1983) Expression of intermediate filaments in normal ovaries and ovarian epithelial, sex cord–stromal, and germinal tumors. Int J Gynecol Pathol 2: 64–71
78. Mikhail G, Allen WM (1967) Ovarian function in human pregnancy. Am J Obstet Gynecol 99: 308–312
79. Mohsin S (1979) The sympathetic innervation of the mammalian ovary. A review of pharmacological and histochemical studies. Clin Exp Pharmacol Physiol 6: 335–354
80. Nelson WW, Greene RR (1953) The human ovary in pregnancy. Int Abstr Surg 97: 1–23
81. Nelson WW, Greene RR (1958) Some observations on the histology of the human ovary during pregnancy. Am J Obstet Gynecol 76: 66–89
82. Nicosia SV (1983) Morphological changes of the human ovary throughout life. In: The Ovary. Serra GB (ed). New York, Raven Press
83. Okamura H, Virutamasen P, Wright KH, Wallach EE (1972) Ovarian smooth muscle in the human being, rabbit, and cat. Am J Obstet Gynecol 112: 183–191
84. Owman C, Rosengren E, Sjoberg N (1967) Adrenergic innervation of the human female reprodutive organs: A histochemical and chemical investigation. Obstet Gynecol 30: 763–773
85. Papadaki L, Beilby JOW (1973) The fine structure of the surface epithelium of the human ovary. J Cell Sci 8: 445–465
86. Pauerstein CJ, Eddy CA, Croxatto JD, Hess R, Siler-Khodr TM, Croxatto HB (1978) Temporal relationships of estrogen, progesterone, and luteinizing hormone levels to ovulation in women and infrahuman primates. Am J Obstet Gynecol 130: 876–886
87. Pedersen PH, Larsen JF (1968) The ultrastructure of the human granulosa lutein cell of the first trimester of gestation. Acta Endocrinol 58: 481–496
88. Pennington GW (1974) The reproductive endocrinology of childhood and adolescence. Clin Obstet Gynaecol 1: 509–531
89. Peters H, Himelstein-Braw R, Faber M (1976) The normal development of the ovary in childhood. Acta Endocrinol 82: 617–630
90. Plentl AA, Friedman EA (1971) Lymphatic System of the female genitalia. Philadelphia, Saunders
91. Plotz EJ, Wiener M, Stein AA, Hahn BD (1967) Enzymatic activities related to steroidogenesis in postmenopausal ovaries of patients with and without endometrial carcinoma. Am J Obstet Gynecol 99: 182–197
92. Pryse-Davies J (1974) The development, structure and function of the female pelvic organs in childhood. Clin Obstet Gynaecol 1: 483–508
93. Rao CV (1982) Receptors for gonadotropins in human ovaries. Recent Advances in Fertility Research, Part A: Developments in Reproductive Endocrinology, pp 123–135
94. Reagan JW (1950) Ceroid pigment in the human ovary. Am J Obstet Gynecol 59: 433–436
95. Reed MJ, Beranek PA, Ghilchik MW, James VHT (1985) Conversion of estrone to estradiol and estradiol to estrone in postmenopausal women. Obstet Gynecol 66: 361–365
96. Reeves G (1971) Specific stroma in the cortex and medulla of the ovary. Cell types and vascular supply in relation to follicular apparatus and ovulation. Obstet Gynecol 37: 832–844
97. Rice BF, Savard K (1966) Steroid hormone formation in the human ovary: IV. Ovarian stromal compartment; formation of radioactive steroids from acetate-1-^{14}C and action of gonadotropins. J Clin Endocrinol 26: 593–609
98. Rice BF, Hammerstein J, Savard K (1964) Steroid hormone formation in the human ovary: II. Action of gonadotropins in vitro in the corpus luteum. J Clin Endocrinol 24: 606–615
99. Scully RE (1979) Tumors of the ovary and maldeveloped gonads. In: Atlas of Tumor Pathology, Second Series, Fascicle 16. Washington, D.C., Armed Forces Institute of Pathology
100. Scully RE (1981) Smooth-muscle differentiation in genital tract disorders (Editorial). Arch Pathol Lab Med 105: 505–507
101. Scully RE, Cohen RB (1964) Oxidative-enzyme activity in normal and pathologic human ovaries. Obstet Gynecol 24: 667–681
102. Stangel JJ, Richart RM, Okagaki T, Cottral G (1970) Nuclear DNA content of luteinized cells of the human ovary. Am J Obstet Gynecol 108: 543–549
103. Starup J, Visfeldt J (1974) Ovarian morphology in early and late human pregnancy. Acta Obstet Gynecol Scand 53: 211–218
104. Sternberg WH (1949) The morphology, androgenic function, hyperplasia, and tumors of the human ovarian hilus cells. Am J Pathol 25: 493–521
105. Sternberg WH, Segaloff A, Gaskill CJ (1953) Influence of chorionic gonadotropin on human ovarian hilus cells (Leydig-like cells). J Clin Endocrinol Metab 13: 139–153
106. Tanabe K, Gagliano P, Channing CP, Nakamura Y, Yoshimura Y, Iizuka R, Fortuny A, Sulewski J, Rezai N (1983) Levels of inhibin-F activity and steroids in human follicular fluid from normal women and women with polycystic ovarian disease. J Clin Endocrinol Metab 57: 24–31
107. Valdes-Dapena MA (1967) The normal ovary of childhood. Ann NY Acad Sci 142: 597–613
108. Vermeulen A (1976) The hormonal activity of the postmenopausal ovary. J Clin Endocrinol Metab 42: 247–253
109. Visfeldt J, Starup J (1974) Dating of the human corpus luteum of menstruation using histological parameters. Acta Pathol Microbiol Scand 82: 137–144
110. Visfeldt J, Starup J (1975) Histology of the human corpus luteum of early and late pregnancy. Acta Path Microbiol Scand 83: 669–677
111. Weiss G, Rifkin I (1975) Progesterone and estrogen secretion by puerperal human ovaries. Obstet Gynecol 46: 557–559
112. Weiss G, O'Byrne EM, Steinetz BG (1976) Relaxin: A

product of the human corpus luteum of pregnancy. Science 194: 948–949

113. Weiss G, O'Byrne EM, Hochman JA, Goldsmith LT, Rifkin I, Steinetz BG (1977) Secretion of progesterone and relaxin by the human corpus luteum at midpregnancy and at term. Obstet Gynecol 50: 679–681

114. White RF, Hertig AT, Rock J, Adams E (1951) Histological and histochemical observations on the corpus luteum of human pregnancy with special reference to corpora lutea associated with early normal and abnormal ova. Contrib Embryol 34: 55–74

115. Wiley CA, Esterly JR (1976) Observations on the human corpus luteum: Histochemical changes during development and involution. Am J Obstet Gynecol 125: 514–519

116. Young RH, Scully RE (1983) Ovarian tumors of probable wolffian origin. Am J Surg Pathol 7: 125–135

117. Yussman MA, Taymor ML (1970) Serum levels of follicle stimulating hormone and luteinizing hormone and of plasma progesterone related to ovulation by corpus luteum biopsy. J Clin Endocrinol 30: 396–399

118. Zhang J, Young RH, Arseneau J, Scully RE (1982) Ovarian stromal tumors containing lutein or Leydig cells (luteinized thecomas and stromal Leydig cell tumors)—a clinicopathological analysis of fifty cases. Int J Gynecol Pathol 1: 270–285

16

Nonneoplastic Lesions of the Ovary

Philip B. Clement, M.D.

Because nonneoplastic lesions of the ovary frequently occur as pelvic masses and are often associated with abnormal hormonal manifestations, they may mimic an ovarian neoplasm on clinical examination, at operation, and on pathologic examination. Many occur in the reproductive years and may be associated with infertility. Their proper recognition is, therefore, important to allow appropriate, usually conservative therapy, thereby avoiding unnecessary oophorectomy.

Congenital Lesions

Absent Ovary

In phenotypic females, absence of both ovaries is usually associated with an abnormal karyotype and a syndrome of gonadal dysgenesis (see Chapter 2, Abnormal Sexual Development). In such cases, bilateral streak gonads or a unilateral streak gonad and contralateral intraabdominal testis are usually found. However, rare cases of truly agonadal people have been reported, usually with a karyotype that is 46XY or, rarely, 46XX.[301,302] Rare patients with ataxia telangiectasia have had no evidence of ovarian tissue at laparotomy.[53]

Rarely, one ovary may be absent in an otherwise normal woman, typically representing an incidental finding at operation or postmortem examination. It is usually associated with agenesis or malformation of the ipsilateral fallopian tube, round ligament, kidney, or ureter, alone or in various combinations.[205,220] The differential diagnosis would include adnexal torsion with atrophy or autoamputation, as well as failure of descent.[369] In the last disorder, the ovary is present but is in an ectopic position, at the level of the liver or close to the kidney.[352]

Lobulated, Accessory, and Supernumerary Ovary

Examples of lobulated, accessory, and supernumerary ovary are among the rarest of gynecologic abnormalities. A lobulated ovary may be divided by one or several fissures into two or more lobes.[420] The lobes may be completely separate, or connected by fibrous or ovarian stroma; rarely, both ovaries may be affected. A closely related anomaly is an accessory ovary, a structure containing normal ovarian tissue located in the vicinity of a normal, eutopic ovary with which it has a direct or ligamentous attachment.[101,133,420] A supernumerary ovary is a similar structure but is located at some distance from, and not connected to, a eutopic ovary.* It may be within the pelvis, attached to the uterus, bladder, or pelvic walls, or retroperitoneal, within the omentum, periaortic area, or mesentery.[352,420] In most cases, the accessory or supernumerary ovary is less than 1 cm in size, and it is likely that smaller examples are unrecognized at operation or autopsy.[101,420] They may be multiple and bilateral.[133,154] The ectopic ovarian tissue possesses the functional potential (as evidenced by persistent menses after bilateral oophorectomy)[213] and the pathologic potential of normal ovaries.[133,170] The presence of a supernumerary ovary is, therefore, one histogenetic mechanism to account for ovarian-type tumors in extraovarian sites. This derivation is even more likely for nonepithelial tumors, such as granulosa–theca tumor within the broad ligament,[137] which are unlikely to have a mesothelial or secondary müllerian origin (see Chapter 17, Endometriosis).[93,312]

Embryologically, lobulated and accessory ovary are closely related. The former results from lobulation of the ovarian anlage, and the latter presumably develops from a slightly separated part of the otherwise normally developing and migrating ovarian anlage. Pathogenetic theories for supernumerary ovary include aberrant migration of part of the gonadal ridge after incorporation of the germ cells or, alternatively, arrest of some of the migrating germ cells in an ectopic location, with inductive transformation of the surrounding tissue into ovarian stroma.[312] As many as one third of patients with lobulated ovaries, accessory ovary, and supernumerary ovary have other congenital genitourinary abnormalities.

Ovarian Remnant Syndrome

Examples of accessory and supernumerary ovary should be distinguished from the so-called ovarian remnant syndrome, a disorder representing a complication of a difficult oophorectomy.* Patients with this syndrome typically have a history of bilateral oophorectomy during which extensive periovarian adhesions were encountered. The adhesions are usually a result of prior pelvic surgery, endometriosis, or pelvic inflammatory disease. The absence of menopausal symptoms and a lack of atrophic changes on cervicovaginal smears after bilateral oophorectomy are clues to persistent estrogen synthesis in some patients. Within weeks to months but occasionally years after oophorectomy, the patient has pelvic pain and a mass. At operation, a cystic mass is found within the pelvis that is bound by dense adhesions to surrounding structures. In approximately 40% of patients, a segment of ureter has been involved, with obstruction of its lumen. In a unique case, an ovarian remnant formed an intussusceptum in the small intestine, with secondary obstruction.[425] Pathologic examination of the mass reveals one or several cysts arising within a remnant of ovarian tissue presumably left at the time of the oophorectomy. In the majority of cases, a corpus luteum cyst is found on histologic examination (Fig. 16.1),

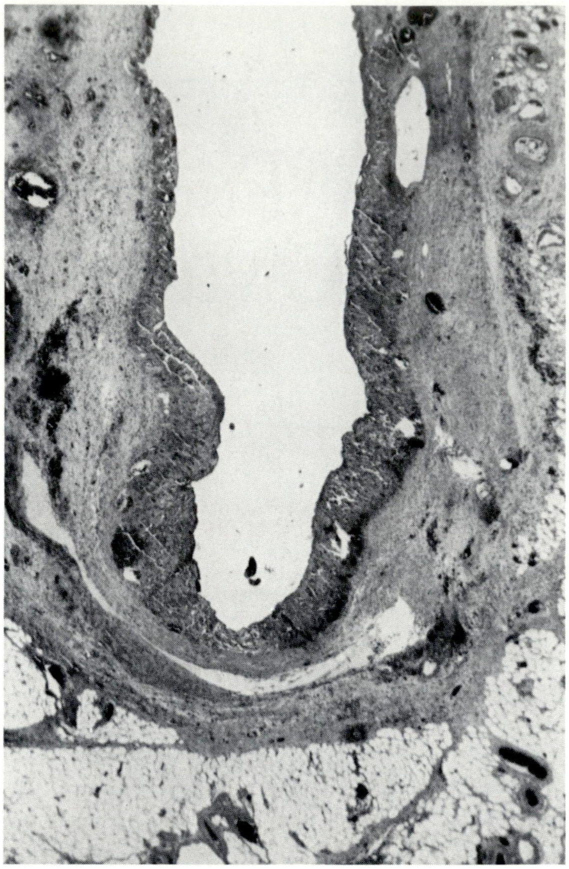

FIG. 16.1. Ovarian remnant syndrome. A corpus luteum cyst is surrounded by congested fibroadipose tissue.

* References 93, 154, 213, 224, 301, 312.

* References 175, 250, 252, 281, 393, 425.

but other pathologic processes, including endometriosis and benign neoplasms, have been documented.

Adrenal Cortical Rests

Although accessory adrenal cortical tissue is frequently observed within the wall of the fallopian tube and the broad ligament, it is an extremely rare finding in the ovary.[394] The adrenal rests typically appear as yellow, spherical, encapsulated nodules measuring several millimeters in size (Fig. 16.2). Adrenal cortical ectopia in these sites can be explained by the close proximity of the anlage of the adrenal cortex to the gonadal ridge during embryonic development. Ovarian adrenal cortical rests may be the origin of rare examples of ovarian steroid (lipid) cell tumors, which resemble adrenal cortical tissue in both their histologic appearance and endocrine manifestations.[352]

Uterus-Like Ovarian Mass

Two examples of a uterus-like ovarian mass have been reported, consisting of a central cavity lined by endometrial tissue surrounded by a thick, smooth muscle wall.[91,313] Although the lesions can be explained on the basis of an ovarian endometriotic cyst with extensive smooth muscle metaplasia of the stromal component, so-called endomyometriosis, a congenital malformation of the ipsilateral müllerian duct has been suggested as a more likely pathogenesis.[313,328] This interpretation is supported by the presence of congenital abnormalities of the urinary tract in both reported patients with this lesion.

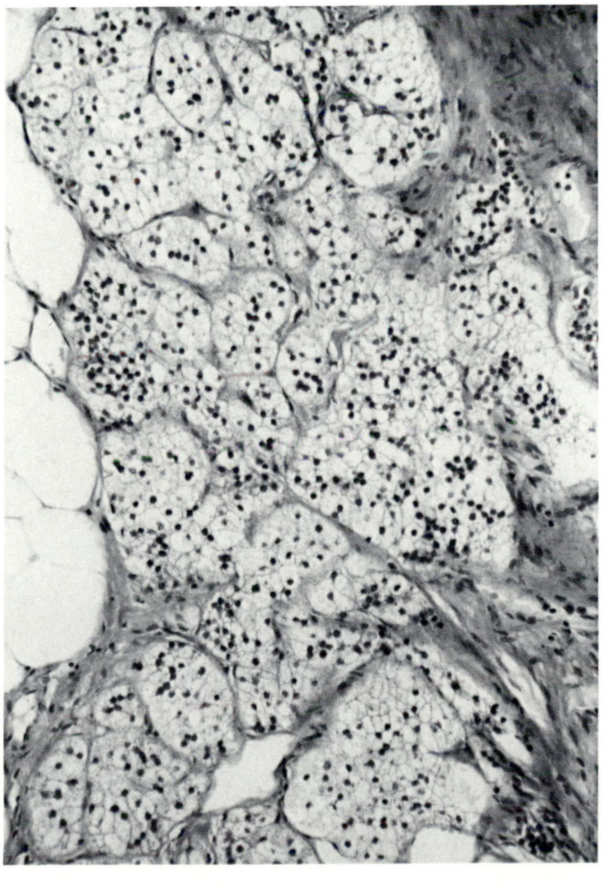

Fig. 16.2. Adrenal cortical rest within mesovarium.

Splenic–Gonadal Fusion

Splenic–gonadal fusion is an extremely rare anomaly resulting from fusion of the anlage of both organs during embryonic development. The male/female ratio is 9:1. Three examples have been described in newborn female infants, two of which were associated with partially undescended ovaries, as well as other, multiple, congenital anomalies.[314] All three cases were of the continuous type in which a cord-like structure connected the spleen to the left ovary or surrounding structures. In one of these infants several intraovarian splenic nodules were found. An additional case has been described in an adult female who was found to have a septate uterus and a cluster of splenic nodules surrounding the otherwise normal left ovary.[12] The differential diagnosis in this patient would include traumatic splenosis, but in such cases there is usually a history of trauma, and the nodules of splenic tissue are more widely dispersed throughout the peritoneal cavity.[19,297,415]

Inflammatory Disorders

Infectious Diseases

Common Bacterial Infections

The majority of acute and chronic inflammatory lesions involving the ovary are infectious, specifically bacterial, in etiology and usually represent a manifestation of sexually transmitted pelvic inflammatory disease (PID). Approximately 20% of cases of PID occur in patients with an intrauterine device, the presence of which increases the risk of infection three- to eightfold.[110,201] Ovarian involvement in PID is almost always secondary to salpingitis and typically takes the form of a unilateral or bilateral tuboovarian abscess (Fig. 16.3). The organism responsible for the acute stages of PID is typically *Neisseria gonorrhoeae*, but *Chlamydia trachomatis*, *Mycoplasma hominis*, or a mixture of aerobic and anerobic organisms that are often present in the normal vagina may also be responsible. A mixed flora with a preponderance of endogenous anaerobic organisms is typically recovered from the contents of a tuboovarian abscess.[109,222]

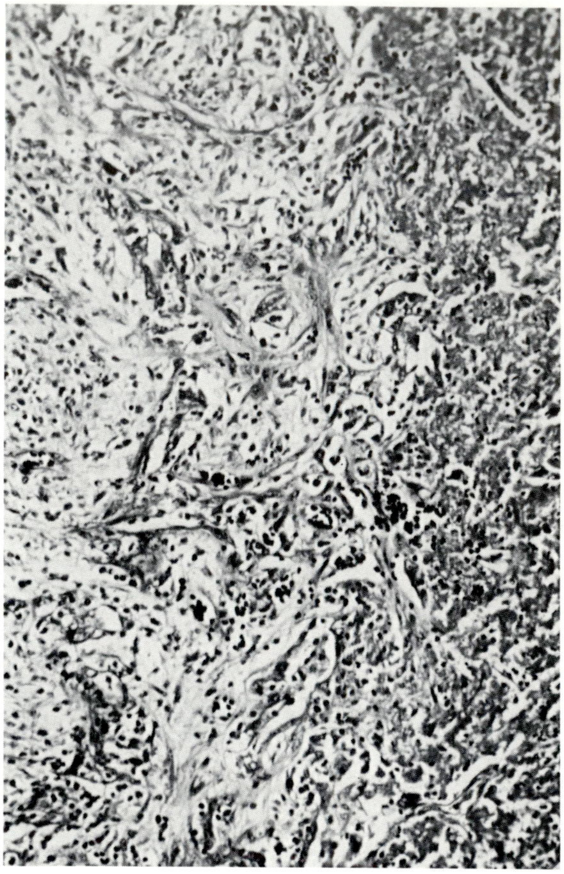

FIG. 16.3. Tuboovarian abscess. Lining consists of inflammatory debris with subjacent granulation tissue.

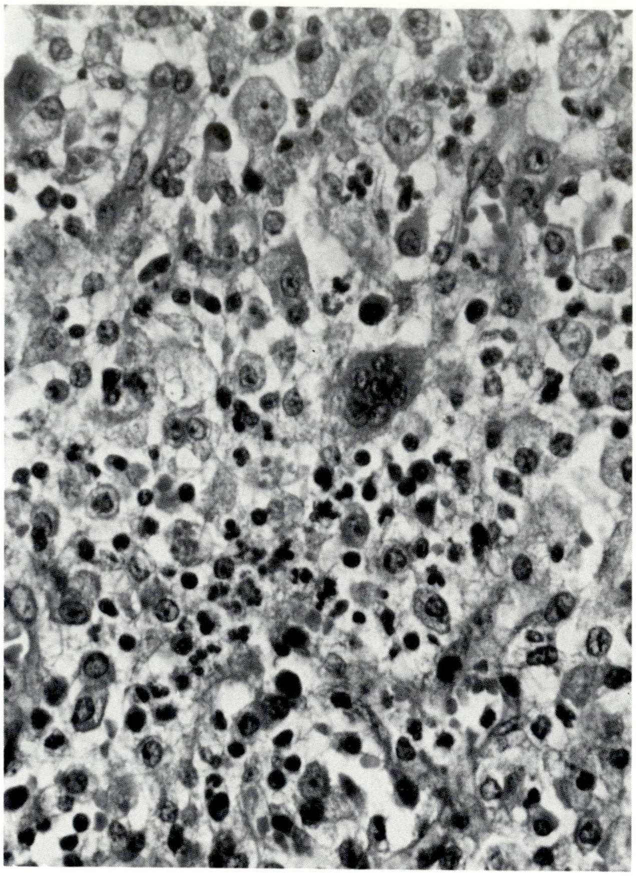

FIG. 16.4. Xanthogranuloma of ovary. Inflammatory reaction consists predominantly of foamy histiocytes, some of which are multinucleated. (Reprinted by permission of Pace et al., Ref. 298.)

The symptoms of patients with tuboovarian abscess are typically abdominal or pelvic pain and, less consistently, fever, vaginal discharge or bleeding, and urinary symptoms.[222] An adnexal mass is palpable, demonstrable with imaging techniques, or visible at laparoscopy. A history of PID is obtained in only one third to one half of patients, suggesting that subclinical infections are common.[222] Much less common than a tuboovarian abscess is an abscess confined to the ovary. An ovarian abscess is typically a result of direct or lymphatic spread of organisms from a nongynecologic pelvic inflammatory process, such as diverticulitis, appendicitis, or following a pelvic operation.[419,428] Rarely, the abscess may be secondary to a blood-borne infection. An uncommon complication of an ovarian or tuboovarian abscess is rupture, typically into the peritoneal cavity, with secondary peritonitis,[80,268,300] or rarely into an adjacent organ (colon,[367] bladder,[232] vagina[14]), with fistula formation.

Milder, chronic or recurrent forms of ovarian involvement by pelvic inflammatory disease may take the form of a chronic perioophoritis, with periovarian and tuboovarian adhesions that may completely surround the ovary. Sclerocystic ovarian changes have been described in such cases.[315] Rarely, a chronic ovarian abscess may result in a solid tumor-like mass, variably designated ovarian *xanthogranuloma*[272] or *xanthogranulomatous oophoritis*.[298] Both of the reported examples of this lesion occurred in patients with recurrent PID. On gross examination, the involved ovary in each case was replaced by a well-circumscribed, solid, yellow, lobulated mass that measured 4 cm in one and 8 cm in the other example. Microscopic examination revealed sheets of foamy histiocytes, admixed with multinucleated giant cells, plasma cells, fibroblasts, neutrophils, and foci of necrosis (Fig. 16.4). No organisms were demonstrable with special stains. Several additional examples of pseudotumorous xanthogranulomatous inflammation with a more diffuse involvement of the adnexa have been described.[219,359]

Rare Bacterial Infections

Actinomycosis. Pelvic actinomyces infection is uncommon and usually represents a complication of an intrauterine device (IUD), although most cases of IUD-

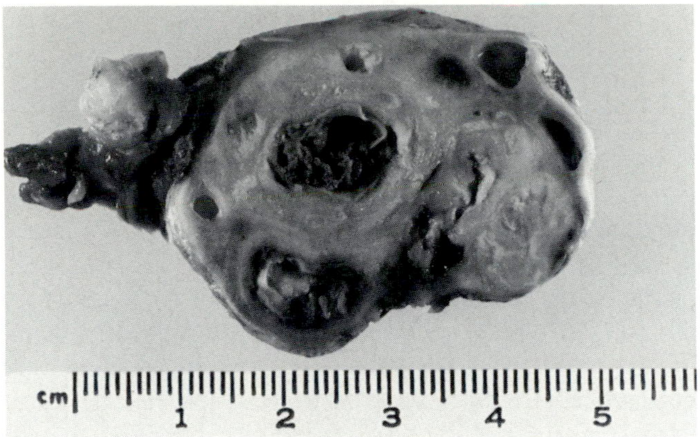

FIG. 16.5. Actinomycosis of ovary. The ovary is enlarged by many confluent abscesses. (Reprinted by permission of Schmidt et al., Ref. 346.)

associated pelvic inflammatory disease are probably nonactinomycotic (Chapter 10, Benign Diseases of Endometrium).* The most common predisposing factor in pelvic actinomycosis is the duration of IUD use; almost 85% of cases have occurred in women who have had an IUD in place for 3 or more years.[345] The infection may also be more common in women using plastic compared to Copper IUDs.[203] There is a high likelihood of subsequent sterility.[345]

Gross examination reveals the adnexal involvement to be typically unilateral, with massively destructive, often multiple, abscesses involving the ovary (Fig. 16.5) and fallopian tube (Chapter 14, Diseases of Fallopian Tube). Rarely the characteristic actinomycotic (sulfur) granules may be grossly visible within the abscess cavities. Microscopic examination reveals a characteristic but nonspecific inflammatory response composed predominantly of neutrophils and foamy histiocytes that may be admixed with lesser numbers of lymphocytes and plasma cells. A specific diagnosis can be made only by finding the granules within the inflammatory exudate. They may be extremely scarce, requiring numerous blocks to demonstrate their presence.[260] The granules are composed of circumscribed masses of basophilic, gram-positive, argyrophilic bacteria growing as branching filaments with a characteristic radial or palisading pattern at the periphery of the granule (Fig. 16.6). A fluorescent antibody stain has been found to be useful in demonstrating the organisms.[305] A diagnosis of actinomycosis may be made before salpingo-oophorectomy in some patients by demonstrating the granules within endometrial curettings and Papanicolaou cervicovaginal smears. In one study, almost 90% of patients with actinomyces demonstrated by the latter method were found to have a tuboovarian abscess.[63,203]

* References 44, 203, 222, 234, 260, 343, 345, 346.

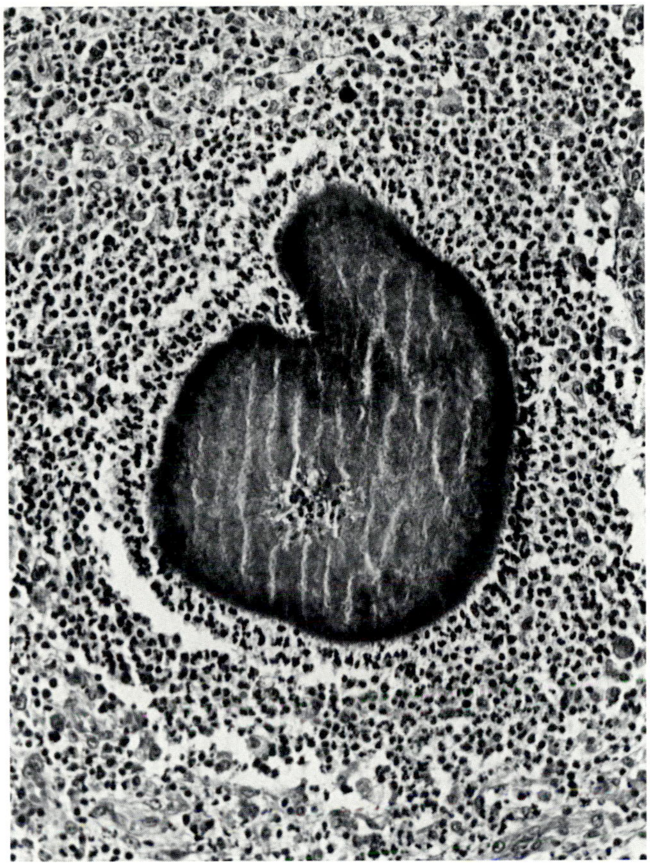

FIG. 16.6. Actinomycosis of ovary. A colony of actinomyces (sulfur granule) is surrounded by a purulent exudate. (Reprinted by permission of the Armed Forces Institute of Pathology, Neg. No. 74–13508.)

Tuberculosis. Tuberculous oophoritis is uncommon and usually secondary to extension from the more frequently involved fallopian tubes (see Chapter 14, Diseases of the Fallopian Tube). Whereas the fallopian tubes are almost always involved in tuberculosis of the female genital tract, the ovarian parenchyma is involved in only 10% of cases.[290] On macroscopic inspection, the ovaries are typically surrounded by ampullary adhesions. Grossly visible caseous ovarian lesions are rare. On histologic examination, ovarian parenchymal tuberculosis is typically confined to the cortex. In some cases, involvement of the surrounding peritoneum with granulomatous nodules in the presence of ovarian enlargement may simulate a neoplasm at the time of surgery.[290,391]

Malacoplakia. Of 17 reported cases of gynecologic malacoplakia (see Chapter 10, Benign Diseases of Endometrium), only 2 have been described in the ovary.[4,70,74] In both cases, friable, hemorrhagic masses involved one or both ovaries and the ipsilateral fallopian tube.[70] Histologic examination revealed the typical features of malacoplakia. Organisms were not demonstrated by culture or histologic examination.

Leprosy. Leprosy may rarely involve the female genital tract, and the ovary appears to be the most common gynecologic site for this disease.[54] In one well-documented case, microscopic examination of the grossly normal ovaries revealed large numbers of vacuolated histiocytes within the ovarian stroma. *Mycobacterium leprae* was demonstrated in these cells with acid-fast stains. In chronic forms of leprous oophoritis, a chronic inflammatory cell infiltrate and fibrosis are seen, and bacilli are usually demonstrable.

Syphilis. For unknown reasons, syphilitic involvement of the ovary is very rare. Luetic oophoritis has been described in congenital, secondary, and tertiary forms of the disease. The pathology of these various stages is similar to that in extraovarian sites.[233]

Parasitic Infections

Parasitic infestations of the ovary in most parts of the world are extremely rare. Ovarian schistosomiasis, however, is relatively common in endemic areas, and the fallopian tube is usually involved simultaneously.[18,25,240,400] The patients typically have lower abdominal pain, a pelvic mass, and, occasionally, irregular menses and infertility. The typical findings at surgery include an enlarged tube and ovary, numerous adhesions, and scattered peritoneal nodules. The gross appearance may, therefore, simulate a malignant tumor. On histologic examination, a granulomatous inflammatory response, often containing eosinophils, is seen in response to the *Schistosoma* eggs. Dense fibrosis is frequently seen in the later stages of the disease.

There have been a number of reports of ovarian involvement by *Enterobius vermicularis.** The lesions are usually an incidental operative finding and are located on the ovarian surface or, rarely, deeper within the ovary. In several cases, there has been simultaneous involvement of the pelvic peritoneum, simulating a metastatic tumor.[124] The granulomas, which frequently contain eosinophils and may exhibit caseous necrosis, surround the adult female worms and ova.[262,370] It is likely that the worms reach the peritoneal cavity by upward migration through the lumen of the female genital tract from the perineum.

Rare cases of ovarian echinococcosis have been described.[22,158] In one, a 12 cm, typical hydatid cyst involved the ovary.

* References 38, 124, 208, 223, 262, 370.

Viral Infections

Oophoritis secondary to cytomegalovirus infection has been described as an incidental finding at autopsy in four immunosuppressed patients.[112,390] In at least three of the patients, ovarian involvement was part of a more generalized infection. On macroscopic examination, the ovaries were of normal size but contained foci of superficial cortical hemorrhagic necrosis measuring 1 to 2 mm in diameter.[390] Microscopic examination revealed foci of coagulative necrosis, with variable numbers of neutrophils, nuclear debris, and hemorrhage. In the surrounding stroma, lymphocytes, plasma cells, and vascular dilatation were present. Ovarian stromal cells, and in one patient, endothelial cells, even at a distance from the necrotic foci, exhibited cytomegaly with typical intranuclear and occasionally intracytoplasmic inclusion bodies (Fig. 16.7). Electron microscopic examination disclosed numerous intranuclear and intracytoplasmic herpes-type viral particles. The presence of necrosis and bizarre cells may mimic a malignant tumor on histologic examination. An additional example of cytomegalovirus oophoritis has

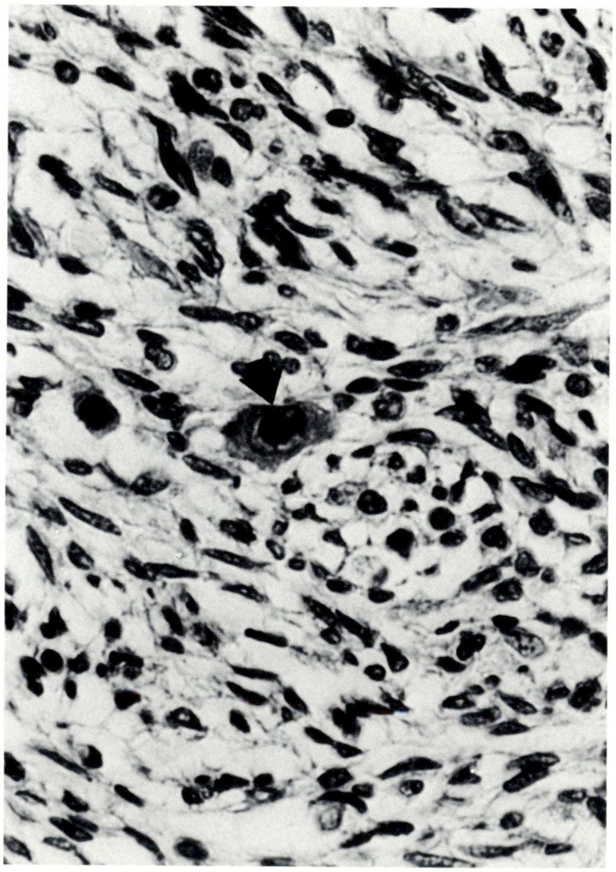

FIG. 16.7. Cytomegalovirus infection of ovary. Ovarian stromal cell contains an intranuclear inclusion (*arrow*). (Reprinted by permission of Subietas et al., Ref. 390.)

been described in which the infection appeared confined to an ovarian thecoma.[230]

Mumps oophoritis as a clinical entity occurs much less commonly than mumps orchitis, with clinical evidence of the lesion in 5% of females with mumps. The pathology of the acute stage, however, has not been well described.[15] It is postulated that germ cell depletion secondary to mumps oophoritis may result in premature menopause and possibly an increased risk of ovarian cancer.[9,92,276]

Fungal Infections

Fungal infections of the ovary are extremely rare, even in patients with disseminated mycoses. Three examples of tuboovarian abscess, as part of pelvic inflammatory disease caused by *Blastomyces dermatitidis*, have been reported.[115,156,282] In one patient, the tuboovarian abscesses were bilateral and associated with multiple miliary nodules involving the pelvic peritoneum.[156] Two of the cases were probably secondary to hematogenous spread from the lungs, and the third was sexually transmitted.

Three cases of ovarian involvement by coccidioidomycosis have been reported.[161] The ipsilateral fallopian tube was involved in each case, with the formation of a tuboovarian abscess in one. In two of the patients, the disease appeared confined to the pelvis, and in the third patient, it was disseminated.

One case of adnexal involvement by *Aspergillus* has been reported in an IUD user.[215] The tuboovarian abscess ruptured, producing generalized peritonitis.

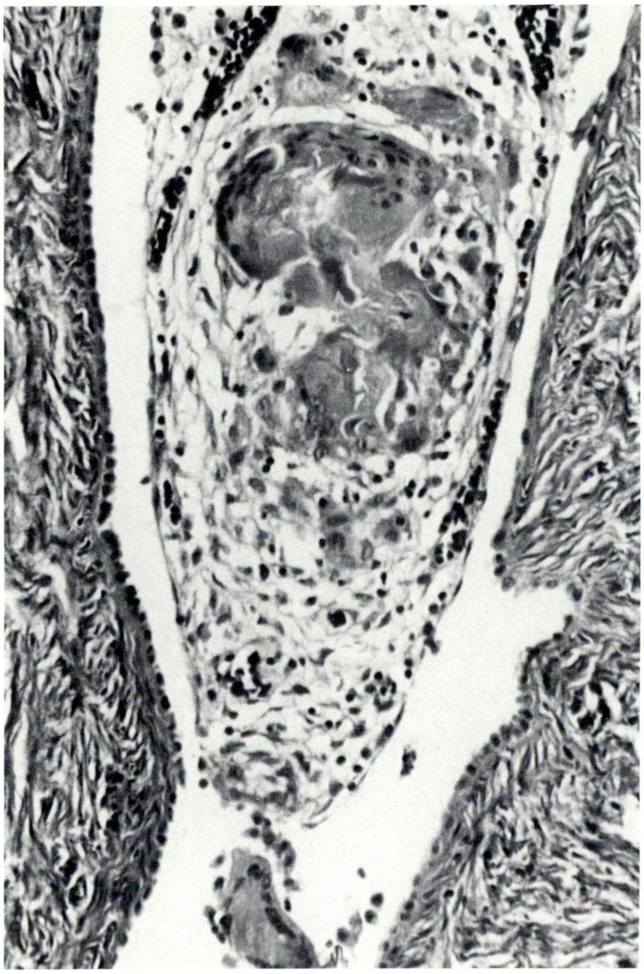

Fig. 16.8. Foreign body reaction to keratin implants on ovarian serosal surface. There was a coexistent endometrial adenoacanthoma confined to the uterus.

Noninfectious Diseases

A variety of noninfectious, typically granulomatous, inflammatory diseases may involve the ovary. In addition, granulomas may be seen rarely in autoimmune oophoritis (see p. 501).

Foreign Body Granulomas

A variety of foreign materials implanting on the ovarian serosa may evoke a granulomatous reaction on the ovarian and peritoneal surfaces, mimicking a malignant tumor at the time of surgery. Examples include lipogranulomatous inflammation secondary to the presence of hysterosalpingographic contrast material[398] and a foreign body reaction to keratin from ruptured cystic teratomas, endometrial adenoacanthomas,[75] and adenosquamous carcinomas (Fig. 16.8).[426] A similar reaction has been described secondary to the presence of starch granules from surgical gloves at the time of pelvic surgery[288] or pelvic examination,[299] and more rarely from starch-containing douche fluid[167] or lubricants.[341] Rarely, the granulomas induced by the presence of starch granules may be of the tuberculoid type, with or without caseous necrosis, rather than of the foreign body type, mimicking tuberculosis on microscopic examination.[288] A unique case of ovarian foreign body granulomatous reaction to vegetable material has been described secondary to colonic perforation.[40]

Isolated Palisading Granulomas

Isolated, noninfectious granulomas of uncertain pathogenesis have been described recently within the ovaries of four premenopausal patients.[164] In three patients, the granulomas were incidental histologic findings. These patients had a history of prior surgery performed on the involved ovary. The fourth patient had no prior surgery and had lower abdominal pain and a pelvic mass; an enlarged ovary was found at laparotomy. In the patients who had undergone prior surgery, the granulomas, most of which were multiple and bilateral, had hyalinized

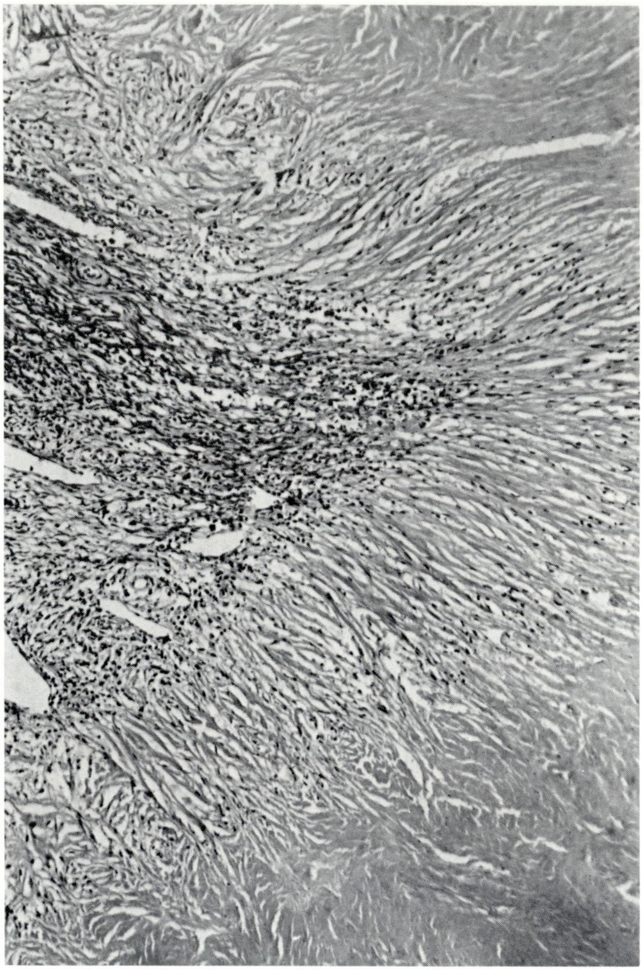

FIG. 16.9. Isolated palisading granuloma of ovary. (Reprinted by permission of Herbold et al., Ref. 164.)

cores surrounded by palisading histiocytes and a fibrous pseudocapsule (Fig. 16.9). In the fourth patient, the ovary was nearly replaced by granulomas with a central necrotic zone surrounded by palisading histiocytes and occasional giant cells. The tissue between the granulomas contained numerous eosinophils. In all four cases, there was no evidence of foreign material, microorganisms, or, with immunoperoxidase staining, immunoglobulins. It was speculated that the pathogenesis of the granulomas in the first three patients was related to prior surgery, but the etiology of the granulomas in the fourth patient was not determined. It is conceivable that the lesions are related to prior surgery in at least some of these patients, since similar palisading granulomas occur postoperatively within the cervix and, in males, in the prostate.[269]

Granulomas Secondary to Systemic Diseases

Granulomatous oophoritis rarely can be due to involvement by sarcoidosis. Three such cases have been reported, but only two have been described in detail.[68,372,430] Both of the latter patients were known to have systemic sarcoidosis, as well as involvement of other gynecologic sites, including the endometrium. The sarcoid granulomas in the ovaries were incidental histologic findings.[68,430] Crohn's disease may also be a rare cause of granulomatous oophoritis, usually by direct extension of the inflammatory process from the bowel. The ipsilateral fallopian tube is also usually involved.[59,171,431]

Cortical Granulomas

These are common, incidental, microscopic findings within the ovarian cortex consisting of spherical, well-circumscribed lesions measuring 100 to 500 μm in diameter. They are composed of spindle cells, epithelioid cells, lymphocytes, and occasional multinucleated giant cells; anisotropic fat crystals may also be seen (Fig. 16.10).* Hughesdon suggests that the granulomas become fibrotic with time, accounting for at least some of the spherical, cloud-like, hyaline scars commonly encountered within the cortical stroma of postmenopausal women.[177,178] These scars resemble corpora fibrosa, but are usually distinguishable from the latter by their more superficial location within the cortex, greater cellularity, weaker eosinophilia, and the presence of a reticulum framework (Fig. 16.10).[178] It has also been suggested that hyaline scars may represent regressed foci of endometrial stromatosis, luteinized stromal cells, or ectopic decidua within the ovary.[177,178]

The frequency of cortical granulomas appears to be related to age. They are not usually encountered before the age of 30, but Hughesdon, using serial sections, demonstrated the presence of active lesions in 40% of women over the age of 40 and that the number of lesions per cross section of ovary increase in successive decades.[178]

The clinical significance, if any, of cortical granulomas is unknown. Possible associations with ovarian stromal hyperplasia, endometrial carcinoma, or both, have been suggested but not demonstrated consistently.[178,326,433]

Surface Proliferative Lesions

Surface Epithelial Inclusion Cysts

Surface epithelial inclusion cysts are believed to arise from cortical invaginations of the ovarian surface epithelium that have lost their connection with the surface. Although most numerous in postmenopausal women, they can be demonstrated on thorough microscopic ex-

---

* References 45, 55, 177, 178, 326, 433.

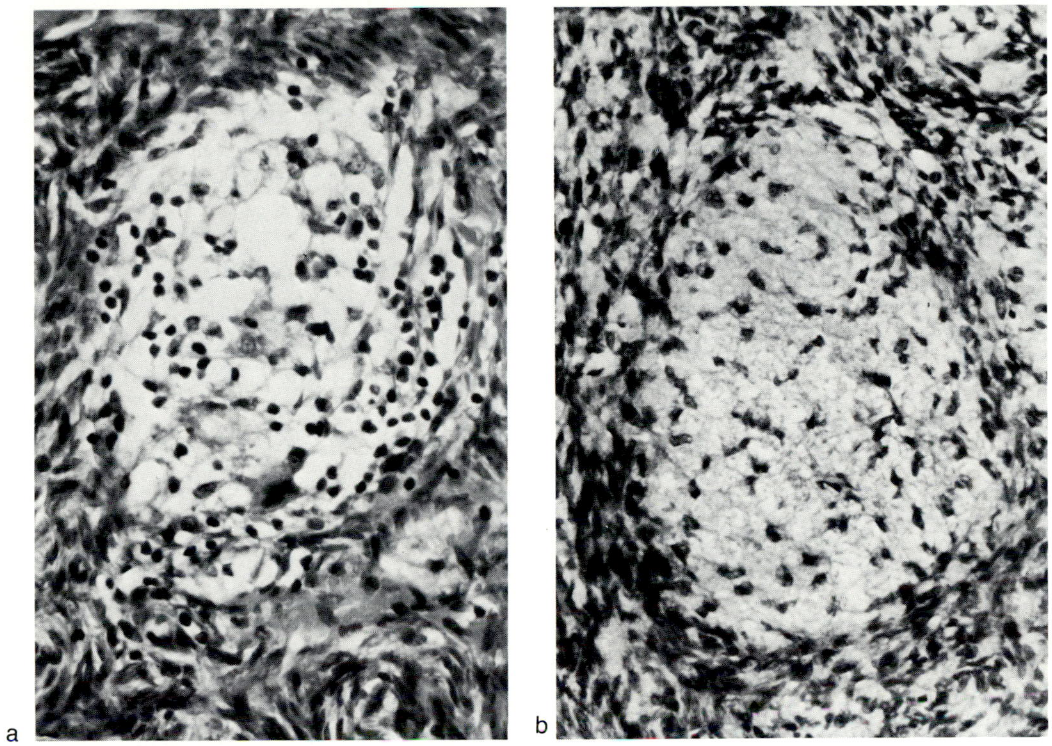

FIG. 16.10. *a*. Cortical granuloma. Circumscribed collection of lymphocytes, spindle cells, and occasional multinucleated giant cells. *b*. Hyaline scar consisting of collagen and spindle cells.

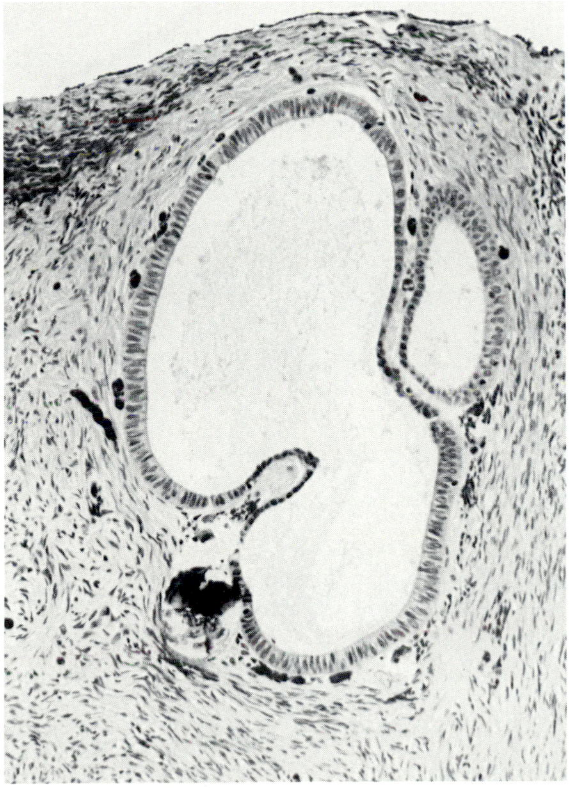

FIG. 16.11. Epithelial inclusion cyst. Cyst beneath ovarian surface epithelium is lined by a single layer of columnar cells. A psammoma body is present within the adjacent stroma.

amination of ovaries from females of all ages, including fetuses, infants, and adolescents.[48,50]

Large inclusion cysts, which may measure up to 1 cm in diameter, may be visible on gross inspection of the ovary, although most will be appreciable only on microscopic examination. They are usually multiple, scattered singly or in small clusters throughout the superficial cortex; less commonly, they may extend into the deeper cortical or medullary stroma. Inclusion cysts are typically lined by a single layer of columnar epithelium. In postmenopausal patients, the epithelium is usually tubal (endosalpingeal) in type. In such cases, psammoma bodies may be seen within the cysts, the adjacent stroma (Fig. 16.11), and very rarely, within cervicovaginal Papanicolaou smears.[236] Less commonly the lining of inclusion cysts may consist of a single layer of endometrioid or endocervical columnar epithelium.[279,412] An Arias–Stella-like reaction has been described within inclusion cysts in pregnant patients.[50] Occasionally in adults, and typically in fetal and premenarcheal ovaries, the cysts have a nonspecific, flat, cuboidal, or columnar lining.

It is generally believed that ovarian epithelial inclusion cysts give rise to the majority of common epithelial tumors of the ovary.[352] Although there are no convincing data to substantiate this view, possible support for this hypothesis has come from immunoperoxidase studies demonstrating the presence of a variety of tumor markers

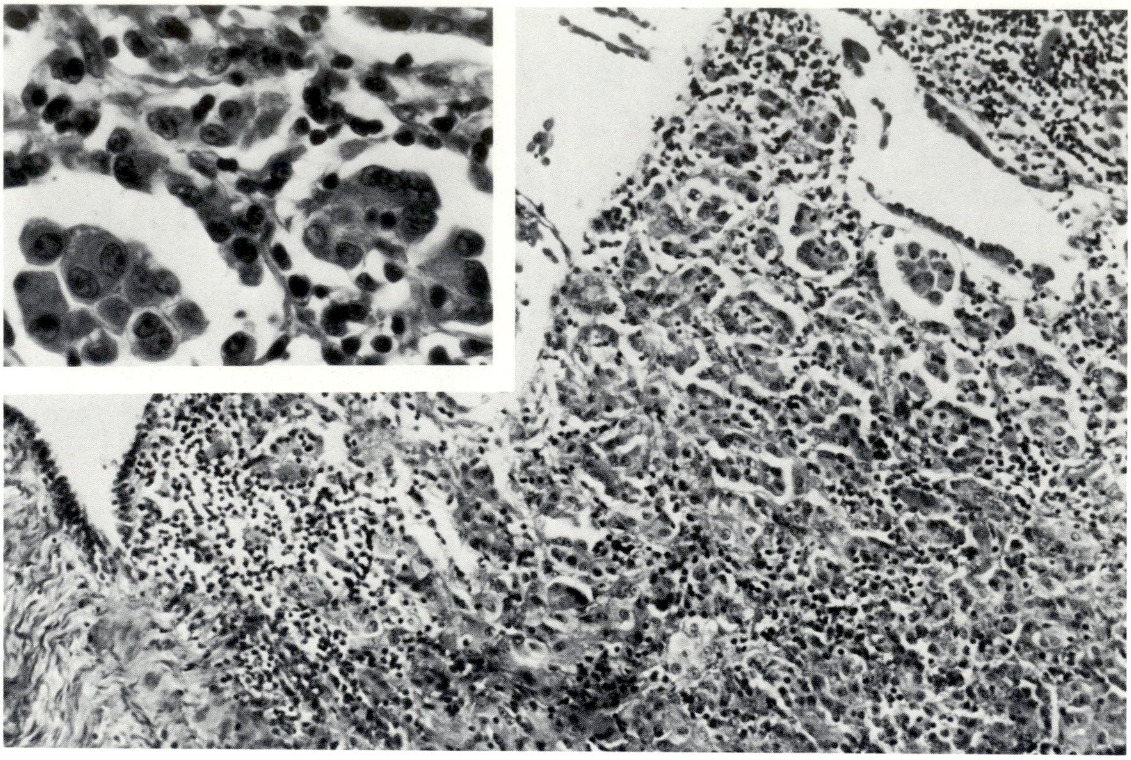

Fig. 16.12. Mesothelial proliferation on ovarian surface. Mesothelial cells, growing in a papillary pattern, are admixed with lymphocytes. The mesothelial cells exhibit mild nuclear pleomorphism and multinucleation (*inset*).

in cells lining inclusion cysts. The markers, which may be seen in the serum of patients with common epithelial carcinomas of the ovary, include carcinoembryonic antigen (CEA), human chorionic gonadotropin (hCG), placental lactogen, alpha-$_2$-glycoprotein, beta-$_1$-glycoprotein, CA125, and placental alkaline phosphatase.[49,195,292]

Mesothelial Proliferations

Proliferation of mesothelial cells on the ovarian surface, within periovarian fibrous adhesions, or elsewhere on the pelvic peritoneum is usually a response to pelvic inflammation (see Chapter 17, Endometriosis). Florid examples may be associated with complex glandular and papillary proliferations of mesothelial cells, which may exhibit focal reactive atypia (Fig. 16.12). Such a process may simulate a metastatic carcinoma or primary serous surface carcinoma.[236,352]

Surface Stromal Proliferations

Nodular and papillary stromal projections from the ovarian surface are common incidental histologic findings in the late reproductive and postmenopausal age groups. They are composed of ovarian stroma exhibiting varying degrees of hyalinization covered by a single layer of surface epithelium (Fig. 16.13).

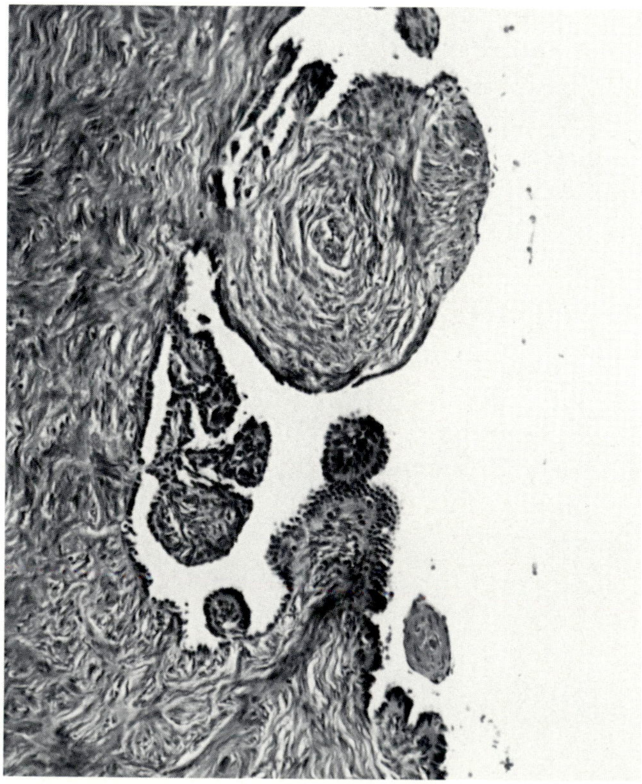

Fig. 16.13. Papillary and nodular stromal proliferation involving ovarian surface.

Nonneoplastic Lesions of the Follicular and Stromal Elements

This section deals with the wide spectrum of nonneoplastic lesions that arise from the ovarian follicles and stroma. Many of them are secondary to ovarian stimulation by pituitary or chorionic gonadotropins and may be associated with excessive production of estrogens, androgens, or both. Included is a discussion of lesions involving nonneoplastic proliferations of Leydig cells. Most of these are not of stromal origin, but as previously discussed (see Chapter 15, Anatomy and Histology of Ovary), Leydig cell differentiation is within the metaplastic potential of the ovarian stromal cell.

Solitary Cysts of Follicular Origin

Solitary (one or occasionally a few) cysts of follicular origin should be distinguished from disorders characterized by multiple, bilateral, follicular cysts.

Follicle and Corpus Luteum Cysts

Gross Appearance. Solitary follicle cysts (FC) and corpus luteum cysts (CLC) are thin-walled and unilocular, ranging from 3 cm to 8 cm in diameter, although larger examples may occur rarely (Fig. 16.14).[3,51,57,61] CLCs are usually distinguishable by the presence of a convoluted yellow lining (Fig. 16.15). Contents of FCs and CLCs vary from a serous or serosanguineous fluid to clotted blood.

Microscopic Appearance. FCs are lined by an inner layer of granulosa cells and an outer layer of theca interna cells. The cells in either layer may be luteinized (Fig. 16.16). Distinction between the two layers can be facilitated by a reticulin stain, which will reveal dense reticulum surrounding the theca cells but sparse or absent reticulum in the granulosa layer (Fig. 16.16). CLCs exhibit a convoluted lining composed of large luteinized granulosa cells and smaller luteinized theca interna cells, with a prominent innermost layer of connective tissue (Fig. 16.17). Those associated with pregnancy may also exhibit characteristic hyaline bodies and foci of calcification within the granulosa cells (Fig. 16.17 inset). Focal infarction of a CLC has been described in association with a tubal pregnancy. It was postulated that the infarction was due to inadequate hCG production by the ectopic trophoblast.[403] Involutional fibrosis of a corpus luteum or CLC usually leads to the formation of a solid corpus albicans, although, rarely, a corpus albicans cyst may result.

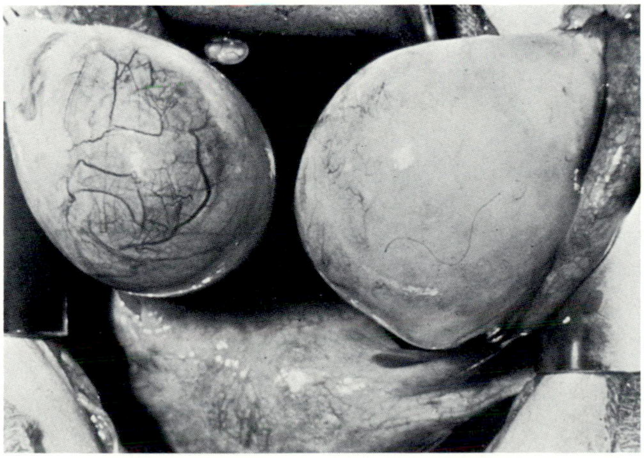

Fig. 16.14. Solitary follicle cyst within each ovary. (Reprinted by permission of *The New England Journal of Medicine*, 292; 199–203, 1975.)

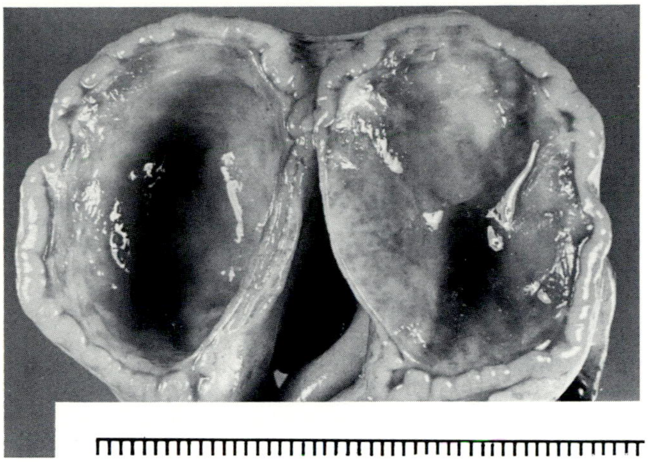

Fig. 16.15. Corpus luteum cyst. Note the convoluted lining.

Clinical Aspects. Solitary FCs are common, occurring during fetal life,[273,405] in newborns,[57,61] throughout childhood,[3] in the reproductive era,[306] and rarely after the onset of the menopause.[387,389] Solitary FCs may be more common in postpubertal patients with cystic fibrosis.[360] CLCs occur during the reproductive era but exceptionally may follow sporadic ovulation in a postmenopausal woman.[352]

The proportion of FCs and CLCs associated with clinical manifestations is unknown, since many are incidentally discovered on pelvic ultrasound, laparoscopy, or laparotomy. Patients with clinically evident FCs and CLCs typically have either a palpable adnexal mass or manifestations related to increased estrogen production, such as sexual precocity,* menstrual disturbances,[306] or endometrial hyperplasia.[387] An uncommon clinical presentation of FCs and CLCs is rupture with hemoperito-

* References 81, 95, 214, 245, 249, 274, 278, 311, 389, 423.

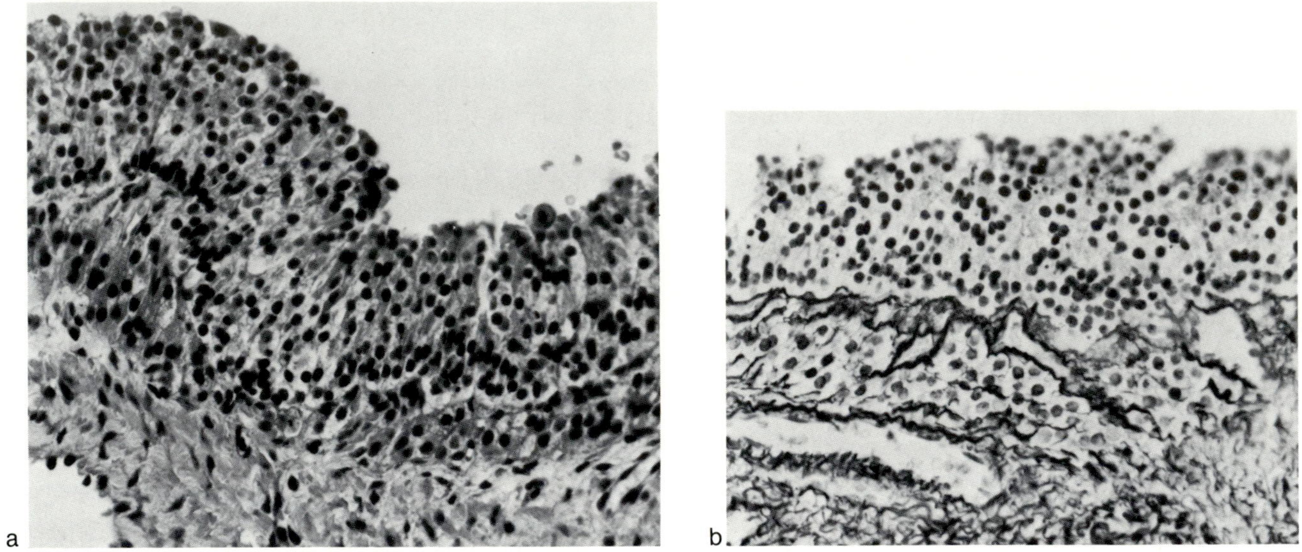

FIG. 16.16. Follicle cyst. *a*. Lining consists of inner layer of granulosa cells and outer layer of theca interna cells. *b*. Distinction between the two layers is enhanced with reticulin stain, showing reticulum network within theca interna layer and an absence of reticulin within the granulosa layer. [Reprinted by permission of Clement (1985) In: Contemporary Issues in Surgical Pathology, Vol 6. Roth, Czernobilsky (eds). New York, Churchill Livingstone.]

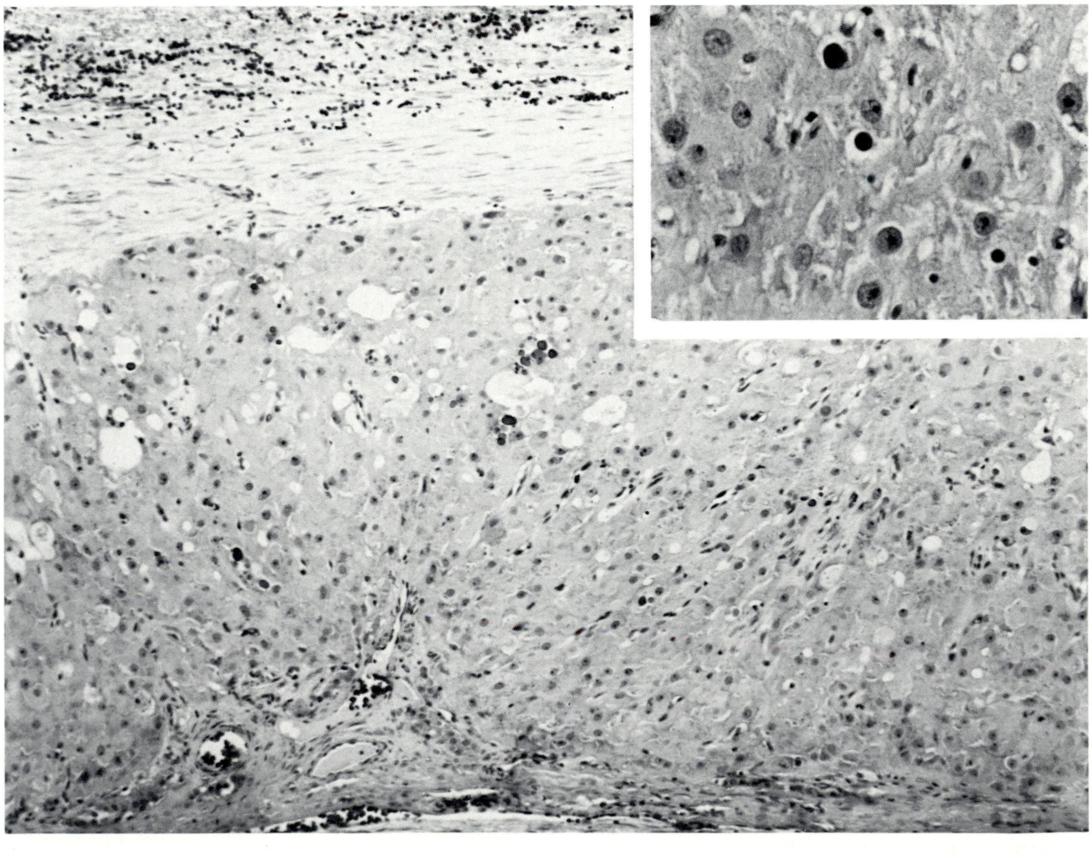

FIG. 16.17. Corpus luteum cyst of pregnancy. The cyst has an inner lining of connective tissue and an outer layer of large luteinized granulosa cells, some of which contain hyaline bodies (*inset*).

neum,[123,155] a complication more likely to occur in patients receiving anticoagulant therapy[225,257,303,304,357] or with bleeding diatheses.[347,417] A rare manifestation of a CLC is ureteric[175,250] or intestinal[425] obstruction as part of the ovarian remnant syndrome.[393]

Most cases of FC and CLC regress spontaneously within 2 months. Thus clinical monitoring of small ovarian cysts in women of reproductive age is justifiable for this period. The process can be accelerated by administration of a combined estrogen–progestogen preparation.[374]

Pathogenesis. The pathogenesis of most FCs is probably related to abnormalities in the release of anterior pituitary gonadotropins. These cysts may be recurrent.[249,278] Others appear to be autonomous primary ovarian lesions that do not recur after removal.[311] Girls with the McCune-Albright syndrome and precocious puberty secondary to an FC may have elevated levels of gonadotropins, whereas in others it appears to be mediated by a gonadotropin-independent mechanism.[81,96,249,424]

Large Solitary Luteinized Follicle Cyst of Pregnancy and Puerperium

A rare type of solitary FC with distinctive clinical and pathologic features occurs during pregnancy and the puerperium and is presumably related to hCG stimulation.[8,78,216] Patients have a palpable adnexal mass or a unilateral ovarian cyst during cesarean section. None have exhibited clinical evidence of an endocrine disturbance. On gross inspection, the cyst resembles a typical follicle cyst except for its large size (median diameter 25 cm). On microscopic examination, it is lined by one to several layers of luteinized cells without recognizable separation into granulosa and theca layers. The luteinized cells typically exhibit focal marked nuclear plemorphism and hyperchromatism (Fig. 16.18). Other cytologic features of malignancy are absent, and the atypical changes are most likely degenerative in nature.

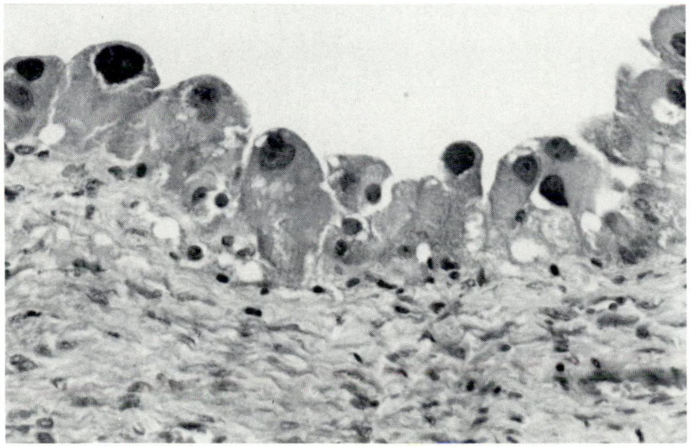

Fig. 16.18. Large solitary luteinized follicle cyst of pregnancy and puerperium. The cyst is lined by a single layer of luteinized cells which exhibit nuclear pleomorphism and hyperchromasia. [Reprinted by permission of Clement (1985) In: Contemporary Issues in Surgical Pathology, Vol 6. Roth, Czernobilsky (eds). New York, Churchill Livingstone.]

Differential Diagnosis of Solitary Follicle Cysts

Solitary cysts of follicular origin should be distinguished from other ovarian cysts that can be solitary and unilocular. Cysts otherwise identical to FCs and CLCs but measuring less than 2.5 cm in diameter are generally regarded as physiological and designated cystic follicles and cystic corpora lutea respectively. Simple cysts have an absent lining or one composed of a layer of nonspecific cuboidal or flattened cells. Most are probably of follicular or surface epithelial origin.

Cysts of surface epithelial origin that are small, incidental microscopic findings are designated inclusion cysts (p. 478). Otherwise similar cysts, but measuring over 1 cm, are considered neoplastic and designated serous, endometrioid, and mucinous cystadenoma depending on the nature of their lining (Chapter 18, Common Epithelial Tumors of Ovary). Ovarian cysts lined exclusively by mature squamous epithelium are referred to as epidermoid cysts.[289,440] Although such cysts have been considered to represent monodermal teratomas, recent reports, including one which demonstrated Walthard-like nests in the walls of some of these cysts,[440] have favored a surface epithelial origin. Endometriotic cysts are readily distinguishable by their characteristic lining of endometrial epithelium and stroma and secondary inflammatory response (see Chapter 17, Endometriosis).

Differentiating large FCs from the rare unilocular cystic granulosa cell tumor may be difficult (see Chapter 19, Sex Cord-Stromal Ovarian Tumors). The latter are usually considerably larger and are lined by several layers of granulosa cells that form Call–Exner bodies; luteinization of the granulosa cells is unusual.

Multiple Cysts of Follicular Origin

This section will deal with disorders characterized by the presence of multiple follicle cysts (excluding polycystic ovary disease, p. 486). These disorders are usually secondary to elevated levels of gonadotropins and are associated with bilateral ovarian enlargement.

Hyperreactio Luteinalis

Hyperreactio luteinalis (HL) is characterized by ovarian enlargement caused by numerous luteinized follicle cysts secondary to hCG stimulation.[67,143,163,339,421]

Pathologic Features. On macroscopic examination, multiple, usually bilateral cysts producing moderate to massive ovarian enlargement (up to 26 cm) are seen (Fig.

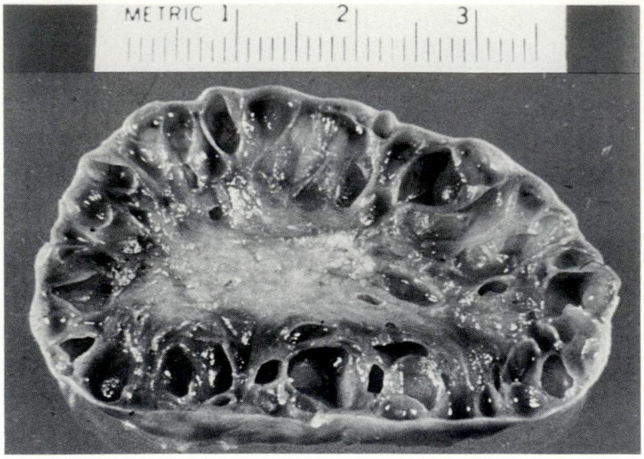

FIG. 16.19. Hyperreactio luteinalis. Multiple thin-walled follicle cysts are present within the cortex. [Courtesy of Dr. R.E. Scully. Reprinted by permission of Clement (1985) In: Contemporary Issues in Surgical Pathology, Vol 6. Roth, Czernobilsky (eds). New York, Churchill Livingstone.]

16.19). The cysts may be filled with clear or hemorrhagic fluid. Microscopic examination reveals FCs with prominent luteinization of the theca interna layer and, in some cases, the granulosa cells (Fig. 16.20). There is usually marked stromal edema and prominent stromal luteinization.

Clinical Aspects. The condition is most commonly seen in association with disorders resulting in high levels of circulating hCG, such as hydatidiform moles, choriocarcinoma, fetal hydrops (usually secondary to Rh sensitization but rarely of nonimmunologic type[162]), and multiple gestations.[67,143] Rarely, it has been preceded by the polycystic ovary syndrome.[41] The presence of HL in patients with gestational trophoblastic disease (GTD) may indicate an increased risk for persistent or metastatic disease (see Chapter 24, Gestational Trophoblastic Disease).[94,211,277] The frequency of HL in women with GTD ranges from 10 to 37%, depending on whether clinical examination or sonography is used for detection.[340] Because HL rarely occurs in patients with otherwise normal pregnancies and normal hCG levels, the pathogenesis of the disorder is probably not related to high levels of hCG alone.[29,67]

HL may become clinically apparent at any time in pregnancy or discovered as an incidental finding during the course of cesarean section. Less commonly, the clinical manifestations occur within the first 10 days postpartum[67] or, exceptionally, late in the puerperium.[32] The patients usually have pain, palpable adnexal masses,

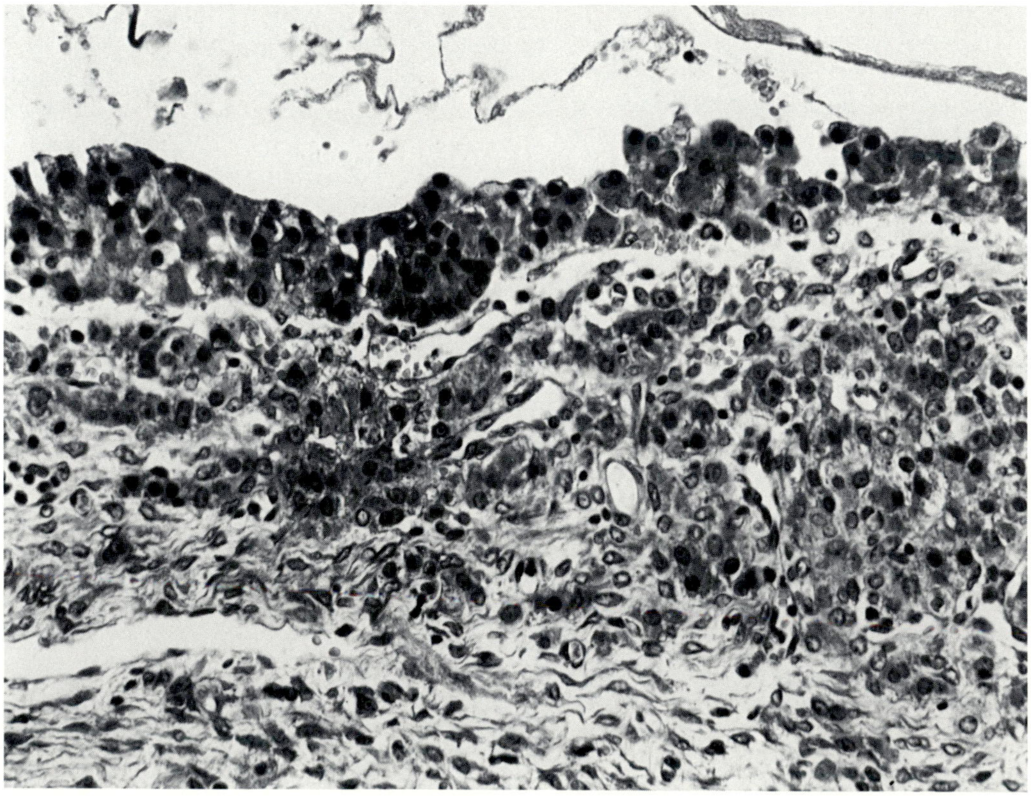

FIG. 16.20. Hyperreactio luteinalis. The cyst lining consists of granulosa and theca layers, both of which exhibit marked luteinization. [Reprinted by permission of Clement (1985) In: Contemporary Issues in Surgical Pathology, Vol 6. Roth, Czernobilsky (eds). New York, Churchill Livingstone.]

or both. In patients with HL secondary to trophoblastic disease, cystic ovarian enlargement is detected at the time of curettage or during the postoperative follow-up period.[277,307]

In approximately 25% of cases unassociated with trophoblastic disease, there has been virilization of the patient but not the female infant, probably because the androgens produced by these cysts are aromatized to estrogens by the placenta.[41,163,193] Elevated plasma testosterone levels have also been demonstrated in nonvirilized patients with trophoblastic disorders, the levels being directly proportional to the magnitude of ovarian enlargement.[339] Complications of HL include hemoperitoneum from cyst rupture, torsion, and ascites.

HL typically regresses in the postpartum period but sometimes requires as long as 6 months.[235] Exceptional cases regress spontaneously during pregnancy.[226] In cases associated with trophoblastic disease, gradual regression occurs 2–12 weeks after uterine evacuation,[277] but occasionally the cysts continue to enlarge before their eventual regression.[307] Because HL is self-limited, operative intervention is needed only to remove infarcted tissue, control hemmorrhage, or reduce ovarian size in order to diminish androgen production in virilized patients.[67] Rarely, HL may recur in subsequent pregnancies.[108,361]

Ovarian Hyperstimulation Syndrome

An iatrogenic form of HL, referred to as the *ovarian hyperstimulation syndrome* (OHS), can develop in as many as 44% of women undergoing ovulation induction, typically with some form of FSH followed by hCG, or rarely clomiphene alone.* OHS occurs only after ovulation and is more severe in patients who conceive.

In severe cases, the ovaries can become massively enlarged and ascites, with or without hydrothorax, can develop due to increased permeability of the peritoneal and pleural surfaces. Elevation of serum estrogens, progesterone, and testosterone typically occur.[159,342,350] Hemoconcentration with secondary oliguria and thromboembolic phenomena is a life-threatening complication. Elevated serum levels of renin, aldosterone, and antidiuretic hormone may occur in such patients.[159] The patients usually respond to conservative therapy, and surgical intervention is necessary only in the rare instance of cyst torsion or rupture. The cysts usually regress within 6 weeks. Pathologic examination of the ovaries reveals changes identical to those seen in HL, with the additional finding of one or more corpora lutea. Careful selection of patients and regulation of dosage of the ovulation-induction drug by monitoring estrogen levels and cyst size has reduced the frequency of OHS.

OHS does not usually occur in women with multiple ovulations undergoing in vitro fertilization despite estrogen levels that exceed the safe range. Aspiration of the multiple follicles appears to prevent the development of the syndrome in most, but not all, patients.[128]

* References 77, 159, 259, 342, 402, 421.

Juvenile Hypothyroidism

Multiple bilateral FCs may occur in girls with juvenile hypothyroidism.* Depending on the method of detection, as many as 75% of girls with hypothyroidism may have multicystic ovaries.[229] Rarely, the ovarian enlargement may be the presenting sign leading to a diagnosis of hypothyroidism.[229,325] The clinical features, in addition to the ovarian enlargement and manifestations of hypothyroidism, include varying degrees of sexual precocity in over half the patients and galactorrhea. Sexual precocity appears to be secondary to elevated estrogen levels resulting from an increased secretion of pituitary gonadotropins, and the galactorrhea due to mildly elevated levels of prolactin.[34,229] Pathologic examination, which has been performed in only a few patients, has revealed FCs, some with luteinization of the theca interna layer. In two cases, a depletion of primordial follicles was also noted.[366,407,435] Treatment with thyroxin has resulted in regression of the hypothyroidism, ovarian cysts, and sexual precocity and a decline in the elevated gonadotropin and prolactin levels.

Prematurity

Multiple, bilateral FCs associated with estradiol production have been described in infants born before the 30th week of gestation.[356] The cysts, which are secondary to elevated levels of FSH and LH, appear at a postconceptional age that slightly precedes the expected time of delivery. It is postulated that marked prematurity is associated with relative insensitivity of the hypothalamus and anterior pituitary to negative feedback by estradiol.[356]

17-Hydroxylase Deficiency

Congenital deficiency of 17-hydroxylase, an enzyme required for both cortisol and estrogen synthesis, results in low estrogen levels and secondarily elevated levels of FSH and LH. The rare patients with this disorder exhibit congenital adrenal hyperplasia, hypokalemia, hypertension, primary amenorrhea, absence of sexual maturation, and ovarian enlargement due to multiple, bilateral FCs.[243]

* References 34, 114, 229, 325, 366, 407, 435.

Polycystic Ovary Disease

Polycystic ovary disease (PCO) is an idiopathic disorder (or possibly a spectrum of related disorders) characterized by chronic anovulation and sclerocystic ovaries associated with inappropriate gonadotropin secretion, hyperandrogenemia, and increased peripheral conversion of androgens to estrogens.[131] The current clinical spectrum of PCO is considerably broader than the syndrome initially defined by Stein and Leventhal in 1935.[82] Stromal hyperthecosis is a closely related disorder that overlaps both clinically and pathologically with PCO.

Gross Appearance. Both ovaries are typically rounded and two to five times normal size, although their size can be normal. Unilateral involvement is rare.[131] They have a white surface through which superficial cortical cysts are visible. Examination of their cut surface reveals a thickened, white, superficial cortex and numerous subjacent cysts, typically measuring less than 1 cm in diameter (Fig. 16.21). There is usually a central zone of stroma with few or no stigmata of ovulation (corpora lutea or albicantia).[46,131,150,352]

Microscopic Appearance. The stroma of the superficial cortex is fibrotic and hypocellular, resembling a capsule (Fig. 16.22).[150,179] Within this zone, prominent venules and arterioles may be seen.[149,179] Tongues of similarly fibrotic stroma may extend from the superficial cortex into the deeper cortex and medulla.[179] The cysts (atretic cystic follicles) have an inner lining composed of several layers of nonluteinized granulosa cells that may be focally exfoliated.[149] An outer layer consists of theca interna cells, which typically exhibit varying degrees of luteinization (Fig. 16.23). Although the latter finding has been referred to as *follicular hyperthecosis*, cystic follicles in women with PCO differ from those in normal women only in their increased number.[150] Maturing follicles (up to midantral stage) and atretic follicles exhibiting prominent luteinization of the theca interna may be twice as numerous as in normal ovaries.[131,149,179] Primordial follicles are normal in number and appearance.[149,179] As noted, stigmata of prior ovulation (corpora lutea and albicantia) are typically absent, but corpora lutea have been described in as many as 30% of otherwise typical cases of PCO, and their presence does not exclude the diagnosis.[150,179] The deeper cortical and medullary stroma may exhibit up to a fivefold increase in volume and exhibit focal luteinization.[179] Focal metaplastic alteration of the stroma into smooth muscle has been reported.[179] Nests of ovarian hilus (Leydig) cells may

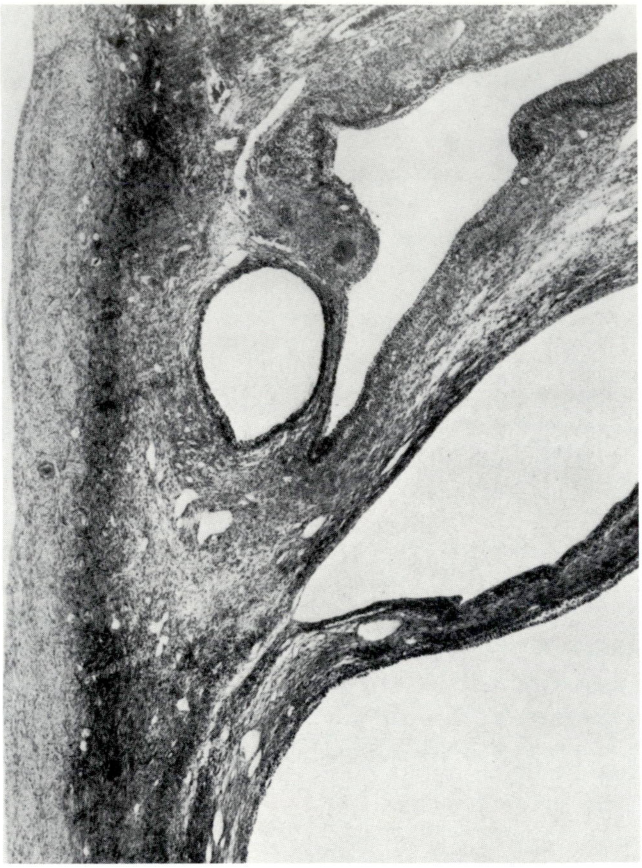

Fig. 16.22. Polycystic ovary disease. Multiple cystic follicles lie beneath the superficially fibrotic cortex. [Reprinted by permission of Clement (1985) In: Contemporary Issues in Surgical Pathology, Vol 6. Roth, Czernobilsky (eds). New York, Churchill Livingstone.]

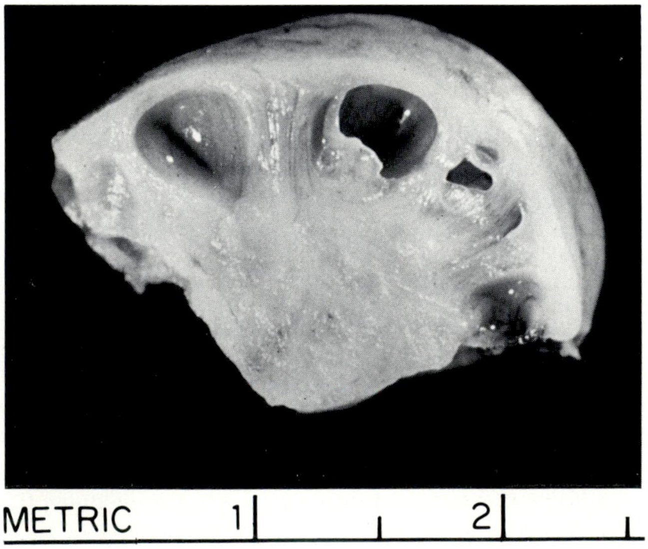

Fig. 16.21. Polycystic ovary disease. Superficial cortical fibrosis and multiple cystic follicles are present. [Courtesy of Dr. R.E. Scully. Reprinted by permission of Clement (1985) In: Contemporary Issues in Surgical Pathology, Vol 6. Roth, Czernobilsky (eds). New York, Churchill Livingstone.]

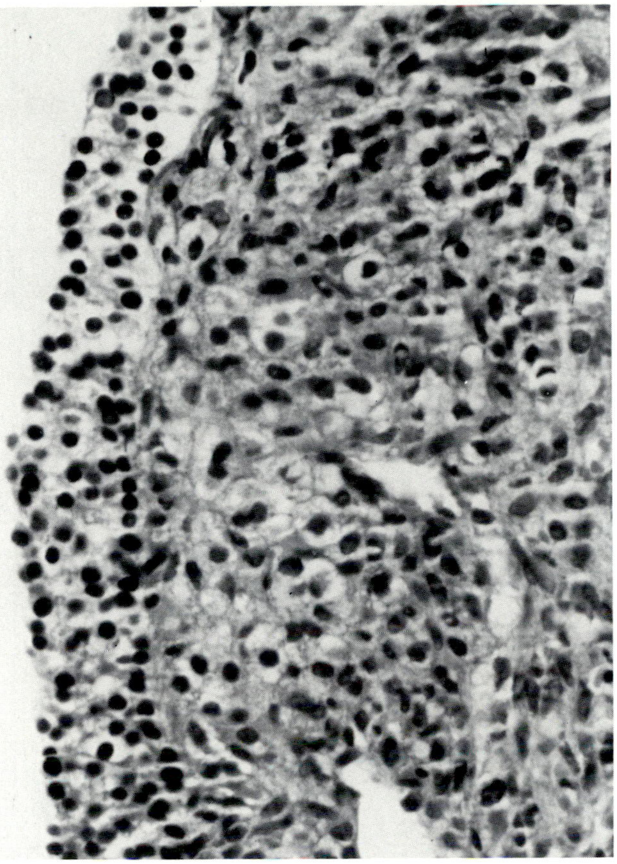

FIG. 16.23. Polycystic ovary disease. A cystic follicle is lined by nonluteinized granulosa cells and an outer, thicker layer of luteinized theca interna cells. [Reprinted by permission of Clement (1985) In: Contemporary Issues in Surgical Pathology, Vol 6. Roth, Czernobilsky (eds). New York, Churchill Livingstone.]

be more numerous in patients with PCO than in age-matched controls.[179]

Clinical Aspects. PCO is not a rare disease and has been estimated to involve 3.5–7.0% of the female population.[131] The affected patients typically are in their third decade with a history of premenarcheal obesity, oligoamenorrhea (rarely primary amenorrhea), infertility, and hirsutism.[46,131,149,439] As previously noted, however, the clinical spectrum of patients with PCO has expanded from that initially described, and some patients with oligomenorrhea, infertility, and the typical biochemical profile of PCO are normal in appearance. Frank virilization (clitoromegaly, deep voice, temporal baldness, male habitus) is rare. The sudden onset of virilization is more likely to be indicative of stromal hyperthecosis or a virilizing ovarian tumor.[131] The ovaries in PCO may be palpably enlarged or normal.

PCO can be familial and may be the most common endocrinopathy causing familial hirsutism.[131] A genetic basis for the disease may, therefore, exist in some patients, although its frequency is unknown.[131] In one study of familial PCO, approximately half of the sisters of patients with PCO were similarly affected, consistent with a dominant, autosomal mode of inheritance.[83] Other studies have suggested an X-linked transmission.[131]

Manifestations of unopposed estrogenic stimulation, including menometrorrhagia, endometrial hyperplasia, and endometrial carcinoma, occur in a significant proportion of patients (see Chapter 12, Endometrial Carcinoma). The tumors typically occur in obese patients under the age of 40. Conversely, up to one quarter of patients with endometrial carcinoma under 40 have PCO.[131] The tumors are almost always well-differentiated adenocarcinomas or adenoacanthomas with absent or only superficial myometrial invasion.* The carcinomas are rarely, if ever, fatal, and many are reversible with progesterone therapy or by induction of ovulation. A wide variety of extrauterine tumors have also been described in patients with PCO,[24,88,132,144,181] but a recent large series of patients with chronic anovulation syndrome showed that the endometrium was the only site at increased risk for neoplasia, with a relative risk of 3.1.[88]

Hyperprolactinemia is present in approximately 27% and galactorrhea in 13% of patients with PCO.[84,130,131] Some hyperprolactinemic patients have been shown to have pituitary adenomas, and therefore tomographic scanning of the sella may be necessary.[130,131,373] Some patients with PCO may exhibit features of the HAIR-AN syndrome of hyperandrogenism (HA), insulin resistance (IR), and acanthosis nigricans (AN),† a syndrome discussed in the section dealing with stromal hyperthecosis.

Pathophysiology. The pathophysiology of PCO is complex and not yet completely understood. The literature on this subject has been reviewed recently by Futterweit.[131] The initiating pathogenetic factors are unknown, but a cardinal disturbance is an increased secretion of luteinizing hormone releasing factor (LHRF), leading to fluctuating raised levels of luteinizing hormone (LH).[46,439] LH stimulates the follicular theca interna cells to produce androstenedione, which is converted to estrone primarily within body fat.[47] Estradiol levels remain normal or low normal, resulting in an elevated estrone/estradiol ratio.[131] Elevated estrone levels appear to selectively inhibit FSH secretion, resulting in low or low normal FSH levels. Inhibin-F, a nonsteroidal peptide produced by granulosa cells, may be increased in patients with PCO and may additionally suppress FSH by a negative feedback mechanism.[396] The raised LH levels and

* References 88, 118, 134, 191, 261, 318, 434.
† References 62, 71, 104, 119, 142, 397.

the decreased FSH levels produce an elevated LH/FSH ratio, a characteristic finding in patients with PCO. The increased circulating estrogens enhance the sensitivity of pituitary LH-producing cells to LHRF, resulting in a self-perpetuating cycle.[46,439]

Androstenedione may also be converted peripherally to testosterone, but the plasma levels of the latter are usually high normal or only slightly elevated in contrast to patients with stromal hyperthecosis.[46,439] Ovarian estrogen production in PCO is markedly diminished, as manifested by almost undetectable estrogens in the follicular fluid and ovarian tissue, probably due to inactivity of the FSH-dependent aromatase system within the granulosa cells.[107,131,264,429] This inadequate intrafollicular estrogen synthesis, together with the elevated LH/FSH ratio, results in cessation of follicle growth at the midantral stage and consequent anovulation.

Obesity may play a role in initiating or perpetuating PCO in some patients.[36,131] The conversion of androstenedione to estrone occurs predominantly in body fat, and the extent of the conversion is significantly correlated with body weight, especially with the amount of adipose tissue.[82] Obesity is also associated with lowered levels of steroid hormone-binding globulin, resulting in increased levels of free serum testosterone.[256] The latter may directly inhibit follicular maturation or be converted peripherally to estrogens, which further enhance LH secretion. Obese patients may also exhibit insulin resistance and hyperinsulinemia. Insulin has been shown to stimulate ovarian androgen production and may also enhance LH secretion from the pituitary.[2,31,364,365,436]

The role of the hypothalamus in the pathogenesis of PCO is not clearly defined. It has been hypothesized that PCO may be initiated during puberty by a primary hypothalamic (or other CNS) defect, producing an increase in secretion of LHRF, possibly effected by an endorphin-mediated reduction in dopaminergic inhibition of LHRF release.* A consequent increased hypophyseal sensitivity to negative and positive feedback by ovarian steroids, so-called decreased hypophyseal gonadostat set-point, results in diminished FSH release, increased pulsatile LH secretion, and an elevated LH/FSH ratio.[131,265] A similar hypothalamic defect in dopaminergic inhibition of prolactin secretion may account for hyperprolactinemia.[131,316] The latter may also be due to stimulation of the pituitary lactotropes by chronic hyperestrogenemia producing basophil hyperplasia or to a basophil adenoma.[130,373,439] The hyperprolactinemia may play a role in initiating or maintaining anovulation in some patients with PCO disease.

The adrenal contribution to the androgen pool appears to be increased in some patients with PCO, as manifested by elevated dehydroepiandrosterone levels and an increase in serum progesterone and 17-alpha-hydroxyprogesterone after ACTH stimulation.* These patients may represent a subset of patients (PCO-II) distinct from patients with typical PCO (PCO-I).[131,265] It has been postulated that in such patients subtle alterations in peripubertal adrenal steroid biosynthesis leading to increased adrenal androgen secretion may be the initiating event in the pathogenesis of PCO.

* References 10, 131, 316, 363, 437–439.

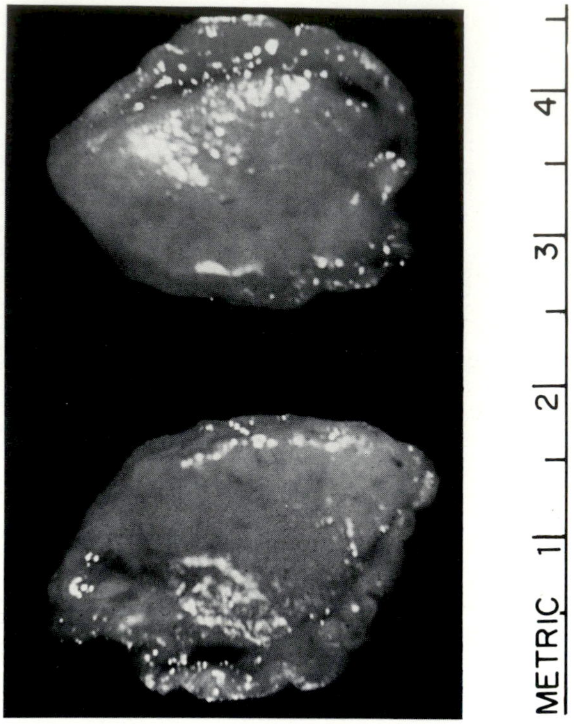

Fig. 16.24. Stromal hyperplasia and hyperthecosis. The ovaries are involved by a solid, homogeneous proliferation that had a yellow color in the unfixed state. (Courtesy of Dr. R.E. Scully.)

Differential Diagnosis. The differential diagnosis includes a wide variety of other disorders that by the disruption of normal cyclic gonadotropin release cause chronic anovulation and sclerocystic ovaries. The latter pathologic finding is, therefore, a nonspecific morphologic expression of chronic anovulation in the premenopausal patient. These include (1) adrenal disorders, such as Cushing's syndrome, congenital adrenal hyperplasia, and virilizing adrenal tumors, (2) primary hypothalamic–pituitary disorders, and (3) ovarian lesions that produce excessive quantities of estrogens or androgens, including such neoplasms as sex cord–stromal tumors and steroid (lipid) cell tumors and such nonneoplastic lesions as Leydig cell hyperplasia and stromal hyperthecosis. As previously noted, in some cases of stromal hyperthecosis, there is an overlap both clinically and pathologically with

* References 21, 131, 221, 231, 270, 375, 439.

PCO, and the two disorders may represent opposite poles of a single disease spectrum.[246–248] Sclerocystic ovaries have also been described in patients after long-term use of oral contraceptives,[308,337] as well as in patients with periovarian adhesions.[315] Finally, it should be noted that the majority of prepubertal ovaries typically exhibit a sclerocystic appearance.[267]

Stromal Hyperplasia and Stromal Hyperthecosis

Stromal hyperplasia (SH) is characterized by varying degrees of nonneoplastic proliferation of ovarian stromal cells. Stromal hyperthecosis (HT) refers to focal luteinization of the stromal cells and is usually accompanied by at least a moderate degree of SH.

Gross Appearance. Both SH and HT result in bilateral ovarian enlargement, with each gonad measuring up to 7 cm in diameter, thus potentially mimicking ovarian neoplasia. Rarely, the ovaries may be of normal size.[55,239,352] Examination of the cut surface reveals parenchymal replacement by homogeneous, firm, white to yellow tissue (Fig. 16.24).[55,284] In premenopausal patients, sclerocystic changes similar to those seen in PCO may also be present.[116,179,247,248,285]

Microscopic Appearance. A varying degree of nodular or diffuse cortical and medullary proliferation of ovarian stromal cells is present (Fig. 16.25). A mild degree of SH cannot be reliably distinguished from the normal appearance.[55] The stromal cells in SH are plumper than the normal postmenopausal ovarian stromal cell, with oval to fusiform, vesicular nuclei and, frequently, cytoplasmic lipid.[352] In HT, focal luteinization of stromal cells appears as small clusters or nodules of polygonal cells with abundant eosinophilic to vacuolated cytoplasm containing variable amounts of lipid. (Fig. 16.26).[55,120,352] The nucleus of the cells is round, with a central small nucleolus. The luteinized cells are most commonly found

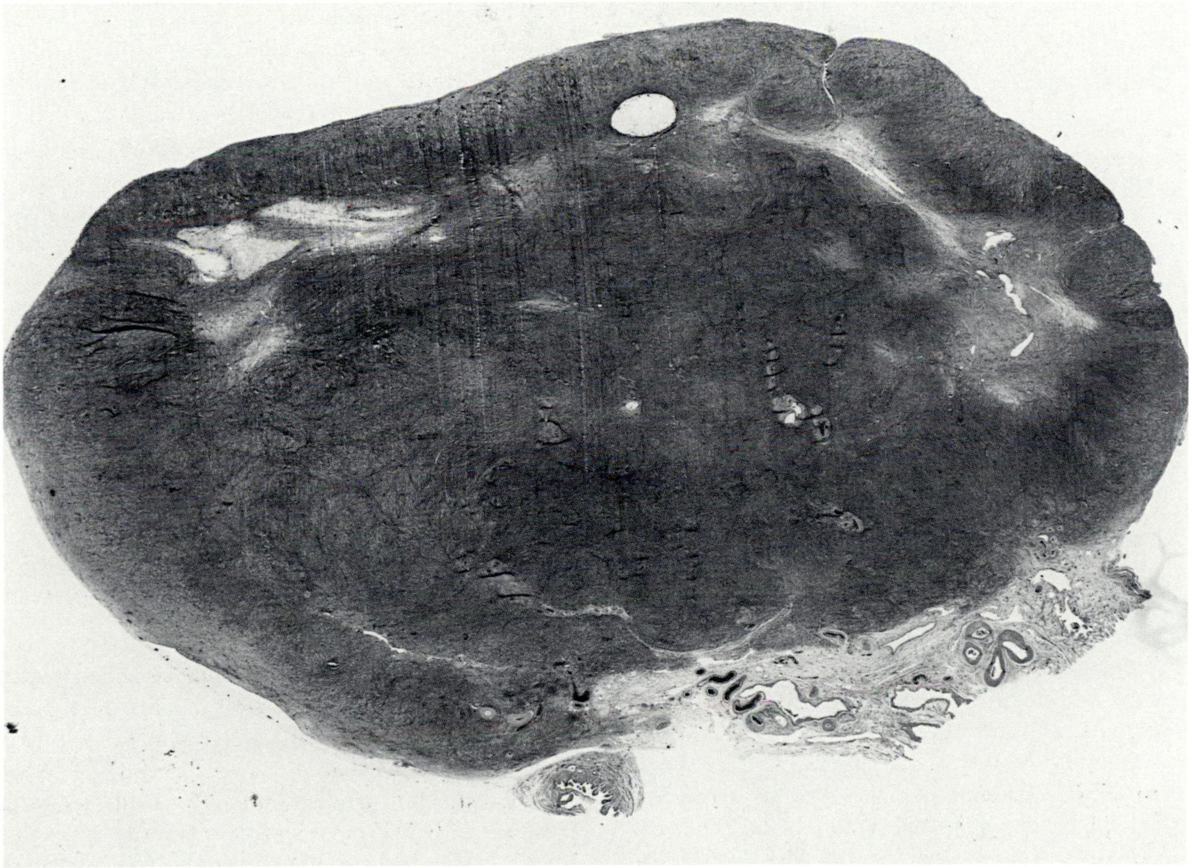

Fig. 16.25. Stromal hyperplasia. A diffuse proliferation of ovarian stromal cells within the cortex and medulla is seen. [Reprinted by permission of Clement (1985) In: Contemporary Issues in Surgical Pathology, Vol 6. Roth, Czernobilsky (eds). New York, Churchill Livingstone.]

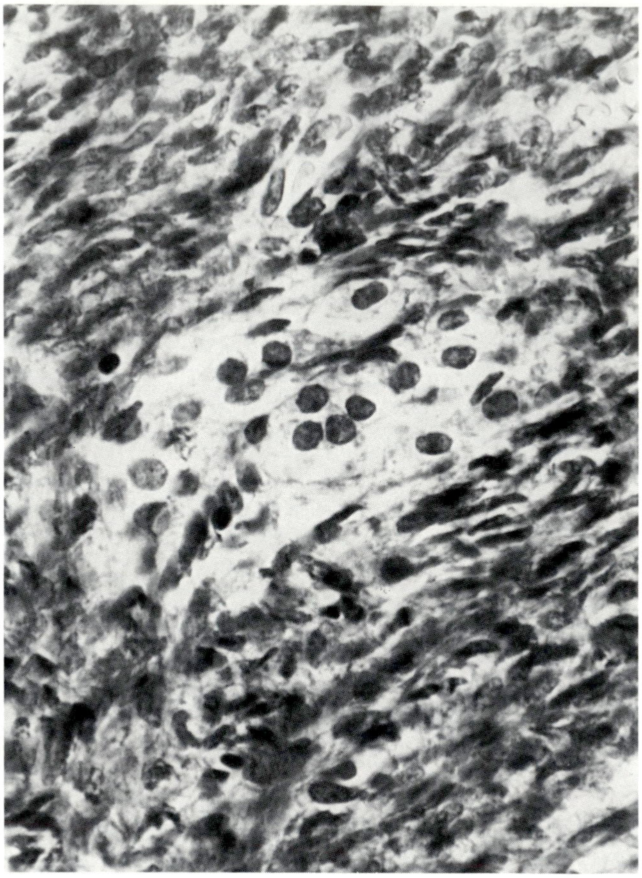

FIG. 16.26. Stromal hyperthecosis. A nest of luteinized stromal cells is present within the ovarian stroma. [Reprinted by permission of Clement (1985) In: Contemporary Issues in Surgical Pathology, Vol 6. Roth, Czernobilsky (eds). New York, Churchill Livingstone.]

in the medulla but may also be present in the cortex. In one case of HT studied with immunoperoxidase techniques, the luteinized stromal cells stained positively for testosterone, estradiol, and FSH but negatively for LH.[239]

Other ovarian findings in cases of HT include small stromal nodules of metaplastic smooth muscle,[353] Leydig cell hyperplasia,[55,385] Leydig cell tumors,[200,330,385] stromal luteomas,[351] and thecomas.[384,444] SH in the absence of HT may also be associated with thecomas.[331,384,444] Some cases of HT may be associated with massive ovarian edema.

Associated pathologic findings in the endometrium in patients with SH and HT may include endometrial hyperplasia and endometrial carcinoma, a reflection of the hyperestrinism present in some of these patients.* One case of HT has been described in which pseudosarcomatous changes in the endometrial stroma were identified, in additon to foci of ectopic decidua within the ovaries.[319] Both of these findings have been associated with hyperprogestational states, thus raising the possibility of progesterone production by the ovarian stroma in this patient.

* References 1, 6, 120, 204, 239, 248, 379.

Clinical Aspects. The clinical manifestations are variable. Moderate to severe SH is most commonly encountered in patients in their sixth and seventh decades and has been documented in over one third of autopsied patients in this age group. Similar degrees of SH were found in only 18% of patients over the age of 71 years, suggesting that it may be a reversible process.[55] There is suggestive evidence that SH of moderate to severe degree is associated with androgen hypersecretion and, to a lesser extent, obesity, hypertension, and glucose intolerance.[55] Similarly, HT is most frequently encountered in patients in the sixth to ninth decades. It has been documented in one third of autopsied patients over the age of 55.[55] In this age group, HT is usually of mild degree and of doubtful clinical significance.[55] Indeed, it has been suggested that exhaustive histologic sampling may indicate that rare luteinized stromal cells may be a normal finding in postmenopausal females (see Chapter 15, Anatomy and Histology of Ovary).[55] Florid examples of HT are more common in patients in the younger reproductive age group, although rare cases may occur in adolescents and postmenopausal patients.[58,239,418] These patients characteristically exhibit marked virilization, obesity, hypertension, and a disturbed glucose tolerance or, less commonly, clinical findings more characteristic of PCO.[33,247,248] Some familial cases have been reported,[146,194] and one case of HT has been described in a patient with acromegaly.[284] Patients with HT may exhibit estrogenic manifestations, such as endometrial hyperplasia or carcinoma,[120,204,239,248,379] whereas the existence of a predisposition to endometrial carcinoma in patients with pure SH is not clear.*

In contrast to patients with PCO, those with HT usually exhibit little or no response to clomiphene treatment and often only a transient response to wedge resection.[116,194,199,285] Many patients require bilateral oophorectomy to halt progressive virilization. Such treatment may also result in disappearance of hypertension and abnormalities in glucose tolerance.[58,248]

Pathophysiology. Ovarian stromal cells, both luteinized and nonluteinized, may exhibit oxidative enzyme activity, so-called enzymatically active stromal cells.[120,323,354] These cells are capable of androgen and, to a lesser extent, estrogen production.[323,354] Hormonal studies in patients with HT have shown markedly increased production rates and serum levels of both ovarian testoster-

* References 45, 55, 244, 293, 326, 327, 348, 379, 433.

one, dihydrotestosterone, and androstenedione, usually in the male range.* One in vitro study indicated that the abnormal androgen production is probably due to an increase in the volume of the ovarian stroma rather than to a biochemical defect in the latter.[39] As noted, the luteinized stromal cells were shown by immunoperoxidase methods to be the probable source of the testosterone in one case of HT.[239]

Unlike patients with PCO, most premenopausal patients with HT have normal gonadotropin levels.[194,284] The possibility that gonadotropins may play a role in some cases, however, is suggested by (1) elevated LH levels in occasional premenopausal and most postmenopausal patients with HT,[146,199] (2) the increase in pituitary amphophils in some cases of marked HT,[65] (3) the often prominent stromal luteinization during pregnancy, (4) positive staining for FSH within the luteinized stromal cells,[239] and (5) in vitro incubation studies indicating gonadotropin responsiveness of the ovarian stromal cells.[99,323]

Estrogen production is noncyclic, with the predominant estrogen being estrone derived from peripheral aromatization of androstenedione.[284] As a result, these patients typically have an increased estrone/estradiol ratio, a pattern similar to that seen in PCO and in postmenopausal women who develop endometrial carcinoma.[6] In some patients with SH and HT, the ovarian stroma appears capable of aromatizing androstenedione to estradiol directly.[99,204,239,264,284]

Differential Diagnosis. The differential diagnosis of HT includes other disorders associated with solid proliferation of luteinized cells, both nonneoplastic and neoplastic, most of which are also virilizing. The former category includes pregnancy luteoma and Leydig cell hyperplasia (hilar and stromal). The neoplasms include luteinized thecoma as well as steroid (lipid) cell tumors, including Leydig tumors and stromal luteoma. These neoplasms, in contrast to HT, are almost always unilateral and typically form distinct tumors or nodules appreciable on gross examination. Luteinized stromal cells, histologically similar to those present in HT, may also be encountered within the nonneoplastic stroma of a variety of benign and malignant ovarian tumors, including primary surface epithelial and germ cell tumors and metastatic tumors, the so-called tumors with functioning stroma (see Chapter 19, Sex Cord-Stromal Ovarian Tumors).[7,237,317]

HAIR–AN Syndrome

Some patients with HT have the HAIR–AN syndrome, a syndrome that has been estimated to be present in as many as 5% of all women with hyperandrogenism.[16,30,104,253] The syndrome consists of hyperandrogenism (HA), typically of early, sometimes premenarcheal, onset, insulin resistance (IR), and acanthosis nigricans (AN).[30] The striking degree of masculinization present in some of these patients may be disproportionate to the degree of HA.[104] The patients may have symptomatic diabetes or a normal glucose tolerance.[196]

The syndrome has also been described in patients with the otherwise typical clinical and biochemical profiles of PCO, although it appears likely that most, if not all, such patients also have significant degrees of HT.[104] Unusual histologic findings described in a patient with HT and the HAIR–AN syndrome include prominent follicular atresia, large numbers of degenerating oocytes, medullary stromal fibrosis, and numerous small nests of granulosa cells forming Call–Exner bodies.[253] Dermoid cysts[183] and stromal luteomas[145] have been rarely described in patients with the HAIR–AN syndrome in association with HT, sclerocystic ovaries, or both.

The typical laboratory findings include hyperinsulinemia and elevated serum levels and increased production rates of testosterone and androstenedione.[30,104,142] In some patients, the severity of IR is proportional to the testosterone elevation.[30,62] Proposed mechanisms of IR have included a decreased number of insulin receptors (type A), anti-insulin receptor antibodies that decrease insulin receptor affinity for insulin (type B), and postreceptor defects in insulin action or clearance (type C).* Incubation studies of ovarian tissue have demonstrated that (1) there is a 50–250-fold increase in testosterone production from the ovarian stroma compared to the ovarian stroma of normal ovaries[264] and (2) insulin alone (and LH alone) can stimulate the accumulation of androstenedione and testosterone in cultures of both the follicular theca interna cells and the ovarian stromal cells.[31] These findings are consistent with recent studies demonstrating specific receptors for insulin in the ovarian stroma.[310] Insulin may act at the ovarian level in synergy with the elevated levels of LH that occur in some of these patients.[31] As noted previously, insulin may also enhance LH secretion from the pituitary. On the basis of these and other findings, it has been postulated that the primary defect in the HAIR–AN syndrome is IR leading to hyperinsulinemia and that the other abnormalities are probably secondary.[30] Thus, any cause of IR leading to hyperinsulinemia can produce the HAIR–AN syndrome.[30] The HA may itself increase the severity of IR, and thus a self-perpetuating cycle that increases in severity may result.[31] The AN is probably an epiphenomenon secondary to HA, hyperinsulinemia, or both.[30]

Bilateral oophorectomy in patients with the HAIR–

* References 1, 6, 33, 116, 117, 199, 239, 284.

* References 28, 30, 119, 125, 196, 397.

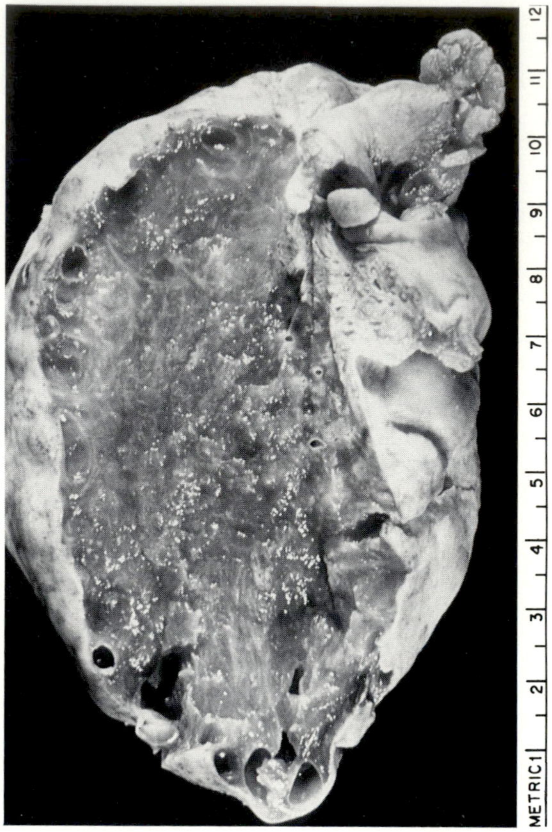

FIG. 16.27. Massive ovarian edema. The ovary is enlarged and markedly edematous. [Courtesy of Dr. R.E. Scully. Reprinted by permission of Clement (1985) In: Contemporary Issues in Surgical Pathology, Vol 6. Roth, Czernobilsky (eds.) New York, Churchill Livingstone.]

AN syndrome results in a decrease in circulating androgens but usually does not ameliorate IR.[30,183,253] Gonadotropin suppression with oral contraceptives has been successful in decreasing ovarian androgen production in some patients.[30] Marked improvement of AN may follow correction of HA.[145]

Massive Ovarian Edema and Ovarian Fibromatosis

Tumor-like enlargement of one or both ovaries secondary to an accumulation of edema fluid within the ovarian stroma is referred to as *massive ovarian edema*. Approximately 50 cases of this disorder have been reported.* A lesion designated *ovarian fibromatosis* by Young and Scully, characterized by diffuse ovarian fibrosis, is closely related to massive edema and is, therefore, considered in this section.[440]

Gross Appearance.

Massive Ovarian Edema. The ovary is enlarged, soft, and fluctuant, ranging in size from 5.5 to 35 cm (mean diameter 11.5 cm). The heaviest ovary has weighed 2400 g.[440] The ovary has a shiny, white, smooth exterior and a cut surface that is solid, tan, homogeneous and gelatinous, exuding a watery fluid (Fig. 16.27). The most superficial cortex appears white and fibrotic, resembling a capsule. Occasional superficial FCs may be present. The ipsilateral fallopian tube may also be edematous.

Ovarian Fibromatosis. Typically there is complete or almost complete ovarian involvement by a fibromatous process.[440] The ovaries measure from 6 to 12 cm in maximum diameter. The external surfaces are white and typically smooth or lobulated. The cut surfaces are firm, white, and solid, although residual cystic follicles surrounded by the fibrous tissue are present in one-third of cases (Fig. 16.28).

Microscopic Appearance.

Massive Ovarian Edema. The striking finding on low magnification is marked, diffuse, stromal edema that separates and sometimes involves the follicular structures but typically spares the superficial cortex (Fig. 16.29). The latter is usually thickened and fibrotic. Higher magnification reveals spindle-shaped ovarian stromal cells separated by abundant pale-staining fluid that focally may have a microcystic appearance.[440] In nonedematous areas, the stroma may have the appearance of normal stroma, hyperplastic stroma, or ovarian fibromatosis similar to that seen in pure ovarian fibromatosis.[440] In approximately 40% of cases, foci of luteinized cells are present

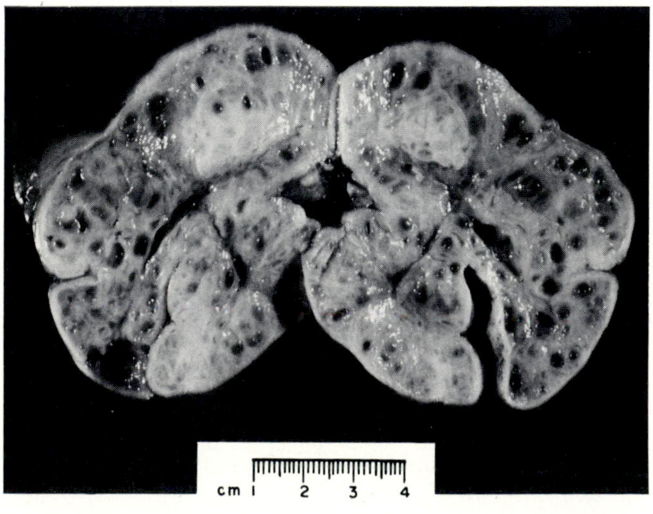

FIG. 16.28. Ovarian fibromatosis. The ovary is enlarged by a diffuse fibrous proliferation that surrounds multiple cystic follicles. (Courtesy of Young and Scully, Ref. 440.)

* References 76, 129, 197, 198, 406, 440.

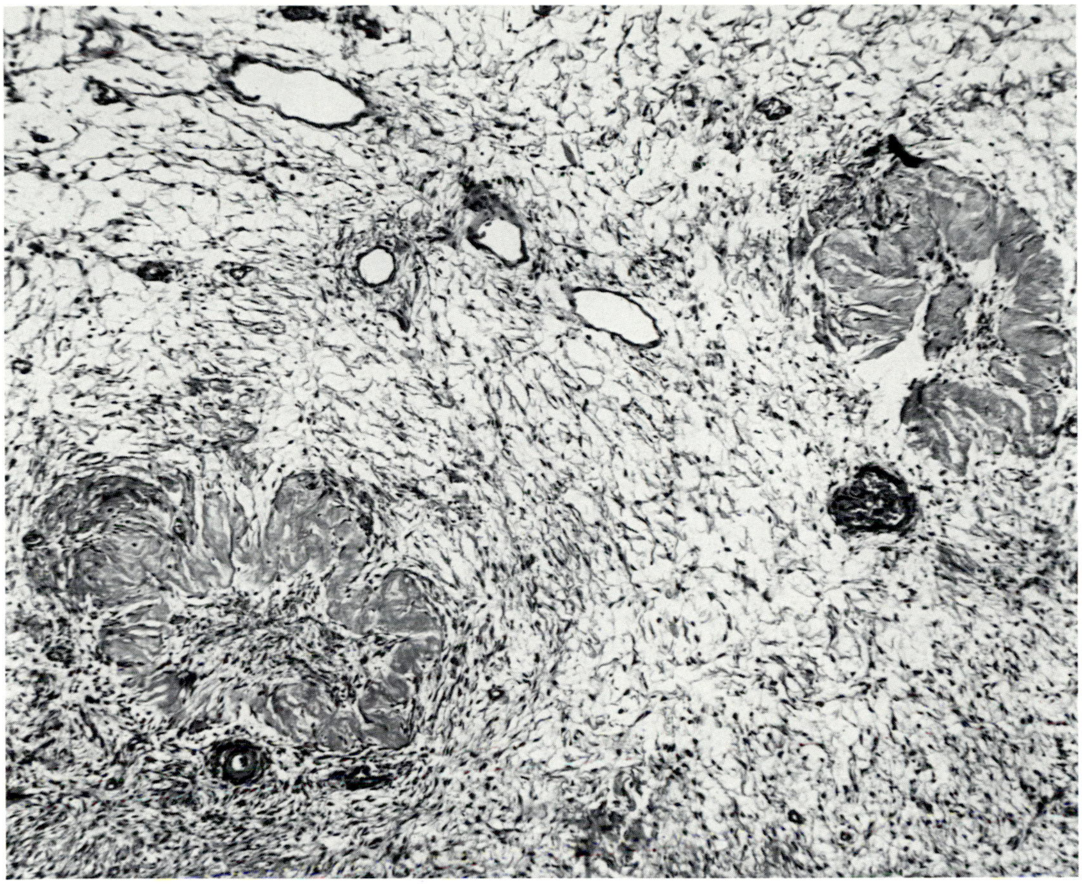

FIG. 16.29. Massive ovarian edema. The edematous ovarian stroma separates several corpora fibrosa. [Reprinted by permission of Clement (1985) In: Contemporary Issues in Surgical Pathology, Vol 6. Roth, Czernobilsky (eds). New York, Churchill Livingstone.]

(Fig. 16.30).[440] Associated nonspecific findings include vascular and lymphatic dilatation within the ovary and occasionally the mesosalpinx, extravasated erythrocytes, hemosiderin-laden macrophages, and mast cells. Foci of necrosis may be seen rarely.[332,440]

The contralateral ovary is normal in over 75% of patients but occasionally is enlarged and also edematous.[246,440] Exceptional cases in which the opposite ovary has been nonedematous and exhibited stromal hyperthecosis or a sclerocystic appearance have been described.[440]

Ovarian Fibromatosis. This disorder is characterized by a proliferation of collagen-producing spindle cells that typically surround normal follicular structures and produce collagenous thickening of the superficial cortex (Fig. 16.31).[440] The process varies from moderately cellular fascicles of spindle cells with a focal storiform pattern to relatively acellular bands of dense collagen. Small foci of uninvolved ovarian stroma are usually present. In rare cases, luteinized cells are seen within the lesion or the adjacent, nonfibrotic stroma. Associated findings include small foci of stromal edema and microscopic foci of sex cord elements within the fibromatous tissue in a minority of cases. Occasionally, the process is bilateral.

Clinical Aspects.

Massive Ovarian Edema. The patients are typically young, with a mean age of 21 years (range 6 to 33 years) and have abdominal or pelvic pain, menstrual irregularities, and abdominal distention. The pain may be of sudden onset and mimic the pain of acute appendicitis. In approximately 20% of patients, androgenic manifestations are present. Of these, two-thirds are virilized, and the rest exhibit only hirsutism.[408,440] The androgenic manifestations have been nearly always associated with the presence of lutein cells. Serum testosterone has been elevated in some cases. Only one patient exhibited estrogenic effects, manifested by precocious puberty.[332] Pelvic examination typically reveals a palpable adnexal mass.[246,440] In approximately one-half of patients, there is evidence of partial or complete torsion of the involved ovary, and in one patient, the contralateral ovary was found to be on a twisted pedicle and infarcted.[197] Intra-

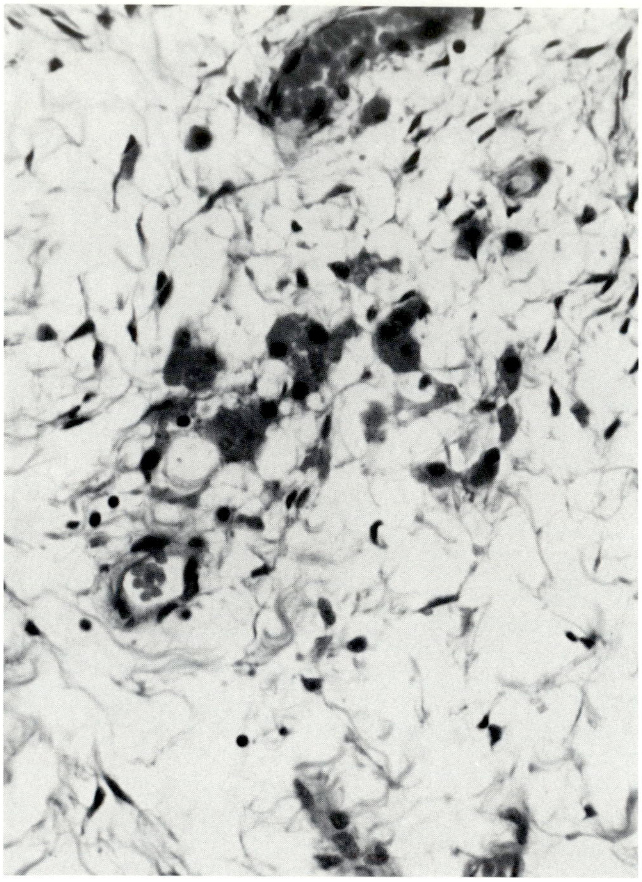

FIG. 16.30. Massive ovarian edema with luteinized stromal cells. [Reprinted by permission of Clement (1985) In: Contemporary Issues in Surgical Pathology, Vol 6. Roth, Czernobilsky (eds). New York, Churchill Livingstone.]

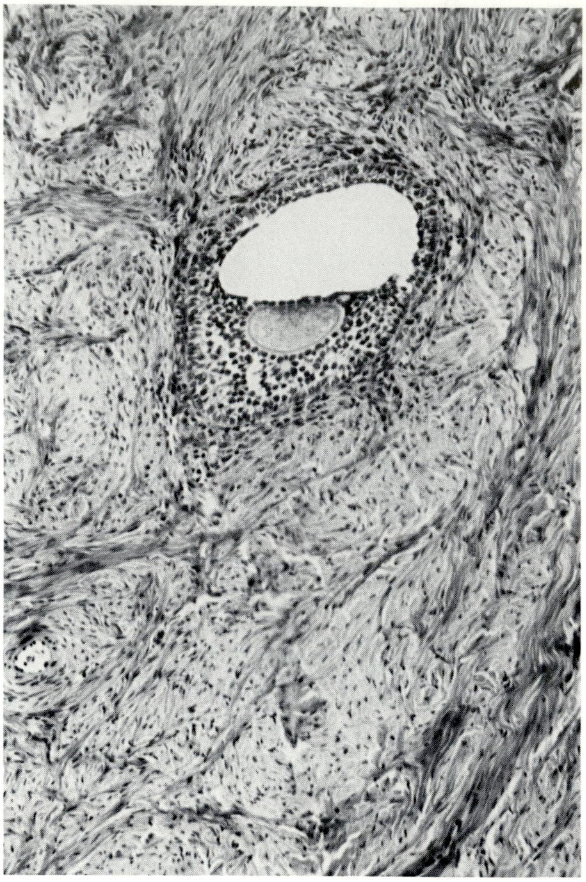

FIG. 16.31. Ovarian fibromatosis. Fibrotic ovarian stroma surrounds an antral follicle.

peritoneal fluid is not usually present, with the exception of two patients who had an associated Meigs' syndrome.[129]

Ovarian Fibromatosis. The patients range in age from 13 to 39 years, with an average of 25 years.[440] Clinical manifestations include menstrual abnormalities, abdominal pain, and, less commonly, virilization and hirsutism. An adnexal mass is palpated in the majority. Occasionally, the ovarian enlargement is an incidental finding late in pregnancy or at the time of cesarean section. In some cases, the involved ovary was found twisted on its pedicle at the time of surgery. The endocrine manifestations, including, in several cases, infertility, disappear after oophorectomy, indicating that the lesion produces steroid hormones.

Pathogenesis. The pathogenesis of massive edema is thought to be intermittent torsion of the ovary on its pedicle, causing partial obstruction of venous and lymphatic drainage. Torsion is observed in half the cases of massive edema, and a few cases have been reported in association with obstruction of ovarian lymphatics secondary to metastatic carcinoma within pelvic and paraaortic lymph nodes.[440] Luteinization of the ovarian stromal cells is considered a secondary phenomenon, possible due to an hCG-like substance within the edema fluid.[197,383]

An alternative theory is that the process begins as a stromal proliferation, either fibromatosis or stromal hyperthecosis, that enlarges the ovary, promoting torsion with subsequent edema.[246,440] This interpretation is supported by the clinical similarities and pathologic overlap between massive edema and ovarian fibromatosis. Young and Scully suggest that massive edema is simply ovarian fibromatosis following torsion and accumulation of edema fluid.[440] Similarly, some examples of massive edema in which luteinized stromal cells are present in the same ovary and in the contralateral, edematous or nonedematous ovary may represent cases of stromal hyperthecosis in which one or both ovaries have undergone torsion.

Most of the reported patients with massive edema have been treated by oophorectomy, but a small number have been successfully managed conservatively by wedge resection, with or without fixation of the involved ovary.

A frozen section should be performed on the removed tissue at the time of surgery to exclude a neoplasm. If the lesion is thought to be a malignant tumor, the involved ovary or the larger ovary in cases of bilateral involvement can be removed to avoid the risk of disseminating tumor.[440]

Differential Diagnosis. The differential diagnosis of massive edema includes ovarian neoplasms that may exhibit an edematous or myxoid appearance, most commonly fibroma but also sclerosing stromal tumor,[69] Krukenberg tumor, and the rare ovarian myxoma.[241] Massive edema and fibromatosis are distinguished from a neoplasm by the presence of follicular derivatives visible on both macroscopic and microscopic examination. A neoplasm may be surrounded by a rim of normal ovarian tissue in contrast to massive edema and fibromatosis, which usually diffusely involve the ovarian tissue. Additionally, ovarian fibromas occur in an older age group and are hormonally inactive.

Pregnancy Luteoma

Pregnancy luteoma (PL) is a nonneoplastic lesion characterized by tumor-like ovarian enlargement during pregnancy secondary to solid proliferations of luteinized cells. Approximately 100 cases have been described.*

Gross Appearance. PL is characterized by soft, fleshy, solid, circumscribed, yellow, brown, or gray nodules ranging up to 20 cm, with a median of 6 cm (Fig. 16.32). They are multiple in at least half of the cases and bilateral in a third.[352] Hemorrhagic foci are common. A separate corpus luteum of pregnancy may also be visible. Examination of ovaries days to weeks postpartum reveals focally infarcted lesions or brown puckered scars.[352]

Microscopic Appearance. The circumscribed nodules are composed of large, polygonal, luteinized cells growing in a diffuse, trabecular, or follicular pattern, the last associated with spaces containing colloid-like material (Fig. 16.33 and 16.34a). The cytoplasm is abundant, eosinophilic, and granular and contains little or no lipid (Fig. 16.34b). Rare cases may exhibit small numbers of intracellular colloid droplets similar to those seen in corpora lutea of pregnancy (see Chapter 15, Anatomy and Histology of Ovary). Although nuclear atypism is minimal, the nuclei are usually somewhat larger and more pleomorphic and hyperchromatic than the adjacent luteinized stromal cells.[291] Nucleoli are usually prominent. The mitotic rate is usually low (range 0 to 7 mitoses/10 HPF), and rare abnormal mitoses may be seen.[291,382] The stroma between the cells is scant, and reticulum fibrils surround groups of cells in an organoid pattern.

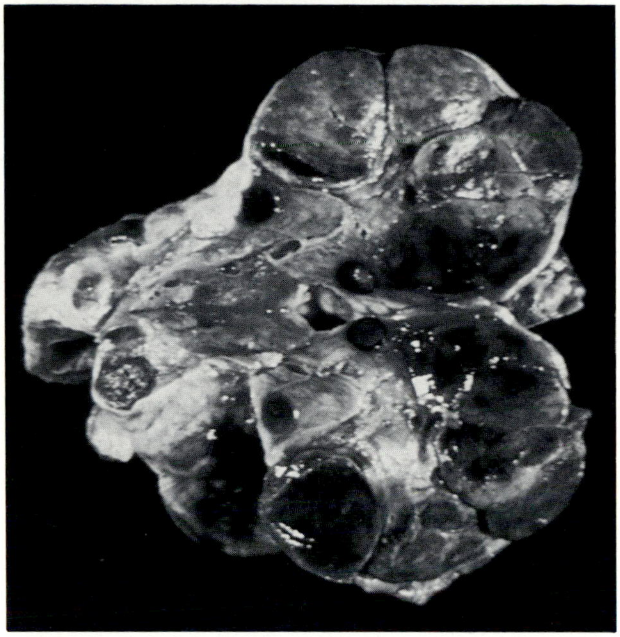

FIG. 16.32. Pregnancy luteoma. Multiple, solid, circumscribed, focally hemorrhagic nodules replace the normal parenchyma. [Courtesy of Dr. R.E. Scully. Reprinted by permission of Clement (1985) In: Contemporary Issues in Surgical Pathology, Vol 6. Roth, Czernobilsky (eds). New York, Churchill Livingstone.]

Ultrastructual examination has shown the characteristic features of steroid-producing cells.[135] Occasional PLs that have been examined several weeks postpartum exhibit cellular degeneration, necrosis, inflammation, and fibrosis.[352,383]

Clinical Aspects. The majority of patients are in their third or fourth decade, black, and multiparous. Most patients are usually asymptomatic, with the ovarian enlargement being discovered incidentally at term during cesarean section or postpartum tubal ligation. Rarely, a pelvic mass may be palpable or cause obstruction of the birth canal. In approximately 25% of patients during the latter half of pregnancy, there is onset of virilization or exacerbation of hirsutism that was present before pregnancy. Two thirds of female infants born to virilized mothers also show virilization, typically manifested by clitoromegaly and labial fusion.[136,410] Regression of the enlarged ovaries usually begins within days after delivery, and they become normal in size within several weeks. In rare cases, PLs may develop during consecutive pregnancies.[136,206] The diagnosis is made by excisional biopsy of one nodule. Since PL is a benign, self-limited condition, no treatment is required.

Plasma testosterone[283,410,432,442] and other androgens[442] may reach levels 70 times above normal in virilized patients. Elevated testosterone has also been

* References 136, 291, 309, 324, 382, 383, 399.

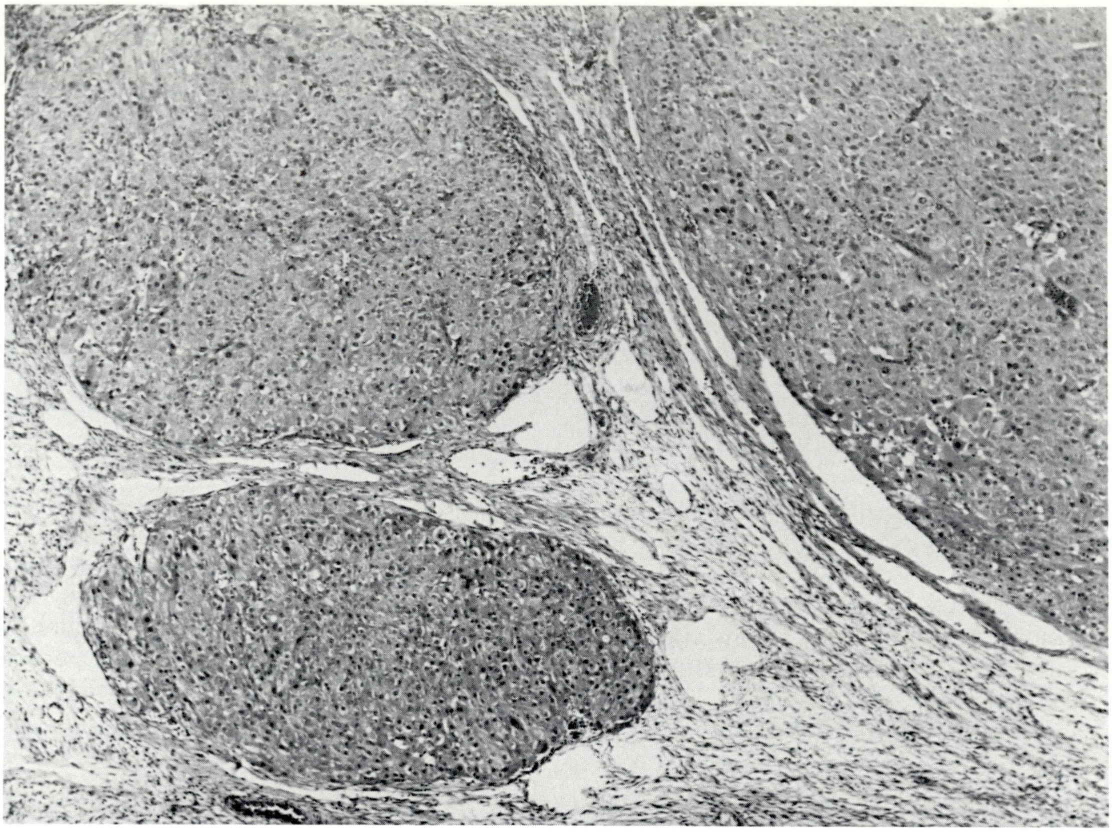

FIG. 16.33. Pregnancy luteoma. Three solid nodules of luteinized cells are present. [Reprinted by permission of Clement (1985) In: Contemporary Issues in Surgical Pathology, Vol 6. Roth, Czernobilsky (eds). New York, Churchill Livingstone.]

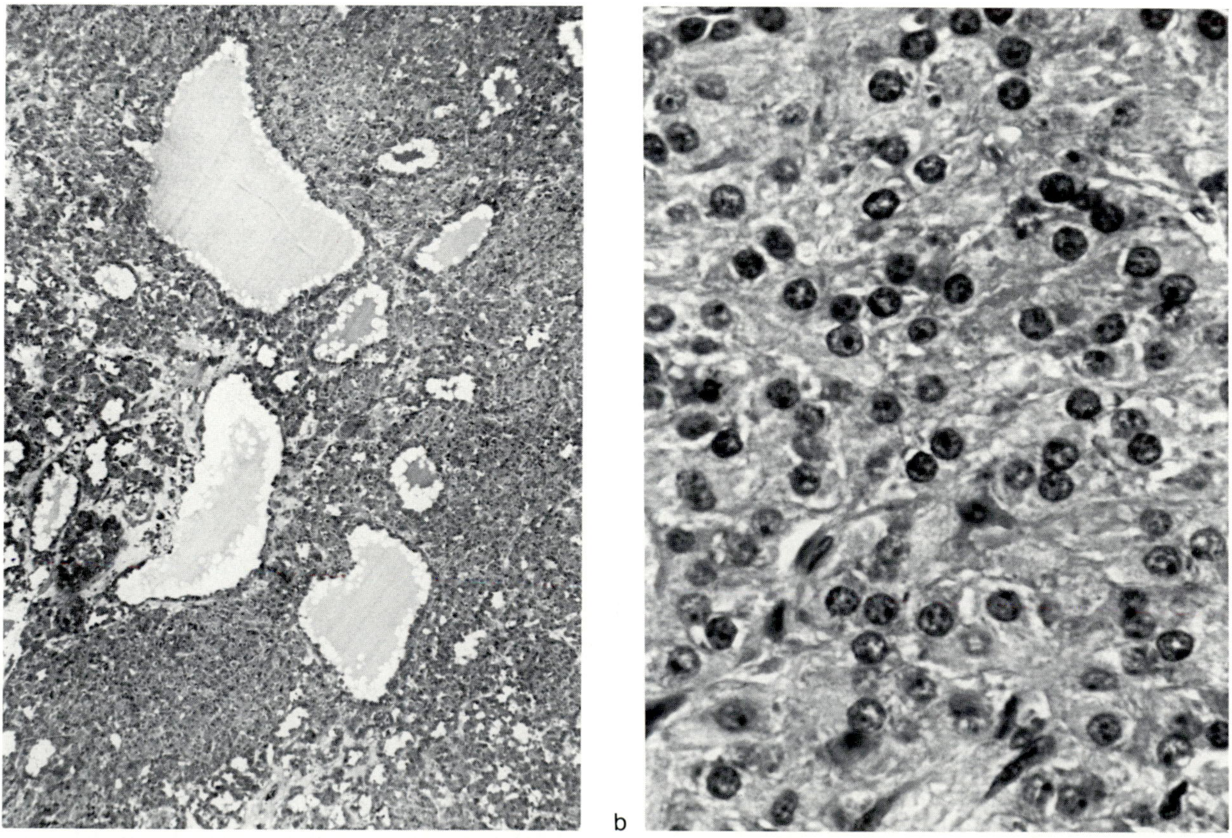

a

b

FIG. 16.34. Pregnancy luteoma. *a*. Follicular pattern. *b*. Solid growth pattern of polygonal luteinized cells.

demonstrated in nonvirilized patients.[283] The hormone levels decrease rapidly after delivery, usually reaching normal concentrations within 2 weeks postpartum. Besides the high circulating levels of testosterone, virilization of the mother may be due to a decrease in testosterone-binding proteins, with a resultant increase in the biologically active unbound fraction.[410,432] Androgen levels in infants may be increased but are usually lower than maternal levels[410] or normal.[283] Since the placenta aromatizes androgens to estrogens, virilization of female infants is unusual. When it does occur, this aromatization may be defective, or the androgen load exceeds the aromatization capacity of the placenta.[163,283]

Pathogenesis. PLs most likely arise from hCG-induced proliferations of luteinized ovarian stromal cells,[382] a conclusion favored by in vitro incubation studies that have shown that luteoma cells resemble ovarian stromal cells in their steroidogenic capacity.[296,324] Some authors, however, have favored origin from luteinized follicular granulosa and theca cells.[291] The condition appears dependent on hCG for its structural and functional integrity, although in contrast to hyperreactio luteinalis, it is not usually found in women with gestational trophoblastic disease. The occasional history of hirsutism antedating the pregnancy suggests the possibility that a preexistent endocrinopathy (such as stromal hyperthecosis or PCO) may predispose to the development of the lesion in some patients.[352]

Differential Diagnosis. Although a number of lesions composed of luteinized cells occurring during pregnancy may resemble PL on microscopic examination, the gross appearance of PL characterized by multiple, bilateral, solid, brown nodules is quite distinctive. Thus, a large, solitary, luteinized follicle cyst of pregnancy and puerperium, hyperreactio luteinalis, and corpus luteum of pregancy are easily identified. Solid primary neoplasms composed partially or entirely of luteinized cells, such as granulosa tumors, thecomas, and steroid cell tumors, may occur during pregnancy and, therefore, should be included in the differential diagnosis. Such tumors will almost always be unilateral and solitary compared to the more frequent bilaterality and multinodularity of the PL. The partly luteinized group, that is, luteinized granulosa cell tumors and luteinized thecomas, will always contain more typical nonluteinized foci and usually have denser reticulum patterns and more abundant intracellular lipid than seen in PL. Entirely luteinized tumors belonging to the steroid (lipid) cell category may closely resemble PL histologically. Features favoring a steroid cell neoplasm include a dense reticulum pattern, intracellular lipid, lipochrome pigment, and, in Leydig cell tumors, a hilar location and the presence of crystals of Reinke (see Chapter 19, Sex Cord–Stromal Ovarian Tumors).

Leydig Cell Hyperplasia

Leydig cells typically occur in the ovarian hilus (hilus cells), where they can be found in virtually all adult ovaries, typically intermingled with nonmyelinated nerves. A minority of cells typically contain specific crystals of Reinke (see Chapter 15, Anatomy and Histology of Ovary).[380] Rarely, Leydig cells can be found in nonhilar locations, either within the ovarian stroma or in extra-ovarian sites, such as the lamina propria or adventitia of the fallopian tube.[172,227]

Hilar Leydig Cell Hyperplasia

On histologic examination, hilar Leydig cell hyperplasia is characterized by an increased number of cells in a nodular or diffuse arrangement, increased cell size, the presence of mitotic figures, cellular and nuclear pleomorphism, hyperchromasia, and multinucleation (Fig. 16.35).[386] Mild hyperplasia, usually unassociated with clinical endocrine disturbance, is found commonly in postmenopausal women.[352] More severe degrees of hyperplasia, often associated with virilization, may occur

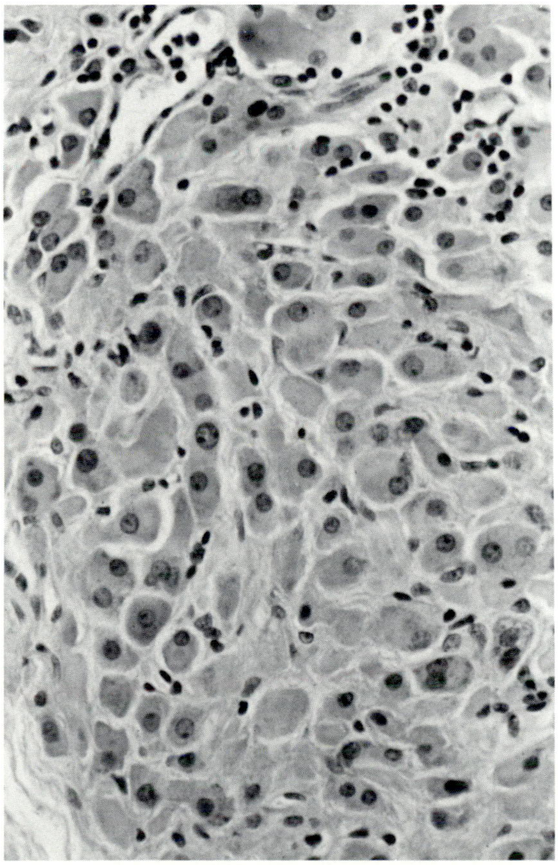

FIG. 16.35. Hilar cell hyperplasia. Cells exhibit mild nuclear pleomorphism and multinucleation. No crystals are seen in this field.

in younger women, with[386] or without[97,266,380] an associated pregnancy. In some cases, elevated serum testosterone levels have been reported.[266]

Hilar Leydig cell hyperplasia may be associated with one or more other ovarian lesions, including stromal hyperplasia, stromal hyperthecosis, stromal Leydig cell hyperplasia, and hilar Leydig cell neoplasia.[97,380,381,385] One case of hilar cell hyperplasia has been associated with the gonadotropin-resistant ovary syndrome.[266]

Stromal Leydig Cell Hyperplasia

Rarely, nonneoplastic transformation of ovarian stromal cells to crystal-containing Leydig cells may be seen (Fig. 16.36). This may occur as a focal microscopic finding in ovaries exhibiting otherwise typical stromal hyperthecosis.[385] In one such case, there was coexistent bilateral hilar Leydig cell hyperplasia and bilateral hilar Leydig cell tumors.[385] It has been suggested that stromal Leydig cells may be the cell of origin for rare stromal neoplasms that contain Leydig cells.[330,385,444] Crystal-containing Leydig cells have also been rarely described within the nonneoplastic stroma of a variety of ovarian neoplasms, including mucinous and serous cystadenomas,[139] Brenner tumors,[157] struma ovarii,[383,444] and strumal carcinoid tumors.[444]

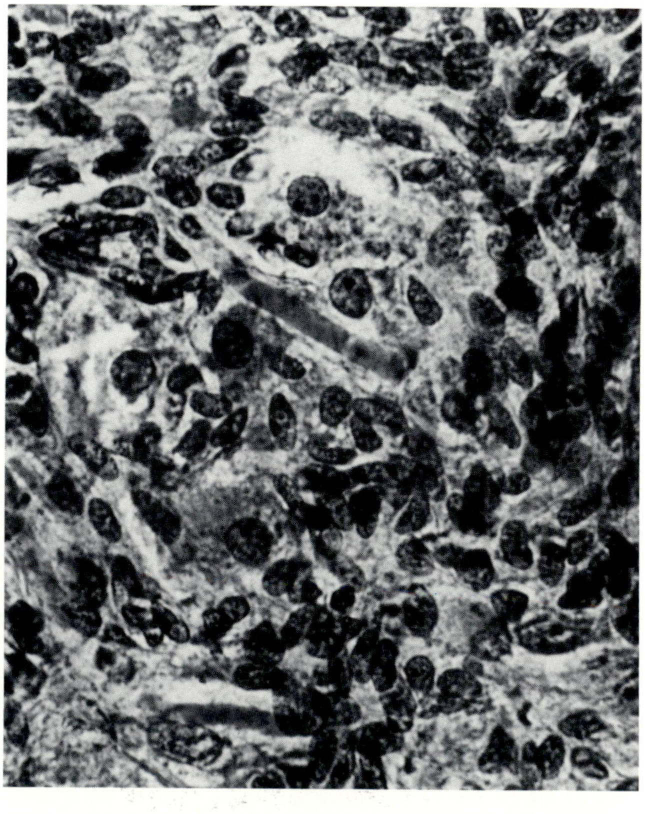

FIG. 16.36. Stromal Leydig cells. Occasional crystal-containing Leydig cells are present within the ovarian stroma. (Reprinted by permission of Sternberg, Roth, Ref. 385.)

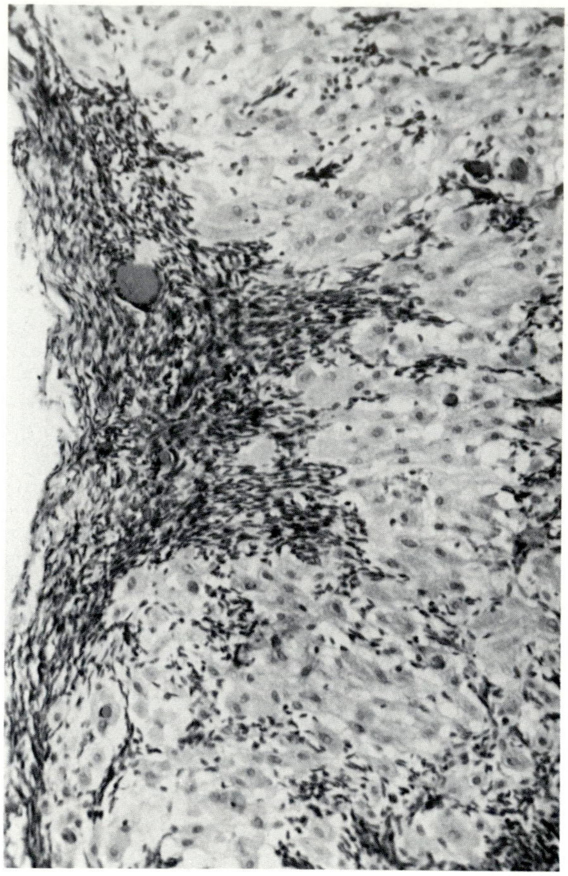

FIG. 16.37. Ovarian decidual reaction within the ovarian stroma.

Ovarian Stromal Metaplasias Including Decidual Reaction

The ovarian stromal cell has the potential to differentiate, presumably by a process of metaplasia, into a variety of other mesenchymal cell types, most commonly decidua but rarely smooth muscle, fat, and bone.

Ovarian Decidual Reaction

An ectopic decidual reaction may be encountered within the ovarian stroma as an isolated finding or as part of a more widespread decidual transformation of the subperitoneal pelvic mesenchyme (Chapter 17, Endometriosis).* The decidual foci may be visible on macroscopic examination as small, soft, reddish subserosal nodules, ridges, or patches that tend to bleed easily on contact.[35,166,189,377] More frequently, however, the decidua is an incidental finding on microscopic examination. The process typically involves the stroma of the superficial cortex beneath the ovarian surface epithelium (Fig. 16.37). The decidualized cells occur singly, as small nodules, or confluent

* References 35, 42, 166, 189, 322, 377.

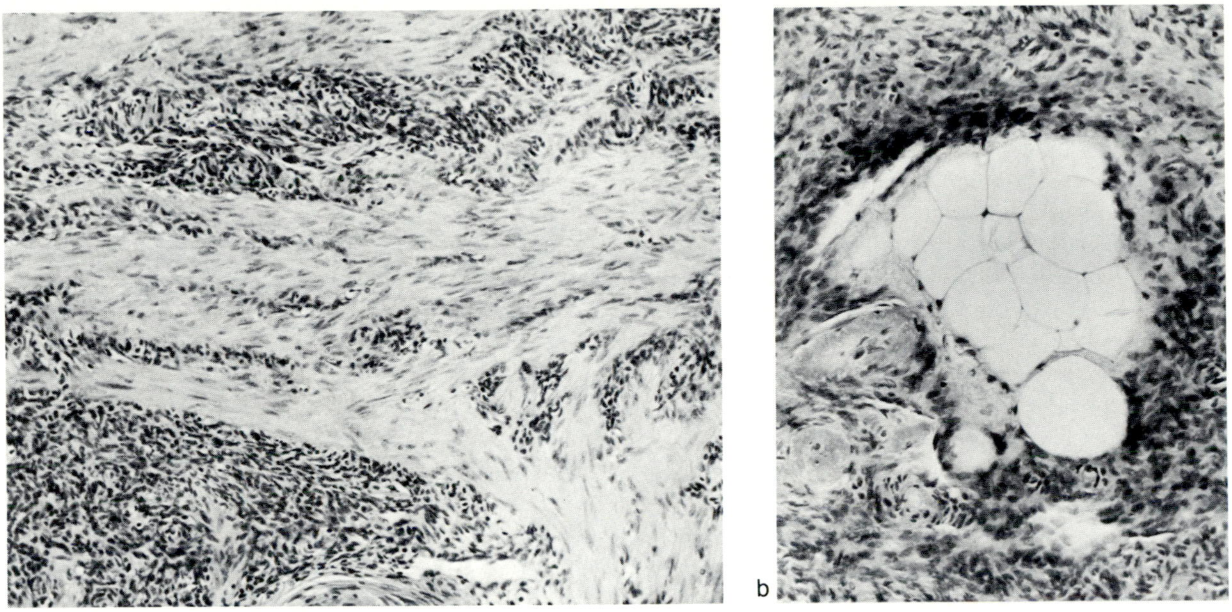

FIG. 16.38. Ovarian stromal metaplasia. *a.* Foci of smooth muscle separated by ovarian stromal cells. *b.* A focus of adipose tissue within the ovarian stroma.

sheets and may form small, polypoid projections from the ovarian surface.[166,189] The cells are indistinguishable from eutopic decidua on light microscopic examination and have a similar ultrastructure (Chapter 9, Anatomy and Histology of Uterine Corpus).[166] Cells transitional in appearance between spindle-shaped ovarian stromal cells and fully decidualized cells are usually present.[35] In some cases, ultrastructural examination has revealed cells exhibiting smooth muscle differentiation and intercellular collagen fibrils.[165] A rich vascular network of distended capillaries and a sprinkling of lymphocytes are typically found within the decidual foci.[189,352] Florid examples, particularly if the decidual cells show focal cytologic atypia, can simulate metastatic carcinoma on histologic examination.[42] Degenerative changes within the decidua are typically seen postpartum.

As in other sites of the secondary müllerian system, an ovarian decidual reaction usually represents a response of the indigenous stromal cells to high circulating or local levels of estrogen and progesterone.[55] The process is seen most commonly during pregnancy, occurring as early as the ninth week of gestation, and by term is a finding present in virtually all ovaries.[42,166,189,377] Less commonly, it may occur in association with trophoblastic disease, in patients treated with progestagens, in the vicinity of a corpus luteum, and in association with hormonally active neoplastic and nonneoplastic lesions of the ovaries and adrenal glands.[35,55,294,352] Prior ovarian radiation may be a predisposing factor by increasing the sensitivity of the stromal cells to the hormonal stimulation.[294] Occasionally foci of ectopic decidua may occur within the ovaries of pre- and postmenopausal women with no obvious cause.[35,294]

Rarer Ovarian Stromal Metaplasias

Foci of metaplastic smooth muscle may be rarely encountered in the ovarian stroma, not only within otherwise normal ovaries, but also within those exhibiting stromal hyperthecosis or sclerocystic changes (Fig. 16.38a).[179,353] Smooth muscle may also be found in the stroma surrounding cysts of various types.[353] Foci of mature fat have been described as a rare incidental histologic finding within the subcapsular ovarian stroma in obese, but otherwise normal women (Fig. 16.38b).[160,173] Heterotopic bone formation in the ovary in the absence of an ovarian neoplasm is also unusual, typically occurring within periovarian adhesions or the walls of endometriotic cysts but rarely within otherwise normal ovaries.[141,362]

Disorders of Premature Ovarian Failure

Premature ovarian failure (POF) is a result of a variety of disorders that lead to the onset of secondary amenorrhea and infertility before the age of 35–40.* POF is uncommon, accounting for only 4–7 % of patients with secondary amenorrhea.[334,336] The ovarian failure is usually permanent, but occasionally subsequent pregnancy

* References 13, 52, 85, 87, 320–321, 336, 376, 401, 404.

occurs.[5,295,321] The patients typically have a 46XX karyotype, although occasional patients with an otherwise typical presentation have had chromosomal abnormalities, usually 47XXX (pure or mosaic), but occasionally 45X0/46XX.[52,334,411] Some authors, however, exclude such cases from the category of POF so that it includes only "chromosomally competent" patients.[13] Individuals with POF typically have normal secondary sexual characteristics. Less commonly, the ovarian failure is complete or nearly complete before puberty, and these patients have primary amenorrhea or oligomenorrhea and incompletely developed secondary sexual features. POF, therefore, probably represents a continuum in which patients may be affected at any age before the expected age of menopause.[321] In contrast to patients with POF, patients with gonadal dysgenesis (see Chapter 2, Abnormal Sexual Development) typically have an abnormal karyotype and an absence of ovarian tissue (streak gonads, abdominal testes), as well as primary amenorrhea, ambiguous internal and external genitalia, and somatic abnormalities.

The absence or decline in follicular activity in patients with POF results in low serum estrogen levels, often accompanied by estrogen withdrawal symptoms. Because of the failure of negative feedback, the low estrogen levels lead to elevated levels of pituitary gonadotropins, a feature that is essential in differentiating POF from central causes of amenorrhea related to hypothalamic or pituitary dysfunction.[336]

If the evaluation of a patient with hypergonadotropic POF is to include microscopic examination of ovarian tissue, the latter should be obtained by bilateral generous wedge biopsies at the time of laparotomy.[321] At least three histologic patterns have been recognized corresponding to true premature menopause, resistant ovary syndrome, and autoimmune oophoritis. It is not known with certainty, however, if each represents a distinct disorder or a nonspecific morphologic manifestation of a number of different disorders.[336]

True Premature Menopause

This disorder is characterized by ovaries that are typically small on gross inspection and may resemble streak gonads. On microscopic examination, the ovaries exhibit premature follicular depletion, resembling normal perimenopausal or postmenopausal ovaries with complete, or nearly complete, absence of primordial and developing follicles (Fig. 16.39).[52,210,336,443] Follicles in varying stages of atresia and stigmata of prior ovulation exclude a streak gonad.

The etiology and pathogenesis of premature menopause are unknown in most cases. Postulated pathogenetic mechanisms include a decreased number of ovarian germ cells at birth, acceleration of normal follicular atresia, or prepubertal or postpubertal destruction of germ cells.[334] The last mechanism accounts for POF secondary to cytotoxic drugs or radiation and previous mumps oophoritis. Because mumps oophoritis is probably clinically occult in the majority of cases, it may be a more frequent cause of premature menopause (including familial cases) than is generally suspected.[9,276] Other familial cases appear to be due to a genetic (probably autosomal dominant) abnormality.[90,258,371] Galactosemia may also play a role in some patients. Finally, there is evidence to implicate immunologic factors in some women. A varying proportion of cases have been associated with antiovarian antibodies, autoimmune disorders, or both. Similar antibodies, however, have been described in premenopausal patients without overt ovarian failure and in women who have undergone menopause at a normal age.[87,335] Some or all of these cases with antiovarian antibodies and a pattern of premature follicular depletion may represent an end-stage of autoimmune oophoritis and are considered further in that section.[335,336] Some patients have a decreased ratio of inducer/helper lymphocytes to suppressor/cytotoxic lymphocytes, as well as a decreased concentration of serum IgA, suggesting a mild suppression of immune competence.[127] Depletion of primordial follicles has been described in several women with ataxia telangiectasia, which may be related to their severe immunosuppression or to their athymic state.[56,127,271] Athymic mice have been shown to have low neonatal gonadotropin levels, an abnormality that is believed to

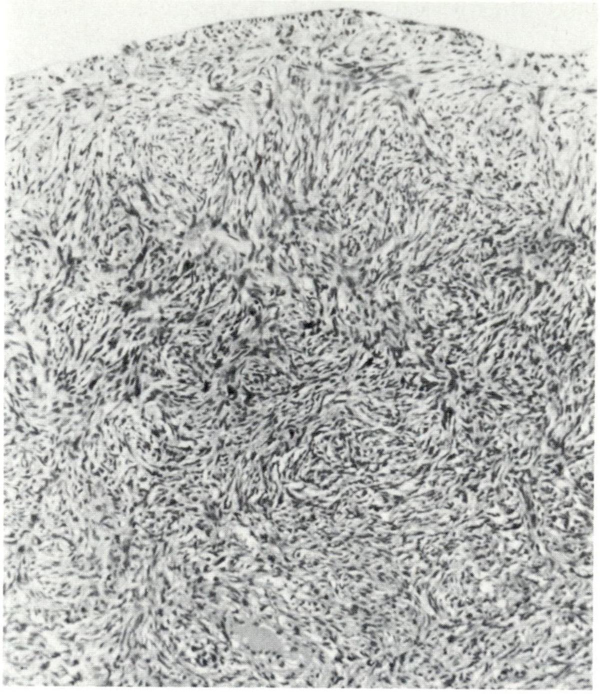

FIG. 16.39. True premature menopause. No primordial or maturing follicles are present within the stroma.

result in the disorganized folliculogenesis and premature follicular depletion seen in these animals. The existence of a thymic–ovarian–pituitary–hypothalamic axis has been suggested in human females.[127]

Resistant Ovary Syndrome

This rare syndrome, which is found in approximately 20% of patients with POF, is characterized by primary or secondary amenorrhea, endogenous hypergonadotropinemia, and resistance to exogenous gonadotropins, often in massive doses.* The resistance to endogenous and exogenous gonadotropins may be relative or absolute, episodic or chronic.

The ovaries typically have a normal prepubertal or adult appearance on macroscopic inspection. Histologic examination reveals an appropriate number of normal-appearing primordial follicles but a complete, or nearly complete, absence of developing follicles. Atretic follicles and stigmata of prior ovulation may be seen. Three patients have been described in whom many of the atretic follicles exhibited central calcification within the space normally occupied by the ovum.[148] A histologic pattern similar to that in the resistant ovary syndrome occurs in morbid obesity,[122] Cushing's syndrome,[182] and hypogonadotropic ovarian failure secondary to hypothalamic–pituitary dysfunction.[329]

The pathogensis of this disorder is not yet established, but a possible deficiency of FSH and LH receptors within the ovary, the presence of antibodies to these receptors, and a postreceptor defect have been postulated.[212,395] In one study, circulating autoimmune antibodies to thyroglobulin and smooth muscle were found.[336] An IgG-like substance that alters FSH receptors and thereby impairs binding of this hormone has been found in the serum of several patients with associated myasthenia gravis.[73,111,218]

The presence of galactosemia in some patients with POF suggests that it may play a pathogenetic role. Approximately two thirds of females with galactosemia in one study had POF. In many such patients, dietary treatment of galactosemia had been delayed.[202] Only one reported patient with galactosemia and POF had an ovarian biopsy performed, and a resistant ovary pattern was found.[336] In one series of galactosemic patients who were not biopsied, however, a number of patients were found to have severely atrophic ovaries, suggesting that in some of these patients, the histologic pattern may be that of true premature menopause (follicular depletion).[202] Galactose or its metabolites may exert a direct toxic effect on the ovary or interfere with gonadotropin-receptor sites or steroidogenesis after binding.[202,336]

Autoimmune Oophoritis

Autoimmune oophoritis is a rare disorder characterized by the presence of a folliculotrophic lymphoid infiltrate that affects atretic follicles, developing follicles, and corpora lutea. The intensity of the infiltrate increases with the degree of follicular maturation (Fig. 16.40).[89,147,186,188,336] The inflammatory infiltrate consists predominantly of lymphocytes and plasma cells, but eosinophils, histiocytes, and, rarely, sarcoid-like granulomas[336] have been described. The theca interna layer of the involved follicles is typically more intensely infiltrated than the granulosa layer and may be focally destroyed. Primordial and preantral follicles are typically present but uninvolved. Lymphoid infiltrates have been found in the ovarian hilus in a perineural distribution in one patient. No Leydig cells were identifiable, and it was postulated that they had been destroyed by the inflammatory process.[147]

Less than a dozen patients with autoimmune oophoritis

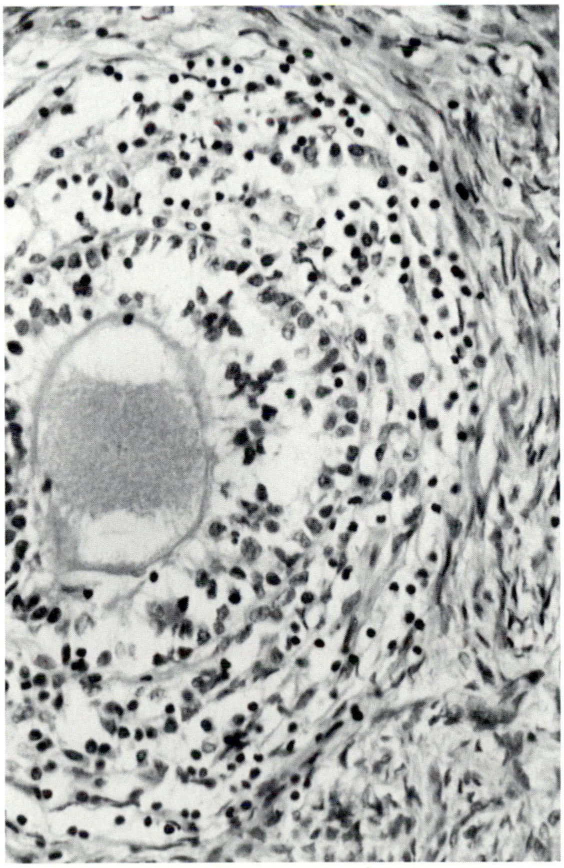

FIG. 16.40. Autoimmune oophoritis. A maturing follicle is infiltrated by mononuclear inflammatory cells.

* References 5, 52, 66, 100, 209, 210, 212, 228, 336, 378, 395.

have been verified histologically.[89,147,186,188,336] Most such patients have had steroid cell antibodies in their sera as well as idiopathic Addison's disease. The latter may arise at the same time or subsequent to the ovarian failure and is associated in at least some patients with lymphocytic adrenalitis. The steroid cell antibodies, which are rare in the general population, belong to a group of antibodies reactive with a range of antigens in steroid-producing cells.[184] They are typically reactive against adrenal cortex, but in some cases also to theca interna, corpus luteum, thyroid epithelium (and thyroglobulin), gastric parietal cells, and thymocytes, alone or in combination.* By their immunofluorescent staining properties with normal tissues and adsorption studies, it has been shown that some of the antiovarian antibodies are cross-reactive with antigens in the adrenal cortex.[184,186–188] Steroid cell antibodies have been shown to be cytotoxic to human granulosa cells in tissue culture.[263] It is likely, however, that cell-mediated immune mechanisms also play a pathogenetic role.[106]

Autoimmune oophoritis may be considerably more common than the small number of histologically documented cases would suggest. In some series of patients with POF who were not biopsied or in whom a biopsy revealed premature follicular depletion, as many as half the patients had one or more associated autoimmune disorders, most frequently Addison's disease. Conversely, as many as 25% of patients with idiopathic Addison's disease may have POF.[13,86,185,186] Other autoimmune diseases that may occur less commonly in these patients include Hashimoto's thyroiditis, Grave's disease, rheumatoid arthritis, hypoparathyroidism, myasthenia gravis, diabetes mellitus, atrophic gastritis, pernicious anemia, alopecia, vitiligo, hemolytic anemia, idiopathic thrombocytopenic purpura, and sicca syndrome.† A family history of an autoimmune disease was found in 18% of patients in one study who had both POF and an autoimmune disease.[13] Most patients with POF and an associated autoimmune disorder and rarely patients with no evidence of an autoimmune disorder had one or more steroid cell antibodies in their sera. A subgroup of patients with POF have chronic mucocutaneous candidiasis (CMCC) or chronic vaginal candidiasis (CVC), suggesting a defect in T-cell function, possibly secondary to circulating antibodies against T-lymphocytes demonstrable in some of these patients.[255] Patients with CMCC and CVC also frequently have anti-*Candida*, antithymocyte, and antiovarian antibodies, suggesting a shared antigen on these cells.[255] These findings suggest that some patients with the pattern of premature follicular depletion on biopsy may represent an end-stage of an autoimmune process, possibly autoimmune oophoritis, which is no longer recognizable on histologic examination.

* References 17, 20, 79, 188, 335, 336, 409, 427.

† References 13, 17, 20, 79, 86, 106, 186, 188, 335, 409, 427.

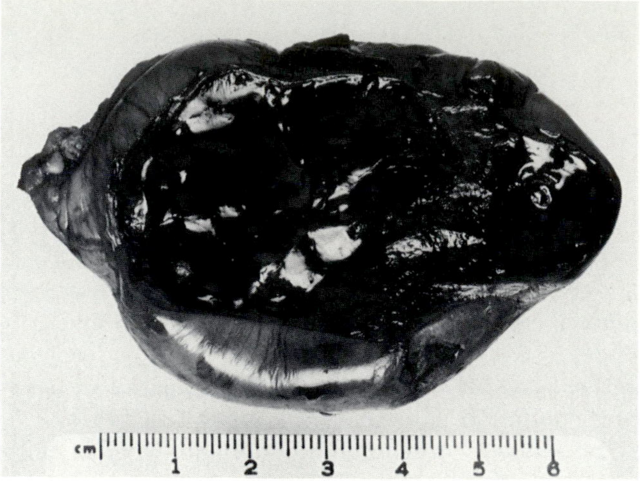

FIG. 16.41. Ovarian hemorrhage. Ovary from a patient being treated with anticoagulation therapy is replaced by a large hematoma.

Vascular Lesions

Ovarian Hemorrhage

Rupture of the normal corpus luteum or a corpus luteum cyst may occasionally result in hemorrhage and, occasionally, fatal hemoperitoneum. Although this may occur in otherwise normal women, it is observed more often in women receiving anticoagulant therapy (Fig. 16.41).[155,257,303,357] The right ovary is the source of the hemorrhage in almost two thirds of patients, and the clinical manifestations frequently resemble those of acute appendicitis.[155]

Ovarian Torsion

Ovarian or adnexal torsion is most frequently a complication of an underlying ovarian lesion, usually a nonneoplastic cyst or benign tumor but rarely a malignant neoplasm.[23,98] Less commonly, torsion of a previously normal ovary may occur, typically in infants or children,[113,152,349] but rarely in adults.[242] The mechanism in such cases is not known, but an unusual degree of adnexal mobility has been noted in children at postmortem examination.[349] Rare examples of bilateral adnexal torsion, synchronous or asynchronous, have been reported.[105]

The patients have clinical findings similar to those of acute appendicitis or recurrent episodes of abdominal pain and, occasionally, a palpable adnexal mass. Laparotomy reveals a swollen, hemorrhagic, and in some cases, infarcted, tuboovarian mass twisted on its pedicle. In rare cases, the torsion and infarction may be asymptomatic.* In such cases, autoamputation may occur, result-

* References 23, 43, 140, 287, 355, 369.

ing in a separate, occasionally calcified, mass lying free or attached to adjacent structures in the peritoneal cavity.

Ovarian Vein Thrombophlebitis

Patients with puerperal ovarian vein thombosis or thrombophlebitis (POVT) typically have, in the first week postpartum, fever and lower abdominal pain and an abdominal mass, almost always on the right side.[11,60,280] The clinical picture may simulate acute appendicitis. At operation, the involved ovarian vein is markedly enlarged, and the thrombus usually extends to the inferior vena cava on the right or to the renal vein on the left. Rarely, one or both of these structures may also be thrombosed.[26] There is marked edema and inflammation of the surrounding retroperitoneal tissues. The ipsilateral ovary is usually congested but not infarcted, although asymptomatic bilateral ovarian infarction in a postpartum patient secondary to massive pelvic venous thrombosis has been reported.[138] Some cases of POVT may be associated with the ovarian vein syndrome.

Most cases of POVT are secondary to bacterial spread from puerperal endomyometritis.[280] The marked right-sided predominance is explained on the basis of retrograde venous flow in the left ovarian vein during the puerperium, protecting that side from bacterial spread from the uterus.[280] One apparently unique case of POVT was proven on histologic examination to be secondary to amniotic fluid embolism.[207]

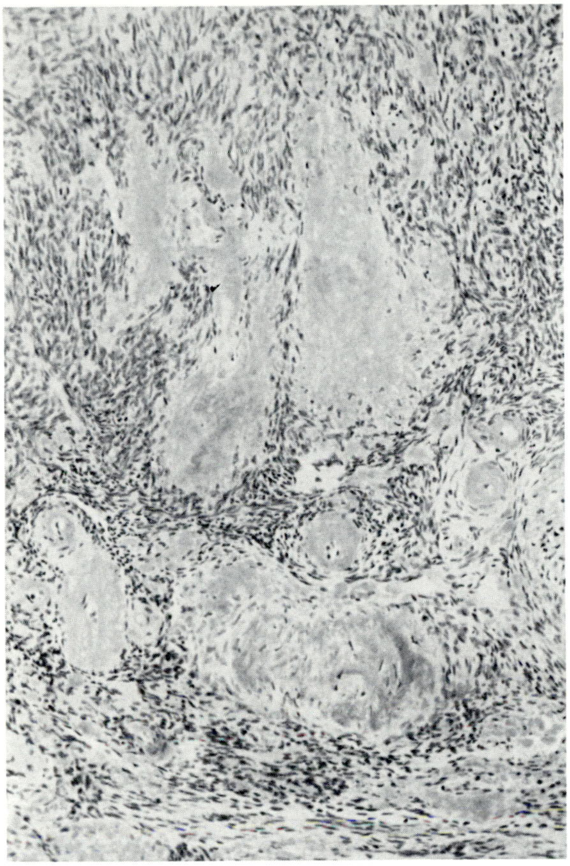

FIG. 16.42. Ovarian amyloidosis. Amyloid deposits in ovarian stroma and vessels.

Rare Vascular Lesions

Rare examples of retroperitoneal hemorrhage secondary to rupture of an ovarian artery or vein, typically during pregnancy or the puerperium, have been reported.[64,153,190] In some cases, the rupture represents a complication of an aneurysm of the ovarian artery.[64,190]

Varicosities of the ovarian vein, almost always on the right side, may occur in pregnant or parous women and cause ipsilateral ureteric compression and pyelonephritis, constituting the so-called ovarian vein syndrome.[176] Other ovarian vascular lesions include ovarian arteritis[180,238] and ovarian arteriovenous fistulas as a complication of gynecologic surgery.[392]

Changes Secondary to Metabolic Diseases

Amyloidosis may rarely involve the ovaries, typically being an incidental histologic finding in patients with systemic amyloidosis (Fig. 16.42).[174,251] There has been a single case of tumorous amyloidosis confined to the ovary that was associated with endometriosis in that site.[338]

Rare cases of ovarian enlargement secondary to involvement by systemic storage disorders (lipidoses, mucopolysaccharidoses) have been reported.[102,414] In such cases, the stored material is typically within macrophages, allowing histologic distinction from a steriod cell tumor and from foci of mature adipose tissue within the ovarian stroma. An autopsy study in patients with diabetes mellitus revealed atrophic and fibrotic changes in the ovaries more frequently than in ovaries from control patients, although the differences were not statistically significant.[126]

In contrast to frequent testicular involvement in hemochromatosis in which hemosiderin is typically seen within walls of testicular vessels,[254] pathologic changes in the ovary secondary to this disorder appear to be rare or nonexistent.

Changes Secondary to Cytotoxic Drugs and Radiation

Cytotoxic Drugs

Cytotoxic drugs used in the treatment of malignant neoplasms (and rarely other disorders) may be associated with a variety of histologic changes in the ovary. These

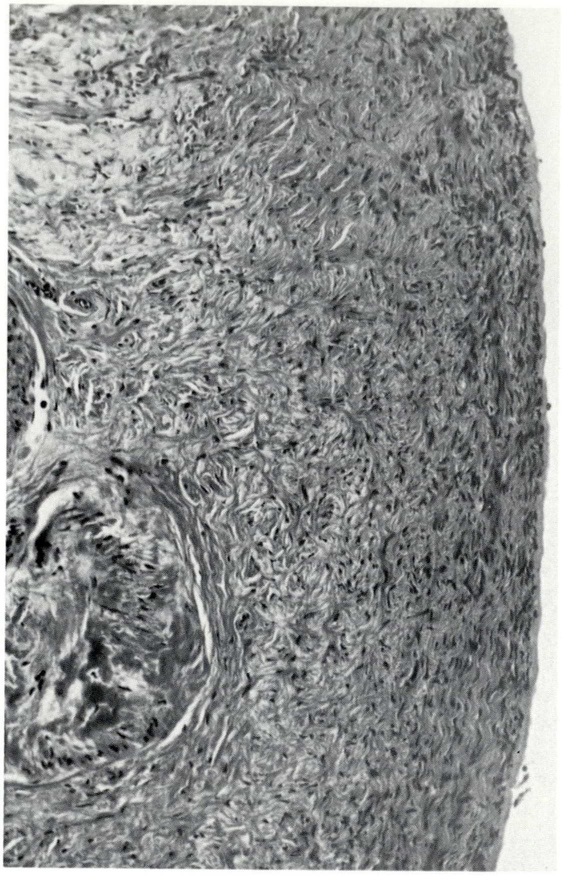

FIG. 16.43. Radiation changes. The ovarian stroma is fibrotic, and blood vessels are hyalinized.

include, in both prepubertal and postpubertal patients, focal or diffuse cortical fibrosis, impaired follicular maturation, and a reduction or depletion in follicle numbers.* Some studies have shown a direct correlation between the severity of these changes and the duration of the chemotherapy, the number of drugs, and malnourishment of the patients.[169,286] These morphologic findings are consistent with clinical observations of diminished ovarian endocrine function or ovarian failure in some of these patients.† The risk of ovarian failure appears to be greater in patients in whom treatment is begun after the age of 25.[37,344] In rare cases, the ovarian failure may be reversible after cessation of the therapy.[368,413]

Radiation

The ovary is among the most radiosensitive of organs. Relatively low doses of radiation (500–600 R) to the ovaries are associated with complete or nearly complete disappearance of primordial and developing follicles, fibrosis of the ovarian stroma, and vascular sclerosis in over 90% of patients (Fig. 16.43).[27,121,151,168,333] Follow-up studies of both adult and pediatric patients who received pelvic radiation have shown that ovarian failure occurs in the majority of such patients.[103,168,358,388] The ovarian stroma appears to be more radioresistant than the follicles and may continue to secrete androgens after radiation.[192]

* References 168, 169, 217, 275, 286, 413, 416.
† References 37, 72, 275, 344, 368, 413, 422.

References

1. Abraham GE, Buster JE (1976) Peripheral and ovarian steroids in ovarian hyperthecosis. Obstet Gynecol 47: 581–586
2. Adashi EY, Hsueh AJW, Yen SSC (1981) Insulin enhancement of luteinizing hormone and follicle-stimulating hormone release by cultured pituitary cells. Endocrinology 108: 1441–1449
3. Adelman S, Benson CD, Hertzler JH (1975) Surgical lesions of the ovary in infancy and childhood. Surg Gynecol Obstet 141: 219–222
4. Aikat BK, Radhakrishnan VV, Rao MS (1973) Malakoplakia—a report of two cases with review of the literature. Ind J Pathol Bacteriol 16: 64–70
5. Aiman J, Smentek C (1985) Premature ovarian failure. Obstet Gynecol 66: 9–14
6. Aiman J, Edman CD, Worley RJ, Vellios F, MacDonald PC (1978) Androgen and estrogen formation in women with ovarian hyperthecosis. Obstet Gynecol 51: 1–9
7. Aiman J, Nalick RH, Jacobs A, Porter JC, Edman CD, Vellios F, MacDonald PC (1977) The origin of androgen and estrogen in a virilized postmenopausal woman with bilateral benign cystic teratomas. Obstet Gynecol 49: 695–704
8. Albukerk JN, Berlin M (1976) Unilateral lutein cyst in pregnancy. NY State J Med 76: 259–261
9. Aleem FA (1981) Familial 46,XX gonadal dysgenesis. Fertil Steril 35: 317–320
10. Aleem FA, McIntosh T (1984) Elevated plasma levels of beta-endorphin in a group of women with polycystic-ovarian disease. Fertil Steril 42: 686–689
11. Allan TR, Miller GC II, Wabrek AJ, Burchell RC (1976) Postpartum and postabortal ovarian vein thrombophlebitis. Obstet Gynecol 47: 525–528
12. Almenoff IA (1966) Splenic–gonadal fusion. NY State J Med 66: 1679–1691
13. Alper MM, Garner PR (1985) Premature ovarian failure: Its relationship to autoimmune disease. Obstet Gynecol 66: 27–30
14. Altman LC (1972) Ovarian abscess and vaginal fistula. Obstet Gynecol 40: 321–322
15. Andreoli C, Vischi F (1961) Parotitis and ovaritis. Panminerva Med 3: 358–361
16. Annos T, Taymor ML (1981) Ovarian pathology associated with insulin resistance and acanthosis nigricans. Obstet Gynecol 58: 662–664
17. Appel GB, Holub DA (1976) The syndrome of multiple endocrine gland insufficiency. Am J Med 61: 129–133
18. Arean VM (1956) Manson's schistosomiasis of the female genital tract. Am J Obstet Gynecol 72: 1038–1053

19. Auerbach RD, Kohorn EI, Cornelius EA, Chambers JT (1985) Splenosis: A complicating factor in total abdominal hysterectomy. Obstet Gynecol 65: 65S–68S
20. Ayala A, Canales ES, Karchmer S, Alarcon D, Zarate A (1979) Premature ovarian failure and hypothyroidism associated with sicca syndrome. Obstet Gynecol 53: 98S–101S
21. Ayers JWT (182) Differential response to adrenocorticotropin hormone stimulation in polycystic ovarian disease with high and low dehydroepiandrosterone sulfate levels. Fertil Steril 37: 645–649
22. Azhar H (1977) Primary echinococcal infection of the ovary. Br J Obstet Gynaecol 84: 633
23. Azoury RS, Chehab RM, Mufarrij IK (1980) The twisted adnexa. A clinical pathological review. Diagn Gynecol Obstet 2: 185–191
24. Babaknia A, Calfopoulos P, Jones HW Jr (1976) The Stein-Leventhal syndrome and coincidental ovarian tumors. Obstet Gynecol 47: 223–224
25. Bahary CM, Ovadia Y, Neri A (1967) *Schistosoma mansoni* of the ovary. Am J Obstet Gynecol 98: 290–292
26. Bahnson RR, Wendel EF, Vogelzang RL (1985) Renal vein thrombosis following puerperal ovarian vein thrombophlebitis. Am J Obstet Gynecol 152: 290–291
27. Baker TG (1971) Radiosensitivity of mammalian oocytes with particular reference to the human female. Am J Obstet Gynecol 110: 746–761
28. Bar RS, Muggeo M, Kahn CR, Gorden PH, Roth J (1980) Characterization of insulin receptors in patients with the syndromes of insulin resistance and acanthosis nigricans. Diabetologia 18: 209
29. Barad DH, Gimovsky ML, Petrie RH, Bowe ET (1981) Diagnosis and management of bilateral theca lutein cysts in a normal term pregnancy. Diagn Gynecol Obstet 3: 27–30
30. Barbieri RL, Ryan KJ (1983) Hyperandrogenism, insulin resistance, and acanthosis nigricans syndrome: A common endocrinopathy with distinct pathophysiologic features. Am J Obstet Gynecol 147: 90–101
31. Barbieri RL, Makris A, Ryan KJ (1984) Insulin stimulates androgen accumulation in incubations of human ovarian stroma and theca. Obstet Gynecol 64: 73S–80S
32. Barclay DL, Leverich EB, Kemmerly JR (1969) Hyperreactio luteinalis: Postpartum persistence. Am J Obstet Gynecol 105: 642–644
33. Bardin CW, Lipsett MB, Edgcomb JH, Marshall JR (1967) Studies of testosterone metabolism in a patient with masculinization due to stromal hyperthecosis. N Engl J Med 277: 399–402
34. Barnes ND, Hayles AB, Ryan RJ (1973) Sexual maturation in juvenile hypothyroidism. Mayo Clin Proc 48: 849–856
35. Bassis ML (1956) Pseudodeciduosis. Am J Obstet Gynecol 72: 1029–1037
36. Bates GW, Whitworth NS (1982) Effect of body weight reduction on plasma androgens in obese, infertile women. Fertil Steril 38: 406–409
37. Beard MEJ, Conder JL, Clark VA (1984) Ovarian failure following cytotoxic therapy. NZ Med J 97: 759–762
38. Beckman EN, Holland JB (1981) Ovarian enterobiasis—A proposed pathogenesis. Am J Trop Med Hyg 30: 74–76
39. Belisle S, Lehoux J-G, Benard B, Ainmelk Y (1981) Ovarian hyperthecosis: in vivo and in vitro correlations of the androgen profile. Obstet Gynecol 57: 70S–75S
40. Benirschke K, Bonin ML, Rost T (1984) Plant material in ovary following barium enema (Letter). Arch Pathol Lab Med 108: 359–360
41. Berger NG, Repke JT, Woodruff JD (1984) Markedly elevated serum testosterone in pregnancy without fetal virilization. Obstet Gynecol 63: 260–262
42. Bersch W, Alexy E, Heuser HP, Staemmler HJ (1973) Ectopic decidua formation in the ovary (so-called deciduoma). Virchows Arch [Pathol Anat] 360: 173–177
43. Beyth Y, Bar-On E (1984) Tuboovarian autoamputation and infertility. Fertil Steril 42: 932–934
44. Bhagavan BS, Gupta PK (1978) Genital actinomycosis and intrauterine contraceptive devices. Hum Pathol 9: 567–578
45. Bigelow B (1958) Comparison of ovarian and endometrial morphology spanning the menopause. Obstet Gynecol 11: 487–513
46. Biggs JSG (1981) Polycystic ovarian disease—Current concepts. Aust NZ J Obstet Gynaecol 21: 26–36
47. Biggs JSG, Thomas FJ (1981) Sites of steroid production in the polycystic ovary. Br J Obstet Gynaecol 88: 42–46
48. Blaustein A (1981) Surface cells and inclusion cysts in fetal ovaries. Gynecol Oncol 12: 222–233
49. Blaustein A, Kaganowicz A, Wells J (1982) Tumor markers in inclusion cysts of the ovary. Cancer 49: 722–726
50. Blaustein A, Kantius M, Kaganowicz A, Pervez N, Wells J (1982) Inclusions in ovaries of females aged day 1–30 years. Int J Gynecol Pathol 1: 145–153
51. Bloomfield RD, Suarez JR, Malangit AC (1979) Giant theca-lutein cyst. Am J Obstet Gynecol 133: 459–460
52. Board JA, Redwine FO, Moncure CW, Frable WJ, Taylor JR (1979) Identification of differing etiologies of clinically diagnosed premature menopause. Am J Obstet Gynecol 134: 936–944
53. Boder E, Sedgwick RP (1958) Ataxia–telangiectasia. A familial syndrome of progressive cerebellar ataxia, oculocutaneous telangiectasia and frequent pulmonary infection. Pediatrics 21: 526–554
54. Bonar BE, Rabson AS (1957) Gynecological aspects of leprosy. Obstet Gynecol 9: 33–43
55. Boss JH, Scully RE, Wegner KH, Cohen RB (1965) Structural variations in the adult ovary—Clinical significance. Obstet Gynecol 25: 747–763
56. Bowden DH, Danis PG, Sommers SC (1963) Ataxia–telangiectasia. A case with lesions of ovaries and adenohypophysis. J Neuropathol Exp Neurol 22: 549–554
57. Bower R, Dehner LP, Ternberg JL (1974) Bilateral ovarian cysts in the newborn. A triad of neonatal abdominal masses, polyhydramnios, and maternal diabetes mellitus. Am J Dig Dis 128: 731–733
58. Braithwaite SS, Erkman-Balis B, Avila TD (1978) Postmenopausal virilization due to ovarian stromal hyperthecosis. J Clin Endocrinol Metab 46: 295–300
59. Brooks JJ, Wheeler JE (1977) Granulomatous salpingitis secondary to Crohn's disease. Obstet Gynecol 49: 31S–37S
60. Brown TK, Munsick RA (1971) Puerperal ovarian vein

thrombophlebitis: A syndrome. Am J Obstet Gynecol 109: 263–273
61. Brune WH, Pulaski EJ, Shuey HE (1957) Giant ovarian cyst. Report of a case in a premature infant. N Engl J Med 257: 876–878
62. Burghen GA, Givens JR, Kitabchi AE (1980) Correlation of hyperandrogenism with hyperinsulinism in polycystic ovarian disease. J Clin Endocrinol Metab 50: 113–116
63. Burkman R, Schlesselman S, McCaffrey L, Gupta PK, Spence M (1982) The relationship of genital tract actinomycetes and the development of pelvic inflammatory disease. Am J Obstet Gynecol 143: 585–589
64. Burnett RA, Carfrae DC (1976) Spontaneous rupture of ovarian artery aneurysm in the puerperium. Two case reports and a review of the literature. Br J Obstet Gynaecol 83: 744–750
65. Burt AS (1954) The human hypophysis in ovarian stromal hyperplasia and pregnancy. Cancer 7: 1227–1234
66. Campenhout JV, Vauclair R, Maraghi K (1972) Gonadotropin-resistant ovaries in primary amenorrhea. Obstet Gynecol 40: 6–12
67. Caspi E, Schreyer P, Bukovsky J (1973) Ovarian lutein cysts in pregnancy. Obstet Gynecol 42: 388–398
68. Chalvardjian A (1978) Sarcoidosis of the female genital tract. Am J Obstet Gynecol 132: 78–80
69. Chalvardjian A, Scully RE (1973) Sclerosing stromal tumors of the ovary. Cancer 31: 664–670
70. Chalvardjian A, Picard L, Shaw R, Davey R, Cairns JD (1980) Malacoplakia of the female genital tract. Am J Obstet Gynecol 138: 391–394
71. Chang RJ, Nakamura RM, Judd HL, Kaplan SA (1983) Insulin resistance in nonobese patients with polycystic ovarian disease. J Clin Endocrinol Metab 57: 356–359
72. Chapman RM (1983) Gonadal injury resulting from chemotherapy. Am J Indust Med 4: 149–161
73. Charreau EH, Chiauzzi V, Cigorraga S, Escobar ME, Rivarola M (1982) Immunoglobulin anti FSH receptor in the resistant ovary syndrome. Rec Adv Fertil Res Part A: 111–121
74. Chen KTK, Hendricks EJ (1985) Malacoplakia of the female genital tract. Obstet Gynecol 65: 84S–87S
75. Chen KTK, Kostich ND, Rosai J (1978) Peritoneal foreign body granulomas to keratin in uterine adenoacanthoma. Arch Pathol Lab Med 102: 174–177
76. Chervenak FA, Castadot MJ, Wiederman J, Sedlis A (1980) Massive ovarian edema: Review of world literature and report of two cases. Obstet Gynecol Surv 35: 677–684
77. Chow KK, Choo HT (1984) Ovarian hyperstimulation syndrome with clomiphene citrate. Case report. Br J Obstet Gynaecol 91: 1051–1052
78. Clement PB, Scully RE (1980) Large solitary luteinized follicle cyst of pregnancy and puerperium. Am J Surg Pathol 4: 431–438
79. Collen RJ, Lippe BM, Kaplan SA (1979) Primary ovarian failure, juvenile rheumatoid arthritis, and vitiligo. Am J Dis Child 133: 598–600
80. Collins CG, Nix FG, Cerha HT (1956) Ruptured tuboovarian abscess. Am J Obstet Gynecol 72: 820–829
81. Comite F, Shawker TH, Pescovitz OH, Loriaux DL, Cutler GB Jr (1984) Cyclical ovarian function resistent to treatment with an analogue of luteinizing hormone-releasing hormone in McCune-Albright syndrome. N Engl J Med 311: 1032–1036
82. Coney P (1984) Polycystic ovarian disease: Current concepts of pathophysiology and therapy. Fertil Steril 42: 667–682
83. Cooper HE, Spellacy WN, Prem KA, Cohen WD (1968) Hereditary factors in the Stein-Leventhal syndrome. Am J Obstet Gynecol 100: 371–387
84. Corenblum B, Taylor PJ (1982) The hyperprolactinemic polycystic ovary syndrome may not be a distinct entity. Fertil Steril 38: 549
85. Coulam CB (1982) Premature gonadal failure. Fertil Steril 38: 645–655
86. Coulam CB (1983) The prevalence of autoimmune disorders among patients with primary ovarian failure. Am J Reprod Immunol 4: 63–66
87. Coulam CB, Ryan RJ (1979) Premature menopause I. Etiology. Am J Obstet Gynecol 133: 639–643
88. Coulam CB, Annegers JF, Kranz JS (1983) Chronic anovulation syndrome and associated neoplasia. Obstet Gynecol 61: 403–407
89. Coulam CB, Kempers RD, Randall RV (1981) Premature ovarian failure: Evidence for autoimmune function. Fertil Steril 36: 238–240
90. Coulam CB, Stringfellow S, Hoefnagel D (1983) Evidence for a genetic factor in the etiology of premature ovarian failure. Fertil Steril 40: 693–695
91. Cozzutto C (1981) Uterus-like mass replacing ovary. Arch Pathol Lab Med 105: 508–511
92. Cramer DW, Welch WR, Cassells S, Scully RE (1983) Mumps, menarche, menopause, and ovarian cancer. Am J Obstet Gynecol 147: 1–6
93. Cruikshank SH, Van Drie DM (1982) Supernumerary ovaries: Update and review. Obstet Gynecol 60: 126–129
94. Curry SL, Hammond CB, Tyrey L, Creasman WT, Parker RT (1975) Hydatidiform mole. Diagnosis, management, and long-term follow-up of 347 patients. Obstet Gynecol 45: 1–8
95. Danon M, Robboy SJ, Kim S, Scully RE, Crawford JD (1975) Cushing syndrome, sexual precocity and polyostotic fibrous dysplasia (Albright syndrome) in infancy. J Pediatr 87: 917–921
96. D'Armiento M, Reda G, Camagna A, Tardella L (1983) McCune-Albright syndrome: Evidence for autonomous multiendocrine function. J Pediatr 102: 584–586
97. Davidson BJ, Waisman J, Judd HL (1981) Long-standing virilism in a woman with hyperplasia and neoplasia of ovarian lipidic cells. Obstet Gynecol 58: 753–759
98. Demopoulos RI, Bigelow B, Vasa U (1978) Infarcted uterine adnexa. Associated pathology. NY State J Med 78: 2027–2029
99. Dennefors BL, Janson PO, Knutson F, Hamberger L (1980) Steroid production and responsiveness to gonadotropin in isolated stromal tissue of human postmenopausal ovaries. Am J Obstet Gynecol 136: 997–1002
100. Dewhurst CJ, de Koos EB, Ferreira HP (1975) The resistant ovary syndrome. Br J Obstet Gynaecol 82: 341–345

101. Dillon WP, Dewey M (1981) A case of accessory ovary. Obstet Gynecol 58: 660–661
102. Dincsoy HP, Rolfes DB, McGraw CA, Schubert WK (1984) Cholesterol ester storage disease and mesenteric lipodystrophy. Am J Clin Pathol 81: 263–269
103. Doll R, Smith PG (1968) The long-term effects of x-irradiation in patients treated for metropathia haemorrhagica. Br J Radiol 41: 362–368
104. Dunaif A, Hoffman AR, Scully RE, Flier JS, Longcope C, Levy LJ, Crowley WF Jr (1985) Clinical, biochemical, and ovarian morphologic features in women with acanthosis nigricans and masculinzation. Obstet Gynecol 66: 545–552
105. Dunnihoo DR, Wolff J (1984) Bilateral torsion of the adnexa: A case report and a review of the world literature. Obstet Gynecol 64: 55S–59S
106. Edmonds M, Lamki L, Killinger DW, Volpe R (1973) Autoimmune thyroiditis, adrenalitis and oophoritis. Am J Med 54: 782–787
107. Erickson GF, Hsueh AJW, Quigley ME, Rebar RW, Yen SSC (1979) Functional studies of aromatase activity in human granulosa cells from normal and polycystic ovaries. J Clin Endocrinol Metab 49: 514–519
108. Erkkola R, Seppala P, Klemi PJ (1985) Virilization during pregnancy due to bilateral hyperthecosis. Hormone Res 21: 83–87
109. Eschenbach DA (1980) Epidemiology and diagnosis of acute pelvic inflammatory disease. Obstet Gynecol 55: 142S–152S
110. Eschenbach DA, Harnisch JP, Holmes KK (1977) Pathogenesis of acute pelvic inflammatory disease: role of contraception and other risk factors. Am J Obstet Gynecol 128: 838–850
111. Escobar ME, Cigorraga SB, Chiauzzi VA, Charreau EH, Rivarola MA (1982) Development of gonadotropin-resistant ovary syndrome in myasthenia gravis: Suggestion of similar autoimmune mechanisms. Acta Endocrinol 99: 431–436
112. Evans DJ, Lampert IA (1978) Ovarian involvement by cytomegalovirus (Letter). Hum Pathol 9: 122
113. Evans, JP (1978) Torsion of the normal uterine adnexa in premenarcheal girls. J Pediatr Surg 13: 195–196
114. Evers JLH, Rolland R (1981) Primary hypothyroidism and ovarian activity: Evidence for an overlap in the synthesis of pituitary glycoproteins. Case report. Br J Obstet Gynaecol 88: 195–202
115. Farber ER, Leahy MS, Meadows TR (1968) Endometrial blastomycosis acquired by sexual contact. Obstet Gynecol 32: 195–199
116. Farber M, Daoust PR, Rogers J (1974) Hyperthecosis syndrome. Obstet Gynecol 44: 35–41
117. Farber M, Madanes A, O'Brian D, Millan VG, Turksoy RN, Rule AH (1981) Asymmetric hyperthecosis ovarii. Obstet Gynecol 57: 521–525
118. Fechner RE, Kaufman RH (1974) Endometrial adenocarcinoma in Stein-Leventhal syndrome. Cancer 34: 444–452
119. Ferrannini E, Muggeo M, Navalesi R, Pilo A (1982) Impaired insulin degradation in a patient with insulin resistance and acanthosis nigricans. Am J Med 73: 148–154
120. Fienberg R (1969) The stromal theca cell and postmenopausal endometrial adenocarcinoma. Cancer 24: 32–38
121. Fisher B, Cheung AYC (1984) Delayed effect of radiation therapy with or without chemotherapy on ovarian function in women with Hodgkin's disease. Acta Radiol Oncol 23: 43–48
122. Fisher ER, Gregorio R, Stephan T, Nolan S, Danowski TS (1974) Ovarian changes in women with morbid obesity. Obstet Gynecol 44: 839–844
123. Fitzgerald JA, Berrigan MV (1959) Accurate diagnosis of "ovarian vascular accidents." Review of 32 instances, with clinical conclusions. Obstet Gynecol 13: 175–180
124. FitzGerald TB, Mainwaring AR, Ahmed A (1974) Pelvic peritoneal oxyuriasis simulating metastatic carcinoma. A case report. Br J Obstet Gynaecol 81: 248–250
125. Flier JS, Kahn CR, Roth J (1979) Receptors, antireceptor antibodies and mechanisms of insulin resistance. N Engl J Med 300: 413–419
126. Fraley DS, Totten RS (1968) An autopsy study of endocrine organ changes in diabetes mellitus. Metabolism 17: 896–900
127. Friedman CI, Neff J, Kim MH (1984) Immunologic parameters in premature follicular depletion: T and B lymphocytes, T-cell subpopulations, cutaneous reactivity, and serum immunoglobulin concentrations. Diagn Immunol 2: 48–52
128. Friedman CI, Schmidt GE, Chang FE, Kim MH (1984) Severe ovarian hyperstimulation following follicular aspiration. Am J Obstet Gynecol 150:436–437
129. Fukuda O, Munemura M, Tohya T, Maeyama M, Iwamasa T (1984) Massive edema of the ovary associated with hydrothorax and ascites. Gynecol Oncol 17: 231–237
130. Futterweit W (1983) Pituitary tumors and polycystic ovarian disease. Obstet Gynecol 62: 74S–79S
131. Futterweit W (1985) In: Polycystic Ovarian Disease. Clinical Perspectives in Obstetrics and Gynecology. New York, Springer-Verlag
132. Futterweit W, Scher J, Nunez AE, Strauss L, Rayfield EJ (1983) A case of bilateral dermoid cysts, insulin resistance and polycystic ovarian disease: The association of ovarian tumors with polycystic ovaries with a review of the literature. Mt Sinai J Med 50: 251–255
133. Gabbay-Moore M, Ovadia Y, Neri A (1982) Accessory ovary with bilateral dermoid cysts. Eur J Obstet Gynaecol Reprod Biol 14: 171–173
134. Gallup DG, Stock RJ (1984) Adenocarcinoma of the endometrium in women 40 years of age or younger. Obstet Gynecol 64: 417–419
135. Garcia-Bunuel R, Brandes D (1976) Luteoma of pregnancy: Ultrastructural features. Hum Pathol 7: 205–214
136. Garcia-Bunuel R, Berek JS, Woodruff JD (1975) Luteomas of pregnancy. Obstet Gynecol 45: 407–414
137. Gardner GH, Greene RR, Peckham B (1957) Tumors of the broad ligament. Am J Obstet Gynecol 73: 536–555
138. Gardstein HF Jr, Ferenczy A, Richart RM (1973) Asymptomatic bilateral ovarian infarction and venous thrombosis. Am J Obstet Gynecol 116: 1164–1166
139. Garneau R, Cabanne F (1968) Dysembryome ovarian de type enteroide et biliohepatoide avec hyperplasie functio-

nelle des cellules sympathicotropes de Berger. Ann Anat Pathol (Paris) 13: 423—432
140. Georgy FM, Viechnicki MB (1974) Absence of an ovary and uterine tube. Obstet Gynecol 44: 441–442
141. Gerbie AB, Greene RR, Reis RA (1958) Heteroplastic bone and cartilage in the female genital tract. Obstet Gynecol 11: 573–578
142. Gibson M, Schiff I, Tulchinsky D, Ryan KJ (1980) Characterization of hyperandrogenism with insulin-resistant diabetes type A. Fertil Steril 33: 501–505
143. Girouard DP, Barclay DL, Collins CG (1964) Hyperreactio luteinalis. Review of the literature and report of 2 cases. Obstet Gynecol 23: 513–525
144. Givens JR, Andersen RN, Wiser WL, Donelson AJ, Coleman SA (1975) A testosterone-secreting gonadotropin-responsive pure thecoma and polycystic ovarian disease. J Clin Endocrinol Metab 41: 845–853
145. Givens JR, Kerber IJ, Wiser WL, Andersen RN, Coleman SA, Fish SA (1974) Remission of acanthosis nigricans associated with polycystic ovarian disease and a stromal luteoma. J Clin Endocrinol Metab 38: 347–355
146. Givens JR, Wiser WL, Coleman SA, Wilroy RS, Andersen RN, Fish SA, Watson BS (1971) Familial ovarian hyperthecosis: A study of two families. Am J Obstet Gynecol 110: 959–972
147. Gloor E, Hurlimann J (1984) Autoimmune oophoritis. Am J Clin Pathol 81: 105–109
148. Gloor E, Juillard E, Curchod A, Legeret J (1982) Ovarian hypoplasia with follicular calcifications. Am J Clin Pathol 78: 857–860
149. Goldzieher JW, Green JA (1962) The polycystic ovary. I. Clinical and histologic features. J Clin Endocrinol Metab 22: 325–338
150. Green JA, Goldzieher JW (1965) The polycystic ovary. IV. Light and electron microscope studies. Am J Obstet Gynecol 91: 173–181
151. Gronroos M, Klemi P, Piiroinen O, Erkkola R, Nikkanen V, Ruotsalainen P (1982) Ovarian function during and after curative intracavitary high dose-rate irradiation: Steroidal output and morphology. Eur J Gynecol Reprod Biol 14: 13–21
152. Grosfeld JL (1969) Torsion of the normal ovary in the first two years of life. Am J Surg 117: 726–727
153. Hager WD (1978) Ruptured utero-ovarian vein syndrome: A case report. Am J Obstet Gynecol 131: 697–698
154. Hahn-Pedersen J, Larsen PM (1984) Supernumerary ovary. Acta Obstet Gynecol Scand 63: 365–366
155. Hallatt JG, Steele CH Jr, Snyder M (1984) Ruptured corpus luteum with hemoperitoneum: A study of 173 surgical cases. Am J Obstet Gynecol 149: 5–9
156. Hamblen EC, Baker RD, Martin DS (1935) Blastomycosis of the female reproductive tract with report of a case. Am J Obstet Gynecol 30: 345–356
157. Hameed K (1972) Brenner tumor of the ovary with Leydig cell hyperplasia. Cancer 30: 945–952
158. Hangval H, Habibi H, Moshref A, Rahimi A (1979) Case report of an ovarian hydatid cyst. J Trop Med Hyg 82: 34–35
159. Haning RV Jr, Strawn EY, Nolten WE (1985) Pathophysiology of the ovarian hyperstimulation syndrome. Obstet Gynecol 66: 220–224
160. Hart WR, Abell MR (1970) Adipose prosoplasia of ovary. Am J Obstet Gynecol 106: 929–930
161. Hart WR, Prins RP, Tsai JC (1976) Isolated coccidioidomycosis of the uterus. Hum Pathol 7: 235–239
162. Hatjis CG (1985) Nonimmunologic fetal hydrops associated with hyperreactio luteinalis. Obstet Gynecol 65: 11S–13S
163. Hensleigh PA, Woodruff JD (1978) Differential maternal—fetal response to androgenizing luteoma or hyperreactio luteinalis. Obstet Gynecol Surv 33: 262–271
164. Herbold DR, Frable WJ, Kraus FT (1984) Isolated noninfectious granuloma of the ovary. Int J Gynecol Pathol 2: 380–391
165. Herr JC, Platz CE, Heidger PM Jr, Curet LB (1979) Smooth muscle within ovarian decidual nodules: A link to leiomyomatosis peritonealis disseminata? Obstet Gynecol 53: 451–456
166. Herr JC, Heidger PM Jr, Scott JR, Anderson JW, Curet LB, Mossman HW (1978) Decidual cells in the human ovary at term. I. Incidence, gross anatomy and ultrastructural features of merocrine secretion. Am J Anat 152: 7–28
167. Hidvegi D, Hidvegi I, Barrett J (1978) Douche-induced pelvic peritoneal starch granuloma. Obstet Gynecol 52: 15S–18S
168. Himelstein-Braw R, Peters H, Faber M (1977) Influence of irradiation and chemotherapy on the ovaries of children with abdominal tumours. Br J Cancer 36: 269–275
169. Himelstein-Braw R, Peters H, Faber M (1978) Morphological study of the ovaries of leukaemic children. Br J Cancer 38: 82–87
170. Hogan ML, Barber DD, Kaufman RH (1967) Dermoid cyst in supernumerary ovary of the greater omentum. Report of a case. Obstet Gynecol 29: 405–408
171. Honore LH (1981) Combined suppurative and noncaseating granulomatous oophoritis associated with distal ileitis (Crohn's disease). Eur J Obstet Gynaecol Reprod Biol 12: 91–94
172. Honore LH, O'Hara KE (1979) Ovarian hilus cell heterotopia. Obstet Gynecol 53: 461–464
173. Honore LH, O'Hara KE (1980) Subcapsular adipocytic infiltration of the human ovary: A clinicopathological study of eight cases. Eur J Obstet Gynaecol Reprod Biol 10: 13–20
174. Hoper PA, Andersson R (1975) Postmortem findings in primary familial amyloidosis with polyneuropathy. Acta Path Microbiol Scand 83: 309–322
175. Horowitz MI, Elguezabal A (1966) Obstruction of the ureter by recent corpus luteum located in the retroperitoneum: Report of 2 cases. J Urol 95: 706–710
176. Hubmer G (1978) The ovarian vein syndrome. Eur Urol 4: 263–268
177. Hughesdon PE (1972) The origin and development of benign stromatosis of the ovary. Br J Obstet Gynaecol 79: 348–359
178. Hughesdon PE (1976) The endometrial identity of benign stromatosis of the ovary and its relation to other forms of endometriosis. J Pathol 119: 201–209

179. Hughesdon PE (1982) Morphology and morphogenesis of the Stein-Leventhal ovary and of so-called "hyperthecosis." Obstet Gynecol Surv 37: 59–77
180. Hugod C, Scheibel M (1978) Kaempecellearteritis i ovarie. Ugeskr Laeg 140: 1093–1094
181. Hutchison JR, Taylor HB, Zimmermann EA (1966) The Stein-Leventhal syndrome and coincident ovarian neoplasms. Obstet Gynecol 28: 700–703
182. Iannaccone A, Gabrilove JL, Sohval AR, Soffer LJ (1959) The ovaries in Cushing's syndrome. N Engl J Med 261: 775–780
183. Imperato-McGinley J, Peterson RE, Sturla E, Darwood Y, Bar RS (1978) Primary amenorrhea associated with hirsutism, acanthosis nigricans, dermoid cysts of the ovaries and a new type of insulin resistance. Am J Med 65: 389–395
184. Irvine WJ (1980) Autoimmunity in endocrine disease. Rec Prog Horm Res 36: 509–556
185. Irvine WJ, Barnes EW (1974) Addison's disease and autoimmune ovarian failure. J Reprod Fertil [Suppl] 21: 1–31
186. Irvine WJ, Barnes EW (1975) Addison's disease, ovarian failure and hypoparathyroidism. Clin Endocrinol Metab 4: 379–434
187. Irvine WJ, Chan MMW, Scarth L (1969) The further characterization of antoantibodies reactive with extra-adrenal steroid-producing cells in patients with adrenal disorders. Clin Exp Immunol 4: 489–503
188. Irvine WJ, Chan MMW, Scarth L, Kolb FO, Hartog M, Bayliss RIS, Drury MI (1968) Immunological aspects of premature ovarian failure associated with idiopathic Addison's disease. Lancet 2: 883–887
189. Israel SL, Rubenstone A, Meranze DR (1954) The ovary at term. I. Decidua-like reaction and surface cell proliferation. Obstet Gyncol 3: 399–407
190. Jafari K, Saleh I (1977) Postpartum spontaneous rupture of ovarian artery aneurysm. Obstet Gynecol 49: 493–494
191. Jafari K, Javaheri G, Ruiz G (1978) Endometrial adenocarcinoma and the Stein-Leventhal syndrome. Obstet Gynecol 51: 97–100
192. Janson PO, Jansson I, Skryten A, Damber J, Lindstedt G (1981) Ovarian endocrine function in young women undergoing radiotherapy for carcinoma of the cervix. Gynecol Oncol 11: 218–223
193. Judd HL, Benirschke K, DeVane G, Reuter SR, Yen SSC (1973) Maternal virilization developing during a twin pregnancy. N Engl J Med 288: 118–122
194. Judd HL, Scully RE, Herbst AL, Yen SSC, Ingersol FM, Kliman B (1973) Familial hyperthecosis: Comparison of endocrinologic and histologic findings with polycystic ovarian disease. Am J Obstet Gynecol 117: 976–982
195. Kabawat SE, Bast RC Jr, Bhan AK, Welch WR, Knapp RC, Colvin RB (1983) Tissue distribution of a coelomic–epithelium-related antigen recognized by the monoclonal antibody OC125. Int J Gynecol Pathol 2: 275–285
196. Kahn CR, Flier JS, Bar RS, Archer JA, Gorden P, Martin MM, Roth J (1976) The syndromes of insulin resistance and acanthosis nigricans: Insulin-receptor disorders in man. N Engl J Med 294: 739–745
197. Kalstone CE, Jaffe RB, Abell MR (1969) Massive edema of the ovary simulating fibroma. Obstet Gynecol 34: 564–571
198. Kanbour AI, Salazar H, Tobon H (1979) Massive ovarian edema. A nonneoplastic pelvic mass of young women. Arch Pathol Lab Med 103: 42–45
199. Karam K, Hajj S (1979) Hyperthecosis syndrome. Acta Obstet Gynecol Scand 58: 73–79
200. Katz M, Hamilton SM, Albertyn L, Pimstone BL, Cohen BL, Tiltman AJ (1977) Virilization with diffuse involvement of ovarian androgen-secreting cells. Obstet Gynecol 50: 623–627
201. Kaufman DW, Shapiro S, Rosenberg L, Monson RR, Miettinen OS, Stolley PD, Slone D (1980) Intrauterine contraceptive device use and pelvic inflammatory disease. Am J Obstet Gynecol 136: 159–162
202. Kaufman FR, Kogut MD, Donnell GN, Goebelsmann U, March C, Koch R (1981) Hypergonadotropic hypogonadism in female patients with galactosemia. N Engl J Med 304: 994–998
203. Keebler C, Chatwani A, Schwartz R (1983) Actinomycosis infection associated with intrauterine contraceptive devices. Am J Obstet Gynecol 145: 596–599
204. Kemmann E, Orenstein D, Smith C, Shelden RM, Jones JR (1980) Estrogenization in women with postmenopausal ovarian hyperthecosis. Int J Obstet Gynecol 18: 188–191
205. Kent BK (1956) Ectopic pregnancy in a congenitally defective tube with absence of the ipsilateral ovary. Am J Obstet Gynecol 72: 1150–1151
206. Kerber IJ, Bell JS, Camacho AM, Fish SA (1969) Luteoma of pregnancy: Recurrent or persistent? South Med J 62: 1343–1348
207. Kern SB, Duff P (1981) Localized amniotic fluid embolism presenting as ovarian vein thrombosis and refractory postoperative fever. Am J Clin Pathol 76: 476–480
208. Khan JS, Steele RJC, Stewart D (1981) *Enterobius vermicularis* infestation of the female genital tract causing generalized peritonitis. Case report. Br J Obstet Gynaecol 88: 681–683
209. Kim MH (1974) "Gonadotropin-resistant ovaries" syndrome in association with secondary amenorrhea. Am J Obstet Gynecol 120: 257–263
210. Kinch RAH, Plunkett ER, Smout MS, Carr DH (1965) Primary ovarian failure. A clinicopathological and cytogenetic study. Am J Obstet Gynecol 91: 630–641
211. Kohorn EI (1983) Theca lutein ovarian cyst may be pathognomonic for trophoblastic neoplasia. Obstet Gynecol 62: 80S–81S
212. Koninckx PR, Brosens IA (1977) The "gonadotropin-resistant ovary" syndrome as a cause of secondary amenorrhea and infertility. Fertil Steril 28: 926–931
213. Kosasa TS, Griffiths CT, Shane JM, Leventhal JM, Naftolin F (1976) Diagnosis of a supernumerary ovary with human chorionic gonadotropin. Obstet Gynecol 47: 236–238
214. Kosloske AM, Goldthorn JF, Kaufman E, Hayek A (1984) Treatment of precocious pseudopuberty associated with follicular cysts of the ovary. Am J Dis Child 138: 147–149
215. Kostelnik FV, Fremount HN (1976) Mycotic tubo-ovarian

abscess associated with the intrauterine device. Am J Obstet Gynecol 125: 272–274
216. Kott MM, Schmidt WA (1981) Massive postpartum corpus luteum cyst: A case report. Hum Pathol 12: 468–470
217. Kuhajda FP, Haupt HM, Moore GW, Hutchins GM (1982) Gonadal morphology in patients receiving chemotherapy for leukemia. Am J Med 72: 759–767
218. Kuki S, Morgan RL, Tucci JR (1981) Myasthenia gravis and premature ovarian failure. Arch Intern Med 141: 1230–1232
219. Kunakemakorn P, Ontai G, Balin H (1976) Pelvic inflammatory pseudotumor: A case report. Am J Obstet Gynecol 126: 286–287
220. Kurcz JA, Sharp MS (1948) Congenital absence of one ovary associated with contralateral tubal pregnancy. Am J Obstet Gynecol 55: 1065–1067
221. Lachelin GCL, Barnett M, Hopper BR, Brink G, Yen SSC (1979) Adrenal function in normal women and women with the polycystic ovary syndrome. J Clin Endocrinol Metab 49: 892–898
222. Landers DV, Sweet RL (1985) Current trends in the diagnosis and treatment of tuboovarian abscess. Am J Obstet Gynecol 151: 1098–1110
223. Lansman HH, Lapin A, Blaustein A (1960) Pelvic oxyuris granuloma associated with endometriosis. Am J Obstet Gynecol 79: 1178–1180
224. Lee B, Gore BZ (1984) A case of supernumerary ovary. Obstet Gynecol 63: 738–740
225. Lee RA, Kazmier FJ (1977) Ovarian hematoma complicating anticoagulant therapy. Mayo Clin Proc 52: 19–23
226. Levine SC, Huffaker J, Jacobson JB, Brodey PA, Fisch AE (1982) Second-trimester spontaneous regression of theca lutein cysts. Obstet Gynecol 60: 124–126
227. Lewis JD (1964) Hilus-cell hyperplasia in ovaries and tubes. Obstet Gynecol 24: 728–731
228. Lim HT, Meinders AE, de Haan LD, Bronkhorst FB (1984) Anovulation presumably due to the gonadotrophin-resistant ovary syndrome. Eur J Obstet Gynaecol Reprod Biol 16: 327–337
229. Lindsay AN, Voorhess ML, MacGillivray MH (1983) Multicystic ovaries in primary hypothyroidism. Obstet Gynecol 61: 433
230. LiVolsi VA, Merino MJ (1979) Cytomegalovirus infection of ovarian thecoma (Letter). Arch Pathol Lab Med 103: 653–654
231. Lobo RA, Geobelsmann U (1981) Evidence for reduced 3-beta-ol-hydroxysteroid dehydrogenase activity in some hirsute women thought to have polycystic ovary syndrome. J Clin Endocrinol Metab 53: 394–400
232. London AM, Burkman RT (1979) Tuboovarian abscees with associated rupture with fistula formation into the urinary bladder. Am J Obstet Gynecol 135: 1113–1114
233. Lubarsch O, Henke F (1937) Handbuch der Speziellen Pathologischen Anatomie und Histologie. Dritter Teil. Die Krankheiten des Eierstockes. Berlin, Springer
234. Luff RD, Gupta PK, Spence MR, Frost JK (1978) Pelvic actinomycosis and the intrauterine contraceptive device. Am J Clin Pathol 69: 581–586
235. Lupien C, Wagar H, Sauerbrei EE (1984) Delayed regression of huge theca lutein cysts monitored by serial sonograms and B-HCG levels. J Can Assoc Radiol 35: 70–72
236. Luzzatto R, Brucker N (1981) Benign inclusion cysts of the ovary associated with psammoma bodies in vaginal smears. Acta Cytol 25: 282–284
237. MacDonald PC, Grodin JM, Edman CD, Vellois F, Siiteri PK (1976) Origin of estrogen in a postmenopausal woman with a nonendocrine tumor of the ovary and endometrial hyperplasia. Obstet Gynecol 47: 644–650
238. Mackler MA, Royster HP (1968) Right ovarian vein thrombophlebitis and ovarian arteritis. J Urol 100: 683–686
239. Madeido G, Tieu TM, Aiman J (1985) Atypical ovarian hyperthecosis in a virilized postmenopausal woman. Am J Clin Pathol 83: 101–107
240. Mahmood K (1975) Granulomatous oophoritis due to *Schistosoma mansoni*. Am J Obstet Gynecol 123: 919–920
241. Majmudar B, Kapernick PS, Phillips RS (1978) Ovarian myxoma. Hum Pathol 9: 723–725
242. Malkary JW, Fenton AN (1964) Torsion of undiseased adnexa. Obstet Gynecol 23: 438–441
243. Mallin SR (1969) Congenital adrenal hyperplasia secondary to 17-hydroxylase deficiency. Two sisters with amenorrhea, hypokalemia, hypertension, and cystic ovaries. Ann Intern Med 70: 69–75
244. Marcus CC (1963) Ovarian cortical stromal hyperplasia and carcinoma of the endometrium. Obstet Gynecol 21: 175–186
245. Massachusetts General Hospital Case Records (1957) Case 43461. Follicle cyst with sexual precocity. N Engl J Med 257: 987–992
246. Massachusetts General Hospital Case Records (1971) Case 24–1971. Ovarian hyperthecosis with massive edema. N Engl J Med 284: 1369–1375
247. Massachusetts General Hospital Case Records (1972) Case 49–1972. Hyperthecosis of ovaries. N Engl J Med 287: 1192–1195
248. Massachusetts General Hospital Case Records (1974) Case 12–1974. Stromal hyperthecosis of ovaries. N Engl J Med 290: 730–736
249. Massachusetts General Hospital Case Records (1975) Case 4–1975. Luteinized follicle cysts of ovary, bilateral. Albright's syndrome. N Engl J Med 292: 199–203
250. Massachusetts General Hospital Case Records (1979) Case 48–1979. Ovarian remnant syndrome. Corpus luteum cyst. N Engl J Med 301: 1228–1233
251. Massachusetts General Hospital Case Records (1980) Case 5–1980. Primary amyloidosis, generalized. Pyelonephritis, bilateral. N Engl J Med 302: 336–344
252. Massachusetts General Hospital Case Records (1980) Case 23–1980. Ovarian remnant syndrome. Endometriosis. N Engl J Med 302: 1354–1358
253. Massachusetts General Hospital Case Records (1982) Case 25–1982. Ovarian stromal hyperthecosis. Acanthosis nigricans. N Engl J Med 306: 1537–1544
254. Massachusetts General Hospital Case Records (1983) Case 25–1983. Hemochromatosis, involving liver and testes, with hypogonadotropic hypogonadism. N Engl J Med 308: 1521–1529
255. Mathur RS, Melchers JT III, Ades EW, Williamson HO, Fudenberg HH (1980) Anti-ovarian and anti-lymphocyte

antibodies in patients with chronic vaginal candidiasis. J Reprod Immunol 2: 247–262
256. Mathur RS, Moody LO, Landgrebe SC, Peress MR, Rust PF, Williamson HO (1982) Sex-hormone-binding globulin in clinically hyperandrogenic women: Association of plasma concentrations with body weight. Fertil Steril 38: 207–211
257. Matseone S, Batts JA Jr, Mandeville EO (1976) Ovarian hemorrhage complicating warfarin sodium anticoagulant therapy. Am J Obstet Gynecol 124: 766–767
258. Mattison DR, Evans MI, Schwimmer WB, White BJ, Jensen B, Schulman JD (1984) Familial premature ovarian failure. Am J Hum Genet 36: 1341–1348
259. McArdle C, Seibel M, Hann LE, Weinstein F, Taymor M (1983) The diagnosis of ovarian hyperstimulation (OHS): The impact of ultrasound. Fertil Steril 39: 464–467
260. McCormick JF, Scorgie RDF (1977) Unilateral tubo-ovarian actinomycosis in the presence of an intrauterine device. Am J Clin Pathol 68: 622–626
261. McDonald TW, Malkasian GD, Gaffey TA (1977) Endometrial cancer associated with feminizing ovarian tumor and polycystic ovarian disease. Obstet Gynecol 49: 654–658
262. McMahon JN, Connolly CE, Long SV, Meehan FP (1984) Enterobius granulomas of the uterus, ovary and pelvic peritoneum. Two case reports. Br J Obstet Gynaecol 91: 289–290
263. McNatty KP, Short RV, Barnes EW, Irvine WJ (1975) The cytotoxic effect of serum from patients with Addison's disease and autoimmune ovarian failure on human granulosa cells in culture. Clin Exp Immunol 22: 378–384
264. McNatty KP, Smith DM, Makris A, DeGrazia C, Tulchinsky D, Osathanondh R, Schiff I, Ryan KJ (1980) The intraovarian sites of androgen and estrogen formation in women with normal and hyperandrogenic ovaries as judged by in vitro experiments. J Clin Endocrinol Metab 50: 755–763
265. Mechanick JI, Futterweit W (1984) Hypothesis: Aberrant puberty and the Stein-Leventhal syndrome. Int J Fertil 29: 35–38
266. Meldrum DR, Frumar AM, Shamonki IM, Benirschke K, Judd HL (1980) Ovarian and adrenal steroidogenesis in a virilized patient with gonadotropin-resistant ovaries and hilus cell hyperplasia. Obstet Gynecol 56: 216–221
267. Merrill JA (1963) The morphology of the prepubertal ovary: Relationship to the polycystic ovary syndrome. South Med J 56: 225–231
268. Mickal A, Sellmann AH, Beebe JL (1968) Ruptured tubo-ovarian abscess. Am J Obstet Gynecol 100: 432–436
269. Mies C, Balogh K, Stadecker M (1984) Palisading prostate granulomas following surgery. Am J Surg Pathol 8: 217–221
270. Milewicz A, Silber D, Mielecki I (1983) The origin of androgen synthesis in polycystic ovary syndrome. Obstet Gynecol 62: 601–604
271. Miller ME, Chatten J (1967) Ovarian changes in ataxia telangiectasia. Acta Paediatr Scand 56: 559–561
272. Minkowitz S, Friedman F, Henniger G (1965). Xanthogranuloma of the ovary. Arch Pathol 80: 209–213
273. Montag TW, Auletta FJ, Gibson M (1983) Neonatal ovarian cyst: Prenatal diagnosis and analysis of cyst fluid. Obstet Gynecol 61: 38S–41S
274. Monteleone JA, Monteleone PL, Danis RK (1973) Pseudoprecocious puberty associated with isolated follicle cyst of the ovary. J Pediatr Surg 8: 949–950
275. Morgenfeld MC, Goldberg V, Parisier H, Bugnard SC, Bur GE (1972) Ovarian lesions due to cytostatic agents during the treatment of Hodgkin's disease. Surg Gynecol Obstet 134: 826–828
276. Morrison JC, Givens JR, Wiser WL, Fish SA (1975) Mumps oophoritis: A cause of premature menopause. Fertil Steril 26: 655–659
277. Morrow CP, Kletzky OA, Disaia PJ, Townsend DE, Mishell DR, Nakamura RM (1977) Clinical and laboratory correlates of molar pregnancy and trophoblastic disease. Am J Obstet Gynecol 128: 424–430
278. Muechler EK, Florack AJ, Cary D, Kapakis M (1982) Isosexual precocious puberty with luteinized follicular cyst. NY State J Med 82: 1353–1356
279. Mulligan RM (1976) A survey of epithelial inclusions in the ovarian cortex of 470 patients. J Surg Oncol 8: 61–66
280. Munslick RA, Gillanders LA (1981) A review of the syndrome of puerperal ovarian vein thombophlebitis. Obstet Gynecol Surv 36: 57–66
281. Muram D, Drouin P (1982) Ovarian remnant syndrome. Can Med Assoc J 127: 399–400
282. Murray JJ, Clark CA, Lands RH, Heim CR, Burnett LS (1985) Reactivation blastomycosis presenting as a tuboovarian abscess. Obstet Gynecol 64: 828–830
283. Nagamani M, Gomez LG, Garza J (1982) In vivo steroid studies in luteoma of pregnancy. Obstet Gynecol 59: 105S–111S
284. Nagamani M, Lingold JC, Gomez JR (1980) Hyperthecosis of the ovaries in acromegaly. Obstet Gynecol 56: 258–262
285. Nagamani M, Lingold JC, Gomez JR, Garza JR (1981) Clinical and hormonal studies in hyperthecosis of the ovaries. Fertil Steril 36: 326–332
286. Nicosia SV, Matus-Ridley M, Meadows AT (1985) Gonadal effects of cancer therapy in girls. Cancer 55: 2364–2372
287. Nissen ED, Kent DR, Nissen SE, Feldman BM (1977) Unilateral tuboovarian autoamputation. J Reprod Med 19: 151–153
288. Nissim F, Ashkenazy M, Borenstein R, Czernobilsky B (1981) Tuberculoid cornstarch granulomas with caseous necrosis. A diagnostic challenge. Arch Pathol Lab Med 105: 86–88
289. Nogales FF, Silverberg SG (1976) Epidermoid cysts of the ovary: A report of five cases with histogenetic considerations and ultrastructural findings. Am J Obstet Gynecol 124: 523–528
290. Nogales-Ortiz F, Tarancon I, Nogales FF (1979) The pathology of female genital tract tuberculosis. Obstet Gynecol 53: 422–428
291. Norris HJ, Taylor HB (1967) Nodular theca-lutein hyperplasia of pregnancy (so-called "pregnancy luteoma"). A clinical and pathologic study of 15 cases. Am J Clin Pathol 47: 557–566
292. Nouwen EJ, Pollet DE, Schelstraete JB, Eerdekens MW,

Hansch C, Van de Voorde A, De Broe ME (1985) Human placental alkaline phosphatase in benign and malignant ovarian neoplasia. Cancer Res 45: 892–902
293. Novak ER, Mohler DI (1953) Ovarian stromal changes in endometrial cancer. Am J Obstet Gynecol 65: 1099–1110
294. Ober WB, Grady HG, Schoenbucker AK (1957) Ectopic ovarian decidua without pregnancy. Am J Pathol 33: 199–217
295. Ohsawa M, Wu M, Masahashi T, Asai M, Narita O (1985) Cyclic therapy resulted in pregnancy in premature ovarian failure. Obstet Gynecol 66: 64S–67S
296. O'Malley BW, Lipsett MB, Jackson MA (1967) Steroid content and synthesis in a virilizing luteoma. J Clin Endocrinol Metab 27: 311–319
297. Overton TH (1982) Splenosis: A cause of pelvic pain. Am J Obstet Gynecol 143: 969–970
298. Pace EH, Voet RL, Melancon JT (1984) Xanthogranulomatous oophoritis: An inflammatory pseudotumor of the ovary. Int J Gynecol Pathol 3: 398–402
299. Paine CG, Smith P (1957) Starch granulomata. J Clin Pathol 10: 51–55
300. Pedowitz P, Bloomfield RD (1964) Ruptured adnexal abscess (tubo-ovarian) with generalized peritonitis. Am J Obstet Gynecol 88: 721–729
301. Peer E, Peretz BA, Makler A, Paldi E (1981) Bilateral adnexal agenesis with an ectopic ovary—Case report and review of the literature. Eur J Obstet Gynaecol Reprod Biol 12: 37–42
302. Penney LL, Betz G (1977) Agonadism. Case report and review. Am J Obstet Gynecol 127: 299–301
303. Perlman JA, Barnes AB, Demirjian Z (1977) Corpus luteum hemorrhages complication chronic anticoagulation. Obstet Gynecol 49: 20S–21S
304. Peters WA, Thiagarajah S, Thornton WN Jr (1979) Ovarian hemorrhage in patients receiving anticoagulant therapy. J Reprod Med 22: 82–86
305. Pine L, Curtis EM, Brown JM (1985) Actinomyces and the intrauterine contraceptive device: Aspects of the fluorescent antibody stain. Am J Obstet Gynecol 152: 287–290
306. Piver MS, Williams LJ, Marcuse PM (1970) Influence of luteal cysts on menstrual function. Obstet Gynecol 35: 740–751
307. Planner RS, Abell DA, Barbaro CA, Beischer NA (1982) Massive enlargement of the ovaries after evacuation of hydatidiform moles. Aust NZ J Obstet Gynaecol 22: 96–100
308. Plate WP (1967) Ovarian changes after long-term oral contraception. Acta Endocrinol 55: 71–77
309. Polansky S, dePapp EW, Ogden EB (1975) Virilization associated with bilateral luteomas of pregnancy. Obstet Gynecol 45: 516–522
310. Poretsky L, Smith D, Seibel M, Pazionos A, Moses AC, Flier JS (1984) Specific insulin binding sites in human ovary. J Clin Endocrinol Metab 59: 809–811
311. Pray LG (1951) Sexual precocity in females: Report of 2 cases, with arrest of precocity in the McCune-Albright syndrome after removal of cystic ovary. Pediatrics 8: 684–692
312. Printz JL, Choate JW, Townes PL, Harper RC (1973) The embryology of supernumerary ovaries. Obstet Gynecol 41: 246–252
313. Pueblitz-Peredo S, Luevano-Flores E, Rincon-Taracena R, Ochoa-Carrillo FJ (1985) Uteruslike mass of the ovary: Endomyometriosis or congenital malformation? A case with a discussion of histogenesis. Arch Pathol Lab Med 109: 361–364
314. Putschar WGJ, Manion WC (1956) Splenic-gonadal fusion. Am J Pathol 32: 15–33
315. Quan A, Charles D, Craig JM (1963) Histologic and functional consequences of periovarian adhesions. Obstet Gynecol 22: 96–101
316. Quigley ME, Rakoff JS, Yen SSC (1981) Increased luteinizing hormone sensitivity to dopamine inhibition in polycystic ovary syndrome. J Clin Endocrinol Metab 52: 231–234.
317. Quinn MA, Baker HWG, Rome R, Fortune D, Brown JB (1983) Response of a mucinous ovarian tumor of borderline malignancy to human chorionic gonadotropin. Obstet Gynecol 61: 121–126
318. Ramzy I, Nisker JA (1979) Histologic study of ovaries from young women with endometrial adenocarcinoma. Am J Clin Pathol 71: 253–256
319. Ravinsky E (1984) Ovarian hyperthecosis associated with pseudosarcomatous changes in the endometrial stroma. Am J Surg Pathol 8: 939–943
320. Rebar RW (1982) Hypergonadotropic amenorrhea and premature ovarian failure. A review. J Reprod Med 27: 179–186
321. Rebar RW, Erickson GF, Yen SSC (1982) Idiopathic premature ovarian failure: Clinical and endocrine characteristics. Fertil Steril 37: 35–41
322. Rewell, RE (1972) Extra-uterine decidua. J Pathol 105: 219–222
323. Rice BF, Savard K (1966) Steroid hormone formation in the human ovary: IV. Ovarian stromal compartment; formation of radioactive steroids from acetate-1-^{14}C and action of gonadotropins. J Clin Endocrinol 26: 593–609
324. Rice FB, Barclay DL, Sternberg WH (1969) Luteoma of pregnancy. Am J Obstet Gynecol 104: 871–878
325. Riddlesberger MM Jr, Kuhn JP, Munschauer RW (1981) The association of juvenile hypothyroidism and cystic ovaries. Radiology 139: 77–80
326. Roddick JW Jr, Greene RR (1957) Relation of ovarian stromal hyperplasia to endometrial carcinoma. Am J Obstet Gynecol 73: 843–852
327. Roddick JW Jr, Greene RR (1958) Relation of ovarian stromal hyperplasia to endometrial carcinoma. II. A comparison of autopsy and surgical controls. Am J Obstet Gynecol 75: 1015–1018
328. Rosai J (1982) Uterus-like mass replacing ovary (Letter). Arch Pathol Lab Med 106: 364–365
329. Ross GT (1976) Hormones and preantral follicle growth in women. Mayo Clin Proc 51: 617–620
330. Roth LM, Sternberg WH (1973) Ovarian stromal tumors containing Leydig cells. II. Pure Leydig cell tumor, non-hilar type. Cancer 32: 952–960
331. Roth LM, Sternberg WH (1983) Partly luteinized theca cell tumor of the ovary. Cancer 51: 1697–1704

332. Roth LM, Deaton RL, Sternberg WH (1979) Massive ovarian edema. A clinicopathologic study of five cases including ultrastructural observations and review of the literature. Am J Surg Pathol 3: 11–21
333. Rubin P, Casarett GW (1968) Clinical Radiation Pathology. Philadelphia, Saunders, Vol I
334. Ruehsen MDM, Jones GS (1967) Premature ovarian failure. Fertil Steril 18: 440–461
335. Ruehsen MDM, Blizzard RM, Garcia-Bunuel R, Jones GS (1972) Autoimmunity and ovarian failure. Am J Obstet Gynecol 112: 693–703
336. Russell P, Bannatyne P, Shearman RP, Fraser IS, Corbett P (1982) Premature hypergonadotropic ovarian failure: Clinicopathological study of 19 cases. Int J Gynecol Pathol 1: 185–201
337. Ryan GM, Craig J, Reid DE (1964) Histology of the uterus and ovaries after long-term cyclic norethynodrel therapy. Am J Obstet Gynecol 90: 715–725
338. Salomonowitz E (1980) Tumorformige Amyloidose des Ovars. Geburtsh Frauenheilk 40: 644–647
339. Samaan NA, Smith JP, Rutledge FN, Barcellona JM (1972) Plasma testosterone levels in trophoblastic disease and the effects of oophorectomy and chemotherapy. J Clin Endocrinol Metab 34: 558–561
340. Santos-Ramos R, Forney JP, Schwarz BE (1980) Sonographic findings and clinical correlations in molar pregnancy. Obstet Gynecol 56: 186–192
341. Saxen L, Kassinen A, Saxen E (1963) Peritoneal foreign-body reaction caused by condom emulsion. Lancet 1: 1295–1296
342. Schenker JG, Weinstein D (1978) Ovarian hyperstimulation syndrome: A current survey. Fertil Steril 30: 255–268
343. Schiffer MA, Elguezabal A, Sultana M, Allen AC (1975) Actinomycosis infections associated with intrauterine contraceptive devices. Obstet Gynecol 45: 67–72
344. Schilsky RL, Sherins RJ, Hubbard SM, Wesley MN, Young RC, Devita VT (1981) Long-term follow-up of ovarian function in women treated with MOPP chemotherapy for Hodgkin's disease. Am J Med 71: 552–556
345. Schmidt WA (1982) IUDs, inflammation, and infection: Assessment after two decades of IUD use. Hum Pathol 13: 878–881
346. Schmidt WA, Bedrossian CWM, Ali V, Webb JA, Bastian FO (1980) Actinomycosis and intrauterine contraceptive devices. Diagn Gynecol Obstet 2: 165–177
347. Schneider D, Bukovsky I, Kaufman S, Sadovsky G, Caspi E (1981) Severe ovarian hemorrhage in congenital afibrinogenemia. Acta Obstet Gynecol Scand 60: 431
348. Schneider GT, Bechtel M (1956) Ovarian cortical stromal hyperplasia. Obstet Gynecol 8: 713–719
349. Schultz LR, Newton WA Jr, Clatworthy HW Jr (1963) Torsion of previously normal tube and ovary in children. N Engl J Med 268: 343–346
350. Schumert Z, Spitz I, Diamant Y, Polishuk WZ, Rabinowitz D (1975) Elevation of serum testosterone in ovarian hyperstimulation syndrome. J Clin Endocrinol Metab 40: 889–892
351. Scully RE (1964) Stromal luteoma of the ovary. Cancer 17: 769–778
352. Scully RE (1979) Tumors of the ovary and maldeveloped gonads. In: Atlas of Tumor Pathology, Second Series, Fascicle 16. Washington, D.C., Armed Forces Institute of Pathology
353. Scully RE (1981) Smooth-muscle differentiation in genital tract disorders (Editorial). Arch Pathol Lab Med 105: 505–507
354. Scully RE, Cohen RB (1964) Oxidative-enzyme activity in normal and pathologic human ovaries. Obstet Gynecol 24: 667–681
355. Sebastian JA, Baker RL, Cordray D (1973) Asymptomatic infarction and separation of ovary and distal uterine tube. Obstet Gynecol 41: 531–535
356. Sedin G. Bergquist C, Lindgren PG (1985) Ovarian hyperstimulation syndrome in preterm infants. Pediatr Res 19: 548–551
357. Semchyshyn S, Zuspan FP (1978) Ovarian hemorrhage due to anticoagulants. Am J Obstet Gynecol 131: 837–844
358. Shalet SM, Beardwell CG, Morris Jones PH, Pearson D, Orrel DH (1976) Ovarian failure following abdominal irradiation in childhood. Br J Cancer 33: 655–658
359. Shalev E, Zuckerman H, Rizescu I (1982) Pelvic inflammatory pseudotumor (xanthogranuloma). Acta Obstet Gynecol Scand 61: 285–286
360. Shawker TH, Hubbard VS, Reichert CM, Guerreiro de Matos OM (1983) Cystic ovaries in cystic fibrosis: An ultrasound and autopsy study. J Ultrasound Med 2: 439–444
361. Shettles LB (1963) Recurrent theca lutein cysts. Obstet Gynecol 21: 339–342
362. Shipton EA, Meares SD (1965) Heterotopic bone formation in the ovary. Aust NZ J Obstet Gynaecol 5: 100–102
363. Shoupe D, Lobo RA (1984) Evidence for altered catecholoamine metabolism in polycystic ovary syndrome. Am J Obstet Gynecol 150: 566–571
364. Shoupe D, Lobo RA (1984) The influence of androgens on insulin resistance. Fertil Steril 41: 385–388
365. Shoupe D, Kumar DD, Lobo RA (1983) Insulin resistance in polycystic ovary syndrome. Am J Obstet Gynecol 147: 588–592
366. Silver HK (1958) Juvenile hypothyroidism with precocious sexual development. J Endocrinol Metab 18: 886–891
367. Simstein NL (1981) Colotuboovarian fistula as complication of pelvic inflammatory disease. South J Med 74: 512–513
368. Siris ES, Leventhal BG, Vaitukaitis JL (1976) Effects of childhood leukemia and chemotherapy on puberty and reproductive function in girls. N Engl J Med 294: 1143–1146
369. Sirisena LA (1978) Unexplained absence of an ovary and uterine tube. Postgrad Med J 54: 423–424
370. Sjovall A, Akerman M (1968) Peritoneal granulomas in women due to the presence of *Enterobius S. Oxyuris vermicularis*. Acta Obstet Gynecol Scand 47: 361–373
371. Smith A, Fraser IS, Noel M (1979) Three siblings with premature gonadal failure. Fertil Steril 32: 528–530
372. Sommers SC (1983) Female genital tract granulomas. In:

Pathology of Granulomas. Ioachim HL (ed). New York, Raven Press, pp. 395–409
373. Sommers SC, Wadman PJ (1956) Pathogenesis of polycystic ovaries. Am J Obstet Gynecol 72: 160–169
374. Spanos WJ (1973) Preoperative hormonal therapy of cystic adnexal masses. Am J Obstet Gynecol 116: 551–554
375. Stahl NL, Teeslink CR, Greenblatt RB (1973) Ovarian, adrenal and peripheral testosterone levels in the polycystic ovary syndrome. Am J Obstet Gynecol 117: 194–200
376. Starup J, Sele V (1973) Premature ovarian failure. Acta Obstet Gynecol Scand 52: 259–268
377. Starup J, Visfeldt J (1974) Ovarian morphology in early and late human pregnancy. Acta Obstet Gynecol Scand 53: 211–218.
378. Starup J, Sele V, Henriksen B (1971) Amenorrhea associated with increased production of gonadotropins and a morphologically normal ovarian follicular apparatus. Acta Endocrinol 66: 248–256
379. Stearns HC, Sneeden VD, Fearl JD (1974) A clinical and pathologic review of ovarian stromal hyperplasia and its possible relationship to common diseases of the female reproductive system. Am J Obstet Gynecol 119: 375–381
380. Sternberg WH (1949) The morphology, androgenic function, hyperplasia, and tumors of the human ovarian hilus cells. Am J Pathol 25: 493–521
381. Sternberg WH (1955) Association of masculinizing ovarian hilus cell tumors, ovarian stromal hyperplasia, and luteinlike cell proliferation (Abstr). Am J Pathol 31: 571
382. Sternberg WH, Barclay DL (1966) Luteoma of pregnancy. Am J Obstet Gynecol 95: 165–181
383. Sternberg WH, Dhurandhar HN (1977) Functional ovarian tumors of stromal and sex cord origin. Hum Pathol 8: 565–582
384. Sternberg WH, Gaskill CJ (1950) Theca-cell tumors: With a report of twelve new cases and observations on the possible etiologic role of ovarian stromal hyperplasia. Am J Obstet Gynecol 59: 575–587
385. Sternberg WH, Roth LM (1973) Ovarian stromal tumors containing Leydig cells. I. Stromal-Leydig cell tumor and nonneoplastic transformation of ovarian stroma to Leydig cells. Cancer 32: 940–951
386. Sternberg WH, Segaloff A, Gaskill CJ (1953) Influence of chorionic gonadotropin on human ovarian hilus cells (Leydig-like cells). J Clin Endocrinol Metab 13: 139–153
387. Stevens ML, Plotka ED (1977) Functional lutein cyst in a postmenopausal woman. Obstet Gynecol 50: 27S–29S
388. Stillman RJ, Schinfeld JS, Schiff I, Gelber RD, Greenberger J, Larson M, Jaffe N, Li FP (1981) Ovarian failure in long-term survivors of childhood malignancy. Am J Obstet Gynecol 139: 62–66
389. Strickler RC, Kelly RW, Askin FB (1984) Postmenopausal ovarian follicle cyst: An unusual cause of estrogen excess. Int J Gynecol Pathol 3: 318–322
390. Subietas A, Deppisch LM, Astarloa J (1977) Cytomegalovirus oophoritis: Ovarian cortical necrosis. Hum Pathol 8: 285–292
391. Sutherland AM (1982) Postmenopausal tuberculosis of the female genital tract. Obstet Gynecol 59: 54S–57S
392. Swenson WM, Tolstedt GE, Romas P, Peters C (1978) Ovarian arteriovenous fistula. An unusal cause of abdominal pain. Obstet Gynecol 51: 62S–63S
393. Symmonds RE, Pettit PDM (1979) Ovarian remnant syndrome. Obstet Gynecol 54: 174–177
394. Symonds DA, Driscoll SG (1973) An adrenal cortical rest within the fetal ovary: Report of a case. Am J Clin Pathol 60: 562–564
395. Talbert LM, Raj MHG, Hammond MG, Greer T (1984) Endocrine and immunologic studies in a patient with resistent ovary syndrome. Fertil Steril 42: 741–744
396. Tanabe K, Gagliano P, Channing CP, Nakamura Y, Yoshimura Y, Iizuka R, Fortuny A, Sulewski J, Rezai N (1983) Levels of inhibin-F activity and steroids in human follicular fluid from normal women and women with polycystic ovarian disease. J Clin Endocrinol Metab 57: 24–31
397. Taylor SI, Dons RF, Hernandez E, Roth J, Gorden P (1982) Insulin resistance associated with androgen excess in women with autoantibodies to the insulin receptor. Ann Intern Med 97: 851–855
398. Teilum G, Madsen V (1950) Endometriosis ovarii et peritonaei caused by hysterosalpingography. Br J Obstet Gynaecol 57: 10–16
399. Thomas E, Mestman J, Henneman C, Anderson G, Hoffman R (1972) Bilateral luteomas of pregnancy with virilization. Obstet Gynecol 39: 577–584
400. Tiboldi T (1978) Involvement of human and primate ovaries in schistosomiasis. A review of the literature. Ann Soc Belge Med Trop 58: 9–20
401. Tulandi T, Kinch RAH (1981) Premature ovarian failure. Obstet Gynecol Surv 36: 521–527
402. Tulandi T, McInnes RA, Arronet GH (1984) Ovarian hyperstimulation syndrome following ovulation induction with human menopausal gonadotropin. Int J Fertil 29: 113–117
403. Turksoy RN, Safaii H, Kappy KA, Schlosser SA, Towne D (1978) Infarction of corpora lutei associated with intrauterine and extrauterine pregnancy. J Reprod Med 21: 102–106
404. Vaidya RA, Aloorkar SD, Rege NR, Joshi UM, Peter J, Sheth AR, Devi PK, Motashaw ND (1977) Premature ovarian failure. J Reprod Med 19: 348–352
405. Valenti C, Kassner EG, Yermakov V, Cromb E (1975) Antenatal diagnosis of a fetal ovarian cyst. Am J Obstet Gynecol 123: 216–219
406. VanWingen T, Upton RT, Cloherty MG, Irwin JR, Linn JG (1984) Bilateral massive edema. A case report. J Reprod Med 29: 875–877
407. Van Wyk JJ, Grumback MM (1960) Syndrome of precocious menstruation and galactorrhea in juvenile hypothroidism: An example of hormonal overlap in pituitary feedback. J Pediatr 57: 416–435
408. Vasquez SB, Sotos JF, Kim MH (1982) Massive edema of the ovary and virilization. Obstet Gynecol 59: 95S–99S
409. Vazquez AM, Kenny FM (1973) Ovarian failure and antiovarian antibodies in association with hypoparathyroidism, moniliasis, and Addison's and Hashimoto's diseases. Obstet Gynecol 41: 414–418
410. Verkauf BS, Reiter EO, Hernandez L, Burns SA (1977)

Virilization of mother and fetus associated with luteoma of pregnancy: A case report with endocrinologic studies. Am J Obstet Gynecol 129: 274–280
411. Villanueva AL, Rebar RW (1983) Triple-X syndrome and premature ovarian failure. Obstet Gynecol 62: 70S–73S
412. von Numers C (1965) Observations on metaplastic changes in the germinal epithelium of the ovary and on the aetiology of ovarian endometriosis. Acta Obstet Gynecol Scand 44: 107–116
413. Warne GL, Fairley KF, Hobbs JB, Martin FIR (1973) Cyclophosphamide-induced ovarian failure. N Engl J Med 289: 1159–1162
414. Wassman ER, Johnson K, Shapiro LJ, Itabashi H, Rimoin DL (1982) Postmortem findings in the Hurler-Scheie syndrome (mucopolyssacharidosis I-H/S). Birth Defects 18 (3B): 13–18
415. Watson WJ, Sundwall DA, Benson WL (1982) Splenosis mimicking endometriosis. Obstet Gynecol 59: 51S–53S
416. Waxman JHX, Terry YA, Wrigley PFM, Malpas JS, Rees LH, Besser GM, Lister TA (1982) Gonadal function in Hodgkin's disease: Long-term follow-up of chemotherapy. Br Med J 285: 1612–1613
417. Weinstein D, Rabinowitz R, Malach D, Mor-Yosef S, Eldor A, Schenker JG (1983) Ovarian hemorrhage in women with Von Willebrand's disease. A report of two cases. J Reprod Med 28: 500–502
418. Wentz AC, Gutai JP, Jones GS, Migeon CJ (1976) Ovarian hyperthecosis in an adolescent patient. J Pediatr 88: 488–493
419. Wetchler SJ, Dunn LJ (1985) Ovarian abscess. Report of a case and a review of the literature. Obstet Gynecol Surv 40: 476–485
420. Wharton LR (1959) Two cases of supernumerary ovary and one of accessory ovary, with an analysis of previously reported cases. Am J Obstet Gynecol 78: 1101–1119
421. White CA, Bradbury JT (1965) Ovarian theca lutein cysts. Experimental formation in women prior to repeat cesarean section. Am J Obstet Gynecol 92: 973–980
422. Whitehead E, Shalet SM, Blackledge G, Todd I, Crowther D, Beardwell CG (1983) The effect of combination chemotherapy on ovarian function in women treated for Hodgkin's disease. Cancer 52: 988–993
423. Wieland RG, Bendezu R, Hallberg MC, Tang P, Webster K (1976) Hormonal evaluation of premature menarche produced by a follicular cyst. Am J Obstet Gynecol 126: 731–733
424. Wierman ME, Beardsworth DE, Mansfield MJ, Badger TM, Crawford JD, Crigler JF Jr, Bode HH, Loughlin JS, Kushner DC, Scully RE, Hoffman WH, Crowley WF Jr (1985) Puberty without gonadotropins. A unique mechanism of sexual development. N Engl J Med 312: 65–72
425. Wilder JR, Barnes WA (1953) Obstruction of the small intestine by corpus luteum cyst. Report of a case. JAMA 151: 730–732
426. Williams WD, Amazon K, Rywlin AM (1984) Peritoneal keratin globules in uterine adenosquamous carcinoma. South Med J 77: 1316–1318
427. Williamson HO, Phansey SA, Mathur RS, Baker ER, Fudenberg HH (1980) Myasthenia gravis, premature menopause, and thyroid antoimmunity. Am J Obstet Gynecol 137: 893–901
428. Willson JB, Black JR III (1964) Ovarian abscess. Am J Obstet Gynecol 90: 34–43
429. Wilson EA, Erickson GF, Zarutski P, Finn AE, Tulchinsky D, Ryan KJ (1979) Endocrine studies of normal and polycystic ovarian tissues in vitro. Am J Obstet Gynecol 134: 56–63
430. Winslow RC, Funkhouser JW (1968) Sarcoidosis of the female reproductive organs. Report of a case. Obstet Gynecol 32: 285–289
431. Wlodarski FM, Trainer TD (1975) Granulomatous oophoritis and salpingitis associated with Crohn's disease of the appendix. Am J Obstet Gynecol 122: 527–528
432. Wolff E, Glasser M, Gordon GG, Olivo J, Southren AL (1973) Virilizing luteoma of pregnancy. Am J Med 54: 229–233
433. Woll E, Hertig AT, Smith GVS, Johnson LC (1948) The ovary in endometrial carcinoma. Am J Obstet Gynecol 56: 617–633
434. Wood GP, Boronow RC (1976) Endometrial adenocarcinoma and the polycystic ovary syndrome. Am J Obstet Gynecol 124: 140–142
435. Wood LC, Olichney M, Locke H, Crispell KR, Thornton WN Jr, Kitay JI (1965) Syndrome of juvenile hypothyroidism associated with advanced sexual development: Report of two new cases and comment on the management of an associated ovarian mass. J Clin Endocrinol Metab 25: 1289–1295
436. Worstman J, Soler NG (1982) Abnormalities of fuel metabolism in the polycystic ovary syndrome. Obstet Gynecol 60: 342–345
437. Wortsman J, Singh KB, Murphy J (1981) Evidence for the hypothalamic origin of the polycystic ovary syndrome. Obstet Gynecol 58: 137–141
438. Wortsman J, Wehrenberg WB, Gavin JR III, Allen JP (1984) Elevated levels of plasma beta-endorphin and gamma$_3$-melanocyte stimulating hormone in the polycystic ovary syndrome. Obstet Gynecol 63: 630–634
439. Yen SSC (1980) The polycystic ovary syndrome. Clin Endocrinol 12: 177–207
440. Young RH, Scully RE (1984) Fibromatosis and massive edema of the ovary, possibly related entities: A report of 14 cases of fibromatosis and 11 cases of massive edema. Int J Gynecol Pathol 3: 153–178
441. Young RH, Prat J, Scully RE (1980) Epidermoid cyst of the ovary. A report of three cases with comments on histogenesis. Am J Clin Pathol 73: 272–276
442. Zander J, Mickan H, Holzmann K, Lohe KH (1978) Androluteoma syndrome of pregnancy. Am J Obstet Gynecol 130: 170–177
443. Zarate A, Karchmer S, Gomez E, Castelazo-Ayala L (1970) Premature menopause. A clinical, histologic, and cytogenetic study. Am J Obstet Gynecol 106: 110–114
444. Zhang J, Young RH, Arseneau J, Scully RE (1982) Ovarian stromal tumors containing lutein or Leydig cells (luteinized thecomas and stromal Leydig cell tumors)—A clinicopathological analysis of fifty cases. Int J Gynecol Pathol 1: 270–285

17

Endometriosis, Lesions of the Secondary Müllerian System, and Pelvic Mesothelial Proliferations

Philip B. Clement, M.D.

This chapter deals primarily with a variety of nonneoplastic and neoplastic lesions that are characterized by müllerian differentiation on histologic examination but a distribution that is predominantly external to structures derived from the müllerian ducts. These lesions typically occur in the pelvis and lower abdomen, involving the peritoneum, the subjacent tissues (including retroperitoneum), and lymph nodes. Their importance to the pathologist, therefore, includes their differentiation on microscopic examination from metastatic tumor.

Although the histogenesis of many of these disorders is not known with certainty, they share a potential origin, by a process of metaplasia, from the secondary müllerian system, a histologically inconspicuous layer composed of the pelvic and lower abdominal mesothelium and subjacent (subcoelomic) mesenchyme in females.[215,270] The putative müllerian potential of this layer is consistent with its close embryologic relationship with the primary müllerian system, the müllerian ducts arising from invaginations of the coelomic epithelium (see Chapter 1, Embryology). Displacement of coelomic epithelium and subcoelomic mesenchyme into lymph nodes during embryonic development could account for the presence of histologically identical lesions within pelvic and abdominal lymph nodes. It should be stressed, however, that the origin of many of these lesions is controversial, and other proposed histogenetic mechanisms will also be discussed.

The most commonly encountered disorder in this group of lesions, both clinically and pathologically, is endometriosis. Endometriosis and neoplasms derived from endometriosis, including the important clinical manifestations such as infertility, are discussed in the first section of this chapter. The second section will be devoted to the rarer nonneoplastic and neoplastic lesions that may potentially originate from the secondary müllerian system. The majority of these are epithelial, histologically mimicking the most common types of primary müllerian epithelia (or neoplasms derived therefrom), namely, endosalpingeal (serous), endocervical (mucinous), and endometrial (endometrioid). Lesions composed of the last type of epithelium lack an endometrial stromal component, allowing their histologic distinction from endometriosis. The metaplastic potential of the pelvic peritoneum also includes differentiation toward cells of transitional (urothelial) type; lesions composed of this type of epithelium, although not strictly müllerian, are also discussed. Pure mesenchymal lesions are much less common, consisting of those composed of smooth muscle or endometrial stromal-type cells. Although the secondary müllerian system as defined includes the ovarian surface epithelium, nonneoplastic and neoplastic lesions derived therefrom are discussed in Chapter 16, Nonneoplastic Lesions of Ovary, and Chapter 18, Epithelial Tumors of Ovary, respectively.

The third section of this chapter briefly considers the various pelvic lesions composed of mesothelial cells lacking müllerian differentiation. They may be confused on microscopic examination with lesions of the secondary müllerian system but should be distinguished from them because of important clinical and pathologic differences.

Endometriosis

Definition

Endometriosis is defined as the presence of endometrial epithelium and stroma in an ectopic site excluding the myometrium; ectopic endometrium within the myometrium is designated *adenomyosis*. Although adenomyosis has been referred to as endometriosis interna, this term is no longer used because endometriosis and adenomyosis are unrelated disorders. Adenomyosis is discussed in Chapter 13, Mesenchymal Tumors of Uterus.

Sites

Common
- Ovaries
- Uterine ligaments (uterosacral, round, broad)
- Rectovaginal septum
- Cul-de-sac
- Pelvic peritoneum covering uterus, tubes, rectosigmoid, and bladder

Less Common
- Cervix, vagina
- Rectosigmoid, appendix
- Bladder, ureter
- Omentum
- Skin (scars, umbilicus, vulva, perineum, inguinal region)
- Pelvic lymph nodes
- Inguinal region (noncutaneous)

Rare
- Lungs and pleura
- Small bowel, cecum
- Skeletal muscle
- Deep soft tissues
- Pancreas, stomach
- Kidney, urethra
- Sciatic nerve
- Subarachnoid space
- Diaphragmatic peritoneum
- Bone, breast

Etiology and Pathogenesis

The pathogenesis of endometriosis remains controversial. The two principal histogenetic theories are (1) metastases of endometrial tissue to its ectopic location (metastatic theory) and (2) metaplastic development of endometrial tissue at the ectopic site (metaplastic theory). Some investigators favor a combination of the metastatic and the metaplastic theories, postulating that endometriosis represents a metaplastic response to the irritative effects of endometrial tissue that has metastasized to the ectopic site.[373] The metastatic theory explains the majority of cases, but there is convincing evidence to support each theory, and as they are not mutually exclusive, it is likely that both are valid.

Metastatic Theory

Menstrual Implantation. Sampson proposed that endometriosis was a consequence of reflux of endometrial tissue through the fallopian tubes by a process of retrograde menstruation, with subsequent implantation and growth on peritoneal surfaces.[333] He also believed that additional foci of endometriosis could arise from periodic rupture of endometriotic cysts and implantation of their contents.[333] Implantation of menstrual endometrium has also been proposed for the origin of endometriosis within abdominal scars after surgery, on traumatized cervical and vaginal mucosa, and within perineal and vulvar scars after vaginal delivery.[117,348] Passage of refluxed menstrual endometrium from the peritoneal cavity through diaphragmatic defects, diaphragmatic lymphatics, or both has been postulated as an explanation for pleural endometriosis.[155]

Observations supporting the menstrual implantation hypothesis include (1) the distribution of pelvic endometriotic lesions, which are most common on the surface of the ovaries and fallopian tubes, (2) retrograde menstruation through the fallopian tubes is a common physiologic process, occurring in 90% of menstruating women with patent tubes,[32,142] (3) menstrual endometrium is viable, capable of growth in tissue culture[187] and after subcutaneous injection in humans,[306] (4) endometriosis frequently occurs in females with congenital obstruction to menstrual flow,[146,151,335,350] (5) endometriosis may follow uteropelvic or uteroabdominal wall fistulas in experimental animals[351,389] and humans,[384] and (6) tubal endometriosis that occurs after tubal ligation originates from the luminal aspect of the tip of the proximal segment.[309,378]

Intraoperative Implantation. Although endometriosis in some scars may be a result of menstrual implantation, it has been proposed that endometriosis within operative scars after uterine operations may be secondary to intraoperative implantation of endometrial tissue.[50,373] Supporting this theory is the greater frequency of scar endometriosis after abdominal hysterotomy than after cesarean section in some studies, consistent with the greater viability of transplanted early-pregnancy endometrium compared to late-pregnancy endometrium.[348] Also, it has been shown that the occurrence of endometriosis within an episiotomy scar is much higher if uterine curettage is performed immediately after delivery than in patients without postdelivery curettage.[282]

Lymphatic and Vascular Spread. The presence of endometriosis in certain distant sites (e.g., lungs, skeletal muscle, subarachnoid space, kidneys) is most easily explained by hematogenous spread from the uterus. Similarly, it has been proposed that endometriosis within lymph nodes is a result of lymphatic spread.[173] Evidence supporting the origin of endometriosis from lymphatic or hematogenous spread includes (1) the presence of normal endometrial tissue within endothelium-lined spaces as an incidental histologic finding within the myometrium,[173,331] (2) the presence of intraluminal vascular involvement in rare endometriotic lesions,[1,417] (3) the presence of intravascular or perivascular trophoblastic tissue and decidua* as an incidental histologic finding within the lungs of pregnant patients,[219] (4) the occurrence of pulmonary endometriosis almost exclusively in women who have had prior uterine surgery that could predispose to the embolization of endometrial tissue,[410] (5) the experimental production of pulmonary endometriosis by intravenous injection of endometrial tissue in rabbits,[157] (6) the postmortem demonstration of desquamated squamous cells in pleural and pulmonary lymphatics in an infant with congenital obstruction of the genital tract similar to those present within the upper vagina, endometrial cavity, and peritoneal cavity,[90] and (7) the observations that tumor cells, blood, dye, and radiographic material can migrate from the pelvis to the umbilicus by retrograde lymphatic flow.[350]

* By current criteria, these intrapulmonary foci of decidua would probably be interpreted as foci of intermediate trophoblast.[202,203]

Metaplastic Theory

The origin of pelvic endometriosis by a process of metaplasia from the pelvic peritoneum is consistent with the putative müllerian potential of this tissue, which has been referred to as the *secondary müllerian system.*[215] Evidence for the metaplastic theory includes (1) the demonstration of endometriosis in subjects in whom metastasis of normally situated endometrium could not occur or is highly unlikely, such as patients with Turner's syndrome and pure gonadal dysgenesis who are amenorrheic and have hypoplastic uteri[31,91,101,286] and in males with endometriosis of the bladder, prostate, scrotum, and abdominal wall,[21,235,342,354] (2) the experimental induction of peritoneal endometriosis adjacent to Millipore filters that contain endometrial tissue but which prevent cellular transfer,[247] (3) the observation that autologous endometrial implants in rabbits degenerate but are associated with the subsequent development of endometriosis in adjacent tissues,[218] (4) the association of endometriosis with a distinctive type of mesothelial proliferation not seen in patients without endometriosis,[191] and (5) the presence of other metaplastic tissues, such as smooth muscle,[313] endocervical and tubal epithelium[213] within endometriotic lesions, and the juxtaposition of endometriosis with other putative metaplastic lesions of the peritoneum, such as disseminated peritoneal leiomyomatosis.[23,181,200]

Other Etiologic Factors

Endometriosis is an idiopathic disease in the vast majority of affected patients, and why only a minority of females develop the disease despite the common occurrence of retrograde menstruation is unknown. Some potential etiologic factors have been discussed (congenital obstruction, iatrogenic implantation); others are summarized in the following section.

Genetic Factors. Familial cases of endometriosis have been reported, and such cases may be more widespread than previously appreciated. In these studies, the prevalence of the disease has been found to be much greater in mothers and sisters of women with endometriosis than in the mothers and sisters of their husbands.[228,305,363] In familial cases, the endometriosis is typically severe. Genetic studies suggest that the mode of the inheritance is most likely polygenic (influenced by several different genes) or multifactorial (a result of interaction between genetic and environmental factors).

Hormonal Factors. Because endometriosis occurs almost exclusively in women of reproductive age, it has been suggested that a disturbance in endocrine function may play an etiologic role.[113] The rare examples of endometriosis in phenotypic females with gonadal dysgenesis and in males have usually been associated with the use of exogenous estrogens.* Experimentally, it has been shown in monkeys that autologous peritoneal transplants of endometrium require no steroid supplementation for initiation, but once implanted, either estradiol or progesterone, alone or in combination, is required for maintenance of the lesion.[82,349] Estrogen levels in human subjects with endometriosis, however, have been normal in several studies.[37,369]

It has been suggested that the progestational milieu of pregnancy may inhibit the development of endometriosis. Many studies have indicated that endometriosis is more likely to occur in women who have delayed pregnancy and is less common in women who have had multiple pregnancies.[79] Similarly, one study found that patients with endometriosis were much less likely to have used oral contraceptives than similar patients without endometriosis.[356]

Recently, some studies found an increased frequency of the luteinized unruptured follicle syndrome (LUFS)[196,232] in patients with endometriosis.[37,52,86–88,296] In normal women, the ruptured corpus luteum releases its progesterone-rich fluid into the peritoneal cavity.[67,196] It has been postulated that this fluid may be inhibitory to the implantation and growth of refluxed endometrial fragments at the time of menstruation.[198] In patients with the LUFS, a corpus luteum is formed, but rupture and fluid release do not occur, resulting in lowered luteal phase levels of progesterone in the peritoneal fluid.[88,196,198] It is hypothesized that this local hormonal imbalance may be critical in allowing endometrial cells to implant on the peritoneum.[198] Other studies, however, have shown no difference in the luteal phase peritoneal fluid hormone values in women with or without endometriosis.

Immune Factors. One study has demonstrated a reduced T-lymphocyte-mediated cytotoxicity to autologous endometrial cells and a decreased lymphocyte stimulation response to autologous endometrial antigens in patients with endometriosis.[374] The degree of the depressed cellular immunity was directly proportional to the severity of the disease. The authors of this study suggested that certain cell-mediated immune mechanisms that may be operative in limiting the growth of endometriotic tissue may be impaired in patients with endometriosis.

Peritoneal Defects. Defects or lacerations of the pelvic peritoneum, concentrated in the region of the broad and uterosacral ligaments, were first described in 1955 by Allen and Masters, who considered them possibly traumatic in origin.[6] More recently, a study of patients with laparoscopically detected pelvic peritoneal defects found that 68% had associated endometriosis.[48] In some cases, the endometriotic foci were located along the edges of the defects. It was concluded that there was a probable relationship between the two processes, although it was not clear whether the defects predisposed to the development of endometriosis or if the defects were a result of the endometriosis.

Pelvic Peritoneal and Ovarian Endometriosis

Gross Appearance

Early endometriotic foci involving pelvic peritoneal surfaces are multiple, punctate, red, blue, or brown lesions, with a slightly raised or puckered contour with the adjacent serosa (Fig. 17.1).[113] The latter may show vascular congestion and ecchymotic or brown discoloration secondary to hemosiderin deposition, so-called powder burns.[83] The endometriotic foci are frequently surrounded by dense fibrous adhesions. The lesions may enlarge to produce nodules, cysts, or both.

Endometriotic cysts (endometriomas) most commonly involve the ovaries, where they may partially or completely replace the normal ovarian tissue; bilateral involvement occurs in one third to one half of patients.[84,97] They rarely exceed 15 cm, and if they are larger, the presence of a neoplasm arising within the cyst should be excluded.[321] The cysts are commonly covered by dense fibrous adhesions that may result in fixation to adjacent structures. Endometriotic cysts typically have a fibrotic wall of variable thickness, with a smooth or granular, brown to yellow lining (Fig. 17.2). The contents of cysts consist of semifluid or inspissated, chocolate-colored material.[113] Any solid areas or intraluminal polypoid projections should be sampled histologically, since they may represent a malignant tumor arising from the cyst lining. Rarely, pelvic peritoneal endometriosis involving the ovaries or extraovarian pelvic sites may appear as multiple, polypoid masses that fill the pelvis, simulating a malignant tumor.[43,106,258,355]

Microscopic Appearance

The diagnosis of endometriosis on microscopic examination requires the presence of ectopic endometrial epithelium associated with endometrial stroma (Figs. 17.3 and 17.4). The appearance of endometriotic tissue can vary

* References 21, 31, 91, 101, 235, 286, 342, 354.

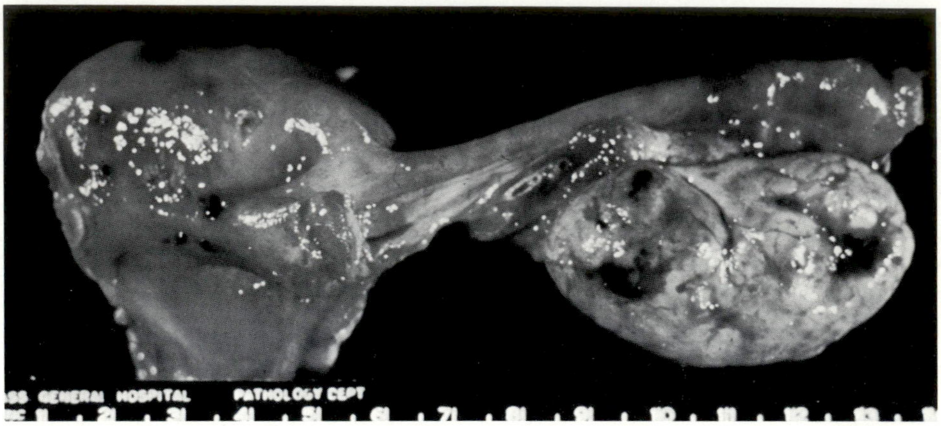

FIG. 17.1. Endometriosis of uterine serosa and ovary. Multiple, hemorrhagic lesions involve the serosal surfaces. (Courtesy of Dr. R. E. Scully.)

depending on the degree of its response to the normal hormonal fluctuations of the menstrual cycle. When the appearance of simultaneous samples of eutopic endometrium and endometriotic foci are compared, it is found that in approximately 80% of patients the latter exhibit cyclic changes, although considerable variability in glandular and epithelial cell morphology may be observed (Fig. 17.5).[25,311] The remaining patients lacked such changes despite well-defined changes in the eutopic endometrium. In one of the latter studies,[25] 70% of foci with a cyclic pattern had changes that were considered synchronous (± 3 days) with the eutopic endometrium, and in 30%, the changes were dyssynchronous. When more than one endometriotic focus was sampled histologically in the same patient, the appearance of the specimens did not differ significantly from one to the other.

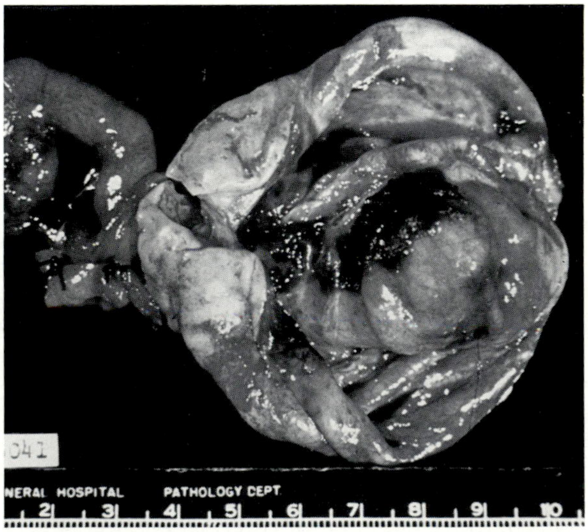

FIG. 17.2. Endometriotic cyst of ovary. The cyst has been opened to reveal a focally hemorrhagic lining. (Courtesy of Dr. R. E. Scully.)

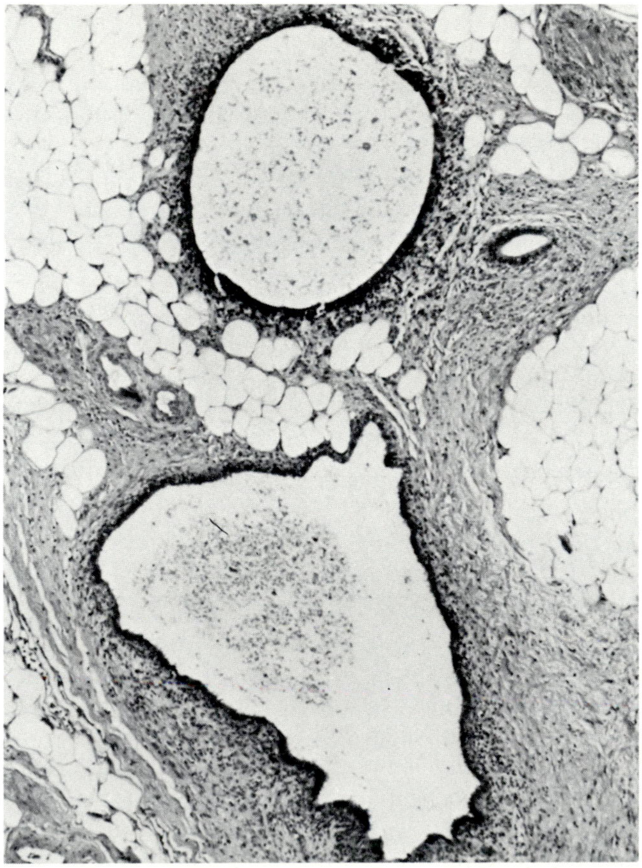

FIG. 17.3. Endometriosis of cul-de-sac. Cystic endometrial glands with a cuff of endometrial stroma are surrounded by fibrous and adipose tissue.

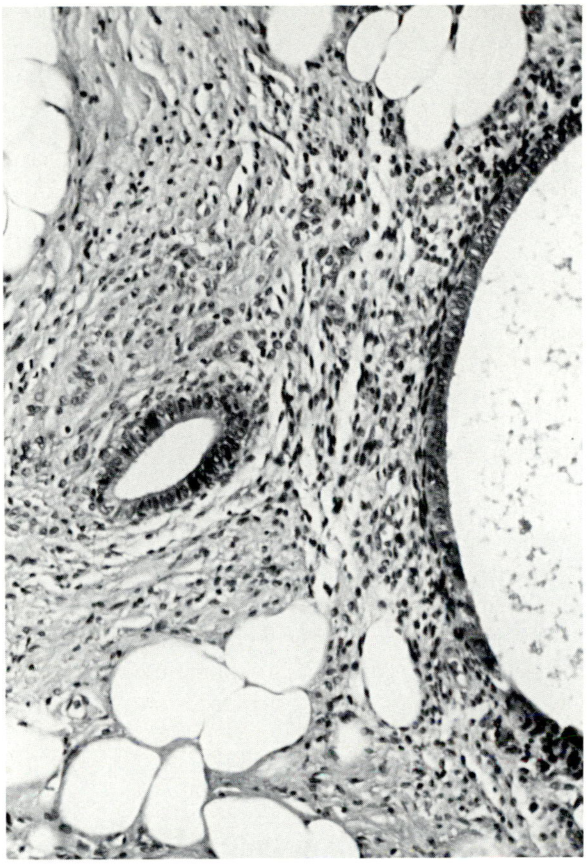

FIG. 17.4. Endometriosis of cul-de-sac (higher magnification of Fig. 17.3). Endometriotic glands are lined by inactive epithelium and surrounded by a thin rim of endometrial stroma.

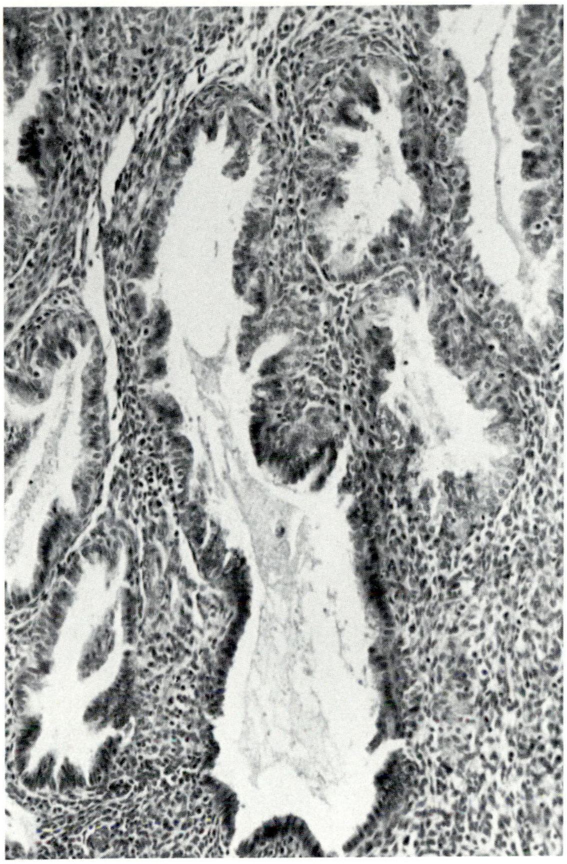

FIG. 17.5. Irregular secretory changes within a focus of endometriosis. The progestational response is less pronounced in the glandular epithelium at bottom of figure.

Other studies, however, have suggested that the degree of hormonal response may vary with the site.[268]

Periodic menstrual changes within the endometriotic focus will result in histologic evidence of recent and remote hemorrhage within the endometriotic stroma and glandular lumens and a secondary inflammatory response. The latter consists predominantly of macrophages, usually containing hemosiderin, ceroid pigment, and lipid (pseudoxanthoma cells) (Fig. 17.6).[267] Occasionally, the pigmented macrophages are of the multinucleated, foreign body type. In addition, variable numbers of neutrophils, lymphocytes, and plasma cells and varying degrees of fibrosis are typically seen. In endometriotic cysts, the epithelial cells lining the cyst are often large and cuboidal, with abundant eosinophilic cytoplasm and large nuclei, which focally may appear atypical (Fig. 17.7).[71,353] Nuclear atypia of this type was recorded in 22% of cases of ovarian endometriosis in one study[71] and probably represents a reactive phenomenon. The epithelial and stromal lining of an endometriotic cyst frequently becomes attenuated, and the former may be reduced to a single layer of cuboidal cells, which may

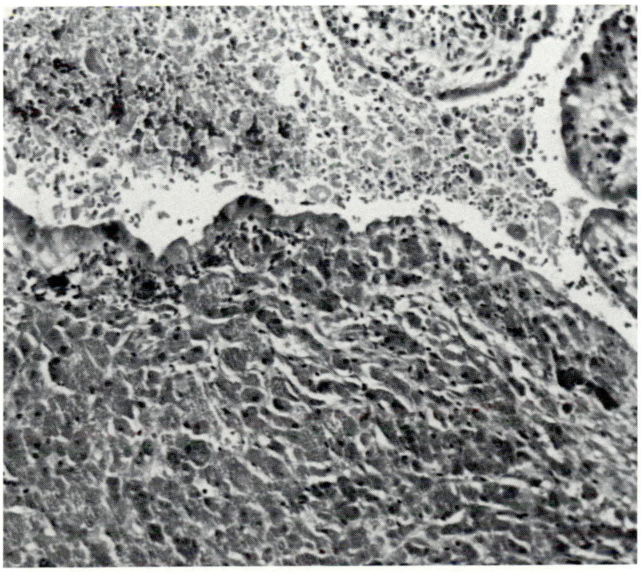

FIG. 17.6. Lining of ovarian endometriotic cyst. The lining consists of endometrial surface epithelium and numerous pigment-laden histiocytes within the subjacent stroma. Menstrual debris is present within the cyst lumen.

retain to some extent endometrial characteristics but which is frequently devoid of specific features.[113] In such circumstances, recognition of the cyst as endometriotic may only be possible if a rim of subjacent endometrial stroma persists. Commonly, the cyst lining of endometrial epithelium and stroma is totally lost and is replaced

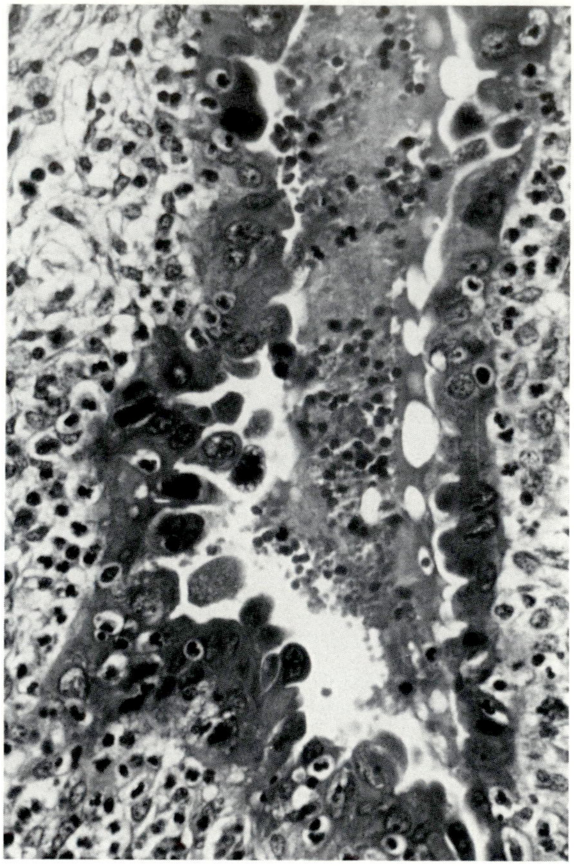

FIG. 17.7. Lining of ovarian endometriotic cyst. The surface epithelial cells show striking nuclear atypia.

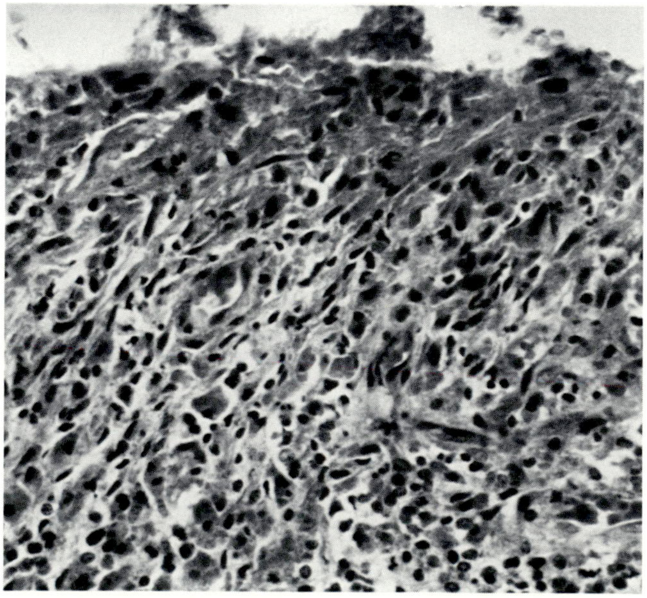

FIG. 17.8. Lining of ovarian endometriotic cyst. In this field, the lining consists only of fibrotic granulation tissue and pigment-laden histiocytes (presumptive endometriosis).

a

b

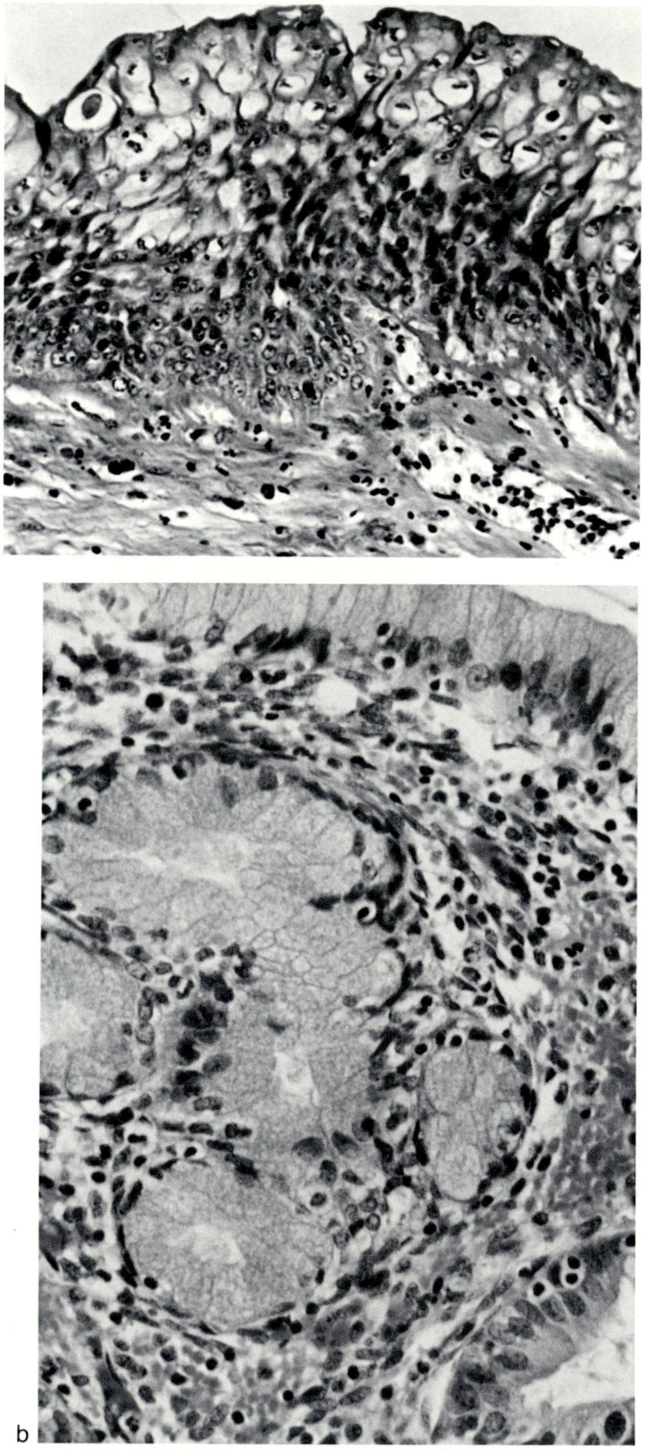

FIG. 17.9. Glandular metaplasia in endometriosis. *a*. Squamous metaplasia in the lining of an endometriotic cyst. *b*. Mucinous metaplasia of endometriotic glands.

by granulation tissue, dense fibrous tissue, and numerous pigmented macrophages (Fig. 17.8). In these cases, a definitive diagnosis of endometriosis cannot be made because a similar appearance can be seen in an old corpus luteum cyst.

Endometriotic foci involving smooth muscle, such as the uterine ligaments, are typically associated with striking proliferation of the smooth muscle, creating an adenomyomatous appearance similar to that of adenomyosis within the myometrium (as in Fig. 17.14).[355] Polypoid endometriosis typically resembles an endometrial polyp on histologic examination.[355] Perineural[318] and vascular invasion[1,417] may occur rarely in otherwise typical, benign endometriotic lesions. Endometriotic tissues may exhibit atrophic changes in postmenopausal patients characterized by cystic glands lined by flattened, epithelial cells surrounded by a dense fibrotic stroma. The appearance is similar to that of simple or cystic atrophy of the endometrium.[188]

Metaplastic Changes. Metaplastic changes similar to those occurring in eutopic endometrial glands (Chapter 11, Endometrial Hyperplasia and Metaplasia) have been described in endometriotic glands. These include tubal (ciliated) metaplasia,[71,214,215] hobnail metaplasia,[71] and, rarely, squamous (Fig. 17.9)[399] and mucinous metaplasia. The latter may be composed of endocervical-type cells (Fig. 17.9) or, more rarely, goblet cells.[213,214,426]

The endometriotic stroma may exhibit smooth muscle metaplasia, most frequently within the walls of ovarian endometriotic cysts.[66,313,315,353,354] The smooth muscle may arise from metaplasia of the ovarian stroma, but a metaplastic origin from the endometriotic stroma is also possible, consistent with the myofibroblastic nature of the endometrial stromal cell.[354] Extensive amounts of smooth muscle within the endometriotic stroma can result in endomyometriosis, uterus-like masses that have been described within an obturator lymph node (Fig. 17.10),[313] ovary,[66,293] broad ligament (mülleroma),[45] lumbosacral region,[201] and in males in the scrotum.[354] In the region of the ovary and broad ligament, these uterus-like masses may represent congenital müllerian duct fusion defects.[45,293,315] An example occurring in the lumbosacral region was considered a choristoma of müllerian

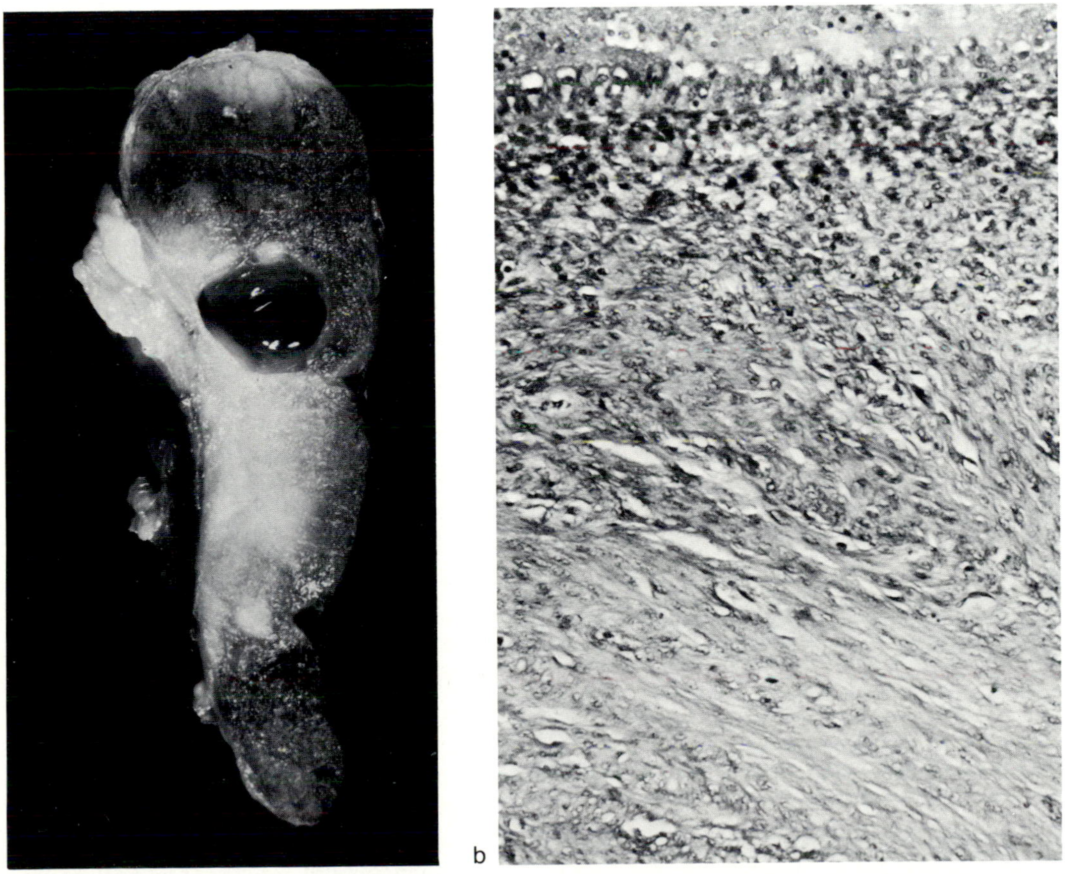

a b

Fig. 17.10. Smooth muscle metaplasia in endometriosis (endomyometriosis of obturator lymph node). *a*. The cut surface of the lymph node is focally replaced by solid, pale tissue that partially surrounds a cystic space. [Reprinted from Arch Pathol Lab Med (1981), 105:556–557. Copyright 1981, American Medical Association.] *b*. The cyst is lined by endometrial epithelium, a thin rim of endometrial stroma, and a thick layer of smooth muscle. (Courtesy of Dr. E. Bossen.)

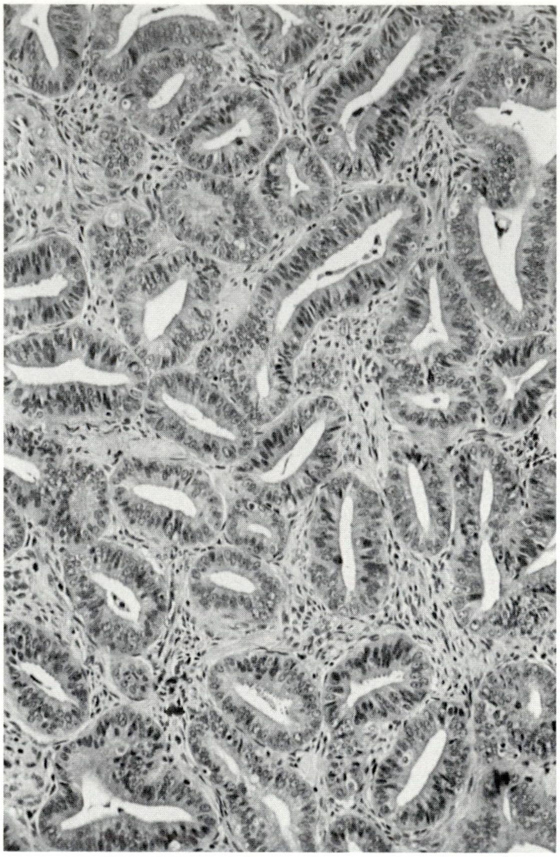

FIG. 17.11. Hyperplasia within endometriosis. Endometriotic glands exhibit architectural and cytologic atypia. Endometrioid carcinoma was found elsewhere in the specimen (see Fig. 17.23).

type.[201] Rarely, foci of ossification and calcification may occur within the endometriotic stroma.[120,355,361]

Unusual Hormonal Effects. A variety of benign or atypical hyperplastic changes similar to those occurring in the endometrium (Chapter 11, Endometrial Hyperplasia and Metaplasia) have been described rarely within endometriotic glands, usually in response to an endogenous or exogenous estrogenic stimulus (Fig. 17.11).[71,103,130,180,353] These hyperplastic changes probably have a premalignant potential similar to those in the endometrium, although there has been little evidence on which to base such a conclusion.[258] Hyperplastic changes, however, have been documented in rare cases within endometriosis that preceded the development of an adenocarcinoma in the same area.[130,424]

Endometriotic tissue may exhibit hyperprogestational changes, typically in pregnancy or due to progestagen treatment.[194,353] In such cases, the endometriotic tissue exhibits a decidual reaction and atrophy of the endometrial glands, which typically are small and lined by cuboidal or flattened epithelial cells (Fig. 17.12a). Rarely, in pregnancy, the glands may exhibit an Arias-Stella reaction (Fig. 17.12b) or optically clear nuclei.[239,252,368] Necrosis of the decidualized cells, foci of marked stromal edema, and infiltration by lymphocytes are additional findings described secondary to exogenous progestational agents.[194] Atrophic changes similar to those seen within endometriotic foci in postmenopausal patients may be seen in premenopausal patients treated with danazol.[283,345] In one study, one third of the endometriotic foci completely disappeared or were replaced by fibrous tissue.[345]

Changes Secondary to Pelvic Inflammatory Disease. Bacterial infection and abscess formation are a rare complication of ovarian endometriotic cysts.[97,337] Microabscesses may be seen on histologic examination of the cyst wall in such cases.[337] There is usually an associated salpingitis, history of a hysterosalpingogram, or both, suggesting the fallopian tubes as the likely portal of the infection.[337]

Histologically documented salpingitis was noted in one third of patients with ovarian endometriosis in one study. Pigmented histiocytes similar to those seen in the walls of endometriotic cysts were noted within the lamina propria of the fallopian tubes in some of these patients. It is unlikely that these inflammatory lesions are a significant factor contributing to infertility in patients with endometriosis, since there is no difference in the fertility rates of patients with endometriosis who do or do not have an associated salpingitis.[110]

Rare Associated Lesions. Rare examples of endometriosis in intimate association with the smooth muscle nodules of peritoneal leiomyomatosis,[162,181,200] glial implants of peritoneal gliomatosis,[5,19] and splenic nodules of splenosis[364] have been described. Endometriosis has also been juxtaposed to peritoneal foci of granulomatous inflammation secondary to hysterosalpingographic contrast material[388] or infestation with *Enterobius vermicularis.*[209]

Differential Diagnosis. Endometriosis may be associated with, and should be distinguished from, endosalpingiosis, a lesion characterized by glands lined by benign endosalpingeal epithelium. Endosalpingiosis lacks endometrial stroma and the typical inflammatory response associated with endometriosis. Endometriotic cysts should not be confused with endometrioid neoplasms. In some cases, the endometrial stroma in the wall of endometriotic cysts can be obliterated by fibrosis over a large area, resulting in an erroneous diagnosis of endometrioid cystadenoma. Conversely, endometrioid neoplasms may contain foci of benign endometrioid epithelium, but endometrioid stroma is absent, and in the vast majority of cases, there is overt histologic malignancy of the epithelial component in other areas of the tumor.[353]

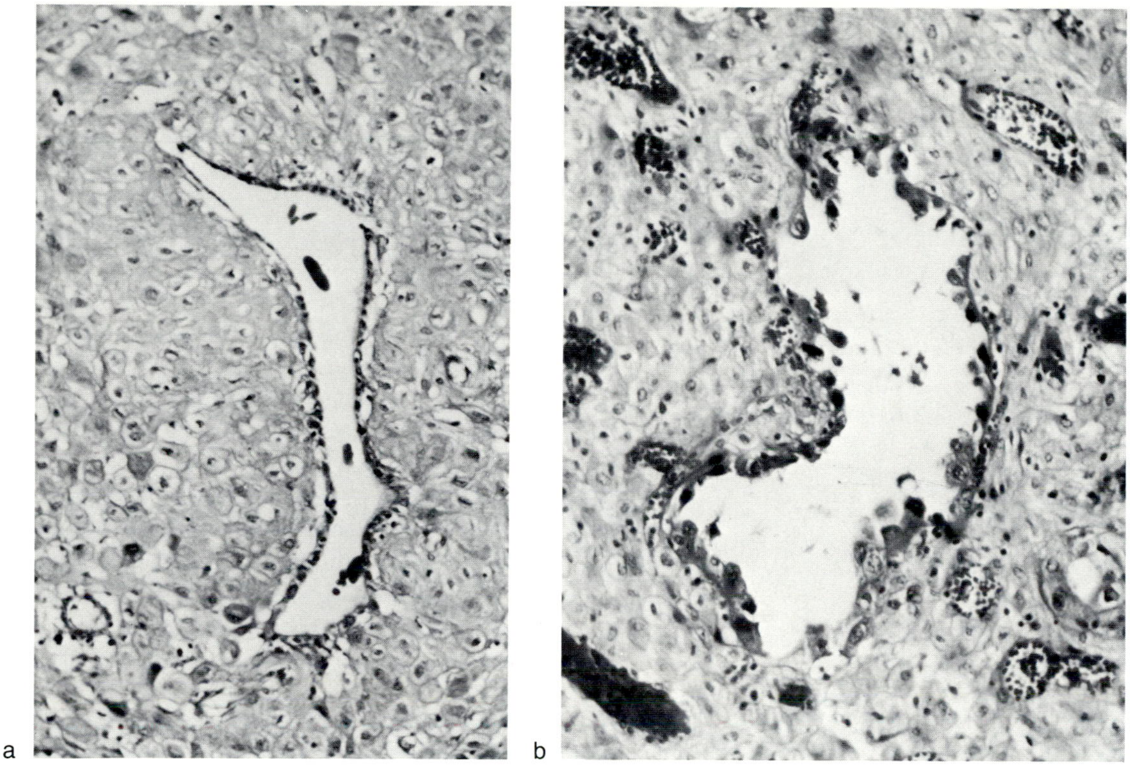

Fig. 17.12. Pregnancy-induced changes within endometriosis. *a*. The endometriotic gland is atrophic, and the stroma exhibits marked decidual transformation. *b*. The endometriotic gland exhibits an Arias–Stella reaction. The stroma is decidualized.

Ultrastructural, Histochemical, and Steroid Receptor Studies

Endometriotic glands typically exhibit ultrastructural features that represent a response, but an incomplete one, to the prevalent hormonal milieu of the particular phase of the menstrual cycle.[344,347] In one study, 25% of the endometriotic foci contained glands that were poorly differentiated and showed no hormonal response ultrastructurally.[347] In the remaining foci, as the proliferative phase progressed, there was an increase in Golgi, mitochondria, rough endoplasmic reticulum, and secretory vesicles, with a further increase in secretory vesicles and intraluminal secretion during the secretory phase. In contrast to eutopic glands, however, it was usually not possible to date the glands precisely within the secretory phase because of marked interglandular and intraglandular variability and the absence of specific ultrastructural characteristics (giant mitochondria, nuclear channel systems) that occurred in the normal endometrium after ovulation. Ultrastructural examination of endometriotic tissue after danazol treatment shows either arrest of the endometriotic glandular epithelium in the early proliferative phase or disorganization of the epithelial cells with atrophic changes, including vacuolization of organelles, especially mitochondria.[345,346] Additional ultrastructural findings secondary to danazol treatment include deep nuclear indentations of the epithelial cells and large numbers of membrane-bound granules filled with a fine fibrillar material within the cytoplasm.[283]

Histochemical studies comparing enzyme profiles of alkaline phosphatase, acid phosphatase, and oxidative enzymes of normal endometrium and endometriotic foci have shown similar but not identical staining reactions in the two sites.[291] One study showed that the normal increase in 17-beta-hydroxysteroid dehydrogenase present in eutopic endometrium during the secretory phase and in response to danazol is absent in endometriotic foci.[398]

Estrogen (ER) and progesterone receptors (PR) have been demonstrated within endometriotic tissue but usually in much lower concentrations than in the normal endometrium.[26,27,172,186,386] In a variable number of cases, one or both receptors are absent.[26] In addition, the normal variation in the quantitity of both receptors exhibited by eutopic endometrium during the menstrual cycle is diminished or absent within foci of endometriosis.[24,129,398] Differences in receptor concentrations between eutopic endometrium and endometriotic epithelium in response to danazol have also been noted.[186,398] No correlation has been found between receptor levels and severity of symptoms. In addition, it has been shown that in contrast to eutopic luteal phase endometrium, endometriotic implants do not appear to secrete measurable quantities of prolactin.[143]

In summary, the findings of these studies are consistent with the incomplete and variable hormonal response of endometriotic foci observed on microscopic examination. They may indicate a greater degree of autonomy of endometriotic tissue from the mechanisms controlling eutopic endometrium and explain the failure of hormonal therapy in some patients.

Clinical Aspects

Epidemiologic Factors. The highest risk of the disease is in the upper socioeconomic levels of developed societies, especially among women who delay pregnancy.[163] In the past, endometriosis was considered to be more common in Caucasians, but recent studies showing a similar frequency of the disease in Orientals[251] and blacks[47] cast doubt on this view. Nonwhites also appear to have an increased risk of the disease as their socioeconomic status improves.[163]

Over 80% of affected patients are in the reproductive age group, typically 25–40 years of age. In this age group, endometriosis is thought to be a common disease, but its true incidence is unknown, since many patients are asymptomatic. Reported incidence figures vary depending on the population studied (low in parous asymptomatic women, higher in patients with infertility or pelvic pain)[137] and whether the diagnosis is made clinically, surgically, or pathologically. Endometriosis has been documented histologically in 18.7–38% of patients of reproductive age undergoing laparotomy.[405,413] According to Houston, true secular trends in the occurrence of endometriosis remain unknown because of an absence of population-based incidence data.[163]

Less than 5% of cases occur in postmenopausal patients, and in such patients, the disease is frequently not diagnosed premenopausally.[188] Endometriosis can be clinically significant in this age group, with 20–30% of affected patients requiring surgery.[188,294] In some postmenopausal patients, an association with obesity and endometrial carcinoma has been noted, suggesting hyperestrinism,[294] but in other series, a majority of patients have had no obvious exogenous or endogenous source of estrogen.[151,188]

Almost 10% of patients with endometriosis are adolescents.[49] Endometriosis has been found at laparoscopy in 47–65% of teenage patients with dysmenorrhea or chronic pelvic pain, suggesting that it is a significant cause of these symptoms in this population.[41,49,124] Some adolescents with endometriosis may have amenorrhea due to a congenital obstruction to menstrual flow.[166,335]

Symptoms and Signs. It is generally believed that the recurrent cyclic menstrual inflammatory and fibrotic changes are responsible for most of the symptomatology of endometriosis. Generally, however, there is little direct relationship between the extent of the disease and the severity of the symptoms, and in some patients, the latter is inversely proportional to the extent of disease.[49,299] Hormonal responsiveness of the lesions as judged histologically also does not correlate with symptoms.[311] Similarly, microscopic examination of symptomatic endometriosis in postmenopausal patients typically reveals atrophic changes.[188]

The typical symptoms that are attributed to pelvic endometriosis are acquired dysmenorrhea, lower abdominal, pelvic, and back pain, dyspareunia, irregular bleeding, and infertility.[83,377] Pelvic examination may reveal tender nodules in the cul-de-sac and uterosacral ligments, tender, semifixed, cystic ovaries, and a fixed, retroverted uterus.[195,299] The rectovaginal septum may be tender and indurated.[257] The endometriotic lesions frequently enlarge and become more painful during menses. As these clinical manifestations are nonspecific, vary widely between patients, and may be absent in a high proportion of patients, a definitive diagnosis requires direct visualization by laparoscopy or laparotomy and biopsy.[83,311] The clinical manifestations also vary according to the site of the endometriosis; these are discussed in subsequent sections.

Effects of Pregnancy. Although rare cases of endometriosis undergo permanent regression during pregnancy, the ameliorative effect of pregnancy noted in many patients with endometriosis is only temporary.[240,401] The behavior of endometriosis during pregnancy is extremely variable among different patients and between one pregnancy and another in the same patient.[240] During pregnancy, visible endometriotic lesions frequently undergo initial enlargement, with occasional ulceration and bleeding, followed by shrinkage. In most sites, there is a decrease in the associated pain.[240]

A rare complication of endometriosis during pregnancy is intrapartum or postpartum rupture of the lesion, most probably due to a softening of the lesion secondary to stromal decidualization, pressure from the expanding uterus, or both. Rupture occurs most frequently in the ovaries or bowel, typically resulting in perforation and an acute abdomen.[8,60,108,317] Hemoperitoneum and death due to hemorrhage from decidualized endometriotic lesions at term have been described.[312]

Rare Complications. Massive, sometimes serosanguineous, ascites may occur in patients with pelvic endometriosis; a right pleural effusion is also present in one third of such patients.[57,138,169,171,175] Seventy percent of the reported cases of this complication have occurred in black women, suggesting a possible racial predilection.[138] If one or both ovaries are involved, the findings at surgery may simulate those of an ovarian carcinoma. The pathogenesis of the ascites is not clear. Possible sources include production by endometriotic cysts, irritated peritoneal mesothelial cells, or the ovarian serosa (Meigs-like syndrome). The ascites typically responds to danazol treatment.[171] Other rare complications include hemorrhage from an endometriotic focus[166,298] and spontaneous rupture of ovarian endometriotic cysts, resulting in an acute abdomen.[151,292]

Pathophysiology of Endometriosis-Related Infertility

Primary or secondary infertility occurs in 30–40% of patients with endometriosis and is the most common manifestation of endometriosis in otherwise healthy, young, married females.[195,377,405] Conversely, it has been estimated that endometriosis is present in 15–25% of infertile women, and in patients with otherwise unexplained infertility, the frequency of endometriosis may be as high as 70–80%.[85,405] The etiology of the infertility, particularly in patients with mild disease, is not fully understood. The following are all possible factors.

Tubal Factors. Both fallopian tubes are usually fully patent in patients with endometriosis, but serosal endometriosis, peritubal adhesions, or both may impair tubal motility. Nonobstructive chronic salpingitis has been found in one third of patients with endometriosis, but no difference has been demonstrated in the prevalence of this lesion between fertile and infertile patients with endometriosis.[72,110]

Ovarian Factors. Traditionally, ovarian function in patients with endometriosis has been regarded as normal, but anovulation,[4,369] luteal phase dysfunction,[51,52,131,149,289,314] LUFS,[37,87–88] and functionally defective oocytes[402] may occur more frequently in patients with endometriosis than in patients without endometriosis. The finding of lower numbers of LH receptors within granulosa cells in patients with endometriosis than in control patients may provide a basis for some of these defects in ovarian function.[314] Very rarely, patients with endometriosis have galactorrhea and hyperprolactinemia.[149,156] In addition, hypersecretion of prolactin in response to thyrotropin-releasing factor has been found in some patients with endometriosis who have normal resting levels of prolactin.[261] It is postulated that the abnormal prolactin levels in these patients may be responsible for one or more of the aforementioned types of ovarian dysfunction.[261]

Prostaglandins. Several studies have indicated that patients with endometriosis may have elevated levels of certain prostaglandins within their endometrium[404,414] and peritoneal fluid.[77,94,199,421] Refluxed menstrual endometrium, pelvic mesothelial cells, peritoneal fluid macrophages, and endometriotic tissue have been suggested as potential sources of the prostaglandins.[94,254,310,357,421] Proposed mechanisms for infertility mediated by prostaglandins include their effects on tubal motility,[414] uterine contractility,[404] and corpus luteum function.[289,422]

In contrast, a number of other studies have shown that there is no difference in prostaglandin levels between patients with and without endometriosis[14,141,310,357,421] indicating that the findings of earlier studies did not consider the significant differences that exist in prostaglandin levels within peritoneal fluid between various phases of the menstrual cycle.[137] Halme has recently concluded that it is unlikely that significant abnormalities exist in local or distant prostaglandin metabolism in patients with endometriosis.[137]

Autoimmune Factors. Elevated levels of immunoglobulin (IgG and IgA) have been demonstrated in the endometrium, sera, and cervical secretions of patients with endometriosis compared to patients without endometriosis, although in some studies the antibody levels did not differ between fertile and infertile patients with the disorder.[238,330,372] Antiendometrial antibodies have been demonstrated in 85% of patients with endometriosis, compared to 2% of patients who did not have demonstrable endometriosis.[409] Similarly, OC-125, a monoclonal antibody against a membrane antigen found in 80% of patients with ovarian carcinoma, has been detected in almost 50% of patients with severe endometriosis.[18] In addition, complement (C3) has been found in eutopic endometrium in patients with endometriosis but not in control patients.[405] Complement factors ($C3_c$ and C4) may be increased in the serum and peritoneal fluid in patients with endometriosis.[14,15] These findings raise the possibility that an autoimmune reaction to endometrial antigens released from menstruating foci of endometriosis could lead to rejection of the conceptus or interference with sperm passage.[405] Antibodies to ovarian tissue, specifically theca and granulosa cells, have been demonstrated in the sera of patients with endometriosis, suggesting a possible autoimmune mechanism for ovarian dysfunction.[238]

Peritoneal Fluid Macrophages. The majority of studies indicate that no significant difference exists either in the peritoneal fluid volume or in the number of peritoneal fluid macrophages between patients with and without endometriosis, allowing for the normal fluctuation in these parameters during the menstrual cycle.* The macrophages, however, may be more enzymatically active and exhibit an increased capacity to phagocytize sperm in vitro than in normal patients.[16,139,141,260] Interference with normal fertilization could result from release of

---

* References 16, 67, 77, 88, 93, 137, 140, 141, 144, 197, 310, 357.

enzymes from the macrophages[141] or their entry into the oviducts with phagocytosis of sperm.[260]

Spontaneous Abortion. An increased rate of first trimester spontaneous abortion varying from 10 to 52% (average 33%) has been reported in patients with endometriosis.[135,262,272,407] In one study, the abortion rate was higher in patients with mild endometriosis (45% of pregnancies) than in patients with severe endometriosis (24% of pregnancies).[407] In most patients, no obvious cause for the abortion is present; in others, an associated inadequate luteal phase may be a causative factor.

Endometriosis in Other Sites

Intestinal Endometriosis

Approximately 10–20% of patients with endometriosis have intestinal involvement; the figure may be as high as 50% in patients with extensive pelvic disease. Only a minority of affected patients, however, will have clinically significant involvement.[132] The intestine was a common site for clinically significant endometriosis in one study of postmenopausal patients with the disease.[188]

The rectosigmoid is involved most often, usually secondary to endometriosis of the rectovaginal septum or cul-de-sac.* Other intestinal sites involved include, in descending order of frequency, the appendix, terminal ileum, cecum, and other parts of the small intestine (including Meckel's diverticulum) and colon.†

Endometriosis of the rectosigmoid is usually a solitary lesion, involving a segment several centimeters or less in length, whereas ileal involvement is frequently multifocal and more extensive.[234] On gross examination, most intestinal lesions are confined to the serosa and subserosa. When the muscularis propria is involved, the segment of bowel is indurated by an ill-defined, noncircumferential mass with a puckered serosal surface. Opening the bowel reveals a gray-white, firm, mural thickening with punctate hemorrhagic areas (Fig. 17.13). On microscopic examination, there is smooth muscle proliferation and fibrosis surrounding endometriotic foci within the muscularis propria (Fig. 17.14). Rare examples of colonic mucosal involvement with a polypoid appearance may simulate a primary carcinoma.[22,106]

Luminal narrowing or obstruction is a common complication of intestinal endometriosis, usually due to marked angulation or kinking of the segment secondary to the thickening of the muscularis (Fig. 17.13). Less commonly, obstruction may be secondary to circumferential mural thickening without kinking, polypoid mucosal involvement, or serosal adhesions. Rarer complications of intestinal involvement include perforation of endometriotic lesions (typically intrapartum or postpartum),[60,108]

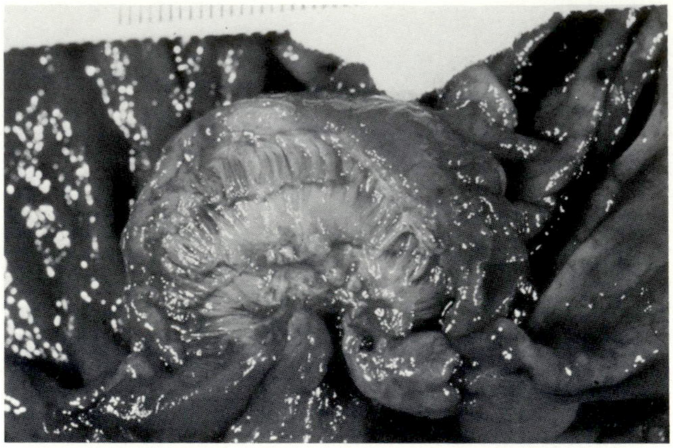

FIG. 17.13. Colonic endometriosis (cut surface). There is marked mural thickening and fibrosis. The serosal surface is retracted, and the overlying mucosa is intact. (Courtesy of Dr. R. D. Croom.)

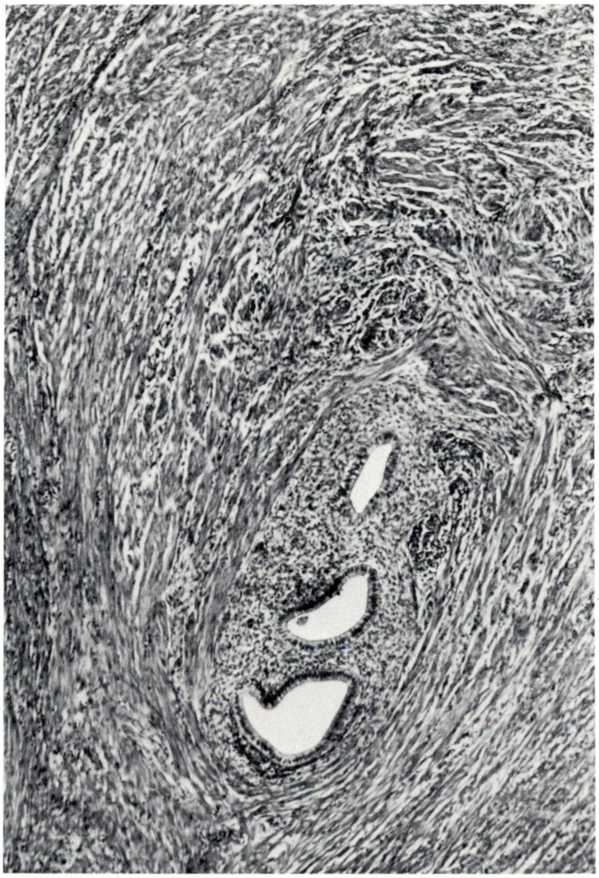

FIG. 17.14. Intestinal endometriosis. The endometriotic tissue within the muscularis propria is surrounded by markedly hyperplastic smooth muscle.

* References 68, 100, 132, 224, 257, 278, 290.

† References 10, 159, 221, 234, 264, 278, 308, 395, 397, 416.

volvulus, intussusception,[10,132,159,207,229,265] acute appendicitis,[264] obstructive mucocele of the appendix,[147,264] and intramural hematoma.[418]

The clinical manifestations are usually nonspecific, but in occasional patients, their catamenial onset may suggest the correct diagnosis. These symptoms include pain, constipation, diarrhea, decreased caliber of the stool, and, rarely, rectal bleeding. Pelvic, endoscopic, and radiologic examination may reveal an obstructing rectosigmoid mass resembling a carcinoma.

Lower Genital Tract Endometriosis

Superficial endometriosis involving the cervix takes the form of small (2–3 mm), solitary to multiple, ecchymotic nodules, cysts, streaks, or patches on the ectocervical mucosa, usually involving areas of prior trauma.[117,268,415] Occasionally, the entire transformation zone is involved, typically in patients who have had a cone biopsy or extensive cautery.[33] Endocervical lesions are less frequently encountered, probably because of their relative inaccessibility to inspection and biopsy. The lesions typically enlarge and change from bright red to blue before menses; during menses they may rupture, leaving an irregular ulcer. Rarely, they may have a papillary or puckered appearance simulating a carcinoma. On histologic examination, the lesions are typically confined to the superficial lamina propria subjacent to the squamous epithelium (Fig. 17.15).[268] Unlike superficial cervical endometriosis, deep cervical endometriosis is usually associated with endometriosis elsewhere in the pelvis. It may be palpable as deep, firm nodules or cysts in the posterior cervix.[117,415] The diagnosis is made by biopsy or pathologic examination of the hysterectomy specimen. The differential diagnosis includes downgrowth of adenomyosis from the uterine corpus. Superficial cervical endometriosis is usually not painful and may be entirely asymptomatic, but usually it presents as premenstrual or postcoital spotting or persistent menorrhagia.

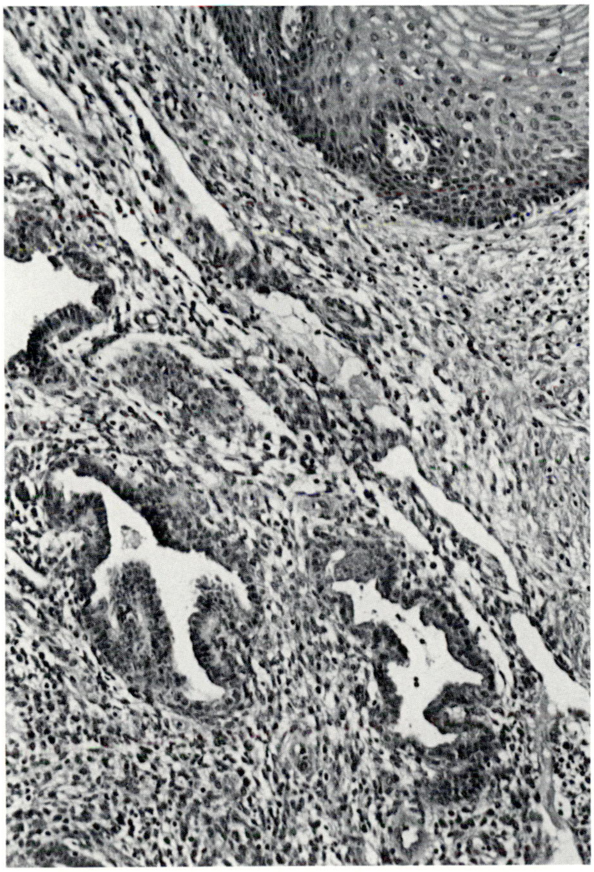

Fig. 17.15. Superficial cervical endometriosis. Endometrial glands (exhibiting secretory changes) and surrounding stroma lie beneath squamous epithelium.

Superficial vaginal endometriosis, which typically involves the vault, is similar to superficial cervical endometriosis in its macroscopic appearance, predilection for involving sites of prior trauma, and lack of associated pelvic endometriosis.[117] Deep vaginal endometriosis associated with pelvic endometriosis is more common, taking the form of nodular or polypoid masses involving the posterior vaginal fornix.[43,117,130,268] The differential diagnosis of vaginal endometriosis, particularly of the superficial type, includes vaginal adenosis of the tuboendometrial variety, but the latter lacks endometrial stroma and the characteristic inflammatory response of endometriosis.

Tubal Endometriosis

The term *endometriosis* has been applied to at least three different, unrelated lesions in the fallopian tube. Most commonly, it refers to serosal or subserosal endometriotic foci associated with endometriosis elsewhere in the pelvis; the myosalpinx is typically not involved.[359]

A second type of lesion is characterized by direct extension of endometrium from the uterine cornua into the interstitial and isthmic segments of the tubes. It has been designated *endometrial colonization* and is typically unassociated with endometriosis elsewhere.[58,78,111,225] The endometrial tissue replaces the normal endosalpingeal mucosa and totally occludes the lumen of the proximal tube (Fig. 17.16); involvement may be bilateral.[58] Endometrial colonization accounts for 15–20% of tubal-related infertility; it may also be associated with tubal pregnancy.[58,225] The etiology of the lesion is not clear, but an association with pelvic inflammatory disease has been noted.[58] Colonization should be differentiated on microscopic examination from focal or diffuse replace-

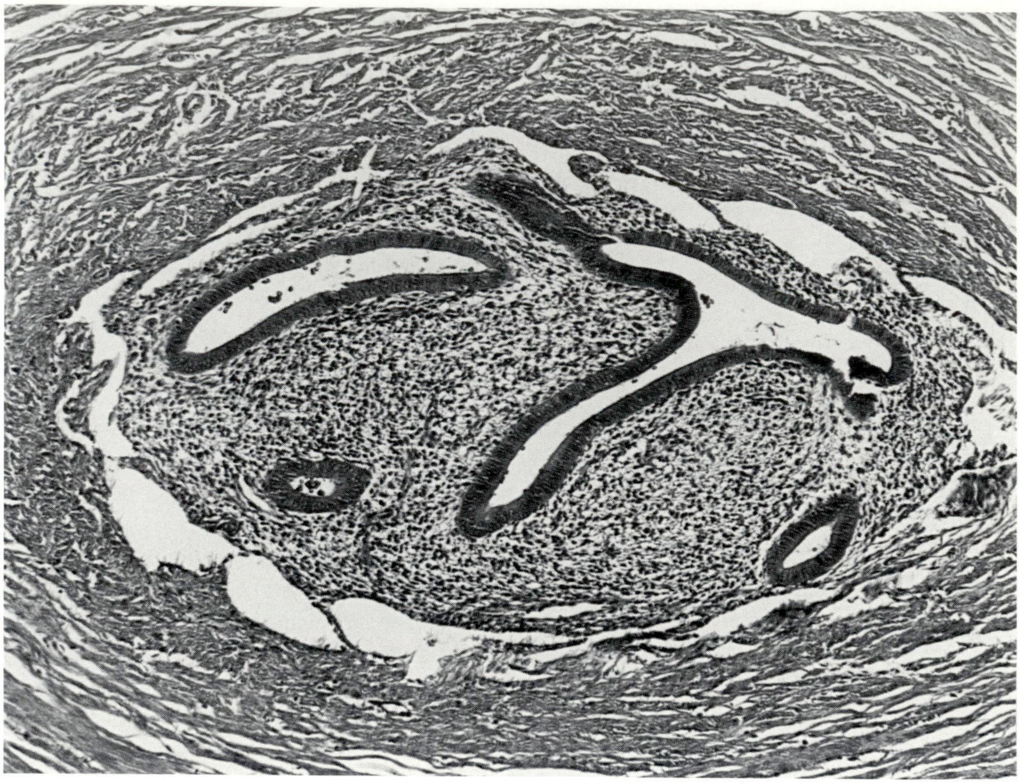

Fig. 17.16. Endometriosis (colonization) of the fallopian tube. The tubal lumen is occluded by endometrial glands and stroma. Spaces at the junction of endometrial tissue and myosalpinx represent dilated lymphatic channels.

ment of the normal endosalpingeal mucosa by endometrium, in which a normal lumen is maintained.[220,322] The latter condition involves the interstitial portion of the tube in 25%[220] and the isthmus in 10%[322] of women with normal fertility and probably represents a normal developmental phenomenon. However, in some of these patients, the ectopic endometrial tissue may give rise to intratubal endometrial-type polyps.[76]

The third type of endometriosis involving the fallopian tube has been designated *postsalpingectomy endometriosis*. It occurs in the tip of the proximal tubal stump, typically 1–4 years after tubal ligation.[309,332,334,378,379] It is closely related to and may be associated with salpingitis isthmica nodosa. The lesion is analogous to uterine adenomyosis, consisting of endometrial glands and stroma extending from the endosalpinx into the myosalpinx, and frequently to the serosal surface. Hysterosalpingography or India ink injection of the specimen may show tuboperitoneal fistulous tracts (Fig. 17.17).[309,379] Postligation pregnancies may result. Postsalpingectomy endometriosis has been documented in 20–50% of tubes examined after ligation. The frequency of this complication is increased with the electrocautery method of ligation, with short proximal stumps, and with increasing postligation intervals.[309,378]

Urinary Tract Endometriosis

Urinary tract involvement is usually associated with endometriosis elsewhere in the pelvis, although rarely it may represent a localized lesion. Approximately 10% of patients with endometriosis have urinary tract involvement, although only 1% have clinically significant lesions. The affected patients are frequently over 40 years of age and may be postmenopausal.[212] The urinary bladder, ureters, kidneys, and urethra, in descending order of frequency, may be involved, although clinically significant involvement is most common in the ureters.*

Bladder involvement is usually an incidental finding on the serosa. Clinically significant bladder endometriosis is usually associated with involvement of the bladder wall, which may represent an extension of serosal or subserosal lesions. In such cases, fibrous adhesions may bind the bladder to the anterior surface of the uterus or other structures. Mural lesions are typically located in the trigone, posterior wall, or floor of the bladder. On gross examination, they are usually solitary, discrete, red-brown, nodular or cystic, polypoid lesions varying in size from several millimeters to 14 cm (Fig. 17.18).

* References 3, 192, 206, 256, 301, 370.

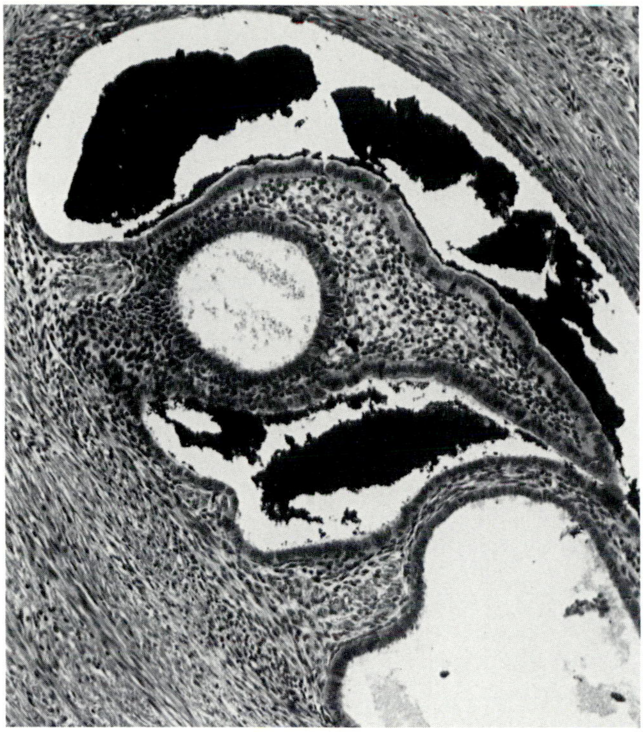

FIG. 17.17. Postsalpingectomy endometriosis of the fallopian tube. Following removal, the lumen of the specimen has been injected with India ink. Endometrial glands and stroma are surrounded by smooth muscle of the myosalpinx. The lumens of the endometrial glands contain India ink. (From Rock JA, Parmley TH, King TM, Laufe LE, Su BC: Endometriosis and the development of tuboperitoneal fistulas after tubal ligation. Fertil Steril 35:16, 1981. Reproduced with permission of the publisher, The American Fertility Society.)

They are covered by intact mucosa, although, occasionally, focal erosion of the overlying mucosa may be seen. The bladder wall may be thickened due to fibrosis and proliferation of the muscularis around the foci of endometriosis. Complications of bladder endometriosis include obstruction of the ureteric orifices and vesicocolic fistula.[3,367]

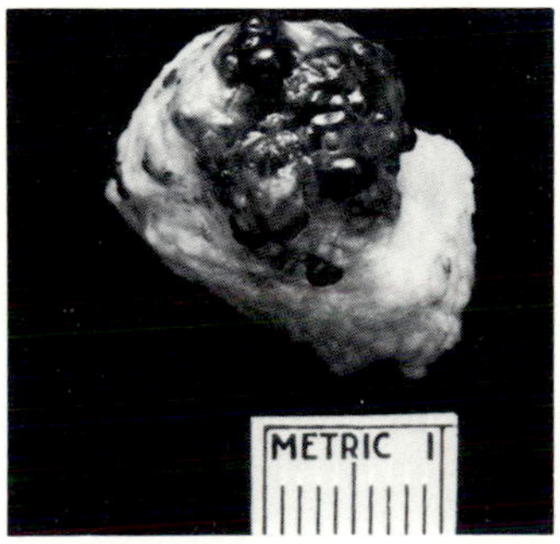

FIG. 17.18. Endometriosis of the bladder. The mucosal surface is replaced by a hemorrhagic, nodular lesion. (Reprinted by permission of Surgery, Gynecology & Obstetrics, Ref. 370.)

Ureteric endometriosis is usually unilateral, confined to the lower one third of the ureter, and associated with endometriosis elsewhere in the pelvis. Involvement of the overlying peritoneum, ureterosacral ligament, or ovary may result in extrinsic compression of the ureteric wall. Less commonly, the endometriosis is intrinsic, resulting in a thickened ureteric wall, with fibrosis and proliferation of the ureteric muscularis. Rarely, the mucosa may also be involved, with a polypoid tumor-like mass projecting into the lumen (Fig. 17.19).[180,206,258,370] Ureteric endometriosis may result in luminal stenosis, hydroureter, hydronephrosis, and, rarely, renal failure.[177,206,212,367,419]

Endometriosis involving the kidney is extremely rare and is usually unassociated with endometriosis elsewhere.[20,136] On gross examination, the endometriotic lesion is a solitary, well-circumscribed, hemorrhagic, solid, and cystic mass that replaces the renal parenchyma.[136] Lesions measuring up to 13 cm in diameter have been reported. Urethral endometriosis is extremely rare and clinically may resemble a caruncle.[126,276]

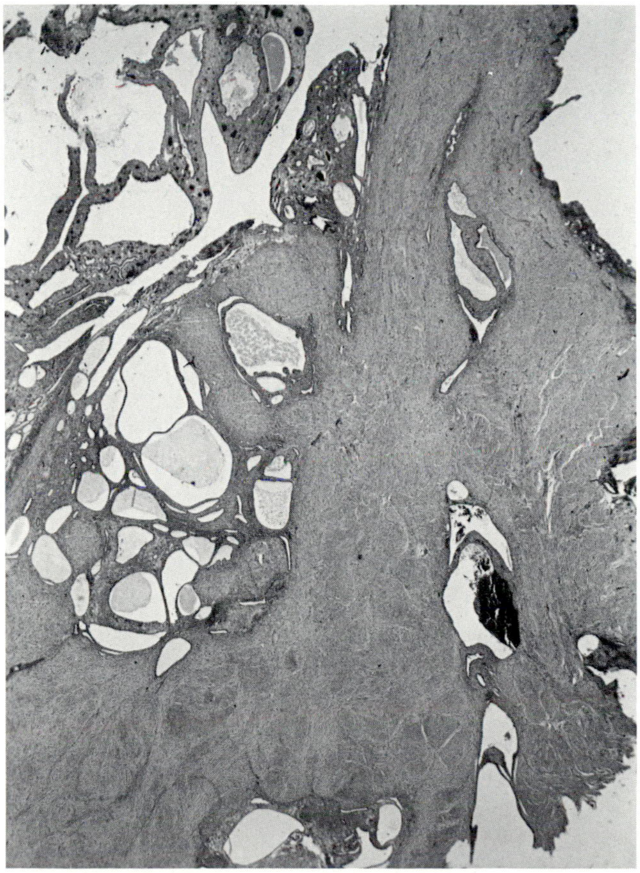

FIG. 17.19. Polypoid endometriosis of the ureter. The endometriosis involves the wall of the ureter and forms a polypoid mass projecting into its lumen (*top left*). (Reprinted by permission of Mostoufizadeh and Scully, Ref. 258.)

A preoperative diagnosis is usually not made because of nonspecific signs and symptoms. Occasionally, the diagnosis may be suspected in a patient with catamenial suprapubic or flank pain or catamenial urinary symptoms. Bladder and kidney involvement may result in a palpable, tender, suprapubic or flank mass, respectively.[3,20]

Cutaneous Endometriosis

Cutaneous endometriosis is typically found within surgical scars after operations on the uterus and tubes and is associated with endometriosis elsewhere in the pelvis in nearly 20% of cases. It occurs less commonly after nongynecologic procedures, such as an appendectomy or inguinal hernia repair.[50,128,213,282,373] Similarly, involvement of scars, typically episiotomy scars, accounts for most cases of endometriosis of the lower vagina, vulva, perineum, and perianal region.[95,96,128,282] Rare cases have occurred within a needle tract after amniocentesis or hypertonic saline abortion.[105,185] Spontaneous, nonscar-related, cutaneous endometriosis generally involves the umbilicus and inguinal region.[373] Rare cases of spontaneous perianal endometriosis have been reported.[250]

The most common symptoms of cutaneous endometriosis are those relating to a mass or nodule that appears in a surgical scar weeks to years after surgery; the average postoperative interval is 30 months.[373] The nodule is frequently painful and tender and, occasionally, may bleed. The patients may notice catamenial enlargement of the lesion and exacerbation of the pain. Patients with perianal lesions may have involvement of the external sphincter, producing anorectal pain and irritation simulating an anal fistula, abscess, or thrombosed hemorrhoid.[128] Umbilical endometriosis may simulate an umbilical hernia on physical examination.[248] In 10% of patients, the cutaneous endometriotic lesions recurred once or twice after their surgical removal.[373]

On macroscopic examination, the endometriotic lesions are firm, solitary, cutaneous nodules varying from a few millimeters to 6 cm in diameter (Fig. 17.20). They range from blue–black to pink depending on the age of the lesion and the depth within the skin.[373] On microscopic examination, the endometriosis is usually in the dermis, less frequently in the subcutis (Fig. 17.21).[373]

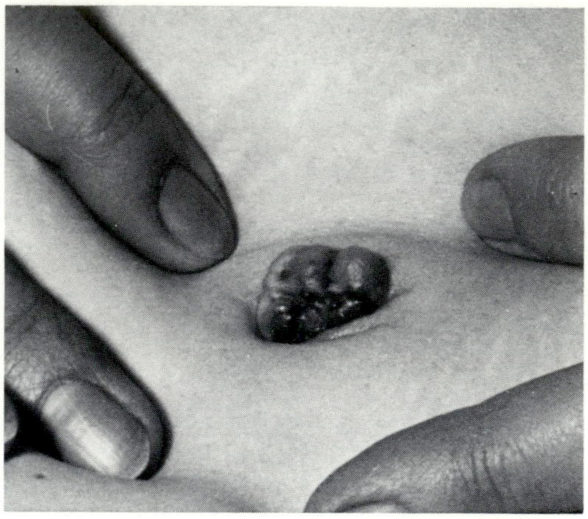

Fig. 17.20. Cutaneous endometriosis. A hemorrhagic, polypoid mass involves the umbilicus. (Reprinted by permission of Steck and Helwig, Ref. 373.)

Endometriosis of Lymph Nodes

Lymph node involvement by endometriosis is unusual. Many examples reported as such in the older literature represent lymph nodes involved by benign müllerian, typically endosalpingiotic, glands.[9] By performing "selective lymphadenectomies," Javert found a 12% frequency of intranodal endometriosis in patients with pelvic endometriosis, adenomyosis, or both.[174] The involved lymph nodes may be visibly or palpably enlarged at the time of surgery. On microscopic examination, in contrast to glandular inclusions, endometriotic foci are characterized by a more central location within the node, an endometrial stromal component, and the frequent presence of erythrocytes and pigmented histiocytes.[174] Decidual transformation of the endometriotic stroma may occur during pregnancy.[323] A unique case of intranodal endomyometriosis has been reported in which there was an extensive smooth muscle component in addition to the endometrial glands and stroma (see Fig. 17.10).[313]

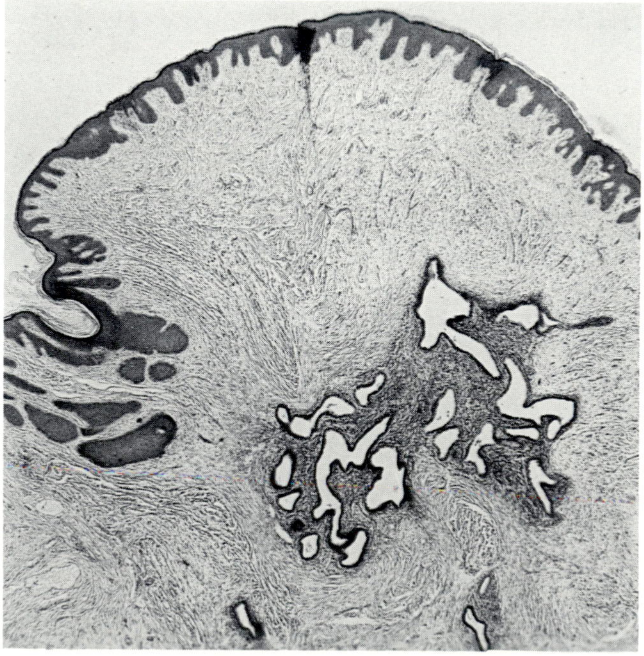

Fig. 17.21. Cutaneous endometriosis. Endometriotic foci are present within the dermis. (Reprinted by permission of Steck and Helwig, Ref. 373.)

Pleuropulmonary Endometriosis

Approximately 25 pathologically documented cases of endometriosis involving the lungs or pleura have been reported, with approximately equal numbers of cases at each site.* Pleural endometriosis, however, is more common, as the pathologically diagnosed cases are estimated to represent only 20% of the purported cases, the remainder being clinically diagnosed.

The vast majority of cases of pleural endometriosis involve the right side, appearing as multiple, dark red to blue nodules or cysts on the diaphragmatic surface. Parietal, visceral, and pericardial pleural surfaces can also be affected, although less commonly. Associated pathologic changes include pleural blebs and multiple, small, diaphragmatic fenestrations.[366] Pulmonary lesions are typically solitary, subpleural nodules or thin-walled cysts measuring several centimeters in diameter, which replace the lung parenchyma. Several lesions have involved bronchial walls. One unique case had a miliary distribution throughout the lungs.[219] In two pregnant patients, the endometriotic lesions exhibited a stromal decidual reaction on histologic examination.

Pleural and pulmonary endometriosis differ in their clinical manifestations. Patients with the former frequently have pelvic endometriosis and typically have recurrent, catamenial pneumothorax. The pathogenesis of the pneumothorax is unclear. Air within the lungs may escape from preexistent blebs or defects in the visceral pleura produced by the endometriotic lesions. Alternatively, air within the peritoneal cavity (probably external air that has passed through the fallopian tubes) may travel through diaphragmatic fenestrations.[366] Rarer clinical manifestations of pleural endometriosis include pleural effusions (which may be bloody),[411] catamenial chest pain, and catamenial hemoptysis.

Patients with pulmonary lesions typically do not have pelvic endometriosis but have a history of prior curettage or hysterectomy. They typically have catamenial hemoptysis or an incidentally discovered radiographic opacity in the lungs.

Inguinal Endometriosis

Noncutaneous inguinal endometriosis may involve the extraperitoneal portion of the round ligament, typically as a painful, right-sided, inguinal, hernia-like mass, exacerbated during the menses.[284,380] The lesion can impinge on the pubic tubercle and appear as arthritis or tendonitis.[284] Rarely, inguinal endometriosis can involve an inguinal hernial sac[40,295] or appear as a femoral hernia.[300]

* References 99, 112, 155, 169, 211, 219, 274, 381, 410.

Endometriosis in Rare Sites

Musculoskeletal. Several cases of endometriosis have involved skeletal muscle or deep soft tissues, including the trapezius,[119] extensor carpi radialis,[263] thigh,[121,269,336] and around the knee.[281] Rare cases of pelvic endometriotic cysts destroying lumbar vertebrae resulting in catamenial lumbar pain have been reported.[75,107]

Upper Abdominal. Rare examples of endometriosis in the upper abdomen have taken the form of implants on the peritoneal surface of the diaphragm[266] as well as endometriomas of the gastric wall[233,285] and tail of the pancreas.[231] One of the patients with gastric endometriosis experienced hematemesis and catamenial melena. The patient with pancreatic involvement had the symptoms of acute pancreatitis.

Rare Miscellaneous Sites. Rare cases of endometriosis of the sciatic nerve sheath at the level of the sciatic notch have resulted in catamenial sciatica.[17,109,154] A case of subarachnoid endometriosis of the lumbar spinal cord has been reported. The patient experienced catamenial radicular pain and recurrent subarachnoid hemorrhage.[222] A rare case of endometriosis appeared as a 1 cm tumor-like mass within the breast in a patient with a 2-year history of catamenial, bloody nipple discharge.[253]

Neoplasms Arising from Endometriosis

Frequency and Predisposing Factors

Rarely, a malignant tumor may arise within a focus of endometriosis.[36,102,258,277,355] This complication has been documented in 0.3–0.8% of patients with ovarian endometriosis.[64,355] The exact frequency of malignancy arising in pelvic endometriosis, however, is unknown because the frequency of endometriosis in the general population is unknown and because the endometriotic focus from which the tumor arose may not be visualized on microscopic examination due to sampling error or obliteration by the tumor.[258] Most studies provide only circumstantial evidence of origin of the tumor within endometriosis, failing to specifically identify how many tumors were proven on histologic examination to arise from endometriotic tissue. Well-documented cases of neoplasms arising within endometriosis are, therefore, rare.[258] The likelihood of a tumor originating within endometriosis is greater if the endometriosis is in the same site as the cancer, if the two processes coexist in an unusual site, or if the patient has had a long history of endometriosis before the appearance of the tumor.[258]

Endogenous or exogenous estrogen may play a role in malignant transformation of endometriosis in occasional cases, a possibility consistent with its known hormonal responsiveness and the presence of estrogen receptors within endometriotic tissue.* In a few of these cases, hyperplastic changes within the endometriotic tissue were documented before the development of an endometrioid carcinoma in the same area.[130,424] There have been rare examples of endometrial stromal sarcoma that have arisen from a focus of endometriosis in patients using exogenous estrogen.[28] Thus, caution is necessary in administering estrogen replacement therapy to patients with known endometriosis, a problem compounded by the relative inaccessibility of most endometriotic tissue to periodic biopsy.[258]

Several endometriosis-related neoplasms have occurred in patients who received prior radiation to their ovaries for treatment of their endometriosis, raising the possibility of radiation-induced neoplasms in these patients.[36]

Sites

The frequency with which a tumor arises within endometriosis in a given site parallels the frequency of endometriosis in that location.[36] Thus, approximately 75% of such tumors arise within the ovary. The remaining 25%, represented by approximately 60 reported cases, arise in extraovarian locations. The most common of the latter sites is the rectovaginal septum, less commonly the vagina, colon and rectum, and urinary bladder.[182] Rare sites include the uterosacral area, parametrium, umbilicus, omentum, uterine corpus, cervix, fallopian tube, vulva, small bowel, cutaneous scar, and pleura.[7,36,134,226,258]

Gross Appearance

Endometrioid and clear cell carcinomas arising from ovarian endometriosis most commonly appear as single or multiple, polypoid masses arising from the lining of an endometriotic cyst or, less commonly, as a solid thickening in the wall of the cyst.[258] The latter is often larger (over 15 cm) than endometriotic cysts unassociated with a neoplasm (Fig. 17.22). No significant differences have been noted in the macroscopic appearance of the rarer tumors arising from endometriosis compared to tumors of the same type arising de novo.

Histologic Types

Endometrioid Carcinoma. This is the most common tumor arising within endometriosis (Fig. 17.23). Ovarian endometrioid carcinoma has been reported to be accompanied by pelvic endometriosis in 11–28% of cases, by ovarian endometriosis of unspecified laterality in 9–20% of cases, and by ipsilateral ovarian endometriosis in 11–17% of cases. A direct origin of endometrioid carcinoma from endometriotic tissue has been demonstrated in as many as 24% of cases in some series.[258] The tumors tend to be better differentiated and are more likely to have squamous components (adenoacanthoma or adenosquamous carcinoma) than is endometrial carcinoma of the uterine corpus.[258] At least 90% of the carcinomas arising from extraovarian endometriosis have been of endometrioid type, including adenoacanthomas and adenosquamous carcinomas.[36,134,258] Rarely, endometrioid tumors arising in ovarian and extraovarian endometriosis may exhibit a benign or borderline adenofibromatous pattern.[130,355]

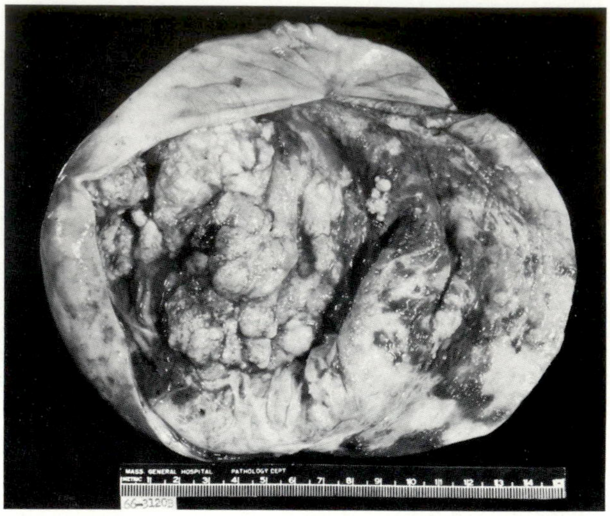

FIG. 17.22. Clear cell carcinoma arising within an endometriotic cyst. Fleshy pale tumor nodules protrude into the cyst lumen. (Reprinted by permission of Scully et al., Ref. 355.)

Clear Cell Carcinoma. This is the second most common tumor arising within endometriosis. In some studies, the frequency of endometriosis coexisting with clear cell carcinomas is even higher than with endometrioid carcinoma; 24–49% of patients with ovarian clear cell carcinoma have had documented concomitant pelvic endometriosis.[13,324] Rare examples of clear cell carcinoma arising within extraovarian endometriosis have also been described (Fig. 17.24).[36,123]

Rare Carcinomas. Very rare examples of ovarian serous tumors (of low malignant potential[133]), benign and malignant mucinous tumors,[64,355] and squamous cell carcinomas[55,217] have been reported in association within ovarian endometriosis. A unique tumor arising from colonic endometriosis was composed of endometrioid adenocarcinoma with focal differentiation resembling choriocarcinoma and endodermal sinus tumor.[208]

Sarcomas. Endometrioid stromal sarcomas and malignant mixed mesodermal tumors, similar on microscopic

* References 28, 36, 130, 216, 358, 424.

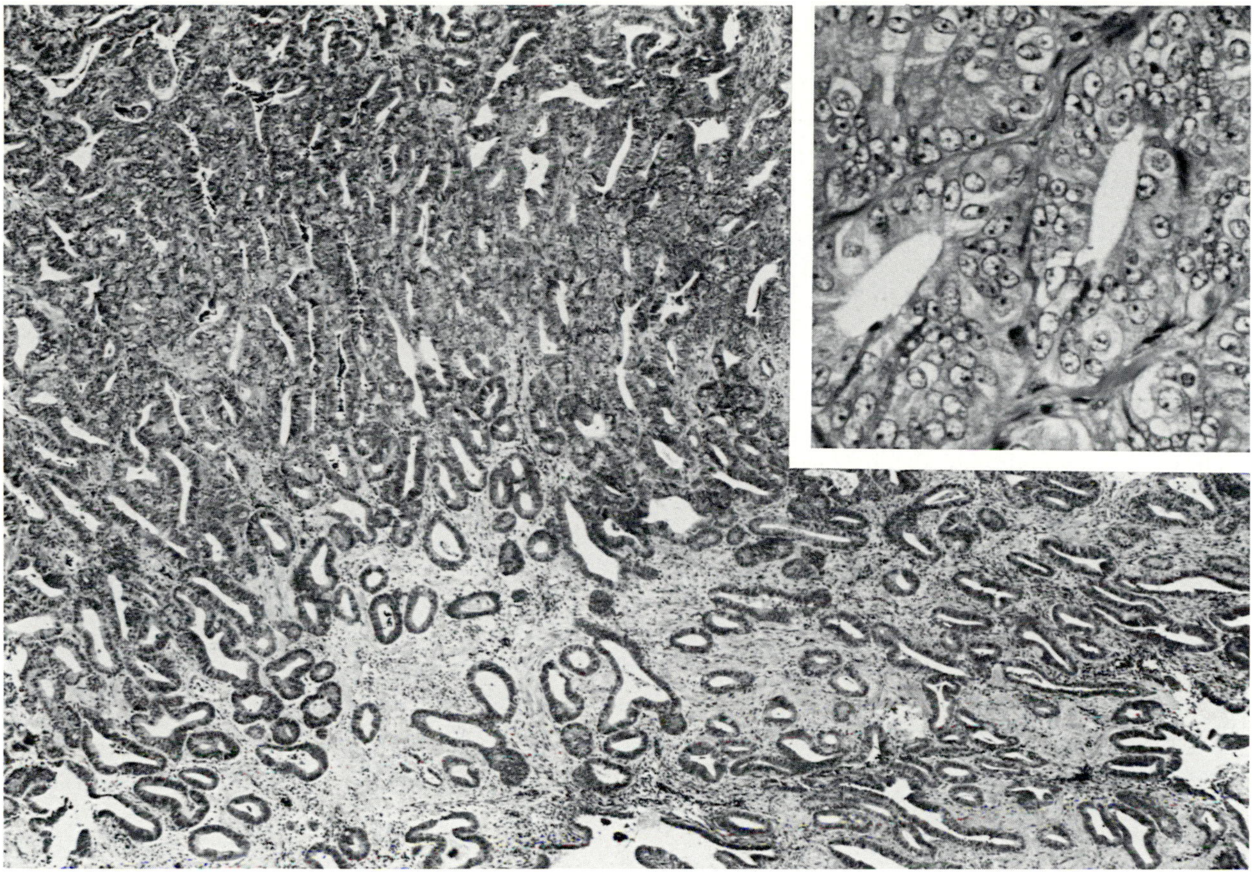

FIG. 17.23. Endometrioid carcinoma arising within endometriosis. Benign endometriotic glands and stroma merge with the carcinomatous glands. *Inset:* High-power view of carcinomatous glands.

examination to those arising in the uterus, may arise within ovarian and extraovarian endometriosis.* Sixty percent of endometrial stromal sarcomas reported in the ovary has been associated with ovarian endometriosis.[426] Vaginal endometriosis was the probable origin for one extrauterine pelvic adenosarcoma.[227]

Clinical Aspects

Patients with endometrioid carcinomas arising within ovarian endometriosis are a decade younger than are patients with ovarian endometrioid carcinoma in general. Only an occasional patient in the former category is postmenopausal. A similar but less striking age distribution is present in patients with ovarian clear cell carcinoma associated with endometriosis.[258] The most common manifestation of endometrioid carcinomas arising in ovarian endometriosis is pain usually of the continuous type compared to the episodic nature of the pain associated with typical endometriosis.[103] Thus, the diagnosis of malignancy should be suspected in patients with known endometriosis when the typical pain pattern changes, including a sudden increase in severity or an onset after the menopause.[103] Increasing size or rupture of an endometriotic cyst may be secondary to malignant changes within the cyst.[103]

Patients with tumors arising from extraovarian endometriosis have a wide age range; those with endometrioid carcinomas range from 30 to 73 years (mean 48 years), and those with endometrioid stromal sarcomas from 20 to 64 years (mean 42 years).[258] Malignancy within extraovarian endometriosis is typically associated with clinical manifestations of hemorrhage, lower abdominal pain, a palpable mass, or combinations thereof.[36]

Because of limited follow-up information and the small number of cases, it is difficult to draw conclusions about any possible differences in the behavior of tumors arising within endometriosis compared to that of tumors of similar histologic type unassociated with endometriosis.[258] It has been suggested, however, that because of their frequent small size and low histologic grade, endometrioid carcinomas arising in ovarian endometriosis are

* References 36, 63, 69, 81, 205, 230, 258, 277, 426.

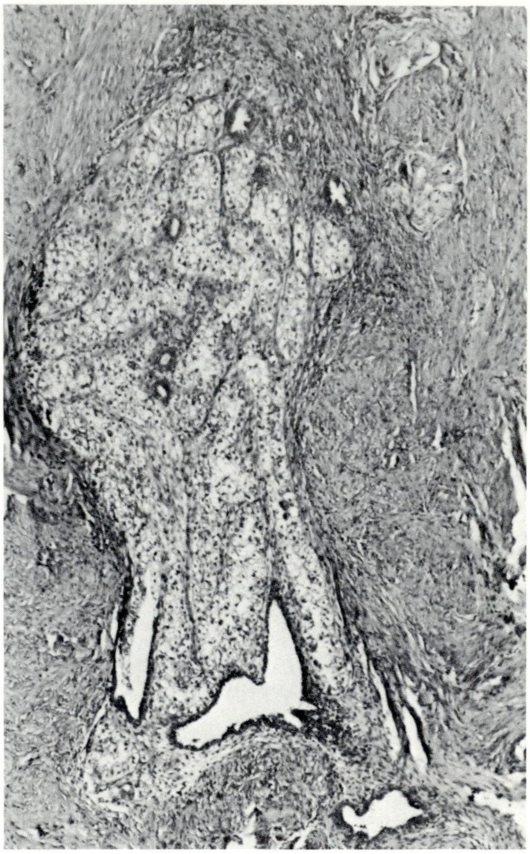

FIG. 17.24. Clear cell carcinoma arising within endometriosis. Benign endometriotic glands and stroma (*bottom*) merge with clear cell carcinoma. (Courtesy of Dr. A. B. P. Ng.)

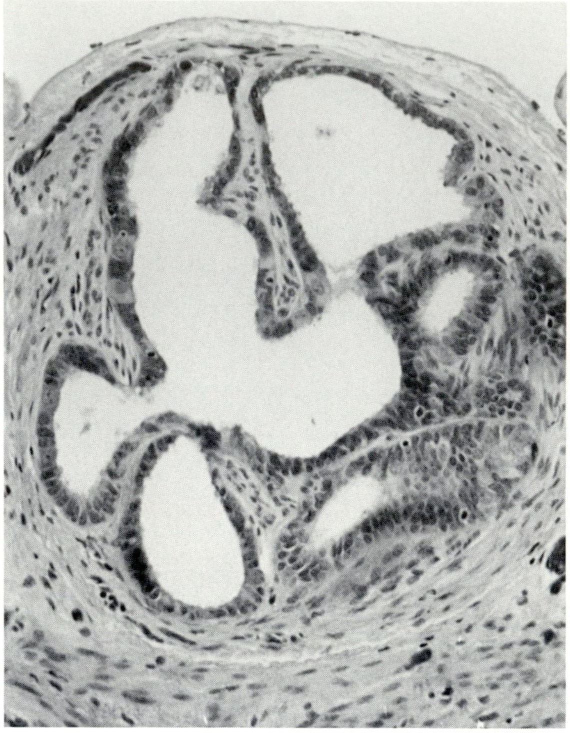

FIG. 17.25. Endosalpingiosis. Complex glandular structure lies beneath uterine serosa. Glands are lined by single layer of benign endosalpingeal epithelium.

less aggressive than are ovarian endometrioid carcinomas in general.[258]

Lesions of the Secondary Müllerian System

Peritoneal Serous Lesions

Lesions arising from the pelvic peritoneum that exhibit serous (endosalpingeal) differentiation on histologic examination include endosalpingiosis (a nonneoplastic process analogous to endometriosis) and serous neoplasms that closely resemble those of ovarian origin.

Endosalpingiosis

Definition. Endosalpingiosis refers to the presence of ectopic, histologically benign epithelium resembling the normal endosalpinx that involves the peritoneum or pelvic and para-aortic lymph nodes. Although the designation *endosalpingiosis* was initially applied to endosalpingeal glands within the myosalpinx,[332] examples of the latter are now designated *salpingitis isthmica nodosa.* The term *endosalpingiosis* is also no longer applied to inclusion cysts within the ovarian cortex.[125] It should be noted that some examples of lesions labeled *endometriosis* in the older literature but that lacked endometrial stroma would be designated *endosalpingiosis* using current criteria.

Pathologic Features. Endosalpingiosis is most commonly encountered on the visceral pelvic peritoneum covering the uterus, fallopian tubes, ovaries, and cul-de-sac.[39,42,53,102,158,391] Less frequent sites include the pelvic parietal peritoneum,[42] omentum,[102,391,427] bladder and bowel serosa,[53,102] periaortic area,[360] and within the skin, including laparotomy scars.[89,332,334] At the time of surgery or on macroscopic inspection of the involved tissues, endosalpingiosis is typically inapparent. Less commonly, it may be visible as multiple, punctate (1–2 mm), white to yellow, opaque or translucent, fluid-filled, cystic lesions that impart a coarsely granular appearance to the involved peritoneal surface. Rarely, larger cysts reaching 1 cm in diameter may be seen.*

On microscopic examination, endosalpingiosis typically consists of multiple, simple, subserosal glands, often cystically dilated, lined by a single layer of epithelium resembling the normal endosalpinx (Fig. 17.25). Irregu-

* References 39, 42, 53, 102, 158, 391.

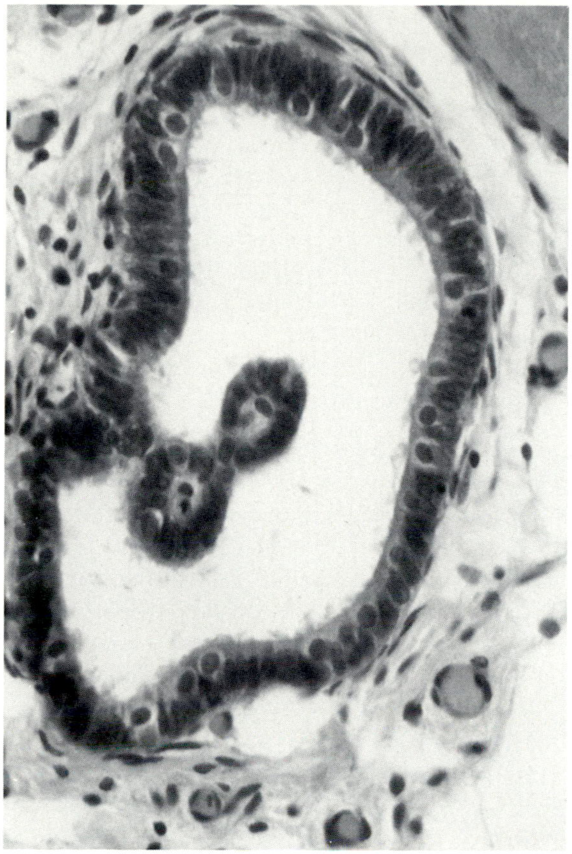

FIG. 17.26. Endosalpingiosis. A gland within the omentum is lined by benign endosalpingeal epithelium composed of multiple cell types.

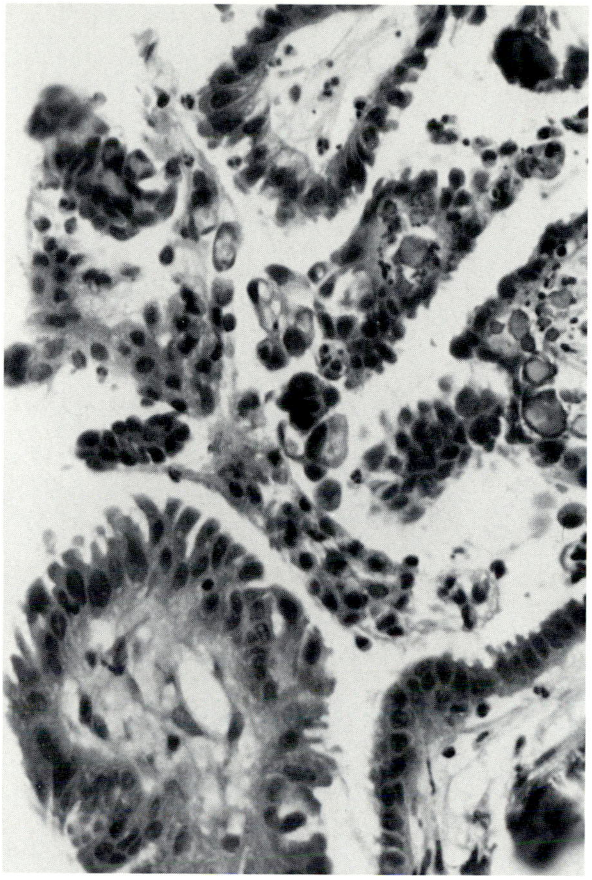

FIG. 17.27. Atypical endosalpingiosis. Papillary formations are lined by stratified, atypical endosalpingeal epithelium; psammoma bodies are present within the stroma. This lesion was an incidental intraoperative finding, appearing as punctate white foci on the uterine serosa. There was no evidence of an ovarian or extraovarian serous neoplasm.

lar glandular contours and crowding can result in complex multiglandular structures with intraluminal papillary stromal projections.[427] The three cell types normally found in the endosalpinx are found to varying degrees: pale ciliated cells, secretory cells, and dark, rod-like, intercalated or peg cells (Fig. 17.26).[42,391,427] The cells have prominent luminal margins, distinct cell borders, and basally situated nuclei. Focal cellular pseudostratification may be present. The nuclei have fine chromatin patterns, delicate nuclear membranes, and typically lack significant nuclear atypia or mitotic activity.[427] Occasionally, however, endosalpingiotic foci can exhibit atypical features on histologic examination, including papillary formations, cribriform patterns, cellular stratification, nuclear pleomorphism, and mitotic activity (Fig. 17.27).[243,353]

Psammoma bodies are frequently present within endosalpingiotic glandular lumens or the adjacent stroma, and in occasional cases, large numbers of psammoma bodies embedded in subserosal connective tissue may be a striking finding (Fig. 17.28). In such cases, a careful search may be required to demonstrate typical foci of endosalpingiotic epithelium.

Staining with the PAS method reveals a basement membrane surrounding each gland and PAS-positive, diastase-resistant material within the luminal tips of some of the lining cells and within the glandular lumens.[427] The glands are frequently surrounded by a loose or dense connective tissue stroma (unlike endometrial stroma) that may contain a sparse mononuclear inflammatory cell infiltrate. Rarely, endosalpingiotic glands may show limited degrees of infiltration of the underlying tissues, exemplified by glands lying within subserosal myometrium.[42] The endosalpingiotic epithelium typically does not exhibit a transition with the overlying surface mesothelial cells, nor do the latter exhibit hyperplastic or reactive changes.[42,427]

The ultimate fate of endosalpingiotic lesions is not known with certainty. Their tendency to undergo calcification, the rarity of endosalpingiosis in postmenopausal women, and the dependence of müllerian epithelia on estrogenic stimulation suggest the probability that the

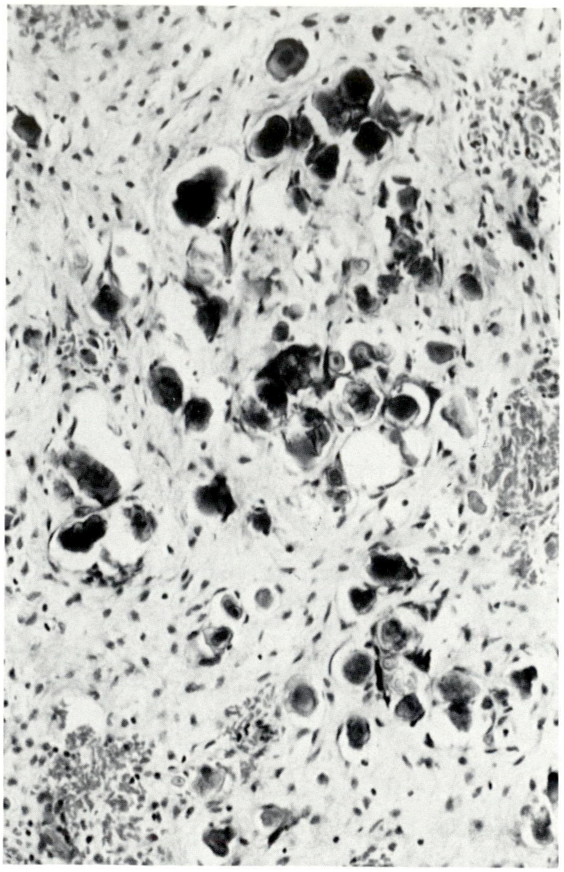

FIG. 17.28. Endosalpingiosis. Numerous psammoma bodies embedded in connective tissue involve pelvic peritoneum. Typical endosalpingiotic glands were sparse, requiring a careful search. The ovarian serosa exhibited similar changes but no evidence of a serous neoplasm.

epithelial component of endosalpingiotic foci undergoes postmenopausal atrophy.[427] No convincing examples of neoplastic transformation of endosalpingiosis have been reported.

Differential Diagnosis. Atypical endosalpingiotic lesions may mimic, on histologic examination, implants associated with an ovarian serous tumor of low malignant potential.[62,324,352,353] When such a tumor is present, histologic features favoring a diagnosis of a metastasis include the presence of an infiltrative pattern, a desmoplastic stromal response, the presence of only one cell type, and the absence of a basement membrane surrounding the glands.[62,427] In occasional cases, however, it may be difficult or impossible to make the distinction reliably on histologic grounds.[62,352] It has also been suggested that at least some peritoneal implants associated with ovarian serous tumors of low malignant potential may represent multifocal autochthonous foci of proliferation arising directly from the peritoneum, possibly in response to the same tumorigenic agents responsible for the ovarian tumor.[324,327]

Endosalpingiotic glands should be differentiated from mesonephric remnants encountered commonly as an incidental microscopic finding within the mesosalpinx. The mesonephric tubules are typically located deeper than endosalpingiosis and are characteristically surrounded by a collar of smooth muscle. In contrast to endosalpingiotic glands, the tubules are lined by a single cell type, usually nonciliated, low columnar to cuboidal epithelial cells lacking mucin secretion. They are unassociated with psammoma bodies. Ultrastructural examination reveals mesonephric, rather than müllerian, differentiation.[34]

Clinical Aspects. Endosalpingiosis occurs exclusively in females, typically during the reproductive years, with a mean age of 29.7 years in one study,[427] although occasional cases have been described in postmenopausal females.[102] Because endosalpingiotic foci do not undergo the cyclical menstrual changes of endometriosis and typically lack the invasiveness of the latter, endosalpingiosis is almost always unassociated with clinical manifestations and is either an incidental finding at the time of surgery or, more commonly, on microscopic examination of the removed tissues. Zinsser and Wheeler found endosalpingiosis in 12.5% of surgically removed omenta examined histologically, a frequency eight times that of omental endometriosis in the population under study. The frequency doubled when omenta were examined prospectively with more thorough histologic sampling.[427]

Rarely, endosalpingiosis may be associated with clinical manifestations. The latter may take the form of multiple fine calcifications throughout the pelvis visible on radiologic examination[391] or psammoma bodies within cul-de-sac fluid,[158,190] peritoneal washings,[54] the lumen of the fallopian tube,[287] or cervical Pap smears.[287,391]

Disorders that may be associated with endosalpingiosis include inflammatory lesions of the fallopian tube, endosalpingiotic glands within lymph nodes, ovarian serous neoplasms,* and endometriosis. In one case, endosalpingiotic glands were intimately admixed with peritoneal nodules of smooth muscle (disseminated peritoneal leiomyomatosis).[56]

Histogenesis. The histogenesis of endosalpingiosis is controversial, but as the proposed theories are not mutually exclusive, more than one origin may be possible. The most commonly held view is that endosalpingiosis represents a multifocal metaplastic process arising from the peritoneal mesothelial cells and, therefore, is of secondary müllerian origin.[42,164,391]

An alternate theory is that endosalpingiosis is a result of peritoneal implantation by sloughed tubal epithelium.[125,218,343,427] The main supportive evidence for this

* References 42, 102, 243, 245, 343, 391, 427.

theory is the frequent association of endosalpingiosis with inflammatory tubal disease, prior tubal lavage, or both.[158,391,427] In one study, all patients with endosalpingiosis had inflammatory tubal disease, and conversely, 42% of patients with tubal disease who had omenta removed had endosalpingiosis.[427] In the same study, almost half the patients had had tubal lavage performed at preoperative intervals of 3–20 months. Proponents of the implantation theory suggest that the absence of endosalpingiosis in males, the absence of reactive or hyperplastic changes in the overlying mesothelial cells, and a lack of histologic transition between the latter and the endosalpingiotic lesions militate against the metaplastic theory.[427]

A rare histogenetic mechanism for endosalpingiosis is direct growth of tubal epithelium onto adjacent tissues from fallopian tube segments involved by salpingitis isthmica nodosa.[332,334] Rare cases may be a result of operative implantation or lymphatic–vascular spread. Either of the latter mechanisms may have explained a unique case of cutaneous endosalpingiosis in a patient who developed multiple endosalpingiotic cutaneous cysts within the umbilicus and surrounding skin after salpingectomy for a ruptured ectopic pregnancy.[89]

Peritoneal Serous Tumors (Extraovarian Serous Neoplasia)

Rare examples of tumors that are indistinguishable on histologic examination from serous surface tumors of low malignant potential or serous surface carcinomas occur in which no ovarian involvement is demonstrable (see Chapter 18, Epithelial Tumors of Ovary). Typically, these tumors diffusely involve the pelvic peritoneum, suggesting a multicentric origin from the latter.[114,242,243,297,328,353] In at least some cases, extraovarian tumor implants associated with serous ovarian tumors of low malignant potential and serous surface ovarian carcinomas may have a similar extraovarian origin.*

Some extraovarian serous tumors lack peritoneal surface involvement and take the form of a localized, typically cystic mass, usually within the broad ligament or, less commonly, the retroperitoneum. Papillary serous cystadenomas (and adenofibromas),[118,161,176,375] serous tumors of low malignant potential,[46,70,73,118,176] and serous carcinomas[118,371,394] have been described in these sites. These extraovarian cystic serous tumors may arise from the pelvic peritoneum, although some of those located in the broad ligament probably arise within cystic remnants of the müllerian duct.[46,70,161,176]

Extraovarian serous tumors are identical to their ovarian counterparts on histologic, histochemical, and ultrastructural examination.[114,243,394] Intracellular amylase, a marker for serous ovarian neoplasia, has also been demonstrated by immunohistochemical methods within the extraovarian forms of serous tumors.[38,392,394] These tumors also resemble primary ovarian serous tumors in their biologic behaviour and response to treatment.[243,394]

Extraovarian serous tumors should be separated from the variety of nonneoplastic and neoplastic mesothelial lesions (discussed later in this chapter) that can involve the pelvic peritoneum, especially diffuse malignant mesotheliomas. Although tumors of intermediate histologic type are rarely encountered, extraovarian serous carcinomas and malignant mesotheliomas are usually morphologically distinguishable.[12,102,114,179,243] This distinction is important because of major differences in the behavior, treatment, and epidemiology between the two groups of neoplasms.

Peritoneal Mucinous Lesions

Benign glands of endocervical type involving the peritoneum, so-called endocervicosis, are extremely rare. Lauchlan mentions several examples involving the posterior uterine serosa and cul-de-sac.[215]

Mucinous neoplasms, similar to those occurring within the ovary, have been described in extraovarian sites, typically in the retroperitoneum.[92,102,215,320,412] A single case has been described in the inguinal region.[382] These tumors form large cystic masses (Fig. 17.29) that resemble ovarian mucinous cystadenomas, mucinous tumors of low malignant potential, or mucinous cystadenocarcinomas on histologic examination (Fig. 17.30). Several of the mucinous cystadenocarcinomas have pursued a clinically malignant course.[92,320] Although some extraovarian mucinous tumors are considered to originate within a supernumerary ovary, the absence of unequivocal ovarian tissue within their walls and the occasional

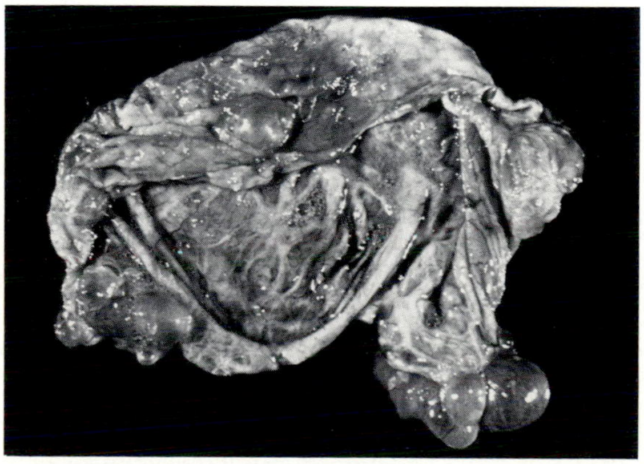

FIG. 17.29. Retroperitoneal mucinous tumor. The specimen has been opened to reveal multiple locules with mucinous contents. (Courtesy of Dr. R. E. Scully.)

* References 12, 127, 242, 243, 279, 324, 328, 408.

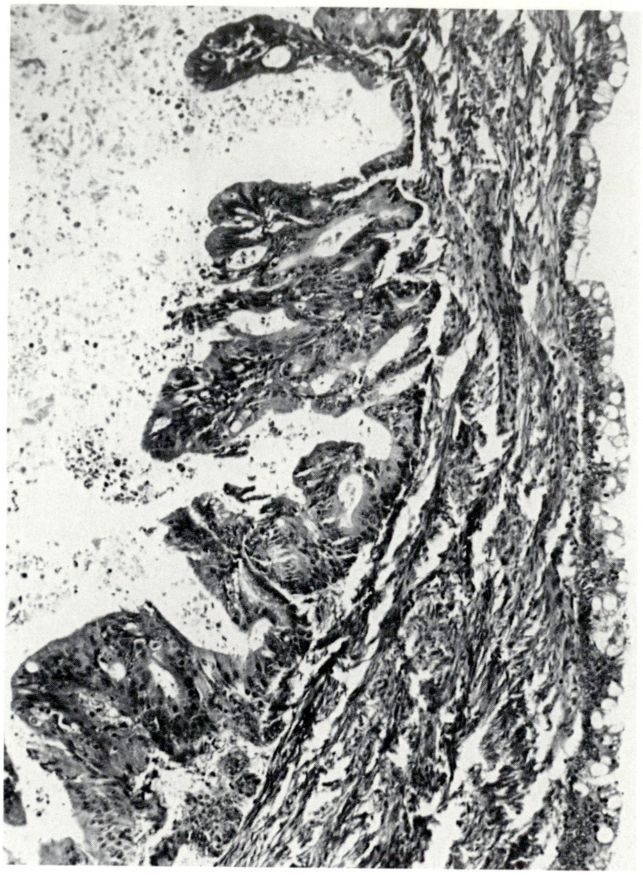

FIG. 17.30. Retroperitoneal mucinous cystadenocarcinoma. Cysts lined by papillary formations composed of atypical mucinous cells. [Reprinted with permission from The American College of Obstetricians and Gynecologists. Roth LM, Ehrlich CE (1977) Mucinous cystadenocarcinoma of the retroperitoneum. Obstetrics and Gynecology 49:486–488.]

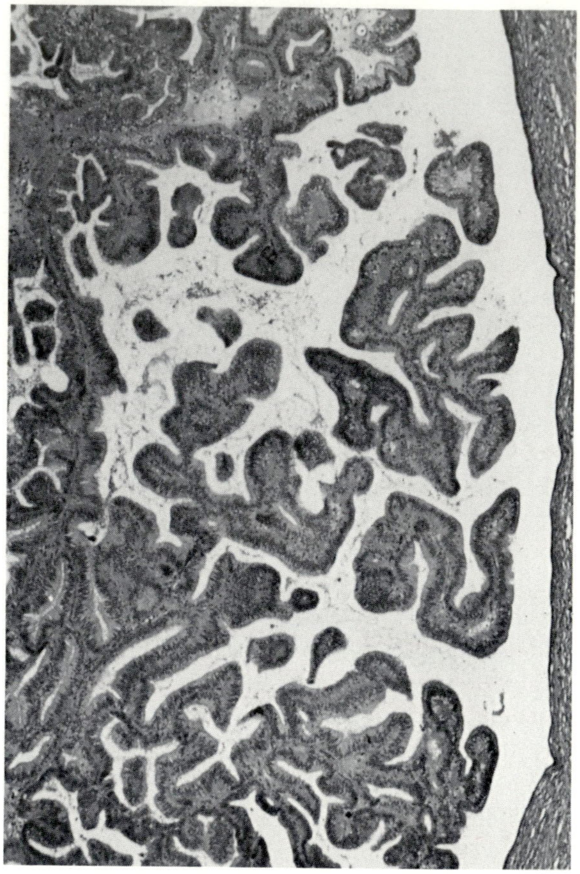

FIG. 17.31. Cystic endometrioid tumor of broad ligament. The low-grade endometrioid carcinoma has a villoglandular pattern.

occurrence of similar tumors in males[320] support a peritoneal origin in the majority of cases.

Peritoneal Endometrioid Lesions

Descriptions of benign, peritoneal, endometrioid glandular lesions lacking an associated endometrial stromal component (i.e., nonendometriotic) are rare. This may be due in part to the histologic similarity between benign glands of tubal and endometrial type and, therefore, a possibility that examples of the latter may be designated *endosalpingiosis*. However, benign glands lined by endometrial epithelium with the peritoneal distribution of endosalpingiosis have been rarely described in the absence of an ovarian endometrioid tumor.[215] In addition, benign endometrioid glandular implants on the peritoneum, lacking an endometrial stromal component, have been reported in association with an ovarian endometrioid tumor of low malignant potential.[324] The peritoneal lesions were interpreted as having arisen in situ directly from the peritoneum. The patient was alive and well 8 years after surgery.[325]

A variety of extrauterine, extraovarian, pelvic, or retroperitoneal neoplasms of endometrioid type may occur in the absence of demonstrable endometriosis. These tumors have generally been considered to arise directly from the peritoneum or subperitoneal stroma. The histologic types have included endometrioid cystadenofibroma,[273] endometrioid tumor of low malignant potential (Fig. 17.31), endometrioid cystadenocarcinoma,[59] endometrial stromal sarcoma,[393] homologous and heterologous types of malignant mixed mesodermal tumor,[150] and adenosarcoma.[61,227,327] The behavior of these tumors based on the small number of reported cases is generally similar to analogous tumors in the ovary and uterus.

Peritoneal Transitional Cell Lesions

Walthard Nests

Walthard nests of transitional (urothelial) epithelium are commonly present on the pelvic peritoneum in women of all ages, typically involving the serosal surfaces of the fallopian tubes, mesosalpinx, and meso-

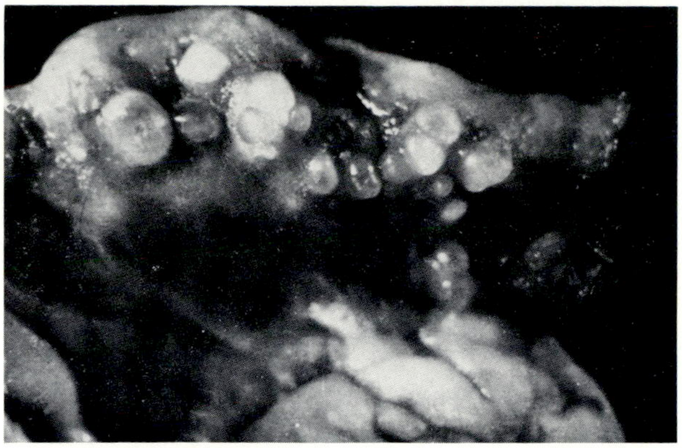

FIG. 17.32. Walthard nests. Multiple small cysts cover the serosa of fallopian tube and mesosalpinx. [From Teoh TB (1953) The structure and development of Walthard nests. J Pathol 66:433–439. Copyright 1953 by John Wiley & Sons, Ltd. Reprinted by permission of John Wiley & Sons, Ltd.]

varium.[35,74,319,390] They are less common on the ovarian surface, where they are usually hilar in location, probably originating from the mesovarium.[74,390] Similar lesions have been described in males on the surfaces of the epididymis, testis, and spermatic cord.[383]

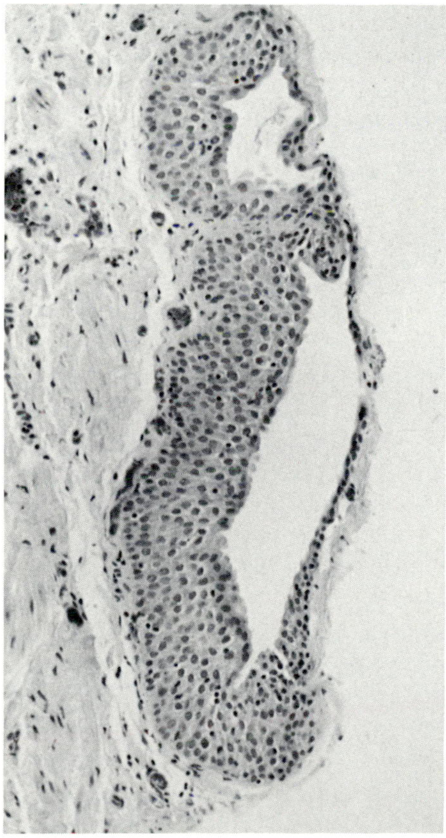

FIG. 17.33. Walthard nests on fallopian tube serosa. Nests with central cystic spaces are formed by benign transitional-type cells.

In females, Walthard nests are usually incidental microscopic findings but, rarely, may be visible macroscopically as white to yellow nodules or cysts measuring several millimeters in diameter on the involved peritoneal surface (Fig. 17.32).[319,390] On histologic examination, they take the form of well-circumscribed, subserosal, solid nests or cysts or, less commonly, surface plaques that focally replace the normal mesothelium (Fig. 17.33). They are composed of cytologically benign, mitotically inactive, transitional-type cells. The nuclei of these cells typically have a fine chromatin pattern, a prominent nuclear groove, and one or two small nucleoli. Less commonly, the cells may have a squamoid appearance, but keratinization is not seen.[319] Flattened or mucinous columnar type cells line the cysts,[74] and mucin may be demonstrable within the cystic spaces.[390] Ultrastructural features of the transitional cells are similar to those of transitional epithelium of the urinary tract and Brenner tumors of the ovary.[35,319] Walthard-like nests have been found in the walls of epidermoid cysts of the ovary, and it has been postulated that the latter may originate within the transitional cell nests.[425]

The serosal location of Walthard nests and their morphologic similarity to ovarian Brenner tumors have led most investigators to favor an origin from transitional cell metaplasia of the peritoneum.

Extraovarian Brenner Tumors

Four examples of extraovarian Brenner tumor have been reported in females, three in the broad ligament and one in the uterus.[400] A direct origin from the pelvic peritoneum was favored in most cases, a derivation similar to that postulated for the majority of ovarian Brenner tumors.[35,319,353] It has been suggested that the extreme rarity of extraovarian Brenner tumors in contrast to the frequency of Walthard nests may indicate an essential role of the ovarian stroma in their development.[376]

Subperitoneal Mesenchymal Lesions

Ectopic Decidua

An ectopic decidual reaction similar to that which may occur within the lamina propria of the fallopian tube, cervix, and vagina also may be seen within the subperitoneal stroma. It has been demonstrated in approximately 90% of patients who have undergone laparotomy during pregnancy.*

Decidual plaques may be found in the superficial cortex of the ovaries (see Chapter 16, Nonneoplastic Lesions of Ovary) and within the subperitoneal stroma of the fallopian tubes, uterus, and uterine ligaments, as well

* References 29, 148, 153, 170, 204, 275, 302, 329.

as on peritoneal surfaces throughout the rest of the pelvis.[271] Similar lesions are much more rarely encountered in the upper abdomen, involving the serosal surfaces of the diaphragm, liver, and spleen.[148,275] Involvement of the renal pelvis has also been described.[30]

Subperitoneal decidua is typically unassociated with clinical manifestations and usually represents an incidental microscopic finding in surgically removed tissues. Rarely, however, florid lesions may be visible at the time of cesarean section or postpartum tubal ligation as multiple, gray to white, focally hemorrhagic nodules studding the involved peritoneal surfaces, simulating a malignant tumor.[204,275] Several cases have been associated with massive and occasionally fatal intraperitoneal hemorrhage occurring during the third trimester, during labor, or postpartum.[167,204,303,329] Other rare clinical presentations include abdominal pain, which may simulate appendicitis, and hydronephrosis and hematuria secondary to renal pelvic involvement.[30,167]

On histologic examination, the lesions are highly vascular and are composed of decidualized cells that appear identical to those found in the endometrium (Fig. 17.34). Smooth muscle cells, probably derived from submesothelial myofibroblasts, may also be admixed.[153] Focal hemorrhagic necrosis and varying degrees of nuclear pleomorphism and hyperchromasia of the decidual cells may suggest a necrotic tumor, but the bland appearance of most of the cells and their mitotic inactivity are inconsistent with a diagnosis of malignancy. More specifically, the differential diagnosis includes rare examples of peritoneal malignant mesothelioma characterized by a solid growth pattern.[385] Although these tumors may bear a superficial resemblance to ectopic decidua on microscopic examination, there are major histologic, histochemical, and ultrastuctural differences between the two lesions, allowing them to be distinguished without difficulty.[385]

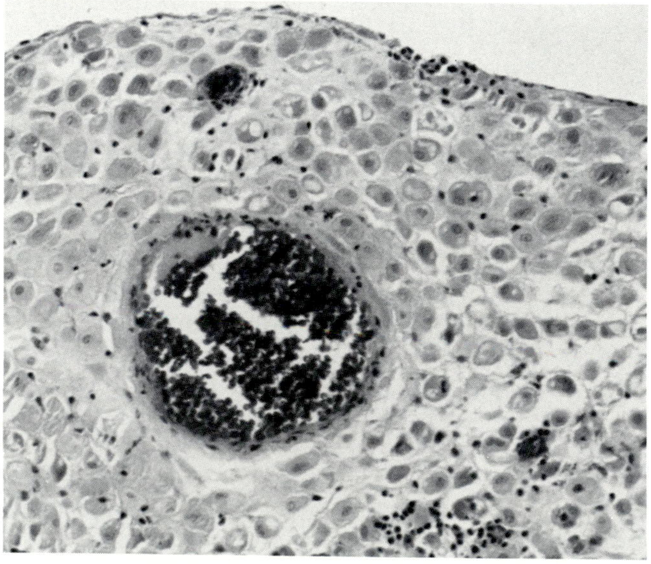

Fig. 17.34. Ectopic decidua beneath pelvic peritoneum. Note the marked vascularity.

Smooth Muscle Proliferations

Disseminated peritoneal leiomyomatosis is a rare disorder characterized by the presence of multiple subperitoneal nodules of cytologically benign smooth muscle, frequently associated with uterine or ovarian leiomyomas (see Chapter 13, Mesenchymal Tumors of the Uterus).* Disseminated peritoneal leiomyomatosis is generally considered to arise from multipotential subperitoneal mesenchymal cells.

Occasional examples of solitary extrauterine leiomyomas[116,160] and leiomyosarcomas,[80,152] typically arising in the broad ligament, may have a histogenesis similar to that of disseminated peritoneal leiomyomatosis or may arise from smooth muscle remnants or vessels within the broad ligament.

Intranodal Lesions

Benign Glands of Müllerian Type

Pathologic Features. Benign glands of müllerian type within lymph nodes are most commonly encountered within pelvic and para-aortic nodes,[9,98,102,164,183,193] and rarely in inguinal and femoral nodes.[338,362] Because the glands are usually identified as an incidental microscopic finding as part of an operative procedure for a pelvic carcinoma, the frequency of their detection depends on the number of lymph nodes removed and the extent of the histologic sampling. Detection rates vary from 2 to 41% of sampled pelvic and para-aortic lymph nodes.

On macroscopic examination of the involved lymph node, the glands are not usually apparent, although rarely they may be recognizable as small cysts measuring several millimeters in diameter.[104,406] The glands are typically located in the periphery of the node, most commonly between the lymphoid follicles in the superficial cortex and within the connective tissue of the node capsule (Fig. 17.35). Rarely, the glands lie free within the subcapsular sinuses.[193] Continuity of the glands with overlying peritoneum has not been demonstrated.[183] In florid cases, they can be diffusely distributed throughout the involved lymph node.[189,193] The glands may be round and cystically dilated or may exhibit an irregular contour due to infolding. They are most commonly lined by a single layer of cuboidal to columnar endosalpingiotic epithelium, with an admixture of ciliated, secretory, and intercalated cell types (Fig. 17.36). With special stains,

* References 153, 181, 280, 288, 387, 396.

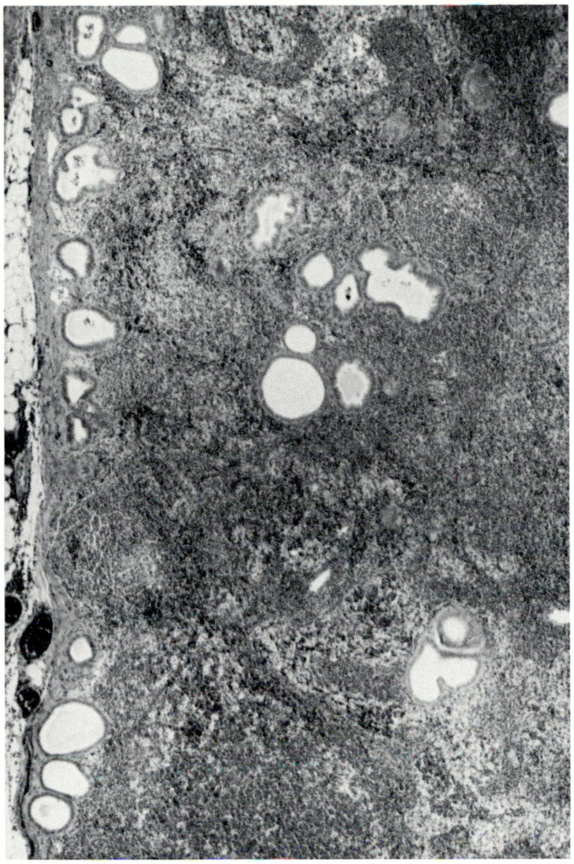

FIG. 17.35. Endosalpingiotic glands within pelvic lymph node. The glands are located immediately beneath the node capsule as well as deeper within the node.

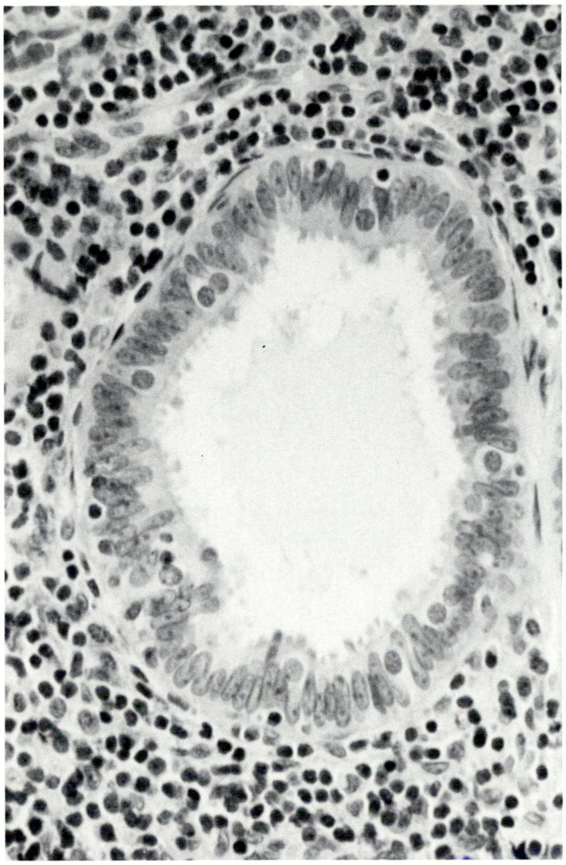

FIG. 17.36. Endosalpingiotic gland within pelvic lymph node. The gland is lined by benign cells of multiple types, including ciliated cells.

mucus can be demonstrated in the luminal aspects of the secretory cells and within the gland spaces.[183,189] The cells are cytologically benign, with regular, basally oriented or pseudostratified, oval to round nuclei, fine nuclear chromatin, and occasional small nucleoli. Mitotic figures are typically absent. In rare cases, the cells can exhibit mild degrees of atypia and stratification; the latter can produce an intraglandular cribriform pattern or luminal obliteration by sheets of cells (Fig. 17.37).[53,98,189] Intraglandular or periglandular psammoma bodies are commonly present. Intranodal glands may be surrounded by a thin rim of fibrous tissue or abut directly on the surrounding lymphoid cells.[183] Acute and chronic inflammatory cells may be present within the glandular lumens.[189] Endometrial stroma, decidua, and evidence of recent or remote hemorrhage are absent.

Rare examples of intranodal glandular inclusions lined by histologically benign endometrioid[102,215,326] and endocervical (mucinous)[104,326] epithelium have been reported. Bland metaplastic squamous epithelium can rarely be identified within benign müllerian glands.[249,338]

Well-documented examples of malignancy arising within intranodal glandular inclusions have not been reported.

Differential Diagnosis. Differentiating the benign glands from metastatic adenocarcinoma is of obvious importance in those patients with a known primary adenocarcinoma in the pelvis. The presence of benign glands, however, does not exclude the possibility of metastatic carcinoma in the same lymph node, since they may coexist.[183,326,341] In most cases, the distinction between the two lesions is not difficult except if a primary ovarian serous tumor of low malignant potential is present, in which case the distinction may be difficult and sometimes arbitrary.[62,98] Features favoring a benign diagnosis include a capsular or interfollicular location of the glands, lining cells of multiple types, including ciliated forms, a lack of significant cellular atypia and mitotic activity, periglandular basement membranes, and absence of a desmoplastic stromal reaction.[62,193]

Similarly, intranodal nests of benign squamous epithelium should not be mistaken for metastatic squamous carcinoma.[249] Features favoring a benign diagnosis in-

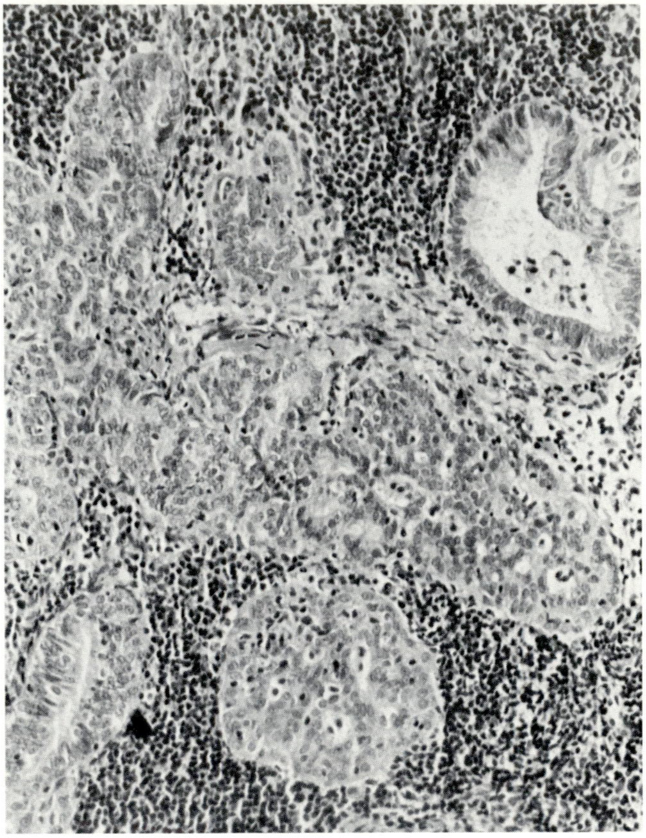

FIG. 17.37. Atypical endosalpingiotic glands within pelvic lymph node. Some of the glands exhibit luminal obliteration by cells growing in solid and cribriform patterns. (Reprinted by permission of Chen, Ref. 53.)

clude their bland cytologic features, mitotic inactivity, and in some, their origin within benign glands.

Rarely, aggregates of benign nevus cells may occur within lymph nodes, typically axillary or cervical. Pelvic or abominal nodal involvement has not been reported, although inguinal nodes may be affected rarely.[102,241] The nevus cells have a distribution within the involved node similar to that of benign müllerian glands. On microscopic examination, the cells resemble their cutaneous counterparts, with bland, uniform, mitotically inactive nuclei and scant cytoplasm that may contain melanin. S-100 protein immunoreactivity of the nevus cells, together with negative staining for cytokeratin and epithelial membrane antigen, may facilitate their distinction from benign müllerian glands and metastatic carcinoma.[420]

Clinical Aspects. Almost all of these patients are in the reproductive and postmenopausal age groups, although rare patients have been of pediatric age.[360] In males, similar lesions have been found in mediastinal lymph nodes[223] but, with the exception of a single case,[168] not in pelvic and abdominal lymph nodes. Although generally without preoperative clinical manifestations, rare cases have resulted in a false positive periaortic lymphangiogram[339] or ureteral obstruction secondary to lymph node enlargement.[406] In occasional cases, visibly enlarged lymph nodes may be encountered at the time of surgery.[189]

A number of patients with intranodal glandular inclusions have had associated endosalpingiosis of the peritoneum,[53,164,360] salpingitis isthmica nodosa, or acute and chronic salpingitis.[164,189,193,360] Other patients have had coexistent ovarian serous tumors, which have been benign,[338] of low malignant potential,[98,102,164] or carcinomas.[98,341]

Histogenesis. Although the origin of benign intranodal glands is uncertain, most investigators have favored a metaplastic origin from remnants of coelomic epithelium entrapped during embryonic development.[104,183] More recently, lymphatic spread of benign tubal epithelium has been postulated as a source.[193] The association of florid intranodal glandular inclusions with inflammatory proliferations of the tubal mucosa and the occasional presence of the endosalpingiotic epithelium within the subcapsular sinuses of the involved lymph nodes are observations that have been used to support this hypothesis.[193] Alternatively, it has been argued that stimuli promoting proliferation of tubal epithelium could also act simultaneously on preexistent nodal inclusions to produce more extensive and easily detectable lesions.[193]

Ectopic Decidua

Ectopic decidua, unassociated with endometriosis, has been described as a rare, incidental microscopic finding in para-aortic and pelvic lymph nodes typically removed as part of a radical hysterectomy for squamous cell carcinoma of the cervix in pregnant patients.[11,65,165,249,423] There may be an associated subserosal ectopic decidual reaction elsewhere in the pelvis.[65] The decidual tissue may be recognized on careful macroscopic examination of the involved lymph node as pinpoint-sized, gray, subcapsular nodules.[65] On microscopic examination, decidual nests occupy the region of the subcapsular sinus and superficial cortex, although more central parts of the lymph node may also be involved (Fig. 17.38). The decidual cells are typically benign in appearance, but focally they may contain bizarre, hyperchromatic nuclei, mimicking metastatic squamous cell carcinoma.[65] The absence of mitotic activity, keratinization, and stromal desmoplasia should facilitate the correct diagnosis.

Leiomyomatosis

Rare cases of lymph node involvement by mitotically inactive, cytologically benign smooth muscle have been described (Fig. 17.39).[2,115,162,165,307] Several of the pa-

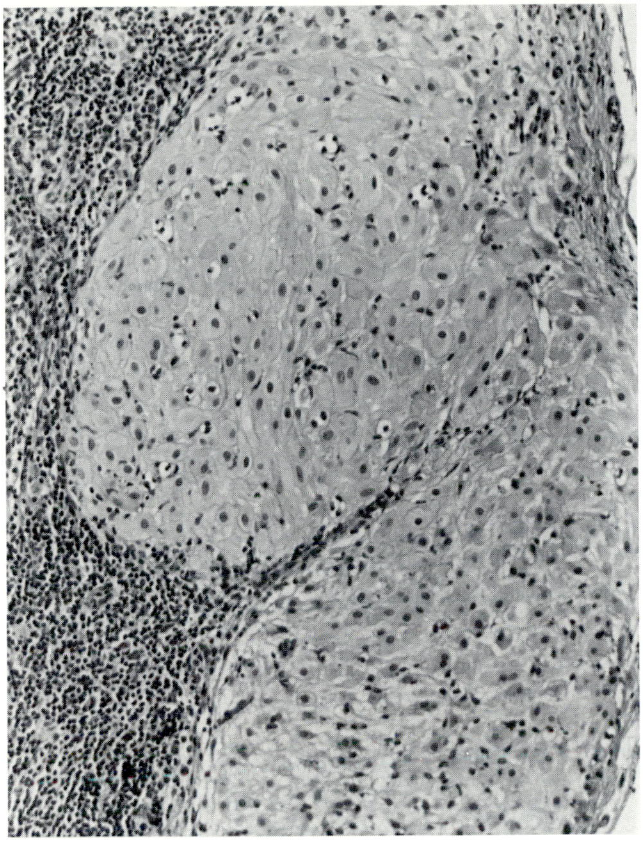

FIG. 17.38. Ectopic decidua within pelvic lymph node. The nodal architecture is focally replaced by sheets of decidualized cells. (Reprinted by permission of Mills, Ref. 249.)

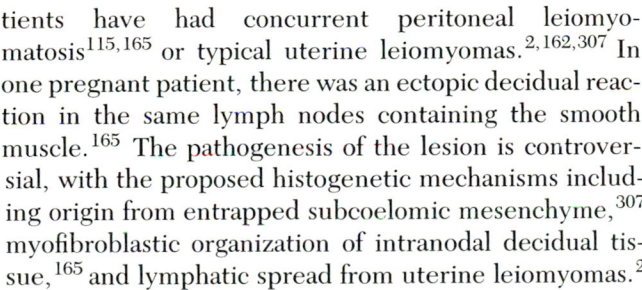

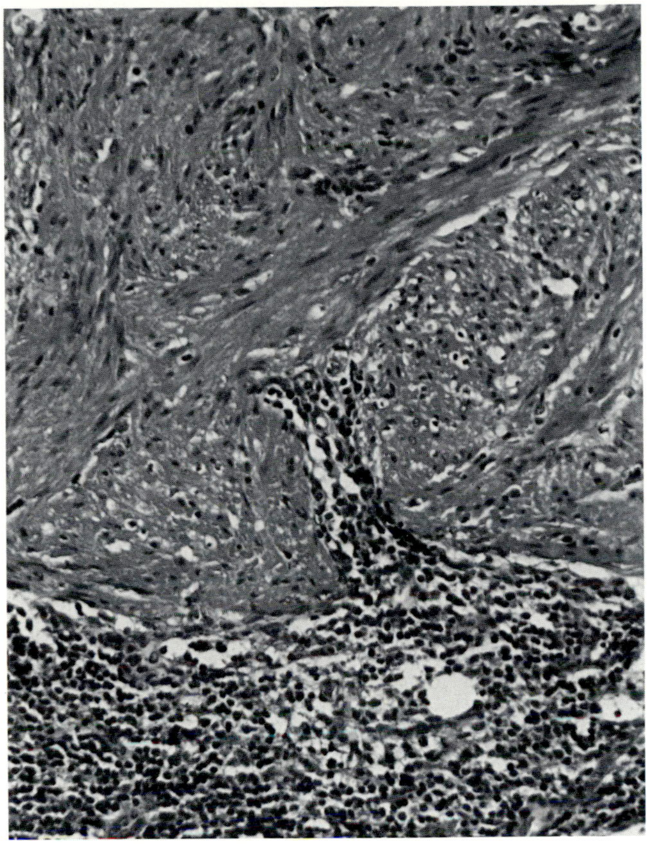

FIG. 17.39. Benign smooth muscle within pelvic lymph node. (Reprinted by permission of Abell and Littler, Ref. 2.)

tients have had concurrent peritoneal leiomyomatosis[115,165] or typical uterine leiomyomas.[2,162,307] In one pregnant patient, there was an ectopic decidual reaction in the same lymph nodes containing the smooth muscle.[165] The pathogenesis of the lesion is controversial, with the proposed histogenetic mechanisms including origin from entrapped subcoelomic mesenchyme,[307] myofibroblastic organization of intranodal decidual tissue,[165] and lymphatic spread from uterine leiomyomas.[2]

Benign intranodal smooth muscle should be distinguished from metastatic, well-differentiated leiomyosarcoma of uterine origin. Patients with the latter condition usually have a large uterine mass, and on histologic examination, the intranodal tumor will usually be more cellular and exhibit evidence of cellular atypicality and mitotic activity.

Pelvic Mesothelial Proliferations

Proliferations of pelvic mesothelial cells lacking müllerian differentiation should be differentiated from the variety of secondary müllerian lesions involving the pelvic peritoneum considered in the preceding section. On histologic examination these mesothelial proliferations are most commonly confused with secondary müllerian lesions of serous type because of the papillary growth patterns typically displayed by both. Mesothelial hyperplasia, cystic mesothelioma (peritoneal inclusion cyst), well-differentiated papillary mesothelioma, and diffuse malignant mesothelioma are discussed in this section. Adenomatoid tumors are also of mesothelial origin but are dealt with in Chapter 13, Mesenchymal Tumors of the Uterus, and Chapter 21, Miscellaneous Tumors of Ovary.

In contrast to the secondary müllerian lesions, these disorders are characterized by cells that resemble, to varying degrees, normal mesothelial cells. A number of them involve, in addition to the pelvic peritoneum in females, the pleura and peritoneum of subjects of either sex. The proliferating cells are typically nonciliated and flat to cuboidal, with a variable amount of eosinophilic cytoplasm. The cytoplasm may contain vacuoles of varying sizes to the extent that occasional signet-ring forms may be present. The vacuoles and extracellular spaces stain negatively with neutral mucin, but characteristically, intracellular and extracellular hyaluronic acid is demonstrable with special stains. In further contrast to peritoneal serous lesions, psammoma bodies are seen only rarely. Preliminary immunohistochemical studies suggest that negative staining for amylase may be helpful in distinguishing a mesothelial process from an extraovarian serous lesion.[394] Ultrastructural differences between mesotheliomas and extraovarian serous tumors may also be useful in distinguishing the two groups of disorders.[403,408] The tumor cells of mesotheliomas, in contrast to those of serous tumors, typically have abundant and long microvilli, numerous tonofilaments, and intracytoplasmic lumens. They typically lack intracellular mucin, and cilia are absent or occur only rarely.[403]

Mesothelial Hyperplasia

Hyperplastic proliferations of pelvic mesothelial cells are a common response to pelvic inflammation and typically represent an incidental finding at the time of surgery (unifocal or multifocal small nodules or granulations) or on microscopic examination.[114,316,353] In some cases, the process may be confined to a hernia sac, reflecting a response to trauma or incarceration.[316] Florid examples may be associated with solid, trabecular, or complex papillary or tubulopapillary patterns, as well as reactive atypia, mitotic activity, multinucleated cells, and limited degrees of infiltration, mimicking a malignant process (see Fig. 16.12).[114,244,316,353] With the exception of those lesions confined to a hernia sac, which are uniformly benign,[316] it may be impossible to reliably distinguish such proliferations from a mesothelial neoplasm. For this reason and because some hyperplastic mesothelial lesions have preceded a mesothelioma, such patients should receive appropriate clinical follow-up.[114,244,304]

Benign Cystic Mesothelioma

This is an uncommon lesion that has been designated *loose cyst of the peritoneal cavity, peritoneal inclusion cyst*, or *cystic mesothelioma*, the variety of diagnostic terms reflecting the uncertainty about its origin and pathogenesis.*

These lesions typically occur in the peritoneal cavity of young adult women (mean age 37 years). Rarely, cystic mesotheliomas may occur in males or in the pleural cavity.[244] The usual clinical manifestations are lower abdominal pain, a palpable mass, or both. In some patients, a history of prior abdominal surgery, pelvic inflammatory disease, or endometriosis is present, suggesting a role for inflammation in the pathogenesis of the cysts in at least some cases.[237] None of these patients have had a history of asbestos exposure. On postoperative follow-

* References 44, 184, 210, 236, 237, 246, 255, 340.

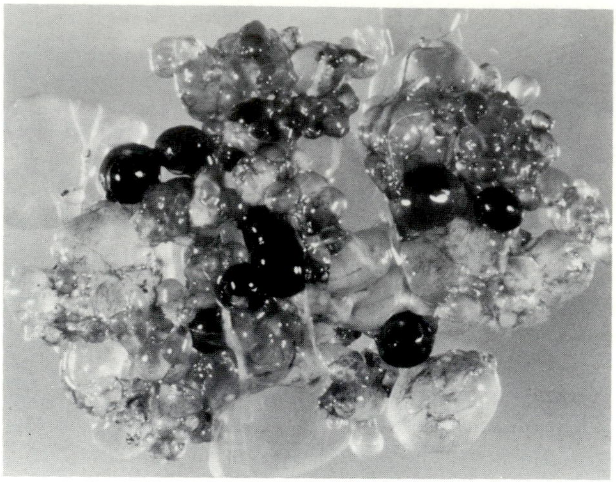

FIG. 17.40. Benign cystic mesothelioma. Multilocular cystic masses consist of thin-walled cysts with a smooth lining. [Reprinted by permission of the Cleveland Clinic Foundation from Miles JM, Hart WR, McMahon JT (1986) Cystic mesothelioma of the peritoneum. Cleve Clin Q 53:109–114.]

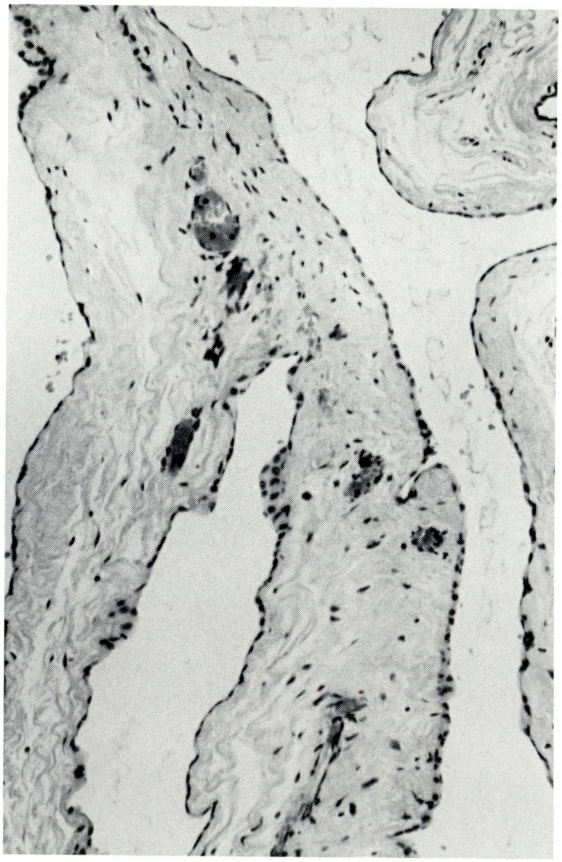

FIG. 17.41. Benign cystic mesothelioma. Cystic spaces are lined by a single layer of flat mesothelial cells and are separated by thin fibrous septae.

up, the lesions do not exhibit malignant behavior, although approximately 40% of the lesions have recurred once or several times at postoperative intervals of several months to many years.[44,184]

At operation, single or multiple, unilocular or multilocular, thin-walled, translucent, cysts measuring up to 20 cm in diameter are found attached to the pelvic and omental peritoneal surfaces (Fig. 17.40). Occasionally, some or all of the cysts may be unattached, lying free in the peritoneal cavity. In florid cases, large numbers of cysts may be present throughout the entire peritoneal cavity.[210] Less commonly, they may form large cystic masses deeply embedded within the retroperitoneum.[237] The cysts have a smooth lining and contain yellow, watery fluid or gelatinous material.

On microscopic examination, the lesions are composed of cysts of varying size, typically lined by a single layer of flat to cuboidal mesothelial cells that lack significant atypia, stratification, or mitotic activity (Fig. 17.41). Microvilli may appear as fuzzy cytoplasmic projections from the luminal cell surfaces.[44] Foci of squamous metaplasia may be seen in a minority of cases.[44,237] In focal areas, the mesothelial cells may exhibit a hobnail appearance, stratification, nuclear pleomorphism, and mitotic activity.[44,184] Some of the cystic spaces typically contain an amorphous, eosinophilic material. The thin septae typically consist of a loose, fibrovascular connective tissue with a sparse inflammatory infiltrate. In occasional cases, however, the cyst walls may exhibit considerable chronic inflammation, fibrosis, and recent and remote hemorrhage.[210,237] The histologic appearance of the cysts is similar in recurrent lesions.

A lesion indistinguishable from the cystic mesothelioma on macroscopic examination is the cystic lymphangioma.[44] However, cystic lymphangiomas more commonly occur in males and children and are most frequently located within the mesentery.[44,184] In contrast to cystic mesotheliomas, they rarely recur, if at all.[44] They are characterized by cells that are more uniformly flat and single-layered, lacking the cuboidal cells, luminal microvilli, and occasional foci of stratification seen in the cystic mesothelioma. Lymphangiomas, in addition, typically contain smooth muscle and sometimes a prominent lymphoid infiltrate within their walls.[44] In some cases, however, the distinction may require histochemical, immunohistochemical, or ultrastructural studies.[184]

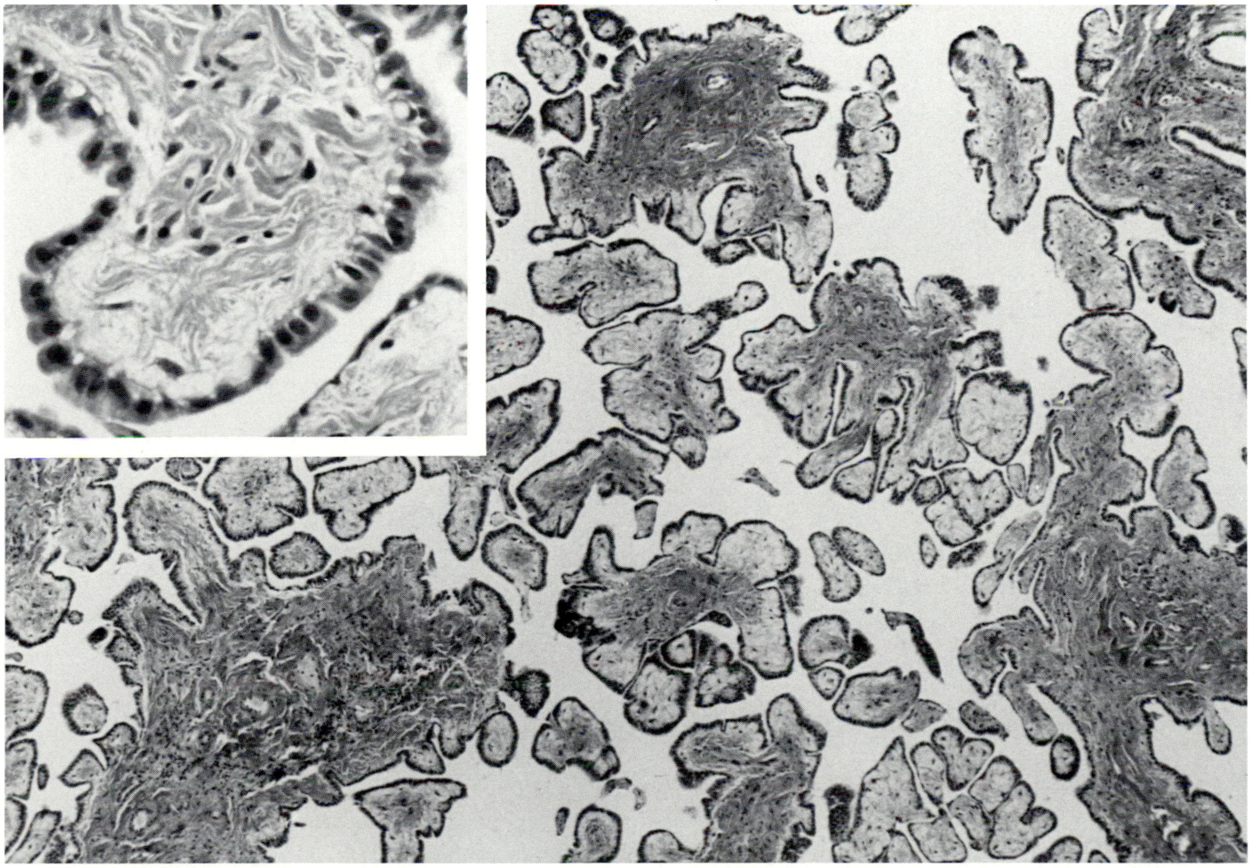

Fig. 17.42. Well-differentiated papillary mesothelioma. Fibrous papillae are lined by a single layer of uniform, flat to cuboidal, mesothelial cells (*inset*).

Well-Differentiated Papillary Mesothelioma

The well-differentiated papillary mesothelioma (WDPM) is a rare lesion that typically involves the peritoneum of females.[114,122,243,244] A few, however, have been encountered in males (tunica vaginalis) and in extraperitoneal (pleural, epicardial) locations.[244] The WDPM usually represents an incidental finding at the time of surgery, although rarely it may be associated with ascites or abdominal pain. None have been asbestos related. All WDPMs reported to date have had a benign clinical course. Because only a few cases have had long-term follow-up, the term *well-differentiated* is preferable to *benign* to qualify these lesions until knowledge of their natural history is more complete.

On gross examination, the tumors are gray to white, firm, single or multiple papillary lesions measuring several centimeters or less. Typically, they involve the peritoneum of the omentum, mesentery, or stomach.[114,122] On microscopic examination, they are better differentiated, both architecturally and cytologically, than diffuse malignant mesotheliomas (DMM).[243] They exhibit a characteristic, uniform, papillary or tubulopapillary pattern composed of fibrous papillae covered by a single layer of uniform, flattened to cuboidal, mesothelial cells (Fig. 17.42).[114,122,243] Rare cases may overlie an otherwise typical adenomatoid tumor, consistent with the mesothelial origin of the latter.[145]

Diffuse Malignant Mesothelioma

This designation refers to the most common type of mesothelioma, a tumor characterized by a diffuse growth pattern, a location in the pleura or peritoneal cavity of either sex, a frequent association with asbestos exposure, and a highly malignant behaviour. Tumors of this type, however, are relatively uncommon within the peritoneal cavity of females, and it appears that the majority of malignant papillary tumors arising from the peritoneum in such patients are examples of extraovarian serous carcinoma.[178,243] DMMs typically exhibit, at least in part, a tubulopapillary pattern (Fig. 17.43), although other epithelial (solid, microcystic) and sarcomatoid patterns may also be seen, typically admixed with the former and rarely as pure patterns.[178,244,385] The tumor cells retain, to a variable degree, a mesothelial appearance, but in contrast to those of a WDPM, they usually exhibit obviously malignant cytologic features (Fig. 17.43, inset).

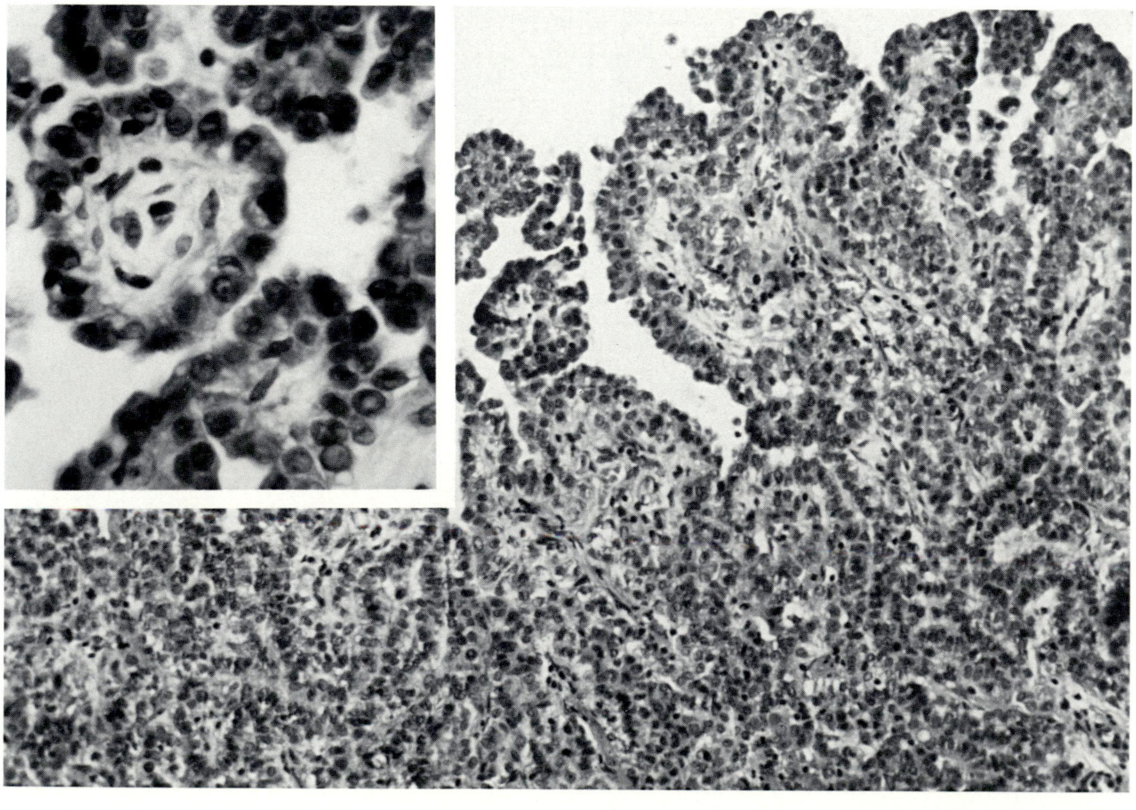

FIG. 17.43. Diffuse malignant mesothelioma. Atypical mesothelial cells (*inset*) are arranged in tubulopapillary and solid patterns.

References

1. Abdel-Shahid RB, Beresford JM, Curry RH (1974) Endometriosis of the ureter with vascular involvement. Obstet Gynecol 43:113–117
2. Abell MR, Littler ER (1975) Benign metastasizing uterine leiomyoma. Multiple lymph nodal metastases. Cancer 36: 2206–2213
3. Abeshouse BS, Abeshouse G (1960) Endometriosis of the urinary tract: A review of the literature and a report of four cases of vesical endometriosis. J Int Coll Surg 34: 43–63
4. Acosta AA, Buttram VC, Besch PK, Malinak LR, Franklin RR, Vanderheyden JD (1973) A proposed classification of pelvic endometriosis. Obstet Gynecol 42: 19–25
5. Albukerk JN, Berlin M, Palladino VC, Silverman J (1979) Endometriosis in peritoneal gliomatosis (Letter). Arch Pathol Lab Med 103: 98–99
6. Allen WM, Masters WH (1955) Traumatic lacerations of uterine support. Am J Obstet Gynecol 70: 500–513
7. Amano S, Yamada N (1981) Endometrioid carcinoma arising from endometriosis of the sigmoid colon: a case report. Hum Pathol 12: 845–848
8. Anderson M, Edmond RM (1974) Rupture of an endometriotic cyst in late pregnancy. Br J Obstet Gynaecol 81: 907–908
9. Aoki M (1967) Endometriosis of the pelvic lymph nodes. Acta Pathol Jpn 17: 217–234
10. Aronchick CA, Brooks FP, Dyson WL, Baron R, Thompson JJ (1983) Ileocecal endometriosis presenting with abdominal pain and gastrointestinal bleeding. Dig Dis Sci 28: 566–572
11. Ashraf M, Boyd CB, Beresford WA (1984) Ectopic decidual reaction in para-aortic and pelvic lymph nodes in the presence of cervical squamous cell carcinoma during pregnancy. J Surg Oncol 26: 6–8
12. August CZ, Murad TM, Newton M (1985) Multiple focal extrovarian serous carcinoma. Int J Gynecol Pathol 4: 11–23
13. Aure JC, Hoeg K, Kolstad P (1971) Carcinoma of the ovary and endometriosis. Acta Obstet Gynecol Scand 50: 63–67
14. Badaway SZA, Marshall L, Gabal AA, Nusbaum ML (1982) The concentration of 13,14-dihydro-15-keto prostaglandin F_{2a} and prostaglandin E_2 in peritoneal fluid of infertile patients with the without endometriosis. Fertil Steril 38: 166–170
15. Badaway SZA, Cuenca V, Stitzel AB, Jacobs RDB, Tomar RH (1984) Autoimmune phenomena in infertile patients with endometriosis. Obstet Gynecol 63: 271–275
16. Badaway SZA, Cuenca V, Marshall L, Munchback R, Rinas AC, Coble DA (1984) Cellular components in peritoneal fluid in infertile patients with and without endometriosis. Fertil Steril 42: 704–708
17. Baker GS, Parsons WR, Welch JS (1966) Endometriosis within the sheath of the sciatic nerve. Report of two patients with progressive paralysis. J Neurosurg 25: 652–655
18. Barbieri RL, Bast RC, Niloff JM, Kistner RW, Knapp RC (1985) Evaluation of a serological test for the diagnosis of endometriosis using a monoclonal antibody OC-125. Presented at the Annual Meeting of the Society of Gynecologic Investigation. March 1985, Abstract 33/P.
19. Bassler R, Theele CH, Labach H (1982) Nodular and tumorlike gliomatosis peritonei with endometriosis caused by a mature ovarian teratoma. Pathol Res Pract 175: 392–403
20. Bazaz-Malik G, Saraf V, Rana BS (1980) Endometrioma of the kidney: Case report. J Urol 123: 422–423
21. Beckman EN, Leonard GL, Pintado SO, Sternberg WH (1985) Endometriosis of the prostate. Am J Surg Pathol 9: 374–379
22. Benz EJ, Dockerty MB, Dixon CF (1952) Polypoid endometrioma of colon: Report of a case in which unusual pathologic features were present. Proc Mayo Clin 27: 201–208
23. Bergen S, Owen J, Snider WR, Lim YC (1981) Disseminated adenomyomas of the abdominal and pelvic cavities. Am Surg 47: 232–235
24. Bergqvist A, Jeppsson S, Ljunberg O (1985) Histochemical demonstration of estrogen and progesterone binding in endometriotic tissue and in uterine endometrium. J Histochem Cytochem 33: 155–161
25. Bergqvist A, Ljungberg O, Myhre E (1984) Human endometrium and endometriotic tissue obtained simultaneously: A comparative histological study. Int J Gynecol Pathol 3: 135–145
26. Bergqvist A, Rannevik G, Thorell J (1981) Estrogen and progesterone cytosol receptor concentration in endometriotic tissue and intrauterine endometrium. Acta Obstet Gynecol Scand [Suppl] 101: 53–58
27. Bergqvist A, Carlstrom K, Jeppsson S, Ljungberg O (1984) Histochemical localization of specific estrogen and progesterone binding in human endometrium and endometriotic tissue. A preliminary report. Acta Obstet Gynecol Scand [Suppl] 123: 15–18
28. Berkowitz RS, Ehrmann RL, Knapp RC (1978) Endometrial stromal sarcoma arising from vaginal endometriosis. Obstet Gynecol 51: 34S–37S
29. Bersch W, Alexy E, Heuser HP, Staemmler HJ (1973) Ectopic decidua formation in the ovary. Virchows Arch [Pathol Anat] 360: 173–177
30. Bettinger HF (1947) Ectopic decidua in renal pelvis. J Pathol Bacteriol 5: 686–687
31. Binns BA, Banerjee R (1983) Endometriosis with Turner's syndrome treated with cyclical oestrogen/progesterone. Case report. Br J Obstet Gynaecol 90: 581–582
32. Blumenkrantz MJ, Gallagher N, Bashore RA, Tenckhoff H (1981) Retrograde menstruation in women undergoing chronic peritoneal dialysis. Obstet Gynecol 57: 667–670
33. Branscomb L (1960) Habitual premenstrual spotting following electrocauterization of the cervix: A newly observed phenomenon. Am J Obstet Gynecol 79: 16–23
34. Bransilver BR, Ferenczy A, Richart RM (1973) Female genital tract remnants. An ultrastructural comparison of hydatid of Morgagni and mesonephric ducts and tubules. Arch Pathol Lab Med 96: 255–261
35. Bransilver BR, Ferenczy A, Richart RM (1974) Brenner tumors and Walthard cell nests. Arch Pathol Lab Med 98: 76–86

36. Brooks JJ, Wheeler JE (1977) Malignancy arising in extragonadal endometriosis. A case report and summary of the world literature. Cancer 40: 3065–3073
37. Brosens IA, Koninckx PR, Corveleyn PA (1978) A study of plasma progesterone, oestradiol-17 beta, prolactin and LH levels and of the luteal phase appearance of the ovaries in patients with endometriosis and infertility. Br J Obstet Gynaecol 85: 246–250
38. Bruns DE, Mills SE, Savory J (1982) Amylase in fallopian tube and serous ovarian neoplasms. Immunohistochemical localization. Arch Pathol Lab Med 106: 17–20
39. Bryce RL, Barbatis C, Charnock M (1982) Endosalpingiosis in pregnancy. Case report. Br J Obstet Gynaecol 89: 166–168
40. Brzezinski A, Durst AL (1983) Endometriosis presenting as an inguinal hernia. Am J Obstet Gynecol 146: 982–983
41. Bullock JL, Massey FM, Gambrell RD (1974) Symptomatic endometriosis in teen-agers. A reappraisal. Obstet Gynecol 43: 896–900
42. Burmeister RE, Fechner RE, Franklin RR (1969) Endosalpingiosis of the peritoneum. Obstet Gynecol 34: 310–318
43. Cantor JO, Fenoglio CM, Richart RM (1979) A case of extensive abdominal endometriosis. Am J Obstet Gynecol 134: 846–847
44. Carpenter HA, Lancaster JR, Lee RA (1982) Multilocular cysts of the peritoneum. Mayo Clin Proc 57: 634–638
45. Chalmers JA (1961) Mulleroma—A rare cause of dysmenorrhoea. Br J Obstet Gynaecol 68: 762–764
46. Chandraratnam E, Leong AS-Y (1983) Papillary serous cystadenoma of borderline malignancy arising in a paraovarian paramesonephric cyst. Light microscopic and ultrastructural observations. Histopathology 7: 601–611
47. Chatman DL (1976) Endometriosis and the black woman. J Reprod Med 16: 303–306
48. Chatman DL (1981) Pelvic peritoneal defects and endometriosis: Allen-Masters syndrome revisited. Fertil Steril 36: 751–756
49. Chatman DL, Ward AB (1982) Endometriosis in adolescents. J Reprod Med 27: 156–160
50. Chatterjee SK (1980) Scar endometriosis: A clinicopathologic study of 17 cases. Obstet Gynecol 56: 81–84
51. Cheesman KL, Ben-Nun I, Chatterton RT Jr, Cohen MR (1982) Relationship of luteinizing hormone, pregnanediol-3-glucuronide, and estriol-16-glucuronide in urine of infertile women with endometriosis. Fertil Steril 38: 542–548
52. Cheesman KL, Cheesman SD, Chatterton RT Jr, Cohen MR (1983) Alterations in progesterone metabolism and luteal function in infertile women with endometriosis. Fertil Steril 40: 590–595
53. Chen KTK (1981) Benign glandular inclusions of the peritoneum and periaortic lymph nodes. Diagn Gynecol Obstet 3: 265–268
54. Chen KTK (1983) Psammoma bodies in pelvic washings (Letter). Acta Cytol 27: 377–379
55. Chen KTK, Weilert M (1982) Squamous cell carcinoma arising in endometriosis. Diagn Gynecol Obstet 4: 343–346
56. Chen KTK, Hendricks EJ, Freeburg B (1982) Benign glandular inclusion of the peritoneum associated with leiomyomatosis peritonealis disseminata. Diagn Gynecol Obstet 4: 41–44
57. Chervenak FA, Greenlee RM, Lewenstein L, Tovell HMM (1981) Massive ascites associated with endometriosis. Obstet Gynecol 57: 379–381
58. Cioltei A, Tasca L, Titiriga L, Maakaron G, Calciu V (1979) Nodular salpingitis and tubal endometriosis. I. Comparative clinical study. Acta Eur Fertil 10: 135–141
59. Clark JE, Wood H, Jaffurs WJ, Fabro S (1979) Endometrioid-type cystadenocarcinoma arising in the mesosalpinx. Obstet Gynecol 54: 656–658
60. Clement PB (1977) Perforation of the sigmoid colon during pregnancy: A rare complication of endometriosis. Br J Obstet Gynaecol 84: 548–550
61. Clement PB, Scully RE (1978) Extrauterine mesodermal (müllerian) adenosarcoma. A clinicopathologic analysis of five cases. Am J Clin Pathol 69: 276–283
62. Colgan TJ, Norris HJ (1983) Ovarian epithelial tumors of low malignant potential: A review. Int J Gynecol Pathol 1: 367–382
63. Cooper P (1978) Mixed mesodermal tumor and clear cell carcinoma arising in ovarian endometriosis. Cancer 42: 2827–2831
64. Corner GW Jr, Hu C-Y, Hertig AT (1950) Ovarian carcinoma arising in endometriosis. Am J Obstet Gynecol 59: 760–774
65. Covell LM, Disciullo AJ, Knapp RC (1977) Decidual change in pelvic lymph nodes in the presence of cervical squamous cell carcinoma during pregnancy. Am J Obstet Gynecol 127: 674–676
66. Cozzutto C (1981) Uterus-like mass replacing ovary. Report of a new entity. Arch Pathol Lab Med 105: 508–511
67. Crain JL, Luciano AA (1983) Peritoneal fluid evaluation in infertility. Obstet Gynecol 61: 159–164
68. Croom RD, Donovan ML, Schwesinger WH (1984) Intestinal endometriosis. Am J Surg 148: 660–667
69. Crum CP, Wible J, Frick HC, Fenoglio CM, Richart RM, Williamson S (1981) A case of extensive pelvic endometriosis terminating in endometrial sarcoma. Am J Obstet Gynecol 140: 718–719
70. Czernobilsky B, Lancet M (1972) Broad ligament adenocarcinoma of müllerian origin. Obstet Gynecol 40: 238–242
71. Czernobilsky B, Morris WJ (1979) A histologic study of ovarian endometriosis with emphasis on hyperplastic and atypical changes. Obstet Gynecol 53: 318–323
72. Czernobilsky B, Silverstein A (1978) Salpingitis and ovarian endometriosis. Fertil Steril 30: 45–49
73. D'Ablaing G III, Klatt EC, DiRocco G, Hibbard LT (1983) Broad ligament serous tumor of low malignant potential. Int J Gynecol Pathol 2: 93–99
74. Danforth DN (1942) Cytologic relationship of Walthard cell rest to Brenner tumor of ovary and the pseudomucinous cystadenoma. Am J Obstet Gynecol 43: 984–996
75. d'Anglejan G, Goutallier, de Lara AC, Ryckewaert A (1970) Radiculalgie par endometriose pelvienne avec lesions osseuses. Rev Rhuma 37: 251–253
76. David MP, Ben-Zwi D, Langer L (1981) Tubal intramural

polyps and their relationship to infertility. Fertil Steril 35: 526–531

77. Dawood MY, Khan-Dawood FS, Wilson L Jr (1984) Peritoneal fluid prostaglandins and prostanoids in women with endometriosis, chronic pelvic inflammatory disease, and pelvic pain. Am J Obstet Gynecol 148: 391–395
78. De Brux J (1975) The contribution of pathological anatomy to the diagnosis and prognosis of different forms of tubal sterility. Acta Eur Fertil 6: 185–195
79. Devereux WP (1963) Endometriosis: Long-term observation, with particular reference to incidence in pregnancy. Obstet Gynecol 22: 444–450
80. Di Domenico A, Stangl F, Bennington J (1982) Leiomyosarcoma of the broad ligament. Gynecol Oncol 13: 412–415
81. Dictor M (1985) Malignant mixed mesodermal tumor of the ovary: A report of 22 cases. Obstet Gynecol 65: 720–724
82. Dizerega GS, Barber DL, Hodgen GD (1980) Endometriosis: Role of ovarian steroids in initiation, maintenance, and suppression. Fertil Steril 33: 649–653
83. Dmowski WP (1984) Pitfalls in clinical, laparoscopic and histologic diagnosis of endometriosis. Acta Obstet Gynecol Scand [Suppl] 123: 61–66
84. Dmowski WP, Radwanska E (1984) Current concepts on pathology, histogenesis and etiology of endometriosis. Acta Obstet Gynecol Scand [Suppl] 123: 29–33
85. Dmowski WP, Radwanska E (1984) Endometriosis and infertility. Acta Obstet Gynecol Scand [Suppl] 123: 73–79
86. Dmowski WP, Rao R, Scommegna A (1980) The luteinized unruptured follicle syndrome and endometriosis. Fertil Steril 33: 30–34
87. Donnez J, Thomas K (1982) Influence of the luteinized unruptured follicle syndrome in fertile women and in women with endometriosis. Eur J Obstet Gynecol Reprod Biol 14: 187–190
88. Donnez J, Langerock S, Thomas K (1983) Peritoneal fluid volume, 17-beta-estradiol and progesterone concentrations in women with endometriosis and/or luteinized unruptured follicle syndrome. Gynecol Obstet Invest 16: 210–220
89. Dore N, Landry M, Cadotte M, Schurch W (1980) Cutaneous endosalpingiosis. Arch Dermatol 116: 909–912
90. Doshi N, Fujikura T (1978) Squamous cell passage from the peritoneal cavity to lymph glands and pulmonary lymphatics in a malformed infant: A mechanism for endometriosis and pulmonary metastasis. Am J Obstet Gynecol 131: 221–223
91. Doty DW, Gruber JS, Wolf GC, Winslow RC (1980) 46XY pure gonadal dysgenesis: Report of 2 unusual cases. Obstet Gynecol 55: 61S–63S
92. Douglas GW, Kastin AJ, Huntington RW Jr (1965) Carcinoma arising in a retroperitoneal müllerian cyst, with widespread metastasis during pregnancy. Am J Obstet Gynecol 91: 210–216
93. Drake TS, Metz SA, Grunert GM, O'Brien WF (1980) Peritoneal fluid volume in endometriosis. Fertil Steril 34: 280–281
94. Drake TS, O'Brien WF, Ramwell PW, Metz SA (1981) Peritoneal fluid thromboxane B_2 and 6-keto-prostaglandin F_{1a} in endometriosis. Am J Obstet Gynecol 140: 401–404
95. Duncan CJ (1934) Endometrioma of Bartholin's gland. N Engl J Med 211: 24–25
96. Duson CK, Zelenik JS (1954) Vulvar endometriosis. Obstet Gynecol 3: 76–79
97. Egger H, Weigmann P (1982) Clinical and surgical aspects of ovarian endometriotic cysts. Arch Gynecol 233: 37–45
98. Ehrmann RL, Federschneider JM, Knapp RC (1980) Distinguishing lymph node metastases from benign glandular inclusions in low-grade ovarian carcinoma. Am J Obstet Gynecol 136: 737–746
99. Elliot DL, Barker AF, Dixon LM (1985) Catamenial hemoptysis. New methods of diagnosis and therapy. Chest 87: 687–688
100. Elliott GB, Christensen RM, Elliott KA (1970) Invasive endometriosis of the intestine: Report of 21 cases. Can J Surg 13: 387–395
101. El-Mahgoub S, Yassen S (1980) A positive proof for the theory of coelomic metaplasia. Am J Obstet Gynecol 137: 137–140
102. Farhi DC, Silverberg SG (1982) Pseudometastases in female genital cancer. Pathol Annu 1: 47–76
103. Fathalla MF (1967) Malignant transformation in ovarian endometriosis. Br J Obstet Gynaecol 74: 85–92
104. Ferguson BR, Bennington JL, Haber SL (1969) Histochemistry of mucosubstances and histology of mixed müllerian pelvic lymph node glandular inclusions. Evidence for histogenesis by müllerian metaplasia of coelomic epithelium. Obstet Gynecol 33: 617–625
105. Ferrari BT, Shollenbarger DR (1977) Abdominal wall endometriosis following hypertonic saline abortion. JAMA 238: 56–57
106. Ferraro LR, Hetz H, Carter H (1956) Malignant endometriosis. Pelvic endometriosis complicated by polypoid endometrioma of the colon and endometriotic sarcoma: Report of a case and review of the literature. Obstet Gynecol 7: 32–39
107. Fischer S (1953) Seltene lokalisation einer endometriosis externa extraperitonealis. Geburtsch Frauenh 13: 240–243
108. Floberg J, Backdahl M, Silfersward C, Thomassen PA (1984) Postpartum perforation of the colon due to endometriosis. Acta Obstet Gynecol Scand 63: 183–184
109. Forrest JS, Brooks DL (1972) Cyclic sciatica of endometriosis. JAMA 222: 1177–1178
110. Forrest J, Buckley CH, Fox H (1984) Pelvic endometriosis and tubal inflammatory disease. Int J Gynecol Pathol 3: 343–347
111. Fortier KJ, Haney AF (1985) The pathologic spectrum of uterotubal junction obstruction. Obstet Gynecol 65: 93–98
112. Foster DC, Stern JL, Buscema J, Rock JA, Woodruff JD (1981) Pleural and parenchymal pulmonary endometriosis. Obstet Gynecol 58: 552–556
113. Fox H, Buckley CH (1984) Current concepts of endometriosis. Clin Obstet Gynaecol 11: 279–287
114. Foyle A, Al-Jabi M, McCaughey WTE (1981) Papillary

peritoneal tumors in women. Am J Surg Pathol 5: 241–249
115. Fujii S, Okamura H, Nakashima N, Bann C, Aso T, Nishimura T (1980) Leiomyomatosis peritonealis disseminata. Obstet Gynecol 55: 79S–83S
116. Gardner GH, Greene RR, Peckham B (1957) Tumors of the broad ligament. Am J Obstet Gynecol 73: 536–555
117. Gardner HL (1966) Cervical and vaginal endometriosis. Clin Obstet Gynecol 9: 358–372
118. Genadry R, Parmley T, Woodruff JD (1977) The origin and clinical behaviour of the parovarian tumor. Am J Obstet Gynecol 129: 873–879
119. Gennari L, Luciani L (1965) A case of endometriosis of the trapezius muscle. Tumori 51: 361–366
120. Gerbie AB, Greene RR, Reis RA (1958) Heteroplastic bone and cartilage in the female genital tract. Obstet Gynecol 11: 573–578
121. Gitelis S, Petasnick JP, Turner DA, Ghiselli RW, Miller AW III (1985) Endometriosis simulating a soft tissue tumor of the thigh: CT and MR evaluation. J Comput Assist Tomogr 9: 573–576
122. Goepel JR (1981) Benign papillary mesothelioma of peritoneum: A histological, histochemical and ultrastructural study of six cases. Histopathology 5: 21–30
123. Goldberg MI, Ng ABP, Belinson JL, Hutson ED, Nordqvist SRB (1978) Clear cell adenocarcinoma arising in endometriosis of the rectovaginal septum. Obstet Gynecol 51: 38S–40S
124. Goldstein DP, deCholnoky C, Emans SJ, Leventhal JM (1980) Laparoscopy in the diagnosis and management of pelvic pain in adolescents. J Reprod Med 24: 251–256
125. Goodall JR (1943) A study in endometriosis, endosalpingiosis, endocervicosis, and peritoneal–ovarian sclerosis. Philadelphia, Lippincott, pp 79–88
126. Goodall JR (1944) Urinary complications of pelvic endometriosis. Ann Surg 120: 891–900
127. Gooneratne S, Sassone M, Blaustein A, Talerman A (1982) Serous surface papillary carcinoma of the ovary: A clinicopathologic study of 16 cases. Int J Gynecol Pathol 1: 258–269
128. Gordon PH, Schottler JL, Balcos EG, Goldberg SM (1976) Perianal endometrioma. Report of five cases. Dis Colon Rectum 19: 260–265
129. Gould SF, Shannon JM, Cunha GR (1983) Nuclear estrogen binding sites in human endometriosis. Fertil Steril 39: 520–524
130. Granai CO, Walters MD, Safaii H, Jelen I, Madoc-Jones H, Moukhtar M (1984) Malignant transformation of vaginal endometriosis. Obstet Gynecol 64: 592–595
131. Grant A (1966) Additional sterility factors in endometriosis. Fertil Steril 17: 514–519
132. Gray LA (1966) The managment of endometriosis involving the bowel. Clin Obstet Gynecol 9: 309–330
133. Gray LA, Barnes ML (1965) Relation of endometriosis to ovarian carcinoma. Am Surg 31: 798–806
134. Grimes DA, Fowler WC Jr (1980) Adenosquamous carcinoma of the cecum arising in endometriosis. Gynecol Oncol 9: 254–255
135. Groll M (1984) Endometriosis and spontaneous abortion. Fertil Steril 41: 933–935
136. Hajdu SI, Koss LG (1970) Endometriosis of the kidney. Am J Obstet Gynecol 106: 314–315
137. Halme J (1985) Basic research in endometriosis. Obstet Gynecol Annu 14: 288–309
138. Halme J, Chafe W, Currie JL (1985) Endometriosis with massive ascites. Obstet Gynecol 65: 591–592
139. Halme J, Becker S, Wing R (1984) Accentuated cyclic activation of peritoneal macrophages in patients with endometriosis. Am J Obstet Gynecol 148: 85–90
140. Halme J, Becker S, Hammond MG, Raj S (1982) Pelvic macrophages in normal and infertile women: The role of patent tubes. Am J Obstet Gynecol 142: 890–895
141. Halme J, Becker S, Hammond MG, Raj MHG, Raj S (1983) Increased activity of pelvic macrophages in infertile women with mild endometriosis. Am J Obstet Gynecol 145: 333–337
142. Halme J, Hammond MG, Hulka JF, Raj SG, Talbert LM (1984) Retrograde menstruation in healthy women and in patients with endometriosis. Obstet Gynecol 64: 151–154
143. Haney AF, Handwerger S, Weinberg JB (1984) Peritoneal fluid prolactin in infertile women with endometriosis: Lack of evidence of secretory activity by endometrial implants. Fertil Steril 42: 935–938
144. Haney AF, Muscato JJ, Weinberg JB (1981) Peritoneal fluid populations in infertility patients. Fertil Steril 35: 696–698
145. Hanrahan JB (1963) A combined papillary mesothelioma and adenomatoid tumor of the omentum. Report of a case. Cancer 16: 1497–1500
146. Hanton EM, Malkasian GD Jr, Dockerty MB, Pratt JH (1966) Endometriosis associated with complete or partial obstruction of menstrual egress. Report of 7 cases. Obstet Gynecol 28: 626–629
147. Hapke MR, Bigelow B (1977) Mucocele of the appendix secondary to obstruction by endometriosis. Hum Pathol 8: 585–589
148. Harbitz HF (1936) Ectopic decidua. Acta Pathol Microbiol Scand [Suppl] 26: 16–20
149. Hargrove JT, Abraham GK (1980) Abnormal luteal function in patients with endometriosis (Abstr). Fertil Steril 34: 302
150. Hasiuk AS, Petersen RO, Hanjani P, Griffen TD (1984) Extragenital malignant mixed müllerian tumor. Case report and review of the literature. Am J Clin Pathol 81: 102–105
151. Henriksen E (1955) Endometriosis. Am J Surg 90: 331–337
152. Herbold DR, Fu YS, Silbert SW (1983) Leiomyosarcoma of the broad ligament. A case report and literature review with follow-up. Am J Surg Pathol 7: 285–292
153. Herr JC, Platz CE, Heidger PM Jr, Curet LB (1979) Smooth muscle within ovarian decidual nodules: A link to leiomyomatosis peritonealis disseminata? Obstet Gynecol 53: 451–456
154. Hibbard J, Schreiber JR (1984) Footdrop due to sciatic nerve endometriosis. Am J Obstet Gynecol 149: 800–801
155. Hibbard LT, Schumann WR, Goldstein GE (1981) Thoracic endometriosis: A review and report of two cases. Am J Obstet Gynecol 140: 227–232

156. Hirschowitz JS, Soler NG, Wortsman J (1978) The galactorrhoea–endometriosis syndrome. Lancet 1: 896–898
157. Hobbs JE, Bortnick R (1940) Endometriosis of the lungs. An experimental and clinical study. Am J Obstet Gynecol 40: 832–843
158. Holmes MD, Levin HS, Ballard LA (1981) Endosalpingiosis. Clevel Clin Q 48: 345–352
159. Honore LH (1980) Endometriosis of Meckel's diverticulum associated with intestinal obstruction—A case report. Am J Proctol 31 (2): 11–12
160. Honore LH (1981) Parauterine leiomyomas in women: A clinicopathologic study of 22 cases. Eur J Obstet Gynecol Reprod Biol 11: 273–279
161. Honore LH, Nickerson KG (1976) Papillary serous cystadenoma arising in a paramesonephric cyst of the parovarium. Am J Obstet Gynecol 125: 870–871
162. Horie A, Ishii N, Matsumoto M, Hashizuma, Kawakami M, Sato Y (1984) Leiomyomatosis in the pelvic lymph node and peritoneum. Acta Pathol Jpn 34: 813–819
163. Houston DE (1984) Evidence for the risk of pelvic endometriosis by age, race and socioeconomic status. Epidemiol Rev 6: 167–191
164. Hsu YK, Parmley TH, Rosenshein NB, Bhagavan BS, Woodruff JD (1980) Neoplastic and non-neoplastic mesothelial proliferations in pelvic lymph nodes. Obstet Gynecol 55: 83–88
165. Hsu YK, Rosenshein NB, Parmley TH, Woodruff JD, Elberfeld HT (1981) Leiomyomatosis in pelvic lymph nodes. Obstet Gynecol 57: 91s–93s
166. Huffman JW (1981) Endometriosis in young teen-age girls. Pediatr Annu 10: 501–506
167. Hulme-Moir I, Ross MS (1969) A case of early postpartum abdominal pain due to hemorrhagic deciduosis peritonei. Br J Obstet Gynaecol 76: 746–749
168. Huntrakoon M (1985) Benign glandular inclusions in the abdominal lymph nodes of a man. Hum Pathol 16: 644–646
169. Irani S, Atkinson L, Cabaniss C, Danovitch SH (1976) Pleuroperitoneal endometriosis. Obstet Gynecol 47: 72S–74S
170. Israel SL, Rubenstone A, Meranze DR (1954) The ovary at term. I. Decidua-like reaction and surface cell proliferation. Obstet Gynecol 3: 399–407
171. Iwasaka T, Okuma Y, Yoshimura T, Kidera Y, Sugimori H (1985) Endometriosis associated with ascites. Obstet Gynecol 66: 72S–75S
172. Janne O, Kauppila A, Kokko E, Lantto T, Ronnberg L, Vihko R (1981) Estrogen and progestin receptors in endometriosis lesions: Comparison with endometrial tissue. Am J Obstet Gynecol 141: 562–566
173. Javert CT (1951) Observations on the pathology and spread of endometriosis based on the theory of benign metastasis. Am J Obstet Gynecol 62: 477–487
174. Javert CT (1952) The spread of benign and malignant endometrium in the lymphatic system with a note on coexisting vascular involvement. Am J Obstet Gynecol 64: 780–806
175. Jenks JE, Artman LE, Hoskins WJ, Miremadi AK (1984) Endometriosis with ascites. Obstet Gynecol 63: 75S–77S
176. Kanbour A, Salazar H, Stock R (1978) Papillary cystadenoma originating in hydatid cyst of Morgagni: Clinicopathologic study and observations on histogenesis (Abstr). Lab Invest 38: 350
177. Kane C, Drouin P (1985) Obstructive uropathy associated with endometriosis. Am J Obstet Gynecol 151: 207–211
178. Kannerstein M, Churg J (1977) Peritoneal mesothelioma. Hum Pathol 8: 83–94
179. Kannerstein M, Churg J, McCaughey WTE, Hill DP (1977) Papillary tumors of the peritoneum in women: Mesothelioma or papillary carcinoma. Am J Obstet Gynecol 127: 306–314
180. Kapadia SB, Russak RR, O'Donnell WF, Harris RN, Lecky JW (1984) Postmenopausal ureteral endometriosis with atypical adenomatous hyperplasia following hysterectomy, bilateral oophorectomy, and long-term estrogen therapy. Obstet Gynecol 64: 60S–63S
181. Kaplan C, Bernirschke K, Johnson KC (1980) Leiomyomatosis peritonealis disseminata with endometrium. Obstet Gynecol 55: 119–122
182. Kapp DS, Merino M, LiVolsi V (1982) Adenocarcinoma of the vagina arising in endometriosis: Long-term survival following radiation therapy. Gynecol Oncol 14: 271–278
183. Karp LA, Czernobilsky B (1969) Glandular inclusions in pelvic and abdominal para-aortic lymph nodes. Am J Clin Pathol 52: 212–218
184. Katsube Y, Mukai K, Silverberg SG (1982) Cystic mesothelioma of the peritoneum. A report of five cases and review of the literature. Cancer 50: 1615–1622
185. Kaunitz A, Di Sant'Agnese PA (1979) Needle tract endometriosis: An unusual complication of amniocentesis. Obstet Gynecol 54: 753–755
186. Kauppila A, Vierikko P, Isotalo H, Ronnberg L, Vihko R (1984) Cytosol estrogen and progestin receptor concentrations and 17-beta-hydroxysteroid dehydrogenase activities in the endometrium and endometriotic tissue. Effects of hormonal stimulation. Acta Obstet Gynecol Scand [Suppl] 123: 45–49
187. Keettel WC, Stein RJ (1951) The viability of the cast-off menstrual endometrium. Am J Obstet Gynecol 61: 440–442
188. Kempers RD, Dockerty MB, Hunt AB, Symmonds RE (1960) Significant postmenopausal endometriosis. Surg Gynecol Obstet 111: 348–356
189. Kempson RL (1978) Consultation case. Am J Surg Pathol 2: 321–325
190. Kern WH (1969) Benign papillary structures with psammoma bodies in culdocentesis fluid. Acta Cytol 13: 178–180
191. Kerner H, Gaton E, Czernobilsky B (1981) Unusual ovarian, tubal, and pelvic mesothelial inclusions in patients with endometriosis. Histopathology 5: 277–282
192. Kerr WS (1966) Endometriosis involving urinary tract. Clin Obstet Gynecol 9: 331–357
193. Kheir SM, Mann WJ, Wilkerson JA (1981) Glandular inclusions in lymph nodes. The problem of extensive involvement and relationship to salpingitis. Am J Surg Pathol 5: 353–359
194. Kistner RW (1966) Current status of the hormonal treatment of endometriosis. Clin Obstet Gynecol 9: 271–292

195. Kistner RW (1979) Endometriosis and infertility. Clin Obstet Gynecol 22: 101–119
196. Koninckx PR, De Moor P, Brosens IA (1980) Diagnosis of the luteinized unruptured follicle syndrome by steroid hormone assays on peritoneal fluid. Br J Obstet Gynaecol 87: 929–934
197. Koninckx PR, Renaer M, Brosens IA (1980) Origin of peritoneal fluid in women: An ovarian exudation product. Br J Obstet Gynaecol 87: 177–183
198. Koninckx PR, Ide P, Vandenbroucke W, Brosens IA (1980) New aspects of the pathophysiology of endometrosis and associated infertility. J Reprod Med 24: 257–260
199. Koskimies AI, Tenhunen A, Ylikorkala O (1984) Peritoneal fluid 6-keto-prostaglandin F_{1a}, thrombaxane B2 in endometriosis and unexplained infertility. Acta Obstet Gynecol Scand [Suppl] 123: 19–21
200. Kuo T, London SN, Dinh TV (1980) Endometriosis occurring in leiomyomatosis peritonealis disseminata. Ultrastructural study and histogenetic consideration. Am J Surg Pathol 4: 197–204
201. Kurman RJ, Funk RL, Kirshenbaum AH (1969) Spina bifida with associated choristoma of müllerian origin. J Pathol 99: 324–327
202. Kurman RJ, Main CS, Chen H (1984) Intermediate trophoblast: A distinctive form of trophoblast with specific morphological, biochemical and functional features. Placenta 5: 349–370
203. Kurman RJ, Young RH, Norris HJ, Main CS, Lawrence WD, Scully RE (1984) Immunocytochemical localization of placental lactogen and chorionic gonadotropin in the normal placenta and trophoblastic tumors, with emphasis on intermediate trophoblast and the placental site trophoblastic tumor. Int J Gynecol Pathol 3: 101–121
204. Kwan D, Pang LSC (1964) Deciduosis peritonei. Br J Obstet Gynecol 71: 804–806
205. Labay GR, Feiner F (1971) Malignant pleural endometriosis. Am J Obstet Gynecol 110: 478–480
206. Langmade CF (1975) Pelvic endometriosis and ureteral obstruction. Am J Obstet Gynecol 122: 463–469
207. Langsam LB, Prasanta KR, Galang CF (1984) Intussusception of the appendix. Dis Col Rectum 27: 387–392
208. Lankerani MR, Aubrey RW, Reid JD (1982) Endometriosis of the colon with mixed "germ cell" tumor. Am J Clin Pathol 78: 555–559
209. Lansman HH, Lapin A, Blaustein A (1960) Pelvic oxyuris granuloma associated with endometriosis. Am J Obstet Gynecol 79: 1178–1180
210. Lascano EF, Villamayor RD, Llauro JL (1960) Loose cysts of the peritoneal cavity. Ann Surg 152: 836–844
211. Lattes R, Shepard F, Tovell H, Wylie R (1956) A clinical and pathological study of endometriosis of the lung. Surg Gynecol Obstet 103: 552–558
212. Laube DW, Calderwood GW, Benda JA (1985) Endometriosis causing ureteral obstruction. Obstet Gynecol 65: 69S–71S
213. Lauchlan SC (1965) Two types of müllerian epithelium in an abdominal scar. Am J Obstet Gynecol 93: 89–90
214. Lauchlan SC (1966) The cytology of endometriosis. Am J Obstet Gynecol 94: 533–535
215. Lauchlan SC (1972) The secondary müllerian system. Obstet Gynecol Surv 27: 133–146
216. Lauslahti K (1972) Malignant external endometriosis. A case of adenocarcinoma of umbilical endometriosis. Acta Pathol Microbiol Scand [A] 80 [Suppl] 233: 98–102
217. Lele SB, Piver S, Barlow JJ, Tsukada Y (1978) Squamous cell carcinoma arising in ovarian endometriosis. Gynecol Oncol 6: 290–293
218. Levander G, Normann P (1955) The pathogenesis of endometriosis. An experimental study. Acta Obstet Gynecol Scand 34: 366–398
219. Lindenberg K, Schmid J, Ruttner J, Sulser H, Schmid M (1975) Endometriosis of the lung. Arch Gynak 218: 219–226
220. Lisa JR, Gioia JD, Rubin IC (1954) Observations on the interstitial portion of the fallopian tube. Surg Gynecol Obstet 99: 159–169
221. LiVolsi VA, Perzin KH (1974) Endometriosis of the small intestine, producing intestinal obstruction or simulating neoplasm. Am J Dig Dis 19: 100–108
222. Lombardo L, Mateos JH, Barroeta FF (1968) Subarachnoid hemorrhage due to endometriosis of the spinal canal. Neurology 18: 423–426
223. Longo S (1976) Benign lymph node inclusions. Hum Pathol 7: 349–354
224. Macafee CHG, Greer HLH (1960) Intestinal endometriosis. Br J Obstet Gynaecol 67: 539–555
225. Madelenat P, De Brux J, Palmer R (1977) L'etiologie des obstructions tubaires proximales et son role dan le pronostic des implantations. Gynecologie 28: 47–53
226. Madsen H, Hansen P, Andersen OP (1980) Endometrioid carcinoma in an operation scar. Acta Obstet Gynecol Scand 59: 475–476
227. Mahoney AD, Waisman J, Zeldis LJ (1977) Adenomyoma. A precursor of extrauterine müllerian adenosarcoma? Arch Pathol Lab Med 101: 579–584
228. Malinak LR, Buttram VC, Elias S, Simpson JL (1980) Heritable aspects of endometriosis. II. Clinical characteristics of familial endometriosis. Am J Obstet Gynecol 137: 332–337
229. Mann WJ, Fromowitz F, Saychek T, Madariaga JR, Chalas E (1984) Endometriosis associated with appendiceal intussusception. A report of two cases. J Reprod Med 29: 625–629
230. Marchevsky AM, Kaneko M (1978) Bilateral ovarian endometriosis associated with carcinosarcoma of the right ovary and endometrioid carcinoma of the left ovary. Am J Clin Pathol 70: 709–712
231. Marchevsky AM, Zimmerman MJ, Aufses Jr AH, Weiss H (1984) Endometrial cyst of the pancreas. Gastroenterology 86: 1589–1591
232. Marik J, Hulka J (1978) Luteinized unruptured follicle syndrome: A subtle cause of infertility. Fertil Steril 29: 270–274
233. Mariscal G, Laynez M (1971) Comentarios sobre un caso de endometriosis gastrica. Rev Esp Enferm Apar Digest 33: 603–604
234. Martimbeau PW, Pratt JH, Gaffey TA (1975) Small-bowel obstruction secondary to endometriosis. Mayo Clinic Proc 50: 239–243

235. Martin JD Jr, Hauck AE (1985) Endometriosis in the male. Am Surg 51: 426–430
236. Massachusetts General Hospital Case Records (1960) Case 46382. Ruptured corpus luteum, right ovary, with hemoperitoneum. Peritoneal cysts, with squamous metaplasia. N Engl J Med 263: 605–609
237. Massachusetts General Hospital Case Records (1965) Case 2-1965. Peritoneal inclusion cysts, loose, attached and retroperitoneal (paracolonic). N Engl J Med 272: 41–46
238. Mathur S, Peress MR, Williamson HO, Youmans CD, Maney SA, Garvin AJ, Rust PF, Fudenberg HH (1982) Autoimmunity to endometrium and ovary in endometriosis. Clin Exp Immunol 50: 259–266
239. Mazur MT, Hendrickson MR, Kempson RL (1983) Optically clear nuclei. An alteration of endometrial epithelium in the presence of trophoblast. Am J Surg Pathol 7: 415–423
240. McArthur JW, Ulfelder H (1965) The effect of pregnancy upon endometriosis. Obstet Gynecol Surv 20: 709–733
241. McCarthy SW, Palmer AA, Bale PM, Hirst E (1974) Naevus cells in lymph nodes. Pathology 6: 351–358
242. McCaughey WTE (1982) Papillary tumors of the ovary (Editorial). Int J Gynecol Pathol 1: 313–314
243. McCaughey WTE (1985) Papillary peritoneal neoplasms in females. Pathol Annu 2: 387–404
244. McCaughey WTE, Kannerstein M, Churg J (1985) Tumors and pseudotumors of the serous membranes. In: Atlas of tumor pathology. Washington, D.C., Armed Forces Institute of Pathology, series 2, fascicle 20
245. McCaughey WTE, Kirk ME, Lester W, Dardick I (1984) Peritoneal epithelial lesions associated with proliferative serous tumours of the ovary. Histopathology 8: 195–208
246. Mennemeyer R, Smith M (1979) Multicystic, peritoneal mesothelioma. A report with electron microscopy of a case mimicking intra-abdominal cystic hygroma (lymphangioma). Cancer 44: 692–698
247. Merrill JA (1963) Experimental induction of endometriosis across Millipore filters. Surg Forum 14: 399–401
248. Michowitz M, Baratz M, Stavorovsky M (1983) Endometriosis of the umbilicus. Dermatologica 167: 326–330
249. Mills SE (1983) Decidua and squamous metaplasia in abdominopelvic lymph nodes. Int J Gynecol Pathol 2: 209–215
250. Minvielle UL, de la Cruz JV (1968) Endometriosis of the anal canal: Presentation of a case. Dis Colon Rectum 11: 32–35
251. Miyazawa K (1976) Incidence of endometriosis among Japanese women. Obstet Gynecol 48: 407–409
252. Moller NE (1959) The Arias-Stella phenomenon in endometriosis. Acta Obstet Gynecol Scand 38: 271–274
253. Moloshok AA, Ivanko AI (1984) Endometriosis of the breast (an observation). Vopr Onkol 30: 88–89
254. Moon YS, Leung PCS, Ho Yuen B, Gomel V (1981) Prostaglandin F in human endometriotic tissue. Am J Obstet Gynecol 141: 344–345
255. Moor JH Jr, Crum CP, Chandler JG, Feldman PS (1980) Benign cystic mesothelioma. Cancer 45: 2395–2399
256. Moore JG, Hibbard LT, Growdon WA, Schifrin BS (1979) Urinary tract endometriosis: Enigmas in diagnosis and management. Am J Obstet Gynecol 134: 162–172
257. Morson BC, Dawson IMP (1979) Gastrointestinal pathology. London, Blackwell Scientific Publications
258. Mostoufizadeh M, Scully RE (1980) Malignant tumors arising in endometriosis. Clin Obstet Gynecol 23: 951–963
259. Mudge TJ, James MJ, Jones WR, Walsh JA (1985) Peritoneal fluid 6-keto-prostaglandin F_{1alpha} levels in women with endometriosis. Am J Obstet Gynecol 152: 901–904
260. Muscato JJ, Haney AF, Weinberg JB (1982) Sperm phagocytosis by human peritoneal macrophages: A possible cause of infertility in endometriosis. Am J Obstet Gynecol 144: 503–510
261. Muse ZK, Wilson EA, Jawad MJ (1982) Prolactin hyperstimulation in response to thyrotropin-releasing hormone in patients with endometriosis. Fertil Steril 38: 419–422
262. Naples JD, Batt RE, Sadigh H (1981) Spontaneous abortion rate in patients with endometriosis. Obstet Gynecol 57: 509–512
263. Navratil E, Kramer A (1936) Endometriose in der armmuskulatur. Klin Wochnschr 15: 1765–1770
264. Nielsen M, Lykke J, Thomsen JL (1983) Endometriosis of the vermiform appendix. Acta Pathol Microbiol Scand [A] 91: 253–256
265. Nissen ED, Goldstein AI (1973) Intussusception of the appendix associated with endometriosis. Int J Gynaecol Obstet 11: 184–189
266. Norenberg DD, Gundersen JH, Janis JF, Gundersen AL (1977) Early pregnancy on the diaphragm with endometriosis. Obstet Gynecol 49: 620–622
267. Novak ER (1960) Pathlogy of endometriosis. Clin Obstet Gynecol 3: 413–428
268. Novak ER, Hoge AF (1958) Endometriosis of the lower genital tract. Obstet Gynecol 12: 687–693
269. Nunn LL (1949) Endometrioma of the thigh. Northwest Med 48:474–475
270. Ober WB, Black MB (1955) Neoplasms of the subcoelomic mesenchyme. Arch Pathol Lab Med 59: 698–705
271. Ober WB, Grady HG, Schoenbucher AK (1957) Ectopic ovarian decidua without pregnancy. Am J Pathol 33: 199–214
272. Olive DL, Franklin RR, Gratkins LV (1982) The association between endometriosis and spontaneous abortion. A retrospective clinical study. J Reprod Med 27: 333–338
273. Ortega I, Nogales F, Gonzalez-Campora R, Matilla A, Galera H (1982) Extragenital endometrioid cystadenofibroma. Acta Obstet Gynecol Scand 61: 283–284
274. Oses AV, Rodriguez EH, Garcia JLS, Sanchez TA, Corral MJ, Serrano LP (1982) Catemenial pneumothorax with pleural endometriosis and hemoptysis. Diagn Gynecol Obstet 4: 295–299
275. O'Sullivan D, Heffernan CK (1960) Deciduosis peritonei in pregnancy. Report of two cases. Br J Obstet Gynaecol 67: 1013–1016
276. Palagiri A (1978) Urethral diverticulum with endometriosis. Urology 11: 271–272
277. Palladino VS, Trousdell M (1969) Extra-uterine müllerian tumors. A review of the literature and the report of a case. Cancer 23: 1413–1422
278. Panganiban W, Cornog JL (1972) Endometriosis of the

intestines and vermiform appendix. Dis Colon Rectum 15: 253–260
279. Parmley T (1982) Papillary tumors of the ovary (Editorial). Int J Gynecol Pathol 1: 314–315
280. Parmley TH, Woodruff JD, Winn K, Johnson JWC, Douglas PH (1975) Histogenesis of leiomyomatosis peritonealis disseminata (disseminated fibrosing deciduosis). Obstet Gynecol 46: 511–516
281. Patel VC, Samuels H, Abeles E, Hirjibehedin PF (1982) Endometriosis at the knee. A case report. Clin Orthop 171: 140–144
282. Paull T, Tedeschi LG (1972) Perineal endometriosis at the site of episiotomy scar. Obstet Gynecol 40: 28–34
283. Pedersen H, Rank F (1984) Morphology of endometriosis before and during treatment with danazol. Acta Obstet Gynecol Scand [Suppl] 123: 13–14
284. Pellegrini VD Jr, Pasternak HS, Macaulay WP (1981) Endometrioma of the pubis: A differential in the diagnosis of hip pain. A report of two cases. J Bone Joint Surg 63A: 1333–1334
285. Pelzer SG (1954) Cystic endometriosis of the epigastrium. J Int Coll Surg 21: 528–531
286. Peress MR, Sosnowski JR, Mathur RS, Williamson HO (1982) Pelvic endometriosis and Turner's syndrome. Am J Obstet Gynecol 144: 474–476
287. Picoff RC, Meeker CI (1970) Psammoma bodies in the cervicovaginal smear in association with benign papillary structures of the ovary. Acta Cytol 14: 45–47
288. Pieslor PC, Orenstein JM, Hogan DL, Breslow A (1979) Ultrastructure of myofibroblasts and decidualized cells in leiomyomatosis peritonealis disseminata. Am J Clin Pathol 72: 875–882
289. Pittaway DE, Wentz AC (1984) Endometriosis and corpus luteum function. Is there a relationship? J Reprod Med 29: 712–716
290. Ponka JL, Brush BE, Hodgkinson CP (1973) Colorectal endometriosis. Dis Colon Rectum 16: 490–499
291. Prakash S, Ulfelder H, Cohen RB (1965) Enzyme–histochemical observations on endometriosis. Am J Obstet Gynecol 91: 990–997
292. Pratt JH, Shamblin WR (1970) Spontaneous rupture of endometrial cysts of the ovary presenting as an acute abdominal emergency. Am J Obstet Gynecol 108: 56–62
293. Pueblitz-Peredo S, Luevano-Flores E, Rincon-Taracena R, Ochoa-Carrillo FJ (1985) Uteruslike mass of the ovary: Endomyometriosis or congenital malformation? A case with a discussion of histogenesis. Arch Pathol Lab Med 109: 361–364
294. Punnonen R, Klemi PJ, Nikkanen V (1980) Postmenopausal endometriosis. Eur J Obstet Gynec Reprod Biol 11: 195–200
295. Quagliarello J, Coppa G, Bigelow B (1985) Isolated endometriosis in an inguinal hernia. Am J Obstet Gynecol 152: 688–689
296. Radwanska E, Dmowski WP (1982) Luteal function in infertile women with endometriosis (Abstr). Fertil Steril 37: 313
297. Raju U, Fine G, Ohorodnik J (1982) Papillary serous peritoneal tumors in women: A light microscopic and ultrastructural study (Abstr). Lab Invest 46: 67A
298. Ranney B (1970) Endometriosis: II. Emergency operations due to hemoperitoneum. Obstet Gynecol 36: 437–442
299. Ranney B (1980) Endometriosis: Pathogenesis, symptoms and findings. Clin Obstet Gynecol 23: 865–874
300. Recalde AL, Majmudar B (1977) Endometriosis involving the femoral vein. South Med J 70: 69–74
301. Reddy AN, Evans AT (1974) Endometriosis of the ureters. J Urol 111: 474–480
302. Rewell RE (1972) Extra-uterine decidua. J Pathol 105: 219–222
303. Richter MA, Choudhry A, Barton JJ, Merrick RE (1983) Bleeding ectopic decidua as a cause of intraabdominal hemorrhage. A case report. J Reprod Med 28: 430–432
304. Riddell RH, Goodman MJ, Moossa AR (1981) Peritoneal malignant mesothelioma in a patient with recurrent peritonitis. Cancer 48: 134–139
305. Ridley JH (1968) The histogenesis of endometriosis. A review of facts and fancies. Obstet Gynecol Surv 23: 1–35
306. Ridley JH, Edwards IK (1958) Experimental endometriosis in the human. Am J Obstet Gynecol 76: 783–790
307. Rigaud C, Bogomoletz WV (1983) Leiomyomatosis in pelvic lymph node (Letter). Arch Pathol Lab Med 107: 153–154
308. Rio FW, Edwards DL, Regan JF, Schmutzer KJ (1970) Endometriosis of the small bowel. Arch Surg 101: 403–405
309. Rock JA, Parmley TH, King TM, Laufe LE, Su BC (1981) Endometriosis and the development of tuboperitoneal fistulas after tubal ligation. Fertil Steril 35: 16–20
310. Rock JA, Dubin NH, Ghodgaonkar RB, Bergquist CA, Erozan YS, Kimball AW Jr (1982) Cul-de-sac fluid in women with endometriosis: Fluid volume and prostanoid concentration during the proliferative phase of the cycle—days 8 to 12. Fertil Steril 37: 747–750
311. Roddick JW, Conkey G, Jacobs EJ (1960) The hormonal response of endometrium in endometriotic implants and its relationship to symptomatology. Am J Obstet Gynecol 79: 1173–1177
312. Rogers WS, Seckinger DL (1965) Decidual tissue as a cause of intraabdominal hemorrhage during labor. Obstet Gynecol 25: 391–397
313. Rohlfing MB, Kao KJ, Woodard BH (1981) Endomyometriosis: Possible association with leiomyomatosis disseminata and endometriosis (Letter). Arch Pathol Lab Med 105: 556–557
314. Ronnberg L, Kauppila A, Rajaniemi H (1984) Luteinizing hormone receptor disorder in endometriosis. Fertil Steril 42: 64–68
315. Rosai J (1982) Uteruslike mass replacing ovary (Letter). Arch Pathol Lab Med 106: 364
316. Rosai J, Dehner LP (1975) Nodular mesothelial hyperplasia in hernia sacs. A benign reactive condition stimulating a neoplastic process. Cancer 35: 165–175
317. Rossman F, D'Ablaing G III, Marrs RP (1983) Pregnancy complicated by ruptured endometrioma. Obstet Gynecol 62: 519–521
318. Roth LM (1973) Endometriosis with perineural involvement. Am J Clin Pathol 59: 807–809
319. Roth LM (1974) The Brenner tumor and the Walthard

cell nest. An electron microscopic study. Lab Invest 31: 15–23
320. Roth LM, Ehrlich CE (1977) Mucinous cystadenocarcinoma of the retroperitoneum. Obstet Gynecol 49: 486–488
321. Roth MS, Goodner DM (1977) Large endometrioma occurring in an adolescent. Obstet Gynecol 49: 364–366
322. Rubin IC, Lisa JR, Trinidad S (1956) Further observations on ectopic endometrium of the fallopian tube. Surg Gynecol Obstet 103: 469–474
323. Russell HB (1945) Decidual reaction of endometrium ectopic in an abdominal lymph node. Surg Gynecol Obstet 81: 218–220
324. Russell P (1979) The pathological assessment of ovarian neoplasms. II. The proliferating epithelial tumours. Pathology 11: 251–282
325. Russell P (1984) Borderline epithelial tumours of the ovary: A conceptual dilemma. Clin Obstet Gynecol 11: 259–277
326. Russell P, Laverty CR (1980) Benign müllerian rests in pelvic lymph node. Pathology 12: 129–130
327. Russell P, Slavutin L, Laverty CR, Cooper-Booth J (1979) Extrauterine mesodermal (müllerian) adenosarcoma. A case report. Pathology 11: 557–560
328. Russell P, Bannatyne PM, Solomon HJ, Stoddard LD, Tattersall MHN (1985) Multifocal tumorigenesis in the upper female genital tract—Implications for staging and management. Int J Gynecol Pathol 4: 192–210
329. Sabatelle R, Winger E (1973) Postpartum intraabdominal hemorrhage caused by ectopic deciduosis. Obstet Gynecol 41: 873–875
330. Saifuddin A, Buckley CH, Fox H (1983) Immunoglobulin content of the endometrium in women with endometriosis. Int J Gynecol Pathol 2: 255–263
331. Sampson JA (1927) Metastatic or embolic endometriosis, due to the menstrual dissemination of endometrial tissue into the venous circulation. Am J Pathol 3: 93–109
332. Sampson JA (1930) Postsalpingectomy endometriosis (endosalpingiosis). Am J Obstet Gynecol 20: 443–480
333. Sampson JA (1940) The development of the implantation theory for the origin of peritoneal endometriosis. Am J Obstet Gynecol 40: 549–557
334. Sampson JA (1945) Pathogenesis of postsalpingectomy endometriosis in laparotomy scars. Am J Obstet Gynecol 50: 597–620
335. Schifrin BS, Erez S, Moore JG (1973) Teen-age endometriosis. Am J Obstet Gynecol 116: 973–980
336. Schlicke CP (1946) Ectopic endometrial tissue in the thigh. JAMA 132: 445–446
337. Schmidt CL, Demopoulos RI, Weiss G (1981) Infected endometriotic cysts: Clinical characterization and pathogenesis. Fertil Steril 36: 27–30
338. Schneider V (1980) Benign glandular lymph node inclusions. Diagn Gynecol Obstet 2: 313–320
339. Schneider V, Walsh JW, Goplerud DR (1980) Benign glandular inclusions in para-aortic lymph nodes: A cause for false positive lymphangiography. Am J Obstet Gynecol 138: 350–352
340. Schneider V, Partridge JR, Gutierrez, Hurt WG, Maizels MS, Demay RM (1983) Benign cystic mesothelioma involving the female genital tract: Report of four cases. Am J Obstet Gynecol 145: 355–359
341. Schnurr RC, Delagado G, Chun B (1978) Benign glandular inclusions in para-aortic lymph nodes in women undergoing lymphadenectomies. Am J Obstet Gynecol 130: 813–816
342. Schrodt GR, Alcorn MO, Ibanez J (1980) Endometriosis of the male urinary system: A case report. J Urol 124: 722–723
343. Schuldenfrei R, Janovski NA (1962) Disseminated endosalpingiosis associated with bilateral papillary serous cystadenocarcinoma of the ovaries. A case report. Am J Obstet Gynecol 84: 382–389
344. Schweppe KW, Wynn RM (1981) Ultrastructural changes in endometriotic implants during the menstrual cycle. Obstet Gynecol 58: 465–473
345. Schweppe KW, Wynn RM (1984) Endocrine dependency of endometriosis: An ultrastructural study. Eur J Obstet Gynecol Reprod Biol 17: 193–208
346. Schweppe KW, Dmowski WP, Wynn RM (1981) Ultrastructural changes in endometriotic tissue during danazol treatment. Fertil Steril 36: 20–26
347. Schweppe KW, Wynn RW, Beller FK (1984) Ultrastructural comparison of endometriotic implants and eutopic endometrium. Am J Obstet Gynecol 148: 1024–1037
348. Scott RB, Te Linde RW (1954) Clinical external endometriosis. Probable viability of menstrually shed fragments of endometrium. Obstet Gynecol 4: 502–510
349. Scott RB, Wharton LR (1957) The effect of estrone and progesterone on the growth of experimental endometriosis in rhesus monkeys. Am J Obstet Gynecol 74: 852–865
350. Scott RB, Nowak RJ, Tindale RM (1958) Umbilical endometriosis and the Cullen sign. A study of lymphatic transport from pelvis to the umbilicus in monkeys. Obstet Gynecol 11: 556–563
351. Scott RB, Te Linde RW, Wharton LR (1953) Further studies on experimental endometriosis. Am J Obstet Gynecol 66: 1082–1103
352. Scully RE (1977) Ovarian tumors. Am J Pathol 87: 686–720
353. Scully RE (1979) Tumors of the ovary and maldeveloped gonads. Atlas of tumor pathology. Washington, D.C., Armed Forces Institute of Pathology, series 2, fascicle 16
354. Scully RE (1981) Smooth-muscle differentiation in genital tract disorders (Editorial). Arch Pathol Lab Med 105: 505–507
355. Scully RE, Richardson GS, Barlow JF (1966) The development of malignancy in endometriosis. Clin Obstet Gynecol 9: 384–411
356. Sensky TE, Liu DTY (1980) Endometriosis: Associations with menorrhagia, infertility and oral contraceptives. Int J Gynaecol Obstet 17: 573–576
357. Sgarlata CS, Hertelendy F, Mikhail G (1983) The prostanoid content in peritoneal fluid and plasma of women with endometriosis. Am J Obstet Gynecol 147: 563–565
358. Shamsuddin AKM, Villa Santa U, Tang CK, Mohamed NC (1979) Adenocarcinoma arising from extragonadal endometriosis 14 years after total hysterectomy and bilateral salpingo-oophorectomy for endometriosis: Report of a case

with ultrastructural studies. Am J Obstet Gynecol 133: 585–586
359. Sheldon RS, Wilson RB, Dockerty MB (1967) Serosal endometriosis of fallopian tubes. Am J Obstet Gynecol 99: 882–884
360. Shen SC, Bansal M, Purrazzella R, Malviya V, Strauss L (1983) Benign glandular inclusions in lymph nodes, endosalpingiosis, and salpingitis isthmica nodosa in a young girl with clear cell adenocarcinoma of the cervix. Am J Surg Pathol 7: 293–300
361. Shipton EA, Meares SD (1965) Heterotopic bone formation in the ovary. Aust NZ J Obstet Gynaecol 5: 100–102
362. Silton RM (1979) More glandular inclusions (letter). Am J Surg Pathol 3: 285–286
363. Simpson JL, Elias S, Malinak LR, Buttram VC (1980) Heritable aspects of endometriosis. I. Genetic studies. Am J Obstet Gynecol 137: 327–331
364. Sinder C, Dochat GR, Wentsler NE (1956) Splenoendometriosis. Am J Obstet Gynecol 92: 883–884
365. Sinykin MB (1960) Endosalpingiosis. Minn Med 43: 759–761
366. Slasky BS, Siewers RD, Lecky JW, Zajko A, Burkholder JA (1982) Catamenial pneumothorax: The roles of diaphragmatic defects and endometriosis. AJR 138: 639–643
367. Slutsky JN, Callahan D (1983) Endometriosis of the ureter can present as renal failure: A case report and review of endometriosis affecting the ureters. J Urol 130: 336–337
368. Sobel HJ, Marquet E, Schwarz R, Mazur MT (1984) Optically clear endometrial nuclei. Ultrastruct Pathol 6: 229–231
369. Soules MR, Malinak LR, Bury R, Poindexter A (1976) Endometriosis and anovulation: A coexisting problem in the infertile female. Am J Obstet Gynecol 125: 412–417
370. Stanley KE, Utz DC, Dockerty MB (1965) Clinically significant endometriosis of the urinary tract. Surg Gynecol Obstet 120: 491–498
371. Stapleton JJ, Haber MH, Lindner LE (1981) Paramesonephric papillary serous cystadenocarcinoma. A case report with scanning electron microscopy. Acta Cytol 25: 310–316
372. Startseva NV (1980) Clinico-immunological aspects in genital endometriosis. Akush Ginekol 56: 23–26
373. Steck WD, Helwig EB (1966) Cutaneous endometriosis. Clin Obstet Gynecol 9: 373–383
374. Steele RW, Dmowski WP, Marmer DJ (1984) Immunologic aspects of human endometriosis. Am J Reprod Immunol 6: 33–36
375. Steinberg L, Rothman D, Drey NW (1970) Müllerian cyst of the retroperitoneum. Am J Obstet Gynecol 107: 963–964
376. Sternberg WH (1963) Nonfunctioning ovarian neoplasms. In: Grady HG, Smith DE, eds. The ovary. International Academy of Pathology Monograph. Baltimore, Williams & Wilkins
377. Stevenson CS, Campbell CG (1960) The symptoms, physical findings, and clinical diagnosis of pelvic endometriosis. Clin Obstet Gynecol 3: 441–455
378. Stock RJ (1982) Postsalpingectomy endometriosis: A reassessment. Obstet Gynecol 60: 560–570
379. Stock RJ (1983) Histopathologic changes in fallopian tubes subsequent to sterilization procedures. Int J Gynecol Pathol 2: 13–27
380. Strasser EJ, Davis RM (1977) Extraperitoneal inguinal endometriosis. Am Surg 43: 421–422
381. Suginami H, Hamada K, Yano K (1985) A case of endometriosis of the lung treated with danazol. Obstet Gynecol 66: 68S–71S
382. Sun CJ, Toker C, Masi JD, Elias EG (1979) Primary low-grade adenocarcinoma occurring in the inguinal region. Cancer 44: 340–345
383. Sundarasivarao D (1953) The müllerian vestiges and benign epithelial tumours of the epididymis. J Pathol 66: 417–432
384. Szlachter NB, Moskowitz J, Bigelow B, Weiss G (1980) Iatrogenic endometriosis: Substantiation of the Sampson hypothesis. Obstet Gynecol 55: 52S–53S
385. Talerman A, Montero JR, Chilcote RR, Okagaki T (1985) Diffuse malignant peritoneal mesothelioma in a 13-year-old girl. Report of a case and review of the literature. Am J Surg Pathol 9: 73–80
386. Tamaya T, Motoyama T, Ohono Y, Ide N, Tsurusaki T, Okada H (1979) Steroid receptor levels and histology of endometriosis and adenomyosis. Fertil Steril 31: 396–400
387. Tavassoli FA, Norris HJ (1982) Peritoneal leiomyomatosis (leiomyomatosis peritonealis disseminata): A clinicopathologic study of 20 cases with ultrastructural observations. Int J Gynecol Pathol 1: 59–74
388. Teilum G, Madsen V (1950) Endometriosis ovarii et peritonaei caused by hysterosalpingography. Br J Obstet Gynaecol 57: 10–16
389. Te Linde RW, Scott RB (1950) Experimental endometriosis. Am J Obstet Gynecol 60: 1147–1173
390. Teoh TB (1953) The structure and development of Walthard nests. J Pathol 66: 433–439
391. Tutschka BG, Lauchlan SC (1980) Endosalpingiosis. Obstet Gynecol 55: 57S–60S
392. Ueda G, Yamasaki M, Inoue M, Tanaka Y, Abe Y, Ogawa M (1985) Immunohistochemical study of amylase in common epithelial tumors of the ovary. Int J Gynecol Pathol 4: 240–244
393. Ulbright TM, Kraus FT (1981) Endometrial stromal tumors of extrauterine tissue. Am J Clin Pathol 76: 371–377
394. Ulbright TM, Morley DJ, Roth LM, Berkow RL (1983) Papillary serous carcinoma of the retroperitoneum. Am J Clin Pathol 79: 633–637
395. Uohara JK, Kobara TY (1975) Endometriosis of the appendix. Am J Obstet Gynecol 121: 423–426
396. Valente PT (1984) Leiomyomatosis peritonealis disseminata. A report of two cases and review of the literature. Arch Pathol Lab Med 108: 669–672
397. Venables JH (1972) Endometriosis of the ileum: Four cases with obstruction. Am J Obstet Gynecol 113: 1054–1055
398. Vierikko P, Kauppila A, Ronnberg L, Vihko R (1985) Steroidal regulation of endometriosis tissue: Lack of induction of 17-beta-hydroxysteroid dehydrogenase activity by progesterone, medroxyprogesterone acetate, or danazol. Fertil Steril 43: 218–224

399. von Numers C (1965) Observations on metaplastic changes in the germinal epithelium of the ovary and on the aetiology of ovarian endometriosis. Acta Obstet Gynecol Scand 44: 107–116
400. Wagner I, Bettendorf U (1980) Extraovarian Brenner tumor. Case report and review. Arch Gynecol 229: 191–196
401. Walton LA (1977) A reexamination of endometriosis after pregnancy. J Reprod Med 19: 341–344
402. Wardle PG, McLaughlin EA, McDermott A, Mitchell JD, Ray BD, Hull MGR (1985) Endometriosis and ovulatory disorder: Reduced fertilization in vitro compared with tubal and unexplained infertility. Lancet 2: 236–239
403. Warhol MJ, Hunter NJ, Corson JM (1982) An ultrastructural comparison of mesotheliomas and adenocarcinomas of the ovary and endometrium. Int J Gynecol Pathol 1: 125–134
404. Weed JC (1980) Prostaglandins as related to endometriosis. Clin Obstet Gynecol 23: 895–900
405. Weed JC, Arquembourg PC (1980) Endometriosis: Can it produce an autoimmune response resulting in infertility? Clin Obstet Gynecol 23: 885–893
406. Weir JH, Janovski NA (1963) Paramesonephric lymph-node inclusions—A cause of obstructive uropathy. Obstet Gynecol 21: 363–367
407. Wheeler JM, Johnson BM, Malinak LR (1983) The relationship of endometriosis to spontaneous abortion. Fertil Steril 39: 656–660
408. White PF, Merino MJ, Barwick KW (1985) Serous surface papillary carcinoma of the ovary: A clinical, pathologic, ultrastructural, and immunohistochemical study of 11 cases. Pathol Annu 1: 403–418
409. Wild RA,Shivers CA (1985) Antiendometrial antibodies in patients with endometriosis. Am J Reprod Immunol 8: 84–86
410. Wilhelm JL, Scommegna A (1977) Catamenial pneumothorax. Bilateral occurrence while on suppressive therapy. Obstet Gynecol 50: 227–231
411. Wilkins SB, Bell-Thomson J, Tyras DH (1985) Hemothorax associated with endometriosis. J Thor Cardiovasc Surg 89: 636–638
412. Williams PP, Gall SA, Prem KA (1971) Ectopic mucinous cystadenoma. A case report. Obstet Gynecol 38: 831–837
413. Williams TJ, Pratt JH (1977) Endometriosis in 1,000 consecutive celiotomies: Incidence and management. Am J Obstet Gynecol 129: 245–250
414. Willman EA, Collins WP, Clayton SG (1976) Studies in the involvement of prostaglandins in uterine symptomatology and pathology. Br J Obstet Gynaecol 83: 337–341
415. Wolfe SA, Mackles A, Greene HJ (1961) Endometriosis of the cervix. Am J Obstet Gynecol 81: 111–123
416. Won KH (1969) Endometriosis, mucocele and regional enteritis of Meckel's diverticulum. Arch Surg 98: 209–212
417. Wurster KH, Leu HJ (1972) Zur frage der hamatogenen Ausbreitung der Endometriose. Geburtshilfe Frauenheilkd 32: 983–986
418. Wynn TE (1971) Endometriosis of the sigmoid colon. Massive intramural hematoma. Arch Pathol Lab Med 92: 24–27
419. Yates-Bell AJ, Molland EA, Pryor JP (1972) Endometriosis of the ureter. Br J Urol 44: 58–67
420. Yazdi HM (1985) Nevus cell aggregates associated with lymph nodes. Immunohistochemical observations. Arch Pathol Lab Med 109: 1044–1046
421. Ylikorkala O, Viinikka L (1983) Prostaglandins and endometriosis. Acta Obstet Gynecol Scand [Suppl] 113: 105–107
422. Ylikorkala O, Koskimies A, Laatkainen T, Tenhunen A, Viinikka L (1984) Peritoneal fluid prostaglandins in endometriosis, tubal disorders, and unexplained infertility. Obstet Gynecol 63: 616–620
423. Yoonessi M, Satchindanand SK, Ortinez CG, Goodell T (1982) Benign glandular elements and decidual reaction in retroperitoneal lymph nodes. J Surg Oncol 19: 81–86
424. Young EE, Gamble CN (1969) Primary adenocarcinoma of the rectovaginal septum arising from endometriosis. Report of a case. Cancer 24: 597–601
425. Young RH, Prat J, Scully RE (1980) Epidermoid cyst of the ovary. A report of three cases with comments on histogenesis. Am J Clin Pathol 73: 272–276
426. Young RH, Prat J, Scully RE (1984) Endometrioid stromal sarcomas of the ovary. A clinicopathologic analysis of 23 cases. Cancer 53: 1143–1155
427. Zinsser KR, Wheeler JE (1982) Endosalpingiosis in the omentum. A study of autopsy and surgical material. Am J Surg Pathol 6: 109–117

18

Common Epithelial Tumors of the Ovary

Bernard Czernobilsky, M.D.

The common epithelial tumors of the ovary constitute about two-thirds of all primary ovarian neoplasms and almost 90% of all malignant ovarian tumors.[151] They are considered to be derived from the surface epithelium (coelomic epithelium or mesothelium) covering the ovary and from the underlying stroma.[157a] Although this histogenesis has been accepted by most authorities, the supporting evidence varies in the individual tumors from fairly conclusive to circumstantial. The histologic heterogeneity encountered in this group of tumors does not contradict their common origin. Although the ovary is not of müllerian origin, the source of these neoplasms, namely, the surface epithelium, is derived from the coelomic epithelium, which in the embryo gives rise to the müllerian ducts. The latter form the fallopian tubes, uterine body, cervix, and possibly the upper part of the vagina with their large variety of epithelia. The presence of different epithelial elements in these tumors can, therefore, be satisfactorily explained. Furthermore, admixtures of histologic elements from various epithelial ovarian tumors within a given tumor are very common and constitute further evidence of their common derivation. The cause for the great neoplastic potential of the ovarian surface epithelium, however, has not yet been elucidated.

Classification

In view of these histogenetic considerations, it is not surprising that for many years the classification of ovarian tumors has been one of the most confusing chapters in pathology. Only with the publication of the "Histologic Classification of Ovarian Tumors by the World Health Organization (WHO),[157b] which is based on histogenetic principles, has some order been established in this field. Table 18.1 represents the WHO listing of the common epithelial tumors that are discussed in this chapter. New concepts and newly identified entities make periodic reappraisals necessary. Thus, for the purpose of the present discussion, the WHO classification has been modified (Table 18.2). In this classification, which reflects my con-

TABLE 18.1 Histologic classification of ovarian tumors: Common "epithelial" tumors.[a]

- A. Serous tumors
  - 1. Benign
    - a. Cystadenoma and papillary cystadenoma
    - b. Surface papilloma
    - c. Adenofibroma and cystadenofibroma
  - 2. Of borderline malignancy (carcinomas of low malignant potential)
    - a. Cystadenoma and papillary cystadenoma
    - b. Surface papilloma
    - c. Adenofibroma and cystadenofibroma
  - 3. Malignant
    - a. Adenocarcinoma, papillary adenocarcinoma, and papillary cystadenocarcinoma
    - b. Surface papillary carcinoma
    - c. Malignant adenofibroma and cystadenofibroma
- B. Mucinous tumors
  - 1. Benign
    - a. Cystadenoma
    - b. Adenofibroma and cystadenofibroma
  - 2. Of borderline malignancy (carcinomas of low malignant potential)
    - a. Cystadenoma
    - b. Adenofibroma and cystadenofibroma
  - 3. Malignant
    - a. Adenocarcinoma and cystadenocarcinoma
    - b. Malignant adenofibroma and cystadenofibroma
- C. Endometrioid tumors
  - 1. Benign
    - a. Adenoma and cystadenoma
    - b. Adenofibroma and cystadenofibroma
  - 2. Of borderline malignancy (carcinomas of low malignant potential)
    - a. Adenoma and cystadenoma
    - b. Adenofibroma and cystadenofibroma
  - 3. Malignant
    - a. Carcinoma
      - i. Adenocarcinoma
      - ii. Adenoacanthoma
      - iii. Malignant adenofibroma and cystadenofibroma
    - b. Endometrioid stromal sarcomas
    - c. Mesodermal (müllerian) mixed tumors, homologous and heterologous
- D. Clear cell (mesonephroid) tumors
  - 1. Benign: adenofibroma
  - 2. Of borderline malignancy (carcinomas of low malignant potential)
  - 3. Malignant: carcinoma and adenocarcinoma
- E. Brenner tumors
  - 1. Benign
  - 2. Of borderline malignancy (proliferating)
  - 3. Malignant
- F. Mixed epithelial tumors
  - 1. Benign
  - 2. Of borderline malignancy
  - 3. Malignant
- G. Undifferentiated carcinoma
- H. Unclassified epithelial tumors

[a] From International Histological Classification of Tumours, No. 9: Histological Classification of Ovarian Tumours, 1973. (Reproduced by permission of the copyright holder, World Health Organization.)

cepts of the common epithelial tumors of the ovary, carcinomas of low malignant potential are emphasized, benign, so-called proliferating tumors are introduced, the subject of endometrioid and clear cell neoplasms has been enlarged, and newly described entities are included. In addition, this chapter includes discussions of enzymatically active stromal cells, immunocytochemistry, and extraovarian peritoneal proliferations. Table 18.3 represents the FIGO staging for ovarian cancer, which is helpful in the evaluation of the clinical behavior of these neoplasms.

Clinicopathologic Features

Serous Tumors

Benign Serous Tumors

SEROUS CYSTADENOMA

It is obvious that the benign serous cystadenomas originate in the surface epithelium of the ovary, since these tumors possess the same histologic features as the common epithelial inclusion cysts, which arise through invaginations of the surface epithelium.[121]

These are common tumors, comprising about 20% of all benign ovarian neoplasms. The majority of these neoplasms are encountered during the reproductive years, although they can occur also in infancy.[112] In 7–12% of patients, the tumors are bilateral.[152a]

Gross Appearance. These neoplasms are usually cystic, unilocular, large, and filled with clear serous fluid, although occasionally one may also encounter more stringy mucinous material.[151] The diagnosis is, therefore, not based on the nature of the fluid but on the histologic features of the epithelial lining cells. The external surface of the cyst is smooth and glistening, often with a marked vascular pattern (Fig. 18.1). The majority of these neoplasms are unilocular, but multilocular forms exist. The inner lining is either entirely smooth or may have areas with grossly visible papillary projections (Fig. 18.2). In the benign serous cystadenoma, the papillary projections practically never cover the entire inner surface of the tumor. Whenever this occurs, the tumor is either frankly malignant or is a carcinoma of low malignant potential.

TABLE 18.2. Common epithelial tumors of the ovary: A modification of the WHO histologic classification.

- A. Serous tumors
  - 1. Benign
    - a. Serous cystadenoma
    - b. Serous adenofibroma and cystadenofibroma
    - c. Proliferating serous adenofibroma and cystadenofibroma
  - 2. Malignant
    - a. Serous carcinoma of low malignant potential (of borderline malignancy)
    - b. Serous carcinoma
    - c. Malignant serous adenofibroma and cystadenofibroma
- B. Mucinous tumors
  - 1. Benign
    - a. Mucinous cystadenoma
    - b. Mucinous adenofibroma and cystadenofibroma
    - c. Proliferating mucinous adenofibroma and cystadenofibroma
  - 2. Malignant
    - a. Mucinous carcinoma of low malignant potential (of borderline malignancy)
    - b. Mucinous carcinoma
    - c. Malignant mucinous adenofibroma and cystadenofibroma
- C. Endometrioid tumors
  - 1. Typical endometrioid tumors
    - a. Benign
      - i. Endometrioid adenofibroma and cystadenofibroma
      - ii. Proliferating endometrioid adenofibroma and cystadenofibroma
    - b. Malignant
      - i. Endometrioid carcinoma of low malignant potential (of borderline malignancy)
      - ii. Endometrioid carcinoma
  - 2. Mesodermal (müllerian) mixed tumors
    - a. Benign
      - i. Adenofibroma
    - b. Malignant
      - i. Adenosarcoma
      - ii. Mesodermal (müllerian) mixed, homologous tumor
      - iii. Mesodermal (müllerian) mixed, heterologous tumor
  - 3. Clear cell tumors
    - a. Benign
      - i. Clear cell adenofibroma and cystadenofibroma
      - ii. Proliferating clear cell adenofibroma and cystadenofibroma
    - b. Malignant
      - i. Clear cell carcinoma of low malignant potential (of borderline malignancy)
      - ii. Clear cell carcinoma
- D. Brenner tumors
  - 1. Benign
    - a. Typical Brenner tumor
    - b. Metaplastic Brenner tumor
    - c. Proliferating Brenner tumor
  - 2. Malignant
    - a. Brenner tumor of low malignant potential (of borderline malignancy)
    - b. Malignant Brenner tumor
- E. Carcinoma not otherwise classifiable

Microscopic Appearance. The predominant lining of both the smooth and papillary areas consists of a single layer of regular cuboidal epithelium, with basally arranged uniform nuclei. As in other ovarian epithelial neoplasms, a variety of cells, such as columnar, cuboidal, mucus-secreting, ciliated, clear, and hobnail, are frequently encountered (Fig. 18.3, 18.4, and 18.5). In large cysts under pressure, the epithelium is usually cuboidal, probably as a result of compression by the fluid. The luminal border of these cells contains diastase-resistant, periodic acid-Schiff (PAS)-positive, mucicarmine-positive, and alcian blue-positive material. Mitoses are not encountered. Psammoma bodies, which are round microscopic calcifications formed most likely as a result of degenerative changes, are frequently present and do not represent evidence of malignancy (Fig. 18.6). The stroma of the cyst wall, as well as that of the papillary projections, consists of connective tissue with scattered blood vessels. It is occasionally edematous and hyalinized.

Ultrastructure. The epithelial lining cells of serous cystadenomas[64] generally contain uniform oval nuclei, with only mild irregularities of nuclear borders and relatively homogeneous central chromatin, which is condensed along the periphery. Microvilli and cilia are present along the luminal border. Interdigitations are prominent and numerous (Fig. 18.7). The absence of prominent nuclear irregularity and the presence of marked complex cell interdigitations distinguish the benign serous cystadenomas from the borderline and frankly malignant lesions.[64]

Behavior and Treatment. Because the serous cystadenomas are benign neoplasms, removal of the involved ovary constitutes adequate therapy, although in postmenopausal women, total abdominal hysterectomy and bilateral salpingo-oophorectomy are usually performed.

Serous Cystadenofibroma

The cystadenofibroma is the one neoplasm among the common epithelial tumors in which the origin from the

TABLE 18.3. FIGO staging of carcinoma of the ovary.

Stage I.	Growth limited to the ovaries
Stage IA.	Growth limited to one ovary; no ascites. No tumor on the external surface; capsule intact
Stage IB.	Growth limited to both ovaries; no ascites. No tumor on the external surfaces; capsules intact
Stage IC.[a]	Tumor either Stage IA or IB but with tumor on the surface of one or both ovaries; or with capsule ruptured; or with ascites present containing malignant cells or with positive peritoneal washings
Stage II.	Growth involving one or both ovaries with pelvic extension
Stage IIA.	Extension and/or metastases to the uterus and/or tubes
Stage IIB.	Extension to other pelvic tissues
Stage IIC.[a]	Tumor either Stage IIA or IIB but with tumor on the surface of one or both ovaries; or with capsule(s) ruptured; or with ascites present containing malignant cells or with positive peritoneal washings
Stage III.	Tumor involving one or both ovaries with peritoneal implants outside the pelvis and/or positive retroperitoneal or inguinal nodes. Superficial liver metastasis equals Stage III. Tumor is limited to the true pelvis but with histologically verified malignant extension to small bowel or omentum
Stage IIIA.	Tumor grossly limited to the true pelvis with negative nodes but with histologically confirmed microscopic seeding of abdominal peritoneal surfaces
Stage IIIB.	Tumor of one or both ovaries with histologically confirmed implants of abdominal peritoneal surfaces, none exceeding 2 cm in diameter. Nodes negative
Stage IIIC.	Abdominal implants >2 cm in diameter and/or positive retroperitoneal or inguinal nodes
Stage IV.	Growth involving one or both ovaries with distant metastasis. If pleural effusion is present there must be positive cytologic test results to allot a case to Stage IV. Parenchymal liver metastasis equals Stage IV

[a] In order to evaluate the impact on prognosis of the different criteria for allotting cases to Stage IC or IIC it would be of value to know if rupture of the capsule was (1) spontaneous or (2) caused by the surgeon and if the source of malignant cells detected was (1) peritoneal washings or (2) ascites.

ovarian surface epithelium and underlying stroma can be most easily traced. Nevertheless, cystadenofibromas occupy an equivocal position among ovarian tumors. Although some look upon them as mere variants of serous cystadenomas,[94] others consider them as separate, fairly

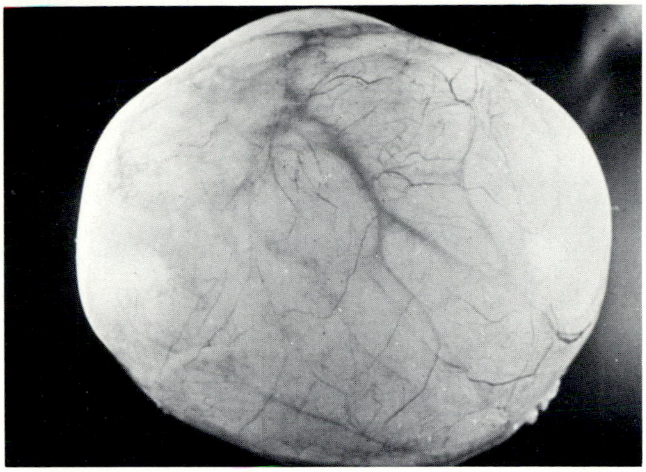

FIG. 18.1. External surface of a serous cystadenoma demonstrating a smooth capsule with prominent vasculature.

common tumors.[103] Cystadenofibromas constitute nearly half of all benign ovarian cystic serous tumors.[31] The patients' ages range from 15 to 65, with a mean of 30.7 years.[37]

Gross Appearance. Because small papillary projections arising from the normal ovarian surface are fairly common, it is advisable not to make a diagnosis of cystadenofibroma if the lesion is less than 1 cm in diameter. The tumors vary in size from 1 to 20 cm, with a mean of 9 cm. These neoplasms are cystic, with small, tight clusters of short, rounded papillary structures (Fig. 18.8). In contrast, the papillary projections of the serous cystadenomas are softer, more elongated, and usually occupy larger areas of the inner cyst lining. Some of the cystadenofibromas are multiloculated. The intracystic fluid is of the serous, clear type. Bilaterality is 5.8%.[37]

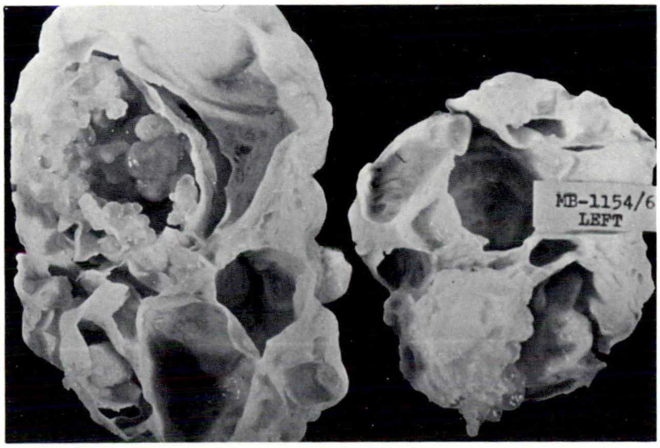

FIG. 18.2. Cut surface of a serous cystadenoma showing a multilocular structure with papillary areas.

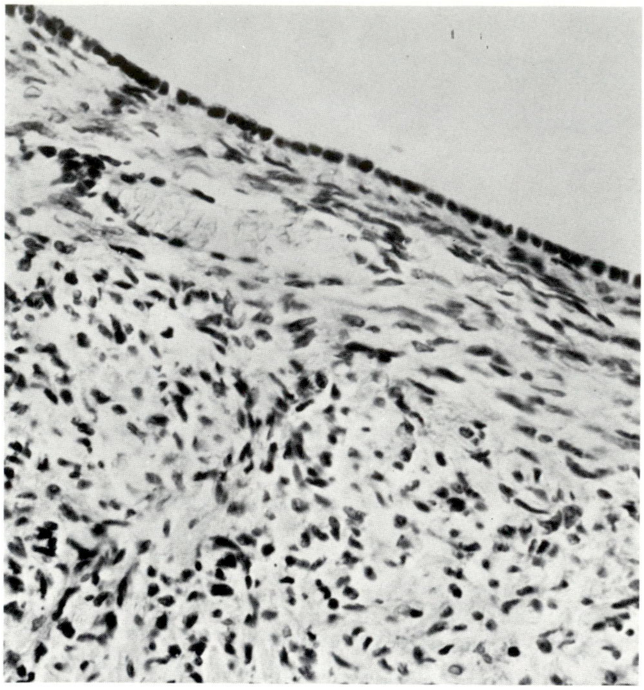

Fig. 18.3. Low cuboidal epithelial lining cells of serous cystadenoma.

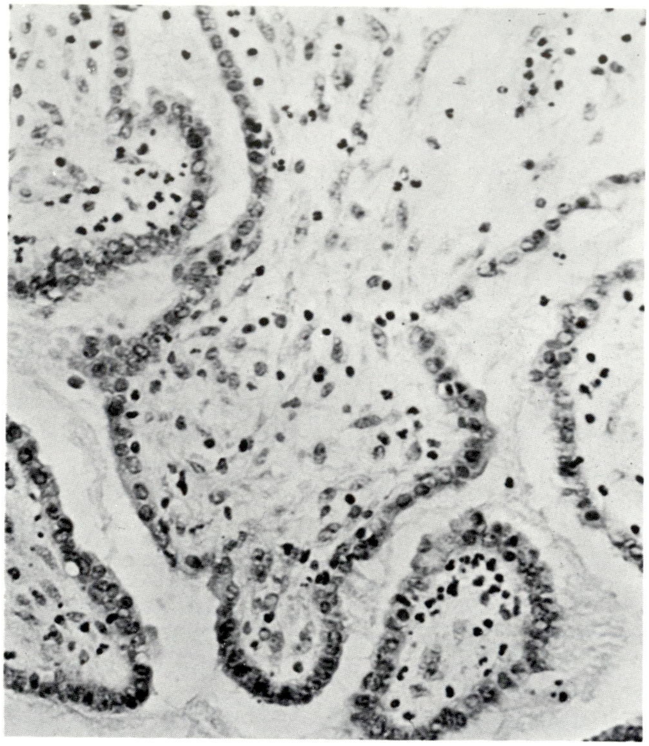

Fig. 18.5. Papillary serous cystadenoma lined by a variety of epithelial cells.

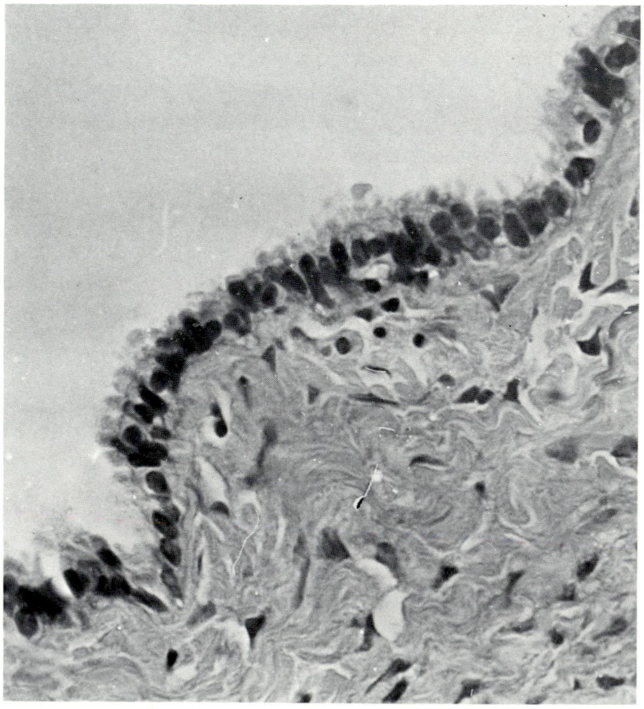

Fig. 18.4. Columnar and ciliated epithelial cells lining a serous cystadenoma.

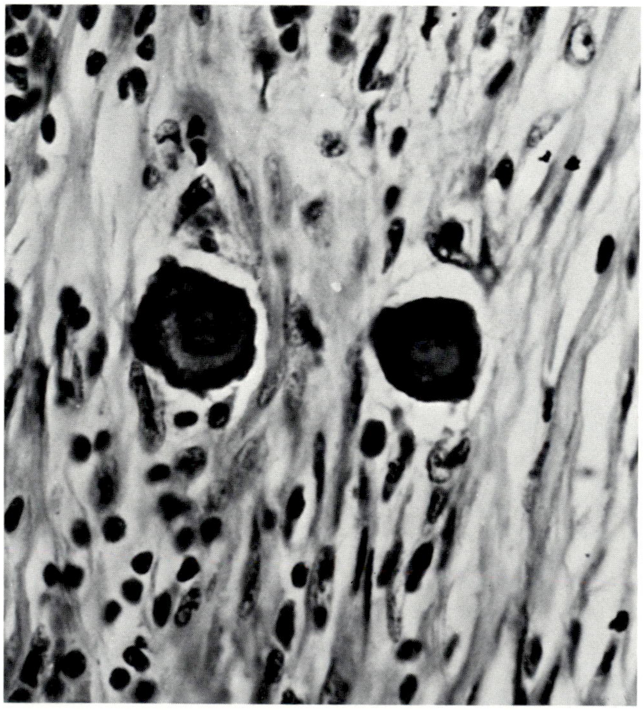

Fig. 18.6. Psammoma bodies in the wall of a serous cystadenoma demonstrating the typical concentric arrangement.

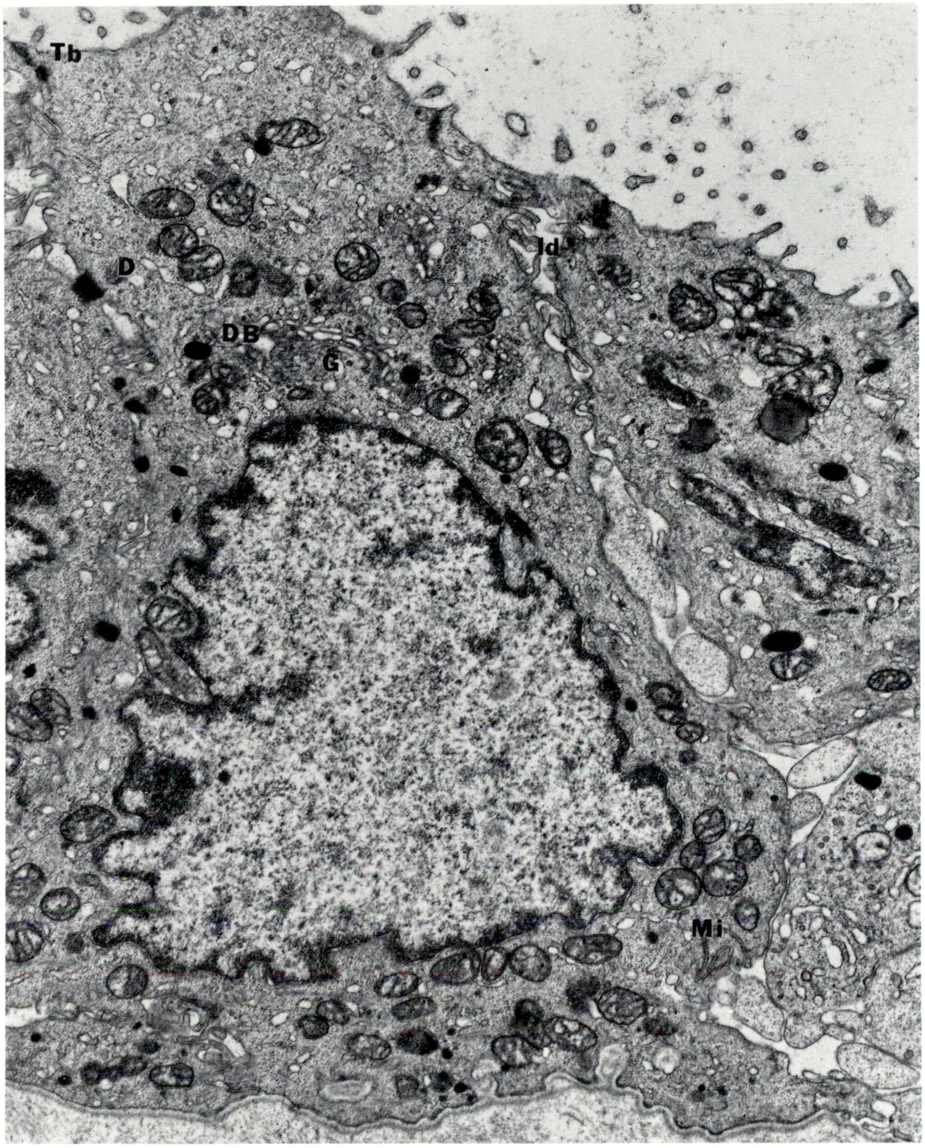

Fig. 18.7. Electron micrograph of serous cystadenoma with slightly irregular nuclear borders, numerous cell membrane interdigitations (Id), desmosomes (D), and terminal bars (Tb). Cytoplasm includes supranuclear Golgi complex (G), round to oval mitochondria (Mi), and dense bodies (DB). ×16,720. (Reprinted by permission of Gondos, Ref. 64.)

Microscopic Appearance. The epithelium lining the cyst wall and its papillary projections is predominantly serous but can also be a variety of other müllerian type epithelia[84] (Figs. 18.9, 18.10, and 18.11). Nevertheless, this lesion is discussed under the heading of serous tumors because, in most instances, the serous cells constitute the predominant epithelial component. As in the other papillary tumors, psammoma bodies are occasionally present.

The stroma of the papillary structures ranges from highly cellular, fibrous to almost acellular, hyalinized tissue. Severe stromal edema is a common finding (Fig. 18.12). A highly characteristic feature is a narrow, acellular zone of connective tissue situated between the epithelial lining cells and the fibrous stroma of the papillae (Fig. 18.13).[37] This same acellular zone is also present in the cortex of the normal ovary. Occasionally, the cyst wall has thickened areas, which are composed of fibrous stroma and glandular spaces lined by the same type of epithelium as the papillary projections. These are still classified as cystadenofibroma because the diagnosis of adenofibroma is reserved for predominantly solid tumors only. The various microscopic features are summarized in Table 18.4.

Ultrastructure. Transmission electron microscopy[52a] demonstrates mature ciliated cells with numerous supra-

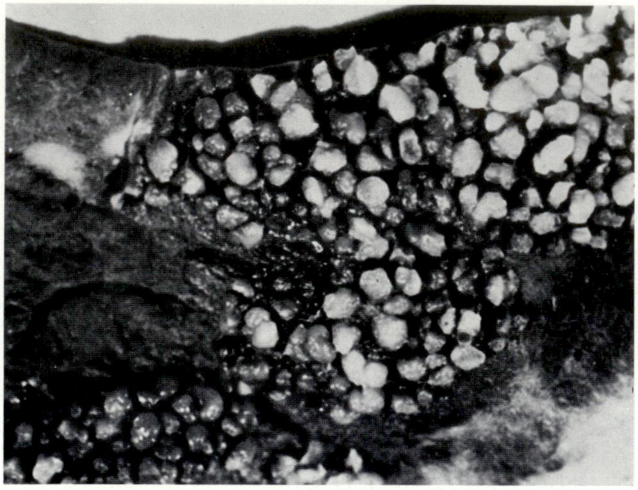

FIG. 18.8. Cystadenofibroma showing tight clusters of firm, short, rounded papillary structures arising from the cyst wall. (Reprinted by permission of Czernobilsky et al., Ref. 37.)

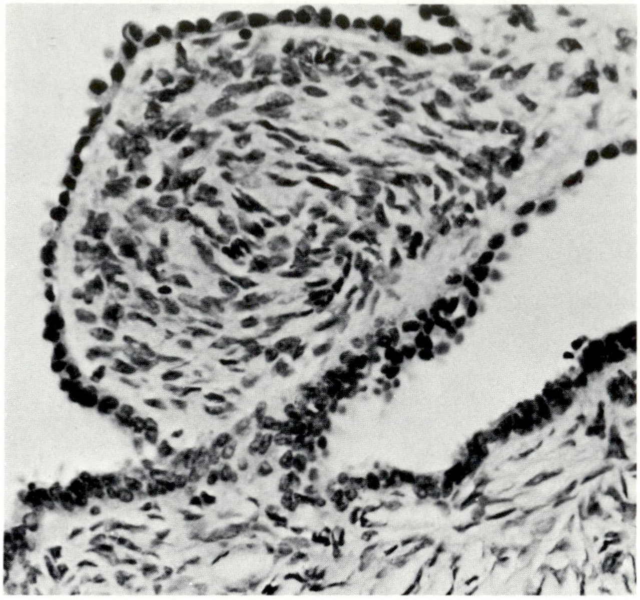

FIG. 18.10. Cuboidal, columnar, and hobnail-type epithelial lining of a cystadenofibroma. (Reprinted by permission of Czernobilsky et al., Ref. 27.)

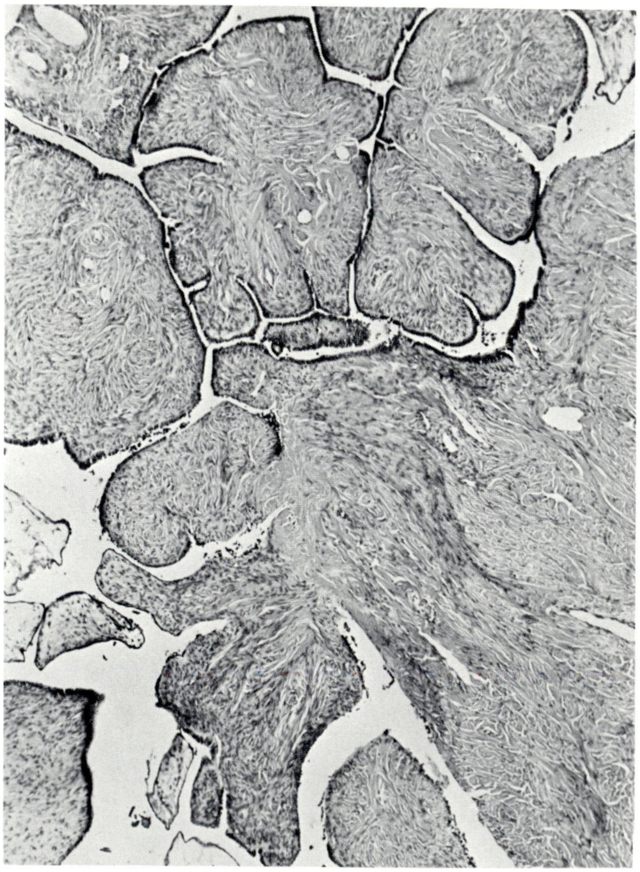

FIG. 18.9. Papillary projections of cystadenofibroma consisting of broad, fibrous structures lined by epithelial cells.

nuclear mitochondria and cross-striated ciliary rootlets (Fig. 18.14).

Behavior and Treatment. Because cystadenofibromas are benign tumors, surgical removal constitutes adequate therapy. Furthermore, because of the characteristic macroscopic and microscopic appearance of these tumors,

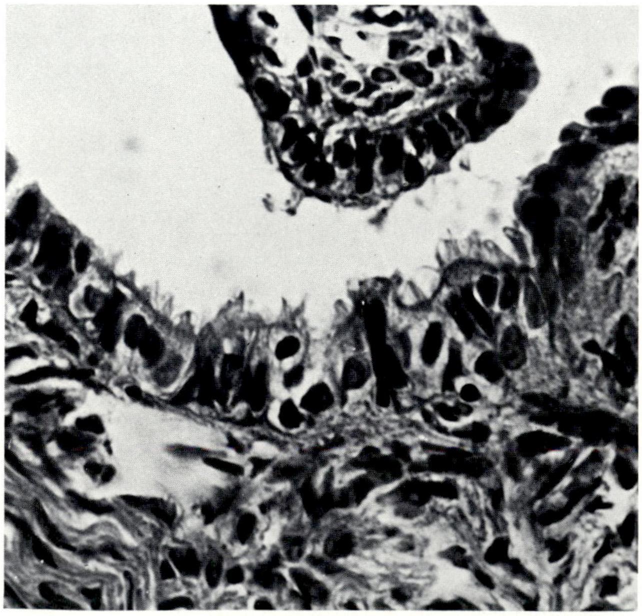

FIG. 18.11. Ciliated cells with interspersed clear cells lining a cystadenofibroma. (Reprinted by permission of Czernobilsky et al., Ref. 37.)

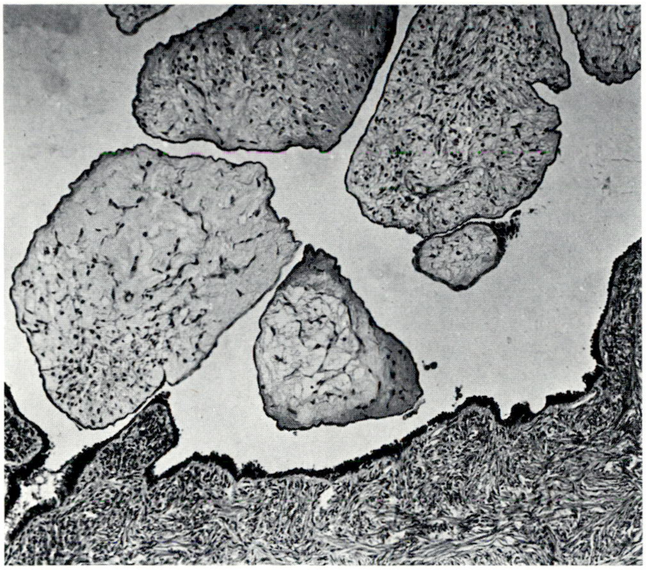

FIG. 18.12. Markedly edematous papillary formations arising in the wall of a cystadenofibroma.

the pathologist should usually be able to arrive at a correct diagnosis when a frozen section is requested, thus saving the patient unnecessary extensive surgery. Kao and Norris[85] described 10 cases of cystadenofibromas with epithelial atypia and suggested that these may be equivalent to other borderline tumors of the ovary. So far, none of these tumors has recurred. They are more extensively discussed in the section on proliferating tumors.

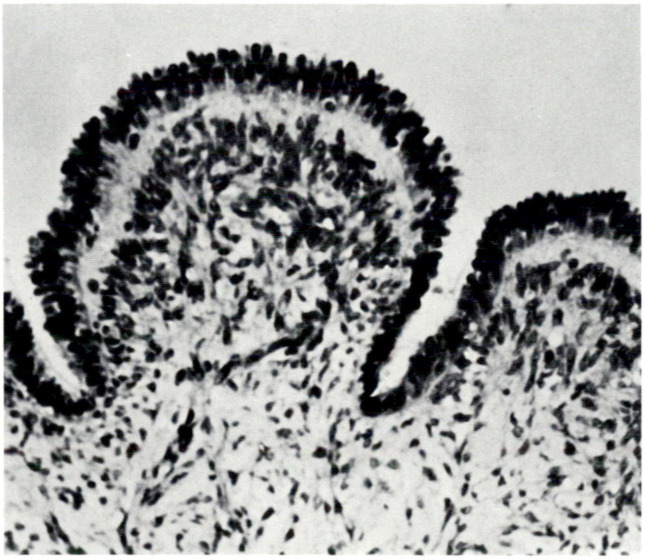

FIG. 18.13. Narrow, acellular zone of connective tissue situated between the epithelial lining and the fibrous stroma of the papillae in a cystadenofibroma. (Reprinted by permission of Czernobilsky et al., Ref. 37.)

TABLE 18.4. Microscopic features of 34 cystadenofibromas and 39 cystadenomas.[a]

Features	Cystadenofibroma (no. of cases)	Cystadenoma (no. of cases)
Papillary projections	34	14
Epithelial lining		
Cuboidal	34	39
Columnar	22	20
Cilia	11	10
Hobnail	7	8
Clear	4	1
Pseudostratification	6	8
Psammoma bodies	10	5
Tufting	0	6
Atypism	0	5
Mitoses	0	5
Borderline malignancy	0	3
Stroma		
Spindle cells	34	32
Collagen	27	28
Hyaline	15	3
Edema	18	10
Subepithelial acellular layer	11	1

[a] Each tumor presenting more than one feature. (Reprinted by permission from Czernobilsky et al., ref. 25.)

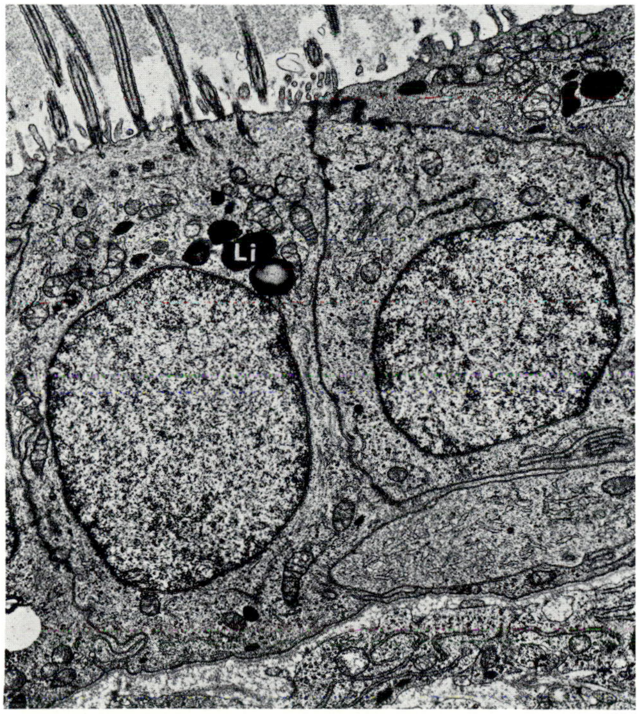

FIG. 18.14. Electron micrograph of mature ciliated cells with supranuclear mitochondria and lipid droplets (Li), similar to those of normal oviductal mucosa, which are characteristic of the lining cells of cystadenofibroma. ×4437. (Courtesy of Dr. A. Ferenczy.)

Serous Adenofibroma

The adenofibroma is a benign, solid, ovarian neoplasm composed of dense, fibrous connective tissue with interspersed glandular spaces of various sizes. Occasionally, the latter may be visible macroscopically. The lesion is often described together with the cystadenofibroma and is considered a solid variant of the latter. We prefer to regard these solid or predominantly solid neoplasms as a separate entity.[31,167] Nevertheless, there seems to be no doubt about the surface epithelium–cortical stromal origin of this tumor, although this is more easily demonstrable in the cystadenofibroma.

Because these tumors are usually discussed together with cystadenofibromas, reliable incidence figures are not available. Nonetheless, the solid adenofibroma is a rare neoplasm. Patients' ages range from 23 to 70 years, with 50% of the tumors occurring after the age of 50.[167]

These tumors are solid or predominantly solid, ranging in size from 1 to about 15 cm. As with cystadenofibroma, we and others[167] do not consider the microscopic or tiny cortical adenofibromas as neoplasms. Except for the presence of tiny scattered cystic foci, the solid adenofibromas are similar to ovarian fibromas. About 20% of the tumors are bilateral, whereas 25% showed microscopic cortical adenofibromas in the contralateral ovary.[167]

The glandular spaces are lined by a variety of epithelia that are similar to those seen in cystadenofibromas, with a predominance of the cuboidal type. Atypism and mitotic figures are not present. The cellularity of the stroma varies, too, from highly cellular, especially in close proximity to the glands, to almost acellular hyalinized areas (Figs. 18.15 and 18.16). The luminal border of the epithelial cells and the intraluminal fluid stain positively with diastase-resistant PAS, mucicarmine, and alcian blue stains.

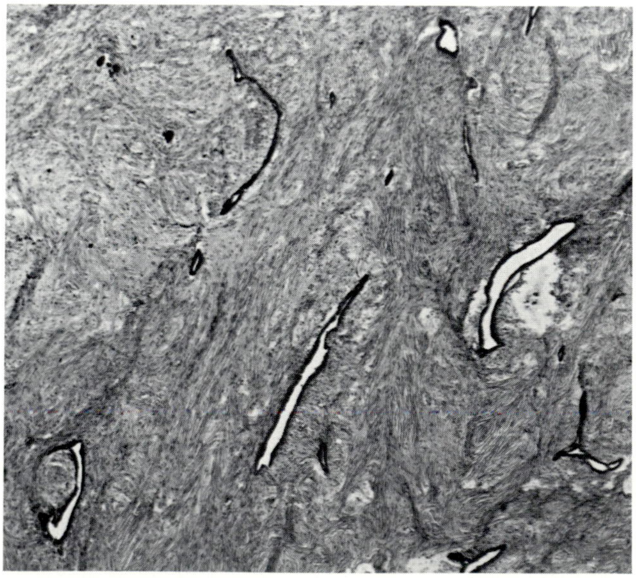

Fig. 18.15. Fibrous stroma with compressed slit-like glandular spaces in an adenofibroma.

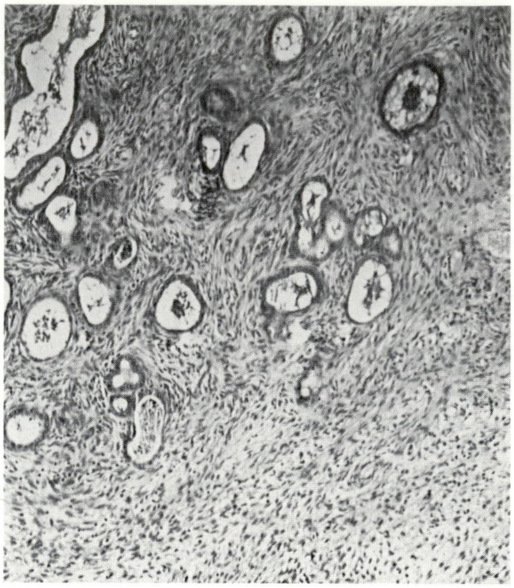

Fig. 18.16. Cellular stroma with rounded glands in adenofibroma.

Proliferating Serous Adenofibroma and Cystadenofibroma

The term *proliferating* was first applied to an ovarian epithelial tumor by Roth and Sternberg in 1971 for a special type of benign Brenner tumor.[132] More recently, this terminology has also been applied to other benign ovarian epithelial neoplasms in which epithelial proliferative activity is more prominent than in the ordinary benign tumors. Some degree of atypia and increased mitotic activity is usually present but much less than in carcinomas of low malignant potential (of borderline malignancy), a term occasionally used erroneously as synonym for proliferating tumors.

The serous proliferating tumors are usually adenofibromas in which the glandular components show crowding and bizarre shapes but lack confluence and appreciable nuclear atypism or mitotic activity (Fig. 18.17).[33] Some of the serous cystadenofibromas with epithelial atypia described by Kao and Norris[85] may also belong to this category. Since follow-up in the reported cases as well as in our cases fail to reveal any instance of recurrence or metastases, it appears that these are indeed benign neoplasms, albeit with more than usual proliferative activity. In a spectrum of ovarian epithelial tumors, they could thus be placed between the ordinary benign lesions and carcinomas of low malignant potential.

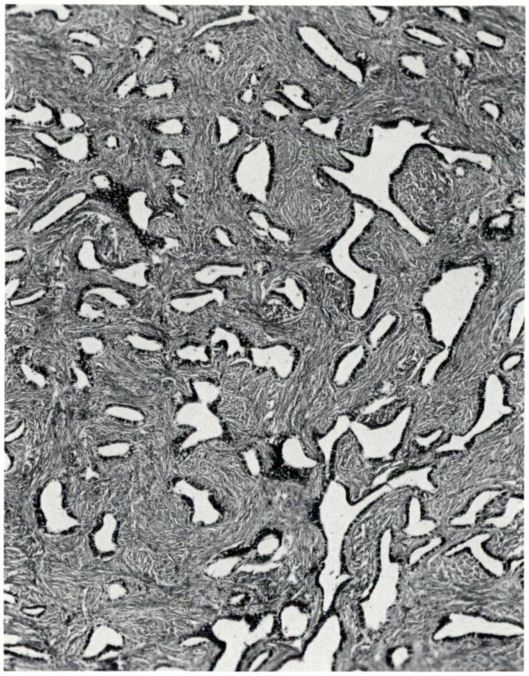

FIG. 18.17. Proliferating serous adenofibroma showing numerous irregularly shaped glandular spaces lined by cuboidal cells in fibrous stroma. (Courtesy of Dr. H. J. Norris.)

Malignant Serous Tumors

SEROUS CARCINOMA OF LOW MALIGNANT POTENTIAL (OF BORDERLINE MALIGNANCY)

The concept of ovarian carcinomas of low malignant potential was first introduced by Taylor, who, in 1929, termed these tumors *semi-malignant*.[165] In the early 1950s, considerable interest was expressed in these types of neoplasms,[91,175] but it was only in 1964 that they were incorporated into the classification of the International Federation of Gynecology and Obstetrics (FIGO)[142] and, subsequently, in the WHO Histological Classification of Ovarian Tumors (Table 18.1).[157b]

The term *of borderline malignancy* that precedes *carcinoma of low malignant potential* in the WHO classification and that is widely used has been a source of misunderstanding about the nature of these tumors. Although they behave much less aggressively than frank carcinomas, they are malignant, which is why the term *borderline* is ambiguous. Colgan and Norris[30] proposed referring to this group of neoplasms as *tumors of low malignant potential*. I prefer using the term *carcinoma of low malignant potential* (LMP), which is in accordance with the WHO classification.

About 15% of all serous tumors are carcinomas of LMP and 33–60% are limited to one ovary.[138] Extraovarian

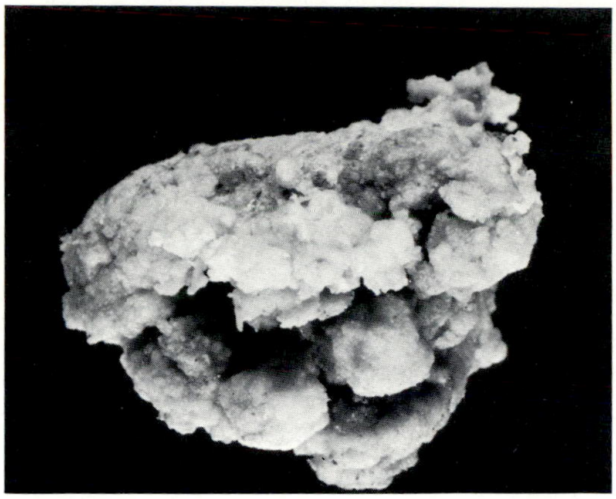

FIG. 18.18. Serous carcinoma of low malignant potential showing exuberant growth of papillary structures arising in inner lining of cyst.

spread is present in 16–18% of serous carcinomas of LMP.[9]

Gross Appearance. Serous carcinoma of LMP is similar to the previously described benign serous cystadenomas with papillary projections, however, the papillary component in the former is usually more abundant than in benign serous cystadenoma[94] (Fig. 18.18).

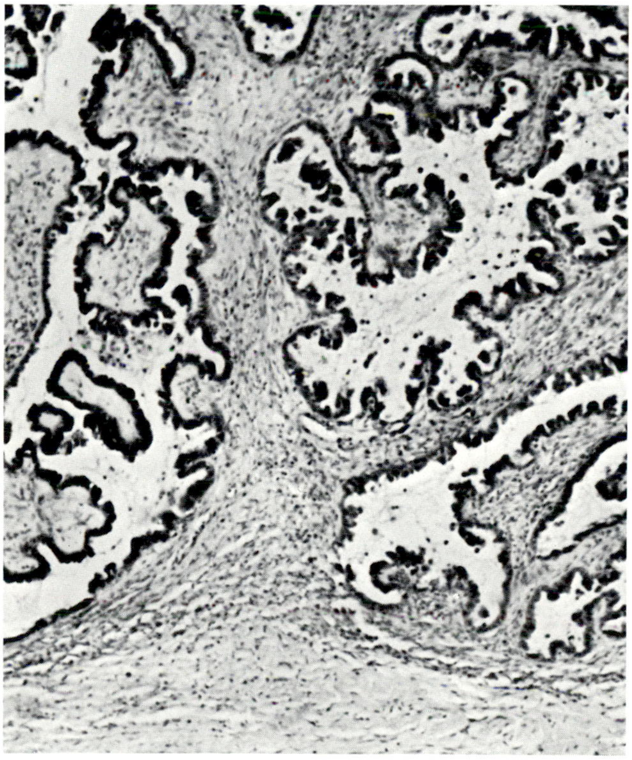

FIG. 18.19. Irregular papillary growth in a serous carcinoma of low malignant potential.

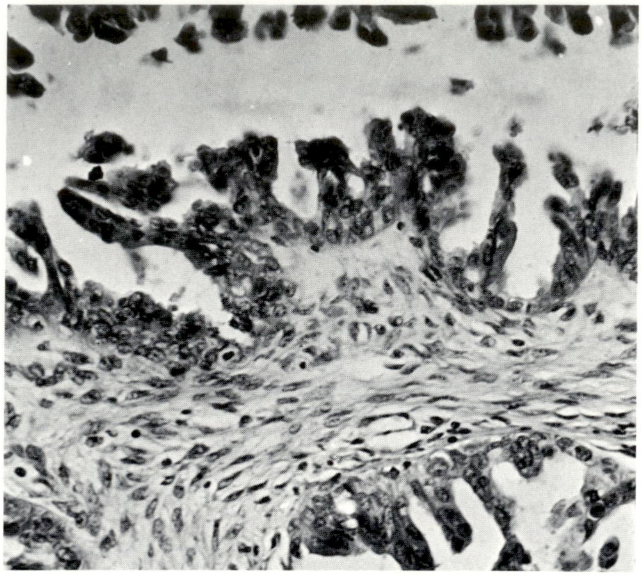

FIG. 18.20. Detail of epithelial lining in a serous carcinoma of low malignant potential, showing stratification, pleomorphism, and tuft formation.

Microscopic Appearance. The histologic criteria for the diagnosis of carcinomas of LMP are as follows: stratification of the epithelial lining of the papillae, formation of microscopic papillary projections or tufts arising from the epithelial lining of the papillae, which often become detached, nuclear atypism, and mitotic activity (Figs. 18.19 and 18.20). The histologic hallmark of serous carcinoma of LMP is the epithelial tufts arising from the papillary projections and the absence of stromal invasion. Deep invaginations should not be confused with invasion. The former have a regular contour, surrounding basement membrane, and similarity to the surface lining epithelium and are not associated with a stromal reaction. Cellular pleomorphism, nuclear atypism, and mitotic activity do not place these tumors in the invasive category. Because of the variability of the histologic picture, especially in large tumors, sampling should be thorough. One block of tissue for every 1–2 cm of maximum tumor diameter generally suffices.[71] In instances where there is tumor spread beyond the ovary, the diagnosis is based on the histologic features of the ovarian neoplasm.

Ultrastructure. Both carcinomas of LMP and invasive serous cystadenocarcinomas (Fig. 18.21) show a marked degree of nuclear infolding. In contrast, the epithelial cells of the tumors of LMP show cilia, which are absent in the invasive malignant neoplasms. Interdigitations are less prominent in tumors of LMP than in benign serous cystadenomas.[64]

Behavior and Treatment. The prognosis of serous carcinomas of LMP is far better than that of invasive carcinoma and is not influenced by the degree of nuclear atypia, cellular stratification, or mitotic activity.[87] In the series of Fisher et al.,[54] the 5-year survival of patients with tumors of LMP was 100%, compared to 50% for patients with serous cystadenocarcinoma. The 10-year survival

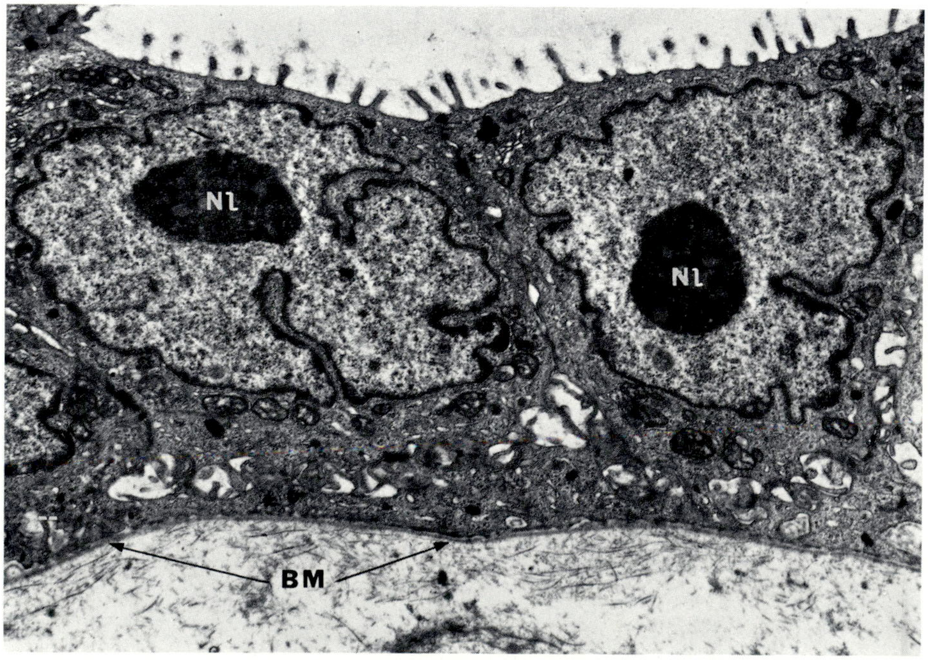

FIG. 18.21. Electron micrograph of a serous carcinoma of low malignant potential, showing deep nuclear indentations, prominent regular nucleoli (NL) and smooth basal lamina (BM). ×6045. (Reprinted with permission of Gondos, Ref 64.)

for serous carcinomas of LMP is approximately 75%, compared to 13% for serous cystadenocarcinoma.[138,143] Recurrences of serous tumors of LMP may appear as late as 10–15 years after the initial surgery.[9] Typically, they spread over the peritoneal surface, without invading.

In summary, the diagnosis of carcinoma of LMP is based on the microscopic appearance of the primary ovarian tumor, irrespective of the clinical stage and subsequent biologic behavior. Diagnostic accuracy and prognostication have not been improved by the application of adjunctive techniques, such as measurements of nuclear DNA and morphometry.[43,58]

Because of the good prognosis for this tumor, a unilateral salpingo-oophorectomy is advocated for stage I disease, especially in young women, in whom this neoplasm is relatively frequent.[9] In more advanced stages, the treatment of choice is total hysterectomy with bilateral salpingo-oophorectomy. Adjuvant chemotherapy for patients with advanced stage disease does not seem to influence survival.[13] Long and careful follow-up is indicated for all patients.

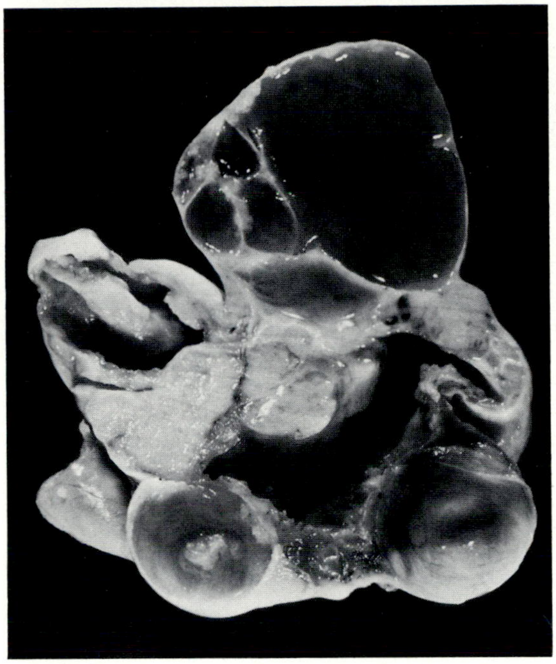

Fig. 18.22. Cut surface of serous carcinoma with cystic, papillary, and solid areas.

Serous Carcinoma

These are the most common malignant ovarian tumors, comprising approximately 40% of the group of common epithelial tumors.[140] They occur most frequently between the ages of 40 and 60 years.

Gross Appearance. They are bilateral in about 50% of patients.[77a] According to Allen and Hertig,[1] 56.2% of these tumors measure over 15 cm in diameter, 39.9% from 5 to 15 cm, and 3.9% less than 5 cm in diameter. They are primarily cystic, multiloculated tumors, with soft, friable papillae that may fill the entire cavity (Fig. 18.22). Fluid, if present, is usually turbid or bloody. The external surface is smooth or may have papillary projections, probably the result of penetration of the tumor through the cyst wall.

Microscopic Appearance. Serous cystadenocarcinomas are graded as well differentiated, moderately differentiated, and poorly differentiated. In well-differentiated serous carcinomas, the papillary structures are well formed, with prominent fibrous stalks. This pattern is less regular in moderately differentiated tumors, where the papillae are more crowded together and individual stalks cannot always be discerned. In poorly differentiated tumors, the papillary pattern is largely obliterated, and the tumor is composed of solid sheets of cells (Figs. 18.23, 18.24, and 18.25). Histologic grading should, therefore, be based primarily on the architectural pattern and not on nuclear characteristics. Nuclei may show various degrees of atypism, pleomorphism, and mitotic activity in all three grades. Capsular invasion can occur regardless of histologic grading. According to Aure et al.,[8] the presence of psammoma bodies in 32.5% of serous cystadenocarcinomas is associated with a higher survival. As in benign and LMP tumors, the luminal border of the epithelial cells stains positively with diastase-resistant PAS, mucicarmine, and alcian blue stains.

Ultrastructure. The epithelium[64] displays marked nuclear irregularity, a decreased amount of cell membrane

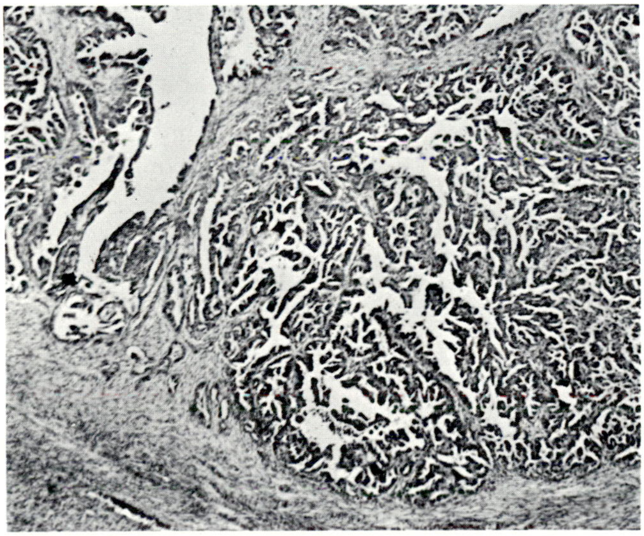

Fig. 18.23. Well-differentiated serous cystadenocarcinoma with crowded, irregular papillary structures pushing and invading into the surrounding stroma.

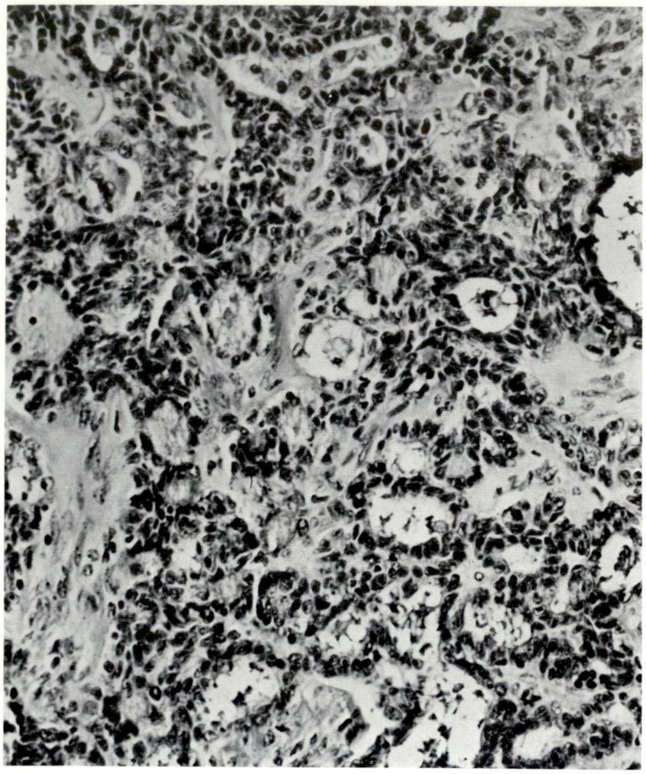

FIG. 18.24. Moderately well-differentiated serous cystadenocarcinoma with a prominent cellular stroma.

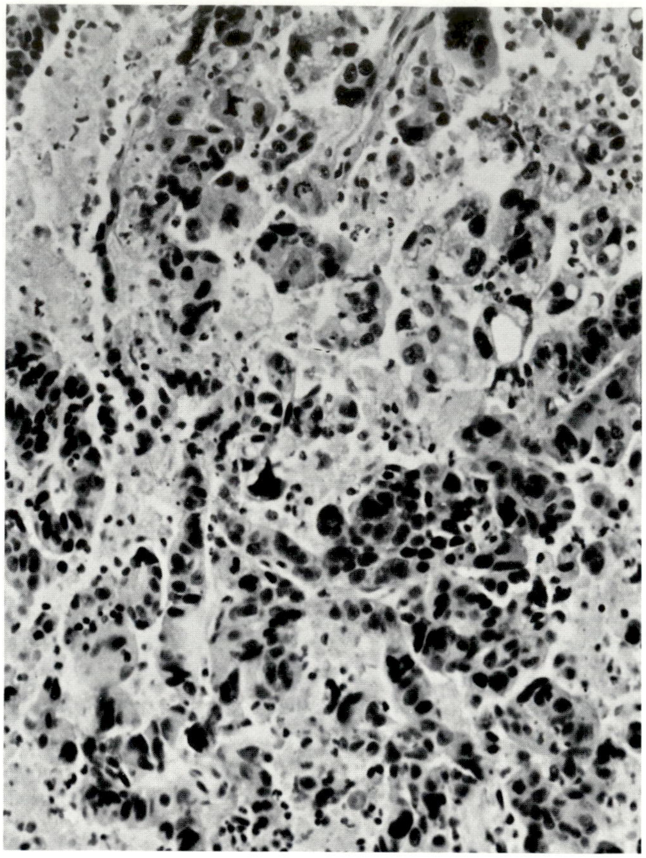

FIG. 18.25. Poorly differentiated serous cystadenocarcinoma, showing highly anaplastic tumor cells with only a suggestion of papillary arrangement.

interdigitation, and reduced cilia (Fig. 18.26). These features differ significantly from those of benign serous cystadenoma but present some similarities to carcinomas of LMP. Ferenczy et al.[52b] described both endometrial-type and endocervical-type cells in the well-differentiated tumors and postulated that the endocervical-type cells are the source of the mucin production occasionally seen in these neoplasms.

Behavior and Treatment. Clinical staging performed at the time of initial surgery is of primary prognostic significance.[11] Furthermore, cytoreductive surgery affects progression-free intervals, survival, and cure rates. Patients with residual tumor masses of less than 1.5 cm diameter have the best survival.[68] Histologic differentiation and grading are of much less value in predicting the outcome of the disease. Pelvic examination continues to be the principal method of detection. Recent surgical staging studies disclose that more than three quarters of serous cystadenocarcinomas are in advanced stages at the time of initial diagnosis, and, consequently, the prognosis remains poor, with an overall 5-year survival rate of less than 20%.[143] A detailed discussion of the various modalities of therapy is beyond the scope of this chapter. Bilateral salpingo-oophorectomy and hysterectomy is the optimal method of treatment in most patients. This can be supplemented by chemotherapy and occasionally by radiotherapy.[48]

Some serous carcinomas grow exophytically from the ovarian surface. Gooneratne et al.[69] described 16 such cases, which were all bilateral and, in most instances, also showed disseminated tumor throughout the abdominal cavity. The problem of ovarian and extraovarian focal papillary and glandular lesions not associated with predominant ovarian common epithelial tumors is discussed in a separate section at the end of this chapter and in Chapter 17, Endometriosis.

Malignant Serous Adenofibroma and Cystadenofibroma

These are extremely rare tumors. Up to 1970, only 30 such cases had been reported.[31,109,137,167] In contrast to the age of patients with benign cystadenofibromas and adenofibromas, patients with the malignant neoplasms are older than 40 years.[31,137,167]

Gross Appearance. These tumors are solid, with focal small cysts, and therefore do not differ significantly from

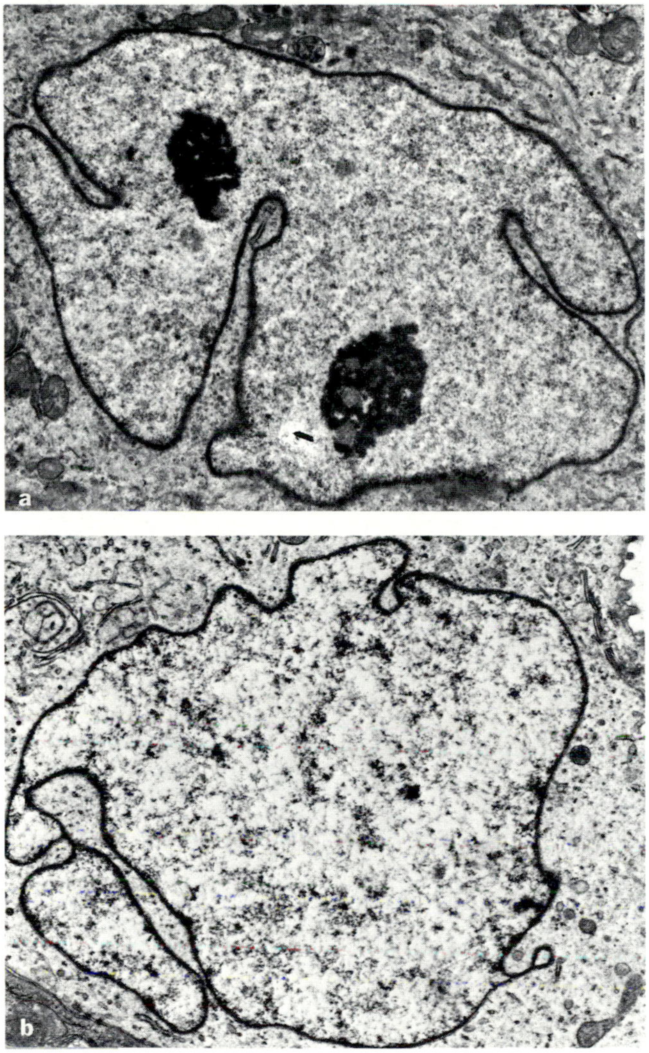

FIG. 18.26. Electron microphotograph of the nuclei of serous cystadenocarcinoma, showing multiple deep indentations and prominent nucleoli (*a*), ×9490, and irregular lobulation (*b*), ×9855. (Reprinted by permission of Gondos, Ref. 64.)

the benign adenofibromas. Nearly one half of the 10 reported cases were bilateral, with the contralateral ovary occasionally containing a benign adenofibroma.[31,167]

Microscopic Appearance. The glandular component of the tumor shows, in addition to cellular atypism, mitotic activity and stratification, invasive features. As in the other epithelial tumors of the ovary, the epithelial element may include various müllerian types of epithelia. The tumor is classified according to the predominant cell type. The diagnosis of malignant adenofibroma should only be made on a tumor that has preserved some of the benign components of an adenofibroma but displays malignant features.

Behavior and Treatment. Treatment is total hysterectomy with bilateral salpingo-oophorectomy followed by chemotherapy.[137] Five patients with malignant adenofibromas died within 1 year after surgical extirpation.[137,167] The clinical stage determines the prognosis.

Mucinous Tumors

Benign Mucinous Tumors

MUCINOUS CYSTADENOMA

Whereas the origin of the serous tumors from the surface epithelium is generally accepted, the histogenesis of mucinous tumors is more problematic.[121,128] The finding of goblet cells, argentaffin cells,[55] Paneth cells,[153] and rarely bile-secreting cells, as well as the presence of cystic teratomas in about 5% of mucinous tumors, suggests that some mucinous neoplasms may represent monomorphic endodermal differentiation of a teratoma.[27] On the other hand, the frequent admixture of elements from other müllerian-type neoplasms[27,151] and the observation that the ovarian surface epithelium may undergo mucinous metaplasia[88,89] support a müllerian origin. In spite of conflicting reports as to the chemical similarities or differences between intestinal mucin and the mucin within ovarian tumors,[27,62] the prefix *pseudo-* for the latter has been abandoned.

Mucinous cystadenomas comprise about 20% of all benign ovarian neoplasms.[88] The tumor is most frequent during the third to fifth decades, although it does occur in young women. In the Jensen and Norris series,[78] mucinous cystadenomas constituted about 47% of benign epithelial tumors in patients less than 20 years of age.

Gross Appearance. These tumors are cystic and frequently multiloculated (Fig. 18.27) and range in diameter from 1 to 50 cm, with the majority measuring 15–30 cm.[27] The external surface is that of an opaque or translucent cyst under pressure. On cut section, the lining is usually smooth, although occasionally raised papillary areas can be identified. The cysts contain thick, stringy material, but as in serous cystadenomas, the diagnosis is established after microscopic examination of the epithelium and not from the gross appearance of the intracystic fluid, which can be misleading.[151] Only about 5% of the tumors are bilateral.[27]

Microscopic Appearance. The characteristic lining of the mucinous cystadenoma is that of a single layer of tall, columnar epithelium with clear, mucin-containing cytoplasm and uniform, basally arranged nuclei (Fig. 18.28). The entire cytoplasm and the luminal content stain positively for mucus. The stromal component is made of fibrous tissue of varying cellularity.

Ultrastructure. Two types of mucinous cells are present.[50,98] In 13 of 17 mucinous cystadenomas studied

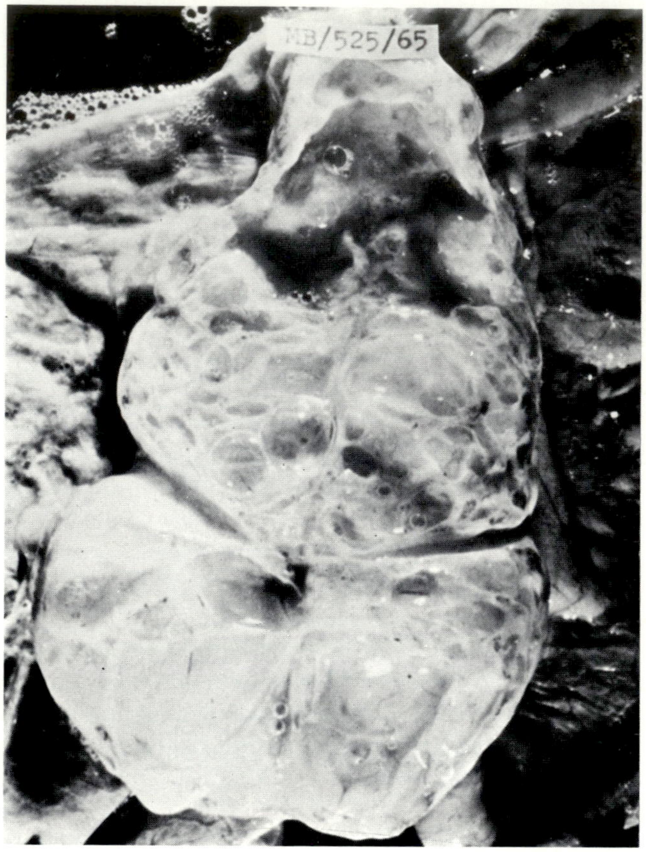

FIG. 18.27. Cystic multiloculated mucinous cystadenoma.

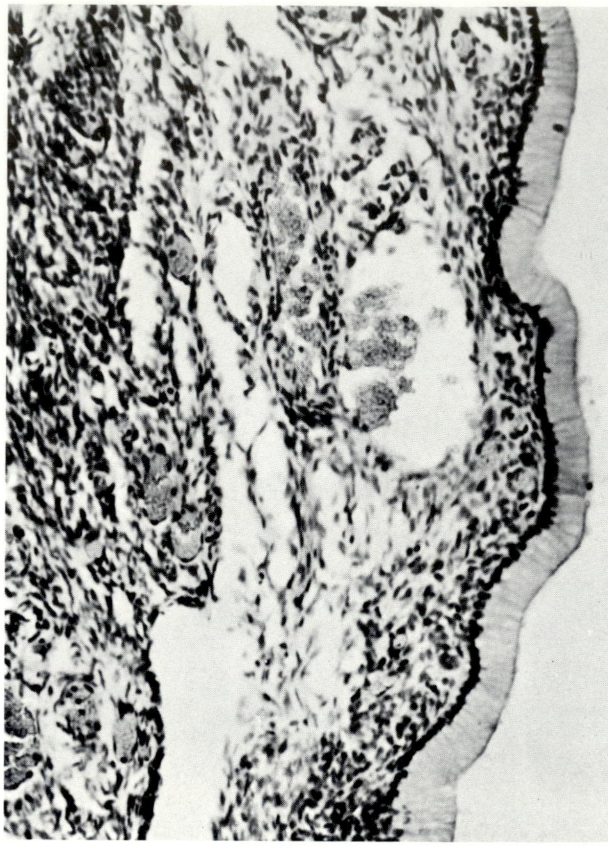

FIG. 18.28. Mucin-containing regular columnar epithelium with basally arranged nuclei lining a mucinous cystadenoma.

by Langley et al.,[98] the epithelium resembled that of the endocervix, whereas in the remaining 4 tumors, it was of gastrointestinal type (Fig. 18.29). Fenoglio et al.[50] reported pure endocervical and mixed intestinal–endocervical type of mucinous cystadenomas, and favored a metaplastic surface epithelial origin for these neoplasms.

Behavior and Treatment. Since the tumors are benign, removal of the involved ovary constitutes adequate therapy provided the opposite ovary is carefully examined to rule out the presence of a bilateral neoplasm.

MUCINOUS ADENOFIBROMA AND CYSTADENOFIBROMA

Pure mucinous cystadenofibromas and adenofibromas are very rare, although occasionally mucinous epithelial elements can be encountered in serous tumors of this variety.

Malignant Mucinous Tumors

MUCINOUS CARCINOMA OF LOW MALIGNANT POTENTIAL (OF BORDERLINE MALIGNANCY)

In the past most reports of borderline malignancy in ovarian neoplasms have dealt with serous tumors.[143,175] In studies of borderline mucinous tumors,[9,54,71,143] the histologic criteria are similar to those used for borderline serous tumors.

According to Aure et al.,[9] 6% of all mucinous tumors are carcinomas of LMP, whereas in the series of Hart and Norris,[71] the frequency is 13%. The age distribution is 9–70 years, with a median of 35 years.[71] About 85% are stage I when diagnosed.[138]

Gross Appearance. These neoplasms do not differ significantly from their benign counterpart, being large, multilocular, cystic tumors with a smooth outer surface. The inner lining is also similar to that of the benign mucinous cystadenomas. Although generally smooth, papillary excrescences and solid thickening of the capsule have been observed in up to 50% of cases.[71] In the same series, bilaterality was present in 8% of patients with borderline mucinous carcinomas, although in 57% of these, the contralateral ovary contained a benign mucinous cystadenoma. Pseudomyxoma peritonei was not observed in these patients.[71] Russell described dissection of mucin through the ovarian stroma in about 25% of carcinomas of LMP.[139]

Microscopic Appearance. As in serous carcinoma of LMP, the diagnosis of mucinous carcinomas of LMP is made on histologic criteria only. In contrast to benign

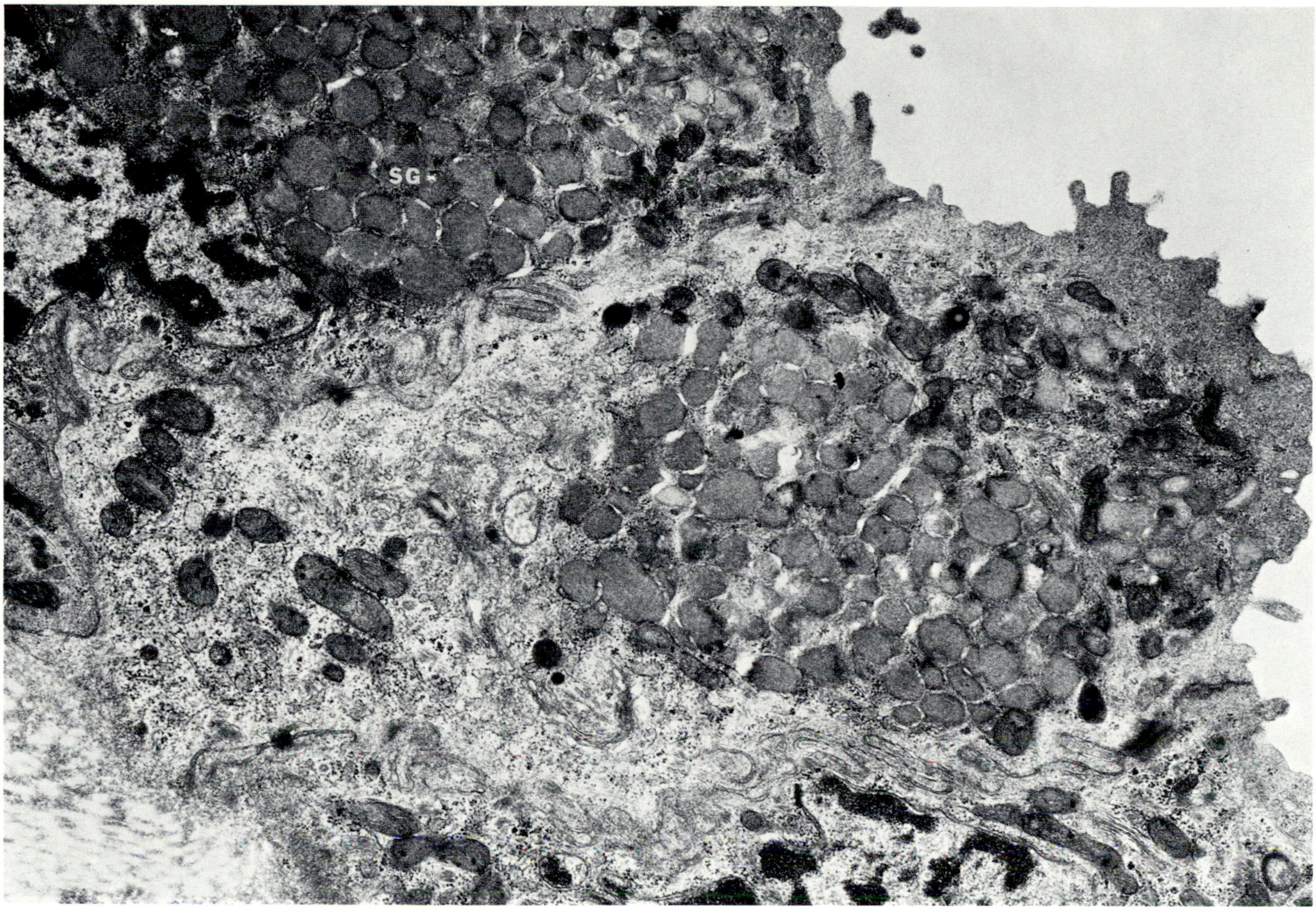

FIG. 18.29. Electron micrograph of the cells of a mucinous cystadenoma packed with mucin-containing secretory granules (SG) compressing the nucleus in the left upper corner of the photograph. These cells are similar to those found in normal endocervix. ×8858. (Courtesy of Dr. A. Ferenczy.)

mucinous cystadenomas, the epithelial lining of carcinomas of LMP is characterized by stratification, cellular atypism with irregular, hyperchromatic nuclei, and enlarged nucleoli. Mitotic figures are also encountered. Gland formation and a filigree pattern similar to the tufting described in borderline serous tumors are characteristic features (Figs. 18.30 and 18.31). The mucinous tumor of LMP is distinguished from mucinous carcinoma by the absence of stromal invasion, but this may be difficult to evaluate.[151] Hart and Norris propose that when epithelial stratification exceeds three cell layers, the tumor should be considered an invasive mucinous carcinoma,[71] a view that is disputed by Russell.[138] Areas of solid or cribriform epithelial growth without intervening connective tissue septae are a manifestation of invasion and are, therefore, diagnostic of invasive carcinoma. Ample sampling (a block of tissue for each 1–2 cm of the tumor's maximal dimension) of the tumor is necessary.[71]

Attempts to achieve a more accurate diagnosis of borderline mucinous tumors have been made by quantitative analysis of nuclear and cytoplasmic features.[10] To date, the results have not been conclusive.

Behavior and Treatment. For tumor confined to one ovary only, unilateral salpingo-oophorectomy appears to be adequate therapy. Santesson and Kottmeier[143] reported 68% 10-year survival in borderline tumors, in contrast to 34% in invasive carcinomas. In the series of Hart and Norris,[71] 94% of patients with tumors of LMP were alive and well from 1.7 to 28.4 years, with a mean of 8.6 years. However, three patients died of metastatic tumor 1, 1.2, and 7.3 years, respectively, after treatment.

Mucinous Carcinoma

Mucinous adenocarcinoma constitutes 6–10% of all malignant primary ovarian neoplasms.[152b] Most patients with this tumor are in their fourth to sixth decades, although the median age in the Hart and Norris series [71] was 35 years.

Gross Appearance. Mucinous cystadenocarcinomas are grossly cystic, multiloculated neoplasms that may reach 50 cm in diameter. Solid areas and papillary projections are more frequent than in the benign and borderline lesions (Fig. 18.32). About 25% are bilateral,[27] although

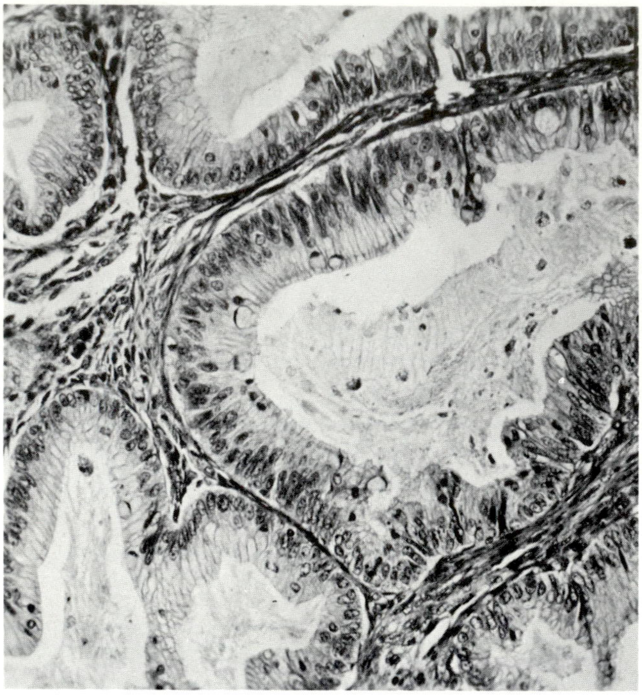

FIG. 18.30. Mucinous carcinoma of low malignant potential, showing stratified mucinous epithelium with atypical nuclei. (Reprinted by permission of Hart and Norris, Ref. 71.)

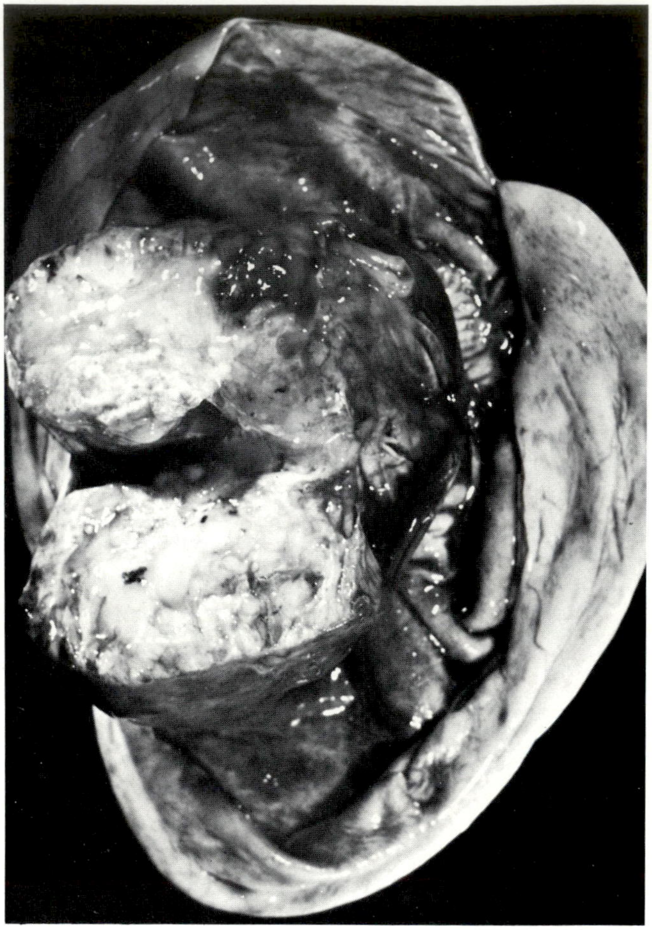

FIG. 18.32. Mucinous cystadenocarcinoma with a large solid tumor arising from the cyst lining.

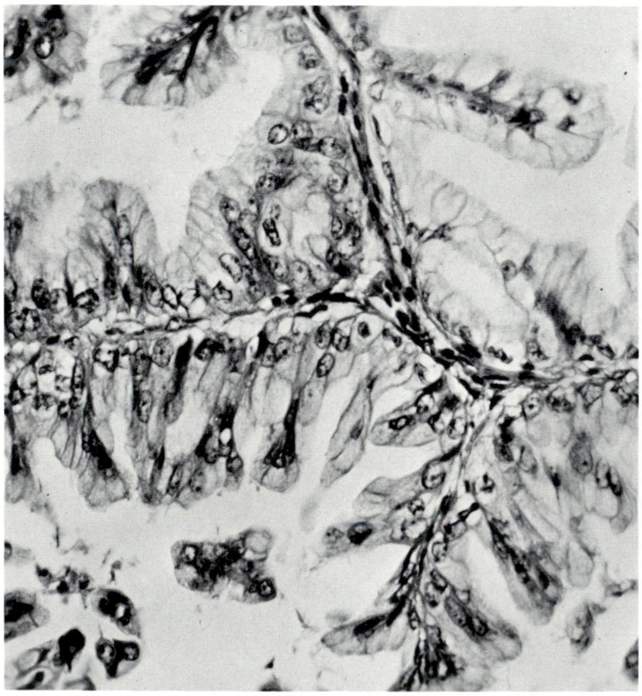

FIG. 18.31. Tufting of cells in a mucinous carcinoma of low malignant potential. (Reprinted by permission of Hart and Norris, Ref. 71.)

this frequency varies from 5% to 50% in different series.[71,176]

Microscopic Appearance. Histologically, mucinous adenocarcinomas can be divided into well differentiated moderately differentiated, and poorly differentiated. In some of the older series,[1,27] well-differentiated or grade 1 carcinomas include lesions that are now generally classified as carcinoma of LMP. The histologic differentiation relates primarily to cysts and gland-like structures of the tumor, which are lined by tall, columnar, mucin-producing cells with few mitoses in the well-differentiated group and lined by atypical epithelium with more numerous mitoses in the moderately differentiated tumors. In the poorly differentiated neoplasms, the epithelium has irregular nests and cords. Stromal invasion is characterized by irregular cords and glands scattered throughout the stroma, sometimes arranged in back-to-back fashion (Fig. 18.33). Primary so-called Krukenberg tumors of the ovary have been described in which no other primary tumor was identified[80] (see Chapter 22, Metastatic Ovarian Tumors).

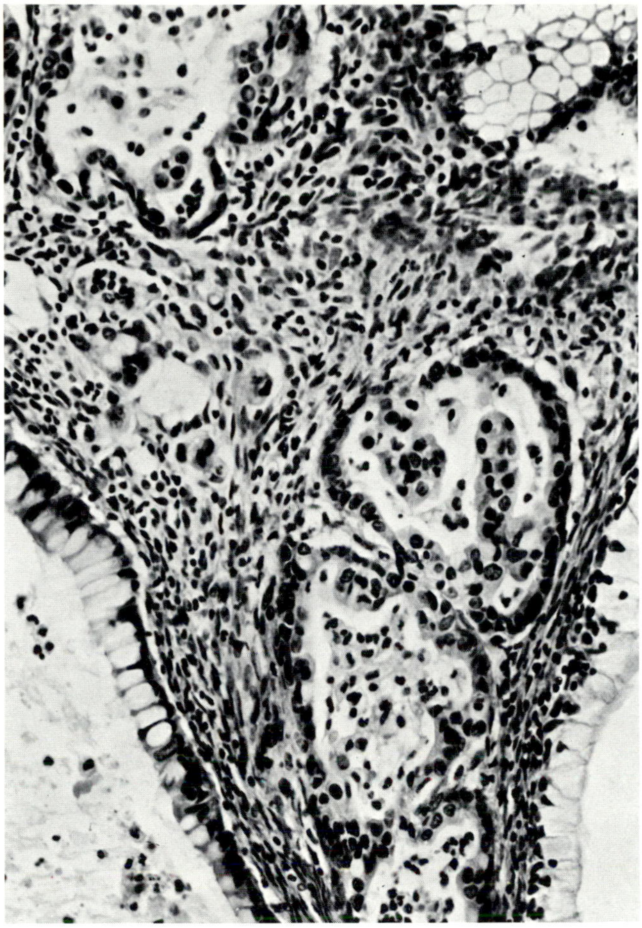

FIG. 18.33. Mucinous cystadenocarcinoma showing benign histologic areas with obvious stromal invasion by malignant elements.

Ultrastructure. Ultrastructural studies of mucinous adenocarcinoma[52c] reveal cells similar to those found in mucin-producing colonic adenocarcinoma. Prat and Scully described benign, LMP, and invasive mucinous tumors with mural nodules, which they diagnosed as sarcomas,[124] and sarcoma-like lesions.[125] Subsequent light microscopic[126] and electron microscopic studies[38] suggest that these nodules are anaplastic carcinomas.

Behavior and Treatment. The treatment of choice for mucinous cystadenocarcinoma is hysterectomy with bilateral salpingo-oophorectomy, which can be followed by chemotherapy. The 5-year survival rate is 40%.[143]

Pseudomyxoma Peritonei

A complication of ovarian mucinous tumors is the appearance of pseudomyxoma peritonei in about 2–5% of cases.[158,176] This consists of massive gelatinous accumulations, often arranged in a locular fashion in the peritoneal cavity, similar to that occasionally observed with mucoceles of the appendix. Appendiceal mucoceles, ovarian mucinous tumors, and pseudomyxomas peritonei occasionally occur together in the same patient,[158] making it difficult, if not impossible, to determine the primary lesion. It is believed that the cells that implant on the peritoneal surfaces and secrete vast amounts of mucus reach the abdominal cavity through the ovarian cyst wall, although a perforation is not always demonstrable. Microscopic dissection of the mucinous material through the cyst wall may constitute another such pathway. The finding of pools of mucin within the stroma of an ovarian mucinous tumor has been termed *pseudomyxoma ovarii* and is often associated with a coexistent pseudomyxoma peritonei.[71] Histologically, extraovarian peritoneal epithelial implants are composed of strips of a single layer of mature cells, with basally arranged regular nuclei filled with mucus (Fig. 18.34). Atypism or mitotic activity is usually not encountered despite the aggressive behavior of these lesions. Individual epithelial cells are also found to be floating free within the gelatinous masses. In many instances, the enormous quantities of mucus present make it difficult to identify cellular elements. It has been suggested that the source of this peritoneal lesion is a more aggressive form of an ovarian mucinous carcinoma of LMP.[100]

Treatment is primarily surgical and, because of the

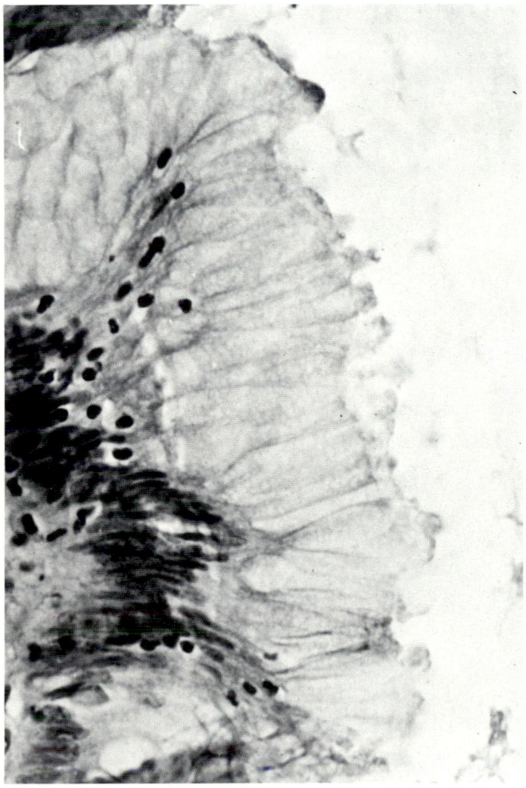

FIG. 18.34. Layer of mucinous cells attached to the peritoneal surface in a case of pseudomyxoma peritonei.

recurrent nature of the lesion, often repetitive. Intraperitoneal alkylating agents have been used with some success, whereas the use of intraperitoneal radioactive materials, abdominal radiation, and mucolytic agents has been disappointing.[100] A 45% 5-year and a 40% 10-year survival rate have been reported.[102]

Malignant Mucinous Adenofibroma and Cystadenofibroma

As is the case with benign mucinous adenofibroma and cystadenofibroma, pure malignant mucinous adenofibromas and cystadenofibromas are extremely rare.

Endometrioid Tumors

Typical Endometrioid Tumors

Benign Typical Endometrioid Tumors

Endometrioid Adenofibroma and Cystadenofibroma. Although the WHO classification lists among benign endometrioid tumors adenoma, cystadenoma, adenofibroma, and cystadenofibroma, this discussion is focused on the latter two, since these are the most common and since, with the exception of the prominent fibrous stroma, their presentation and behavior are similar to those of endometrioid adenomas and cystadenomas. In a series of cystadenofibromas studied by Kao and Norris,[84] 10% of the tumors were of the endometrioid type. Roth et al.[133] described two endometrioid adenofibromas. The tumors are similar to the common, serous adenofibromas and cystadenofibromas and vary from the latter only by their epithelial elements, which are of endometrioid nature and frequently show squamous metaplasia.

Proliferating Endometrioid Adenofibroma and Cystadenofibroma. For a more detailed discussion of the concept of proliferating ovarian tumors, the reader is referred to the section dealing with proliferating serous adenofibroma and cystadenofibroma.

Proliferating endometrioid adenofibromas have histologic features similar to those of atypical endometrial hyperplasia.[15,85,133] In these neoplasms, the endometrioid glands embedded in the fibrous stroma show increased proliferation, complexity, and crowding, as well as some atypism, occasional mitoses, and squamous metaplasia (Fig. 18.35). The biologic behavior of all of these tumors has been benign, and thus they should not be confused with carcinomas of LMP.

Occasionally, foci of invasive endometrioid carcinoma may be present within an ordinary benign or proliferating adenofibromatous tumor. In these cases, the carcinomatous areas differ from the proliferating variant by confluence and stromal invasion.[133]

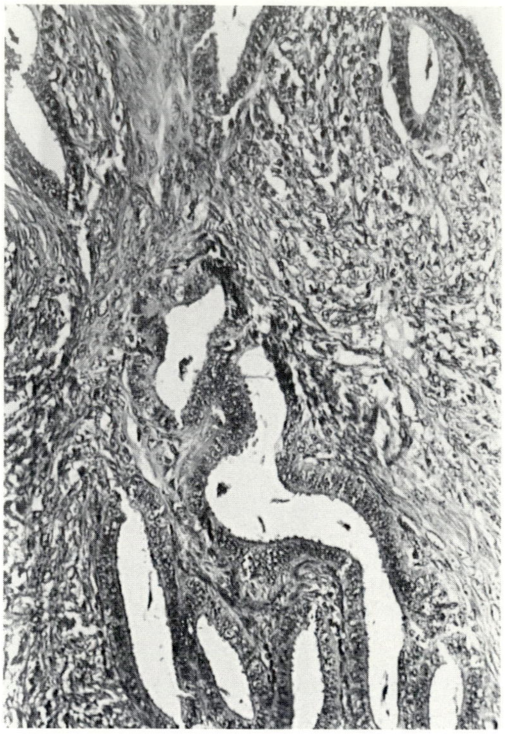

Fig. 18.35. Proliferating endometrioid adenofibroma showing irregularly shaped, crowded, endometrial-type glands in fibrous stroma.

Malignant Typical Endometrioid Tumors

Endometrioid Carcinoma of Low Malignant Potential (of Borderline Malignancy). Although endometrioid carcinoma of the ovary is common, there is a paucity of endometrioid carcinomas of LMP, perhaps due to the lack of well-defined histologic criteria. Endometrioid adenofibromas with unusual proliferative activity have been classified by Roth et al.[133] and by Czernobilsky[34] as benign proliferating rather than borderline neoplasms, whereas a group of endometrioid adenofibromas, some with similar features as those described above, were designated as showing atypia by Kao and Norris.[85] Bell and Scully[15] defined a borderline endometrioid adenofibroma as showing "closely packed glands or epithelial islands with a cribriform pattern composed of cells with low-grade malignant nuclear characteristics embedded in an abundant fibromatous stroma without evidence of invasion." It appears that the only legitimate nonadenofibromatous endometrioid carcinoma of low-grade potential is that described by Colgan and Norris,[30] in which the glands are crowded, back-to-back, and irregular, and the epithelium displays some atypia and low mitotic activity. The tumor is usually cystic, and the epithelial processes are attached to a fibrous wall without evidence of invasion (Fig. 18.36).

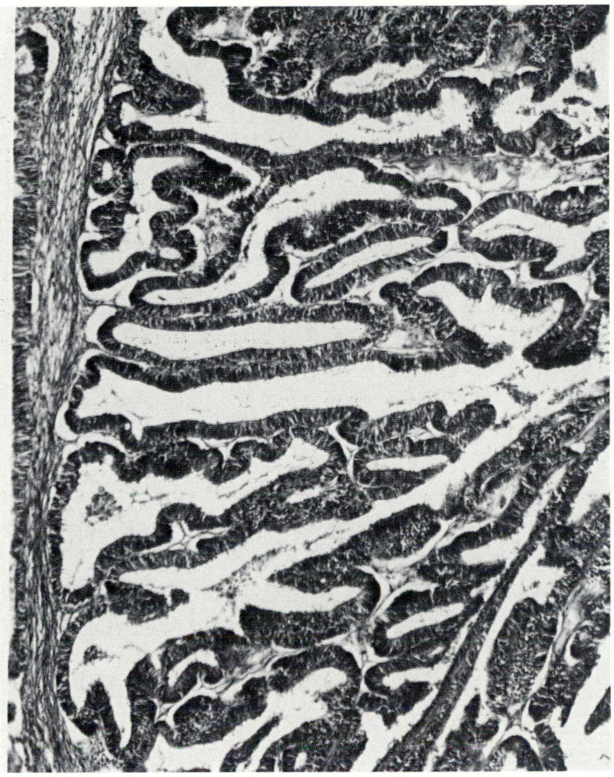

FIG. 18.36. Cystic endometrioid carcinoma of low malignant potential with papillary processes lined by endometrial-type glands. No obvious invasion or cyst wall is present. (Reprinted by permission from Colgan and Norris, Ref. 30.)

At this writing, none of the reported endometrioid tumors of LMP have recurred or metastasized.[15,85] Treatment has varied from removal of the involved adnexa to hysterectomy with bilateral salpingo-oophorectomy.

Endometrioid Carcinoma. Endometrioid carcinoma of the ovary is defined as a primary ovarian carcinoma that is histologically identical to typical endometrial adenocarcinoma. This entity was described in 1925 by Sampson,[141] who insisted that the origin of this tumor from preexisting ovarian endometriosis must be demonstrable. Since then, endometriosis has repeatedly been implicated as the source of this neoplasm, although this cannot be proved in each case.[47,49,65] In the series of Czernobilsky et al. of 75 cases of endometrioid carcinoma,[41] 17% had endometriosis in the ovary harboring the neoplasm. However, in only 3 of these was there continuity between the endometriosis and the endometrioid carcinoma. It is possible that the tumor destroys the preexisting endometriosis, making a direct transition to the neoplasm impossible to identify. Furthermore, because the surface epithelium of the ovary is considered by most as the source of ovarian endometriosis,[73] endometrioid carcinoma can arise directly from it without first passing through a benign endometrioid stage.

The frequency of endometrioid carcinoma is about 20% ranging from 10 to 24.4%, of all primary ovarian adenocarcinomas.[41,101,156] It is the second most common primary ovarian adenocarcinoma after serous cystadenocarcinoma. The mean age of the patients with this neoplasm is about 53 years.[41,101]

Gross Appearance. Most endometrioid carcinomas are cystic, ranging in size from 2 to 35 cm. Frequently, friable, soft, or papillary structures partly fill the lumen. In some instances, the neoplasm is completely solid, with necrotic or hemorrhagic areas (Fig. 18.37). About 30–50% of the tumors are bilateral, with about half of the patients having stage I and II disease.[41,151]

Microscopic Appearance. When the same histologic grading that is used for endometrial adenocarcinoma is applied, endometrioid carcinoma is graded from well differentiated (grade 1) to poorly differentiated (grade 3) according to the extent of the glandular formation (Figs. 18.38 and 18.39). Over 50% of these neoplasms are grades 1 and 2.[41,101] Although the endometrial-like character is most readily recognizable in the well-differentiated tumors, it may be difficult, if not impossible, to identify in poorly differentiated neoplasms. In such cases, a diagnosis of "adenocarcinoma not otherwise classifiable" is preferable.

As in endometrial adenocarcinoma, squamous elements in endometrioid carcinomas are common. The term *adenoacanthoma*, which, as in the case of uterine adenocarcinoma with squamous elements, was used for

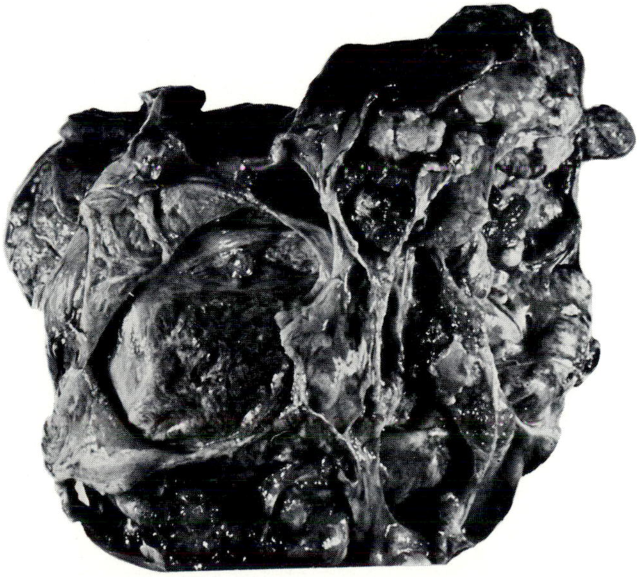

FIG. 18.37. Endometrioid carcinoma with multilocular cystic structures partly filled with soft and papillary tumor tissue. (Courtesy of Dr. H. T. Enterline.)

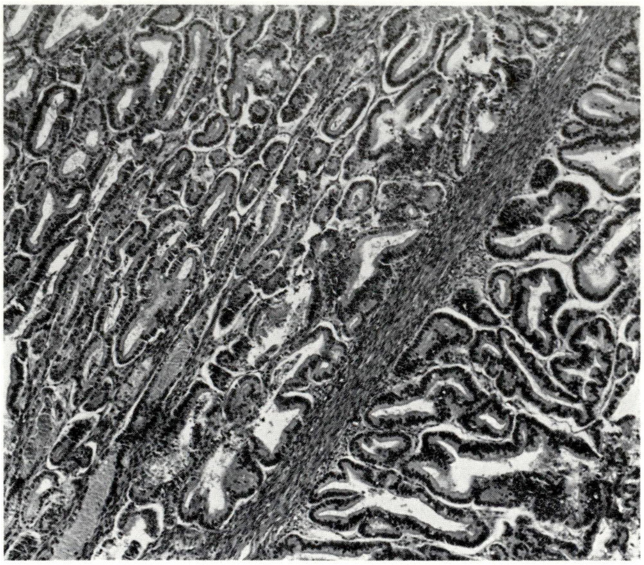

FIG. 18.38. Well-differentiated endometrioid carcinoma. (Reprinted by permission of Czernobilsky et al., Ref. 40.)

the equivalent ovarian neoplasms, is now being replaced by *adenocarcinoma with squamous differentiation* with the addition of the histologic grading[96] (see Chapter 12, Endometrial Carcinoma). This appears to be preferable to *adenoacanthoma*, meaning benign squamous metaplasia, and *adenosquamous carcinoma*, in which the squamous elements are histologically malignant. These terms are not clearly defined, which explains the wide range of frequency that has been reported in the literature[41,49,65] (Fig. 18.40). In contrast to those who restricted the term *adenoacanthoma* to histologically benign squamous areas within an adenocarcinoma,[116] it can be used in a broader sense, to include tumors that showed squamous, squamoid, and atypical, possible malignant nests.[41,169] Fu et al.[59] have shown that in patients in whom the squamous component of the endometrioid carcinoma was histologically malignant, so-called adenosquamous carcinoma, the 5-year survival was much lower than in those with benign squamous elements. A pure squamous endometrioid carcinoma also exists but is very rare. Other conditions, such as squamous carcinoma aris-

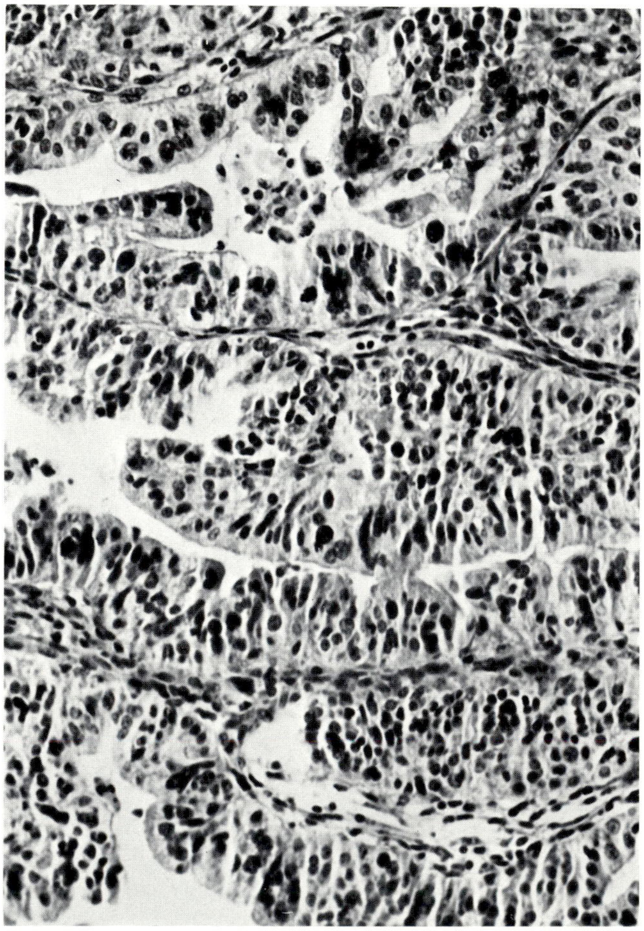

FIG. 18.39. Moderately well to poorly differentiated endometrioid carcinoma.

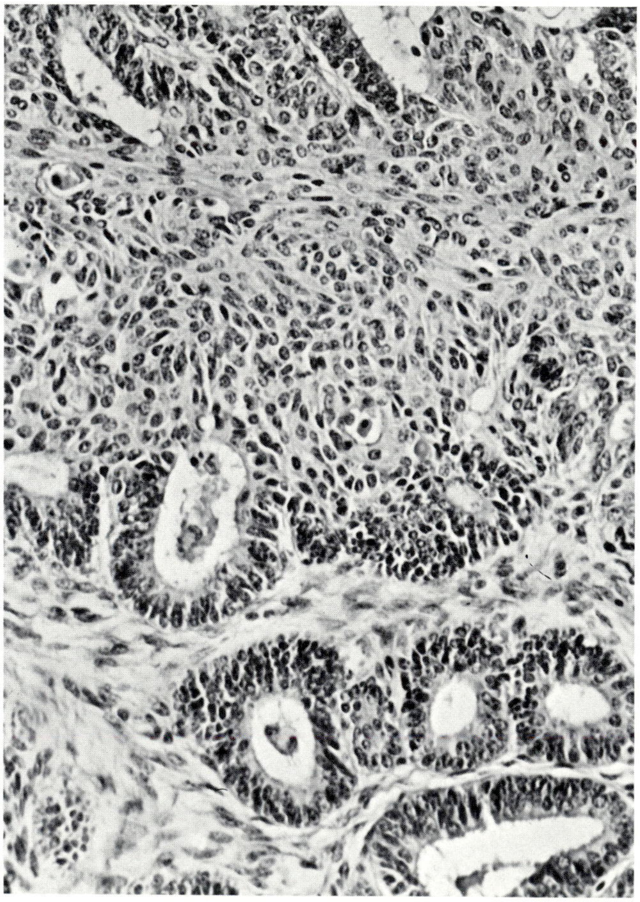

FIG. 18.40. Adenoacanthoma demonstrating typical endometrioid carcinomatous glands with large area of squamous epithelium.

ing in a cystic teratoma, metastases, and a malignant Brenner tumor, must be ruled out before accepting such a diagnosis.

There are many instances in which endometrioid carcinomas contain additional histologic elements clearly belonging to other types of müllerian neoplasms. Thus, among the 75 cases of endometrioid carcinoma described by Czernobilsky et al.,[41] 18 showed elements of clear cell carcinoma, 7 of serous cystadenocarcinomas, and 1 of anaplastic carcinoma (Fig. 18.41).

One of the interesting features of this neoplasm is the frequent finding of a concomitant endometrial carcinoma (see Chapter 12, Endometrial Carcinoma, and Chapter 22, Metastatic Ovarian Tumors). This was observed in 14.6% of the patients in the Czernobilsky et al. series[41] and in more than 50% by Dockerty.[47] It is often difficult to establish whether these ovarian and endometrial cancers are independent primaries or metastatic from each other. The good survival of these patients, which is not consistent with metastatic disease,[92] and the focal, noninvasive nature of the endometrial carcinoma (Fig. 18.42) suggest that the two neoplasms are independent rather than metastatic.[26,41] The FIGO ruling that, for purposes of cancer reporting and staging, a carcinoma involving both the endometrium and the ovary should be classified as originating in the organ to which the symptoms are related[152c] is not entirely satisfactory, since even small endometrial lesions can have bleeding before a large ovarian carcinoma manifests itself.

Papillary endometrioid carcinoma can occasionally contain psammoma bodies[41] and be difficult to distinguish from papillary serous carcinomas. Special stains do not help in differentiating these tumors because the luminal border of the epithelium in both of these tumors stains positively with diastase-resistant PAS, mucicarmine, and alcian blue stains. The epithelial cells lining the papillary structures of endometrioid carcinomas, in contrast to those of serous cystadenocarcinomas, are predominantly columnar and pseudostratified, with prominent elongated hyperchromatic nuclei. Ultrastructural studies can be of help because in endometrioid carcinoma the cells show features indistinguishable from those of endometrial adenocarcinoma but different from those of serous cystadenocarcinoma.[32]

A histologic variant of endometrioid carcinoma mimicking Sertoli and Sertoli-Leydig cell tumors has been described[135,179] (see Chapter 19, Sex Cord-Stromal Tumors). These tumors show tubular structures with interlacing lining cells similar to those of Sertoli-Leydig cell tumors (Fig. 18.43). The nuclei, however, lack the typical paired or antipodal arrangement seen in Sertoli cells. The presence of typical endometrioid areas, mucin at the apical borders of the epithelial cells, and particularly

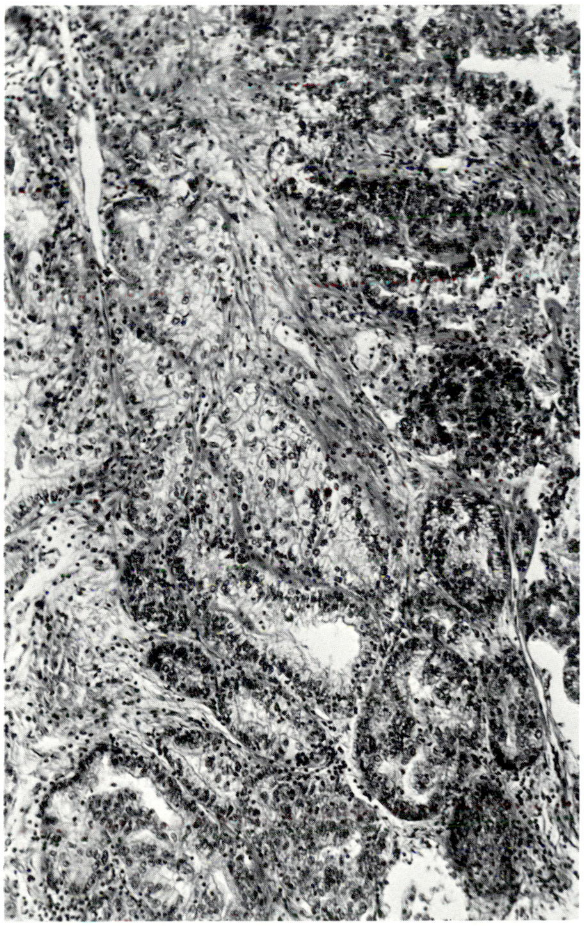

FIG. 18.41. Endometrioid carcinoma (*right* of photograph) mixed with clear cell carcinoma elements (*left*). (Reprinted by permission from Czernobilsky et al., Ref. 41.)

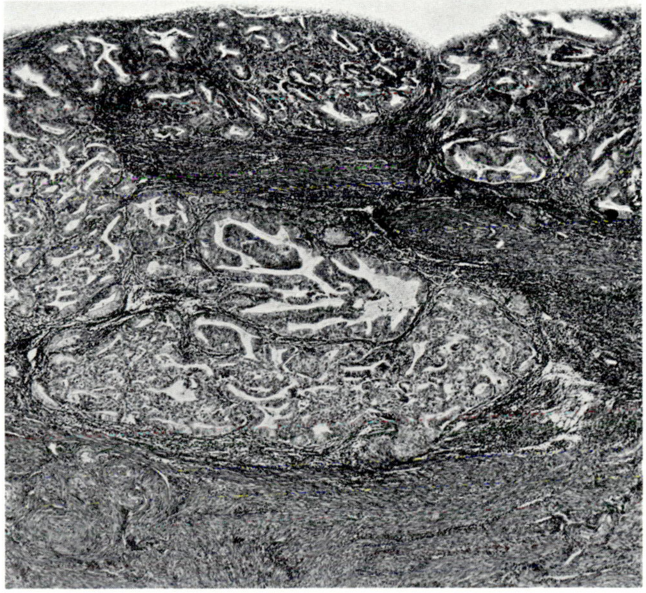

FIG. 18.42. Superficial small fundal endometrial adenocarcinoma in a patient with endometrioid carcinoma of the ovary.

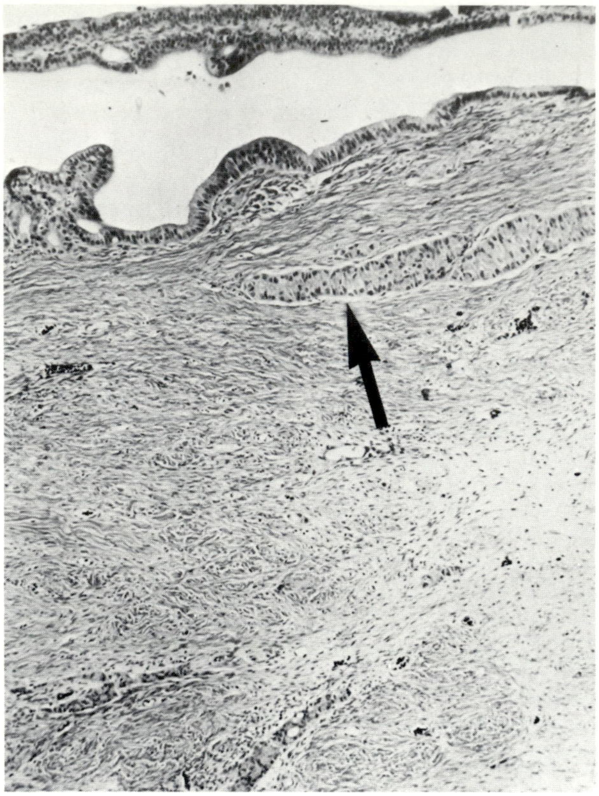

FIG. 18.43. Solid tubules (*arrow*) in an endometrioid carcinoma, mimicking a Sertoli tumor.

areas of squamous differentiation point to an endometrioid rather than a sex cord–stromal tumor.

Differential diagnosis between endometrioid carcinoma and metastatic colonic adenocarcinoma may be problematic. In these instances, even minute areas of squamous differentiation or mixtures of other müllerian-type epithelia point to a primary ovarian carcinoma. Goblet cells or a multinodular growth pattern favor metastatic intestinal cancer[171] (see Chapter 22, Metastatic Ovarian Tumors).

Ultrastructure. Cells have abundant intermediate filaments and lack membrane-bound, electron-dense granules that characterize its serous counterpart.[32] In tumors with squamous differentiation, tonofilament–desmosomal complexes can be seen (Fig. 18.44).

Behavior and Treatment. Total hysterectomy with bilateral salpingo-oophorectomy is the treatment of endometrioid carcinoma. Survival does not seem to be affected by the addition of radiation.[41]

Most authors have stressed the better prognosis of endometrioid carcinoma as compared to that of other ovarian cancers.[101,150] According to Santesson and Kottmeier,[143] the 5-year and 10-year survival is 55% and 40%, respectively, whereas the 5-year survival of patients with serous cystadenocarcinoma is less than 20%. The 5-year and 10-year cumulative survival rates of endometrioid carcinoma reported by Czernobilsky et al.[41] were 40% and 32.7%, respectively. In stage I, the 5-year survival was 92.5%, which dropped to 27.8% in stage II for all histologic grades, and even lower in more advanced clinical stages (Table 18.5). There was no good correlation between survival rates and histologic grading, nor was the prognosis influenced by an admixture with other tumors of müllerian origin or by the presence of a synchronous endometrial carcinoma (Tables 18.5 and 18.6). These data again emphasize that in ovarian carcinomas the most important prognostic features are the extent of the tumor and the amount of residual tumor after surgical treatment.

Mesodermal (Müllerian) Mixed Tumors

This group includes a number of rare biphasic tumors made up of epithelial and stromal elements, all of which occur more frequently in the endometrium than in the ovary.[117,118] Rare pure ovarian stromal sarcomas, probably arising in stroma of endometriosis have also been reported[156] (see Chapter 13, Mesenchymal Tumors of Uterus). Although endometrioid elements are prominent in the epithelial components of the biphasic neoplasms, other types of müllerian epithelia are frequently encountered. These tumors have nevertheless been classified by WHO under the heading of "endometrioid tumors" because of their occurrence as primary uterine neoplasms. These neoplasms can also arise from preexisting ovarian endometriosis[144] or from the multipotential surface epithelium of the ovary. Since endometriosis is rarely identified in ovaries harboring these neoplasms and because of the advanced age of these patients, in whom endometriosis is usually not active, the majority of these tumors most likely arise from coelomic epithelial with stromal participation. They can be considered to represent a histologic spectrum in which the epithelial and stromal components show a variety of proliferative or malignant characteristics.

The benign representatives of these biphasic tumors, namely, endometrioid adenofibroma and cystadenofibroma, were discussed previously.

MALIGNANT MESODERMAL MIXED TUMORS

Adenosarcoma. These neoplasms are characterized by benign neoplastic glands lined by benign, often atypical müllerian-type epithelial cells with a sarcomatous stroma resembling endometrial stromal sarcoma (Fig. 18.45). These lesions were first described in the uterus but were subsequently reported in the ovary as well.[29,39] The overall pattern of growth is reminiscent of the previously described cystadenofibroma and is usually a large cystic neoplasm with solid areas. According to Clement and

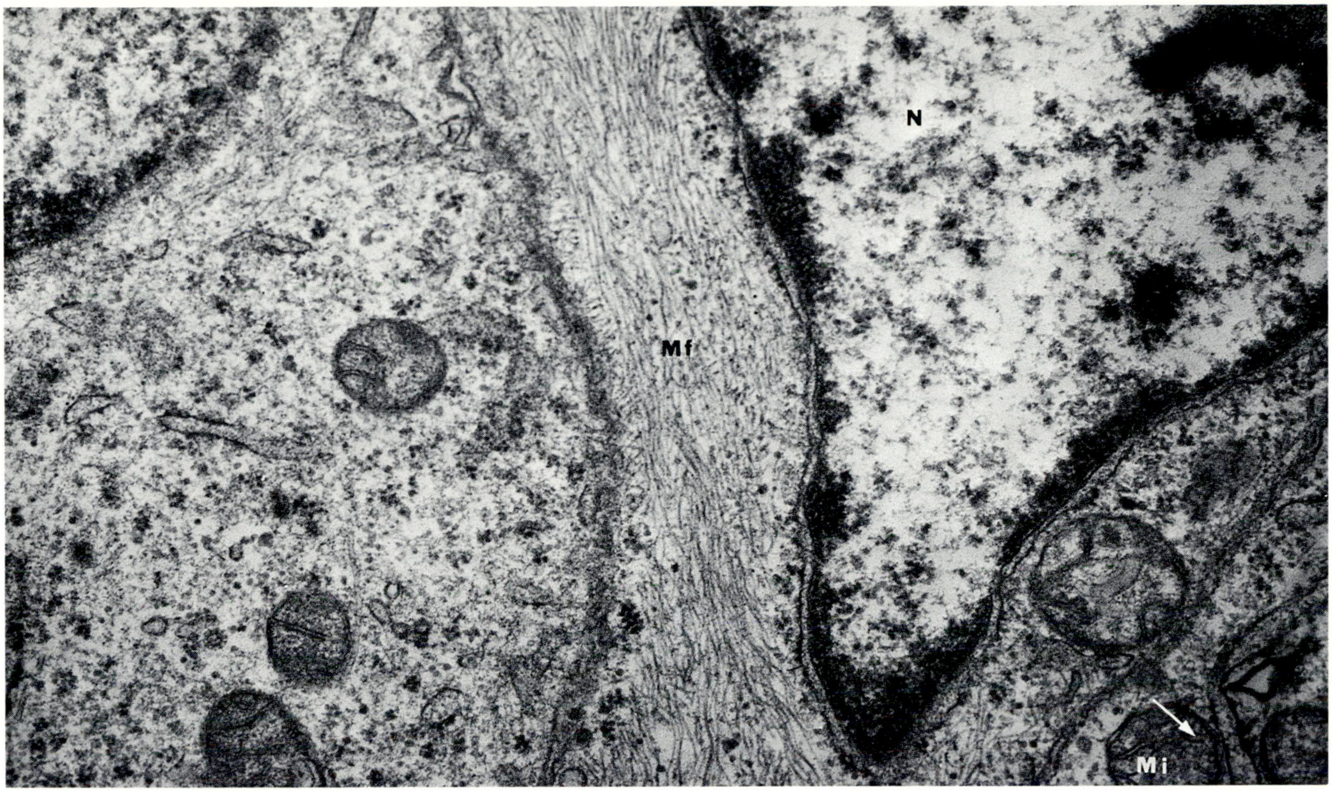

FIG. 18.44. Electron micrograph of a well-differentiated endometrioid carcinoma showing the characteristic perinuclear (N) microfilament (Mf). Note the mitochondria (Mi) in close apposition (*arrow*) with parallel membranes of granular endoplasmic reticulum. ×25,750. (Courtesy of Dr. A. Ferenczy.)

TABLE 18.5. Five-year cumulative survival figures of all the patients with endometrioid carcinoma of the ovary as compared to their various subdivisions.[a]

Clinical stage	Entire series	"Mixed" endometrioid	"Pure" endometrioid	Adenoacanthoma	Endometrioid without squamous	Endometrioid with endometrial carcinoma	Endometrioid without endometrial carcinoma
I	92.5% (31)	88.9% (10)	93.8% (21)	93.3% (19)	90.9% (12)	80% (5)	94.9% (26)
II	27.8% (5)	25% (4)	100% (1)	50% (2)	0% (3)	—	27.8% (5)
III	3.7% (33)	11% (9)	0% (24)	0% (11)	5.5% (22)	25% (4)	3.5% (29)
IV	0% (6)	0% (3)	0% (3)	0% (4)	0% (2)	0% (2)	0% (4)
All stages combined	40.5% (75)	40.8% (26)	39.9% (49)	51.5% (36)	29.8% (39)	45.5% (11)	29.7% (64)

[a] Numbers in parentheses indicate number of patients in each clinical stage. (Reprinted by permission from Czernobilsky et al., Ref. 24.)

TABLE 18.6. Comparison of cumulative 5-year survival of patients with endometrioid carcinoma of the ovary by histologic grading and clinical staging.[a]

Clinical stage	Histologic grading 1	2	3	4	All histologic grades combined
I	100% (11)	83.6% (15)	100% (3)	100% (2)	92.5% (31)
II	—	100% (1)	0% (4)	—	27.8% (5)
III	0% (5)	0% (12)	0% (9)	21.4% (7)	3.7% (33)
IV	—	0% (1)	0% (4)	0% (1)	0% (6)
All stages combined	67.3% (16)	44.5% (29)	13.2% (20)	37.5% (10)	40.5% (75)

[a] Numbers in parentheses indicate number of patients. (Reprinted by permission from Czernobilsky et al., Ref. 24.)

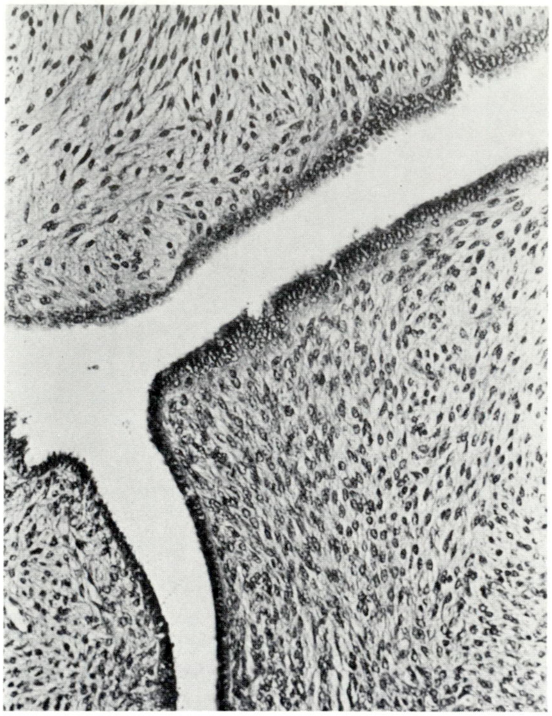

FIG. 18.45. Adenosarcoma with club-shaped projections lined by benign cuboidal and columnar epithelium. The stroma is cellular and composed of spindle cells.

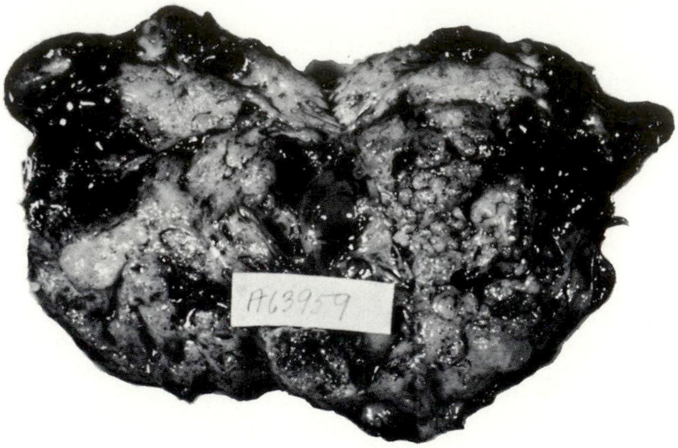

FIG. 18.46. Cross-section of a carcinosarcoma showing solid, cystic, and hemorrhagic areas. (Reprinted by permission of The American College of Obstetricians and Gynecologists. (Obstetrics and Gynecology, 31:21, 1968).]

Scully,[29] the prognosis for patients with this tumor is better than for those in whom both the epithelial and stromal components are malignant.

A review of the literature of these neoplasms by Czernobilsky et al.[39] revealed that patients with this tumor are in the late reproductive and menopausal age groups, compared to older patients with uterine adenosarcomas. The mitotic count of the stromal component of adenosarcoma has less value in the assessment and prognosis than has been reported in uterine stromal tumors of various types. Kao and Norris[86] described similar neoplasms in which the stroma was atypical and cellular rather than sarcomatous. They considered some of these as cellular adenofibromas and others as low-grade adenosarcomas.

Mesodermal (Müllerian) Mixed Homologous Tumor (Carcinosarcoma). Because of the rarity of this neoplasm, its true frequency is unknown. This is a tumor of the elderly, the ages ranging from 43 to 78 years, with a median age of 57 years.

Gross Appearance. Most of the tumors are unilateral, large, partly cystic neoplasms, with a median diameter of 14 cm. The solid portions often demonstrate necrotic areas and hemorrhage[44] (Fig. 18.46).

Microscopic Appearance. The typical microscopic appearance is that of an admixture of malignant epithelial and stromal elements. The epithelial component is most frequently an adenocarcinoma of varying differentiation, occasionally with intracellular mucinous material. It can also demonstrate papillary and squamous features (Fig. 18.47). The epithelial component is usually sharply de-

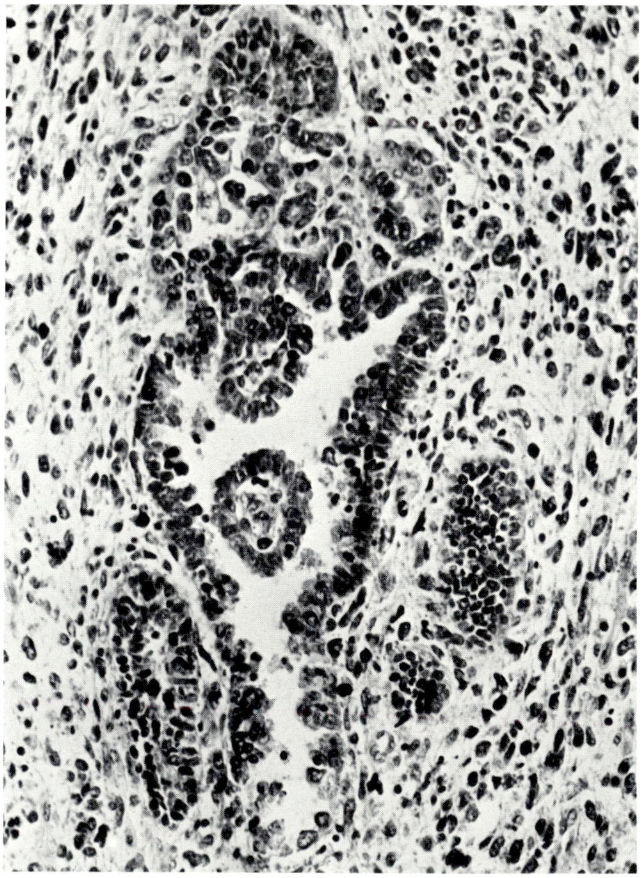

FIG. 18.47. Adenocarcinoma with a surrounding sarcomatous stroma in a carcinosarcoma.

marcated from the surrounding stroma, although transition between the epithelial and sarcomatous components of the tumor can occasionally be observed. The stroma in carcinosarcomas is predominantly composed of tightly packed hyperchromatic spindle cells with numerous mitoses without heterologous elements (Fig. 18.48).

Carcinosarcomas must be differentiated from ovarian adenocarcinomas with prominent cellular stroma. In the latter lesions the stroma may be extremely cellular but does not show the marked pleomorphism and mitotic activity that characterizes the stromal sarcomatous element of carcinosarcoma.

Behavior and Treatment. Treatment consists of total hysterectomy with bilateral salpingo-oophorectomy and chemotherapy.

One of the reasons justifying a separate discussion of homologous and heterologous mesodermal mixed tumors is the allegedly somewhat better prognosis for the former.[44] This difference in prognosis was first observed by Norris et al.,[117,118] who studied similar tumors arising in the endometrium. In the series by Czernobilsky and Labarre,[36] behavioral differences between these two types of neoplasms in the ovary could not be established, possibly because of the small number of patients. However, it does appear that when stratified by stage there is no statistically significant difference in the clinical behavior of homologous and heterologous mesodermal mixed tumors. Both are highly malignant tumors with a median survival of 6 months (heterologous) to 12 months (homologous). The tumors disseminate widely, mostly by peritoneal seeding.[44] At autopsy, the sarcomatous element is usually the predominating one in the various sites in which the tumor is found.[36,44]

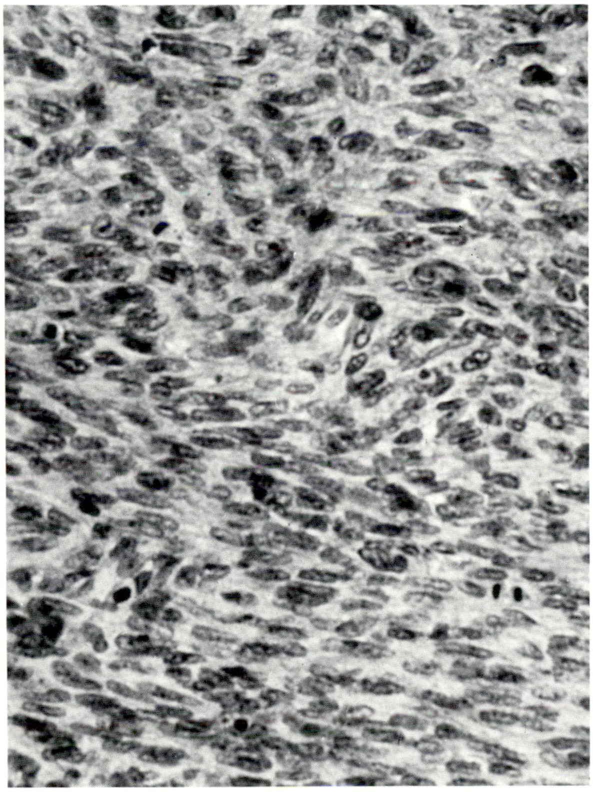

Fig. 18.48. Area of pure stromal sarcoma in a carcinosarcoma. [Reprinted with permission from The American College of Obstetricians and Gynecologists. (Obstetrics and Gynecology, 31:21, 1968).]

Mesodermal (Müllerian) Mixed Heterologous Tumor. Because of the rarity of this tumor, no reliable figures of its incidence are available. According to Dehner et al.[44] the mean age is 53 years. Only 1 of their 14 patients was below the age of 40. Most women are nulliparous.[3,36,44]

Gross Appearance. The appearance of mixed mesodermal tumors is similar to that of carcinosarcoma, namely, unilateral, large, partly cystic neoplasms with a median diameter of about 15 cm[44] (Fig. 18.49).

Microscopic Appearance. The microscopic feature that distinguishes heterologous from homologous tumors is the stromal component. In the heterologous tumors, the stroma presents a variety of malignant, mesenchymal elements in addition to nonspecific spindle cell areas. These consist most commonly of cartilage, striated muscle, and osteoid.[44] The epithelial component is similar to that of carcinosarcoma (Figs. 18.50 and 18.51). Hyaline droplets containing alpha$_1$-antitrypsin have been described in both epithelium and mesenchyme of these tumors.[45]

Because of the mixture of epithelial and heterologous elements, the tumors must be distinguished from immature teratomas (see Chapter 20, Germ Cell Tumors of Ovary). In mixed heterologous tumors, there is complete absence of any orderly or organized arrangement of the

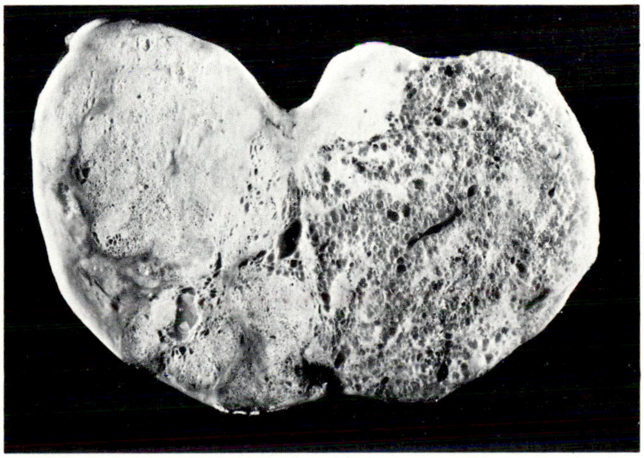

Fig. 18.49. Mixed mesodermal tumor showing a mixture of solid and cystic areas. (Courtesy of Dr. H. J. Norris.)

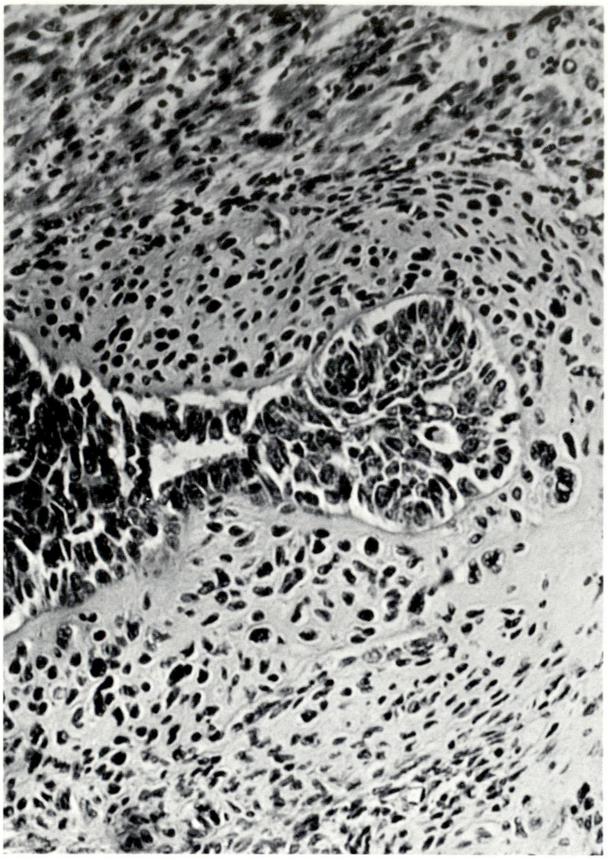

FIG. 18.50. Mixed mesodermal tumor with a malignant glandular structure surrounded by highly atypical cartilage and smooth muscle (*upper field* of photomicrograph). [Reprinted with permission from The American College of Obstetricians and Gynecologists. (Obstetrics and Gynecology, 31:21, 1968).]

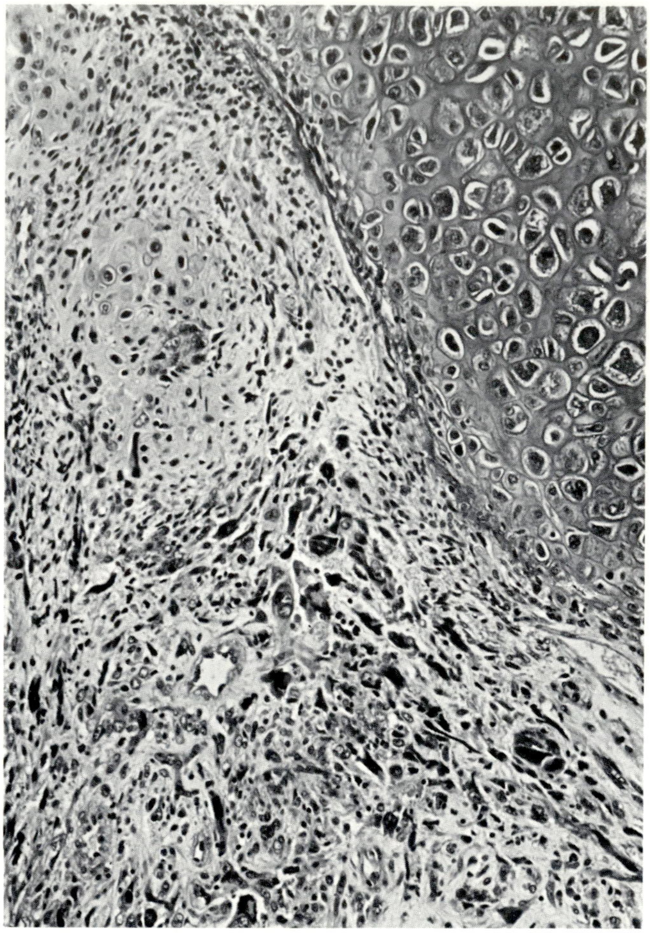

FIG. 18.51. Detail of sarcomatous elements in mixed mesodermal tumor showing chondrosarcoma and anaplastic sarcoma.

stromal elements, whereas in immature teratomas, an organoid pattern is at least partially preserved. In addition, neuroepithelial elements, which are commonplace in immature teratomas, have never been described in mixed heterologous tumors. Finally, immature teratomas are tumors of young women, in contrast to the mesodermal mixed tumors, which typically appear after menopause.

Behavior and Treatment. Treatment of these lesions is hysterectomy and bilateral salpingo-oophorectomy and adjuvant multiagent chemotherapy. The actuarial survival at 15 months is 50% for patients with carcinosarcomas, compared to only 14% for those with mixed mesodermal tumors.[44] The presence of cartilage and absence of striated muscle does not appear to influence the prognosis.

Clear Cell Tumors

The histogenesis of these tumors has been the subject of considerable controversy. For many years, they were thought to be of mesonephric origin and termed *mesonephroma*[119,120,145] because the clear cells that make up the majority of these tumors resemble those that line the renal tubules. The occasional presence of structures suggesting primitive glomeruli in these tumors gave further support to the mesonephric theory. Teilum[166] eventually reclassified some of these neoplasms as *endodermal sinus tumors*, which belong to the germ cell category of ovarian neoplasms (see Chapter 20, Germ Cell Tumors of Ovary). The mesonephric histogenetic theory continued to be questioned over the years by many authors who favored a müllerian rather than a mesonephric origin.[101,163,164] Scully and Barlow[154] in 1967 established the relationship of clear cell tumors to müllerian-type neoplasms on the following basis: (1) the high frequency of pelvic endometriosis in patients with ovarian clear cell carcinoma, (2) the coexistence of endometrioid and clear cell carcinomas, (3) the observation that clear cell carcinoma occasionally arises from the epithelium of endometriosis, and (4) the fact that a clear cell-type carcinoma of the uterine corpus originates in the endometrium, which is of obvious müllerian derivation. Other authors have subsequently confirmed these observations.[40] Furthermore, ultrastructural studies[52d,140,161] have provided additional data to support the müllerian origin of clear cell carcinoma. Finally, various authors have commented on the similar prognosis of clear cell and endometrioid carcinomas.[40,95] Thus, on the basis of this evidence, it appears that clear cell tumors of the ovary, although histologically distinctive, represent a form of endometrioid neoplasia.[34] True mesonephric ovarian tumors are very rare lesions and, as has been shown in other sites in the female genital tract, are not composed of clear cells.[104]

Benign Clear Cell Tumors

Clear Cell Adenofibroma and Cystadenofibroma. Until recently, there were not any well-documented cases of benign clear cell tumors, although these have been mentioned in a few series.[4,72] The two cases that Roth et al.[136] described as clear cell adenofibroma are probably the first well-defined examples of such neoplasms. The series of Bell and Scully[16] is the largest one in the literature. These tumors are similar to the other adenofibromas described previously in this chapter, with the exception of their epithelial components. These consist of tubular or cystic glands lined by clear or hobnail cells in addition to indifferent appearing epithelial cells. There is little or no cytologic atypism and no mitotic activity (Fig. 18.52).

Proliferating Clear Cell Adenofibroma and Cystadenofibroma. Although the existence of this tumor has been proposed on theoretical grounds (Table 18.2), it has not yet been documented. One would expect it to be an adenofibromatous tumor in which the epithelial component consists of irregular complex glands lined by clear or hobnail cells showing minimal atypism and little mitotic activity. This is a hypothetical description of a neoplasm that, as has been the case with a number of other ovarian common epithelial tumors, were first listed in the WHO classification of ovarian tumors and only subsequently proven to exist.

Malignant Clear Cell Tumors

Clear Cell Carcinoma of Low Malignant Potential. This is an adenofibromatous tumor in which the clear cell elements show moderate to marked nuclear atypia with some mitoses.[16,136] Occasional solid groups or cords of cells can also occur among the tubules. However, there is no confluence of the epithelial components and no invasion of the stroma (Fig. 18.53). There have been no recurrences or metastases so far in the small series reported by Roth et al.[136] However, of the 12 borderline clear cell adenofibromas reported by Bell and Scully,[16] 1 had a questionable lung metastasis 4 years after it

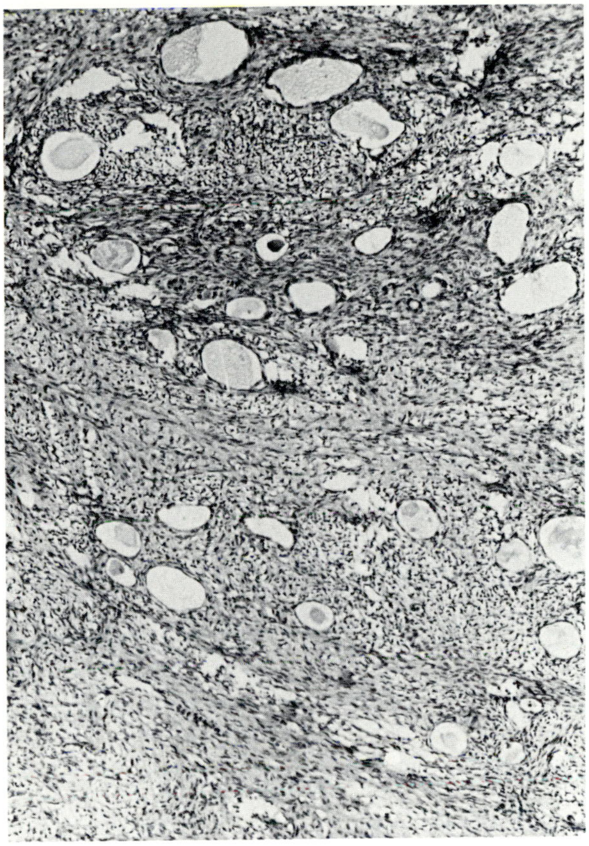

Fig. 18.52. Benign clear cell adenofibroma with scattered, nonconfluent glandular structures lined by benign-appearing clear, hobnail, and indifferent epithelial cells.

appeared. Similar cases termed *unusual cystadenofibromas* were also described by Kao and Norris.[84] The case illustrated in the Armed Forces Institute of Pathology fascicle on ovarian tumors[152d] also seems to fit into this category.

In both benign clear cell tumors and clear cell carcinomas of LMP, the pattern is similar to what Schiller[146] described as *parvilocular tumors or cystomas.* However, this appellation referred to a growth pattern of a heterogeneous group of tumors and not to a specific entity. Thus, *parvilocular* should not be used as a diagnostic term.

Clear Cell Carcinoma. Clear cell carcinomas of the ovary constitute about 5%[95] to 11%[40] of all primary ovarian carcinomas. The mean age of patients with this tumor is 54 years, with a range from about 40 to 78 years.[40,95]

Gross Appearance. These tumors vary in size from 2 to 30 cm in diameter.[40] Most are partially cystic, with yellow, white, gray, and hemorrhagic areas. Forty percent are bilateral.[40,53]

Microscopic Appearance. The predominant histologic pattern is that of tubules, glandular areas, papillae, and

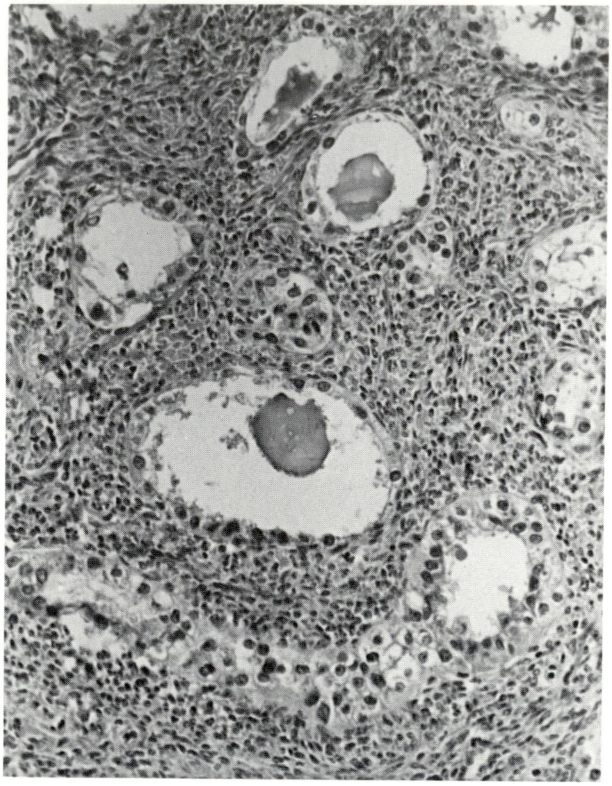

Fig. 18.53. Clear cell carcinoma of LMP in which the glands and tubules within the fibrous stroma are lined by clear and hobnail cells with nuclear atypia.

cysts scattered within varying amounts of stroma. The characteristic epithelial cells lining these structures consist of so-called hobnail cells, with large prominent nuclei and scant cytoplasm near the enlarged apex of the cell, clear cells that are cuboidal, columnar, or pavement-shaped with completely clear cytoplasm, and scattered darker granular cells (Figs. 18.54 and 18.55). In certain areas, the tumor may resemble the Arias-Stella type reaction seen within gestational endometrium[40] (see Chapter 9, Anatomy and Histology of Uterus.) Occasionally, one encounters areas of frank clear cell carcinoma in an otherwise clear cell adenofibromatous tumor of LMP. Of the 11 patients in this category, 2 died of their tumor.[136] Occasional clear cells demonstrate intracytoplasmic PAS-positive, diastase-resistant material, but in most instances, there is intraluminal and luminal border positive staining with mucicarmine, diastase-resistant PAS, and alcian blue. Klemi et al.[90] described hyaline globules in these neoplasms that are similar to those found in endodermal sinus tumor and thus can no longer be considered pathognomonic of the latter tumor.

One of the interesting features of clear cell carcinoma is the frequent admixture with elements from other

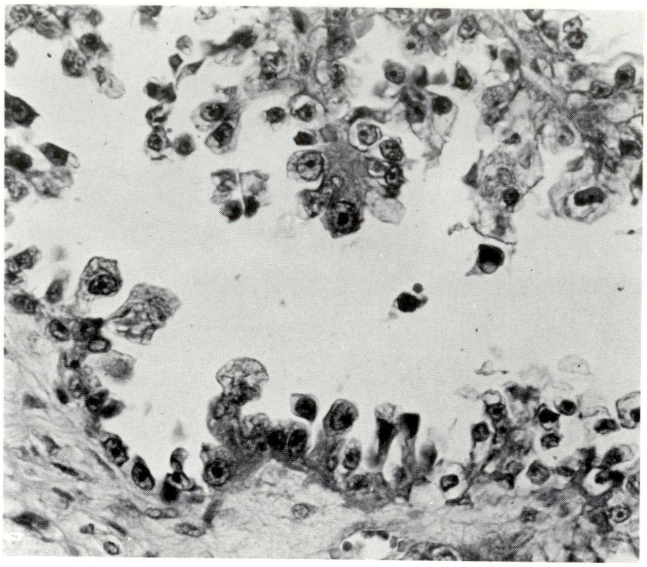

Fig. 18.54. Hobnail-shaped clear cells in a clear cell carcinoma. (Reprinted by permission of Czernobilsky et al., Ref. 40.)

müllerian-type neoplasms, which seem to be even more prominent in this neoplasm than in the other tumors of surface epithelial origin. The most frequent association is with endometrioid and serous carcinomas[40,95,154] (Fig. 18.56).

Ultrastructure. Electron microscopic studies of the clear cells from this tumor[52,140,161] reveal prominent aggregates of glycogen particles in close relationship with stacked granular endoplasmic reticulum and other features that

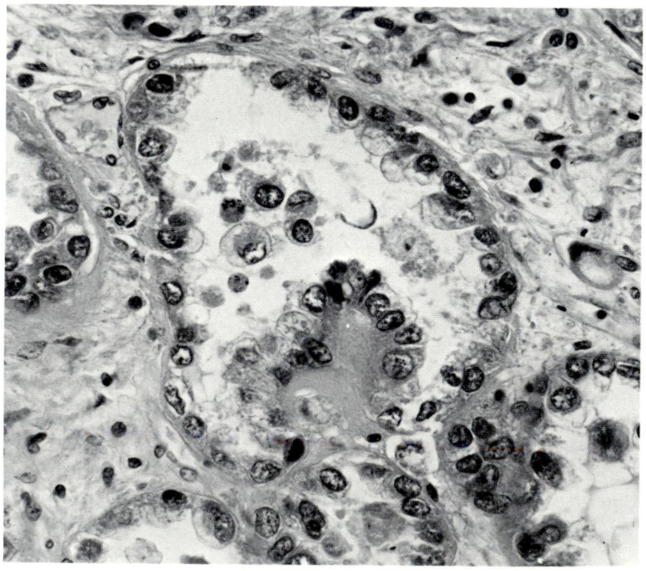

Fig. 18.55. Glandular structure with intraluminal projection referred to as glomerular body in clear cell carcinoma. (Reprinted by permission of Czernobilsky et al., Ref. 40.)

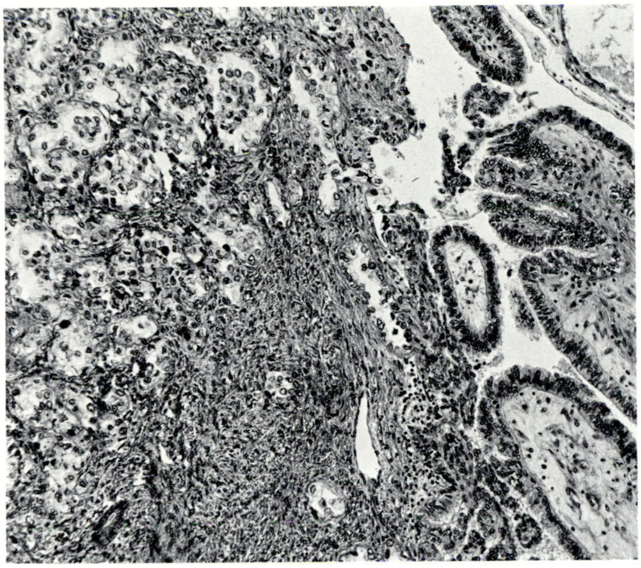

FIG. 18.56. Clear cell carcinoma (*left side* of photomicrograph) with associated papillary serous cystadenocarcinoma. (Reprinted by permission of Czernobilsky et al., Ref. 40.)

are common to clear cell carcinomas of endometrial, cervical, and vaginal origin (Figs. 18.57 and 18.58).

Behavior and Treatment. Treatment is total hysterectomy with bilateral salpingo-oophorectomy. Postoperative irradiation, and intraperitoneal radioactive gold, phosphorus, or nitrogen do not appear to significantly affect the course of the disease.[53]

The 5-year survival of patients with pure and mixed clear cell carcinoma is 41% and 34%, respectively, with 10-year survival figures of 32% and 28%.[40] These figures do not differ significantly from those of a group of patients with endometrioid carcinomas (Fig. 18.59). The clinical stage, however, plays a significant role in the prognosis. Those patients with tumors limited to one ovary had a 5-year survival of 80%, as compared to a 11% survival for those with more extensive neoplasms. Similar observations were made by Kottmeier[93] and by Kurman and Craig,[95] with overall 5-year survival figures ranging from 39% to 27%, respectively. The prognosis of clear cell carcinoma is superior to that of serous cystadenocarcinomas and approaches that of endometrioid carcinoma.

Brenner Tumors

In 1907, Dr. Fritz Brenner described an ovarian tumor that he named *oophoroma folliculare*,[24] postulating a granulosa cell origin. Since then, numerous histogenetic theories have been advanced, probably more so than for any other single ovarian neoplasm.

The granulosa cell theory, first mentioned by Brenner himself, was based on a superficial resemblance of the epithelial elements of the neoplasm to granulosa cells, but it has been refuted by ultrastructural studies.[22,129] Greene[67] suggested a possible origin from ovarian stroma, a theory that is not tenable because of the lack of similarity between the epithelial and stromal elements of the tumor in spite of the apparent continuity between the reticulum fibers of the stroma and those present within the epithelial nests. Schiller's mesonephric theory[17,147] was supported by the frequent occurrence of this tumor near the rete ovarii and its histologic similarity to urinary tract epithelium. Here too, however, ultrastructual studies revealed no similarities between the epithelium of Brenner tumors and that of mesonephric remnants.[23] The latter study also refuted a possible origin of the Brenner tumor from müllerian remnants.[63] Another theory, that of metaplasia of mucinous epithelium,[147] was based on the association of mucinous cystadenomas and Brenner tumors. However, careful observations suggest that mucinous cells present within epithelial nests of Brenner tumors are the result of mucinous metaplasia rather than the source of the Brenner epithelium. Because of the occasional presence of heterologous epithelia in Brenner tumors, a teratomatous origin has also been suggested,[79] but the metaplastic theory seems to be more tenable.

The Walthard cell nest theory was advanced by Meyer in 1932.[105] These nests are most commonly found on the surface of the fallopian tubes, mesosalpinx, mesovarium, and occasionally in the ovarian hilus, where Brenner tumors are not usually located. Nevertheless, there exists a striking histologic similarity among the Walthard cell nests, urothelium, and the epithelium of the Brenner tumor on both light and electron microscopic examination.[22,129] These observations do not contradict the current view that Brenner tumors arise from the surface epithelium of the ovary, a theory based on observations of continuity between this epithelium and that of the Brenner tumor.[5] It is, therefore, assumed that Brenner tumors are derived from the coelomic epithelium of the ovary, which through a metaplastic process forms the typical urothelial-like epithelial elements of the neoplasm as well as Walthard cell nests, providing a common denominator for the morphologic similarities among these seemingly unrelated epithelial elements.[23,129,163]

Benign Brenner Tumors

TYPICAL BRENNER TUMOR

According to Jondahl et al.,[79] Brenner tumors constitute 1.7% of all ovarian neoplasms, although some consider it to be even less frequent. Bilaterality occurred in 6.5%, and patients' ages ranged from 6 to 81 years, half the patients being over 50 years. In Silverberg's series,[162]

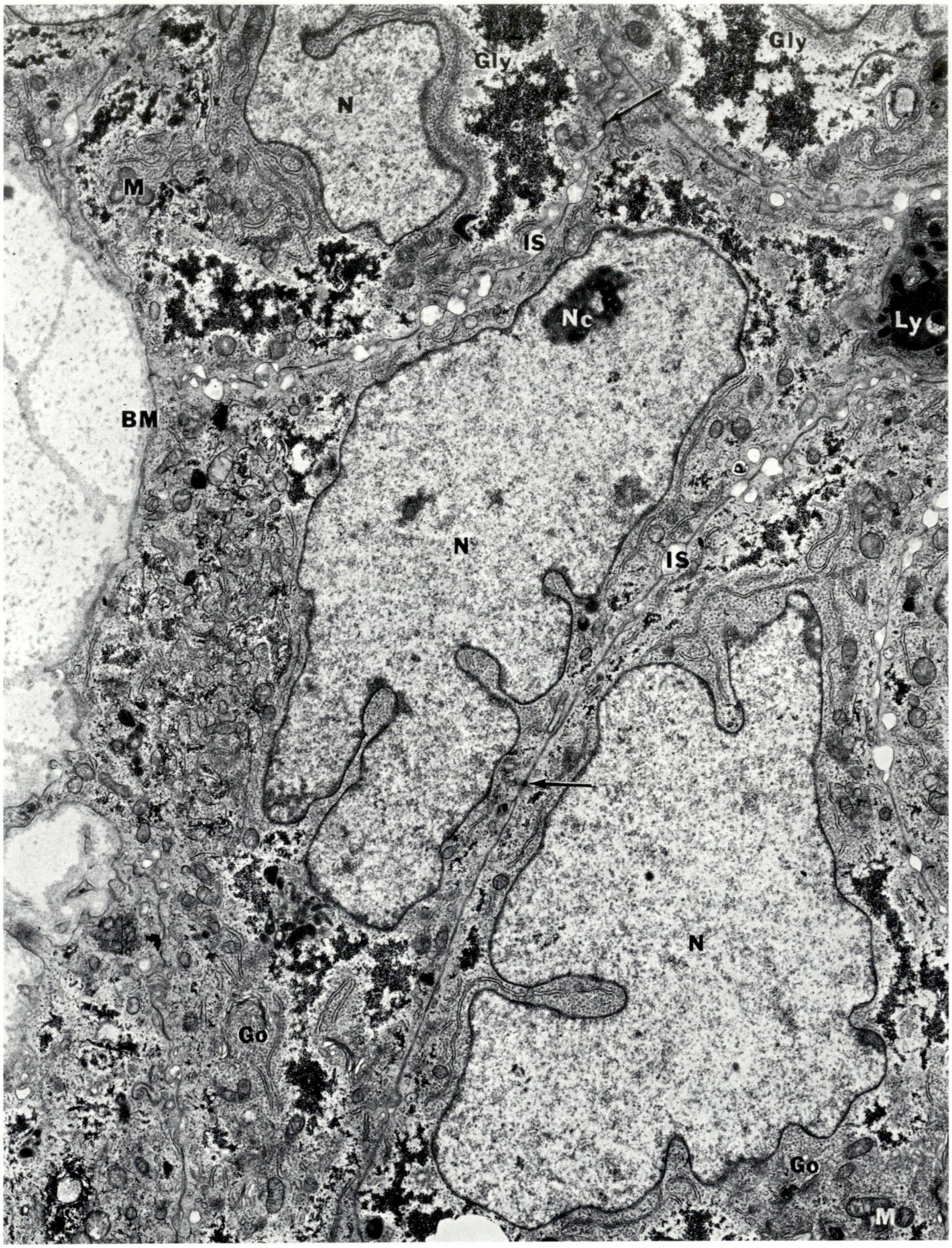

FIG. 18.57. Survey electron micrograph of clear cell carcinoma. Basement membrane (BM) separates the neoplastic cells from the stroma. Desmosomes are frequent (*arrows*). Clusters of glycogen (Gly), lysosomes (Ly), Golgi complexes (Go), mitochondria (M), and numerous intercellular spaces (IS) are noted. Nuclei (N) are rather large and lobular and sometimes contain a coiled nucleous (Nc). ×5580. [Reprinted with permission from The American College of Obstetricians and Gynecologists. (Obstetrics and Gynecology, 44:551, 1974).]

the tumors had a left-sided predominance, bilaterality was 3.7%, and only 31.5% of the patients were postmenopausal.

Gross Appearance. The majority of Brenner tumors are solid and firm, with a gray-white and whorled cut surface (Fig. 18.60). They vary in size from microscopic tumors to huge masses, most of the larger ones measuring 2–8 cm in diameter. The frequency of microscopic lesions explains the common incidental discovery of this tumor. Frequently, small cystic structures can be identified in these solid tumors, and occasionally the entire neoplasm

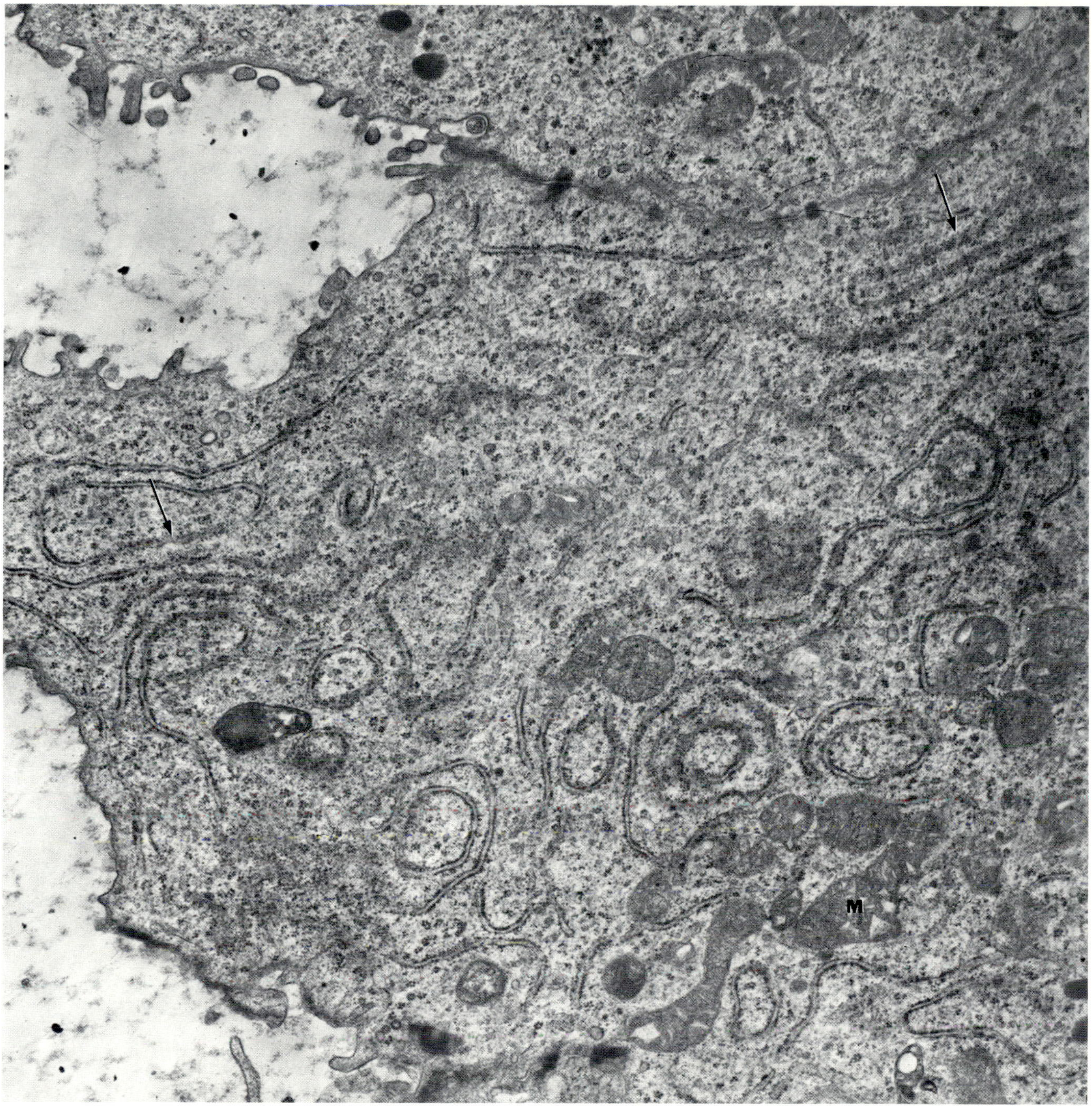

FIG. 18.58. Electron micrograph of the luminal aspect (*left*) of three cells lining a tubule of clear cell carcinoma. Note the hobnail arrangement of cells and the short, thick microvilli. Terminal tight junctions and desmosomes are seen between the cells. Mitochondria (M) and lamellae of granular endoplasmic reticulum, some of which are stacked in parallel rows (*arrows*), are prominent, as are ribosomes and glycogen granules. ×20,000. (Reprinted by permission of Silverberg, Ref. 161.)

is grossly cystic. Brenner tumors are not encapsulated but do produce compression of the surrounding ovarian tissue.

Microscopic Appearance. Brenner tumors are comprised of solid to partly cystic epithelial nests surrounded by a stroma composed of bundles of tightly packed, spindle-shaped cells. The epithelial cells are polygonal and of squamoid type, with pale, eosinophilic cytoplasm and oval nuclei that have distinct nucleoli and longitudinal grooving, the so-called coffee-bean appearance (Figs. 18.61 and 18.62). The nuclear grooving is also present

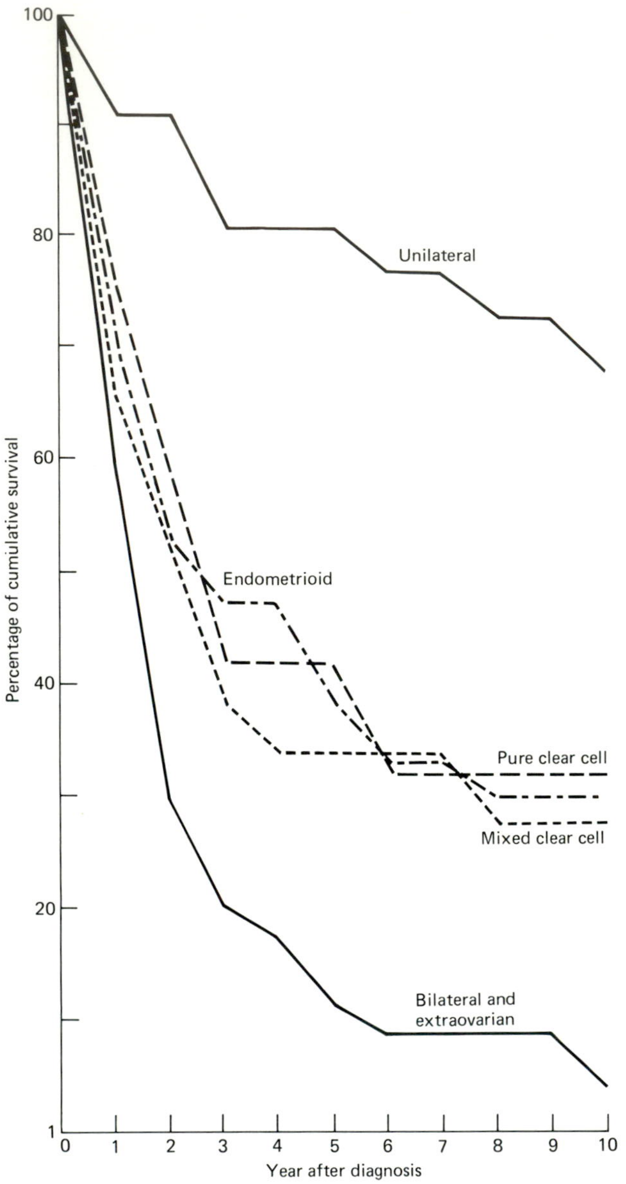

FIG. 18.59. Cumulative survival of patients with pure clear cell carcinoma, mixed clear cell carcinoma (a combination of focal and predominant clear cell groups), and endometrioid carcinoma of the ovary. The unilateral line refers to a combination of all types of neoplasms confined to one ovary. Bilateral and extraovarian group includes tumors of all types either unilateral with spread beyond the ovary, or bilateral with or without spread beyond the ovary. (Reprinted by permission of Czernobilsky et al., Ref. 40.)

in Walthard cell nests. It is caused by a peculiar infolding of the nuclei[6] and can be observed in other epithelial or mesothelial cells as well. Mitotic figures and epithelial atypism are not identified.

The association of Brenner tumors with other cystic neoplasms, especially mucinous cystadenomas and cystic teratomas, is well known. In Silverberg's study,[162] such

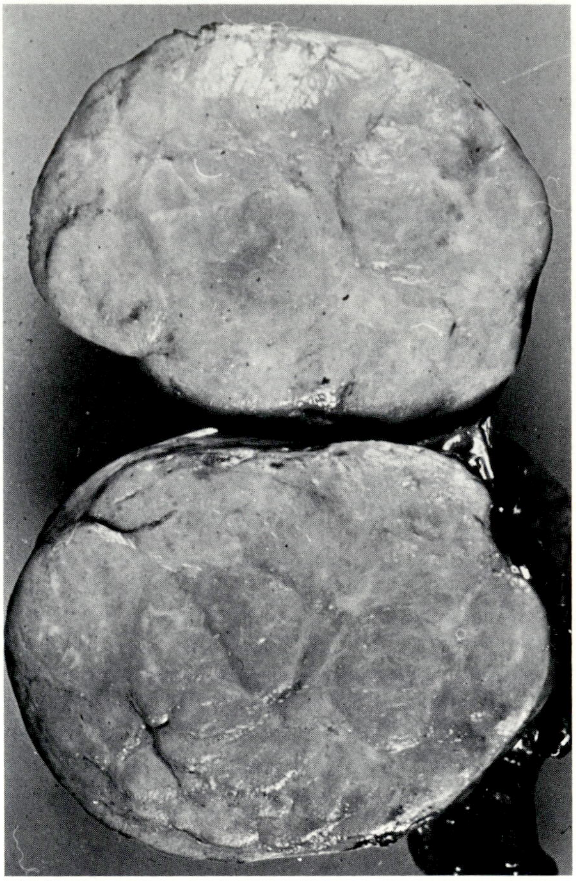

FIG. 18.60. Cut section of a solid, nodular Brenner tumor. (Courtesy of Dr. H. T. Enterline.)

an association was observed in the ipsilateral ovary in 19 (33%) of 60 patients. Six of the neoplasms was mucinous cystadenomas and three were cystic teratomas.

Ultrastructure. Electron microscopic studies of Brenner tumors[22,129,130] show similarities between their epithelial elements and those of urothelium and Walthard cell nests (Figs. 18.63 and 18.64), an observation that is consistent with the origin of the Brenner tumor from metaplastic coelomic epithelium.

Behavior and Treatment. Treatment of the benign Brenner tumor is oophorectomy.

METAPLASTIC BRENNER TUMOR

This variant described by Roth et al.[134] shows an unusual degree of cyst formation. The epithelial nests of transitional type demonstrate prominent mucinous metaplasia (Fig. 18.65). In areas, the metaplasia is of a ciliated, columnar, nonmucinous type. Although the glandular pattern is complex, nuclear atypia is not present, and there is no stromal invasion. Areas of typical Brenner tumor are always present. This variant differs from Bren-

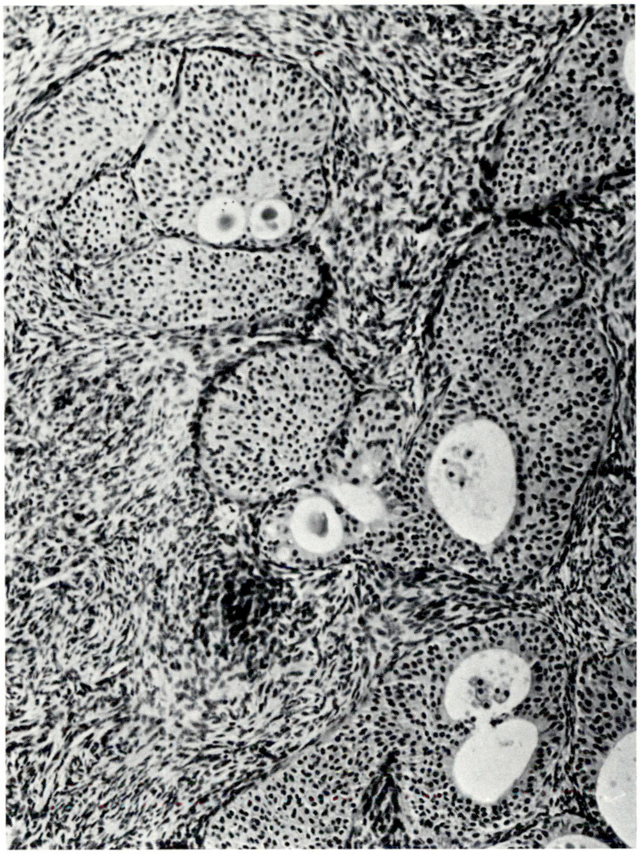

Fig. 18.61. Brenner tumor showing a solid and partly cystic epithelial nest in the dense fibrous stroma.

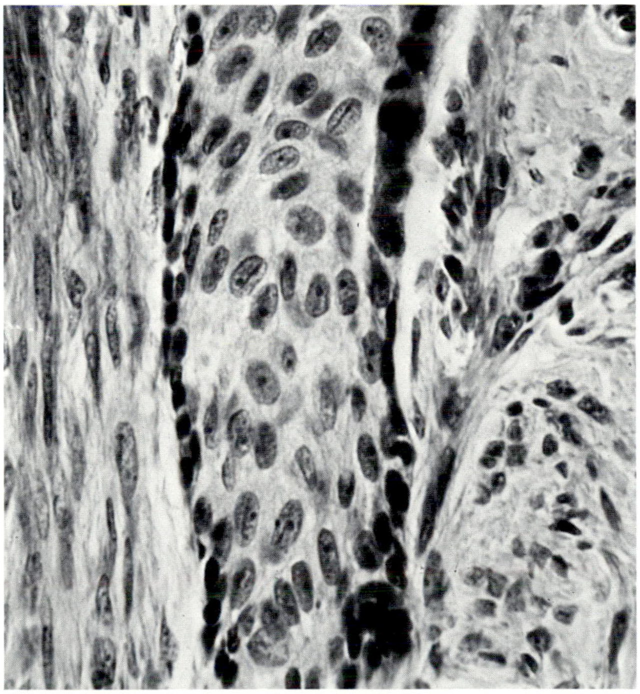

Fig. 18.62. Detail of an epithelial nest of a Brenner tumor demonstrating typical longitudinal grooving, or coffee-bean appearance, of the nuclei.

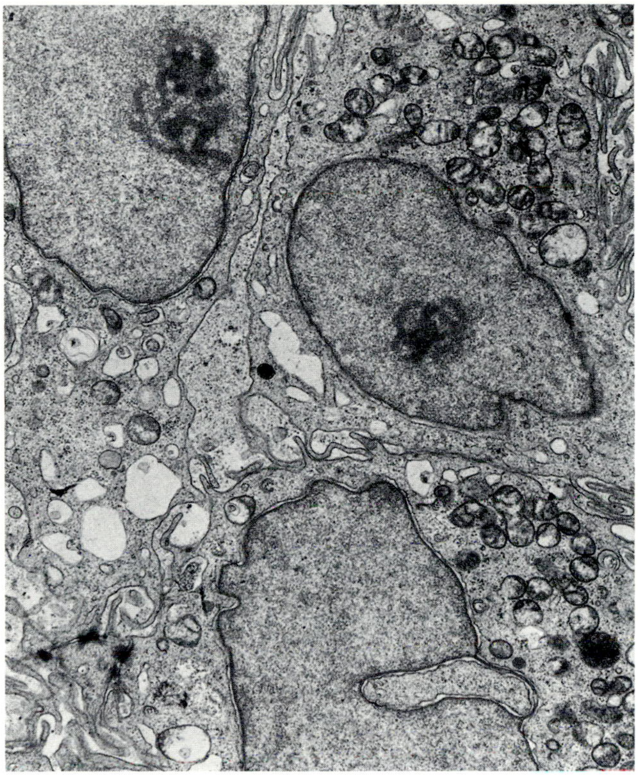

Fig. 18.63. Electron micrograph of the epithelial cells of a Brenner tumor. The nuclei are irregular and have evenly distributed chromatin and a prominent nucleolus. A cytoplasmic invagination into the nucleus is present in the cell on the *right*. Intercellular spaces are abundant. ×10,800. (Reprinted by permission from Roth, Ref. 135.)

ner tumors with associated mucinous cystadenoma, which forms a distinct, separate cystic neoplasm.

The mean age of the four patients described by Roth et al.[134] was 65. All tumors were unilateral and ranged in size from 8 to 32 cm in maximum dimension. The 5-year follow-up of these patients was 100%.

Proliferating Brenner Tumor

In 1971, Roth and Sternberg[132] described three unusual Brenner tumors, which on the basis of histologic characteristics were designated "proliferating" and placed in an intermediate category between the benign and malignant forms. The patients were 78, 66, and 59 years old.

The ovarian tumors were all unilateral and cystic and measured from about 12 to 25 cm in diameter. Papillary projections into the lumen of the cyst could be grossly recognized in two of the cases.

The papillary portions of the tumors, as well as parts of the cystic areas, were lined by 8–20 layers of well-differentiated transitional-type epithelium, with only mild focal atypia (Figs. 18.66 and 18.67). A few mitotic figures were observed. There was no stromal invasion.

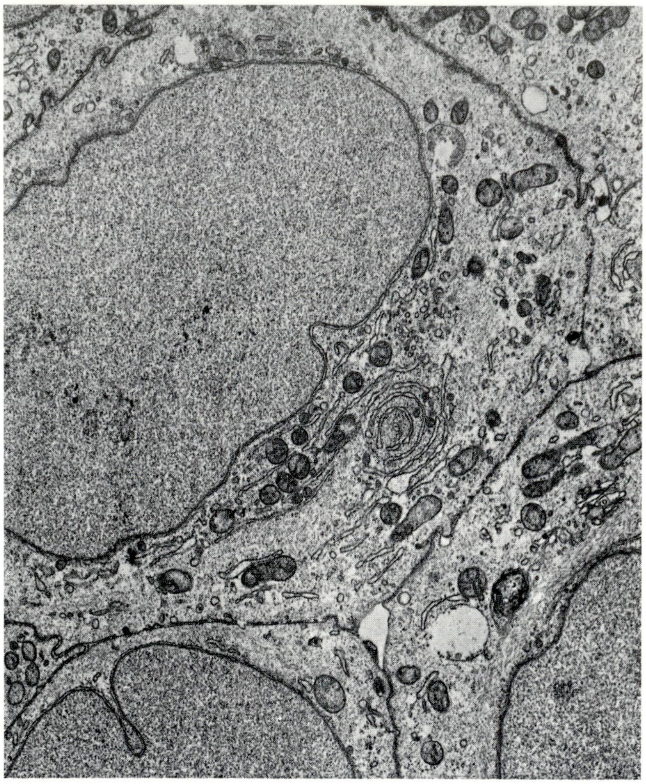

FIG. 18.64. Electron micrograph of the urothelial cells of the human urinary bladder. Note the general similarity to the epithelium of the Brenner tumor. The cells show a greater uniformity. Intercellular spaces, less abundant than in the Brenner tumor, are present at the angles between adjacent cells. A cytoplasmic invagination into the nucleus is present in the *lower left hand corner*. ×9200. (Reprinted by permission from Roth, Ref. 130.)

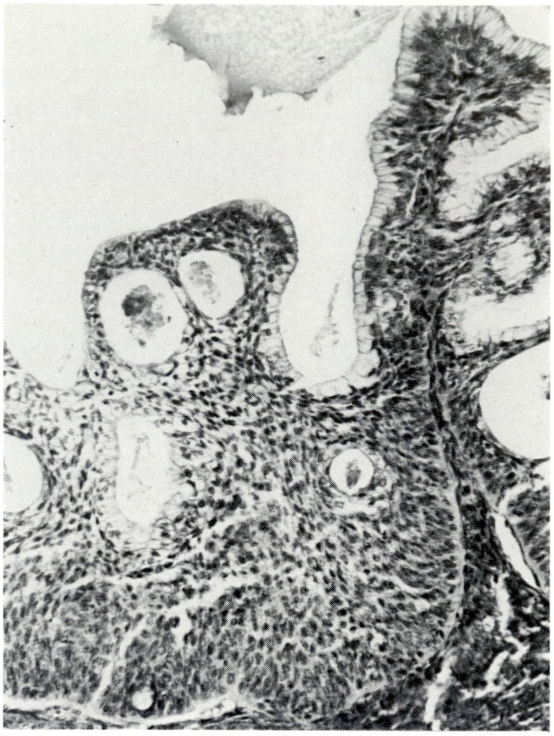

FIG. 18.65. Metaplastic Brenner tumor with a layer of mucinous columnar epithelium overlying the transitional epithelium. (Reprinted by permission of Roth et al., Ref. 134.)

Adjacent to these areas, typical Brenner tumors were observed in all three patients. Because of the close association with Brenner tumors and the urothelial characteristics of the proliferating elements, Roth and Sternberg[132] considered these lesions to represent a proliferating variant of Brenner tumors and found a few additional cases among previously reported malignant Brenner tumors. None of these patients developed recurrences.

Miles and Norris[107] and Hallgrimson and Scully[70] reported additional cases of proliferating Brenner tumors. Most of these tumors were also large and cystic, with polypoid masses projecting into the lumen. Treatment in these cases consisted of total abdominal hysterectomy with unilateral or bilateral salpingo-oophorectomy. Follow-up, which ranged from 1 month to 18 years, revealed no recurrences in any of the patients.

Proliferating Brenner tumors are histologically and clinically benign neoplasms. A reevaluation of a so-called proliferating Brenner tumor with metastases[127] revealed that the tumor was most likely malignant at the time

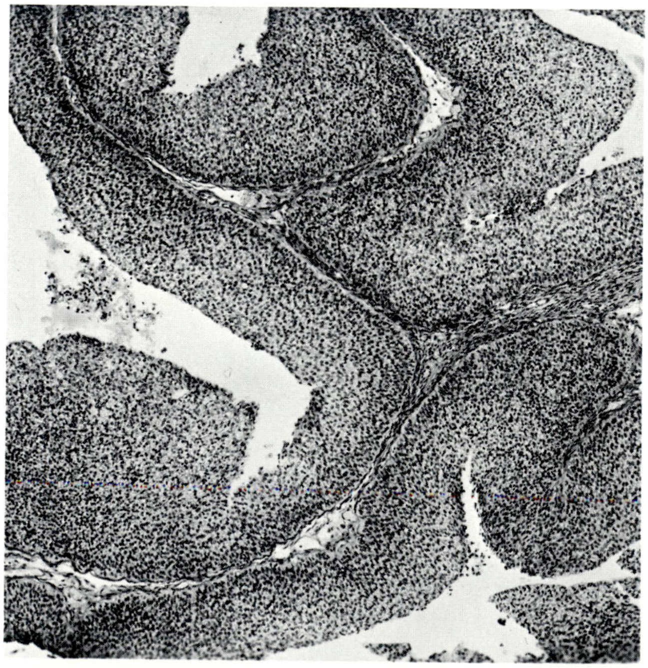

FIG. 18.66. Multilayered epithelium lining the cystic areas of a proliferating Brenner tumor. (Courtesy of Dr. H. J. Norris.)

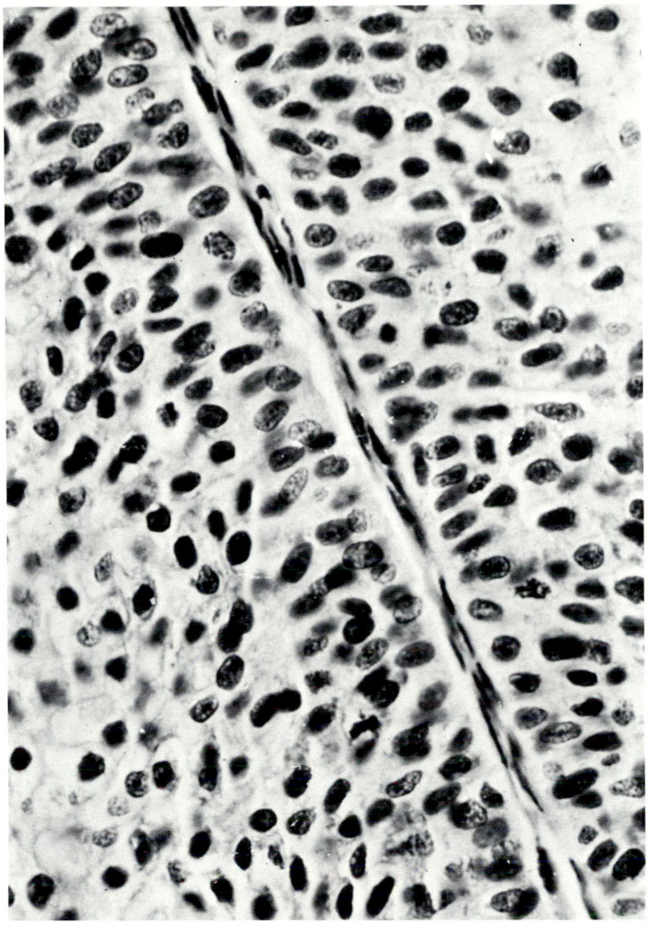

FIG. 18.67. Atypism of the epithelial elements of a proliferating Brenner tumor.

of its discovery.[131] Another case originally classified as borderline has also subsequently been placed in the malignant category.[152] Although these tumors were classified at one time as "borderline tumors" in an effort to comply with the WHO classification of ovarian tumors (Table 18.1), this does not seem justifiable on the basis of current experience.

Malignant Brenner Tumors

BRENNER TUMOR OF LOW MALIGNANT POTENTIAL (OF BORDERLINE MALIGNANCY)

Roth et al.[134] described four patients with this type of tumor. Their mean age was 61 years. All of the tumors were unilateral and varied from 8 to 20 cm in maximum dimension. Follow-up was inadequate in this small series.

As in proliferating Brenner tumors, tumors of LMP are cystic, with papillary fronds. However, in contrast to proliferating tumors, the epithelium resembles that of noninvasive papillary transitional cell carcinoma of the urinary bladder grade 3 or squamous cell carcinoma in situ (Fig. 18.68). Areas of proliferating, metaplastic, or typical benign Brenner tumor must be identified. On a morphologic basis, it appears from the study of Roth et al.[134] that Brenner tumors of LMP may develop from proliferating tumors by progressive anaplasia of the papillary epithelium. Because of the small number of reported cases of this entity and the absence so far of clinical evidence of malignant behavior, it should be emphasized that this category of Brenner tumors is based entirely on histologic criteria.

Malignant Brenner Tumor. This is a rare neoplasm, with only about 41 cases reported up to 1973.[107] Malignant Brenner tumors constituted 5% of all Brenner tumors in the Miles and Norris[107] series, but this probably does not represent its true frequency because of the consultative nature of AFIP material. Early reports of malignant Brenner tumors may possibly be reclassified now as proliferating or LMP Brenner tumors, whereas others may have been carcinomas arising in associated cystadenomas and not in the Brenner tumor itself.[76,174]

The average age of patients with malignant Brenner tumor is 60–65 years.[76,131]

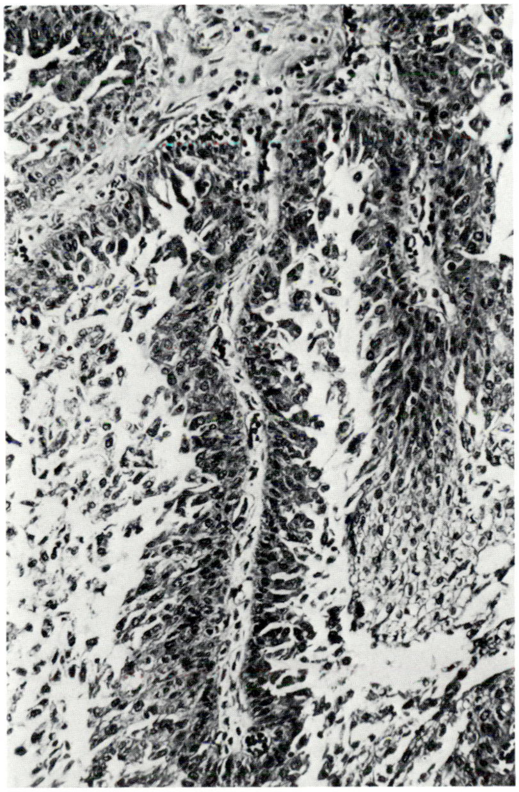

FIG. 18.68. Brenner tumor of LMP showing papillary areas with epithelial disarray, loss of cohesion, nuclear crowding, and atypia resembling high-grade noninvasive transitional cell carcinoma. (Reprinted by permission of Roth et al., Ref. 134.)

Gross Appearance. These are usually large, partly cystic, unilateral tumors. The cystic portions are frequently lined by friable, polypoid masses.

Microscopic Appearance. Because of the controversial aspects of this tumor, it is important to adopt strict histologic criteria before making the diagnosis. The criteria proposed by Hull and Campbell[75] are as follows: (1) frankly malignant histologic features must be present, (2) there must be intimate association between the malignant element and a benign Brenner tumor, (3) mucinous cystadenomas should preferably be absent or must be well separated from both the benign and the malignant Brenner tumor, and (4) stromal invasion by epithelial elements of the malignant Brenner tumor must be demonstrated.

It is of interest that in the series by Roth et al.,[131] well-differentiated tumors often occurred in close relationship to proliferating Brenner tumor and occasionally to areas of LMP. The malignant component consisted of transitional cell, squamous, or undifferentiated carcinoma or an admixture of these. In well-differentiated Brenner tumors, the degree of epithelial atypism was less than that of a grade 3 invasive transitional cell carcinoma, whereas in poorly differentiated tumors, the predominant cell type was high-grade transitional, squamous, glandular, or undifferentiated (Fig. 18.69).

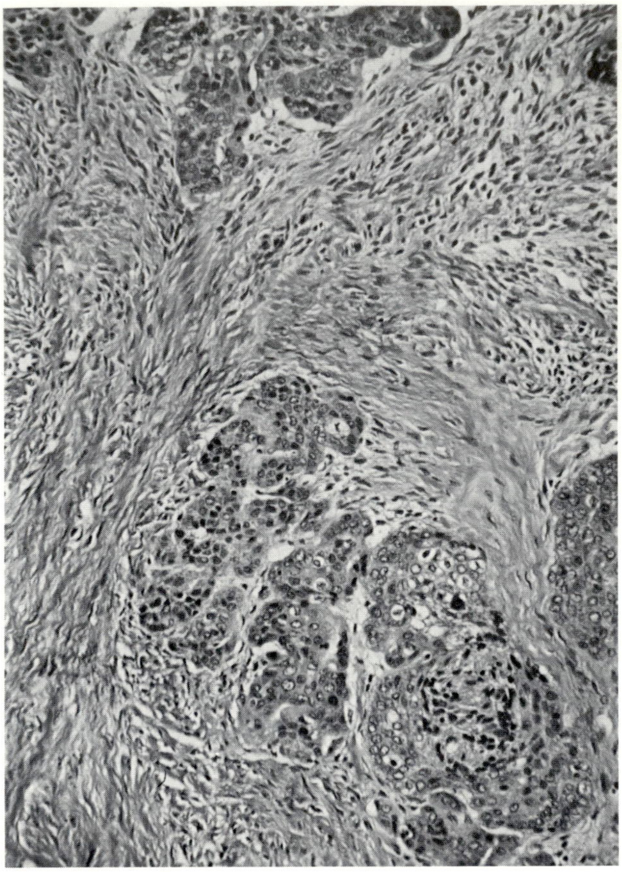

Fig. 18.69. Well-differentiated malignant Brenner tumor showing irregular confluent clusters of tumor cells infiltrating the stroma. (Reprinted by permission of Roth and Czernobilsky, Ref. 131.)

Behavior and Treatment. Treatment consists in most instances of total hysterectomy with bilateral salpingo-oophorectomy. Of 16 patients with follow-up in Idelson's series,[76] 4 were alive and well 1–3 years after the diagnosis was established. Of the 8 patients with malignant Brenner tumors in the Hallgrimson and Scully publication,[70] 2 died and 1 was alive with residual cancer. Three of seven patients in the study by Miles and Norris[107] died of their disease 3 months to 2 years after removal. Two of the eight patients reported by Roth et al.[131] died of metastases 10 months and 5 years after diagnosis.

Carcinoma Not Otherwise Classifiable

In contrast to the preceding categories of primary epithelial tumors of the ovary, each of which represents a distinct type of neoplasm, this last group is of malignant epithelial tumors that, because of a lack of any characteristic microscopic features or lack of differentiation cannot be classified under any of the previously discussed headings. Because the microscopic appearance of these neoplasms is adenocarcinomatous, they are classified as epithelial tumors. Many of these tumors are highly undifferentiated, and, therefore, the differential diagnosis between these adenocarcinomas and tumors of other origins, especially poorly differentiated granulosa cell tumors, can be difficult.[151] The major clinical and pathologic points of distinction between these two commonly misinterpreted tumors have been summarized by Young and Scully[178] as follows: 5% of granulosa cell tumors, but 25% of undifferentiated carcinomas are bilateral; 90% of granulosa cell tumors are stage I, whereas most anaplastic carcinomas are stages III and IV; nuclei of granulosa cell tumors are round to angular, pale, and commonly grooved, compared to the nuclei of undifferentiated carcinomas, which are hyperchromatic and pleomorphic, with many mitoses. Both intracellular and extracellular mucin are more characteristic for carcinoma than for granulosa cell tumors (see Chapter 19, Sex Cord–Stromal Ovarian Tumors).

The majority of nonclassifiable carcinomas represent poorly differentiated serous cystadenocarcinomas and endometrioid carcinomas, since these two neoplasms constitute about 50% of all malignant primary epithelial tumors of the ovary. Papillary or solid glandular patterns predominate in the tumors. In the Santesson and Kottmeier series,[143] they constituted 5.2% of all primary malignant epithelial ovarian neoplasms. As are most highly malignant ovarian neoplasms, the unclassifiable adenocarcinomas are usually large, partly cystic masses with areas of necrosis and hemorrhage. According to Kottmeier,[92] 54% of these tumors are bilateral. At the time of diagnosis many of these carcinomas have spread beyond the ovaries, resulting in a very poor prognosis.

Luteinized and Enzymatically Active Stromal Cells in Common Epithelial Tumors

A careful histologic examination of the stroma adjacent to or forming part of the various ovarian epithelial tumors reveals, in many instances, single or groups of lipid-containing luteinized cells (Fig. 18.70). It was speculated that the ovarian tumor stimulated the stromal cells to differentiate into such thecal or luteinized elements.[114] In 1958, Hughesdon[74] described serous, mucinous, clear cell, and endometrioid tumors, associated with what he termed "a thecal reaction" of the stroma. In four of six cases in which the uterus was available, the endometrium showed cystic hyperplasia. One of the patients demonstrated mild virilism. Such observations, as well as the high frequency of vaginal bleeding and the association of endometrial hyperplastic conditions in patients with ovarian epithelial neoplasms, suggest that some of these hitherto nonfunctioning tumors do demonstrate endocrine activity, which in most instances is of the estrogenic type and may originate in the luteinized stromal cells. The disappearance in a number of patients of the endocrine manifestations after surgical removal of the ovarian tumors[18,,27,159] further indicated that the hormonal synthesis originated in the epithelial neoplasms.

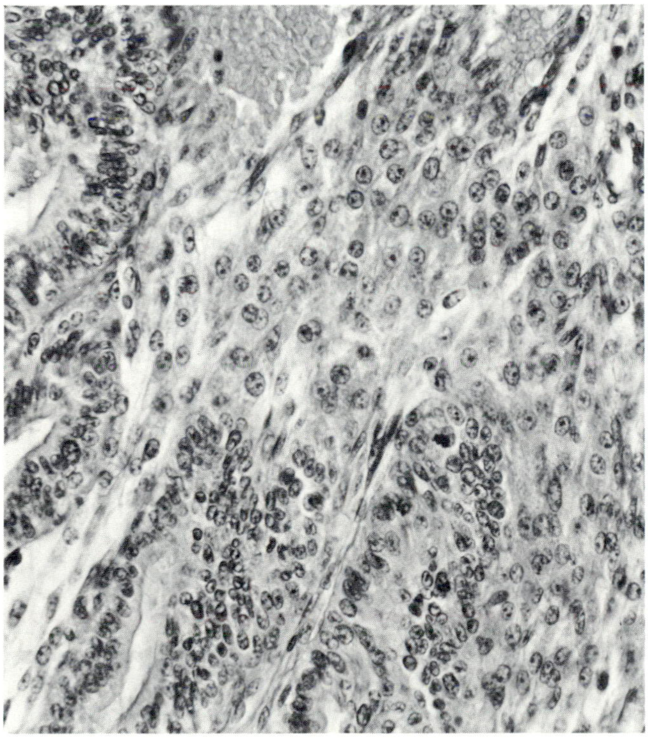

Fig. 18.70. Glands of endometrioid carcinoma surrounded by luteinized cells. (Reprinted by permission of Czernobilsky (1970) Utero-ovarian pathology in dysfunctional uterine bleeding. Clin Obstet Gynecol 13:416.)

Histochemical investigations of the luteinized stromal cells demonstrated that, in addition to their lipid content, these cells showed reduced diphosphopyridine nucleotidase (DPNH), glucose-6-phosphate (G6P) dehydrogenase, and 6-phosphogluconic acid (6PGA) dehydrogenase activity, possibly indicating steroid hormone synthesis.[177] Scully and Cohen[155] coined the term "enzymatically active stromal cells" (EASC) to describe stromal ovarian cells not necessarily containing lipid but showing strong oxidative enzyme activity. The enzymes demonstrated included isocitric dehydrogenase, G6P dehydrogenase, and lactic acid dehydrogenase. These cells, which can be present in the stroma of normal ovaries as well as in most epithelial ovarian neoplasms, probably represent a stage in the development of stromal lutein cells. A study by Pfleiderer and Teufel[123] revealed that EASC were detectable in 37% of 85 ovarian tumors, 66 of which were tumors of epithelial origin.

According to Janovski and Paramanandhan,[77b] who summarized the subject, EASC have been described in almost all the epithelial ovarian neoplasms but occurred most often in mucinous tumors. The observation by Ming and Goldman,[108] based on a review of the literature, that almost 50% of patients with Brenner tumors have had either endometrial hyperplasia, polyps, or carcinoma, all indicating hyperestrinism, is surprising, since this neoplasm has not been considered as hormonally active. Stromal theca cells were identified in only 7 of the 69 cases reviewed.

In conclusion, the correlation between hormonal activity and the presence of luteinized and enzymatically active stromal cells in ovarian epithelial neoplasms is far from perfect. In contrast to the occurrence of such cells in many ovarian epithelial tumors, the number of cases that clinically manifest endocrine activity, proven to be related to these neoplasms, is quite small.

Immunocytochemistry of Common Epithelial Tumors

Immunocytochemical methods have been used in common epithelial tumors as an adjuvant tool to conventional diagnostic techniques and for the purpose of achieving a better understanding of the origin and the nature of the neoplasms. The topics discussed include intermediate filaments, carcinoembryonic antigen (CEA), amylase, mucin antigens, and tumor-associated antigens.

Intermediate Filaments

The cytoplasm of vertebrate cells is composed, to a large extent, by the cytoskeleton, which includes actin-containing microfilaments, tubulin-containing microtubules, and filaments of an intermediate size. The last can be divided into five types: cytokeratin characteristic of epithelial cells, vimentin that occurs in mesenchymally derived cells, desmin typical of myogenic cells, neurofilaments found in neuronal cells, and glial filaments that are found in astrocytes.[57] During tumor development, the cell type specificity of intermediate filaments is largely conserved.[57,60] This property has made it possible to make use of immunohistochemical techniques to identify intermediate filaments as an aid in the differential diagnosis.[60,122]

In addition to being able to distinguish epithelial, mesenchymal, myogenic, neuronal, and glial neoplasms even in highly anaplastic neoplasms, the identification of the type of cytokeratin present in the tumor cell allows for an even more subtle distinction between epithelial neoplasms of different origins. This is due to the fact that, in contrast to the other intermediate filaments, the cytokeratin filaments are a complex family of at least 19 different polypeptides, which differ in their isoelectric pH values and their molecular weights.[110] A given epithelium can, therefore, be characterized by the specific pattern of its cytokeratin components.[173]

These methods of study have been applied, albeit in a limited way, to the study of ovarian neoplasms. Results have been variable mainly because of the mode of fixation, type of antibody used, and so on.[97] Altmannsberger et al.[2] demonstrated that formalin is the least suitable fixative, whereas alcohol is the most suitable for the demonstration of cytokeratins by the immunoperoxidase technique. This was also shown by Miettinen et al.,[106] who identified expression of cytokeratin in a variety of ethanol-fixed ovarian common epithelial tumors. Reproducibility can only be achieved when using cryostat sections of freshly frozen tissues[2,115] (preferably in isopentane precooled in liquid nitrogen) and with the use of specifically characterized antibodies. For example, Ganjei et al.[61] found in nonpredigested paraffin sections of formalin-fixed material that positive staining for cytokeratin was limited to Brenner tumors and to squamous components of endometrioid carcinoma, whereas a large variety of other ovarian common epithelial tumors did not stain. It has been unequivocally established that all epithelial cells, both benign and malignant, including those of the female genital tract, can be stained for cytokeratins, which are also identified in two-dimensional gels.[111,173] The results of Ganjei et al.[61] were probably due to alteration of the antigenicity of keratin by formalin as well as the use of an antibody that reacted with cytokeratins found in squamous-type epithelium only. This may also explain the results of Schlegel et al.,[148,149] who achieved strong positive staining for cytokeratin only in formalin-fixed, paraffin-embedded histologic sections of squamous and transitional epithelium, as well as in mesothelium.

Studies with fresh snap frozen tissue samples from the female genital tract, including ovarian epithelial neoplasms,[42,111] have shown that in all cases the epithelial components of the neoplasms were decorated by monoclonal broad-spectrum antibodies to cytokeratins as well as by monoclonal antibodies to cytokeratins staining simple, nonstratified epithelia (Fig. 18.71). In addition, two-

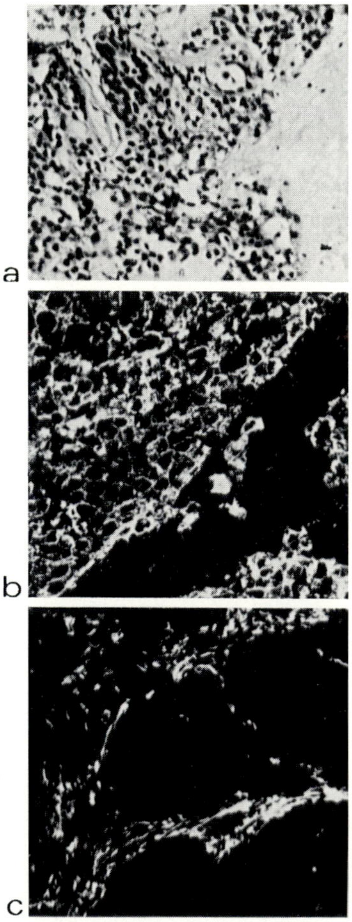

FIG. 18.71. *a*. Anaplastic tumor of ovary with sheets of tumor cells lacking architectural pattern. *b*. Cytokeratin staining of tumor cells with monoclonal cytokeratin antibody $K_G8.13$. Stroma is negative. *c*. Positive staining limited to stroma of tumor with guinea pig antibody to human vimentin. Tumor itself is negative. *b*. and *c*. Immunofluorescent photomicrographs of frozen sections of the neoplasm. This staining pattern established the epithelial nature of this neoplasm. (Reprinted by permission of Czernobilsky et al., Ref. 42.)

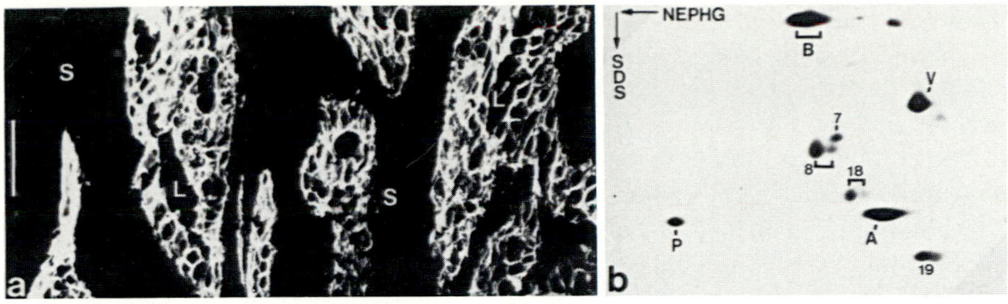

FIG. 18.72. *a*. Monoclonal cytokeratin antibody $K_G8.13$ staining tumor cells of serous adenocarcinoma of ovary. Immunofluorescent microscopy of frozen section. S, stroma; *bar* = 40 μm. *b*. Two-dimensional gel electrophoresis of cystosketal proteins of microdissected region from same tumor as *a*, showing presence of cytokeratin polypeptides Nos. 7, 8, 18, and 19. NEPHG, direction of first dimension using nonequilibrium pH gradient electrophoresis (basic polypeptides are to the left, acidic ones to the right); SDS, direction of second dimension in the presence of sodium dodecyl sulfate. Brackets indicate major isoelectric variants of the same polypeptide. V, vimentin from stromal area. Polypeptides added as internal markers for coelectrophoresis are P, 3-phosphoglycerokinase; B, bovine serum albumin; A, rabbit alpha-actin. Highly sensitive silver staining. [Reprinted from Moll R, Levy R, Czernobilsky B, Hohlweg-Majert P, Dallenbach, Hallweg G, France WW (1983) Cytokeratins of normal epithelia and some neoplasms of the female genital tract. Lab Invest 49: 599, © by US and Canadian Academy of Pathology.]

dimensional gel electrophoresis of normal ovarian surface epithelium and of a variety of common epithelial tumors of the ovary[42,111] has shown that these contained cytokeratin polypeptides Nos. 7, 8, 18, and 19 (numbered according to the catalogue of Moll et al.[110]) (Fig. 18.72). These data add additional support to the view that common epithelial tumors of the ovary do indeed originate from the surface epithelium.

The practical application of the demonstration of intermediate filaments in ovarian tumors is manifold. Anaplastic carcinomas that express only cytokeratins can be differentiated from sarcomas that are characterized by vimentin and, in the case of myogenic sarcomas, by desmin.[21,42] Granulosa cell tumors, as well as certain germ cell tumors that can mimic anaplastic carcinomas, may also be correctly diagnosed by this method. For example, granulosa cell tumors may contain vimentin[106] or show expression of both vimentin and cytokeratin.[35] Furthermore, the identification of intermediate filaments, particularly the type of cytokeratin protein present in tumor cells, may be used to determine the source of metastatic tumors to the ovary.

Carcinoembryonic Antigen

Although carcinoembryonic antigen (CEA) is neither organ nor tumor specific, its detection in tissue sections may be important for follow-up because it makes it possible to evaluate response to treatment by measurements of CEA serum levels. All common epithelial tumors of the ovary, except serous tumors and some anaplastic carcinomas, contain CEA, especially mucinous tumors[28] (Fig. 18.73). Of primary mucinous tumors studied by Charpin et al.[28] with a monoclonal antibody to CEA,

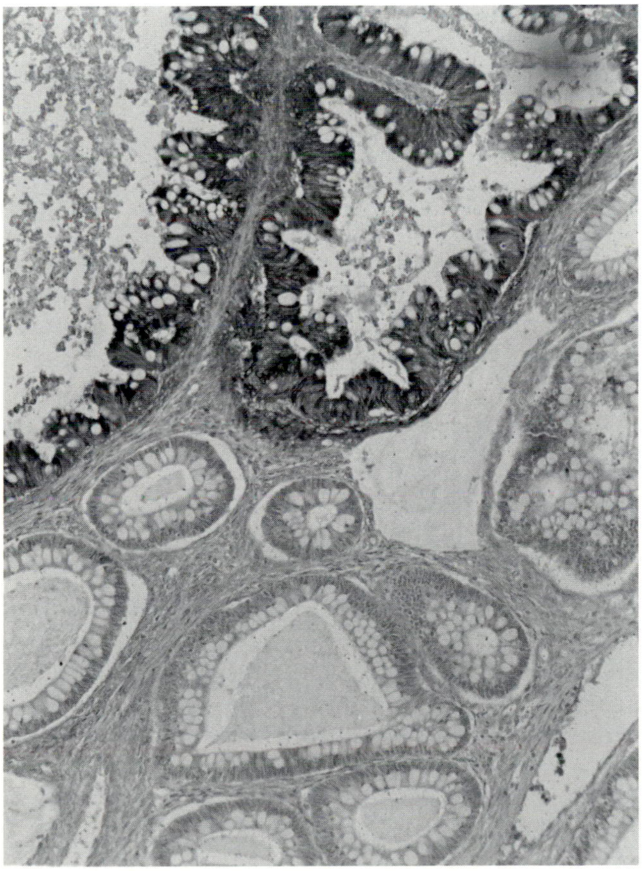

FIG. 18.73. Mucinous cystadenoma showing positive staining of tumor cells with CEA identified by black intracytoplasmic deposit. Not all of the neoplastic glands contain CEA. (Courtesy of Dr. R. Kurman.)

62% were CEA positive, and of these 15% of benign, 80% of carcinomas of LMP, and 100% of carcinomas showed CEA positivity. In the same series, 30% of endometrioid carcinomas, 50% of mesodermal mixed tumors, 14% of clear cell carcinomas, and 36% of Brenner tumors were CEA positive. Similar results were obtained by Shevchuk et al.[160] and Fenoglio et al.[51] It is of interest that the cellular localization of CEA in benign mucinous and Brenner tumors differs from that seen in their malignant counterparts.[28] Thus, in the benign tumors, CEA is localized on the luminal surface of the cells, probably because of its presence in the glycocalyx, whereas in carcinomas of LMP and in carcinomas, it is found throughout the cytoplasm in a diffuse fashion. Attempts have been made to make use of CEA activity as a diagnostic tool in the differential diagnosis of carcinomas of LMP and carcinoma. Dietel[46] found that 70% of ovarian adenocarcinomas but only 10% of borderline tumors showed CEA positivity. Unfortunately CEA cannot be used to differentiate primary from metastatic ovarian adenocarcinoma, since the latter is frequently from the breast or gastrointestinal tract, where CEA is prominent.[28,51]

Amylase

Alpha-amylase has been identified in secretions of the fallopian tube and tube-like epithelia of müllerian origin.[66] Subsequently, it was also found in benign ovarian serous tumors as well as in serous carcinomas of LMP and serous carcinomas[25,172] (Fig. 18.74). The relationship of amylase to fallopian tube as well as to tube-like epithelium, such as is encountered in serous tumors, is further borne out by the staining of carcinoma of the fallopian tube and of serous type papillary carcinoma of the endometrium with antiamylase.[172]

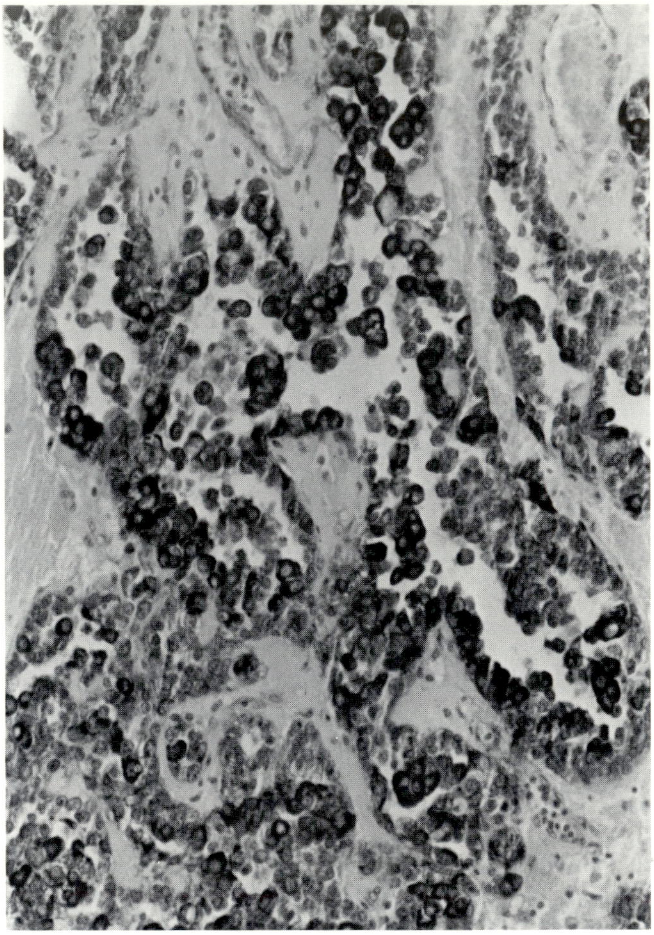

FIG. 18.74. Alpha-amylase staining of tumor cells of a serous adenocarcinoma. (Courtesy of D. M. Nadji.)

Mucin Antigens

Ueda et al.[170] stained benign mucinous tumors, mucinous carcinomas of LMP, and mucinous carcinomas for intestinal mucin antigens (IMA), which are specific for goblet cells of the normal intestinal mucosa,[113] and for mucin antigen M_1, which is associated primarily with ovarian mucinous cystadenoma.[12] Their results showed that in all the various types of mucinous tumors examined, many cells were positive for M_1 mucin antigen. IMA was positive only in a few goblet cells regardless of argyrophil cells and not in all of the neoplasms. Although it was hoped that studies such as this might settle the issue of müllerian versus monophyletic teratomatous origin of ovarian mucinous tumors, the results obtained with these antibodies have so far not contributed to elucidating their histogenesis.

Tumor-Associated Antigens

As in other neoplasms, tumor-associated antigens are also expressed in ovarian epithelial tumors. Bast et al.[14] described OC 125, a murine IgG_1 monoclonal antibody that was raised against an ovarian carcinoma cell line derived from ascites of a patient with serous cystadenocarcinoma. Kabawat et al.[81,82] demonstrated the reactivity of this antibody with ovarian serous, endometrioid, undifferentiated carcinomas, and one of four clear cell tumors. No reactivity was found in mucinous tumors or in any of the nonepithelial ovarian tumors tested. In fetal and adult tissues, this antibody reacted with the peritoneal lining, pleura, and pericardium, whereas in adults, it also reacted with epithelium of fallopian tubes, endometrium, endocervix, and tumors derived thereof. Only occasional nongynecologic tumors showed a positive reaction. Another monoclonal antibody that is specific for mucinous tumors only has been reported by Bhattacharaya et al.[19] These antibodies, although not exclusively specific for ovarian carcinomas, can occasionally be of some diagnostic help. In addition, tumor-associated antigens supply the clinician with a tool for monitoring the course of treatment with serologic immunoassays.

Extraovarian Peritoneal Papillary and Glandular Lesions Not Associated with Predominant Ovarian Common Epithelial Tumors

Multiple extraovarian papillary and glandular lesions on the peritoneum in association with a primary serous papillary carcinoma of the ovaries raise the question of whether this represents metastatic spread or synchronous tumor formation (Fig. 18.75), since it is known that multiple peritoneal lesions may arise in the absence of ovarian neoplasms (see Chapter 17, Endometriosis). Foyle et al.[56] described 25 such cases, which presented a spectrum ranging from well-differentiated mesotheliomas to serous papillary carcinomas. Fifteen of these patients died a few months to 29 years after the diagnosis was established. In a series of 9 cases, August et al.[7] found histologic evidence of malignancy that resembled serous ovarian tumors, showing papillary and glandular components with prominent psammoma bodies. These foci also displayed some ultrastructural features shared by both serous ovarian tumors and malignant mesotheliomas. The authors concluded that the peritoneal tumors probably arose from stimulated mesothelial cells. The patients' ages ranged from 53 to 87 years, three showed progressive disease, and a fourth patient died of abdominal malignancy within 2 months of diagnosis. The question of whether or not these peritoneal lesions should be classified as mesotheliomas was also raised by Kannerstein et al.,[83] who reported 15 such cases and preferred not to group them with mesothelial tumors.

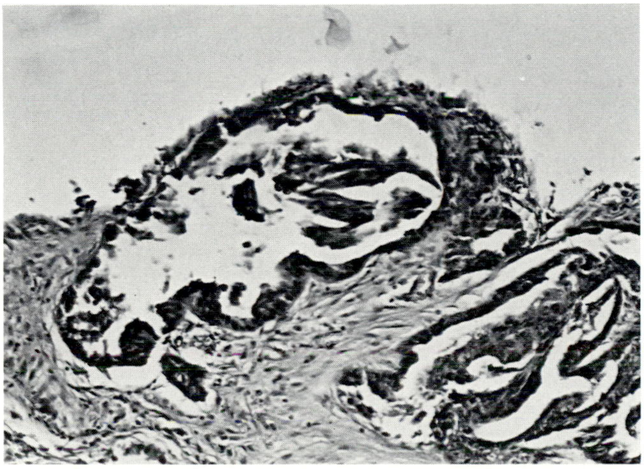

FIG. 18.75. Foci of crowded irregular glands with some papillary projections on peritoneal surface. In this case, no ovarian or other abnominal neoplasms were present.

The arguments favoring or opposing the classification of peritoneal papillary lesions in women as "mesotheliomas" as opposed to "serous surface papillary carcinoma" appear to be mainly semantic, since it has been established that the ovarian surface epithelium and the peritoneal mesothelium are structurally similar.[20] Thus, it can be surmised that stimuli responsible for proliferation and metaplasia of the ovarian surface epithelium culminating in the development of the common epithelial tumors can also affect extraovarian mesothelium in a similar manner. The association of ovarian endometriosis with unusual ovarian and peritoneal epithelial glandular inclusions may constitute an example of such a common stimulus.[89]

Aside from the multiple focal extraovarian peritoneal lesions that fulfil histologic criteria for malignancy and may also behave in a malignant fashion,[7,56] it is not unusual to find, during laparotomies, tiny peritoneal proliferations that histologically are consistent with benign or so-called borderline serous lesions or cannot be accurately classified because of their minute size. These may in some cases involve the ovarian surface to some extent, and some have designated these as "endosalpingiosis"[152f] (see Chapter 17, Endometriosis). In such cases, if a primary ovarian tumor can be ruled out, no further treatment is indicated, but patients should be followed. Most of these cases have a benign clinical course.

Acknowledgment. I thank Ms. Rene Satanower for excellent secretarial assistance in the preparation of this chapter.

References

1. Allen MS, Hertig AT (1949) Carcinoma of the ovary. Am J Obstet Gynecol 58: 640
2. Altmannsberger M, Osborn M, Schauer A, Weber K (1981) Antibodies to different intermediate filament proteins. Cell-type specific markers in paraffin-embedded tissues. Lab Invest 45: 427
3. Anderson C, Cameron HM, Neville AM, Simpson HW (1967) Mixed mesodermal tumors of the ovary. J Pathol Bacteriol 93: 301
4. Anderson MC, Langley FA (1970) Mesonephroid tumors of the ovary. J Clin Pathol 23: 210
5. Arey LB (1961) The origin and form of the Brenner tumor. Am J Obstet Gynecol 81: 743
6. Arey LB (1943) Nature and significance of grooved nuclei of Brenner tumors and Walthard cell islands. Am J Obstet Gynecol 45: 614
7. August CZ, Murad TM, Newton M (1985) Multiple focal extraovarian serous carcinoma. Int J Gynecol Pathol 4: 11

8. Aure JC, Høeg K, Kalstad P (1971) Psammoma bodies in serous carcinoma of the ovary. A prognostic study. Am J Obstet Gynecol 109: 113
9. Aure JC, Høeg K, Kalstad P (1971) Clinical and histologic studies of ovarian carcinoma. Long-term follow-up of 990 cases. Obstet Gynecol 37: 1
10. Baak JPA, Blanco AA, Kurver PHY, Langley FA, Boon ME, Lindeman J, Overdiep SH, Nieuwlaat A, Brekelmans E (1981) Quantitation of borderline and malignant mucinous ovarian tumors. Histopathology 5: 353
11. Bagley CM, Young RD, Canellos GP, DeVita VT (1972) Treatment of ovarian carcinoma: Possibilities for progress. N Engl J Med 287: 856
12. Bara J, Malarewicz A, Loisillier F, Burton P (1977) Antigens common to human ovarian mucinous cyst fluid and gastric mucosa. Br J Cancer 36: 49
13. Barnhill D, Heller P, Brzozowski P, Advani H, Gallup D, Park R (1985) Epithelial ovarian carcinoma of low malignant potential. Obstet Gynecol 65: 53
14. Bast RC, Fenny M, Lazarus H, Nadler LM, Colvin RB, Knapp RC (1981) Reactivity of a monoclonal antibody with human ovarian carcinoma. J Clin Invest 68: 1351
15. Bell DA, Scully RE (1985) Atypical and borderline endometrioid adenofibromas of the ovary. A report of 27 cases. Am J Surg Pathol 9: 205
16. Bell DA, Scully RE (1985) Benign and borderline clear cell adenofibroma of the ovary. Cancer 56: 2922
17. Berge T, Borglin NE (1967) Brenner tumors: Histogenetic and clinical studies. Cancer 20: 308
18. Bettinger HF, Jacobs J (1946) A contribution to the problem of masculinization. Med J Aust 1: 10
19. Bhattacharaya M, Chatterjee SK, Barlow JJ, Fugi H (1982) Monoclonal antibodies recognizing tumor-associated antigen in human ovarian mucinous cystadenocarcinoma. Cancer Res 42: 1650
20. Blaustein A (1984) Peritoneal mesothelium and ovarian surface cells—Shared characteristics. Int J Gynecol Pathol 3: 361
21. Bonazzi del Pogetto C, Virtanen F, Lehto V-P, Wahlström T, Saksela E (1983) Expression of intermediate filaments in ovarian and uterine tumors. Int J Gynecol Pathol 1: 359
22. Bransilver BR, Ferenczy A, Richart RM (1974) Brenner tumors and Walthard cell nests. Arch Pathol 98: 76
23. Bransilver BR, Ferenczy A, Richart RM (1973) Female genital tract remnants: An ultrastructural comparison of hydatid of Morgagni and mesonephric ducts and tubules. Arch Pathol 96: 255
24. Brenner F (1907) Das oophoroma folliculare. Frankfurt Z Pathol 1: 150
25. Bruns DE, Mills SE, Savory J (1982) Amylase in fallopian tube and serous ovarian neoplasm. Immunohistochemical localization. Arch Pathol Lab Med 106: 617
26. Campbell JS, Magner D, Fournier P (1961) Adenoacanthoma of ovary and uterus occurring as coexistent or sequential primary neoplasms. Cancer 14: 817
27. Cariker M, Dockerty MB (1954) Mucinous cystadenomas and mucinous cystadenocarcinomas of the ovary: A clinical pathologic study of 355 cases. Cancer 7: 302
28. Charpin C, Bhan AK, Zurawski VR Jr, Scully RE (1982) Carcinoembryonic antigen (CEA) and carbohydrate determinant 19–9 (CA 19–9) localization in 121 primary and metastatic ovarian tumors: An immunohistochemical study with the use of monoclonal antibodies. Int J Gynecol Pathol 1: 231
29. Clement PB, Scully RE (1978) Extrauterine mesodermal (müllerian) adenosarcoma. A clinicopathologic analysis of five cases. Am J Clin Pathol 69: 276
30. Colgan JY, Norris HJ (1983) Ovarian epithelial tumors of low malignant potential: A review. Int J Gynecol Pathol 1: 367
31. Compton HL, Fink FM (1970) Serous adenofibroma and cystadenofibroma of the ovary. Obstet Gynecol 36: 636
32. Cummins PA, Fox H, Langley FA (1974) An electron microscopic study of the endometrioid adenocarcinoma of the ovary and a comparison of its fine structure with that of normal endometrium and of adenocarcinoma of the endometrium. J Pathol 113: 165
33. Czernobilsky B (1977) Cystadenofibroma, adenofibroma and malignant adenofibroma of the ovary. Pathol Ann 12: 207–212
34. Czernobilsky B (1982) Endometrioid neoplasia of the ovary: A reappraisal. Int J Gynecol Pathol 1: 203
35. Czernobilsky B, Moll R, Leppien G, Schweikhart G, Franke WW. Desmosomal plaque-associated vimentin filaments in human ovarian granulosa cell tumors of various histologic patterns. Am J Pathol (In press)
36. Czernobilsky B, LaBarre GC (1968) Carcinosarcoma and mixed mesodermal tumor of the ovary. A clinicopathologic analysis of 9 cases. Obstet Gynecol 31: 21
37. Czernobilsky B, Borenstein R, Lancet M (1974) Cystadenofibroma of the ovary. A clinicopathologic study of 34 cases and comparison with serous cystadenoma. Cancer 34: 1971
38. Czernobilsky B, Dgani R, Roth LM (1983) Ovarian mucinous cystadenocarcinoma with mural nodules of carcinomatous derivation. A light and electron microscopic study. Cancer 51: 141
39. Czernobilsky B, Gillespie JT, Roth LM (1982) Adenosarcoma of the ovary. A light and electron microscopic study with a review of the literature. Diagn Gynecol Obstet 4: 25
40. Czernobilsky B, Silverman BB, Enterline HT (1970) Clear-cell carcinoma of the ovary. A clinicopathologic analysis of pure and mixed forms and comparison with endometrioid carcinoma. Cancer 25: 762
41. Czernobilsky B, Silverman BB, Mikuta JJ (1970) Endometrioid carcinoma of the ovary. A clinicopathologic study of 75 cases. Cancer 26: 1141
42. Czernobilsky B, Moll R, Franke WW, Dallenbach-Hellweg G, Hohlweg-Majert P (1984) Intermediate filaments of normal and neoplastic tissues of the female genital tract with emphasis on problems of differential tumor diagnosis. Pathol Res Pract 179: 31
43. Dallenbach F, Komitowski D (1982) Digital picture analysis of borderline papillary serous cystadenomas of the ovary. In: Dallenbach G (ed) Ovarialtumoren. New York, Springer-Verlag, pp 158–166
44. Dehner LP, Norris HJ, Taylor HB (1971) Carcinosarcomas

and mixed mesodermal tumors of the ovary. Cancer 27: 207
45. Dictor M (1982) Ovarian malignant mixed mesodermal tumor: The occurrence of hyaline droplets containing α_1-antitrypsin. Hum Pathol 13: 930
46. Dietel M (1985) Discrimination between benign, borderline, and malignant epithelial ovarian tumors using tumor markers: An immunohistochemical study. Cancer Detect Prevent 6: 255
47. Dockerty MB (1954) Primary and secondary ovarian adenoacanthoma. Surg Gynecol Obstet 99: 392
48. Ehrlich CE (1985) Clinical management of ovarian cancer. In: Roth LM, Czernobilsky B (eds) Tumors and tumorlike conditions of the ovary. New York, Churchill Livingstone, pp 247–256
49. Fathalla MF (1967) Malignant transformation in ovarian endometriosis. J Obstet Gynaecol Br Commonw 74: 85
50. Fenoglio CM, Ferenczy A, Richart RM (1975) Mucinous tumors of the ovary. Ultrastructural studies of mucinous cystadenomas with histogenetic considerations. Cancer 36: 1709
51. Fenoglio CM, Crum CP, Pascal RR, Richart RM (1981) Carcinoembryonic antigen in gynecologic patients. II. Immunohistological expression. Diagn Gynecol Obstet 4: 291
52. Ferenczy A, Richart RM (1974) The female reproductive system. Dynamics of scan and transmission electron microscopy. New York, John Wiley and Sons, a: p 287, b: 291, c: pp 301–303, d: 308–309
53. Fine G, Clarke HD, Horn RC (1973) Mesonephroma of the ovary. A clinical, morphological, and histogenetic appraisal. Cancer 31: 398
54. Fisher ER, Krieger JS, Skirpan PJ (1955) Ovarian cystoma. Clinicopathologic observations. Cancer 8: 437
55. Fox H, Kazzaz B, Langley FA (1964) Argyrophil and argentaffin cells in the female genital tract and ovarian mucinous cysts. J Pathol Bacteriol 88: 479
56. Foyle A, Al-Yabi M, McCaughey WT (1981) Papillary peritoneal tumors in women. Am J Surg Pathol 5: 241
57. Franke WW, Schmid E, Osborn M, Weber K (1978) Different intermediate-sized filaments distinguished by immunofluorescence microscopy. Proc Natl Acad Sci USA 75: 5034
58. Friedlander ML, Taylor IW, Russell P, Musgrove EA, Hedley DH, Tattersall MHN (1983) Ploidy as a prognostic factor in ovarian cancer. Int J Gynecol Pathol 2: 55
59. Fu YS, Stock RJ, Reagan JW, Storaasli JP, Wentz WBC (1979) Significance of squamous components in endometrioid carcinoma of the ovary. Cancer 44: 614
60. Gabbiani G, Kapanci Y, Barrazone P, Franke WW (1981) Immunochemical identification of intermediate-sized filaments in human neoplastic cells: A diagnostic aid for the surgical pathologist. Am J Pathol 104: 206
61. Ganjei P, Nadji M, Penneys NS, Averette HE, Morales AR (1983) Immunoreactive prekeratin in Brenner tumors of the ovary. Int J Gynaecol Pathol 1: 353
62. Garcia-Bunnel R, Morris B (1964) Histochemical observation on mucin in human ovarian neoplasms. Cancer 17: 1108
63. Goldman RL (1970) A Brenner tumor of the testis. Cancer 26: 853
64. Gondos B (1971) Electron microscopic study of papillary serous tumors of the ovary. Cancer 27: 1455
65. Gray LA, Barnes ML (1967) Endometrioid carcinoma of the ovary. Obstet Gynecol 29: 694
66. Green CL (1957) Identification of alpha-amylase as a secretion of the human fallopian tube and "tube-like" epithelium of müllerian and mesonephric duct origin. Am J Obstet Gynecol 73: 402
67. Greene RR (1952) The diverse origins of Brenner tumors. Am J Obstet Gynecol 64: 878
68. Griffiths CT (1974) Surgical resection of tumor bulk in the primary treatment of ovarian carcinoma. In: Symposium on ovarian carcinoma. Natl Cancer Inst Monogr 42: 101
69. Gooneratne S, Sassone M, Blaustein A, Talerman A (1982) Serous surface papillary carcinoma of the ovary. A clinicopathologic study of 16 cases. Int J Gynecol Pathol 1: 258
70. Hallgrimson J, Scully RE (1972) Borderline and malignant Brenner tumors of the ovary. A report of 15 cases. Acta Pathol Microbiol Scand A [Suppl 80] 233: 56
71. Hart WR, Norris HJ (1973) Borderline and malignant mucinous tumors of the ovary. Histologic criteria and clinical behaviour. Cancer 31: 1031
72. Hayes D (1972) Mesonephroid tumors of the ovary. J Obstet Gynaecol Br Commonw 79: 728
73. Hertig AT, Gore H (1961) Atlas of tumor pathology, Section IX, Vol 33. Tumors of the female sex organs. Part 3: Tumors of the ovary and fallopian tube. Washington, DC, Armed Forces Institute of Pathology, pp 106–109
74. Hughesdon PE (1958) Thecal and allied reactions in epithelial ovarian tumors. J Obstet Gynaecol Br Commonw 65: 702
75. Hull MGR, Campbell CR (1973) The malignant Brenner tumor. Obstet Gynecol 42: 527
76. Idelson MG (1963) Malignancy in Brenner tumors of the ovary, with comments on histogenesis and possible estrogen production. Obstet Gynecol Surv 18: 246
77. Janovski NA, Paramanandhan TL (1973) Ovarian tumors. Tumors and tumor-like conditions of the ovaries, fallopian tubes and ligaments of the uterus. Stuttgart, Georg Thieme, a: p 32, b: pp 119–123
78. Jensen RD, Norris HJ (1972) Epithelial tumors of the ovary. Occurrence in children and adolescents less than 20 of age. Arch Pathol 94: 29
79. Jondahl WH, Dockerty MD, Randall CM (1950) Brenner tumors of the ovary: A clinicopathologic study of 31 cases. Am J Obstet Gynecol 60: 160
80. Joshi VV (1968) Primary Krukenberg tumor of the ovary. Review of literature and case report. Cancer 22: 1199
81. Kabawat SE, Bast RC, Welch WR, Knapp RC, Colvin RB (1983) Immunopathologic characterization of a monoclonal antibody that recognizes common surface antigens of human ovarian tumors of serous endometrioid and clear cell types. Am J Clin Pathol 79: 98
82. Kabawat SE, Bast RC, Bhan AK, Welch WR, Knapp RC, Colvin RB (1983) Tissue distribution of a coelomic-epithelium-related antigen recognized by the monoclonal antibody OC 125. Int J Gynecol Pathol 2: 275

83. Kannerstein M, Churg J, McCaughey WTE, Hill DP (1977) Papillary tumors of the peritoneum in women: Mesothelioma or papillary carcinoma. Am J Obstet Gynecol 127: 306
84. Kao GF, Norris HJ (1979) Unusual cystadenofibromas: Endometrioid, mucinous, and clear cell types. Obstet Gynecol 54: 729
85. Kao GF, Norris HJ (1978) Cystadenofibromas of the ovary with epithelial atypia. Am J Surg Pathol 2: 357
86. Kao GF, Norris HJ (1978) Benign and low grade variants of mixed mesodermal tumor (adenosarcoma) of the ovary and adnexal region. Cancer 42: 1314
87. Katzenstein A-LA, Mazur MT, Morgan TE, Kao MS (1978) Proliferative serous tumors of the ovary. Histologic features and prognosis. Am J Surg Pathol 2: 339
88. Kent SW, McKay DG (1960) Primary cancer of the ovary. Am J Obstet Gynecol 80: 430
89. Kerner H, Gaton E, Czernobilsky B (1981) Unusual ovarian, tubal and pelvic mesothelial inclusions in patients with endometriosis. Histopathology 5: 277
90. Klemi PJ, Meurman L, Grönroos M, Talerman A (1982) Clear cell (mesonephroid) tumors of the ovary with characteristics resembling endodermal sinus tumor. Int J Gynecol Pathol 1: 95
91. Kottmeier HL (1952) The classification and treatment of ovarian tumors. Acta Obstet Gynecol Scand 31: 313
92. Kottmeier HL (1968) Surgical management—Conservative surgery. Indications according to the type of the tumor. In: Gentil F, Junqueira AC (eds) Ovarian cancer. UICC Monograph Series, New York, Springer-Verlag, Vol 11, pp 157–164
93. Kottmeier HL (1965) The diagnosis and treatment of ovarian malignancies. Arch Pathol 37: 51
94. Kraus FT (1967) Gynecologic pathology. St. Louis, CV Mosby, p 333
95. Kurman RJ, Craig JM (1972) Endometrioid and clear cell carcinoma of the ovary. Cancer 29: 1653
96. Kurman RJ, Norris HJ (1982) Endometrial neoplasia: Hyperplasia and carcinoma. In: Blaustein A (ed) Pathology of the female genital tract, 2nd ed. New York, Springer-Verlag, pp 331–333
97. Kurman RJ, Ganjei P, Nadji M (1984) Contributions of immunocytochemistry to the diagnosis and study of ovarian neoplasms. Int J Gynecol Pathol 3: 3
98. Langley FA, Cummins PA, Fox H (1972) An ultrastructural study of mucin-secreting epithelia in ovarian neoplasms. Acta Pathol Microbiol Scand [Suppl 80] 233: 76
99. Lauchlan SL (1966) Histogenesis and histogenetic relationship of Brenner tumors. Cancer 19: 1628
100. Limber GK, King RE, Silverberg SG (1973) Pseudomyxoma peritonaei. A report of ten cases. Ann Surg. 178: 587
101. Long ME, Taylor HC (1964) Endometrioid carcinoma of the ovary. Am J Obstet Gynecol 90: 936
102. Long RT, Spratt JS, Dowling E (1969) Pseudomyxoma peritonaei: New concepts in management with a report of 17 patients. Am J Surg 117: 162
103. Malloy JJ, Dockerty MB, Welch JS, Hunt AB (1965) Papillary ovarian tumors. I. Benign tumors and serous and mucinous cystadenocarcinomas. Am J Obstet Gynecol 93: 867
104. McGee CT, Cromer DW, Greene RR (1962) Mesonephric carcinoma of the cervix—Differentiation from endocervical adenocarcinoma. Am J Obstet Gynecol 84: 358
105. Meyer R (1932) Über verschiedene Erscheinungsformen der als typus Brenner bekannten Eierstockgeschwulst, ihre Absonderung von den Granulosa-Zell Tumoren und Zuordnung unter andere Ovarialgeschwülste. Arch Gynaek 148: 541
106. Miettinen M, Lehto V-P, Virtanen I (1983) Expression of intermediate filaments in normal ovaries and ovarian epithelial, sex cord–stromal, and germinal tumors. Int J Gynecol Pathol 2: 64
107. Miles PA, Norris HJ (1972) Proliferative and malignant Brenner tumors of the ovary. Cancer 30: 174
108. Ming SC, Goldman H (1962) Hormonal activity of Brenner tumors in postmenopausal women. Am J Obstet Gynecol 83: 666
109. Minkowitz S, Cohen HM (1966) Adenocarcinoma within serous cystadenofibroma of the ovary. NY State J Med 66: 529
110. Moll R, Franke WW, Schiller DL, Geiger B, Krepler R (1982) The catalog of human cytokeratins: Patterns of expression in normal epithelia, tumors and cultured cells. Cell 31: 11
111. Moll R, Levy R, Czernobilsky B, Hohlweg-Majert P, Dallenbach-Hellweg G, Franke WW (1983) Cytokeratins of normal epithelia and some neoplasms of the female genital tract. Lab Invest 49: 599
112. Moore JG, Schifrin BS, Erez S (1965) Ovarian tumors in infancy, childhood and adolescence. Am J Obstet Gynecol 93: 850
113. Mori T, Inaji H, Nakajo Y, Ikenaka T, Kosaki G (1979) Immunochemical studies of intestinal mucus antigen (IMA) and CEA-related antigens (NCA-2, NCA) in normal intestinal mucosa. Proc VII Intern Soc Oncodevelopmental Biology 179
114. Morris JM, Scully RE (1958) Endocrine pathology of the ovary. St. Louis, CV Mosby, pp 131–139
115. Nagle RB, Clark VA, McDaniel KM, Davis JR (1983) Immunohistochemical demonstration of keratins in human ovarian neoplasms. A comparison of methods. J Histochem Cytochem 31: 1010
116. Ng ABP (1968) Mixed carcinoma of the endometrium. Am J Obstet Gynecol 102: 506
117. Norris HJ, Taylor HB (1966) Mesenchymal tumors of the uterus. III. A clinical and pathologic study of 31 carcinosarcomas. Cancer 19: 1459
118. Norris HJ, Roth E, Taylor HB (1966) Mesenchymal tumors of the uterus. II. A clinical and pathologic study of 31 mixed mesodermal tumors. Obstet Gynecol 28: 57
119. Novak E, Woodruff JD, Novak ER (1954) Probable mesonephric origin of certain female genital tumors. Am J Obstet Gynecol 68: 1222
120. Novak ER, Woodruff JD (1959) Mesonephroma of the ovary—Thirty-five cases from the ovarian tumor registry of the American Gynecological Society. Am J Obstet Gynecol 77: 632
121. Novak ER, Woodruff JD (1979) Novak's gynecologic and

obstetric pathology with clinical and endocrine relations. Philadelphia, WB Saunders, pp 394–395
122. Osborn M, Weber K (1983) Tumor diagnosis by intermediate filament typing: A novel tool for surgical pathology. Lab Invest 48: 372
123. Pfleiderer A, Teufel G (1968) Incidence and histochemical investigation of enzymatically active cells in stroma of ovarian tumors. Am J Obstet Gynecol 102: 997
124. Prat J, Scully RE (1979) Sarcomas in ovarian mucinous tumors. A report of two cases. Cancer 44: 1327
125. Prat J, Scully RE (1979) Ovarian mucinous tumors with sarcoma-like mural nodules. A report of seven cases. Cancer 44: 1332
126. Prat J, Young RH, Scully RE (1982) Ovarian mucinous tumors with foci of anaplastic carcinoma. Cancer 50: 3007
127. Pratt-Thomas HR, Kreutner A, Underwood PB, Dowdeswell H (1976) Proliferative and malignant Brenner tumors of ovary. Report of two cases, one with Meigs' syndrome, review of literature and ultrastructural comparisons. Gynecol Oncol 4: 176
128. Reagan JW (1949) Histopathology of ovarian pseudomucinous cystadenoma. Am J Pathol 25: 689
129. Roth LM (1974) The Brenner tumor and the Walthard cell nest. An electron microscopic study. Lab Invest 31: 15
130. Roth LM (1971) Fine structure of the Brenner tumor. Cancer 27: 1482
131. Roth LM, Czernobilsky B (1985) Ovarian Brenner tumors. II. Malignant. Cancer 56: 592
132. Roth LM, Sternberg WH (1971) Proliferating Brenner tumors. Cancer 27: 687
133. Roth LM, Czernobilsky B, Langley FA (1981) Endometrioid adenofibromatous and cystadenofibromatous tumors. Benign, proliferating and malignant. Cancer 48: 1838
134. Roth LM, Dallenbach-Hellweg G, Czernobilsky B (1985) Ovarian Brenner tumors. I. Metaplastic, proliferating and of low malignant potential. Cancer 56: 582
135. Roth LM, Liban E, Czernobilsky B (1982) Ovarian endometrioid tumors mimicking Sertoli and Sertoli–Leydig cell tumors (sertoliform variant of endometrioid carcinoma). Cancer 50: 1322
136. Roth LM, Langley FA, Fox H, Wheeler JE, Czernobilsky B (1984) Ovarian clear cell adenofibromatous tumors: Benign, of low malignant potential, and associated with invasive clear cell carcinoma. Cancer 53: 1156
137. Rothman D, Blumenthal HT (1959) Serous adenofibroma and cystadenofibroma of the ovary. Report of five cases with malignant change in one. Obstet Gynecol 14: 389
138. Russell P (1979) The pathological assessment of ovarian neoplasms. I. Introduction to the common "epithelial" tumors and analysis of benign "epithelial" tumors. Pathology 11: 5
139. Russell P (1979) The pathological assessment of ovarian neoplasms. II. The proliferating "epithelial" tumors. Pathology 11: 251
140. Salazar H, Merkow LP, Walter WS, Pardo M (1974) Human ovarian neoplasms: Light and electron microscopic correlations. II. The clear cell tumor. Obstet Gynecol 44: 551
141. Sampson JA (1925) Endometrial carcinoma of the ovary arising in endometrial tissue in that organ. Arch Surg 10: 1
142. Santesson L (1961) Suggested classification of ovarian tumors. Meeting of the Cancer Committee of the International Federation of Gynecologists and Obstetricians. Stockholm, Sweden, August 24–26
143. Santesson L, Kottmeier HL (1968) General classification of ovarian tumors. In: Gentils F, Junqueira AC (eds) Ovarian cancer, UICC Monograph Series, New York, Springer-Verlag, Vol II, pp 1–8
144. Saunders P, Price AB (1970) Mixed mesodermal tumor of the ovary arising in pelvic endometriosis. Proc R Soc Med 63: 1050
145. Schiller W (1939) Mesonephroma ovarii. Am J Cancer 35: 1
146. Schiller W (1943) Parvilocular tumors of the ovary. Arch Pathol 35: 391
147. Schiller W (1934) Zur histogenese der Brennerschen ovarial Tumoren. Arch Gynaekol 157: 65
148. Schlegel R, Banks-Schlegel S, Pinkus GS (1980) Immunohistochemical localization of keratin in normal human tissues. Lab Invest 42: 91
149. Schlegel R, Banks-Schlegel S, McLeod JA, Pinkus GS (1980) Immunoperoxidase localization of keratin in human neoplasms. A preliminary survey. Am J Pathol 101: 41
150. Schuller EF, Kirol PM (1966) Prognosis in endometrioid carcinoma of the ovary. Obstet Gynecol 27: 850
151. Scully RE (1970) Recent progress in ovarian cancer. Hum Pathol 1: 73
152. Scully RE (1979) Atlas of tumor pathology. Second series. Fascicle 16. Tumors of the ovary and maldeveloped gonads. Washington, DC, Armed Forces Institute of Pathology, a: p 55, b: p 75, c: p 102, d: p 127, e: pp 132–135, f: pp 63–64
153. Scully RE (1970) Germ cell tumors of the ovary. In: Sturgis SH, Taymor ML (eds) Progress in gynecology. New York, Grune & Stratton, Vol V, p 343
154. Scully RE, Barlow JF (1967) "Mesonephroma" of ovary. Tumor of müllerian nature related to the endometrioid carcinoma. Cancer 20: 1405
155. Scully RE, Cohen RB (1964) Oxidative-enzyme activities in normal and pathologic human ovaries. Obstet Gynecol 24: 667
156. Scully RE, Richardson GS, Barlow JF (1966) The development of malignancy in endometriosis. Clin Obstet Gynecol 9: 384
157. Serov SF, Scully RE, Sobin LH (1973) International histological classification of tumours, No. 9. Histological typing of ovarian tumours. Geneva, World Health Organization, a: p 37, b: pp 17–18
158. Shanks HGI (1961) Pseudomyxoma peritonei. J Obstet Gynaecol Br Commonw 68: 212
159. Sharman A, Sutherland AM (1947) A case of serous adenofibroma of the ovary. J Obstet Gynaecol Br Emp 54: 382
160. Shevchuk MM, Fenoglio CM, Richart RM (1980) Histogenesis of Brenner tumors. II. Histochemistry and CEA. Cancer 46: 2617
161. Silverberg SC (1973) Ultrastructure and histogenesis of

clear cell carcinoma of the ovary. Am J Obstet Gynecol 115: 394

162. Silverberg SC (1971) Brenner tumor of the ovary. A clinicopathologic study of 60 tumors in 54 women. Cancer 28: 588
163. Sternberg W (1963) Nonfunctioning ovarian neoplasms. In: Grady HC, Smith DE (eds) The ovary. International academy of pathology monograph. Baltimore, Williams & Wilkins, pp 209–254
164. Tarridge J, Kingsley WB (1968) "Mesonephroma" of the ovary. A report of five cases. Cancer 22: 1208
165. Taylor HC (1929) Malignant and semimalignant tumors of the ovary. Surg Gynecol Obstet 48: 702
166. Teilum G (1969) Endodermal sinus tumors of the ovary and testis. Comparative morphogenesis of the so-called mesonephroma ovarii (Schiller) and extra embryonic (yolk sac-allantoic) structures of the rat's placenta. Cancer 12: 1092
167. Timonen S, Purola E (1967) Adenofibroma and cystadenofibroma of the ovary. Ann Chir Gynaecol Fenn [Suppl. 56] 154: 5
168. Towers RP (1956) A note on the origin of the pseudomucinous cystadenoma of the ovary. J Obstet Gynaecol Br Emp 63: 253
169. Tweeddale DN, Early LS, Goodsitt ES (1964) Endometrial adenoacanthoma. A clinical and pathologic analysis of 82 cases with observations on histogenesis. Obstet Gynecol 23: 611
170. Ueda G, Tanaka Y, Hiramatsu K, Inoue Y, Yamasaki M, Inoue M, Kurachi K, Mori T (1982) Immunohistochemical study of mucous antigens in gynecologic tumors with special reference to argyrophil cells. Int J Gynecol Pathol 1: 41
171. Ulbright TM, Roth LM, Stehman FB (1984) Secondary ovarian neoplasia. A clinicopathologic study of 35 cases. Cancer 53: 1164
172. Van Kley H, Cramer SF, Bruns De (1981) Serous ovarian neoplastic amylase (SONA): A potentially useful marker for serous ovarian tumors. Cancer 48: 1444
173. Winter S, Yarrasch ED, Schmid E, Franke WW, Denk H (1980) Differences in polypeptide composition of cytokeratin filaments, including filaments from different epithelial tissues and cells. Eur J Cell Biol 22: 371
174. Woodruff JD, Acosta AA (1962) Variations in the Brenner tumors. Am J Obstet Gynecol 83: 657
175. Woodruff JD, Novak ER (1954) Papillary serous tumors of the ovary. Am J Obstet Gynecol 67: 1112
176. Woodruff JD, Bie LS, Sherman RJ (1960) Mucinous tumors of the ovary. Obstet Gynecol 16: 699
177. Woodruff JD, Williams TJ, Goldberg B (1963) Hormone activity of the common ovarian neoplasm. Am J Obstet Gynecol 87: 679
178. Young RH, Scully RE (1982) Ovarian sex cord–stromal tumors. Recent progress. Int J Gynecol Pathol 1: 101
179. Young RH, Prat J, Scully RE (1982) Ovarian endometrioid carcinomas resembling sex cord–stromal tumors. A clinicopathological analysis of 13 cases. Am J Surg Pathol 6: 513

19

Sex Cord-Stromal, Steroid Cell, and Other Ovarian Tumors with Endocrine, Paraendocrine, and Paraneoplastic Manifestations

Robert H. Young, M.D., and Robert E. Scully, M.D.

Sex Cord–Stromal Tumors

This category of ovarian neoplasms includes all those that contain granulosa cells, theca cells and their luteinized derivatives, Sertoli cells, Leydig cells, and fibroblasts of gonadal stromal origin, singly or in various combinations, and in varying degrees of differentiation.[247–250,311,316,320] The generic terms that have been most widely applied to these tumors reflect differing views of gonadal embryology. Those investigators who are convinced that all the cell types listed above are derived from the mesenchyme, or specialized stroma, of the genital ridge have proposed the terms *mesenchymomas*[44] and *gonadal stromal tumors* for these neoplasms.[197,198,204] In contrast, other investigators, recognizing that many embryologists favor the participation of coelomic and mesonephric epithelium in the formation of the sex cords, which are the proximal precursors of granulosa and Sertoli cells, have preferred the terms *sex cord–mesenchyme tumors*[187,244] and *sex cord–stromal tumors*.[257]

In the developing testis, the sex cords are clearly distinguishable by the fifth week of embryonic life as slender columns of primitive Sertoli cells, but similar cords, at least in the sense of thin columns, are not encountered in the developing ovary. Instead, packets of small pregranulosa cells enveloping germ cells become evident later in embryonic life. For that reason, the term *sex cords* has been criticized as inaccurate to describe the progenitors of granulosa cells. Nevertheless, the long-established usage of this designation by embryologists and the lack of a better term justify its retention. The term *sex cord–stromal tumors,* which has been adopted by the World Health Organization (WHO),[257] has the advantage of acknowledging the presence, in tumors in this general category, of derivatives of either or both the sex cords and the stroma. The components derived from the sex cords (granulosa and Sertoli cells) are typically arranged in epithelial configurations, whereas those derived from the stroma have the appearance of cellular gonadal stroma or its specialized derivatives, the theca and Leydig cells.

Most sex cord–stromal tumors (granulosa–stromal cell tumors) are composed of ovarian cell types but some (Sertoli–stromal cell tumors) contain only cells of testicular type. Occasionally, cells and patterns of growth characteristic of both gonads are present in single tumors (gynandroblastomas). When the neoplastic cells are immature and their appearance is intermediate between those of testicular and ovarian cell types, or when the architectural patterns of the tumor are not specific for either the testis or ovary, it may be impossible to determine whether the tumor belongs in the granulosa–stromal or Sertoli–stromal cell category. In such cases the term *sex cord–stromal tumor, unclassified,* is used. The classification of sex cord–stromal tumors used in this chapter is that of WHO expanded slightly to allow separate designation of several tumors recognized since that classification was adopted (Table 19.1).

Sex cord–stromal tumors make up approximately 8% of all ovarian tumors,[22,107,148,310] with fibromas, which are almost never associated with endocrine manifestations, accounting for approximately half. Most of the other tumors in this category are granulosa cell tumors, which are usually of a low grade of malignancy.*

* References 28–30, 102, 198, 265, 270.

TABLE 19.1. Classification of sex cord–stromal tumors

Granulosa–stromal cell tumor
Granulosa cell tumor
Adult type
Juvenile type
Tumors in the thecoma–fibroma group
Thecoma
Typical
Luteinized
Fibroma–fibrosarcoma
Fibroma
Cellular fibroma
Fibrosarcoma
Stromal tumor with minor sex cord elements
Sclerosing stromal tumor
Unclassified
Sertoli–stromal cell tumors
Sertoli cell tumor
Leydig cell tumor
Sertoli-Leydig cell tumors
Well differentiated
Of intermediate differentiation
Poorly differentiated
With heterologous elements
Gynandroblastoma
Sex cord tumor with annular tubules
Unclassified

Granulosa–Stromal Cell Tumors

This group includes all ovarian tumors composed of granulosa cells, theca cells, and fibroblasts, singly or in any combination, and in varying degrees of differentiation. Granulosa cell tumors that occur typically in middle-aged and older women differ in several important respects from those that usually arise in children and young adults, and these two subtypes, referred to as *adult* and *juvenile granulosa cell tumors,* are discussed separately.

Tumors in the thecoma–fibroma group are composed exclusively or almost exclusively of theca cells, fibroblasts of ovarian stromal origin, or both. The presence of occasional small nests of granulosa cells or of tubules lined by Sertoli cells does not exclude tumors from this category; such tumors have been referred to as fibromas or thecomas with minor sex cord elements.[312]

Granulosa Cell Tumor (Adult Type)

Clinical Aspects. Adult granulosa cell tumors* account for approximately 1–2% of all ovarian tumors and 95% of all granulosa cell tumors. They occur more often in postmenopausal than premenopausal women and are the most common clinically estrogenic ovarian tumors. The

* References 28–30, 102, 198, 265, 270.

precise proportion of adult granulosa cell tumors that secrete hormones is difficult to establish because a specimen of endometrium to evaluate the effects of estrogenic stimulation is often unavailable. The typical endometrial alteration associated with functioning tumors in this category is cystic hyperplasia, usually accompanied by varying degrees of precancerous atypicality.[122] Carcinoma of the endometrium, which is almost always well differentiated, has been reported in from slightly less than 5% to slightly more than 25% of patients. The wide variation in these figures is attributable, at least in part, to differing views of the dividing line between markedly atypical hyperplasia and grade 1 adenocarcinoma. If strict criteria for the diagnosis of carcinoma are used and if all patients with a granulosa cell tumor, not just those who have had an endometrial curettage or hysterectomy, are considered, the correct figure for the frequency of associated endometrial carcinoma is under 5%.[270]

The endometrial changes associated with adult granulosa cell tumors are manifested clinically in women in the reproductive age group by metropathia hemorrhagica, which is characterized by irregular, excessive uterine bleeding, but amenorrhea, lasting from months to years, may precede the abnormal bleeding or may be the only hormonal manifestation.[90,270] Postmenopausal bleeding is the most common endocrine symptom in older women, in whom carcinoma of the endometrium is encountered about twice as often as it is in younger patients.[122] Occasionally, swelling and tenderness of the breasts are prominent symptoms. Elevated levels of estrogens have been reported in the blood and urine,[285] and vaginal cytologic smears typically show an increased maturation of squamous epithelial cells.[140] Alterations resembling those seen in a secretory endometrium have been observed rarely in association with granulosa cell tumors, suggesting the possibility of significant production of progesterone as well as estrogen by the neoplasm.

Rarely, androgenic changes are the sole endocrine manifestation of adult granulosa cell tumors; 22 androgen-secreting tumors have been reported.[121,139,191,199] Most of the patients have been frankly virilized, but some have been only hirsute. The tumors in these 22 patients were solid or solid and cystic in 12 patients and cystic in 10. The cysts are typically thin-walled and may be single or multiple, resembling serous cystadenomas.[191,199] Since granulosa cell tumors in general are composed exclusively of thin-walled cysts in only 3% of patients,[259] the almost 50% frequency of a cystic gross appearance of tumors associated with androgenic manifestations is of great interest. From another viewpoint, 17% of granulosa cell tumors composed of thin-walled cysts seen in consultation by one of us (RES) have been androgenic, in contrast to only 1.5% of solid or solid and cystic granulosa cell tumors. The nature of the association of androgen production with the formation of thin-walled cysts remains an enigma.

Gross Appearance. Adult granulosa cell tumors vary in size from those that are too small to be felt on pelvic examination (10–15%)[92] to very large masses that distend the abdomen. One of the largest recorded tumors weighed 15.4 kg;[81] the average diameter is approximately 12 cm. At operation the tumor may appear predominantly solid or predominantly cystic (Fig. 19.1. Plate 3) and is unilateral in over 95% of cases. Sectioning a solid tumor reveals a gray-white or yellow color, depending on its lipid content, and a soft or firm consistency, depending on its relative content of neoplastic cells and fibrothecomatous stroma. Areas of necrosis and massive areas of hemorrhage are common. Most characteristically, however, the tumor is predominantly cystic, with numerous compartments that are typically filled with fluid or clotted blood (Fig. 19.1a, Plate 3) and separated by solid tissue. An interesting clinical corollary of the hemorrhage in both solid and cystic granulosa cell tumors is that 10–12% of them present as an acute abdominal disorder caused by rupture and hemoperitoneum.[28–30,270]

Microscopic Appearance. Microscopic examination of an adult granulosa cell tumor reveals only granulosa cells or, more often, an additional component of theca cells, fibroblasts, or both; in some cases, the latter cell types predominate. The granulosa cells grow in a wide variety of patterns, which are very commonly admixed (Fig. 19.2). The better differentiated tumors typically have microfollicular, macrofollicular, insular, trabecular, solid-

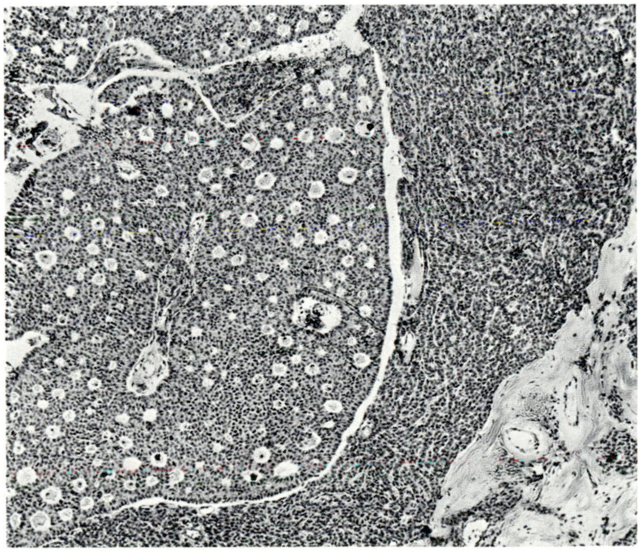

Fig. 19.2. Granulosa cell tumor. Microfollicular pattern (*left*) and watered-silk pattern (*right*) are present. (Reproduced by permission from Morris J McL, Scully RE: Endocrine Pathology of the Ovary, St. Louis, 1958, The C. V. Mosby Co.)

tubular, and rarely hollow-tubular patterns (Figs. 19.2, 19.3, 19.4, 19.5, and 19.6). The microfollicular pattern is characterized by the presence of numerous small cavities simulating the Call-Exner bodies of the developing graafian follicle (Figs. 19.2, 19.3, and 19.4). These cavities may contain eosinophilic fluid and, often, one or a few degenerating nuclei, hyalinized basement membrane material, or rarely basophilic fluid. The microfollicles are separated typically by well-differentiated granulosa cells that contain scanty cytoplasm and pale, angular or oval, often grooved nuclei arranged haphazardly in relation to one another and to the follicles (Fig. 19.3).

It is important to distinguish the Call-Exner bodies of adult granulosa cell tumors from the glands of adenocarcinomas and carcinoids (Tables 19.2 and 19.3) and from the hyaline bodies that are seen in gonadoblastomas[246] and sex cord tumors with annular tubules[245,330] because all four of these tumors have clinical implications that differ considerably from those of granulosa cell tumors. The glands of adenocarcinomas and carcinoids are generally lined by cells that have a more orderly arrangement than that of neoplastic granulosa cells. The lumens in adenocarcinomas are often filled with mucin whereas those of carcinoids typically contain dense eosinophilic secretion, which is sometimes calcified. The nuclei of adenocarcinomas almost always appear more highly malignant than those of granulosa cell tumors, whereas those of carcinoids are characteristically round and contain coarse chromatin. The hyaline bodies of gonadoblastomas and sex cord tumors with annular tubules are typically larger than Call-Exner bodies and can sometimes be observed to be continuous with hyaline thickenings of the basement membrane along the periphery of the tumor cell nests. These bodies also often undergo calcification.

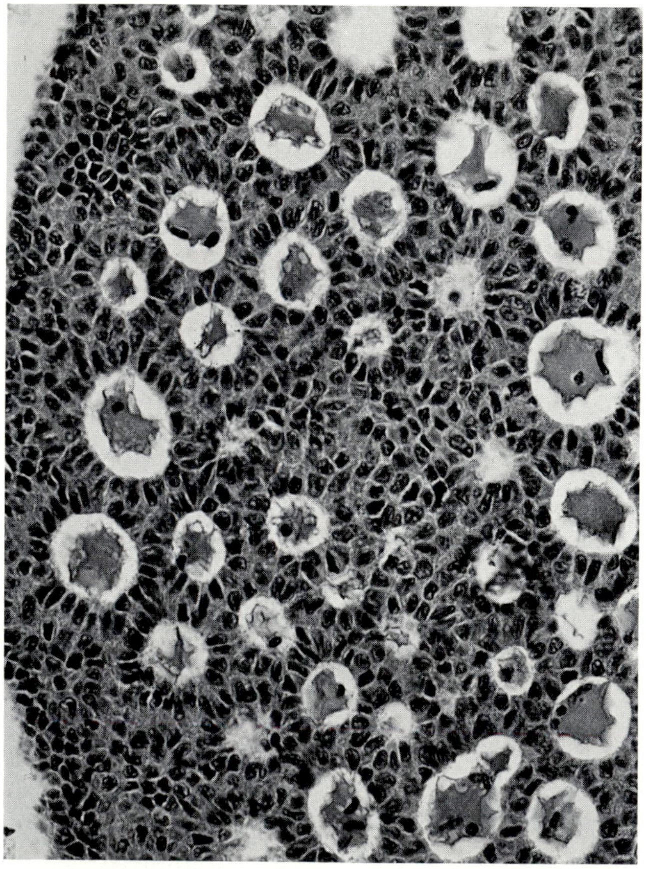

FIG. 19.3. Granulosa cell tumor, microfollicular pattern. Call–Exner bodies are surrounded by granulosa cells with angular nuclei in haphazard arrangement. (Reprinted by permission of Scully and Morris, Ref. 253.)

The macrofollicular pattern (Fig. 19.5) is characterized by cysts lined by well-differentiated granulosa cells, beneath which theca cells are usually present. The degree of differentiation in the walls of the cysts may be so marked that high-power distinction from nonneoplastic follicle cysts may be different. In practice, however, this problem rarely exists, since the cysts are viewed in the context of the clinical, gross, and other microscopic findings. Cystic granulosa cell tumors are occasionally difficult to distinguish from other cystic tumors and even nonneoplastic cysts when the granulosa cells lining the cysts are extensively denuded.[191] In such cases, thorough sampling may be necessary to identify diagnostic foci of granulosa cell tumor.

The trabecular (Fig. 19.6) and insular forms of granulosa cell tumor are characterized by bands and islands of granulosa cells separated by a fibromatous or thecomatous stroma. In the solid tubular pattern, the tubules may be uniformly cellular or contain peripheral nuclei and central masses of cytoplasm. Occasionally, a few hollow tubules or glandlike structures are encountered. The various tubular patterns encountered in granulosa cell tumors are indistinguishable from those of well-differentiated Sertoli cell tumors. Their presence is ignored as a diagnostic criterion unless they are present in significant portions of the tumor, and, in such cases, a diagnosis of mixed granulosa cell and Sertoli cell tumor, or gynandroblastoma,[257] is warranted.

The less well differentiated forms of granulosa cell tumor typically have a watered-silk (moiré silk) (Fig. 19.2), gyriform (Fig. 19.7), or diffuse (sarcomatoid) pattern (Fig. 19.8), alone or in combination. The first two patterns are manifested by undulating or zigzag rows of granulosa cells, generally in single file, whereas the diffuse pattern is characterized by a monotonous cellular growth resembling a low-grade round cell sarcoma. Mitoses may be numerous. The misinterpretation of an undifferentiated carcinoma as a diffuse granulosa cell tumor is one of the most frequent errors in ovarian tumor pathology. If the clinical course of the patient is atypically malignant for a granulosa cell tumor, the possibility of

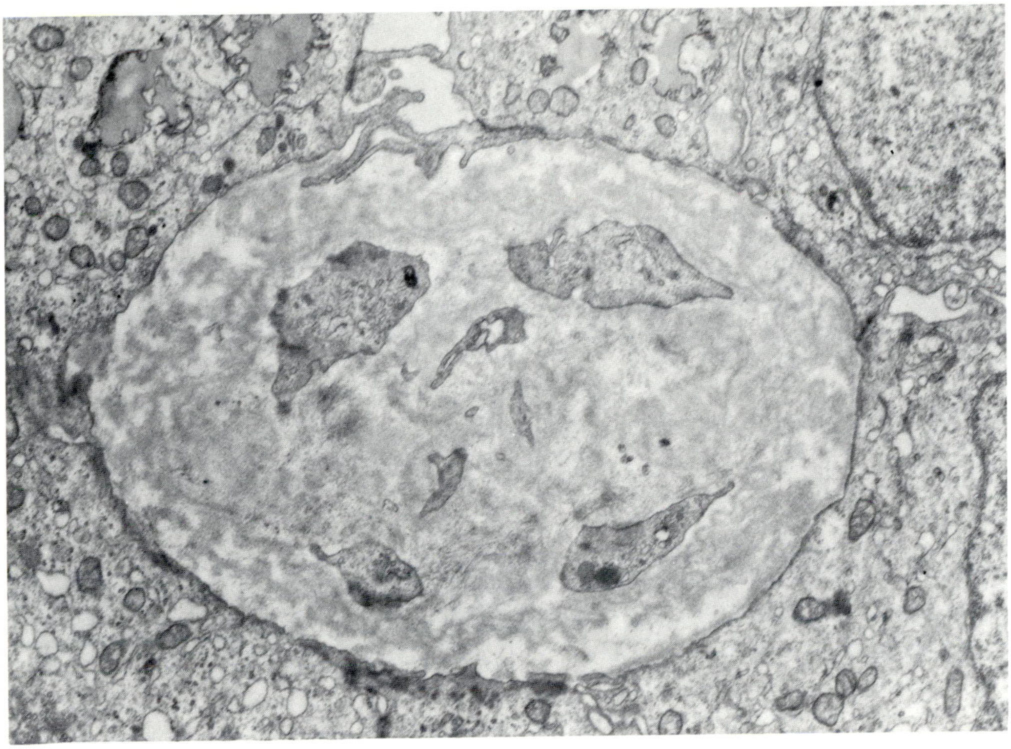

FIG. 19.4. Granulosa cell tumor. A Call–Exner body contains cellular fragments and amorphous debris. The surrounding cells show prominent microvilli and junctional complexes. ×12,000. (Reprinted with permission from The American College of Obstetricians and Gynecologists. From Gondos B, Monroe SA. Cystic granulosa cell tumor with massive hemoperitoneum. Light and electron microscopic study. Obstet Gynecol 38:683–689, 1971.)

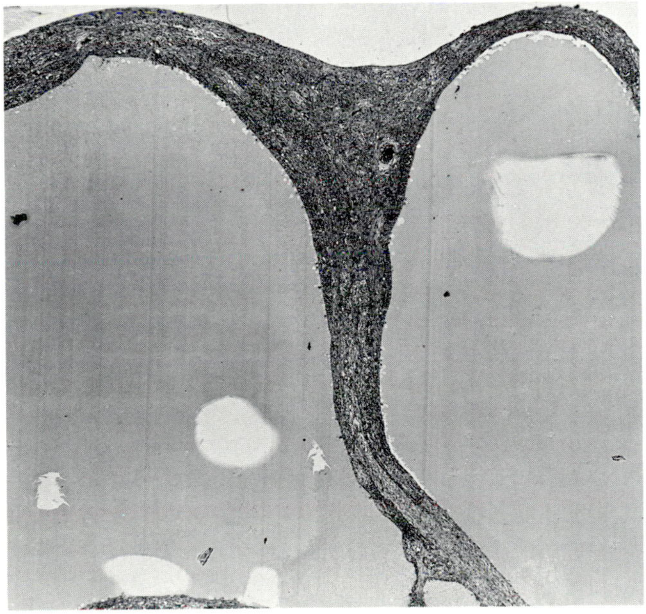

FIG. 19.5. Granulosa cell tumor, macrofollicular pattern. [Reprinted by permission of The New England Journal of Medicine, 265:1213, 1961.] General Hospital (1961) Case 89–1961. N Engl J Med 265:1213.]

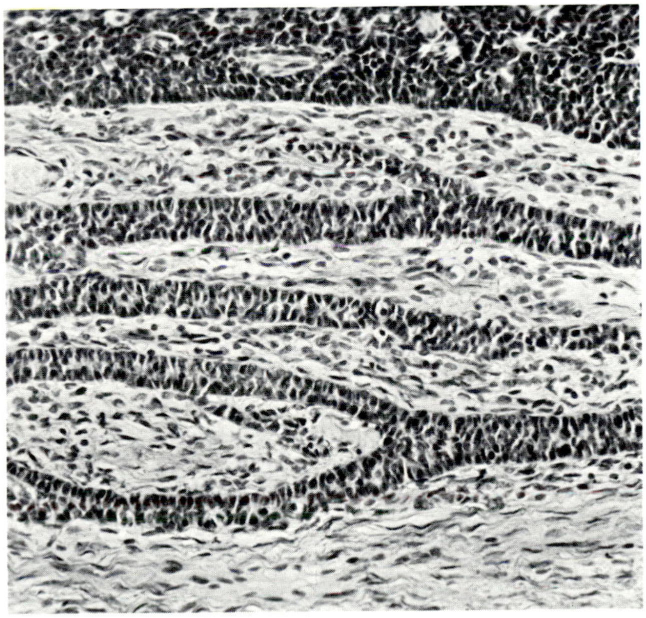

FIG. 19.6. Granulosa cell tumor, trabecular pattern. (Reprinted by permission of Serov et al., Ref. 257.)

TABLE 19.2. Granulosa cell tumor versus undifferentiated carcinoma and poorly differentiated adenocarcinoma.

Granulosa cell tumor	Carcinoma
Bilateral in less than 5%	Bilateral in over 25%
Stage I in 90% of cases	Stage III or IV in most cases
Nuclei round to angular, pale, and commonly grooved[a]	Nuclei hyperchromatic, often bizarre with atypical mitoses
Mucin occasionally in follicles (mainly in juvenile type)	Intracellular droplets or extracellular pools of mucin, psammoma bodies or glands may be present
Good prognosis	Poor prognosis
Indolent course, when clinically malignant[b]	Rapid course

[a] Exception: dark, ungrooved nuclei of juvenile granulosa cell tumor.
[b] Exception: rare juvenile granulosa cell tumors.

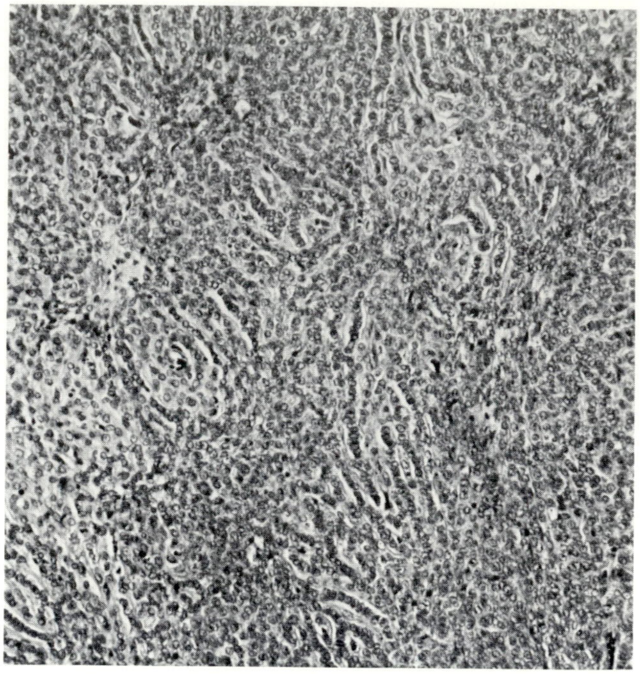

FIG. 19.7. Granulosa cell tumor, gyriform pattern.

such a misdiagnosis must be considered. The single best criterion for distinguishing these two tumors is the appearance of the nuclei, which are typically uniform, pale, and often grooved in granulosa cell tumors (Figs. 19.9 and 19.10) and are hyperchromatic, usually of unequal size and shape, and rarely grooved in undifferentiated carcinomas. Abnormal mitotic figures are often found in the latter as well. Other features helpful in the differential diagnosis are summarized in Table 19.2. The highly malignant small cell carcinoma, which is often associated with hypercalcemia,[77] may also be misdiagnosed as a granulosa cell tumor. The differential features of these

TABLE 19.3. Granulosa cell tumor versus carcinoid.

Granulosa cell tumor	Insular carcinoid
Variety of patterns	Islands, round acini, solid tubules, and ribbons
Call-Exner bodies, ill defined, with watery to dense eosinophilic content, occasionally pyknotic nuclei	Acini sharply outlined with dense content, sometimes calcified
Nuclei round to angular, pale, often grooved, haphazardly oriented	Nuclei round with coarse chromatin and regular orientation
Thecomatous stroma common, at least focally	Fibromatous or hyalinized stroma, may be focally luteinized
Usually uninodular and almost always unilateral, no teratomatous elements	Often multinodular and almost always bilateral if metastatic, always unilateral and usually associated with other teratomatous elements if primary
Cells nonargentaffin, may contain fine argyrophilic granules	Cells usually argentaffin, almost always argyrophilic

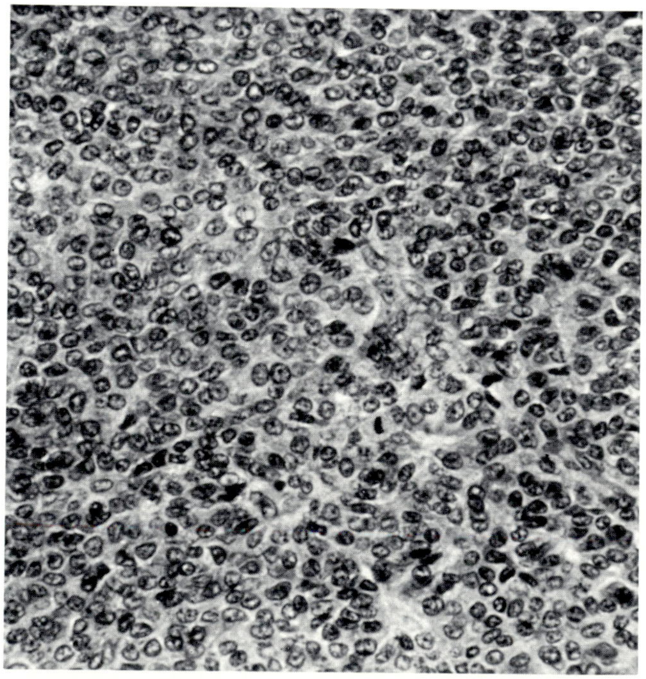

FIG. 19.8. Granulosa cell tumor, diffuse pattern. The nuclei are pale and oval. [Reprinted by permission of The New England Journal of Medicine, 261:146, 1959.]

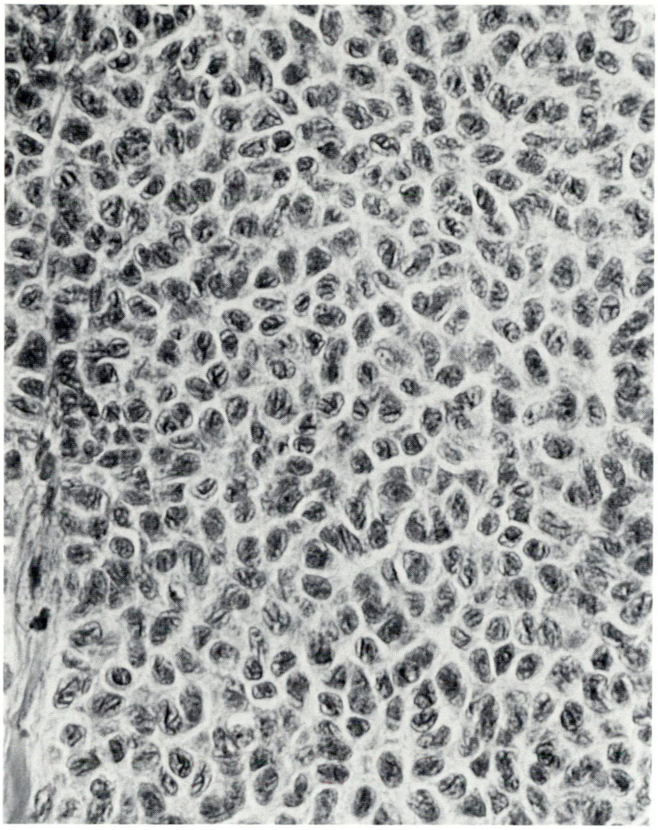

FIG. 19.9. Granulosa cell tumor. The nuclei are pale and have prominent grooves. (Reprinted by permission of Young RH, Scully RE: Ovarian sex cord-stromal and steroid cell tumors. In: Roth LM, Czernobilsky B, eds., Tumors and Tumor-Like Conditions of the Ovary. Churchill Livingstone Inc, New York, 1985.)

tumors are presented in Table 19.4. Finally, a diffuse granulosa cell tumor is occasionally confused with an endometrioid stromal sarcoma or metastatic endometrial stromal sarcoma of the ovary,[329] but a variety of features, including the frequent high stage and bilaterality of the latter, their typical content of numerous arterioles, and their rich reticulum content, aid in this differential diagnosis. In this, as in other problems in the diagnosis of granulosa cell and other sex cord–stromal tumors, extensive sampling of the specimen is often helpful.

In some granulosa cell tumors, the neoplastic cells contain abundant dense or vacuolated cytoplasm (Fig. 19.11), approaching to varying degrees the appearance of the granulosa cells of the corpus luteum. In such cases, the term *luteinized granulosa cell tumor* is appropriate.

The presence of theca cells in varying quantities in most granulosa cell tumors has led to the occasional use of the term *granulosa–theca cell tumor*. Although this designation accurately describes the cellular content of many of these neoplasms, the term *granulosa cell tumor* is more widely accepted for tumors containing both cell types. One reason for this preference is the probability that the presence of theca cells in some cases reflects a response of the ovarian stroma to the growth of granulosa cells rather than the coexistence of a truly neoplastic component. Evidence favoring such an interpretation includes the nonspecific presence of thecalike cells in a variety of ovarian tumors, both benign and malignant and both primary and metastatic, and the observation that theca cells are usually absent in granulosa cell tumors that have extended beyond the ovary.[93] It seems likely, however, that some tumors in which the theca cell element is prominent or even greatly preponderant are truly mixed neoplasms.

The theca cells in granulosa cell tumors may resemble theca externa or theca interna cells and may be luteinized. In some tumors, particularly those with a diffuse pattern, differentiation of granulosa and theca cells with routine staining may be difficult or impossible. In such cases, a reticulum stain may be helpful. Just as in a developing graafian follicle, so in a granulosa cell tumor the fibrils typically invest theca cells individually. In contrast, the granulosa cell layer of a follicle, which is not vascularized, contains no fibrils, and in a granulosa cell tumor the reticulum is usually sparse, being typically confined to perivascular zones (Fig. 19.12). In occasional tumors, an intermediate pattern of fibril distribution is present, and the reticulum stain is not useful in the differentiation of the two cell types.

Several histochemical reactions that are characteristic of steroid hormone-producing cells, particularly those that demonstrate various types of lipid content or oxidative enzyme activity, are usually positive in the theca cells and negative or weakly positive in the granulosa cells of a tumor containing both cell types.[114,173,174,252,309] This finding and ultrastructural observations[96,104,110,115] have led some observers to conclude that the theca cell component of granulosa cell tumors produces the hormones responsible for estrogenic manifestations. Additional evidence in favor of this conclusion is the observation that granulosa cell tumors that recur outside ovarian tissue and lack theca cells are typically not obviously estrogenic. In some cases, however, histochemical and other evidence[104,165] has suggested a role for the granulosa cells in estrogen secretion. Likewise, Kurman et al.[157] have demonstrated immunohistochemically the presence of a variety of steroid hormones in granulosa cells. Whether these findings reflect production, storage, or binding of these hormones, however, has not been established. Possibly the theca cells in granulosa cell tumors produce androgens, and aromatase in the granulosa cells converts these hormones to estrogens according to the two-cell theory of estrogen production by the normal graafian follicle.[12,83]

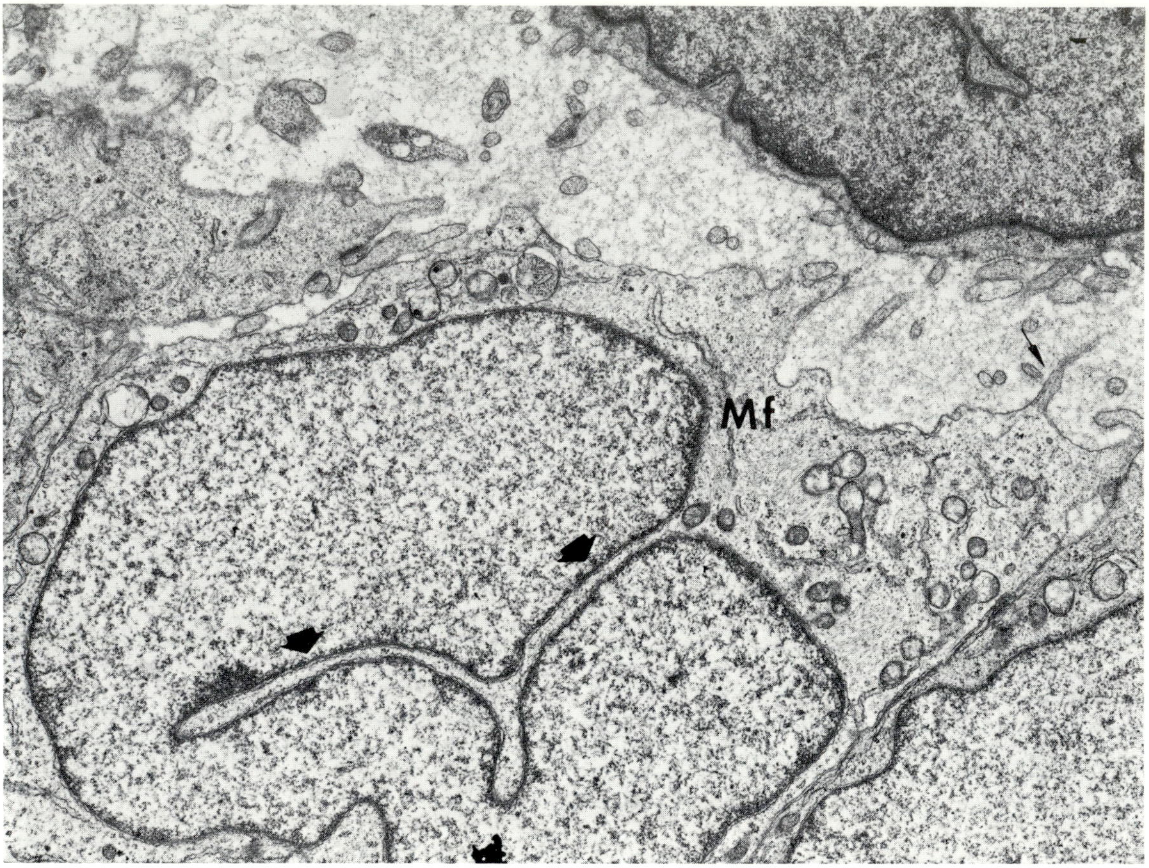

FIG. 19.10. Granulosa cell tumor. The deep indentation of the nuclear membrane (*large arrows*) corresponds to the nuclear wrinkling on light microscopic examination. The sparse cytoplasm contains clusters of small mitochondria and numerous microfibrils (Mf). The plasma membrane has hair-like microvillous processes (*small arrow*) projecting into the intercellular space. ×8000. (Courtesy of Dr. A. Ferenczy, Montreal, Canada. Reprinted by permission of Scully, Ref. 248.)

Behavior and Treatment. After the removal of a granulosa cell tumor, the manifestations of hyperestrinism typically regress. If the uterus has been conserved in a young woman, estrogen withdrawal bleeding usually occurs in 1 or 2 days and regular menses ensue shortly thereafter. Granulosa cell tumors of all patterns have a malignant potential, with a capacity to extend beyond the ovary or recur after apparently successful removal. Spread is largely within the pelvis and lower abdomen. Distant metastases are rare, but have been reported in many sites.[169,276] Although recurrences may appear within 5 years, they are often not evident until a much longer postoperative interval has elapsed, and numerous cases have been reported in which the tumor has reappeared 2 or even 3 or more decades after the initial therapy. The 10-year survival figures that have been recorded in the literature have varied widely from under 60% to more than 90%, and progressive declines in survival have been documented after longer follow-up periods.*

The optimal treatment of a granulosa cell tumor in menopausal or postmenopausal women is total hysterectomy with bilateral salpingo-oophorectomy. In younger women, in whom the preservation of fertility is an important consideration, however, removal of only the tumor and the adjacent fallopian tube is justifiable if spread beyond the ovary is not demonstrable and examination of the contralateral ovary shows no suggestion of involvement. Recurrence is usually fatal, but some recurrent tumors have been treated successfully by reoperation, radiation therapy, or a combination thereof.[146,240,264] Too little information is available on the chemotherapy of granulosa cell tumors to evaluate the comparative merits of various agents, but several of them have been used with varying degrees of success.†

Ninety percent of granulosa cell tumors are stage I,[28–30,270] and these tumors have a considerably better prognosis than higher stage tumors, as shown by an 86% versus a 49% relative survival at 10 years, respec-

* References 10, 28–30, 43, 44, 79, 90, 102, 198, 265, 270.

† References 80, 138, 163, 167, 194, 240, 266.

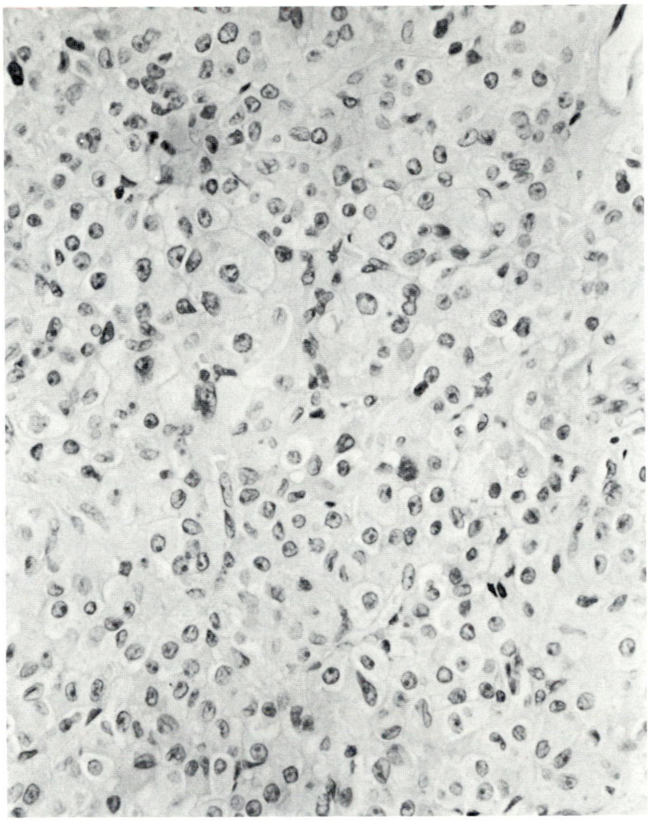

FIG. 19.11. Granulosa cell tumor, luteinized.

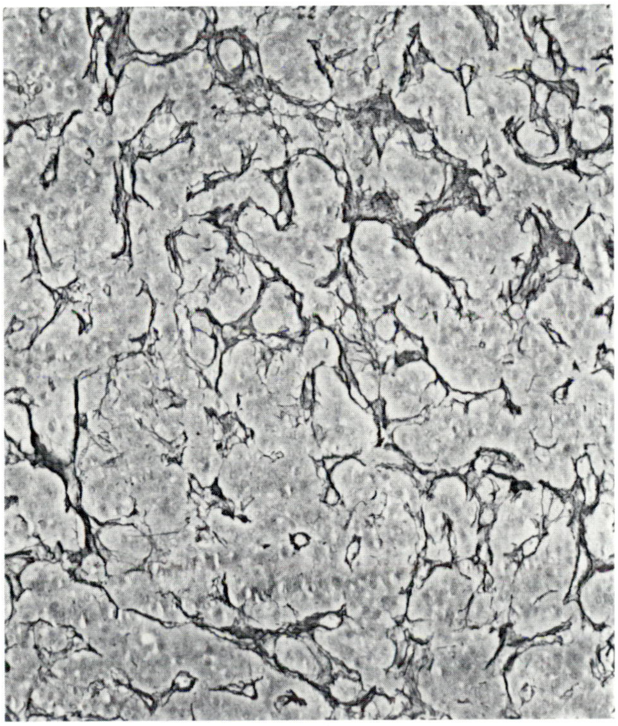

FIG. 19.12. Granulosa cell tumor (*reticulum stain*). Reticulum surrounds aggregates of granulosa cells. Contrast with Fig. 19.21.

tively, in one large series[270] and a 96% versus a 26% survival in another.[30] Rupture also adversely affects the outlook, with an 86% relative 25-year survival of patients with intact stage I tumors compared to only a 60% survival of those with ruptured tumors that are otherwise in the same stage.[30]

The size of granulosa cell tumors has also been related to their prognosis. In one series, all the patients with tumors 5 cm or less in diameter survived 10 years, but only 57% of those with tumors 6 to 15 cm in diameter and 53% of those with even larger tumors survived for that period of time.[102] Another investigation reported a 73% crude overall survival of patients with tumors under 5 cm in diameter, a 63% survival of those with tumors between 5 and 15 cm, and a 34% survival of those with a tumor over 15 cm in diameter.[270] In another series, stage I tumors 5 cm or less in diameter were associated with a 100% relative 10-year survival in contrast to a 92% survival of patients with larger stage I tumors.[30] The last series is the only one in which the survival rate was corrected for stage, and on that basis the improvement in prognosis for the smaller stage I tumors was not statistically significant. Therefore, a relation between tumor size and prognosis independent of stage has not been clearly established.

Attempts to correlate the histologic pattern and the degrees of nuclear atypia and mitotic activity with prognosis have met with varying success. Kottmeier[152] reported a significantly better prognosis if the tumor was well differentiated (with a follicular or cylindromatous pattern) than if it was more poorly differentiated (sarcomatoid). This difference was reflected in 5-year survival figures of 87% and 64%, respectively, but was more obvious in the figures for 10 years, which were 82% versus 29%. The latter figures emphasize that very long follow-up is necessary before survival data for any series of granulosa cell tumors becomes meaningful. Several other investigators have failed to confirm the prognostic importance of pattern alone in granulosa cell tumors.[30,102,198,265,270]

The degree of nuclear atypicality within granulosa cell tumors has also been correlated with their prognosis. In one study, the 5-year survival of patients whose tumors showed no atypia was 92% compared to 80% for those with slight atypicality and 30% for those with moderate atypicality.[270] In another study, there was an 80% relative 25-year survival in cases with grade 1 nuclear atypicality in contrast to only a 60% survival in those with grade 2 atypia.[30] In both of these studies, nuclear atypicality was the most reliable prognostic index in patients with stage I tumors. For higher stage tumors, nuclear atypicality and mitotic rate were of similar significance. With regard to the relation of nuclear atypicality to prognosis, it should be noted that assessment of its degree is somewhat subjective. Also, approximately 2% of granulosa cell tumors contain mononucleate and multinucleate cells with large, bizarre, hyperchromatic nuclei (Fig. 19.13), the presence of which does not appear to worsen the prognosis.[313] These nuclear changes, which resemble those seen in uterine leiomyomas with bizarre nuclei, may also be encountered in Sertoli–Leydig cell tumors and thecomas and are probably degenerative. In a recent study of eight granulosa cell tumors, seven Sertoli–Leydig cell tumors, and two thecomas with bizarre nuclei, follow-up was obtained on 11 patients, all of whom were alive without evidence of disease from 3 to 21 years postoperatively.[313]

The mitotic activity of granulosa cell tumors has also been correlated with their prognosis. In one study, there was a 70% 10-year survival associated with tumors that had two or fewer mitotic figures per 10 high-power fields (HPF) compared to only a 37% survival for those with three or more.[270] In another investigation,[102] tumors with many mitotic figures were associated with a worse prognosis than those with few, but most of the tumors with high mitotic rates were also at a higher stage than those with low mitotic rates, and differences in mitotic rate did not have a statistically significant effect on the prognosis of stage I tumors.

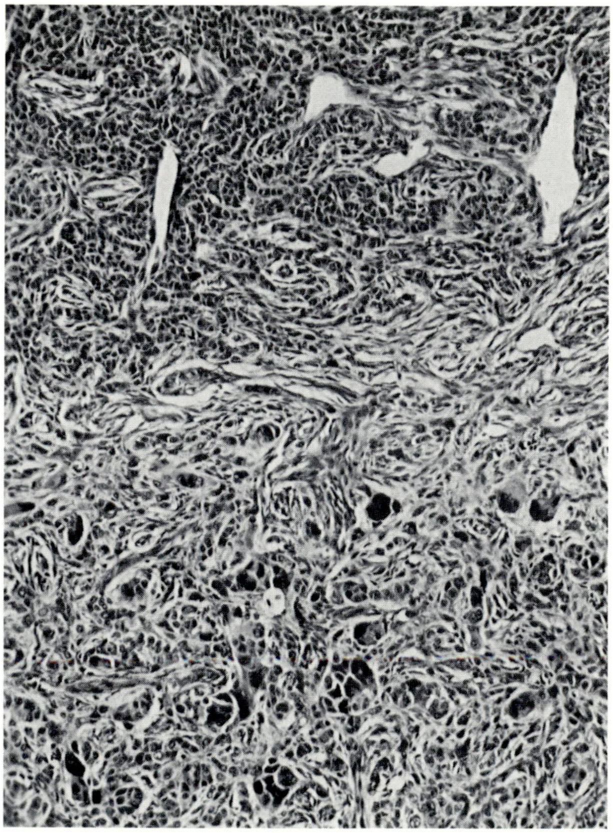

FIG. 19.13. Typical granulosa cell tumor (*top*) adjacent to area with bizzare nuclei (*bottom*). (Reprinted by permission of Young and Scully, Ref. 313.)

Granulosa Cell Tumor (Juvenile Type)

Clinical Aspects. Somewhat under 5% of granulosa cell tumors are diagnosed before the age of normal puberty. The great majority of these tumors as well as many granulosa cell tumors in young adults differ histologically from adult granulosa cell tumors (Table 19.4), and the designation *juvenile* has been selected for such tumors because 97% of them occur in the first three decades.[323] Approximately 80% of juvenile granulosa cell tumors occurring in children result in isosexual precocity,[323] accounting for 10% of cases of that syndrome in the female.[137,141,196] (The more common form of isosexual precocity is of central origin, with premature release of gonadotropins from the anterior pituitary gland; it is usually constitutional or idiopathic.) The precocity caused by granulosa cell tumors is more specifically designated *pseudoprecocity* because there is no associated ovulation or progesterone production, precluding the possibility of pregnancy, which exists, in contrast, in cases of true sexual precocity. Typically, pseudoprecocity is heralded by development of the breasts, followed by the appearance of pubic and axillary hair, stimulation and enlargement of the external and internal secondary sex organs, irregular uterine bleeding, and a whitish vaginal discharge believed to originate in the endocervical glands. Somatic and skeletal development are typically accelerated as well. Androgenic manifestations, such as clitoromegaly, occasionally occur.[26,323]

When it occurs after puberty, the juvenile granulosa cell tumor usually causes abdominal pain or swelling, sometimes associated with menstrual irregularities or amenorrhea. Approximately 6% of all the patients have acute abdominal symptoms due to rupture of the tumor and hemoperitoneum.[323] An interesting clinical association of the juvenile granulosa cell tumor has been its association with Ollier's disease (enchondromatosis) in three patients[282,323] and with Maffucci's syndrome (enchondromatosis and hemangiomatosis) in two patients.[159,161,323]

The juvenile granulosa cell tumor is bilateral in only about 2% of patients.[214,323] It appears ruptured at operation in approximately 10% of patients, and ascites is present in a similar percentage. Spread beyond the ovary is unusual; in our series only 2% of the tumors were stage II, and we have seen a single case recently in which the tumor was stage III on the basis of omental spread. The diameter of the tumor has ranged from 3.0 to 32.0 cm, with an average of 12.5 cm. Because of the usual moderate to large size of the tumor, an adnexal mass is almost always detectable clinically. Rarely, however, a mass has not been palpable preoperatively even on bimanual rectal examination.[55]

Gross Appearance. The range of gross appearances of the juvenile granulosa cell tumor is similar to that of

TABLE 19.4. Granulosa cell tumors (GCTs) versus small cell carcinoma.

Juvenile GCT	Adult GCT	Small cell CA
Almost always before 30	All ages but mostly postmenopausal	Always premenopausal
Rarely malignant	Indolent course if malignant	Highly malignant
No hypercalcemia	No hypercalcemia	Hypercalcemia common
Usually estrogenic	Usually estrogenic	Never estrogenic
Follicles, large, irregular, often contain mucin	Follicles, usually small (Call–Exner bodies), typically round	"Follicles," usually large and rounded
Thecomatous component common	Fibrothecomatous component common	Stroma scanty or nonspecific
Cytoplasm usually abundant	Cytoplasm usually scanty	Cytoplasm usually scanty but may be focally abundant
Nuclei dark, ungrooved, and often pleomorphic	Nuclei pale and often grooved	Nuclei dark and uniform
Mitoses usually numerous	Mitoses variable	Mitoses numerous

the adult form. Like the latter, the single most common presentation is as a solid and cystic neoplasm, in which the cysts may contain hemorrhagic fluid. Uniformly solid and uniformly cystic neoplasms are also encountered; the latter may be multilocular or, rarely, unilocular. The solid component is typically yellow-tan or gray and occasionally exhibits extensive necrosis, hemorrhage, or both (Fig. 19.14, Plate 3).

Microscopic Appearance. Microscopic examination typically reveals a solid cellular neoplasm, with focal follicle formation (Figs. 19.15 and 19.16), but the tumor may also be uniformly solid or uniformly follicular. In the solid areas, the neoplastic cells may be arranged diffusely or divided into nodules by fibrous septa. Occasionally, small clusters of tumor cells are present in a fibrous stroma. In the solid foci, the granulosa cells usually predominate, but often there is an admixture of theca cells and in some areas the latter may predominate. Occasionally the granulosa cells and theca cells are admixed together in a haphazard fashion. In such cases, reticulum stains may aid in their differentiation. Foci resembling typical thecoma with hyaline bands are encountered rarely but are usually minor in extent. Areas of sclerosis and calcification may also be seen.

The follicles usually vary in size and shape (Fig. 19.15) but may be regular and round to oval (Fig. 19.16). They generally do not reach the large size of the follicles in the macrofollicular form of the adult granulosa cell tumor. Their lumens contain eosinophilic or basophilic secretion, which stains with mucicarmine in approximately two thirds of the cases. Granulosa cells of varying layers of thickness line the follicles and are occasionally surrounded by mantles of theca cells. More often, however, the granulosa cells lining the follicles blend into the

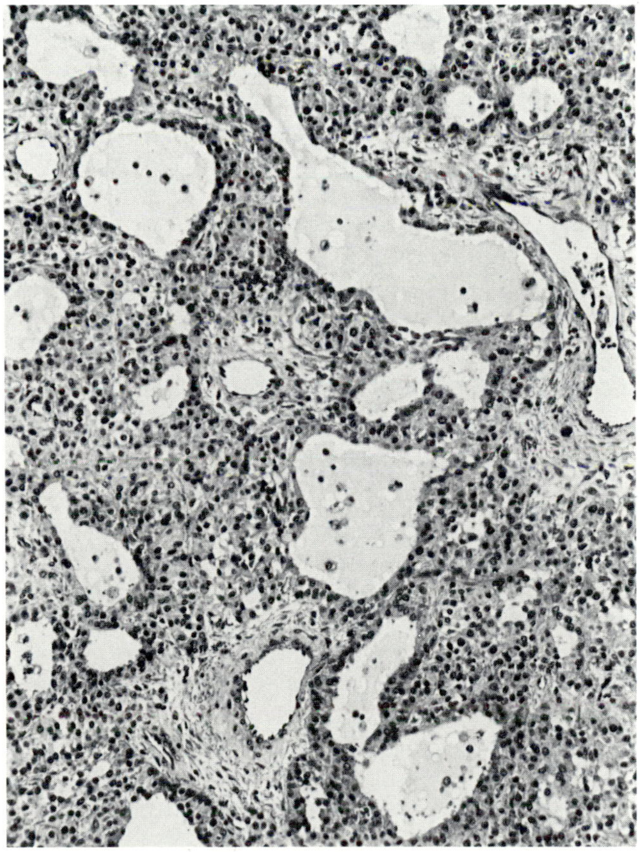

FIG. 19.15. Juvenile granulosa cell tumor. Follicles of varying sizes and shapes are separated by cellular areas. (Reprinted by permission of Young et al., Ref. 323.)

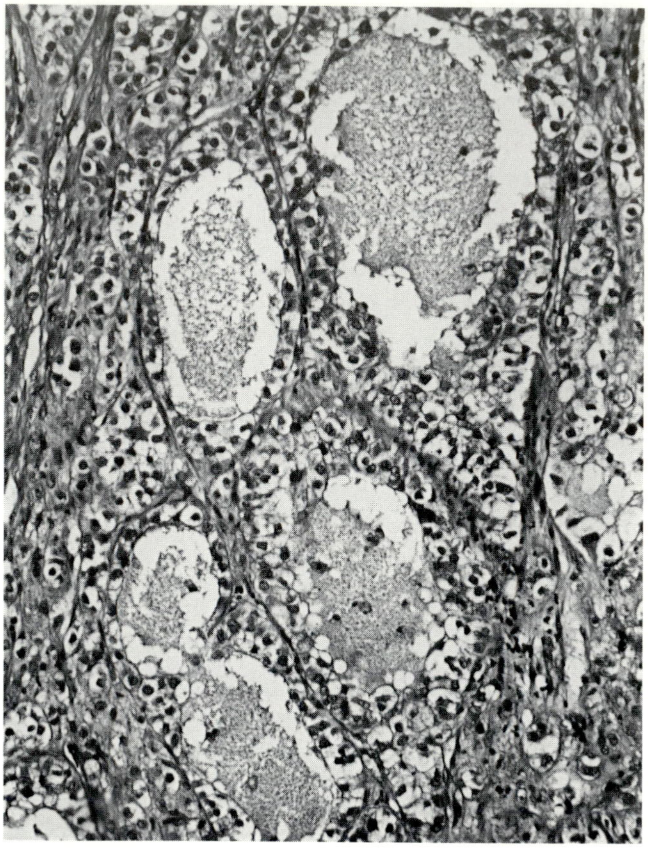

FIG. 19.16. Juvenile granulosa cell tumor. Round to oval follicles lined by cells with abundant pale cytoplasm enclose secretion that was basophilic. (Reprinted by permission of Young and Scully, Ref. 311.)

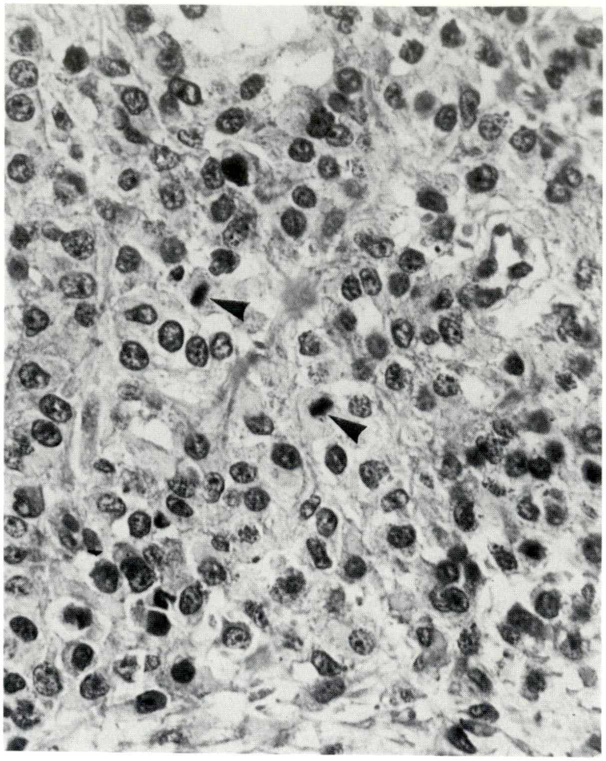

FIG. 19.17. Juvenile granulosa cell tumor. The cells have abundant cytoplasm; their nuclei are hyperchromatic, lack grooves, and exhibit mitotic activity (*arrows*). (Reprinted by permission of Young RH, Scully RE: Ovarian sex cord-stromal and steroid cell tumors. In: Roth LM, Czernobilsky B, eds., Tumors and Tumor-Like Conditions of the Ovary. Churchill Livingstone Inc, New York, 1985.)

intervening diffusely cellular areas. Rarely, the lining cells resemble hobnail cells.

The two characteristic cytologic features of the neoplastic granulosa cells that distinguish them from those of adult granulosa cell tumors are their generally rounded, hyperchromatic nuclei, which lack grooves in most cases, and their frequent abundant content of eosinophilic (luteinized) cytoplasm (Fig. 19.17). The theca cell component of the tumors is also usually luteinized, and lipid stains typically disclose moderate to large amounts of lipid within the cytoplasm of both the granulosa and theca cells. The theca cells are more often spindle-shaped than are the granulosa cells, and, like the latter, usually contain hyperchromatic nuclei. In rare juvenile granulosa cell tumors, small foci more characteristic of the adult granulosa cell tumor are encountered.

Nuclear atypicality in juvenile granulosa cell tumors varies from minimal to marked. In approximately 13% of the cases, severe degrees are present (Fig. 19.18). The mitotic rate (Fig. 19.17) also varies greatly but is generally greater than that seen in adult granulosa cell tumors.[270] In our series of juvenile granulosa cell tumors,[323] the average count was 7 per 10 HPF, and in the series from the Armed Forces Institute of Pathology,[332] it was 5.5 per 10 HPF.

Behavior and Treatment. Although the juvenile granulosa cell tumor usually appears less well differentiated than the adult type, follow-up data in our series of 125 cases and in the series of Lack et al.,[160] Roth et al.,[227] and Zaloudek and Norris,[332] which contain in combination an additional 38 cases, indicate a high cure rate. Seven of the tumors in our series and one in that of Zaloudek and Norris[332] were clinically malignant. In contrast to the adult granulosa cell tumors, which often recur late, however, all the clinically malignant juvenile tumors have reappeared within 3 years, and several have had a relatively rapid course.[279,323]

In our series of juvenile granulosa cell tumors, the feature of greatest prognostic significance was the stage of the tumor.[323] Only 2 of the 80 stage I tumors for which follow-up information was available were clinically malignant. Rupture did not have an adverse effect on prognosis. Two of the 10 stage IC tumors were malignant;

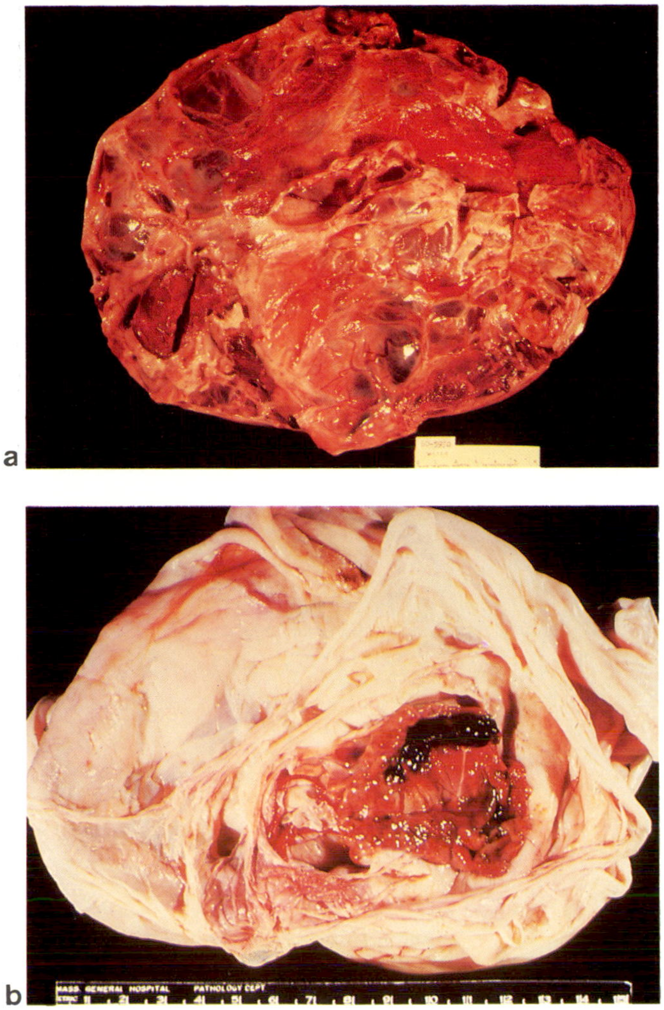

FIG. 19.1.*a*. Adult granulosa cell tumor, multicystic. (Reprinted by permission of The New England Journal of Medicine 265:1213, 1961.) *b*. Opened unilocular–cystic granulosa cell tumor resembling serous cystadenoma.

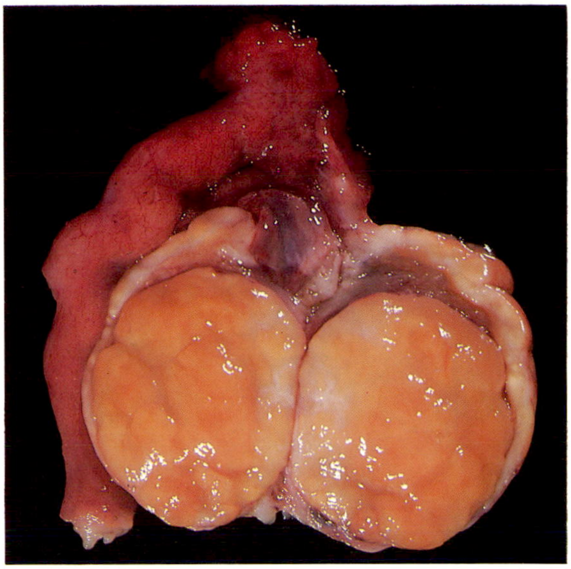

FIG. 19.19. Luteinized thecoma. 1 cm

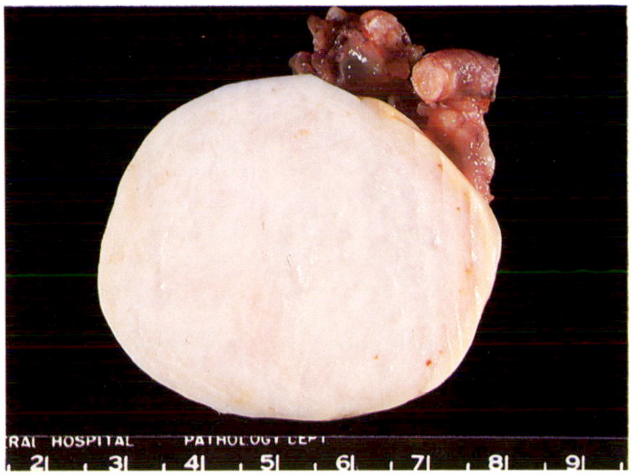

FIG. 19.25. Fibroma. Metric scale.

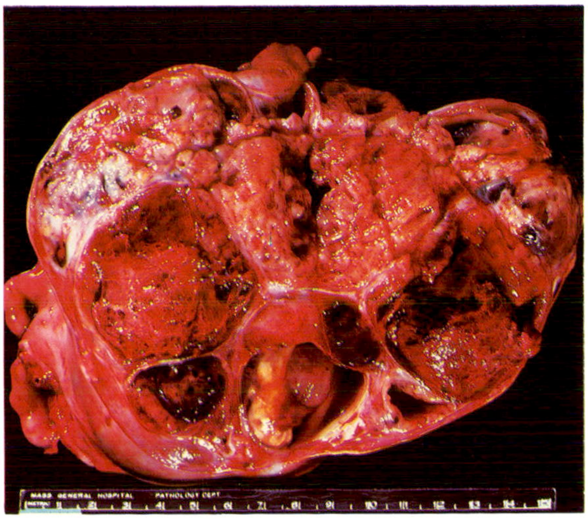

FIG. 19.14. Juvenile granulosa cell tumor. (Reprinted with permission from Ref. 323.)

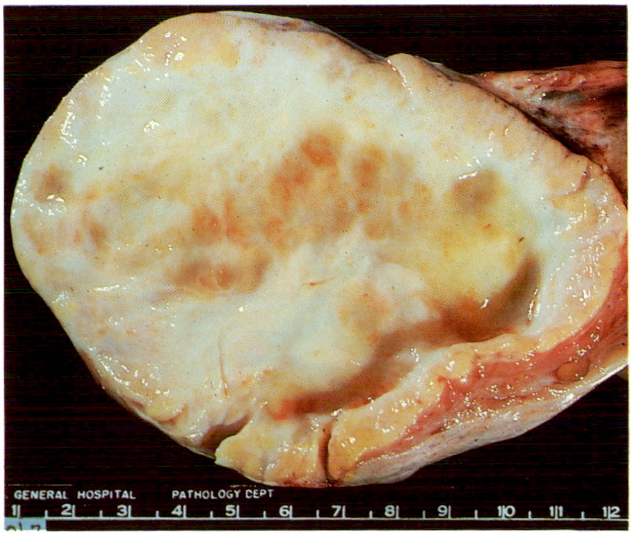

FIG. 19.31. Sclerosing stromal tumor. Metric scale.

Plate 4

a
b

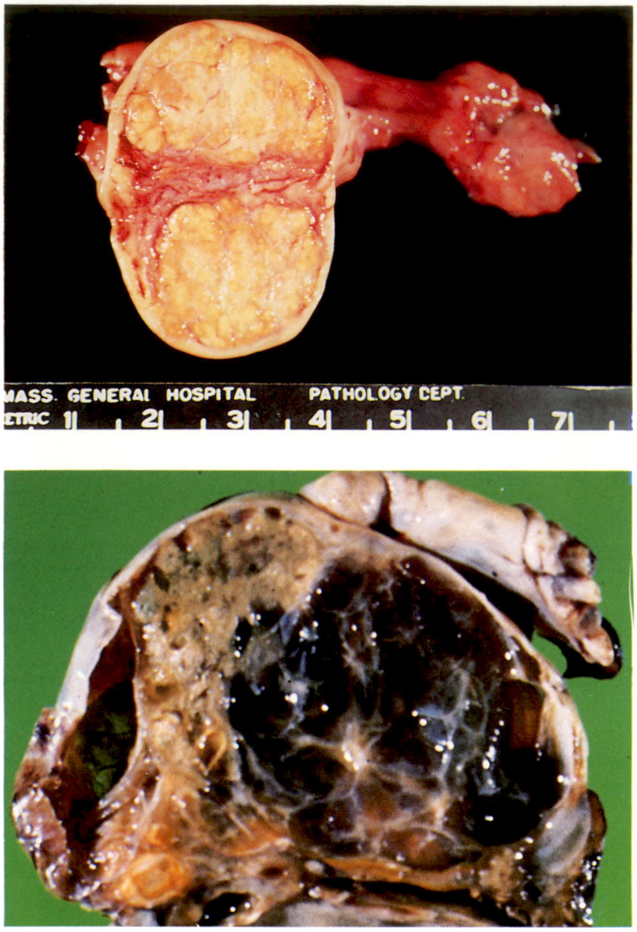

Fig. 19.38.*a*. Well-differentiated Sertoli–Leydig cell tumor. *b*. Sertoli–Leydig cell tumor with heterologous elements. The sectioned surface shows mucinous cysts and a minor component of lobulated yellow tissue. (Reprinted by permission of Young and Scully, Ref. 316.)

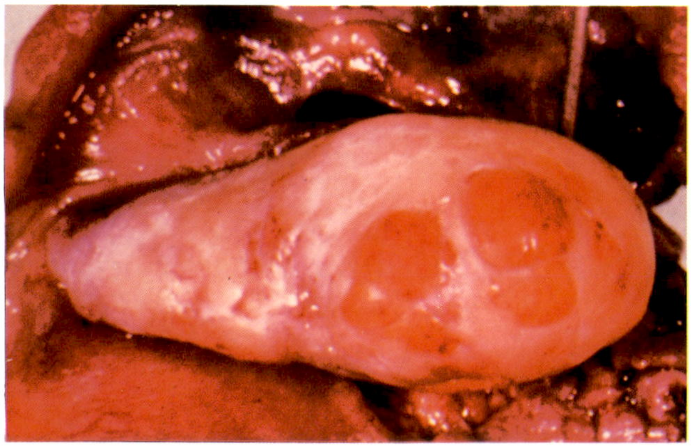

Fig. 19.62. Stromal luteoma.

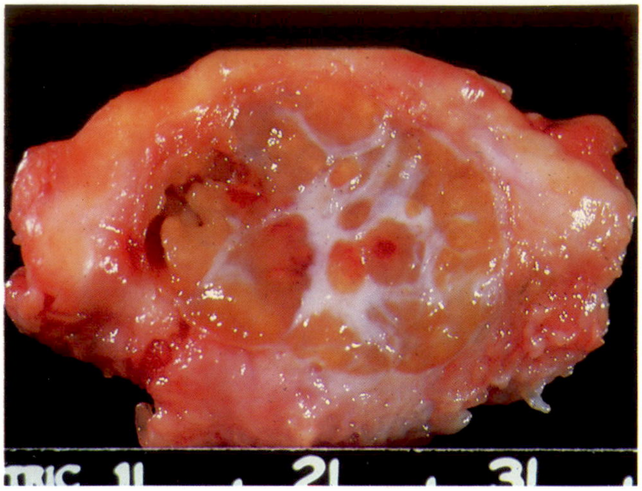

Fig. 19.68. Hilus cell tumor.

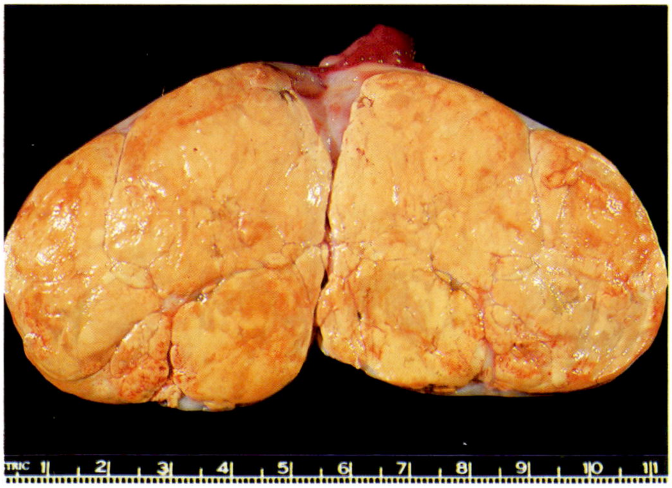

Fig. 19.69. Steroid cell tumor, unclassified (lipid cell tumor).

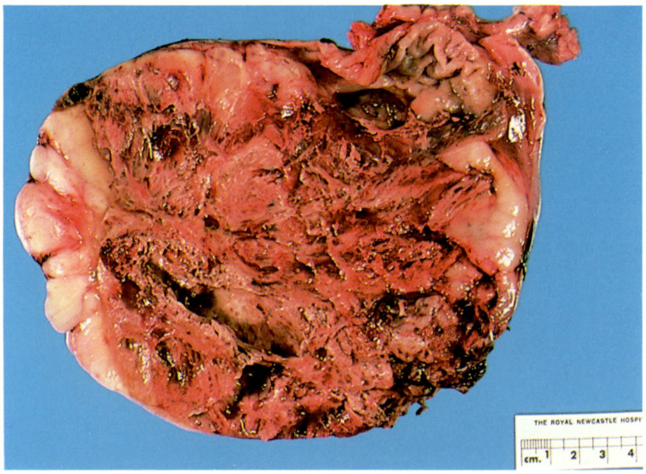

Fig. 19.79. Small cell carcinoma associated with hypercalcemia.

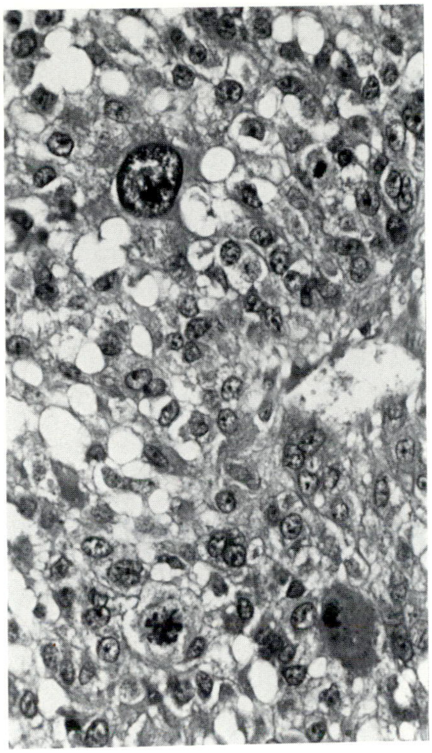

FIG. 19.18. Juvenile granulosa cell tumor. Marked nuclear atypicality and an abnormal mitotic figure are visible. This tumor was clinically malignant. (Reprinted by permission of Young and Scully, Ref. 311.)

in one of them, malignant cells were present on cytologic examination of the ascitic fluid. All 3 stage II tumors were fatal. Although both the mitotic rate and the degree of nuclear atypicality correlated with the prognosis when tumors of all stages were considered, no such correlation was evident when only stage I tumors were evaluated. In conclusion, despite the frequent presence of disquieting features, such as severe nuclear atypicality and very high mitotic rates, a juvenile granulosa cell tumor that is confined to the ovary appears to have an excellent prognosis.

In view of the rarity of bilateral ovarian involvement and their excellent prognosis, stage 1A granulosa cell tumors can be treated by a unilateral operation. Very little experience has accumulated on the role of radiation therapy and chemotherapy in the management of persistent or recurrent tumor, but isolated examples of the efficacy of these modes of therapy have been recorded.[323]

Thecoma

Thecomas can be divided into typical[17,108] and luteinized forms.[135,225,335] The typical thecoma is composed of swollen, lipid-laden stromal cells resembling theca cells; varying numbers of fibroblasts are usually present as well. Although differing criteria for the differential diagnosis of thecoma and fibroma have resulted in varying estimates of the frequency of these tumors, thecomas are approximately one-third as common as granulosa cell tumors if one includes in the former category only those tumors containing moderate to abundant lipid or associated with evidence of estrogen secretion. The thecoma occurs at an older average age than the granulosa cell tumor, being very rare before puberty and uncommon before the age of 30 years. In a recent large series, 84% of the patients were postmenopausal, with a mean age of 59 years; only 10% of the patients were under 30 years of age.[31] In that series, 60% of the postmenopausal women had uterine bleeding, and 21% of the patients had endometrial carcinoma.

Thecomas range in size from small, impalpable tumors to large, solid masses. Most of them are 5–10 cm in diameter.[17,108] Sectioning typically discloses a solid yellow mass (Fig. 19.19, Plate 3), but in some cases, the tumor is white with only focal tinges of yellow. Cysts and foci of hemorrhage and necrosis are uncommon. Microscopic examination reveals masses of cells, most of which are ill-defined and oval or rounded. The cytoplasm is pale and vacuolated, containing moderate to abundant amounts of lipid (Fig. 19.20). The nuclei vary from round to spindle-shaped and exhibit little or no atypia. Mitoses are absent or infrequent. Hyaline plaques are often conspicuous (Fig. 19.20). In thecomas, in contrast to granulosa cell tumors, reticulum fibrils typically surround individual tumor cells (Fig. 19.21).

Tumors that are predominantly fibromatous or thecomatous but also contain collections of steroid-type cells resembling luteinized theca and stromal cells have been called *luteinized thecomas* (Fig. 19.22). In our series of 46 cases of these tumors, half of them were estrogenic, 39% were nonfunctioning, and 11% were androgenic.[335] Two of the four patients with tumors of this type described by Roth and Sternberg[225] were also virilized. This relatively high frequency of masculinization contrasts with its great rarity in association with nonluteinized thecomas. Luteinized thecomas also occur in a younger age group than typical thecomas. Although they are most frequent in postmenopausal women, 30% of them have occurred in patients under 30 years of age. When, on rare occasions, crystals of Reinke are identified in the steroid-type cells (Fig. 19.23),[241] the term *stromal Leydig cell tumor* is appropriate.[273] Only six such tumors have been reported; three of them were virilizing.[273,335]

Both typical and luteinized thecomas are unilateral in 97% of the cases and are almost never malignant. Several tumors have been reported as malignant thecomas, but some of them are better interpreted as endocrinologically inactive fibrosarcomas or diffuse granulosa cell tumors.[307] In patients in whom the preservation of fertility is important, a thecoma can be treated adequately

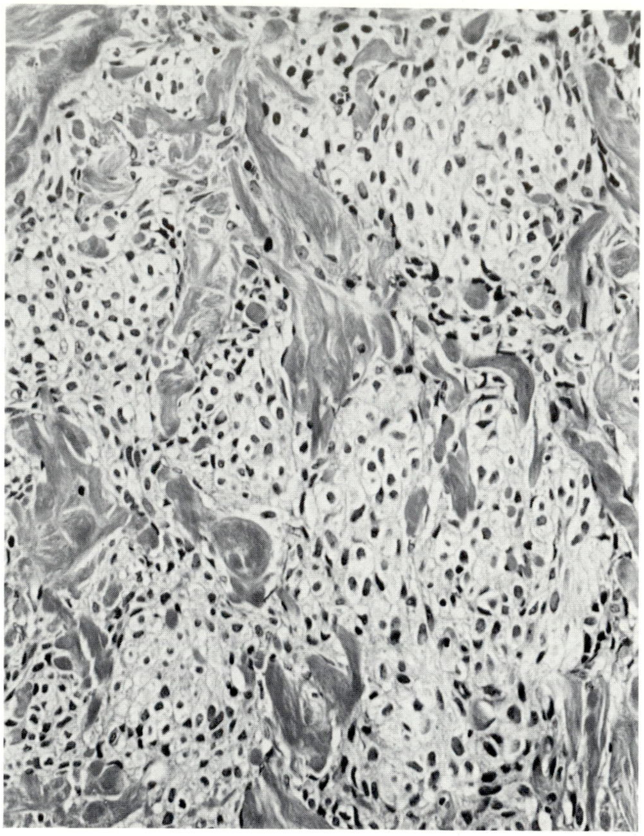

FIG. 19.20. Thecoma. The tumor cells have abundant pale cytoplasm. Hyaline plaques are conspicuous. (Reprinted by permission of Young and Scully, Ref. 316.)

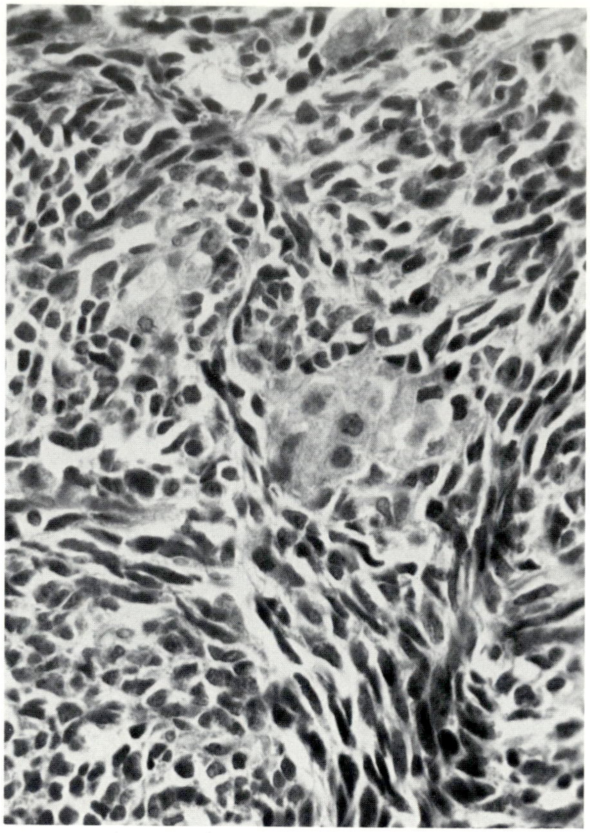

FIG. 19.22. Luteinized thecoma. Luteinized cells are present within fibromatous background. (Reprinted by permission of Young and Scully, Ref. 311.)

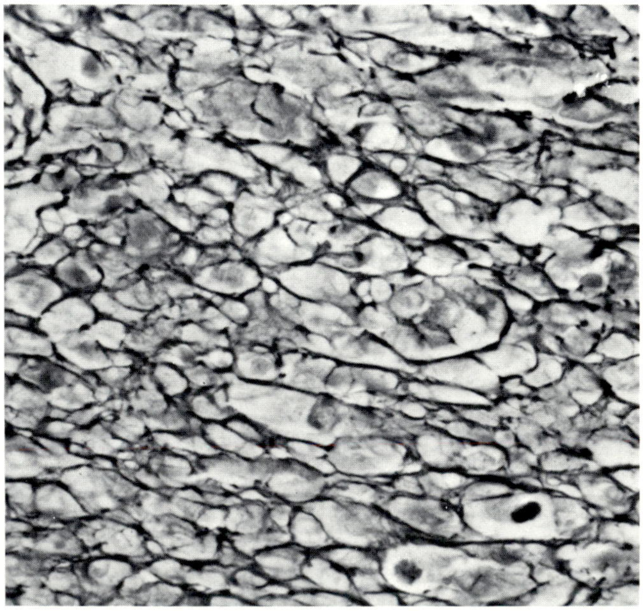

FIG. 19.21. Thecoma (reticulum stain). Contrast with reticulum pattern of granulosa cell tumor in Fig. 19.12. (Reprinted by permission of Serov et al., Ref. 257.)

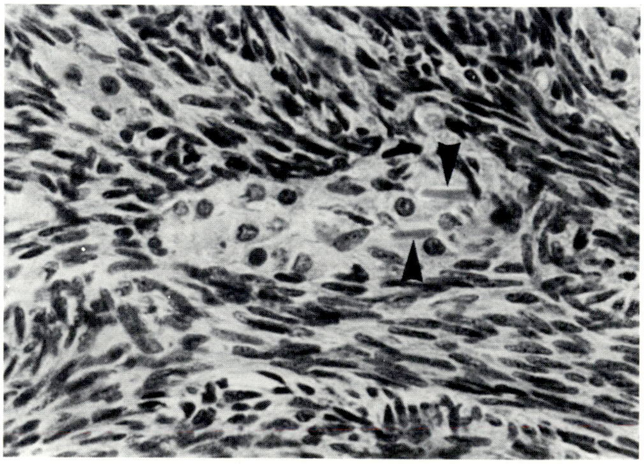

FIG. 19.23. Stromal Leydig cell tumor. Crystals of Reinke (*arrows*) are present within steroid type cells. (Reprinted by permission of Scully RE: An unusual ovarian tumor containing Leydig cells but associated with endometrial hyperplasia, in a postmenopausal woman. J Clin Endocr Metab 13:1254–1263, 1953, © by The Endocrine Society.)

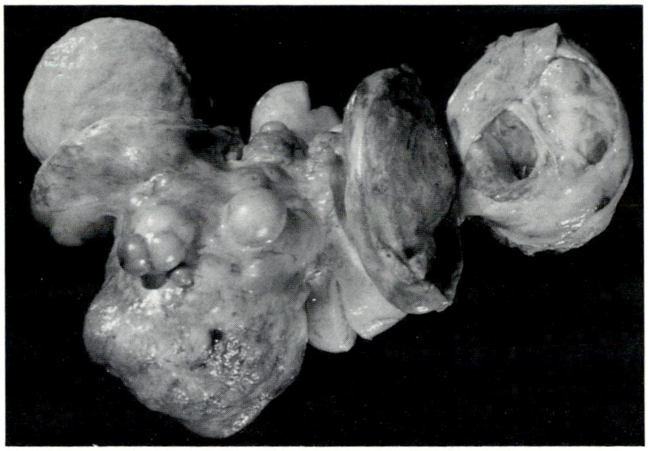

FIG. 19.24. Multinodular, partly sectioned fibroma from patient with basal cell nevus syndrome. (Reprinted by permission of Case Records of the Massachusetts General Hospital, Ref. 52.)

by oophorectomy. Total hysterectomy with bilateral salpingo-oophorectomy is indicated, however, in most patients who are menopausal or postmenopausal.

Fibroma

This tumor, which is composed of spindle cells forming variable amounts of collagen, accounts for 4% of all ovarian tumors. It occurs at all ages but is most frequent during middle age, with an average age of 48 years. Fewer than 10% of these tumors are encountered under the age of 30 years.[36,145,188,298] The fibroma is not associated with steroid hormone production but may be accompanied by two unusual clinical syndromes, Meigs' syndrome[177] and the basal cell nevus syndrome (Gorlin's syndrome).[23,42,116,117,216] The former, which complicates about 1% of ovarian fibromas, is defined as ascites and pleural effusion accompanying a fibrous ovarian tumor, usually a fibroma, and disappearing after the removal of the tumor. Ascites alone is present in association with 10–15% of ovarian fibromas over 10 cm in diameter.[237] The most widely accepted explanation of Meigs' syndrome is seepage of fluid from the tumor through its serosal surface into the peritoneal cavity, with subsequent passage into one or both pleural cavities either via lymphatics or through a communication between the abdominal and pleural cavity, such as the foramen of Bochdalek.[177]

The hereditary basal cell nevus syndrome is characterized by one or more of the following findings: basal cell carcinomas appearing early in life, keratocysts of the jaw, calcification of the dura, mesenteric cysts, and other less common abnormalities,[116,117] as well as ovarian fibromas, which are typically bilateral, multinodular, and calcified (Fig. 19.24).[52] A case of fibrosarcoma of the ovary in a child with the basal cell nevus syndrome was reported recently.[153]

Fibromas range in size from microscopic to very large.[82] Very small tumors are not uncommon, and their occurrence probably accounts for the high frequency of such tumors in some series of ovarian neoplasms. For statistical purposes, a fibromatous nodule less than 3 cm in diameter should not be considered a true neoplasm. Sectioning of fibromas typically reveals hard, flat, chalky-white surfaces that have a whorled appearance (Fig. 19.25, Plate 3). Areas of edema, occasionally with cyst formation, are relatively common. Focal or diffuse calcification and bilaterality are each observed in fewer than 10% of the cases,[268] but, as mentioned previously, these features are characteristic of the fibromas associated with the basal cell nevus syndrome (Fig. 19.24). Microscopic examination reveals intersecting bundles of spindle cells producing collagen (Figs. 19.26 and 19.27), and a storiform pattern is often encountered (Fig. 19.26).

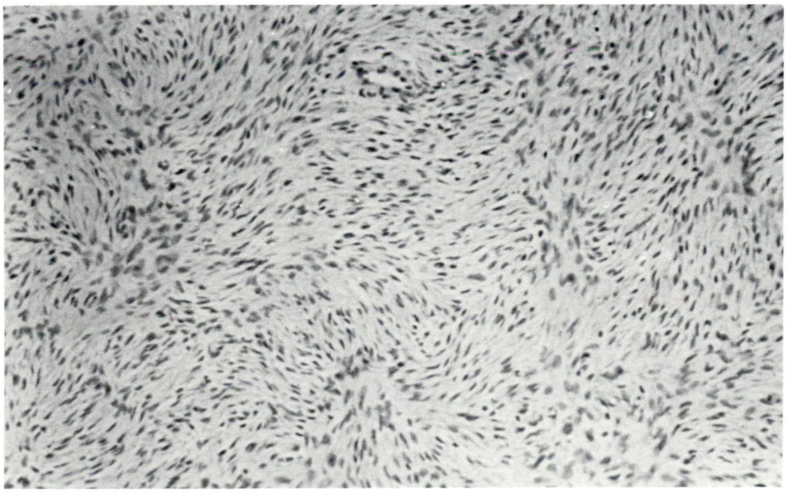

FIG. 19.26. Fibroma with storiform pattern.

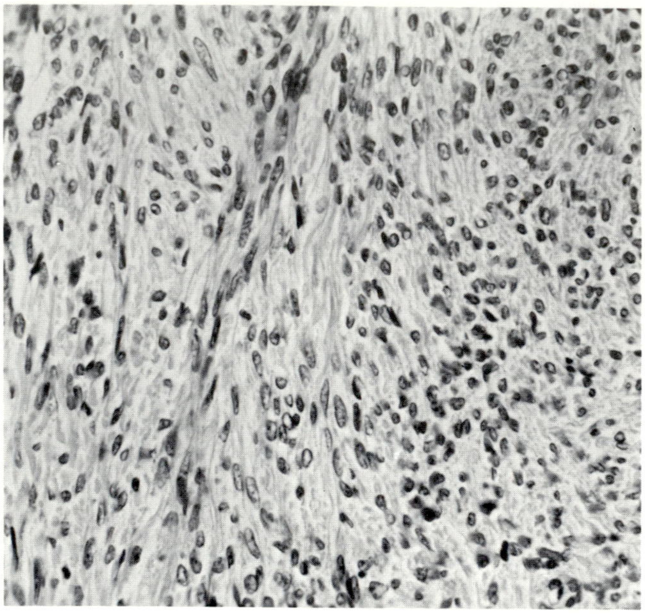

FIG. 19.27. Fibroma. The cells have small, spindle-shaped nuclei lacking atypia or mitotic activity. (Reprinted by permission of Serov et al., Ref. 257.)

The presence of bands of hyalinized fibrous tissue is not uncommon. Many tumors show varying degrees of intercellular edema (Fig. 19.28), which may have a myxoid appearance.[237] The cytoplasm of the neoplastic cells may contain small quantities of lipid. An occasional fibroma contains a minor component of sex cord elements (Fig. 19.29).

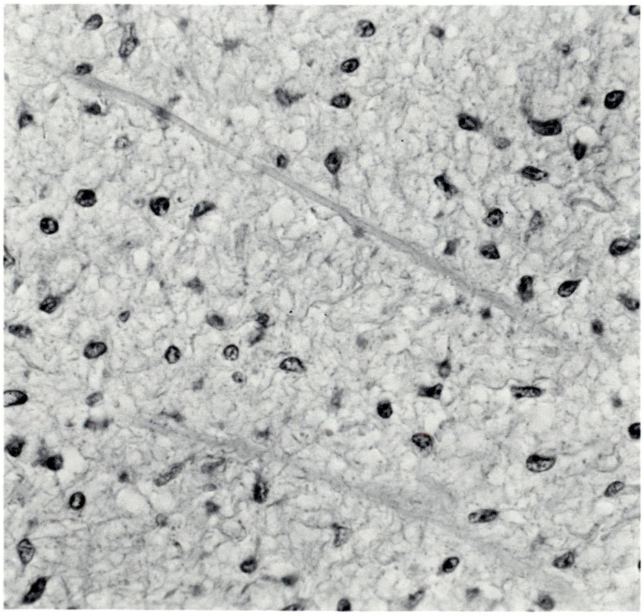

FIG. 19.28. Edematous fibroma. (Reprinted by permission of Serov et al., Ref. 257.)

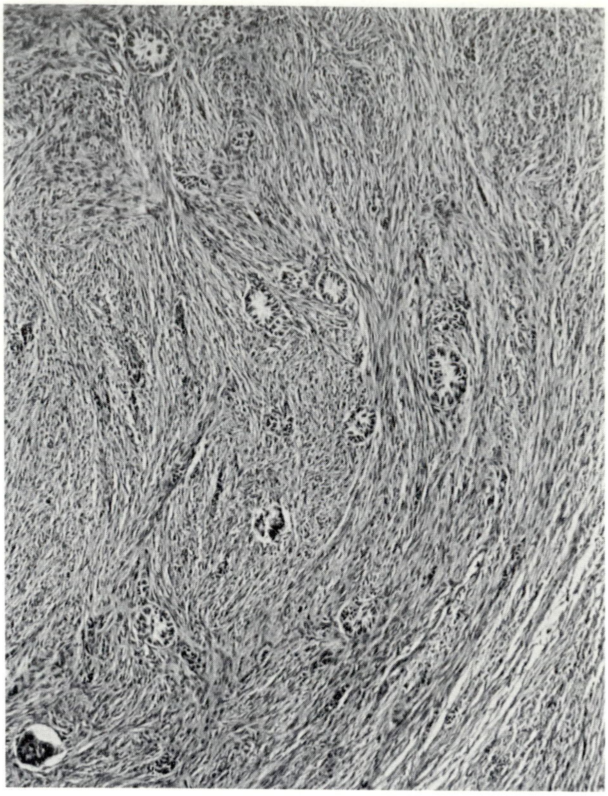

FIG. 19.29. Fibroma with minor sex cord elements. Sertoliform tubules are scattered within a fibromatous tumor. (Reprinted by permission of Young and Scully, Ref. 312.)

The fibroma must be distinguished from several non-neoplastic ovarian processes, specifically massive edema, fibromatosis, and stromal hyperplasia. The first two disorders are usually unilateral but may be bilateral and are characterized by proliferation of ovarian stromal cells, with marked intercellular edema and the production of abundant dense collagen, respectively.[317] Unlike fibromas, which almost always displace follicles, corpora lutea, and corpora albicantia, massive edema and fibromatosis encompass these structures. Stromal hyperplasia, in contrast to an ovarian fibroma, is bilateral and is characterized by a multinodular or diffuse proliferation of closely packed, small stromal cells with minimal collagen formation.[35]

Ovarian fibromas are almost always benign, but cellular forms containing 1–3 mitotic figures per 10 HPF and showing no more than slight nuclear atypicality are of low malignant potential (LMP) (Fig. 19.30), occasionally recurring, particularly if they are adherent or have ruptured.[210] Very rarely, fibromas without any atypical features are associated with peritoneal implants.[164,311] Tumors with 4 or more mitotic figures per 10 HPF and significant nuclear atypicality are almost always associated with a malignant course and warrant the designation *fibrosarcoma*.[210]

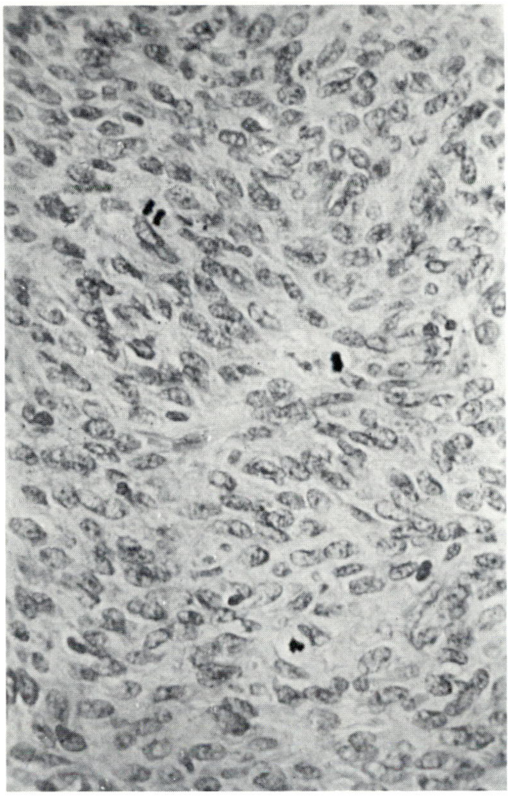

FIG. 19.30. Cellular fibroma with mitotic figures.

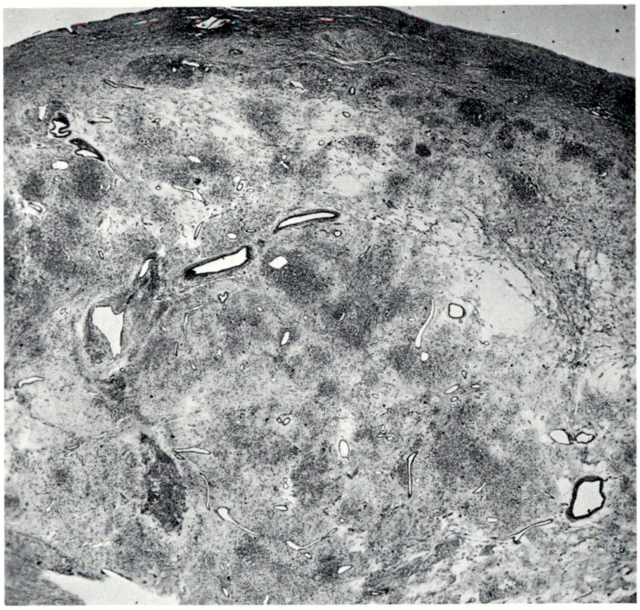

FIG. 19.32. Sclerosing stromal tumor. Cellular pseudolobules are separated by edematous hypocellular tumor. (Reprinted by permission of Chalvardjian and Scully, Ref. 59.)

Sclerosing Stromal Tumor

This tumor was within the unclassified category in the 1973 WHO classification but has subsequently been established as a distinct entity.[59] It differs from the fibroma and the thecoma both clinically and pathologically. Whereas the latter tumors are uncommon in the first 3 decades, over 80% of sclerosing stromal tumors have been encountered during the second and third decades, with an average age at diagnosis of 27 years.[311] In contrast to the thecoma, the sclerosing stromal tumor has been associated with evidence of estrogen secretion in only a few cases.[106,284] In two cases, there was evidence of both estrogen and androgen production,[70,331] and in two, only androgenic manifestations were present.[171,215] All the sclerosing stromal tumors encountered to date have been benign.*

Gross examination reveals a unilateral, discrete, sharply demarcated mass. Its sectioned surface is basically solid and white but often shows areas of edema and cyst formation and foci of yellow discoloration (Fig. 19.31, Plate 3). A rare specimen occurs as a unilocular cyst.[132,294] Microscopic examination discloses a number of distinctive features: a pseudolobular pattern (Fig. 19.32),

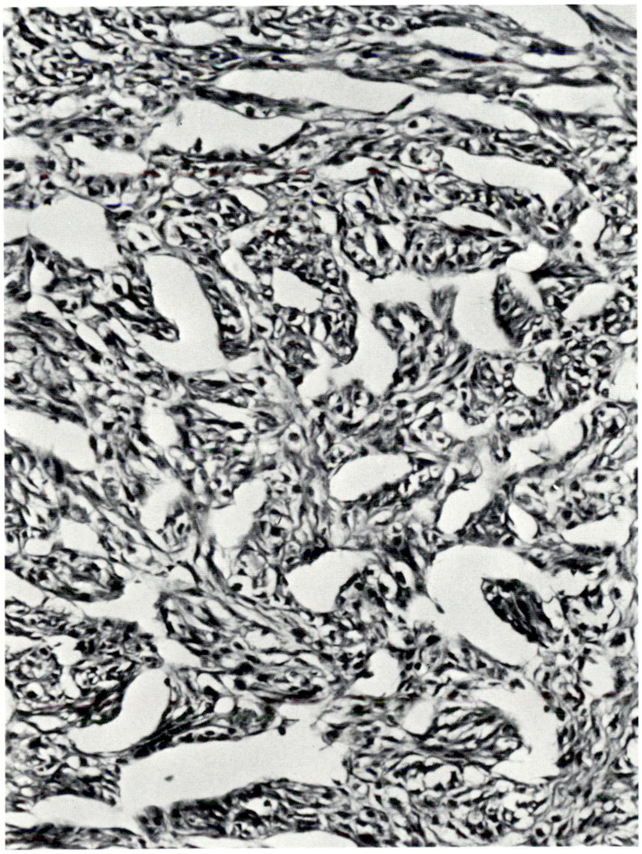

FIG. 19.33. Sclerosing stromal tumor. Pseudolobule is richly vascularized. (Reprinted by permission of Chalvardjian and Scully, Ref. 59.)

* References 59, 70, 106, 132, 171, 215, 258, 284, 296.

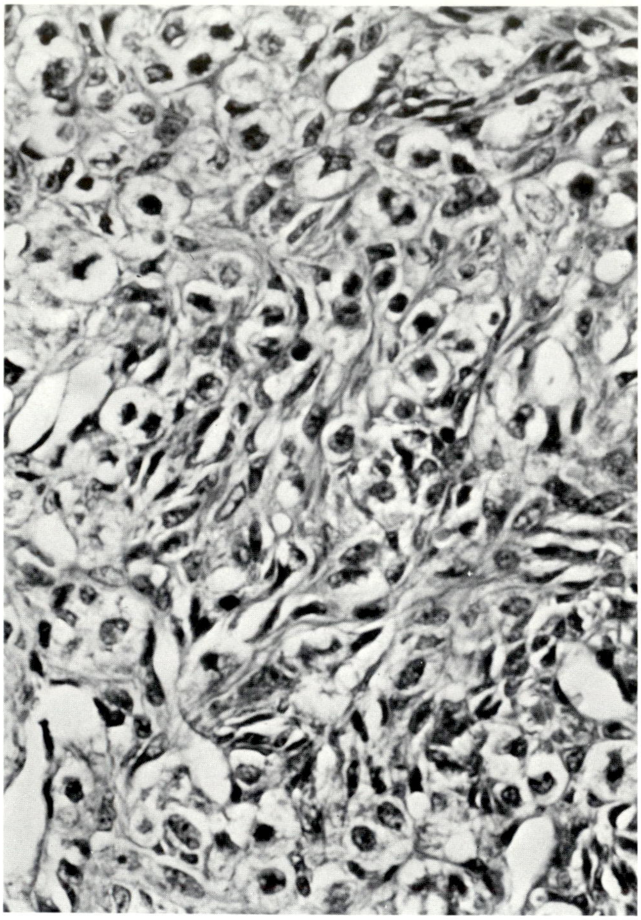

FIG. 19.34. Sclerosing stromal tumor. Spindle cells are mixed with large rounded vacuolated cells. (Reprinted by permission of Chalvardjian and Scully, Ref. 59.)

in which cellular nodules are separated by less cellular areas of densely collagenous or edematous connective tissue, sclerosis within the nodules, prominent thin-walled vessels in some of the nodules (Fig. 19.33), and a disorganized admixture of fibroblasts and rounded, vacuolated cells within the nodules (Fig. 19.34). Occasionally, the vacuolated cells have a signet cell appearance, creating some confusion with the signet cells of a Krukenberg tumor, but the vacuolated cells contain lipid instead of mucin. The lipid-laden cells appear to be inactive or weakly active lutein cells. In the rare functioning tumors, the lutein cells resemble more closely those encountered in a luteinized thecoma. Although overlap exists among fibromas, thecomas, sclerosing stromal tumors, and even steroid cell tumors, the presence of various distinctive features of these four tumors, presented in Table 19.5, almost always allows a specific diagnosis.

Unclassified Tumors

Rare tumors in the intermediate zone between fibromas and thecomas are impossible to classify more specifically. Such tumors are made up of cells having some but not all the features of theca cells, containing small to moderate amounts of lipid, and being associated with equivocal evidence of estrogen secretion.

In 1976, Ramzy[217] described an unusual ovarian tumor, which he designated signet ring stromal tumor, from a 28-year-old woman. Microscopic examination disclosed signet ring cells that failed to stain for lipid or mucin. Reticulum stains suggested that the neoplastic cells were mesenchymal in origin. No additional examples of this entity have been reported, but we have seen one such tumor from a 34-year-old woman. The nature of the tumor and its vacuoles remains unclear.

TABLE 19.5. Sclerosing versus other stromal tumors and steroid cell tumors.

Parameter	Sclerosing stromal tumor	Fibroma	Thecoma	Steroid cell tumor
Age	80% under 30 years	10% under 30 years		25% under 30 years
Function	Almost always absent	Absent	Typically estrogenic[a]	Typically androgenic
Gross variegation	Yes	No	No	No
Pseudolobulation	Yes	Rare	Rare	No
Prominent ectatic vessels	Yes	Rare	Rare	Rare
Two cell types	Yes	No	Only in luteinized form	No
Hyaline plaques	No	Common	Common	No
Behavior	Benign	Almost always benign	Almost always benign	Often malignant

[a] Luteinized form androgenic in 11% of cases.

Sertoli–Stromal Cell Tumors (Androblastomas)

These tumors contain Sertoli cells, Leydig cells, fibroblasts, or all of these cells in varying proportions and varying degrees of differentiation. Because the less well-differentiated neoplasms within this category may recapitulate the development of the testis, the terms *androblastoma* and *arrhenoblastoma* have been used as synonyms. However, the connotation of masculinization associated with those terms is misleading because many tumors in this category have no endocrine manifestations and a few are estrogenic or progestagenic. Nevertheless, WHO has selected *androblastoma* as an alternative term for these tumors.[257] We prefer the designation *Sertoli–stromal cell tumor* over WHO's *Sertoli–Leydig cell tumor* for this general category of neoplasms because the latter term is also used for the subtypes that contain both Sertoli and Leydig cells, leading to confusion. Other tumors within this group are pure Sertoli cell tumors, pure Leydig cell tumors, and stromal Leydig cell tumors. The last have already been mentioned in the discussion of luteinized thecomas, and pure Leydig cell tumors will be considered in the section on steroid cell tumors, since they may be confused with other tumors in that category.

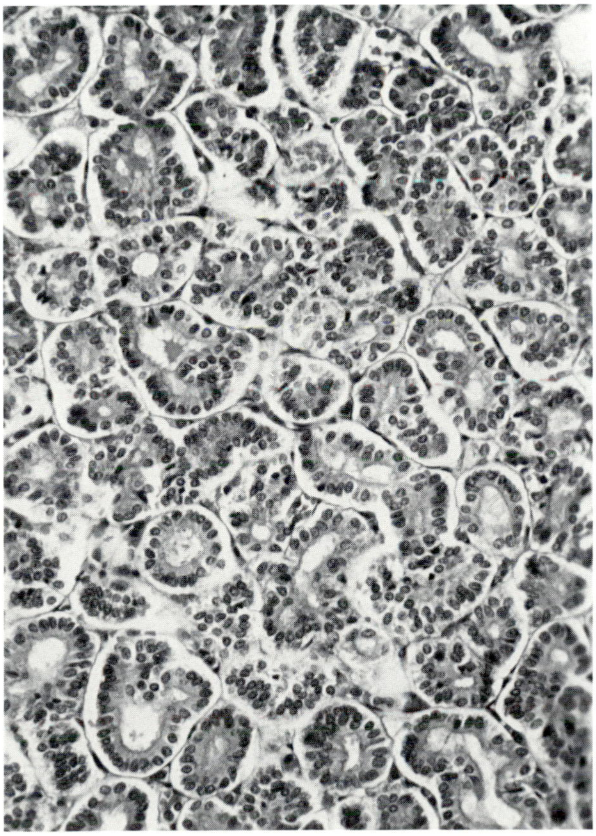

FIG. 19.35. Sertoli cell tumor. Closely packed hollow tubules lined by well-differentiated cuboidal to columnar epithelial cells. (Reprinted by permission of Young and Scully, Ref. 315.)

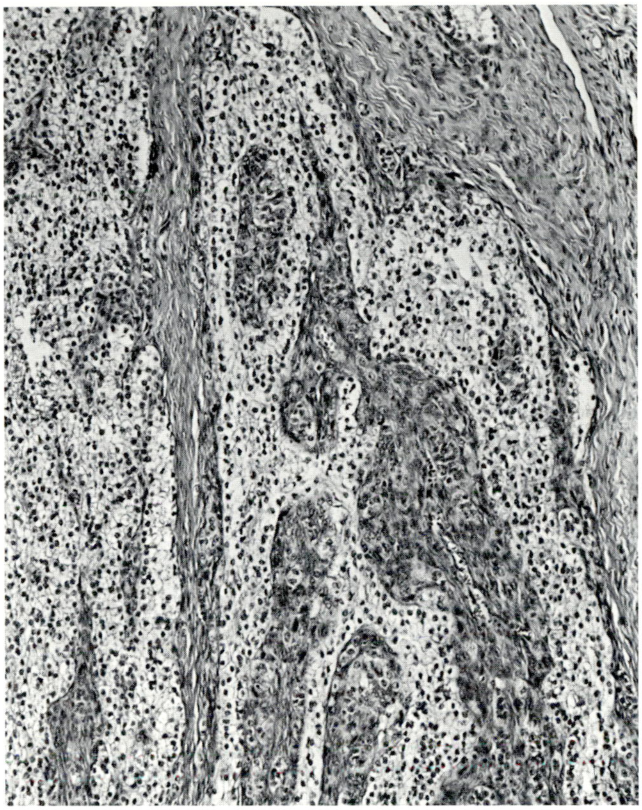

FIG. 19.36. Sertoli cell tumor, lipid rich. (Reprinted by permission of Serov et al., Ref. 257.)

Sertoli Cell Tumor

These tumors account for approximately 4% of Sertoli–stromal cell tumors.[286,288–290,315] They are characterized by a predominant pattern of hollow (Fig. 19.35) or solid tubules (Figs. 19.36 and 19.37), usually dispersed within a fibrous stroma that contains no Leydig cells or very few of them. When the Sertoli cells contain abundant cytoplasmic lipid (Figs. 19.36 and 19.37), the term *lipid-rich Sertoli cell tumor* is appropriate. This tumor had been interpreted initially as a lipid-rich granulosa cell tumor and designated *folliculome lipidique*.[61] Seven Sertoli cell tumors, most or all of which appear to have been of the lipid-rich type, have resulted in isosexual pseudoprecocity. Two of these tumors were from patients with the Peutz–Jeghers syndrome.[267,315] One Sertoli cell tumor was associated with progesterone as well as estrogen production.[295] All the Sertoli cell tumors encountered to date have been unilateral and stage I. They have averaged approximately 9 cm in diameter and typically formed lobulated, solid, yellow or brown masses. Microscopic examination usually discloses little if any nuclear atypia or mitotic activity, and the prognosis is

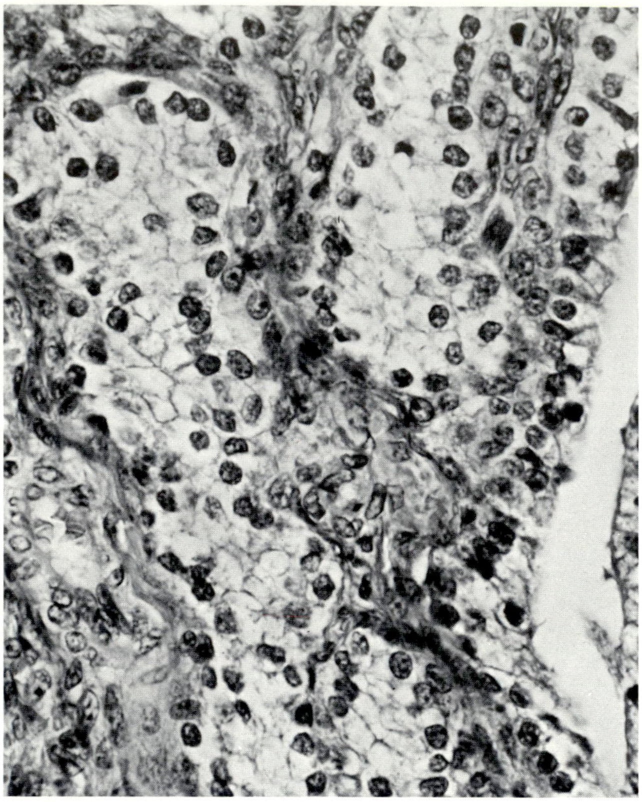

FIG. 19.37. Sertoli cell tumor, lipid rich. (Reprinted by permission of Serov et al., Ref. 257.)

excellent. Rare tumors exhibiting moderate degrees of nuclear atypia have been reported, however, and we have seen one tumor in a sexually precocious child that was focally poorly differentiated, metastasized distantly, and was rapidly fatal.[315]

Sertoli–Leydig Cell Tumor

These tumors account for less than 0.5% of all ovarian tumors but are among the most fascinating from both pathologic and clinical viewpoints.[109,202,206,229,333] They have been divided into four categories by WHO: well differentiated, of intermediate differentiation, poorly differentiated, and with heterologous elements.[257] In addition, tumors with a retiform pattern of significant extent merit separate consideration.[314] Sertoli–Leydig cell tumors occur in all age groups but are encountered most often in young women. In our series of over 200 cases the average age was 25 years, 75% of the patients were 30 years of age or younger, and only 9.5% were over 50 years of age. The average age in two other large series was 24 and 24.5 years.[319] The well-differentiated tumors occur on average a decade later, and tumors with a retiform pattern occur a decade earlier than other tumors in this category. Tumors with a retiform pattern are more common than any other subtype in the first decade.

Clinical Aspects. Although the most striking mode of presentation of Sertoli–Leydig cell tumors is virilization, this develops in only about one third of the patients.[319] In such cases, a patient who has been having normal periods typically begins to have oligomenorrhea, followed within a few months by amenorrhea. There is a concomitant loss of female secondary sex characteristics, with atrophy of the breasts and disappearance of normal bodily contours. Progressive masculinization is heralded by acne, with hirsutism, temporal balding, deepening of the voice, and enlargement of the clitoris following in its wake. The androgen secretion by the tumor may also result in erythrocytosis. Although two studies[206,229] reported an increased frequency of androgenic changes in association with less well differentiated tumors, there was no significant difference in the frequency of these manifestations among the various subtypes in our series, except that it was lower with tumors containing heterologous elements and lowest with tumors having a prominent retiform component.[319]

Plasma levels of testosterone, androstenedione, and other androgens, alone or in combination, may be elevated in patients with Sertoli–Leydig cell tumors.[207,213] The urinary 17-ketosteroid values are usually normal or only slightly raised, although occasionally a high level has been recorded.[333] These findings are in contrast to those associated with virilizing adrenal tumors, which are often accompanied by high urinary levels of 17-ketosteroids.[112] The values for plasma androgens and urinary 17-ketosteroids are not reliable, however, in the differentiation of ovarian and adrenal virilizing tumors, since the latter are often accompanied by elevated testosterone and normal urinary 17-ketosteroid levels.[3] Tests involving attempted stimulation by tropic hormones and suppression by gonadal and adrenocortical steroids have not proved decisive in differentiating these tumors.[144] Seven Sertoli–Leydig cell tumors associated with elevated plasma levels of alpha fetoprotein have been reported,[20,62,168,281,292] but values as high as those accompanying endodermal sinus tumors were recorded in only two cases.[281,326]

Approximately 60% of patients with Sertoli–Leydig cell tumors have no endocrine manifestations and usually complain of abdominal swelling or pain.[319] Occasional tumors have been associated with various estrogenic syndromes, including irregular menses, menorrhagia, or menometrorrhagia in women in the reproductive age group and postmenopausal bleeding in older women.[76,319] No well-documented case of a Sertoli–Leydig cell tumor associated with isosexual precocity has been reported. At laparotomy almost all Sertoli–Leydig cell tumors are unilateral; in our series only 1.5% were bilateral.[319] The tumors are stage IAi in about 80% of the cases, in 12% the tumor has either ruptured or involved the external surface of the ovary, and in 4% ascites is present. Only about 2.5% of the tumors have spread beyond the ovary, usually within the pelvis and rarely into the upper abdomen. All the well-differentiated tumors in our series were stage IAi. The poorly differentiated tumors were more often ruptured or were at a higher stage than the tumors of intermediate differentiation.

Gross Appearance. Sertoli–Leydig cell tumors vary as greatly in their gross appearance as granulosa cell tumors, and these neoplasms cannot be distinguished on macroscopic examination alone. There are, however, a few general differences. Sertoli–Leydig cell tumors contain cysts filled with blood less often than do granulosa cell tumors and, unlike the latter, almost never have the appearance of a unilocular, thin-walled cyst. Sertoli–Leydig cell tumors vary in size from microscopic to huge masses, but the majority are between 5 and 15 (average 13.5) cm in diameter (Fig. 19.38, Plate 4). Poorly differentiated tumors tend to be larger than those of better differentiation and contain areas of hemorrhage and necrosis more frequently. Tumors with heterologous or retiform components are more often cystic than are tumors without these elements. The heterologous tumors occasionally simulate mucinous cystic tumors on gross examination, and retiform tumors may contain large, edematous papillae, resembling serous papillary tumors.

Microscopic Appearance. Well-differentiated Sertoli–Leydig cell tumors are characterized by a predominantly tubular pattern (Fig. 19.39).[318] On low power examination, a nodular architecture is often conspicuous, with fibrous bands intersecting lobules composed of hollow or, less often, solid tubules. In some tumors, tubules of both types are present. The hollow tubules are typically round to oval and small but may be cystically dilated and may even resemble the tubular glands of a well-differentiated endometrioid adenocarcinoma.[71] The lumens are usually devoid of conspicuous secretion, but in some cases eosinophilic fluid, which may occasionally be mucicarminophilic, is present. The solid tubules are typically elongated but may be round or oval and occasionally resemble prepubertal or atrophic testicular tubules. The tubules contain cuboidal to columnar epipthelial cells with round or oblong nuclei without prominent nucleoil. Nuclear atypia is usually absent or minimal, and mitotic figures are rare. The cells lining the hollow tubules and filling the solid tubules typically contain moderate amounts of dense cytoplasm, but in some cases varying numbers of them have abundant pale cytoplasm rich in lipid. The stromal component consists of bands of mature fibrous tissue containing variable but usually conspicuous numbers of Leydig cells. These cells may contain abundant lipochrome pigment. In our series, crystals of Reinke were identified in some of the Leydig cells in approximately 20% of the cases (Fig. 19.40).[318]

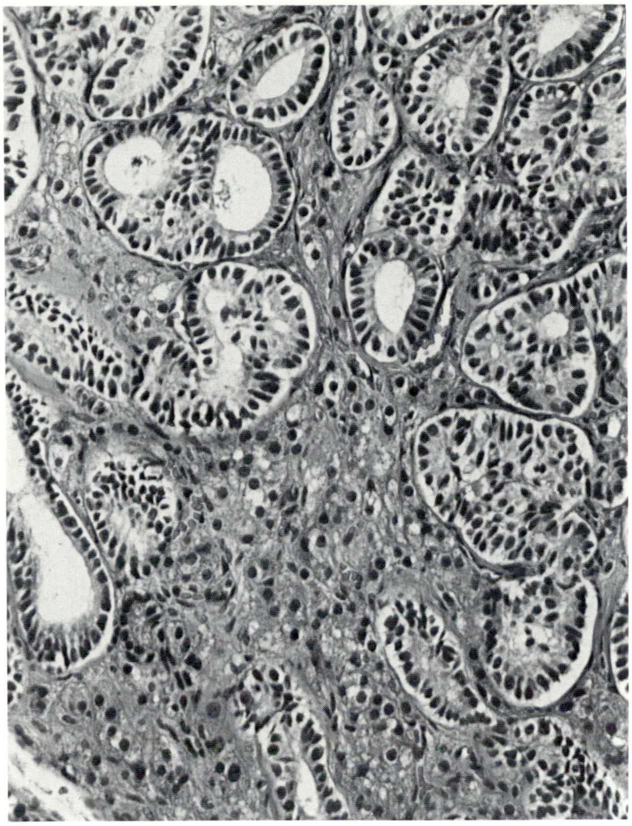

Fig. 19.39. Sertoli–Leydig cell tumor, well differentiated. Hollow tubules separated by Leydig cells in intervening stroma. (Reprinted by permission of Young and Scully, Ref. 318.)

Sertoli–Leydig cell tumors of intermediate and poor differentiation form a continuum characterized by a variety of patterns and combinations of cell types. Some tumors exhibit intermediate differentiation in some areas and poor differentiation in others, and, less commonly, tumors of intermediate differentiation contain well-differentiated foci. Both the Sertoli cells and Leydig cells may exhibit varying degrees of immaturity. In the tumors of intermediate differentiation (grades 2 and 3), immature Sertoli cells with small, round, oval, or angular nuclei are arranged typically in ill-defined masses, often creating a lobulated appearance on low power (Fig. 19.41). Solid and hollow tubules (Fig. 19.42), nests, thin cords resembling the sex cords of the embryonic testis (Fig. 19.43), and broad columns (Fig. 19.44) are often present. These structures are separated by stroma, which ranges from fibromatous to densely cellular to edematous and typically contains clusters of well-differentiated Leydig cells. Occasionally, part or all of the stromal component is made up of immature, cellular mesenchymal tissue resembling a nonspecific sarcoma. Cysts containing eosino-

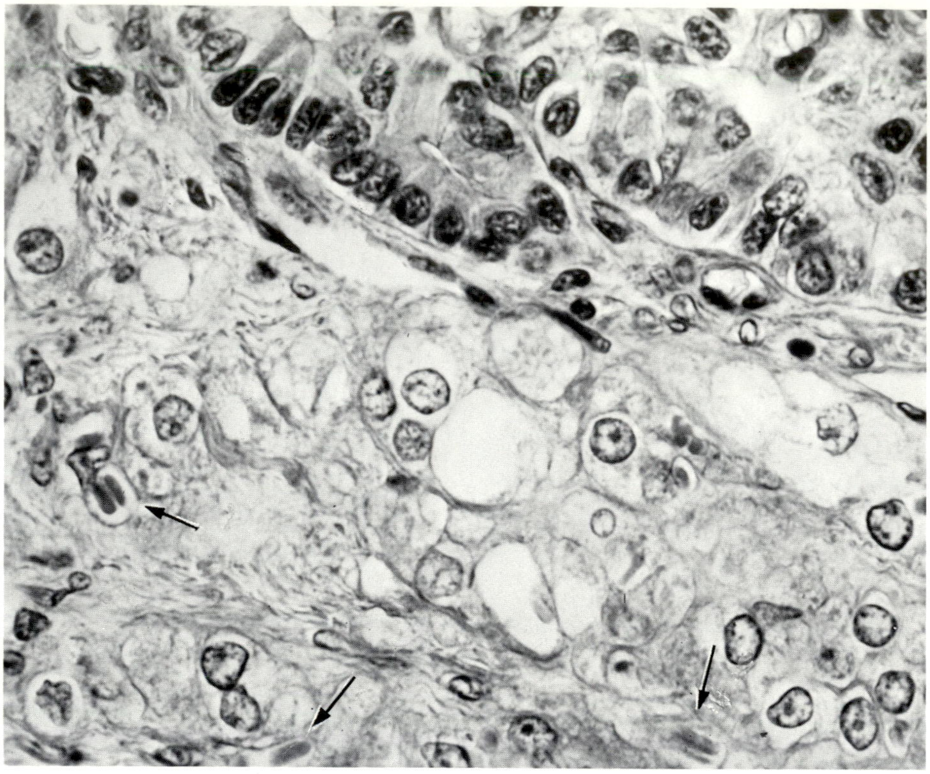

FIG. 19.40. Sertoli–Leydig cell tumor, well differentiated. *Arrows* point to crystals of Reinke. (Reprinted by permission of Scully, Ref. 242.)

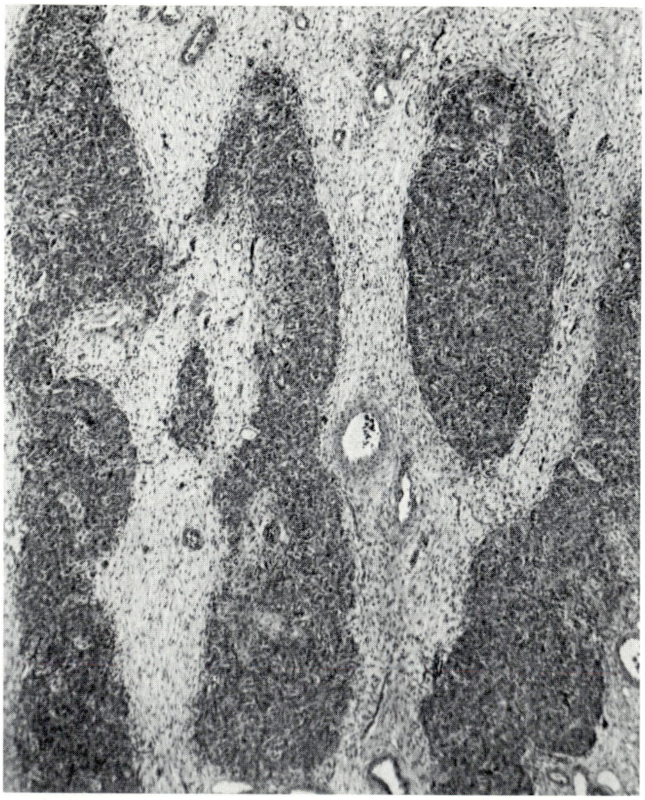

FIG. 19.41. Sertoli–Leydig cell tumor of intermediate differentiation. Cellular lobules are intersected by slightly edematous stromal component. (Reprinted by permission of Young and Scully, Ref. 319.)

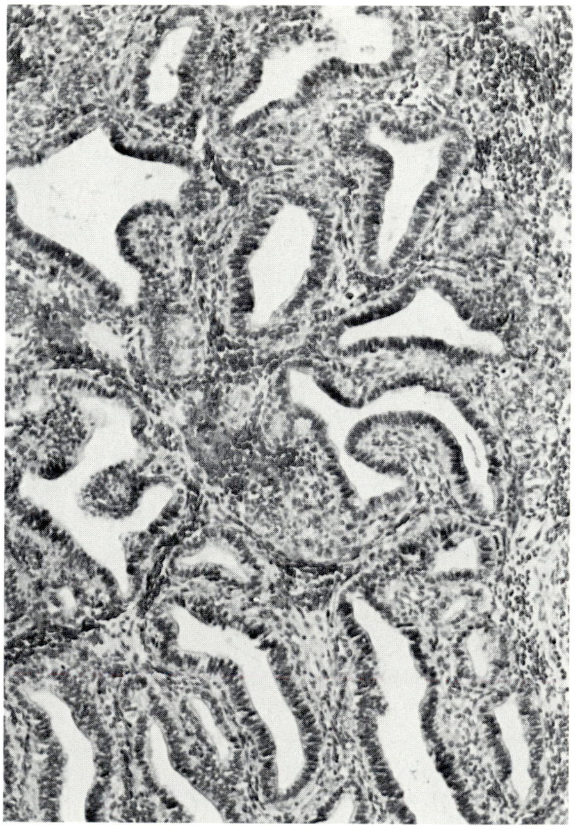

FIG. 19.42. Sertoli–Leydig cell tumor of intermediate differentiation. The tubules in this neoplasm resemble those of an endometrioid tumor.

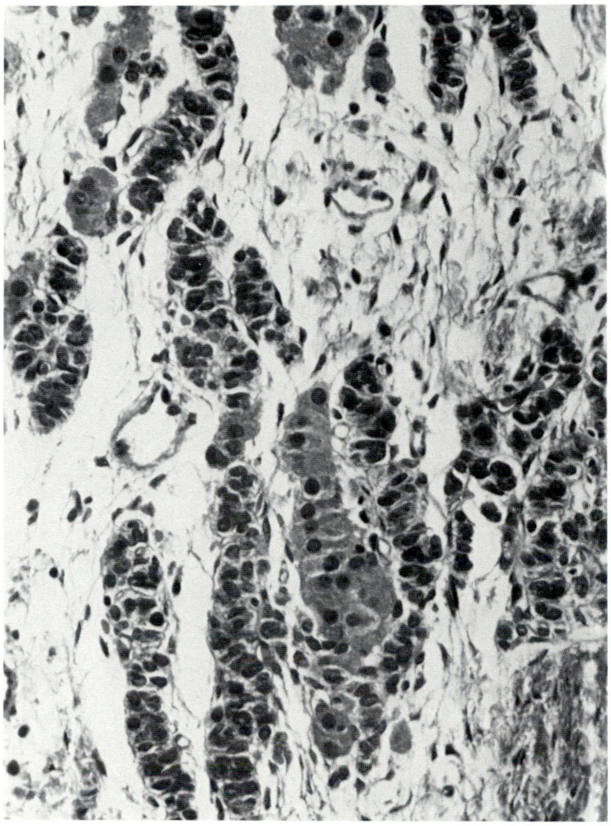

FIG. 19.43. Sertoli–Leydig cell tumor of intermediate differentiation. Cords of immature Sertoli cells and clusters of Leydig cells with abundant cytoplasm. (Reprinted by permission of Young and Scully, Ref. 314.)

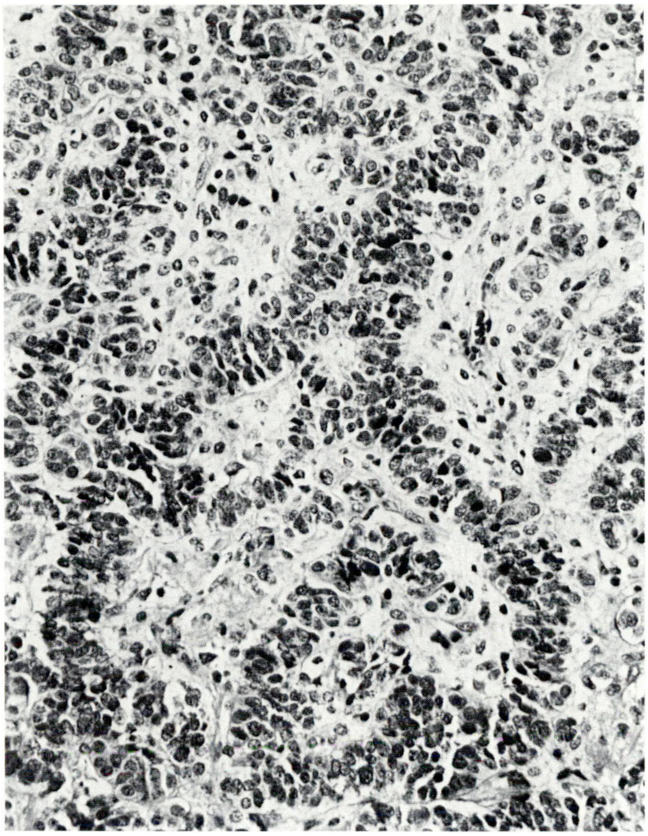

FIG. 19.44. Sertoli–Leydig cell tumor of intermediate differentiation. Anastomosing columns of immature Sertoli cells. (Reprinted by permission of Young and Scully, Ref. 319.)

philic secretion may be present and create a thyroid-like appearance, and follicle-like spaces are encountered rarely.

The Sertoli and Leydig cell elements, singly or together, may contain varying and sometimes large amounts of lipid in the form of small or large droplets (Fig. 19.45). Poorly differentiated (grade 4) Sertoli–Leydig cell tumors were originally classified as sarcomatoid because, aside from the presence of specifically diagnostic elements, they resemble fibrosarcomas (Fig. 19.46). However, they often have a diffuse pattern that is not clearly recognizable as that of a fibrosarcoma. Talerman et al.[282] have described a group of tumors containing diffuse fibrothecomatous and granulosa cell-type proliferation as well as areas of tubular differentiation in most of the cases. These authors have interpreted these tumors, which differ in appearance from the usual forms of Sertoli–Leydig cell tumor, as diffuse nonlobular androblastomas.

Fifteen percent of Sertoli–Leydig cell tumors are composed usually partially but occasionally entirely of tubular structures arranged in a pattern resembling that of the rete testis.[228,244,314] When 5% or more of a specimen is characterized by such a pattern, important clinical correlations warrant adding the term *retiform* to the designation of the tumor (Fig. 19.47).[314] So far a retiform pattern has been encountered only in tumors that are otherwise intermediate, poorly differentiated, or heterologous. Microscopic examination reveals a network of irregularly branching, elongated, narrow, often slit-like tubules and cysts, into which papillae or polypoid structures may project (Fig. 19.48). The tubules and cysts may contain eosinophilic secretion. They are lined by epithelial cells that exhibit varying degrees of stratification and nuclear atypicality. The papillae and polyps are of three types. Most commonly, they are small and rounded or blunt, often containing hyalinized cores (Fig. 19.49). Sometimes they are large and bulbous, containing edematous cores. Finally, in some cases they are delicate and branch extensively and may be lined by stratified cells, simulating the papillae of a serous tumor of borderline or invasive type (Fig. 19.50). The stroma within a retiform area may be hyalinized or edematous, moderately cellular or densely cellular, and immature.

Heterologous elements occur in approximately 20% of Sertoli–Leydig cell tumors, most of which are other-

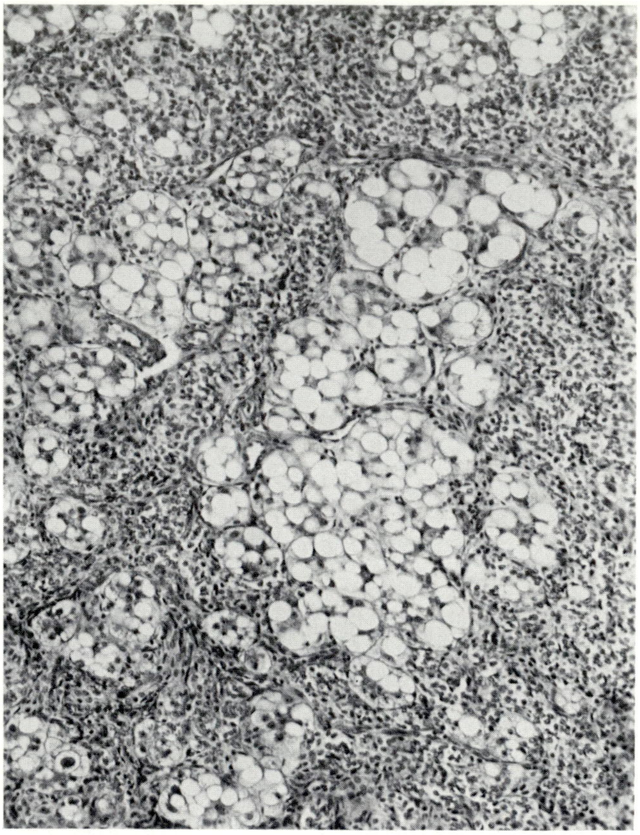

FIG. 19.45. Sertoli–Leydig cell tumor of intermediate differentiation. Nests of Leydig cells with large lipid vacuoles. (Reprinted by permission of Young and Scully, Ref. 319.)

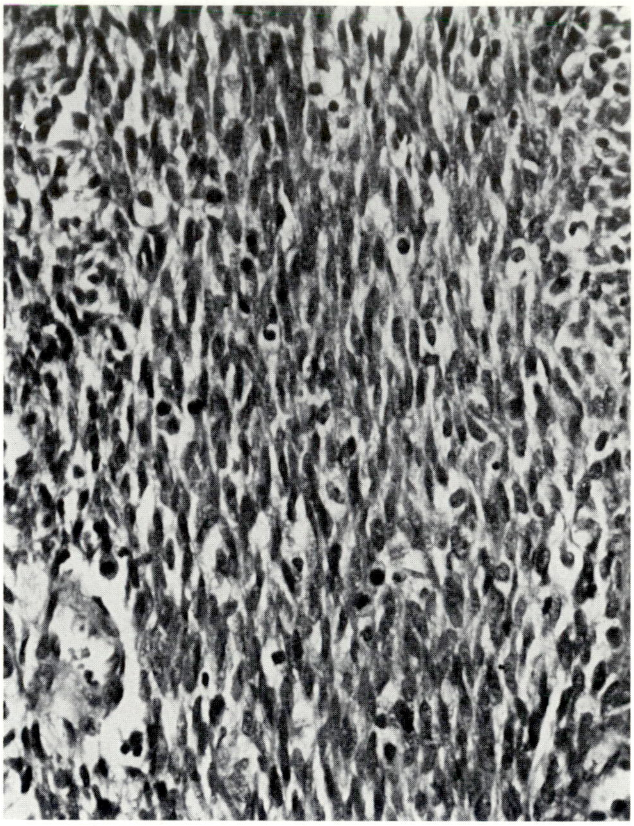

FIG. 19.46. Sertoli–Leydig cell tumor, poorly differentiated. The tumor cells are spindle-shaped and exhibit nuclear atypia and mitotic activity. (Reprinted by permission of Young and Scully, Ref. 319.)

wise of intermediate differentiation, but some of which are poorly differentiated.[211,328] In our series of over 200 tumors, 18% contained glands and cysts lined by moderately to well-differentiated intestinal-type epithelium (Fig. 19.51), which included goblet cells, argentaffin cells, and rarely Paneth cells. Sixteen percent of the heterologous Sertoli–Leydig cell tumors had one or a few microscopic foci of carcinoid (Fig. 19.52).[306,328] Stromal heterologous elements, encountered in 5% of Sertoli–Leydig cell tumors,[120,136,211] include islands of cartilage arising on a sarcomatous background, areas of embryonal rhabdomyosarcoma, or both (Fig. 19.53). We have also seen one heterologous tumor that contained cells resembling hepatocytes,[326] one containing retinal tissue, and another with neuroblastoma in a recurrent tumor.[211] Despite the variety of unexpected tissues in heterologous Sertoli–Leydig cell tumors, it appears unlikely that such neoplasms are of germ cell origin, inasmuch as neither Sertoli nor Leydig cells have ever been identified in gonadal tumors clearly recognizable as teratomas. The alternative concept of neometaplasia of cells of mesodermal derivation[325] is, in our opinion, a more attractive explanation for the existence of these tumors, although other investigators have considered these neoplasms teratomatous.[99,218]

Differential Diagnosis. Because of their many patterns, Sertoli–Leydig cell tumors are often difficult to differentiate from tumors outside the sex cord–stromal category as well as granulosa cell tumors. The small hollow tubular structures, solid tubular aggregates, and cords that are occasionally seen in endometrioid carcinomas may closely mimic structures characteristically encountered in Sertoli–Leydig cell tumors.[226,327] The former tumors may also contain luteinized stromal cells that resemble Leydig cells, creating an even greater problem in differentiation. At least some of the glands of endometrioid carcinomas, however, are usually larger than the tubules of Sertoli–Leydig cell tumors and are lined by epithelium that is less well differentiated. In addition, mucin secretion, areas of squamous differentiation, which range from nests of uniform immature spindle-shaped epithelial cells to morules to keratinizing foci, and an adenofibromatous component of common epithelial type are present in many endometrioid carcinomas, facilitating their diagnosis. Clinical features, such as the much older age of

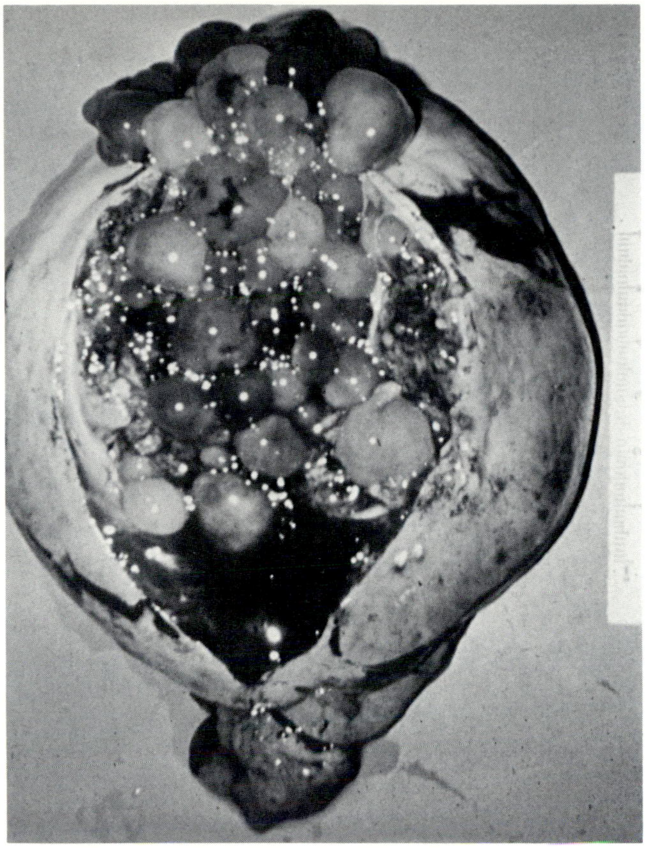

FIG. 19.47. Sertoli–Leydig cell tumor with retiform pattern. Edematous polypoid structures project into lumen of cystic neoplasm. (Reprinted by permission of Young and Scully, Ref. 314.)

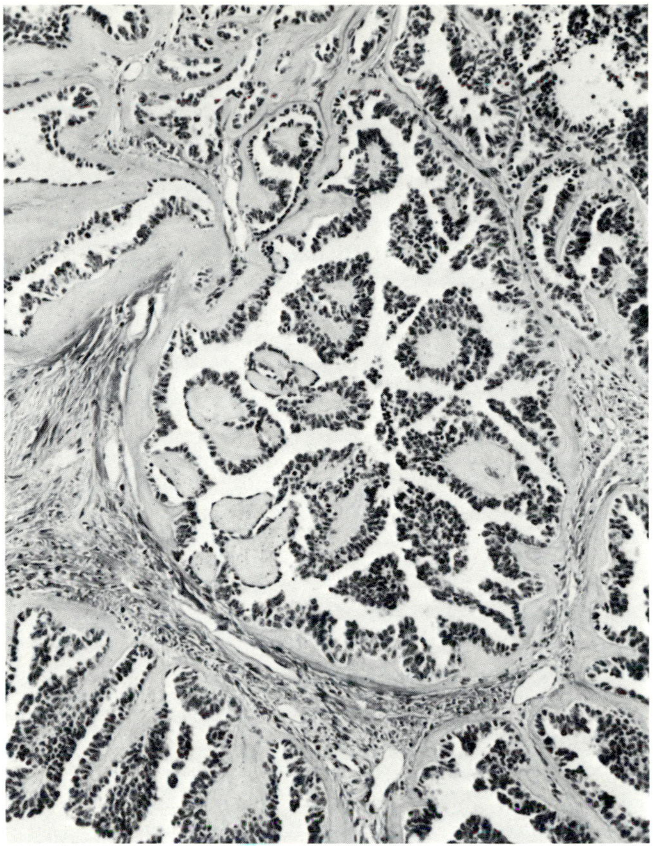

FIG. 19.49. Sertoli–Leydig cell tumor with retiform pattern. The papillae have prominent hyalinized cores and are lined by stratified epithelial cells. (Reprinted by permission of Young RH, Scully RE: Ovarian sex cord-stromal and steroid cell tumors. In: Roth LM, Czernobilsky B, eds., Tumors and Tumor-Like Conditions of the Ovary. Churchill Livingstone Inc, New York, 1985.)

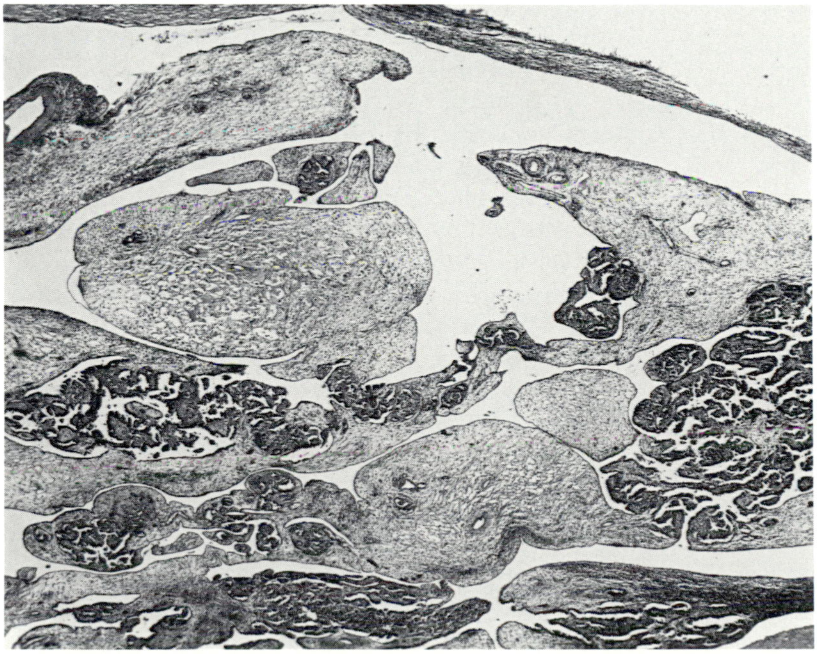

FIG. 19.48. Sertoli–Leydig cell tumor with retiform pattern. Large edematous polypoid structures and many small papillae. (Reprinted by permission of Young and Scully, Ref. 314.)

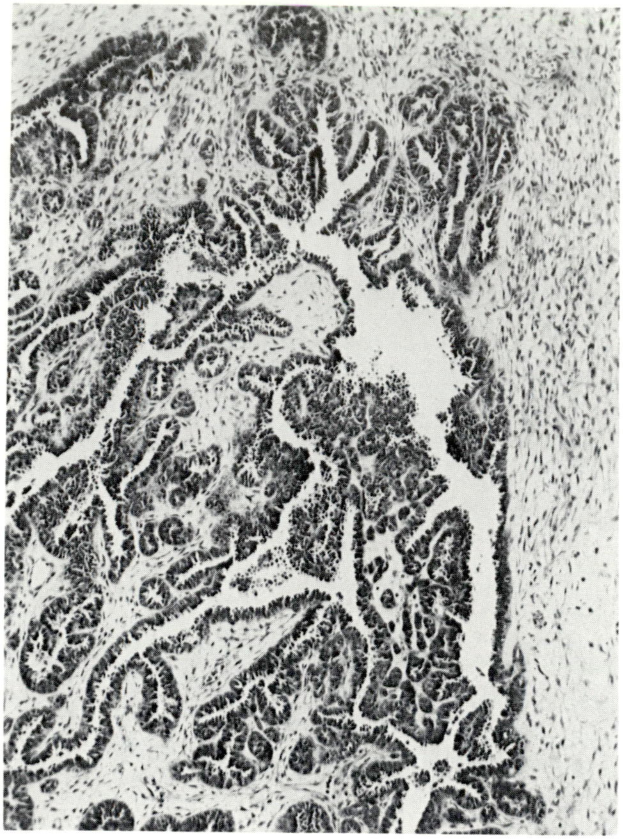

FIG. 19.50. Sertoli–Leydig cell tumor with retiform pattern. A complex papillary pattern simulates a serous papillary adenocarcinoma.

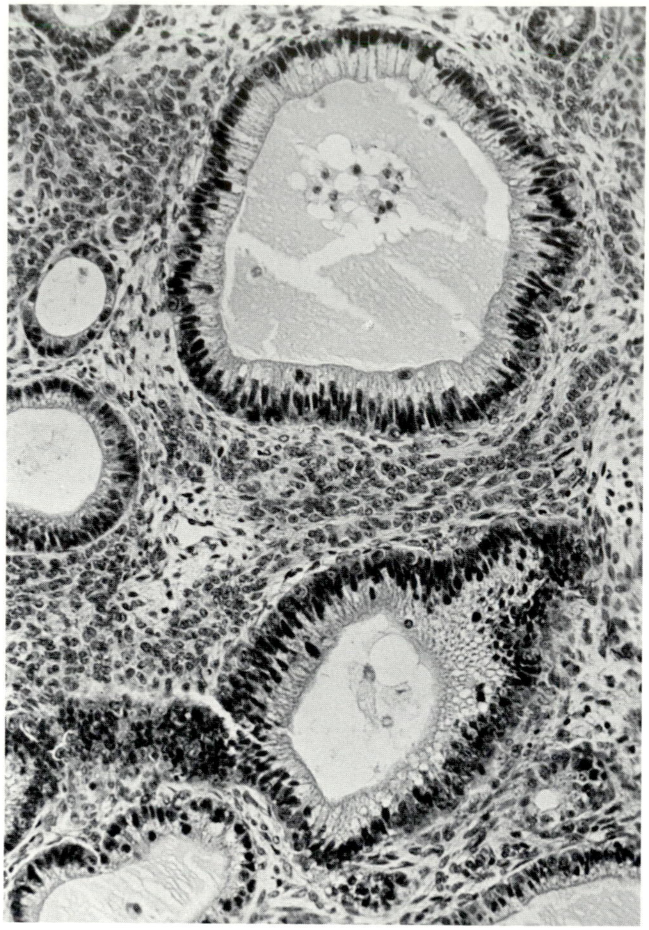

FIG. 19.51. Sertoli–Leydig cell tumor with heterologous elements. Mucinous glands are separated by intermediate form of tumor. (Reprinted by permission of Serov et al., Ref. 257.)

the patient and the absence of androgenic manifestations, support the diagnosis of endometrioid carcinoma,[327] but it must be emphasized that the latter occasionally has a functioning stroma, which is sometimes manifested clinically by estrogenic changes and, rarely, by virilization.

The tubular Krukenberg tumor may mimic a Sertoli–Leydig cell tumor, especially if luteinization of the stroma is present.[41] Further confusion arises in the rare case in which the tumor is associated with virilization. Tubular Krukenberg tumors have been reported to be bilateral, however, in 50% of cases and contain markedly atypical cells, including signet ring cells that contain mucin, easily demonstrable by special stains.[41]

Carcinoid tumors, especially those of the trabecular type, may be confused with intermediate Sertoli–Leydig cell tumors. The ribbons of the former, however, are longer, thicker, and more uniformly distributed than the sex cord-like formations of the latter. Also, rare carcinoid tumors with a solid tubular pattern[311] can be difficult to distinguish from well-differentiated Sertoli cell tumors. Examination of the stroma of carcinoid tumors may be helpful in the differential diagnosis. It is typically less cellular and more fibromatous than that of Sertoli–Leydig cell tumors and does not contain Leydig cells. The most specific diagnostic criterion is the presence of argyrophil granules in almost all carcinoid tumors and of argentaffin granules in many of them. In contrast, only heterologous Sertoli–Leydig cell tumors with glands and cysts lined by gastrointestinal-type epithelium contain such granules. Finally, primary carcinoid tumors are associated with teratomatous elements in 70% of cases,[219–221] whereas metastatic carcinoids are almost always bilateral and are usually associated with a primary tumor of the intestine and metastases elsewhere in the abdomen (see Chapter 22, Metastatic Ovarian Tumors).

The retiform variant of Sertoli–Leydig cell tumor causes specific problems in differential diagnosis. The most common misdiagnosis is endodermal sinus tumor, which is suggested clinically by the young age of the patient and pathologically by the presence of papillae within cystic spaces. The occurrence of androgenic manifestations with about one-quarter of retiform Sertoli–Ley-

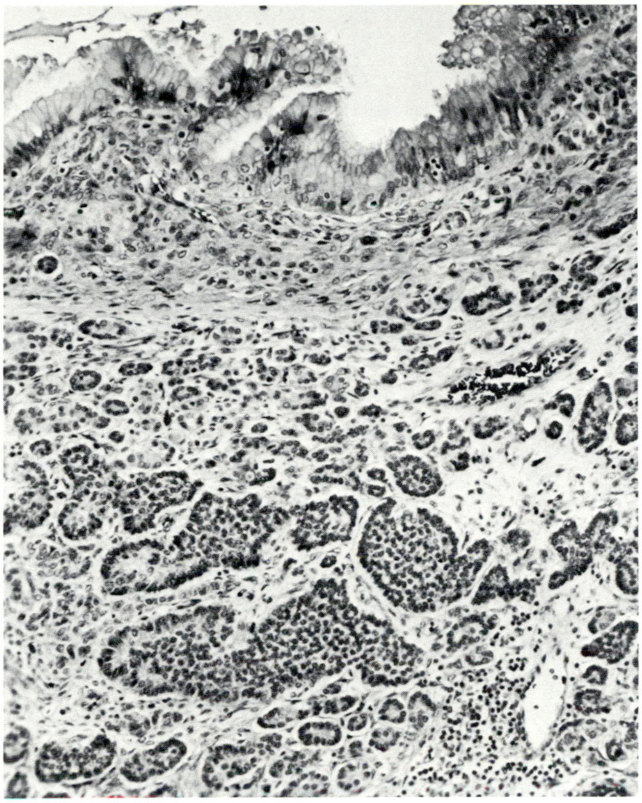

FIG. 19.52. Sertoli–Leydig cell tumor with heterologous elements. Insular carcinoid adjacent to mucinous epithelium.

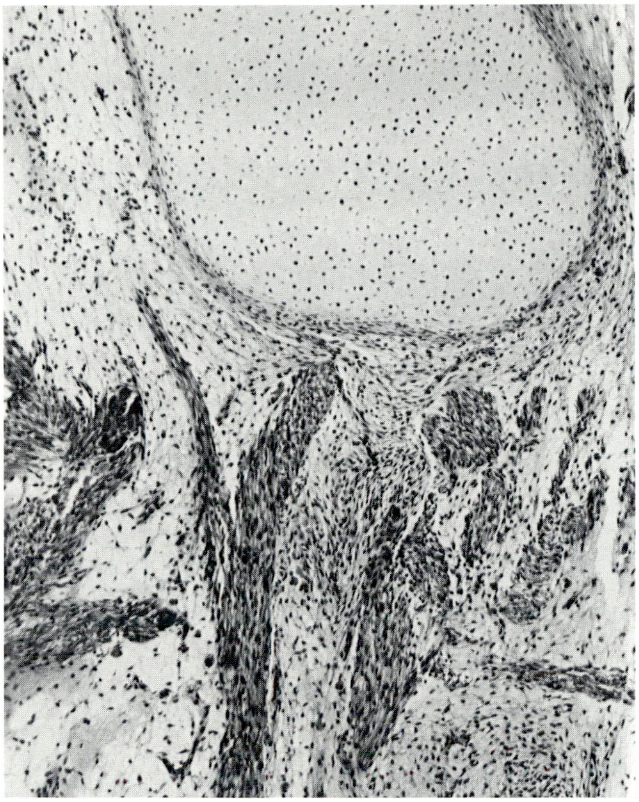

FIG. 19.53. Sertoli–Leydig cell tumor with heterologous elements. Nodule of fetal type cartilage and bundles of strap cells. (Reprinted by permission of Prat, et al., Ref. 211.)

dig cell tumors, however, contrasts with their rare association with endodermal sinus tumors that have a functioning stroma.[275] On gross examination, the retiform tumors generally appear less malignant than endodermal sinus tumors, and microscopic examination reveals less primitive-appearing cells. The presence of other distinctive patterns of either tumor and immunohistochemical staining for alpha-fetoprotein in the endodermal sinus tumor almost always facilitate the diagnosis. A greater problem in differential diagnosis arises because of the characteristic papillary pattern and the frequent presence of cellular stratification on the papillae in retiform tumors, particularly if these features predominate in the specimen. Under such circumstances, a misdiagnosis of a serous cystadenoma of borderline malignancy or a serous or endometrioid carcinoma is often made. A variety of clinical and pathologic features, including the young age of the patient, the association with virilization, and the presence of other, more easily recognizable patterns of Sertoli–Leydig cell tumor, are helpful clues to the correct diagnosis. Finally, the juxtaposition of epithelial and immature mesenchymal elements in some retiform tumors has caused confusion with a malignant mesodermal mixed tumor, but the features outlined previously also serve to exclude the latter diagnosis.

Because occasional sex cord–stromal tumors have a morphologic appearance intermediate between granulosa cell tumors and Sertoli–Leydig cell tumors or exhibit features of both tumors, it is sometimes difficult to decide whether a given tumor should be placed in the granulosa, Sertoli–Leydig cell, or mixed category. This problem is discussed in the sections on gynandroblastoma and unclassified sex cord–stromal tumors. Major criteria that help to differentiate granulosa cell tumors and Sertoli–Leydig cell tumors are listed in Table 19.6.

Behavior and Treatment. After the removal of a virilizing Sertoli–Leydig cell tumor, normal menses characteristically resume in about 4 weeks. The excessive hair almost always diminishes to some extent. Clitoromegaly and deepening of the voice are less apt to regress. The prognosis in cases of Sertoli–Leydig cell tumor is closely related to its stage and degree of differentiation. The rare tumors that occur at a stage higher than I have a poor prognosis, with a mortality rate of 100% in our series.[319] The survival rates of patients with stage I tumors correlates with the degree of differentiation. In our series, none of the well-differentiated tumors, 11% of those of intermediate differentiation, 59% of the poorly differentiated tumors, and 19% of those with heterolo-

TABLE 19.6. Adult granulosa cell tumor versus Sertoli-Leydig cell tumor.

Granulosa cell tumor	Sertoli-Leydig cell tumor
All age groups, mostly postmenopausal	Mainly young women
Usually estrogenic, rarely androgenic	Usually androgenic, occasionally estrogenic
Microfollicular, macrofollicular, trabecular, insular, and diffuse patterns	Hollow or solid tubules, cords, diffuse patterns
Granulosa cells usually mature with pale, often grooved nuclei	Sertoli cells often immature
Fibrothecomatous component common	Fibromatous component uncommon; mesenchyme often immature and cellular
Steroid-type cells (lutein cells) usually not prominent and uncommonly clustered	Steroid-type cells (Leydig cells) tend to cluster; rarely contain crystals of Reinke
Heterologous elements absent	Heterologous elements in 20% of cases
Retiform elements absent	Retiform elements in 15% of cases

gous elements were clinically malignant. The homologous component of the tumor was poorly differentiated in all 8 clinically malignant tumors in the heterologous category, and in 7 of them the heterologous elements included skeletal muscle, cartilage, or both. Earlier studies in the literature failed to establish a relation between the degree of differentiation of Sertoli–Leydig cell tumors and their prognosis,[202,206] but later investigations have supported the findings in our series. The only clinically malignant tumor in the series of Roth et al.[229] was poorly differentiated, and 4 of the 20 poorly differentiated tumors reported by Zaloudek and Norris[333] were malignant, in contrast to only 1 of the 44 tumors of intermediate differentiation and none of the 7 well-differentiated tumors. In our series, there was also evidence that the presence of a retiform pattern had an adverse effect on the prognosis; 25% of stage I tumors of intermediate differentiation that had a significant retiform component were malignant as opposed to 10% of those with no retiform component.[319] It is noteworthy that the only stage III tumor of intermediate differentiation in our series had an almost completely retiform pattern, and we have recently seen an additional Sertoli–Leydig cell tumor with a predominantly retiform pattern that was stage III. Rupture also adversely affected the outcome of stage I tumors. Thirty percent of the tumors of intermediate differentiation that had ruptured were clinically malignant, in contrast to only 7% of those that were intact. In the poorly differentiated category, 86% of the ruptured tumors were malignant, compared to 45% of those that had not ruptured.

In contrast to granulosa cell tumors, which often recur many years after primary therapy, Sertoli–Leydig cell tumors typically reappear relatively early. Sixty-six percent of the malignant tumors in our series recurred within 1 year, and only 6.6% recurred after 5 years.[319] The recurrent tumor is usually confined to the pelvis and abdomen, but distant metastases to the lung, scalp, and supraclavicular lymph nodes have been reported. Three of the patients in our series had parenchymal liver metastases.

The treatment of a patient with a Sertoli–Leydig cell tumor depends on her age, the stage of her tumor, the presence or absence of rupture, and the degree of differentiation. In young women, the low frequency of bilaterality justifies the performance of a unilateral salpingo-oophorectomy if the tumor is stage IA and preservation of fertility is desired. More aggressive surgical therapy and adjuvant therapy are indicated for tumors higher than stage I. Adjuvant therapy may also be advisable for stage I tumors that are poorly differentiated, contain mesenchymal heterologous elements, or are ruptured tumors of intermediate differentiation. Experience with the adjuvant therapy of Sertoli–Leydig cell tumors is relatively limited. Radiation therapy, combination chemotherapy, or both seem to have been of benefit in occasional reported cases.[240,319]

Other Types of Sex Cord–Stromal Tumor

Gynandroblastoma

This extremely rare tumor[9,58,89,193,201] has been greatly overdiagnosed. According to WHO, the term should be used only if well-differentiated ovarian and testicular-type cells are clearly recognizable within the neoplasm (Fig. 19.54). Since small foci of ovarian cell types are often encountered in well-sampled, otherwise typical Sertoli–Leydig cell tumors, and, conversely, testicular cell types are demonstrable focally in occasional granulosa–stromal cell tumors, the diagnosis of gynandroblastoma should be restricted to the very rare tumors that contain significant components of both forms of neoplasia. According to our criteria, the minor component should account for at least 10% of a tumor in the sex cord–stromal category to warrant a diagnosis of gynandroblastoma. The nature of the hormones secreted by a sex cord–stromal tumor should not, of course, determine its morphologic diagnosis in view of the proven capacity of tumors of testicular cell types to secrete estrogens and of those of ovarian cell types to produce androgens.

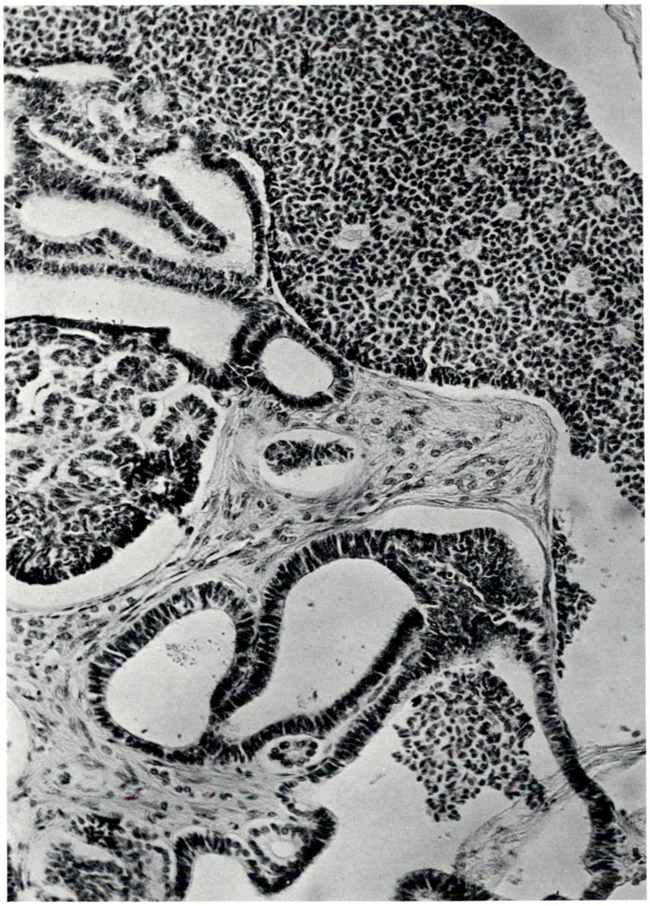

FIG. 19.54. Gynandroblastoma. (Reprinted by permission of Scully, Ref. 242.)

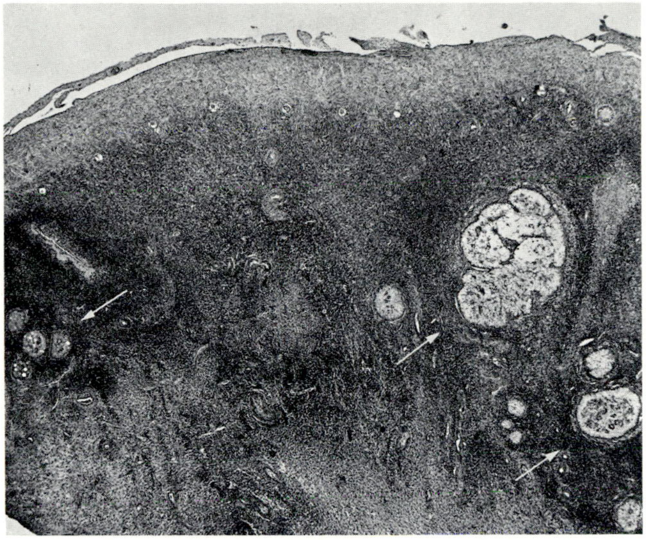

FIG. 19.55. Sex cord tumor with annular tubules. Multicentric foci are present within ovary from patient with Peutz–Jeghers syndrome. (Reprinted by permission of Scully, Ref. 245.)

Sex Cord Tumor with Annular Tubules

This tumor (Figs. 19.55, 19.56, 19.57, and 19.58), which was originally included within the category of sex cord–stromal tumors, unclassified, has been established as a distinctive entity since formulation of the WHO classification.[245,330] It is characterized basically by the presence of simple and complex annular tubules (Figs. 19.56 and 19.58). The simple tubules have the shape of a ring, with the nuclei oriented around the periphery and around a central hyalinized body composed of basement membrane material. An intervening anuclear cytoplasmic zone forms the major component of the ring. The much more numerous complex tubules are rounded structures made up of intercommunicating rings revolving around multiple hyaline bodies. Tumors containing annular tubules have been interpreted as Sertoli cell tumors by some observers[286] and granulosa cell tumors by others,[127] but the pattern of growth has features intermediate between these two tumors, and focal differentiation into both typical Sertoli cell tumor with elongated tubules and typical granulosa cell tumor with Call-Exner

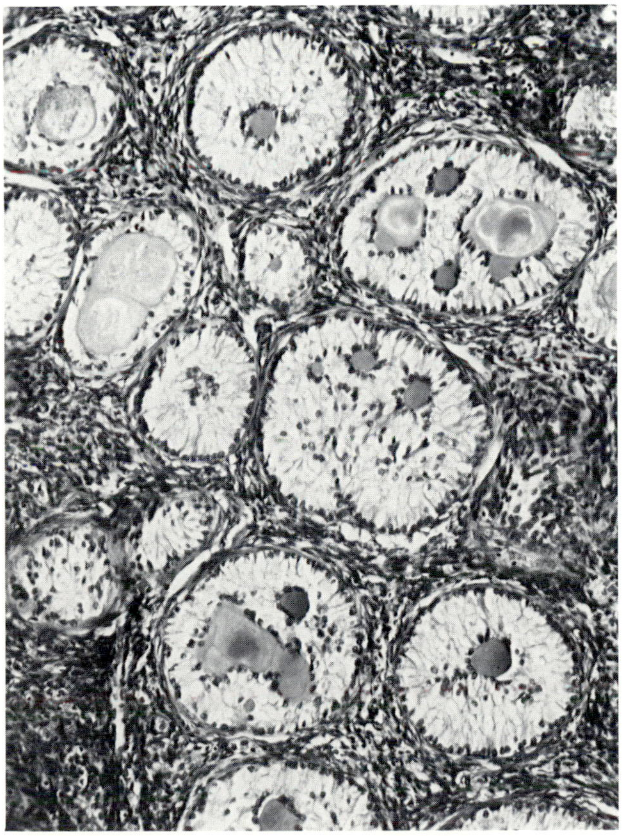

FIG. 19.56. Sex cord tumor with annular tubules. Simple and complex annular tubules encircle hyaline material.

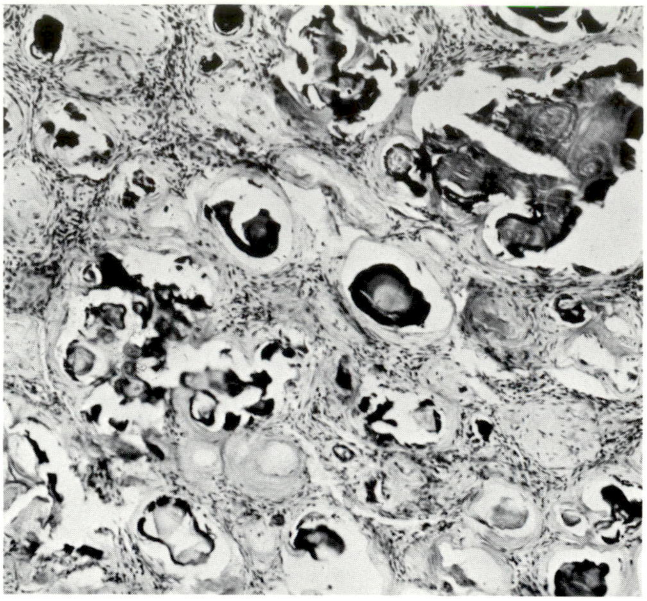

FIG. 19.57. Sex cord tumor with annular tubules. Extensive calcification of the epithelial nests has occurred in this tumor from a patient with the Peutz–Jeghers syndrome.

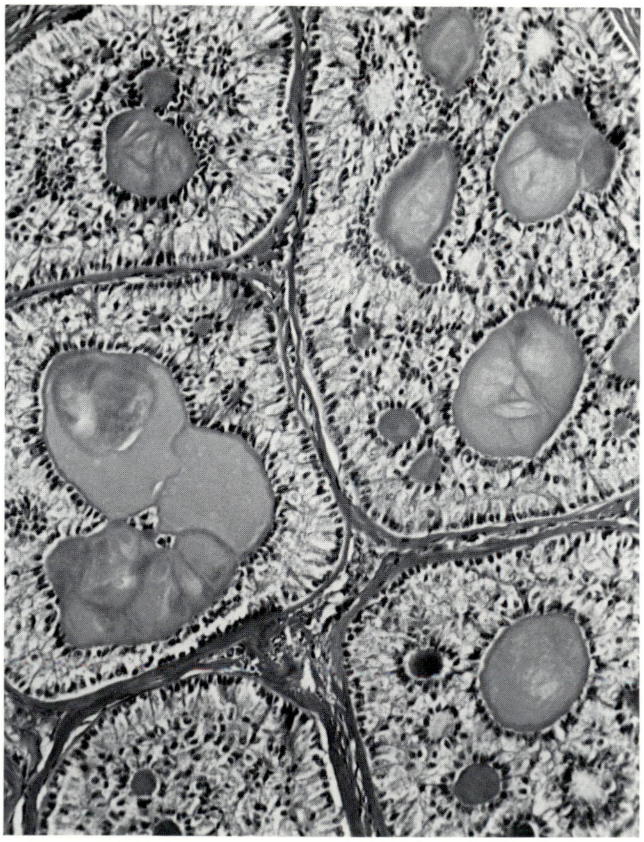

FIG. 19.58. Sex cord tumor with annular tubules. There was no evidence of Peutz–Jeghers syndrome in the patient with this neoplasm.

bodies is seen in some of the cases. Cells of the Sertoli type have been identified ultrastructurally by the demonstration of Charcot–Böttcher filaments (Fig. 19.59),[4,14,286] which are considered specific cytoplasmic inclusions of Sertoli cells. A study of small tumors of this type suggests an origin in the ovarian cortex from the granulosa cells of follicles. Other evidence of such an origin is the well-known tubular differentiation of follicles that occurs in the canine ovary.

Sex cord tumors with annular tubules vary both clinically and pathologically, depending on whether or not the patient has the Peutz-Jeghers syndrome (mucocutaneous melanin pigmentation, gastrointestinal hamartomatous polyposis, and occasionally adenoma malignum of the cervix)[172] (Table 19.7). Almost all female patients with this syndrome whose ovaries have been examined microscopically have had sex cord tumorlets with annular tubules, which have been multifocal (Fig. 19.55) and bilateral in at least two thirds of the patients. The largest reported lesion in a patient with this syndrome was 3 cm in diameter. Focal calcification has been seen in over half the cases (Fig. 19.57). In almost all the patients, the lesions have been incidental findings in ovaries removed for other reasons. All the tumorlets associated with the Peutz–Jeghers syndrome have been benign, warranting conservative treatment.

In patients without the Peutz–Jeghers syndrome (Fig. 19.58), in contrast, the tumors are almost always unilateral and usually form palpable masses. Transitions to typical granulosa cell tumor and typical Sertoli cell tumor are much more common than in the tumorlets associated with the Peutz–Jeghers syndrome. Forty percent of the patients have had manifestations of estrogen secretion, and at least one-fifth of the tumors have been clinically malignant.[330]

Four ovarian tumors from girls with the Peutz–Jeghers syndrome have caused sexual precocity. Two of them, occurring in sisters, had the features of Sertoli cell tumor with lipid storage,[267,318] whereas the other two had microscopic features that were unique in our experience, including diffuse areas, tubular differentiation, microcysts and papillae, and the presence of two distinctive cell types, one containing abundant eosinophilic cytoplasm, and the other containing scanty cytoplasm (Figs. 19.60 and 19.61).[322] All four tumors appeared to be clinically benign. The occurrence of these unusual neoplasms in association with the Peutz–Jeghers syndrome suggests an association.

Unclassified Sex Cord–Stromal Tumors

This ill-defined group of tumors, which accounts for less than 10% of those in the sex cord–stromal category, includes those in which a predominant pattern of testicular or ovarian differentiation is not clearly recognizable.

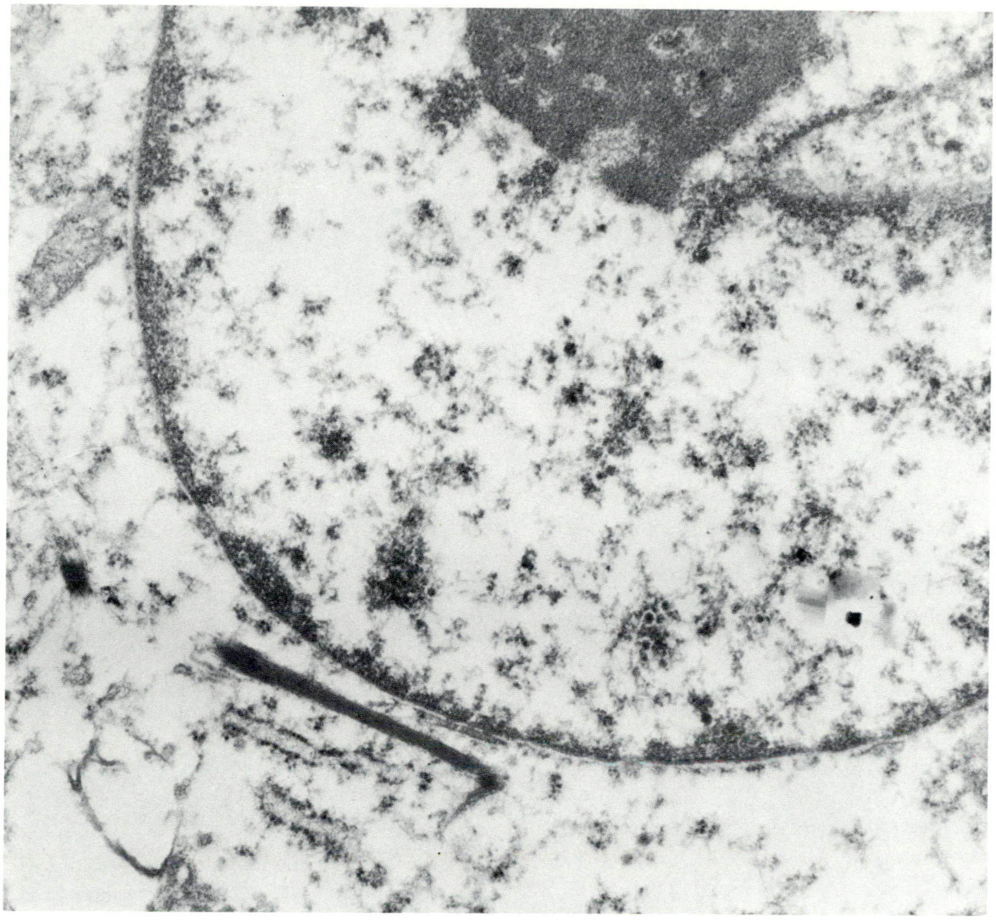

Fig. 19.59. Charcot–Böttcher filament in characteristic paranuclear location. (Reprinted by permission of Tavassoli and Norris, Ref. 286.)

The boundary lines between these tumors and those of both ovarian and testicular cell types are vague because interpretations of intermediate patterns of growth and closely similar cell types are inevitably subjective.

Sex Cord–Stromal Tumors During Pregnancy

Sex cord–stromal cell tumors may be particularly difficult to subclassify when they occur in pregnant patients[324] because of alterations of their usual clinical and pathologic features. Their diagnosis is rarely suggested clinically, since estrogenic manifestations are not recognizable during pregnancy, and androgenic manifestations are rare, possibly because of the ability of the placenta to aromatize androgens to estrogens. Indeed, virilization of a pregnant patient is much more likely to be due to a nonneoplastic lesion, such as the pregnancy luteoma and hyperreactio luteinalis, or to a tumor with functioning stroma than to a sex cord–stromal tumor.

In a recent study, 17% of 36 sex cord–stromal tumors that were removed during pregnancy were placed in the unclassified group, and many of those that were classified in the granulosa cell or Sertoli–Leydig cell category had large areas with an indifferent appearance.[324] The features that led to difficulty in classification were the presence of prominent intercellular edema, increased luteinization in the granulosa cell tumors, and marked degrees of Leydig cell maturation in one-third of the Sertoli–Leydig cell tumors. All of these changes, which were most common in tumors removed during the third trimester, tended to obscure the underlying

Table 19.7. Sex cord tumor with annular tubules with and without Peutz-Jeghers syndrome.

	With	Without
Bilateral	62%	5%
Grossly visible	27%	75%
Size	3 cm or less	Usually large
Multifocal	82%	6%
Calcification	62%	12%
Clinically malignant	0	20%[a]
Adenoma malignum cervix	15%	4%

[a] Only grossly visible tumors used in this evaluation.

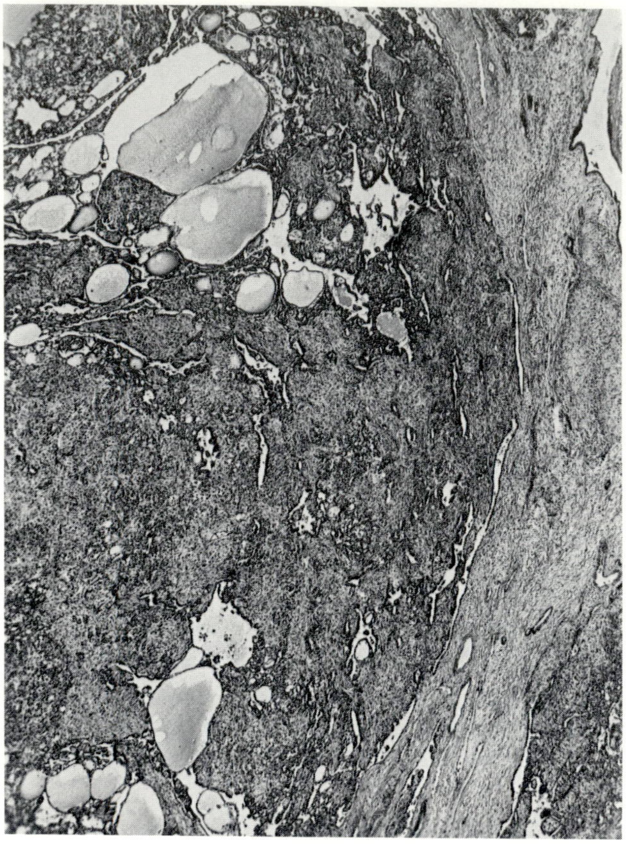

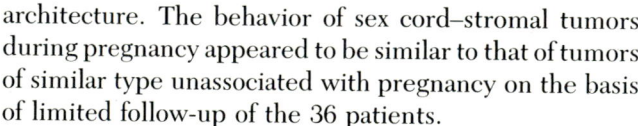

FIG. 19.60. Ovarian sex cord tumor from patient with sexual precocity and Peutz–Jeghers syndrome. Solid areas interrupted by cysts of varying sizes. (Reprinted by permission of Young et al., Ref. 322.)

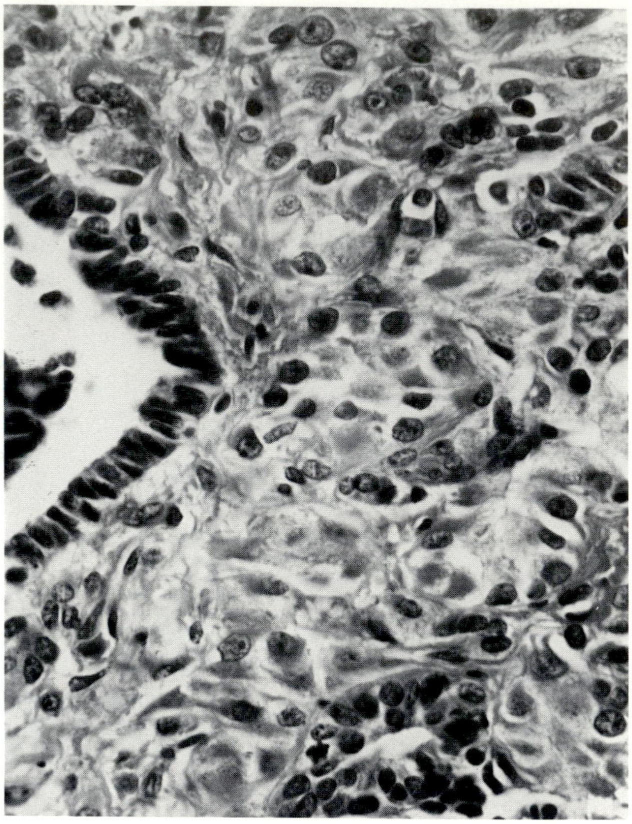

FIG. 19.61. Ovarian sex cord tumor from patient with sexual precocity and Peutz–Jeghers syndrome. Tubules separated by cells with abundant cytoplasm and vesicular nuclei. (Reprinted by permission of Young et al., Ref. 322.)

architecture. The behavior of sex cord–stromal tumors during pregnancy appeared to be similar to that of tumors of similar type unassociated with pregnancy on the basis of limited follow-up of the 36 patients.

Immunohistochemistry of Sex Cord–Stromal Tumors

Only small numbers of tumors in the sex cord–stromal category have been examined by immunohistochemical techniques to date.[156,182,183] The largest published experience has been that of Miettinen et al.[182,183] Sixteen fibromas, 2 thecomas and 12 granulosa cell tumors in their series were positive for vimentin and negative for cytokeratin. A small number of tumors in these categories were negative for desmin. In one report, however, granulosa cells of primordial and developing follicles were said to contain cytokeratin.[67]

The cells lining the tubules of Sertoli–Leydig cell tumors have stained positively for cytokeratin but, with one exception, have been negative for epidermal keratin antigens. These cells failed to stain for vimentin, which, however, was demonstrable in cells interpreted as stromal in origin. Because Sertoli cells of the normal testis are negative for cytokeratin,[103] the staining of the putative Sertoli cells in Sertoli–Leydig cell tumors raises the question whether these cells may not be more closely related to other cells of testicular type, such as those lining the straight tubules or rete testis. It is of interest that in one sex cord tumor with annular tubules, the tubular cells were positive for vimentin and negative for cytokeratin.[183]

The argyrophil cells of mucinous and carcinoid components of heterologous Sertoli–Leydig cell tumors have reacted for serotonin and one or more polypeptide hormones on immunohistochemical examination.[255] In one Sertoli–Leydig cell tumor associated with elevated levels of alpha-fetoprotein in the serum, immunohistochemical staining for this antigen was localized in cells resembling liver cells within the tumor.[326] In other cases, there was staining of the Leydig cell component of the neoplasm.[62,168,292]

Kurman et al.[157,158] have demonstrated immunohistochemically a variety of steroid hormones, including estrogens, androgens, and progesterone, in the granulosa, theca, Sertoli, and Leydig cells of sex cord–stromal tumors. It is not clear whether their presence reflects local secretion or binding of these hormones to cellular receptors.

Steroid Cell Tumors

The terms *lipid cell tumor* and *lipoid cell tumor* have been applied to ovarian neoplasms composed entirely of cells resembling typical steroid hormone-secreting cells, that is, lutein cells, Leydig cells, and adrenal cortical cells.[99,287] These terms are nonspecific and inaccurate, however, since many ovarian tumors contain lipid and some of those in this category contain little or none. One of us (RES) previously proposed the designation *steroid cell tumors* for these neoplasms,[248,250] which can be subdivided into several subtypes according to their presumed cell of origin or other distinctive features (Table 19.8).

Stromal Luteoma

This designation[243] has been applied to small steroid cell tumors that lie within the ovarian stroma (Fig. 19.62, Plate 4; Fig. 19.63) and are, therefore, presumed to arise from it. Such an origin is supported by the capacity of the ovarian stroma to differentiate into lutein cells in the nonneoplastic disorder designated *stromal hyperthecosis*.[273] Adrenal rest cells and Leydig cells, the other possible sources of tumors of this type, on the other hand, have been identified within the ovarian stroma on only extremely rare occasions.[273,277] The diagnosis of stromal luteoma is supported in almost all the cases by the finding of stromal hyperthecosis elsewhere in the ovary. In some cases, the nests of lutein cells in stromal hyperthecosis may form grossly recognizable nodules (nodular hyperthecosis). The dividing line between a large hyperthecotic nodule and a stromal luteoma is arbitrary; we reserve the former designation for the presence of large nodular foci of lutein cells of microscopic dimensions and the latter for an even larger nodule that is grossly visible, clearly outstripping other foci of stromal luteinization. Microscopic examination of a stromal luteoma reveals a more or less rounded nodule of cells of lutein type, which generally contain relatively little lipid. One occasional confusing feature of this tumor is focal degeneration with the formation of irregular spaces that may simulate glands or vessels (Fig. 19.64).[243] Many large steroid cell tumors may have begun their development as stromal luteomas, but cannot be diagnosed specifically as such because their confinement to the ovarian stroma can no longer be demonstrated microscopically.

Table 19.8. Steroid cell tumors.

Stromal luteoma
Leydig cell tumor
Hilus cell tumor
Non-hilus cell type
Not otherwise specified

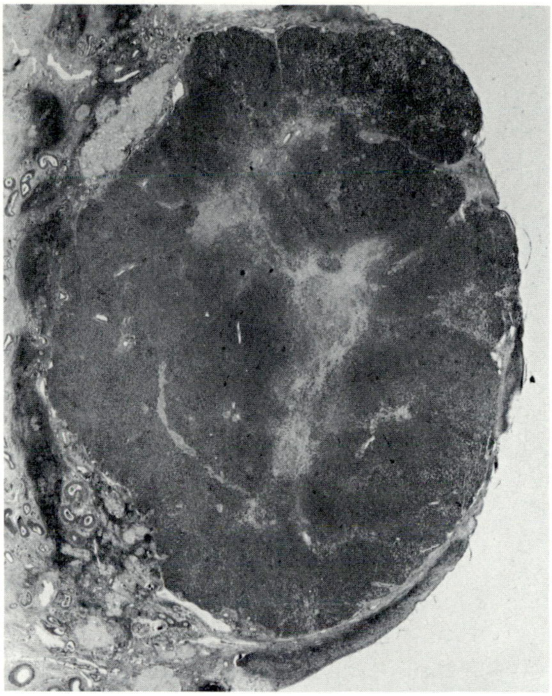

Fig. 19.63. Stromal luteoma, partly surrounded by ovarian stroma.

The stromal luteoma is usually estrogenic, but may be androgenic or both. Underlying stromal hyperthecosis may contribute to the clinical picture, which is sometimes one of long-standing endocrine manifestations. One stromal luteoma has been described in a patient with acanthosis nigricans and the insulin resistance syndrome.[113] All the reported cases have been benign.

Leydig Cell Tumors

A Leydig cell nature of a steroid cell tumor (Figs. 19.65, 19.66, and 19.67) can be proven only by the identification of the more or less specific crystals of Reinke in the cytoplasm of the neoplastic cells on either light microscopic (Fig. 19.66) or electron microscopic examination (Fig. 19.67).* Since only 35–40% of Leydig cell tumors of the testis contain crystals of Reinke on light-microscopic examination[150,189] and Leydig cells cannot be differentiated from lutein cells or adrenal cortical cells in

* References 7, 8, 32, 85, 133, 203, 233, 234, 239, 272.

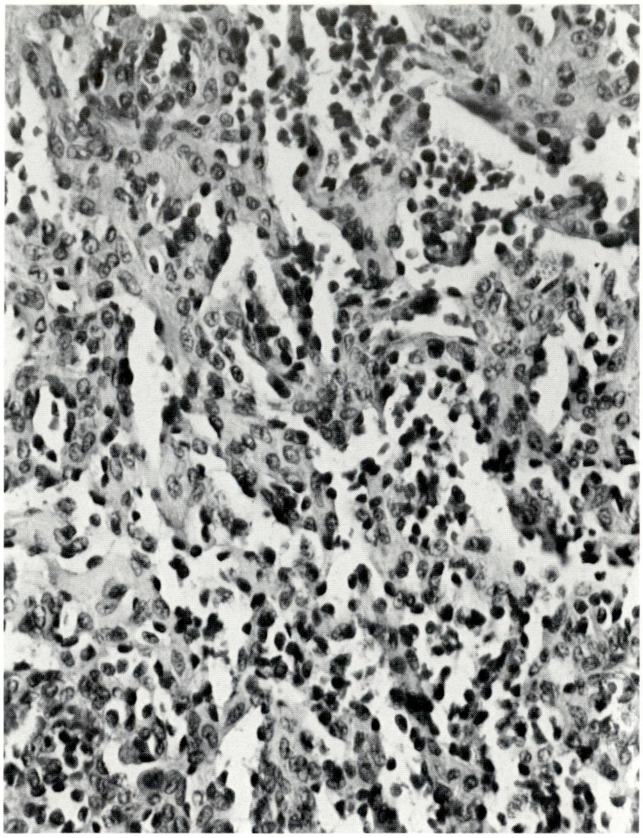

Fig. 19.64. Stromal luteoma. Degenerative changes have produced irregular spaces.

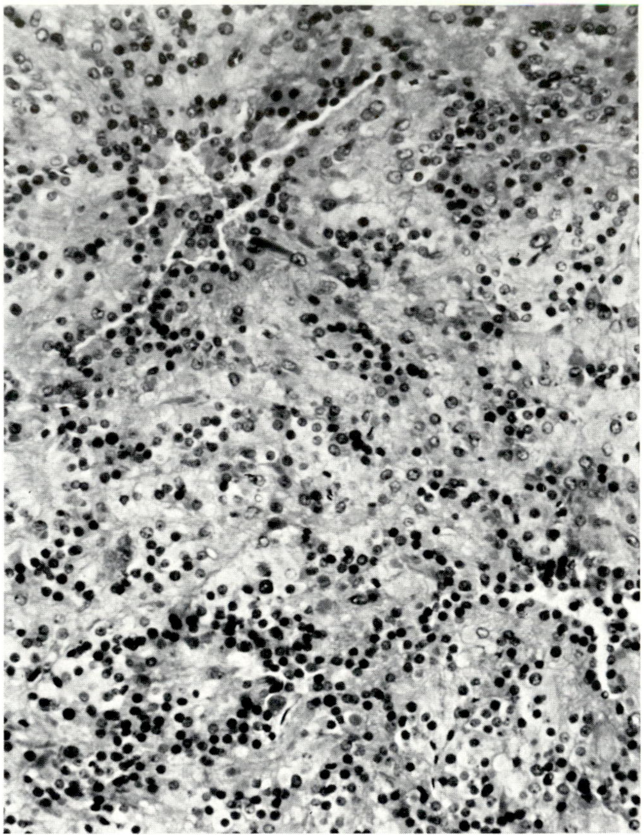

Fig. 19.65. Hilus cell tumor. (Reprinted by permission of Scully, Ref. 248.)

the absence of these inclusions, it is probable that a number of unclassified steroid cell tumors are Leydig cell tumors that cannot be specifically identified as such.

Ovarian Leydig cell tumors have been divided into two subtypes by Roth and Sternberg,[224] the hilus cell tumor and the Leydig cell tumor, nonhilar type. The former, which are much more common, originate in the ovarian hilus from hilar Leydig cells, which have been identified in 80–85% of adult ovaries, usually lying in relation to nonmedullated nerve fibers.[271] Hilus cell tumors occur at an average age of 58 years and cause hirsutism or virilization in three quarter of patients.[85] Rarely, they are associated with estrogenic manifestations.[133] The androgenic changes typically have a less abrupt onset and are milder than those associated with Sertoli–Leydig cell tumors. The urinary 17-ketosteroid levels are usually normal or only slightly elevated because these tumors produce predominantly the potent androgen, testosterone, which is not a 17-ketosteroid, instead of the weaker androgens, androstenedione and dehydroepiandrosterone, elevations of which are typically associated with high values of urinary 17-ketosteroids. Almost all the hilus cell tumors recorded in the literature have been benign. Only one case of malignant hilus cell tumor merits serious consideration, but the presence of crystals of Reinke in the neoplastic cells in that case was not convincingly documented in the illustrations.[86]

Hilus cell tumors are usually reddish-brown to yellow, are centered in the hilar region, and are rarely of large size (Fig. 19.68, Plate 4). Microscopic examination typically reveals a circumscribed mass of steroid cells with abundant eosinophilic cytoplasm and little intracellular lipid. Cytoplasmic lipochrome pigment may be abundant. The cells are usually diffusely distributed, but occasionally their nuclei cluster and are separated by nucleus-free eosinophilic zones (Fig. 19.65). This pattern is highly suggestive of a hilus cell tumor even in the absence of crystals of Reinke. The diagnosis of hilus cell tumor is also favored if a crystal-free steroid cell tumor located in the hilus has a background of hilus cell hyperplasia or, like normal hilus cells, is associated with nonmedullated nerve fibers.

The Leydig cell tumor of nonhilar type is thought to arise directly from ovarian stromal cells. Only four examples of this tumor have been reported,[224] and except for their location, their clinical and pathologic features have not differed from those of hilus cell tumors. An ovarian stromal cell derivation of these tumors is sup-

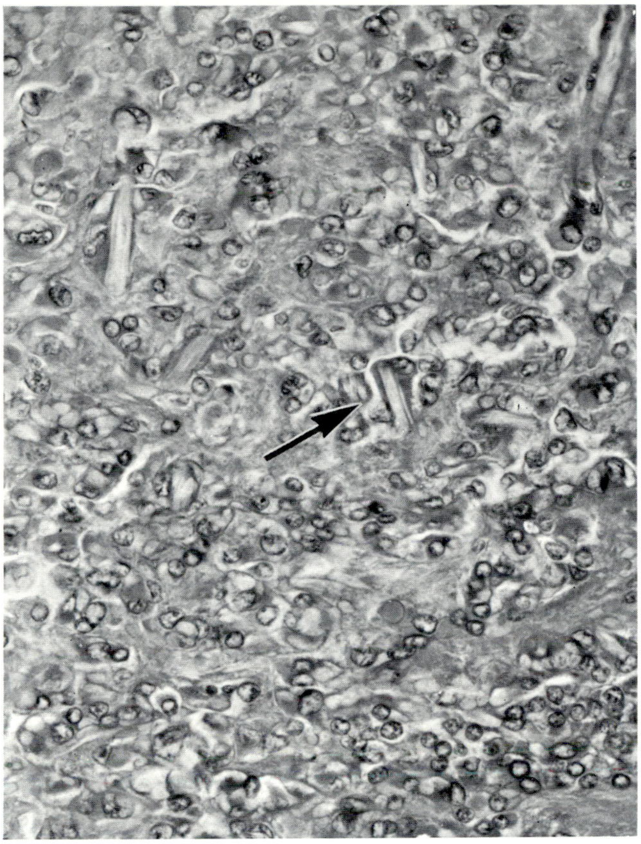

FIG. 19.66. Hilus cell tumor. *Arrow* points to crystals of Reinke. [Reproduced by permission from: Morris J McL, Scully RE (1958) Endocrine Pathology of the Ovary. St. Louis, 1958. The C.V. Mosby Co. Courtesy of Dr. Somers Sturgis.]

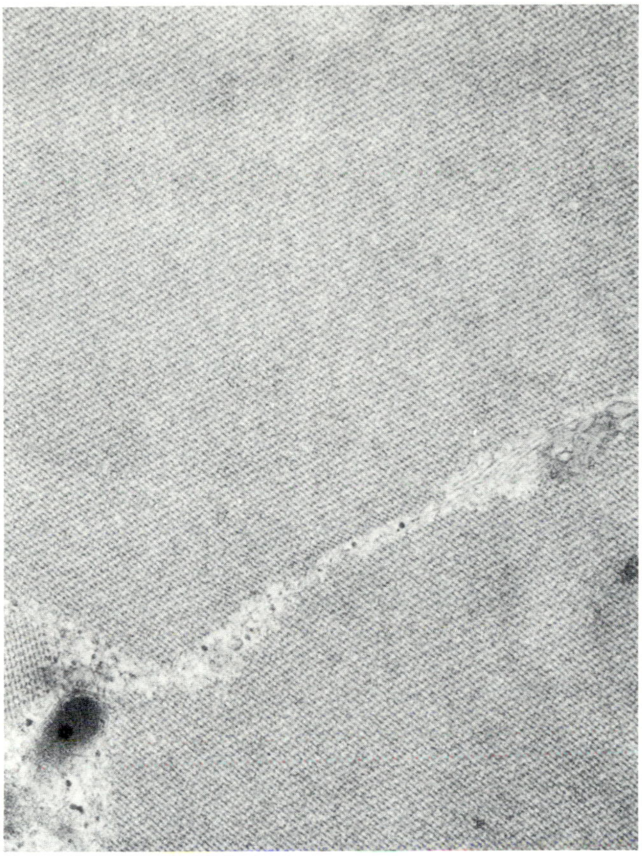

FIG. 19.67. Hilus cell tumor. Reinke crystal is composed of protein-containing, tightly apposed 300 Å-wide hexagonal microtubular units. (Courtesy of Dr. A. Ferenczy, Montreal, Canada. Reprinted by permission of Scully, Ref. 248.)

ported by the very rare finding of Leydig cells containing crystals in the steroid cell nests of ovaries that otherwise have the typical appearance of stromal hyperthecosis.[273]

Steroid Cell Tumor of Adrenal Cortical Type

The striking resemblance of many steroid cell tumors to adrenal cortical tumors has suggested that some of them may arise from adrenal cortical rests. Although such rests are extremely rare within the ovary,[277] they have been identified in the broad ligament and, occasionally, within the ovarian hilus in about one-quarter of women.[91] In a few patients with steroid cell tumors, the responses of elevated levels of urinary 17-ketosteroids and 17-hydroxycorticosteroids to ACTH stimulation and dexamethasone suppression have been more suggestive of an origin from cells of adrenal cortical than gonadal type, but such responses are not specifically diagnostic.[149,291] The strongest evidence that rare steroid cell tumors arise from adrenal cortical rests is their association with either the adrenogenital syndrome or Cushing's syndrome. In one case, cortisol and corticosterone were produced in vitro by a virilizing steroid cell tumor of the ovary from an 8-year-old girl, who was said to have had the adrenogenital syndrome due to adrenal cortical hyperplasia.[190] We have seen three malignant ovarian steroid cell tumors, including the case reported in detail by Marieb et al.,[170] that were associated with clinical and laboratory features diagnostic of Cushing's syndrome, including elevated cortisol levels in the plasma or urine.[321] All three patients had extensive metastatic disease within the abdomen at the time of operation. Although these tumors might have arisen from adrenal cortical rests, an alternative explanation for their occurrence is the assumption of adrenal cortical function by tumors arising from lutein or Leydig cells. Because of the latter possibility, the term *steroid cell tumor, adrenal cortical type* is preferable to *adrenal rest tumor* for tumors of this type.

Steroid Cell Tumor, Not Otherwise Specified

Tumors in this category, which are the most common of the steroid cell tumors, yield no clue to their cell of origin. They may occur at any age and are most often virilizing, but they may be estrogenic or unassociated with endocrine manifestations.[33,46] In a review of the cases at the Armed Forces Institute of Pathology (AFIP), Taylor and Norris found that at least one quarter of them were clinically malignant.[287] Gross examination discloses well-circumscribed masses that are orange or yellow if their cells contain large amounts of intracytoplasmic lipid (Fig. 19.69, Plate 4), red to brown if they are lipid-poor or lipid-free, or dark brown to black if they contain abundant intracytoplasmic lipochrome. Necrosis and cystic degeneration are occasionally observed. All the malignant tumors in the AFIP series were 8 cm in diameter or larger, although we have seen one malignant tumor in this category that was only 7 cm in diameter.[128a] In our series 78% of those with a diameter of 7 cm or greater were malignant.[287] Microscopic examination typically shows cells arranged in a diffuse pattern (Fig. 19.70) or in nests or columns separated by a rich vascular network. A minor fibromatous component and areas of hyalinization are seen rarely. In most cases, nuclear atypia is slight (Fig. 19.70), but it may be moderate or marked and may be associated with considerable mitotic activity. Indeed, over 90% of those tumors in our series with 2 or more mitotic figures per 10 HPF were clinically malignant. Occasional tumors lacking nuclear atypia and containing only rare mitotic figures may metastasize, however. Other microscopic features strongly associated with a malignant behavior are necrosis and hemorrhage.

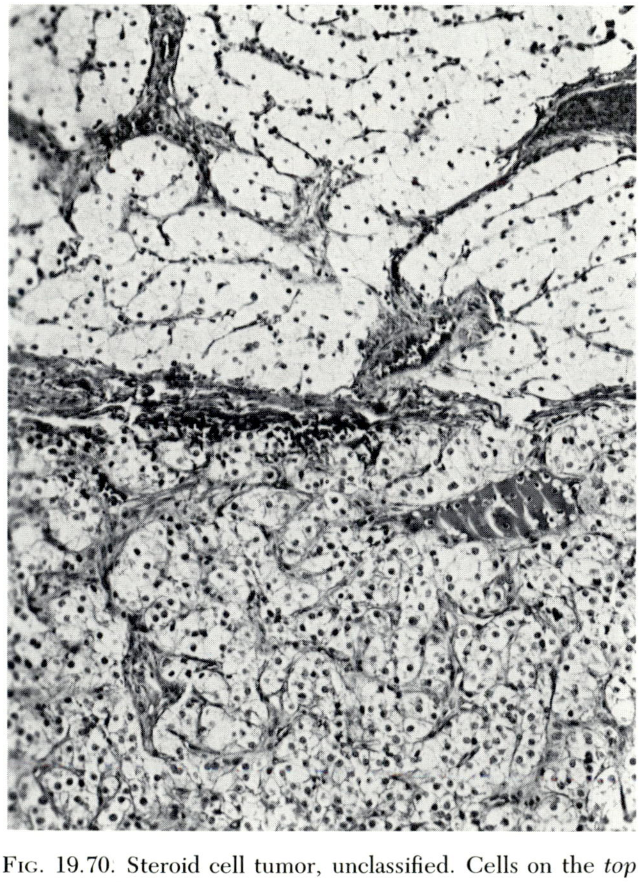

FIG. 19.70. Steroid cell tumor, unclassified. Cells on the *top* have abundant pale cytoplasm, whereas those on the *bottom* have less abundant cytoplasm. (Reprinted by permission of Young RH, Scully RE: Ovarian sex cord-stromal and steroid cell tumors. In: Roth LM, Czernobilsky B, eds., Tumors and Tumor-Like Conditions of the Ovary. Churchill Livingstone Inc, New York, 1985.)

Steroid cell tumors may be confused with other neoplasms, particularly highly luteinized granulosa cell tumors and thecomas, clear cell carcinomas composed entirely of either clear cells or cells with abundant eosinophilic cytoplasm, metastatic renal cell carcinomas, and, rarely, lipid-rich Sertoli cell tumors. The rare granulosa cell tumor or thecoma that is markedly luteinized can be distinguished from a steroid cell tumor by the focal presence of nonluteinized granulosa cells in the former and the finding of abundant intercellular reticulum in the latter. Clear cell carcinomas that are composed exclusively of clear cells have glycogen-rich cytoplasm and typically eccentric nuclei, in contrast to the characteristic lipid-filled cytoplasm and central nuclei of steroid cell tumors containing clear cells. Clear cell carcinomas composed largely of cells with dense, eosinophilic cytoplasm tend to exhibit epithelial arrangements of their cells and almost always contain foci of more typical clear cell carcinoma. A very rare steroid cell tumor, however, may be difficult to distinguish from a clear cell carcinoma or a metastatic renal cell carcinoma,[2] just as some adrenal cortical carcinomas may be difficult to distinguish from renal cell carcinomas. The distinction of a lipid-rich Sertoli cell tumor with a prominent diffuse pattern from a steroid cell tumor depends on identifying areas with a tubular pattern in the former.

Pregnancy luteomas, which are hyperplastic nodules composed of lutein cells that develop during pregnancy, may form large masses that resemble steroid cell tumors grossly and microscopically (see Chapter 16, Nonneoplastic Lesions of Ovary). Like the latter, they may also be virilizing (in about one-quarter of the cases). Unlike steroid cell tumors, however, approximately one-third of pregnancy luteomas are bilateral and approximately one-half are multiple. Microscopic examination reveals masses of cells with abundant eosinophilic cytoplasm containing little or no lipid. Mitotic figures may be numerous, sometimes up to 2 or 3 per 10 HPF. In contrast, a steroid cell tumor with minimal cytologic atypia that resembles a pregnancy luteoma usually contains only rare mitotic figures. Although it may be impossible to distinguish a lipid-poor or lipid-free steroid cell tumor from a solitary pregnancy luteoma, a lesion encountered during the third trimester of pregnancy is presumed to be the latter unless clear-cut evidence indicates otherwise.

Other Ovarian Tumors with Endocrine Function

Ovarian Tumors with Functioning Stroma

A wide variety of ovarian tumors other than those in the sex cord–stromal and steroid cell categories may be hormonally active as a result of steroid hormone production by their stromal cells (Figs. 19.71, 19.72, 19.73, 19.74, 19.75, and 19.76). These tumors, which have been designated ovarian tumors with functioning stroma,[253] may be benign or malignant and, if in the latter category, primary or metastatic. Almost every ovarian tumor has been reported to be associated with stromal hormone production, but this phenomenon is seen much more often with some neoplasms than others.

Ovarian tumors with functioning stroma are infrequently associated with overt endocrine manifestations but commonly accompanied by subclinical elevations of steroid hormone values.[222,223] In one early investigation,[230] 39% of postmenopausal women with ovarian cancer were reported to have increased cornification of their cervical and vaginal squamous cells on cytologic smears. In a more recent study, Rome et al.[223] demonstrated a 50% frequency of elevation of total urinary estrogens in patients with common epithelial tumors or metastatic carcinomas in the ovary. The stromal cells responsible for the hormone secretion in ovarian tumors with functioning stroma typically resemble lutein or Leydig cells and have been referred to as *luteinized stromal cells*. These cells almost always lie within the tumor singly, diffusely, or in clusters (Figs. 19.71, 19.72, 19.73, 19.74, and 19.75), but on rare occasions they are mainly distributed just outside the tumor, sometimes forming a peripheral band (Fig. 19.76).[231] Very rarely, crystals of Reinke can be identified in the lutein-like cells, warranting their interpretation as Leydig cells. It must be emphasized, however, that steroid-type cells may be prominent in the absence of clinical evidence of hormone overproduction, and, conversely, evidence of function may exist in the absence of fully developed cells of steroid type.

Ovarian tumors with functioning stroma can be divided into three major categories.[251] In the first two, germ cell tumors that contain syncytiotrophoblast cells and tumors in pregnant patients, the luteinized stromal cells probably develop as a result of stimulation by chorionic gonadotropin (hCG). The cause of the stromal alteration in the third (idiopathic) group, which accounts for the majority of cases, is unclear, but ectopic production of

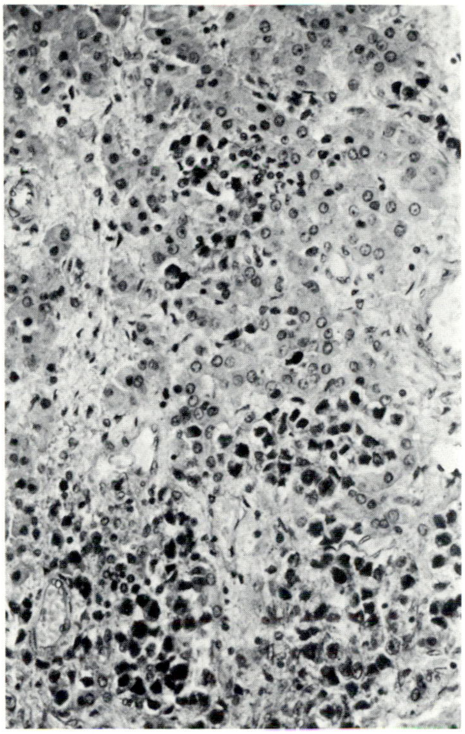

FIG. 19.72. Dysgerminoma with syncytiotrophoblast cells. Degenerating dysgerminoma cells are separated by steroid-type cells with pale nuclei and abundant dense cytoplasm in the peripheral portion of the tumor.

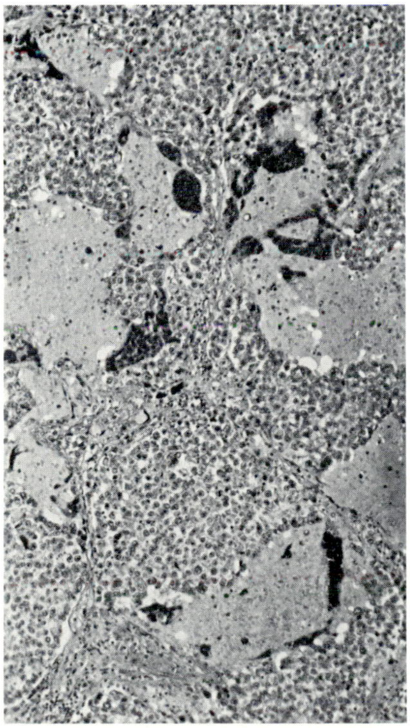

FIG. 19.71. Dysgerminoma with syncytiotrophoblast cells. Multinucleated syncytiotrophoblast cells surround pools of blood in otherwise typical dysgerminoma.

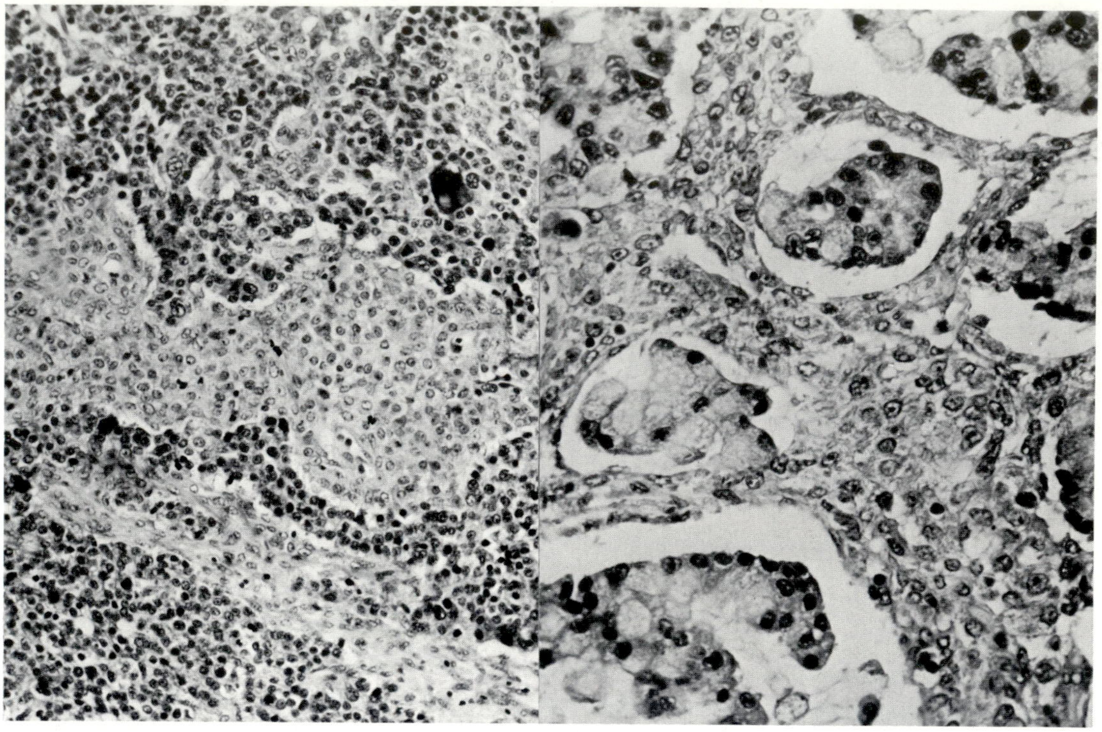

FIG. 19.73. Krukenberg tumor with luteinization of stroma. At *left*, cords of carcinoma cells are separated by masses of luteinized cells. At *right*, clusters of mucin-filled cells are separated by luteinized stromal cells. This tumor was associated with virilization and decidual change of the endometrium. (Reprinted by permission of Scully and Richardson, Ref. 254.)

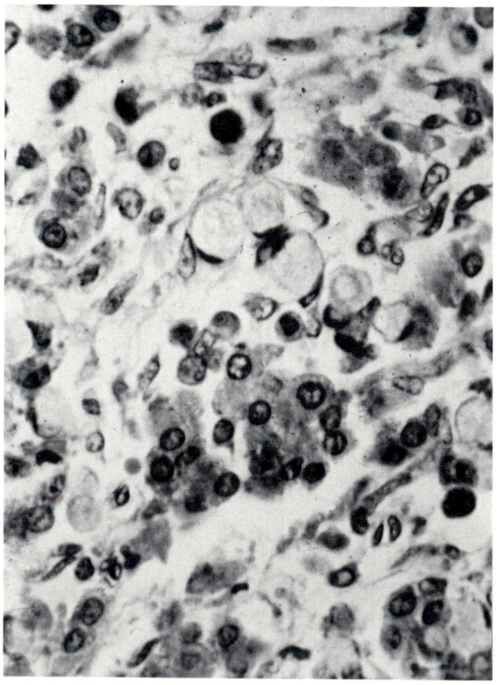

FIG. 19.74. Krukenberg tumor. Signet cells are separated by luteinized stromal cells. This tumor was associated with virilization. (Reprinted by permission of Scully, Ref. 251.)

hCG or some other stromal stimulant by the neoplastic cells may be responsible.

Germ Cell Tumors Containing Syncytiotrophoblast Cells

Two dysgerminomas with syncytiotrophoblast cells have been associated with luteinization of the stroma and endocrine manifestations (Figs. 19.71 and 19.72). One was accompanied by isosexual precocity[300] and the other by postpubertal virilization.[50]

Germ cell tumors that produce hCG, including dysgerminomas with syncytiotrophoblast giant cells,[147,334] may also be responsible for manifestations of steroid hormone secretion in the absence of recognized stromal luteinization.[34,154,155] In these cases and possibly as an additional mechanism in cases with stromal luteinization, high plasma levels of hCG may stimulate the ovary contralateral to the tumor to form luteinized follicles and corpora lutea that secrete steroid hormones. This mechanism may account for the endocrine manifestations, which are mostly estrogenic, that occur in patients with choriocarcinoma[256] and have been reported in 60% of patients with embryonal carcinoma and 40% of those with malignant mixed germ cell tumors in the series of Kurman and Norris.[154,155]

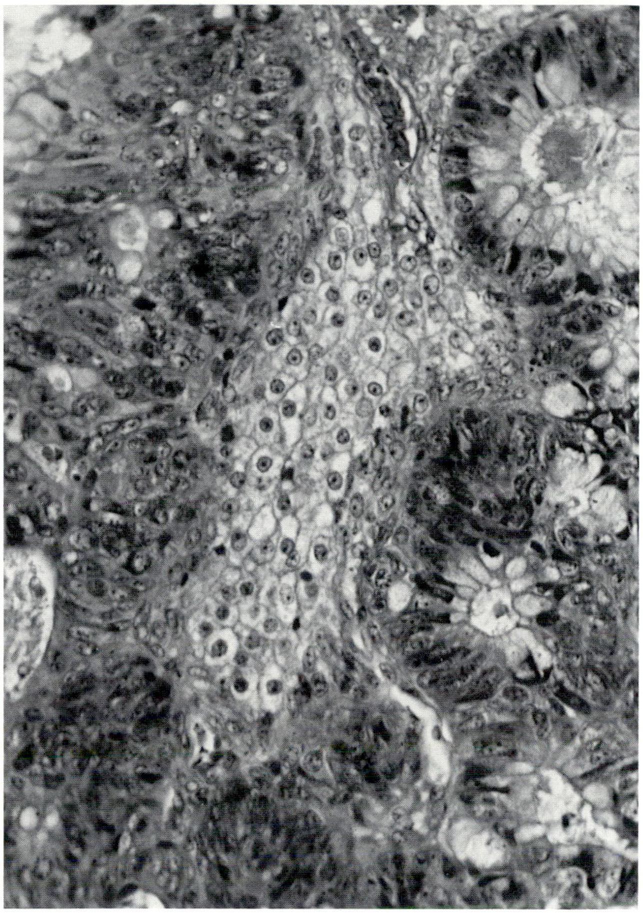

FIG. 19.75. Metastatic adenocarcinoma from colon. The neoplastic glands are separated by vacuolated luteinized stromal cells. (Reprinted by permission of Scully and Richardson, Ref. 254.)

Tumors with Functioning Stroma Occurring During Pregnancy

Although it is logical to speculate that ovarian tumors with functioning stroma in pregnant patients may secrete estrogens, this possibility has not been investigated by hormone assay, and clinical manifestations of estrogen excess are not expected to be present during gestation. In contrast, 19 examples of virilization caused by ovarian tumors with functioning stroma during pregnancy have been reported. These tumors have included 9 Krukenberg tumors,[19,98,100,235,304,305] 5 mucinous cystic tumors,[38,60,200,235,242,304] 2 Brenner tumors,[25,126,178,187] and single examples of serous cystadenoma,[94] endodermal sinus tumor,[242] and dermoid cyst.[49] The onset of the virilization in these patients has ranged from the third to the ninth month of gestation. The endocrine status of the offspring is known in 10 cases: the child was a normal male in 3, a normal female in 2, and a virilized female in 5 cases.

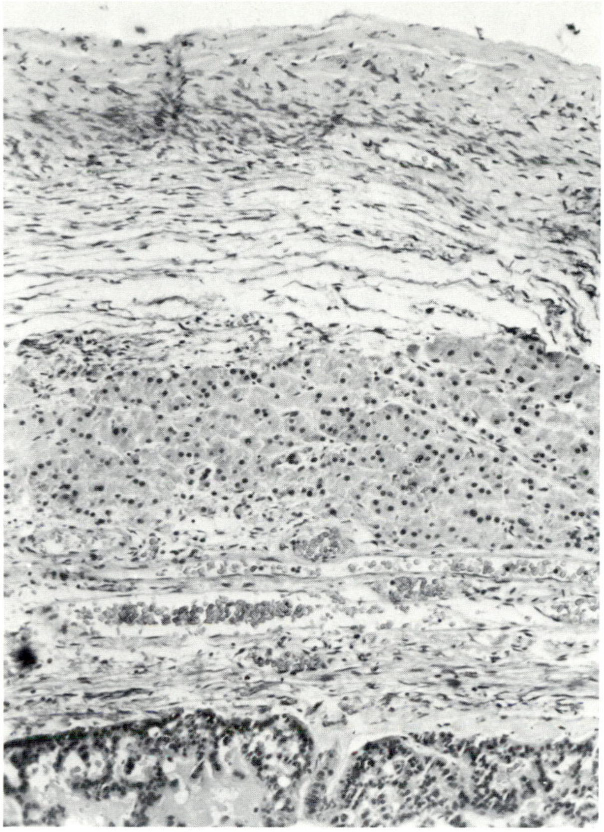

FIG. 19.76. Strumal carcinoid with peripheral band of steroid-type cells.

Idiopathic Group of Tumors

Whereas ovarian tumors with functioning stroma in the first two categories are encountered in young females, patients with tumors in the idiopathic group are usually postmenopausal, reflecting the higher prevalence of ovarian tumors, both primary and metastatic, and possibly the higher levels of circulating luteinizing hormone in this age group. A wide variety of ovarian tumors has been associated with an idiopathic functioning stroma, but its frequency has varied from one type of neoplasm to another.

Mucinous tumors often contain functioning stroma, resulting in either estrogenic or androgenic manifestations. In one series,[87] approximately one quarter of both mucinous cystadenomas and cystadenocarcinomas were accompanied by evidence of an "active endometrium" in postmenopausal women. In another study, approximately two-thirds of patients with mucinous tumors of various types had elevated total estrogen levels in the urine.[223] Three mucinous tumors have been responsible for virilization of nonpregnant patients.[27,68,105]

Occasional cases of endometrioid carcinoma have been reported to be associated with endometrial hyperplasia in postmenopausal women,[134,253,327] and in one patient, virilization and breast secretion developed.[253] We have recently seen a well-differentiated endometrioid carcinoma from a patient with an elevated serum testosterone level and the recent development of hirsutism.[316] Rome et al.[223] found that urinary estrogen levels were elevated in five of six patients with endometrioid carcinoma, indicating that these tumors may be associated with function more often than had been realized. Clear cell carcinomas have been accompanied only exceptionally by endometrial hyperplasia,[134] and Rome et al.[223] found that the urinary estrogens were normal in all four of their patients with tumors of this type. Serous tumors have also been associated only rarely with evidence of hyperestrinism.[87,175] Two of three patients with undifferentiated carcinoma of the ovary studied by Rome et al.[223] had elevated urinary total estrogen excretion. Brenner tumors have been accompanied by endometrial hyperplasia in 10–16% of the cases.[16,101,142,263,293] In one case,[124] Leydig cells were identified in the stroma. These studies indicate that all types of common epithelial tumor may be associated with stromal activation but that endocrine manifestations are seen with significant frequency only in patients with mucinous tumors.

Germ cell tumors of various types lacking trophoblastic cells have rarely been associated with stromal luteinization and evidence of steroid hormone secretion in the absence of pregnancy.[130] The germ cell tumors within the idiopathic category that have been accompanied by androgenic or estrogenic manifestations have included a variety of subtypes, such as dermoid cyst,[5] struma ovarii,[308] carcinoid tumors,[78,219,220] embryonal carcinoma,[1] and endodermal sinus tumor.[212,275] The steroid cells that are stimulated in cases of germ cell tumor are peripheral (Fig. 19.76) rather than within the tumor in many if not most of the cases.[231] Solid mature teratomas and immature teratomas have not been accompanied by evidence of steroid hormone production, to the best of our knowledge.

Metastatic carcinomas that contain mucinous cells, like primary mucinous tumors of the ovary, are frequently associated with luteinization of the stroma (Figs. 19.73, 19.74, and 19.75) and, in a significant proportion of cases, with clinical evidence of elevated steroid hormone levels. Scully and Richardson[254] found clinical evidence of excess estrogens, as manifested by irregular premenopausal bleeding or postmenopausal bleeding, in one quarter of patients with metastatic adenocarcinoma from the large intestine and stomach. One metastatic adenocarcinoma from the colon was responsible for masculinization[254] and another for both virilizing and estrogenic changes.[51] Seven Krukenberg tumors from nonpregnant patients have been associated with virilization (Figs. 19.73 and 19.74). The majority of these tumors were of gastric origin,[19,98,235,304,305] but one arose in the breast[269] and another, a tubular Krukenberg tumor, in the appendix.[41] One Krukenberg tumor of gastric origin[40] and a metastatic adenocarcinoma of colonic origin[205] have been associated with decidual changes in the endometrium in addition to virilization.

Ovarian Tumors Associated with Thyroid Hyperfunction

Although strumas of the ovary have been demonstrated by immunohistochemical staining to contain triiodothyronine and thyroxine[128] and, therefore, probably produce thyroid hormones at subclinical levels in many cases, clinical evidence suggestive of hyperthyroidism has rarely been confirmed by modern laboratory tests.[99] Rare strumal carcinoids (see Chapter 20, Germ Cell Tumors of Ovary) have been accompanied by evidence of hypersecretion of thyroid hormone in the form of postoperative thyroid storm or hypothyroidism,[219] and thyroglobulin has been demonstrated in the colloid within tumors of this type.[118,299]

Ovarian Tumors Associated with Carcinoid Syndrome

Of the three major categories of primary carcinoid tumor of the ovary (see Chapter 20, Germ Cell Tumors of Ovary), insular, trabecular, and strumal, one third of the insular tumors[220] and a single example of strumal carcinoid[301] have been associated with the carcinoid syndrome. This disorder occurs in the absence of hepatic or other metastases in cases of ovarian carcinoid because the hormonal effluent of the tumor enters the systemic circulation directly, bypassing the portal venous system and avoiding inactivation in the liver. The carcinoid syndrome caused by a primary ovarian carcinoid is, therefore, curable if the tumor is confined to the ovary and irreversible damage to cardiac valves has not occurred.

Ovarian Tumors Associated with Zollinger–Ellison Syndrome

Three mucinous tumors, two cystadenomas, and one cystadenocarcinoma have caused the Zollinger–Ellison syndrome.[64,162,186] In two of these cases, gastrin-containing cells were identified immunohistochemically in neuroendocrine cells within the cyst lining.

Ovarian Tumors Associated with Paraendocrine Disorders

A variety of paraendocrine disorders have been described in association with numerous types of ovarian tumor, some manifested by signs and symptoms of a well-known endocrine disease and others by subclinical laboratory

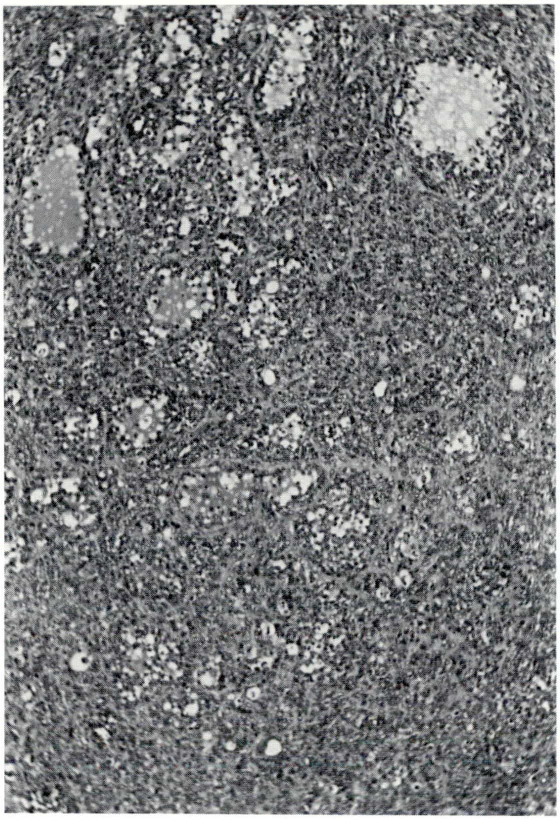

FIG. 19.77. Small cell carcinoma. Many small follicles are present within an otherwise densely cellular neoplasm.

abnormalities, indicating ectopic production of hormones or hormone-like substances by the tumor cells. In some of these cases, the hormone being produced has been identified, whereas in others, such as cases of hypercalcemia, the mechanism of the disorder remains unclear. In all the cases included within this category of neoplasms, successful therapy of the tumor has led to disappearance of the paraendocrine state.

Hypercalcemia

Fifty-six ovarian tumors (37 in the literature and 19 unreported in our files) have been reported to be associated with paraendocrine hypercalcemia. Most have not been accompanied by recognizable clinical manifestations of hypercalcemia.* Approximately half the tumors have been a distinctive type of small cell carcinoma. The rest have included clear cell carcinomas (12 cases), serous carcinomas (7 cases), undifferentiated carcinomas (2 cases), and miscellaneous neoplasms (6 cases).

Small Cell Carcinoma

The small cell carcinoma that is often associated with hypercalcemia was first described by Dickersin et al. 1981[77] (Figs. 19.77 and 19.78). This tumor, of which we have now seen 80 examples, is, in our experience, the most common form of undifferentiated carcinoma of the ovary in females under 40 years of age and has been accompanied by elevated levels of calcium in two-thirds of the patients in whom it has been measured. The age of the patients has ranged from 10 to 42 (average 22) years. The symptoms, abdominal pain and swelling, have been those associated with ovarian tumors in general.

At laparotomy the tumors have, with one exception, been unilateral. Spread beyond the ovary has occurred in approximately one quarter of the cases. Gross examination reveals fleshy white to pale tan masses, often containing large areas of hemorrhage and necrosis (Fig. 19.79, Plate 4). The most common microscopic appearance is a diffuse arrangement of closely packed epithelial cells with scanty cytoplasm and small nuclei that typically contain single small nucleoli. Mitotic figures are numerous. The tumor cells also grow in nests, cords, and irregular groups. Distinctive follicle-like structures containing eosinophilic fluid are present in most of the cases (Fig. 19.77). In about 25% of the tumors, large cells with abundant eosinophilic cytoplasm resembling luteinized

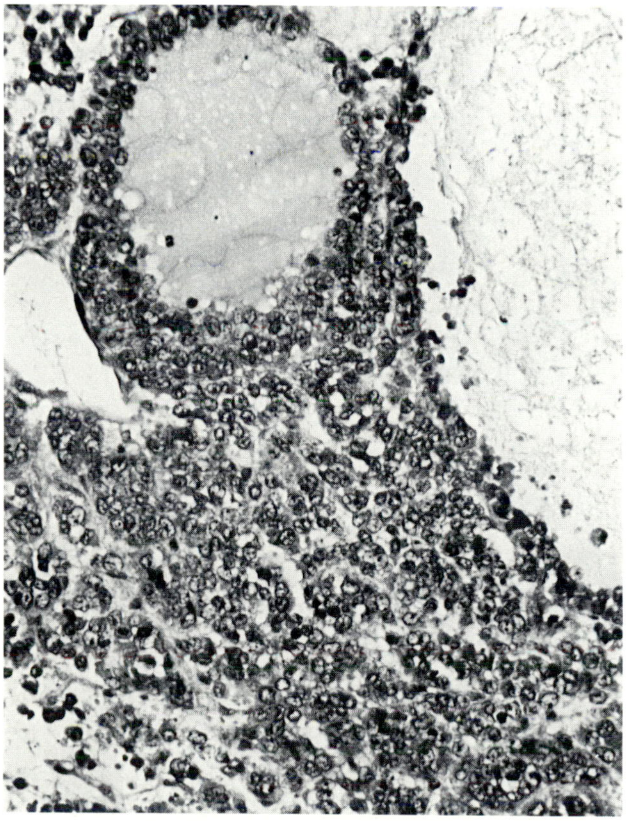

FIG. 19.78. Small cell carcinoma. Follicle-like structures lined by and surrounded by small cells with scanty cytoplasm and hyperchromatic nuclei.

* References 2, 6, 47, 77, 97, 131, 143, 274, 278.

cells have been present focally (Fig. 19.80); rarely, these cells have predominated. The stroma is generally scanty and consists of nonspecific fibrous tissue.

Special staining and ultrastructural examination have not revealed any features that identify the cell type of this tumor. Although it is composed of relatively small cells, dense core granules have not been found. The age distribution and the characteristic presence of uniform small cells and follicle formation suggest a sex cord derivation, but transitions to recognizable forms of sex cord tumors have not been observed. No unquestionable teratomatous elements have been found, but in 7 of our 80 cases occasional glands lined by mucinous epithelium were present. Unfortunately, this finding does not establish the origin of the tumor, since mucinous epithelium may be seen in common epithelial tumors, germ cell neoplasms, and Sertoli-Leydig cell tumors. Immunoperoxidase staining has shown that the tumor cells are positive for keratin and vimentin in the majority of cases so studied.

The small cell carcinoma is often confused with a granulosa cell tumor of either adult or juvenile type. The features of these three types of tumor are contrasted in Table 19.4. Diffuse small cell carcinomas may also resemble malignant lymphomas, particularly on low-power examination, but adequate sampling reveals patterns of growth that indicate the epithelial nature of the tumor. Also, the cytologic features of the neoplastic cells are incompatible with any form of malignant lymphoma. We have seen one case in which a primitive neuroectodermal tumor of the ovary with a diffuse pattern and follicle-like spaces resembled a small cell carcinoma. Extensive sampling, however, disclosed a few teratomatous elements, and the diagnosis was confirmed by the immunohistochemical demonstration of glial fibrillary acidic protein. Exceptionally, the differential diagnosis of a small cell carcinoma includes the rare embryonal rhabdomyosarcoma of the ovary.

The small cell carcinoma has a very poor prognosis. Ten of the eleven patients described in the initial report died of their tumor, and follow-up in subsequent patients has confirmed the dismal prognosis. We have seen two patients in whom recurrence has involved the contralateral ovary, suggesting that despite the almost invariable appearance of unilateral involvement at the time of exploration, hysterectomy and bilateral salpingo-oophorectomy may be indicated as the initial surgical procedure. There has been little or no experience with successful chemotherapy or radiation therapy for this tumor.

The mechanism of the hypercalcemia associated with small cell carcinoma and other ovarian cancers is unknown. Stewart et al.[274] have suggested that it results from the production of a parathormone-like substance. Roles for osteoclast-activating factor, prostaglandins, and a vitamin D-like steroid have been proposed by others.[143,151]

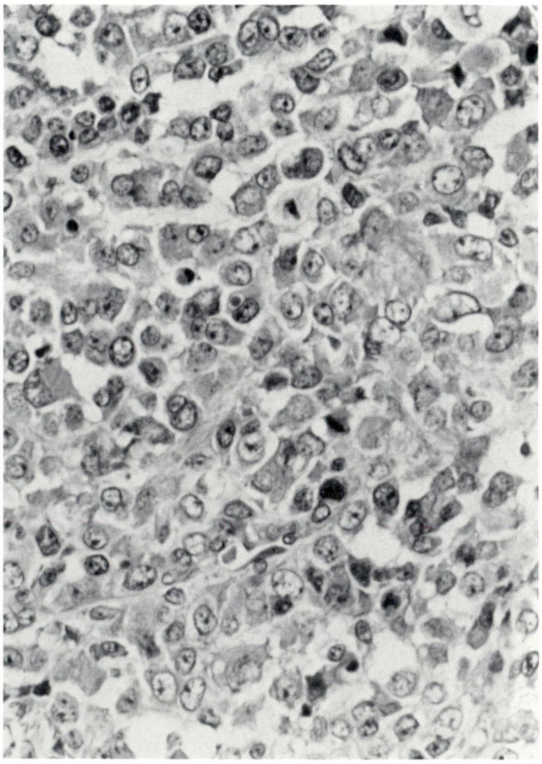

FIG. 19.80. Small cell carcinoma. Focal area is composed of large cells with abundant dense cytoplasm.

Cushing's Syndrome

As mentioned earlier, three cases of Cushing's syndrome have resulted from cortisol production by a metastasizing steroid cell tumor.[170,321] In an additional remarkable case, a pituitary adenoma composed of cells that stained immunohistochemically for ACTH arose within a dermoid cyst, secreted ACTH, and caused Cushing's syndrome.[179] Sporadic other examples of this syndrome appear to have resulted from ectopic ACTH production by ovarian tumors, which have included an adenocarcinoma,[208] a small cell carcinoma presumably primary in the ovary,[39] and a tumor interpreted as a Sertoli cell tumor.[195] Immunohistochemical staining for ACTH has revealed its frequent presence in a variety of ovarian tumors,[255] which helps to explain the occasional production of ACTH by these neoplasms.

Ectopic Chorionic Gonadotropin Production

Ectopic chorionic gonadotropin (hCG) production was reported by Civantos and Rywlin in three women with serous papillary or mucinous adenocarcinomas of the ovary.[63] All had elevated urinary hCG levels ranging from 1000 to 25,000 IU per 24 hours. Each of the tumors contained poorly differentiated areas, with cells resembling syncytiotrophoblast cells. These cells were positive for hCG on immunofluorescence staining. In one of these patients, the contralateral ovary contained numerous lutein cells, and a decidual reaction was present in the endometrium. This patient had vaginal bleeding, but no endocrine effects were present in the other two patients. Vaitukaitis[302] reported that 10 of 28 ovarian tumors of various types were associated with the presence of immunoreactive hCG in the plasma, and Samaan et al.[236] found the beta-subunit of hCG in the plasma of 41% of women with common eipthelial carcinomas. Immunohistochemical staining of common epithelial tumors for hCG has yielded varying results.[57,94,184] One group[184] found an approximately 40% frequency of staining, with no significant differences among benign, borderline, and invasive tumors, whereas another group[94] found only a 10% frequency of staining of carcinomas and no staining of benign tumors. Because of its presence in a wide variety of tumors, including one granulosa cell tumor,[94] immunohistochemical identification of hCG is of relatively little help in differential diagnosis. The subject of ectopic hCG production by ovarian tumors overlaps with that of ovarian tumors with idiopathic functioning stroma. In spite of the possible interrelation of these subjects, no correlation among plasma hCG elevation, immunohistochemical demonstration of hCG in ovarian tumors, luteinization of the stroma of ovarian tumors, and endocrine manifestations has as yet been published.

Hypoglycemia

Four patients have been reported in whom an ovarian neoplasm has been associated with hypoglycemia. The tumors have been a serous cystadenocarcinoma, a dysgerminoma, a fibroma, and a malignant schwannoma.[180,181,260] In the case of the malignant schwannoma, insulin and proinsulin were recovered from the tumor tissue.[260]

Renin Production

Korzets et al.[151] reported a case of renin-producing Sertoli cell tumor of the ovary with secondary hyperaldosteronism, hypertension, and hypokalemia. These authors interpreted the Sertoli cell tumor that Ehrlich et al.[88] considered to be an aldosterone-secreting tumor as probably belonging in the category of a renin-producing tumor.

Ovarian Tumors Associated with Paraneoplastic Syndromes

Nervous System Disorders

Ovarian cancer is among the most common malignant tumors associated with nervous system disorders; in one series, the frequency was 16%.[66] A variety of lesions affecting both the gray matter and white matter of the cerebrum, cerebellum, and spinal cord, the peripheral nerves, and the myoneural junction, accompanied by myasthenia gravis, may occur.[37,129,297] Paraneoplastic subacute cerebellar degeneration is one of the most common lesions, with ovarian cancer accounting for 16% of the cases.[129] The cerebellar manifestations usually antedate recognition of the cancer, and typically there is no improvement after removal of the tumor.[123] In one recently reported patient, manifestations of the cerebellar degeneration partially regressed after plasmapheresis,[65] and in two patients, circulating antibodies to Purkinje cells were identified.[119] Limbic encephalitis has also been associated with ovarian carcinoma,[56] and necrotizing myelopathy, a rare paraneoplastic complication of cancer, accompanied an ovarian adenosquamous carcinoma in one patient at our hospital.[53]

Connective Tissue Disorders

The connective tissue disorder most commonly associated with ovarian cancer is dermatomyositis.[18,280,303] In one review of 25 women with this disease, 5 were found to have malignant tumors, 3 of which were ovarian carcinomas.[238] In another study of 10 patients with dermatomyositis or polymyositis and a malignant tumor of the female genital tract, 5 had ovarian cancer.[303] The onset of the dermatomyositis usually precedes recognition of the ovarian tumor, which becomes evident within 2 years in most cases.[303] The dermatologic and, to a lesser extent, the myopathic symptoms typically regress after removal of the tumor and return if it recurs.

Medsger et al.[176] have described six patients with high stage ovarian carcinoma in whom polyarthritis and palmar fasciitis preceded the diagnosis of carcinoma by 5–25 months. The arthritic symptoms were similar to those of rheumatoid arthritis. Four of the ovarian tumors were endometrioid carcinomas, one was a serous carcinoma, and one was an undifferentiated carcinoma. An additional example of this syndrome associated with serous carcinoma was subsequently described.[261] One woman with ovarian carcinoma had hypertrophic pulmonary osteoarthropathy,[166] and occasional patients have had rheumatoid arthritis, scleroderma, or systemic lupus erythematosus.[21,45,84,166]

Hematologic Disorders

Approximately 30 ovarian tumors have been reported to be associated with autoimmune hemolytic anemia, which is usually Coombs-positive.[48] Most of these tumors have been dermoid cysts,[15,24,48,74,209] but occasional examples of carcinoma[48] and a single case of granulosa cell tumor[73] have also been reported. In the last case, the patient also had splenic angiomas. In many cases, corticosteroid therapy, splenectomy, or both have resulted in little or no improvement, but removal of the ovarian tumor has produced a rapid remission of the hemolytic disorder. Payne et al.[209] have listed several mechanisms proposed to explain the relation of the dermoid cyst to the anemia: (1) liberation by the tumor of a substance that alters the surfaces of red cells, making them antigenic to the host, (2) stimulation of production of an antibody that cross-reacts with the red cells by an antigen in the wall or lumen of the cyst, and (3) direct production of a red cell antibody by the tumor. Support for the last theory is provided by the finding of immunoglobulin in the cyst fluid in several cases.[209]

Ovarian tumors are commonly associated with laboratory evidence of disseminated intravascular coagulation (DIC), but clinical manifestations of this disorder are uncommon. In one study,[13] 72% and, in another,[11] 94% of women with ovarian cancer had fibrin degradation products in their serum. In their review of cases of clinically evident DIC, however, Sack et al.[232] cited seven that were associated with ovarian cancer. At least three other cases have been reported subsequently.[54,75,262] Nonbacterial thrombotic endocarditis has also been recorded as a complication of ovarian cancer.[75]

Erythrocytosis may develop as a result of androgen production by an ovarian tumor but rarely accompanies an ovarian neoplasm as an isolated laboratory abnormality.[111,125] In one patient, a virilizing steroid cell tumor was accompanied by an unusually high red cell count, which was attributed in part to erythropoietin production by the tumor.[185] Other hematologic abnormalities rarely associated with ovarian tumors include nonthrombocytopenic purpura,[69] granulocytosis,[278] and pancytopenia.[192]

References

1. Abell MR (1986) Undifferentiated malignant germ cell neoplasm (embryonal carcinoma) of ovary with stromal luteinization. Am J Obstet Gynecol 101: 570–572
2. Abouav J, Berkowitz SB, Kolb FO (1959) Reversible hypercalcemia in masculinizing hypernephroid tumor of the ovary. Report of a case. N Engl J Med 260: 1057–1062
3. Aguirre P, Scully RE (1983) Testosterone-secreting adrenal ganglioneuroma containing Leydig cells. Am J Surg Pathol 7: 699
4. Ahn GH, Chi JG, Lee SK (1986) Ovarian sex cord tumor with annular tubules. Cancer. 57: 1066
5. Aiman J, Nalick RH, Jacobs A, Porter JC, Edman CD, Vellios F, MacDonald PC (1977) The origin of androgen and estrogen in a virilized postmenopausal woman with bilateral benign cystic teratomas. Obstet Gynecol 49: 695–704
6. Allan SG, Lockhart SP, Leonard RCF, Smyth JF (1984) Paraneoplastic hypercalcemia in ovarian carcinoma. Br Med J 288: 1714–1715
7. Allander E, Wagermark J (1969) Leydig cell tumors of the ovary. Report of three cases. Acta Obstet Gynecol Scand 48: 433
8. Anderson MC (1972) Hilar cell tumour of the ovary. J Clin Pathol 25: 106
9. Anderson MC, Rees DA (1975) Gynandroblastoma of the ovary. Br J Obstet Gynaecol 82: 68
10. Anikwue C, Dawood MY, Kramer E (1979) Granulosa and theca cell tumors. Obstet Gynecol 51: 214–220
11. Anstey JT, Blythe JG (1978) Fibrin degradation products and the diagnosis of ovarian carcinoma. Obstet Gynecol 52: 605–608
12. Armstrong DT, Papkoff H (1976) Stimulation of aromatization by endogenous and exogenous androgens in ovaries of hypophysectomized rats in vivo by FSH. Endocrinology 99: 1144–1151
13. Astedt B, Svanberg L, Nilsson IM (1971) Fibrin degradation products and ovarian tumours. Br Med J 4: 458
14. Astengo-Osuna C (1984) Ovarian sex cord tumor with annular tubules. Case report with ultrastructural findings. Cancer 54: 1070–1075
15. Baker LRI, Brain MC, Azzopardi JG, Worlledge SM (1968) Autoimmune haemolytic anaemic associated with ovarian dermoid cyst. J Clin Pathol 21: 626
16. Balasa RW, Adcock LL, Prem KA, Dehner LP (1977) The Brenner tumor. Obstet Gynecol 50: 120–128
17. Banner EA, Dockerty MB (1945) Theca cell tumors of the ovary. A clinical and pathological study of twenty-three cases (including thirteen new cases) with a review. Surg Gynecol Obstet 81: 234–242
18. Barnes BE (1976) Dermatomyositis and malignancy. A review of the literature. Ann Intern Med 84: 68–76
19. Bell RJM (1977) Fetal virilisation due to maternal Krukenberg tumour. Lancet 1: 1162–1163
20. Benfield GFA, Tapper-Jones L, Stout TV (1982) Androblastoma and raised serum alpha-fetoprotein with familial multinodular goitre. Case report. Br J Obstet Gynaecol 89: 323
21. Bennett RM, Ginsberg MH, Thomsen S (1976) Carcinomatous polyarthritis. Arthritis Rheum 19: 953–959
22. Bennington JL, Ferguson BR, Haber SL (1968) Incidence and relative frequency of benign and malignant ovarian neoplasms. Obstet Gynecol 32: 627–732
23. Berlin NI, Van Scott EJ, Clendenning WE, Archard HO, Block JB, Witkop CJ, Haynes HA (1966) Basal cell nevus syndrome. Ann Intern Med 64: 403
24. Bernstein D, Naor S, Rikover M, Menahem H (1974) Hemolytic anemia related to ovarian tumor. Obstet Gynecol 43: 276–280
25. Besch PK, Byron RC, Barry RD, Teteris NJ, Hamwi GJ, Vorys N, Ullery JC (1963) Testosterone synthesis by a Brenner tumor. Part II. In vitro biosynthetic steroid conversion of a Brenner tumor. Am J Obstet Gynecol 86: 1021–1026
26. Betta P, Bellingeri D (1985) Androgenic juvenile granulosa cell tumor. Case report. Eur J Gynaecol Oncol 6: 71–74
27. Bettinger HF, Jacobs H (1946) A contribution to the problem of masculinization. Med J Aust 1: 10–13
28. Björkholm E (1980) Granulosa cell tumors: A comparison of survival in patients and matched controls. Am J Obstet Gynecol 138: 329–331

29. Björkholm E, Pettersson F (1980) Granulosa-cell and theca-cell tumors. The clinical picture and long-term outcome for the Radiumhemmet series. Acta Obstet Gynecol Scand 59: 361
30. Björkholm E, Silfverswärd C (1981) Prognostic factors in granulosa cell tumors. Gynecol Oncol 11: 261
31. Björkholm E, Silfverswärd C (1980) Theca-cell tumors. Clinical features and prognosis. Acta Radiol Oncol Radiat Phys Biol 19: 241
32. Boivin Y, Richart RM (1965) Hilus cell tumors of the ovary. A review, with a report of 3 new cases. Cancer 18: 231
33. Bonaventura LM, Judd H, Roth LM, Cleary RE (1978) Androgen, estrogen, and progesterone production by a lipid cell tumor of the ovary. Am J Obstet Gynecol 131: 403
34. Borushek S, Berger I, Echt C, Gold JJ (1965) Functioning malignant germ cell tumor of the ovary in a 4½-year-old girl. Cancer 18: 1485–1488
35. Boss JH, Scully RE, Wegner KH, Cohen RB (1965) Structural variations in the adult ovary—Clinical significance. Obstet Gynecol 25: 747–764
36. Bower JF, Erickson ER (1967) Bilateral ovarian fibromas in a 5-year-old. Am J Obstet Gynecol 99: 880
37. Brain L (1963) The neurological complications of neoplasms. Lancet 1: 179–184
38. Bronstein R, Hardouin G, Henrion R (1972) Kyste mucoide virilisant au cours de la grossesse. J Gynecol Obstet Biol Reprod 1: 891–899
39. Brown H, Lane M (1965) Cushing's and malignant carcinoid syndromes from ovarian neoplasm. Arch Intern Med 115: 490–494
40. Bruno MS, Ober WB (1959) Clinicopathologic Conference. NY State J Med 59: 4001–4007
41. Bullon A, Arseneau J, Prat J, Young RH, Scully RE (1981) Tubular Krukenberg tumor. A problem in histopathologic diagnosis. Am J Surg Pathol 5: 225–232
42. Burket RL, Rauh JL (1976) Gorlin's syndrome: Ovarian fibromas at adolescence. Obstet Gynecol 47: 43s–44s
43. Burslem RW, Langley FA, Woodcock AS (1954) A clinicopathological study of oestrogenic ovarian tumours. Cancer 7: 552
44. Busby T, Anderson GW (1954) Feminizing mesenchymomas of the ovary. Am J Obstet Gynecol 68: 1391
45. Calabro JJ (1967) Cancer and arthritis. Arthritis Rheum 10: 553–567
46. Campbell PE, Danks DM (1963) Pseudoprecocity in an infant due to a luteoma of the ovary. Arch Dis Child 38: 519
47. Cannon PM, Smart CR, Wilson ML, Edwards CB (1975) Hypercalcemia with ovarian granulosa cell carcinoma. Rocky Mountain Med J 72: 72–74
48. Carreras Vescio LA, Toblli JE, Rey JA, Assaf ME, De Maria HE, Marletta J (1983) Autoimmune hemolytic anemia associated with an ovarian neoplasm. Medicina 43: 415–424
49. Case Records of the Massachusetts General Hospital (1970) Case 13–1970. N Engl J Med 282: 676–681
50. Case Records of the Massachusetts General Hospital (1972) Case 11–1972. N Engl J Med 286: 594–600
51. Case Records of the Massachusetts General Hospital (1975) Case 10–1975. N Engl J Med 292: 521
52. Case Records of the Massachusetts General Hospital (1976) Case 14–1976.
53. Case Records of the Massachusetts General Hospital (1976) Case 26–1976. N Engl J Med 294: 1447–1454
54. Case Records of the Massachusetts General Hospital (1978) Case 13–1978. N Engl J Med 298: 786–792
55. Case Records of the Massachusetts General Hospital (1983) Case 21–1983. N Engl J Med 308: 1279–1284
56. Case Records of the Massachusetts General Hospital (1985) Case 30–1985. N Engl J Med 313: 249–257
57. Casper S, van Nagell JR, Powell DF, Dubilier LD, Donaldson ES, Hanson MB, Pavlik EJ (1981) Immunohistochemical localization of tumor markers in epithelial ovarian cancer. Am J Obstet Gynecol 149: 154–158
58. Chalvardjian A, Derzko C (1982) Gynandroblastoma. Its ultrastructure. Cancer 50: 710
59. Chalvardjian A, Scully RE (1973) Sclerosing stromal tumors of the ovary. Cancer 31: 664
60. Chan LKC, Prathap K (1970) Virilization in pregnancy associated with an ovarian mucinous cystadenoma. Am J Obstet Gynecol 108: 946–949
61. Christian E (1910) Un cas d'epitheliome a granulations de lutéine d'origine probablement ovarienne. Soc Anat Ann 12: 639–641
62. Chumas JC, Rosenwaks Z, Mann WJ, Finkel G, Pastore J (1984) Sertoli-Leydig cell tumor of the ovary producing alpha-fetoprotein. Int J Gynecol Pathol 3: 213–219
63. Civantos F, Rywlin AM (1972) Carcinomas with trophoblastic differentiation and secretion of chorionic gonadotrophins. Cancer 29: 789–798
64. Cocco AE, Conway SJ (1975) Zollinger-Ellison syndrome associated with ovarian mucinous cystadenocarcinoma. N Engl J Med 293: 485–486
65. Cocconi G, Ceci G, Juvarra G, Minopoli MR, Cocchi T, Fiaccadori F, Lechi A, Boni P (1985) Successful treatment of subacute cerebellar degeneration in ovarian carcinoma with plasmapheresis. A case report. Cancer 56: 2318–1320
66. Croft PB, Wilkinson M (1965) The incidence of carcinomatous neuromyopathy in patients with various types of carcinoma. Brain 88: 427–434
67. Czernobilsky B (1984) Immunohistochemistry of normal tissues of the female genital tract. Presentation at XVth International Congress of International Academy of Pathology, Miami Beach, FL
68. DaCosta CC (1938) Tumor masculinizante. Rev Gynecol Obstet 2: 3–9
69. Dales M (1965) Purpura associated with ovarian tumor. Br Med J 1: 127
70. Damjanov I, Drobnjak P, Grizelj V, Longhino N (1975) Sclerosing stromal tumor of the ovary. A hormonal and ultrastructural analysis. Obstet Gynecol 45: 675–679
71. Dardi LE, Miller AW, Gould VE (1982) Sertoli-Leydig cell tumor with endometrioid differentiation. Case report and discussion of histogenesis. Diagn Gynecol Obstet 4: 227–234
72. Davidson BJ, Waisman J, Judd HL (1981) Long-standing

virilism in a woman with hyperplasia and neoplasia of ovarian lipidic cells. Obstet Gynecol 58: 753
73. Dawson MA, Talbert W, Yarbro JW (1971) Hemolytic anemia associated with an ovarian tumor. Am J Med 50: 552
74. DeBruyere M, Sokal G, Devoitille JM, Fauchet-Dutrieux MC, De Spa V (1971) Autoimmune haemolytic anaemia and ovarian tumour. Br J Haematol 20: 83
75. Delgado G, Smith JP (1975) Gynecological malignancy associated with nonbacterial thrombotic endocarditis (NBTE). Gynecol Oncol 3: 205–209
76. DeTorres EF (1974) Feminization in tumors of Sertoli-Leydig cells. Acta Cytol 18: 187
77. Dickersin GR, Kline IW, Scully RE (1982) Small cell carcinoma of the ovary with hypercalcemia. A report of eleven cases. Cancer 49: 188
78. Dickman SH, Toker C (1971) Strumal carcinoid of the ovary with masculinization. Cancer 27: 925–930
79. Diddle AW (1951) Granulosa- and theca-cell ovarian tumors: Prognosis. Cancer 15: 215–228
80. Disaia PJ, Saltz A, Kagan AR, Rich W (1978) A temporary response of recurrent granulosa cell tumor to adriamycin. Obstet Gynecol 52: 355
81. Dockerty MB, MacCarty WC (1939) Granulosa cell tumors, with the report of a 34-lb. specimen and a review. Am J Obstet Gynecol 37: 425
82. Dockerty MB, Masson JC (1944) Ovarian fibromas: A clinical and pathologic study of two hundred and eighty-three cases. Am J Obstet Gynecol 47: 741
83. Dorrington JH, Moon YS, Armstrong DT (1975) Estradiol 17-β biosynthesis in cultured granulosa cells from hypophysectomized immature rats: Stimulation by FSH. Endocrinology 97: 1328–1331
84. Duncan SC, Winkelmann RK (1979) Cancer and scleroderma. Arch Dermatol 115: 950–955
85. Dunnihoo DR, Grieme DL, Woolf RB (1966) Hilar-cell tumors of the ovary. Report of 2 new cases and a review of the world literature. Obstet Gynecol 27: 703
86. Echt CR, Hadd HE (1968) Androgen excretion patterns in a patient with a metastatic hilus cell tumor of the ovary. Am J Obstet Gynecol 100: 1055
87. Eddie DAS (1967) Hormonal activity with ovarian tumours. J Obstet Gynaecol Br Commonw 74: 283–285
88. Ehrlich EN, Dominguez OV, Samuels LT, Lynch D, Oberhelman H, Warner NE (1963) Aldosteronism and precocious puberty due to an ovarian androblastoma (Sertoli cell tumor). J Clin Endocrinol Metab 23: 358–367
89. Emig OR, Hertig AT, Rowe FJ (1959) Gynandroblastoma of the ovary. Review and report of a case. Obstet Gynecol 13: 135
90. Evans AT, Gaffey TA, Malkasian GD Jr., Annegers JF (1980) Clinicopathologic review of 118 granulosa and 82 theca cell tumors. Obstet Gynecol 55: 231
91. Falls JL (1955) Accessory adrenal cortex in the broad ligament. Incidence and functional significance. Cancer 8: 143
92. Fathalla MF (1967) The occurrence of granulosa and theca tumors in clinically normal ovaries. A study of 25 cases. J Obstet Gynaecol Br Commonw 74: 279
93. Fathalla MF (1968) The role of the ovarian stroma in hormone production by ovarian tumors. J Obstet Gynaecol Br Commonw 75: 78–83
94. Fayez JA, Bunch TR, Miller GL (1974) Virilization in pregnancy associated with an ovarian serous cystadenoma. Am J Obstet Gynecol 120: 341–346
95. Fenoglio CM, Hayata T, Crum CP, Richart RM (1982) The expression of human chorionic gonadotrophin in the female genital tract. Localization by the immunoperoxidase technique. Diagn Gynecol Obstet 4: 94–97
96. Ferenczy A, Richart RM (1974) Female Reproductive System: Dynamics of Scan and Transmission Electron Microscopy. New York, John Wiley & Sons
97. Ferenczy A, Okagaki T, Richart RM (1971) Para-endocrine hypercalcemia in ovarian neoplasms. Report of mesonephroma with hypercalcemia and review of literature. Cancer 27: 427–433
98. Forest MG, Orgiazzi J, Tranchant D, Mornex R, Bertrand J (1978) Approach to the mechanism of androgen overproduction in a case of Krukenberg tumor responsible for virilization during pregnancy. J Clin Endocrinol Metab 47: 428–434
99. Fox H, Langley FA (1976) Tumors of the Ovary. Chicago, Year Book Medical Publishers
100. Fox LP, Stamm WJ (1965) Krukenberg tumor complicating pregnancy. Report of a case with androgenic activity. Am J Obstet Gynecol 92: 702–710
101. Fox H, Agrawal K, Langley FA (1972) The Brenner tumour of the ovary: A clinicopathologic study of 54 cases. J Obstet Gynaecol Br Commonw 79: 661–665
102. Fox H, Agrawal K, Langley FA (1975) A clinicopathological study of 92 cases of granulosa cell tumor of the ovary with special reference to the factors influencing prognosis. Cancer 35: 231
103. Franke WW, Grund C, Schmid E (1979) Intermediate-sized filaments in Sertoli cells are of vimentin-type. Eur J Cell Biol 19: 269–275
104. Gaffney EF, Majmudar B, Hertzler GL, Zane R, Furlong B, Breding E (1983) Ovarian granulosa cell tumors—Immunohistochemical localization of estradiol and ultrastructure, with functional correlations. Obstet Gynecol 61: 311
105. Garneau R, Cabanne F (1968) Dysembryome ovarien de type entéroide et bilio-hépatoide avec hyperplasie fonctionnelle des cellules sympathicotropes de Berger. A propos d'une observation. Ann Anat Pathol 13: 423–432
106. Gee DC, Russell P (1979) Sclerosing stromal tumours of the ovary. Histopathology 3: 367–376
107. Gee DC, Russell P (1981) The pathological assessment of ovarian neoplasms. IV: The sex cord stromal tumors. Pathology 13: 235–255
108. Geist SH, Gaines JA (1938) Theca cell tumors. Am J Obstet Gynecol 35: 39–51
109. Genton CY (1980) Ovarian Sertoli-Leydig cell tumors. A clinical, pathological and ultrastructural study with particular reference to the histogenesis of these tumors. Arch Gynecol 230: 49–75
110. Genton CY (1980) Some observations on the fine structure of human granulosa cell tumors. Virchows Arch [Pathol Anat] 387: 353–369
111. Ghio R, Haupt E, Ratti M, Boccaccio P (1981) Erythrocytosis associated with a dermoid cyst of the ovary and

erythropoietic activity of the tumour fluid. Scand J Haematol 27: 70–74
112. Givens JR (1976) Hirsutism and hyperandrogenism. Adv Int Med 21: 221–247
113. Givens JR, Kerber IJ, Wiser WL, Anderson RW, Coleman SA, Fish SA (1974) Remission of acanthosis nigricans associated with polycystic ovarian disease and a stromal luteoma. J Clin Endocrinol Metab 38: 347
114. Goldberg B, Seegar Jones GE, Woodruff JD (1963) A histochemical study of steroid 3-β-ol dehydrogenase activity in some steroid-producing tumors. Am J Obstet Gynecol 86: 1003–1014
115. Gondos B, Monroe SA (1971) Cystic granulosa cell tumor with massive hemoperitoneum. Light and electron microscopic study. Obstet Gynecol 38: 683–689
116. Gorlin RJ, Sedano HO (1971) The multiple nevoid basal cell carcinoma syndrome revisited. Birth Defects 7: 140
117. Gorlin RJ, Vickers RA, Kelln E, Williamson JJ (1965) The multiple basal cell nevi syndrome. Cancer 18: 89
118. Greco MA, LiVolsi VA, Pertschuk LP, Bigelow B (1979) Strumal carcinoid of the ovary. An analysis of its components. Cancer 43: 1380–1388
119. Greenlee JE, Brashear HR (1983) Antibodies to cerebellar Purkinje cells in patients with paraneoplastic cerebellar degeneration and ovarian carcinoma. Ann Neurol 14: 609–613
120. Guerard MJ, Ferenczy A, Arguelles MA (1982) Ovarian Sertoli-Leydig cell tumor with rhabodomyosarcoma: An ultrastructural study. Ultrastruct Pathol 3: 347
121. Guintoli RL, Celebre JA, Wu CH, Wheeler JE, Mikuta JJ (1976) Androgenic function of a granulosa cell tumor. Obstet Gynecol 47: 77
122. Gusberg SB, Kardon P (1967) Proliferative endometrial response to theca-granulosa cell tumors. Am J Obstet Gynecol 111: 633
123. Hall DJ, Dyer ML, Parker JC (1985) Ovarian cancer complicated by cerebellar degeneration: A paraneoplastic syndrome. Gynecol Oncol 21: 240–246
124. Hameed H (1972) Brenner tumor of the ovary with Leydig cell hyperplasia. A histologic and ultrastructural study. Cancer 30: 945–952
125. Hammond D, Winnick S (1974) Paraneoplastic erythrocytosis and ectopic erythropoietins. Ann NY Acad Sci 230: 219–227
126. Hamwi GJ, Byron RC, Besch PK, Vorys N, Teteris NJ, Ullery JC (1963) Testosterone synthesis by a Brenner tumor. Part I. Clinical evidence of masculinization during pregnancy. Am J Obstet Gynecol 86: 1015–1020
127. Hart WR, Kumar N, Crissman JD (1980) Ovarian neoplasms resembling sex cord tumors with annular tubules. Cancer 45: 2352–2363
128. Hasleton PS, Kelehan P, Whittaker JS, Burslen RW, Turner L (1978) Benign and malignant struma ovarii. Arch Pathol Lab Med 102: 180–184
128a. Hayes MC, Scully RE (1987) Ovarian steroid cell tumors, not otherwise specified (lipid cell tumors): A clinicopathological analysis of 63 cases (In preparation)
129. Henson RA, Urich H (1982) Cancer and the Nervous System: The Neurological Manifestations of Systemic Malignant Disease. Boston, Blackwell Scientific Publications
130. Herrington JB, Scully RE (1983) Endocrine aspects of germ cell tumors. In: The Human Teratomas, Damjanov I, Knowles B, Solter D (eds). Humana Press, Clifton, New Jersey
131. Holtz G, Johnson TR Jr, Schrock ME (1979) Paraneoplastic hypercalcemia in ovarian tumors. Obstet Gynecol 54: 483
132. Hsu C, Ma L, Mak L (1983) Sclerosing stromal tumor of the ovary: Case report and review of the literature. Int J Gynecol Pathol 2: 192–200
133. Huang TY, Holaday WJ (1970) An ovarian hilus cell tumor associated with endometrial carcinoma: Report of a case. Am J Clin Pathol 54: 147
134. Hughesdon PE (1958) Thecal and allied reactions in epithelial ovarian tumours. J Obstet Gynaecol Br Commonw 65: 702–709
135. Hughesdon PE (1983) Lipid cell thecomas of the ovary. Histopathology 7: 681–692
136. Hughesdon PE, Fraser IT (1953) Arrhenoblastoma of ovary. Case report and historical review. Acta Obstet Gynecol Scand [Suppl 4] 32: 1
137. Iturzaeta N, Kenny FM, Sieber W (1967) Precocious pseudopuberty due to granulosa cell tumor in three girls. Am J Dis Child 114: 39
138. Jacobs AJ, Deppe G, Cohen CJ (1982) Combination chemotherapy of ovarian granulosa cell tumor with Cis-platinum and doxorubicin. Gynecol Oncol 14: 294
139. Jarabak J, Talerman A (1983) Virilization due to a metastasizing granulosa cell tumor. Int. J Gynecol Pathol 2: 316–324
140. Johnston WW, Goldston WR, Montgomery MS (1971) Clinicopathologic studies in feminizing tumors of the ovary. III. The role of genital cytology. Acta Cytol 15: 334
141. Jolly H (1955) Sexual Precocity. A Personal Study of 69 Patients. American Lecture Series. Springfield, Ill, Charles C Thomas
142. Jorgensen EO, Dockerty MB, Wilson RB (1970) Clinicopathologic study of 53 cases of Brenner tumors of the ovary. Am J Obstet Gynecol 108: 122–127
143. Josse RG, Wilson DR, Heersche JNM, Mills JRF, Murray TM (1981) Hypercalcemia with ovarian carcinoma: Evidence of a pathogenetic role for prostaglandins. Cancer 48: 1233–1241
144. Judd HL, Spore WW, Talner LB, Rigg LA, Yen SSC, Benirschke K (1974) Preoperative localization of a testosterone-secreting ovarian tumor by retrograde venous catherization and selective sampling. Am J Obstet Gynecol 120: 91
145. Junaid TA, Nkposong EO, Kolawole TM (1972) Cutaneous meningiomas and an ovarian fibroma in a 3-year-old girl. J Pathol 108: 165
146. Kalavathi N (1971) Granulosa cell tumor—Hormonal aspects and radiosensitivity. Clin Radiol 22: 524–527
147. Kaplan C, Hawley R (1981) Dysgerminoma with giant cells. A case report with immunoperoxidase. Diag Gynecol Obstet 3/4: 325–329
148. Katsube Y, Berg JM, Silverberg SG (1982) Epidemiologic pathology of ovarian tumors: A histopathologic review of primary ovarian neoplasms diagnosed in the Denver standard metropolitan statistical area, 1 July–31 December

1969 and 1 July–31 December 1979. Int J Gynecol Pathol 1: 3–16
149. Kempson RL (1968) Ultrastructure of ovarian stromal cell tumors. Sertoli-Leydig cell tumor and lipid cell tumor. Arch Pathol 86: 492
150. Kim I, Young RH, Scully RE (1985) Leydig cell tumors of the testis. A clinicopathological analysis of 40 cases and review of the literature. Am J Surg Pathol 9: 177
151. Korzets A, Nouriel H, Steiner Z, Griffel B, Kraus L, Freund U, Klajman A (1986) Resistant hypertension associated with a renin-producing ovarian Sertoli cell tumor. Am J Clin Pathol 85: 242–247
152. Kottmeier HL (1953) Carcinoma of the Female Genitalia. The Abraham Flexner Lectures, Series No. 11. Baltimore, Williams & Wilkins
153. Kraemer BB, Silva EG, Sneige N (1984) Fibrosarcoma of the ovary. A new component in the nevoid basal-cell carcinoma syndrome. Am J Surg Pathol 8: 231–236
154. Kurman RJ, Norris HJ (1976) Malignant mixed germ cell tumors of the ovary. Obstet Gynecol 48: 579–589
155. Kurman RJ, Norris HJ (1976) Embryonal cell carcinoma of the ovary. A clinicopathologic entity distinct from endodermal sinus tumor resembling embryonal carcinoma of the adult testis. Cancer 38: 2420–2433
156. Kurman RJ, Ganjei P, Nadjii M (1984) Contributions of immunocytochemistry to the diagnosis and study of ovarian neoplasms. Int J Gynecol Pathol 3: 3–26
157. Kurman RJ, Goebelsmann U, Taylor CR (1979) Steroid localization in granulosa-theca tumors of the ovary. Cancer 43: 2377
158. Kurman RJ, Andrade D, Goebelsmann U, Taylor CR (1978) An immunohistochemical study of steroid localization in Sertoli-Leydig tumors of the ovary and testis. Cancer 42: 1772
159. Kuzma JF, King JM (1948) Dyschondroplasia with hemangiomatosis (Maffucci's syndrome) and teratoid tumor of the ovary. Arch Pathol 46: 74
160. Lack EE, Perez-Atayde AR, Murthy ASK, Goldstein DP, Crigler JF, Vawter GF (1981) Granulosa theca cell tumors in premenarchal girls. A clinical and pathologic study of ten cases. Cancer 48: 1846
161. Lewis RJ, Ketcham AS (1973) Maffucci's syndrome: Functional and neoplastic significance. Case report and review of the literature. J Bone Joint Surg 55-A: 1465
162. Long TT, Barton TK, Draffin R, Reeves WJ, McCarty KS (1980) Conservative management of the Zollinger-Ellison syndrome. Ectopic gastrin production by an ovarian cystadenoma. JAMA 243: 1837–1839
163. Lusch CJ, Mercurio TM, Runyeon WK (1978) Delayed recurrence and chemotherapy of a granulosa cell tumor. Obstet Gynecol 51: 505
164. Lyday RO (1952) Fibroma of the ovary with abdominal implants. Am J Surg 84: 737
165. MacAulay MA, Weliky I, Schulz RA (1967) Ultrastructure of a biosynthetically active granulosa cell tumor. Lab Invest 17: 562–570
166. MacKenzie AH, Scherbel AL (1963) Connective tissue syndromes associated with carcinoma. Geriatrics 18: 745
167. Malkasian GD Jr, Webb MJ, Jorgensen EO (1974) Observations on chemotherapy of granulosa cell carcinomas and malignant ovarian teratomas. Obstet Gynecol 44: 885
168. Mann WJ, Chumas J, Rosenwaks Z, Merrill JA, Davenport D (1986) Elevated serum alpha-fetoprotein associated with Sertoli-Leydig cell tumors of the ovary. Obstet Gynecol 67: 141–144
169. Margolin KA, Pak HY, Esensten ML, Doroshow JH (1985) Hepatic metastasis in granulosa cell tumor of the ovary. Cancer 56: 691–695
170. Marieb HJ, Spangler S, Kashgarian M, Heiman A, Schwartz ML, Schwartz PE (1983) Cushing's syndrome secondary to ectopic cortisol production by an ovarian carcinoma. J Clin Endocrinol Metab 57: 737–740
171. Martinelli G, Govoni E, Pileri S, Grigioni FW, Doglioni C, Pelusi G (1983) Sclerosing stromal tumor of the ovary. Virchows Arch [Pathol Anat] 402: 155–161
172. McGowan L, Young RH, Scully RE (1980) Peutz-Jeghers syndrome with adenoma malignum of cervix. A report of two cases. Gynecol Oncol 10: 125
173. McKay DG, Hertig AT, Hickey WF (1953) The histogenesis of granulosa and theca tumors of the human ovary. Obstet Gynecol 1: 125–136
174. McKay DG, Robinson D, Hertig AT (1949) Histochemical observations on granulosa cell tumors, thecomas, and fibromas of the ovary. Am J Obstet Gynecol 58: 625–639
175. McNulty JR (1959) The ovarian serous cystadenofibroma. A report of 25 cases. Am J Obstet Gynecol 77: 1338
176. Medsger TA, Dixon JA, Garwood VF (1982) Palmar fasciitis and polyarthritis associated with ovarian carcinoma. Ann Intern Med 96: 424–431
177. Meigs JV (1954) Fibroma of the ovary with ascites and hydrothorax. Meigs' syndrome. Am J Obstet Gynecol 67: 962
178. Meiling RL, Bouselis JG, Teteris NJ, Ullery JC, George OT (1963) Histochemical observations of a Brenner cell tumor with masculinization. Am J Obstet Gynecol 87: 463–470
179. Merino M (1984) Corticotroph cell pituitary adenoma within an ovarian teratoma. Case presentation, Evening Seminar on Gynecologic Pathology, International Academy of Pathology, San Francisco
180. Meyer-Hofmann G, Schwarzkopf H, Hartmann H (1960) Spontaneous hypoglycemia with extrapancreatic tumors. Dtsch Med Wochenschr 85: 2106–2108
181. Michael CA (1967) Pelvic fibroma causing recurrent attacks of hypoglycemia. J Obstet Gynaecol Br Commonw 74: 301–303
182. Miettinen M, Lehto V-P, Virtanen I (1983) Expression of intermediate filaments in normal ovaries and ovarian epithelial, sex cord-stromal, and germinal tumors. Int J Gynecol Pathol 2: 64–71
183. Miettinen M, Talerman A, Wahlstrom T, Astengo-Osuna C, Virtanen I (1985) Cellular differentiation in ovarian sex cord–stromal and germ cell tumors studied with antibodies to intermediate-filament proteins. Am J Surg Pathol 9: 640–651
184. Mohabeer J, Buckley CH, Fox H (1983) An immunohistochemical study of the incidence and significance of human chorionic gonadotrophin synthesis by epithelial ovarian neoplasms. Gynecol Oncol 16: 78–84

185. Montag TW, Murphy RE, Belinson JL (1984) Virilizing malignant lipid cell tumor producing erythropoietin. Gynecol Oncol 19: 98–103
186. Morgan DR, Wells M, MacDonald RC, Johnston D (1985) Zollinger-Ellison syndrome due to a gastrin-secreting ovarian mucinous cystadenoma. Case report. Br J Obstet Gynaecol 192: 867–869
187. Morris J McL, Scully RE (1958) Endocrine Pathology of the Ovary. St. Louis, CV Mosby
188. Morrison CW, Woodruff JD (1964) Fibrothecoma and associated ovarian stromal neoplasia. Obstet Gynecol 23: 344
189. Mostofi FK, Price EB Jr (1973) Tumors of the male genital system. Atlas of Tumor Pathology, Second Series, Fascicle 8, Washington, D.C., Armed Forces Institute of Pathology
190. Motlik K, Starka L (1973) Adrenocortical tumour of the ovary. (A case report with particular stress upon morphological and biochemical findings.) Neoplasma 20: 97
191. Nakashima N, Young RH, Scully RE (1984) Androgenic granulosa cell tumors of the ovary. A clinicopathological analysis of seventeen cases and review of the literature. Arch Pathol Lab Med 108: 786
192. Napoli VM, Wallach H (1976) Pancytopenia associated with a granulosa cell tumor of the ovary. Report of a case. Am J Clin Pathol 65: 344–350
193. Neubecker RD, Breen JL (1962) Gynandroblastoma. A report of five cases with a discussion of the histogenesis and classification of ovarian tumors. Am J Clin Pathol 38: 60
194. Neville AJ, Gilchrist KW, Davis TE (1984) The chemotherapy of granulosa cell tumors of the ovary: Experience of the Wisconsin Clinical Cancer Center. Med Pediatr Oncol 12: 397–400
195. Nichols J, Warren JC, Mantz FA (1962) ACTH-like excretion from carcinoma of the ovary. JAMA 182: 713–718
196. Niswander KR, Courey NG, Woodward T (1965) Precocious pseudopuberty caused by ovarian tumors. Obstet Gynecol 26: 381
197. Norris HJ, Chorlton I (1974) Functioning tumors of the ovary. Clin Obstet Gynecol 17: 189
198. Norris HJ, Taylor HB (1968) Prognosis of granulosa-theca tumors of the ovary. Cancer 21: 255
199. Norris HJ, Taylor HB (1969) Virilization associated with cystic granulosa tumors. Obstet Gynecol 34: 629
200. Novak DJ, Lauchlan SC, McCawley JC, Faiman C (1970) Virilization during pregnancy. Case report and review of literature. Am J Med 49: 281–290
201. Novak ER (1967) Gynandroblastoma of the ovary. Review of 8 cases from the Ovarian Tumor Registry. Obstet Gynecol 30: 709
202. Novak ER, Long JH (1965) Arrhenoblastoma of the ovary. A review of the Ovarian Tumor Registry. Am J Obstet Gynecol 92: 1082
203. Novak ER, Mattingly RF (1960) Hilus cell tumor of the ovary. Obstet Gynecol 15: 425
204. Novak ER, Kutchmeshgi J, Mupas RS, Woodruff JD, et al. (1971) Feminizing gonadal stromal tumors. Obstet Gynecol 38: 701
205. Ober WB, Pollak A, Gerstmann KE, Kupperman HS (1962) Krukenberg tumor with androgenic and progestational activity. Am J Obstet Gynecol 84: 739–744
206. O'Hern TM, Neubecker RD (1962) Arrhenoblastoma. Obstet Gynecol 19: 758
207. Osborn RH, Yannone ME (1971) Plasma androgens in the normal and androgenic female. A review. Obstet Gynecol Surv 26: 195
208. Parsons V, Rigby B (1958) Cushing's syndrome associated with adenocarcinoma of the ovary. Lancet 2: 992–994
209. Payne D, Muss HB, Homesley HD, Jobson VW, Baird FG (1981) Autoimmune hemolytic anemia and ovarian dermoid cysts: Case report and review of the literature. Cancer 48: 721–724
210. Prat J, Scully RE (1981) Cellular fibromas and fibrosarcomas of the ovary: A comparative clinicopathologic analysis of seventeen cases. Cancer 47: 2663
211. Prat J, Young RH, Scully RE (1982) Ovarian Sertoli-Leydig cell tumors with heterologous elements (ii) cartilage and skeletal muscle. A clinicopathologic analysis of twelve cases. Cancer 50: 2465
212. Prat J, Bhan AK, Dickersin GR, Robboy SJ, Scully RE (1982) Hepatoid yolk sac tumor of the ovary (endodermal sinus tumor with hepatoid differentiation). A light microscopic, ultrastructural and immunohistochemical study of seven cases. Cancer 50: 2355–2368
213. Prunty FTG (1967) Hirsutism, virilism and apparent virilism and their gonadal relationship. Part I. J Endocrinol 38: 85
214. Pysher TJ, Hitch DC, Krous HF (1981) Bilateral juvenile granulosa cell tumors in a 4-month old dysmorphic infant. A clinical, histologic, and ultrastructural study. Am J Surg Pathol 5: 789
215. Quinn MA, Oster AO, Fortune D, Hudson B (1981) Sclerosing stromal tumor of the ovary. Case report with endocrine studies. Br J Obstet Gynaecol 88: 555–558
216. Raggio M, Kaplan AL, Harberg JF (1983) Recurrent ovarian fibromas with basal cell nevus syndrome (Gorlin syndrome). Obstet Gynecol 61: 95s–96s
217. Ramzy I (1976) Signet-ring stromal tumor of ovary. Histochemical, light, and electron microscopic study. Cancer 38: 166–172
218. Reddick RL, Walton LA (1982) Sertoli-Leydig cell tumor of the ovary with teratomatous differentiation. Clinicopathologic considerations. Cancer 50: 1171
219. Robboy SJ, Scully RE (1980) Strumal carcinoid of the ovary. Cancer 46: 2019–2034
220. Robboy SJ, Norris HJ, Scully RE (1975) Insular carcinoid primary in the ovary. A clinicopathologic analysis of 48 cases. Cancer 36: 404–418
221. Robboy SJ, Scully RE, Norris HJ (1977) Primary trabecular carcinoid of the ovary. Obstet Gynecol 49: 202–207
222. Rome RM, Laverty CR, Brown JB (1973) Ovarian tumours in postmenopausal women. Clinicopathological features and hormonal studies. J Obstet Gynaecol Br Commonw 80: 984–991
223. Rome RM, Fortune DW, Quinn MA, Brown JB (1981) Functioning ovarian tumors in postmenopausal women. Obstet Gynecol 57: 705–710
224. Roth LM, Sternberg WH (1973) Ovarian stromal tumors

containing Leydig cells. II. Pure Leydig cell tumor, non-hilar type. Cancer 32: 952
225. Roth LM, Sternberg WH (1983) Partly luteinized theca cell tumor of the ovary. Cancer 51: 1697
226. Roth LM, Liban E, Czernobilsky B (1982) Ovarian endometrioid tumors mimicking Sertoli and Sertoli-Leydig cell tumors. Sertoliform variant of endometrioid carcinoma. Cancer 50: 1322
227. Roth LM, Nicholas TR, Ehrlich CE (1979) Juvenile granulosa cell tumor. A clinicopathologic study of three cases with ultrastructural observations. Cancer 44: 2194
228. Roth LM, Slayton RE, Brady LW, Blesdsing JA, Johnson G (1985) Retiform differentiation in ovarian Sertoli-Leydig cell tumors. A clinicopathologic study of six cases from a gynecologic oncology study group. Cancer 55: 1093
229. Roth LM, Anderson MC, Govan ADT, Langley FA, Gowing NFC, Woodcock AS (1981) Sertoli-Leydig cell tumors. A clinicopathologic study of 34 cases. Cancer 48: 187
230. Rubin DK, Frost JK (1963) The cytologic detection of ovarian cancer. Acta Cytol 7: 191–195
231. Rutgers J, Scully RE (1986) Functioning ovarian tumors with peripheral steroid cell proliferation: A report of twenty-four cases . Int J Gynecol Pathol 5: 319–337
232. Sack GH, Levin J, Bell WR (1977) Trousseau's syndrome and other manifestations of chronic disseminated coagulopathy in patients with neoplasms: Clinical, pathophysiologic and therapeutic features. Medicine 56: 1–37
233. Salm R (1967) Pure and mixed hilus cell tumours of ovary. Ann Roy Coll Surg Engl 41: 344
234. Salm R (1974) Ovarian hilus-cell tumours: Their varying presentations. J Pathol 113: 117
235. Salomon-Bernard Y, Thibaud E, Vignal J, Musset R (1975) Tumeurs a stroma fonctionnel. In: Tumeurs de l'Ovaire, Cabanne F (ed). Paris, Masson et Cie, Ch 11, p 309
236. Samaan NA, Smith JP, Rutledge FN, Schultz PN (1976) The significance of measurement of human placental lactogen, human chorionic gonadotropin, and carcinoembryonic antigen in patients with ovarian carcinoma. Am J Obstet Gynecol 126: 186–189
237. Samanth KK, Black WC (1970) Benign ovarian stromal tumors associated with free peritoneal fluid. Am J Obstet Gynecol 107: 538
238. Scaling ST, Kaufman RH, Patten BM (1979) Dermatomyositis and female malignancy. Obstet Gynecol 54: 474–477
239. Schnoy N (1982) Ultrastructure of a virilizing ovarian Leydig-cell tumor. Virchows Arch [Pathol Anat] 397: 17
240. Schwartz PE, Smith JP (1976) Treatment of ovarian stromal tumors. Am J Obstet Gynecol 125: 402
241. Scully RE (1953) An unusual ovarian tumor containing Leydig cells but associated with endometrial hyperplasia, in a postmenopausal woman. J Clin Endocrinol Metab 13: 1254–1263
242. Scully RE (1962) Androgenic lesions of the ovary. In: The Ovary, Grady HG, Smith DE (eds). International Academy of Pathology Monograph No. 3, Baltimore, Williams & Wilkins, Ch 9, p 143
243. Scully RE (1964) Stromal luteoma of the ovary. A distinctive type of lipoid-cell tumor. Cancer 17: 769
244. Scully RE (1968) Sex cord–mesenchyme tumours. Pathologic classification and its relation to prognosis and treatment. In: Ovarian Cancer, Junqueira AC, Gentil F (eds). IUCC Monograph Series. Heidelberg, Springer-Verlag, Vol II, pp 40–56
245. Scully RE (1970) Sex cord tumor with annular tubules. A distinctive ovarian tumor of the Peutz-Jeghers syndrome. Cancer 25: 1107
246. Scully RE (1970) Gonadoblastoma. A review of 74 cases. Cancer 25: 1340
247. Scully RE (1977) Sex cord–stromal tumors. Pathology of the Female Genital Tract, Blaustein A (ed). New York, Springer-Verlag, Chap 25
248. Scully RE (1979) Tumors of the ovary and maldeveloped gonads. In: Atlas of Tumor Pathology, 2nd series, Fascicle No. 16, Washington, D.C., Armed Forces Institute of Pathology
249. Scully RE (1980) Sex cord-stromal, lipid cell, and germ cell tumors. In: Gynecology and Obstetrics, Gynecologic Oncology, Sciarra JJ (ed). Hagerstown, MD, Harper and Row
250. Scully RE (1986) The ovary. In: Endocrine Pathology, Wolfe HJ (ed). New York, Springer-Verlag
251. Scully RE (1987) Ovarian tumors with functioning stroma. In: Haines and Taylor's Gynaecological and Obstetrical Pathology, 3rd ed, Fox H (ed). Edinburgh, Churchill-Livingstone
252. Scully RE, Cohen RB (1964) Oxidative-enzyme activity in normal and pathologic human ovaries. Obstet Gynecol 24: 667–681
253. Scully RE, Morris JMcL (1957) Functioning ovarian tumors. In: Progress in Gynecology III, Meigs J, Sturgis SH (eds). New York, Grune & Stratton, Ch 2, p 20
254. Scully RE, Richardson GS (1961) Luteinization of the stroma of metastatic cancer involving the ovary and its endocrine significance. Cancer 14: 827–840
255. Scully RE, Aguirre P, DeLellis RA (1984) Argyrophilia, serotonin, and peptide hormones in the female genital tract and its tumors. Int J Gynecol Pathol 3: 51–70
256. Serment HL, Laffargue P, Piana L, Blanc B (1970) Ovarian hormone tumors of female children. Int J Gynaecol Obstet 8: 409
257. Serov SF, Scully RE, Sobin LH (1973) International Histological Classification of Tumours, No. 9. Histological Typing of Ovarian Tumours. Geneva, World Health Organization
258. Shah KH, Steele HD (1981) Sclerosing stromal tumor of the ovary. A case report and further observations. Diag Gynecol Obstet 3: 155–159
259. Sher J, Marsh M (1963) Multilocular cystic granulosa cell tumor. Am J Clin Pathol 40: 72
260. Shetty MR, Boghossian HM, Duffell D, Freel R, Gonzalez JC (1982) Tumor-induced hypoglycemia. A result of ectopic insulin production. Cancer 49: 1920–1923
261. Shiel WC, Prete PE, Jason M, Andrews BS (1985) Palmar fasciitis and arthritis with ovarian and non-ovarian carcinomas. New syndrome. Am J Med 79: 640–644
262. Siegman-Igra Y, Flatau E, Deligdish L (1977) Chronic diffuse intravascular coagulation (DIC) in nonmetastatic ovarian cancer. Report of a case and review of the literature. Gynecol Oncol 5: 92–100
263. Silverberg SG (1971) Brenner tumor of the ovary: A clini-

copathologic study of 60 tumors in 54 women. Cancer 28: 588–596
264. Simmons RL, Sciarra JJ (1967) Treatment of late recurrent granulosa cell tumors of the ovary. Surg Gynecol Obstet 124: 65
265. Sjöstedt S, Wahlen T (1961) Prognosis of granulosa cell tumors. Acta Obstet Gynecol Scand 40: 1
266. Smith JP, Rutledge F (1970) Chemotherapy in the treatment of cancer of the ovary. Am J Obstet Gynecol 107: 691
267. Solh HM, Azoury RS, Najjar SS (1983) Peutz-Jeghers syndrome associated with precocious puberty. J Pediatr 103: 593–595
268. Sotto LSJ, Postoloff AV, Carr F (1956) A case of calcified ovarian fibroma with ossification. Am J Obstet Gynecol 71: 1355
269. Spadoni LR, Lindberg MC, Mottet NK, Herman WL (1965) Virilization coexisting with Krukenberg tumor during pregnancy. Am J Obstet Gynecol 92: 981–991
270. Stenwig JT, Hazekamp JT, Beecham JB (1979) Granulosa cell tumors of the ovary. A clinicopathological study of 118 cases with long-term follow-up. Gynecol Oncol 7: 136
271. Sternberg WH (1949) The morphology, endocrine function, hyperplasia and tumors of the human ovarian hilus cells. Am J Pathol 25: 493
272. Sternberg WH, Dhurandhar HN (1977) Functional ovarian tumors of stromal and sex cord origin. Hum Pathol 8: 565
273. Sternberg WH, Roth LM (1973) Ovarian stromal tumors containing Leydig cells. 1. Stromal-Leydig cell tumor and non-neoplastic transformation of ovarian stroma to Leydig cells. Cancer 32: 940
274. Stewart AF, Romero R, Schwartz PE, Kohorn EI, Broadus AE (1982) Hypercalcemia associated with gynecologic malignancies. Biochemical characterization. Cancer 49: 2389–2394
275. Stewart KR, Casey MJ, Gondos B (1981) Endodermal sinus tumor of the ovary with virilization. Light and electron microscopy study. Am J Surg Pathol 5: 385–391
276. Sweeney EC, Lee G (1979) Granulosa cell tumour of the ovary metastasizing to the heart: A light and electron microscopic study. Ir J Med Sci 148: 11–12
277. Symonds DA, Driscoll SG (1973) An adrenal cortical rest within the fetal ovary. Report of a case. Am J Clin Pathol 60: 562
278. Takeda A, Suzumoria K, Sugimoto Y, Yagami Y, Miyazawa T, Yamada C, Matsuyama M (1984) Clear cell carcinoma of the ovary with colony-stimulating factor production. Occurrence of marked granulocytosis in a patient and nude mice. Cancer 54: 1019–1023
279. Takeuchi H, Hamada H, Sodemoto Y, Ushigome S (1983) Juvenile granulosa cell tumor with rapid distant metastases. Acta Pathol Jpn 33: 537
280. Talbott JH (1977) Acute dermatomyositis-polymyositis and malignancy. Semin Arthritis Rheum 6: 305–360
281. Talerman A, Haije WG (1985) Letter to the Editor. Int J Gynaecol Pathol 4: 171–172
282. Talerman A, Hughesdon PE, Anderson MC (1982) Diffuse nonlobular ovarian androblastoma usually associated with feminization. Int J Gynaecol Pathol 1: 155–171
283. Tamini HK, Bolen J (1984) Enchondromatosis (Ollier's disease) and ovarian juvenile granulosa cell tumor. Cancer 53: 1605–1608
284. Tang M, Liu T (1982) Ovarian sclerosing stromal tumors. Clinocopathologic study of 10 cases. Chin Med J 95: 186
285. Targett CS (1974) Estrogen excretion in a case of thecagranulosa cell tumor. Am J Obstet Gynecol 119: 859
286. Tavassoli FA, Norris HJ (1980) Sertoli tumors of the ovary. A clinicopathologic study of 28 cases with ultrastructural observations. Cancer 46: 2282
287. Taylor HB, Norris HJ (1967) Lipid cell tumors of the ovary. Cancer 20: 1953
288. Teilum G (1958) Classification of testicular and ovarian androblastoma and Sertoli cell tumors. Cancer 11: 769
289. Teilum G (1949) Homologous ovarian and testicular tumors. III. Estrogen-producing Sertoli cell tumors (androblastoma tubulare lipoides) of the human testis and ovary. J Clin Endocrinol 9: 301
290. Teilum G (1971) Special Tumors of Ovary and Testis. Comparative Pathology and Histological Identification. Philadelphia, J.B. Lippincott
291. Teter J, Bulski T, Wasilewska B (1962) A virilizing adrenal rest tumor of the ovary with postmenopausal uterine hypertrophy. Bull Pol Med Sci Hist 5: 144
292. Tetu B, Ordonez NG, Silva EG (1986) Sertoli-Leydig cell tumor of the ovary with alpha-fetoprotein production. Arch Pathol Lab Med 110: 65–68
293. Tighe JR (1961) Brenner tumours of the ovary: A clinicopathological study. J Obstet Gynaecol Br Commonw 68: 292–296
294. Tiltman AJ (1985) Sclerosing stromal tumor of the ovary: Demonstration of Ligandin in three cases. Int J Gynaecol Pathol 4: 362–369
295. Tracy SL, Askin FB, Reddick RL, Jackson B, Kurman RJ (1985) Progesterone-secreting Sertoli cell tumor of the ovary. Gynecol Oncol 22: 85–96
296. Tsukamoto N, Nakamura M, Ishikawa H (1976) Sclerosing stromal tumor of the ovary. Gynecol Oncol 4: 335–339
297. Tyler HR (1974) Paraneoplastic syndromes of nerve, muscle, and neuromuscular junction. Ann NY Acad Sci 230: 348–357
298. Tytle T, Rosin D (1984) Bilateral calcified ovarian fibromas. South Med J 77: 1178–1180
299. Ueda G, Sato Y, Yamasaki M, Inoue M, Hiramatsu K, Kurachi K, Amino N, Miyai K (1978) Strumal carcinoid of the ovary. Histological, ultrastructural and immunohistological studies with anti-human thyroglobulin. Gynecol Oncol 6: 411–419
300. Ueda G, Nobuaki H, Hayakawa K, Tanizawa O, Ichii H, Nakagawa H, Mineda H, Furuyama J, Matsumoto K, Mori M (1972) Clinical histochemical and biochemical studies of an ovarian dysgerminoma with trophoblasts and Leydig cells. Am J Obstet Gynecol 114: 748–754
301. Ulbright TM, Roth LM, Ehrlich CE (1982) Ovarian strumal carcinoid. An immunocytochemical and ultrastructural study of two cases. Am J Clin Pathol 77: 622–631
302. Vaitukaitis JL (1974) Human chorionic gonadotropin as a tumor marker. Ann Clin Lab Sci 4: 276–280

303. Verducci MA, Malkasian GD, Friedman SJ, Winkelmann RK (1984) Gynecologic carcinoma associated with dermatomyositis-polymyositis. Obstet Gynecol 64: 695–698
304. Verhoeven ATM, Mastboom JL, Van Leusden HAIM, Van Der Velden WHM (1973) Virilization in pregnancy coexisting with an (ovarian) mucinous cystadenoma: A case report and review of virilizing ovarian tumors in pregnancy. Obstet Gynecol Surv 28: 597–622
305. Vicens E, Martinez-Mora J, Potau N, Sans M, Boix-Ochoa J (1980) Masculinization of a female fetus by Krukenberg tumor during pregnancy. J Pediatr Surg 15: 188–190
306. Waxman M, Damjanov I, Alpert L, Sardinsky T (1981) Composite mucinous ovarian neoplasms associated with Sertoli-Leydig and carcinoid tumors. Cancer 47: 2044
307. Waxman M, Vuletin JC, Urcuyo R, Belling CG (1979) Ovarian low-grade stromal sarcoma with thecomatous features. A critical reappraisal of the so-called malignant thecoma. Cancer 44: 2206
308. Woodruff JD, Rauh JT, Markley RL (1966) Ovarian stroma. Obstet Gynecol 27: 194–201
309. Woodruff JD, Williams TJ, Goldberg B, Lawterbach M, Preece E (1973) Hormonal activity of the common ovarian neoplasms. Am J Obstet Gynecol 87: 679
310. Yaker A, Benirschke K (1975) A ten-year study of ovarian tumors. Virchows Arch [Pathol Anat] 366: 275–286
311. Young RH, Scully RE (1982) Ovarian sex cord–stromal tumors. Recent progress. Int J Gynaecol Pathol 1: 101
312. Young RH, Scully RE (1983) Ovarian stromal tumors with minor sex cord elements: A report of seven cases. Int J Gynaecol Pathol 2: 227
313. Young RH, Scully RE (1983) Ovarian sex cord–stromal tumors with bizarre nuclei. A clinicopathologic analysis of seventeen cases. Int. J Gynaecol Pathol 1: 325
314. Young RH, Scully RE (1983) Ovarian Sertoli-Leydig cell tumors with a retiform pattern: A problem in histopathologic diagnosis. A report of 25 cases. Am J Surg Pathol 77: 755
315. Young RH, Scully RE (1984) Ovarian Sertoli cell tumors. A report of ten cases. Int J Gynaecol Pathol 2: 349
316. Young RH, Scully RE (1984) Ovarian sex cord–stromal tumors: Recent advances and current status. Clin Obstet Gynecol 11: 93
317. Young RH, Scully RE (1984) Fibromatosis and massive edema of the ovary, possibly related entities. A report of 14 cases of fibomatosis and 11 cases of massive edema. Int J Gynecol Pathol 3: 153
318. Young RH, Scully RE (1984) Well-differentiated ovarian Sertoli-Leydig cell tumors. A clinicopathological analysis of 23 cases. Int J Gynecol Pathol 3: 277
319. Young RH, Scully RE (1985) Ovarian Sertoli-Leydig cell tumors. A clinicopathological analysis of 207 cases. Am J Surg Pathol 9: 543–569
320. Young RH, Scully RE (1985) Ovarian sex cord–stromal and steroid cell tumors. In: Tumors and Tumor-like Conditions of the Ovary, Roth LM, Czernobilsky B (eds). Contemporary Issues in Surgical Pathology. New York, Churchill-Livingstone, Vol 6, pp 43–73
321. Young RH, Scully RE (1987) Ovarian steroid cell tumors associated with Cushing's syndrome. A report of three cases. Int J Gynecol Pathol 6: 40
322. Young RH, Dickersin GR, Scully RE (1983) A distinctive ovarian sex cord–stromal tumor causing sexual precocity in the Peutz-Jeghers syndrome. Am J Surg Pathol 7: 223
323. Young RH, Dickersin GR, Scully RE (1984) Juvenile granulosa cell tumor of the ovary. A clinicopathologic analysis of 125 cases. Am J Surg Pathol 8: 575
324. Young RH, Dudley AG, Scully RE (1984) Granulosa cell, Sertoli-Leydig cell and unclassified sex cord-stromal tumors associated with pregnancy. A clinicopathological analysis of thirty-six cases. Gynecol Oncol 18: 181
325. Young RH, Kleinman GM, Scully RE (1981) Glioma of the uterus. Report of a case with comments on histogenesis. Am J Surg Pathol 5: 695–699
326. Young RH, Perez-Atayde AR, Scully RE (1984) Ovarian Sertoli-Leydig cell tumor with retiform and heterologous components. Report of a case with hepatocytic differentiation and elevated serum alpha-fetoprotein. Am J Surg Pathol 8: 709
327. Young RH, Prat J, Scully RE (1982) Ovarian endometrioid carcinomas resembling sex cord–stromal tumors. A clinicopathological analysis of 13 cases. Am J Surg Pathol 6: 513–522
328. Young RH, Prat J, Scully RE (1982) Ovarian Sertoli-Leydig cell tumors with heterologous elements (i) mucinous epithelium and carcinoid. Cancer 50: 2448
329. Young RH, Prat J, Scully RE (1983) Endometrioid stromal sarcomas of the ovary. A clinicopathological analysis of twenty-three cases. Cancer 53: 1143
330. Young RH, Welch WR, Dickersin GR, Scully RE (1982) Ovarian sex cord tumor with annular tubules: Review of 74 cases including 27 with Peutz-Jeghers syndrome and 4 with adenoma malignum of the cervix. Cancer 50: 1384
331. Yuen BH, Robertson I, Clement PB, Mincey EK (1982) Sclerosing stromal tumor of the ovary. Obstet Gynecol 60: 252
332. Zaloudek C, Norris HJ (1982) Granulosa tumors of the ovary in children. A clinical and pathologic study of 32 cases. Am J Surg Pathol 6: 503
333. Zaloudek C, Norris HJ (1984) Sertoli-Leydig tumors of the ovary. A clinicopathologic study of 64 intermediate and poorly differentiated neoplasms. Am J Surg Pathol 8: 405–418
334. Zaloudek CJ, Tavassoli FA, Norris HJ (1981) Dysgerminoma with syncytiotrophoblastic giant cells. A histologically and clinically distinctive subtype of dysgerminoma. Am J Surg Pathol 5: 361–367
335. Zhang J, Young RH, Arseneau J, Scully RE (1982) Ovarian stromal tumors containing lutein or Leydig cells (luteinized thecomas and stromal Leydig cell tumors). A clinicopathological analysis of fifty cases. Int J Gynecol Pathol 1: 270

20

Germ Cell Tumors of the Ovary

A. Talerman, M.D., Ph.D., F.R.C. Path.

This group of ovarian neoplasms is composed of a number of histologically different tumor types and embraces all the neoplasms considered to be ultimately derived from the primitive germ cells of the embryonic gonad. The concept of germ cell tumors as a specific group of gonadal neoplasms has evolved in the last three decades. It is based on (1) the common histogenesis of these neoplasms, (2) the relatively frequent presence of histologically different neoplastic elements within the same tumor mass, and (3) the presence of histologically similar neoplasms in extragonadal locations along the line of migration of the primitive germ cells from the wall of the yolk sac to the gonadal ridge,[332] as well as on the remarkable homology between the various tumors in the male and the female.

In no other group of gonadal neoplasms is this homology better illustrated. Although the strong morphologic resemblance between the testicular seminoma and its ovarian counterpart, the dysgerminoma, was noted soon after these neoplasms were first described, for a long time there was no agreement as to their histogenesis. Nevertheless, these were the first neoplasms to become accepted as originating from germ cells. It was not until the studies by Teilum[292,293] on the homology of ovarian and testicular neoplasms, the studies by Friedman and Moore[81] and Dixon and Moore[63] on testicular tumors, and those by Friedman[80] on related extragonadal neoplasms that the germ cell origin of other neoplasms belonging to this group was suggested. These views were supported by the embryologic studies of Witschi[332] and Gillman,[90] and later by the experimental work of Stevens[262–264] and Pierce et al.[207,208,210,211,213] on germ cell tumors in rodents.

Although occasional unusual neoplasms composed of germ cells and sex cord derivatives had been noted previously,[167,238] it was not until Scully's detailed description of gonadoblastoma[238] that these neoplasms were recognized. More recently, another neoplasm composed of germ cells and sex cord derivatives, the mixed germ cell–sex cord stroma tumor, has been described in detail.[270,271]

This chapter, therefore, is devoted not only to neoplasms of germ cell origin but also to those composed of germ cells and sex cord derivatives.

Histogenesis

The histogenesis and interrelationships of the various types of germ cell neoplasms, as suggested by Teilum,[298] are shown in Fig. 20.1.

According to Teilum,[298] dysgerminoma (seminoma) is a primitive germ cell neoplasm that has not acquired the potential for further differentiation. Embryonal carcinoma is regarded as a conceptual as well as a morphologic entity and represents a germ cell neoplasm composed of multipotential cells, which are capable of further differentiation. This can take place in an embryonal or somatic direction, resulting in teratomatous neoplasms showing various degrees of maturity, or in an extraembryonal direction along either of two pathways: vitelline, differentiating toward endodermal sinus (yolk sac) tumor, or trophoblastic, differentiating toward a choriocarcinoma. The process of differentiation is dynamic, and, therefore, the resulting neoplasms may be composed of different elements showing various stages of development. Although according to this view,[298] dysgerminoma is considered incapable of further differentiation, recent immunocytochemical evidence indicates that some seminoma or dysgerminoma cells can differentiate into embryonal carcinoma and further. Although the great majority of

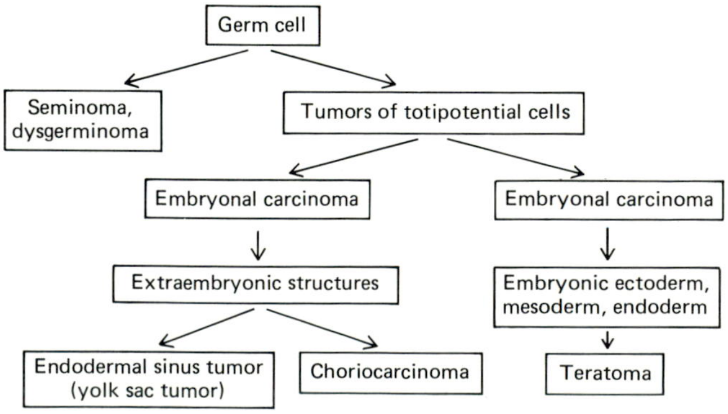

FIG. 20.1. The histogenesis and interrelationship of tumors of germ cell origin. (Modified from Teilum, Ref. 298.)

seminoma or dysgerminoma cells are cytokeratin-negative, whereas embryonal carcinoma, endodermal sinus tumor, and choriocarcinoma are composed entirely of cytokeratin-positive cells,[21,172,173] some seminomas and dysgerminomas contain cytokeratin-positive cells.[172] The very intimate admixture of dysgerminoma cells with other neoplastic germ cell elements seen in some germ cell tumors also supports this view.

Classification

A number of classifications of germ cell neoplasms of the ovary have been proposed over the years,* each one becoming more detailed and encompassing newly established entities. Some years ago, a panel of pathologists was established under the auspices of the World Health Organization to formulate a histologic classification of ovarian neoplasms to be used throughout the world. The classification proposed[250] divides the germ cell tumors into a number of groups and also includes neoplasms composed of germ cells and sex cord–stromal derivatives. The classification used in this text is a slight modification of this classification[250] and is as follows:

- I. *Germ cell tumors*
  - A. Dysgerminoma
  - B. Endodermal sinus tumor
  - C. Embryonal carcinoma
  - D. Polyembryoma
  - E. Choriocarcinoma
  - F. Teratomas
    - 1. Immature (solid, cystic, or both)
    - 2. Mature
      - a. Solid
      - b. Cystic
        - i. Mature cystic teratoma (dermoid cyst)
        - ii. Mature cystic teratoma (dermoid cyst) with malignant transformation
    - 3. Monodermal or highly specialized
      - a. Struma ovarii
      - b. Carcinoid
      - c. Strumal carcinoid
      - d. Others
  - G. Mixed forms (tumors composed of types A through F in any possible combination)
- II. *Tumors composed of germ cells and sex cord–stromal derivatives*
  - A. Gonadoblastoma
  - B. Mixed germ cell–sex cord–stromal tumor

* References 110, 123, 239–241, 296, 299.

Clinical and Pathologic Features of Germ Cell Tumors

Germ cell tumors constitute the second largest group of ovarian neoplasms after the common epithelial tumors and comprise approximately 20% of all ovarian neoplasms. This is observed in Europe and North America, whence most reports concerning the incidence of ovarian neoplasms emanate. In countries in Asia and Africa where the incidence of common epithelial tumors is much lower, germ cell tumors constitute a much larger proportion of ovarian neoplasms. Germ cell tumors are encountered at all ages from infancy to old age but are seen most frequently from the first to the sixth decades. They have been observed during fetal life. In children and adolescents, more than 60% of ovarian neoplasms are of germ cell origin, and one third of them are malignant.[2,36,38,183] In adults, the great majority of germ cell tumors (95%) are benign and consist of mature cystic teratomas (dermoid cysts).

Dysgerminoma

Synonyms

Germinoma, disgerminoma,[171] ovarian seminoma,[166] gonocytoma,[294] embryonal carcinoma with lymphoid stroma.[72]

Although the term dysgerminoma was first introduced by Meyer[171] in 1931, ovarian neoplasms showing this histologic pattern had been recognized earlier. Chenot[44] in 1911 was the first to note their occurrence and their similarity to the testicular seminoma described some years earlier.[45] In view of the strong resemblance to their testicular counterpart, the tumor was named ovarian seminoma by Masson,[166] and this became the most popular term until its replacement by dysgerminoma. It is still widely used in the French literature. The term disgerminoma, as originally suggested by Meyer[171] and which later became dysgerminoma, has over the years gained almost universal acceptance.

Histogenesis. Dysgerminoma is composed entirely of germ cells that show morphologic, including ultrastructural,[114,130,152,192] and histochemical[157,158] similarity to primordial germ cells. The cells of dysgerminoma are considered to be in an early and sexually indifferent stage of differentiation. They are arrested at a developmental stage at which they have not yet gained the ability for further differentiation.[298] However, there is now evidence that occasional cells may acquire this ability and may differentiate to embryonal carcinoma and further.[172] These cells are sexually and hormonally inert. An origin from the primordial germ cells that migrate to the ovary during early embryogenesis from their site of origin in the wall of the yolk sac[332] is the most widely accepted view of the histogenesis of dysgerminoma. It is supported by the occurrence of homologous neoplasms in the testis (seminoma) and along the route of migration of the primordial germ cells from the wall of the yolk sac to the primitive gonad, in the mediastinum, retroperitoneum, posterior abdominal wall, and parapineal and sacrococcygeal regions.[80,90]

The presence of sex chromatin bodies (Barr bodies) in the cells of dysgerminoma is a matter of controversy. Sex chromatin bodies were said to be present in the cells of a number of dysgerminomas by some investigators,[307] whereas others[12] could not identify them. The latter view is more in accordance with an origin from the primordial germ cells. The finding of twice the amount of DNA in the nuclei of dysgerminoma cells as compared with the nuclei of lymphocytes in all the cases studied[12] further supports the origin from primordial germ cells, which have the same amount of DNA in their nuclei (twice the amount present in normal diploid cells).

Incidence. Dysgerminoma is an uncommon tumor accounting for 1–2% of primary ovarian neoplasms and for 3–5% of ovarian malignancies.[175,189,229] Although until 1950 only 427 cases had been recorded in the literature,[175] at least as many cases have been reported since, and dysgerminoma is considered the most common malignant ovarian germ cell neoplasm occurring in pure form. The exact incidence of dysgerminoma in different parts of the world is not known, since most cancer registry reports do not differentiate between the various types of ovarian neoplasms.[149] In some countires there are considerable regional variations.[24] Although the majority of reports emanate from Europe and North America, dysgerminoma has been encountered in all parts of the world and in all races. A high incidence has been reported from Japan[110] and in a study from Bombay, India.[124]

Clinical Aspects. Although Meyer[171] emphasized the frequent occurrence of dysgerminoma in pseudohermaphrodites and in patients with other forms of sexual maldevelopment, the great majority of patients with dysgerminoma are normally developed and sexually normal adolescent or young adult females.

The tumor may occur at any age from infancy to old age; the reported cases range between the age of 7 months[37] and 70 years,[175] but the majority of cases occur in adolescence and early adult life.* In view of this, the tumor has been called *carcinoma puellarum.*[185] Dys-

* References 4, 12, 40, 60, 79, 100, 110, 125, 135, 136, 175, 186, 199, 225, 240, 241, 246, 287, 322.

germinoma occurs not infrequently before puberty[37] but is rare after menopause.[60,240] Most cases occur in the second and third decades; nearly half the patients are under 20 years of age and 80% are under 30 years.* Therefore, dysgerminoma is one of the most common malignant ovarian neoplasms of childhood, adolescence, and early adult life.† Dysgerminoma has been reported in siblings,[287] as well as in mother and daughter.[122]

The symptomatology of dysgerminoma is not distinctive and is similar to that observed in patients with other solid ovarian neoplasms.‡ The duration of symptoms is usually short; despite this, the tumor is often large, indicating a rapid growth.[229,287] The most common presenting symptoms are abdominal enlargement and presence of a mass in the lower abdomen, sometimes associated with abdominal pain that may be caused by torsion. Loss of weight may also be an accompanying symptom. In a number of cases, the tumor has been found incidentally; in these cases, the tumor is usually small. Sometimes the tumor may be detected during pregnancy.§ In such cases it may be discovered as an incidental finding or may be obstructing labor.[229] Dysgerminoma is one of the two most common ovarian neoplasms observed in pregnancy—the other being serous cystadenoma.[109,136] The relatively common finding of dysgerminoma in pregnant patients is nonspecific and relates to the age of the patients.

Dysgerminoma may also be discovered incidentally in patients investigated for primary amenorrhea; in these cases it is not infrequently associated with gonadoblastoma.[232,233,242,328] Occasionally, menstrual and endocrine abnormalities may be the presenting symptom,[60] but this tends to be more common in patients with dysgerminoma combined with other neoplastic germ cell elements, especially choriocarcinoma. In children, precocious sexual development may occur.[2,32,36,109]

Macroscopic Appearance. Dysgerminoma is usually unilateral. It tends to occur more often in the right ovary,[175,229,246,287] which is affected in approximately 50% of cases, whereas the left is affected in 33–35% and bilateral involvement occurs in 15–17%.[175,229] More frequent bilateral involvement has been reported in some series[190,199,287] and less frequent in others.[12,60,168] Much higher frequency of bilateral tumors is observed in patients with dysgerminoma associated with gonadoblastoma, the dysgerminoma arising from and overgrowing the gonadoblastoma.‖

Pure dysgerminomas are solid tumors that are round, oval, or lobulated, with a smooth, gray-white, slightly glistening fibrous capsule. They vary in size from small lesions a few centimeters in diameter to large masses measuring 50 cm across[12,37] and filling the pelvic and abdominal cavities. Tumors weighing in excess of 5 kg have been described.[175] Compressed ovarian tissue may be seen surrounding small tumors, but in large tumors it is not discernible. The capsule is usually intact but may be ruptured, especially in large tumors. This may lead to the formation of adhesions between the tumor and the surrounding structures. The consistency of dysgerminoma varies from firm and rubbery in the small and medium-sized tumors, to soft in the large ones. On cut surface (Fig. 20.2), the tumor is solid and varies in color from gray-pink to pink and from yellow to light tan. Red, brown, or yellow discoloration caused by hemorrhage or necrosis is also seen, especially in large tumors. This may sometimes lead to the formation of small cysts, but cystic areas are only occasionally seen in pure dysgerminoma. Presence of cystic areas should alert the observer to the possibility that other neoplastic elements may be present in association with the dysgerminoma. In view of the important prognostic implications concerning the presence of other neoplastic germ cell elements, judicious sampling of different parts of the tumor, especially of the less typical areas, is recommended.

Microscopic Appearance. Dysgerminoma exhibits very distinctive histologic appearances. It is histologically identical with the classic seminoma of the testis. It is composed of aggregates, islands or strands, of large uniform cells surrounded by varying amounts of connective tissue stroma containing lymphocytes (Figs. 20.3 and 20.4). The cells are large and measure from 15 to 25 μm across. They are oval or round and usually have distinguishable cytoplasmic borders (Fig. 20.5). In well-fixed material, the cell boundaries are well defined. The cells contain an ample amount of pale, slightly granular eosinophilic or clear cytoplasm. The centrally located

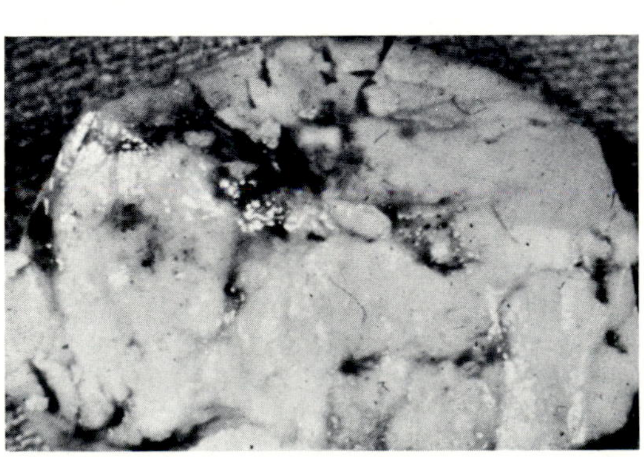

FIG. 20.2. Dysgerminoma. The cut surface is solid. There is some hemorrhage present.

* References 12, 38, 100, 111, 175, 229, 287, 308, 322.
† References 4, 12, 38, 40, 79, 100, 111, 136, 175, 183, 229, 322.
‡ References 12, 60, 100, 175, 229, 322.
§ References 12, 60, 136, 199, 229, 287, 308.
‖ References 87, 107, 232, 233, 242, 269.

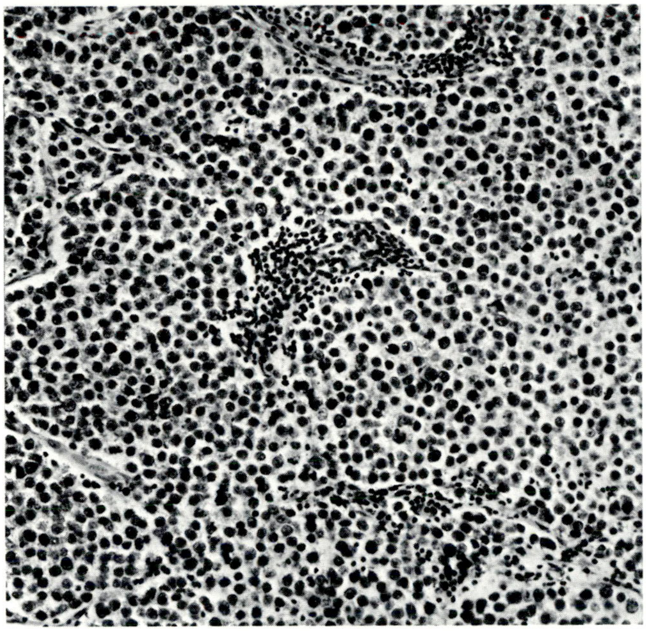

FIG. 20.3. Dysgerminoma composed of large aggregates of uniform cells surrounded by delicate strands of connective tissue containing lymphocytes.

vesicular nucleus is large, occupying nearly half the cell. The nucleus is oval or round, has a sharp nuclear membrane with unevenly dispersed finely granular chromatin, and contains usually one, but sometimes two, prominent eosinophilic nucleoli. Some variation in the size of the cells and nuclei and in the amount of nuclear chromatin is usually seen. Large or giant uninucleate tumor cells, which in all other respects resemble typical dysgerminoma cells, may be seen (Fig. 20.6). Mitotic activity is almost always detectable (Figs. 20.5 and 20.6) and may vary from slight to brisk. This difference in mitotic activity may be observed not only in different tumors but also in different parts of the same tumor.

The cytoplasm of the tumor cells contains glycogen, which can be demonstrated with the periodic acid–Schiff (PAS) reaction, and this can be used as an aid in diagnosis. The amount of glycogen in tumor cells is variable, and glycogen is lost from the cytoplasm on prolonged fixation in formalin. In view of this, the PAS reaction may vary from strong to very weak. The majority of dysgerminoma cells do not show positive immunocytochemical staining for cytokeratin, although occasional cells may show a positive reaction.[172,173] In view of this, immunocytochemical staining for cytokeratin provides a useful diagnostic test that distinguishes between dysgerminoma and embryonal carcinoma or endodermal sinus tumor, which show a uniformly positive staining reaction for cytokeratin.[172,173]

Lipid is also present in the cytoplasm of the tumor cells and can be demonstrated in frozen tissue with the aid of lipid stains. The cells of dysgerminoma, like the primordial germ cells, show a positive alkaline phosphatase reaction beneath the cytoplasmic rim[157] and, in general, show similar histochemical reactions to those of primordial germ cells. An increased amount of DNA,

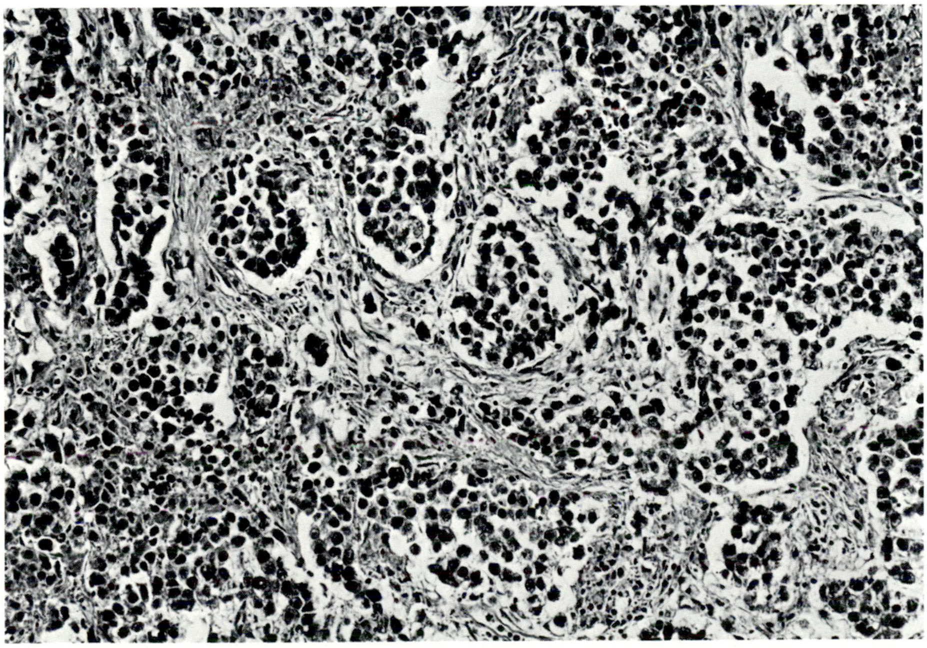

FIG. 20.4. Dysgerminoma composed of islands of tumor cells surrounded by connective tissue stroma containing lymphocytes.

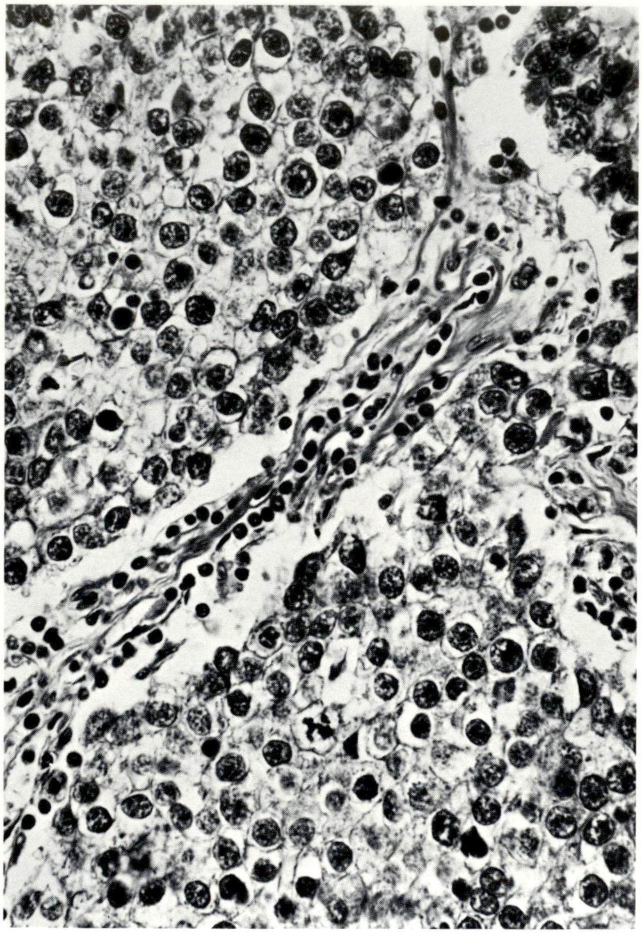

FIG. 20.5. Dysgerminoma showing the cellular composition and a connective tissue septum infiltrated by lymphocytes. An abnormal mitosis is seen just below the *center*.

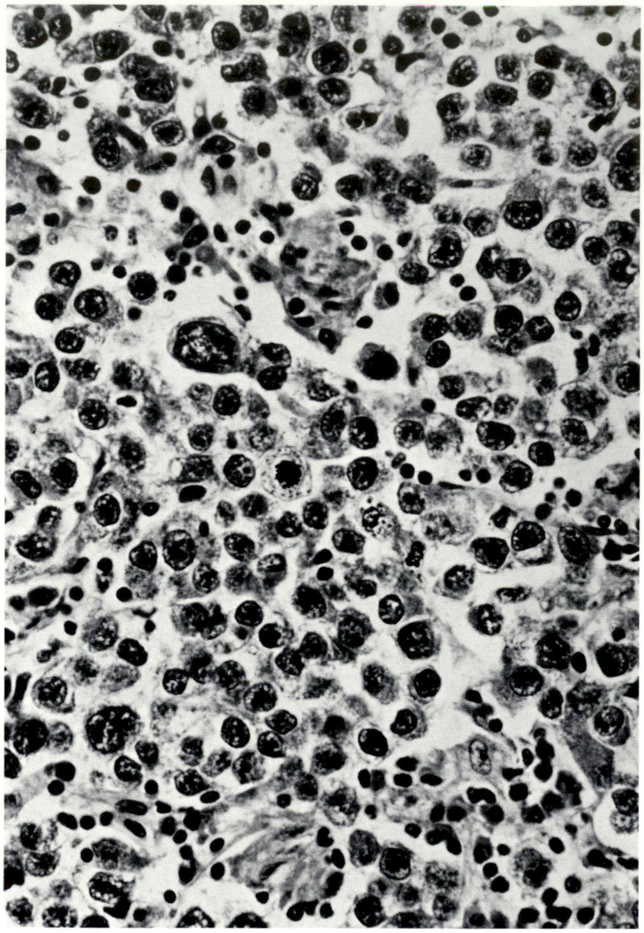

FIG. 20.6. Dysgerminoma showing a slight variation in size of the cells, a large uninucleate cell, and a mitosis in the center.

double the amount present in normal somatic cells, has been observed in the nuclei of dysgerminoma using densitometry.[12]

The stroma that surrounds the tumor cells is composed of connective tissue that may be hyalinized. It is almost always infiltrated by lymphocytes. The lymphocytic infiltration may vary from slight to marked, and large collections of lymphocytes may be present (Fig. 20.7). Occasionally, lymphoid follicles containing germinal centers may be seen. Plasma cells and eosinophils are not infrequently seen within the connective tissue stroma. Granulomatous reaction is also not infrequently seen; this manifests itself as collections of histiocytes surrounded by lymphocytes, plasma cells, and occasional giant cells of both the Langhans and foreign body types (Fig. 20.8). The connective tissue stroma shows considerable variation in its appearance and amount. The latter tends to determine the pattern of the tumor; thus, depending on the amount of stroma, the tumor cells form large aggregates, smaller nests, islands, cords, or strands. The stroma varies from a fine, delicate fibrovascular network to large, fibrous strands or broad, fibrous, often hyalinized septa. It can be loose and edematous or dense and hyalinized. Occasionally, the amount of stroma may be very large, and this leads to wide separation of the nests of tumor cells (Fig. 20.4). At the opposite end of the spectrum, there are tumors that are very cellular and contain only an imperceptible amount of stroma. There may be a considerable variation in the amount of stroma in various parts of the same tumor.

Foci of necrosis and hemorrhage are frequently found and may be of considerable size in large tumors or in tumors affected by torsion. Small foci of hyalinization may also be present, but large hyalinized areas sometimes observed in testicular seminoma are uncommon. Calcification is only occasionally seen in dysgerminoma. It occurs as small untidy spots or flecks of calcified material that are found in association with necrosis, hemorrhage, fibrosis, or hyalinization. Occasionally, relatively large, round, or ovoid calcified bodies are found, which may

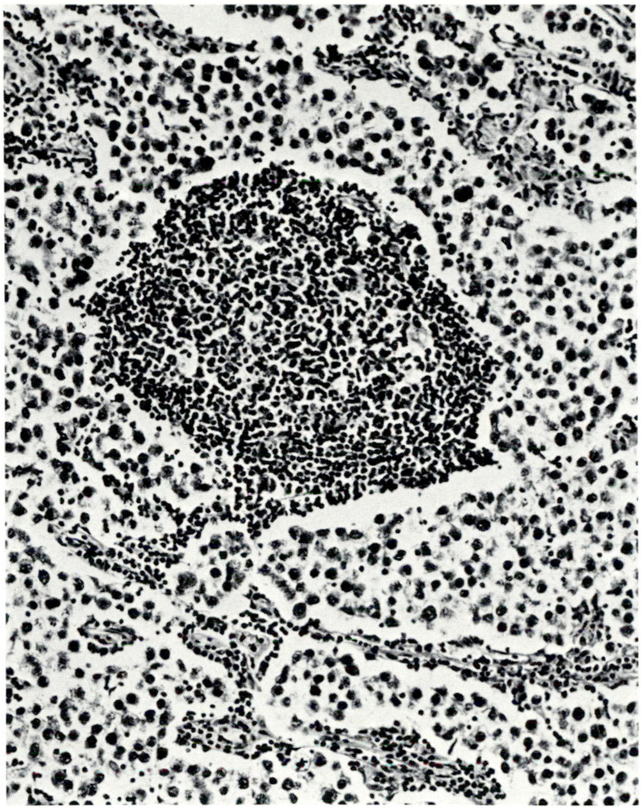

FIG. 20.7. Dysgerminoma showing a large collection of lymphocytes and a fine connective tissue septa surrounding the tumor cells.

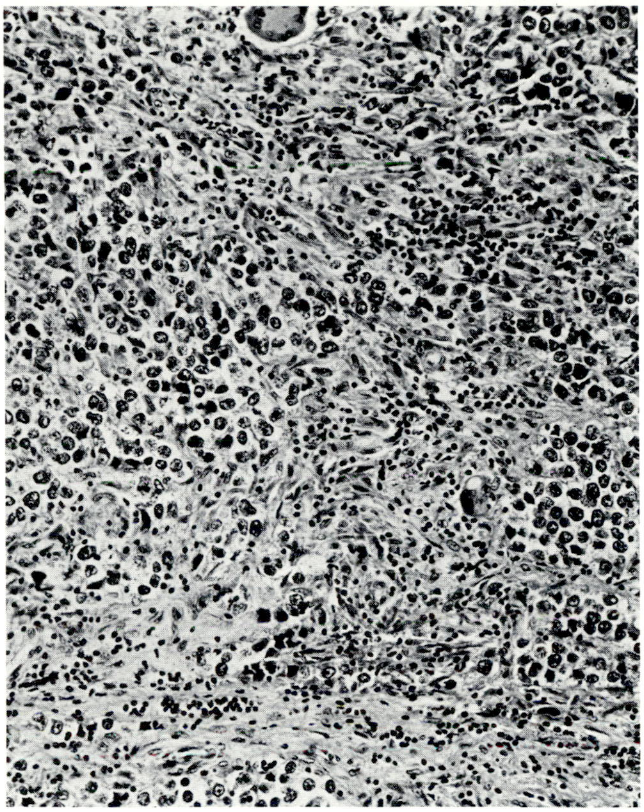

FIG. 20.8. Dysgerminoma showing a granulomatous reaction with foreign body and Langhans giant cells.

indicate the presence of a burnt-out gonadoblastoma[242] (Fig. 20.9).

In 6–8% of dysgerminomas, there are individual or collections of syncytiotrophoblastic giant cells, that produce human chorionic gonadotropin (hCG). The presence of these cells is associated with elevation of serum hCG levels; hCG can also be demonstrated in tissue sections by immunofluorescent and immunoperoxidase techniques. The syncytiotrophoblastic giant cells may form large syncytial masses resembling the syncytiotrophoblast of a choriocarcinoma but differing from the latter in the complete absence of a cytotrophoblast (Fig. 20.10). The syncytiotrophoblastic cells must also be differentiated from foreign body and Langhans giant cells, which are not infrequently seen in association with a granulomatous reaction, and from uninucleate and multinucleate tumor giant cells, which are seen in some dysgerminomas. There is no evidence that dysgerminomas containing syncytiotrophoblastic giant cells are associated with worse prognosis.[340] The serum hCG level can be monitored as a tumor marker in the same way as in patients with gestational trophoblastic disease (see Chapter 24, Gestational Trophoblastic Disease) or with mixed germ cell tumors containing choriocarcinoma.

Dysgerminoma may be associated with other neoplastic germ cell elements. Recent studies indicate a greater frequency of these mixed tumors* as compared to earlier reports.[175] This change is considered to result from a more detailed examination of the tumors and from a better recognition of the fact that germ cell tumors may be composed of histologically different neoplastic elements occurring in combination. For example, dysgerminoma may be combined with teratoma (Fig. 20.11), endodermal sinus tumor (Fig. 20.12), embryonal carcinoma, and choriocarcinoma. Some tumors may contain all these neoplastic germ cell elements. The association of dysgerminoma with gonadoblastoma is frequent, occurring in 50% of cases of gonadoblastoma.[242] Histologically, the other neoplastic germ cell elements may be intimately admixed with the dysgerminoma (Fig. 20.11) or may be found adjacent to the dysgerminoma and separated from it by a fibrous septum (Fig. 20.12). Endodermal sinus tumor elements and choriocarcinoma may be affected by hemorrhage and necrosis; a thorough search

* References 12, 37, 76, 122, 127, 140, 199, 229, 287, 308.

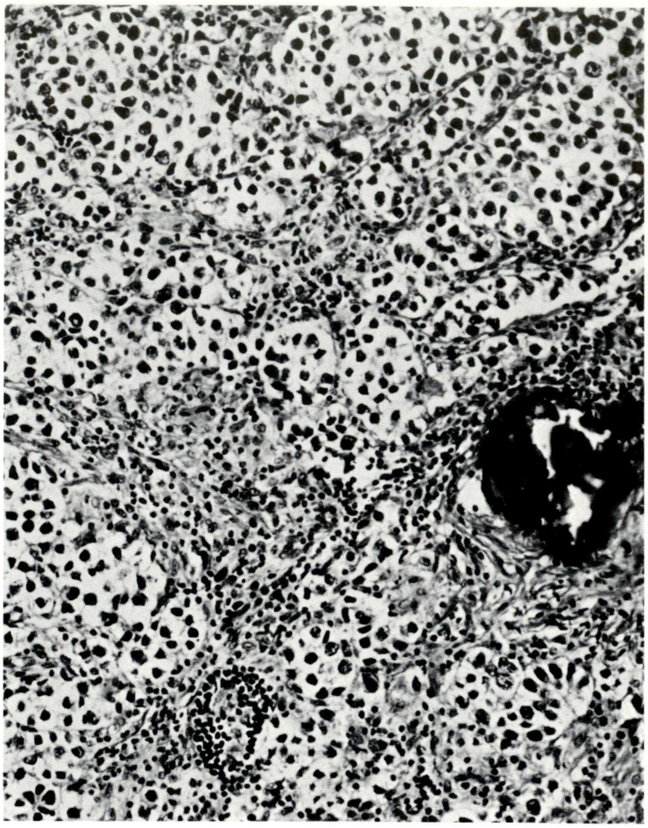

FIG. 20.9. Dysgerminoma containing a large calcified concretion. Nests of gonadoblastoma were found in other parts of the tumor.

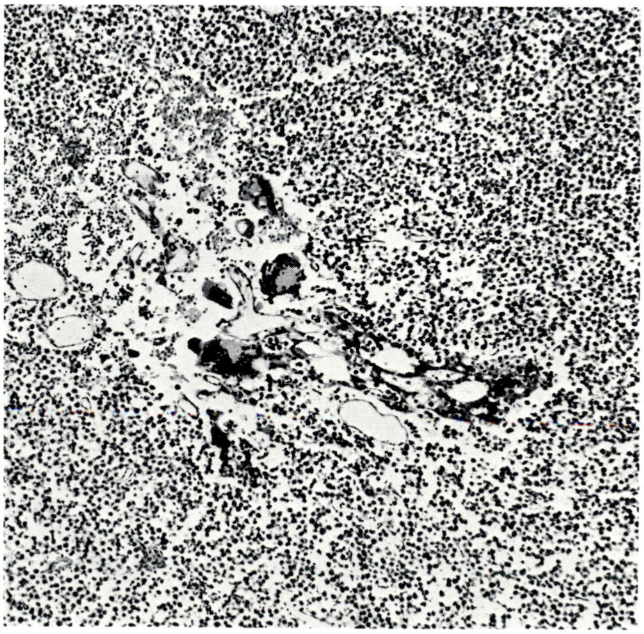

FIG. 20.10. Dysgerminoma containing collections of giant cells forming large syncytial masses resembling syncytiotrophoblast.

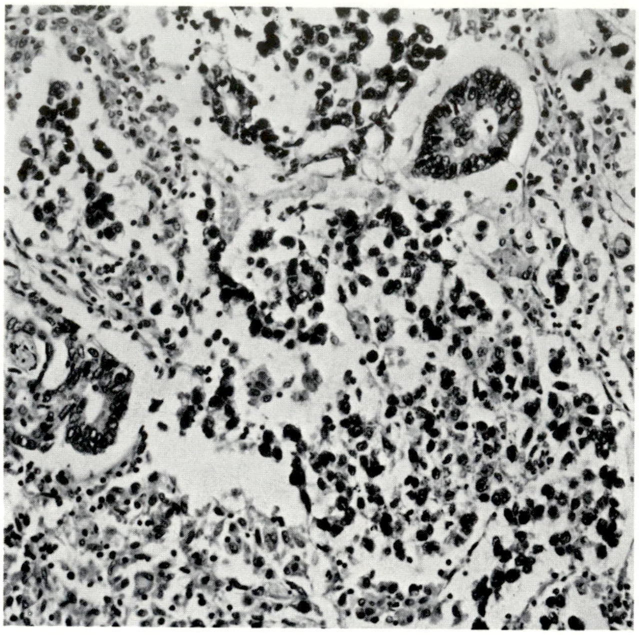

FIG. 20.11. Dysgerminoma intimately admixed with immature teratoma composed of primitive glandular epithelium. (Reprinted by permission of Talerman et al., Ref. 289.)

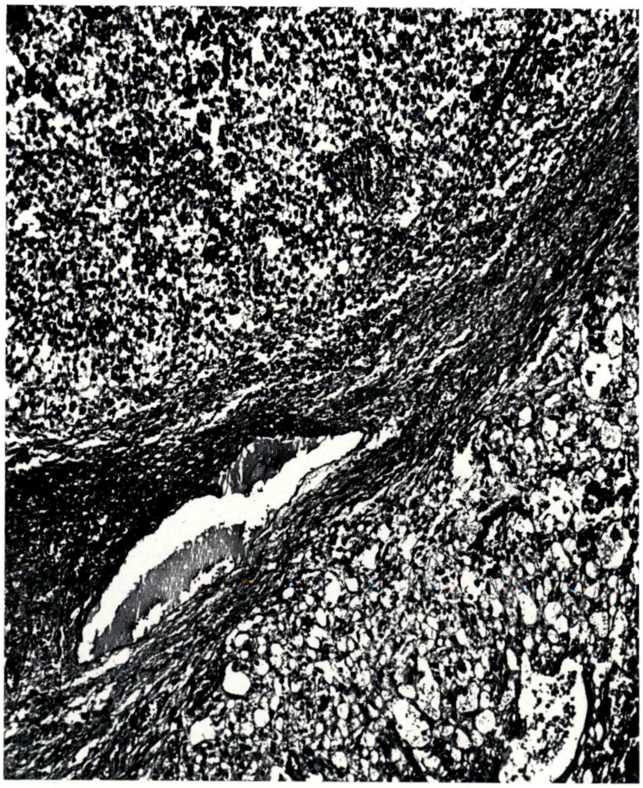

FIG. 20.12. Dysgerminoma admixed with endodermal sinus tumor. Note the fibrous septum separating the two elements.

by extensive sampling may be necessary to confirm their presence.

The cells of dysgerminoma, when studied with the electron microscope,[53,114,130,152,192] have been found to closely resemble the cells of classic testicular seminoma;[204] when studied with the light microscope, they resemble germ cell neoplasms in other locations showing a similar histologic pattern,[143,215] as well as normal maturing germ cells in the ovary.[95,108] Slight ultrastructural differences have been noted between individual germ cells present within a tumor, as well as between those present in the different tumors studied. It is likely that some of these differences are related to the degree of differentiation and maturity of the tumor cells.

Behavior. Dysgerminoma is a malignant neoplasm capable of metastatic and local spread. Despite its less aggressive behavior and its marked radiosensitivity as compared with other malignant germ cell neoplasms, the malignant potential of dysgerminoma should not be minimized. Dysgerminoma is a rapidly growing neoplasm, but metastatic spread does not occur very early in the course of the disease, although it is not possible to predict this in individual cases. When the tumor is small and freely mobile, its capsule is usually intact, but large tumors may be adherent to the surrounding structures or may rupture.[60,229] Rupture may occur either spontaneously, or at operation. This leads to spillage of the tumor contents and peritoneal implantation, causing serious prognostic consequences.[60,229] Penetration of the ovarian surface by the tumor and formation of adhesions to surrounding structures may lead to direct extension by the tumor.

Metastatic spread occurs via the lymphatic system; the lymph nodes in the vicinity of the common iliac arteries and the terminal part of the abdominal aorta are first affected. Occasionally, there may be marked enlargement of these lymph nodes, with formation of large masses. Usually the enlargement is slight to moderate and can be detected by lymphangiography and computerized tomography (CT) scanning. From the abdominal lymph nodes, the tumor spreads to the mediastinal and supraclavicular lymph nodes. Hematogenous spread to distant organs occurs later, and any organ may be affected, although involvement of the liver, lungs, and bones tends to be most common.* In cases of pure dysgerminoma, the metastases usually present a similar histologic appearance to the primary tumor, but occasionally, tumors composed of pure dysgerminoma may be associated with metastases composed of other neoplastic germ cell elements. This metastatic pattern is much more commonly observed in combined tumors. It has been suggested that cellular tumors with small amounts of stroma, slight lymphocytic infiltration, and associated with cellular atypia and high mitotic activity tend to be more aggressive.[12,60] However, in view of the inconstancy of these findings—marked histologic variations within the same tumor and its radiosensitivity—there is at present no good evidence that the behavior of an individual tumor can be assessed from its histologic appearance.[71,229,287] This does not apply to dysgerminomas admixed with other, more malignant germ cell elements; in these cases the outcome is less favorable.*

* References 4, 12, 40, 60, 79, 110, 175, 229.

Dysgerminoma, like its testicular counterpart the seminoma, is associated with elevated levels of serum lactic dehydrogenase (LDH) and its isoenzyme-1 (LDH-1), and these substances can be used as tumor markers.[13,82,341] There is a good correlation between the volume of tumor tissue present and the serum levels of the enzymes. Also because a considerable amount of tumor tissue is needed to produce elevated serum levels, these enzymes are better tumor markers in patients with dysgerminomas, than seminomas. The latter are usually smaller.

It has been shown recently that patients with testicular seminoma have elevated levels of serum placental alkaline phosphatase (Regan isoenzyme) (PLAP) and that this isoenzyme may be used as a tumor marker.[141] Although PLAP has not been satisfactorily studied in patients with dysgerminoma, it is very likely that similar results would be obtained in patients with this neoplasm and that PLAP could also be used as a tumor marker in patients with dysgerminoma.

Prognosis. The prognosis of patients with pure dysgerminoma is now considered to be favorable. Although earlier reports indicated that the prognosis was poor and that the 5-year survival was only 27%,[73,175] more recent studies have reported a much better prognosis for pure dysgerminoma, with a 5-year survival of 75–90%.† At the same time, the 5-year survival of patients with unilateral encapsulated dysgerminoma has been reported in excess of 90%,[12,38,60,136,160] although patients who were treated by unilateral salpingo-oophorectomy had 18–52% recurrence rates. The recurrences were treated successfully with radiation therapy. The unfavorable prognostic parameters include presence of metastases at the time of diagnosis, presence of adhesions and spread into adjacent structures and organs, bilaterality, and large size of the tumor.‡ It should be noted that none of these parameters is by itself considered to indicate a hopeless outcome, and many patients with these findings have been cured with radiotherapy. Some investigators consider patients younger than 20 years[38,60,168,199] as well as patients older

* References 12, 37, 60, 76, 127, 135, 140, 199, 230, 287, 308.

† References 4, 12, 37, 38, 60, 100, 136, 159, 308.

‡ References 37, 38, 60, 136, 199, 287.

than 40 years[38,168,199] to have a worse prognosis. Others[12,37] do not regard age as important in this connection.

There is general agreement that the presence of other neoplastic germ cell elements has an adverse effect on prognosis.* Eighty percent of recurrences occur in the first 2 years after diagnosis,[199] and it has been reported that more than 75% occur in the first year.[38,60]

Therapy. Dysgerminoma, like its testicular counterpart, the classic seminoma, is a highly radiosensitive tumor. Patients with bilateral or disseminated dysgerminoma, as well as patients with unilateral encapsulated tumors no longer desirous of having children, are treated by hysterectomy and bilateral salpingo-oophorectomy followed by radiation therapy to the abdominal and, in some centers, to the mediastinal lymph nodes.

For young women with unilateral encapsulated pure dysgerminoma, two different therapeutic approaches have been advocated. One consists of unilateral oophorectomy, or salpingo-oophorectomy, wedge biopsy of the remaining ovary, careful follow-up of the patient, and treatment by radiotherapy of any metastases or recurrences if these occur.† The arguments in favor of this mode of therapy are based on very much better 5-year survival figures exceeding 90% described in recent series dealing solely with similar cases.[12,60,159] The advantages of this mode of treatment are that fertility is preserved and there are no genetic hazards associated with administration of radiotherapy, a factor that at present is impossible to assess accurately. If metastases or recurrences develop, they can be controlled successfully by radiotherapy. The second approach also advocates conservative therapy similar to that mentioned above, but in order to decrease and prevent the formation of metastases and recurrences, radiotherapy is administered to the abdominal lymph nodes on the ipsilateral side while the remaining ovary is shielded. There is evidence that this approach tends to decrease the risk of metastases and recurrences.[38,136,287] It is suggested by the advocates of conservative surgery without radiotherapy that this risk is not very serious, especially as the metastases or recurrences can be treated by radiotherapy when they develop.[4,12,40,60,240,308] The conservative approach to the therapy of unilateral encapsulated dysgerminoma has been gaining ground over the years, and this approach is strongly recommended, but each individual case should be considered on its merits. It should be noted that before this mode of treatment can be considered, the opposite ovary must be normal, there should be no evidence of spread of the tumor in the abdominal cavity, and the abdominal and pelvic lymph nodes must be free from metastases on inspection, CT scanning, and lymphangiography. In addition, the patient must be chromatin positive and have a normal female 46XX karyotype.

The treatment of patients with dysgerminoma occurring in dysgenetic gonads must be hysterectomy and bilateral salpingo-gonadectomy in view of the high risk of development of bilateral neoplasms in these patients and in view of the fact that the gonads are hormonally and functionally inactive (see Chapter 2, Abnormal Sexual Development). Therefore, determination of the karyotype of all patients with dysgerminoma, especially those with evidence of virilization or developmental and menstrual abnormalities, is strongly recommended. This is very important in prepubertal patients, for in these patients other signs of abnormal function, such as primary amenorrhea, virilization, and absence of normal sexual development, are lacking. It must be emphasized that in patients who are sexually and genetically abnormal, the excision of the tumor is not associated with reversion to a normal state, and substitution hormonal therapy must be administered. Adequate treatment in these cases prevents development of a tumor in the opposite gonad or leads to the removal of a clinically inapparent lesion that may subsequently prove lethal.[82]

Because of the marked radiosensitivy of dysgerminoma, chemotherapy is only occasionally employed in the treatment of this tumor. Chemotherapy provides effective treatment and can be used either in conjunction with radiotherapy or in cases that cannot be controlled with radiotherapy, as well as in cases of disseminated disease. The chemotherapeutic agents that have been employed include chlorambucil, cyclophosphamide, methotrexate, dactinomycin and combinations of these agents.

Endocrine Aspects. In the great majority of cases, dysgerminoma is not associated with endocrine manifestations. Occasional cases have been described where the tumor was associated with elevated urinary chorionic gonadotropins, positive pregnancy tests, or signs of precocious puberty, and these manifestations have disappeared following excision of the tumor. Although in these cases the tumor has been said to be a pure dysgerminoma,[105,176] the possibility of admixture with choriocarcinomatous elements that have not been detected, perhaps because of inadequate sampling, is the most likely explanation.[40,70,110,199,229]

The presence of choriocarcinoma in association with dysgerminoma is not frequent, but most of the reported series contain cases of this type.[122,199,230,287,308] Recently, occasional cases of pure dysgerminoma, containing multinucleate syncytiotrophoblastic giant cells but lacking cytotrophoblastic elements, have been noted to be associated with gonadotropin production. Although some cases

* References 12, 37, 199, 229, 230, 287, 308.
† References 4, 12, 40, 79, 136, 240, 241.

of dysgerminoma showing these histologic appearances were recognized previously, evidence of gonadotropin production by the syncytiotrophoblastic giant cells was obtained only recently. This provides another possible explanation, apárt from the presence of true choriocarcinomatous elements, for the occasional presence of endocrine activity in cases of dysgerminoma. However, there remains a very small group of cases where, in spite of a careful search, trophoblastic elements have not been found. In some of these cases, the dysgerminoma has been associated with an increase in luteinized stromal or Leydig-like cells and it is likely that these cells may be responsible for the feminizing side effects. These cells may also be responsible for the virilizing side effects observed in occasional cases of dysgerminoma.[315] Dysgerminoma associated with evidence of virilization is mostly found in association with gonadoblastoma in patients with pure or mixed gonadal dysgenesis.

Genetic Aspects. When Meyer[171] described dysgerminoma, he observed that the tumor frequently occurred in hermaphrodites, pseudohermaphrodites, and patients with underdeveloped or malformed genitalia. In fact, 27 of 48 cases collected by Meyer[171] occurred in sexually abnormal patients, and this relationship was strongly emphasized. It is considered that most of these reports described patients with gonadal dysgenesis and dysgerminoma that had originated from a gonadoblastoma. Although subsequent authors supported Meyer's contention about the very close association between dysgerminoma and developmental and sexual abnormalities, later reports suggested that it is not as close as had been postulated. These later reports stated that the majority of patients with dysgerminoma were normally developed females without any sexual abnormalities.* Most patients with dysgerminoma do not exhibit any menstrual abnormalities and are either capable of bearing or have actually borne children.[12,38,60] In a number of cases, the diagnosis has been made during pregnancy.† A number of patients have become pregnant and have had normal offspring following therapy.[12, 36, 86, 278, 321] The majority of recent reports emphasize the occurrence of dysgerminoma in normal female patients,‡ and some have even cast doubt on the relationship with developmental and sexual abnormalities.[12]

The common association of dysgerminoma with gonadoblastoma, a tumor that nearly always occurs in patients with dysgenetic gonads,§ indicates that there is a relationship between dysgerminoma and genetic and somatosexual abnormalities (see Chapter 2, Abnormal Sexual Development).

* References 12, 40, 79, 175, 186, 199, 225, 246, 253.
† References 12, 38, 60, 135, 136, 229, 287, 308.
‡ References 12, 38, 40, 60, 122, 287, 308.
§ References 86, 107, 232, 233, 242, 328.

Endodermal Sinus Tumor

Synonyms

Yolk sac tumor, mesonephroma,[235] embryonal carcinoma, mesoblastoma vitellinum, mesoblastoma, Teilum tumor.

Histogenesis. Endodermal sinus tumor is a malignant germ cell neoplasm that is considered to arise from the undifferentiated and multipotential embryonal carcinoma by selective differentiation toward yolk sac or vitelline structures, in the same way as nongestational choriocarcinoma differentiates toward trophoblastic structures. The concept of endodermal sinus tumor, its morphologic identity, and its establishment as a specific entity in the classification of germ cell neoplasms have resulted from the studies by Teilum, stretching over nearly three decades.* This concept has received strong support from the experimental studies of the neoplastic rodent yolk sac by Pierce et al.[206,208,209,211]

An ovarian neoplasm that showed the histologic appearances of endodermal sinus tumor and another, quite different, ovarian neoplasm composed of clear and hobnailed cells that showed papillary pattern in places were grouped together by Schiller[235] and designated as a mesonephroma of the ovary because of the presence of structures resembling immature glomeruli. Other investigators,[240] in spite of careful studies, were unable to demonstrate the mesonephric origin of this tumor and have considered it as an endothelioma of the ovary, as suggested earlier.[237] In 1946, Teilum[294] indicated that the tumor described as mesonephroma[235,236] included two distinct entities with different histogenesis, histologic pattern, age incidence, and clinical behavior. One of these entities was highly malignant, occurred in young patients, was homologous with certain testicular neoplasms, and was considered to be of germ cell origin.[294] In addition to the terms *mesonephroma*[64,235,236] and *endothelioma*,[131,237] these tumors have been designated as *embryonal carcinoma*[2,176] because of certain similarities to the embryonal carcinoma of the testis.[63] Although embryonal carcinoma showing the histologic patterns resembling the typical embryonal carcinoma of the testis[63] is occasionally seen in ovarian tumors,[139] the majority of ovarian tumors of this type show a distinctive pattern with differentiation toward yolk sac or vitelline structures[117,119,297,298,300] and should be termed *endodermal sinus* or *yolk sac tumor*. These tumors differ from the undifferentiated embryonal carcinoma,[63] although they resemble closely the endodermal sinus or yolk sac tumor of both infantile[37,209,300] and adult testes.† It is

* References 294, 295, 297, 298, 300.
† References 209, 273, 297, 298, 300, 336.

now generally accepted that the term *embryonal carcinoma* should be used only to designate ovarian neoplasms showing the typical histologic patterns of the embryonal carcinoma as described in testicular tumors.[63,139]

The not infrequent combination of endodermal sinus tumor elements in ovarian tumors with other neoplastic germ cell elements* is one of the arguments in favor of the germ cell origin of this neoplasm. Endodermal sinus tumor, either pure or combined with other neoplastic germ cell elements, has been encountered in extragonadal locations where germ cell tumors are known to occur—in the mediastinum,[118,182,284,292,300] the sacrococcygeal region,[46,118,121,217,300] the pineal gland,[6,28,300] and the vagina.[121,300,317]

Incidence. Endodermal sinus tumor is an uncommon ovarian neoplasm, although more than 350 cases have been reported.† Its exact incidence is difficult to assess because it has relatively recently been established as an entity. Over the years, it has been diagnosed under a variety of names and has been occasionally misinterpreted as a benign neoplasm. Because of its specific age incidence, however, it may be considered as one of the most common malignant ovarian neoplasms of childhood, adolescence, and early adult life. It is being diagnosed with much greater frequency nowadays and is considered the second most common malignant ovarian germ cell neoplasm occurring in pure form. Although most reports deal with Caucasians, endodermal sinus tumor has been encountered in other races.‡ The reported age distribution of patients with endodermal sinus tumor ranges from 16 months[117] to 46 years,[121] but most patients have been under 30 years of age.§ Endodermal sinus tumor of the ovary has been encountered in two patients, aged 57[39] and 67 years,[245] but these cases are considered exceptional.

Clinical Aspects. The symptomatology is nonspecific and is usually that associated with the presence of a lower abdominal or pelvic mass.‖ The majority of patients have symptoms of abdominal enlargement and pain. Occasionally, the symptoms are acute and severe and may lead to the diagnosis of acute abdominal emergency.[23,126,127,138,177,230] This is usually caused by torsion of the tumor[117,177,230] A number of cases have been encountered during pregnancy.** The presence of endodermal sinus tumor is not associated with endocrine symptoms,[37,117,177,230] although endocrine symptoms may be present if the tumor is combined with choriocarcinoma.[76,138,230] Such neoplasms are classified as mixed germ cell tumors. On clinical examination, a tumor mass is usually palpable and is frequently of considerable size.* In recent years increased levels of α-fetoprotein (AFP) have been found in sera of patients with endodermal sinus tumor,† and this is now considered a very useful diagnostic test for the presence of endodermal sinus tumor elements in a primary tumor, its metastases, and recurrences.

Macroscopic Appearance. Endodermal sinus tumors are usually unilateral.‡ Bilaterality must be differentiated from metastatic spread to the contralateral ovary, which is not infrequent. Endodermal sinus tumor shows a certain predilection for the right ovary.[37,117,138,177,230] The tumor is usually large, varying in size from 3 to 30 cm in diameter, with the majority of tumors being in excess of 10 cm.§ It frequently weighs in excess of 500 g, and tumors weighing 5 kg are recorded.[126] The tumors are usually encapsulated round, oval, or globular; firm, smooth, or somewhat lobulated; and gray-yellow, with areas of hemorrhage and cystic or gelatinous changes (Fig. 20.13). It may form adhesions to the surrounding structures and invade them. On sectioning, it is mainly solid, but cystic spaces are frequently present. The fluid present in the cysts may also be gelatinous. Necrosis and hemorrhage and the presence of other neoplastic germ cell elements, especially teratoma, may alter the appearance of the tumor.

Microscopic Appearance. Endodermal sinus tumors exhibit a range of histologic patterns that differ considerably from each other, and although all the different patterns are frequently observed in the same tumor, one or two may predominate. The following histologic patterns may be observed in endodermal sinus tumor:

1. Microcystic
2. Endodermal sinus
3. Solid
4. Alveolar–glandular
5. Polyvesicular vitelline
6. Myxomatous
7. Papillary
8. Macrocystic
9. Hepatoid
10. Primitive endodermal (intestinal)

---

* References 29, 37, 117, 127, 140, 177, 230, 284, 285, 287, 300.
† References 75, 88, 126, 127, 138, 285.
‡ References 87, 117, 126, 138, 145, 177.
§ References 88, 117, 126, 138, 177, 230, 285, 300.
‖ References 37, 88, 117, 126, 138, 177, 230.
** References 36, 117, 126, 127, 138, 177.

* References 23, 37, 88, 117, 126, 127, 138, 145, 177, 230, 285.
† References 16, 17, 88, 121, 182, 247, 278, 285, 302, 325.
‡ References 37, 88, 117, 126, 127, 138, 177, 230, 247, 285, 300.
§ References 23, 37, 117, 126, 127, 138, 177, 230, 285.

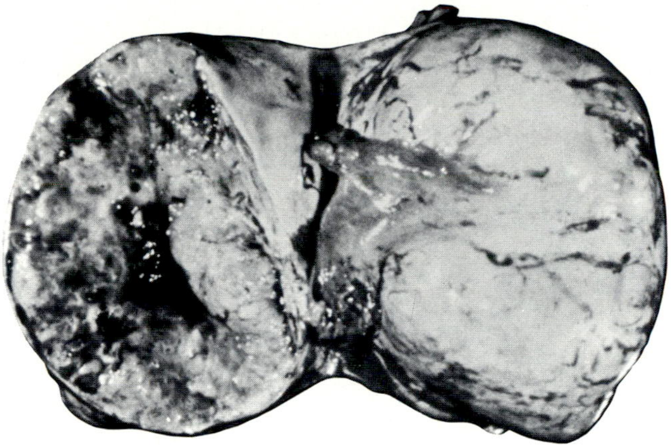

Fig. 20.13. Endodermal sinus tumor. It is oval shaped, encapsulated, with a central area of cystic degeneration. (Courtesy of R. Scully, M.D.)

The first five histologic patterns were described by Teilum[298–300] and were considered by him as the principal microscopic patterns of endodermal sinus tumor.

1. *Microcystic* (Fig. 20.14) and *myxomatous* (Fig. 20.15) *patterns* composed of a loose vacuolated network, with small cystic spaces or microcysts forming a honeycomb pattern. The microcysts are lined by flat, pleomorphic, mesothelial-like cells, with large hyperchromatic or vesicular nuclei that show brisk mitotic activity. There is usually some variation in the

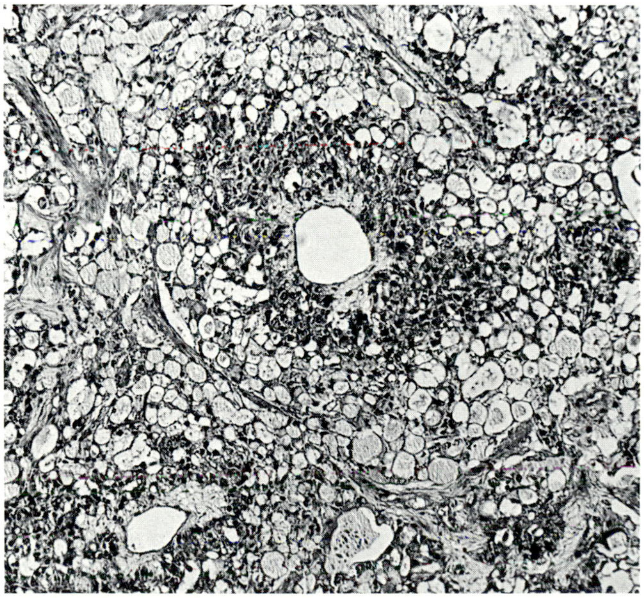

Fig. 20.14. Endodermal sinus tumor showing microcystic pattern. A labyrinthine structure composed of tumor cells radiating around a blood vessel resembling a perivascular formation is seen in the center.

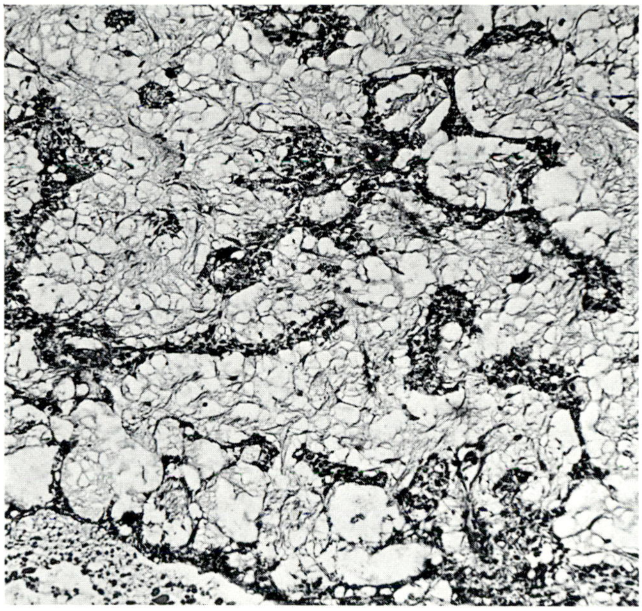

Fig. 20.15. Endodermal sinus tumor showing myxomatous pattern. Small collections of epithelial-like cells forming strands or gland-like structures are seen within the myxomatous tissue.

size of the cysts (Fig. 20.14). In the underlying capillary spaces, hematopoiesis may be seen. The vacuolated network may contain pale, PAS-positive, mucinous material, forming small lakes or precipitates, as well as small, round, brightly eosinophilic PAS-positive and diastase-resistant globules or droplets. These globules are also found within the cytoplasm of the tumor cells (Fig. 20.16). Hyaline, eosinophilic, PAS-positive, basement membrane material may also be seen in places and may be conspicuous in some tumors, the bands of hyaline material being surrounded by tumor cells. Areas composed of fine, loose myxomatous tissue containing alveolar spaces (Fig. 20.17), occasional gland-like structures lined by cuboidal epithelium (Fig. 20.18), and small cellular aggregates, often merging with the microcystic or other patterns, are also present (Fig. 20.19). The loose myxomatous pattern was considered to be analogous to the magma reticulare or the extraembryonic mesoderm of the exocoelom,[302] and the presence of this pattern led to the recognition of the mesoblastic nature of this tumor.[295] These two histologic patterns should be considered as separate principal patterns.
2. *Endodermal sinus pattern* composed of perivascular formations (Fig. 20.20), consisting of a narrow band of connective tissue with a capillary blood vessel in the center and lined by a layer of cuboidal or low columnar embryonal epithelial-like cells. The cells have large, slightly vesicular nuclei and prominent

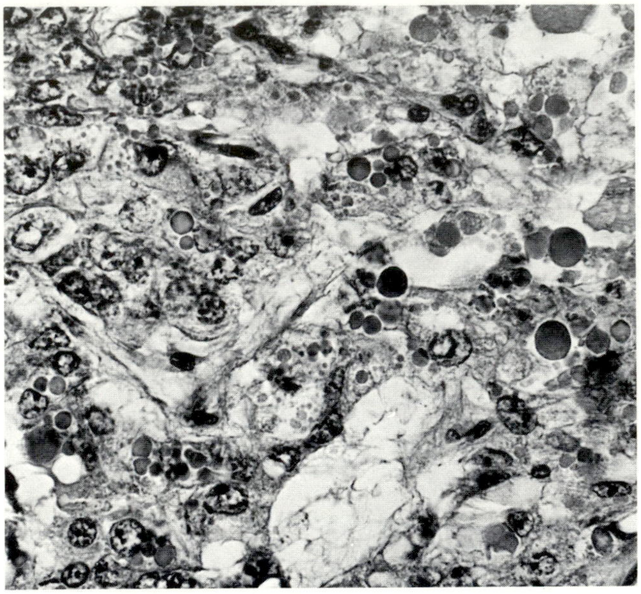

FIG. 20.16. Endodermal sinus tumor showing numerous round hyaline globules present both inside and outside the cells. Larger precipitates of this material are seen at the upper right.

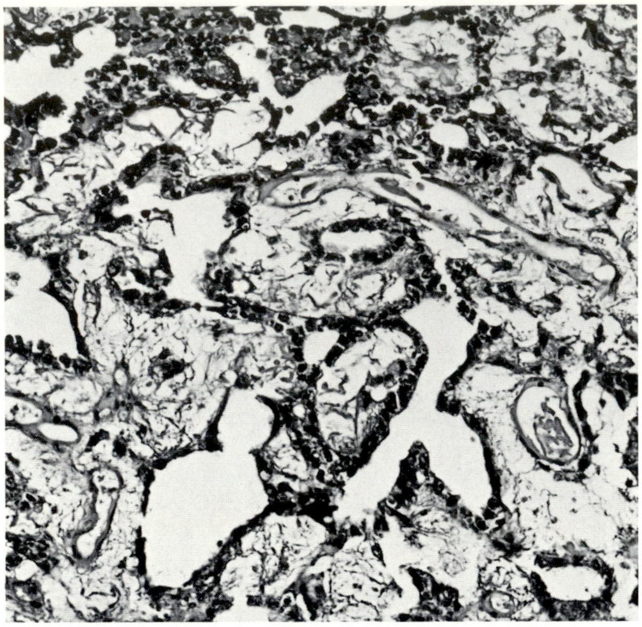

FIG. 20.18. Endodermal sinus tumor showing loose myxomatous pattern containing numerous cavities and channels. Note hyaline material at top left.

nucleoli and show mitotic activity. The surrounding capsular sinusoid space is lined by a single layer of flat cells with prominent hyperchromatic nuclei. These characteristic perivascular formations are said to recapitulate the so-called endodermal sinuses,[297,298,300] which, although not conspicuous in the human placenta, are well-defined embryologic structures in the rat placenta.[65] These typical structures are also known as sinuses of Duval, Schiller–Duval bodies,[117,209] or glomerulus-like structures and resemble superficially immature renal glomeruli. When sectioned longitudinally, the perivascular

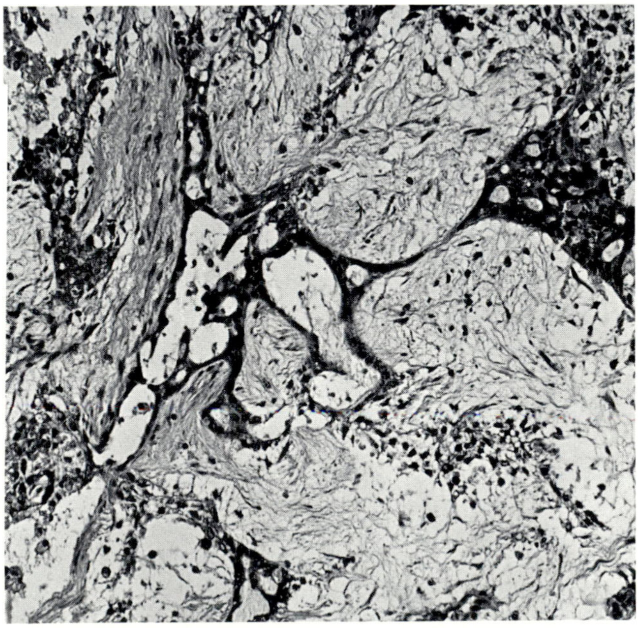

FIG. 20.17. Endodermal sinus tumor composed of myxomatous tissue containing glandular and alveolar spaces and channels.

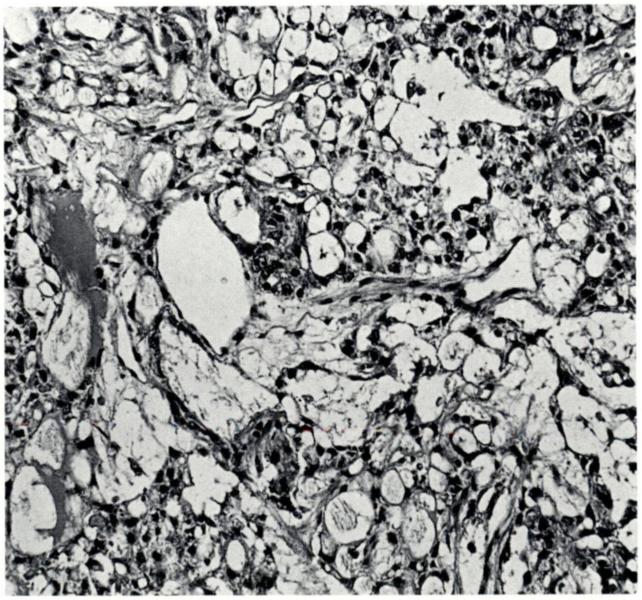

FIG. 20.19. Endodermal sinus tumor showing small cellular aggregates, microcysts, and myxomatous tissue. Mucinous material is also seen.

structures consist of a central connective tissue core containing a longitudinal vessel surrounded by epithelial-like cells that often form small papillary formations projecting into the surrounding capsular sinusoid space. The presence of these perivascular formations can be considered diagnostic of endodermal sinus tumor, but in some tumors they may be poorly represented, somewhat atypical, or absent. Although the tumor should always be carefully examined and searched in order to identify these structures, their absence does not preclude the diagnosis if the appearances of the tumor are typical in all other respects. Apart from the presence of the perivascular structures, the general pattern consists of a complicated labyrinth of communicating cavities and channels. In addition, there are papillary processes and blood vessels surrounded by narrow connective tissue cores and epithelial-like cells radiating into the surrounding stroma, resembling the typical perivascular formations but differing from them by the absence of the sinusoid space[300] (Fig. 20.14).

3. *Solid pattern* (Fig. 20.21) composed of aggregates of small epithelial-like polygonal cells with clear cytoplasm, large vesicular or pyknotic nuclei, prominent nucleoli, and exhibiting brisk mitotic activity. The tumor cells in the solid aggregate may resemble dysgerminoma cells, but they usually show greater cellular and nuclear pleomorphism and presence of at least occasional microcysts (Fig. 20.21). The presence of the latter helps to differentiate between these two entities. The presence of other patterns of endodermal sinus tumor is also helpful in this respect, as is diffuse or focal staining for AFP and uniformly positive staining for cytokeratin (Fig. 20.22), which are observed in endodermal sinus tumor and not in dysgerminoma.

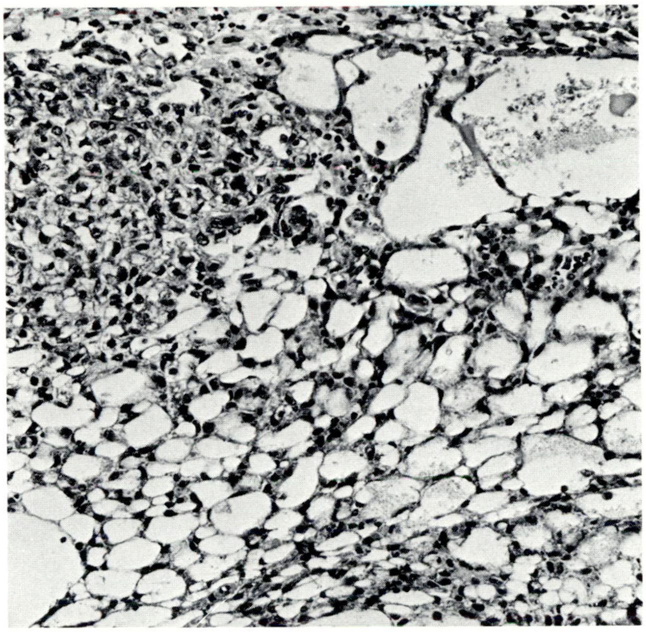

Fig. 20.21. Endodermal sinus tumor showing solid and microcystic patterns. Some larger cysts (macrocysts) are seen at *top right*.

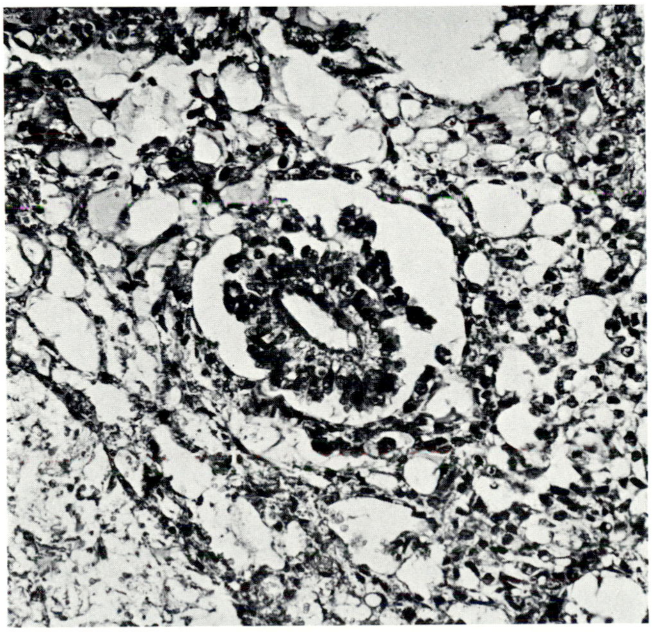

Fig. 20.20. Endodermal sinus tumor showing a typical perivascular formation (Schiller–Duval body).

4. *Alveolar-glandular pattern* (Fig. 20.18 and 20.23) composed of alveolar, glandlike, or larger cystic spaces and cavities lined by flat or cuboidal epithelial-like cells with large, prominent nuclei and surrounded by myxomatous stroma or cellular aggregates. Some of these spaces may be lined by more than one layer of cells, and sometimes the lining cells form small papillary projections protruding into the lumen. The layer of cells lining these spaces may be continuous with the lining of the perivascular sinusoid spaces.[297] Gland-like formations lined by columnar or cuboidal epithelial-like cells may be seen and in some tumors may be prominent and may form bizarre patterns (Fig. 20.18).
5. *The polyvesicular vitelline tumor pattern*[180,298–300] is composed of numerous cysts or vesicles surrounded by compact connective tissue stroma (Figs. 20.24 and 20.25). The vesicles are lined partly by columnar or cuboidal epithelial cells, frequently showing basal or paraluminal vacuolation, and partly by flat mesothelial-like cells (Fig. 20.25). The individual vesicles or cysts vary in size and shape and contain invagi-

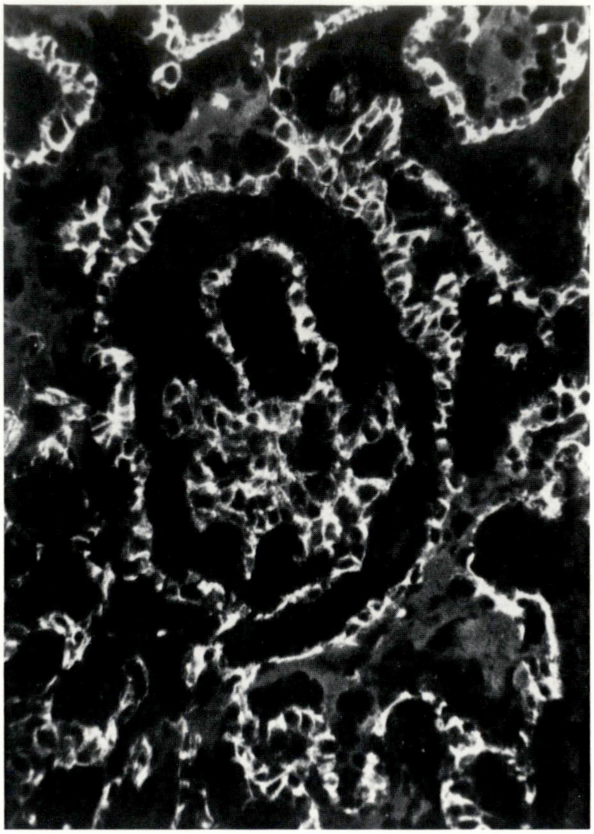

FIG. 20.22. Endodermal sinus tumor stained for low molecular weight cytokeratin. Note the uniformly positive staining of all the tumor cells. The intervening connective tissue cells are unstained.

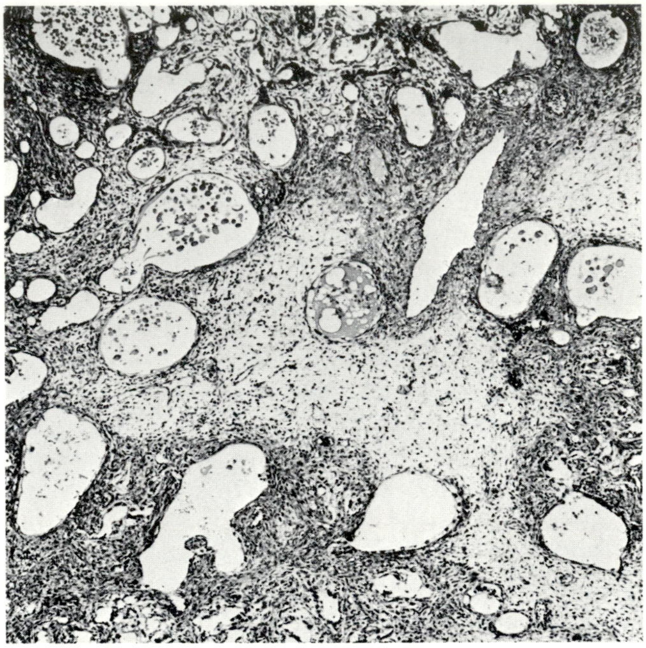

FIG. 20.24. Endodermal sinus tumor showing polyvesicular vitelline pattern.

nated protrusions into the lumen. The wall of the cyst may show a constriction dividing the part lined by the mesothelial cells from that lined by the columnar or cuboidal epithelium (Fig. 20.25). This is considered to reflect the embryologic conversion

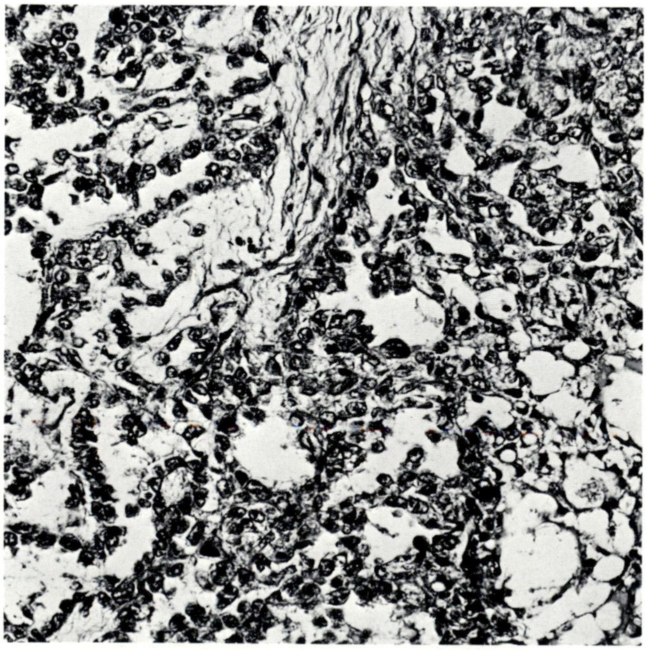

FIG. 20.23. Endodermal sinus tumor showing glandular alveolar pattern.

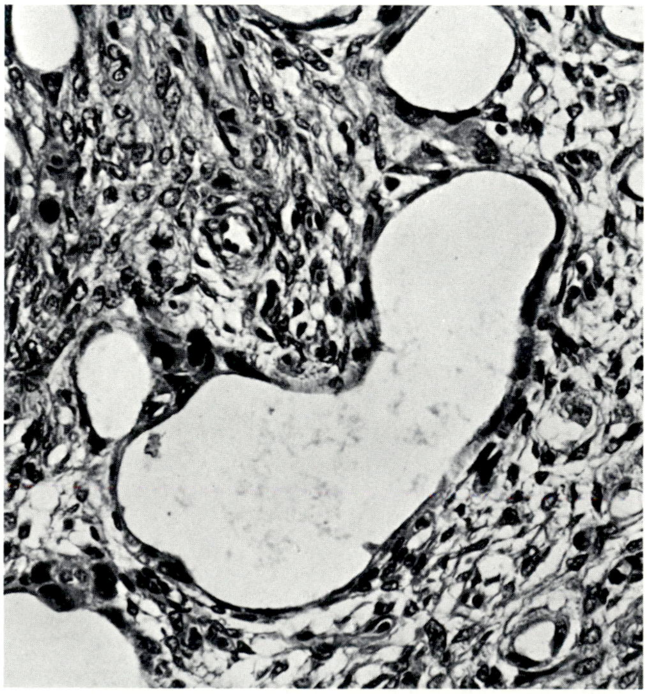

FIG. 20.25. Endodermal sinus tumor with polyvesicular vitelline pattern showing a typical vesicle.

of the primary yolk sac into the secondary yolk sac.[298–300] Occasionally, the whole tumor may exhibit the polyvesicular vitelline pattern; such tumors have been designated as polyvesicular vitelline tumors.[180,298–300]

Small eosinophilic, PAS-positive, diastase-resistant droplets or globules may be present either within the tumor cells or outside them; they may be numerous and prominent in some tumors (Fig. 20.16). They may be observed in tumors exhibiting all the histologic patterns described above, and their identification is a helpful diagnostic feature. However, their presence is not diagnostic of endodermal sinus tumor, since they are observed in many malignant, often poorly differentiated neoplasms. The droplets are considered to be secreted by the tumor cells and accumulate within the cytoplasm. As the amount of secretion increases, the cell becomes distended and ruptures, discharging its contents into the surrounding tissue. This explains the presence of these glob ules outside the cells and the presence of pale, eosinophilic, slightly PAS-positive material. Recently, the significance of these globules in endodermal sinus tumor has been further enhanced by demonstrating with immunofluorescent and immunoperoxidase techniques that some contain AFP[121,138,252,301] (Fig. 20.26). Other globules may contain alpha$_1$-antitrypsin, and other plasma proteins, such as transferrin.[193,252,311] The presence of hyaline, PAS-positive material forming bands or connective tissue cores surrounded by tumor cells is not an infrequent finding in endodermal sinus tumor; in some tumors, it may be a prominent feature, with the tumor cells resting on and surrounding the bands of hyaline material (Fig. 20.27). There may be an increased amount of the eosinophilic, PAS-positive globules described above in the vicinity of the hyaline bands, suggesting a relationship between these two features and a possibility of common origin.[298,300] The hyaline, PAS-positive material in endodermal sinus tumor has been found to be similar to the hyaline material produced by mouse teratocarcinoma during its conversion to ascitic form, and this is considered to be a strong argument in favor of the yolk sac origin of the tumor.[205,206,209,211] The cells of endodermal sinus tumor, when examined with the electron microscope, resemble the ultrastructural appearance of the normal human yolk sac.[98,121,180,181,300]

In addition to the five histologic patterns described above, five additional patterns observed in this tumor merit consideration as specific patterns.

6. *Myxomatous pattern* (Fig. 20.15), which Teilum[298–300] combined with the microcystic, may be observed on its own or may predominate.

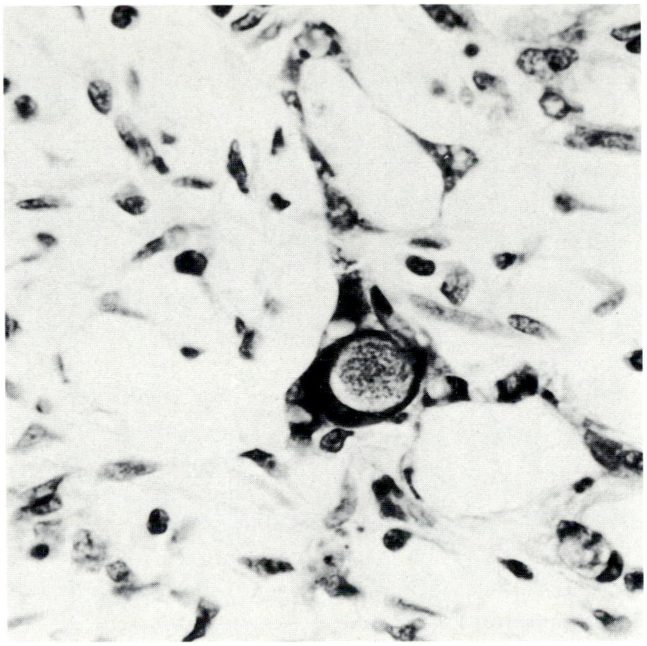

FIG. 20.26. Endodermal sinus tumor showing positive staining for AFP. The AFP forms a granular deposit within the cytoplasm of the large tumor cell (*center*).

7. *Papillary pattern* (Fig. 20.27) is composed of papillary structures consisting of connective tissue cores lined by epithelial-like cells showing a considerable degree of cellular and nuclear pleomorphism and mitotic activity. The connective tissue may show extensive

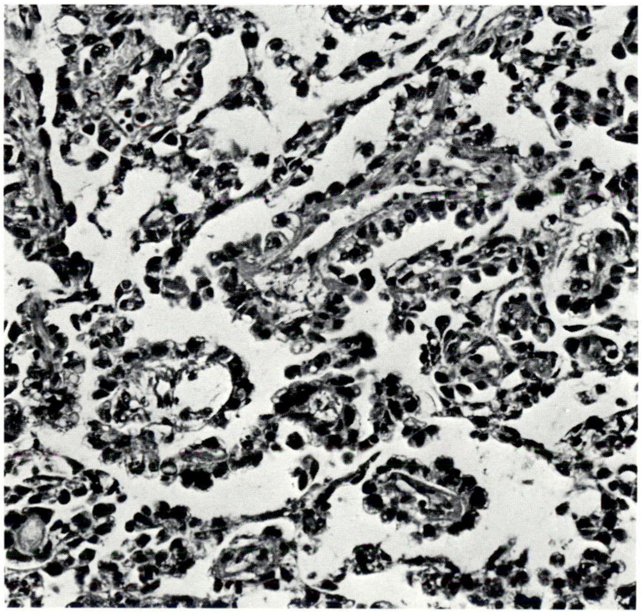

FIG. 20.27. Endodermal sinus tumor showing papillary pattern. The papillae are composed of hyaline material lined by tumor cells.

hyalinization. This pattern may be the predominant pattern within a tumor.

8. *Macrocystic pattern* is observed when endodermal sinus tumor exhibits larger cysts in contrast to microcysts or alveolar spaces. In some tumors, this pattern may predominate.
9. *Hepatoid pattern* is composed of cells with eosinophilic, even, or granular cytoplasm, showing a solid pattern and considerable resemblance to hepatocytes. This pattern was considered by Teilum[298–300] as a variant of the solid pattern. Such tumors have been designated as hepatoid endodermal sinus tumors[213] or endodermal sinus tumor with hepatoid pattern (Fig. 20.28). These tumors are only infrequently admixed with other histologic patterns of endodermal sinus tumor or other neoplastic germ cell elements. The rarity of the tumor may cause diagnostic problems, but the presence of a solid ovarian tumor composed of hepatocyte-like cells surrounded by connective tissue and forming solid aggregates, cords, or clusters and associated with elevated serum AFP in a young patient would strongly favor a diagnosis of endodermal sinus tumor with hepatoid pattern.
10. *Primitive endodermal (intestinal) pattern* in which the tumor is composed entirely of primitive endodermal glands is encountered occasionally (Fig. 20.29). The tumor in these cases is composed of nests or collections of primitive endodermal glands surrounded by connective tissue, which varies from loose and edematous to dense and hyalinized. The degree of differentiation varies from primitive to relatively well differentiated. The glands may contain inspissated secretion within the lumen, and the tumor may resemble a mucin-secreting adenocarcinoma. Ultrastructurally, the nuclei are large and show prominent nucleolonema, whereas the cytoplasm contains many ribosomes, rough endoplasmic reticulum, and mitochondria. Dense amorphous intracellular material is also present. Endodermal sinus tumors showing this pattern have been associated with very high levels of serum AFP. This pattern has been designated as primitive endodermal (intestinal) pattern. The presence of primitive endodermal glandular tissue, lobular or nest-like pattern, and high levels of serum AFP differentiate this type of endodermal sinus tumor from mucinous tumors of the ovary.

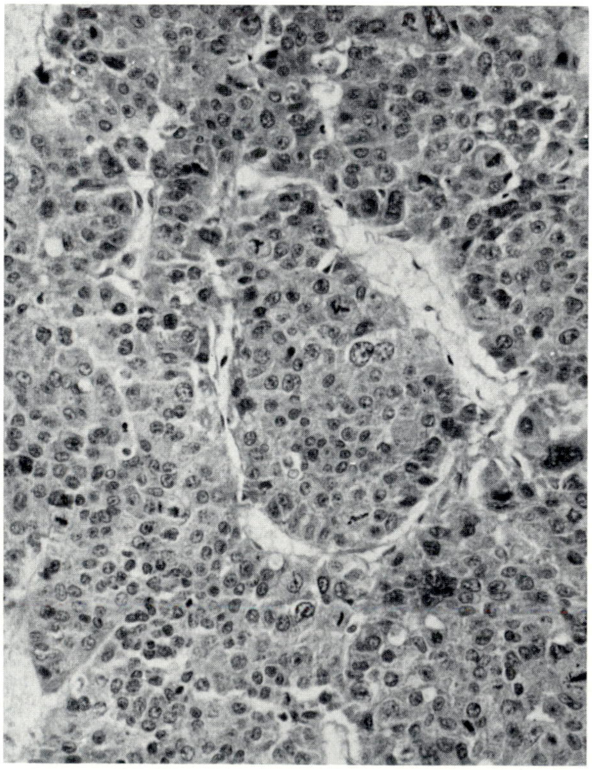

Fig. 20.28. Endodermal sinus tumor showing hepatoid pattern. The tumor is composed of solid aggregates or cords of polygonal cells with even or granular eosinophilic cytoplasm resembling hepatocytes. Note the brisk mitotic activity.

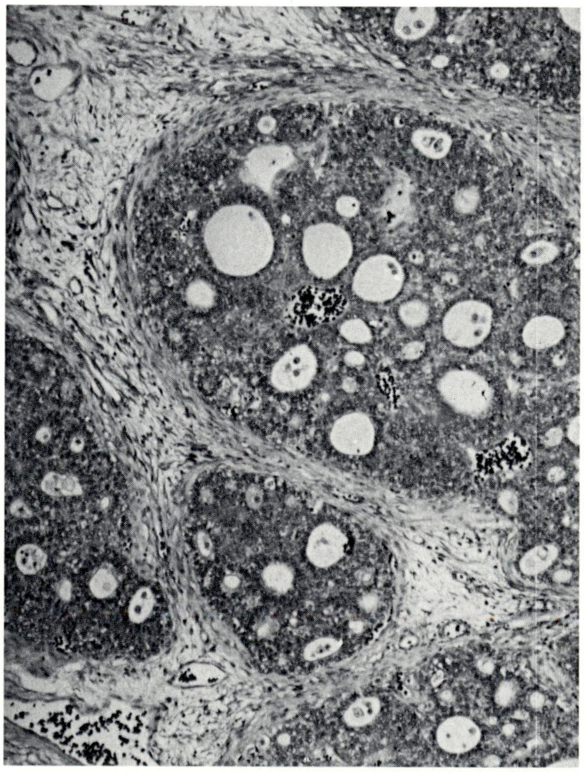

Fig. 20.29. Endodermal sinus tumor showing the endodermal (intestinal) pattern. The tumor is composed of nests of primitive endodermal cells forming glands or solid aggregates, which are surrounded by connective tissue.

Differential Diagnosis. Before it was recognized as a specific entity, endodermal sinus tumor was included with neoplasms composed of clear or parvilocular cells in the group of neoplasms of the ovary designated as mesonephroma,[235,236] or it was grouped together with embryonal carcinoma of the ovary.[2,37,177] It is with these two histogenetically different neoplasms that the endodermal sinus tumor may be confused. The clear cell tumors of the ovary show much more regular tubular patterns, lack the honeycomb network composed of microcysts, and have papillary frond-like projections that are often lined by clear or hobnail cells. The typical perivascular formations, endodermal sinuses, or Schiller-Duval bodies present in endodermal sinus tumor are absent. The epithelial cells lining the tubules are cuboidal with clear cytoplasm or are hobnailed with nuclei bulging into the lumen. Areas composed of large polygonal cells with clear cytoplasm and small, dark, uniform, centrally situated nuclei resembling those of renal carcinoma are present. Since these cells line cystic spaces, they frequently proliferate in a papillary fashion or form solid aggregates. When the clear cell carcinoma is composed entirely of tubules or spaces, confusion may arise with the polyvesicular vitelline pattern. However, the epithelial lining is usually composed of the projecting hobnail cells and not of the two types of epithelia seen in the vesicles forming the polyvesicular vitelline pattern. The cystic spaces are more tubular and less vesicle-like. The clear cell tumors occur also in other parts of the female genital tract, usually occur in older patients, and are associated with a more favorable prognosis.[177,187,300]

The embryonal carcinoma, which is uncommon in the ovary,* lacks the specific patterns observed in the endodermal sinus tumor. In its undifferentiated form, it is composed of aggregates of primitive embryonal cells. The tumor cells are frequently larger than those seen in the solid cellular aggregates in endodermal sinus tumor. The cytoplasm is more granular, there is more marked cellular and nuclear pleomorphism, and the nucleoli are more prominent. Even when the tumor is somewhat more differentiated, with the embryonal cells forming cords, tubules, or papillae and lining clefts or spaces, it still lacks the typical patterns associated with endodermal sinus tumor.

The cells of endodermal sinus tumor are uniformly cytokeratin positive[172,173] (Fig. 20.22). The presence of this feature as well as positive staining for AFP differentiates between endodermal sinus tumor showing solid pattern and dysgerminoma, with which it may be confused and which shows only occasional cytokeratin-positive cells.[172]

Endodermal sinus tumor, because of its cystic pattern and presence of numerous small blood vessels, has been confused with vascular tumors, but careful examination reveals that the pattern is more cystic and the absence of a true vascular pattern is confirmed by reticulum stains. The presence of positive immunocytochemical staining for vimentin and for factor VIII further confirms the presence of vascular tissue, whereas positive staining for cytokeratin (Fig. 20.22) favors endodermal sinus tumor. Confusion may occasionally arise, with some Sertoli–Leydig cell tumors showing a retiform pattern.[337] The presence of more marked cellular and nuclear pleomorphism, brisk mitotic activity, the presence of other histologic patterns observed in endodermal sinus tumor and their absence in Sertoli–Leydig cell tumors aid in the differential diagnosis.

Behavior. Endodermal sinus tumor of the ovary is a highly malignant neoplasm, metastasizing early and invading the surrounding structures and organs. Local invasion and intracoelomic spread frequently lead to extensive involvement of the abdominal cavity by tumor deposits. Endodermal sinus tumor metastasizes first via the lymphatic system to the paraaortic and common iliac lymph nodes and then to the mediastinal and supraclavicular lymph nodes. Hematogenous spread occurs later, and metastases are found in the lungs, liver, and other organs. The tumor is very aggressive locally, and spread beyond the ovary is observed in a number of patients at the time of operation.* Recurrences in the pelvis are very frequent, even when the tumor and the affected adnexa have been excised completely.[117,126,138,177,285] They usually appear within a few weeks or months following excision of the primary tumor.

Therapy. Until recent years, the treatment of patients with endodermal sinus tumor was disappointing. The treatment was primarily surgical,† since endodermal sinus tumor is not sensitive to radiation therapy.[23,230] Extensive surgery is of little avail and is not justified, since it does not improve prognosis.[117,126,138] The small number of long-term survivors were mainly patients with tumors confined to the ovary, most of whom were treated by unilateral adnexectomy.‡ Although single-agent chemotherapy or a combination of two agents has been tried without success, in recent years there has been marked improvement in prognosis with conservative surgery (unilateral salpingo-oophorectomy) and adjuvant multiagent combination chemotherapy.§ The combination chemotherapy most frequently used has been dactinomycin, vincristine, and cyclophosphamide[84,89,257,] or dacti-

* References 117, 139, 177, 240, 285, 297–300.

* References 37, 88, 126, 127, 138, 177, 230, 285, 300.
† References 37, 117, 126, 138, 177, 230, 240, 300.
‡ References 37, 117, 126, 127, 138, 177, 240.
§ References 33, 66, 75, 84, 89, 228, 257, 258, 285, 291.

nomycin, 5-fluorouracil, and cyclophosphamide.[75,258] More recently, a combination of *cis*platinum, bleomycin, and vinblastine has been found to be even more effective and has produced remissions in patients with advanced stage disease and in patients in whom other combinations of multiagent chemotherapy have failed.[33,66,89,291] The new adjuvant combination chemotherapy has revolutionized the treatment of patients with endodermal sinus tumor.

Alpha-Fetoprotein and Other Tumor Markers. Alpha-fetoprotein (AFP), an alpha$_1$-globulin, was first identified as a specific constituent of normal human fetal serum by Bergstrand and Czar[26] in 1956. In the human embryo, serum AFP reaches its maximum concentration of approximately 3000 mg/liter at about 12–13 weeks of gestation. Its level then decreases slowly until birth, when the concentration is in the region of 55 mg/liter. After birth, AFP disappears rapidly from the serum, and 3 weeks after full-term delivery, it can be detected only in very small amounts (0–15 ng/ml) by radioimmunoassay or very sensitive enzyme immunoassays.

The sites of AFP synthesis in the human fetus and in other mammalian species have been studied by Gitlin et al.,[91–93] who demonstrated conclusively that during fetal life AFP is produced by the yolk sac, liver, and upper gastrointestinal tract. They also demonstrated that AFP synthesis commences in the yolk sac. In recent years there has been considerable interest in the histologic aspects of germ cell neoplasms associated with elevated serum AFP, and it has been demonstrated that germ cell tumors in patients with elevated serum AFP either are composed entirely of or contain endodermal sinus tumor elements.* Table 20.1 shows the results of preoperative serum AFP determinations in patients with ovarian germ cell tumors. Elevation of serum AFP has not been observed in patients with pure dysgerminoma or seminoma of the testis,† mature cystic teratoma of the ovary,[16,278,286] immature teratoma of the ovary or testes, and pure gonadoblastoma.[278,284,286]

Although very occasional Sertoli–Leydig cell tumors, especially those showing retiform pattern,[337] may be associated with elevated levels of serum AFP,[47,279,338] this has not been observed in patients with other ovarian or testicular tumors that are not of germ cell origin.[278,284,286] Slightly elevated levels of serum AFP up to 60 ng/ml (upper limit of normal serum AFP—20 ng/ml) have been observed in some cases of embryonal carcinoma of the testis.[284,286] This can be explained on the basis of early biochemical differentiation of the embryonal carcinoma in the vitelline direction toward endodermal sinus tumor. Using immunofluorescent and immunoperoxidase techniques, AFP has been identified in the cells of endodermal sinus tumor and in the eosinophilic, PAS-positive, diastase-resistant globules present both inside and outside the tumor cells.[121,126,138,252,301] Large amounts of AFP have been extracted from tumor tissue in endodermal sinus tumors of the ovary and testis.[285,301,325] The results of these studies indicate that endodermal sinus tumor elements are associated with AFP synthesis. In view of the fact that normal yolk sac in the human and other mammalian species has been shown to be associated with AFP synthesis,[93] it is reasonable to assume that tumors differentiating toward yolk sac or vitelline structures, such as endodermal sinus tumor, may also be capable of AFP synthesis in the same way as choriocarcinoma is capable of producing chorionic gonadotropin. This hypothesis[121,138,278,286,302] not only explains the selective synthesis of AFP by some germ cell tumors but also gives further support to the view that endodermal sinus tumor is a germ cell neoplasm resulting from differentiation of primitive malignant germ cell elements in the direction of yolk sac or vitelline structures. The immunocytochemical localization of AFP in embryonal carcinoma and in areas of endodermal sinus tumor showing no morphologic evidence of yolk sac differentiation suggests that the biochemical manifestations of yolk sac differentiation, like AFP synthesis, precede morphologic differentiation.[139]

From a practical point of view, serum AFP determination is considered to be a very useful diagnostic test in patients with endodermal sinus tumor. It is also of value in monitoring the results of therapy and for early detection of metastases and recurrences, although it should be noted that a normal result may not always imply the absence of active disease but only the absence of the tumor element associated with AFP synthesis. Preoperatively, if the tumor contains endodermal sinus tumor elements, the AFP can be detected in the serum and

TABLE 20.1. Serum AFP in patients with ovarian germ cell tumors measured by radioimmunoassay.[a]

	Number of cases	Serum AFP
Mixed germ cell tumors containing EST	39	Elevated
Pure EST	23	Elevated
Pure dysgerminoma	25	Normal
Dysgerminoma with syncytiotrophoblastic giant cells	4	Normal
Teratoma (immature and mature)	12	Normal
Teratoma (immature and mature) with dysgerminoma	8	Normal
Mature cystic teratoma (dermoid cyst)	15	Normal

AFP, alpha-fetoprotein; EST, endodermal sinus tumor.
[a] Unpublished data.

* References 16, 17, 74, 121, 145, 182, 247, 278, 284–286, 292, 300, 326.

† References 256, 278, 284–286, 300.

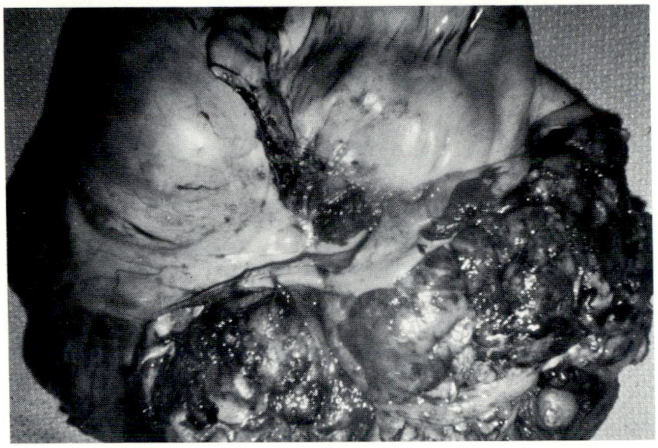

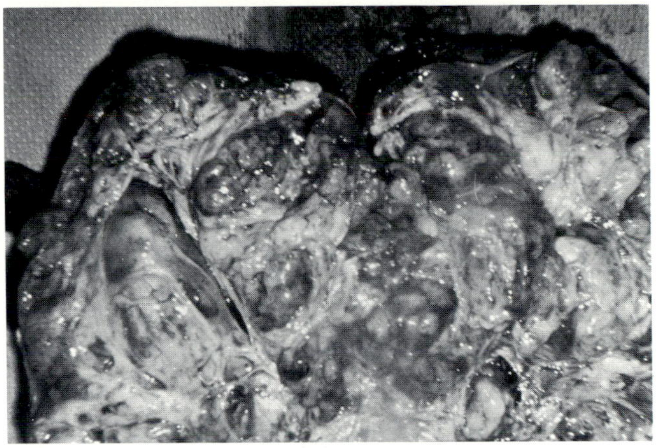

FIG. 20.34. *Left:* Embryonal carcinoma. A large lobular mass that is partially encapsulated. *Right:* The cut surface is red-gray to gray-white in color corresponding to areas of hemorrhage and necrosis.

have a large, prominent, centrally situated, and somewhat irregular vesicular or hyperchromatic nucleus with a fine nuclear membrane and frequently more than one nucleolus. Mitotic activity is usually brisk, and abnormal mitoses are frequently seen. Cellular and nuclear pleomorphism is usually marked. Giant cells and multinucleated cells may be seen. In the slightly better-differentiated tumors, the cells, apart from forming solid areas, also tend to line clefts and spaces and form papillae (Fig. 20.36). The cells appear more epithelial than those of the most undifferentiated type, being more cuboidal or columnar in shape and showing more regular arrangement, mutual orientation, and a suggestion of a formation of a cellular layer (Fig. 20.36). Although there is a suggestion of glandular differentiation, true glandular formations are absent. The papillae are composed of solid collections of cells or may contain a cystic space or a small vessel surrounded by tumor cells. They must be differentiated from perivascular formations observed in endodermal sinus tumor. Very primitive mesenchymal tissue may be present in conjunction with the epithelial-like component.

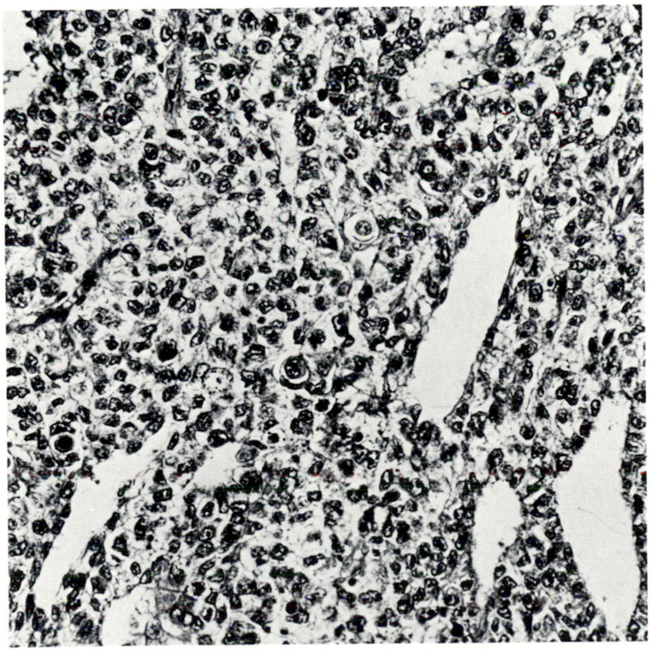

FIG. 20.35. Embryonal carcinoma showing a mainly solid pattern. The tumor was admixed with teratoma and endodermal sinus tumor.

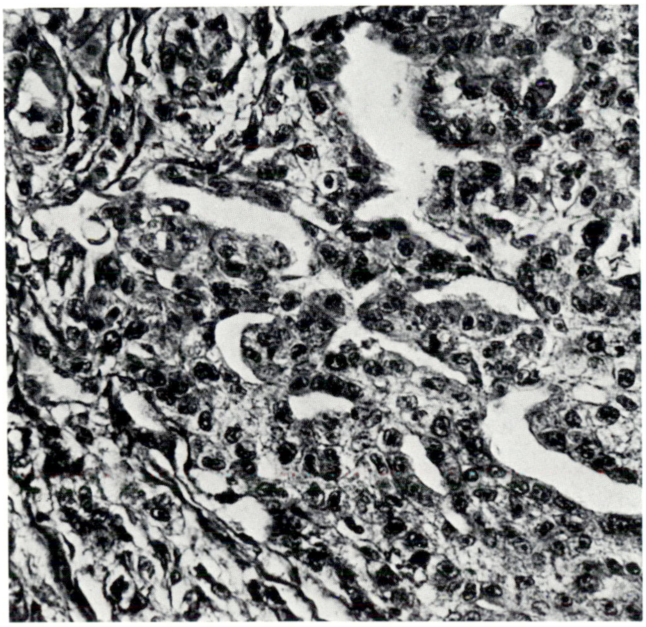

FIG. 20.36. Embryonal carcinoma forming clefts and spaces. [Reprinted with permission from The American College of Obstetricians and Gynecologists. (Obstetrics and Gynecology, 43:138, 1974).]

Syncytiotrophoblastic giant cells immediately adjacent to aggregates of embryonal carcinoma cells or lying isolated in the stroma are found very frequently. Foci of necrosis and hemorrhage are frequently seen.

Differential Diagnosis. Embryonal carcinoma may be present in the form of small solid aggregates or of pseudoglandular or cleftlike formations surrounded by better-differentiated malignant teratomatous elements showing somatic differentiation. It may coexist with other neoplastic germ cell elements, such as endodermal sinus tumor, immature or mature teratoma, choriocarcinoma, polyembryoma, or dysgerminoma. It may be occasionally confused with the last. Differentiation from dysgerminoma is very important because of a totally different prognosis and response to treatment. It is usually the solid primitive type of embryonal carcinoma that is more likely to be confused with dysgerminoma, since the presence of clefts, alveoli, or cell-lined spaces militates against the diagnosis of dysgerminoma. The cells of embryonal carcinoma are usually larger and show much more marked cellular and nuclear pleomorphism. Mitotic activity is usually more prominent, and bizarre mitoses are more frequent. The nuclear membrane is less sharp and the nuclei are more irregular, are larger, and usually contain more than one dark hyperchromatic nucleolus, in contrast to the rounded, prominent, usually single, and frequently eosinophilic nucleolus of dysgerminoma. The presence of connective tissue stroma infiltrated by lymphocytes and granulomatous reaction are prominent features of dysgerminoma. Their usual, although not invariable, absence in embryonal carcinoma is an important differentiating feature.

Cells of embryonal carcinoma stain positively for cytokeratin, whereas the great majority of dysgerminoma cells are negative. In addition, the majority of embryonal carcinomas show at least some positive staining for AFP, whereas dysgerminoma cells are invariably negative. Immunocytochemical localization of AFP and cytokeratin provides a useful method for differentiating between these two neoplasms.[21,172,173]

Behavior and Therapy. Embryonal carcinoma of the ovary, as its testicular counterpart, is a highly malignant neoplasm. It is aggressive locally, spreads extensively in the abdominal cavity, and metastasizes early. The metastatic spread is similar to that observed with other germ cell neoplasms, taking place first via the lymphatic system and later by hematogenous spread. The primary treatment of embryonal carcinoma is surgical. Since the tumors are usually unilateral, conservative treatment is advocated if the tumor is localized to the ovary. Embryonal carcinoma is not radiosensitive. The prognosis in the past has been unfavorable, but introduction of the various forms of combination chemotherapy effective in the treatment of malignant germ cell tumors has led to marked improvement. The response to combination chemotherapy using vincristine, dactinomycin, and cyclophosphamide or preferably bleomycin, vinblastine, and cisplatin is probably similar to that observed in patients with embryonal carcinoma of the testis.[10,66,95,228,259]

Polyembryoma

Synonyms

Polyembryonic embryoma,[254] malignant teratoma with embryoid bodies.[22]

Polyembryoma is a very rare ovarian germ cell neoplasm composed of numerous embryoid bodies resembling morphologically normal presomite embryos. Similar homologous neoplasms occur more frequently in the human testis,[22,70,71,300] although pure polyembryoma is altogether very rare. Only eight cases of ovarian polyembryoma have been recorded.[22,268] In all these cases, the polyembryoma was associated with other neoplastic germ cell elements, mainly immature, or with mature teratoma.[22,254,268] All these tumors occurred in young patients or in patients in the reproductive age group.[22,202,254,268] The oldest patient was 38 years old.[254] The clinical findings are similar to those observed in patients with other malignant germ cell neoplasms of the ovary.

Histogenesis. There are conflicting views of the origin of embryoid bodies. It has been suggested that they arise by parthenogenic development from primitive germ cells present in malignant teratoma, indicating the mode of origin of teratomatous tumors, and therefore this may be considered as a model of their histogenesis.[164,203,254] Other investigators question this view as well as the entire concept that embryoid bodies bear a close similarity to early human embryos, since embryoid bodies never appear to develop beyond the 18-day stage.[22,329,330] They consider that embryoid bodies probably develop transiently by bizarre differentiation, possibly in response to local release of organizers in malignant teratomas of the gonads. Another view that has been advanced accepts the morphologic similarities between the early embryo and the embryoid bodies but disputes their parthenogenic origin.[70,205,206,262,263] It maintains that embryoid bodies are formed after initiation of teratogenesis, most likely from multipotential malignant embryonal cells present in a tumor and not directly from germ cells.[264] This is supported by the observations of the development of embryoid bodies from undifferentiated embryonal cells in strain-129 mice. The tumor, a teratoma that had been serially transplanted for many years, was considered to be devoid of germ cells.[205,206,262,263] These findings are in accordance with the view that embryoid bodies probably persist only transiently within the tumor, and while new embryoid bodies are being formed others lose their identity and their multipotential cells undergo further differentiation.[71] Although the origin and development of embryoid bodies are still a matter of dispute, the view that they originate from multipotential malignant embryonal cells, which is supported by experimental observations,[205,206,262,263] is most favored at present.

Macroscopic Appearance. Polyembryoma is usually unilateral. Macroscopically, the tumor resembles other malignant germ cell tumors, varying in size from relatively small (9.5 cm in longest diameter)[22] to tumors filling almost the whole abdominal cavity and invading the surrounding structures.[254] The tumor is usually solid and contains hemorrhagic and necrotic areas.

Microscopic Appearance. Polyembryoma is composed of numerous embryoid bodies, and the better-differentiated ones are composed of an embryonic disk, amniotic cavity, and yolk sac surrounded by primitive extraembryonic mesenchyme (Fig. 20.37). Sometimes trophoblastic differentiation may be seen in the vicinity of the embryoid body. When the embryoid bodies are less well-formed, they are composed of a medullary plate and amnion associated with a blastocystic space or with extraembryonic mesenchyme. They may have two or more amniotic cavities and share a single yolk sac cavity or vice versa. There may be a considerable disproportion between the two cavities, and the cavities may be malformed. There may be a considerable variation in size between the different embryoid bodies; some may be more primitive and others appear to be better developed. Some embryoid bodies may be severely malformed and show bizarre appearances (Fig. 20.38). None of the embryoid bodies appear to have developed beyond the 18-day stage. The embryonic disk of a classic embryoid body is lined on one side by cuboidal epithelial cells of uniform size, resembling endoderm, and on the other by tall columnar epithelium, resembling ectoderm. The latter merges with low cuboidal epithelium lining the rest of the cavity, which resembles the amnion. The cavity resembling the yolk sac is on the opposite side of the embryonic disk from the amnion (Fig. 20.37). The embryoid bodies are surrounded by extraembryonic mesenchyme, which is composed of either closely or more loosely packed spindle-shaped cells of regular appearance (Fig. 20.37) and showing occasional mitotic figures. Loose myxomatous areas may be present (Fig. 20.38). Teratomatous structures in various stages of differentiation are frequently seen interspersed among the embryoid bodies. In one reported case,[22] hCG and human placental lactogen were demonstrated within syncytiotrophoblastic cells that were present in the vicinity of the embryoid bodies. Cytotrophoblastic cells were not identified in this tumor. In another reported case, there was elevation of serum AFP and hCG. AFP was demonstrated by immunoperoxidase within the cells lining the yolk sac cavities and hCG within the syncytiotrophoblastic giant cells that were present in the vicinity of the embryoid bodies.[268]

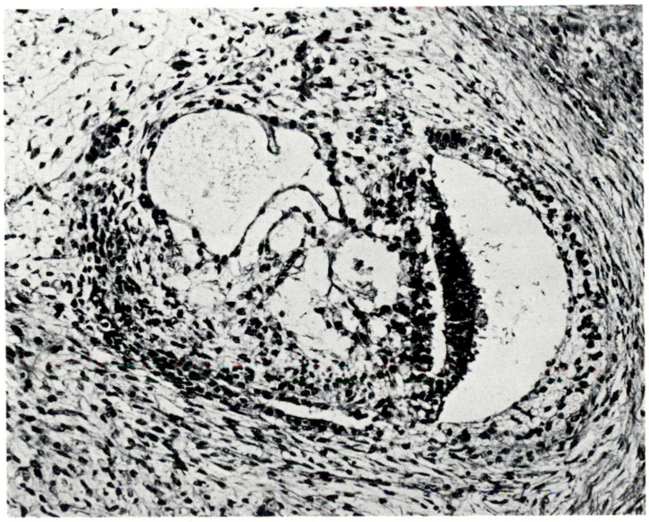

FIG. 20.37. Polyembryoma. Embryoid body showing amniotic cavity (*right*), embryonic disk (*center*), and atypical yolk sac (*left*).

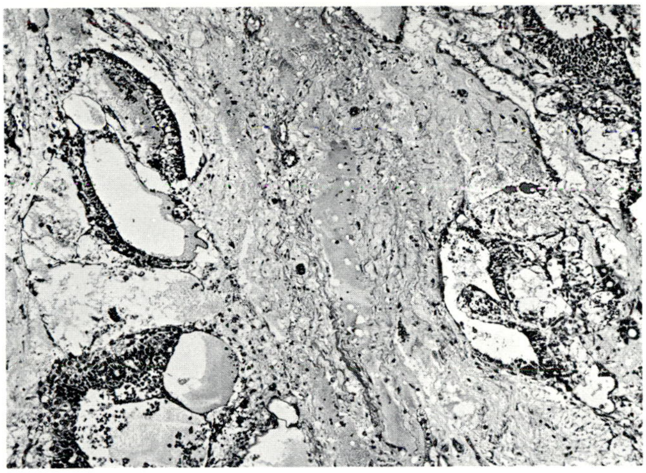

FIG. 20.38. Polyembryoma. Embryoid bodies showing bizarre appearances.

Behavior and Therapy. Polyembryoma is a highly malignant germ cell neoplasm. In the majority of cases, it has been associated with invasion of adjacent structures and organs and extensive metastases, which were mainly confined to the abdominal cavity.[254] One patient with a relatively small mobile tumor, absence of capsular penetration, and no evidence of metastases has survived more than 5 years.[22] Another patient was well and disease free 6 months after diagnosis,[268] but the other patients with polyembryoma have died of their disease.

The primary treatment of polyembryoma is surgical, and since the tumor is usually unilateral unless there is spread beyond the ovary, excision of the tumor and the adjoining adnexa is the treatment of choice. The tumor is not sensitive to radiotherapy, but responds to the combination chemotherapy used in treatment of malignant germ cell tumors.[268]

Choriocarcinoma

Synonyms

Chorioncarcinoma, chorionepithelioma, teratomatous choriocarcinoma.

Pure ovarian choriocarcinoma of germ cell origin is a very rare neoplasm,[316] and even the presence of choriocarcinomatous elements admixed with other neoplastic germ cell elements is considered to be rare in ovarian tumors.[71] In the majority of cases, the tumor is admixed with other neoplastic germ cell elements, and their presence is diagnostic of nongestational choriocarcinoma, except for the remote possibility of the tumor being a gestational choriocarcinoma metastatic to an ovarian germ cell tumor. The presence of other neoplastic germ cell elements is a particularly helpful diagnostic feature in postmenarchal patients, in whom exclusion of gestational origin of the tumor may be difficult. In view of this, it is considered that nongestational choriocarcinoma may be diagnosed with confidence in postmenarchal patients and not only in young children, as had been considered earlier.[191] At least 50 cases of ovarian germ cell tumors containing choriocarcinoma have been reported.* The tumor, in common with other malignant germ cell neoplasms, occurs in children and young adults. Its occurrence in children has been emphasized; in some series, 50% of cases occurred in children who had not reached puberty.[165] This high incidence in children may result from the previous reluctance of making the diagnosis in adults.

Histogenesis. Choriocarcinoma of the ovary may originate in three different ways:

1. As a primary gestational choriocarcinoma associated with ovarian pregnancy
2. As metastatic choriocarcinoma from a primary gestational choriocarcinoma arising in other parts of the genital tract, mainly the uterus
3. As a germ cell tumor differentiating in the direction of trophoblastic structures, usually admixed with other neoplastic germ cell elements

In each case it is very important to ascertain the mode of origin of the tumor, as apart from the histogenetic aspects there are important practical therapeutic and prognostic considerations. Alternatively, choriocarcinoma of the ovary may be divided into two broad groups: (1) gestational choriocarcinoma encompassing the first two groups mentioned above and (2) nongestational choriocarcinoma, a germ cell tumor differentiating toward trophoblastic structures. As this chapter deals solely with germ cell tumors, only the nongestational choriocarcinoma is discussed here.

Clinical Aspects. The clinical findings in patients with ovarian nongestational choriocarcinoma are similar to those observed in patients with other malignant ovarian germ cell neoplasms, except that they may be modified by the endocrine activity of the tumor, which secretes hCG. This is particularly noticeable in prepubertal children who show evidence of isosexual precocious puberty, with mammary development, growth of pubic and axillary hair, and uterine bleeding. Adult patients may have signs of ectopic pregnancy. Because the nongestational choriocarcinoma, like its gestational counterpart, is associated with increased production of hCG, estimation of urinary or plasma hCG is a very useful diagnostic test. Serum hCG levels are also useful in monitoring the progress of the disease and its response to therapy, as well as in detecting metastases and recurrences containing choriocarcinomatous tissue. It should be noted that normal levels of hCG do not exclude the presence of metastases or recurrences composed of other neoplastic germ cell elements. Chorionic gonadotropin can be extracted from tumor tissue, and its presence within tumor tissue can be demonstrated by immunofluorescent and immunoperoxidase techniques. In view of this, the determination of serum or plasma hCG is strongly recommended in all cases of malignant germ cell tumors, especially in those in which choriocarcinomatous elements or syncytiotrophoblastic giant cells are present. Table 20.2 shows the results of preoperative serum hCG and beta-hCG determinations in patients with ovarian germ cell tumors.

Macroscopic Appearance. The tumor is usually unilateral, solid, gray-white, and hemorrhagic. Necrosis may be in evidence. The tumors are usually of considerable size. Since most of these tumors are composed of a combination of neoplastic germ cell elements, the appearances tend to vary according to the elements present in the tumor.

Microscopic Appearance. Choriocarcinoma is composed of two types of cells, the cytotrophoblast and the syncytiotrophoblast, and both should be present if a definite diagnosis is to be made (Fig. 20.39). The cytotrophoblast is composed of medium-sized polygonal, round, or oval cells with clear cytoplasm, sharp nuclear borders, and centrally situated, small, round, and hyperchromatic nuclei or larger vesicular nuclei containing nucleoli and

* References 32, 59, 76, 142, 165, 191, 230, 312.

TABLE 20.2. Serum hCG and beta-hCG in ovarian germ cell tumors measured by radioimmunoassay.[a]

	Number of cases	Serum hCG
Mixed germ cell tumors containing choriocarcinoma	8	Elevated
Mixed germ cell tumors containing EST	26	Normal
Pure EST	15	Normal
Pure dysgerminoma	18	Normal
Dysgerminoma with syncytiotrophoblastic giant cells	3	Elevated
Teratoma (immature and mature)	8	Normal
Teratoma (immature and mature) and dysgerminoma	7	Normal
Mature cystic teratoma (dermoid cyst)	11	Normal

hCG, human chorionic gonadotropin; EST, endodermal sinus tumor.
[a] Unpublished data.

showing brisk mitotic activity. The syncytiotrophoblast is composed of large basophilic, vacuolated cells with irregular outlines, and although frequently elongated, they may vary in shape. These cells contain multiple hyperchromatic nuclei, varying in shape and size, or large masses of chromatin. The cytotrophoblastic cells are usually disposed centrally within a tumor mass and are partly or completely surrounded by irregular collections or layers of the syncytiotrophoblastic cells (Fig. 20.39). There is a considerable variation in the pattern and in the ratio of the two components in different parts of the same tumor and in different tumors. The tumor cells form solid aggregates, nearly always associated with hemorrhage and necrosis, which may be so extensive that the tumor tissue is hardly recognizable. The tumor tissue may be seen on the outside of a hemorrhagic area and may form a projection into the hemorrhagic mass. When the tumor is combined with other germ cell elements, the choriocarcinoma may form small nodules associated with hemorrhage and surrounded by other germ cell elements. The presence of other germ cell elements within the tumor is a frequent finding.

It appears that the cytotrophoblast is the more primitive element, and the syncytiotrophoblast is formed from it either directly or indirectly. The syncytiotrophoblast is the differentiated, nondividing, hormone-secreting component. These findings are supported by electron microscopic and immunohistochemical studies[207,210] (Fig. 20.40).

Behavior and Therapy. Nongestational choriocarcinoma of the ovary is a highly malignant germ cell neoplasm. It invades adjacent structures, spreads widely throughout

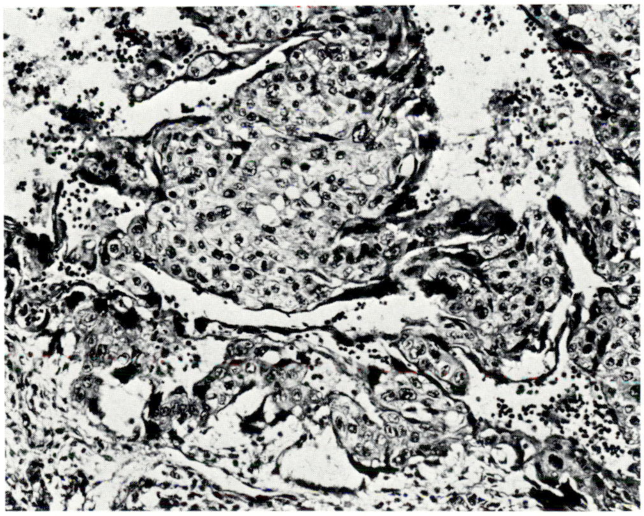

FIG. 20.39. Choriocarcinoma showing cytotrophoblast composed of medium-sized cells, situated centrally, and syncytiotrophoblast composed of very large multinucleated cells, situated peripherally.

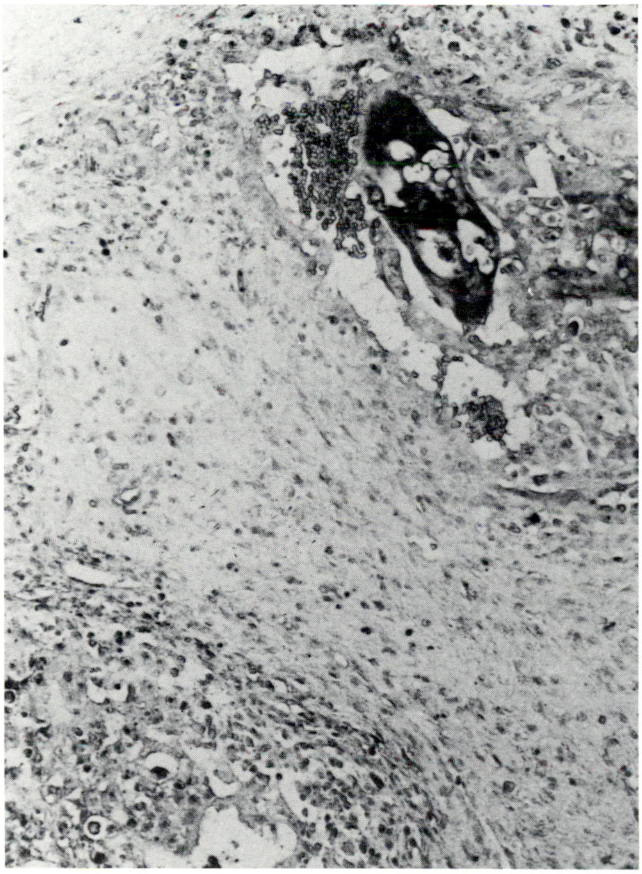

FIG. 20.40. Mixed germ cell tumor containing choriocarcinoma. The syncytiotrophoblastic element of the latter shows strong positive staining for beta-hCG. The cytotrophoblast is negative. Note the hemorrhage that is usually associated with this tumor.

the abdominal cavity, and metastasizes via both the lymphatics and the blood vessels. Although gestational choriocarcinoma tends to spread primarily via the bloodstream, nongestational choriocarcinoma shows lymphatic and intraabdominal spread and hematogenous spread may not be so marked. The prognosis of patients with choriocarcinoma is unfavorable but may be somewhat better than of patients with endodermal sinus tumor. In one large series there were 4 survivors out of 12 patients with tumors containing choriocarcinoma, as compared to 5 out of 35 patients with tumors containing endodermal sinus tumor.[127,334]

Unlike gestational choriocarcinoma, the treatment of which has been revolutionized by the discovery that it responds to methotrexate, nongestational choriocarcinoma does not respond to this drug.[127,144,240,300] Since these tumors are also not radiosensitive, the treatment has been primarily surgical. Although occasional therapeutic successes have been achieved,[59,127] these usually have been in patients with small tumors, and the successful treatment has consisted of unilateral ovariectomy or adnexectomy. More recently, in spite of the lack of success with single-agent chemotherapy using methotrexate, a combination therapy using three or more chemotherapeutic agents including vinblastine, cisplatin, and bleomycin, has been tried with some success in a number of cases.[32,33,89,95,291,323]

Teratoma

Histogenesis. The origin of teratomas has been a matter of interest, speculation, and dispute for centuries. In the past, many theories have been advanced to explain their origin, including witchcraft, nightmares, and many other bizarre causes.[30] In more recent times, three main theories have been put forward. Of these, the most recently propounded is the parthenogenic theory, which suggests an origin from the primordial germ cell. It has been steadily gaining support and is now generally accepted. The other two theories, one suggesting an origin from blastomeres segregated at an early stage of embryonic development and the second suggesting an origin from embryonal rests, have few adherents nowadays.[71,190] Support for the germ cell theory has come from the anatomic distribution of the tumors, which occur along the line of migration of the primordial germ cells from the yolk sac to the primitive gonad, and from the fact that the tumors occur most commonly during the years of reproductive activity. Support also comes from animal experiments in which cystic teratomas can be produced only during the period of reproductive activity of the gonad, as in roosters injected with zinc and copper salts,[15,42] and from the nuclear sexing and karyotyping of teratomas. It has been shown that cells of ovarian teratomas are always chromatin-positive, unlike the cells of testicular teratomas, which may be chromatin-negative, chromatin-positive, or mixed in this order.[307] The karyotypes of all benign ovarian teratomas studied have been found to be 46XX.[51,85,148,218] Further support for the germ cell theory of origin has come from the recent work of Linder et al.[146–148] They studied the histogenesis of mature cystic teratoma of the ovary using both cytogenetic techniques and the electrophoretic variants of four enzymes in normal as well as in tumor cells. They have demonstrated that these tumors are of germ cell origin and arise from a single germ cell after the first meiotic division.[148]

Classification. Ovarian teratomas have usually been divided into two main groups. One includes the great majority of cases (99%) composed of the cystic and mature forms, also known as dermoid cysts; the remaining very small group is composed of the solid and immature forms.* Tumors composed entirely or to a large extent of thyroid tissue known as *struma ovarii* were included in the larger group of dermoid cysts or were sometimes classified separately. In recent years, more detailed classifications of ovarian teratoma have been proposed, taking into account new information that has come to light concerning the morphology and behavior of this group of neoplasms.[123,239–241,250]

The classification adopted in this chapter is the one recently proposed by the WHO Ovarian Tumor Panel,[250] and the ovarian teratomas have been divided into the following subgroups:

1. Immature
2. Mature
   a. Solid
   b. Cystic
      i. Mature cystic teratoma (dermoid cyst)
      ii. Mature cystic teratoma (dermoid cyst) with malignant transformation
3. Monodermal and highly specialized
   a. Struma ovarii
   b. Carcinoid
   c. Strumal carcinoid
   d. Others

Immature Teratoma

Immature teratomas are composed of tissues derived from the three germ layers—ectoderm, mesoderm, and endoderm—and, in contrast to the very much more common mature teratoma, they contain immature or embryonal structures. Mature tissues are frequently present and sometimes may predominate. In these cases, the tumor should be differentiated from a mature teratoma with malignant transformation. The presence of immature or embryonal elements as opposed to the neoplastic

* References 71, 110, 185, 189, 299, 334.

transformation of mature tissues differentiates between these two types of neoplasm.

Clinical Aspects. The immature teratoma of the ovary is an uncommon tumor, comprising less than 1% of teratomas of the ovary.[36,43,161,188,334] In contrast to the mature cystic teratoma, which is encountered most frequently during the reproductive years but occurs at all ages, the immature teratoma has a very specific age incidence, occurring most commonly in the first two decades of life and being almost unknown after the menopause.[36,37,161,334] In view of this, teratomas occurring in childhood, adolescence, and early adult life should always be very carefully examined and thoroughly sampled.

The tumor is usually asymptomatic until it reaches a considerable size. It tends to grow rapidly and may manifest itself as a pelvic or lower abdominal mass. It may cause pressure symptoms, abdominal heaviness, or dull pain, or it may undergo torsion, causing acute abdominal pain.

Macroscopic Appearance. The tumor is usually unilateral[36,37,43,189,330,334] but may coexist with a benign cystic teratoma in the opposite ovary.[331] The tumors are usually large, varying in size from 9 to 28 cm in the longest diameter.[37] They may form a round, oval, or lobulated soft or firm mass (Fig. 20.41). The tumor is often prone to perforate its capsule, which is not always well-defined.[36,37,331] It tends to form adhesions to the surrounding structures and to invade locally.[36,37] The tumor is predominantly solid but frequently contains cystic structures.[36,37,43,161,331] Occasionally, it may be predominantly cystic, with solid areas present in the cyst wall.[37,154,309] The cut surface is usually variegated, trabeculated, and lobulated, varying in color from gray to dark brown. Occasionally, foci of cartilage or bone may be recognizable and hair may be present. The cystic areas are usually filled with serous or mucinous fluid, colloid, or fatty material.

Microscopic Appearance. The tumor is composed of a variety of immature and mature tissues derived from the three germ layers. Occasionally, the tumor may be composed of a small number of tissues, although usually derivatives of all the three germ layers are present. Ectoderm is usually represented by neural tissue. Glia, ganglion cells, neuroblastic tissue (Fig. 20.42), neuroepithelium, nerve trunks, and ocular structures are often represented. Skin elements (Fig. 20.42), including pilosebaceous units, sweat glands, and hair, are not infrequently present. Mesodermal elements include fibrous connective tissue, cartilage (Fig. 20.42), bone, muscle, usually smooth but occasionally striated, lymphoid tissue, and undifferentiated embryonic mesenchyme. Endodermal elements are usually represented by tubules lined by columnar, sometimes ciliated, epithelium. Occasionally, gastrointestinal or bronchial epithelium may be present. All these tissues, which may be in stages of maturity varying from embryonic to mature, are scattered haphazardly throughout the tumor and so differ from the orderly organoid arrangement seen in a mature teratoma. In cases where the tumor is composed mainly of mature tissues, differentiation from mature teratoma may be difficult, and patients have been diagnosed as having a benign lesion only to return within a short time with recurrence. In a number of such cases, review of the material taken from the original tumor has revealed immature elements. Therefore, careful examination and thorough sampling of the tumor are strongly recommended. Immature teratoma may be combined with other neoplastic germ cell elements, such as endodermal sinus tumor, dysgerminoma, embryonal carcinoma, choriocarcinoma, and polyembryoma. It can therefore form a part of a malignant germ cell tumor composed of two or more neoplastic germ cell elements (mixed germ cell tumor). Immature teratoma has been reported to develop from the germ cell element of gonadoblastoma.[242]

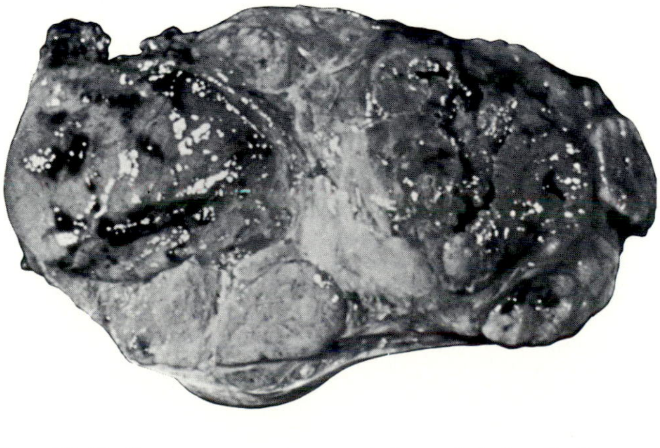

FIG. 20.41. Immature teratoma. A large lobulated, firm to soft tumor mass with areas of hemorrhage and necrosis.

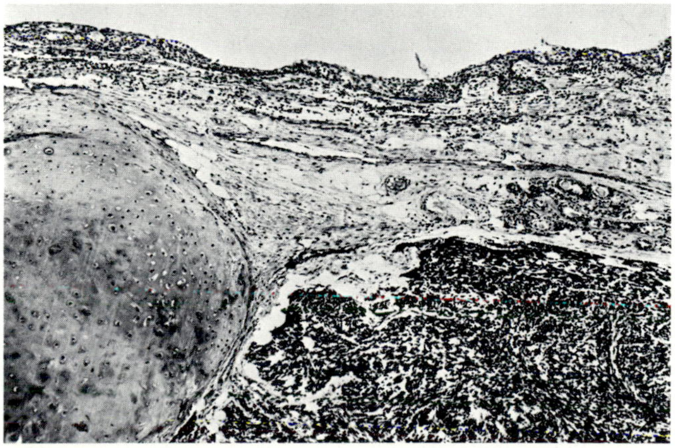

FIG. 20.42. Immature teratoma showing both solid and cystic areas. The tumor was mainly composed of neuroblastic tissue (*right*). Note the squamous epithelium, adnexal glands, and cartilage.

Differential Diagnosis. Immature solid teratoma must be differentiated from the malignant mixed müllerian (mesodermal) tumor, which although occurring most frequently in the uterus also occurs in the ovary. Malignant mixed müllerian (mesodermal) tumor is composed of derivatives of müllerian mesoderm, a primitive structure that gives rise both to the stroma and epithelium of the endometrium. The monodermal origin of malignant mixed müllerian (mesodermal) tumor distinguishes it from teratoma.[290] Malignant mixed müllerian (mesodermal) tumor occurs most frequently in postmenopausal women between the ages of 50 and 70 years and, unlike solid immature teratoma, only occasionally occurs in younger patients. The tumor is composed of sarcomatous and carcinomatous tissue. The carcinoma is invariably an adenocarcinoma, squamous cell carcinoma, or adenosquamous carcinoma, and the sarcomatous elements may be composed of a wide variety of tissues, including leiomyosarcoma, chondrosarcoma, rhabdomyosarcoma, fibrosarcoma, undifferentiated sarcomatous tissue, and myxomatous tissue. Derivatives of the three germ layers are absent in malignant mixed müllerian (mesodermal) tumor; neuroectodermal derivatives, prominent in solid immature teratoma, are never seen. Malignant mixed müllerian (mesodermal) tumor does not exhibit the great variety of tissues present in teratoma, and the tissues present in malignant mixed müllerian (mesodermal) tumor generally form more typical sarcomatous or carcinomatous patterns (see Chapter 13, Mesenchymal Tumors of Uterus).

Behavior and Therapy. Immature teratoma is a malignant neoplasm that usually grows rapidly, penetrates its capsule, and forms adhesions to the surrounding structures. It spreads throughout the peritoneal cavity by implantation. It metastasizes first to the retroperitoneal, paraaortic, and more distant lymph nodes and later to the lungs, liver, and other organs. Peritoneal implants and metastases are not infrequently present at operation for the removal of the primary tumor.[36,37,331] Excision of the tumor is usually followed by a local recurrence, which occurs within a few weeks or months. Recurrences usually occur within the first year following the primary treatment, and patients free from recurrence for 12–18 months survive.[36,37] Rupture of the tumor with spillage of the contents during operation is not infrequent and tends to be associated with poor outcome. The metastases and peritoneal implants may be composed of different tissues, and thus their teratomatous nature is readily apparent, but they may also be composed of a single tissue. The histologic appearances of the metastases and of the peritoneal implants may or may not reflect the appearances of the primary tumor.

In the past treatment has been unsatisfactory and prognosis was poor, with less than 20% of patients surviving 5 years after the operation.[36,43,161] Better results have been claimed in cases where the only immature element was neurogenic.[161,334] It has been noted that there is a good correlation between the histologic appearances of the tumor and prognosis.[184,309] Very immature and poorly differentiated tumors have been found to be associated with worse prognosis, whereas a more favorable outcome has been observed in patients with more mature and better differentiated tumors.[184,309,331]

A histologic grading has been proposed and is of value for prognostic purposes. This grading,[309] is based on the relative amounts of immature and mature tissues present within the tumor and differentiation and mitotic activity within the immature components, is as follows:

Grade 0	All tissues mature; no mitotic activity
Grade 1	Minor foci of abnormally cellular or embryonal tissue mixed with mature elements; slight mitotic activity
Grade 2	Moderate quantities of embryonal tissue mixed with mature elements; moderate mitotic activity
Grade 3	Large quantities of embryonal tissue present; high mitotic activity

Although the value of this grading has not been accepted by some investigators,[36,37] there is good evidence that in uncomplicated cases such a relationship exists.[309] The value of this histologic grading based on the mitotic activity and maturation of the tissue as a prognostic index has been supported recently by some investigators,[184] and its use is strongly recommended.

The recommended treatment for patients with immature teratoma has been bilateral adnexectomy and hysterectomy,[35,110] but it has become apparent that since the tumors are very rarely bilateral, there is no advantage in performing a radical operation unless the opposite ovary and uterus are involved.[36,240,331,334] Although radiation therapy has frequently been used to treat immature teratoma, the tumor does not respond to radiotherapy.[36,37,162] It shows a good response to combination therapy using either vincristine, dactinomycin, and cyclophosphamide (VAC), or vinblastine, bleomycin, and cisplatin (VBP) regimens. Therapy with VAC is the treatment of choice,[89,184,257,258,291] since the results obtained are similar to those with VBP and the latter is more toxic.

Mature Solid Teratoma

Synonyms

Solid adult teratoma, benign solid teratoma.

Solid mature teratoma is a very rare ovarian neoplasm and a very uncommon type of ovarian teratoma. The age incidence is similar to that of solid immature teratoma, the tumor occurring mainly in children and young adults.[200,309,325] The majority of solid ovarian teratomas are composed at least partly of immature tissues and are therefore considered to be malignant. The occasional cases of solid ovarian teratoma composed entirely of mature tissues have usually been included in this group and thus misinterpreted as malignant. At the same time, this practice has improved the survival statistics, which were generally very poor in patients with immature ovarian teratoma. Solid mature teratoma is composed entirely of mature tissues derived from the three germ layers. Very rigid diagnostic criteria must be strictly adhered to, and the examination and sampling of the tumor must be very thorough, since inclusion of cases with immature elements completely changes the prognosis of this neoplasm, which otherwise is excellent.[189,200,309,331,334] Neurogenic elements, which are one of the most common tissues present in this tumor, may often be the cause of difficulties.[240] The presence of immature neural elements immediately excludes the tumor from this group, as by definition only tumors composed entirely of mature tissues may be included.

Macroscopic Appearance. The tumors are usually large, do not show any specific features, and show similar appearance to the majority of solid teratomas, which are composed of immature tissues. They grow slowly in comparison with immature solid teratoma, but since they are usually discovered after they have reached a considerable size, this feature is of little help in diagnosis. In all reported cases of solid mature teratoma, the tumor has been unilateral.[188,200,309,331,334]

Microscopic Appearance. The tumor is composed of a variety of tissues derived from the three germ layers and arranged in an orderly manner resembling the much more common mature cystic teratoma, except that they form a solid pattern or at least a predominantly solid pattern. The tumor is composed entirely of mature tissues (Figs. 20.43 and 20.44). Sometimes neurogenic elements may predominate (Fig. 20.44).

Occasionally, solid mature teratoma may be associated with peritoneal implants composed entirely of mature glial tissue. (Fig. 20.45). In spite of extensive involvement that may be present and irrespective of the mode of therapy employed, the prognosis is excellent.[219] Presence of peritoneal implants composed entirely of mature glial tissue may occasionally be observed in patients with immature solid teratoma and with mature cystic teratoma. The prognosis is likewise excellent.[178,219]

Behavior and Therapy. Since the tumor is unilateral, oophorectomy or unilateral adnexectomy is the treatment of choice, resulting in a complete cure.[200,309,331,334]

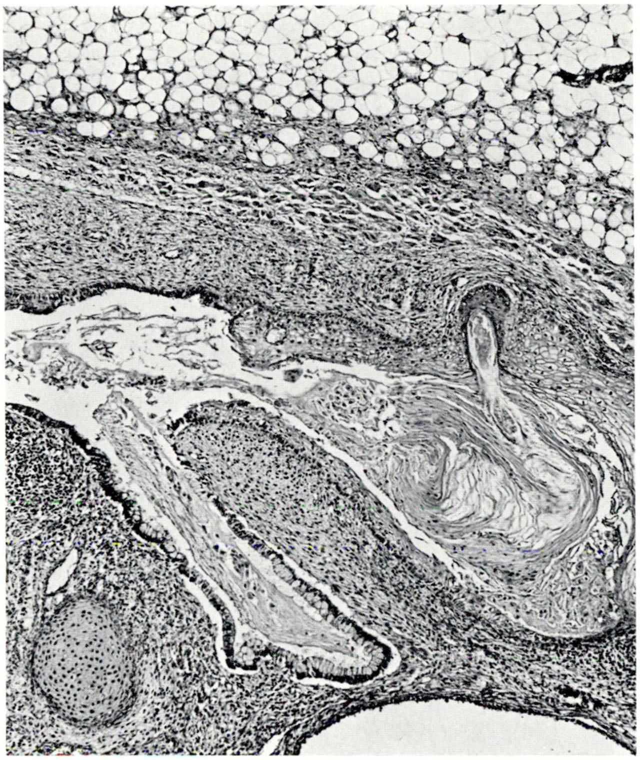

Fig. 20.43. Mature solid teratoma composed of squamous and glandular epithelium, adipose and fibrous tissue, and cartilage.

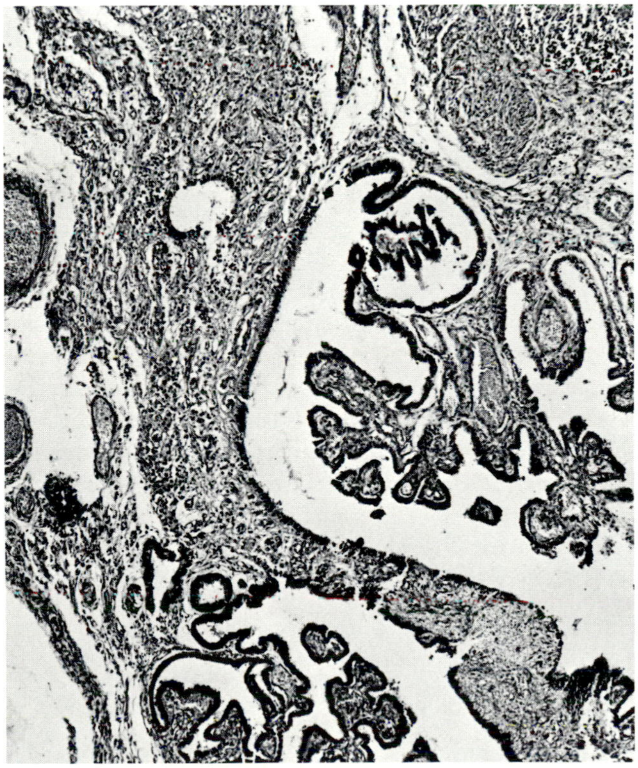

Fig. 20.44. Mature solid teratoma composed of mature neural tissue and choroid plexus.

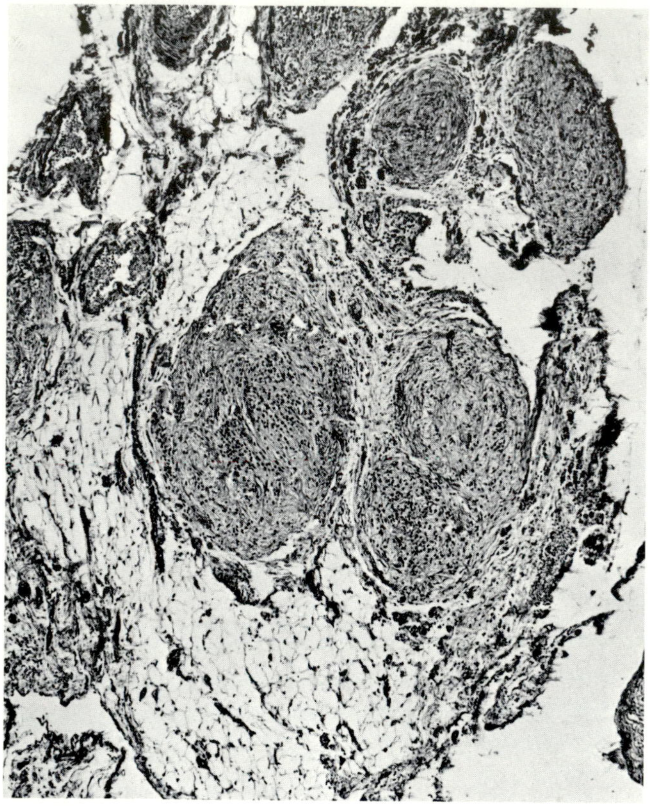

Fig. 20.45. Mature solid teratoma. Mature glial implants on omentum.

Mature Cystic Teratoma

Synonyms

Dermoid cyst, dermoid, adult cystic teratoma, benign cystic teratoma.

Mature cystic teratoma of the ovary, or dermoid cyst, has been known since antiquity. The tumor is composed of well-differentiated derivatives of the three germ layers—ectoderm, mesoderm, and endoderm—with ectodermal elements predominating. In its pure form, mature cystic teratoma is always benign, but occasionally it may undergo malignant change in one of its elements. It may also form a part of a germ cell neoplasm composed of a number of different neoplastic germ cell elements (mixed germ cell tumor).

Clinical Aspects. Mature cystic teratoma is the most common type of ovarian teratoma and the most common type of ovarian germ cell neoplasm. It occurs relatively frequently and comprises from 5 to 25% of all ovarian neoplasms,[202] usually in excess of 10%.[30,109,169,202] Mature cystic teratoma occurs most commonly during the reproductive years, but, unlike other germ cell tumors of the ovary, it has a wider age distribution and may be encountered at any age from infancy to old age.[43,202] In some series, more than 25% of cases have been observed in postmenopausal women.[160]

Mature cystic teratoma is often discovered as an incidental finding on physical examination, radiologic examination, or at abdominal operation performed for other indications. When symptoms are present, they are usually abdominal pain (47.6%), abdominal mass, or swelling (15.4%), and abnormal uterine bleeding (15.1%).[202] The abdominal pain is usually constant, slight, or moderate but, in a number of cases, may be severe and acute because of torsion or rupture of the tumor. This tends to occur more commonly when the tumor is large. The abnormal uterine bleeding and its relief after excision of the tumor may suggest the presence of endocrine imbalance. Histologic examination of the neoplasms in such cases has failed to reveal any explanation for the endocrine imbalance.[160] Decreased fertility has been observed in patients with mature cystic teratoma of the ovary,[30,109] but in most cases there is no satisfactory explanation of this finding. In 10% of cases, however, the tumor is diagnosed during pregnancy.[43] Mature cystic teratoma may be diagnosed radiologically because of the presence of teeth, bone, and cartilage (Fig. 20.46). A number of cases have been diagnosed preoperatively in this manner.[160,202]

Macroscopic Appearance. Mature cystic teratoma does not have any special predilection for either ovary. In 7.9–15% of cases it is bilateral.[202] The tumor varies in size from very small (0.5 cm across) to very large (measuring in excess of 40 cm) and weighing many kilograms. Approximately 60% of mature cystic teratomas measure from 5 to 10 cm across, and more than 90% measure less than 15 cm across.[202] The tumor is round, oval, or globular, with a smooth, gray-white, glistening surface (Fig. 20.46). It is usually freely mobile but occasionally may form adhesions to the surrounding structures, especially if there has been leakage of the contents. On palpation, the tumor is soft and fluctuant, with firm or hard areas. This is usually observed immediately after its removal from the body, since at room temperature the tumor tends to solidify. The contents of the tumor are liquid at temperatures above 34°C and become solid at temperatures below 25°C.[30] The cut surface of the tumor reveals a cavity filled with fatty material and hair and surrounded by a firm capsule of varying thickness. The fatty material is similar in constitution to normal sebum.[320] The tumor is usually unilocular but may be multilocular, being divided by septa into a number of compartments. Several tumors may be present in the same ovary. Within the tumor, arising from its wall and projecting into its cavity, there is a protuberance composed of a mass of tissue that may vary in size from a small nodule to a rounded elevated mass. It is usually single but may be multiple, and, although it is frequently solid, it may be partly cystic. It has been variously termed

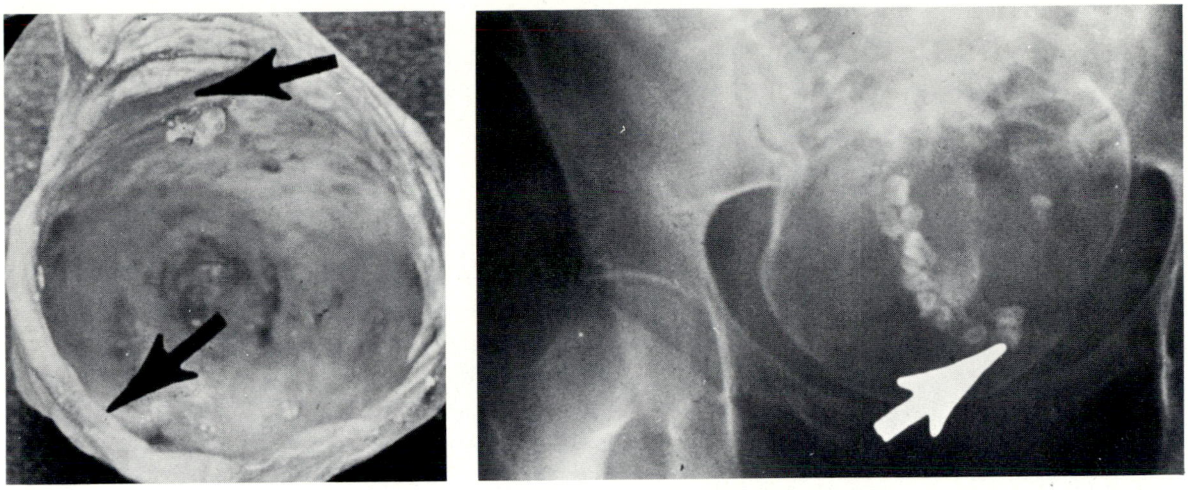

FIG. 20.46. *Left:* Benign cystic teratoma. Well-encapsulated spherical cystic mass. *Arrows* point to teeth. *Right:* Tumor produced dystocia and was diagnosed by pelvimetry. A row of teeth is seen at *arrow tip*. (Courtesy of A. Blaustein, M.D.)

dermoid mamilla, dermoid protuberance, Rokitansky's protuberance, embryonic node, dermoid nipple, and so on. The hair pressure in the tumor arises from this protuberance, and when bone or teeth are present, they tend to be located within this area, which is composed of a variety of different tissues and is one of the sites that should always be carefully sampled when the tumor is being examined. Mature cystic teratomas contain macroscopically recognizable and well-formed teeth in 31% of cases.[30] Phalanges, long and other bones, parts of the rib cage, loops of intestine, and even fetus-like structures are occasionally encountered.[1,14,319]

Microscopic Appearance. The outer side of the cyst wall is composed of ovarian stroma that may often be fibrosed and hyalinized, making its recognition difficult. The cavity of the cyst is lined mainly by skin, and in small tumors, cutaneous structures may form the entire lining. The skin is lined by keratinized squamous epithelium (Figs. 20.47 and 20.48) and contains usually abundant sebaceous and sweat glands (Fig. 20.47). Hair and other dermal appendages are usually present. Occasionally, the cyst wall may be lined by bronchial or gastrointestinal epithelium or epithelium of columnar or cuboidal type, and the squamous epithelium may be present only in the region of the dermoid protuberance. Sometimes, there may be loss of the lining epithelium caused by desquamation, and this may be associated with foreign body giant cell reaction. The latter may be seen in other parts of the tumor as a reaction to the contents of the tumor. Foreign body giant cell reaction may also be seen when the contents of the tumor are spilled, leading to the formation of adhesions. The area around the dermoid protuberance may contain a large variety of tissues derived from the three germ layers. Ectodermal tissue is usually most abundant and is usually represented by squamous epithelium and other skin derivatives, brain tissue, glia, neural tissue, retina, choroid plexus, and ganglia. Mesodermal tissue is represented by bone, cartilage (Fig. 20.48), smooth muscle, and fibrous and fatty tissue. Endodermal tissue is represented by gastrointes-

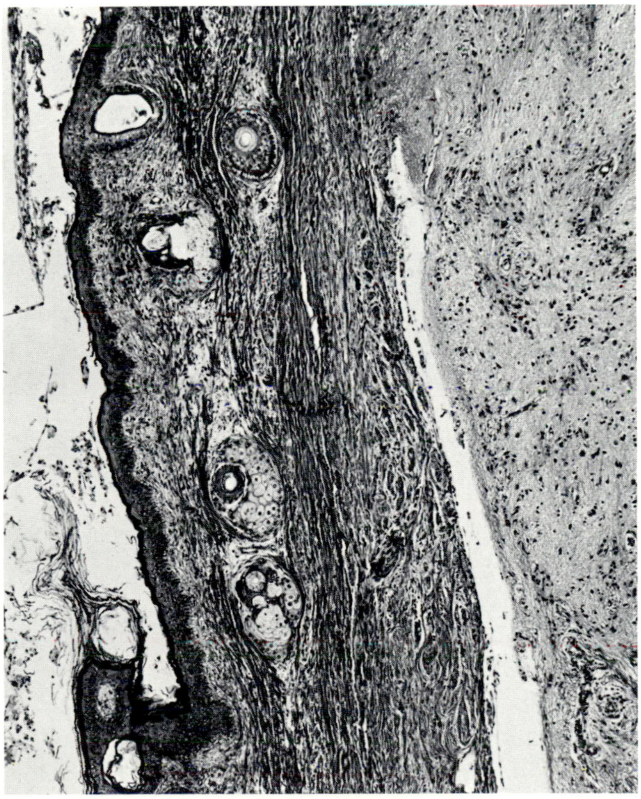

FIG. 20.47. Mature cystic teratoma. The lining of the cyst is composed of skin with its appendages. Mature neural tissue is seen beneath the cutaneous structures.

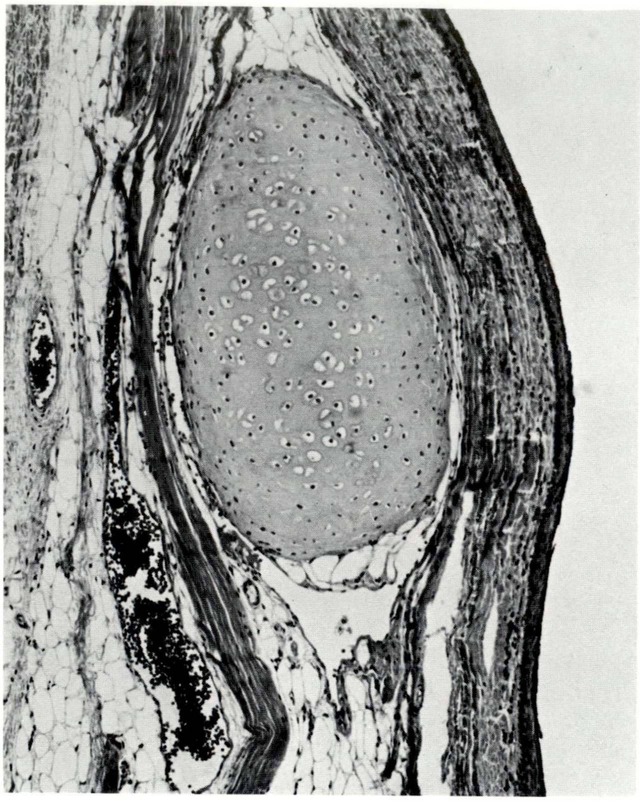

FIG. 20.48. Mature cystic teratoma lined by squamous epithelium and containing cartilage, muscle, and fatty tissue.

tinal and bronchial epithelium and glands, thyroid, and salivary gland tissue. In a careful study of 100 cases, ectodermal structures were found in 100%, mesodermal in 93%, and endodermal in 71% of cases. It was thought that the presence of mesodermal and endodermal derivatives would have been higher had more sections been examined.[30] The various tissues present in mature cystic teratoma show an orderly organoid arrangement forming cutaneous, bronchial, and gastrointestinal tissues, as well as bone and other structures. Although these tissues may be scattered diffusely, they do not exhibit the disorderly haphazard arrangement that is observed in immature teratoma.

Mature cystic teratoma must be differentiated from the rare cases of fetus in fetu, considered most likely to be caused by an inclusion of a monozygotic diamniotic twin. Fetus in fetu can be distinguished from a teratoma by its location in the retroperitoneal space, presence of vertebral organization with formation of limb buds, and a well-developed organ system. Fetus in fetu shows better organization than the most differentiated teratomas.[103,151] Like mature cystic teratoma, fetus in fetu is a benign lesion.

Complications. Mature cystic teratoma of the ovary may be associated with various complications. In view of the fact that in many of these cases the condition is amenable to cure, their recognition is of considerable importance. These complications can be classified as follows:

1. Torsion
2. Rupture
3. Infection
4. Hemolytic anemia
5. Development of malignancy

Torsion is the most frequent complication.[43,194,202] It has been observed in 16.1% of cases in one large series.[202] This complication tends to be more common during pregnancy and puerperium.[160,202] Mature cystic teratoma is said to comprise from 22% to 40% of ovarian tumors in pregnancy, and from 0.8% to 12.8% of reported cases of mature cystic teratoma have occurred in pregnancy.[43,202] The fact that these tumors when they occur during pregnancy are more liable to be associated with this complication is of considerable importance. Torsion is also more common in children and younger patients.[194,202] The patients usually have severe acute abdominal pain, and the condition is considered as an acute abdominal emergency. Excision of the affected ovary or salpingo-oophorectomy is the treatment of choice.

Torsion tends to predispose to rupture of the tumor. Rupture of mature cystic teratoma is an uncommon complication,[3] occurring in approximately 1% of cases.[160,202] It is much more common during pregnancy and may manifest itself during labor.[160,194] The immediate result of the rupture may be shock or hemorrhage, especially during pregnancy or labor, but the prognosis even in these cases is usually favorable. Rupture of the tumor into the peritoneal cavity may be followed by chemical peritonitis caused by the spillage of the contents of the tumor. It produces a marked granulomatous reaction and leads to the formation of dense adhesions throughout the peritoneal cavity. Rupture of the tumor may occasionally be followed by the development of glial implants on the peritoneum. This occurs when the tumor contains mature neuroglial elements, and spillage leads to deposition of numerous small nodules composed of mature glia in the peritoneal cavity. In spite of the wide dissemination of these deposits throughout the peritoneal cavity, the prognosis is favorable, and simple surgical excision of the primary tumor is considered to be adequate therapy.[219] Mature cystic teratoma may rupture not only into the peritoneal cavity but also into the adjacent organs, usually into the bladder or the rectum. More than 30 such cases have been reported.[55]

Infection is an uncommon complication of mature cystic teratoma and occurs in approximately 1% of cases.[160] The infecting organism is usually a coliform, but *Salmonella* infection causing typhoid fever has also been reported.[111]

Autoimmune hemolytic anemia has been occasionally noted in patients with teratoma of the ovary, mainly mature cystic teratoma. Excision of the tumor in these cases resulted in the disappearance of the anemia and a complete cure.[19,27,56,57,198] Nineteen cases of benign cystic teratoma and seven other cystic ovarian tumors associated with this complication have been reported.[27,198] The patients have symptoms and signs of progressive anemia, which may be moderate or severe. It is accompanied by reticulocytosis, spherocytosis, and increased osmotic fragility. Normoblasts may be present in the peripheral blood. The indirect serum bilirubin is elevated, and the direct antiglobulin test (Coombs test) is positive, indicating the presence of autoantibodies that react with the patient's red blood cells. The platelets are normal in number. The spleen may be palpable but is only slightly enlarged. Steroids are only transiently effective in treating the disease, and splenectomy has no effect on the progress of the disease.[27,198] Excision of the ovarian tumor leads to the permanent disappearance of the anemia.[27,56,57,198] The following possible pathogenetic mechanisms have been suggested[27]:

1. Presence in the tumor of substances that are antigenically different from the host and that stimulate the production by the host of antibodies, which cross-react with her own red blood cells.
2. Antibody production by the tumor directed specifically against the host's red blood cells resembling the graft-versus-host reaction.
3. Coating of red blood cells with products secreted by the tumor, resulting in changed red blood cell antigenicity.

In view of this, pelvic and radiologic examinations are indicated in a young woman with autoimmune hemolytic anemia that does not respond to steroid treatment, as it may help to detect an ovarian teratoma and prevent an unnecessary splenectomy.[56,198,240]

Therapy. The treatment of choice for an uncomplicated mature cystic teratoma is excision of the affected ovary. In young patients, if the tumor is small and conservation of a part of the ovary is possible, excision of the tumor may be the treatment of choice, usually resulting in a complete cure. Local recurrences following conservative treatment for mature cystic teratoma are very uncommon and occur in less than 1% of cases.[68]

Mature Cystic Teratoma (Dermoid Cyst) with Malignant Transformation

Clinical Aspects. Malignant transformation is an uncommon complication of mature cystic teratoma. It occurs in approximately 2% of cases,[48,137,160,201,202] although in one report the incidence was almost 4%.[195] The age of patients with this complication as reported in the literature ranges from 19 to 88 years[202] but this tumor is usually observed in postmenopausal patients.*

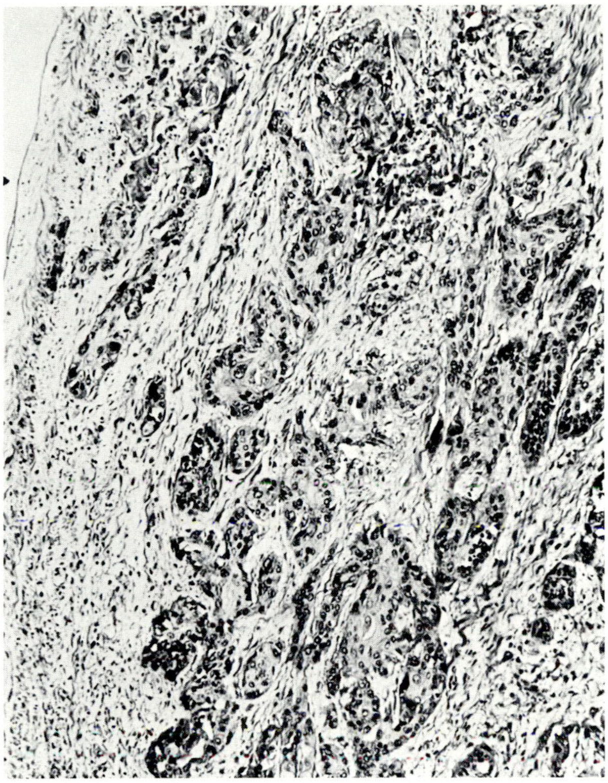

Fig. 20.49. Squamous cell carcinoma arising in and invading a mature cystic teratoma. Surface of the ovary is seen at *top left*.

Clinically, this tumor cannot be readily differentiated from an uncomplicated mature cystic teratoma or other ovarian tumor, although evidence of its rapid growth, pain, loss of weight, and other systemic symptoms suggest the presence of a malignant tumor. Sometimes, the tumor may be found as an incidental observation. We have encountered, at autopsy, a large mature cystic teratoma containing a squamous cell carcinoma (Fig. 20.49) in the left ovary of a 56-year-old woman.

Macroscopic Appearance. The tumor is frequently larger than an average mature cystic teratoma.[43,137] It may exhibit a more solid appearance, but differentiation cannot be made on macroscopic grounds. Malignant transformation in mature cystic teratoma tends to occur in patients with unilateral tumors.[137,201,202]

Microscopic Appearance. The tumor exhibits malignant transformation in one of its constitutent tissues, most frequently the squamous epithelium (Fig. 20.49),

* References 48, 132, 137, 160, 195, 201, 202.

with formation of a typical squamous cell carcinoma.[43,48,137,195,201] Any of the tissues present in a mature cystic teratoma may undergo malignant transformation, and a variety of malignant tumors have been reported, including carcinoid tumor, thyroid carcinoma, basal cell carcinoma (Fig. 20.50), adenocarcinoma of the intestinal epithelium, malignant melanoma, leiomyosarcoma, and chondrosarcoma.* The malignant element invades other parts of the tumor and its wall (Fig. 20.49), which it tends to perforate. Invariably, only one tissue element becomes malignant, and the presence of many different malignant elements indicates that the tumor is an immature teratoma and not a mature cystic teratoma that has undergone malignant transformation.

Behavior and Therapy. The mode of spread of the malignant tumor differs from that observed in other tumors of germ cell origin. The tumor spreads by direct invasion and peritoneal implantation and generally does not metastasize to the lymph nodes.[137,201] Extensive local invasion and absence of lymph node involvement is usually observed at laparotomy.[195] Hematogenous dissemination is uncommon.

The prognosis of patients with mature cystic teratoma with malignant transformation is unfavorable.[48,137,195,201,202] There are only 15–30.8% 5-year survivors.[137,201,202] Better prognosis has been reported when the malignant element is a squamous cell carcinoma confined to the ovary and is excised without spillage of the contents. In such cases the 5-year survival is 63%.[201] There have been no 5-year survivors when the malignant element was an adenocarcinoma or a sarcoma.[201]

Treatment is hysterectomy and bilateral adnexectomy.[110,137] Since the tumors are usually unilateral, however, in cases where there is no penetration of the capsule and no involvement of the adjacent structures, a more conservative surgical procedure may be just as effective. However, since malignant transformation of a mature cystic teratoma almost always occurs in postmenopausal women, total abdominal hysterectomy and bilateral salpingo-oophorectomy is the treatment of choice. If the tumor has spread beyond the confines of the ovary and there is involvement of the adjacent structures, a more radical procedure with resection of the tumor and the involved structures or viscera is advocated.[195] Response to radiation and chemotherapy is unsatisfactory.[137,195]

Struma Ovarii

Thyroid tissue is a relatively frequent constituent of mature cystic teratoma and has been demonstrated in 5–20% of cases.[240,241] Struma ovarii is considered as a one-sided development of a teratoma, as a tumor in which the thyroid tissue has overgrown all other tissues, or one in which only the thyroid tissue has developed. The term *struma ovarii* should be reserved only for tumors composed either entirely or predominantly of thyroid tissue or for those in which thyroid tissue can be recognized macroscopically.

Clinical Aspects. Struma ovarii is uncommon and comprises 2.7% of ovarian teratomas.[103] The age distribution of patients with struma ovarii is generally the same as that of patients with benign cystic teratoma and ranges from 6 to 74 years. The majority of patients are in the reproductive years.[53,179,255,333,335] There are usually no specific symptoms; the clinical findings are similar to those observed in patients with benign cystic teratoma. The only differences are that in some cases struma ovarii was associated with enlargement of the thyroid gland, and in other cases there was clinical evidence that the struma ovarii was responsible for the development of thyrotoxicosis, although this was not confirmed by laboratory tests, since these were not performed preoperatively.[179,240,255,335] Some cases of thyrotoxicosis have been associated with struma ovarii, which has also shown changes of thyroid hyperactivity.[103,226] The ectopic thyroid tissue present within struma ovarii may, therefore, be the subject of the same physiologic and pathologic

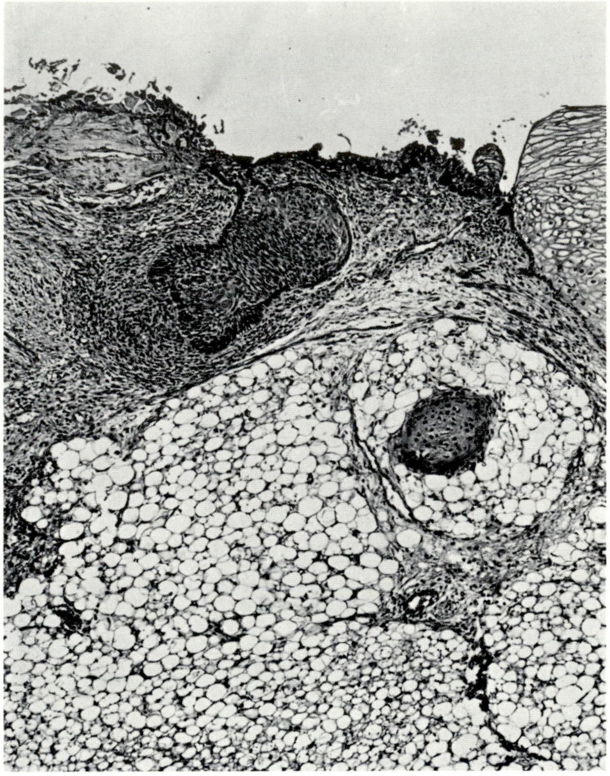

FIG. 20.50. Basal cell carcinoma arising in a mature cystic teratoma.

* References 48, 71, 110, 132, 160, 163, 201, 202, 330.

changes as thyroid gland. Although the true thyroid nature of the tissue present in struma ovarii was not accepted initially, its true thyroid composition has been demonstrated conclusively.[67,212,255]

Macroscopic Appearance. Struma ovarii is usually unilateral,[53,179,335] but, in one report, in 15% of cases the contralateral ovary also contained a teratoma and this tumor contained thyroid tissue in some of the cases.[255] Earlier reports have stated that in 50% of cases struma ovarii has been associated with a mature cystic teratoma, in 31% with a cystadenoma, and only in 17% was thyroid tissue the sole constituent.[255] More recent reports indicate a predominance of pure struma ovarii over those associated with mature cystic teratoma and a paucity of cases associated with cystadenoma.[179,335]

Struma ovarii may vary in size but usually measures less than 10 cm in diameter. It tends to be larger if it is associated with other elements. The surface is usually smooth, and prior to sectioning, the tumor shows similar appearances to mature cystic teratoma. Occasionally, adhesions may be present. The cut surface of the tumor may be composed entirely of light tan, glistening thyroid (Fig. 20.51) tissue or may consist of thyroid tissue associated with other tissues. Hemorrhage, necrosis, and foci of fibrosis may be present. Solid tumors with small amounts of colloid appear less glistening and more fleshy.

Microscopic Appearance. The tumor is composed of mature thyroid tissue consisting of acini of various sizes, lined by a single layer of columnar or flattened epithelium (Fig. 20.52). The acini contain eosinophilic, PAS-positive colloid. The intensity of the staining may vary. There may be a considerable variation in the size of the acini, which may be large containing a large amount of colloid or may be small. Occasionally, the lining of the acini may be columnar, containing small papillary projections not unlike those seen in hyperactive thyroid gland. Sometimes the appearances may resemble a nodular adenomatous goiter. Adenoma-like lesions may also be observed. Struma ovarii showing appearances suggestive of Hashimoto's thyroiditis has also been reported.[69]

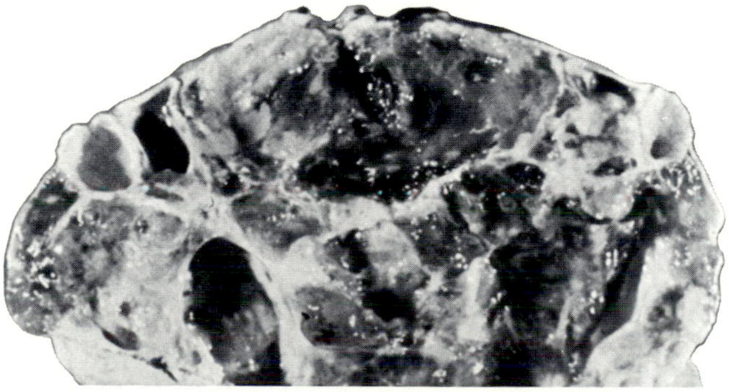

Fig. 20.51. Struma ovarii. The cut surface shows compartments of amber-colored thyroid tissue separated by thick fibrous septae. (Courtesy of B. Bigelow, M.D.)

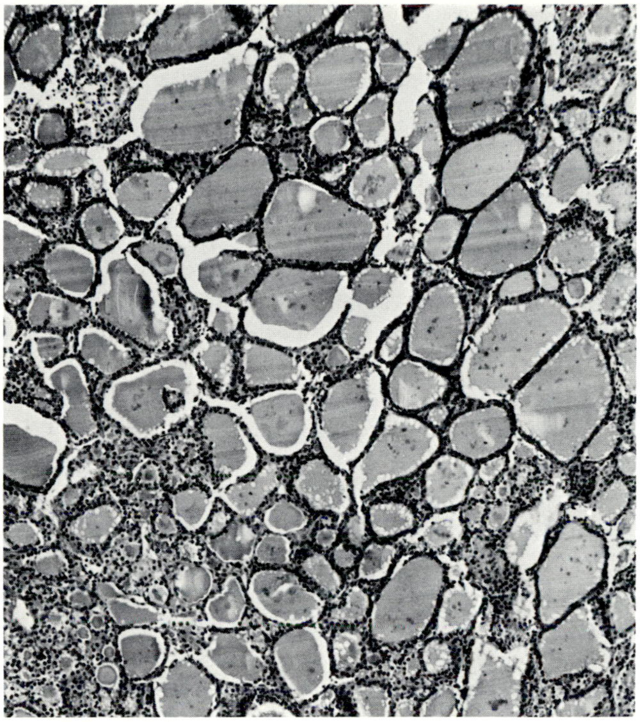

Fig. 20.52. Struma ovarii. The tumor is composed of normal thyroid tissue.

Behavior and Therapy. Most cases of struma ovarii are benign and can be treated by excision of the ovary or by unilateral salpingo-oophorectomy. In a small number of cases, there are complications, the most important being the development of malignancy and the presence of ascites or ascites associated with pleural effusion producing a pseudo-Meigs' syndrome.[129,240] Ascites may be found in 17% of cases of struma ovarii, and its presence does not indicate that the tumor is malignant.[255] The cause of the ascites and pleural effusion has not been fully elucidated. In the majority of reported cases, excision of the tumor led to complete remission.[240]

Malignant change in struma ovarii is uncommon. In a number of reported cases, the diagnosis was based on the histology of the tumor, and there were no metastases or other features of malignancy. A number of other reported cases were examples of strumal carcinoid.[240,241] Only 17 of 45 reported cases of malignant struma ovarii were associated with metastases.[97,179,240,241,335] The presence of metastases is unequivocal proof of the malignant nature of the tumor. The malignant struma ovarii usually shows follicular pattern, but papillary carcinoma is also observed. We have encountered a 26-year-old patient with a mature cystic teratoma containing thyroid tissue and a typical well-differentiated papillary adenocarcinoma of the thyroid (Fig. 20.53), which was associated with metastases in the paraaortic lymph nodes. The patient was well and symptom-free 3½ years after excision of the tumor followed by laparotomy and dissection of the paraaortic lymph nodes, as well as a course of radiation therapy. There was no evidence of metastases elsewhere.

Malignant struma ovarii may involve the peritoneum. The tumor deposits, which are composed of malignant thyroid tissue, should not be confused with deposits of benign thyroid tissue representing peritoneal spread of nonmalignant struma ovarii (benign strumosis).[240,241] Occasionally, the distinction between these entities may pose considerable difficulties, especially when the malignant neoplasm is of the well-differentiated follicular type. Other routes of spread are via the lymphatics to the paraaortic and other lymph nodes and via the bloodstream to the lungs and bones. The prognosis in cases unassociated with metastases is generally good, but when metastases are present, it is less favorable. Treatment consists of surgery and administration of radioactive iodine (^{131}I) and other agents used in the treatment of thyroid malignancy, including radiation therapy.

Occasionally, struma ovarii may be associated with extraovarian extension caused either by rupture of the tumor or by local spread. In such cases, the peritoneal cavity contains tumor deposits, which may be numerous and are composed of mature thyroid tissue. The condition is benign and is termed *benign strumosis*.[240,241] It is only rarely associated with untoward side effects, which are mainly due to the formation of adhesions. Benign strumosis may be treated by excision of the tumor deposits or by administration of radioactive iodine (^{131}I).

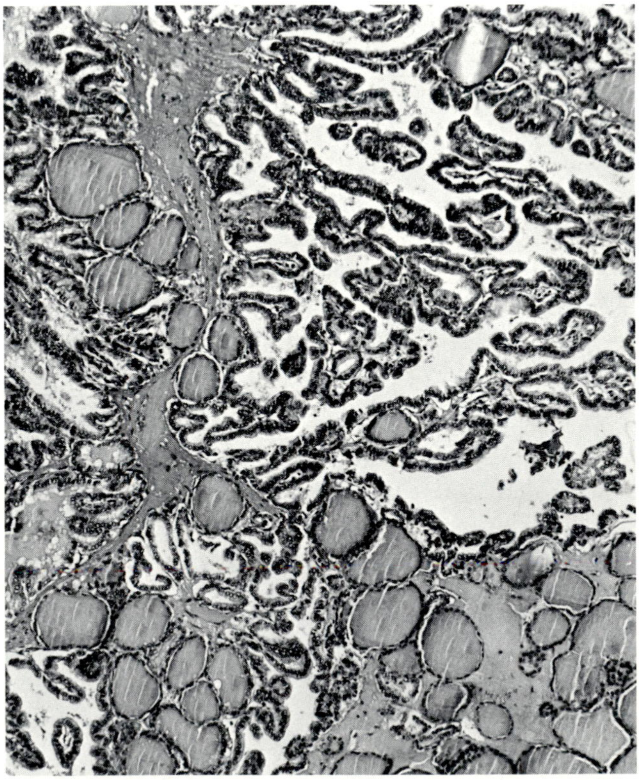

FIG. 20.53. Papillary carcinoma arising in thyroid tissue present in a mature cystic teratoma.

Carcinoid

Carcinoid tumors of the ovary are classified as follows:[275]

1. Primary
   a. Insular or islet carcinoid (carcinoid tumors of midgut origin)
   b. Trabecular carcinoid (carcinoid tumors of foregut and hindgut origin)
   c. Mucinous (goblet, adenocarcinoid) carcinoid
2. Metastatic

The insular carcinoid tumor is the most common, followed by the trabecular and mucinous types. The metastatic carcinoid tumors of the ovary, of which the insular type is the most common, are discussed with other metastatic tumors of the ovary in Chapter 22, Metastatic Ovarian Tumors.

Insular or Islet Carcinoid

Insular carcinoid tumor, considered to be of midgut derivation, is the most common type of primary ovarian carcinoid tumor. It usually arises in association with gastrointestinal or respiratory epithelium present in a mature cystic teratoma. It may also be observed within a solid teratoma, a mucinous tumor, in association with a Sertoli-Leydig cell tumor,[339] or may occur in a pure form.[221,240,244,275,310] The latter is considered to arise either as a one-sided development of a teratoma or from enterochromaffin cells present within the ovary. Approximately 40% of ovarian insular carcinoids occur in pure form, and the remaining 60% are combined.[275]

Clinical Aspects. More than 70 cases of primary ovarian insular carcinoid tumors have been reported,[221] and many unreported cases are known to the author. The age of patients ranges from 31 to 79 years, but most patients are either postmenopausal or perimenopausal.[221,244] One third of the reported cases have been associated with the typical carcinoid syndrome, in spite of the absence of metastases.[214,221] This is in contrast to intestinal carcinoids, which are associated with the syndrome only when there is metastatic spread to the liver. One reason for this difference is that the blood flow from the ovary goes directly into the systemic circulation and does not pass through the liver, which inactivates the serotonin produced by the tumor. The presence

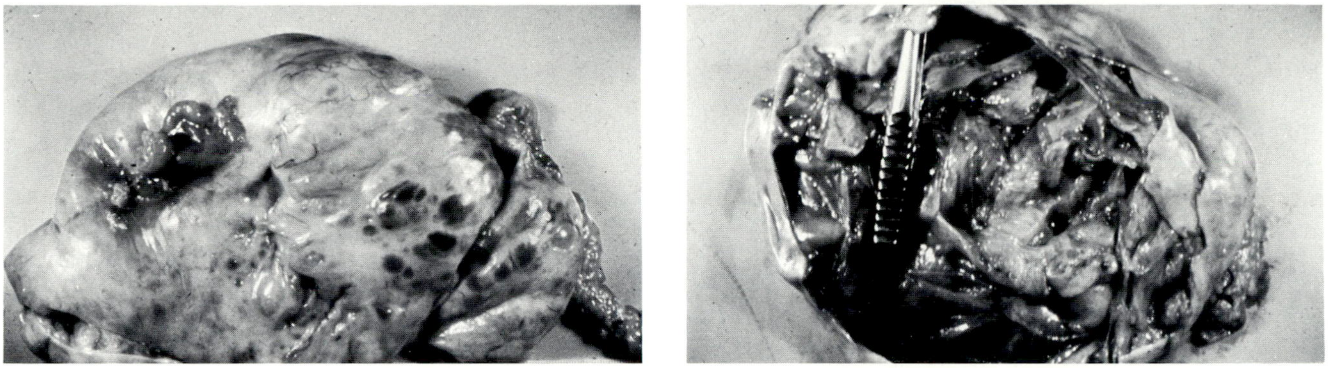

FIG. 20.54. *Left:* Carcinoid of the ovary. It is oval-shaped and encapsulated. *Right:* The cut surface is yellow to brown and largely cystic. (Courtesy of B. Bigelow, M.D.)

or absence of symptoms of carcinoid syndrome is also dependent on the number of secreting tumor cells. Functioning ovarian carcinoid tumors have all measured approximately 10 cm in diameter (with only one exception[231]) whereas intestinal carcinoids are usually smaller. Thus, there is a good correlation between the size of the tumor and the presence of carcinoid syndrome. The excision of the tumor has been associated with rapid remission of the symptoms in all the described cases, the disappearance of 5-hydroxyindole acetic acid (5-HIAA) from the urine,[221] and marked decrease of serum serotonin. Determination of serum serotonin and urinary 5-HIAA may be used to monitor disease activity and response to therapy and for early detection of metastases. Therefore they may be used as tumor markers in patients with insular carcinoid tumor. If the tumor is nonfunctioning, there are no specific features, and the presentation is the same as in cases of mature cystic teratoma.

Macroscopic Appearance. The tumor shows similar appearances to those of mature cystic teratoma within which it is usually found. The same applies if the tumor is associated with a solid teratoma or a mucinous tumor. If the carcinoid is not associated with other tissue elements, the tumor is solid. The carcinoid may vary in size from microscopic to 20 cm in longest diameter and is solid and homogeneous (Fig. 20.54a,b). Its color may vary from light brown to yellow or pale gray. Primary ovarian carcinoids are practically always unilateral, although they may be associated with a benign cystic teratoma in the contralateral ovary.

Microscopic Appearance. The primary ovarian carcinoid usually shows the typical appearances associated with midgut carcinoids.[221,327] The tumor is composed of collections of small acini and solid nests of uniform polygonal cells with ample amounts of cytoplasm and round or oval, centrally located hyperchromatic nuclei (Fig. 20.55). Mitotic activity is low. The cytoplasm is basophilic or amphophilic and may contain red, brown, or orange argentaffin (Fig. 20.56) or argyrophil granules, which are demonstrated in the great majority of cases of primary ovarian carcinoids.[221] Ultrastructurally, the cells of the ovarian insular carcinoid show similar appearances to those of insular carcinoid tumors from other locations[275,310] and show abundant neurosecretory granules, which exhibit marked variation in size and shape, being round, oval, or elongated. Serotonin may be demonstrated within the cytoplasm of the tumor cells by

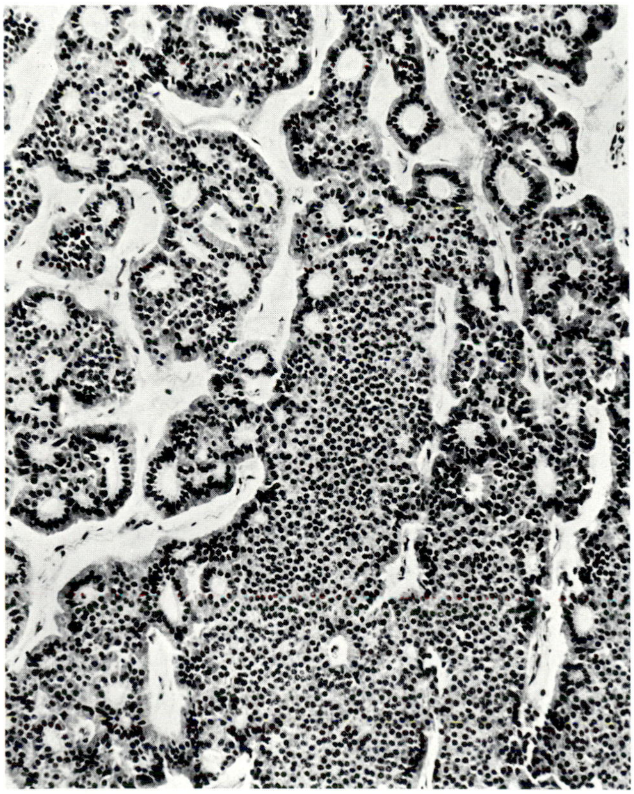

FIG. 20.55. Primary ovarian carcinoid showing the typical solid and acinar patterns of midgut carcinoids.

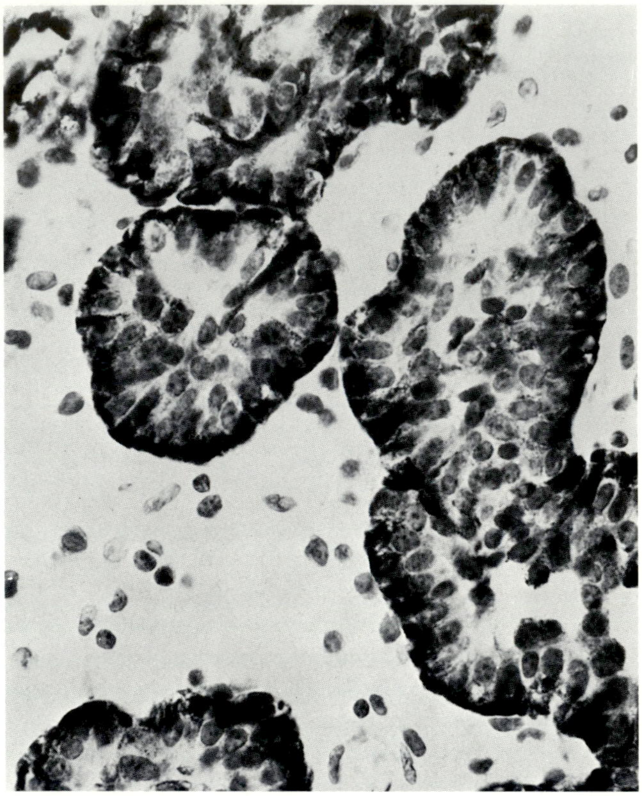

FIG. 20.56. Ovarian carcinoid. The tumor cells contain numerous argentaffin granules stained black.

immunofluorescence and immunoperoxidase techniques.[260] Occasionally, other neurohormonal peptides may also be demonstrated within the cytoplasm of the tumor cells, but their finding is much less frequent than in trabecular or strumal carcinoids.[260] The connective tissue surrounding the tumor nests is frequently dense and hyalinized due to the fibrogenic effect of the serotonin produced by the tumor.

Differential Diagnosis. Primary carcinoid of the ovary must be differentiated from metastatic carcinoid of the ovary, which is usually of gastrointestinal origin and practically always affects both ovaries,[222,251] unlike the primary ovarian carcinoid, which is unilateral.[221] Macroscopically, the metastatic carcinoid is composed of tumor nodules, whereas primary ovarian carcinoid forms a single homogeneous mass. When other teratomatous elements are associated with primary ovarian carcinoid, they are a very helpful distinguishing feature.[221] Primary ovarian carcinoid may sometimes be confused with Brenner tumor, but the appearances of the cell nests and the grooved coffee-bean nuclei of the cells of Brenner tumor are against the diagnosis of a carcinoid, whereas the typical small acinar pattern and the presence of argyrophil- and argentaffin-positive cells are in favor of a carcinoid. Confusion with granulosa cell tumor may also arise because Call–Exner bodies may be confused with carcinoid acini, but the cells of the carcinoid tumor usually show an acinar pattern and contain more cytoplasm and argentaffin granules.[221,310] Cystic areas that may be present in a granulosa cell tumor are nearly always absent in a carcinoid. Occasionally, ovarian carcinoid may be confused with a Krukenberg tumor, but the latter is usually bilateral and may be larger, and the cellular appearances are different. The cells of Krukenberg tumor tend to merge with the stroma, are larger, and show greater pleomorphism, a signet-ring appearance, and more brisk mitotic activity. Acinar pattern is less evident. Demonstration of argyrophil and argentaffin granules, which can be detected in the majority of ovarian carcinoids, confirms the diagnosis. These granules can be identified even more easily with the aid of the electron microscope, manifesting themselves as numerous pleomorphic neurosecretory granules present within the cytoplasm.[221,251,275,310]

Behavior and Therapy. Although insular carcinoid tumors of the ovary are considered to be malignant, they are slow growing and are only occasionally associated with metastases. Metastasis has been observed only in five patients, and four of these patients died with metastatic disease.[76,221,244,248] In occasional patients, features of carcinoid syndrome, such as tricuspid incompetence resulting in right-sided heart failure, may progress after the excision of the tumor and lead to the death of the patient. This has been observed in two cases.[221] In the great majority of patients with the carcinoid syndrome, the symptoms and signs of the syndrome observed preoperatively disappear or regress during the postoperative period.[221] The treatment is the same as for ovarian tumors of low malignant potential. Since nearly all patients with this tumor are postmenopausal or perimenopausal, bilateral salpingo-oophorectomy and hysterectomy is the treatment of choice. Surgical excision of foci of extraovarian spread or of metastases if present is indicated. The tumor does not respond to radiation therapy, and there is at present little experience with chemotherapy. Estimation of serum serotonin and 5-HIAA in the urine may be used to monitor the progress of the disease.

Trabecular Carcinoid

Trabecular carcinoid includes carcinoid tumors of hindgut or foregut derivation. Primary trabecular or ribbon carcinoid usually arises in association with teratomatous elements,[223] but of four cases of trabecular carcinoid seen by the author, two were pure and not associated with teratomatous elements.[277]

Clinical Aspects. Trabecular carcinoid is rare, and only 21 cases have been reported. The age varies from 24 to 74 years, with most patients being postmenopausal.[223,277] Trabecular carcinoid is a slowly growing neoplasm that can reach a large size. None of the known cases have been associated with the carcinoid syndrome. In three patients whose urine was examined immediately after the operation, 5-HIAA was normal.[223]

Macroscopic Appearance. The appearances of trabecular carcinoid depend on whether the tumor is associated with teratomatous elements or not. When associated with teratoma, the appearances are similar to those of a mature cystic teratoma, but when the tumor is in a pure form, it is a solid, firm to hard, round or oval mass with a smooth outline and tan to yellow in color on cross-section (Fig. 20.57). The tumors have always been unilateral[223,277] but occasionally have been associated with mature cystic teratoma in the opposite ovary.[223] In the reported cases, the tumors measured from 4 to 25 cm in the longest diameter.[223,277]

Microscopic Appearance. The tumor is composed of long, usually wavy ribbons, cords, or trabeculae running parallel and surrounded by fibromatous connective tissue stroma that is usually dense (Fig. 20.58). The ribbons, cords, or trabeculae are composed of cells that are usually one but sometimes two cells thick (Fig. 20.58). The nuclei are elongated or ovoid and contain finely dispersed chromatin. The cytoplasm is abundant and often contains orange to red-brown granules, which usually stain positively with argyrophil and argentaffin stains. Ultrastructurally, the neurosecretory granules are round or oval and show slight variation in size.[223,251,275,280]

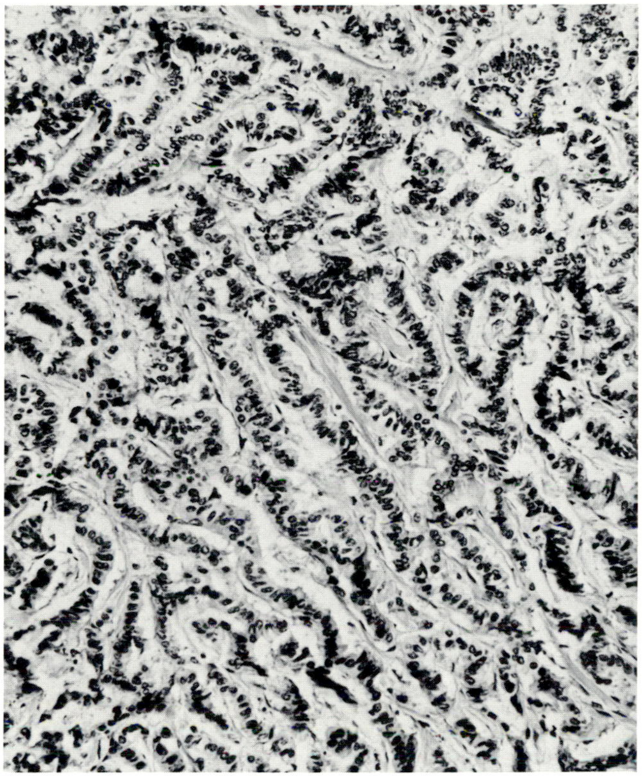

FIG. 20.58. Trabecular carcinoid tumor of the ovary composed of long ramifying cords of tumor cells surrounded by dense fibrous stroma.

Differential Diagnosis. Primary trabecular carcinoid must be distinguished from metastatic trabecular carcinoid, which is usually bilateral and frequently associated with metastases elsewhere in the body. The presence of teratomatous elements, which are frequently found in the primary lesion, helps to distinguish the primary from a metastatic lesion. Trabecular carcinoid may sometimes exhibit an insular pattern in places, but this is usually a minor feature and the trabecular pattern predominates. Presence of thyroid follicles indicates that the tumor is a struma ovarii and carcinoid (strumal carcinoid), and their presence must be excluded before a diagnosis of trabecular carcinoid is made. Occasionally, trabecular carcinoid must be distinguished from a Sertoli–Leydig cell tumor (androblastoma) showing a cord-like pattern, but the presence of occasional tubules as well as different cellular and nuclear appearances differentiate between these two entities. Presence of argyrophil and argentaffin granules or neurosecretory granules ultrastructurally confirms the diagnosis.

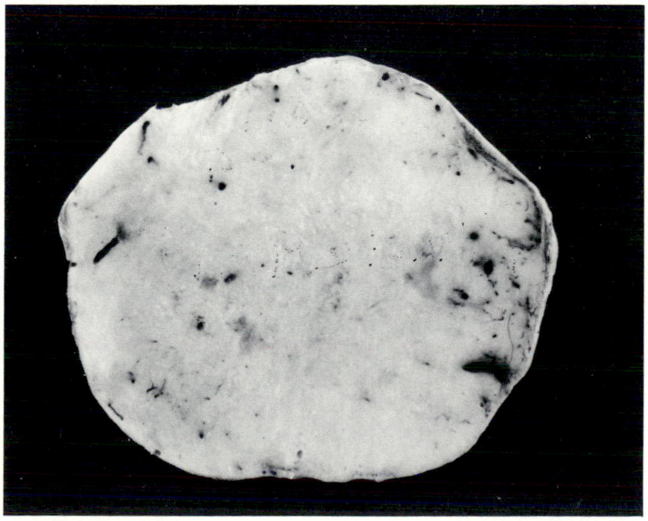

FIG. 20.57. Pure trabecular carcinoid tumor of the ovary. The cut surface is solid, uniform, and yellow. The outer surface is smooth.

Behavior and Prognosis. The prognosis of patients with trabecular carcinoid of the ovary is very favorable, since these tumors are not associated with metastases. In one case, only a peritoneal implant was found 2 years following bilateral salpingo-oophorectomy and hysterectomy.[223]

The optimal treatment is the excision of the affected

adnexa, which results in a complete cure, but follow-up of the patient is advisable.

Mucinous Carcinoid

Synonyms
Goblet cell carcinoid, adenocarcinoid

Primary mucinous carcinoid is a relatively recently described variant of carcinoid tumor, which has been encountered mainly in the vermiform appendix[134,266,318] and occasionally has been observed in the ovary.[275] However, it should be noted that at least some of the tumors described as primary Krukenberg tumors of the ovary may have been examples of this entity. A number of cases of mucinous carcinoid tumor metastatic to the ovary have been reported.[113]

Clinical Aspects. The age of patients ranges from 14 to 53 years. Mucinous carcinoid is usually observed in pure form but may be seen in association with mature cystic teratoma. The tumor is unilateral but may be associated with metastases in the contralateral ovary.[275]

Macroscopic Appearance. Macroscopically, the tumor is usually of considerable size, and most of the tumors have been in excess of 8 cm in the longest diameter. The tumor is gray-yellow, firm, and usually solid but may contain cystic areas even when it is seen in pure form.[275]

Microscopic Appearance. Microscopically, it is composed of numerous small glands or acini with very small lumens lined by uniform columnar or cuboid cells containing small round or oval nuclei or goblet cells distended with mucin and containing nuclei varying from signet ring to round or oval (Fig. 20.59). Some cells may be disrupted by excessive distention with mucin, which may result in the formation of small pools of mucin within the glands or even in the obliteration of the gland, resulting in the presence of pools of mucinous material within the connective tissue (Fig. 20.60). The glands are surrounded by connective tissue, which may vary from loose and edematous to dense fibrous or hyalinized. Some of the glands or acini may be larger and occasionally may be cystic (Fig. 20.60). In some areas the tumor cells tend to invade the surrounding connective tissue, often assuming signet-ring appearance, and in these areas the tumor resembles a classical Krukenberg tumor. In some tumors, such appearances may predominate. The tumor cells may form large solid aggregates and show a less uniform appearance and more atypical features, with large hyperchromatic nuclei and brisk mitotic activity. The cytoplasm may exhibit orange-red granules and may even be bright red. Argyrophil and argentaffin granules are present and, in some tumors, may be abundant,

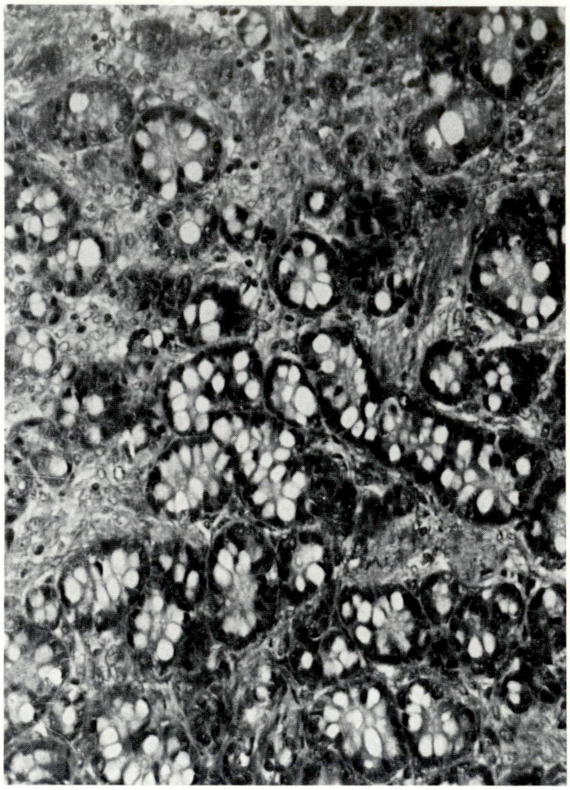

FIG. 20.59. Mucinous carcinoid tumor of the ovary. The tumor is composed of numerous small glands and acini with imperceptible or very small lumens. Numerous goblet cells distended with mucin are present.

although in general they are seen less frequently than in other types of carcinoid tumors.[28,275]

Ultrastructurally, neurosecretory granules are present in some cells and absent in others. The tumor cells may contain both neurosecretory granules and mucinous material. Using immunocytochemical techniques, some of the tumor cells have been shown to contain serotonin and gastrin, and these substances may be present within the same tumor cell.[281] Other neurohormonal peptides have not been detected in the tumor cells. CEA can also be demonstrated within the cytoplasm of the tumor cells.

Differential Diagnosis. Primary mucinous carcinoid tumor of the ovary must be differentiated from its metastatic counterpart. The latter, in common with other types of carcinoid metastatic to the ovary, is nearly always bilateral and instead of forming a single tumor mass shows scattered tumor deposits involving ovarian tissue. Depending on their size, these deposits may form tumor nodules observed macroscopically or may only be detectable microscopically. Histologically, they may have appearances indistinguishable from the primary tumor.

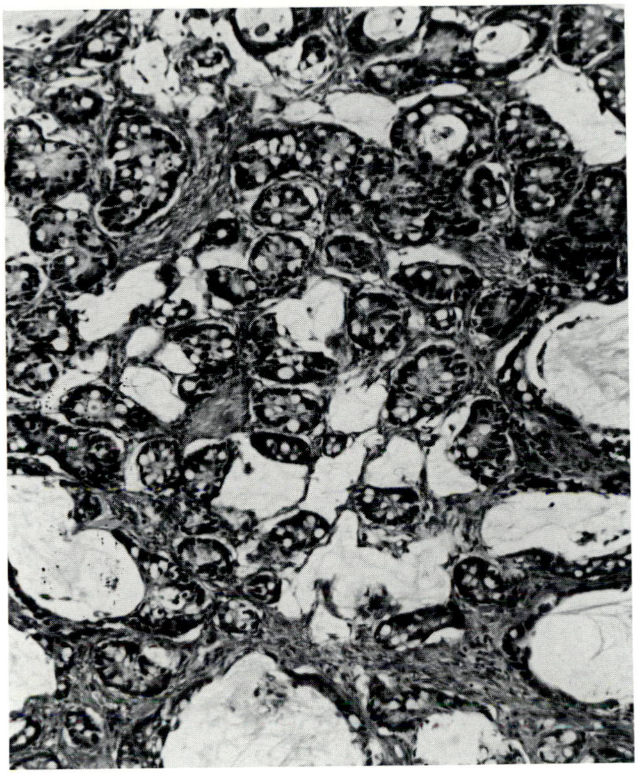

FIG. 20.60. Mucinous carcinoid tumor of the ovary composed of small glands and acini. Many acini are disrupted by excessive distention with mucin, resulting in the formation of pools of mucin within the surrounding connective tissue. Larger glands distended with mucin are also present.

Mucinous carcinoid must be distinguished from mucinous tumors of the ovary, especially when the carcinoid tumor is composed of large acini, shows increased mucin production, and exhibits a pleomorphic pattern. Occasionally, confusion may arise with well-differentiated endometrioid tumors of the ovary, which may resemble mucinous tumors.

Mucinous carcinoid must be distinguished from a Krukenberg tumor. The differentiation between these two entities may be very difficult, especially if the mucinous carcinoid assumes a predominantly Krukenberg-like pattern or if the Krukenberg tumor contains numerous argentaffin and argyrophil granules. The presence of these granules as well as of the neurosecretory granules observed ultrastructurally cannot be used for differentiation between these two entities. Involvement of both ovaries and the presence of primary extraovarian signet-ring or mucinous adenocarcinoma are indicative of Krukenberg tumor.

Behavior and Treatment. The primary mucinous carcinoid of the ovary behaves in a more aggressive manner than other types of primary ovarian carcinoid tumors.[275] This is similar to the behavior of mucinous carcinoid tumors of the vermiform appendix.[135,266,318] The tumor tends to spread mainly via the lymphatics, and metastases may be present at the time of initial laparotomy. Patients who do not exhibit metastatic disease at the time of diagnosis have much better prognosis compared with those who have metastases, however small, at the time of diagnosis.[275]

The treatment is surgical depending on the extent of the disease, but in postmenopausal patients, those with involvement of the contralateral ovary, and patients who do not want children, hysterectomy, bilateral salpingo-oophorectomy, and omentectomy, as well as excision of all the tumor deposits present, are indicated. Paraaortic lymph node dissection may be indicated, since metastatic tumor deposits may be present. Surgery may be followed by combination chemotherapy, including 5-fluorouracil, although the efficacy of this mode of therapy is so far not proven. Radiation therapy does not appear to be effective. Premenopausal patients with tumors localized to the ovary may be treated by unilateral salpingo-oophorectomy and carefully followed-up.

Strumal Carcinoid

Synonyms

Struma ovarii and carcinoid.

Strumal carcinoid is an uncommon ovarian tumor composed of thyroid tissue intimately admixed with carcinoid tumor, showing a ribbon or cordlike pattern. Other teratomatous elements are also present in most of the tumors.[220,241] It has become recognized as a separate entity only in recent years.[240,241,250] The histologic pattern of struma ovarii, merging imperceptibly with carcinoid tumor that exhibits the ribbon-like pattern observed in hindgut carcinoids,[327] had been recognized previously.* However, it was usually interpreted as a carcinoma developing in a struma ovarii, although the resemblance to a carcinoid tumor was noted in some cases.[97,132]

Clinical Aspects. More than 50 cases have been reported.[220] The age incidence is similar to struma ovarii, ranging from 21 to 77 years.[21] The tumor is usually not associated with any specific clinical findings. In one reported case it was associated with virilization.[61] Like hindgut carcinoids and unlike the primary ovarian insular carcinoid, strumal carcinoid is not associated with the carcinoid syndrome.[220,244]

Macroscopic Appearance. Macroscopically, this tumor, if pure, may be similar to struma ovarii or carcinoid. If

* References 97, 115, 132, 212, 333, 335.

the tumor is a part of a teratoma it manifests as a yellow nodule within the teratoma.[220]

Microscopic Appearance. Microscopically, the tumor is composed of thyroid follicles containing colloid that merge with ribbons of neoplastic cells usually set in dense fibrous tissue stroma similar to the trabecular carcinoid (Figs. 20.61 and 20.62). The thyroid follicles are often small in size at the junction between the two types of tissue. The carcinoid is usually composed of long, winding or straight ribbons of columnar cells with elongated hyperchromatic nuclei (Fig. 20.60). It may also be composed of small islands of tumor cells separated by dense fibrous tissue stroma from each other, from the long ribbons of carcinoid cells, and from the thyroid follicles (Fig. 20.61). Slight mitotic activity is present in the carcinoid part of the lesion. In some cases, argyrophil and argentaffin granules have been identified in the carcinoid cells.[11,240,241,249] The latter have been found to exhibit similar ultrastructural appearances to those seen in medullary carcinoma of the thyroid, including the presence of neurosecretory granules.[11] In two tumors, amyloid deposits were identified and were verified both histochemically and ultrastructurally.[11,58] This ultrastructural similarity between the cells of medullary carcinoma of the thyroid and carcinoid tumors has been noted previously.[34,98] One case of medullary carcinoma of the thyroid has been associated with the carcinoid syndrome.[174] It is considered by some investigators that the whole lesion represents a carcinoid, and the thyroid tissue is only thyroid-like and represents a carcinoid.[108,150,216]

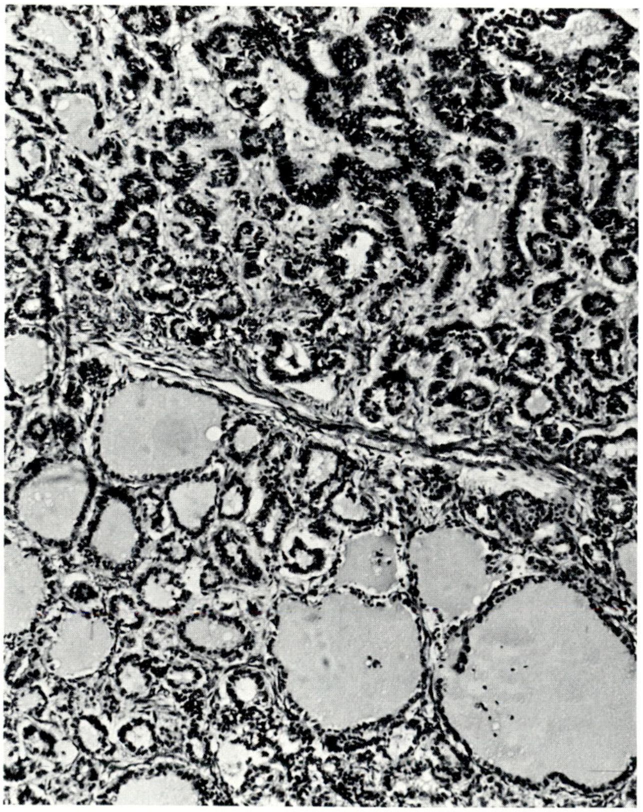

FIG. 20.61. Struma ovarii and carcinoid. The carcinoid forms long narrow cords and ribbons (*top*) merging with thyroid follicles (*bottom*).

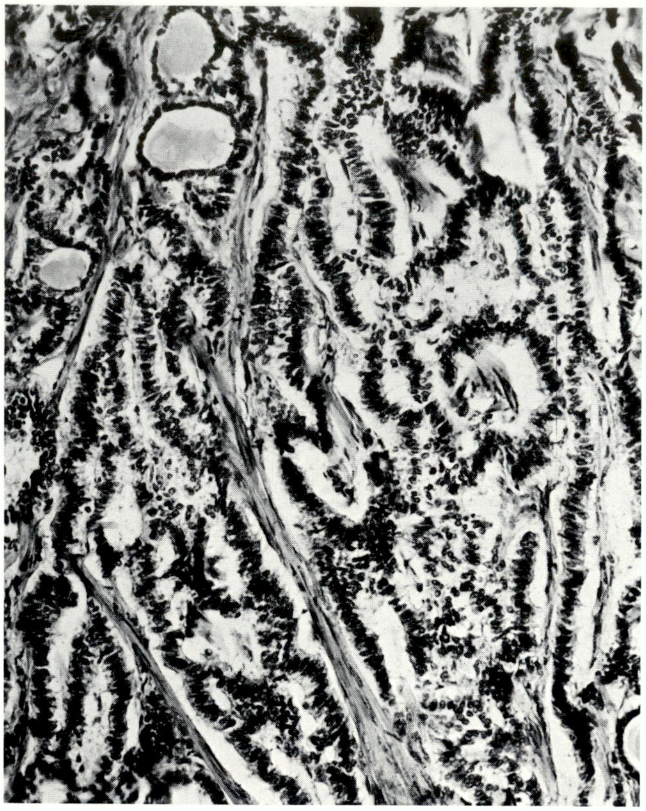

FIG. 20.62. Struma ovarii and carcinoid. The carcinoid is composed of columnar or cuboidal epithelial cells forming narrow winding cords and ribbons. Thyroid follicles are also seen.

Other investigators have demonstrated thyroglobulin within the thyroid component of the tumor, thus indicating its thyroid nature.[100,220,249,313,314] It is, therefore, considered that in verified cases of strumal carcinoid the tumor consists of thyroid tissue intimately admixed with a carcinoid. Strumal carcinoid should be distinguished from carcinoma of the thyroid arising in struma ovarii, with which it has often been confused. The latter has the typical appearances observed in carcinoma of the thyroid and usually exhibits the follicular or papillary pattern.

Behavior and Therapy. Strumal carcinoid has been only once associated with metastases, and even in this case the patient was apparently cured by a combination of surgery and radiation therapy.[335] All other cases have followed a benign course.[240,241,244] It is of interest that carcinoid tumors of hindgut origin are not associated with metastases and follow a benign course.[326]

Other Types of Monodermal Teratoma

The mucinous tumors of the ovary are usually described with the epithelial neoplasms and are considered to be derived from the germinal epithelium of the ovary. They are usually grouped together with the epithelial and not with the germ cell neoplasms of the ovary. However, there are undoubtedly some cases where the tumor is of germ cell origin, forming a monodermal teratomatous neoplasm in which the mucinous element (of intestinal derivation) has overgrown all the other tissues in the same manner that in a pure struma ovarii the thyroid tissue has overgrown all the other tissues. The presence of occasional teratomatous tumors composed mainly of mucinous (intestinal type) epithelium of endodermal derivation and only a small amount of other tumor elements, as well as a 5% association of mature cystic teratoma with mucinous cystadenoma, lends to support this mode of origin for at least some mucinous tumors. Mucinous epithelium resembling intestinal epithelium has been observed in association with struma ovarii and with strumal carcinoid. In these cases, it was the only other tissue element present. The mucinous epithelium frequently contains goblet cells and so shows greater resemblance to intestinal than to endocervical epithelium. In 21% of cases, the epithelium lining mucinous tumors of the ovary contains argyrophil and argentaffin granules.[77] In occasional cases, Paneth cells are also present.[240] These findings are considered to be a strong argument in favor of the derivation of at least some mucinous ovarian tumors from intestinal type of epithelium and their teratomatous (germ cell) origin. It is possible that studies of the type undertaken by Linder et al., using both chromosomal and isoenzyme techniques,[148] may help to clarify the origin of mucinous tumors of the ovary and confirm that some of these are of germ cell origin. Mucinous tumors of the ovary are discussed fully with tumors of epithelial derivation (see Chapter 18, Epithelial Tumors of Ovary).

Other rare examples of monodermal teratomatous neoplasms observed in the ovary include the epidermoid cyst, which is lined by epidermis without appendages, the sebaceous gland tumor,[265] the malignant neuroectodermal tumor of the ovary,[5] the melanotic tumor, resembling the retinal anlage tumor,[105,133] and the possible benign cystic counterpart of the latter.[9] Monodermal teratomatous origin of some malignant connective tissue tumors is very difficult to prove because of the occurrence of connective tissue neoplasms derived from normal ovarian tissue. Monodermal teratomatous origin of tumors derived from ectodermal or endodermal tissues is more easily acceptable, and there may be as yet undescribed tumors of this type.

Mixed Germ Cell Tumors

Mixed germ cell tumors are tumors composed of more than one neoplastic germ cell element, such as dysgerminoma combined with teratoma, endodermal sinus tumor, choriocarcinoma, embryonal carcinoma, or polyembryoma, as well as any other possible combination of these tumor types. This group includes only neoplasms composed entirely of neoplastic germ cell elements and does not include the gonadoblastoma and mixed germ cell–sex cord stroma tumor, which in addition to germ cells contains sex cord–stromal derivatives as an integral component. The relatively frequent finding of different neoplastic germ cell elements in gonadal tumors of germ cell origin is considered to be a strong argument in favor of the common histogenesis of this group of neoplasms. The various tumor elements present in these tumors may be intimately admixed (Fig. 20.11) or may form separate areas adjacent to each other and separated by fibrous septa (Fig. 20.12). Although many ovarian tumors belonging to this group are classified according to the predominant element present, it is emphasized that when these tumors are examined, all areas of varying appearance should be carefully sampled and thoroughly analyzed. All the neoplastic germ cell elements observed within the tumor, however small, should be reported and described and, if possible, their relative size estimated. The importance of this practice is by no means only academic, since the behavior and treatment of neoplasms belonging to this group vary considerably, and the presence of a small area composed of a more malignant element may alter the therapeutic approach and the prognosis. The presence of more malignant elements within a tumor is usually associated with a more aggressive behavior, an unsatisfactory response to therapy, and a poor prognosis.* However, it should be noted that the clinical course in the majority of patients with tumors composed of endodermal sinus tumor associated with dysgerminoma or other germ cell elements usually does not differ materially from that observed in patients with pure endodermal sinus tumor.[37,117,127,177,230] The different response to treatment and the different behavior of some cases of dysgerminoma described in the past may have been a result of the presence of other germ cell elements that were not identified. Although, in the past, mixed germ cell tumors were considered to be uncommon,[177] they tend to figure much more frequently in recent reports† probably because of more careful and extensive examination of the tumor.

* References 12, 140, 199, 230, 287, 308.

† References 12, 36, 37, 74, 76, 111, 117, 140, 177, 182, 230, 285, 287, 308, 334.

Clinical and Pathologic Features of Tumors Composed of Germ Cells and Sex Cord–Stromal Derivatives

Gonadoblastoma

Synonyms

Dysgenetic gonadoma,[170] gonocytoma,[303] tumor of dysgenetic gonad.[49]

In 1953, Scully[238] described two patients with a distinctive gonadal tumor, which he named *gonadoblastoma*. The tumor was composed of germ cells and sex cord–stromal derivatives, resembling immature granulosa, and Sertoli cells. One of the tumors also contained stromal elements indistinguishable from lutein or Leydig cells. Both tumors occurred in phenotypic females who showed abnormal sexual development. The older patient who was postpubertal showed virilization and it was considered that the tumor was capable of steroid hormone secretion. The tumors were located at the site of normal ovaries, but normal ovarian tissue was not discernible and the exact nature of the gonads in which the tumors had originated could not be determined. Both patients had bilateral tumors that were partly overgrown by dysgerminoma. It was subsequently demonstrated that both patients were chromatin-negative. The tumor was named *gonadoblastoma* because it appeared to recapitulate the development of the gonads and because it occurred in individuals with abnormal sexual development and in gonads, the nature of which could not be determined.[242]

In 1960, Teter[303] proposed a new classification of neoplasms containing germ cells and their endocrine relationships based on the term *gonocytoma*, which had been introduced previously.[294] This classification was an attempt to correlate the histologic, endocrine, clinical, and genetic aspects of this group of neoplasms. Unfortunately, the histologic findings did not always correlate well with the endocrine, genetic, and clinical aspects of the cases. In 1970, Scully[242] in an extensive study of the subject presented convincing arguments against Teter's classification and considered it unjustifiable on both pathologic and clinical grounds. Further support for Scully's views came from other investigators[116,270,271] and from the present concept that the classification of gonadal neoplasms should be based on the morphologic features and histogenesis and not on endocrine, clinical, and genetic considerations.

In view of its distinctive histologic appearance which distinguishes it from any other gonadal neoplasm, gonadoblastoma is considered to be a separate and specific entity. The neoplastic nature of gonadoblastoma has been questioned because some lesions are very small and may undergo complete regression by hyalinization and calcification. Furthermore, when malignancy supervenes, it manifests itself as germ cell neoplasia in spite of the fact that gonadoblastoma is composed of two or three different cell types. When the tumor has metastasized, gonadoblastoma as such has never been observed in the metastases. Nevertheless, gonadoblastoma shows exactly the same pattern in the very small lesions—bisexual formations[306]—as in the large ones, including mitotic activity in the germ cell element and early overgrowth by dysgerminoma. The association with dysgerminoma is seen in 50% of cases[106,242] and with other more malignant germ cell neoplasms in an additional 10%.[242,272] In view of this, the concept that gonadoblastoma represents an in situ germ cell malignancy[242] is considered to be justified.

Clinical Aspects. The exact incidence of gonadoblastoma is not known. Although more than 150 cases have been reported, it is considered to be uncommon. Gonadoblastoma is usually seen in young patients, occurring most frequently in the second and somewhat less frequently in the third and first decades, in that order. All the reported cases occurred in patients under 30 years of age. Gonadoblastoma is much more common in phenotypic females than in phenotypic males, the ratio being 4:1.[242]

Patients with gonadoblastoma usually have primary amenorrhea, virilization, or developmental abnormalities of the genitalia (see Chapter 2, Abnormal Sexual Development). The discovery of gonadoblastoma is made in the course of investigations of these conditions. Another mode of presentation is the presence of a gonadal tumor. The gonadoblastoma, forms part of the tumor in these cases and is discovered on histologic examination. The majority of patients with gonadoblastoma (80%) are phenotypic females, and the remainder are phenotypic males with cryptorchidism, hypospadias, and female internal secondary sex organs. Among the phenotypic females, 60% are virilized and the remainder are normal in appearance.[242] The majority of the phenotypic female patients exhibit abnormal genital development, and breast development is often diminished even among the nonvirilized females. Although primary amenorrhea is a very common presenting symptom among phenotypic females with gonadoblastoma, a few patients have episodes of spontaneous cyclical bleeding, but in the majority of these patients the episodes are sporadic and the bleeding scanty. Occasional patients menstruate normally.[242] The virilization present in phenotypic female patients with gonadoblastoma does not usually regress after excision of the tumor, although this has been seen in occasional cases, and in a few additional cases there was partial regression. Although most patients have gonadal dysgenesis, gonadoblastoma has been described in one patient who has had two normal pregnancies following the excision of a dysgerminoma containing a small focus of gonadoblastoma. This patient was chromatin-positive and had a 46XX karyotype.[25] Gonadoblastoma has also been observed in four true hermaphrodites, two of whom had 46XX karyotype[155,288] and the other two 46XY.[196,267] It was also seen in two males with normally descended testes,[116,276] one of whom fathered two children subsequent to the excision of the testis bearing the lesion.[116]

Macroscopic Appearance. Gonadoblastoma has been found more often in the right gonad than in the left and has been bilateral in 38% of cases.[242] Recent reports suggest an even higher frequency of bilateral involvement. Although many tumors are recognized on gross examination, in a number of cases the lesion is detected only on histologic examination. This may be the case with bilateral tumors, only one of which may be recognized macroscopically. In the majority of cases, the gonad of origin is indeterminate because it is overgrown by the tumor. When the nature of the gonad can be identified, it is usually a streak or a testis. The contralateral gonad in these cases may be a streak or a testis, and the former is more likely to harbor a gonadoblastoma.[242]

Pure gonadoblastoma varies in size from a microscopic lesion to 8 cm in diameter, with most tumors measuring a few centimeters. When gonadoblastoma becomes overgrown by dysgerminoma (Fig. 20.63) or other malignant germ cell elements, much larger tumors may be observed.[242,272] The macroscopic appearance of the tumor varies to some extent according to the presence of hyalinization and calcification, as well as overgrowth by dysgerminoma. Gonadoblastoma is a solid tumor and presents a smooth or slightly lobulated surface. It varies from soft and fleshy to firm and hard. It is speckled with calcific granules and may be almost completely calcified. Calcification has been recognized on gross examination in 45% of cases, and in more than 20% it has been detected radiologically.[242] The tumor varies in color from gray or yellow to brown, and on cut-section it appears to be somewhat granular.

Although the external sex organs in patients with gonadoblastoma present a wide variety of appearances ranging from normal to completely ambiguous, the secondary internal sex organs consist almost always of a uterus, which is hypoplastic in the majority of cases, and two or occasionally one normal fallopian tube. This is also seen in the phenotypic males. Male secondary internal sex organs, such as the epididymis, vas deferens, and prostate, are found occasionally in the virilized phenotypic females and are always found in the phenotypic male pseudohermaphrodites.[242]

Microscopic Appearance. Gonadoblastoma is composed of collections of cellular nests surrounded by connective tissue stroma (Fig. 20.64). The nests are solid, usually small, and oval or round but occasionally may be larger and elongated. The cellular nests contain a mixture of germ cells and sex cord derivatives resembling immature Sertoli and granulosa cells (Fig. 20.65). The germ cells are large and round, with pale or slightly granular cytoplasm and large round vesicular nuclei, often with prominent nucleoli showing histologic and ultrastructural ap-

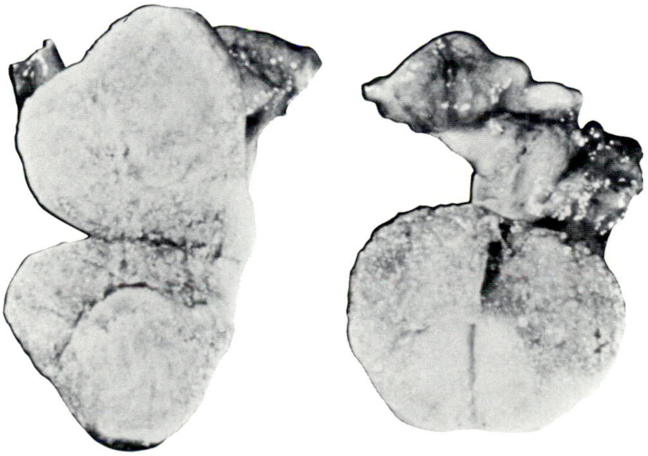

FIG. 20.63. Gonadoblastoma with dysgerminoma. The outer surface is smooth, the cut surface solid, granular, and yellow-brown in color. (Courtesy of R. Scully, M.D.)

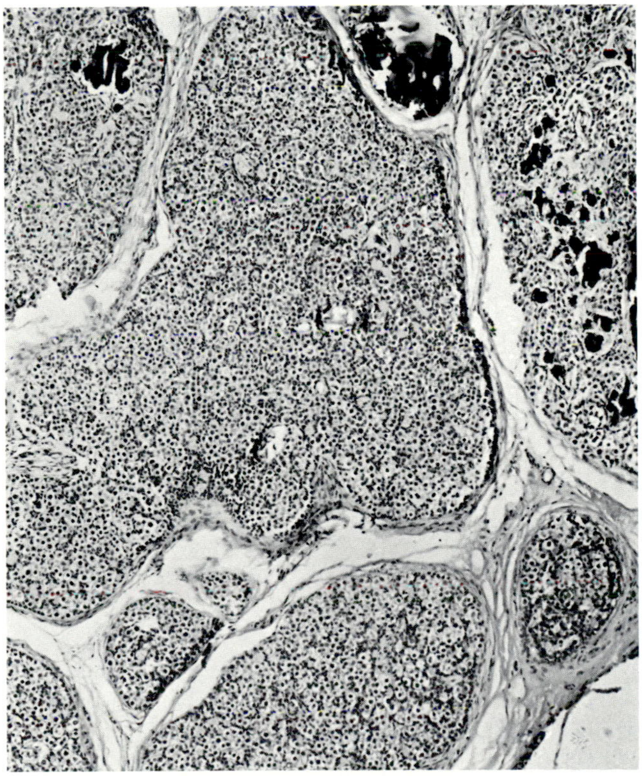

FIG. 20.64. Gonadoblastoma showing the cellular nests surrounded by connective tissue stroma. Note foci of calcification (*heavy black areas*).

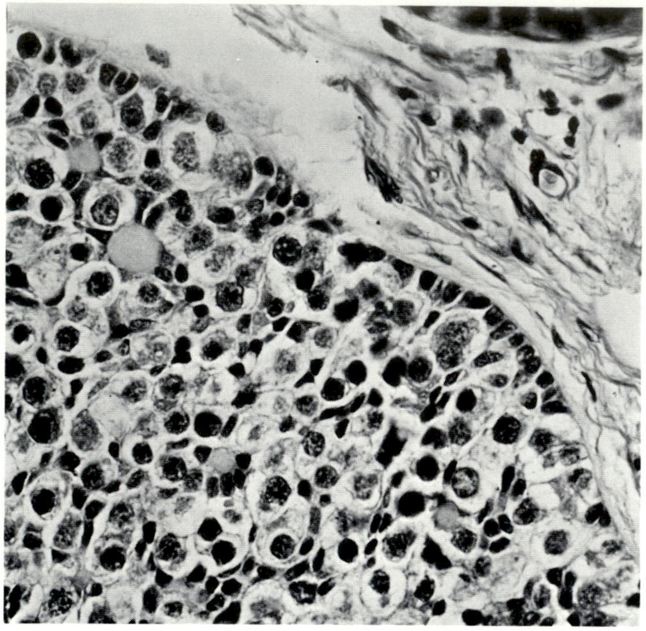

FIG. 20.65. Gonadoblastoma nest composed of large germ cells intimately admixed with smaller sex cord derivatives. Hyaline Call–Exner-like bodies are also seen.

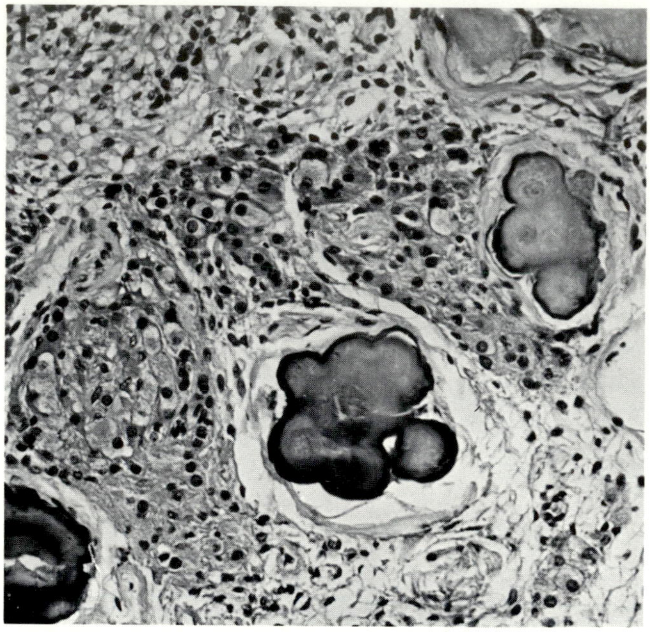

FIG. 20.66. Gonadoblastoma. Calcified nest surrounded by connective tissue containing numerous Leydig or lutein-like cells. Same case as in Figure 20.65.

pearances and histochemical reactions similar to the germ cells of dysgerminoma or seminoma. The germ cells show mitotic activity, which may be marked in some cases. They are intimately admixed with immature Sertoli and granulosa cells, which are smaller and epithelial-like. The latter are round or oval and have dark, oval or slightly elongated carrot-shaped nuclei. Mitotic activity is not seen in these cells. The immature Sertoli and granulosa cells are arranged within the cell nests in three typical patterns (Fig. 20.65):

1. They line the periphery of the nests in a coronal pattern.
2. They surround individual or collections of germ cells in the same way as the follicular epithelium surrounds the ovum of the primary follicle.
3. They surround small round spaces containing amorphous hyaline, eosinophilic, and PAS-positive material that resemble Call–Exner bodies.

The connective tissue stroma surrounding the cellular nests frequently contains collections of cells indistinguishable from Leydig cells or luteinized cells of ovarian stromal origin (Fig. 20.66). There is considerable variation in the number of these cells from case to case; in some cases they are numerous, in others they are identified with difficulty.

Although in many cases the cells are indistinguishable from Leydig cells and may contain lipochrome granules, Reinke crystals, which are specifically diagnostic of Leydig cells, have never been identified in their cytoplasm. The Leydig or lutein-like cells are identified in 66% of cases, and they are present nearly twice as frequently in older patients as in those 15 years of age or younger.[242] The presence of Leydig or lutein-like cells is not necessary for the diagnosis of gonadoblastoma. The connective tissue stroma surrounding the cellular nests may be scanty or abundant and may vary from dense and hyalinized to cellular, resembling ovarian stroma. These latter appearances are more common in tumors that either have arisen in or are suspected to originate in a gonadal streak.[242] Occasionally, the stroma may be loose and edematous. The basic composition of gonadoblastoma, consisting of the two cell types present within the cellular nests and with the Leydig or lutein-like cells present in the stroma, has been confirmed by electron microscopy.[54,87,114,120,153] Although there is full agreement concerning the nature of the germ cells, the nature of the stromal cells is in dispute. They are considered by some to be Sertoli cells or their precursors,[153] whereas others consider them as primitive sex cord–stromal cells and are unable to differentiate them further.[54,114,242,274] The nature of the amorphous, hyaline, eosinophilic material forming Call–Exner-like bodies is also a matter of dispute. It is considered to be either of basement membrane origin[54,120,153] or composed of fibrillar material formed by the stromal cells before they undergo fragmentation and cell death.[114] The former view is supported by the majority of investigators.

The basic histologic appearances of gonadoblastoma may be altered and distorted by three processes: hyalinization, calcification, and overgrowth by dysgerminoma.[87,242,327] Hyalinization takes place by coalescence and extension of the hyaline Call–Exner-like bodies within the nests and of the basement membrane-like band of similar material present around the nest. The hyaline material replaces the tumor cells, and the whole nest may be affected and replaced. Calcification is a common feature (Figs. 20.64 and 20.66) and is seen microscopically in 81% of cases; it usually begins in the Call–Exner-like bodies with formation of small calcific spherules that are frequently laminated, resembling psammoma bodies (Fig. 20.66). The process continues with enlargement and fusion of the calcified bodies and calcification of the hyalinized material, resulting in formation of a calcified mass embracing the whole nest. The process may extend to the stroma, which may also undergo hyalinization and calcification. In such cases, tumor cells become very scarce or absent, and the presence of smooth, rounded, calcified masses may be the only evidence that gonadoblastoma was present (Fig. 20.9). Although this finding is not considered to be diagnostic of gonadoblastoma—it has been called a *burned-out gonadoblastoma*[242,269]—it is a strong argument in favor of the diagnosis and indicates that a careful search for more viable areas of the tumor should be made.

Gonadoblastoma is frequently overgrown by dysgerminoma (Fig. 20.67). This is seen in 50% of cases.[242] The overgrowth of dysgerminoma may vary from the presence of a small collection of germ cells in the stroma outside the gonadoblastoma nests to massive overgrowth of the whole tumor, in which occasional nests of gonadoblastoma may be seen. The dysgerminoma in these cases shows the typical appearances of pure dysgerminoma or seminoma, histologically, histochemically, and ultrastructurally.[54,114,120] Gonadoblastoma may be associated with and overgrown by other more malignant germ cell neoplasms, such as immature teratoma, endodermal sinus tumor, embryonal carcinoma, and choriocarcinoma. This occurs in 10% of cases.[272]

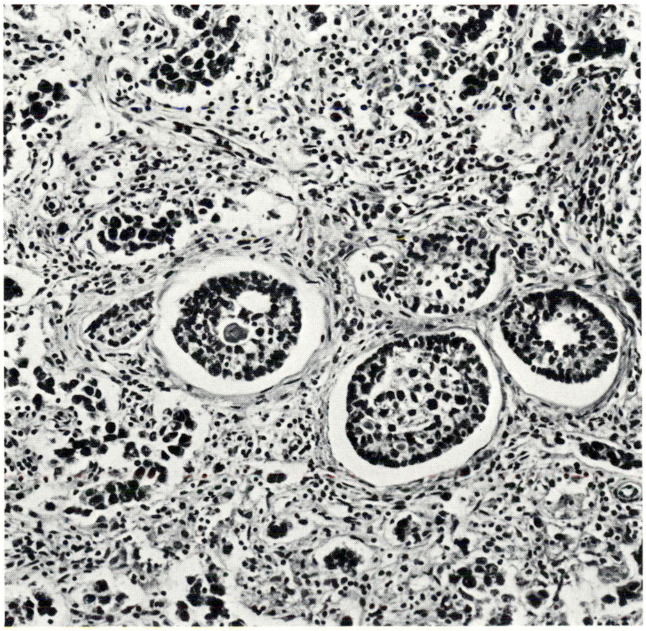

FIG. 20.67. Gonadoblastoma nests surrounded by dysgerminoma. [Reprinted with permission from The American College of Obstetricians and Gynecologists. (Obstetrics and Gynecology, 38:416, 1971).]

Differential Diagnosis. Gonadoblastoma, because of its distinctive histologic appearance and its cellular composition, cannot be easily confused with any of the well-recognized gonadal neoplasms. The gonadal tumors with which confusion may arise are all newly recognized entities and may be related to it. Gonadoblastoma may be confused with the mixed germ cell–sex cord–stromal tumor,[270,271,282] which shares with gonadoblastoma the unique distinction of being composed of germ cells and sex cord–stromal derivatives. The mixed germ cell–sex cord–stromal tumor shows less uniform appearance, absence of nest-like pattern, absence of calcification and hyalinization, a more pronounced proliferative activity involving also the sex cord–stromal derivatives, the tendency to occur in normal gonads, and other genetic, endocrine, and somatic differences. The other lesion resembling gonadoblastoma is the ovarian sex cord tumor with annular tubules,[243,244] which is usually found in patients with Peutz–Jeghers syndrome. This lesion is composed of tubules lined by Sertoli and granulosa-like cells, contains similar round, eosinophilic, and hyaline Call–Exner-like bodies, and tends to calcify in the same manner as gonadoblastoma. The basic difference from gonadoblastoma is the absence of germ cells (see Chapter 19, Sex Cord–Stromal Ovarian Tumors).

Behavior and Therapy. The prognosis of patients with pure gonadoblastoma is excellent, provided the tumor and the contralateral gonad, which may be harboring a macroscopically undetectable gonadoblastoma, are excised. When gonadoblastoma is associated with dysgerminoma, the prognosis is still very good. Metastases tend to occur later and more infrequently than in dysgerminoma arising de novo. All patients with gonadoblastoma and dysgerminoma with known follow-up, including the occasional cases with metastases,[2,107,234] are alive and well following treatment, with the exception of two patients who died with disseminated dysgerminoma.[106,305] The prognosis is totally different when gonadoblastoma is associated with more malignant germ cell neoplasms, such as embryonal carcinoma, endodermal sinus tumor, choriocarcinoma, and immature teratoma. In the past, none of these patients survived longer than 18 months.[272] More recently, the administration of combination chemotherapy used in the treatment of malignant germ cell tumors has improved this dismal prognosis.

Gonadoblastoma occurs almost entirely in patients with dysgenetic gonads, which are not capable of normal function. Moreover, since the gonadoblastoma may act as a source from which malignant germ cell neoplasms may originate, there is general agreement that excision of the gonads is the treatment of choice.* This applies not only to the gonad that appears to be abnormal but also to the contralateral gonad, however normal or small it may be. If one of the gonads is not excised, the risk of a malignant neoplasm developing is considerable, although the time interval may vary.[232] There is no complete agreement whether the uterus should be excised together with the gonads. It has been considered that for psychologic reasons it should be left in situ so that periodic bleeding simulating menstruation can take place on estrogen–progesterone substitution therapy. However, since estrogen administration is associated with a risk of development of endometrial carcinoma,[52] excision of the uterus together with the gonads has been advocated.[233]

Endocrine Aspects. The association of gonadoblastoma with certain endocrine abnormalities was noted in one of the two cases first reported.[239] In view of the fact that gonadoblastoma occurs almost entirely in patients with gonadal dysgenesis, the defective gonadal development present in these patients should not be confused with the presence of endocrine effects that are associated with the tumor and are not a result of the abnormal gonadal development. Although the virilization produced by the tumor may regress following the excision of the tumor, there is no further gonadal development and the gonadal abnormalities remain.

Although the exact source of the steroid hormone production was not originally known, the interstitial cells resembling Leydig or lutein cells were considered to be the most likely source of the androgens.[239] Further observations have shown that the presence of Leydig or luteinlike cells is not always associated with the presence of virilization, although they are more frequently encountered in tumors from virilized phenotypic female patients than in those from nonvirilized patients. The possibility that the tumor may secrete estrogens, as evidenced by complaints of hot flushes and other menopausal symptoms following the excision of the tumor, has also been noted.[242] Originally, the evidence of hormone secretion was mainly clinical, usually evidenced by virilization occurring after puberty and manifesting itself as masculine body contour, hirsutism, and clitoromegaly. Slight elevation of the urinary 17-ketosteroid excretion was noted in some cases.[50,156] The gonadotropins, when estimated, were usually elevated.[303]

In recent years it has been shown that gonadoblastoma is capable of producing testosterone from progesterone in vitro.[8,18,19,101,153,224] Production of estrogens from progesterone by gonadoblastoma has also been observed.[101,153] Evidence of testosterone secretion in vivo in patients with gonadal dysgenesis has been presented.[128,324] Androgen and estrogen formation from progesterone in vitro has been demonstrated in a streak gonad that did not contain any Leydig and lutein cells microscopically but from the description may have contained a small burned-out gonadoblastoma.[153] Although in vitro testosterone formation has been ascribed to the Leydig or lutein-like cells present in the gonadoblastoma,[19,224] the demonstration of steroid production by a streak gonad that did not contain Leydig or lutein cells indicates that the stromal tissue also has the capability of steroid synthesis.[153]

In spite of all these advances in the study and understanding of the hormonal aspects of gonadoblastoma and dysgenetic gonads, considerable problems remain, the most important being why some patients become virilized and others do not. Although there is a relationship between the virilization of patients with gonadoblastoma and the presence of Leydig or lutein-like cells, this relationship is not constant. It may be that the reason is quantitative and that the amount of the steroid secretion may be inadequate to produce virilization because of a small cell mass. Another possible reason is that the steroid metabolic pathways may be different and that gonadoblastoma may produce different steroid hormones or different quantities of various steroid hormones. Some of these hormones may be metabolically nonfunctioning and therefore unassociated with endocrine side effects, whereas the metabolically active steroids may be associated with evidence and visible signs of endocrine activity.[153]

Genetic Aspects. Gonadoblastoma occurs almost entirely in patients with pure or mixed gonadal dysgenesis or in male pseudohermaphrodites (see Chapter 2, Abnormal Sexual Development). Occasional patients are of short stature and may have other stigmata of Turner's syndrome.[232] The majority of patients are chromatin-negative; this has been observed in 89% of cases.[242] Nearly all patients with gonadoblastoma whose karyotype was recorded (96%) were found to have a Y chromosome.[232] Three patients had a 46XX karyotype,[25,94,227] and one of these was fertile;[25] one patient had a 45X/46XX mosaicism.[197] The most frequently encountered karotype was 46XY, which was seen in half the cases; this was followed by 45X/46XY mosaicism, which was seen in a quarter of the cases. The remainder showed many different forms of mosaicism.[232] Six patients had morphologic abnormalities of the Y chromosome. Of 25 patients with gonadal dysgenesis and dysgerminoma, 96% had a Y

* References 87, 107, 233, 242, 272, 305, 328.

chromosome. The karyotype was 46XY in 60%, followed by 45X/46XY in 24%. The remainder showed various forms of mosaicism.[232] One patient had 45X monosomy and Turner's syndrome. All other patients with features of Turner's syndrome had various forms of mosaicism containing a Y chromosome. The similarity between the distribution of the karyotypes in the gonadoblastoma group and patients with dysgerminoma and gonadal dysgenesis is striking, and 62% of the former group and 45% of the latter had clitoral hypertrophy.[232]

Family history of gonadal dysgenesis has been noted in at least 10 reports of patients with gonadoblastoma.[7,8,269] Evidence of gonadal dysgenesis affecting three generations of the family of a patient with gonadoblastoma was obtained in two instances.[7,21] Gonadoblastoma has been reported in one pair of twins[78] and in four pairs of siblings.[7,8,31,269] All these patients had 46XY karyotype. It has been postulated that the mode of inheritance is either an X-linked recessive gene or an autosomal sex-linked mutant gene.[21,232,233,261]

Mixed Germ Cell–Sex Cord–Stromal Tumor

Synonyms

Epithelioma Pflügerien,[167] Pflügerome,[41] mixed germ cell tumor,[116] gonocytoma II.[305,304]

The descriptive term *mixed germ cell–sex cord–stromal tumor* was originally intended to embrace all the tumors composed of these cell types, including the gonadoblastoma. In view of the fact that the latter term is now so well established, it is considered that the term *mixed germ cell–sex cord–stromal tumor* should be reserved for tumors composed of these cell types that exhibit distinctive histologic appearances differing from those of gonadoblastoma.[270,271] This term is considered to be preferable to the term *Pflügerome*[41] or *epithelioma Pflügerien*[167] because these terms imply a possible origin from Pflüger's tubes (germ cell clusters in a granulosal envelope that are formed during gonadal embryogenesis and may persist into infancy). Since there is no good evidence for this mode of origin and there is some doubt as to the formation of Pflüger's tubes during human embryogenesis, the term *Pflügerome* is not considered to be satisfactory. The term *mixed germ cell tumor*[116] is considered to be unsatisfactory because it implies a tumor composed of a mixture of different types of germ cell elements without the presence of sex cord–stromal elements, and this term is used in this context in the classification of ovarian tumors proposed by the WHO ovarian tumor panel.[250]

Clinical Aspects. These neoplasms are rare, and only a few adequately documented cases have been recorded, although it is likely that some cases may not have been recognized and have been classified with tumors of germ cell origin or with sex cord–stromal tumors. This is supported by the fact that since this neoplasm has been recognized as a specific entity, additional well-documented and so far unreported cases have been encountered. Tumors of this type have been observed more frequently in normal phenotypic female patients but have also been encountered in normal adult males. Most of the known cases in females, were encountered in children in the first decade. Ten cases occurred in infants under 1 year of age.[62,271,274] In one case, the tumor occurred in a 31-year-old woman who has had a normal pregnancy. Therefore, the age incidence of patients with this neoplasm, differs from that of patients with gonadoblastoma.[274]

In contrast to patients with gonadoblastoma, patients with this neoplasm are normal phenotypic females, usually children. The main presenting symptom has been the presence of an abdominal tumor mass sometimes complicated by torsion and symptoms of acute abdominal emergency. One 8-year-old patient exhibited signs of precocious puberty for 3 years before the discovery of a large ovarian tumor.[282] Signs of precocious puberty were also seen in two infants aged under 1 year. The other patients did not have endocrine abnormalities. The somatosexual development of all the patients has been normal, and there was no evidence of any abnormalities affecting the gonads or the external genitalia.

Macroscopic Appearance. The tumors encountered have been relatively large (Fig. 20.68), varying in size from 7.5 to 18 cm in diameter and weighing from 100 to 1050 g. The tumor was found to be unilateral in all cases but one, and the contralateral gonad has always been described as a normal ovary. In some cases where biopsy was performed, this was confirmed on microscopic examination.

The tumor is usually round or oval, firm in consistency, and surrounded by a smooth, slightly glistening gray or gray-yellow capsule. In most cases the tumor was solid[270,271] (Fig. 20.68), but in some cases it was partly solid and partly cystic, containing a number of cystic spaces that varied in size.[282] The cut surface of the tumor is uniformly gray to gray-pink or yellow to pale brown. Neither calcified areas nor foci of necrosis have been observed on gross examination. The fallopian tubes and the uterus have always been found to be normal. There have been no abnormalities affecting the external genitalia.

Microscopic Appearance. The tumor is composed of germ cells and sex cord derivatives, intimately admixed with each other. The tumor cells form three different histologic patterns, which in places intermingle with each other. One is composed of long, narrow ramifying cords or trabeculae (Fig. 20.69), which in places expand to form wider columns and larger round or oval cellular

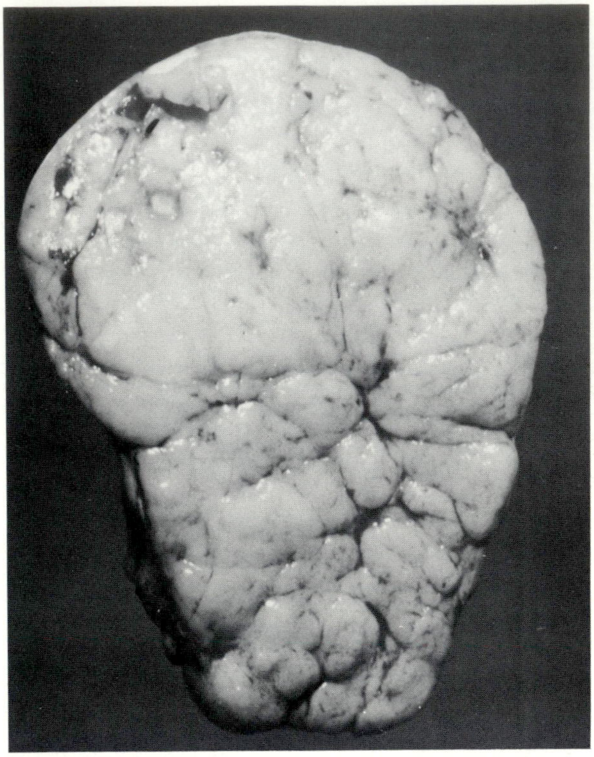

FIG. 20.68. Mixed germ cell–sex cord–stromal tumor of the ovary from a 9-month-old normal female child. The tumor is large, and the external surface is lobulated. The cut surface is solid, bulging, uniform, and gray-yellow. (Courtesy H. W. Oechler, M.D.)

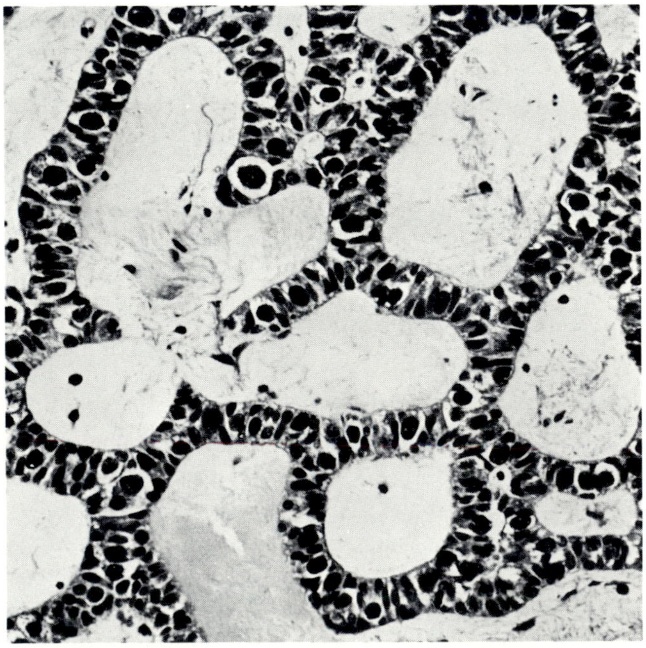

FIG. 20.69. Mixed germ cell–sex cord–stromal tumor composed of long ramifying cords. Note the large germ cells and smaller sex cord derivatives and the loose connective tissue stroma.

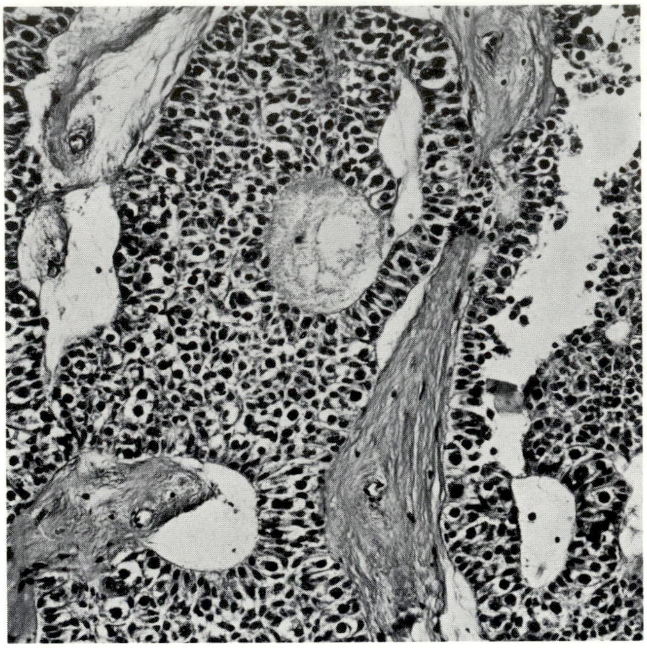

FIG. 20.70. Mixed germ cell–sex cord–stromal tumor composed of large cellular aggregates and more slender cords. Note the hyaline connective tissue stroma.

aggregates surrounded by connective tissue stroma (Fig. 20.70). The second consists of tubular structures devoid of a lumen and surrounded by a fine connective tissue network (Figs. 20.71 and 20.72). In some places, the tubular pattern is less obvious, and the tumor forms small clusters or larger round or oval cellular masses

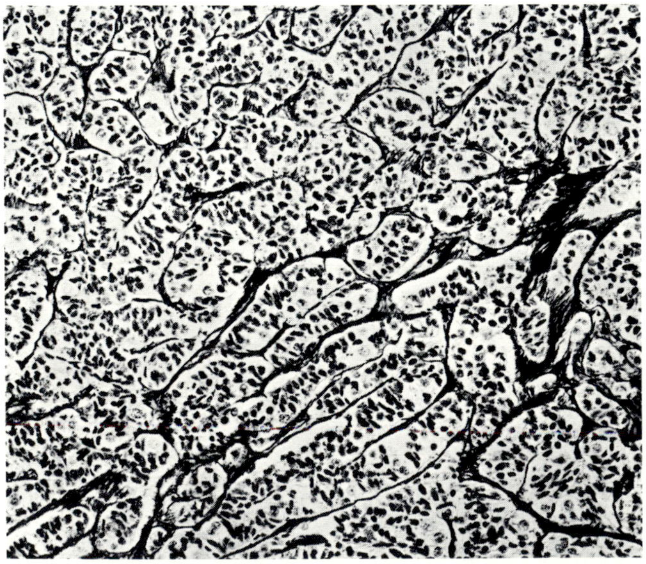

FIG. 20.71. Mixed germ cell–sex cord–stromal tumor composed of solid tubules surrounded by fine connective tissue septa. [Reprinted with permission from The American College of Obstetricians and Gynecologists. (Obstetrics and Gynecology, 40:473, 1972).]

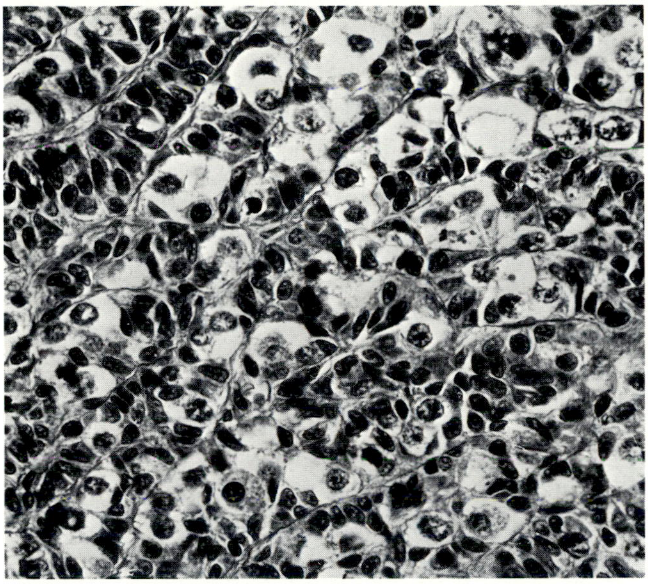

FIG. 20.72. Mixed germ cell–sex cord–stromal tumor showing the tubular pattern and cellular composition. [Reprinted with permission from The American College of Obstetricians and Gynecologists. (Obstetrics and Gynecology, 40:473, 1972).]

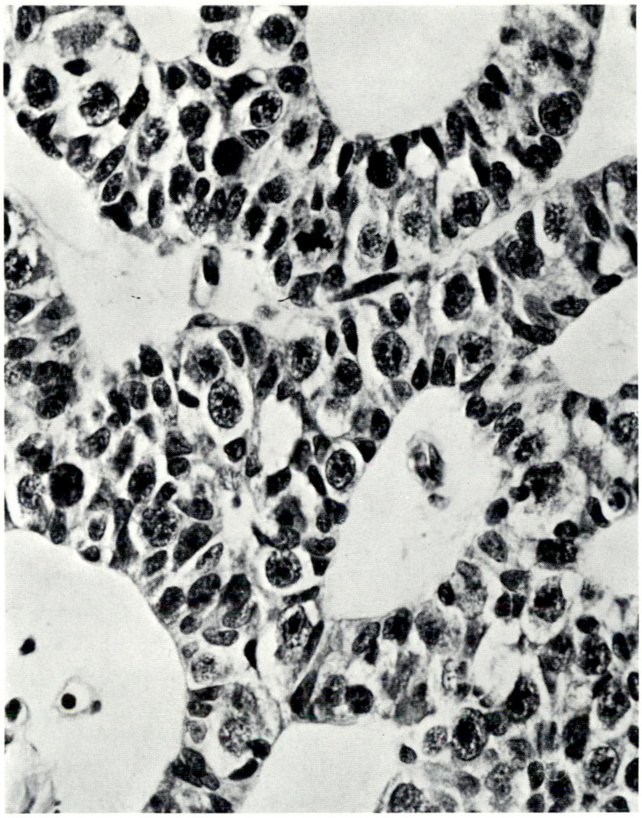

FIG. 20.73. Mixed germ cell–sex cord–stromal tumor showing the cord-like pattern and cellular composition. Tripolar mitosis is seen above *center*.

surrounded by connective tissue stroma. The latter varies in amount and appearance and tends to be more abundant in tumors showing mainly the cordlike or trabecular pattern (Fig. 20.69), whereas the tubular variety tends to be more cellular and contains less connective tissue (Figs. 20.71 and 20.72). The stroma may vary from loose and edematous (Fig. 20.69) to dense fibrous and hyalinized (Fig. 20.70). The former is seen more often where the cord-like pattern is most prominent, whereas the latter surrounds the larger cellular aggregates. The third pattern consists of scattered collections of germ cells surrounded by sex cord elements that may be very abundant. The germ cells admixed with sex cord derivatives may also be scattered individually and in small groups within connective tissue stroma. Admixture between the above-described patterns is often seen. The typical nest-like pattern present in gonadoblastoma is not observed. In one case, only a few very small collections of Leydig or lutein-like cells were observed,[270] but in all the remaining cases, these cells were not identified.

The two cellular elements present in the tumor, the germ cells and the sex cord derivatives, are intimately admixed together. The sex cord derivatives are arranged peripherally in a single file, forming long rows at the periphery of the cords (Figs. 20.69 and 20.73) or peripherally lining the tubular structures (Fig. 20.72) as well as surrounding individual or groups of germ cells within the small clusters or larger aggregates. The germ cells resemble those observed in dysgerminoma and gonadoblastoma in all respects, including histochemical reactions. In some cases, a number of the germ cells present in this tumor appear more mature than the germ cells observed in gonadoblastoma or dysgerminoma and tend to resemble primordial germ cells. In view of this, it is possible that they may represent a later stage in the maturation of the germ cell than that seen in gonadoblastoma or dysgerminoma. They show brisk mitotic activity (Fig. 20.73). The sex cord derivatives tend to resemble Sertoli cells more than granulosa cells. They show variable degrees of mitotic activity. The tumor does not show hyalinization, calcification, or the regressive changes observed in gonadoblastoma and appears to be actively proliferative. There is some variation in the cellular content in some parts of the tumor; in some areas there is a preponderance of germ cells, whereas in others the sex cord derivatives predominate. However, the intimate admixture of these two cell types is seen everywhere. Most tumors show a solid pattern, although occasional small clefts may be present. Cystic spaces of varying size either lined by flattened epithelial-like cells, devoid of lining, or lined by sex cord derivatives may be observed. They resemble the cystic spaces observed in some retiform Sertoli-Leydig cell tumors[337] or cystic sex cord–stromal tumors.

Normal ovarian tissue as evidenced by the presence

of normal ovarian stroma, and at least some primordial follicles has been identified in all cases, including a case where it could not be identified in the original sections available.[270] In some cases, graafian follicles are also present.[271,282] In other cases, tumor deposits are found very close to the surface of the ovary. Mixed germ cell–sex cord–stromal tumor has never been observed in metastatic lesions or seen in tumors present in extragonadal sites. The histologic appearances of this tumor were described in detail some years ago.[270,271] Originally, it was considered that the tumor might consist of two specific varieties, each with a different histologic pattern. Subsequently, it has become apparent that not only two but three histologic patterns may be present in the same tumor and can be seen to intermingle and merge with each other.[274,282]

Differential Diagnosis. Histologically, this tumor is most likely to be confused with gonadoblastoma. It can be differentiated from it by the absence of the nest-like pattern, greater proliferative activity, including that of the sex cord derivatives, absence of calcification and hyalinization within the tumor, and in the majority of cases by the absence of Leydig or lutein-like cells. Macroscopically, the tumors are larger. The gonad of origin is a normal ovary, and there is no evidence of gonadal dysgenesis or any somatosexual abnormalities. The patients are chromatin-positive and have a normal female 46XX karyotype. There is no evidence of virilization, and if there are signs of abnormal endocrine activity, they manifest themselves as feminization. Occasionally, if the germ cells are relatively scanty, the tumor may be confused with the sex cord–stromal tumors of the ovary, but the presence of germ cells should alert the observer to the true identity of the tumor. If the sex cord derivatives either are few in number, are missed, or are disregarded, the tumor may be included with the germ cell tumors, but the presence of sex cord elements intimately admixed with the germ cells should indicate its true identity. The presence of prominent clefts and cystic spaces, especially when the latter contain papillary projections, may cause confusion with Sertoli-Leydig cell tumors showing the retiform pattern or even with serous papillary tumors. The presence of germ cells admixed with sex cord derivatives indicates that the tumor is a mixed germ cell–sex cord–stromal tumor.

Behavior and Therapy. Although the biologic behavior of this neoplasm is not known with certainty, the prognosis of patients with mixed germ cell–sex cord–stromal tumor of the ovary seems to be very favorable. In the majority of cases when the tumor was not associated with other malignant neoplastic germ cell elements, there has been no recurrence or metastases following excision of the affected adnexa, and the patients are well and free of disease for periods varying from 1 to 15 years. In all these cases the tumor was confined to the ovary, was fully mobile, and was excised completely. In one case the patient probably had the tumor for 3 years prior to its excision, and there was no evidence of metastases in the abdominal cavity and the biopsy of the contralateral ovary was normal. The patient is well and disease-free 9 years following the excision of the tumor.[282] In two patients in their 20s and one in her early 30s, the mixed germ cell–sex cord–stromal tumor was associated with dysgerminoma. There was no evidence of metastases. The patients are well and disease-free from 2 to 7 years after one-sided adnexectomy and radiation therapy. In three children aged 5, 6, and 15 years, the tumor was overgrown by other malignant germ cell elements, including choriocarcinoma and endodermal sinus tumor. In these cases, the tumor metastasized and resulted in the death of the patients. The metastases were composed of the malignant germ cell elements. When the tumor is associated with the latter, the patient should be treated with the appropriate combination chemotherapy used in treatment of malignant nondysgerminomatous germ cell tumors.

Since the patients with this tumor are young, normally developed female children and since the prognosis is generally favorable, the treatment of choice is conservative. If there is no involvement of adjacent organs and structures, oophorectomy or excision of the affected adnexa is adequate. Careful examination of the abdomen and a biopsy of the contralateral ovary are recommended. Following this procedure, the patient should be fully investigated, and this should include chromosome studies. If the karyotype is 46XX and if no other abnormalities are detected, further therapy is not necessary, although careful long-term follow-up is essential.

Endocrine Aspects. The majority of patients with mixed germ cell–sex cord–stromal tumor do not exhibit any endocrine abnormalities as observed clinically. In the majority of cases, tests of hormonal function have not been performed preoperatively. In cases where they have been performed postoperatively, they have been found to be normal. In one case, the patient, an 8-year-old girl, exhibited signs of precocious puberty manifesting as mammary development and menstrual bleeding for 3 years prior to the diagnosis of a large ovarian tumor. There was an increased urinary estrogen excretion. Following excision of the ovarian tumor, the uterine bleeding ceased and the urinary estrogens became normal.[282] Isosexual precocious puberty has been seen in two other patients under 1 year of age, who exhibited mammary development and vaginal bleeding. The urinary estrogens were elevated, and vaginal smears showed estrogen effect. Following the excision of the tumor, there was a complete return to normality. There was no evidence of virilization in any of the patients. These findings indicate that female patients with this neoplasm do not have any associated endocrine abnormalities or if these are present they manifest themselves as feminization. One of the patients, who had mixed germ cell–sex cord–stromal tumor excised at the age of 10 years,[270] has developed normally and commenced menstruating at the age of 15 years. She is well and disease-free 12 years after excision of the tumor.

Genetic Aspects. Nearly all female patients with this neoplasm have had genotype and karyotype determinations and have been found chromatin-positive and to have the normal female chromosome complement of 46XX. All the patients with this tumor showed normal somatosexual development. Therefore, there is no evidence that patients with this tumor have chromosomal abnormalities or gonadal dysgenesis.

References

1. Abbot TM, Herman WJ Jr, Scully RE (1984) Ovarian fetiform teratoma (homunculus) in a 9-year-old girl. Int J Gynecol Pathol 2: 392
2. Abell MR, Johnson VJ, Holtz F (1965) Ovarian neoplasms in childhood and adolescence. Part 1. Tumors of germ cell origin. Am J Obstet Gynecol 92: 1059
3. Abitol MM, Pomerance W, Mackles A (1959) Spontaneous intraperitoneal rupture of benign cystic teratomas. Review of literature and report of two cases. Obstet Gynecol 13: 198
4. Afridi MA, Vongtama V, Tsukada Y, Piver MS (1976) Dysgerminoma of the ovary. Radiation therapy for recurrence and metastases. Am J Obstet Gynecol 126: 190
5. Aguirre P, Scully RE (1982) Malignant neuroectodermal tumor of the ovary: A distinctive form of monodermal teratoma. Report of five cases. Am J Surg Pathol 6: 283
6. Albrechtsen R, Klee JG, Moller JE (1972) Primary intracranial germ cell tumours, including five cases of endodermal sinus tumour. Acta Pathol Microbiol Scand [80A Suppl] 233: 32
7. Allard S, Cadotte M, Boivin Y (1972) Dysgenesie gonadique pure familiale et gonadoblastome. L'Union Medicale du Canada 101: 448
8. Anderson CT Jr, Carlson IH (1975) Elevated plasma testosterone and gonadal tumors in two 46XY "sisters." Arch Pathol 99: 360
9. Anderson MC, McDicken IW (1971) Melanotic cyst of the ovary. J Obstet Gynaecol Br Commw 78: 1047
10. Ansfield FJ, Korbitz BC, Davis HL, Ramirez G (1969) Triple drug therapy in testicular tumors. Cancer 24: 442
11. Arhelger RB, Kelly B (1974) Strumal carcinoid. Report of a case with electron microscopical observations. Arch Pathol 97: 323
12. Asadourian LA, Taylor HB (1969) Dysgerminoma. An analysis of 105 cases. Obstet Gynecol 33: 370
13. Awais GA (1983) Dysgerminoma and serum lactic dehydrogenase levels. Obstet Gynecol 61: 99
14. Azoury RS, Jubayli NW, Barakat BY (1973) Dermoid cyst of the ovary containing fetus-like structure. Obstet Gynecol 42: 887
15. Bagg HJ (1936) Experimental production of teratoma testis in a fowl. Am J Cancer 26: 69
16. Ballas M (1972) Yolk sac carcinoma of the ovary with alpha-fetoprotein in serum and ascitic fluid demonstrated by immunoosmophoresis. Am J Clin Pathol 57: 511
17. Ballas M (1974) The significance of alpha-fetoprotein in the serum of patients with malignant teratomas and related gonadal neoplasms. Am J Clin Lab Sci 4: 267
18. Bardin CW, Rosen S, Le Maire WJ, Tjio JH, Gallup J, Marshall J, Savard K (1968) In vivo and in vitro studies of androgen metabolism in a patient with pure gonadal dysgenesis and Leydig cell hyperplasia. J Clin Endocrinol Metab 29: 1429
19. Barry KG, Crosby WH (1957) Autoimmune hemolytic anemia arrested by removal of ovarian teratoma: Review of the literature and report of a case. Ann Int Med 47: 1002
20. Bartlett DJ, Grant JK, Pugh MA, Aherne W (1968) A familial feminizing syndrome. A family showing intersex characteristics with XY chromosomes in three female members. J Obstet Gynaecol Br Commw 75: 199
21. Battifora H, Sheibani K, Tubbs RR, Kopinski MI, Sun TT (1984) Antikeratin antibodies in tumor diagnosis. Distinction between seminoma and embryonal carcinoma. Cancer 54: 843
22. Beck JS, Fulmer HF, Lee ST (1969) Solid malignant ovarian teratoma with "embryoid bodies" and trophoblastic differentiation. J Pathol 99: 67
23. Beilby JOW, Todd PJ (1974) Yolk sac tumour of the ovary. J Obstet Gynaecol Br Commw 81: 90
24. Berg JW, Baylor SM (1973) The epidemiologic pathology of ovarian cancer. Hum Pathol 4: 537
25. Bergher de Bacalao E, Dominguez I (1969) Unilateral gonadoblastoma in a pregnant woman. Am J Obstet Gynecol 105: 1279
26. Bergstrand CG, Czar B (1956) Demonstration of a new protein fraction in serum from human fetus. Scand J Lab Invest 8: 174
27. Bernstein D, Naor S, Rikover M, Manahem H (1974) Hemolytic anemia related to ovarian tumor. Obstet Gynecol 43: 276
28. Bestle J (1968) Extragonadal endodermal sinus tumours originating in the region of the pineal gland. Acta Pathol Microbiol Scand 74: 214
29. Bettinger HF, Jacobs H (1948) Mesonephroma ovarii. Med J Aust 1: 100
30. Blackwell WJ, Dockerty MB, Masson JC, Mussey RD (1946) Dermoid cysts of the ovary; clinical and pathological significance. Am J Obstet Gynecol 51: 151
31. Boczkowski K, Teter J, Sternadel Z (1972) Sibship occurrence of XY gonadal dysgenesis with dysgerminoma. Am J Obstet Gynecol 113: 952
32. Borushek S, Berger I, Echt C, Gold JJ (1965) Functioning malignant germ cell tumor of the ovary in a 4½ year old girl. Cancer 18: 1485
33. Bradof JE, Hakes TB, Ochoa M, Golbey R (1982) Germ cell malignancies of the ovary. Treatment with vinblastine,

actinomycin D, bleomycin and cisplatin containing chemotherapy combinations. Cancer 50: 1070
34. Braunstein H, Stephens CL, Gibson RL (1968) Secretory granules in medullary carcinoma of the thyroid. Electron microscopic demonstration. Arch Pathol 85: 306
35. Breen JL, Maxson WS (1977) Ovarian tumors in children and adolescents. Clin Obstet Gynecol 20: 607
36. Breen JL, Neubecker RD (1963) Malignant teratoma of the ovary. An analysis of 17 cases. Obstet Gynecol 21: 669
37. Breen JL, Neubecker RD (1967) Ovarian malignancy in children with special reference to the germ cell tumors. Ann NY Acad Sci 142: 658
38. Brody S (1961) Clinical aspects of dysgerminoma of the ovary. Acta Radiol (Stockholm) 56: 209
39. Brown JR, Green JD (1976) Yolk sac carcinoma. South Med J 69: 728
40. Burkons DM, Hart WR (1978) Ovarian germinomas (dysgerminomas). Obstet Gynecol 51: 221
41. Cabanne F (1971) Gonadoblastomes et tumerus de l'ebauche gonadique. Ann Anat Pathol (Paris) 16: 387
42. Carleton RL, Friedman NB, Bomze EJ (1953) Experimental teratomas of testis. Cancer 6: 464
43. Caruso PA, Marsh MR, Minkowitz S, Karten G (1971) An intense clinicopathologic study of 305 teratomas of the ovary. Cancer 27: 343
44. Chenot M (1911) Contribution à l'étude des épithéliomas primitifs de l'ovaire. Thesis, Paris
45. Chevassu M (1906) Tumeurs du Testicule. Thesis, Steinhall Paris
46. Chretien PB, Milam JD, Foote FW, Miller TR (1970) Embryonal adenocarcinomas (a type of malignant teratoma) of the sacrococcygeal region. Clinical and pathologic aspects of 21 cases. Cancer 26: 522
47. Chumas JC, Rosenwaks Z, Mann JW, Finkel G, Pastore J (1984) Sertoli-Leydig cell tumor of the ovary producing alpha-fetoprotein. Int J Gynecol Pathol 3: 213
48. Climie AR, Heath LP (1968) Malignant degeneration of benign cystic teratoma of the ovary. Review of the literature and report of a chondrosarcoma and a carcinoid tumor. Cancer 22: 824
49. Collins DH, Symington T (1965) Sertoli cell tumour. In: Collins DH, Pugh RCB (eds) The pathology of testicular tumours. Edinburgh and London, Livingstone Ltd., pp 52–61
50. Cooperman LR, Hamlin J, Elmer N (1968) Gonadoblastoma: A rare ovarian tumor with characteristic roentgen appearance. Radiology 90: 322
51. Corfman PA, Richart RM (1964) Chromosome number and morphology of benign cystic teratomas. N Engl J Med 271: 1241
52. Cutler BS, Forbes AP, Ingersoll FM, Scully RE (1972) Endometrial carcinoma after stilbestrol therapy in gonadal dysgenesis. N Engl J Med 287: 628
53. Dalgaard JB, Wetteland P (1956) Struma ovarii. A follow-up study of 20 cases. Acta Chir Scand 112: 1
54. Damjanov I, Drobnjak P, Grizelj V (1975). Ultrastructure of gonadoblastoma. Arch Pathol 99: 25
55. Dandia SD (1967) Rectovesical fistula following an ovarian dermoid with recurrent vesical calculus. A case report. J Urol 97: 85
56. Davidsohn I, Kovarik S, Stejskal R (1968) Immunological aspects. Influence of prognosis and treatment. In: Gentil F, Junqueira AC (eds) Ovarian cancer U.I.C.C. Monograph Series, Vol 11. Berlin, Heidelberg, New York, Springer-Verlag, pp 105–121
57. Dawson MA, Wilimer T, Yarbro JW (1971) Hemolytic anemia associated with an ovarian tumor. Am J Med 50: 552
58. Dayal Y, Tashjian AH Jr, Wolfe HJ (1979) Immunocytochemical localization of calcitonin-producing cells in a strumal carcinoid with amyloid stroma. Cancer 43: 1331
59. De Haan QC (1965) Non-gestational choriocarcinoma of the ovary. Obstet Gynecol 26: 708
60. De Lima FAO (1966) Disgerminoma do Ovario, contribucao para o seo estudo anatomo-clinico. Thesis, Sao Paulo, Brazil
61. Dikman SH, Toker C (1971) Strumal carcinoid of the ovary with musculinization. Cancer 27: 925
62. Diligent E (1971) Gonadoblastomes et dysgenesies pseudogonadoblastiques. Thesis. Nancy
63. Dixon FJ, Moore RA (1952) Tumors of the male sex organs. Atlas of Tumor Pathology, Sect VIII, Fasc 31b and 32. Washington, D.C., Armed Forces Institute of Pathology
64. Duhig JT (1959) An unusual adenocarcinoma of the ovary. A case simulating Schiller's mesonephroma. Am J Obstet Gynecol 77: 201
65. Duval M (1891) Le placenta de rongeurs. J Anat Physiol (Paris) 27: 515
66. Einhorn LH, Donohue J (1977) Cisdiammine dichloroplatinum, vinblastine, and bleomycin combination chemotherapy in disseminated testicular cancer. Ann Intern Med 87: 293
67. Emge LA (1940) Functional and growth characteristics of struma ovarii. Am J Obstet Gynecol 40: 738
68. Engel T, Greeley AV, Sweeney WJ III (1965) Recurrent dermoid cysts of the ovary. Report of 2 cases. Obstet Gynecol 26: 757
69. Erez SE, Richart RM, Shettles LB (1965) Hashimoto's disease in a benign cystic teratoma of the ovary. Am J Obstet Gynecol 92: 273
70. Evans RW (1957) Developmental stages of embryo-like bodies in teratoma testis. J Clin Pathol 10: 321
71. Evans RW (1966) Histological appearances of tumours, 2nd ed. Edinburgh and London, Livingstone
72. Ewing J (1940) Neoplastic diseases, 4th ed. Philadelphia, Saunders, pp 641, 672
73. Felmus LB, Pedowitz P (1968) Clinical malignancy of endocrine tumors of the ovary and dysgerminoma. Obstet Gynecol 29: 344
74. Flamant F, Caillou B, Pejovic MH, Gerard-Marchant R, Gout M, Lemerle J, Sarrazin D, Zucker JM, Schweisguth O (1978) Prognostic factors in malignant germ cell tumors of the ovary in children excluding pure dysgerminoma. Eur J Cancer 14: 901
75. Forney JP, Di Saia PJ, Morrow CP (1975) Endodermal sinus tumor. A report of two sustained remissions treated postoperatively with a combination of actinomycin D, 5-

fluorouracil and cyclophosphamide. Obstet Gynecol 45: 186

76. Fox H, Langley FA (1976) Tumours of the ovary. London, William Heinemann Medical Books
77. Fox H, Kazzaz B, Langley FA (1964) Argyrophil and argentaffin cells in the female genital tract and in ovarian mucinous cysts. J Pathol Bacteriol 88: 479
78. Frazier SD, Bashore RA, Mosier HD (1964) Gonadoblastoma associated with pure gonadal dysgenesis in monozygous twins. J Pediatr 64: 740
79. Freel JH, Cassir JF, Pierce VK, Woodruff J, Lewis JL Jr (1979) Dysgerminoma of the ovary. Cancer 43: 798
80. Friedman NB (1951) The comparative morphogenesis of extragenital and gonadal teratoid tumors. Cancer 4: 265
81. Friedman NB, Moore RA (1946) Tumors of the testis. A report of 922 cases. Mil Surgeon 99: 573
82. Fujii S, Konishi I, Suzuki A, Okamura H, Okazaki T, Mori T (1985) Analysis of serum lactic dehydrogenase levels and its isoenzymes in ovarian dysgerminoma. Gynecol Oncol 22: 65
83. Galager HS, Lewis RP (1973) Sequential gonadoblastoma and choriocarcinoma. Obstet Gynecol 41: 123
84. Gallion H, Van Nagell JR, Powell DF, Donaldson ES, Hanson M (1979) Therapy of endodermal sinus tumor of the ovary. Am J Obstet Gynecol 135: 447
85. Galton M, Benirschke K (1959) 46 chromosomes in an ovarian teratoma. Lancet 2: 761
86. Gans B, Bahary C, Levie B (1963) Ovarian regeneration and pregnancy following massive radiotherapy for dysgerminoma. Report of a case. Obstet Gynecol 22: 596
87. Garvin AJ, Pratt-Thomas HR, Spector M, Spicer SS, Williamson HO (1976) Gonadoblastoma: Histologic, ultrastructural and histochemical observations in five cases. Am J Obstet Gynecol 125: 459
88. Gershenson DM, Del Junco G, Herson J, Rutledge FN (1983) Endodermal sinus tumor of the ovary. The M.D. Anderson experience. Obstet Gynecol 61: 194
89. Gershenson DM, Copeland LJ, Kavanagh JJ, Cangir A, Del Junco G, Saul PB, Stringer CA, Freedman RS, Edwards CL, Wharton JT (1985) Treatment of malignant nondysgerminomatous germ cell tumors of the ovary with vincristine, dactinomycin and cyclophosphamide. Cancer 56: 2756
90. Gillman J (1948) The development of the gonads in man with consideration of the role of fetal endocrines and the histogenesis of ovarian tumors. Contrib Embryol 32: 83
91. Gitlin D, Boesman M (1967) Sites of serum alpha-fetoprotein synthesis in the human and in the rat. J Clin Invest 46: 1010
92. Gitlin D, Pericelli A (1970) Synthesis of serum albumin, prealbumin, alpha-fetoprotein, alpha-1-antitrypsin and transferrin by the human yolk sac. Nature 228: 995
93. Gitlin D, Pericelli A, Gitlin G (1972) Synthesis of alphafetoprotein by liver, yolk sac and gastrointestinal tract of the human conceptus. Cancer Res 32: 979
94. Goldsmith CI, Hart WR (1975) Ataxia–telangiectasia with ovarian gonadoblastoma and contralateral dysgerminoma. Cancer 36: 1838
95. Goldstein DP, Piro JA (1972) Combination chemotherapy in the treatment of germ cell tumors containing choriocarcinoma. Surg Gynecol Obstet 134: 61
96. Gondos B, Bhiraleus P, Hobel CJ (1971) Ultrastructural observations on germ cells in human fetal ovaries. Am J Obstet Gynecol 110: 644
97. Gonzalez-Angulo A, Kaufman R, Braungardt CD, Chapman FC, Hinshaw AJ (1963) Adenocarcinoma of thyroid arising in struma ovarii (malignant struma ovarii). Report of two cases and review of the literature. Obstet Gynecol 21: 567.
98. Gonzalez-Crussi F, Roth LM (1976) The human yolk sac and yolk sac carcinoma. Hum Pathol 7: 675
99. Gonzalez-Licea A, Hartman WH, Yardley JH (1968) Medullary carcinoma of the thyroid. Ultrastructural evidence of its origin from the parafollicular cell and its possible relation to carcinoid tumors. Am J Clin Pathol 49: 512
100. Gordon A, Lipton D, Woodruff JD (1981) Dysgerminoma: A review of 158 cases from the Emil Novak Ovarian Tumor Registry. Obstet Gynecol 58: 497
101. Greco MA, LiVolsi VA, Pertschuk LP, Bigelow B (1979) Strumal carcinoid of the ovary; an analysis of its components. Cancer 43: 1380
102. Griffiths K, Grant JK, Browning NCK, Whyte WG, Sharp JL (1966) Steroid synthesis in vitro by tumor tissue from dysgenetic gonad. J Endocrinol 34: 155
103. Grosfeld JL, Stepita DS, Nance WE, Palmer CG (1974) Fetus-in-fetu. An unusual cause for an abdominal mass in infancy. Ann Surg 180: 80
104. Gusberg SB, Danforth DN (1944) Clinical significance of struma ovarii. Am J Obstet Gynecol 48: 537
105. Hain AM (1949) An unusual case of precocious puberty associated with ovarian dysgerminoma. J Clin Endocrinol 9: 1349
106. Hameed K, Burslem MRG (1970) A melanotic ovarian neoplasm resembling the "retinal anlage" tumor. Cancer 25: 564
107. Hart WR, Burkons DM (1979) Germ cell neoplasms arising in gonadoblastomas. Cancer 34: 669
108. Hart WR, Regezi JA (1978) Strumal carcinoid of the ovary. Ultrastructural observations and long-term follow-up study. Am J Clin Pathol 69: 356
109. Hertig AT, Adams CE (1967) Studies on the human oocyte and its follicle. 1. Ultrastructural and histochemical observations on primordial follicle stage. J Cell Biol 34: 647
110. Hertig AT, Gore H (1961) Tumors of the female sex organs. Part 3. Tumors of the ovary and fallopian tube. Atlas of Tumor Pathology, Sec 9, Fasc 33. Washington D.C., Armed Forces Institute of Pathology
111. Higuchi K, Kato T (1958) Dysgerminoma of the ovary. J Jpn Obstet Gynecol Soc 5: 206
112. Hingorani V, Narula RK, Bhalla S (1963) *Salmonella typhi* infection in an ovarian dermoid. Report of a case. Obstet Gynecol 22: 118
113. Hirschfield LS, Kahn LB, Winkler B, Bochner RZ, Gibstein AA (1985) Adenocarcinoid of the appendix presenting as bilateral Krukenberg's tumor of the ovaries. Arch Pathol Lab Med 109: 930
114. Hou-Jensen K, Kempson RL (1974) The ultrastructure

of gonadoblastoma and dysgerminoma. Hum Pathol 5: 79
115. Hughesdon PE (1955) Two cases of struma ovarii showing the histogenesis of thyroid and thymus in ovarian teratoma. J Pathol Bacteriol 70: 35
116. Hughesdon PE, Kumarasamy T (1970) Mixed germ cell tumors (gonadoblastomas) in normal and dysgenetic gonads. Virchows Arch [Pathol Anat] 349: 258
117. Huntington RW Jr., Bullock WK (1970) Yolk sac tumors of the ovary. Cancer 25: 1357
118. Huntington RW Jr., Bullock, WK (1970) Yolk sac tumors of extragonadal origin. Cancer 25: 1368
119. Huntington RW Jr., Morgenstern NL, Sargent JA, Giem RN, Richards A, Hanford KC (1963) Germinal tumors exhibiting the endodermal sinus pattern of Teilum in young children. Cancer 16: 34
120. Ishida T, Tagatz GE, Okagaki T (1976) Gonadoblastoma. Ultrastructural evidence of testicular origin. Cancer 37: 1770
121. Itoh T, Shirai T, Naka A, Matsumoto S (1974) Yolk sac tumor and alpha-fetoprotein: Clinicopathological study of four cases. Gann 65: 215
122. Jackson SM (1967) Ovarian dysgerminoma. Br J Radiol 40: 459
123. Janovski NA, Paramanandhan TL (1973) Ovarian tumors. Tumors and tumor-like conditions of the ovaries, fallopian tubes and ligaments of the uterus. Stuttgart, Georg Thieme
124. Jatoi AF (1959) Dysgerminoma of the ovary (a study of 23 cases). J Postgrad Med 5: 22
125. Jedberg H (1949) Some clinical aspects of dysgerminoma ovarii. Acta Obstet Gynecol Scand 28: 194
126. Jimerson GK, Woodruff JD (1977) Ovarian extraembryonal teratoma: 1. Endodermal sinus tumor. Am J Obstet Gynecol 127: 73
127. Jimerson GK, Woodruff JD (1977) Ovarian extraembryonal teratoma: 2. Endodermal sinus tumor mixed with other germ cell tumors. Am J Obstet Gynecol 127: 302
128. Judd HL, Scully RE, Atkins L, Neer RM, Kliman B (1970) Pure gonadal dysgenesis with progressive hirsutism. N Engl J Med 282: 881
129. Kawahara H (1963) Struma ovarii with ascites and hydrothorax. Am J Obstet Gynecol 85: 85
130. Kay S, Silverberg SG, Schatzki PF (1972) Ultrastructure of an ovarian dysgerminoma. Report of a case featuring neurosecretory-type granules in stromal cells. Am J Clin Pathol 58: 458
131. Kazancigil TR, Laquer W, Ladewig P (1940) Papilloendothelioma of the ovary; report of three cases and discussion of Schiller's "mesonephroma ovarii." Am J Cancer 40: 199
132. Kelley RR, Scully RE (1961) Cancer developing in dermoid cysts of the ovary. A report of 8 cases including a carcinoid and a leiomyosarcoma. Cancer 14: 989
133. King ME, Mouradian JA, Micha JP, Chaganti RSK, Allen SL (1985) Immature teratoma of the ovary with predominant malignant retinal anlage tumor. A parthenogenetically derived tumor. Am J Surg Pathol 9: 221
134. Klein HZ (1974) Mucinous carcinoid tumor of the vermiform appendix. Cancer 33: 770
135. Koller O, Gjonnes H (1964) Dysgerminoma of the ovary. Acta Obstet Gynecol Scand 43: 268
136. Krepart G, Smith JP, Rutledge F, Declos L (1978) The treatment for dysgerminoma of the ovary. Cancer 41: 986
137. Krumerman MS, Chung A (1977) Squamous carcinoma arising in benign cystic teratoma of the ovary. Cancer 39: 1237
138. Kurman RJ, Norris HJ (1976) Endodermal sinus tumor of the ovary. A clinical and pathologic analysis of 71 cases. Cancer 38: 2404
139. Kurman RJ, Norris HJ (1976) Embryonal carcinoma of the ovary. A clinicopathologic entity distinct from endodermal sinus tumor resembling embryonal carcinoma of the adult testis. Cancer 38: 2420
140. Kurman RJ, Norris HJ (1976) Malignant mixed germ cell tumors of the ovary. A clinical and pathologic analysis of 30 cases. Obstet Gynecol 48: 579
141. Lange PH, Millan JL, Stigbrand T, Vessella RL, Ruoslahti E, Fishman WH (1982) Placental alkaline phosphatase as a tumor marker for seminoma. Cancer Res 42: 3244
142. Larson NE, Dockerty MB, Pratt JH (1958) Primary mixed choriocarcinoma and dysgerminoma of the ovary. Report of a case. Proc Mayo Clin 33: 341
143. Levine GD (1973) Primary thymic seminoma—A neoplasm ultrastructurally similar to testicular seminoma and distinct from epithelial thymoma. Cancer 31: 729
144. Liebert KI, Stent L (1960) Dysgerminoma of the ovary with chorionepithelioma. J Obstet Gynaecol Br Emp 77: 627
145. Lien L (1979) Determination of serum AFP for the diagnosis and treatment of ovarian endodermal sinus tumor. Zhonghua Fuchanke Zazhi 14: 22 (in Chinese)
146. Linder D (1969) Gene loss in human teratomas. Proc Natl Acad Sci USA 63: 699
147. Linder D, Power J (1970) Further evidence for postmeiotic origin of teratomas in the human female. Ann Hum Genet 34: 21
148. Linder D, McCaw BK, Hecht F (1975) Parthenogenic origin of benign ovarian teratoma. N Engl J Med 292: 63
149. Lingeman CH (1974) Etiology of cancer of the human ovary. A review. J Natl Cancer Inst 53: 1603
150. Livnat EJ, Scommegna A, Recant W, Jao W (1977) Ultrastructural observations of the so-called strumal carcinoid of the ovary. Arch Pathol Lab Med 101: 585
151. Lord JM (1956) Intra-abdominal foetus in fetu. J Pathol Bacteriol 72: 627
152. Lynn JA, Varon HH, Kingsley WB, Martin JH (1967) Ultrastructure and biochemical studies of estrogen-secreting capacity of a "non-functional" ovarian neoplasm (dysgerminoma). Am J Pathol 51: 639
153. Mackay AM, Pattigrew N, Symington T, Neville AM (1974) Tumors of dysgenetic gonads (gonadoblastoma). Ultrastructural and steroidogenic aspects. Cancer 34: 1108
154. McCullough CD, Hardart F (1963) Neuroblastomatous transformation in a benign cystic teratoma. Obstet Gynecol 21: 259
155. McDonough PG, Byrd JR, Tho PT, Otken L (1976) Gona-

doblastoma in a true hermaphrodite with 46XX karyotype. Obstet Gynecol 47: 355
156. McDonough PG, Greenblatt RB, Byrd JR, Hastings EV (1967) Gonadoblastoma (gonocytoma III). Report of a case. Obstet Gynecol 29: 54
157. McKay DG, Hertig AT, Adams EC, Danziger S (1953) Histochemical observations on the germ cells of human embryos. Anat Rec 117: 201
158. McKay DG, Pinkerton JHM, Hertig AT, Danziger S (1961) The adult human ovary: A histochemical study. Obstet Gynecol 18: 13
159. Malkasian GD Jr., Symmonds RE (1964) Treatment of the unilateral encapsulated germinoma. Am J Obstet Gynecol 90: 379
160. Malkasian GD Jr., Dockerty MB, Symmonds RE (1967) Benign cystic teratomas. Obstet Gynecol 29: 719
161. Malkasian GD Jr., Symmonds RE, Dockerty MB (1965) Malignant ovarian teratomas. Report of 31 cases. Obstet Gynecol 25: 810
162. Malkasian GD Jr., Webb MJ, Jorgensen EO (1974) Observations on chemotherapy of granulosa cell carcinoma and malignant ovarian teratoma. Obstet Gynecol 44: 885
163. Marcial-Rojas RA, de Arellano RGA (1956) Malignant melanoma arising in a dermoid cyst of the ovary. Cancer 9: 523
164. Marin-Padilla M (1965) Origin, nature and significance of the "embryoids" of human teratomas. Virchow's Arch [Pathol Anat] 340: 105
165. Marrubini G (1949) Primary chorionepithelioma of the ovary. Report of two cases. Acta Obstet Gynecol Scand 28: 251
166. Masson P (1912) Seminomes ovariennes. Bull Soc Anat (Paris) 87: 402
167. Masson P (1923) Epitheliomas pflügeriens. In: Diagnostics de laboratoire. Les tumeurs. Paris, Maloine
168. Mathieu J, Planchu M (1950) Le prognostic et le traitement du seminome de l'ovaire. Les oestrogenes out-ils place dans le traitement du seminome en general? Lyon Chir 45: 76
169. Matz MH (1961) Benign cystic teratomas of the ovary. Obstet Gynecol Surv 16: 591
170. Melicow MM, Uson AC (1959) Dysgenetic gonadomas and other gonadal neoplasms in intersex. Cancer 12: 552
171. Meyer R (1931) The pathology of some special ovarian tumors and their relation to sex characteristics. Am J Obstet Gynecol 22: 697
172. Miettinen M, Virtanen I, Talerman A (1985) Intermediate filament proteins in human testis and testicular germ-cell tumors. Am J Pathol 120: 402
173. Miettinen M, Talerman A, Wahlstrom T, Astengo-Osuna C, Virtanen I (1985) Cellular differentiation in ovarian sex cord–stromal and germ-cell tumors studied with antibodies to intermediate-filament proteins. Am J Surg Pathol 9: 640
174. Moertel CG, Beahrs OH, Woolner LB, Tyce GM (1965) "Malignant carcinoid syndrome" associated with noncarcinoid tumors. N Engl J Med 273: 244
175. Mueller CW, Topkins P, Lapp WA (1950) Dysgerminoma of the ovary. An analysis of 427 cases. Am J Obstet Gynecol 60: 153
176. Neigus I (1952) Ovarian dysgerminoma with chorionepithelioma. Am J Obstet Gynecol 64: 422
177. Neubecker RD, Breen JL (1962) Embryonal carcinoma of the ovary. Cancer 15: 546
178. Nielsen SNJ, Scheithauer BW, Gaffey TA (1985) Gliomatosis peritonei. Cancer 56: 2499
179. Nieminen I, Von Numers C, Widholm O (1964) Struma ovarii. Acta Obstet Gynecol Scand 42: 399
180. Nogales FF Jr, Matilla A, Nogales-Ortiz F, Galera-Davidson HL (1978) Yolk sac tumors with pure and mixed polyvesicular vitelline patterns. Hum Pathol 9: 553
181. Nogales FF Jr, Silverberg SG, Bloustein PA, Martinez-Hernandez A, Pierce GB (1977) Yolk sac carcinoma (endodermal sinus tumor). Ultrastructure and histogenesis of gonadal and extragonadal tumors in comparison with normal human yolk sac. Cancer 39: 1462
182. Norgaard-Pedersen B, Albrechtsen R, Teilum G (1975) Serum alpha-fetoprotein as a marker for endodermal sinus tumor (yolk sac tumor), or a vitelline component of teratocarcinoma. Acta Pathol Microbiol Scand (A) 83: 573
183. Norris HJ, Jensen RD (1972) Relative frequency of ovarian neoplasms in children and adolescents. Cancer 30: 713
184. Norris HJ, Zirkin HJ, Benson WL (1976) Immature (malignant) teratoma of the ovary. A clinical and pathologic study of 58 cases. Cancer 37: 2359
185. Novak E (1952) Gynecologic and obstetric pathology, 3rd ed. Philadelphia, Saunders
186. Novak E, Gray LA (1938) Dysgerminoma of the ovary. Am J Obstet Gynecol 35: 925
187. Novak E, Woodruff JD, Novak ER (1954) Probable mesonephric origin of certain female genital tumors. Am J Obstet Gynecol 68: 1224
188. Novak ER (1948) Solid teratoma of the ovary, with report of five cases. Am J Obstet Gynecol 56: 300
189. Novak ER, Woodruff JD (1967) In: Novak ER (ed) Gynecologic and obstetric pathology, 6th ed. Philadelphia, Saunders, p 367
190. Nystrom C (1956) Dysgerminoma of the ovary. Acta Obstet Gynecol Scand 35: 385
191. Oliver HM, Horne EO (1948) Primary teratomatous chorionepithelioma of the ovary. Report of a case. N Engl J Med 239: 14
192. Overbeck L, Philipp E (1969) Die Ultrastruktur des Disgerminoms im Ovar. Zugleich ein Beitrag zur Histogenese des Tumors. Z Geburtschilfe Gynaekol 170: 125
193. Palmer PE, Safaii H, Wolfe HJ (1976) Alpha-1-antitrypsin and alpha-fetoprotein markers in endodermal sinus (yolk sac) tumors. Am J Clin Pathol 65: 575
194. Pantoja E, Noy MA, Axtmayer RW, Colon FE, Pelegrina I (1975) Ovarian dermoids and their complications. Comprehensive historical review. Obstet Gynecol Surv 30: 1
195. Pantoja E, Rodriguez-Ibanez I, Axtmayer RW, Noy MA, Pelegrina I (1975) Complications of dermoid tumors of the ovary. Obstet Gynecol 45: 89
196. Park IJ, Pyeatte JC, Jones HW, Woodruff JD (1972) Gonadoblastoma in a true hermaphrodite with 46XY genotype. Obstet Gynecol 40: 466
197. Patel SK, Prentice SA (1972) Gonadoblastoma—Distinctive ovarian tumor. Arch Pathol 94: 165
198. Payne D, Muss HB, Homesley HD, Jobson VM, Baird

FG (1981) Autoimmune hemolytic anemia and ovarian dermoid cysts. Case report and review of the literature. Cancer 48: 721
199. Pedowitz P, Felmus LB, Grayzel DM (1955) Dysgerminoma of the ovary. Prognosis and treatment. Am J Obstet Gynecol 70: 1284
200. Peterson WF (1956) Solid histologically benign teratomas of the ovary. A report of four cases and review of the literature. Am J Obstet Gynecol 72: 1094
201. Peterson WF (1957) Malignant degeneration of benign cystic teratomas of the ovary: A collective review of the literature. Obstet Gynecol Surv 12: 793
202. Peterson WF, Prevost EC, Edmunds FT, Huntley JM Jr., Morris FK (1955) Benign cystic teratomas of the ovary. A clinico-statistical study of 1007 cases with review of the literature. Am J Obstet Gynecol 70: 368
203. Peyron A (1939) Faits nouveaux relatifs à l'origine et à l'histogenese des embryomes. Bull Assoc Franc Cancer 28: 658
204. Pierce GB Jr. (1966) Ultrastructure of human testicular tumors. Cancer 19: 1963
205. Pierce, GB Jr., Dixon FJ (1959) Testicular teratomas. 1. Demonstration of teratogenesis by metamorphosis of multipotential cells. Cancer 12: 573
206. Pierce GB Jr., Dixon FJ (1959) Testicular teratomas. 2. Teratocarcinoma as ascitic tumor. Cancer 12: 584
207. Pierce GB Jr., Midgley AR (1963) The origin and function of human syncytiotrophoblastic giant cells. Am J Pathol 43: 153
208. Pierce GB Jr., Verney EL (1961) An in vitro and in vivo study of differentiation in teratocarcinomas. Cancer 14: 1017
209. Pierce GB Jr., Bullock WK, Huntington RW Jr. (1970) Yolk sac tumors of the testis. Cancer 25: 644
210. Pierce GB Jr., Midgley AR, Beals TF (1962) An ultrastructural study of differentiation and maturation of trophoblast of the monkey. Lab Invest 13: 451
211. Pierce GB Jr., Midgley AR, Sri Ram J, Feldman JD (1964) Parietal yolk sac carcinoma. Clue to the histogenesis of Reichert's membrane of the mouse embryo. Am J Pathol 41: 549
212. Plaut A (1933) Ovarian struma: A morphologic, pharmacologic, and biologic examination. Am J Obstet Gynecol 25: 351
213. Prat J, Bhan AK, Dickersin GR, Robboy SJ, Scully RE (1982) Hepatoid yolk sac tumor of the ovary (endodermal sinus tumor with hepatoid differentiation). A light microscopic ultrastructural and immunohistochemical study of seven cases. Cancer 50: 2355
214. Qizilbash AH, Trebilcock RG, Patterson MC, Lamont KG (1974) Functioning primary carcinoid tumor of the ovary. A light and electron microscopic study with review of the literature. Am J Clin Pathol 62: 629
215. Ramsey HJ (1965) Ultrastructure of a pineal tumor. Cancer 18: 1014
216. Ranchod M, Kempson RL, Dorgeloh JR (1976) Strumal carcinoid of the ovary. Cancer 37: 1913
217. Rao NR, Veliath GD, Srinivasan M (1964) An unusual case of sacrococcygeal mesonephroma (Schiller). Cancer 17: 1604
218. Rashad MH, Fathalla MF, Kerr MC (1966) Sex chromatin and chromosome analysis in ovarian teratomas. Am J Obstet Gynecol 96: 461
219. Robboy SJ, Scully RE (1970) Ovarian teratoma with glial implants on the peritoneum. An analysis of 12 cases. Hum Pathol 1: 643
220. Robboy SJ, Scully RE (1980) Strumal carcinoid of the ovary. An analysis of 50 cases of a distinctive tumor composed of thyroid tissue and carcinoid. Cancer 46: 2019
221. Robboy SJ, Norris HJ, Scully RE (1975) Insular carcinoid primary in the ovary—A clinicopathologic analysis of 48 cases. Cancer 36: 404
222. Robboy SJ, Scully RE, Norris HJ (1974) Carcinoid metastatic to the ovary. A clinicopathologic analysis of 35 cases. Cancer 33: 798
223. Robboy SJ, Scully RE, Norris HJ (1977) Primary trabecular carcinoid of the ovary. Obstet Gynecol 49: 202
224. Rose LI, Underwood RH, Williams GH, Pincus GS (1974) Pure gonadal dysgenesis. Studies of in vitro androgen metabolism. Am J Med 57: 957
225. Sailer S (1940) Ovarian dysgerminoma. Am J Cancer 38: 473
226. Sailer S (1943) Struma ovarii. Am J Clin Pathol 13: 271
227. Salet J, de Gennes LJ, de Grouchy J, Musset R, Pelissier C, Yaneva H, Sebaoun M, Netter A (1970) A propos d'un cas de gonadoblastome 46XX. Ann Endocrinol (Paris) 31: 927
228. Samuels ML, Lanzotti VJ, Holoye PY, Boyle LY, Smith TL, Johnson DE (1976) Combination chemotherapy of germinal cell tumors. Cancer Treat Rev 3: 185
229. Santesson L (1947) Clinical and pathological survey of ovarian tumours treated at the Radiumhemmet. 1. Dysgerminoma. Acta Radiol (Stockholm) 28: 643
230. Santesson L, Marrubini G (1957) Clinical and pathological survey of ovarian embryonal carcinomas, including so-called "mesonephreomas" (Schiller) or "mesoblastomas" (Teilum) treated at the Radiumhemmet. Acta Obstet Gynecol Scand 36: 399
231. Saunders AM, Hertzman VO (1960) Malignant carcinoid teratoma of the ovary. Can Med Assoc J 83: 602
232. Schellhas HF (1974) Malignant potential of the dysgenetic gonad. Part 1. Obstet Gynecol 44: 298
233. Schellhas HF (1974) Malignant potential of the dysgenetic gonad. Part 2. Obstet Gynecol 44: 455
234. Schellhas HF, Trujillo JM, Rutledge FN, Cork A (1971) Germ cell tumors associated with XY gonadal dysgenesis. Am J Obstet Gynecol 109: 1197
235. Schiller W (1939) Mesonephroma ovarii. Am J Cancer 35: 1
236. Schiller W (1942) Histogenesis of ovarian mesonephroma. Arch Pathol 33: 443
237. Schmitz EF (1925) Malignant endothelioma of perithelioma type in the ovary. Am J Obstet Gynecol 9: 247
238. Scully RE (1953) Gonadoblastoma. A gonadal tumor related to dysgerminoma (seminoma) and capable of sex hormone production. Cancer 6: 455
239. Scully RE (1963) Germ cell tumors of the ovary and Fallopian tube. In: Meigs JV, Sturgis SH (eds) Progress in gynecology, Vol 4. New York, Grune and Stratton, pp 335–347

240. Scully RE (1970) Germ cell tumors of the ovary. In: Sturgis SH, Taymor ML (eds) Progress in gynecology, Vol 5. Grune and Stratton, New York, pp. 329–348
241. Scully RE (1970) Recent progress in ovarian cancer. Hum Pathol 1: 73
242. Scully RE (1970) Gonadoblastoma. Cancer 25: 1340
243. Scully RE (1970) Sex cord tumor with annular tubules. A distinctive ovarian tumor of the Peutz-Jeghers syndrome. Cancer 25: 1107
244. Scully RE (1979) Tumors of the ovary and maldeveloped gonads. In: Atlas of tumor pathology, 2nd series, Fasc 16. Washington, D.C., Armed Forces Institute of Pathology
245. Scully RE (1980) Personal communication
246. Seegar GE (1938) Ovarian dysgerminomas. Arch Surg 37: 697
247. Sell A, Sogaard H, Norgaard-Pedersen B (1976) Serum alpha-fetoprotein as a marker for the effects of postoperative radiation therapy and/or chemotherapy in 8 cases of ovarian endodermal sinus tumor. Int J Cancer 18: 574
248. Sens MA, Levenson TB, Metcalf JS (1982) A case of metastatic carcinoid arising in an ovarian teratoma. Cancer 49: 2541
249. Senterman MK, Cassidy PN, Fenoglio CM, Ferenczy A (1984) Histology, ultrastructure and immunocytochemistry of strumal carcinoid. A case report. Int J Gynecol Pathol 3: 232
250. Serov SF, Scully RE, Sobin LH (1973) Histological typing of ovarian tumors. International histological classification of tumors. No 9. Geneva, World Health Organization
251. Serratoni FT, Robboy SJ (1975) Ultrastructure of primary and metastatic ovarian carcinoids—Analysis of 11 cases. Cancer 36: 157
252. Shirai T, Itoh T, Yoshiki T, Noro T, Tomino Y, Hayasaka T (1976) Immunofluorescent demonstration of alpha-fetoprotein, and other plasma proteins in yolk sac tumor. Cancer 38: 1661
253. Sjovall A (1943) Disgerminome des Ovariums. Acta Obstet Gynecol Scand 23: 585
254. Simard LC (1957) Polyembryonic embryoma of the ovary of parthenogenetic origin. Cancer 10: 215
255. Smith FG (1946) Pathology and physiology of struma ovarii. Arch Surg 53: 603
256. Smith JB, O'Neill RT (1971) Alpha-fetoprotein. Occurrence in germinal cell and liver malignancies. Am J Med 51: 767
257. Smith JP, Rutledge F (1975) Advances in chemotherapy for gynecologic cancer. Cancer 36: 669
258. Smith JP, Rutledge FN, Sutow WW (1963) Malignant gynecologic tumors in children. Current approaches to treatment. Am J Obstet Gynecol 116: 261
259. Solomon J, Steinfeld JL, Bateman JR (1967) Chemotherapy of germinal tumors. Cancer 26: 747
260. Sporrong B, Falkmer S, Robboy SJ, Alumets J, Hakanson R, Ljungberg O, Sundler F (1982) Neurohormonal peptides in ovarian carcinoids. An immunohistochemical study of 81 primary carcinoids and of intraovarian metastases from six midgut carcinoids. Cancer 49: 68
261. Sternberg WH, Barclay DL, Kloepfer HW (1968) Familial XY gonadal dysgenesis. N Engl J Med 278: 695
262. Stevens LC (1959) Embryology of testicular teratomas in strain 129 mice. J Natl Cancer Inst 23: 1249
263. Stevens LC (1960) Embryonic potency of embryoid bodies derived from a transplantable testicular teratoma of the mouse. Develop Biol 2: 285
264. Stevens LC (1962) The biology of teratomas including evidence indicating their origin from primordial germ cells. Ann Biol 1: 585
265. Strauss AF, Gates HS (1964) Giant sebaceous gland tumor of the ovary. Am J Clin Pathol 41: 78
266. Subbuswamy SG, Gibbs NM, Ross CF, Morson BC (1974) Goblet cell carcinoid of the appendix. Cancer 34: 338
267. Szokol M, Kondrai G, Papp, Z (1977) Gonadal malignancy and 46XY karyotype in a true hermaphrodite. Obstet Gynecol 49: 358
268. Takeda A, Ishizuka T, Goto T, Goto S, Ohta M, Tomoda Y, Hoshino M (1982) Polyembryoma of ovary producing alpha-fetoprotein and HCG. Immunoperoxidase and electron microscopic study. Cancer 49: 1878
269. Talerman A (1971) Gonadoblastoma and dysgerminoma in two siblings with dysgenetic gonads. Obstet Gynecol 38: 416
270. Talerman A (1972) A distinctive gonadal neoplasm related to gonadoblastoma. Cancer 30: 1219
271. Talerman A (1972) A mixed germ cell–sex cord stroma tumor in a normal female infant. Obstet Gynecol 40: 473
272. Talerman A (1974) Gonadoblastoma associated with embryonal carcinoma. Obstet Gynecol 43: 138
273. Talerman A (1975) The incidence of yolk sac tumor (endodermal sinus tumor) elements in germ cell tumors of the testis in adults. Cancer 36: 211
274. Talerman A (1980) The pathology of gonadal neoplasms composed of germ cells and sex cord stroma derivatives. Pathol Res Pract 170: 24
275. Talerman A (1984) Carcinoid tumors of the ovary. J Cancer Res Clin Oncol 107: 125
276. Talerman A, Delemarre JFM (1975) Gonadoblastoma associated with embryonal carcinoma in an anatomically normal male. J Urol 113: 355
277. Talerman A, Evans MI (1982) Primary trabecular carcinoid tumor of the ovary. Cancer 50: 1407
278. Talerman A, Haije WG (1974) Alpha-fetoprotein and germ cell tumors. A possible role of yolk sac tumor in production of alpha-fetoprotein. Cancer 34: 1722
279. Talerman A, Haije WG (1985) Ovarian Sertoli cell tumor with retiform and heterologous elements. Am J Surg Pathol 9: 459
280. Talerman A, Okagaki T (1985) Ultrastructural features of primary trabecular carcinoid tumor of the ovary. Int J Gynecol Pathol 4: 153
281. Talerman A, Okagaki T (unpublished observations)
282. Talerman A, van der Harten JJ (1977) A mixed germ cell–sex cord stroma tumor of the ovary associated with isosexual precocious puberty in a normal female child. Cancer 40: 889
283. Talerman A, Haije WG, Baggerman L (1977) Alpha-1-antitrypsin (AAT) and alpha-foetoprotein (AFP) in sera of patients with germ cell neoplasms. Value as tumor markers in patients with endodermal sinus tumour (yolk sac tumour). Int J Cancer 19: 741

284. Talerman A, Haije WG, Baggerman L (1978) Histological patterns in germ cell neoplasms associated with raised serum alphafoetoprotein (AFP). Scand J Immunol 8[Suppl]: 97
285. Talerman A, Haije WG, Baggerman L (1978) Serum alphafetoprotein in diagnosis and management of endodermal sinus (yolk sac) tumor and mixed germ cell tumor of the ovary. Cancer 41: 272
286. Talerman A, Haije WG, Baggerman L (1980) Serum alphafetoprotein (AFP) in patients with germ cell tumors of the gonads and extragonadal sites. Correlation between endodermal sinus (yolk sac) tumor and raised serum AFP. Cancer 46: 340
287. Talerman A, Huyzinga WT, Kuipers T (1973) Dysgerminoma. Clinicopathologic study of 22 cases. Obstet Gynecol 41: 137
288. Talerman A, Jarabak J, Amarose A (1981) Gonadoblastoma and dysgerminoma in a true hermaphrodite with 46,XX karyotype. Am J Obstet Gynecol 140: 175
289. Talerman A, van der Pompe WB, Haije WG, Baggerman L, Boekestein-Tjahjadi HM (1977) Alpha-fetoprotein and carcinoembryonic antigen in germ cell neoplasms. Br J Cancer 35: 288
290. Taylor CW (1972) Müllerian mixed tumor. Acta Pathol Microbiol Scand [80A Suppl] 233: 48
291. Taylor MH, Depetrillo AD, Turner AR (1985) Vinblastine, bleomycin, and cisplatin in malignant germ cell tumors of the ovary. Cancer 56: 1341
292. Teilmann I, Kassis H, Pietra G (1967) Primary germ cell tumour of the anterior mediastium with features of endodermal sinus tumour (mesoblastoma vitellinum). Acta Pathol Microbiol Scand 70: 267
293. Teilum G (1944) Homologous tumours in ovary and testis: Contribution to classification of gonadal tumours. Acta Obstet Gynecol Scand 24: 480
294. Teilum G (1946) Gonocytoma; homologous ovarian and testicular tumours. 1. With discussion of "mesonephroma ovarii" (Schiller: Am J Cancer 1939). Acta Pathol Microbiol Scand 23: 242
295. Teilum G (1950) "mesonephroma ovarii" (Schiller) extraembryonic mesoblastoma of germ cell origin in ovary and testis. Acta Pathol Microbiol Scand 27: 249
296. Teilum G (1952) Classification of ovarian tumours. Acta Obstet Gynecol Scand 31: 292
297. Teilum G (1959) Endodermal sinus tumors of the ovary and testis. Comparative morphogenesis of the so-called mesonephroma ovarii (Schiller) and extraembryonic (yolk sac-allantoic) structures of the rat's placenta. Cancer 12: 1092
298. Teilum G (1965) Classification of endodermal sinus tumour (mesoblastoma vitellinum) and so-called embryonal carcinoma of the ovary. Acta Pathol Microbiol Scand 64: 407
299. Teilum G (1968) Tumours of germinal origin. In: Gentil F, Junqueira AC (eds) Ovarian cancer, U.I.C.C. Monograph Series, Vol 11. Berlin, Heidelberg, New York, Springer-Verlag, pp 58–73
300. Teilum G (1976) Special tumors of the ovary and testis. Comparative histology and identification, 2nd ed. Copenhagen, Munksgaard
301. Teilum G, Albrechtsen R, Norgaard-Pedersen B (1974) Immunofluorescent localization of alpha-fetoprotein synthesis in endodermal sinus tumor (yolk sac tumor). Acta Pathol Microbiol Scand 82A: 586
302. Teilum G, Albrechtsen R, Norgaard-Pedersen B (1975) The histogenetic–embryologic basis for reappearance of alpha-fetoprotein in endodermal sinus tumors and teratomas. Acta Pathol Microbiol Scand 83A: 80
303. Teter J (1960) A new concept of classification of gonadal tumors arising from germ cell (gonocytoma) and their histogenesis. Gynaecologia (Basel) 150: 84
304. Teter J (1962) A mixed form of feminizing germ cell tumor (gonocytoma II). Am J Obstet Gynecol 84: 722
305. Teter J (1970) Prognosis, malignancy and curability of the germ cell tumor occurring in dysgenetic gonads. Am J Obstet Gynecol 108: 894
306. Teter J, Boczkowski K (1967) Occurrence of tumors in dysgenetic gonads. Cancer 20: 1301
307. Theiss EA, Ashley DJB, Mostofi FK (1959) Nuclear sex of testicular tumors and some related ovarian and extragonadal neoplasms. Cancer 13: 323
308. Thoeny RH, Dockerty MB, Hunt AB, Childs DS Jr. (1961) Study of ovarian dysgerminoma with emphasis on the role of radiation therapy. Surg Gynecol Obstet 113: 692
309. Thurlbeck WM, Scully RE (1960) Solid teratoma of the ovary. Cancer 13: 804
310. Toker C (1969) Ovarian carcinoid. A light and electron microscopic study. Am J Obstet Gynecol 103: 1019
311. Tsuchida Y, Kaneko M, Yokomori K, Saito S, Urano Y, Endo Y, Asaka T, Takeuchi T (1978) Alpha-fetoprotein, prealbumin, albumin, alpha-1-antitrypsin, and transferrin as diagnostic and therapeutic markers for endodermal sinus tumors. J Pediatr Surg 13: 25
312. Turner HB, Douglas WM, Gladding TC (1964) Choriocarcinoma of the ovary. Obstet Gynecol 24: 918
313. Ueda G, Sato Y, Yamasaki M, Inoue M, Hiramatsu J, Kurachi K, Amino N, Miyai K (1978) Strumal carcinoid of the ovary. Histological, ultrastructural, and immunohistological studies with anti-human thyroglobulin. Gynecol Oncol 6: 411
314. Ulbright TM, Roth LM, Erlich CE (1982) Ovarian strumal carcinoid. An immunocytochemical and ultrastructural study of two cases. Am J Clin Pathol 77: 622
315. Uzisima H (1956) Ovarian dysgerminoma associated with virilization. Report of a case. Cancer 9: 736
316. Vance RP, Geisinger KR (1985) Pure nongestational choriocarcinoma of the ovary. Report of a case. Cancer 56: 2321
317. Vawter GF (1965) Carcinoma of the vagina in infancy. Cancer 18: 1479
318. Warkel RL, Cooper PH, Helwig EB (1978) Adenocarcinoid, a mucin-producing carcinoid of the appendix. Cancer 42: 2781
319. Weldon-Linne CM, Rushovich AM (1983) Benign ovarian cystic teratomas with homunculi. Obstet Gynecol 61: 88S
320. Wheatley VR (1957) Further observations on the nature of the dermoid cyst fat. J Invest Dermatol 29: 445
321. Whelton JA, Fallon RJ (1964) Successful pregnancy after surgery and supervoltage therapy for metastatic dysgerminoma. N Engl J Med 271: 145

322. Wider JA, O'Leary JA (1968) Dysgerminoma: A clinical review. Obstet Gynecol 31: 560
323. Wider JA, Marshall JR, Bardin CW, Lipsett MB, Rose GT (1969) Sustained remissions after chemotherapy for primary ovarian cancers containing choriocarcinoma. N Engl J Med 280: 1439
324. Wieland RG, Ekstrom B, Vorijs N (1968) $C_{19}O_2$ Steroid secretion by dysgenetic gonads. Obstet Gynecol 32: 643
325. Wilkinson EJ, Friedrich EG, Hosty TA (1973) Alpha-fetoprotein and endodermal sinus tumor of the ovary. Am J Obstet Gynecol 116: 711
326. Williams ED (1966) Histogenesis of medullary carcinoma of the thyroid. J Clin Pathol 19: 114
327. Williams ED, Sandler M (1963) Classification of carcinoid by embryologic grouping. Lancet 1: 238
328. Williamson HO, Underwood PB Jr, Kreutner A Jr, Rogers JF, Mathur RS, Pratt-Thomas HR (1976) Gonadoblastoma: Clinicopathologic correlation in six patients. Am J Obstet Gynecol 126: 579
329. Willis RA (1958) The borderland of embryology and pathology. London, Butterworth
330. Willis RA (1967) Pathology of tumours, 4th ed. London, Butterworth
331. Wisniewski M, Deppisch LM (1973) Solid teratomas of the ovary. Cancer 32: 440
332. Witschi E (1948) Migration of the germ cells of human embryos from the yolk sac to the primitive gonadal folds. Contrib Embryol 32: 69
333. Woodruff JD, Markley RL (1957) Struma ovarii. Demonstration of both pathologic change and physiologic activity; report of four cases. Obstet Gynecol 9: 707
334. Woodruff JD, Protos P, Peterson WF (1968) Ovarian teratomas. Relationship of histologic and ontogenic factors to prognosis. Am J Obstet Gynecol 102: 702
335. Woodruff JD, Rauh JT, Markley RL (1966) Ovarian struma. Obstet Gynecol 27: 194
336. Wurster K, Hedinger C, Meienberg O (1972) Orchioblastomatous foci in testicular teratoma of adults. Virchow's Arch [Pathol Anat] 357: 231
337. Young RH, Scully RE (1983) Ovarian Sertoli-Leydig cell tumors with a retiform pattern. A problem in histopathologic diagnosis. A report of 25 cases. Am J Surg Pathol 7: 755
338. Young RH, Perez-Atayde AR, Scully RE (1984) Ovarian Sertoli-Leydig cell tumor with retiform and heterologous elements. Report of a case with hepatocytic differentiation and elevated serum alpha-fetoprotein. Am J Surg Pathol 8: 709
339. Young RH, Prat J, Scully RE (1982) Ovarian Sertoli-Leydig cell tumors with heterologous elements (1) gastrointestinal epithelium and carcinoid: A clinicopathologic analysis of thirty six cases. Cancer 50: 2448
340. Zaloudek C, Tavassoli FA, Norris HJ (1981) Dysgerminoma with syncytiotrophoblastic giant cells. A histologically and clinically distinctive subtype of dysgerminoma. Am J Surg Pathol 5: 361
341. Zondag HA (1964) Enzyme activity in dysgerminoma and seminoma. A study of lactic dehydrogenase isoenzymes in malignant diseases. Rhode Island Med J 47: 273

21

Nonspecific Tumors of the Ovary, Including Mesenchymal Tumors and Malignant Lymphoma

Aleksander Talerman, M.D., Ph.D., F.R.C.Path.

The tumors discussed in this chapter comprise a heterogeneous group of neoplasms that are not specific to the ovary. They are uncommon in this location, occurring much more frequently in other parts of the body. Consequently, whenever they are encountered in the ovary, these tumors pose difficult problems in diagnosis, histogenesis, behavior, and therapy for the pathologist and clinician. These neoplasms must be differentiated from primary ovarian neoplasms containing mesenchymal tissue, as well as from metastatic and disseminated neoplasms affecting the ovary. Thus, mesenchymal neoplasms nonspecific to the ovary must be differentiated primarily from teratomatous neoplasms containing large amounts of mature or immature mesenchymal elements and from the mixed müllerian (mesodermal) tumors, composed of different malignant connective tissue elements. In contrast, the primary malignant lymphomas must be differentiated from the much more common disseminated malignant lymphoma and leukemia, which not infrequently affect the ovary. These two different groups of neoplasms—the connective tissue neoplasms nonspecific to the ovary and malignant lymphoma of the ovary—although included under the same heading, are discussed separately because of their different nature, behavior, and histogenesis. In addition, the adenomatoid tumor, which is of mesothelial origin, the ovarian tumor of probable wolffian origin, and ovarian neoplasms of neural origin are also included.

Mesenchymal Tumors Nonspecific to the Ovary

Mesenchymal neoplasms nonspecific to the ovary include all primary ovarian neoplasms of connective tissue origin found in the ovary that are nonspecific to it but considered to originate from ovarian tissue, and not of teratomatous or surface epithelial (müllerian) origin. However, this mode of origin cannot be excluded in a number of cases. The neoplasms discussed here are composed of a single neoplastic mesenchymal element, either benign or malignant, in contrast to teratomatous or mixed müllerian tumors, which are usually composed of a number of tissue elements.

Problems concerning classification and histogenesis do arise and can be insurmountable when considering the possibility of one-sided differentiation of a teratoma or of a mixed müllerian tumor of the ovary. In view of this, although some of these neoplasms can be shown to originate directly from ovarian tissue, a considerable number of cases are of indeterminate histogenesis and origin. Mesenchymal neoplasms nonspecific to the ovary can be classified as benign or malignant, and are discussed here in terms of the tissue of origin.

Tumors of Fibrous Tissue Origin

Fibroma

Fibroma is the most common ovarian neoplasm of connective tissue origin and comprises 3 to 5% of ovarian neoplasms. An even higher frequency occurs when fibrosed thecomas are included in this category.

The histogenesis of ovarian fibroma in common with most other ovarian neoplasms of connective tissue origin is controversial. The neoplasm most likely arises from mesenchymal cells of the ovarian stroma, that differentiate in the fibroblastic direction. Some investigators postulate that it arises from a fibrosed thecoma or a Brenner tumor, whereas others believe that it originates from the connective tissue within the ovary, primarily within the ovarian cortex or in the walls of blood and lymphatic vessels. It has also been postulated that ovarian fibroma may originate as a reaction to the hemorrhage that occurs during ovulation, but evidence for this mode of origin is not convincing. Although it can be difficult or even impossible to differentiate between fibroma and fibrosed thecoma, it is worthwhile to make the attempt.

Ovarian fibroma is bilateral in 4–8% of patients, and in 10% of patients, the tumors are multiple.[17] Ovarian fibroma is usually encountered in menopausal and postmenopausal women, but it is seen at all ages. It is very rare in children, and only three examples have been reported.[8,13,47]

Clinically, patients with ovarian fibroma are frequently asymptomatic, mainly because of the tumor's small size. When symptoms do occur, they manifest themselves as abdominal enlargement, urinary symptoms, and abdominal pain, sometimes acute because of torsion of the tumor. Ascites is a relatively common associated finding and is seen in 50% of cases of fibromas measuring in excess of 5 cm in diameter. Ascites and hydrothorax (Meigs's syndrome) is seen in 1–3% of cases.[7,17,35] Excision of the tumor results in resolution of the ascites and hydrothorax. In one case,[51] the tumor was associated with hypoglycemia, that resolved following excision of the fibroma. An increased frequency of ovarian fibroma was noted in subjects with hereditary basal cell nevus syndrome.[30]

Macroscopically, the tumors vary from small round nodules 1–2 cm in diameter to large masses weighing up to 13 kg.[35] The tumor usually forms a round or oval solid mass that is gray-white and firm in consistency. It may sometimes be bosselated or lobulated, but usually the external surface is smooth. The cut surface is uniformly white or gray-white, solid, and smooth, but a whorled pattern similar to that observed in leiomyoma is also seen. In large tumors, foci of hemorrhage or necrosis, sometimes resulting in cyst formation, may be seen.

Microscopically, the tumor is composed of short spindle-shaped cells having narrow or ovoid spindle-shaped nuclei. Mitotic activity is absent or very low. The cells form bundles frequently intersected by hyalinized tissue. Hyalinization and myxomatous change are frequently present. Calcification, edema, hemorrhage, and necrosis may also be seen. Fat is absent except in necrotic areas. The absence of fat differentiates between a fibroma and a thecoma, but it cannot distinguish between a fibroma and a fibrosed thecoma. Thus, these two entities cannot always be distinguished satisfactorily. Massive edema of the ovary[36,89] and the newly described entity of fibromatosis, which may be related to massive edema and usually affects the entire ovary, may resemble an edematous fibroma and must be differentiated from it (see Chapter 16, Nonneoplastic Lesions of Ovary). Cellular fibroma of the ovary must be differentiated from fibrosarcoma. Although in well-differentiated examples of the latter the distinction may be difficult, the presence of mitotic activity tends to be the best distinguishing feature, and the presence of more than 4 mitoses/10 HPF places the tumor in the fibrosarcoma category.[66,71]

Fibroma of the ovary is a benign neoplasm, and the treatment of choice is excision of the affected ovary. This results in resolution of all symptoms. In the occasional patient, ovarian fibroma may be associated with implants in the peritoneum.[44] The presence of these implants should not be taken as evidence of malignancy. The prognosis in these, as in other cases of ovarian fibroma, is excellent.

Fibrosarcoma

Primary fibrosarcoma of the ovary is uncommon.[2,66,71] In a series of 283 ovarian tumors of fibrous tissue origin, there were 4 primary fibrosarcomas.[17] Although some fibrosarcomas of the ovary may have been classified as malignant thecomas and as spindle-cell sarcomas,[26] fully documented tumors of this type are uncommon, although they occur more frequently than do other pure primary sarcomas of the ovary. Fibrosarcoma is usually seen in menopausal and postmenopausal patients.[2,52,56] This tumor may arise de novo from ovarian stroma or may originate as a result of malignant change in a preexistent fibroma. Occasional cases have been observed in children.[1] In one case the tumor was associated with nevoid basal cell carcinoma syndrome.[39]

Macroscopically, fibrosarcoma of the ovary resembles ovarian fibroma, but the tumor is usually larger and is more likely to be associated with hemorrhage and necrosis.[52,66]

Microscopically, ovarian fibrosarcoma shows typical appearances of fibrosarcoma seen in other locations and usually shows marked cellular pleomorphism and brisk mitotic activity.[52,66] The prognosis is generally poor, the tumor metastasizing early via the bloodstream to the lungs. Occasionally, the course of the disease is more protracted, with patients surviving up to 9 years from time of diagnosis.[2,52,56] Tumors showing less marked mitotic activity tend to be less aggressive.[66]

Myxoma of the Ovary

Primary myxoma of the ovary is a very rare neoplasm; only three cases have been reported in the literature.[20,45,48] The patients were aged 14, 25, and 43 years and in each case had an adnexal mass. The other adnexa was normal.[20,45,48] Macroscopically, the tumors were medium size, encapsulated, gray-white, and soft; on cut section they were found to be partly cystic, partly solid. The solid areas were slimy and mucinous, whereas the cystic spaces contained a viscous, glassy, gelatinous material. Microscopically, the tumors showed the typical appearances of myxoma as described by Stout.[78] They were composed of a large amount of loose myxomatous stroma within which there were scattered stellate or spindle-shaped cells, some of which contained hyperchromatic nuclei. There was no nuclear pleomorphism, and mitotic activity was absent. The tumors were poorly vascularized, containing only a few capillary blood vessels and showing absence of plexiform vessels. The myxomatous stroma stained positively with alcian blue stain and contained a network of fine reticulum fibers. Stains for fat proved negative. In some areas, fibrosis was present. There were no other connective tissue elements, and the tumors showed similar appearances throughout.

Most myxomas originate within connective tissue, and the origin of the tumor is still a matter of dispute.[20,78,86] The histogenesis of ovarian myxomas is unknown. Although myxoma is a benign neoplasm, owing to its viscous nature, it is difficult to excise completely and recurrences are not uncommon.[20,78] In contrast, the patients who were treated by unilateral adnexectomy and the two patients for whom there is follow-up information did not show evidence of recurrence 1 year following surgery.[45,48] Although the follow-up in these cases was short, it appears that excision of the tumor, or unilateral adnexectomy, is the treatment of choice for patients with ovarian myxoma.

Myxoma must be differentiated from fibroma with myxoid degeneration, which contains normal fibrous tissue in some areas. More importantly, it must be differentiated from myxomatous liposarcoma, which contains fat, is more vascularized, and shows lipoblasts at least in some areas. It must also be differentiated from mucinous cystadenomas and carcinomas—either primary or metastatic—which contain epithelial cells, show absence of stellate and spindle-shaped cells, and may show glandular differentiation. Myxoma should also be distinguished from embryonal rhabdomyosarcoma, which shows less uniform appearances, cellular and nuclear pleomorphism, and rhabdomyoblasts.

Tumors of Muscle Origin

Leiomyoma

Primary leiomyoma of the ovary is rare.[23] More than 30 cases are on record, but it is likely that some cases are not reported, especially when the tumor is small and is discovered incidentally. At least 5 unreported cases are known to the author.

Primary ovarian leiomyoma must be differentiated from pedunculated subserosal (parasitic) uterine leiomyoma, which has lost its attachment and instead has become attached to the ovary, from which it draws its blood supply. Primary ovarian leiomyoma probably originates from smooth muscle present in the walls of blood vessels in the cortical stroma, in the corpus luteum,[61] and in the ovarian ligaments at their point of attachment to the ovary; its precise histogenesis is uncertain, however. This tumor is usually found in menopausal and postmenopausal women but sometimes occurs in young women. The age of patients ranges from 20 to 65 years.[26] Clinically, many patients are asymptomatic, and the tumor is discovered incidentally. When symptoms are present, they are related to the presence of an adnexal mass, becoming manifest as abdominal swelling and abdominal pain. The latter may be acute, due to torsion. Ascites is rare, and hydrothorax has not been reported. The uterus usually contains leiomyomata. Macroscopically, the tumors are unilateral, solid, firm, round, or oval masses having a smooth surface. On cut-section, they have a white or gray-white solid whorled surface. Hemorrhage and necrosis may be in evidence, altering the appearance. Cyst formation caused by necrosis may occur, and calcification may also be present.

Microscopically, the tumor shows typical appearances of a leiomyoma, as observed in the uterus, the tumor being composed of smooth muscle cells that are uniformly spindle-shaped or elongated and contain elongated blunt-ended or cigar-shaped nuclei. Palisading of the nuclei may be present and may be prominent. Mitotic activity is absent or very low, and cellular and nuclear pleomorphism is not a feature. The tumor cells form bundles intersected by fibrous septa that may be wide and show marked hyalinization. Other degenerative changes seen in uterine leiomyomas may also be present. Connective tissue stains confirm the leiomyomatous nature of the tumor. In two tumors that I studied, this was further confirmed ultrastructurally.

Leiomyosarcoma

Primary leiomyosarcoma of the ovary is very rare, and there are fewer than 10 cases reported in the literature. They are usually found in postmenopausal women.[2,56] A few unreported cases are known to me. The tumors are usually large and solid, and patients have symptoms and signs related to the presence of an abdominal or pelvic mass. The tumors are gray-yellow, soft, fleshy, and frequently associated with hemorrhage and necrosis. Microscopically, they differ from a leiomyoma by the presence of mitotic activity and cellular and nuclear pleomorphism (Figs. 21.1. and 21.2.). In well-differentiated tumors, the mitotic activity may be the only distinguishing feature from a cellular leiomyoma and is considered to be far more important in this respect than cellular and nuclear pleomorphism. Primary leiomyosarcoma of the ovary metastasizes via the bloodstream; the prognosis is generally unfavorable, although the use of combination chemotherapy may improve it. Primary leiomyosarcoma of the ovary must be distinguished from mixed müllerian (mesodermal) tumors containing a prominent leiomyosarcomatous component combined with other malignant mesenchymal and epithelial elements and from immature teratomas with a prominent leiomyomatous tissue component. It must also be distinguished from metastatic leiomyosarcoma of uterine or other origin, as well as from poorly differentiated sarcomas and carcinosarcomas, both primary and metastatic to the ovary.

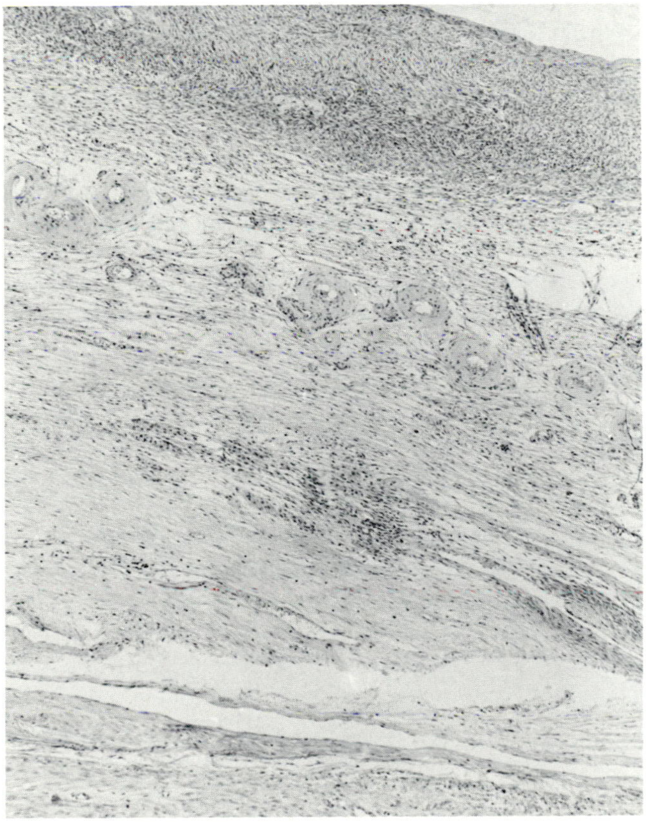

Fig. 21.1. Primary ovarian leiomyosarcoma. The tumor is seen beneath normal ovarian cortex (*top*).

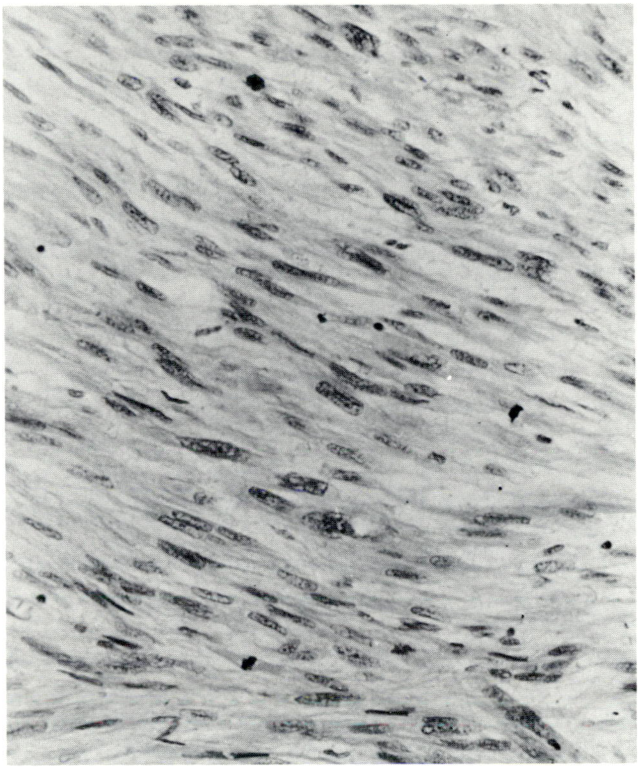

Fig. 21.2. Primary ovarian leiomyosarcoma. Higher magnification of tumor shown in Fig. 21.1. Note brisk mitotic activity and cellular and nuclear pleomorphism.

Rhabdomyoma

No well-documented case of ovarian rhabdomyoma has been recorded.

Rhabdomyosarcoma

Primary rhabdomyosarcoma of the ovary occurs rarely; only 10 well-documented cases have been reported in the literature, and 9 unreported cases are known to me. A careful review of the literature shows that some cases, such as the frequently quoted case reported by Sandison,[69] were not pure rhabdomyosarcomas but rather examples of mixed müllerian (mesodermal) tumor or teratomas with a marked rhabdomyoblastic component. Therefore, before a diagnosis of primary ovarian rhabdomyosarcoma can be made, the tumor must be very carefully and extensively sampled to exclude the presence of other neoplastic elements, the presence of which would preclude a diagnosis of a pure rhabdomyosarcoma of the ovary.

The histogenesis of primary rhabdomyosarcoma of the ovary, like that of other ovarian sarcomas composed of a single neoplastic tissue element, is uncertain. These tumors may originate from the connective tissue of the ovary, as a one-sided development of teratoma, as a result of malignant transformation of a mature cystic teratoma with the malignant element overgrowing the tumor, or as a one-sided development of a mixed müllerian (mesodermal) tumor. Any of these possibilities may be the most likely for a given case.

The age of patients with ovarian rhabdomyosarcoma falls within a wide range of 2.5 to 84 years. The small number of cases makes it impossible to state whether there is a predilection for any particular age group, but, as with rhabdomyosarcomas occurring in other locations, the pleomorphic type occurs in older patients, whereas the embryonal and alveolar types occur in young subjects. Patients with ovarian rhabdomyosarcoma usually have symptoms associated with the presence of a large, usually rapidly growing, abdominal mass, frequently associated with hemorrhagic ascites. Metastases are frequently seen at presentation.

Macroscopically, the tumors are unilateral, but metastatic involvement of the contralateral ovary may be present and should be differentiated from bilateral involvement. The tumors are usually large, exceeding 10 cm in diameter. They are solid, soft, fleshy, and gray-pink to yellow-tan, with areas of hemorrhage and necrosis that may be prominent.

Microscopically, the tumors are composed entirely of rhabdomyoblasts, either of the embryonal type (Figs. 21.3. and 21.4.) admixed with the alveolar (Fig. 21.5.) or even botryoid types, or of the pleomorphic type. Tumors composed of the former types occur in children and young adults, whereas those of the pleomorphic type are observed in older subjects. Whereas the diagnosis of pleomorphic rhabdomyosarcoma should not present undue difficulty, owing to the presence of at least some typical rhabdomyoblasts showing cross-striation, the diagnosis of embryonal rhabdomyosarcoma is much more difficult because the tumor cells are poorly differentiated, making rhabdomyoblastic differentiation discernible only with difficulty. Furthermore, it is necessary to recognize the distinctive alveolar (Fig. 21.5.) or botryoid patterns, which may not be easy. The embryonal rhabdomyosarcoma is composed of rhabdomyoblasts in various stages of differentiation (Figs. 21.3. and 21.4.) and is at least partly composed of collections of small round cells having

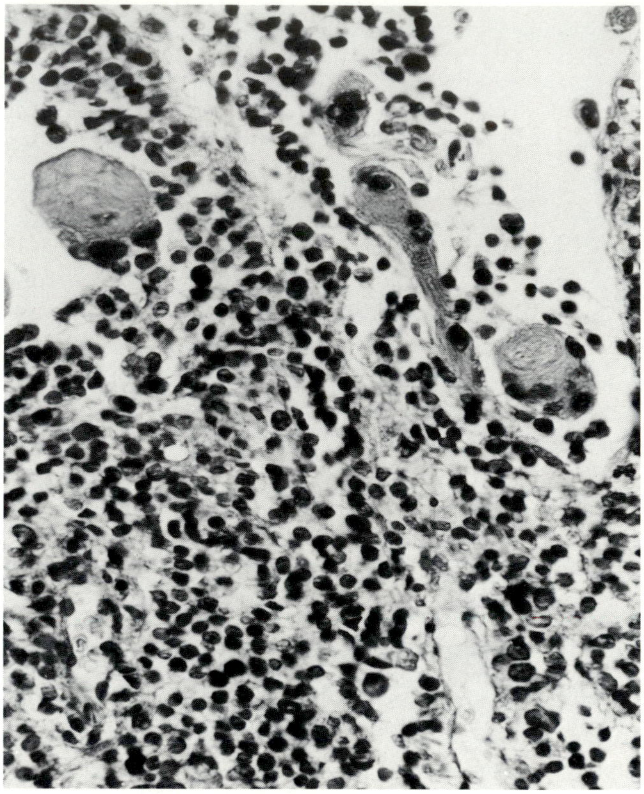

FIG. 21.3. Primary rhabdomyosarcoma of ovary of embryonal type. Most tumor cells are of small round type, but occasional large rhabdomyoblasts, some exhibiting cross-striations, are seen.

a narrow rim of cytoplasm (Fig. 21.3.) that are poorly differentiated. Therefore, the lesion is difficult to distinguish from poorly differentiated small cell carcinoma, malignant lymphoma, or even neuroblastoma or leukemia.[58] Among the small round cells, there are scattered occasional better-differentiated cells with bright eosinophilic cytoplasm and eccentric nuclei (Fig. 21.4.). Occasionally, large, more typical rhabdomyoblasts are seen. The presence of cross-striations is not necessary for diagnosis, but the cells comprising the tumor may be well enough differentiated to exhibit cross-striations (Fig. 21.3.). Demonstration of Z-bands or their precursors by electron microscopy is helpful in making the diagnosis.[31] Immunocytochemical demonstration of myoglobin and desmin is also helpful in this respect. The tumor is frequently affected by edema, hemorrhage, and necrosis, making the diagnosis even more difficult. Therefore, thorough examination and sampling of the tumor are essential in order to make the correct diagnosis. The tumor may be more common than has been hitherto believed, but because of its poor differentiation, it may have been either assigned to the group of undifferentiated ovarian tumors or misdiagnosed. It is, therefore, emphasized that embryonal rhabdomyosarcoma must be consid-

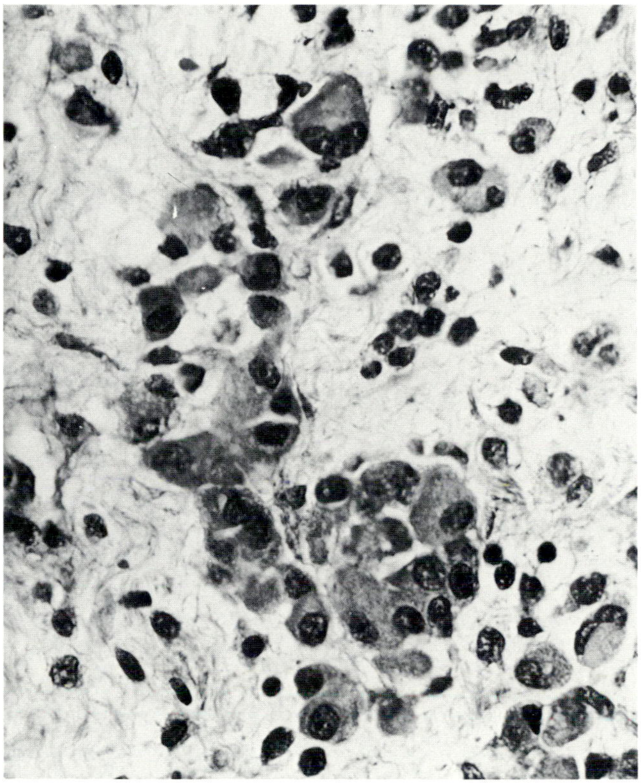

FIG. 21.4. Primary rhabdomyosarcoma of ovary of embryonal type composed of primitive rhabdomyoblasts with ample amount of bright eosinophilic cytoplasm and eccentric nuclei.

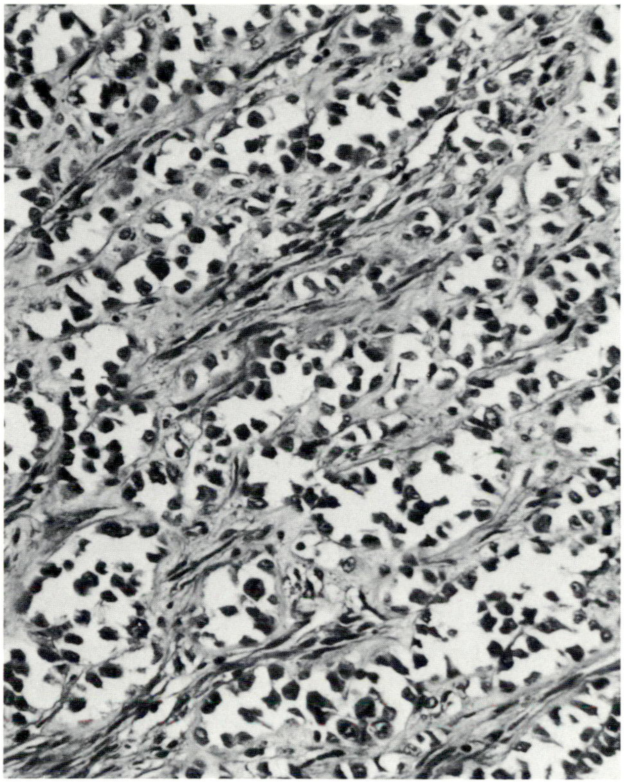

FIG. 21.5. Primary rhabdomyosarcoma of ovary, showing pronounced alveolar pattern.

ered in the differential diagnosis of *undifferentiated small round cell tumor* of the ovary in a young patient. The presence of other neoplastic elements must always be excluded when making this diagnosis. The importance of making the correct diagnosis is not only academic but practical, in view of the advances that have been made in the therapy of embryonal rhabdomyosarcoma during the last two decades. In the past, the prognosis was considered poor, and in most reported cases, the patients died of extensive metastatic disease within 1 year of diagnosis. Recently, two patients with embryonal rhabdomyosarcoma, one of whom had metastases, are well and disease-free following surgery, chemotherapy, and radiotherapy. The combination chemotherapy advocated in such patients consists of dactinomycin, vincristine, and cyclophosphamide. The addition of methotrexate with folinic acid rescue and doxorubicin to this combination may also be of value.

Tumors of Vascular Origin

Hemangioma

Hemangioma is only occasionally found in the ovary; the number of well-documented cases does not exceed 40. Although some cases may not have been recognized or recorded, all investigators consider ovarian hemangioma rare.[21,26,28,29,80] This is somewhat surprising, since the ovary has a very rich and complex vasculature.

The origin of ovarian hemangioma in common with hemangioma in general is a matter of controversy; it is considered either a hamartomatous malformation[86] or a true neoplasm.[22] It is likely that both modes of origin are responsible for their formation. The age of patients with ovarian hemangioma ranges from 4 months to 63 years[26,80] and does not show a predominance in any decade. In most patients, ovarian hemangioma has been noted as an incidental finding at operation or autopsy.[26,80] In a few cases, the lesion was large and the patient had abdominal enlargement due to the presence of an ovarian mass[21,28,49,74] or had acute abdominal pain associated with torsion of the tumor.[46,73] In one case, there was ascites.[49] The lesions are usually unilateral, although in four patients they were bilateral.[9,27,40,77] Ovarian hemangiomas have been noted in patients with generalized hemangiomatosis[40,77] and in patients with hemangiomas in other parts of the genital tract.[40,80] One patient with bilateral ovarian hemangiomas and diffuse abdominopelvic hemangiomatosis had thrombocytopenia. The platelet count returned to normal after excision of the affected ovaries.[16]

Macroscopically, the lesions are small, red or purple, round or oval nodules, measuring from a few millimeters to 1.5 cm in diameter. Larger lesions have also been encountered measuring up to 11.5 cm in the largest diameter.[46] On cut section, they are usually spongy and show a honeycomb appearance. Although they have been found in different parts of the ovary, the medulla and the hilar region appear to be the most common sites.[80]

Microscopically, ovarian hemangioma is of the cavernous or mixed capillary–cavernous type. It consists of collections of vascular spaces, which may vary in size but are usually small, lined by a single layer of endothelial cells, and usually contain red blood cells in their lumen (Fig. 21.6.). Occasionally, thrombosis may be seen. A small amount of connective tissue may be present within the lesion. The treatment of choice is oophorectomy or adnexectomy, which results in a complete cure. Hemangioma must be differentiated from proliferations of dilated blood vessels, frequently seen in the hilar region of the ovary. Although a very small hemangioma may not be easily distinguished from such vascular proliferations, the hemangioma usually forms a nodule or a small mass; the presence of a circumscribed nodule composed of vascular spaces tends to distinguish hemangioma from vascular proliferations, which are usually smaller and more diffuse. The presence of numerous blood cells within the vascular spaces and the absence of pale eosinophilic homogeneous material usually distinguish hemangioma from lymphangioma. Hemangioma must also be distinguished from teratoma with a prominent vascular component. In such cases, careful sampling will detect other teratomatous elements, the presence of which will distinguish the lesion from a hemangioma.

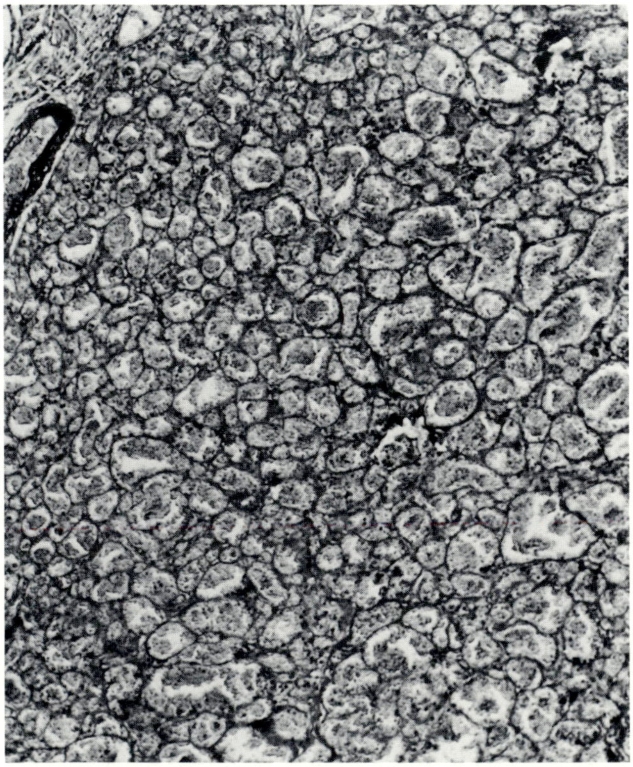

FIG. 21.6. Hemangioma of the ovary composed of numerous small vascular spaces lined by a single layer of endothelial cells. Elastic van Gieson.

Hemangioendothelial Sarcoma (Hemangioendothelioma, Hemangiosarcoma, Angiosarcoma)

Hemangioendothelial sarcoma is a very rare ovarian neoplasm, only nine examples have been recorded.[26,62,65] Five unreported cases have been seen by me. The age incidence varies from 19 to 77 years. This tumor is encountered at all ages, therefore, the statement that it usually occurs in childhood and adolescence[35] is incorrect and may indicate the inclusion of immature teratomas with a prominent vascular component. The tumor is usually unilateral, but one case of bilateral tumors has been recorded.[26] Bilaterality must be differentiated from metastatic spread to the contralateral ovary, which was seen in one personally observed case. The histogenesis of the tumor is uncertain, but it may originate from the vascular tissue present in the ovary, or as a one-sided development of a teratoma. Patients usually have symptoms related to the presence of a lower abdominal mass, which may be associated with torsion and rupture of the tumor and hemorrhage.

Macroscopically, the tumors are usually large, blue-brown, hemorrhagic, soft, and friable. They may be confined to the ovary but are also associated with invasion of the surrounding structures.

Microscopically, they are composed of vascular spaces of varying size and appearance, lined by endothelial cells that are usually large, showing atypical appearance, bizarre nuclei, and mitotic activity (Figs. 21.7. and 21.8.). In some areas, the tumor may contain a considerable amount of connective tissue interspersed between the vascular spaces (Fig. 21.7.). The tumor invades locally and metastasizes via the bloodstream. Prognosis is poor, especially in patients who have metastases at the time of presentation. Hemangioendothelial sarcoma of the ovary must be distinguished from immature teratomatous neoplasms with a prominent vascular component. The presence of other neoplastic germ cell elements distinguishes teratoma from primary hemangioendothelial sarcoma. It must also be distinguished from the very occasional lymphangiosarcoma, which is composed of lymphatic and not of blood vessels, as well as from malignant hemangiopericytoma, which is composed of a proliferation of pericytes and shows a different histologic pattern. Hemangiopericytoma can be further distinguished from hemangioendothelial sarcoma with the help of reticulum stains.

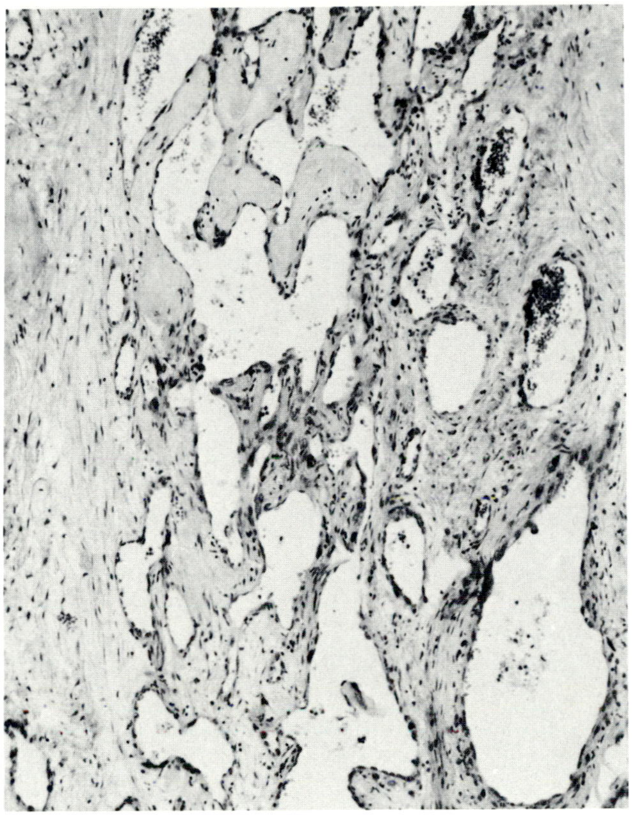

FIG. 21.7. Primary hemangioendothelial sarcoma of ovary. The tumor is composed of vascular spaces surrounded by connective tissue.

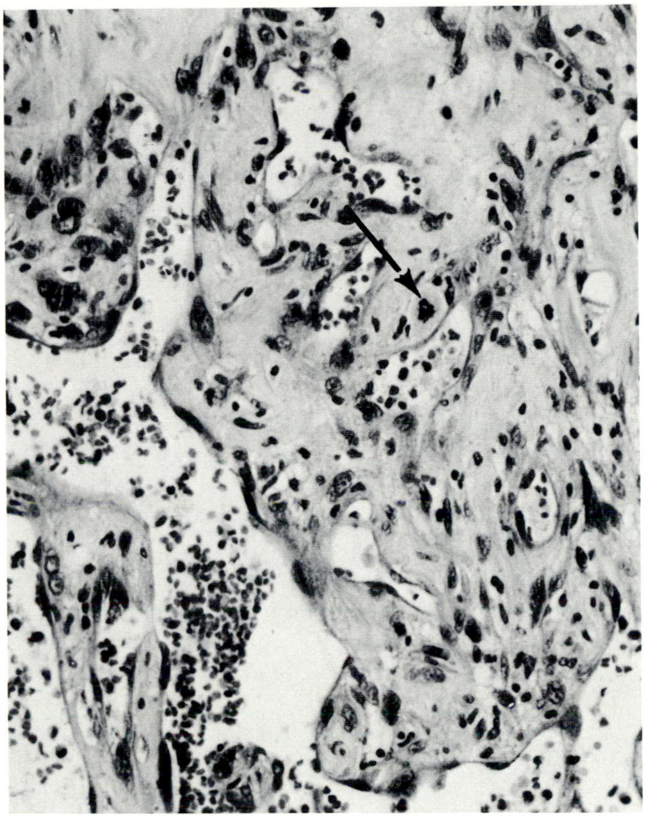

FIG. 21.8. Primary hemangioendothelial sarcoma of ovary. Note the large endothelial cells lining vascular spaces. Large abnormal mitosis is seen to right of center (*arrow*).

Lymphangioma

Lymphangioma of the ovary is very rare, with fewer than 10 documented cases reported.[26] I have seen 2 cases. In both cases, the tumor was small and was found incidentally. Macroscopically, the tumor is unilateral and small, having a smooth, gray surface. On cut section, it is yellow, honeycombed, and composed of numerous small cystic spaces exuding clear yellow fluid.

Microscopically, lymphangioma of the ovary, is composed of closely packed, thin-walled vascular spaces lined with flattened endothelial cells and containing pale homogeneous eosinophilic fluid. As in the case of hemangioma, the histogenesis is a matter of controversy. Some investigators consider these lesions as malformations or hamartomas[86] and some as neoplasms.[22]

Lymphangioma is differentiated from a teratoma with a prominent vascular component by the absence of other germ cell elements. Lymphangioma must also be distinguished from hemangioma and an adenomatoid tumor that contains thin-walled, vessel-like spaces. In contrast to hemangioma, lymphangioma does not contain blood cells in the vascular spaces. The adenomatoid tumor has solid areas, and the cells lining the vessel-like spaces stain positively with PAS and alcian blue stains.

Lymphangiosarcoma

Only one case of lymphangiosarcoma of the ovary has been reported.[68] The tumor, which measured 15 cm in diameter, was found in a 31-year-old woman who had symptoms of a rapidly enlarging abdominal mass. The tumor was composed of proliferating, closely packed lymphatic vessels, which, in one area, showed cellular and nuclear atypia. There was extensive necrosis and hemorrhage. The patient died 1 year following diagnosis, of extensive metastatic disease.[68]

Hemangiopericytoma

No well-documented case of ovarian hemangiopericytoma has been recorded.

Tumors of Cartilage Origin

Chondroma

Only a few reports of ovarian chondroma are available, and documentation in most cases is unsatisfactory. A well-documented case considered to originate from the ovarian stroma has been reported.[57] The tumor, which measured 4 × 3 × 3 cm and was composed entirely of mature cartilage, was found incidentally. Although chondroma may originate from the connective tissue of the ovary by a process of metaplasia, it is more likely that most ovarian tumors described as chondroma were either fibromas showing cartilaginous metaplasia or teratomas having a prominent cartilaginous component.[26]

Chondrosarcoma

A single example of pure chondrosarcoma of the ovary has been reported[81] (Fig. 21.9). A 61-year-old woman had an abdominal mass, which, on extensive microscopic examination, proved to be a pure, well-differentiated chondrosarcoma (Figs. 21.10. and 21.11.). The patient is well and disease-free 6 years after one-sided adnexectomy. The histogenesis of this tumor is uncertain, but the age of the patient and the histologic appearances of the tumor point to an origin in a dermoid cyst with malignant transformation and overgrowth by the malignant cartilaginous component.[81] A well-documented case of mature cystic teratoma (dermoid cyst) with malignant transformation of the cartilaginous element has been reported; the patient died of extensive metastatic disease.[15]

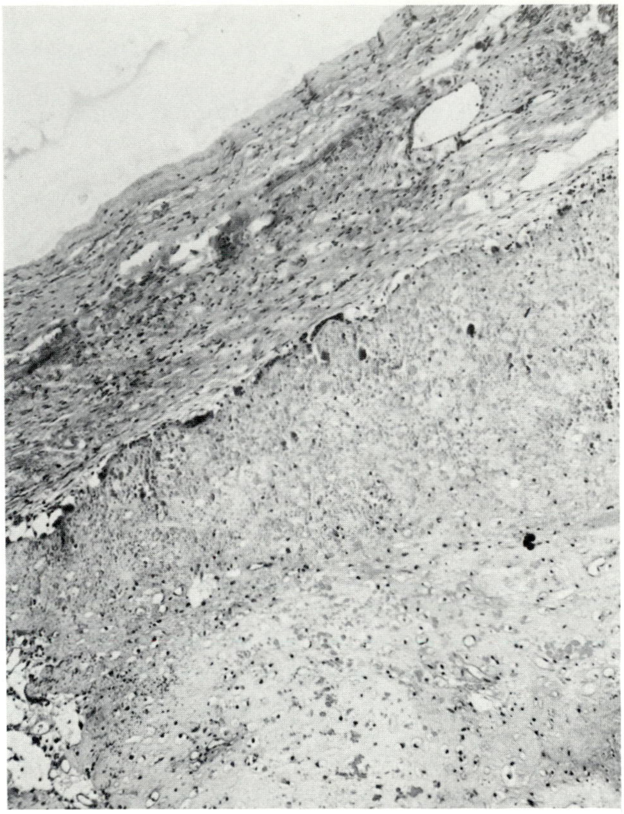

FIG. 21.10. Primary ovarian chondrosarcoma. Tumor is seen beneath normal ovarian cortex.

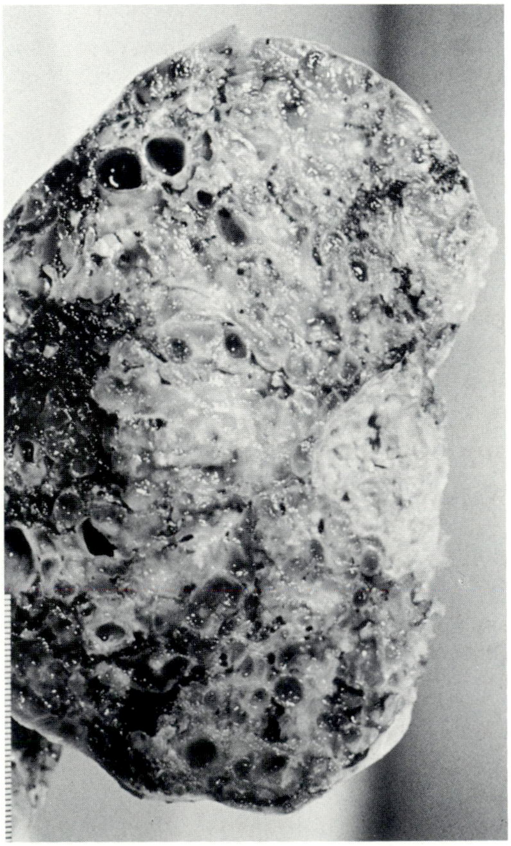

FIG. 21.9. Primary ovarian chondrosarcoma.

Tumors of Bone Origin

Osteoma

Few documented examples of osteoma occurring in the ovary exist, and although an origin from ovarian stroma is possible, most such lesions were probably examples of osseous metaplasia occurring in fibromas or leiomyomas,[35] or possibly examples of metaplasia or heterotopia and not neoplasia occurring in the connective tissue of the ovary.[75] The lesions are usually small but may be large and are histologically composed of dense cortical bone.[35]

Osteosarcoma

Only one example of pure osteosarcoma of the ovary has been reported.[2] The tumor occurred in a 41-year-old woman in whom there was associated metastatic disease. The patient died 5 months after diagnosis. Histologically, the tumor showed typical appearances of osteosarcoma occurring in the skeleton. Although it was believed that the tumor originated directly from ovarian stroma, the histogenesis of this tumor, in common with other pure sarcomas of the ovary, is uncertain. Occasional cases

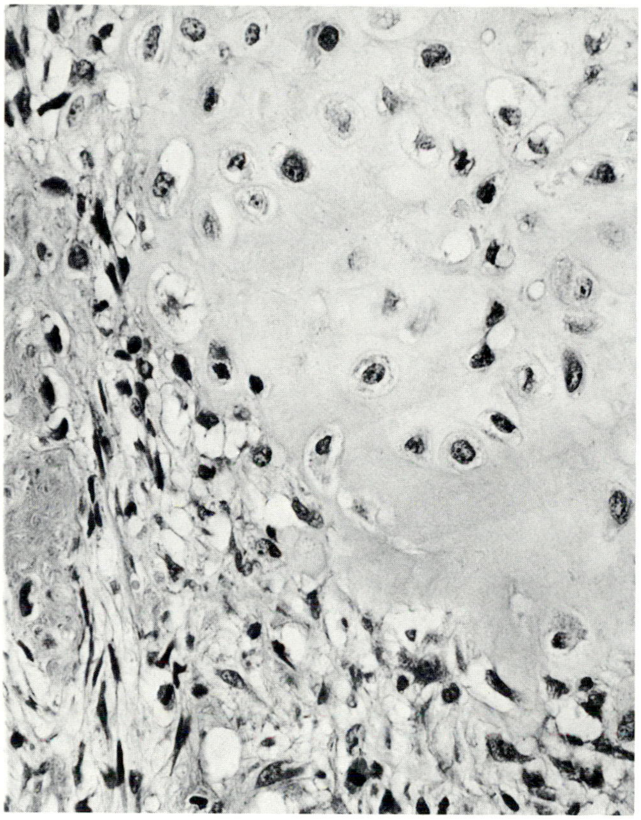

FIG. 21.11. Primary ovarian chondrosarcoma. Higher magnification showing well-differentiated tumor.

of osteosarcoma originating in ovarian teratoma have been recorded,[79] but such cases should not be confused with pure ovarian osteosarcoma, nor should cases of mixed müllerian (mesodermal) tumor with a prominent osteosarcomatous component.

Giant Cell Tumor of the Ovary

A single case of giant cell tumor of the ovary histologically indistinguishable from a giant cell tumor of bone has been reported.[42] The tumor was found incidentally in an ovary of a 31-year-old woman. It was composed of small ovoid or spindle-shaped stromal cells admixed with multinucleated giant cells, many of which contained between 50 and 100 small hyperchromatic nuclei. In places, there was brisk mitotic activity. The patient was well and disease-free 4½ years after excision of the affected adnexa.

Tumors of Neural Tissue Origin

Ovarian tumors originating from neural tissue are rare. The presenting symptoms are usually related to the presence of an intraabdominal mass. The tumors are solid and are usually small. The histogenesis is uncertain and is probably similar to that of mesenchymal tumors of the ovary.

Neurofibroma

A single case of neurofibroma of the ovary was encountered as an incidental finding in a patient with generalized neurofibromatosis (von Recklinghausen's disease).[76] Histologically, the tumor showed appearances similar to those of a neurofibroma occurring elsewhere.

Neurilemmoma

Three cases of ovarian neurilemmoma (schwannoma) have been reported.[16,50,53] In one case, the tumor was large.[53] The tumors were solid and the patients were well and disease-free following the excision of the tumor. Histologically, the tumors showed the typical appearances of a neurilemmoma occurring in other locations.

Neurofibrosarcoma

One case of neurofibrosarcoma occurring in a 38-year-old woman with generalized neurofibromatosis (von Recklinghausen's disease) has been described.[19] The tumor was an incidental finding and had replaced the ovary. It was solid and histologically showed typical appearances of a neurofibrosarcoma with a moderate degree of cellular and nuclear pleomorphism and mitotic activity. There was no evidence of metastases, and the patient was well and disease-free 1 year following diagnosis.[19]

Ganglioneuroma

A single case of ovarian ganglioneuroma occurring in a 4-year-old girl has been reported.[70] The child had abdominal enlargement. The tumor was solid, weighing 200 g, and replaced nearly the whole ovary. Histologically, the tumor was composed of well-differentiated ganglion cells. There was a recurrence following the excision of the tumor. True ganglioneuroma must be differentiated from teratomas showing prominence of ganglion cells and from proliferations of ganglion cells occasionally seen in the hilar region of the ovary; the latter are nonneoplastic and probably hamartomatous in nature.

Pheochromocytoma

A single case of ovarian pheochromocytoma occurring in a 15-year-old girl has been reported.[24] The patient had hypertension, convulsions, and a large, left-sided abdominal tumor mass. The tumor had undergone torsion and weighed 970 g. It was solid, and microscopic examination showed typical appearances of pheochromocytoma. Epinephrine and norepinephrine were extracted from tumor tissue. The symptoms disappeared following excision of the tumor, and the patient was well and disease-free 15 months following the operation.[24]

Tumors of Adipose Tissue Origin

There are no well-documented cases of tumors of adipose tissue origin in the ovary. Some reports relating to the presence of both benign and malignant neoplasms composed of adipose tissue in the ovary exist, but they are not well substantiated. Collections of adipose cells forming islands of fatty tissue that are not encapsulated are seen occasionally within ovarian tissue and are attributed to metaplasia of connective tissue of the ovary. These collections have been described as adipose prosoplasia.[32] Benign adipose tissue seen in the ovary may be part of a teratoma with a prominent adipose tissue component. Malignant adipose tissue may be a part of a mixed müllerian (mesodermal) tumor with a prominent liposarcomatous component, or it may represent metastases from a liposarcoma occurring at another location.[26]

Tumors of Mesothelial Origin

Adenomatoid Tumor

The adenomatoid tumor, which in the female is most frequently found in the fallopian tubes and broad ligament and occasionally in the uterus near the serosal surface, is only rarely found in the ovary (see Chapter 13, Mesenchymal Tumors of Uterus, and Chapter 14, Diseases of Fallopian Tube). Although its histogenesis has been a matter of dispute for a long time, it is now considered to be of mesothelial origin. This is supported by morphologic, histochemical, and ultrastructural observations.[25,83] Adenomatoid tumor is benign and is, therefore, considered a benign mesothelioma.

Six cases of ovarian adenomatoid tumor have been recorded, most of which occurred in patients in the third and fourth decades. The lesions, which are small, round or oval, measuring from 0.5 to 1.5 cm in diameter, are usually found in the hilus of the ovary as incidental findings. Histologically they show similar appearances to adenomatoid tumors occurring in other locations and are composed of clefts and spaces lined by cuboidal, low columnar, or flattened epithelial-like cells (Fig. 21.12) and of solid aggregates of similar cells surrounded by connective tissue that varies from loose and edematous to dense and hyalinized. The epithelial-like cells may exhibit marked vacuolation. They exhibit positive staining with alcian blue, which is digestible with hyaluronidase, and similarly staining material is present in the clefts and spaces. Occasionally, the cells may show weak PAS staining. Ultrastructural observations support the mesothelial origin of this lesion and show an abundance of microvilli, bundles of cytoplasmic filaments, tight junctional complexes, and intercellular spaces (Fig. 21.13). The lesion is benign, and its excision results in a complete cure.

Peritoneal Mesothelioma

Occasionally, peritoneal mesothelioma may involve the surface of the ovary (see Chapter 17, Endometriosis). When the tumor affects the ovary, confusion with primary ovarian neoplasms or benign conditions may occur.[82] The histologic pattern, ultrastructural and immunohistochemical observations, and the behavior and distribution of the lesion are helpful in making the correct diagnosis.[37,82,85] The majority of patients with malignant peritoneal mesothelioma are middle-aged or elderly

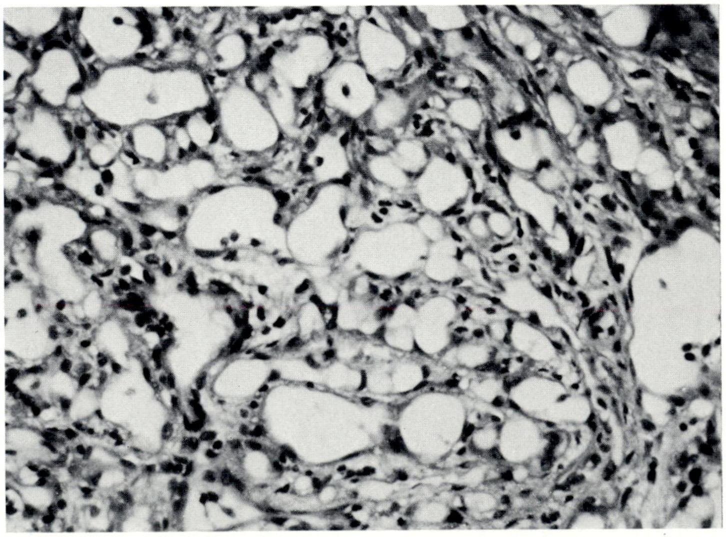

FIG. 21.12. Adenomatoid tumor showing numerous clefts and spaces lined by a single layer of flattened endothelial-like or low cuboid cells.

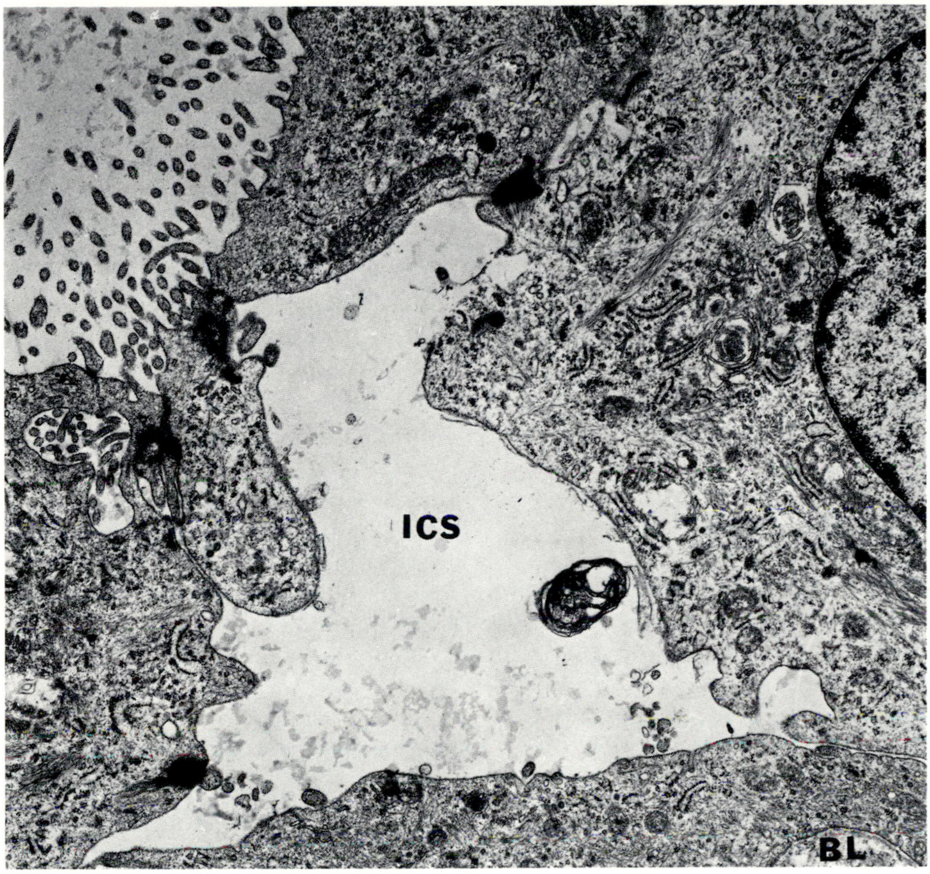

FIG. 21.13. Electron micrograph of an ovarian mesothelioma showing intercellular spaces (ICS) with apical tight junctional complexes. ×16,000. (Reprinted by permission of Ferenczy et al., Ref. 25.)

adults, and the tumor shows a considerable male predominance.[37] Very rarely, it may occur in children.[82]

Other Tumors

Other mesenchymal tumors occurring in the ovary include the sclerosing stromal tumor of the ovary described in detail in Chapter 19, Sex Cord–Stromal Ovarian Tumors. Tumors of teratomatous origin containing mesenchymal tissue are described in Chapter 20, Germ Cell Tumors of Ovary, and mixed müllerian (mesodermal) tumors, carcinosarcomas, endometrial stromal sarcomas, and adenosarcoma are discussed in Chapter 18, Epithelial Tumors of Ovary.

Undifferentiated Sarcomas

Some ovarian tumors are poorly differentiated, and although a diagnosis of sarcoma can be made, the tumor does not exhibit further differentiation beyond showing its mesenchymal origin. Careful and extensive histologic examination in such cases is helpful and may result in finding better-differentiated areas, which will yield a more accurate diagnosis. It is always worthwhile to undertake such examination, although for some cases a more precise diagnosis cannot be made despite extensive sampling.

Tumors of Hematopoietic Origin

Malignant Lymphoma of the Ovary

Malignant lymphoma affecting the ovary can be divided into two types: *primary extranodal malignant lymphoma* of the ovary, and *disseminated malignant lymphoma* affecting the ovary. Primary malignant lymphoma of the ovary is rare and, in turn, can be divided into two different types: (1) first manifestation of generalized malignant lymphoma and (2) localized extranodal malignant lymphoma. Disseminated malignant lymphoma is far more common than the primary type. It too can be divided into two specific types: (1) the ovarian tumor being either the initial or predominant presenting manifestation of the disease and (2) ovarian involvement occurring during the course of the disseminated disease, only discovered histologically following surgery or autopsy.

One specific type of malignant lymphoma, that is, Burkitt's lymphoma, frequently affects the ovary—which is the second most common site after the jaws. The ovary may be the site of primary disease as well as of disseminated disease, and the manifestations of Burkitt's lymphoma may accord with any of the specific types described for both primary and disseminated disease. Patients with primary disease localized to the ovary and with disseminated disease discovered only by histologic examination at surgery or autopsy are uncommon. Consequently, Burkitt's lymphoma is the most common malignant lymphoma in which involvement of the ovary manifests itself clinically and is an important feature of the disease.

Other hematopoietic neoplasms affecting the ovary, such as leukemia, myelomatosis, or plasmacytoma, can also be classified in a similar manner to malignant lymphoma. It should be noted, however, that their primary manifestation in the ovary is rare, even when compared with primary malignant lymphoma, which is itself very uncommon.

Primary Extranodal Malignant Lymphoma of the Ovary

Before the diagnosis of primary extranodal malignant lymphoma can be made, the presence of lymph node, as well as blood and bone marrow involvement by the disease, must be carefully excluded, and the involvement of the affected organ must be the first manifestation of the disease. This is of considerable importance because there is now good evidence that primary extranodal malignant lymphoma tends to run a less aggressive course than does malignant lymphoma affecting the lymph nodes. Although primary extranodal malignant lymphoma is not uncommon, the ovary is an infrequent site, and the number of well-documented cases reported in the literature is fewer than 50.[14,26,63,64]

The diagnosis of primary malignant lymphoma of the ovary can only be made if, in addition to the general criteria for the diagnosis of extranodal malignant lymphoma mentioned earlier, the tumor is confined to the ovary at the time of diagnosis. If, in addition to the ovarian involvement, only the lymph nodes immediately draining the ovary are affected or if local spread from the ovary to the adjacent structures is present, this should not preclude the diagnosis. Primary malignant lymphoma of the ovary shows a wide age range but tends to occur more frequently before menopause. The most common symptoms are abdominal enlargement or abdominal pain. Primary malignant lymphoma of the ovary has also been noted as an incidental finding. On examination, ovarian enlargement is nearly always present and is often bilateral. The tumors range in size from 5 to 27 cm.[14,26,63] They are usually soft, white to gray-white, with lobulated or nodular external surface, and solid and white to gray-pink on cut section, with evidence of hemorrhage and necrosis.

Microscopically, the ovarian tissue is almost completely replaced by a diffuse proliferation of malignant lymphoma cells forming a diffuse pattern, although occasionally a nodular (follicular) pattern, which may be pure or associated with the diffuse pattern, is also seen.[64] Normal ovarian structures, for example, corpora lutea and corpora albicantia, are sometimes present and are surrounded by the neoplastic cells, which may invade them.[14,63,64] The malignant lymphoma is usually of a poorly differentiated type and may be difficult to classify (Fig. 21.14). It is usually of the lymphoblastic or histiocytic type[67] of the large cleaved or noncleaved type.[43,63] Reticulum stains are sometimes helpful in making the diagnosis, but because of the poor differentiation of the tumor, the reticulum network may not be in evidence.

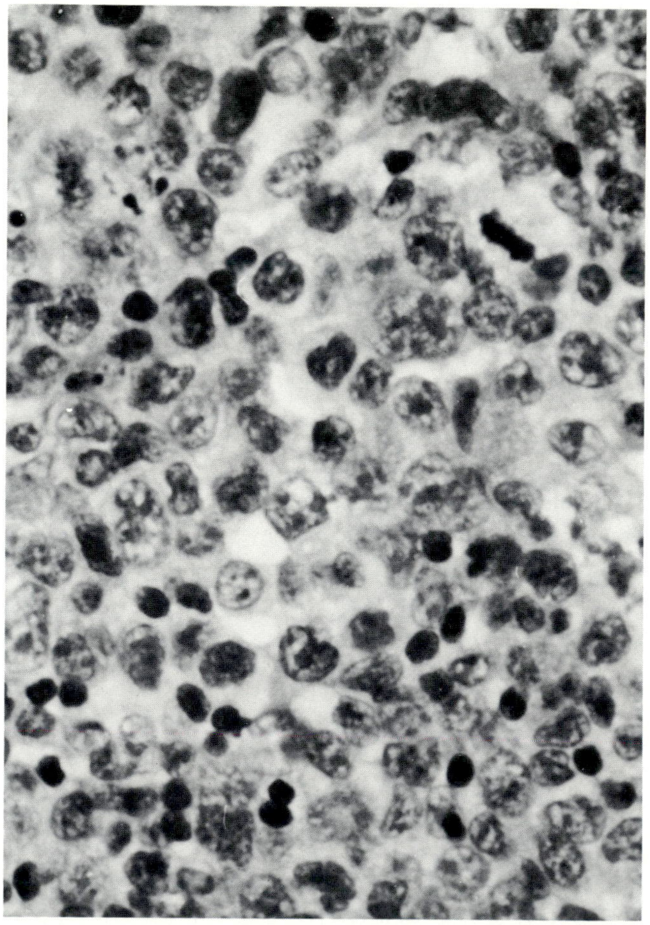

Fig. 21.14. Primary malignant lymphoma of ovary of poorly differentiated type. Note brisk mitotic activity and infiltration by inflammatory cells.

Acute inflammatory cells, plasma cells, and normal lymphocytes may be admixed with the tumor cells (Fig. 21.14), causing diagnostic difficulties. Malignant lymphoma of the ovary must be distinguished from other small round cell tumors composed of diffuse or nodular proliferations of small uniform tumor cells. Malignant lymphoma, especially of the lymphoblastic or poorly differentiated lymphocytic (small cell and large cell cleaved) types, must be distinguished from poorly differentiated metastatic carcinoma, most frequently of mammary origin. The carcinoma cells tend to be less uniform, show usually less marked mitotic activity, may be associated with evidence of fibroblastic reaction, and may in places exhibit an attempt at acinar formation. The presence of or a history of mammary carcinoma confirms the diagnosis. Similar features, except for the last two, differentiate malignant lymphoma from metastatic small (oat) cell carcinoma of the lung. Ultrastructural studies also help distinguish carcinoma from malignant lymphoma.

Histochemical demonstration of mucin and positive immunocytochemical staining for cytokeratin, which indicate carcinoma, are also helpful in distinguishing between these two entities. The presence of occasional, better-differentiated rhabdomyoblasts and of rosette formation helps to distinguish embryonal rhabdomyosarcoma and metastatic neuroblastoma, respectively, from malignant lymphoma. The presence of positive staining for leukocyte common antigen (LCA) distinguishes malignant lymphoma from neoplasms that are not composed of lymphoreticular cells and is a valuable diagnostic aid. Malignant lymphoma must also be distinguished from ovarian involvement by leukemia, and in such cases, blood and bone marrow studies are obviously helpful. The presence of red granular staining in the cytoplasm of the tumor cells when using naphthol-AS-D-chloroacetate esterase (Leder's) stain distinguishes malignant lymphoma cells, which do not stain by this method, from myeloid series cells, which stain positively. Malignant lymphoma must also be distinguished from granulosa cell tumors showing diffuse pattern, but other patterns seen in granulosa cell tumor may be evident, at least in some parts of the tumor. Mitotic activity is less brisk in granulosa cell tumor, and the cellular and nuclear appearances are different. Malignant lymphoma of the histiocytic (large cell noncleaved) type, which sometimes contains normal lymphocytes, must be distinguished from dysgerminoma. The dysgerminoma cells are more uniform in size and appearance and usually contain larger amounts of cytoplasm, which tends to be clear or pale and granular. The cytoplasm typically contains abundant glycogen, which stains postively with PAS stain and is removed by diastase digestion. The nuclei of dysgerminoma cells are more uniform and do not display the marked variation in shape and size seen in the nuclei of the malignant lymphoma cells.

The course of the disease of patients with primary malignant lymphoma of the ovary, is variable. Whereas generalized disease develops in most patients within a few months of the excision of the ovarian neoplasm, in some patients generalized disease does not develop for years. An occasional patient does not show any further involvement, and in some patients the only further involvement is enlargement of paraaortic and parailiac lymph nodes, the lymph nodes that provide lymphatic drainage of the ovary. Although some patients in whom generalized disease develops might not have been examined carefully enough to detect the presence of further disease, on presentation, there is little doubt that in some patients with malignant lymphoma confined to the ovary generalized disease will develop within a few months. Unfortunately, at present, it is not possible to determine which patients will and which will not develop generalized disease. Therefore, all patients should be staged properly and be given adequate therapy, which should include radiation to the regional lymph nodes and chemotherapy. Occasional patients have been reported[14,63,64] who were well and disease-free for periods of 2–5 years following initial treatment; some further unreported cases are known as well.

Hodgkin's Disease Localized to the Ovary. Two cases of Hodgkin's disease localized to the ovary have been reported.[5,41] In both cases, the tumor was unilateral. Microscopically, the ovary was replaced by a malignant cellular infiltrate consisting of lymphocytes, eosinophils, plasma cells, atypical histiocytic cells, and typical Sternberg–Reed cells. Fibrosis and necrosis were also in evidence. Both patients were well and disease-free for periods of 2 and 6 years following diagnosis. Although it is difficult to draw any conclusions from only two cases, it appears that Hodgkin's disease, when localized to the ovary, has a better prognosis than does primary non-Hodgkin's lymphoma of the ovary.

Disseminated Malignant Lymphoma Affecting the Ovary

As mentioned earlier, this entity must be divided into two types: (1) the ovarian tumor being either the initial or predominant presenting manifestation of the disease and (2) ovarian involvement occurring during the course of the disease and being noted at surgery or autopsy, either grossly or microscopically.

The first type of disseminated malignant tumor is uncommon; the second type is common and is becoming even more so because of the longer survival of patients with malignant lymphoma as a result of recent therapy. Since the first type is more relevant to the theme of this book, it is discussed first. The initial finding of an ovarian tumor as the presenting sign of disseminated malignant lymphoma is uncommon, although it is more common than primary malignant lymphoma of the ovary, with more than 50 examples recorded.[26,55,63,87] The age of patients ranges from childhood to old age, but most are 20–50 years of age.[26,55,63,87] The symptoms in these patients are largely similar to those observed in patients with primary malignant lymphoma of the ovary, the most common being abdominal enlargement often associated with abdominal pain. In contrast to women with primary malignant lymphoma of the ovary, these patients frequently complain of malaise, weight loss, pallor, and fatigue. On physical examination, in addition to the finding of an adnexal mass, which is frequently bilateral, lymph node enlargement—either widespread or localized—may be noted. There may be enlargement of the spleen and the liver. The blood count may show anemia. A leukemic blood picture or pancytopenia may be observed. The macroscopic and microscopic appearances of the ovarian tumor are similar to those described in cases of malignant lymphoma localized to the ovary. The malignant lymphoma is usually of a poorly differentiated cell type, either lymphoblastic, poorly differentiated lymphocytic, or reticulum cell sarcoma,[67] or large or small cleaved or noncleaved cell type.[43,63] It is extremely uncommon for generalized Hodgkin's disease to present in this manner. The course of the disease and the prognosis are similar to those observed in patients with generalized non-Hodgkin's malignant lymphoma of the poorly differentiated cell type, which are, at best, very guarded despite recent advances in treatment of these conditions.

Ovarian involvement is observed nowadays in 25–30% of cases of disseminated malignant lymphoma examined at autopsy, but it occurs rarely in patients with disseminated Hodgkin's disease. Patients with malignant lymphoma live longer with the disease because of the improved therapy, and this contributes to the wider dissemination once response to therapy is lost. In such cases, the lymphoma affects many sites that did not become affected in the past, when patients died earlier, with the disease involving mainly the lymphoreticular system. The involvement of the ovaries is usually bilateral, and the ovaries may be of normal size or only slightly enlarged. Microscopically, extensive infiltration by malignant lymphoma cells is usually present, but sometimes the infiltration may be slight.

Burkitt's Lymphoma

Burkitt's lymphoma is a specific type of malignant lymphoma showing a typical age prevalence, clinical and histologic picture, and having a specific geographic distribution. It is observed primarily in East and West Africa south of the Sahara desert and in Papua and New Guinea.[6,11] These are considered the endemic areas, where the tumor is common. The tumor also occurs sporadically outside the endemic areas.[18,60]

Burkitt's lymphoma is a poorly differentiated malignant lymphoma, showing multicentric or multifocal origin. Clinically, it is seen affecting the jaw, ovary, orbit, kidney, thyroid, testis, and other sites, with involvement of the lymph nodes a minor feature. Frequent ovarian involvement by the disease was first noted in West Africa[10] and was also found in the East African cases.[11,59] Relatively frequent involvement of the ovary is also observed in cases from outside the endemic areas.[18,60]

Abdominal pain and swelling caused by ovarian enlargement represent the principal symptoms in 38% of patients with Burkitt's lymphoma. Burkitt's lymphoma occurs mainly in children, with a peak incidence at 4–7 years. Young adults are also affected. Occasionally, the tumor is localized to the ovary without involvement of other sites.[72]

Macroscopically, ovarian involvement by Burkitt's lymphoma is usually bilateral. The ovarian tumors are large, white, and solid with slightly lobulated surface and on cut section have a solid, white, firm surface that can be altered by the presence of necrosis and hemorrhage.

Microscopically, the ovary is completely or nearly completely replaced by proliferation of primitive lymphoreticular cells (Fig. 21.15 and 21.16) that appear round, oval, or indented with a narrow rim of basophilic cytoplasm, exhibiting strong pyroninophilia. The nuclei are large, prominent, and usually round but sometimes oval or reniform (Fig. 21.16). The nuclear membrane is sharp and well defined, and the chromatin is coarse, containing a few small nucleoli. Mitotic activity is brisk. The cytoplasm of the tumor cells contains numerous small vacuoles that contain lipid material. This is more obvious in imprint preparations from the tumor, a procedure that should always be undertaken, since it provides a very good diagnostic aid. Interspersed among the tumor cells are numerous nonneoplastic macrophages (histiocytes) containing phagocytosed material that stains positively with PAS and lipid stains. It is the presence of these macrophages scattered between the tumor cells that gives the tumor its typical *starry sky* appearance (Fig. 21.15). It should be noted that this starry sky appearance is not pathognomonic of Burkitt's lymphoma and may be observed in other types of poorly differentiated neoplasms. The histologic appearance of the cells and the histochemical reactions mentioned earlier are the main features leading to the diagnosis of Burkitt's lymphoma. Burkitt's lymphoma progresses quickly and, in the absence of therapy, is rapidly fatal. It responds dramatically to chemotherapy with antimetabolites and alkylating agents, leading to long remissions, and to complete cure in approximately 20% of cases. Radiotherapy can be used in conjunction with chemotherapy. The behavior of the tumor and its response to therapy are

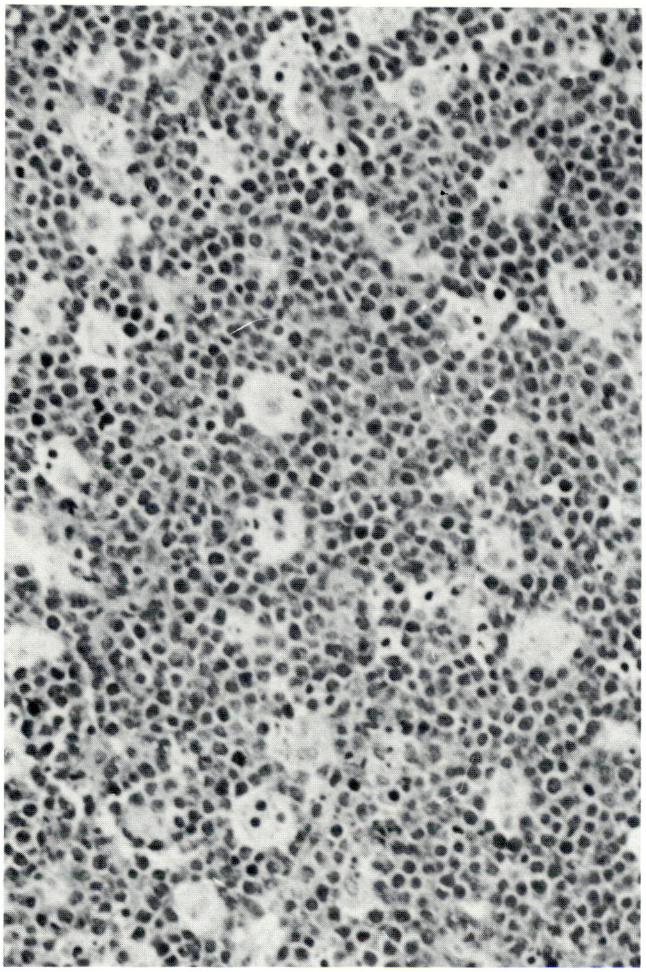

FIG. 21.15. Burkitt's lymphoma affecting ovary showing typical starry sky appearance.

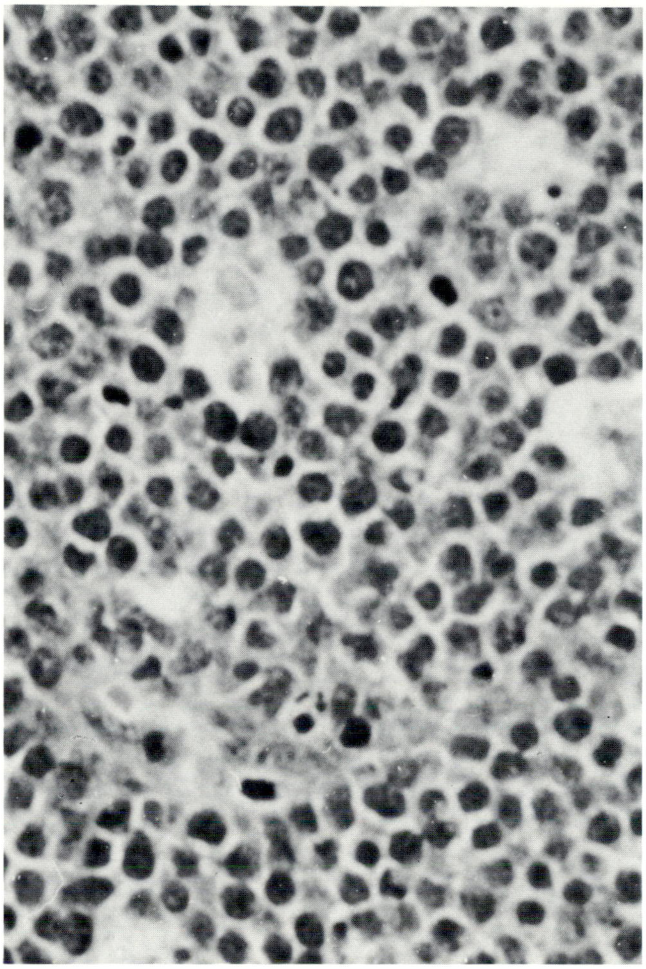

FIG. 21.16. Burkitt's lymphoma affecting ovary. Higher magnification of tumor shown in Fig. 21.15.

similar, whether it is encountered in the endemic or nonendemic areas.[90]

Involvement of the Ovary by Leukemia

Ovarian involvement by leukemia as seen at autopsy is common and is observed in 30–50% of cases. Recent reports indicate more frequent involvement than earlier studies. This may be due to longer containment of the disease by chemotherapy and radiotherapy, such as that observed in malignant lymphoma of the non-Hodgkin's type.

Lymphocytic and Granulocytic Leukemia

Occasionally, the ovary has been found to be the site of a relapse of childhood acute lymphocytic leukemia, although this course of events is by far not as common as in the case of the testes.[12] At times, ovarian enlargement may be the first sign of granulocytic leukemia, the ovarian tumor being designated *ovarian granulocytic sarcoma* or *chloroma*, the latter term due to the green color of the tumor mass. Such cases are usually observed in children[3,54,63] but occasionally are seen in adults.[14] On examination, the peripheral blood or the bone marrow usually shows evidence of leukemia. Occasionally, the presence of an ovarian mass precedes the leukemia by a number of months.[3,54,63] The tumors are frequently bilateral, although one ovary may be larger than the other. Microscopically, the tumor may resemble malignant lymphoma, especially if it is composed of early and primitive hematopoietic cells (Figs. 21.17 and 21.18). The presence of myeloblasts and better-differentiated cells (Fig. 21.18) that may be seen in places is helpful in making the diagnosis. The application of naphthol-AS-D-chloroacetate esterase (Leder's) stain confirms the diagnosis. Electron microscopy is also helpful in making

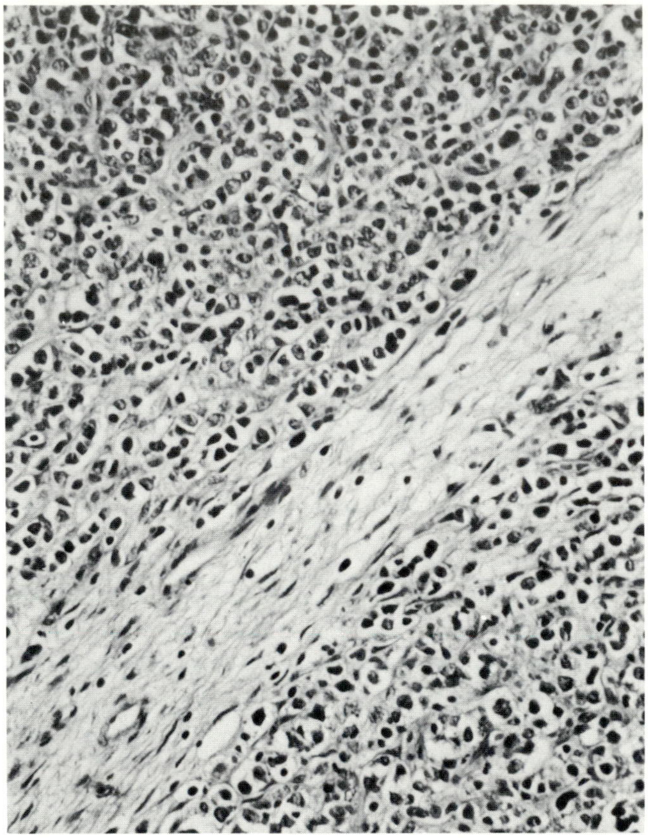

FIG. 21.17. Myelocytic sarcoma of ovary. Tumor is composed of collections of small round cells separated by bands of unaffected connective tissue.

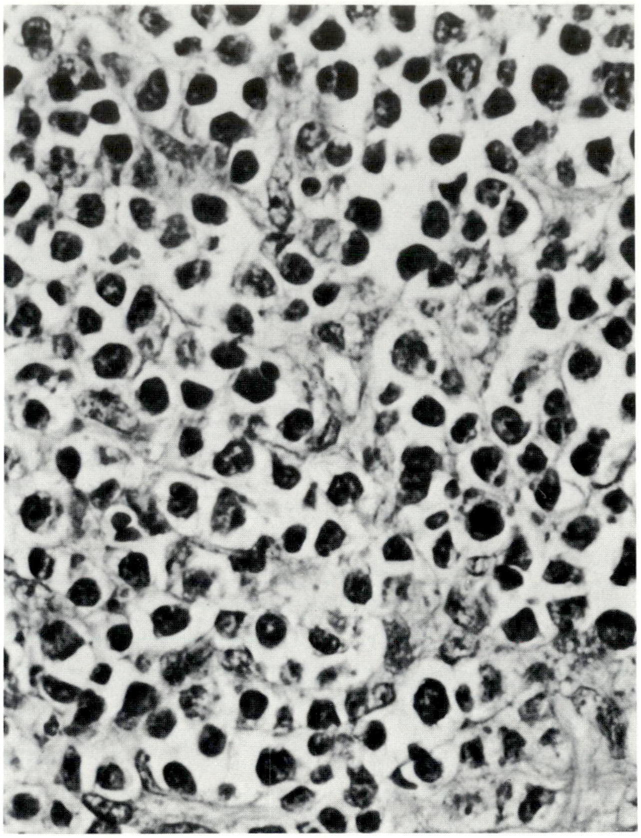

FIG. 21.18. Myelocytic sarcoma of ovary. Tumor is composed of primitive myeloid series cells. In places, slightly better differentiation indicates the myelocytic nature of the lesion.

the diagnosis. The prognosis of the patients is generally poor, but some patients survive a few years.[14] The treatment of choice in patients with granulocytic sarcoma is the combination chemotherapy used in patients with acute or subacute myelocytic leukemia.

Plasma Cell Dyscrasia

Involvement of the ovary by malignant disorders of plasma cells is very rare. It can manifest itself either as involvement of the ovary by multiple myeloma, usually observed at autopsy, although one case in a 44-year-old living woman has been reported,[4] or rarely as a primary extranodal plasmacytoma similar to primary malignant lymphoma of the ovary. One such case, which I observed, occurred in a 35-year-old woman, who had a painful lower abdominal mass. The tumor was unilateral, solid, firm, and gray-white. It measured 15 × 12 × 9 cm and showed ovarian tissue replaced by diffuse proliferation of plasma cells, including many immature forms. There was no evidence of biochemical abnormalities, including monoclonal gammopathy, and no evidence of bone or bone marrow involvement. The patient was well and disease-free 9 months after the operation, when she was lost to follow-up. Two similar cases have been reported in the literature.[33,84] Plasmacytoma must be differentiated from malignant lymphoma affecting the ovary as well as from granulocytic sarcoma. The appearance of the tumor cells, aided by special stains, such as methyl green–pyronin, and electron microscopy are helpful in differentiating these lesions. Biochemical studies including electrophoresis, full blood, and radiologic examinations are necessary to differentiate between the disseminated disease and primary plasmacytoma. Owing to the rarity of primary plasmacytoma of the ovary, it is only possible to speculate about the prognosis, but in common with extramedullary plasmacytoma found in other locations, it is probably better than in cases of multiple myeloma. The treatment of choice is excision of the lesion and careful follow-up of the patient. Chemotherapy used in cases of multiple myeloma may be administered prophylactically.

Tumors of Probable Wolffian Origin

In the original report describing tumors of this type,[38] all the tumors were located within the leaves of the broad ligament or were attached to it or to the fallopian tube. This also applied to subsequent reports dealing with this entity. More recently, 12 ovarian tumors of probable wolffian origin have been reported,[34,88] indicating that tumors of this type also occur in the ovary. The age of the patients ranged from 28 to 79 years. Five patients had abdominal enlargement, and in the remaining seven patients, the tumor was found on physical examination.[34,88] At laparotomy, all the tumors were found to be unilateral. In 11 patients, they were confined to the ovary, and in the remaining patient, there were metastatic deposits in the abdominal cavity.[34,88] In the latter case, the tumor contained foci of undifferentiated carcinoma.[88]

The tumors range in size from 2 to 20 cm in the largest diameter. They are smooth and often lobulated and are either solid or solid and cystic. The cysts vary in size and may range up to 11 cm.[88] Microscopically, the tumor is composed of relatively uniform epithelial cells that line cysts and tubules, sometimes forming a sieve-like pattern (Fig. 21.19). The tumor cells may also form closely packed tubules (Fig. 21.20), grow in a diffuse pattern, or fill tubules or tubular spaces. They have uniform round or oval nuclei, and there is low mitotic activity. The tumor cells do not contain mucin but occasionally may contain glycogen. The amount of intervening connective tissue varies from imperceptible to considerable, forming fibrous bands separating the islands of tumor cells and producing a lobular pattern.[88] In two patients in whom the tumors were associated with aggressive behavior, there was brisk mitotic activity with 10 or more mitoses/10 HPF, and in one of the these patients, there was cellular and nuclear pleomorphism.

Two patients have subsequently developed metastases.[88] Eight patients were known to be alive and disease-free from 1 to 15 years postoperatively, and one was lost to follow-up,[88] indicating that in the majority of cases the tumor is not associated with an aggressive course. It is also of note that there is a good correlation between the mitotic activity and the behavior of this neoplasm. Ovarian tumor of probable wolffian origin may be confused with sex cord–stromal tumors, especially various types of Sertoli–Leydig cell tumors and common epithelial tumors from which it must be differentiated (see Chapter 19, Sex Cord–Stromal Ovarian Tumors). The presence of the typical features of this tumor described above and the absence of the various patterns observed in Sertoli-Leydig cell tumors differentiate it from the latter. The tumor of probable wolffian origin

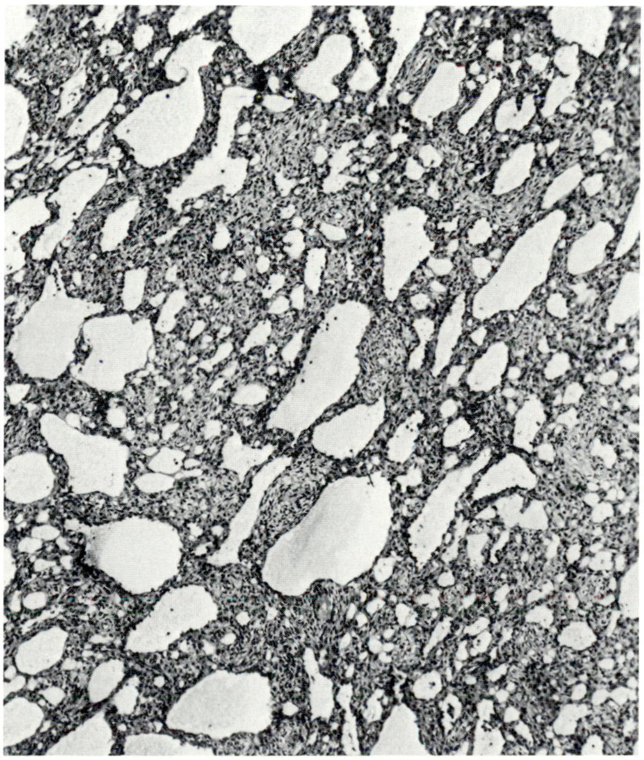

FIG. 21.19. Ovarian tumor of probable wolffian origin. The tumor shows a sieve-like pattern. The tumor cells line clefts and spaces and form solid aggregates. (Reprinted by permission of Young and Scully, Ref. 88.)

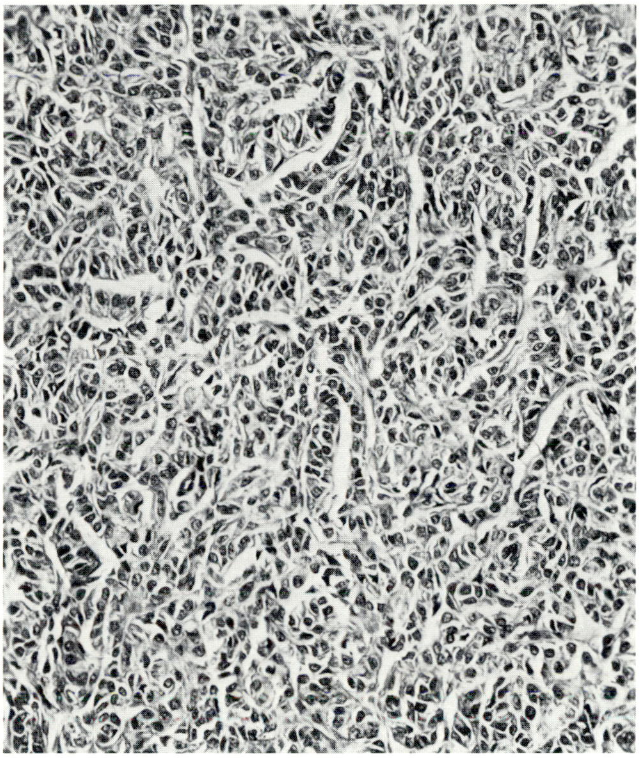

FIG. 21.20. Ovarian tumor of probable wolffian origin. The tumor is composed of closely packed tubules with compressed lumens and is lined by cuboid epithelial cells. (Reprinted by permission of Young and Scully, Ref. 88.)

is distinguished from the various common epithelial tumors of the ovary by the absence of cellular and nuclear pleomorphism, a papillary pattern, and intraluminal and intracellular mucin.

References

1. Abell MR, Holtz F (1965) Ovarian neoplasms in childhood and adolescence. 2. Tumors of non-germ cell origin. Am J Obstet Gynecol 93: 850.
2. Azoury RS, Woodruff, JD (1971) Primary ovarian sarcomas. Report of 43 cases from the Emil Novak Ovarian Tumor Registry. Obstet Gynecol 37: 920
3. Ballon SC, Donaldson RC, Berman ML, Swanson GA, Byron RL (1978) Myeloblastoma (granulocytic sarcoma) of the ovary. Arch Pathol Lab Med 102: 474
4. Bambirra EA, Miranda D, Magalhaes GMC (1982) Plasma cell myeloma simulating Krukenberg's tumor. South Med J 75: 511.
5. Bare WW, McCloskey JF (1961) Primary Hodgkin's disease of the ovary. Obstet Gynecol 17: 447
6. Berard C, O'Conor GT, Thomas LB, Torloni H (1969) Histopathological classification of Burkitt's tumour. Bull WHO 40: 601
7. Biggart JH, Macafee CHG (1955) Tumours of ovarian mesenchyme. A clinico-pathological survey. J Obstet Gynaecol Br Emp 62: 829
8. Bower JF, Erikson ER (1967) Bilateral ovarian fibroma in a 5 year old. Am J Obstet Gynecol 99: 880
9. Braithwaite J (1894) On atrophy with collapse (cirrhosis), fibroid degeneration, angioma of the ovaries. Trans Obstet Soc London 36: 235
10. Brew DS, Jackson JG (1960) Lymphosarcoma of the ovary in young African girls. Br J Cancer 14: 621
11. Burkitt DP, Wright DH (1970) Burkitt's lymphoma. Edinburgh. Livingstone
12. Cecalupo AJ, Frankel LS, Sullivan MP (1982) Pelvic and ovarian extramedullary leukemic relapse in young girls. A report of four cases and review of the literature. Cancer 50: 587
13. Charache H (1959) Ovarian tumors in childhood. Arch Surg 79: 573
14. Chorlton I, Norris HJ, King FM (1974) Malignant reticuloendothelial disease involving the ovary as a primary manifestation. A series of 19 lymphomas and 1 granulocytic sarcoma. Cancer 34: 397
15. Climie AR, Heath LP (1968) Malignant degeneration of benign cystic teratoma of the ovary. Review of the literature and report of a chondrosarcoma and a carcinoid tumor. Cancer 22: 824
16. De Franchis M, Galliani F (1964). Neurinoma del ovario. Riv Patol Clin 19: 567
17. Dockerty MB, Masson JC (1944) Ovarian fibromas: A clinical and pathologic study of two hundred eighty three cases. Am J Obstet Gynecol 47: 741
18. Dorfman FR (1965) Childhood lymphoma in St. Louis, Missouri, clinically and histologically resembling Burkitt's tumor. Cancer 18: 418
19. Dover H (1950) Neurofibrosarcoma of the ovary, associated with neurofibromatosis. Can Med Assoc J 63: 488
20. Dutz W, Stout AP (1961) The myxoma in childhood. Cancer 14: 629
21. Ebrahimi T, Goldsmith JW, Okagaki T (1971) Hemangioma of the ovary. A case report. Obstet Gynecol 38: 677
22. Ewing J (1940) Neoplastic diseases, 4th ed. Philadelphia, Saunders
23. Fallahzadeh H, Dockerty MB, Lee RA (1972) Leiomyoma of the ovary. Report of five cases and review of the literature. Am J Obstet Gynecol 113: 394
24. Fawcett FJ, Kimbell NKB (1971) Phaeochromocytoma of the ovary. J Obstet Gynaecol Br Commonw 78: 458
25. Ferenczy A, Fenoglio CM, Richart RM (1972) Observations on benign mesothelioma of the genital tract (adenomatoid tumor) Cancer 30: 244
26. Fox H, Langley FA (1976) Tumours of the ovary. London, William Heinemann
27. Fundaro P (1969) Emangioma cavernoso bilaterale dell ovaia: Presentazione di un caso e rassegna della literatura. Folia Hered Patol 18: 45
28. Gay RM, Janovski NA (1969) Cavernous hemangioma of the ovary. Gynaecologia 168: 248
29. Gerbie AB, Hirsch MR, Greene RR (1955) Vascular tumors of the female genital tract. Obstet Gynecol 6: 499
30. Glendenning WE, Herdt JR, Black JB (1963) Ovarian fibromas and mesenteric cysts. Their association with hereditary basal cell cancer of the skin. Am J Obstet Gynecol 87: 1008
31. Guérard MJ, Arguelles MA, Ferenczy A (1983) Rhabdomyosarcoma of the ovary. Ultrastructural study of a case and review of the literature. Gynecol Oncol 15: 325
32. Hart WR, Abell MR (1970) Adipose prosoplasia of the ovary. Am J Obstet Gynecol 106: 929
33. Hautzer NW (1984) Primary plasmacytoma of ovary. Gynecol Oncol 18: 115
34. Hughesdon PE (1982) Ovarian tumors of wolffian or allied nature. Their place in ovarian oncology. J Clin Pathol 35: 526
35. Janovski NA, Paramanandhan TL (1973) Ovarian tumors. Tumors and tumor-like conditions of the ovaries, fallopian tubes, and ligaments of the uterus. Philadelphia, WB Saunders
36. Kalstone CE, Jaffe RB, Abell MR (1969) Massive edema of the ovary simulating fibroma. Obstet Gynecol 34: 564
37. Kannerstein M, Churg J (1977) Peritoneal mesothelioma. Hum Pathol 8: 83
38. Kariminejad MH, Scully RE (1973) Female adnexal tumor of probable wolffian origin. Cancer 31: 671
39. Kraemer BB, Silva EG, Sneige N (1984) Fibrosarcoma of the ovary. A new component in the nevoid basal-cell carcinoma syndrome. Am J Surg Pathol 8: 231
40. Lawhead RA, Copeland LJ, Edwards CL (1985) Bilateral ovarian hemangiomas associated with diffuse abdominopelvic hemangiomatosis. Obstet Gynecol 65: 597
41. Long JP, Patchefsky AS (1971) Primary Hodgkin's disease of the ovary. Obstet Gynecol 38: 680
42. Lorentzen M (1980) Giant cell tumor of the ovary. Virchows Arch [Pathol Anat] 388: 113
43. Lukes RJ, Collins RD (1974) Immunologic characterization of human malignant lymphomas. Cancer 34: 1488
44. Lyday RO (1952) Fibroma of the ovary with abdominal implants. Am J Surg 84: 737

45. Majmudar B, Kapernick PS, Phillips RS (1978) Ovarian myxoma. Hum Pathol 9: 723
46. Mann LS, Metrick S (1961) Hemangioma of the ovary. Report of a case. J Int Colleg Surg 36: 500
47. Martins SM, Klinger OJ (1964) Bilateral ovarian fibromas before the menarche. Am J Obstet Gynecol 87: 386
48. Masubuchi K, Kimura M, Suzuki H, Suzuki P, Aoki M (1970) Case of ovarian myxoma. Jpn J Cancer Clin 16: 156
49. McBurney RC, Trumbull M (1955) Hemangioma of the ovary with ascites. Miss Doct 32: 271
50. Meyer R (1943) Nerve tumors of the female genitals and pelvis. Arch Pathol 36: 437
51. Michael CA (1966) Pelvic fibroma causing recurrent attacks of hypoglycaemia in a post-menopausal patient. Proc R Soc Med 59: 835
52. Miles PA, Kiley KC, Mena H (1985) Giant fibrosarcoma of the ovary. Int J Gynecol Pathol 4: 83
53. Mishura VI (1963) Report of large benign tumor—Report of three cases. Vopr Onkol 9: 103
54. Morgan ER, Labotka RJ, Gonzalez-Crussi F, Wiederhold M, Sherman JO (1981) Ovarian granulocytic sarcoma as a primary manifestation of acute infantile myelomonocytic leukemia. Cancer 48: 1819
55. Nelson GA, Dockerty MB, Pratt JH, Re-Mine WH (1958) Malignant lymphoma involving the ovaries. Am J Obstet Gynecol 76: 861
56. Nieminen U, von Numers C, Purola E (1969) Primary sarcoma of the ovary. Acta Obstet Gynecol Scand 48: 423
57. Nogales FF (1982) Primary chondrosarcoma of the ovary. Histopathology 6: 376
58. Nunez C, Abboud SL, Lemon NC, Kemp JA (1983) Ovarian rhabdomyosarcoma presenting as leukemia. Case report. Cancer 52: 297
59. O'Conor GT (1961) Malignant lymphoma in African children. II. A pathological entity. Cancer 14: 270
60. O'Conor GT, Rappaport H, Smith EB (1965) Childhood lymphoma resembling "Burkitt tumor" in the United States. Cancer 18: 411
61. Okamura H, Virutamasen P, Wright KH, Wallach EE (1972) Ovarian smooth muscle in the human being, rabbit, and cat: Histochemical and electron microscopic study. Am J Obstet Gynecol 112: 183
62. Ongkasuwan C, Taylor JE, Tang CK, Prempree T (1982) Angiosarcomas of the uterus and ovary. Clinicopathologic report. Cancer 49: 1469
63. Osborne BM, Robboy SJ (1983) Lymphomas or leukemia presenting as ovarian tumors. An analysis of 42 cases. Cancer 52: 1933
64. Paladugu RR, Bearman RM, Rappaport H (1980) Malignant lymphoma with primary manifestation in the gonad. A clinicopathologic study of 38 patients. Cancer 45: 561
65. Prat J (1979) Sarcomas of the ovary. Pathol Res Pract 165: 146
66. Prat J, Scully RE (1981) Cellular fibromas and fibrosarcomas of the ovary. A comparative clinicopathologic analysis of seventeen cases. Cancer 47: 2663
67. Rappaport H (1966) Tumors of the hematopoietic system. Atlas of tumor pathology, Sect 3, Vol. 8. Washington DC, Armed Forces Institute of Pathology
68. Rice M, Pearson B, Treadwell WB (1943) Malignant lymphangioma of the ovary. Am J Obstet Gynecol 45: 884
69. Sandison AT (1955) Rhabdomyosarcoma of the ovary. J Pathol Bacteriol 70: 433
70. Schmeisser HC, Anderson WAD (1938) Ganglioneuroma of the ovary. JAMA 111: 2005
71. Scully RE (1979) Tumors of the ovary and maldeveloped gonads, Vol 16, 2nd ser. Washington DC, Armed Forces Institute of Pathology
72. Seed PG (1966) Burkitt's tumour in Britain. J Obstet Gynecol Br Commonw 73: 808
73. Shaeffer MD, Cancelmo JJ (1939) Cavernous hemangioma of the ovary in a girl twelve years of age. Am J Obstet Gynecol 38: 722
74. Shearer JP (1935) Hemangioma of the ovary. Reported in a child 3½ years of age. Med Ann DC 4: 223
75. Shipton EA, Meares SD (1965) Heterotopic bone formation in the ovary. Aust NZ J Obstet Gynecol 5: 100
76. Smith FR (1931) Neurofibroma of the ovary associated with Recklinghausen's disease. Am J Cancer 15: 859
77. Stamm C (1891) Beitrag zur Lehre von Blutgefassgeschwulsten. Thesis. University of Gottingen
78. Stout AP (1948) Myxoma, tumor of primitive mesenchyme. Ann Surg 127: 706
79. Stowe LM, Watt JY (1952) Osteogenic sarcoma of the ovary. Am J Obstet Gynecol 64: 422
80. Talerman A (1967) Hemangiomas of the ovary and the uterine cervix. Obstet Gynecol 30: 108
81. Talerman A, Auerbach WM, Van Meurs AJ (1981) Primary chondrosarcoma of the ovary. Histopathology 5: 319
82. Talerman A, Montero JR, Chilcote RR, Okagaki T (1985) Diffuse malignant peritoneal mesothelioma in a 13-year-old girl. Am J Surg Pathol 9: 73
83. Taxy JB, Battifora H, Oyasu R (1974) Adenomatoid tumors. A light microscopic, histochemical and ultrastructural study. Cancer 34: 306
84. Voegt H (1938) Extramedullary plasmacytoma. Virchows Arch [Pathol Anat] 302: 497
85. Warhol MJ, Hunter NJ, Carson JM (1982) An ultrastructural comparison of mesotheliomas and adenocarcinomas of ovary and endometrium. Int J Gynecol Pathol 1: 125
86. Willis RA (1967) Pathology of tumours, 4th ed. London, Butterworths
87. Woodruff JD, Noll Castillo RD, Novak ER (1963) Lymphoma of the ovary. Am J Obstet Gynecol 85: 912
88. Young RH, Scully RE (1983) Ovarian tumors of probable wolffian origin. A report of 11 cases. Am J Surg Pathol 7: 125
89. Young RH, Scully RE (1984) Fibromatosis and massive edema of the ovary, possibly related entities. A report of 14 cases of fibromatosis and 11 cases of massive edema. Int J Gynecol Pathol 3: 153
90. Ziegler JL (1977) Treatment results of 54 American patients with Burkitt's lymphoma are similar to the African experience. N Engl J Med 297: 75

22

Metastatic Tumors of the Ovary

Robert H. Young, M.D., and Robert E. Scully, M.D.

Tumors may metastasize to the ovary from many organs and tissues outside the female genital tract, but neoplasms arising in the intestine, stomach, and breast and hematopoietic tumors, some of which are also primary in the ovary, are the most common forms encountered by the pathologist.* Hematopoietic tumors are discussed in Chapter 21, Nonspecific Ovarian Tumors, and are not considered further in this chapter. Tumors that extend to the ovary directly from adjacent organs or tissues are also included in the broad category of metastatic or secondary tumors; determination of the origin of the tumor in such cases may be impossible when both ovarian and extraovarian involvement is extensive. Metastasis of tumors originating in other organs of the genital tract is discussed in this chapter, but ovarian involvement as part of diffuse neoplasms of the peritoneum is not considered.

It is difficult to establish the frequency of metastatic tumors among all ovarian tumors from the available literature for a variety of reasons. Some studies have been based on autopsy findings, others on surgical specimens, and still others on both. In addition, some series have included clinically silent metastases of breast carcinoma found in specimens from therapeutic oophorectomy and small metastases detected incidentally during operations for gastric or intestinal carcinoma, whereas in other series the cases have been restricted to metastatic tumors that presented clinically as pelvic or abdominal masses. Finally, some investigations have included as metastases ovarian carcinomas associated with uterine cancers of

* References 95, 99, 102, 125, 137, 190, 203.

similar histologic type, whereas it is now thought that in many, if not most, such cases the ovarian tumors are independent primary tumors.

The frequency of metastases to the ovary varies from one country to another because of wide differences in the prevalence of the various cancers that are associated with high rates of ovarian spread.[96] For example, metastatic carcinoma was reported to account for approximately 40% of all ovarian cancers in one series from Japan where gastric carcinoma is common[87] but for fewer than 3% in a series from Uganda, where this form of cancer is relatively rare.[96] The frequency of metastases has also varied greatly in series where differences in the prevalence of the primary tumors do not adequately explain the discrepant results. For example, in an autopsy study from Brazil,[117] metastases to the ovary were found in 29% of cancer patients, whereas in a similar but older investigation from the United States,[211] the frequency was only 5%, and in another from the United Kingdom, it was 4.4%.[62] Such variations may be related, in part, to the frequency and thoroughness of microscopic examination of the ovaries, since gross inspection may not reveal evidence of involvement in from one third to one half of the cases.

The figure for the frequency of ovarian metastases that is most meaningful to the gynecologist is one that expresses the probability that an ovarian cancer found on exploration of a pelvic or abdominal mass is metastatic. This figure was about 6% in the experience of Santesson and Kottmeier[170] and 7% in the series of Ulbright et al.[203]

The age distribution of patients with ovarian metastases depends to a great extent on that of the corresponding primary tumors, but for each of the most common types (intestinal, gastric, and breast) the average age of the patients with ovarian involvement is significantly lower than that of those without ovarian spread. This suggests that the richly vascularized ovaries of young women are more receptive to metastases than are those of older patients, in whom ovarian activity has ceased.[117,163,211]

Tumors spread to the ovary by several routes. Direct spread is an important pathway for carcinomas of the fallopian tube and uterus and for occasional colonic carcinomas, mesotheliomas, and retroperitoneal sarcomas. A second mechanism of spread of genital tract carcinomas is through the lumen of the fallopian tube and onto the surface of the ovary; this route is taken most often by carcinomas of the uterine corpus.[41] Spread from more distant sites is mainly via other routes, including blood vessels and lymphatics. The frequent association of ovarian metastases with other blood-borne metastases, the common finding of tumor within ovarian blood vessels on microscopic examination in cases of metastasis, and the higher frequency of ovarian metastases in young patients are consistent with the important role of hematogenous spread. Retrograde flow within lymphatics is an unlikely route of spread except in the presence of extensive involvement of the lymph nodes draining the ovaries. Such a mechanism of spread also seems inconsistent with the sporadic reports of prolonged survival after a primary cancer and its apparently solitary ovarian metastasis have been removed. Finally, transcoelomic dissemination with surface implantation is an important route by which intraabdominal cancers spread to the ovary. This is supported by the common association of ovarian involvement with generalized peritoneal spread. Also, the pathologist often encounters foci of metastatic carcinoma on the surface of the ovary or so superficially located within its cortex that any explanation other than implantation seems improbable. It is possible that ovulation, by creating a defect in the ovarian surface, provides a portal of entry for cancer cells floating in the peritoneal cavity in premenopausal patients.

Recognition of the metastatic nature of an ovarian tumor depends on several factors: (1) an awareness of the frequency with which metastases occur and simulate a variety of primary tumors, (2) a detailed clinical history, (3) a thorough clinical and operative search by the gynecologist for a primary tumor outside the ovary and for other sites of tumor spread, and (4) a careful evaluation of the gross and microscopic features of the ovarian tumor by the pathologist. It is surprising how often the diagnosis of a metastatic tumor is missed by the pathologist because the existence of a present or prior tumor in another organ is either not known or, if known, disregarded. The surgical and pathologic findings from previous operations should be reviewed if there is any possibility that they could be related to the ovarian tumor being evaluated. In some cases, a search for an extraovarian primary tumor must be conducted postoperatively on the basis of the suspicion of the pathologist that the ovarian tumor is metastatic. Even if an extraovarian primary tumor is not confirmed, a diagnosis of ovarian metastasis must be strongly considered if the distribution of the disease is atypical for primary ovarian cancer or if pathologic examination is highly suggestive of metastasis. For example, the presence of pulmonary or hepatic metastases in the absence of extensive peritoneal spread would be very unusual for an ovarian cancer but not for other cancers that are prone to metastasize to the ovary. It must also be emphasized that an association of an ovarian tumor with clinical or pathologic evidence of excess estrogens, androgens, or progesterone does not exclude the diagnosis of a metastatic tumor, which may have a functioning stroma (see Chapter 19, Sex Cord–Stromal Tumors of Ovary).

The gross features of tumors metastatic to the ovary vary greatly and may resemble those of a variety of primary ovarian tumors. Because of the relatively high fre-

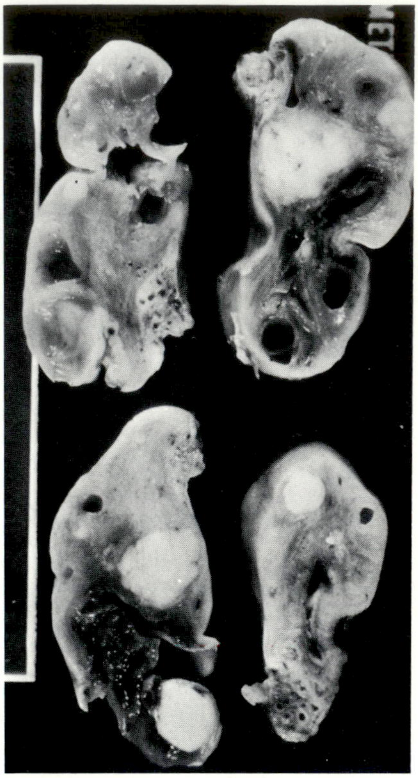

FIG. 22.1. Metastatic carcinoma from the breast. Multiple nodules are seen on the sectioned surfaces of both ovaries.

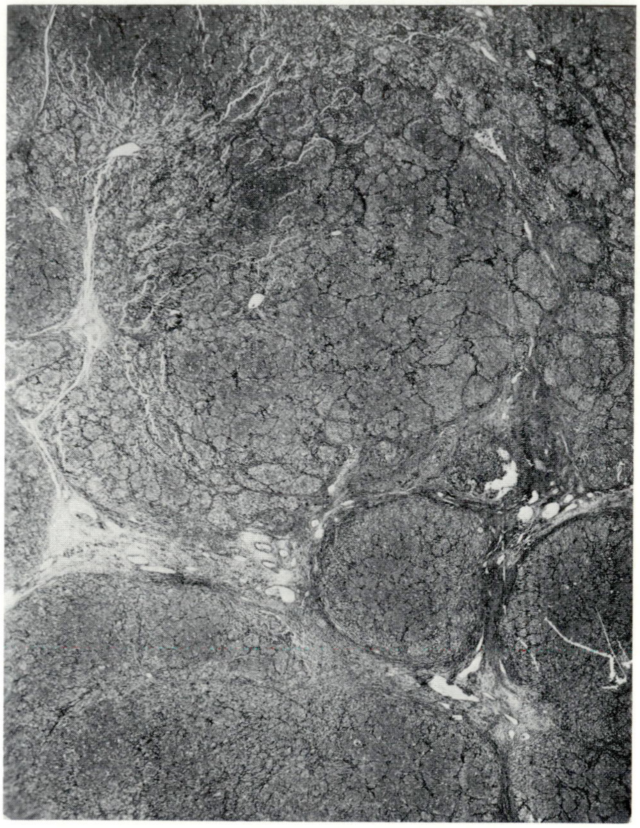

FIG. 22.2. Metastatic carcinoma from the lung. The tumor is growing in the form of multiple nodules.

quency with which metastases are bilateral (two-thirds to three-quarters of cases), the possibility of metastasis should be considered particularly in evaluating bilateral tumors. In general, approximately 15–20% of bilateral ovarian cancers prove to be metastatic on careful evaluation. Two other gross findings that are highly suggestive, but not pathognomonic, of metastasis are the presence of multiple nodules (Fig. 22.1) and the location of nodules on the surface of the ovary without significant involvement of the underlying parenchyma. Conversely, a gross feature of some metastasic tumors, which should not be regarded as establishing the primary nature of the tumor, is the presence of cysts, which may be large, despite the absence of cysts in the primary neoplasm.

The microscopic appearance of a metastatic tumor obviously varies with the appearance of the primary neoplasm. In addition to recognition of specific features of various primary tumors, the presence of implants on the surface of the ovary, growth in the form of multiple nodules (Fig. 22.2), and lymphatic or blood vessel invasion strongly suggest metastasis. A confusing microscopic feature of some metastases is the presence of cysts, some of which simulate follicles on low-power examination. Such cysts may be encountered in a variety of metastatic tumors, including gastric and intestinal carcinomas, carcinoids, small cell carcinomas and malignant melanomas.

Carcinoma of the Fallopian Tube

The ovary is involved secondarily in approximately 13% of tubal carcinomas, usually by direct extension, which is sometimes facilitated by adhesions of inflammatory origin between the two organs.[176] In some cases, there is clinical or pathologic evidence of salpingitis and salpingo-oophoritis, but often it is unclear whether the associated inflammation preceded or followed the development of the carcinoma. If the involvement of the tube and the ovary is extensive, the primary site of the tumor may not be established with certainty; the term *tubo-ovarian carcinoma* has been suggested for these cases. Green and Scully[74] encountered 6 such tumors in an investigation of 24 carcinomas initially considered to be of tubal origin. The tuboovarian carcinomas formed solid or cystic masses; at least one of the cystic tumors appeared to have developed in a postinflammatory tuboovarian cyst.

Since most tubal carcinomas closely resemble serous or undifferentiated carcinomas of the ovary, microscopic examination often fails to establish whether a carcinoma involving both organs is primary in one or the other. Because of the great rarity of primary mucinous, endometrioid, or clear cell carcinoma of the fallopian tube, a tumor of any of these cell types involving equally both organs is probably primary in the ovary. It should be emphasized that mucosal implants from an ovarian carcinoma may replace the tubal epithelium and erroneously suggest a primary tumor of the fallopian tube.

Uterine Tumors

Endometrial Carcinoma

Ovarian involvement in cases in which a diagnosis of endometrial carcinoma has been made has been reported in 34–40% of autopsies[17,31] and 5–15% of specimens obtained by hysterectomy and bilateral salpingo-oophorectomy[173] (see Chapter 12, Endometrial Carcinoma). Conversely, in approximately one third of cases in which a diagnosis of endometrioid carcinoma of the ovary has been made, an endometrial carcinoma has also been found.[47,168] When the uterine corpus and the ovary are both involved by carcinomas, which are usually of the endometrioid type, the question arises whether both cancers are primary or one is metastatic from the other. A number of studies, many of them recent, have addressed this issue.* If the endometrial carcinoma extends deeply into the myometrium with lymphatic or vascular invasion, if tumor is present in the lumen of the fallopian tube, or if tumor is on the ovarian surface or within its lymphatics or blood vessels, it is usually reasonable to conclude that the ovarian involvement is secondary. On the other hand, if lymphatic or hematogenous spread is absent, if the corpus carcinoma is small and limited to the endometrium or superficial myometrium, if it arises on a background of atypical hyperplasia, and if there is a centrally located ovarian tumor, sometimes accompanied by endometriosis, the tumors are probably independently primary. Criteria that are helpful in the determination of primary versus metastatic concomitant ovarian and endometrial carcinomas are presented in Table 22.1. Although the ovarian and uterine tumors are of the endometrioid type in most cases, occasionally they are similar but of other cell types, and rarely the histologic type of tumor is different in the two organs.[56]

In some cases of combined involvement, it is impossible to establish the site of origin even after consideration of the features described above and listed in Table 22.1. In our experience and that of most series, the great majority of synchronous ovarian and corpus carcinomas are independent primary tumors. In one recent study, however, the ovarian tumors were interpreted as metastatic from the corpus in most of the cases.[201] An independent primary explanation for the majority of concomitant ovarian and corpus carcinomas is supported by the survival rates associated with these tumors, which have generally been high. These results would be surprising if either the ovarian or corpus carcinoma were metastatic from the other tumor in most of the cases.

Rarely, ovarian spread from an adenoacanthoma of the uterine corpus takes the form of deposits of keratin associated with a foreign body response on the serosal surface of one or both ovaries.[38] In this small series of cases as well as in our limited experience, this finding does not appear to worsen the prognosis even when associated with similar deposits elsewhere on the peritoneum.

* References 34, 49, 53, 56, 60, 75, 201, 218, 228.

Carcinoma of the Cervix

Squamous cell carcinoma of the cervix metastasizes to the ovary in less than 1% of cases (if examples of direct spread of high-stage tumors are excluded)[14,102,125,180] (see Chapter 8, Cervical Carcinoma). In the series of Mazur et al.,[125] 10 of 14 cases of cervical carcinoma that had spread to the ovary were diagnosed as such in exenteration specimens for central pelvic recurrences. In 2 of the other 4 cases, the metastasis to the ovary mimicked an ovarian primary tumor. The rare association of squamous cell carcinoma of the ovary with squamous cell carcinoma in situ of the cervix suggests the possibility that, in exceptional cases, invasive squamous cell carcinomas of both organs may also be separate primary tumors.[21,178]

Recent data suggest that mucinous adenocarcinomas of the cervix metastasize to the ovary more frequently than squamous cell carcinomas and other adenocarcinomas. In the Armed Forces Institute of Pathology series, 10% of mucinous adenocarcinomas were reported to metastasize to the ovary.[101] At least one other example[69] is recorded in the literature, and we have seen several additional examples.[223] When a cervical mucinous adenocarcinoma and an ovarian mucinous adenocarcinoma coexist, however, difficulties may be encountered in deciding whether they are independent primary tumors or metastatic from one organ to the other.[116,125] Consideration of a variety of criteria similar to those used in dealing with coexistent ovarian and corpus carcinomas often enables one to reach a conclusion, but in some cases it is impossible.[223]

Uterine Sarcomas

Pure uterine sarcomas spread to the ovary infrequently. Only occasional reports mention ovarian metastases of uterine leiomyosarcoma.[83] Ovarian involvement in cases

TABLE 22.1. Criteria for interpretation of nature of concomitant uterine corpus and ovarian carcinomas.

Corpus primary ovarian metastasis	Ovarian primary corpus metastasis	Ovarian primary corpus primary	Ovarian metastasis corpus metastasis	Uncertain primary
Direct extension to ovary from large corpus tumor	Direct extension to corpus from large ovarian primary	No direct extension of either tumor	Usually no direct extension of tumors	Massive involvement of both organs or conflicting findings listed in first four columns
Deep myometrial invasion from endometrium	Myometrial invasion from serosal surface	Myometrial invasion usually absent or superficial	Tumor characteristically in endometrial stroma; myometrial invasion may be present	
Lymphatic or blood vessel invasion in corpus, ovary, or both	Lymphatic or blood vessel invasion in corpus, ovary, or both	No lymphatic or blood vessel invasion	Lymphatic or blood vessel invasion frequent in ovary and corpus	
Atypical hyperplasia of endometrium frequent	Atypical hyperplasia of endometrium usually absent	Atypical hyperplasia of endometrium frequent	Atypical hyperplasia of endometrium absent	
Tumor present in fallopian tube	Tumor present on peritoneal surfaces and sometimes in fallopian tube	Usually both tumors confined to primary sites or have spread minimally	Tumor usually evident outside female genital tract	
Tumor predominant on surface of ovary	Tumor predominant within ovary	Tumor predominant within ovary and endometrium	Ovarian tumor usually bilateral; ovarian surface involvement frequent	
Usually no endometriosis in ovary	Endometriosis sometimes present in ovary	Endometriosis sometimes present in ovary	Endometriosis absent	
Histologic types uniform and consistent with corpus primary	Histologic types uniform and consistent with ovarian primary	Histologic types uniform or dissimilar	Type of tumor inconsistent with or unusual for either organ	

of endometrial stromal sarcoma is more common.* When there is synchronous or asynchronous involvement of the uterus and one or both ovaries by a sarcoma of endometrial stromal type, it may be difficult or impossible to decide whether the tumors are independently primary or whether the ovarian tumor is metastatic from the uterus.[227] The finding of endometriosis in continuity with an ovarian sarcoma indicates its primary nature.

Malignant müllerian mixed tumors of the uterus have been documented to spread to the ovary uncommonly in most reports,[144,145] but in one, 14%[54] and in another, 33%[206] of these tumors were found to be associated with ovarian spread at the time of exploration. Ovarian involvement in cases of müllerian adenosarcoma of the uterus is very uncommon.[172]

* References 13, 98, 125, 131, 142, 197, 218, 221.

Trophoblastic Tumors

The frequency of spread of choriocarcinoma of the uterus to the ovary has varied from one series to another. In an autopsy study of 44 patients, Ober et al.[146] found no examples of ovarian metastasis. However, in other series, 6–22% of the cases were associated with ovarian metastases.[2,153,213] Although a choriocarcinoma that develops in a prepubertal girl is obviously of germ cell origin, the occurrence of a similar tumor in a woman of childbearing age that is not clearly metastatic from a uterine or tubal choriocarcinoma requires thorough sampling in an attempt to demonstrate the presence of teratomatous elements, thereby establishing the germ cell origin of the tumor. If such elements are not found, it may be difficult or impossible to differentiate between a primary choriocarcinoma of the ovary of either gestational or germ cell origin and a metastasis from a choriocarcinoma of the uterus that has regressed. Ovarian enlargement in a patient with a uterine choriocarcinoma is more likely to be due to hyperreactio luteinalis (see Chapter 16, Nonneoplastic Lesions of Ovary) than to involvement by metastatic disease. Invasive hydatidiform mole has been documented to spread to the ovary,[213] and one placental site trophoblastic tumor has spread through the uterine wall to involve one ovary.[111]

Carcinoma of the Vulva and Vagina

Only very rare examples of vulvar and vaginal carcinoma that have spread to the ovary have been reported.[117] Occasional examples of clear cell adenocarcinoma of the vagina have metastasized to the ovary, but in most cases, this is associated with extensive pelvic spread.[164,199]

Breast Carcinoma

In four series from the United States, the frequency of ovarian involvement at autopsy in cases of breast cancer has ranged from 15 to 29%.[1,50,171,207] In contrast, the figure was much lower, only 6.4%, in a recent study from the United Kingdom[82] but much higher, 40%, in an older study from Brazil.[117] The average figure from the literature is about 10%. In the Brazilian study, metastatic breast carcinoma accounted for 29% of all ovarian metastases at autopsy.[117] Metastases from the breast are bilateral at autopsy in approximately 80% of cases.

Most surgical pathologic experience with ovarian metastases of mammary carcinoma has resulted from examination of ovaries removed to decrease the estrogen level in patients with known spread of the tumor.[113] In such cases, ovarian involvement has been reported in from 25 to almost 50% of the cases,[104,118,160,200] with bilateral involvement in approximately 60%.[160] About two-thirds of the affected ovaries were considered normal on gross examination in one series.[118] In contrast, only 2–11% of ovaries obtained by prophylactic oophorectomy for breast cancer (oophorectomy performed in the absence of clinical evidence of distant spread) contain metastases.[26,99]

It is unusual for metastatic carcinoma of the breast to produce signs or symptoms of an ovarian tumor, and only rarely is the ovarian metastasis evident before the primary tumor is detected.* In a series of 79 ovarian metastases presenting as pelvic or abdominal masses, Johansson found 11 (14%) to be of mammary origin.[99] In only 1 of those was the ovarian involvement discovered before diagnosis of the primary tumor. In the remaining 10 cases in Johansson's series, the ovarian tumors became evident clinically at subsequent intervals ranging from less than 1 year to 16 years.[99] Death occurred within 1 year of the detection of ovarian involvement in all but 1 of the 11 patients in that series. In contrast, Osborne and Pitts[152] recorded a mean survival of over 20 months after the diagnosis of metastasis in therapeutic oophorectomy specimens.

On gross examination, the visibly involved ovaries often have irregular, nodular surfaces and typically contain firm or gritty, white nodules of various sizes (Fig. 22.1). When the organ is replaced by tumor, it is transformed into a smooth-surfaced or bosselated mass. Exceptionally, it contains cysts, and very rarely it is entirely cystic.[203]

Microscopic examination may reveal the same variety of patterns and cell types that are observed in primary breast carcinomas (Figs. 22.3 and 22.4). In early examples, small cords of cells may be found in the ovarian cortex. In premenopausal women, small deposits are often situated in the highly vascular theca interna of a graafian follicle or in the granulosa or theca layer of a corpus luteum. The stroma of the tumor varies from

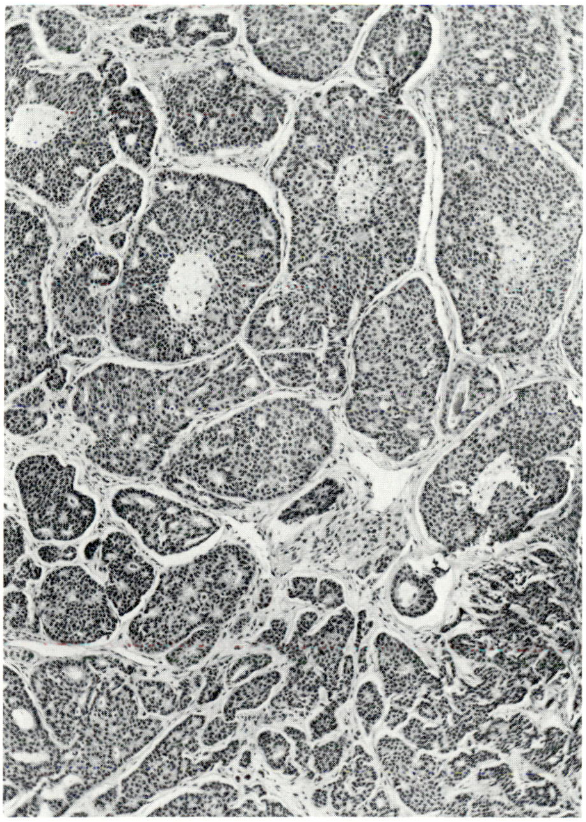

FIG. 22.3. Metastatic ductal carcinoma from the breast. A cribriform pattern is present.

* References 110, 171, 185, 203, 212, 226.

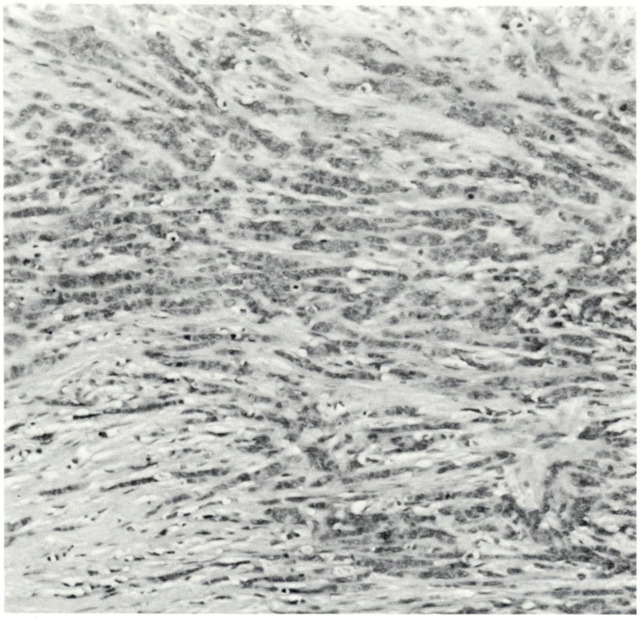

Fig. 22.4. Metastatic lobular carcinoma from the breast. An Indian-file pattern is present.

sparse to abundant. It rarely shows luteinization, in contrast to the stroma of metastatic carcinomas of intestinal origin. Lobular carcinomas spread to the ovary more frequently than those of ductal type. In a recent autopsy study, 36% of the former metastasized to the ovaries in contrast to only 2.6% of the latter.[82] Signet cells are usually not a conspicuous feature of metastatic breast carcinoma unless the primary tumor is of the relatively uncommon signet-ring type.[171] In a recent series, 20% of the patients with that type of tumor had ovarian metastases.[127] Rarely, the features of a metastatic breast cancer are those of a typical Krukenberg tumor,[118] as will be described.

The differential diagnosis of metastatic breast carcinoma may be difficult, particularly if the primary tumor is not apparent. Rare, predominantly glandular tumors may resemble common epithelial tumors, particularly those of endometrioid type, and an insular pattern may mimic a carcinoid tumor (Fig. 22.3). Exceptionally, a diffuse pattern simulates that of a lymphoma or granulocytic sarcoma (chloroma), and the differential diagnosis may be further complicated by an Indian-file arrangement of the cells, which may be exhibited by all three of these tumors. The characteristics of the neoplastic cells and the clinical features, however, almost always permit a correct diagnosis. Metastatic breast carcinomas have also been misinterpreted as granulosa cell tumors, but the contrasting features of the neoplastic cells, especially those of their nuclei, the differing patterns of growth, and the clinical findings facilitate the differential diagnosis in almost all cases.

Carcinoma of the Stomach Including Krukenberg Tumor

The great majority of metastatic gastric carcinomas to the ovary are Krukenberg tumors, which are defined as tumors characterized by the presence of mucin-filled signet-ring cells, typically lying within a cellular stroma derived from the ovarian stroma.[51,78,91,219] The source of Krukenberg tumors in 76–100% of reported cases is a gastric carcinoma, usually arising in the pylorus. Carcinomas of the large intestine, appendix, and breast are the next most common primary sites. The gallbladder, biliary tract, cervix, and urinary bladder are rare sources of these tumors. Saphir[171] demonstrated in an autopsy study that signet-ring cell carcinomas of various organs are more often associated with ovarian metastasis than carcinomas of other histologic types by a ratio of about 4:1. More recent studies have supported his observation; gastric signet-ring cell carcinomas metastasize to the ovary in 41% of cases, whereas intestinal-type carcinomas of the stomach do so in only 17%.[55] Signet-ring cell carcinoma of the colon also metastasizes to the ovaries more frequently than does the usual colonic adenocarcinoma.[5]

The frequency of the Krukenberg tumor varies with that of gastric carcinoma in the population analyzed. At the Radiumhemmett, 39% of ovarian metastases presenting as ovarian tumors were of gastric origin, although not specified to be of the Krukenberg type.[99] In a similar series, Krukenberg tumors of gastric origin accounted for approximately 30% of clinically apparent ovarian metastases.[174] In countries, such as Japan, with a high prevalence of gastric carcinoma and a low prevalence of primary ovarian carcinoma, the Krukenberg tumor accounts for a large proportion of all ovarian cancers. The average age of patients with Krukenberg tumors is about 45 years.[78,91,219] From 28 to 44% of the patients have been under the age of 40 years,[78,91,99] and only

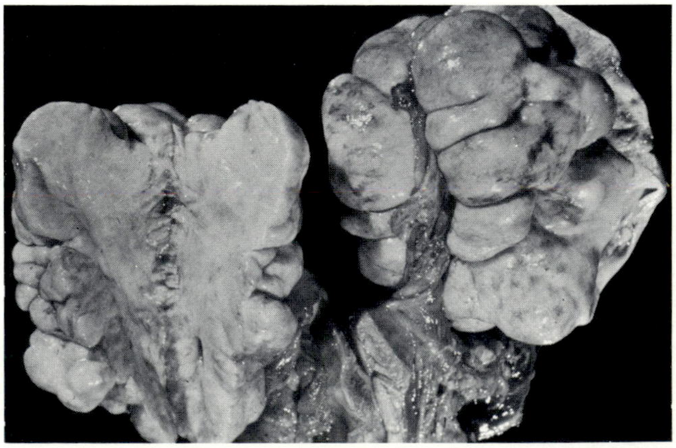

Fig. 22.5. Krukenberg tumor. Bilateral bosselated masses are composed of solid white tissue.

slightly more than 10% of them have been over 60 years of age.[78,99] This age distribution is related in part to the disproportionate frequency of gastric signet-ring cell carcinomas in young women.

Krukenberg tumors typically form rounded or reniform, firm, white masses that may be bosselated and may attain a large size. The sectioned surfaces are usually yellow or white (Fig. 22.5), but areas of purple, red, or brown discoloration and extensive hemorrhage are also encountered (Fig. 22.6). The consistency is characteristically firm, but fleshy, gelatinous, or spongy areas are common. Occasionally, the gross presentation is atypical, with large, thin-walled cysts containing mucinous or watery fluid, separated by relatively small amounts of solid tissue. Both ovaries are involved in 80% or more of the cases. The occasional metastatic gastric carcinoma that is not a Krukenberg tumor may be predominantly solid or predominantly cystic (Fig. 22.7).

Microscopic examination of a Krukenberg tumor reveals mucin-laden, signet-ring cells strewn individually and in small clusters within a cellular ovarian stroma (Figs. 22.8 and 22.9). Occasionally the stroma has a storiform pattern.[91] Frequent variations from the classic appearance include small glands, a prominent tubular architecture (Fig. 22.10),[30] mucin-poor tumor cells in trabeculae and large masses, abundant collagen formation, marked stromal edema (Fig. 22.11), and cell-free pools of mucin in the stroma. Occasionally, small or large cysts lined by slightly atypical appearing mucinous epithelium form a conspicuous component of the tumor, with more characteristic areas lying between the cysts. The cytoplasm of the signet ring cells is occasionally granular and eosinophilic rather than pale and vacuolated, and the cytoplasm sometimes has a bull's-eye ap-

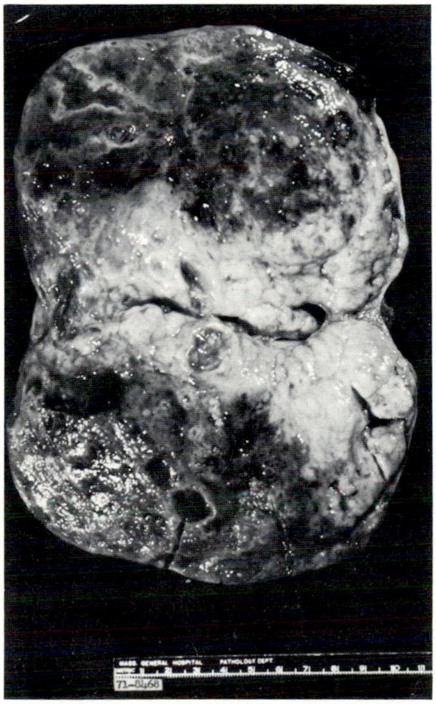

Fig. 22.6. Krukenberg tumor showing extensive hemorrhage.

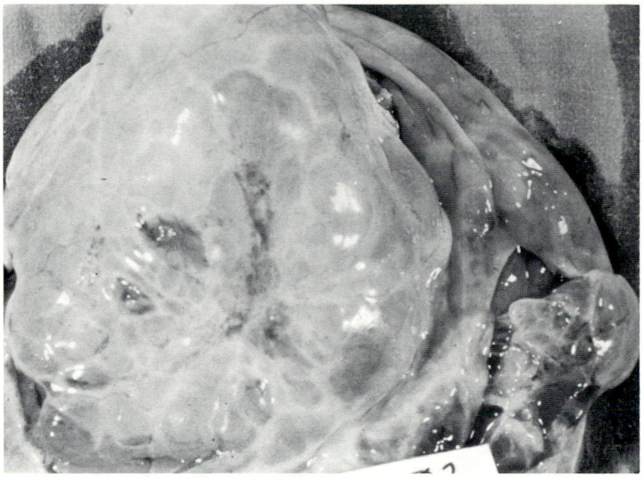

Fig. 22.7. Metastatic adenocarcinoma from the stomach. Multiloculated cystic neoplasm simulating a mucinous cystadenoma.

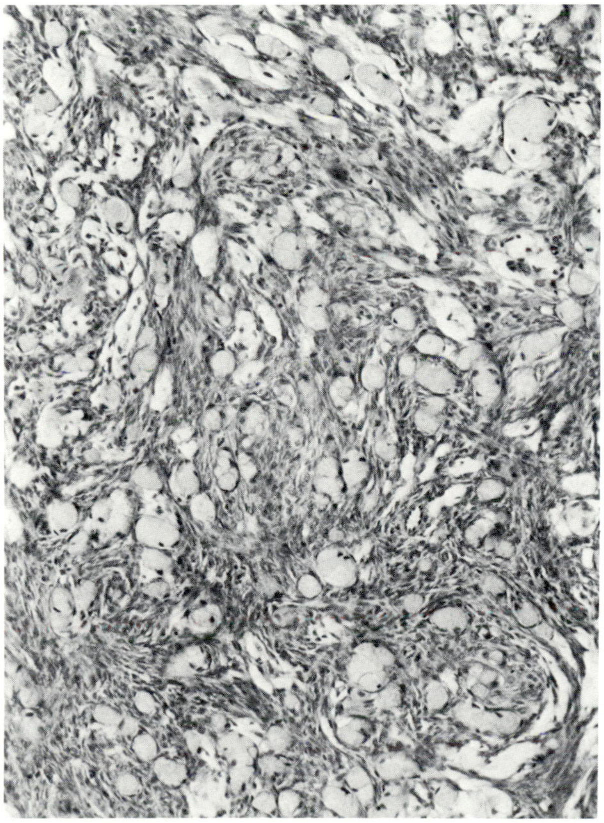

Fig. 22.8. Krukenberg tumor. Numerous signet ring cells are present within a cellular stroma.

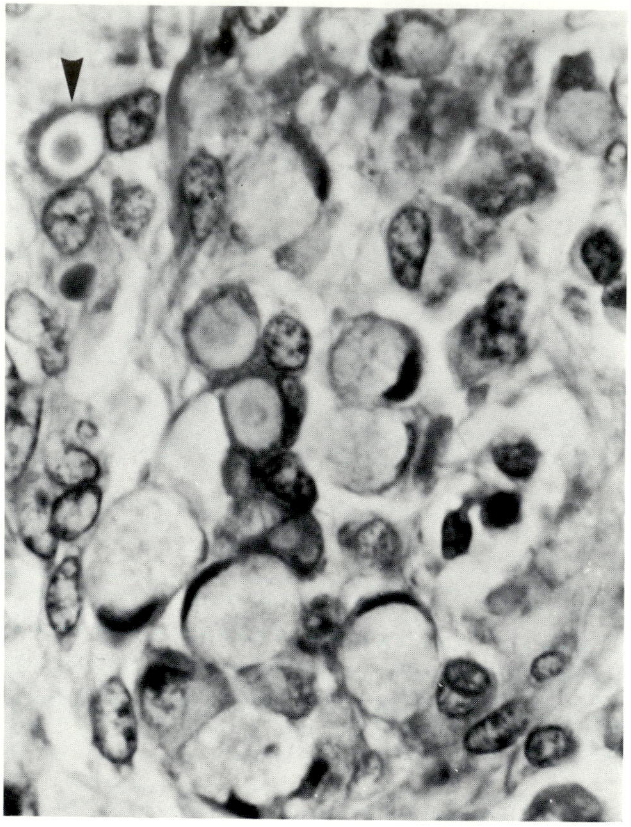

FIG. 22.9. Krukenberg tumor. Signet ring cells with eccentric nuclei and abundant pale cytoplasm. In one cell, a droplet of mucin with a targetoid appearance is present (*arrow*). (Reprinted by permission of Scully, Ref. 173.)

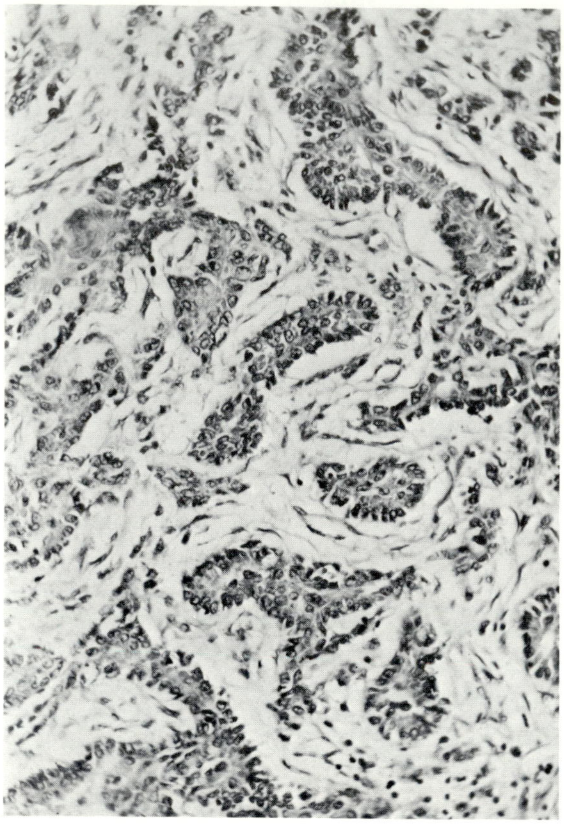

FIG. 22.10. Tubular Krukenberg tumor. The tubules simulate those of a Sertoli–Leydig cell tumor. Signet ring cells are not evident in this illustration.

pearance, containing a large vacuole with a central eosinophilic body (Fig. 22.9). As with metastases in general, blood vessel and lymphatic invasion is common. Lutein cells are occasionally present in the stroma, particularly if the patient is pregnant (see Chapter 19, Sex Cord–Stromal Tumors of Ovary).

The Krukenberg tumor may resemble a fibroma or any other type of solid ovarian tumor on gross examination. Its appearance may also occasionally be deceptive on frozen section or low-power examination[91] but should be readily diagnosable on high-power microscopic examination, especially with the aid of mucin stains. A frequent misdiagnosis is a Sertoli–Leydig cell tumor, particularly when a prominent tubular component (Fig. 22.10) and luteinization of the stroma are encountered. Signet ring cells, however, are not a feature of Sertoli–Leydig cell tumors.[30,225] The sclerosing stromal tumor may contain cells resembling signet cells as well as a proliferating fibroblastic component, but such cells contain lipid rather than mucin. In clear cell carcinomas, the clear cells contain glycogen; mucin, when present, is typically luminal and extracellular. In rare cases, portions of the tumor contain aggregates of signet ring cells, but the presence of other characteristic features of this tumor permit its identification. Mucinous carcinoid tumors that contain large numbers of signet ring cells are distinguished from Krukenberg tumors by their additional component of carcinoid, the presence of which can be confirmed by argyrophil staining. These tumors are discussed further in the section on metastatic carcinoids.

Almost 90% of patients with Krukenberg tumors have symptoms related to ovarian involvement, the most common of which are abdominal pain and swelling. Occasionally, there is abnormal uterine bleeding and rarely overt signs of excess hormone production, such as virilization (see Chapter 19, Sex Cord–Stromal Tumors of Ovary). The remainder of the patients have gastrointestinal or miscellaneous symptoms or are asymptomatic. A history of prior carcinoma of the stomach or, rarely, another organ can be obtained in 20–30% of cases.[78,99] The interval between the diagnosis of a gastric carcinoma and the subsequent discovery of ovarian involvement is usually 6 months or less,[99] but periods as long as 12 years have been reported.[78] In most cases, diagnosis of the gastric carcinoma is made preoperatively, during the operation for the ovarian metastasis, or within a few

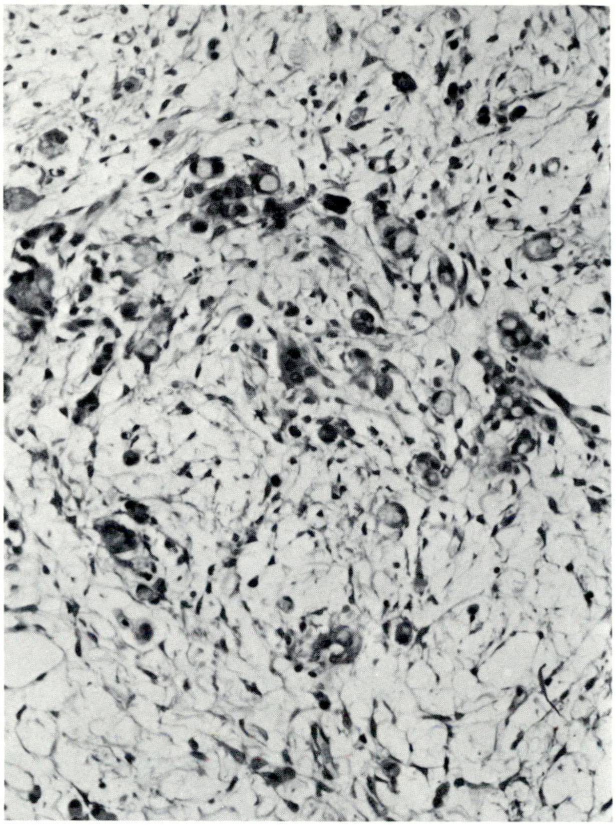

FIG. 22.11. Krukenberg tumor. Signet ring cells are dispersed in an edematous stroma.

of intestinal type in varying degrees of differentiation (Fig. 22.12), which occasionally are cystically dilated (Fig. 22.13), as well as sheets and irregular aggregates of poorly differentiated carcinoma cells.[55,94]

Almost all tumors with the microscopic features of the Krukenberg tumor are metastatic, but very rare examples may be primary. Joshi[100] has accepted as primary 18 reported cases, including 11 in which autopsy examination revealed no evidence of an extraovarian source, and 7 in which the patient survived for 5–13 years after removal of the ovarian tumor. These tumors occurred in patients ranging in age from 16 to 61 years, with an average of 38 years. Although a primary Krukenberg tumor probably exists, one should exercise considerable caution before making such a diagnosis or accepting reported cases as valid. Primary carcinomas, particularly those arising in the breast and stomach, may be very small, requiring exhaustive sectioning to detect them, despite the presence of metastases in some cases. It is possible that tiny primary tumors were missed in these or other organs in the reported autopsied cases of primary Krukenberg tumors. Ulbright and Roth[202] cite a case observed by Kraus in which a primary tumor in the stomach was detected only after microscopic sections months thereafter. Occasionally, the primary tumor is too small to be detected at operation,[91] and radiographic examination of the upper gastrointestinal tract may also fail to reveal evidence of a tumor even after the diagnosis of Krukenberg tumor has been established.[78,91] Rarely, the gastric carcinoma may not be detected until 5 or more years after discovery of the ovarian metastatic tumor.

Almost all the patients die within a year of the diagnosis of the ovarian metastasis, with an average duration of 7 months from diagnosis to death,[78] but a rare patient has survived, apparently free of tumor, for as long as 6 years after gastrectomy and bilateral oophorectomy.[91] Such a result, even though exceptional, justifies removal of both the stomach and the ovarian metastases for possible cure in patients in whom the tumor appears limited to those organs. It is prudent for the surgeon to remove the ovaries routinely in menopausal and postmenopausal women who are having a gastric resection for carcinoma to prevent the later complication of ovarian metastasis and avoid another operation.

Although most metastatic gastric carcinomas to the ovary have the characteristics of a Krukenberg tumor, occasional tumors do not and may be composed of glands

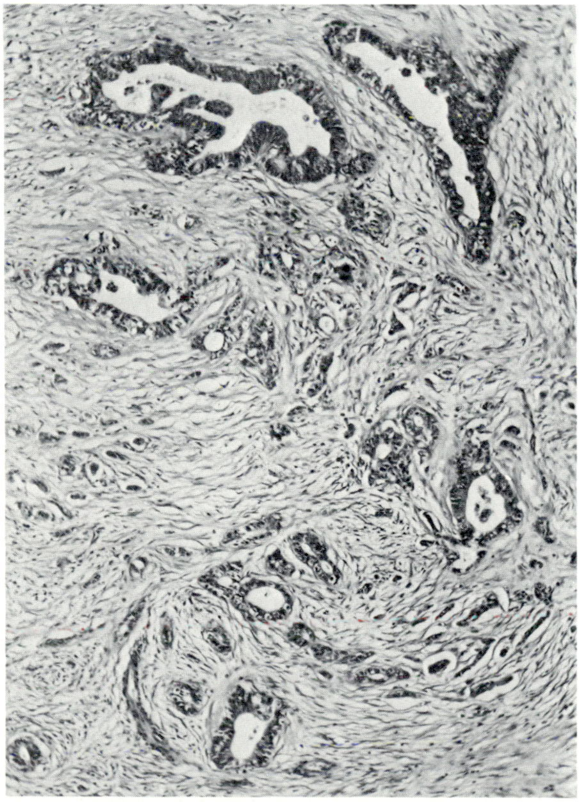

FIG. 22.12. Metastatic adenocarcinoma from the stomach. Glands of varying sizes and shapes and small clusters of tumor cells lie in a fibrous stroma.

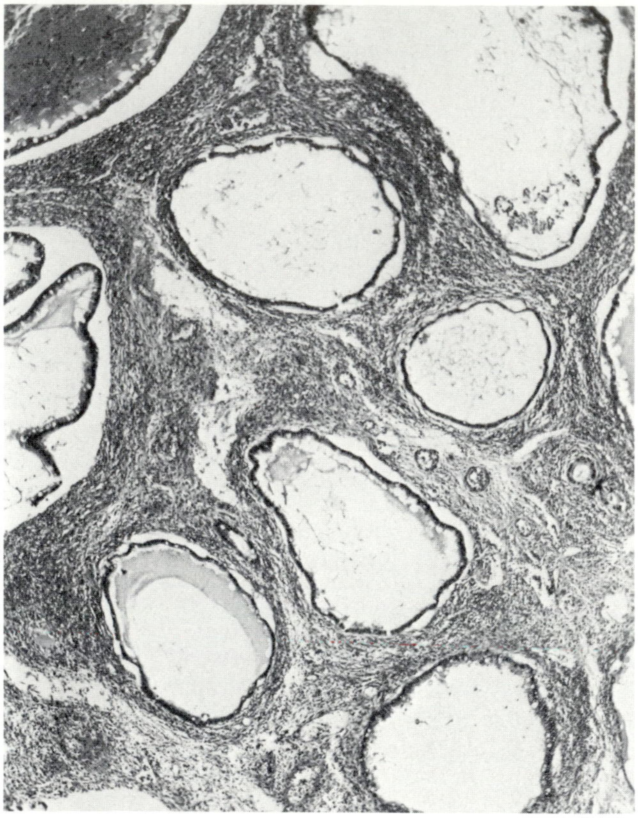

FIG. 22.13. Metastatic adenocarcinoma from the stomach containing cystic glands separated by stroma lacking tumor cells. Same patient as in Fig. 22.12.

prepared from 200 blocks had been examined. Also, it is well known that mammary and gastric carcinomas may remain silent for many years.[129,134] We have seen one case of a Krukenberg tumor in which a primary gastric carcinoma did not become apparent until 5½ years after the ovarian tumor had been removed. Thus, clinical dormancy of the primary tumor probably accounts for some of the cases of Krukenberg tumor with long survival.

Intestinal Carcinoma

Most metastatic ovarian tumors of intestinal origin are from the large intestine, with occasional tumors of small intestinal derivation.[99] Ovarian metastases from intestinal carcinomas have been reported to be less common than those from gastric carcinomas at autopsy, 14 versus 38%, respectively,[171] but when malignant ovarian tumors encountered at the time of operation are evaluated, metastases from intestinal carcinomas are almost five times as frequent as those from gastric carcinomas.[99,174,212,216]

From 2 to 10% of women with intestinal cancer have ovarian metastases at some time during the course of their disease.* The average figure from the literature is 3.8%[72] but was as high as 10% in a study in which the ovaries were cut into 2-mm slices.[72] Four of the six metastatic tumors in that series of 58 cases were not recognized on gross examination of the ovaries. Metastases from the large intestine to the ovary occur relatively more frequently in women under 40 years of age; they occur in from 18 to 27% of the patients in this age group.[119,132,149,157] The mean age of the patients with carcinoma of the large intestine at the Memorial Sloan–Kettering Cancer Center in whom ovarian metastases developed was 51 years, in contrast to 62 years for all the patients with large intestinal cancer.[136]

From a clinical viewpoint, patients with this type of metastatic carcinoma fall into three categories: (1) patients who have an intestinal carcinoma (50–75% of patients)[85,99,136,147] that antedates recognition of the ovarian tumor by up to 3 years in 90% of patients, (2) patients in whom ovarian involvement is found unexpectedly during an operation for resection of an intestinal carcinoma, (3) patients whose initial manifestations are those of an ovarian tumor (3–20% of patients).[81,86,108] Ovarian metastases have been found in up to 8% of patients who have bilateral prophylactic oophorectomy because of intestinal carcinoma.[119,162,188] It has been estimated that routine preoperative barium x-ray examination of the large intestine in women suspected of having an ovarian tumor would be positive for carcinoma in approximately 1–2 of 1000 patients.[173]

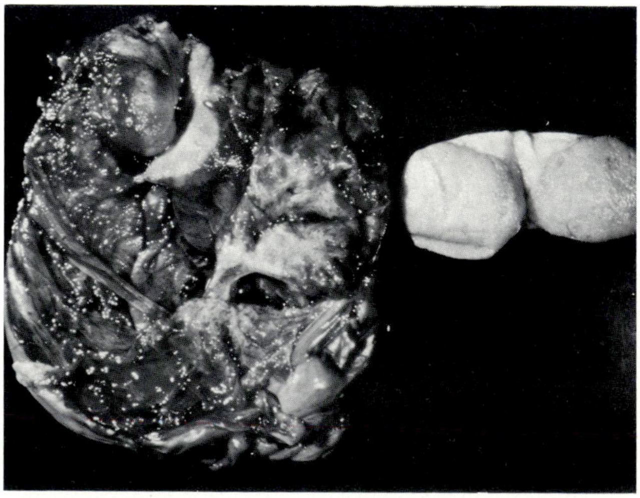

FIG. 22.14. Metastatic carcinoma from the colon. The smaller tumor is solid and buff-colored. The larger tumor is cystic with extensive hemorrhage and necrosis. (Reprinted by permission of Scully, Ref. 173.)

* References 8, 32, 45, 72, 81, 147, 189.

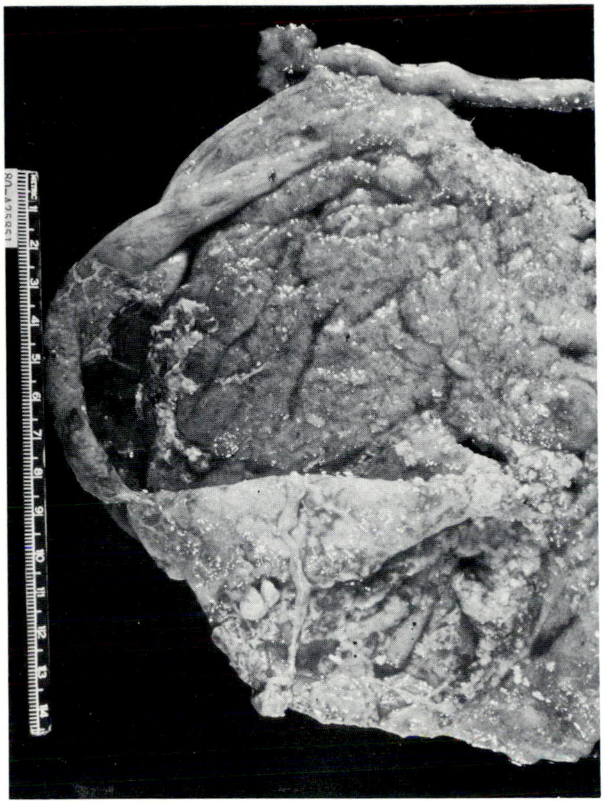

FIG. 22.15. Cystic metastatic carcinoma from the colon. The cyst is lined by shaggy necrotic tumor tissue.

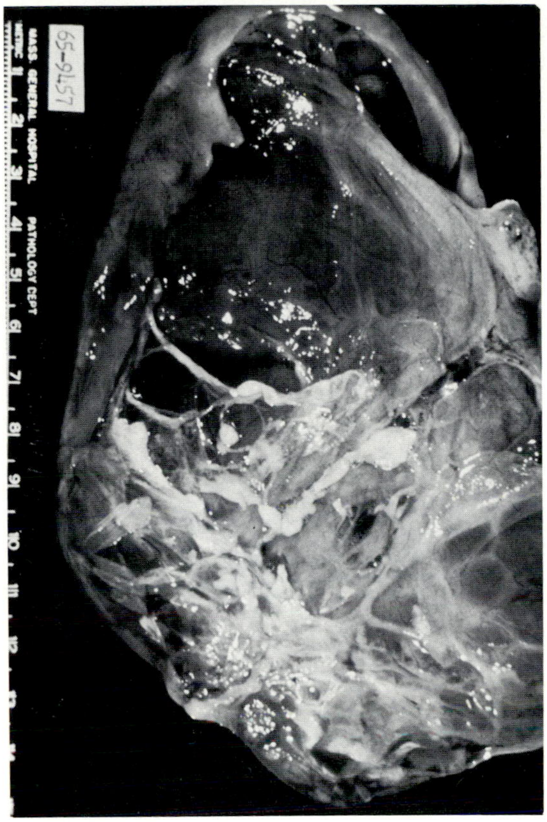

FIG. 22.16. Multicystic metastatic carcinoma from the rectum simulating mucinous cystadenoma.

Metastatic ovarian carcinomas of large intestinal origin, which are bilateral in approximately two-thirds of cases, may form solid masses (Fig. 22.14) but are more often predominantly cystic (Figs. 22.14, 22.15, and 22.16). They are frequently large and may simulate closely primary carcinomas of the ovary. Sectioning typically reveals friable or mushy yellow, red, or gray tissue with cystic compartments that contain necrotic tumor (Fig. 22.15), mucinous or clear fluid, or fresh or old blood. Approximately 10% of the tumors rupture spontaneously during pelvic examination or removal. A very rare example is composed of multiple, thin-walled cysts filled with clear fluid (Fig. 22.16)[202] or has the typical gross features of a Krukenberg tumor.

The neoplastic cells characteristically grow in patterns similar to those of primary intestinal carcinomas (Figs. 22.17 and 22.18), typically forming small or large glands. Mucin-containing goblet cells may be scattered among the mucin-free cells. Occasionally, cystic glands lined by well-differentiated mucin-rich neoplastic cells form a prominent component of the tumor,[202] the tumor is of the Krukenberg type or has the pattern of colloid carcinoma. Necrosis is common and often extensive (Fig.

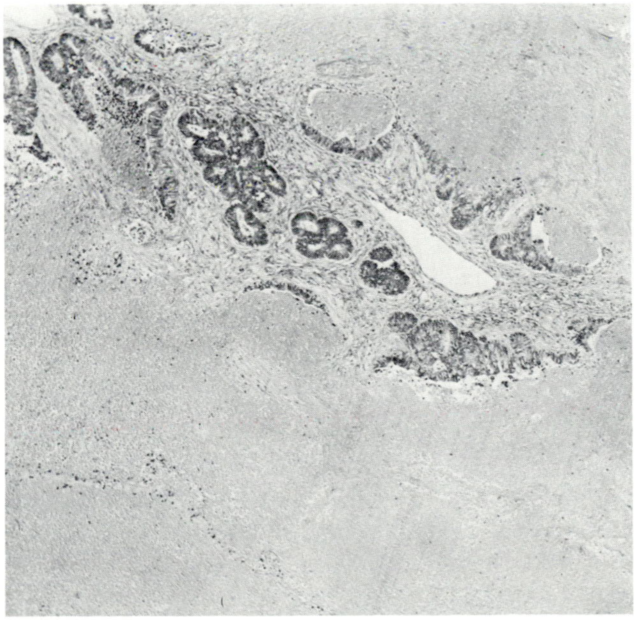

FIG. 22.17. Metastatic adenocarcinoma from the colon with extensive necrosis.

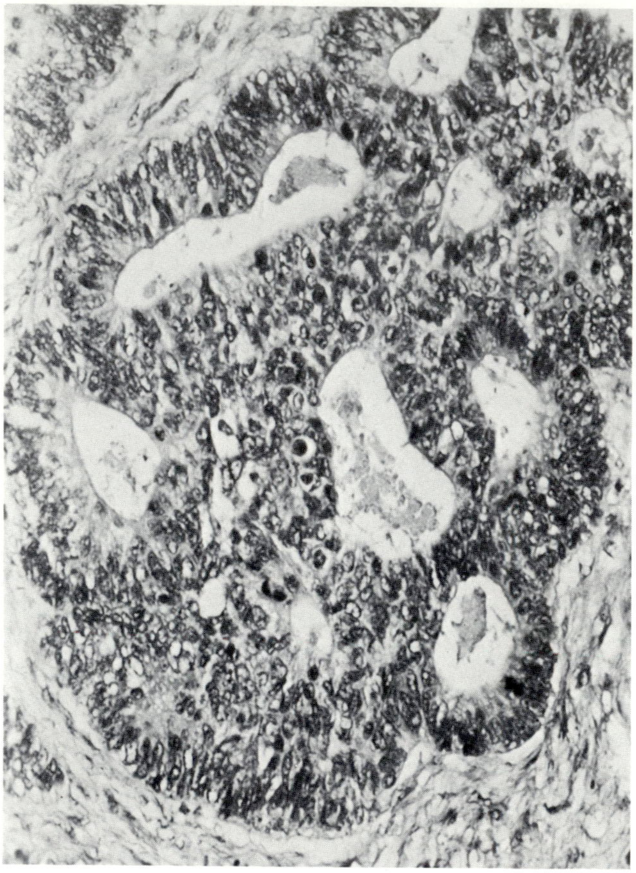

FIG. 22.18. Metastatic adenocarcinoma from the colon. Glands lined by poorly differentiated stratified epithelial cells.

22.17). The stroma varies from negligible to abundant. It may be desmoplastic, edematous, or mucoid but often resembles ovarian stroma, containing cells resembling theca externa cells or theca-lutein cells in about one-third of the cases.[203]

In one series, over two-thirds of the cases of metastatic intestinal carcinoma were initially misinterpreted as primary ovarian adenocarcinomas.[203] The most difficult tumors to exclude on microscopic examination are primary mucinous and endometrioid carcinomas. Aside from clinical clues, the frequent presence of glands and cysts lined by endocervical-type mucinous cells with basal nuclei strongly favors a primary mucinous carcinoma, although as mentioned above, differentiated glands and cysts are encountered in some metastatic intestinal carcinomas. Although goblet cells are more commonly encountered in primary mucinous carcinomas, they may also be seen in metastatic mucinous tumors. In occasional cases, it may be impossible to make a differential diagnosis of metastatic versus primary mucinous adenocarcinoma on the basis of examination of the ovarian tumor alone. With regard to the differential diagnosis of metastatic intestinal adenocarcinoma and endometrioid adenocarcinoma, the glands of the former are typically lined by more poorly differentiated and more highly stratified cells (Fig. 22.18) than those of endometrioid adenocarcinomas with similar degrees of glandular differentiation. In addition, extensive necrosis is common in metastatic intestinal carcinomas (Fig. 22.17) but uncommon in gland-forming endometrioid carcinomas. Foci of squamous differentiation are frequent in endometrioid carcinomas but extremely rare in association with intestinal carcinomas.

Almost all patients with intestinal cancer metastatic to the ovary die within 3 years of detection of the ovarian involvement,[22,85,99] more than half of them within 1 year.[99,174] The mean survival in one series was 16½ months.[136] Webb et al.[212] reported a 5-year survival rate of 5% after treatment of ovarian metastases from gastrointestinal carcinomas and a survival of 9% if the primary tumor was grade 1 or 2. Six of 169 patients (4%) were still alive at 10 years. These results justify removal of both the primary tumor and the metastases whenever feasible. Routine removal of the ovaries in menopausal and postmenopausal women having intestinal resections for carcinoma is also indicated in order to prevent the later development of symptoms of ovarian metastasis and avoid another operation, which has been necessary in from 1 to 7% of these patients in various series.[22,108,136] In some patients, even a third operation has been necessary when only a unilateral oophorectomy has been performed during the second operation.[136] There is no evidence, however, that prophylactic oophorectomy enhances the overall survival rate of patients with intestinal carcinoma.[186] Because young women are more likely to have ovarian metastases than older women,[85] an argument could be made for oophorectomy in these patients as well, but other factors, such as the patient's desire to retain her reproductive capacity, make the decision difficult and one that must be made on an individual basis.

Tumors of the Appendix

Metastases to the ovary from appendiceal tumors are uncommon partly because of the rarity of the latter.[49,90,103,128] In approximately one-third of the 31 reported cases, the ovarian involvement accounted for the presenting symptom. Most of the tumors have been adenocarcinomas, including occasional signet-ring cell and colloid subtypes, but approximately one-quarter have been mucinous carcinoids (goblet cell carcinoids, adenocarcinoids). Very rare appendiceal carcinoids of the typical type have spread to the ovary.[92] In cases of signet-ring cell carcinoma, the metastases may be of the Krukenberg type.

An unknown percentage of patients with low-grade

mucinous cystadenocarcinomas of the appendix, which typically appear as mucoceles on gross examination, have similar tumors in one or both ovaries, accompanied by pseudomyxoma peritonei.[35,126,177] The tumors at both sites characteristically have the microscopic features of ovarian tumors of borderline malignancy. It is probable that the ovarian tumors in these cases are metastatic from the appendiceal tumors, although for purposes of classification and management by gynecologists they are generally included among the primary common epithelial tumors (see Chapter 19, Sex Cord–Stromal Tumors of Ovary). In a minority of cases of ovarian mucinous tumors accompanied by pseudomyxoma peritonei, the appendix has appeared normal at operation and has not been removed or, if removed, has been free of tumor on microscopic examination.

Carcinoid Tumors

Carcinoid tumors account for approximately 2% of metastases that form ovarian masses.[174,220] Although the vast majority of these tumors are of small intestinal origin, rarely the primary tumor is from another site. From another viewpoint, about 2% of small intestinal carcinoids greater than 1 cm in diameter spread to the ovary. Metastatic carcinoids may be large and are typically predominantly solid, with smooth or bosselated surfaces (Fig. 22. 19). Sectioning reveals single or confluent firm, white or yellow nodules, which may resemble ovarian fibromas or thecomas. Cysts of varying size (Fig. 22.20) are occasionally present and are typically filled with clear, watery fluid, resulting in a gross appearance similar to that of a cystadenofibroma (Fig. 22.19). Focal necrosis and hemorrhage may occur (Fig. 22.20). The majority of tumors are bilateral in contrast to primary ovarian carcinoids, which are unilateral.

The microscopic features of metastatic carcinoids are similar to those of primary ovarian carcinoids except that teratomatous elements are not encountered, multinodularity is often prominent, and vascular invasion is occasionally observed (Table 22.2). An insular pattern is the most common type (Figs. 22.21 and 22.22), but trabecular, mixed, and, rarely, solid tubular patterns (Fig. 22.23) are also encountered. Acini, which are typically uniformly small and round, are common (Fig. 22.21); they often contain a homogeneous eosinophilic secretion that may undergo calcification (Fig. 22.22), sometimes in the form of psammoma bodies. Large glands and cysts lined by one or a few layers of neoplastic cells are sometimes seen (Fig. 22.24). With rare exceptions, the carcinoid is the only ovarian metastatic tumor that elicits a stromal proliferation that closely resembles an ovarian fibroma. Occasionally, this stroma becomes extensively hyalinized (Fig. 22.25). A final microscopic

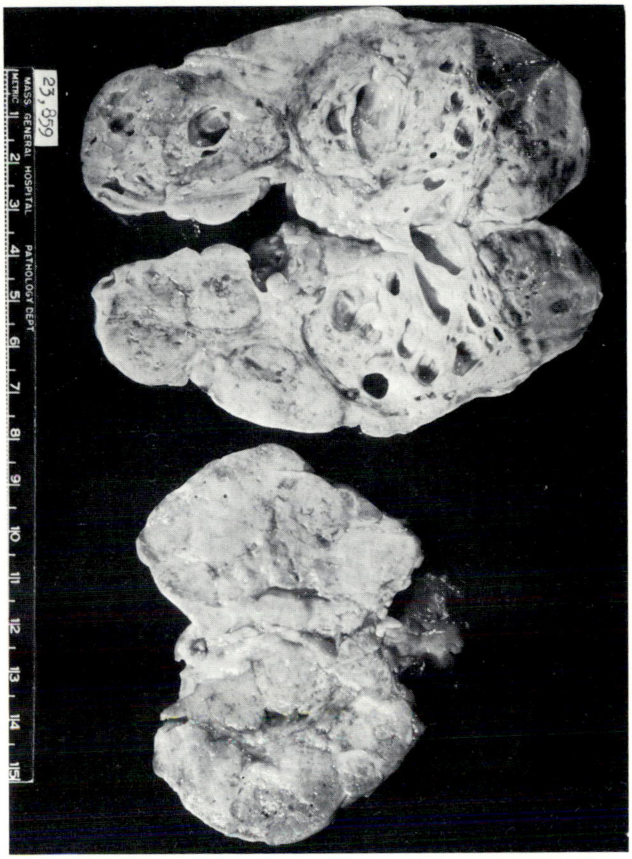

FIG. 22.19. Metastatic carcinoid. The larger tumor contains multiple cysts simulating a cystadenofibroma. (Reprinted by permission of Scully, Ref. 173.)

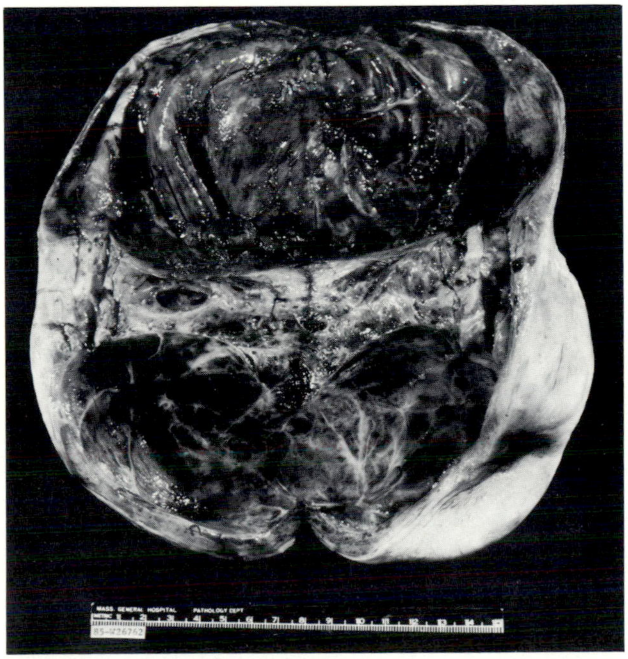

FIG. 22.20. Metastatic carcinoid. The tumor is predominantly cystic with extensive hemorrhage.

TABLE 22.2. Criteria for distinguishing primary and metastatic ovarian carcinoids.

	Primary	Metastatic
Laterality	Unilateral	Most often bilateral
Sectioned surface	Single mass	Multiple nodules
Peritoneal spread	Absent	Common
Teratomatous elements	Usual	Absent
Vascular invasion	Absent	Occasional
Postoperative 5-HIAA	Negative	Usually positive

pattern of metastatic carcinoid is that of a mucinous or goblet cell carcinoid (adenocarcinoid),[106,192,209] in which rounded nests containing goblet cells and argentaffin or argyrophil cells are present (Fig. 22.26). These tumors may also have foci resembling a Krukenberg tumor as well as cystic glands filled with mucin.[196]

Metastatic carcinoids may be confused with a number of tumors other than primary carcinoid tumors, including granulosa cell tumors, Sertoli or Sertoli–Leydig cell tumors, Brenner tumors, adenofibromas and cystadenofibromas, benign, borderline, and malignant, and adenocarcinomas of various types. The microfollicular granulosa cell tumor is often confused with a metastatic

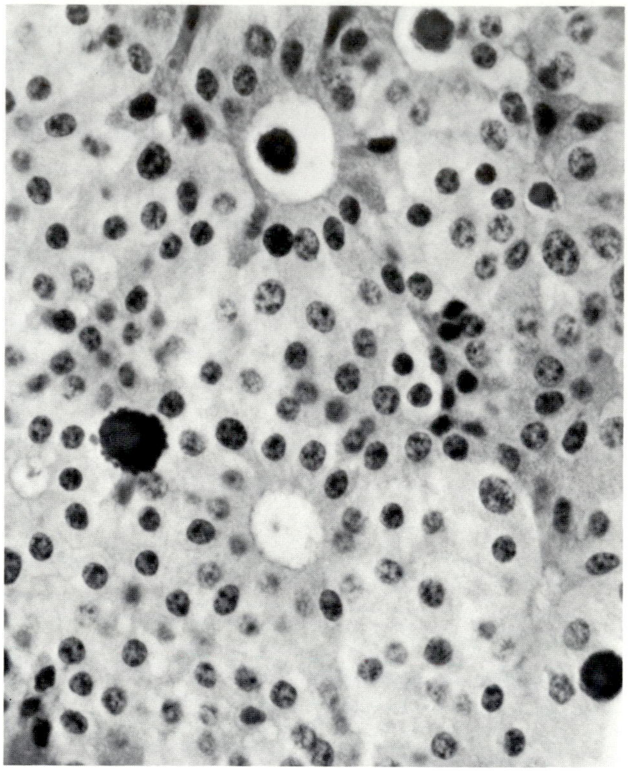

FIG. 22.22. Metastatic insular carcinoid. Several lumens contain dark calcified secretion.

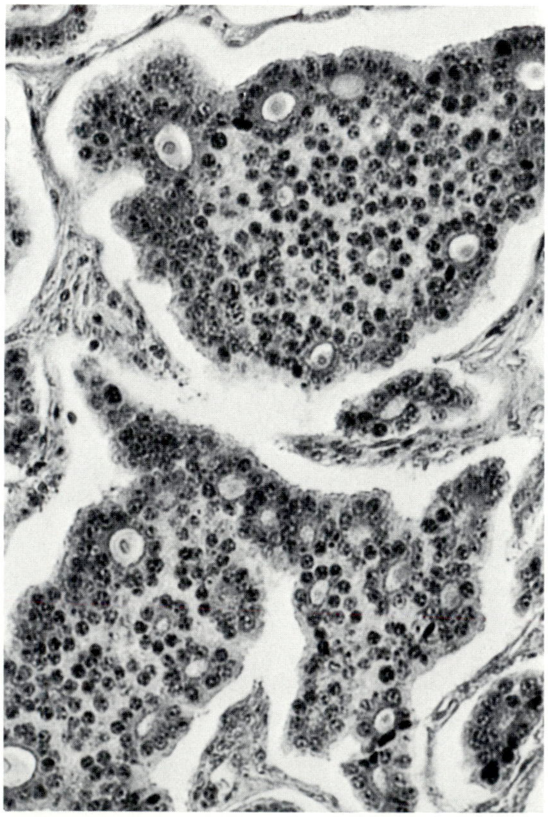

FIG. 22.21. Metastatic insular carcinoid. The gland lumens have smooth, rounded outlines. The nuclei are rounded with evenly distributed, coarse chromatin.

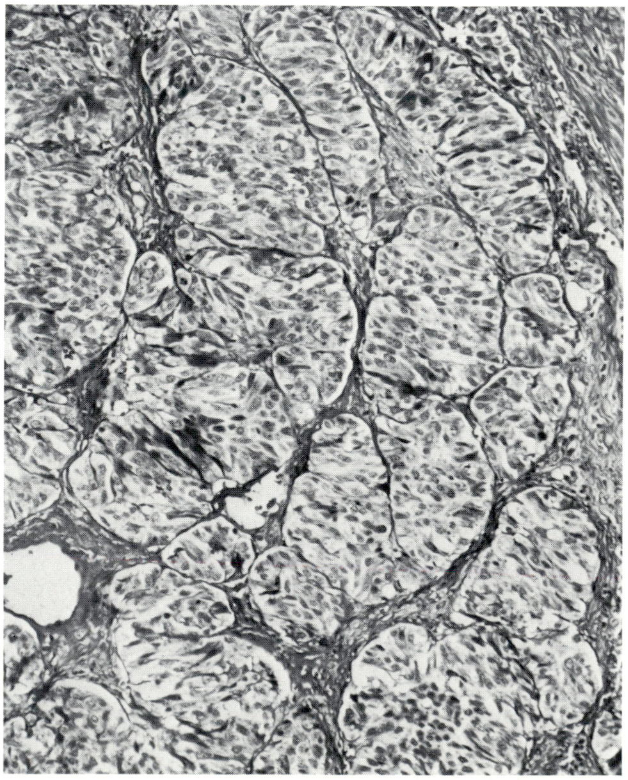

FIG. 22.23. Metastatic carcinoid with solid tubular pattern simulating Sertoli cell tumor.

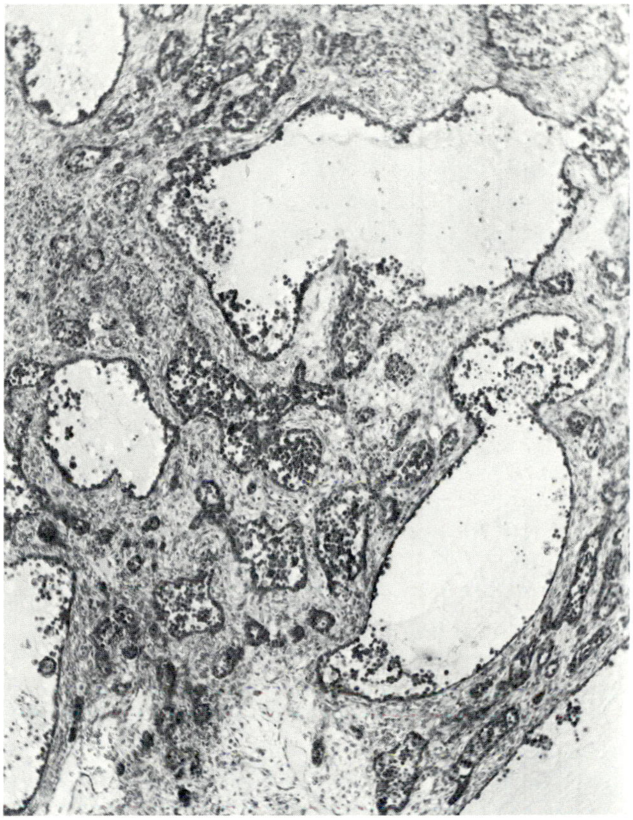

FIG. 22.24. Metastatic carcinoid with cysts lined by one or a few layers of neoplastic cells.

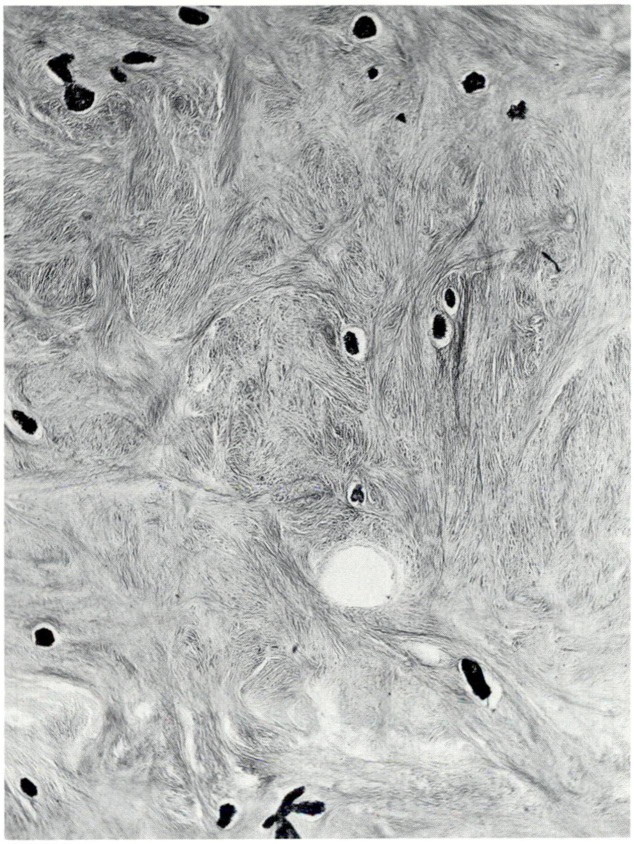

FIG. 22.25. Metastatic carcinoid with abundant hyalinized stroma.

carcinoid. The Call–Exner body of the granulosa cell tumor may resemble the acinus of the carcinoid when it is filled with eosinophilic dense basement membrane material, but it often differs by containing watery, eosinophilic fluid and shrunken nuclei in its lumen. Examination of the neoplastic cells is the most helpful clue to the correct diagnosis. Granulosa cells usually have scanty cytoplasm, and ovoid, angular, or round nuclei that are typically pale and grooved. The cells are commonly haphazardly oriented with respect to one another and the cavities of the Call–Exner bodies. In contrast, the cells of carcinoid tumors typically have round nuclei with coarse chromatin, and their cytoplasm often contains prominent red or red-brown argentaffin granules. The sex cord-like formations of Sertoli–Leydig cell tumors may resemble the ribbons of the trabecular carcinoid, but the latter are usually longer and thicker and have a more orderly architecture. The tubules of Sertoli or Sertoli–Leydig cell tumors may simulate the acini of insular carcinoids. Further confusion may be caused by the presence of a carcinoid component, which is typically minor in extent, in a Sertoli–Leydig cell tumor with heterologous elements. The presence of other distinctive patterns of Sertoli–Leydig cell tumor and attention to the characteristic cytologic features of carcinoid cells, however, should enable one to make the correct diagnosis.

The fibromatous stroma of a Brenner tumor is often indistinguishable from that of a carcinoid, but the epithelial nests of the former contain cells of urothelial type with oval, pale, grooved nuclei rather than cells with the characteristic features of carcinoid tumors. Benign and malignant adenofibromatous tumors and endometrioid adenocarcinomas containing small tubules and acini are generally readily distinguished from carcinoids by recognition of the differing patterns and cytologic features of these tumors. As mentioned earlier, a metastatic breast carcinoma with a prominent insular pattern may simulate a carcinoid tumor (Fig. 22.3). We have seen one case of microadenocarcinoma of the pancreas that metastasized to the ovary and, in the absence of a known pancreatic primary tumor, prompted an initial diagnosis of probable metastatic carcinoid. If the diagnosis of a carcinoid tumor is difficult, more thorough sampling, histochemical staining for argentaffin and argyrophil granules, immunohistochemical staining for chromogranin, neuron-specific enolase, peptide hormones, and serotonin, and electron microscopy for dense core granules should

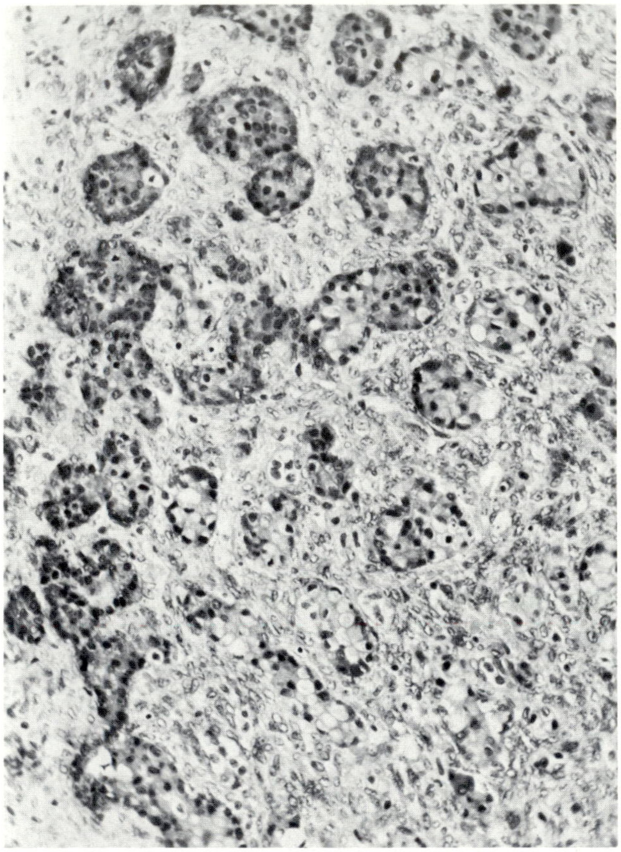

FIG. 22.26. Metastatic mucinous carcinoid. Nests composed of cells with dense cytoplasm containing argentaffin granules and signet-ring cells.

resolve the differential diagnosis. It must be emphasized, however, that some of the other tumors mentioned may, on occasion, contain scattered cells that stain positively for these substances and may contain dense core granules.

Metastatic mucinous carcinoids may contain foci of adenocarcinoma and be difficult to distinguish from pure metastatic adenocarcinomas unless the characteristic pattern of the mucinous carcinoid is recognized and the presence of argentaffin or argyrophil cells is confirmed by special staining. Adenocarcinomas of the stomach, intestine, and ovary may contain scattered argentaffin or argyrophil cells,[109,175,194] and the diagnosis of mucinous carcinoid should be reserved for cases in which the distinctive pattern of that tumor predominates. Distinction of a metastatic mucinous carcinoid from the rare primary mucinous carcinoid of the ovary[196] may be difficult and depends on knowledge of the distribution of disease and the presence or absence of teratomatous elements; bilaterality strongly favors a metastasis (Table 22.2).

In the largest series of carcinoids metastatic to the ovary, the ages of the 35 patients ranged from 21 to 82, with a median of 57 years; almost all of them were older than 40 years.[165] Ten of the tumors in that series were not diagnosed until autopsy. Forty percent of the women whose metastases were discovered at operation had preoperative manifestations of the carcinoid syndrome. Some of them also had signs and symptoms referable to intestinal or ovarian involvement. Extraovarian metastases were found in at least 90% of the patients. The primary site was usually in the ileum, but the cecum, jejunum, appendix, and pancreas were sources in occasional patients.[165] One-third of the patients died within 1 year, and three-fourths died within 5 years after unilateral or bilateral salpingo-oophorectomy, which was accompanied by a hysterectomy and an intestinal operation in some of the patients. Six of the 25 patients, however, were asymptomatic for a median period of 5½ years postoperatively; all 4 patients with the carcinoid syndrome had postoperative relief, 2 for periods of over 3 years after the removal of the ovarian tumors. Metastatic carcinoids in the ovary may also originate in the colon,[20] stomach,[124] and lung.[28,203,224] Almost all examples of metastatic mucinous carcinoid originate in the appendix.

In view of the occasional complication of ovarian metastasis, menopausal or postmenopausal patients with gastrointestinal carcinoids should have a bilateral oophorectomy even in the absence of obvious ovarian involvement to prevent the subsequent growth of occult metastases or the appearance of new metastases. Whenever bilateral ovarian carcinoids are detected, a careful search for an extraovarian primary tumor should be instituted. Both the metastases and the primary tumor, if found, should be excised whenever feasible. In a young woman with a unilateral neoplasm, careful examination of the intestine and other organs for a primary tumor, biopsy of the opposite ovary if enlarged, a thorough search for teratomatous elements in the tumor, and postoperative radiologic studies and measurement of 5-hydroxyindole acetic acid in the urine may be necessary before a determination of the primary or metastatic nature of the tumor and selection of appropriate therapy are made.

Tumors of the Pancreas, Gallbladder, Liver, and Esophagus

Metastases to the ovary from these organs are rare. In an autopsy study of 119 patients of both sexes with pancreatic cancer, Cubilla and Fitzgerald[43] reported metastasis to the ovary in 7 patients. In another autopsy study from Poland of almost 200 patients,[46] no metastases to the ovary were recorded. It is very uncommon for a tumor metastatic from the pancreas to present as an ovarian mass,[44] but we have seen two examples of this phenomenon. In each case the primary tumor was discovered shortly after the operation. In the first case, the

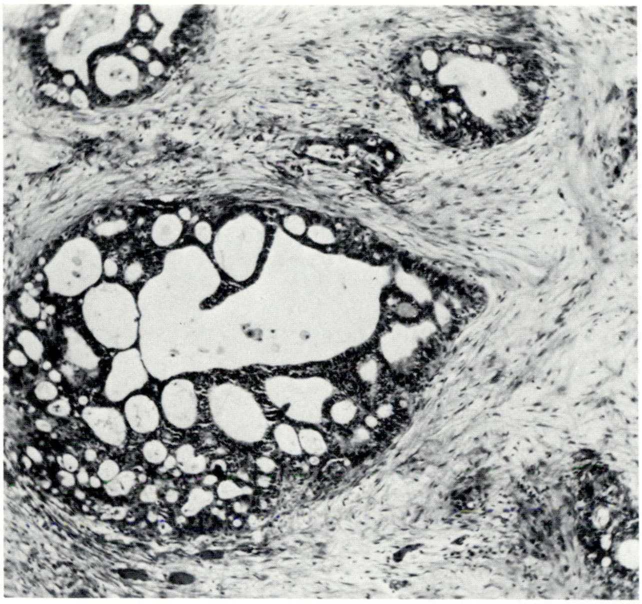

Fig. 22.27. Metastatic adenocarcinoma from the pancreas.

patient had bilateral mucinous cystic tumors (Figs. 22.27 and 22.28) interpreted initially as primary cystadenocarcinomas. The second patient had bilateral solid ovarian tumors that were subsequently discovered to be metastases from a microadenocarcinoma of the pancreas.[42,44] A tumor interpreted as a probable example of islet cell carcinoma metastatic to the ovaries has been reported.[215]

In a review of cases of gallbladder carcinoma encountered at autopsy at Columbia Presbyterian Medical Center over a 35-year period, 4 of 34 women were found to have metastases to the ovary.[24] Cases of hepatocellular carcinoma metastatic to the ovary are exceptionally rare.[159] Two examples have been reported, one in a large autopsy study[141] and the other as a case report.[150] There is one report in the literature of a cholangiocarcinoma metastasizing to the ovaries,[102] and we have seen an additional example.[172] A review of three recent autopsy studies on esophageal carcinoma failed to disclose any examples of metastasis to the ovary.[6,121,184] In a fourth study, "gonadal" spread was described in 2 of 73 patients who came to autopsy.[195]

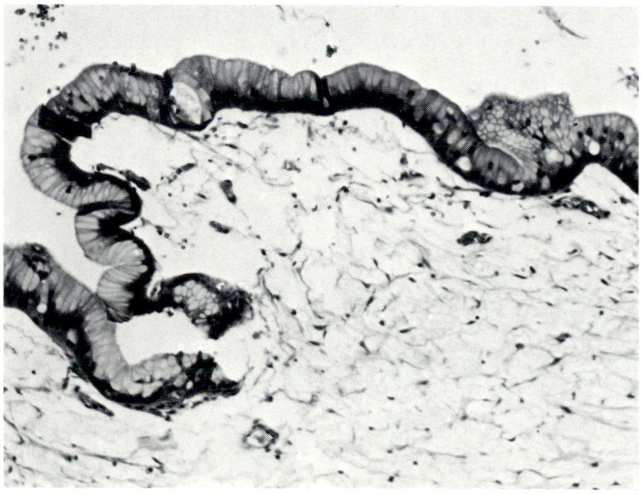

Fig. 22.28. Metastatic adenocarcinoma from the pancreas in the same patient as in Fig. 22.27. Cysts lined by only slightly atypical mucinous epithelium were a prominent component of this neoplasm.

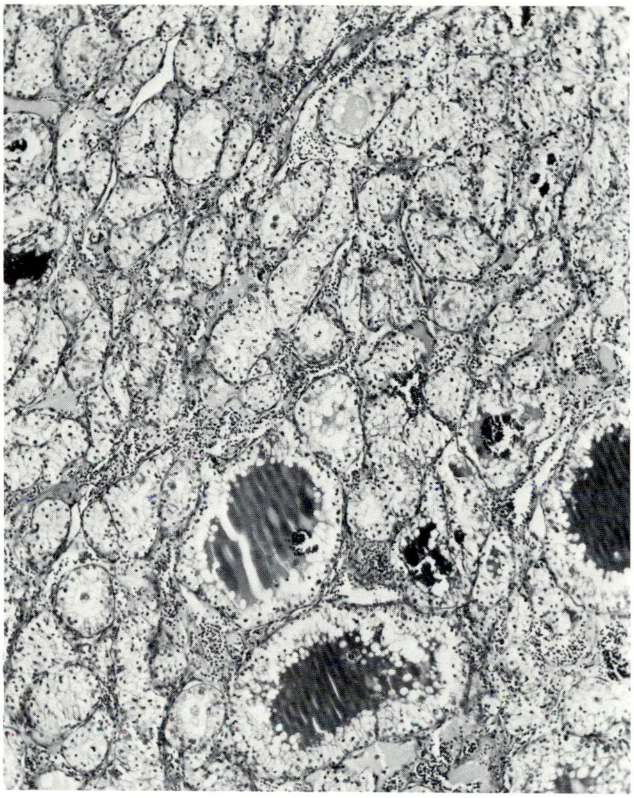

Fig. 22.29. Metastatic renal cell carcinoma, clear cell type. The primary tumor in this patient was not diagnosed until 8 years after the removal of the metastasis.

Renal Tumors

Renal cell carcinoma spreads to the ovary very rarely.* In a review of 324 cases of renal cell carcinoma in women examined at autopsy,[169] no metastases to the ovary were encountered. Clinically detectable ovarian masses, however, have been reported to result from metastasis of renal cell carcinoma. Ovarian involvement has appeared 5–11 years after nephrectomy,[123,187,208] coincident with[29]

* References 99, 102, 155, 169, 208, 216, 220.

or prior to the discovery of the renal tumor.[64,112,175] In one case initially misdiagnosed as a primary clear cell carcinoma of the ovary, the primary renal cell carcinoma became apparent 8 years after oophorectomy (Fig. 22.29).[175]

Metastatic renal cell carcinoma can be indistinguishable from the rare primary clear cell carcinoma of the ovary that is composed exclusively of clear cells. In most cases of ovarian clear cell carcinoma, however, the additional presence of well-developed hobnail cells and conspicuous extracellular mucin in the lumens of the tubules and cysts permits microscopic differentiation.

Ovarian metastases from Wilms tumor of the kidney must be very rare, since no examples are given in three large studies of this neoplasm[9,25,114] and the Armed Forces Institute of Pathology Fascicle on tumors of the kidney.[19]

Tumors of the Urinary Bladder, Ureter, and Urethra

Tumors from these sites uncommonly metastasize to the ovaries. Only occasional cases are mentioned in reports of large series of metastatic tumors.[203] In two combined autopsy studies, only 1 of 42 women with bladder cancer had ovarian metastases,[12,105] and in an older review of the literature, no cases of ovarian involvement were recorded.[59] Two examples of signet-ring cell carcinoma metastatic from the bladder have been reported[40,167]; these tumors had the appearance of a Krukenberg tumor. There is little information about the spread to the ovary of ureteral and urethral cancers. In one study, 2 of 12 women with ureteral cancer had ovarian metastases,[16] and occasional other examples have been recorded.[102] No cases of ovarian metastasis were included in a study of 79 women with urethral cancer,[71] although isolated examples can be found in the literature.[73,158]

It may be difficult to distinguish between a metastatic tumor from the urinary bladder or ureter and a borderline or malignant Brenner tumor.[7,61,193] In almost all the cases of borderline or malignant Brenner tumors, however, foci of typical benign Brenner tumor can also be found,[79] and the presence of associated benign mucinous elements also favors the diagnosis of a Brenner tumor. The metastatic transitional cell carcinoma in the series of Ulbright et al.[203] was cystic, exemplifying the propensity of ovarian metastases from various sites to undergo cystic change.

Adrenal Gland Tumors

Adrenal cortical carcinomas metastasize to the ovary in no more than 6% of cases, and the ovarian involvement is usually not apparent until autopsy.[52,138] We are not aware of a case in which an ovarian metastatic tumor from the adrenal cortex was the presenting manifestation of the disease. Pheochromocytomas spread to the ovary even less commonly; a review of the literature has failed to disclose a documented case. Very rarely, a pheochromocytoma is primary in the ovary.[58,172]

Neuroblastoma spreads to the ovary more frequently than other tumors of the adrenal gland. In one study, 25%[88] and, in another, 28.6%[130] of patients with neuroblastoma had ovarian involvement at autopsy. In one reported case, there was bilateral ovarian involvement at presentation,[130] and one patient had a metastasis in the left ovary.[191] Rarely, neuroblastoma is the predominant or possibly sole constituent of an immature teratoma of the ovary.[3,23] Such tumors must be distinguished from metastatic ovarian neuroblastomas.

Malignant Melanoma

At least 36 cases of malignant melanoma metastatic to the ovary (Fig. 22.30) have been reported. Most of them originated in the skin, but occasional tumors arose in the choroid or elsewhere.[18,122,135,181,198] The metastatic tumor may not be detected for many years after the removal of the primary lesion.[18] Autopsies of patients who died of malignant melanoma have revealed ovarian involvement in 18%, and 95% of these tumors were bilateral.[48,80] Metastatic melanoma must be distinguished from the rare primary melanoma that usually arises in the wall of a dermoid cyst and sometimes is accompanied by junctional activity beneath the squamous lining of the cyst. Recognition of teratomatous elements is important in establishing the primary nature of a melanoma, and the pathologist should accordingly sample the specimen extensively. In cases of apparently pure ovarian melanomas without obvious evidence of a pri-

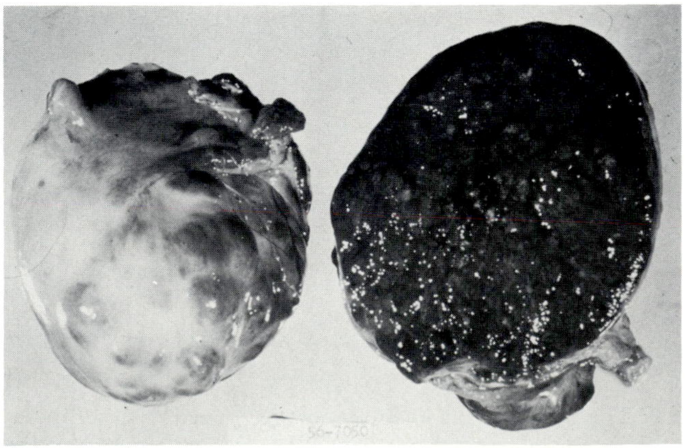

FIG. 22.30. Metastatic malignant melanoma. The tumor has a bosselated external surface; the sectioned surface is black.

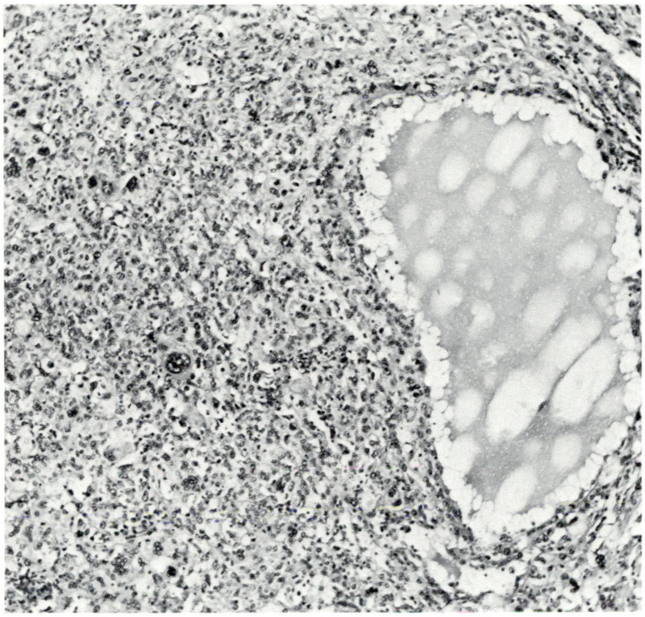

FIG. 22.31. Metastatic malignant melanoma. A follicle-like space is present adjacent to sheets of cells exhibiting conspicuous nuclear atypicality.

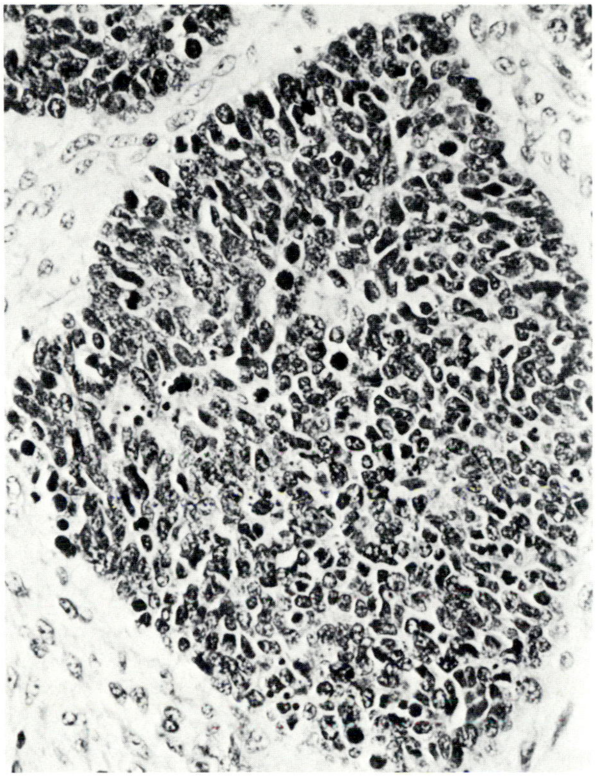

FIG. 22.32. Metastatic oat cell carcinoma from the lung. (Reprinted by permission from Young and Scully, Ref. 224.)

mary tumor elsewhere, a meticulous search for an occult primary tumor should be conducted. If there is no evidence of a primary tumor elsewhere, it is possible that a primary cutaneous melanoma that has regressed[11,76,133] was the source of the ovarian tumor.[122]

Metastatic melanoma, particularly if it is amelanotic, may resemble closely a lipid-poor steroid cell tumor or, if it is found during pregnancy, a pregnancy luteoma. Without special staining, melanin can be misinterpreted as lipochrome pigment, the presence of which may be a feature of steroid cell tumors and impart a dark green or almost black color to the neoplastic tissue. Like a variety of other metastases, occasional cases of metastatic melanoma contain follicle-like spaces (Fig. 22.31). The diagnosis of metastatic melanoma to the ovary may be suggested or confirmed in problem cases by the immunohistochemical demonstration of S100 protein and negative staining for keratin and other antigens.[57,139,140,205]

Lung Tumors

Only approximately 5% of women with lung cancer have ovarian metastases at autopsy,[10,65,115,148,210] and the surgical pathologist rarely encounters an ovarian tumor of this type. Exceptionally, an ovarian metastatic tumor either precedes the discovery of a pulmonary cancer or is found simultaneously.[120,166,224] It may be difficult in some cases to determine which tumor is primary. When the histologic features are typical of a lung carcinoma, such as an oat cell or squamous cell carcinoma, however, a pulmonary origin can be assumed (Fig. 22.32). Oat cell carcinomas, squamous cell carcinomas, adenocarcinomas, large cell undifferentiated carcinomas, and bronchial carcinoids have all been documented to spread to the ovary.[224]

Mediastinal Tumors

Thymomas, which spread beyond the thorax in no more than 20% of cases,[15] involve the ovary very rarely.[27,222] Two reports about the more aggressive thymic carcinoma do not mention metastases to the ovary.[183,217] We have recently seen a patient with an oat cell carcinoma, apparently of thymic origin, that had metastasized to the ovary at the time of presentation. An additional case in the literature of an ovarian tumor that was associated with Cushing's syndrome was probably an example of a metastatic oat cell carcinoma from the thymus.[143]

Miscellaneous Rare Tumors

Metastases to the ovary other than those discussed are of great rarity and generally only relevant to autopsy pathology. Carcinomas of the thyroid only exceptionally spread to the ovary,[63] even when they are of the anaplastic variety.[36] At least five examples are mentioned in the literature[70,93,117,220] and we have seen one example of follicular carcinoma that had metastasized to the ovaries by the time of autopsy.[172] A review of the literature on parathyroid carcinoma has not disclosed any examples of metastasis to the ovary. Rare examples of head and neck carcinoma metastatic to the ovary are documented,[151] and we have seen one patient in whom the primary tumor was an undifferentiated carcinoma of the ethmoid sinus. Salivary gland tumors also spread to the ovary with extreme rarity.[117] Mazur et al.[125] described a rhabdomyosarcoma of the parotid gland that was associated with ovarian spread. We have seen a young woman who had had an adenoid cystic carcinoma of the parotid gland excised at the age of 12 years, followed by local recurrence, lung metastasis, and bilateral symptomatic ovarian metastases 11 years after presentation.[172] This case emphasizes that a history of neoplasia of any type, even relatively remote, may be relevant in the evaluation of an unusual ovarian tumor.

Tumors of the central nervous system and cranium uncommonly metastasize distantly. Although pelvic spread has been documented in a considerable number of patients,[33,68,107,154] we are aware of only two reports in which ovarian spread is mentioned specifically. One was a case of metastatic meningioma to the ovary in Karsh's series,[102] and the other was a metastatic medulloblastoma in a 4-year-old girl, in whose ovary "a cleft near the hilum was full of tumor cells."[156] Tumors of the skin, other than malignant melanoma, rarely spread to the ovary. However, we have recently seen a case of Merkel cell tumor primary in the skin of the groin that metastasized to the ovary, producing a large, symptomatic mass; a similar case has been reported.[66]

Sarcomas, whether from the viscera or the soft tissues, uncommonly metastasize to the ovary,[214] except in late stages of the disease. Only occasional cases are mentioned in the literature.[77,212] We have seen one woman who had severe abdominal pain and at operation was found to have a leiomyosarcoma of the small intestine that had ruptured and was associated with bilateral ovarian metastases. Peritoneal spread of gastrointestinal leiomyosarcomas is relatively common[4,161,179] and undoubtedly has involved the ovarian surfaces in some other cases. Two cases of hemangiosarcoma that metastasized to the ovaries have been documented.[37,84] Metastases of bone tumors to the ovary are very rare[67,204]; a case of Ewing's sarcoma that spread to the ovary is included in one report,[220] and we have seen a primary osteosarcoma of the maxilla that produced a large metastatic tumor in the ovary.[172]

Very rarely, a metastatic tumor involves an ovary that contains a primary ovarian neoplasm.[89,97,125,182] One of these metastatic tumors was a cystosarcoma phyllodes of the breast metastatic to a Brenner tumor.[89] We have seen one Krukenberg tumor of gastric origin in an ovary containing a granulosa cell tumor and another involving an ovarian fibroma.[172]

References

1. Abrams HL, Spiro R, Goldstein N (1950) Metastases in carcinoma. Cancer 3: 74–85
2. Acosta-Sison H (1958) The relative frequency of various anatomic sites as the point of first metastasis in 32 cases of chorionepithelioma. Am J Obstet Gynecol 75: 1149–1152
3. Aguirre P, Scully RE (1982) Malignant neuroectodermal tumor of the ovary, a distinctive form of monodermal teratoma. Report of five cases. Am J Surg Pathol 6: 283–292
4. Akwari OE, Dozois RR, Weiland LH, Beahrs OH (1978) Leiomyosarcoma of the small and large bowel. Cancer 42: 1375–1384
5. Amorn Y, Knight WA (1978) Primary linitis plastica of the colon: Report of two cases and review of the literature. Cancer 41: 2420–2425
6. Anderson LL, Lad TE (1982) Autopsy findings in squamous-cell carcinoma of the esophagus. Cancer 50: 1587–1590
7. Andriole GL, Garnick MB, Richie JP (1985) Unusual behavior of low-grade, low-stage transitional cell carcinoma of bladder. Urology 25: 524–526
8. Antoniades K, Spector HB, Hecksher RH (1977) Prophylactic oophorectomy in conjunction with large-bowel resection for cancer. Report of two cases. Dis Colon Rectum 20: 506–510
9. Aron BS (1974) Wilms' tumor—A clinical study of eighty-one patients. Cancer 33: 637–646
10. Ask-Upmark E (1932) On the location of malignant metastases with special regard to the behavior of the primary malignant tumours of the lung. Acta Pathol Microbiol Scand 9: 239–248
11. Baab GH, McBride CM (1975) Malignant melanoma. The patient with an unknown site of primary origin. Arch Surg 110: 896–900
12. Babaian RJ, Johnson DE, Llamas L, Ayala AG (1980) Metastases from transitional cell carcinoma of urinary bladder. Urology 16: 142–144
13. Baggish MS, Woodruff JD (1972) Uterine stromatosis. Clinicopathologic features and hormone dependency. Obstet Gynecol 40: 487–498
14. Baltzer J, Lohe KJ, Lopcke W, Zander J (1981) Metastatischer befall der ovarien beim operierten plattenepithelkarzinom der zervix. Geburtsh Frauenheilk 41: 672–673
15. Batata MA, Martini N, Huvos AG, Aguilar RJ, Beattie EJ. (1974) Thymomas: Clinicopathological features, therapy and prognosis. Cancer 34: 389–396
16. Batata MA, Whitmore WF, Hilaris BS, Tokita N, Grabstald H. (1975) Primary carcinoma of the ureter. A prognostic study. Cancer 35: 1616–1632
17. Beck RP, Latour JPA (1963) Necropsy reports on 36 cases

of endometrial carcinoma. Am J Obstet Gynecol 85: 307–311

18. Ben David M, Feldberg D, Dicker D, Kessler H, Goldman JA (1984) Ovarian melanoma. An interesting case. Int J Gynaecol Obstet 22: 77–79
19. Bennington JL, Beckwith JB (1975) Tumors of the kidney, renal pelvis, and ureter. Atlas of Tumor Pathology, Second Series, Fascicle 12. Washington, DC, Armed Forces Institute of Pathology
20. Berardi RS (1972) Carcinoid tumors of the colon (exclusive of the rectum). Review of the literature. Dis Colon Rectum 15: 383–391
21. Black WC, Benitez RE (1964) Nonteratomatous squamous-cell carcinoma in situ of the ovary. Obstet Gynecol 24: 865–868
22. Blamey SL, McDermott FT, Pihl E, Hughes SR (1981) Resected ovarian recurrence from colorectal adenocarcinoma. A study of 13 cases. Dis Colon Rectum 24: 272–275
23. Block M, Gilbert E, Davis C (1984) Metastatic neuroblastoma arising in an ovarian teratoma with long-term survival. Case report and review of the literature. Cancer 54: 590–595
24. Brandt-Rauf PW, Pincus M, Adelson S (1982) Cancer of the gallbladder. A review of forty-three cases. Hum Pathol 13: 48–53
25. Breslow NE, Palmer NF, Hill LR, Buring J, D'Angio GJ (1978) Wilms' tumor. Prognostic factors for patients without metastasis at diagnosis. Results of the National Wilms' Tumor Study. Cancer 41: 1577–1589
26. Brickman M, Ferreira B (1967) Metastasis of breast carcinoma to the ovaries—incidence, significance, and relationship to survival. A preliminary study. Grace Hosp Bull 45: 44–49
27. Briese VV, Rohde E (1984) Ovarielle metastasierung eines thymoms. Zentralbl Gynakol 106: 473–476
28. Brown BL, Scharifker DA, Gordon R, Deppe GG, Cohen CJ (1980) Bronchial carcinoid tumor with ovarian metastasis. A light microscopic and ultrastructural study. Cancer 46: 543–546
29. Buller RE, Braga CA, Tanagho EA, Miller T (1983) Renal-cell carcinoma metastatic to the ovary. A case report. J Reprod Med 28: 217–220
30. Bullon A, Arseneau J, Prat J, Young RH, Scully RE (1981) Tubular Krukenberg tumor. A problem in histopathologic diagnosis. Am J Surg Pathol 5: 225–232
31. Bunker ML (1959) The terminal findings in endometrial carcinoma. Am J Obstet Gynecol 77: 530–538
32. Burt CAV (1951) Prophylactic oophorectomy with resection of the large bowel for cancer. Am J Surg 82: 571–577
33. Campbell AN, Chan HSL, Becker LE, Daneman A, Park TS, Hoffman HJ (1984) Extracranial metastases in childhood primary intracranial tumors. A report of 21 cases and review of the literature. Cancer 53: 974–981
34. Campbell JS, Magner D, Fournier P (1961) Adenocarcinoma of ovary and uterus occurring as coexisting or sequential primary neoplasms. Cancer 14: 817–826
35. Campbell JS, Lou P, Ferguson JP, Krongold I, Kemeny T, Mitton DM, Allan N (1973) Pseudomyxoma peritonei et ovarii with occult neoplasms of appendix. Obstet Gynecol 42: 897–902
36. Carcangiu ML, Steeper T, Zampi G, Rosai J (1985) Anaplastic thyroid carcinoma. A study of 70 cases. Am J Clin Pathol 83: 135–158
37. Case Records of the Massachusetts General Hospital (1975) Case 35–1975. N Engl J Med 293: 494–499
38. Chen KTK, Kostich ND, Rosai J (1978) Peritoneal foreign body granulomas to keratin in uterine adenoacanthoma. Arch Pathol Lab Med 102: 174–177
39. Choo YC, Naylor B (1982) Multiple primary neoplasms of the ovary and uterus. Int J Gynaecol Obstet 20: 327–334
40. Corwin S, Tassy F, Malament M, Grady H (1971) Rare signet-ring variant of mucinous adenocarcinoma of the bladder. J Urol 106: 697–700
41. Creasman WT, Lukeman J (1972) Role of the fallopian tube in dissemination of malignant cells in corpus cancer. Cancer 20: 456–457
42. Cubilla AL, Fitzgerald PJ (1979) Classification of pancreatic cancer (nonendocrine). Mayo Clin Proc 54: 449–458
43. Cubilla AL, Fitzgerald PJ (1978) Pancreas Cancer. I. Duct adenocarcinoma. A clinical–pathologic study of 380 patients. Pathol Ann 1:241–289
44. Cubilla AL, Fitzgerald PJ (1984) Tumors of the exocrine pancreas. In: Atlas of Tumor Pathology, Second Series, Fascicle 19. Washington, DC, Armed Forces Institute of Pathology
45. Cutait R, Lesser ML, Enker WE (1983) Prophylactic oophorectomy in surgery for large-bowel cancer. Dis Colon Rectum 26: 6–11
46. Cylwik B, Nowak HF, Glowinska L (1984) Malignant neoplasms of the pancreas. A study based on autopsy data from 1953 to 1982 in Bialystok, Poland. II. A survey of 195 cases. Neoplasma 31: 605–613
47. Czernobilsky B, Silverman BB, Mikuta JJ (1970) Endometrioid carcinoma of the ovary: A clinicopathologic study of 75 cases. Cancer 26: 1141–1152
48. Das Gupta T, Brasfield R (1964) Metastatic melanoma: A clinicopathological study. Cancer 17: 1323–1339
49. De Graaff J, Puyenbroek JI, VanDer Harten JJ (1984) Primary mucinous adenocarcinoma of the appendix with bilateral Krukenberg tumors of the ovary and primary adenocarcinoma of the endometrium. Gynecol Oncol 19: 358–364
50. de la Monte S, Hutchins GM, Moore GW (1984) Endocrine organ metastases from breast carcinoma. Am J Pathol 114: 131–136
51. Diddle AW (1955) Krukenberg tumors: Diagnostic problem. Cancer 8: 1026–1034
52. Didolkar MS, Bescher RA, Elias EG, Moore RH (1981) Natural history of adrenal cortical carcinoma: A clinicopathologic study of 42 patients. Cancer 47: 2153–2161
53. Dockerty MB (1954) Primary and secondary ovarian adenoacanthoma. Surg Gynecol Obstet 99: 392–400
54. Doss LL, Llorens AS, Henriquez EM (1984) Carcinosarcoma of the uterus: A 40-year experience from the state of Missouri. Gynecol Oncol 18: 43–53
55. Duarte I, Llanos O (1981) Patterns of metastases in intesti-

nal and diffuse types of carcinoma of the stomach. Hum Pathol 12: 237–242
56. Eifel P, Hendrickson M, Ross J, Ballon S, Martinez A, Kempson R (1982) Simultaneous presentation of carcinoma involving the ovary and the uterine corpus. Cancer 50: 163–170
57. Erlandson RA (1984) Diagnostic immunohistochemistry of human tumors. An interim evaluation. Am J Surg Pathol 8: 615–624
58. Fawcett FJ, Kimbell NKB (1971) Phaeochromocytoma of the ovary. J Obstet Gynaecol Br Commonw 78: 458–459
59. Fetter TR, Bogaev JH, McCuskey B, Seres JL (1959) Carcinoma of the bladder: Sites of metastases. J Urol 81: 746–748
60. Finn WF (1951) The diagnostic confusion of ovarian metastases from endometrial carcinoma with primary ovarian carcinoma. Am J Obstet Gynecol 62: 403–408
61. Fosså SD, Schjølseth SA, Miller A (1977) Multiple urothelial tumours with metastases to uterus and left ovary. A case report. Scand J Urol Nephrol 11: 81–84
62. Fox H, Langley FA. (1976) Metastatic tumors. In: Tumours of the Ovary. Chicago, Year Book Medical Publishers, pp 300–306
63. Franssila KA (1973) Is the differentiation between papillary and follicular thyroid carcinoma valid? Cancer 32: 853–864
64. Gadd C-B, Hellsten H, Knutson F (1960) Masculinovoblastoma (adrenal-like tumor). A rare virilizing ovarian tumor. Acta Obstet Gynecol Scand 39: 239–258
65. Galluzzi S, Payne PM (1955) Bronchial carcinoma: A statistical study of 741 necropsies with special reference to the distribution of blood-borne metastases. Br J Cancer 9: 511–527
66. George TK, di Sant'Agnese PA, Bennett JM (1985) Chemotherapy for metastatic Merkel cell carcinoma. Cancer 56: 1034–1038
67. Giuliano AE, Feig S, Eilber FR (1984) Changing metastatic patterns of osteosarcoma. Cancer 54: 2160–2164
68. Glasauer FE, Yuan RHP (1963) Intracranial tumors with extracranial metastases. Case report and review of the literature. J Neurosurg 20: 474–493
69. Gloor E (1978) Un cas de syndrome de Peutz-Jeghers associé à un carcinome mammaire bilatéral à un adénocarcinome du col utérin et à des tumeurs des cordons sexuels à tubules annelés bilatérales dans les ovaires. Schweiz Med Wochenschr 108: 717–721
70. Gordon PR, Huvos AG, Strong EW (1973) Medullary carcinoma of the thyroid gland. A clinicopathologic study of 40 cases. Cancer 31: 915–923
71. Grabstaldt H, Hilaris B, Henschke U, Whitmore WF Jr (1966) Cancer of the female urethra. JAMA 197: 113–120
72. Graffner HOL, Alm POA, Oscarson JEA (1983) Prophylactic oophorectomy in colorectal carcinoma. Am J Surg 146: 233–235
73. Graves RC, Guiss LW (1941) Tumors of the urethra. J Urol 46: 925–947
74. Green TH Jr, Scully RE (1962) Tumors of the fallopian tube. Clin Obstet Gynecol 5: 886–906
75. Greene HJ, Grusetz MW, Mackles A (1969) Subsequent second primary and metastatic cancer of the ovary. Clin Obstet Gynecol 12: 972–979
76. Gromet MA, Epstein WL, Blois MS (1978) The regressing thin malignant melanoma. A distinctive lesion with metastatic potential. Cancer 42: 2282–2292
77. Hajdu SI, Shiu MH, Fortner JG (1977) Tendosynovial sarcoma. A clinicopathological study of 136 cases. Cancer 39: 1201–1217
78. Hale RW (1968) Krukenberg tumor of the ovaries. A review of 81 records. Obstet Gynecol 32: 221–225
79. Hallgrimsson J, Scully RE (1972) Borderline and malignant Brenner tumours of the ovary. A report of 15 cases. Acta Pathol Microbiol Scand [A Suppl] 233: 56–66
80. Hameed K (1973) Melanotic ovarian neoplasms. Prog Clin Cancer 5: 209–217
81. Harcourt KF, Dennis DL (1968) Laparotomy for "ovarian tumors" in unsuspected carcinoma of the colon. Cancer 21: 1244–1246
82. Harris M, Howell A, Chrissohou M, Swindell RIC, Hudson M, Sellwood RA (1984) A comparison of the metastatic pattern of infiltrating lobular carcinoma and infiltrating duct carcinoma of the breast. Br J Cancer 50: 23–30
83. Hart WR, Billman JK (1978) A reassessment of uterine neoplasms originally diagnosed as leiomyosarcomas. Cancer 41: 1902–1910
84. Hermann GG, Fogh J, Graem N, Hansen OP, Hippe E (1984) Primary hemangiosarcoma of the spleen with angioscintigraphic demonstration of metastases. Cancer 53: 1682–1685
85. Herrera LO, Ledesma EJ, Natarajan N, Lopez GE, Tsukada Y, Mittelman A (1982) Metachronous ovarian metastases from adenocarcinoma of the colon and rectum. Surg Gynecol Obstet 154: 531–533
86. Herrera-Ornelas L, Natarajan N, Tsukada Y, Prado-Alcala E, Gutierrez-Garcia CJ, Piver S, Mittelman A (1983) Adenocarcinoma of the colon masquerading as primary ovarian neoplasia. An analysis of ten cases. Dis Colon Rectum 26: 377–380
87. Higuchi K, Kato T (1958) Dysgerminoma of the ovary. J Jpn Obstet Gynecol Soc 5: 206–215
88. Himelstein-Braw R, Peters H, Faber M (1977) Influence of irradiation and chemotherapy on the ovaries of children with abdominal tumors. Br J Cancer 36: 269–275
89. Hines JR, Gordon RT, Widger C, et al. (1976) Cystosarcoma phyllodes metastatic to a Brenner tumor of the ovary. Arch Surg 111: 299–300
90. Hirschfield LS, Kahn LB, Winkler B, Bochner RZ, Gibstein AA (1985) Adenocarcinoid of the appendix presenting as bilateral Krukenberg's tumor of the ovaries. Arch Pathol Lab Med 109: 930–933
91. Holtz F, Hart WR (1982) Krukenberg tumors of the ovary. A clinicopathologic analysis of 27 cases. Cancer 50: 2438–2447
92. Hopping RA, Dockerty MB, Masson JC (1942) Carcinoid tumor of the appendix. Report of a case in which extensive intra-abdominal metastases occurred, including involvement of the right ovary. Arch Surg 45: 613–622
93. Ibanez ML, Cole VW, Russell WO, Clark RL (1967) Solid

carcinoma of the thyroid gland. Analysis of 53 cases. Cancer 20: 706–723
94. Ishii T, Ikegami N, Hosoda Y, Koide O, Kaneko M (1981) The biological behaviour of gastric cancer. J Pathol 134: 97–115
95. Israel SL, Helsel EV, Hausman DH (1965) The challenge of metastatic ovarian carcinoma. Am J Obstet Gynecol 93: 1094–1101
96. James PD, Taylor CW, Templeton AC (1973) Tumors of the female genitalia. In: Tumours in a tropical country, Templeton AC (ed). New York, Springer-Verlag
97. Janovski NO, Paramanandhan TL (1973) Major problems in obstetrics and gynecology. In: Ovarian tumors. Tumors and tumor-like conditions of the ovaries, fallopian tubes and ligaments of the uterus. Philadelphia, WB Saunders, Vol 4, 134–135
98. Jensen PA, Dockerty MB, Symmonds RE, Wilson RB (1966) Endometrioid sarcoma ("stromal endometriosis"). Report of 15 cases including 5 with metastases. Am J Obstet Gynecol 95: 79–90
99. Johansson H (1960) Clinical aspects of metastatic ovarian cancer of extragenital origin. Acta Obstet Gynecol Scand 39: 681–697
100. Joshi VV (1968) Primry Krukenberg tumor of ovary. Review of literature and case report. Cancer 22: 1199–1207
101. Kaminski PF, Norris HJ (1984) Coexistence of ovarian neoplasms and endocervical adenocarcinoma. Obstet Gynecol 64: 553–556
102. Karsh J (1951) Secondary malignant disease of the ovaries. A study of 72 autopsies. Am J Obstet Gynecol 61: 154–160
103. Kashani M, Levy M (1983) Primary adenocarcinoma of the appendix with bilateral Krukenberg ovarian tumors. J Surg Oncol 22: 101–105
104. Kasilag FB, Jr, Rutledge FN (1957) Metastatic breast carcinoma in ovary. Am J Obstet Gynecol 74: 989–992
105. Kishi K, Hirota T, Matsumoto K, Kakizo ET, Murase T, Fujita J (1981) Carcinoma of the bladder: A clinical and pathological analysis of 87 autopsy cases. J Urol 125: 36–39
106. Klein HZ (1974) Mucinous carcinoid tumor of the vermiform appendix. Cancer 33: 770–777
107. Kleinman GM, Hochberg FH, Richardson EP Jr (1981) Systemic metastases from medulloblastoma: Report of two cases and review of the literature. Cancer 48: 2296–2309
108. Knoepp LF, Ray JE, Overby I (1973) Ovarian metastases from colorectal carcinoma. Dis Colon Rectum 16: 305–311
109. Kubo T, Watanabe H (1971) Neoplastic argentaffin cells in gastric and intestinal carcinomas. Cancer 27: 447–454
110. Kumar NB, Hart WR (1982) Metastases to the uterine corpus from extragenital cancers. A clinicopathologic study of 63 cases. Cancer 50: 2163–2169
111. Kurman RJ, Scully RE, Norris HJ (1976) Trophoblastic pseudotumor of the uterus. An exaggerated form of "syncytial endometritis" simulating a malignant tumor. Cancer 38: 1214–1226
112. Lasaponara F, Pagliano GL, Rizzello N (1983) Metastasi rivelatrici de neoplasia renale. Minerva Urol 35: 195–200
113. Lee YN, Hori JM (1971) Significance of ovarian metastases in therapeutic oophorectomy for advanced breast cancer. Cancer 27: 1374–1378
114. Lemerle J, Tournade M-F, Gerard-Marchant R, Flamant R, Sarrazin D, Flamant F, Lemerle M, Jundt S, Zucker J-M, Schweisguth O. (1976) Wilms' tumor: Natural history and prognostic factors. A retrospective study of 248 cases treated at the Institut Gustave-Roussy 1952–1967. Cancer 37: 2557–2566
115. Line DH, Deeley TJ (1971) The necropsy findings in carcinoma of the bronchus. Br J Dis Chest 65: 238–242
116. LiVolsi VA, Merino MJ, Schwartz PE (1983) Coexistent endocervical adenocarcionoma and mucinous adenocarcinoma of ovary: A clinicopathological study of four cases. Int J Gynecol Pathol 1: 391–402
117. Luisi A (1968) Metastatic ovarian tumours. In: UICC Monograph Series. Ovarian cancer, Gentil F, Junqueira AC (eds). Berlin, Heidelberg, New York, Springer-Verlag, Vol II, pp 87–104
118. Lumb G, Mackenzie DH (1959) The incidence of metastases in adrenal glands and ovaries removed for carcinoma of the breast. Cancer 12: 521–526
119. MacKeigan JM, Ferguson JA (1979) Prophylactic oophorectomy and colorectal cancer in premenopausal patients. Dis Colon Rectum 22: 401–405
120. Malviya VK, Bansal M, Chahinian P, Deppe G, Lauresen N, Gordon RE (1982) Small cell anaplastic lung cancer presenting as an ovarian metastasis. Int J Gynaecol Obstet 20: 487–493
121. Mandard AM, Chasle J, Marnay J, Villedieu B, Bianco C, Roussel A, Elie H, Vernhes JC (1981) Autopsy findings in 111 cases of esophageal cancer. Cancer 48: 329–335
122. Martinelli G, Tapparelli E, Merz R, Aldovini D, Zumiani G (1984) Case of bilateral ovarian metastasis from regressed melanoma. Eur J Gynaecol Oncol 5: 150–153
123. Martzloff KH, Manlove CH (1949) Vaginal and ovarian metastases from hypernephroma. Case report and review of the literature. Surg Gynecol Obstet 88: 145–154
124. Masson P, Martin JF (1928) Sur la présence des cellules de Kultschitzky dans un épithelioma cylindrique de l'estomac et ses metastases. Bull Assoc Franç Etude Cancer 17: 139–145
125. Mazur MT, Hsueh S, Gersell DJ (1984) Metastases to the female genital tract. Analysis of 325 cases. Cancer 53: 1978–1984
126. McKenna H, Ritchie G, Monks P (1978) Pseudomyxoma peritonei et ovarii with an occult neoplasm of appendix: Case report. Pathology 10: 157–160
127. Merino MJ, Livolsi VA (1981) Signet-ring carcinoma of the female breast: A clinicopathological analysis of 24 cases. Cancer 48: 1830–1837
128. Merino MJ, Edmonds P, LiVolsi VA (1985) Appendiceal carcinoma metastatic to the ovaries and mimicking primary ovarian tumors. Int J Gynecol Pathol 4: 110–120
129. Merlo M, Brown CH, Hazard JB (1960) Gastric carcinoma: Report of twelve patients surviving longer than fifteen years. Cleve Clin Q 27: 235–239
130. Meyer WH, Yu GW, Milvenan ES, Jeffs RD, Kaizer H, Leventhal BG (1979) Ovarian involvement in neuroblastoma. Med Pediatr Oncol 7: 49–54
131. Michaels L, Langley FA (1957) Mesenchymal tumours

of the uterus resembling the haemangiopericytoma. J Obstet Gynaec Br Commonw 64: 561–565
132. Mills SE, Allen MS (1979) Colorectal carcinoma in the first three decades of life. Am J Surg Pathol 3: 443–448
133. Milton GW, Lane Brown MM, Gilder M (1967) Malignant melanoma with an occult primary lesion. Br J Surg 54: 651–658
134. Moertel CG (1968) The natural history of advanced gastric cancer. Surg Gynecol Obstet 126: 1071–1074
135. Morrow CP, DiSaia PJ (1976) Malignant melanoma of the female genitalia: A clinical analysis. Obstet Gynecol Surv 31: 233–271
136. Morrow M, Enker WE (1984) Late ovarian metastases in carcinoma of the colon and rectum. Arch Surg 119: 1385–1388
137. Munnell EW, Taylor HC Jr (1949) Ovarian carcinoma. A review of 200 primary and 51 secondary cases. Am J Obstet Gynecol 58: 943–959
138. Nader S, Hickey RC, Sellin RV, Samaan NA (1983) Adrenal cortical carcinoma. A study of 77 cases. Cancer 52: 707–711
139. Nakajima T, Watanabe S, Sato Y, Kameya T, Hirota T, Shimosato Y (1982) An immunoperoxidase study of S100 protein distribution in normal and neoplastic tissues. Am J Surg Pathol 6: 715–727
140. Nakajima T, Watanabe S, Sato Y, Kameya T, Shimosato Y, Ishihara K (1982) Immunohistochemical demonstration of S100 protein in malignant melanoma and pigmented nevus, and its diagnostic application. Cancer 50: 912–918
141. Nakashima T, Okuda K, Kojiro M, Jimi A, Yamaguchi R, Sakamoto K, Ikari T (1983) Pathology of hepatocellular carcinoma in Japan: 232 consecutive cases autopsied in ten years. Cancer 51: 863–877
142. Nelson HM, Hagerty JR (1962) Endolymphatic stromal myosis. Report of 2 cases and review of the literature. Obstet Gynecol 20: 180–188
143. Norris EH (1938) Arrhenoblastoma. A malignant ovarian tumor associated with endocrinological effects. Am J Cancer 32: 1–29
144. Norris HJ, Taylor HB (1966) Mesenchymal tumors of the uterus. III. A clinical and pathologic study of 31 carcinosarcomas. Cancer 19: 1459–1465
145. Norris HJ, Roth E, Taylor HB (1966) Mesenchymal tumors of the uterus. II. A clinical and pathologic study of 31 mixed mesodermal tumors. Obstet Gynecol 28: 57–63
146. Ober WB, Edgcomb JH, Price EB Jr (1970) The pathology of choriocarcinoma. Ann NY Acad Sci 172: 299–426
147. O'Brien PH, Newton BB. Metcalf JS, Rittenbury MS (1981) Oophorectomy in women with carcinoma of the colon and rectum. Surg Gynecol Obstet 153: 827–830
148. Ochsner A, DeBakey M (1942) Significance of metastasis in primary carcinoma of the lungs. Report of two cases with unusual site of metastasis. J Thorac Surg 11: 357–387
149. Odone V, Chang L, Caces J, George SL, Pratt CB (1982) The natural history of colorectal carcinoma in adolescents. Cancer 49: 1716–1720
150. Ootman EH, Elliott JP (1983) Hepatocellular carcinoma metastatic to the ovary: A case report. Am J Obstet Gynecol 146: 715–718
151. Orr JW, Grizzle WE, Huddleston JF (1982) Squamous cell carcinoma metastatic to placenta and ovary. Obstet Gynecol 59: 81S–83S
152. Osborne MP, Pitts RM (1961) Therapeutic oophorectomy for advanced breast cancer. The significance of metastases to the ovary and of ovarian cortical stromal hyperplasia. Cancer 14: 126–130
153. Park WLH, Lees JC (1950) Choriocarcinoma. A general review, with an analysis of five hundred sixteen cases. Arch Pathol 49: 205–241
154. Pasquier B, Pasquier D, N'Golet A, Panh MH, Couderc P (1980) Extraneural metastases of astrocytomas and glioblastomas. Clinicopathological study of two cases and review of the literature. Cancer 45: 112–125
155. Patel NP, Lavengood RW (1978) Renal cell carcinoma: Natural history and results of treatment. J Urol 119: 722–726
156. Paterson E (1961) Distant metastases from medulloblastoma of the cerebellum. Brain 84: 301–309
157. Pitluk H, Poticha SM (1983) Carcinoma of the colon and rectum in patients less than 40 years of age. Surg Gynecol Obstet 157: 335–337
158. Posso MA, Berg GA, Murphy AI, Totten RS (1961) Mucinous adenocarcinoma of the urethra: Report of a case associated with urethritis glandularis. J Urol 85: 944–948
159. Prat J, Bhan AK, Dickersin GR, Robboy SJ, Scully RE (1982) Hepatoid yolk sac tumor of the ovary (endodermal sinus tumor with hepatoid differentiation). A light microscopic, ultrastructural and immunohistochemical study of seven cases. Cancer 50: 2355–2368
160. Puga FJ, Gibbs CP, Williams TJ (1973) Castrating operations associated with metastatic lesions of the breast. Obstet Gynecol 41: 713–719
161. Ranchod M, Kempson RL (1977) Smooth muscle tumors of the gastrointestinal tract and retroperitoneum. A pathologic analysis of 100 cases. Cancer 39: 255–262
162. Rendelman DF, Gilchrist RK (1959) Indications for oophorectomy in carcinoma of the gastrointestinal tract. Surg Gynecol Obstet 109: 364–366
163. Richardson GS (1967) Case Records of the Massachusetts General Hospital Case 10–1067. N Engl J Med 276: 519–523
164. Robboy SJ, Herbst AL, Scully RE (1974) Clear-cell adenocarcinoma of the vagina and cervix in young females: Analysis of 37 tumors that persisted or recurred after primary therapy. Cancer 34: 606–614
165. Robboy SJ, Scully RE, Norris HJ (1974) Carcinoid metastatic to the ovary. A clinicopathologic analysis of 35 cases. Cancer 33: 798–811
166. Rogers WL (1932) Primary cancer of the lung. A clinical and pathologic survey of fifty cases. Arch Intern Med 49: 1058–1077
167. Rosas-Uribe A, Luna M (1969) Primary signet-ring cell carcinoma of the urinary bladder. Arch Pathol 88: 294–297
168. Russell P, Bannatyne PM, Solomon HJ, Stoddard LD, Tattersall MHN (1985) Multifocal tumorigenesis in the

upper female genital tract—Implications for staging and management. Int J Gynecol Pathol 4: 192–210
169. Saitoh H (1981) Distant metastasis of renal adenocarcinoma. Cancer 48: 1487–1491
170. Santesson L, Kottmeier HL (1968) General classification of ovarian tumours. In: UICC Monograph Series, Ovarian cancer, Gentil F, Junqueira AC (eds). Berlin, Heidelberg, New York, Springer-Verlag, Vol II, pp 1–8
171. Saphir O (1951) Signet-ring cell carcinoma. Mil Surg 109: 360–369
172. Scully RE Personal observations
173. Scully RE (1979) Tumors of the ovary and maldeveloped gonads. In: Atlas of Tumor Pathology, Second Series, Fascicle 16. Washington, DC, Armed Forces Institute of Pathology, pp 323–352
174. Scully RE, Richardson GS (1961) Luteinization of the stroma of metastatic cancer involving the ovary and its endocrine significance. Cancer 14: 827–840
175. Scully RE, Aguirre P, DeLellis RA (1984) Argyrophilia, serotonin and peptide hormones in the female genital tract and its tumors. Int J Gynecol Pathol 3: 51–70
176. Sedlis A (1961) Primary carcinoma of the fallopian tube. Obstet Gynecol Surv 16: 209–226
177. Shanks HGI (1961) Pseudomyxoma peritonei. J Obstet Gynaecol Br Commonw 68: 212–224
178. Shingleton HM, Middleton FF, Gore H (1974) Squamous cell carcinoma in the ovary. Am J Obstet Gynecol 120: 556–560
179. Shiu MH, Farr GH, Papachristou DN, Hajdu SI (1982) Myosarcomas of the stomach: Natural history, prognostic factors and management. Cancer 49: 177–187
180. Silva TF, Friedell GH, Parsons L (1959) Pelvic exenteration for carcinoma of the cervix. Clinicopathological study of sixty operations. N Engl J Med 260: 519–525
181. Silveira E, Badan-Palhares FA, Antunes de Oliveira Filho J, et al (1977) Peritonitis following rupture of metastatic malignant melanoma of the ovary. Gynecol Oncol 5: 304–307
182. Smale L (1980) Metastatic breast adenocarcinoma to Brenner tumors. Gynecol Oncol 9: 251–253
183. Snover D, Levine GD, Rosai J (1982) Thymic carcinoma: Five distinct histological variants. Am J Surg Pathol 6: 451–470
184. Sons HU, Borchard F (1984) Esophageal cancer. Autopsy findings in 171 cases. Arch Pathol Lab Med 108: 983–988
185. Spadoni LR, Lindberg MC, Mottet NK, et al (1965) Virilization co-existing with Krukenberg tumor during pregnancy. Am J Obstet Gynecol 92: 981–991
186. Spratt JS (1983) What to do about ovarian metastases from colonic adenocarcinomas. Am J Surg 146: 286
187. Stadiem ML (1937) An ovarian hypernephroma. Am J Surg 37: 312–318
188. Stearns MW, Deddish MR (1959) Five-year results of abdominal pelvic lymph node dissection for carcinoma of the rectum. Dis Colon Rectum 2: 169–172
189. Stensberg AJ (1964) Ovariemetastaser fra tumorer i colon og rectum. Ugeskrift Laeger 126: 343–346
190. Stone WS (1916) Metastatic carcinoma of ovaries. Surg Gynecol Obstet 22: 407–423
191. Sty JR, Kun LE, Casper JT (1980) Bone scintigraphy in neuroblastoma with ovarian metastasis. Wis Med J 79: 28–29
192. Subbuswamy SG, Gibbs NM, Ross CF, Morson BC (1974) Goblet cell carcinoid of the appendix. Cancer 34: 338–344
193. Svenes KB, Eide J (1984) Proliferative Brenner tumor or ovarian metastases? A case report. Cancer 53: 2692–2697
194. Tahara E, Ito H, Nakagami K, Shimamoto F, Yamamoto M, Sumii K (1982) Scirrhous argyrohpil cell carcinoma of the stomach with multiple production of polypeptide hormones, amine, CEA, lysozyme, and HCG. Cancer 49: 1904–1915
195. Takita H, Vincent RG, Caicedo V, Gutierrez AC (1977) Squamous cell carcinoma of the esophagus: A study of 153 cases. J Surg Oncol 9: 547–554
196. Talerman A (1984) Carcinoid tumors of the ovary. J Cancer Res Clin Oncol 107: 125–135
197. Thatcher SS, Woodruff JD (1982) Uterine stromatosis: A report of 33 cases. Obstet Gynecol 59: 428–434
198. Thiery M, Willighagen R (1966) Melanoma of the female genital tract. Gynaecologia 161: 466–480
199. Tsukada Y, Hewett WJ, Barlow JJ, Pickren JW (1972) Clear-cell adenocarcinoma (mesonephroma) of the vagina. Three cases associated with maternal synthetic nonsteroid estrogen therapy. Cancer 29: 1208–1214
200. Turksoy N (1960) Ovarian metastasis of breast carcinoma. A surgical surprise. Obstet Gynecol 15: 573–578
201. Ulbright TM, Roth LM (1985) Metastatic and independent cancers of the endometrium and ovary: A clinicopathologic study of 34 cases. Hum Pathol 16: 28–34
202. Ulbright TM, Roth LM (1985) Secondary tumors of the ovary. In: Tumors and tumor-like conditions of the ovary. Contemporary issues in surgical pathology, Roth LM, Czernobilsky B (eds). New York, Churchill-Livingstone, No 6, pp 129–152
203. Ulbright TM, Roth LM, Stehman FB (1984) Secondary ovarian neoplasia. A clinicopathologic study of 35 cases. Cancer 53: 1164–1174
204. Uribe-Botero G, Russell WO, Sutow WW, Martin RG (1977) Primary osteosarcoma of bone. A clinicopathologic investigation of 243 cases, with necropsy studies in 54. Am J Clin Pathol 67: 427–435
205. van Duinen SG, Ruiter DJ, Hageman P, Vennegoor C, Dickersin GR, Scheffer E, Rumke P (1984) Immunohistochemical and histochemical tools in the diagnosis of amelanotic melanoma. Cancer 53: 1566–1573
206. Varela-Duran J, Nochomovitz LE, Prem KA, Dehner LP (1980) Postirradiation mixed müllerian tumors of the uterus. A comparative clinicopathologic study. Cancer 45: 1625–1631
207. Viadana E, Bross IDJ, Pickren JW (1973) An autopsy study of some routes of dissemination of cancer of the breast. Br J Cancer 27: 336–340
208. Vorder-Bruegge CG, Hobbs JE, Wegner CR, Wintemute RW (1957) Bilateral ovarian metastases from renal adenocarcinoma: Report of a case and discussion of pathogenesis. Obstet Gynecol 9: 198–205
209. Warkel RL, Cooper PH, Helwig EB (1978) Adenocarci-

noid, a mucin-producing carcinoid tumor of the appendix. A study of 39 cases. Cancer 42: 2781–2793
210. Warren S, Gates O (1964) Lung cancer and metastasis. Arch Pathol 78: 467–473
211. Warren S, Macomber WB (1935) Tumor metastasis. VI. Ovarian metastasis of carcinoma. Arch Pathol 19: 75–82
212. Webb MJ, Decker DG, Mussey E (1975) Cancer metastatic to the ovary. Factors influencing survival. Obstet Gynecol 45: 391–396
213. Wei P-Y, Ouyang P-C (1963) Trophoblastic disease in Taiwan. A review of 157 cases in a 10-year period. Am J Obstet Gynecol 85: 844–849
214. Weiss SW, Enzinger FM (1978) Malignant fibrous histiocytoma. An analysis of 200 cases. Cancer 41: 2250–2266
215. Weitberg AB, Weitzman SA (1983) Metastatic islet cell carcinoma: A potentially treatable cause of "carcinoma of unknown origin." CA 33: 167
216. Wheelock MC, Putong P (1959) Ovarian metastases from adenocarcinomas of colon and rectum. Obstet Gynecol 14: 291–295
217. Wick M, Scheithauer BW, Weiland LH, Bernatz PE (1982) Primary thymic carcinomas. Am J Surg Pathol 6: 613–630
218. Woodruff JD, Julian CG (1969) Multiple malignancy in the upper genital canal. Am J Obstet Gynecol 103: 810–822
219. Woodruff JD, Novak ER (1960) The Krukenberg tumor. Study of 48 cases from the Ovarian Tumor Registry. Obstet Gynecol 15: 351–360
220. Woodruff JD, Murthy YS, Bhaskar TN, Bordbar F, Tseng S-S (1970) Metastatic ovarian tumors. Am J Obstet Gynecol 107: 202–209
221. Yoonessi M, Hart WR (1977) Endometrial stromal sarcomas. Cancer 40: 898–906
222. Yoshida A, Shigematsu T, Mori H, Yoshida H, Fukunishi R (1981) Non-invasive thymoma with widespread blood-borne metastasis. Virchows Arch [Pathol Anat] 390: 121–126
223. Young RH, Scully RE (1987) Mucinous ovarian tumors associated with mucinous adenocarcinomas of the cervix. A clinicopathological analysis of 16 cases. Submitted for publication.
224. Young RH, Scully RE (1985) Ovarian metastases from cancer of the lung: Problems in interpretation. A report of seven cases. Gynecol Oncol 21: 337–350
225. Young RH, Scully RE (1985) Ovarian Sertoli-Leydig cell tumors. A clinicopathological analysis of 207 cases. Am J Surg Pathol 9: 543–569
226. Young RH, Carey RW, Robboy SJ (1981) Breast carcinoma masquerading as a primary ovarian neoplasm. Cancer 48: 210–212
227. Young RH, Prat J, Scully RE (1984) Endometrioid stromal sarcomas of the ovary. A clinicopathologic analysis of 23 cases. Cancer 53: 1143–1155
228. Zaino RJ, Unger ER, Whitney C (1984; 1985) Synchronous carcinomas of the uterine corpus and ovary. Gynecol Oncol 19: 329–335; 21: 337–350

23

Diseases of the Placenta

Deborah J. Gersell, M.D., Frederick T. Kraus, M.D., and Maureen Burke Riffle, M.D.

Development and Anatomy

The placenta, unfortunately, is often ignored, not only by gynecologists and pediatricians but by pathologists as well. The evaluation of a diseased or dead fetus is really incomplete without the examination of its most accessible organ, the placenta. During intrauterine life, the mother, fetus, umbilical cord, membranes, and placenta are all components of a single system, and disease in any one part may profoundly affect the others. Opportunities for examination of the maternal component are limited, since maternal tissue is scant, consisting only of a small amount of decidua adherent to the fetal membranes or basal plate. The placenta, however, is readily available for study, and its examination may provide significant information relating to intrauterine or perinatal death, intrauterine growth retardation, malformations, infections, and the effects of maternal disease on fetal growth and development. As in any organ, appreciation of pathologic changes demands a sound knowledge of normal structure and development. Unlike more static tissues, the placenta undergoes a series of profound morphologic changes during its short life span, making an understanding of the normal somewhat more difficult.

Development

Among the many excellent treatises devoted to the description of implantation and the various stages in the development of the placenta, the monograph by Boyd and Hamilton[51] provides exhaustive and beautifully detailed illustrations and thorough coverage of the historical aspects of human implantation.

The ovum is fertilized in the fallopian tube. After rapid conversion to a blastocyst, the outer cell layer differentiates into the trophoblast, which completely envelops the previllous blastocyst. The embryo will ultimately be derived from the inner cell mass. The trophoblastic cell mass attaches to and penetrates the endometrium on the 6th to 7th postovulatory day. By the 10th to 11th day, the ovum is totally embedded in the endometrial stroma, and the superficial endometrial epithelium has reestablished its continuity. The trophoblastic cell mass differentiates into an inner layer of cytotrophoblast, characterized by uniform cells with clear cytoplasm, distinct cell membranes, and vesicular nuclei, and an outer layer of syncytiotrophoblast, multinucleated cells with dense pyknotic nuclei suspended in abundant amphophilic cytoplasm. Between the cytotrophoblast and syncytiotrophoblast are large mononucleate cells with abundant amphophilic cytoplasm. These cells have some features of both cytotrophoblast and syncytiotrophoblast and have been designated *intermediate trophoblast*[148] (see Chapter 24, Gestational Trophoblastic Disease).

Between the 9th and 13th postovulatory day, blood-filled lacunae form within the rapidly growing trophoblastic mass and separate it into trabecular columns (Fig. 23.1). Thereafter (14th to 20th day), the syncytiotrophoblast of the columns becomes radially oriented around central solid cores of cytotrophoblast. The cytotrophoblast continues to grow peripherally and, at the same time, is penetrated by extraembryonic mesenchyme within which small vessels form. These vessels eventually establish continuity with other vessels forming in the inner chorionic mesenchyme and body stalk, and by

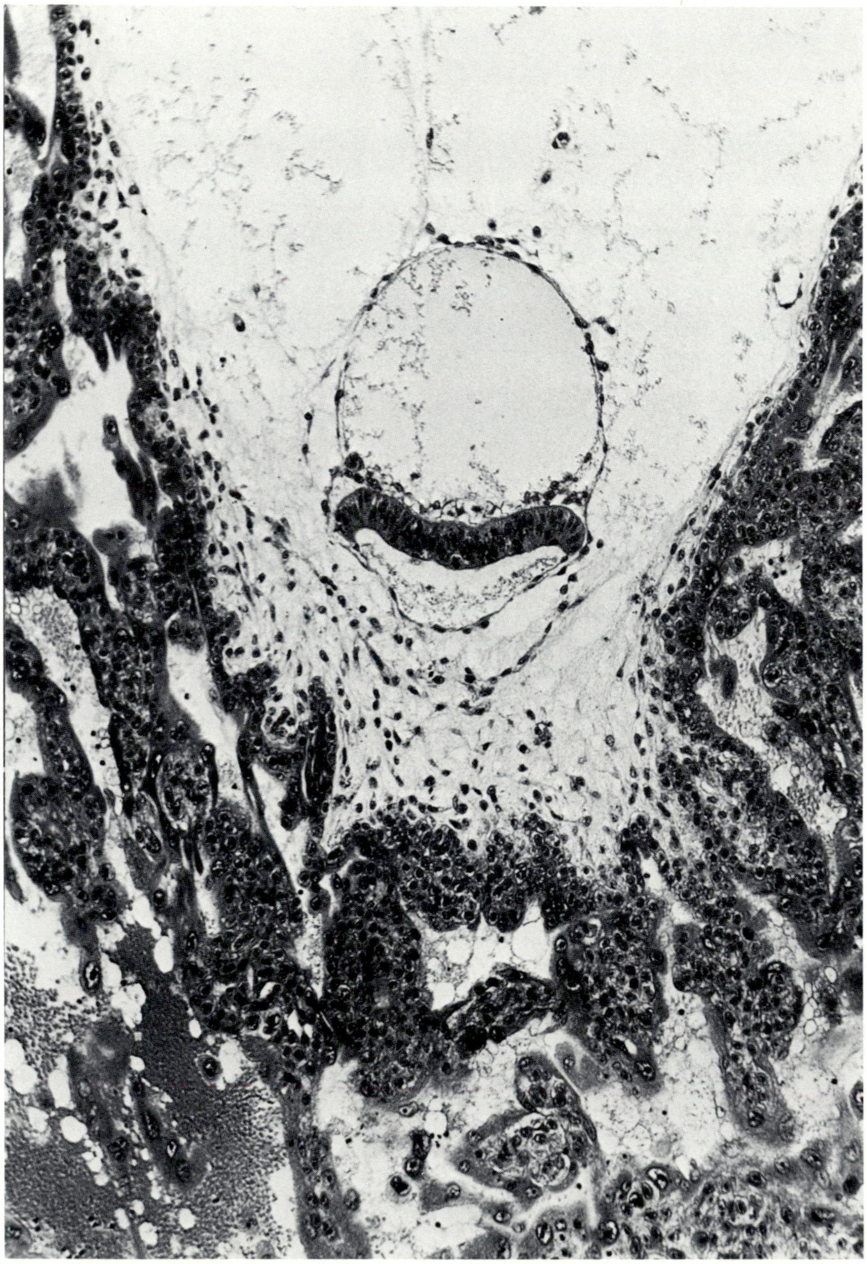

FIG. 23.1. Implantation at 13 days. Trophoblast has differentiated into inner (cytotrophoblast) and outer (syncytiotrophoblast) layers. Focally, the cytotrophoblast has proliferated to form projections, the forerunners of the primary villi. The germ disc is located near the center. (Reprinted courtesy of Department of Embryology, Davis Division, Carnegie Institute of Washington.)

21 days, the placenta is a vascularized, villous organ. Branching and growth of new villi from the primary villous stems follow the same sequence, sprouting of syncytiotrophoblast, intrusion of a cytotrophoblastic core, ingrowth of mesenchyme, and eventual vascularization. This process may continue throughout gestation.[227]

The most peripheral portions of the primary stem villi consist of solid aggregates of cytotrophoblast and intermediate trophoblast, which anchor the villi to the basal plate (Fig. 23.2). The masses of intermediate and cytotrophoblast grow laterally and circumferentially to form a complete shell, which continues to expand and enlarge the intervillous space (Fig. 23.3). The decidua and myometrium at the placental site are diffusely infiltrated by trophoblast. This mingling of trophoblast and decidua is so intimate that it may be difficult to characterize any particular cell as being maternal or fetal in origin with the light microscope. Intermediate trophoblast appears to be the predominant form of trophoblast in the implantation site. In this location, intermediate trophoblastic cells vary greatly in appearance from mononucleate to multinucleate to spindle shaped.

The intermediate trophoblast is also responsible for a remarkable sequence of structural modifications that occurs in the maternal circulation in pregnancy. This process is detailed in the discussion of preeclampsia but basically involves trophoblastic invasion and destruction of the decidual and myometrial segments of the spiral arteries by the intermediate trophoblast (Fig. 23.4). The vascular dilatation that occurs as a consequence of these alterations both increases blood flow to the placenta and effects a considerable blood pressure drop.

Continued growth and enlargement of the chorion result in eventual obliteration of the uterine cavity through fusion of the decidua capsularis and the decidua vera of the opposite uterine wall. This is usually achieved by 20 weeks. During this time, the villi that are oriented toward the uterine cavity undergo progressive atrophy to form the *chorion laeve* (smooth chorion). Remnants of these atrophic villi are still apparent in sections of the extraplacental membranes of the mature placenta (Fig. 23.5). The chorion frondosum, those villi on the embryonic aspect of the chorion that directly contact the decidua basalis, continue to proliferate and form

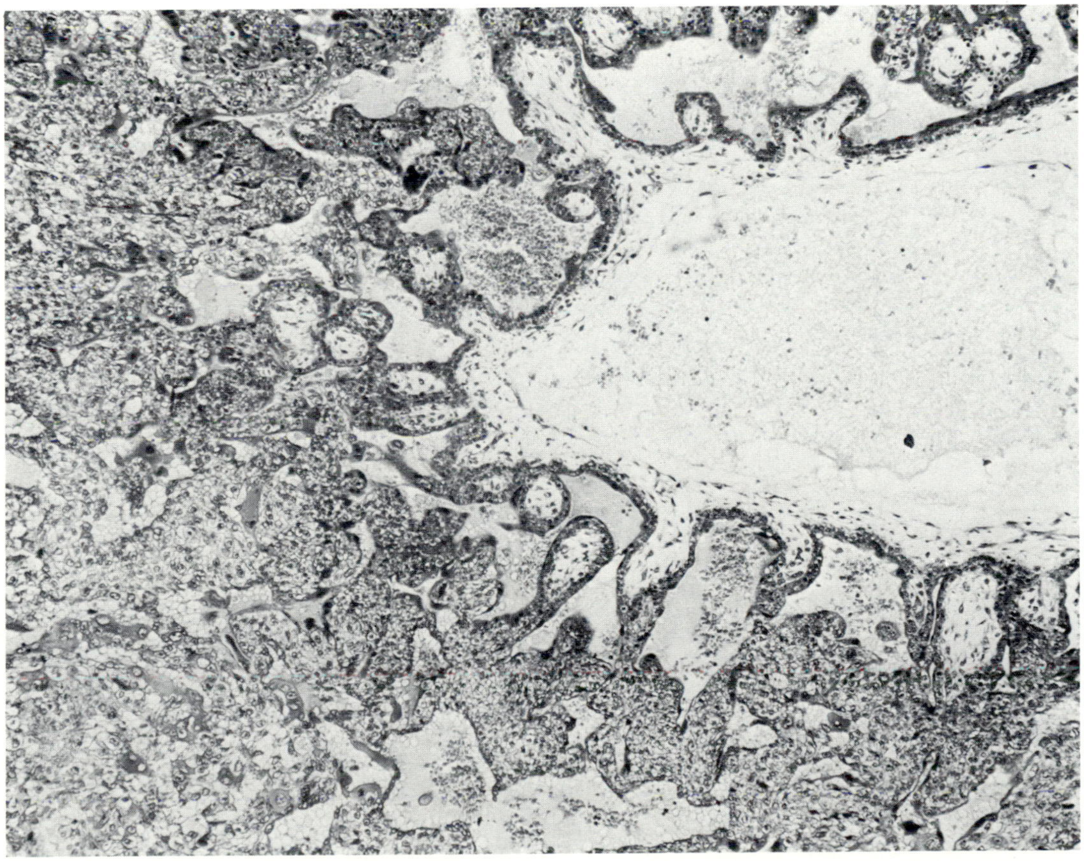

FIG. 23.2. Solid cytotrophoblastic cores are penetrated by mesenchyme, forming secondary villi. (Reproduced by permission from Kraus, Frederick T.: Female Genitalia. In Kissane, John M., editor: Anderson's Pathology, ed. 8, St. Louis, 1985, The C.V. Mosby Co.)

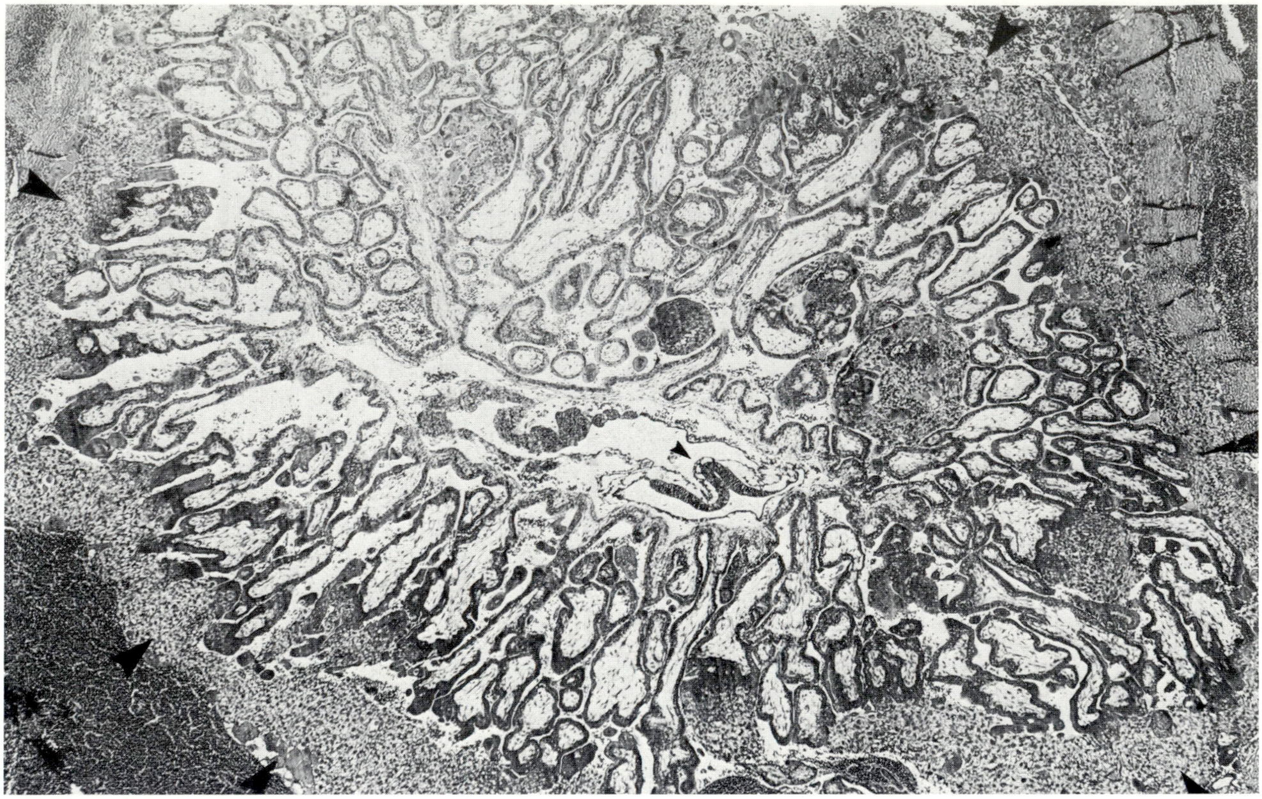

FIG. 23.3. Complete cytotrophoblastic shell (*large arrows*) surrounds the entire conceptus. Portions of the germ disk and yolk sac are present at center (*small arrow*).

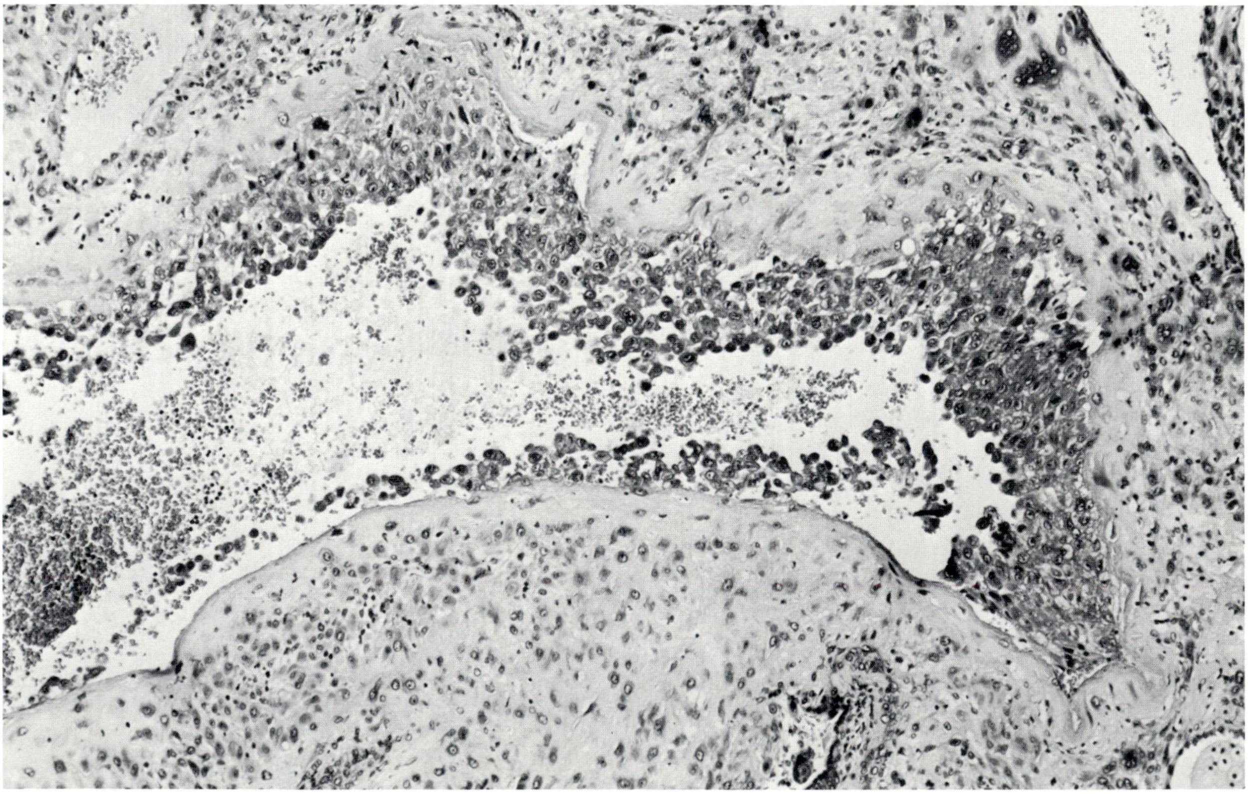

FIG. 23.4. Normal physiologic changes in a spiral artery include the replacement of maternal endothelium by intermediate trophoblast and destruction of the media, with deposition of fibrinoid material resulting in marked vascular dilatation. (Reproduced by permission from Kraus, Frederick T.: Female Genitalia. In Kissane, John M., editor: Anderson's Pathology, ed. 8, St. Louis, 1985, The C.V. Mosby Co.)

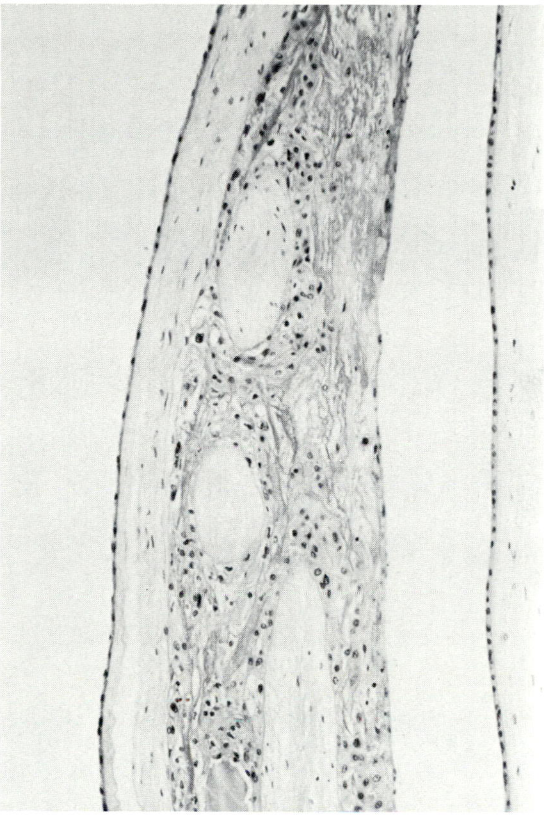

FIG. 23.5. Remnants of atrophic villi (chorion laeve) in the fetal membranes of a normal term gestation.

the definitive placenta. Departure from this orderly process of growth and regression is thought to result in some of the abnormal forms of placentation described below.

In time, the chorionic cavity is obliterated by progressive enlargement of the amnion. The umbilical cord, which originates as a mass of extraembryonic mesoblast at the caudal end of the embryo at about the 15th day, shifts to a more ventral location as the embryo grows. Eventually, cord and embryo prolapse into the amnionic cavity.

Septae appear in the placenta at about 3 months. These are composed of irregular folds of the basal plate that are drawn into the intervillous space by the relatively slowly growing anchoring villi. The cell islands that occur in the septae have been referred to as *X cells* but more recently have been identified as intermediate trophoblast. The septae partition the maternal surface incompletely and irregularly into 15–20 divisions that have no physiologic significance.

The identification and immunocytochemical localization of pregnancy-specific (human chorionic gonadotropin, hCG; human placental lactogen, hPL; pregnancy-specific beta 1-glycoprotein, SP_1) and pregnancy-associated (pregnancy-associated plasma protein A, PAPP-A) hormones have resulted in some interesting observations about the process of normal development and maturation of the placenta.[127,148,149,229,268] Not only have these studies confirmed the existence of and characterized the third type of trophoblast (intermediate trophoblast), but they have also defined a changing ratio and pattern of distribution of these hormones in various stages of development, suggesting a linkage between hormone biosynthesis and degree of trophoblastic differentiation.[127,149] In normal placentas, all hormones (hCG, hPL, and SP_1) are most widely distributed in the syncytiotrophoblast. The intermediate trophoblast, however, contains a considerable amount of both hPL and SP_1 throughout pregnancy as well as a small amount of hCG early in gestation. After the first trimester, there is a marked diminution of hCG in both the syncytiotrophoblast and intermediate trophoblast. In contrast, both hPL and SP_1 increase during the second and third trimesters. None of these hormones is localized in the cytotrophoblast. Similar studies of hormone expression and distribution have been extended to some types of abnormal gestations (diabetes mellitus,[146] preeclampsia[81]) and trophoblastic disease.[54,127,149]

Anatomy and Circulation

The primary stem villi divide into secondary stem villi, which in turn give rise to the tertiary stem villi. These grow downward, insert onto the basal plate, and then reenter the intervillous space, where they branch to form the terminal villi. A smaller number of terminal villi may originate from the tertiary stem villi as they course toward the basal plate. The functional subunit composed of villous parenchyma derived from a single secondary stem villus is called a *lobule*. The aggregate of villi derived from a primary stem villus defines the fetal cotyledon.

Deoxygenated fetal blood reaches the placenta through the two arteries of the umbilical cord. These branch and redivide in the stem villi until they ultimately terminate in the complex anastomosing capillary network of the terminal villi. It is at this interface, across capillary endothelium and attenuated trophoblast, that gas and nutrient exchange occurs. Oxygenated blood returns via venous tributaries to the umbilical vein.

Maternal blood enters the intervillous space through arterial inlets in the basal plate. The maternal blood streams toward the chorionic plate, disperses laterally, percolates around the villi, and exits through venous outlets in the placental floor. The exact anatomic relationship between the maternal arterial inlets in the basal plate and the fetal placental lobules is a matter of debate.

Maturation

The terminal villi are the functional units of the placenta. Their appearance changes dramatically over the course of a normal gestation. Immature first trimester villi are large (170 μ in diameter) and are covered by two distinct layers of trophoblast, an inner layer of cytotrophoblast and an outer layer of syncytiotrophoblast. The villous stroma is very loose and mucoid in appearance. Hofbauer cells, the placental macrophages, are numerous. Vessels are small and centrally placed (Fig. 23.6).

Second trimester villi average 70 μ in diameter. The syncytiotrophoblastic layer is thinner, and the nuclei are less evenly dispersed. The cytotrophoblast does not form a continuous layer and is, in fact, difficult to find with the light microscope after 16 weeks. The villous stroma is more compact and contains some collagen. Hofbauer cells are less conspicuous. Villous capillaries are larger and more numerous (Fig. 23.7).

Mature villi are smaller still (average 40 μ in diameter). The syncytiotrophoblastic nuclei are irregularly aggregated to form knots, leaving between them stretches of anucleate and attenuated syncytiotrophoblastic cytoplasm (Fig. 23.8). Syncytial knots are normally found in about 30% of mature terminal villi. Dilated fetal capillaries protrude beneath and appear to fuse with the thinned syncytiotrophoblast, forming vasculosyncytial membranes (Fig. 23.9). It is in these areas that the closest approximation of the fetal and maternal circulations occurs. Toward term, the stroma of the terminal villi is reduced to thin strands compressed between the numerous dilated capillaries, which constitute almost the entire cut surface of such villi.

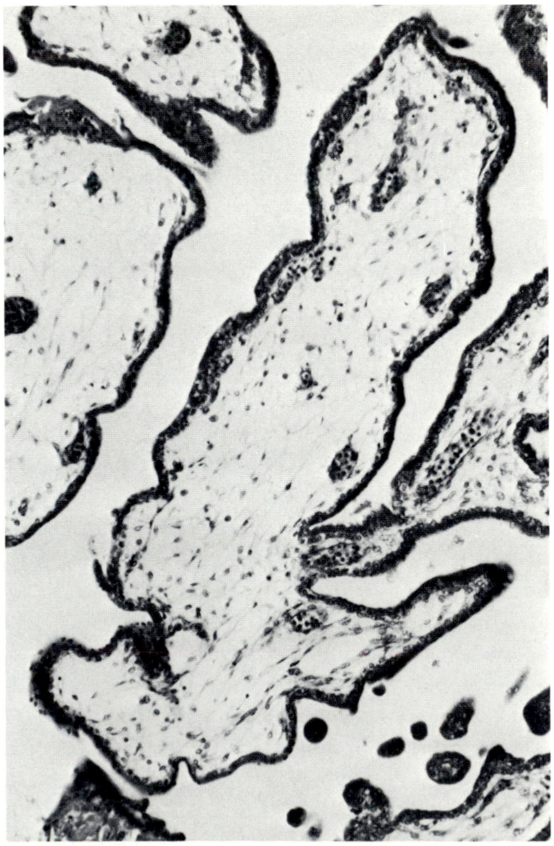

FIG. 23.6. Large, immature first trimester villi (8 weeks). The villous stroma is loose, Hofbauer cells are numerous, and the villous vessels are small and central in location. Two distinct layers of trophoblast are apparent.

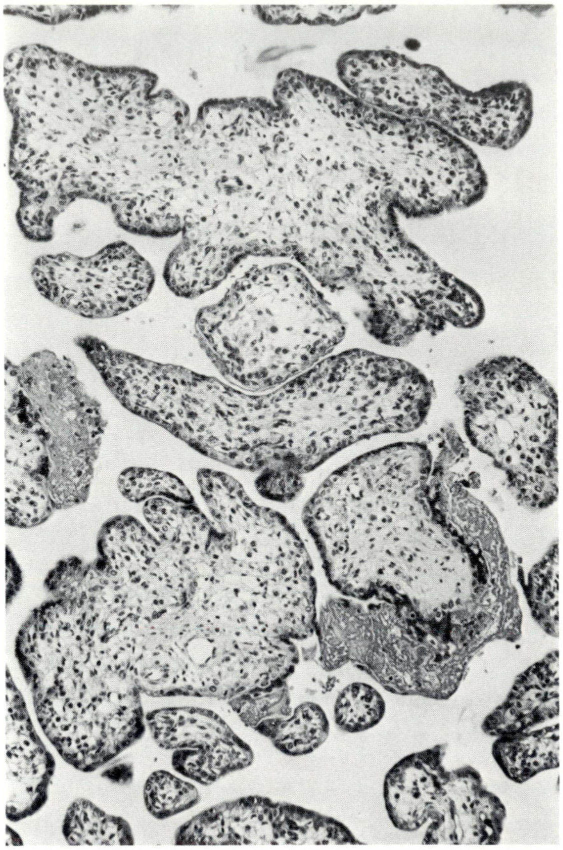

FIG. 23.7. Smaller, second trimester villi. The villous stroma is more compact. Villous capillaries are larger and more numerous. The syncytiotrophoblastic nuclei are less evenly dispersed, and the cytotrophoblast is inconspicuous.

The villi within any one placenta are not homogeneous in appearance. The peripheral villi and those located near the chorionic plate tend to be smaller, with more collagenous stroma and a thicker trophoblastic basement membrane. The villi located in the central portion of the fetal lobule tend to look less mature than those at its periphery. Little is known about the factors that influence placental maturation.

Physiology

Placental functions are numerous and varied. Not only does the placenta play a vital role in the transfer of oxygen and nutrients to the fetus and of fetal metabolites back to the mother, but it synthesizes a wide variety

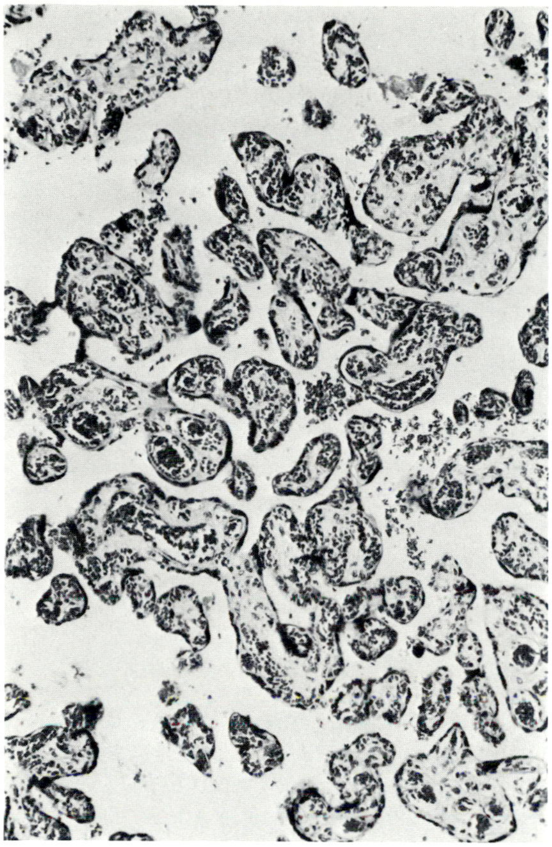

FIG. 23.8. Third trimester villi in cross-section are composed primarily of fetal capillaries with only a small amount of compressed intervening stroma.

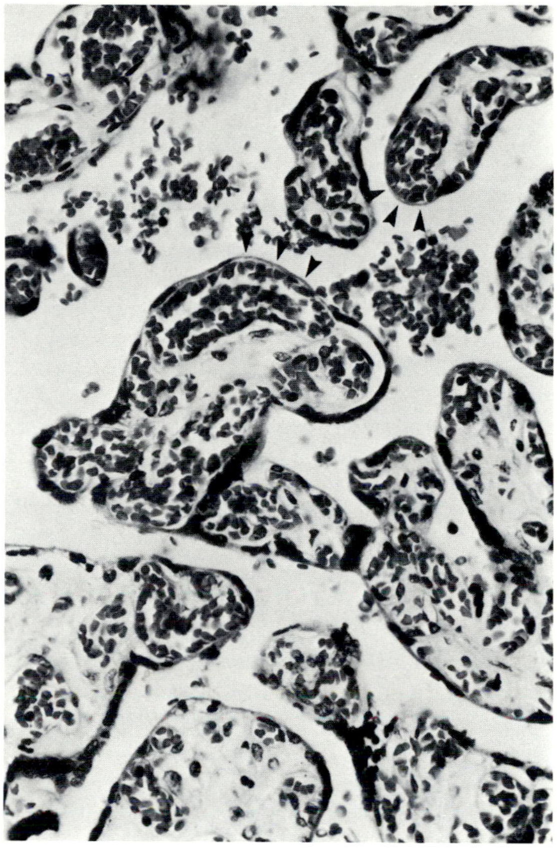

FIG. 23.9. Third trimester villi, vasculosyncytial membranes. Syncytiotrophoblastic nuclei aggregate to form knots. Fetal capillaries protrude beneath and fuse with the anucleate syncytiotrophoblast to form vasculosyncytial membranes (*arrows*).

of peptide and steroid hormones as well. Some of the substances produced require interaction of both fetal and placental tissue (e.g., estriol). Most of the endocrine activities of the placenta are attributed to the syncytiotrophoblast.

Abnormalities of Placentation

Abnormalities of Shape

Accessory (Succenturiate) Lobe

Occasionally, the placenta may deviate from its usual round or oval discoid shape. One of the most common of these variations is the accessory or succenturiate lobe, a condition in which usually one mass but occasionally multiple discrete masses of placental tissue are separated from the main placenta (Fig. 23.10). The accessory lobe may be attached to the main placenta by a narrow isthmus of chorionic tissue or may be separated from it by only fetal membranes. The umbilical cord generally inserts onto the main placental mass. The vascular supply to the accessory lobe runs on the fetal surface, in many cases through fetal membranes unsupported by any underlying villous parenchyma. If these large intramembranous vessels are traumatized during delivery, severe fetal hemorrhage may result. Occasionally, the accessory lobe may be retained in utero after delivery, resulting in postpartum bleeding or infection. The reported frequency of the accessory lobe is variable; Fox estimates that it occurs in about 3% of placentas.[98]

Other Anomalous Shapes

The *bilobate* or *bipartite* placenta consists of two equally sized placental lobes that may be separated by fetal membranes or connected to each other by a narrow isthmus of placental tissue. The umbilical cord usually inserts centrally between the lobes, either into the placental bridge or into the membranes. The clinical significance of this abnormality has not been extensively studied. Fugikura et al. have noted that bilobate placentas occur more frequently in older women of high gravidity and in patients with a history of infertility. They also found

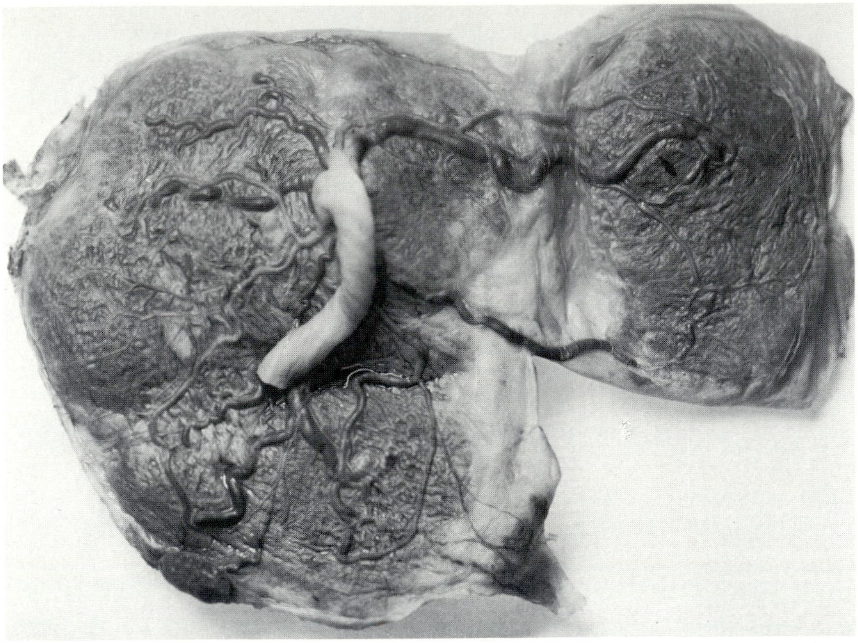

FIG. 23.10. Accessory (succenturiate) lobe. Discrete mass of placental tissue attached to the main placental mass by fetal membranes. Vascular supply to the accessory lobe must traverse unsupported membranes.

a higher frequency of first trimester bleeding and undue placental adherence requiring manual extraction in association with bipartite placentation.[105]

A variety of other anomalous shapes occurs, but these are very uncommon and are rarely encountered. The *multilobate* placenta is one consisting of three or more lobes of roughly equal size. *Placenta membranacea* is a large, thin placenta in which functional chorionic villi diffusely cover the entire gestational sac. The placental tissue may vary in thickness, but only exceptionally is there a dominant area resembling a placental disk. In the human, the placenta normally assumes this configuration in the first few weeks of development, but ultimately the villi oriented toward the uterine cavity atrophy (chorion laeve), leaving the chorion frondosum as the definitive placenta. In some animal species, the placenta is normally of this membranous type. Placenta membranacea in humans is extremely rare. In the few cases reported, obstetric complications, such as antepartum bleeding, have been frequent, undoubtedly relating to the obligate placenta previa that accompanies this form of placentation. *Ring-shaped placenta* is also a very rare occurrence, in which the placenta is annular or cylindrical in shape. A *fenestrate placenta* is distinguished by a focal absence of villous parenchyma in the center of the placenta. The resulting defect may be a through-and-through hole, or the chorionic plate may remain intact over the parenchymal defect.

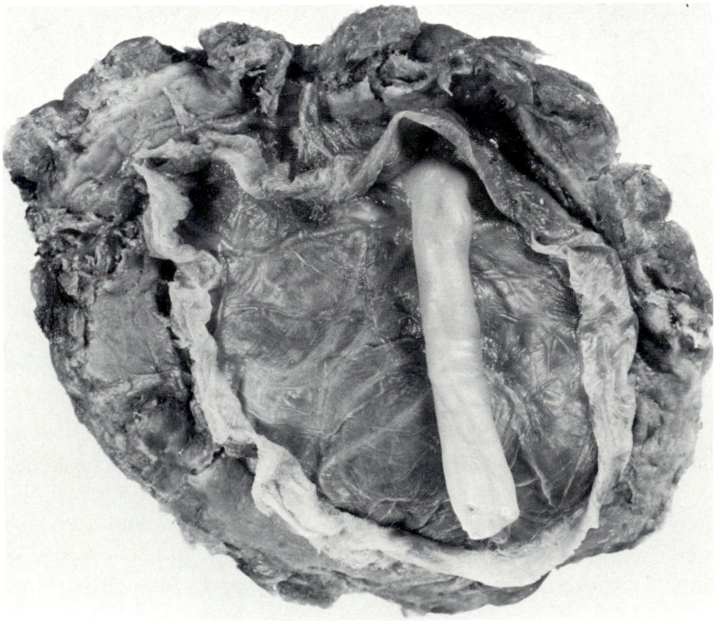

FIG. 23.11. Extrachorial placenta. The fetal membranes do not extend to the peripheral margin of the placenta, leaving a ring of placental tissue extending beyond the chorionic plate. (Reproduced by permission from Kraus, Frederick T.: Gynecologic Pathology, St. Louis, 1967, The C.V. Mosby Co.)

The pathogenesis of these variations in shape is not understood. Among the many theories proposed is that these anomalies reflect a focal failure or disturbance of the normal process of orderly villous atrophy that occurs early in gestation.

Gross Structural Abnormalities

Placenta Extrachorialis

This condition is a common gross structural deviation in which the chorionic plate of the placenta is smaller than its basal plate. The transition from membranous to villous chorion occurs not at the placental margin as in a normal placenta but inside its circumference, some distance from the peripheral edge of the placenta. A ring of bare placental tissue (extrachorial portion) extends submerged into the decidua beyond the limits of the chorionic plate (Fig. 23.11). The two types of extrachorial placenta, circummarginate and circumvallate, are categorized based on the nature of the transition from the membranous to the villous chorion. Grossly, in circummarginate placentas, the transition is flat, whereas in circumvallate placentas, the marginal membrane ring is folded or rolled back upon itself (Fig. 23.12). In both varieties, the fetal vessels appear to terminate at the margin of the chorionic plate (Fig. 23.13) but actually continue their course peripherally in the deeper villous tissue. Histologically, the ring in circummarginate placentas consists only of amnion, decidua, and submerged placenta. The fold in circumvallate placentas is composed of a double layer of reflected amnion, a thin layer of decidua, fibrin, possibly blood clot, and underlying placenta. These two forms of extrachorial placentas may

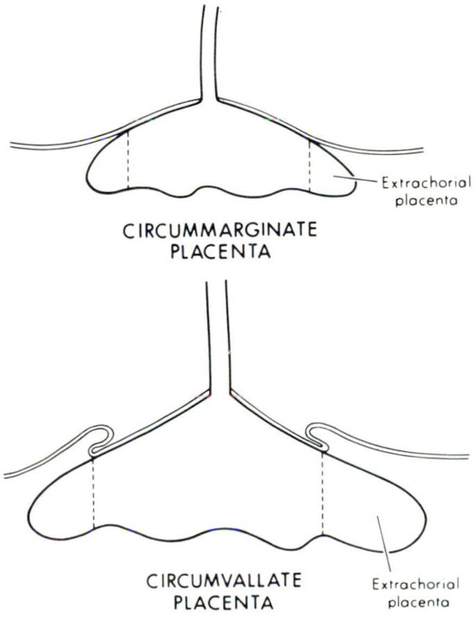

Fig. 23.12. Diagram comparing the rolled membrane ring in the circumvallate placenta to the flat transition in the circummarginate placenta. (After Fox, Ref. 98.)

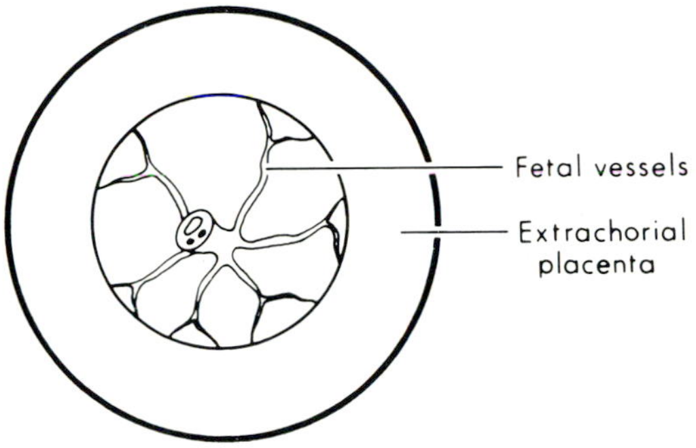

Fig. 23.13. Diagram of an extrachorial placenta, fetal side. Vessels appear to terminate at the margin of the chorionic plate but actually continue peripherally in the extrachorial portion. (After Fox, Ref. 98.)

be partial or complete (circumferential) and may occur in combination with one another.

The many theories attempting to explain the etiology and pathogenesis of extrachorial placentation have been summarized by Scott.[233] Estimates of the frequency of the condition vary widely, and there is considerable disagreement concerning its clinical relevance. Most agree that extrachorial placentas are more common in multigravidas.[33,100,277] An increased frequency of antepartum bleeding, premature labor, fetal hypoxia, and perinatal mortality has been reported in white women with totally circumvallate placentas.[33,100,233] Both partial and complete forms of circumvallate placentas are associated with an unduly high proportion of low birth weight babies.[100]

Abnormalities of Implantation

Placenta Accreta

This condition as defined clinically is an abnormal adherence of the placenta to the uterine wall so that separation does not occur after delivery of the newborn. The pathologic anatomy of this condition is a partial or complete absence of the decidua resulting in an abnormal form of implantation in which placental villi adhere directly to (placenta accreta), invade into (placenta increta), or penetrate through (placenta percreta) the myometrium. Commonly, the degree of placental invasiveness is not uniform, and as a practical matter, the term *placenta accreta* is often used to encompass all degrees of abnormal placental adherence or invasiveness. Customarily, these cases are further subdivided into total (involving the entire placenta), partial (involving one or more cotyledons), or focal (involving isolated foci of the placenta) involvement.

Microscopically, the cardinal feature is absence of the decidua basalis.[166] The region normally occupied by decidua is replaced by loose connective tissue. The decidua parietalis may be normal but is commonly absent as well. Placental villi adhere directly to or actually invade

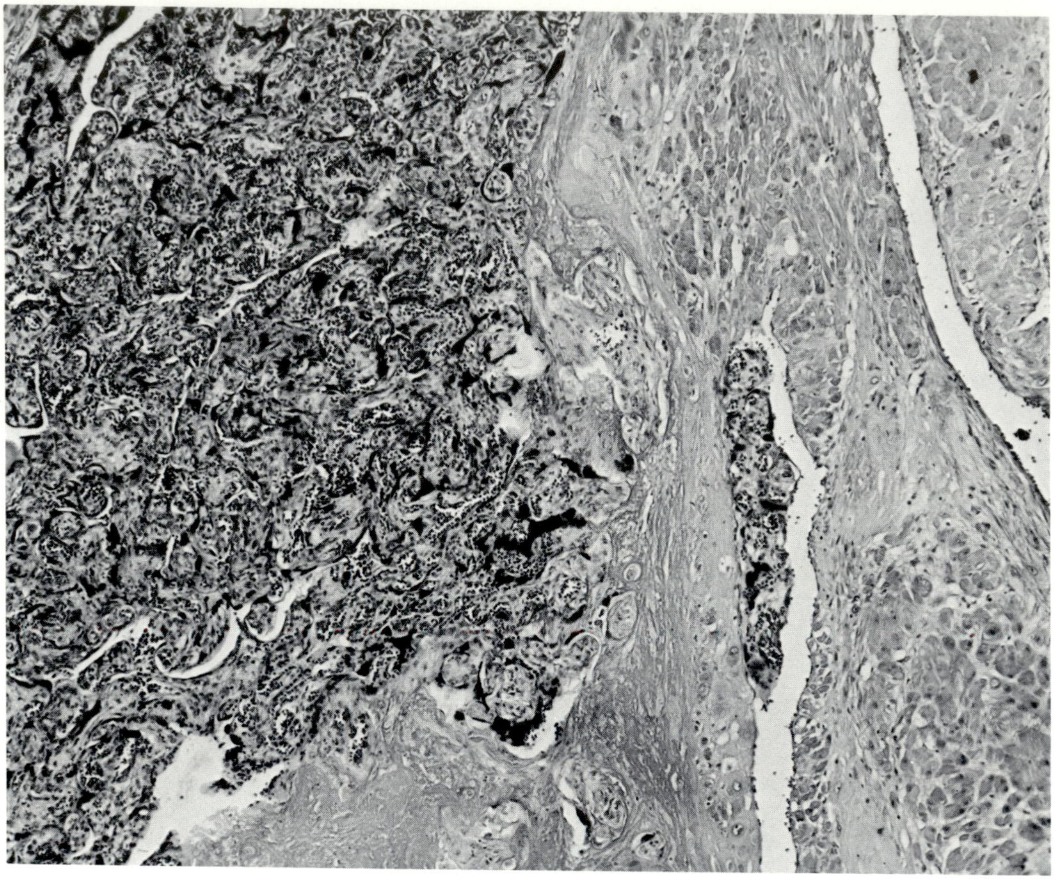

FIG. 23.14. Placenta accreta. Chorionic villi adherent to myometrium without intervening decidua.

the myometrium without intervening decidua (Fig. 23.14). The villi are usually partially separated from focally hyalinized myometrial smooth muscle cells by a layer of fibrin. Blanc has reported the presence of numerous large, thick-walled vessels showing no fibrinoid change or trophoblastic invasion in the superficial myometrium adherent to the placenta.[40] The diagnosis is most often made in a hysterectomy specimen but rarely may be confirmed by examining the placenta itself. In either situation, evaluation is difficult, since the specimen is usually markedly distorted by the disruptive effects of attempts to remove the adherent placenta at the time of delivery.

The true frequency of placenta accreta is difficult to determine. Reported figures have varied widely from 1 in 1667 to 1 in 70,000 pregnancies.[53] In studying a large number of cases reported in the literature, Fox emphasized the particular tendency for placenta accreta to occur in multigravid and obstetrically elderly women.[97] There is a frequent reference to previous placental retention requiring manual removal in these patients. A number of predisposing factors have been related to this condition, the two most significant being placenta previa and previous cesarean section (Fig. 23.15). As many as 64% of patients with placenta accreta have had associated placenta previa in some reports,[53] and many placenta previa accretas occur in cesarean section scars.[171,255] In some cases of partial placenta accreta, only that portion of the placenta implanted over the lower uterine segment or cesarean section scar has been abnormally adherent.[267] A smaller number of patients have a history of previous uterine curettage,[108] uterine sepsis, previous manual removal of the placenta, cornual implantation, leiomyomas, or uterine malformation. The common endpoint in all these conditions is presumably a deficiency in or absence of the decidua. Alternatively, some authors have suggested that placenta accreta is due to an abnormal invasiveness of the placenta rather than to an inadequate decidua.

Clinically, the condition is compatible with normal fetal development and most commonly is suspected only after delivery. Failure of separation of the placenta in the third stage of labor and postpartum bleeding, often life threatening, are the cardinal clinical signs of placenta accreta. Antepartum bleeding and premature labor are also common; these are due principally to the high frequency of associated placenta previa. Uterine rupture may occur at any stage of pregnancy or during labor.[48,255] The overall maternal mortality has dropped from 37%[130] to 2–3% in more recent series.[53,171] Hysterectomy is

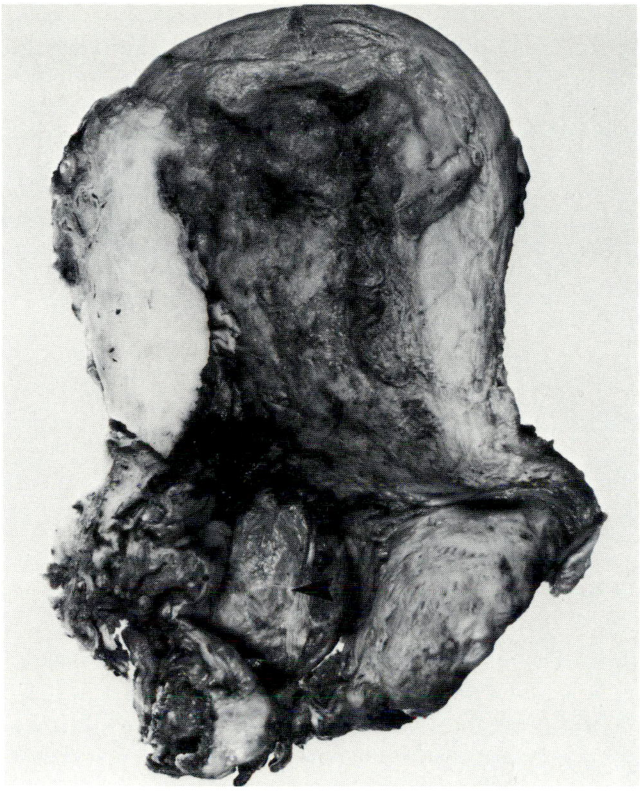

FIG. 23.15. Placenta percreta. Penetration of the placenta through the myometrium at the site of three previous cesarean sections (*lower left* portion of the specimen). A portion of the chorionic plate is indicated by the *arrow*.

the usual treatment, although conservative treatment has been successful in some cases.[164,267]

Multiple Pregnancy

There are a number of excellent and detailed accounts of the phenomenon of multiple pregnancy.[4,29;30,31] These are recommended to supplement the abbreviated discussion of the topic given here.

Twin Gestation

Twins may arise from the fertilization of two separate ova (dizygotic or fraternal twins) or from the division of a single fertilized ovum (monozygotic or identical twins). Although genetically and almost always phenotypically identical, monozygotic twins may occasionally be phenotypically quite discordant.[114,132] Dizygotic twins are no more genetically similar than other singleton siblings.

The frequency of monozygous twinning is relatively constant worldwide (about 3.5 in 1000 pregnancies). The marked geographical differences in total twinning rate reflect the greater predisposition for multiple ovulation in some populations and families than in others. There is a strong hereditary element in dizygous twinning, and there is some evidence that this may be related to increased endogenous levels of follicle-stimulating hormone (FSH). Multiple ovulation has been induced by the administration of clomiphene or a combination of FSH with luteinizing hormone (LH) or hCG. The occurrence of twins in Caucasians in the United States is about 1 in 80 pregnancies, and about one-third of these are monozygotic.

There are basically two types of placentas in twin gestations, monochorionic and dichorionic. All dizygotic twins have dichorionic placentas; in double ovulation, two blastocysts implant, each generating a separate placenta with chorion and amnion (diamnionic–dichorionic, DiDi). If these implantations occur close together, varying degrees of fusion are common (DiDi fused). Otherwise, diamnionic–dichorionic placentas are entirely separate. Monozygotic twins may show any type of placentation depending on the stage at which splitting occurs. If the single fertilized ovum divides very early, before differentiation of the trophoblast (first 2 or 3 days), two separate embryos, each with its own placenta (diamnionic–dichorionic), will develop. If splitting occurs in the blastocyst stage, after formation of the chorion but before formation of the amnion (3rd to 8th day after fertilization), the twins will develop a single placenta with two amnionic sacs (diamnionic–monochorionic, DiMo). A split between the 8th and 13th days after fertilization will result in one placenta and only one amnionic cavity (monoamnionic–monochorionic, MoMo). Later splitting will result in conjoined twins (Fig. 23.16).

An important feature of monochorionic placentas is the presence of vascular communications between the two fetal circulations. Although estimates of the frequency of this phenomenon differ somewhat, it is generally agreed that they occur in essentially all monochorionic placentas. These vascular communications may be superficial, between the large vessels on the fetal surface, or deep, within the placental substance. The majority of superficial anastomoses are between the ar-

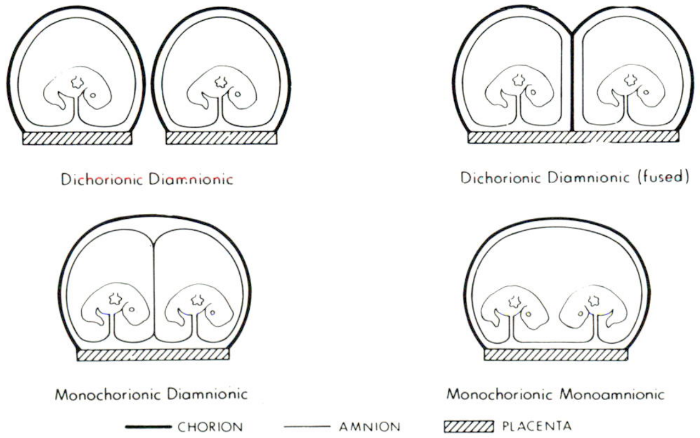

FIG. 23.16. Diagrammatic representation of the various types of twin placentation and their membrane relationships.

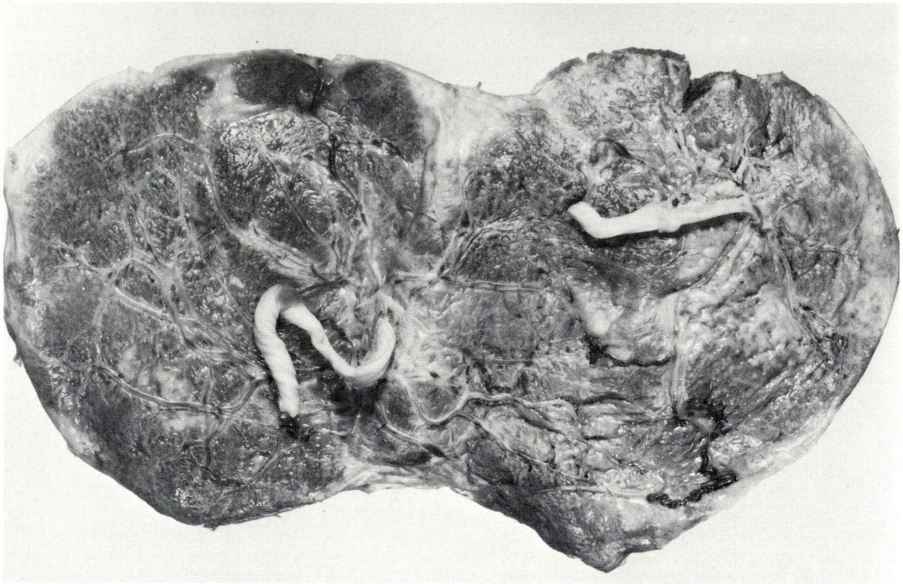

Fig. 23.17. Diamnionic–monochorionic twin placenta. Central merging of the two vascular districts with anastomoses of superficial vessels. (Reproduced by permission from Kraus, Frederick T.: Gynecologic Pathology, St. Louis, 1967, The C.V. Mosby Co.)

teries. Vein-to-vein anastomoses are much less common (Fig. 23.17). Of greater physiologic importance are the arteriovenous anastomoses that occur deep within the capillary bed of a shared cotyledon. Arteriovenous anastomoses are very common, but the physiologic consequences of these communications vary greatly depending on their size, number, and overall balance of blood flow. There is some debate concerning the occurrence of vascular communications in diamnionic–dichorionic fused placentas. As a rule, they are absent, but vascular anastomoses of various types have been reported rarely.[64,208]

All twins with a monochorionic placenta are monozygotic. Dichorionic placentation, however, may result from either dizygous or monozygous twinning. Obviously, different fetal sex establishes a dizygous relation. Blood group analysis or HLA typing may be necessary to determine zygosity in like-sex dichorionic twins. The frequency of different types of twin placentation in a study of 250 consecutive twin deliveries is summarized in Table 23.1.[29]

Establishment of the type of placentation is important, not only as the initial step in the determination of zygosity but also because of its significant impact on perinatal morbidity and mortality. In examining the twin placenta, the pathologist should attempt to (1) define the type of placentation (dichorionic versus monochorionic) and (2) demonstrate the type and number of vascular anastomoses if they are present. If two entirely separate placentas are delivered, they are obviously dichorionic and require only routine examination. Practically speaking, the principal task for the pathologist is to distinguish between a diamnionic–monochorionic placenta and a diamnionic–dichorionic fused placenta. In dichorionic placentas, chorionic tissue is present in the septum between the amnionic cavities. This is absent in the diamnionic–monochorionic placenta. Grossly, the chorionic tissue makes the septum appear opaque (DiDi fused); in its absence, the septum appears more translucent (DiMo). Histologic examination of a roll of the membranous septum will show two layers of amnion separated by two layers of chorion in dichorionic placentas (Fig. 23.18). The septum will consist solely of two layers of amnion in monochorionic placentas (Fig. 23.19). Identical information may be obtained by examination of a section including the T-zone, that portion of the placenta where the septum meets the fetal surface. This is an alternative method for examining the septum in cases in which the septal membranes have been torn or otherwise distorted and cannot be rolled (see Chapter 27, Processing of Gynecologic and Obstetric Tissue).

Table 23.1. Frequency of different types of placentation in 250 consecutive twin deliveries.

77 Monochorionic (31%)	173 Dichorionic (69%) By blood group analysis
3 MoMo (1%)	33 Monozygotic (13%)
74 DiMo (30%)	140 Dizygotic (56%)

Reprinted by permission of Benirschke, Driscoll, Ref. 29.

When the dividing membranes are peeled apart, the two amnions are readily stripped from one another in the diamnionic–monochorionic placenta, leaving no trace of the T-zone on the fetal surface. On the other hand, there is always a separate layer of chorion inserting at the base of the septum in the diamnionic–dichorionic fused placenta that persists after the amnions are stripped away.

To demonstrate the possible presence of vascular communications, the amnionic membranes should be stripped from the placenta. This facilitates the study of all vessels on the fetal surface. The distribution of the fetal blood vessels does not necessarily conform to the

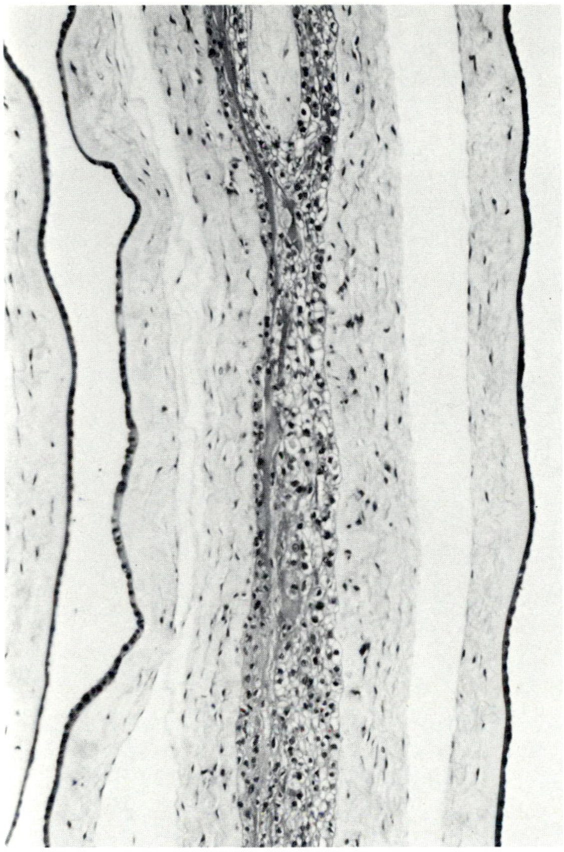

FIG. 23.18. Diamnionic–dichorionic fused twin placenta. Histologic section of the septal membranes shows separation of the two amnions by a central layer of chorionic tissue.

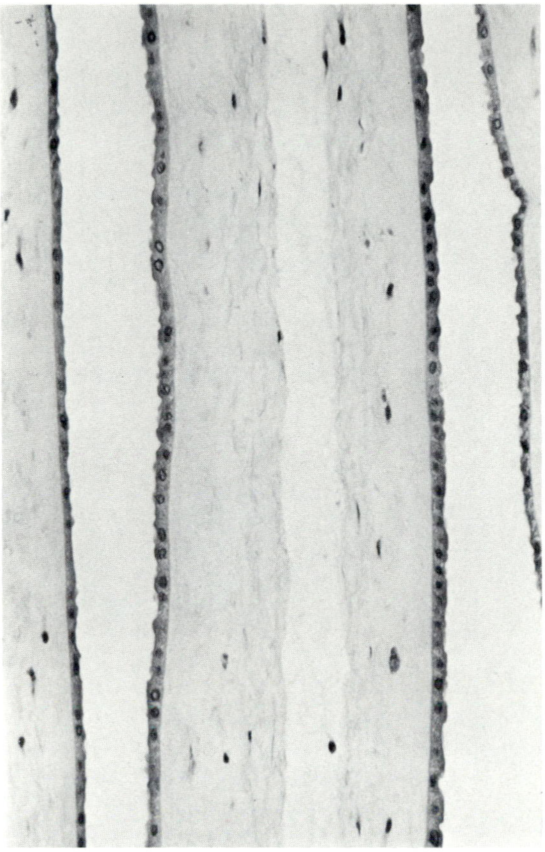

FIG. 23.19. Diamnionic–monochorionic twin placenta. Septal membranes are composed only of two amnions without intervening chorionic tissue.

division of placental tissue indicated by the line of insertion of the dividing membranes. Anastomoses, therefore, do not always lie directly beneath the insertion of the septal membranes. In the majority of diamnionic–monochorionic placentas, the villous tissues of the two vascular districts are imperceptibly merged, and portions are shared by both fetuses. Large, superficial anastomoses are often evident on the fetal surface (Fig. 23.17). Identification of the deep arteriovenous anastomoses is more important and more difficult. Various methods have been used to document these communications, including radiologic examination after the vascular injection of radiopaque dye[64] or injection of colored plastic followed by preparation of a corrosion specimen. These techniques are relatively difficult and time consuming. A simpler method is to inject colored saline or a colloidal dye solution[215] into an arterial branch of one twin's vascular territory and see whether it returns to the same infant or to its partner. This procedure should be repeated at multiple sites in an attempt to document the nature and number of anastomoses. Unfortunately, areas of villous disruption will cause leakage of fluid and compromise the usefulness of this technique. The perfusion pressure is also important. False positive anastomoses may be created by unphysiologically high perfusion pressure, whereas lower pressures may fail to demonstrate existing communications.[215] It should be emphasized that such studies are merely qualitative. The physiologic significance of the anastomoses in vivo is usually better assessed by examining the twins themselves. In diamnionic–dichorionic placentas, vessels do not approach the area of fusion of the two placental masses, and anastomoses are not seen (Fig. 23.20).

Perinatal mortality is much higher in twins than in single pregnancies. An overall mortality of 14% was documented in one study of 250 consecutive twin births.[29] In the same study, twins with monochorionic placentation had a higher perinatal mortality (25.9%) than those with dichorionic placentas (8.9%), and monoamnionic–monochorionic twins had the highest perinatal mortality rate of all (about 50%). The most important factor contributing to this increased death rate is premature onset of labor and delivery. The increased frequency of hydramnios, maternal hypertension, and congenital fetal anomalies also contributes to the excessive perinatal death rate in twin gestations.

Twin–Twin Transfusion Syndrome

A major cause of perinatal mortality in monochorionic twins is the twin–twin transfusion syndrome. This phe-

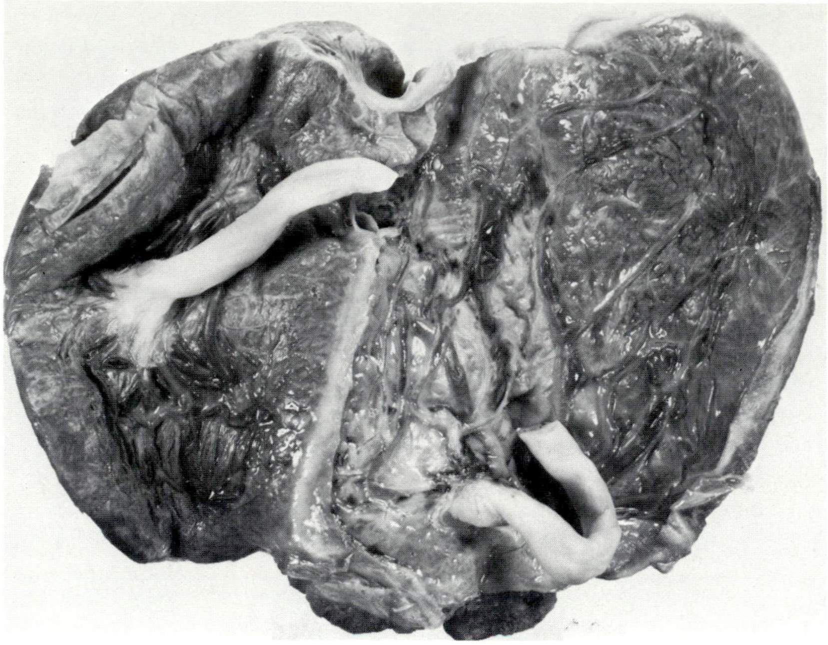

FIG. 23.20. Diamnionic–dichorionic fused twin placenta. The two placental masses are fused but discrete. Fetal vessels do not approach or cross the area of fusion.

nomenon is characterized by a marked discrepancy in the size and appearance of the infants and their corresponding placental segments. The donor twin is smaller, pale, and anemic, whereas the recipient is heavier, edematous, plethoric, and polycythemic. Classically, there is also a marked discordance in the size and weight of the fetal organs, the organs of the recipient being larger and heavier than those of the donor. Microscopically, there is myocardial hyperplasia involving all chambers of the heart, as well as increased smooth muscle mass in the media of the pulmonary and systemic arteries and arterioles in the recipient twin. The heart of the donor twin is usually subnormal in size, and the arterial muscle mass is decreased. Glomeruli are enlarged, up to twice normal size, in the recipient twin, and they are either reduced or normal in size in the donor.[177] Hydramnios is a frequent finding in the recipient twin, whereas oligohydramnios and amnion nodosum may be found in the sac of the donor member.[177]

The placental territory of the donor twin is larger, bulky, and pale. The villi are large and edematous, with numerous Hofbauer cells and small capillaries containing nucleated red blood cells. The donor portion of the placenta greatly resembles the placenta in Rh incompatibility both grossly and microscopically. The recipient placental territory is generally smaller, firm, and deep red. The villous capillaries are somewhat dilated and intensely congested, but otherwise the recipient villi are normal.[4,67]

Schatz proposed the now widely accepted concept that the twin–twin transfusion syndrome results when significant amounts of blood are diverted from the donor twin to the recipient twin through arteriovenous anastomoses deep within shared placental lobules.[29] There is evidence that the concomitant presence of superficial large vessel anastomoses may modify or compensate for the hemodynamic imbalance created by deep arteriovenous shunts.[29]

The clinical definition of the syndrome is not precise. A combination of hematologic and anatomic criteria is generally used. A difference in hemoglobin concentration of greater than 5 g per 100 ml between the twins was considered valid for definitive diagnosis by Rausen et al.[208] The lack of a uniform, clear definition explains, in part, the discrepancies in frequency with which the twin–twin transfusion syndrome is reported to complicate monochorionic–diamnionic placentation; estimates vary from 15 to 30%.[208,254] Whatever the true frequency, the twin–twin transfusion syndrome obviously does not occur as often as one would anticipate given the universal presence of vascular communications in monochorionic twin pregnancies.

The consequences of the twin–twin transfusion syndrome are grave. Mortality rates may be as high as 70%.[208] Both twins are at great risk. The recipient twin is subject to cardiac failure, hemolytic jaundice, kernicterus, and thrombosis due to hemoconcentration. The donor twin may be severely anemic. Disseminated intravascular coagulation has been reported in twins with placental communications. Thromboplastin-rich blood from a dead twin may reach the survivor through the vascular anastomoses.[29] Overall, the twin–twin transfusion syndrome contributes significantly to the increased perinatal mortality in monochorionic twins. Rausen et al. found the twin–twin transfusion syndrome in 34% of monochorionic twin deaths.[208]

In contrast to the chronic intrauterine transfusion characterizing the twin–twin transfusion syndrome, occasionally acute shifts of blood may occur through large superficial anastomoses during delivery. This is a rare occurrence but may result in such emergencies as exsanguination of the second twin through the unligated umbilical cord of the first twin via large anastomoses.

Acardia

The development of acardiac fetuses (monsters) has also been attributed to the twin–twin transfusion syndrome. This anomaly occurs only in monozygotic multiple pregnancies with monochorionic placentation. It occurs in about 1% of monozygotic twin gestations. The acardius is a bizarre and grossly malformed fetus that is perfused and sustained entirely by its normal twin (Fig. 23.21).[47,109,190,235,283] It may be small or large (up to 3500 g) and is attached to the placenta by an umbilical cord, usually containing one artery and one vein. These fetuses differ greatly in gross appearance and degree of organogenesis. One complicated classification system is based on the state of development of the body: (1) acephalus—truck and extremities are developed, but the head is absent, (2) acormus—development of head only, (3) amorphus—a shapeless mass without recognizable structure, (4) myelacephalus—a suggestion of one or more extremities, and (5) anceps—a rudimentary head is present.

Although all acardiac fetuses lack a functioning heart, elements of myocardial tissue may or may not be present. This difference is the basis for the further subdivision of acardiacs into two categories: (1) holoacardius—denoting complete absence of myocardial elements, and (2) hemiacardius—indicating the presence of some myocardial tissue.

Regardless of the state of cardiac and bodily development, circulation to all acardiacs is accomplished by the cotwin. Blood flows to the acardius in a reverse course, from the heart of the normal twin, through a large placental artery–artery anastomosis, and into the umbilical artery of the acardius. After coursing through the acardius, blood returns via its umbilical vein and into the circulatory system of the normal twin through a large placental vein–vein anastomosis. There are two main theories of pathogenesis: (1) the reversal of the circulation may be etiologically responsible for regression or resorption of a previously formed heart in the acardiac, or (2) the anomaly may result from primary agenesis of the heart, the acardiac fetus surviving only when maintained by these very specific types of vascular anastomoses with a twin.

When karyotyped, the acardius and its cotwin have been isosexual. Chromosomal abnormalities have been documented in some acardiacs, all of whom have been associated with a genotypically normal cotwin.[16,70]

Fetus Papyraceus

Fetus papyraceus results from the early intrauterine death of one twin that is compressed against the membranes by the growth of the other twin. The dead fetus shrinks and flattens, eventually resembling amorphous necrotic tissue (Fig. 23.22). Its size and shape depend on the time of death, and, undoubtedly, many are overlooked. Fetus papyracei occur in both monochorial and dichorial placentation and perhaps occasionally result from the twin–twin transfusion syndrome. The frequency with which twin pregnancies are converted to single pregnancies by the death of one twin is unknown.

Monoamnionic–Monochorionic Twins

Monoamnionic–monochorionic twin placentas are the least common type of twin placentation. Estimates of

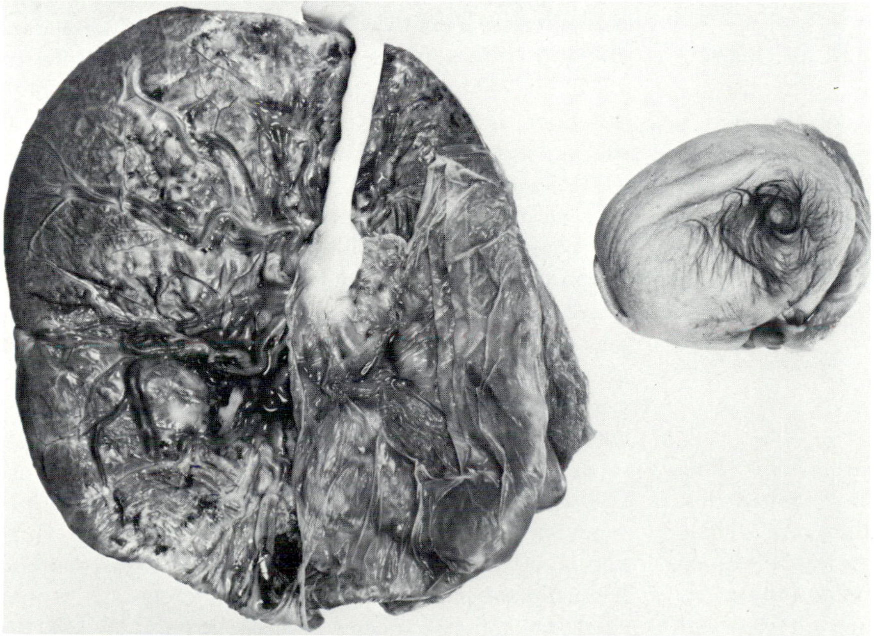

Fig. 23.21. Acardiac fetus. Holoacardius (amorphus).

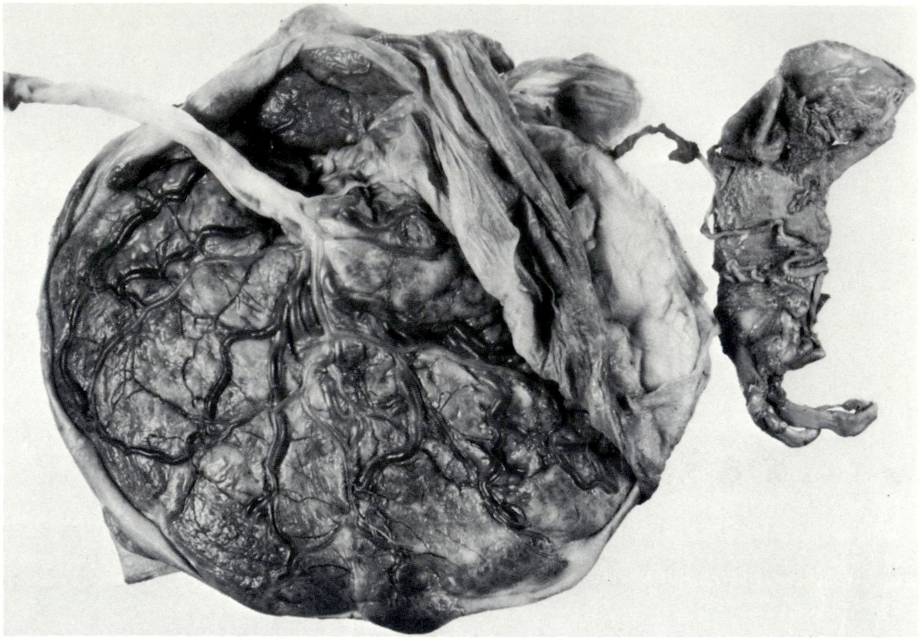

FIG. 23.22. Fetus papyraceus. Necrotic fetus compressed by the growth of its normal twin.

its frequency vary considerably. In one series of twin pregnancies investigated by Wharton et al., 18 of 581 were monoamnionic.[281] Monoamnionic placentation is associated with high fetal mortality.[29,197,265,281] Reported perinatal mortality rates range from 33% to nearly 70%.[281] A significant factor in this mortality rate is the high frequency of cord complications. Twisting and knotting of the two umbilical cords is a very common occurrence.[197,265] An unusual, almost joint type of cord insertion has been documented to occur in monochorionic–monoamnionic twins. The twin–twin transfusion syndrome is not a significant cause of fetal mortality in monoamnionic twins.[281]

Higher Multiple Births

The principles of monozygotic and dizygotic placentation apply equally to triplet, quadruplet, and other higher multiple births. For example, triplets may be trizygotic, dizygotic, or monozygotic. Trizygotic triplets have trichorionic–triamnionic placentation but may be separate or variably fused. Dizygotic triplets may be dichorionic or trichorionic. Monozygotic triplets may be monochorionic, dichorionic, or trichorionic.

Placental Inflammation and Intrauterine Infections

Inflammation and infection of the placenta and fetus are important but controversial subjects. Debate has centered on the definition of inflammation, its etiologic relation to infectious agents, and the clinical relevance of the histologic findings. A great deal of attention has been focused on the consequences of intrauterine and intrapartum infections. At worst, some well-defined infections can result in abortion, stillbirth, prematurity, or multiply handicapped, severely disabled children who are mentally retarded, blind, deaf or suffer from numerous other congenital malformations. In addition to the obvious and identified toll, many more subtle, late sequelae, including learning disabilities, school failure, and especially deafness, are being identified in children whose infections were asymptomatic at birth. The social and financial burden posed by the support of these children is enormous, not to mention the long-term grief and emotional cost to the families involved.

The placenta and fetus are infected via two major pathways: (1) ascending amniotic (transcervical) infection and (2) hematogenous (transplacental) infection. Combinations of these pathways (i.e., ascending deciduoplacentofetal) or other pathways (transfallopian, transuterine via amniocentesis or intrauterine transfusion) have been described or proposed, but for practical purposes, only the first two are of major importance. The pattern of the inflammatory response in the placenta is entirely different for these two entities. In ascending infections, microorganisms in the amniotic fluid produce an acute inflammatory reaction in the fetal membranes (chorioamnionitis), the umbilical cord (funisitis), and ultimately may be aspirated into the lungs of the fetus. The etiologic agents are usually bacterial, but fungi and possibly viruses are occasionally involved. In hematogenous infections, the infectious agent produces an inflammatory response in the villi (villitis) and intervillous space. Viruses are believed to be the most common agents involved, but some bacteria (spirochetes, *Listeria*) and protozoa (*Toxoplasma gondii*) also infect the placenta in this manner. A third important route by which infectious agents may reach the fetus is during passage through an infected birth canal (intrapartum infection). The placenta, of course, is not involved in this process.

Ascending Infection and Chorioamnionitis

Chorioamnionitis is by far the commonest form of placental inflammation in humans. The exact frequency varies depending on the population studied. The incidence of chorioamnionitis is increased in patients of low socioeconomic status and in black women.[180,185,219] Recently, Naeye has emphasized the role of coitus in increasing the frequency and severity of ascending amniotic infection.[175,182] The role of the incompetent cervix has been stressed by Russell.[220]

In most cases of chorioamnionitis, the placenta and fetal membranes appear macroscopically normal. Occasionally, the membranes may be opaque, friable, or foul smelling in cases of particularly severe, long-standing bacterial infection. In rare instances of *Candida* infection, tiny white foci of colonization, 2–3 mm in size, may be seen on the amniotic surface of the umbilical cord.

Histologically, there is evidence of maternal and usually fetal response to amniotic infection.[38,43,44,98] The earliest reaction is maternal and is manifested by an accumulation of neutrophils in the decidua. Next, leukocytes invade the fetal membranes at the lower pole of the amniotic sac, either at the site of membrane rupture or where intact membranes are exposed by the dilating cervix. These leukocytes come from maternal decidual vessels and migrate progressively through the chorion, amnion, and into the amnionic fluid in response to chemotactic factors released by the infecting agent or cells in the inflammatory exudate (Fig. 23.23). Various terms, including membranous deciduitis, membranous chorionitis, and membranous chorioamnionitis, have been applied to distinguish these stages in the progression of the inflammatory response (Fig. 23.24). In the placenta, also at an early stage in the progression of chorioamnionitis, maternal polymorphonuclear leukocytes migrate out of the intervillous space and accumulate immediately beneath the chorionic plate (subchorial intervillositis), often in a deposit of subchorionic fibrin (Fig. 23.25). These neutrophils eventually extend across the chorionic plate and migrate toward the amniotic cavity in response to the same leukotactic stimuli.

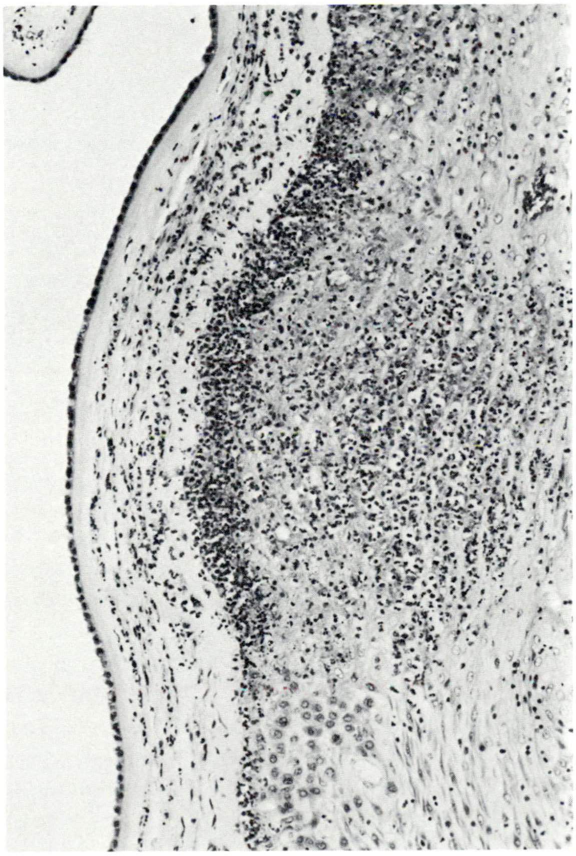

Fig. 23.23. Ascending infection, extraplacental membranes. Maternal neutrophils migrate from decidual vessels through the chorion and amnion toward the source of infection in the amnionic cavity.

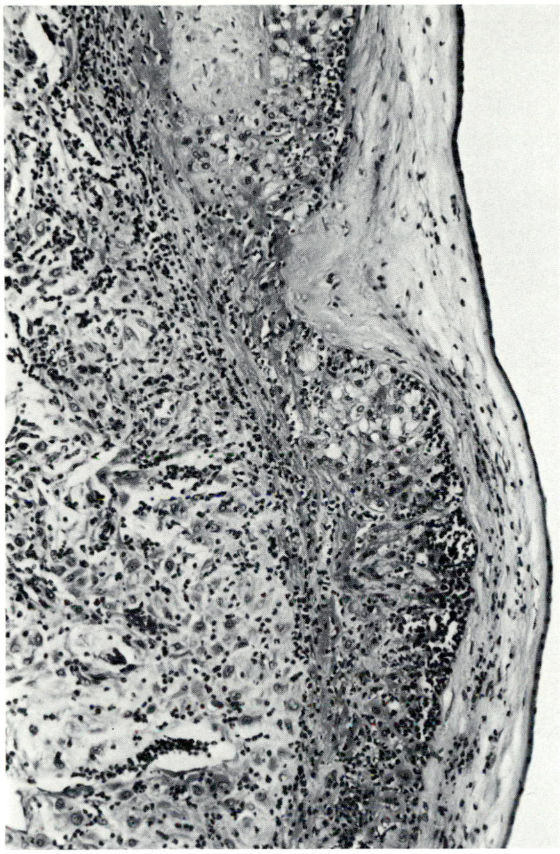

Fig. 23.24. Ascending infection, extraplacental membranes. The progression of the inflammatory response is illustrated here. Neutrophilic infiltration that involves the decidua and chorion on the *top* has extended into the amnion on the *bottom* as well.

The fetal leukocytes also respond to the amniotic infection. This reaction is less marked and somewhat delayed

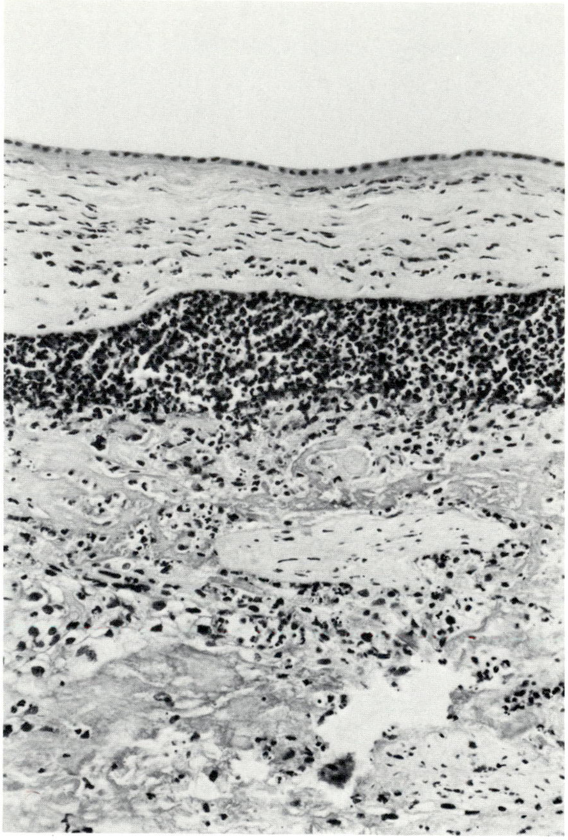

FIG. 23.25. Ascending infection, chorionic plate. Maternal neutrophils migrate out of the blood in the intervillous space and accumulate beneath the chorionic plate.

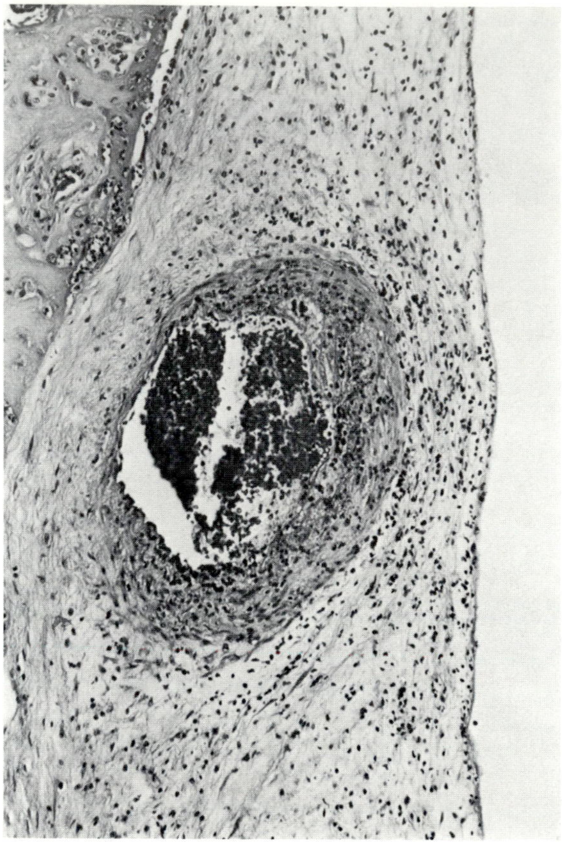

FIG. 23.26. Ascending infection, chorionic plate. Fetal neutrophils migrate through large fetal vessels of the chorionic plate. Orientation toward the source of infection in the amnionic cavity results in crescentic migration pattern.

when compared to the maternal response. In the chorionic plate of the placenta and in the umbilical cord, fetal leukocytes first marginate against vascular endothelium and then migrate through the walls of the large chorionic and umbilical arteries and veins into the chorionic plate or Wharton's jelly, respectively. This vasculitis is not concentric. The migration of inflammatory cells is crescent shaped, oriented toward the source of infection in the amniotic cavity (Figs. 23.26, 23.27 and 23.28). Inflammation of the umbilical cord tends to be segmental, perhaps sometimes caused by proximity to the cervical os or localized to zones affected by pressure, and may be found, therefore, in only one of multiple sections of umbilical cord in this circumstance.

Amniotic infection, then, is a unique situation in which two individuals, mother and fetus, respond to the same infectious stimulus. The overwhelming majority of leukocytes that participate in this process are maternal. This is not unexpected given the great discrepancy in surface area available for stimulation and migration of maternal (free membranes and chorionic plate) versus fetal (chorionic plate, umbilical cord) leukocytes and has been confirmed by analyzing the sex chromatin of the inflammatory cells in the amnionic exudate.[43] The fetal leukocytic response is generally absent in gestations of less than 19–20 weeks (fetal weight less than 500 g). Therefore, in very early abortions, the inflammatory response may be solely maternal. If infection occurs after fetal death, the fetal component will be absent.

In ascending infections, the inflammatory process is characteristically confined to the fetal membranes, chorionic plate, and umbilical cord. Villous tissue is not involved unless fetal infection and bacteremia result secondarily in villitis, an expression of inflammation that may occur in any other fetal organ under these circumstances. The character of the inflammatory infiltrate is usually not specific enough to identify a particular offending agent. In fact, it is relatively unusual to find bacteria in histologic sections even when they have been demonstrated on smears of the amnion. Notable exceptions to this include infections with group B β-hemolytic streptococci, in which colonies of the organism are frequently found without difficulty (Fig. 23.29). This type of infection may occur so rapidly that histologic evidence of chorioamnionitis may be absent even when bacterial colonies are numerous.[44] Hyphal and yeast forms of *Candida*

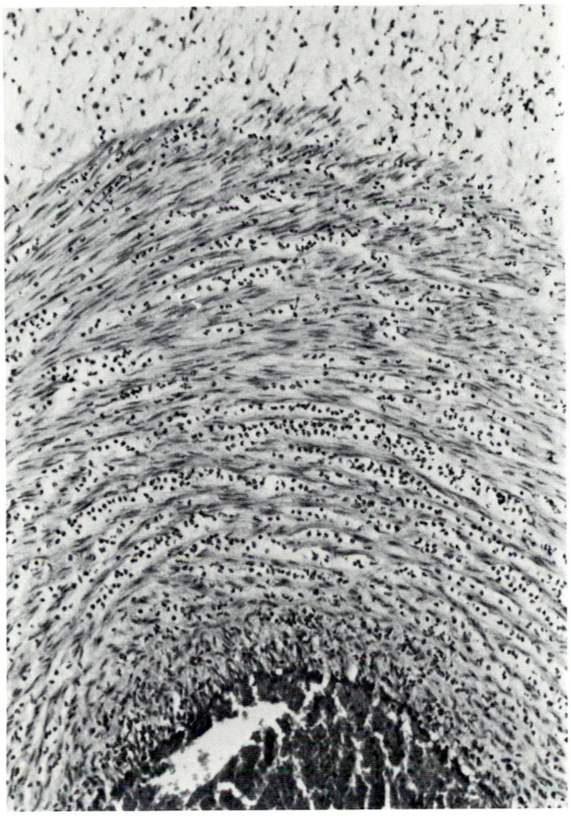

FIG. 23.27. Ascending infection, umbilical cord. Migration of fetal leukocytes from the umbilical artery.

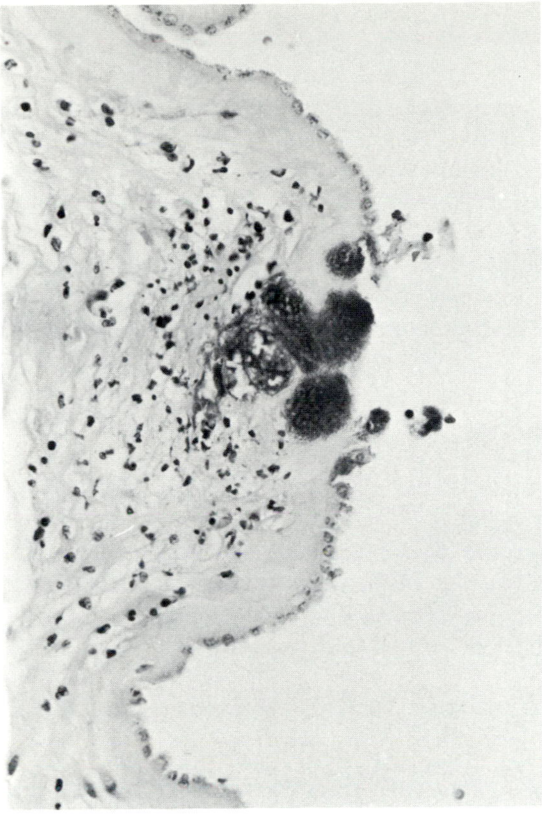

FIG. 23.29. Ascending infection. Colonies of group B β-hemolytic streptococci in amnion.

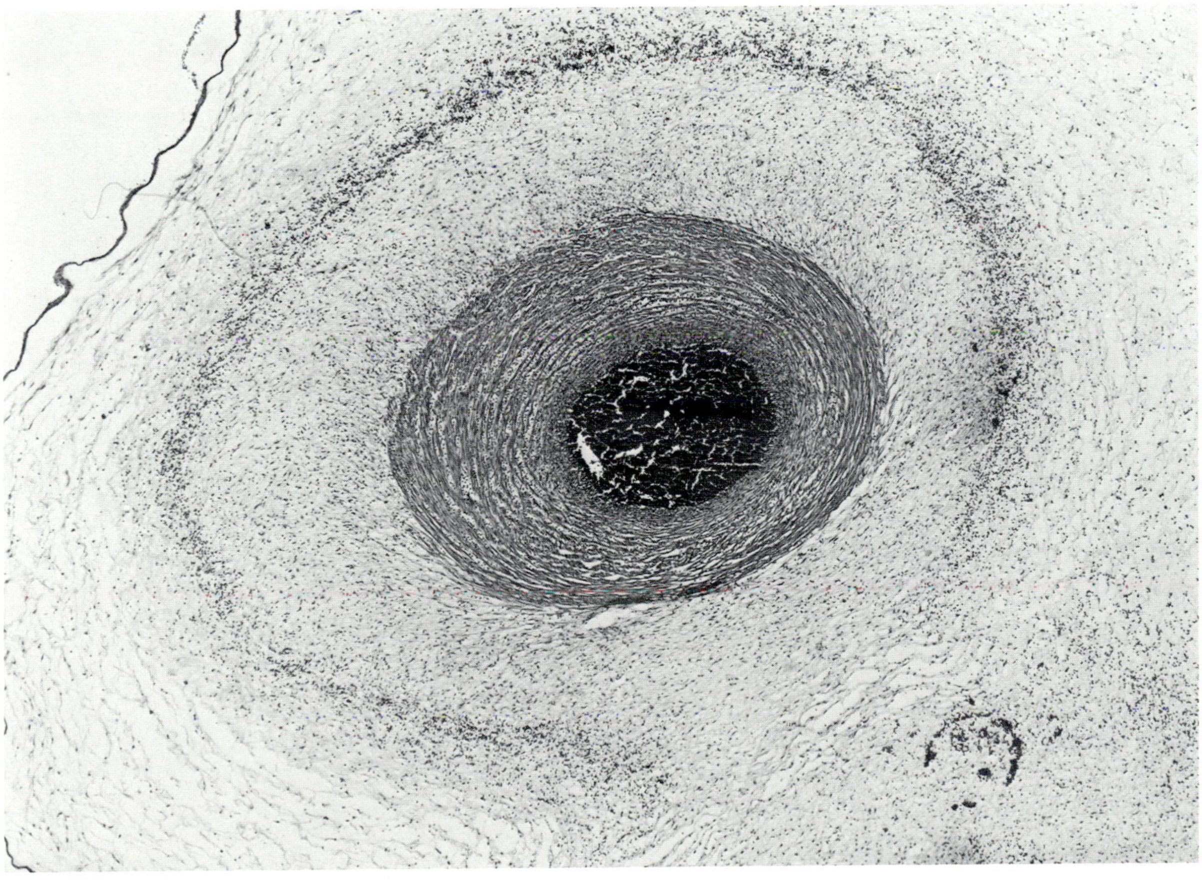

FIG. 23.28. Ascending infection, umbilical cord. Prominent crescentic band of leukocytes is accompanied by continued migration of neutrophils from the umbilical artery. This particular pattern of inflammation has been called *subacute necrotizing (healed) funisitis* and is thought to result from prolonged low-grade or spontaneously healed amnionic infection.

may also be identified, usually in small, superficial, crescentic microabscesses under the amniotic surface of the umbilical cord (Fig. 23.30).[125] The rarity of ascending candidal infection is surprising in view of the frequency with which it is found in the vagina. Natural defenses against *Candida* may help control its spread.[19]

Although there are maternal hazards associated with chorioamnionitis (maternal sepsis), the principal clinical impact of chorioamnionitis is the potential spread of infection to the fetus, which greatly outweighs any risk to the mother. Actually, in most cases of chorioamnionitis, neither mother nor neonate is overtly ill. Nevertheless, neonatal infection and sepsis are the leading cause of perinatal death in the United States as well as in developing countries,[174,220] and such serious neonatal infection very often is associated with chorioamnionitis.[85,220,289]

Inflammation of the placental tissues implies only that the fetus has been exposed to infection, not necessarily that the fetus is infected. In cases of chorioamnionitis, the exposed fetus may be infected in one of two ways: by (1) orificial or (2) hematogenous spread. Microorganisms may gain access to the respiratory or gastrointestinal tracts via aspiration or swallowing of infected amniotic fluid. A distinction should be made between aspiration of amniotic exudate and true pneumonia. In the former, the bronchioles and alveoli contain a mixture of amniotic elements, including a large number of neutrophils, many degenerating. These are confined to the bronchoalveolar tree, and there is no evidence of fetal response to infection (Fig. 23.31). True congenital pneumonia differs in that there is a definite pulmonary interstitial leukocytic infiltrate characteristic of bronchopneumonia. Similarly, swallowing of infected amniotic fluid may result in actual gastritis, ileitis, or gastrointestinal perforation with peritonitis. The fetal skin, eyes, or ear canals may also be contaminated by direct contact with infected amniotic fluid. Hematogenous spread of organisms from the infected amniotic fluid directly to the fetal circulation via the superficial chorionic vessels is another possible mechanism of fetal infection. Certainly, orificial contamination of the fetus does occur in a significant number of cases of chorioamnionitis.[38,183] However, in cases of actual fetal

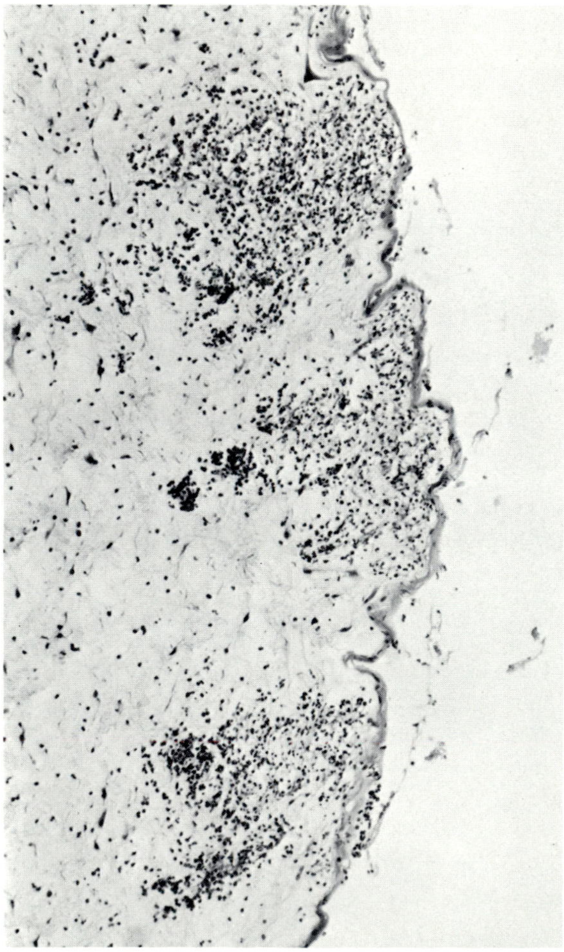

FIG. 23.30. *Candida* infection of umbilical cord. Small candidal microabscesses beneath the amnion of the umbilical cord. Gomori methenamine silver stain showed yeast and hyphae.

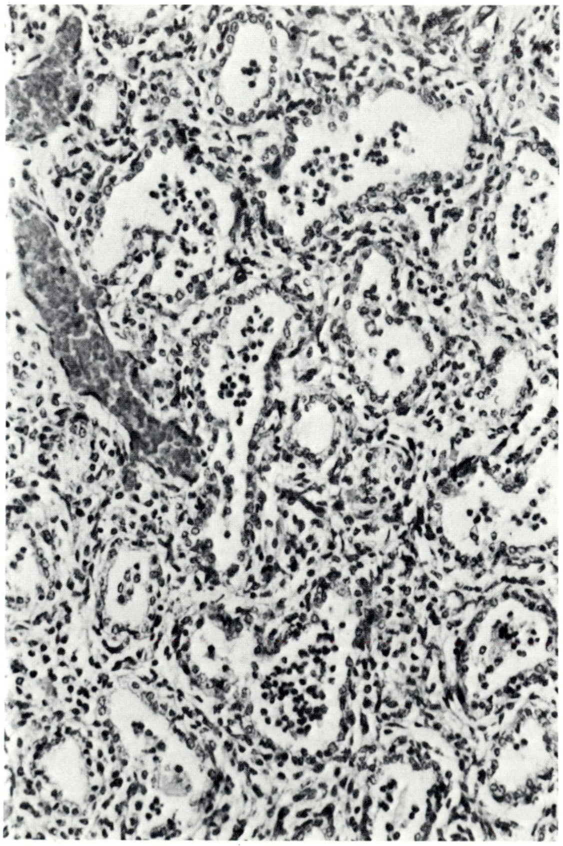

FIG. 23.31. Chorioamnionitis, fetal lung. Neutrophils aspirated from amnionic fluid are accumulated in the fetal bronchoalveolar tree. True fetal pneumonia is not present.

or neonatal sepsis, the relative importance of orifical versus direct spread of microorganisms to fetal chorionic vessels has not yet been clarified.

The etiology and pathogenesis of chorioamnionitis is only partially understood. Certainly, there is a consistent and well-documented relationship between chorioamnionitis and prolonged rupture of membranes:[66,110] the longer the membranes have been ruptured, the greater the likelihood that amniotic infection will occur. This sequence of events, membrane rupture followed by infection, seems to be operative in many term gestations, and in these circumstances, the threat of infection is universally recognized. However, it is not correct to ascribe chorioamnionitis solely to rupture of membranes. The same histologic findings, culture data, and clinical syndromes can be seen in the absence of membrane rupture.[89,167,181,182] In this situation, the cause and effect relationship between membrane rupture and chorioamnionitis may actually be reversed, chorioamnionitis preceding and being the cause, rather than a complication, of ruptured membranes.

Microorganisms, especially bacteria, have been cultured from the amniotic surface and amniotic fluid in many cases of chorioamnionitis. This fact, in addition to the experimental production of chorioamnionitis and congenital pneumonia in animals receiving intraamniotic injections of bacteria, support the widespread although not universal view that chorioamnionitis is caused by amniotic contamination with bacteria and other microorganisms. Similar injections of sterile exogenous irritants, such as gastric juice, acid, or India ink, do not result in chorioamnionitis.[153] The bacteria recovered from the amniotic fluid, fetal membranes, fetal tissues, and cord blood include a variety of anaerobes and aerobes, frequently as mixed flora. The most commonly recovered bacteria are *Escherichia coli,* coagulase-positive staphylococci, streptococci, *Proteus mirabilis, Klebsiella,* and *Pseudomonas.* These bacteria, inhabitants or contaminants of the vagina and cervix, are thought to ascend into the amniotic cavity, a process facilitated by membrane rupture. A perplexing observation has been the relatively high frequency of negative bacterial cultures when there are obvious histologic changes of chorioamnionitis.[162,195,289] This may be explained by the inability of routine culture techniques to detect mycoplasmas, chlamydiae, viruses, or even some organisms, such as *Listeria monocytogenes* or *Clostridium difficile.** In fact, when specifically sought, genital mycoplasmas are emerging with significant regularity in association with chorioamnionitis.[63] The demonstrated antibacterial effect of amniotic fluid itself may interfere with growth in culture.[19,228,264] Many studies have ignored the so-called saprophytic or nonpathogenic organisms, which may in fact be able to produce an inflammatory reaction in the fetal membranes or infection in the fetus. The possibility that many cases of chorioamnionitis are actually noninfective in nature has been cogently disputed by Fox.[98]

* References 79, 147, 161, 173, 239, 260.

A combination of histologic and clinical parameters may be used to predict fetal outcome in cases of chorioamnionitis. The absence of chorioamnionitis is an important finding. This virtually excludes intrauterine ascending infection and significant clinical sepsis in the first 48 hours of life.[220] Infants whose placentas show evidence of chorioamnionitis are at increased risk to develop sepsis and die in the neonatal period.[140,289] The magnitude of the risk has been correlated with the severity of the inflammatory reaction. Neonatal morbidity and mortality are significantly greater when the inflammatory response is graded moderate or severe than when it is mild in degree.[289] The frequency of positive cultures also increases with the severity of the inflammatory response, although the histologic identification of moderate to severe chorioamnionitis alone, even in the absence of a positive culture, is a useful indicator of infection in both the mother and the newborn.[220,289]

Acute chorioamnionitis is strongly correlated with prematurity; its occurrence is inversely proportional to gestational age.[220] This association between chorioamnionitis and preterm labor and delivery is well known, but the nature of the link between the two is still a matter of debate. Nevertheless, the combination of chorioamnionitis and prematurity is definitely associated with a high incidence of perinatal death. In one study, infants born at less than 36 weeks to febrile mothers whose membranes had been ruptured more than 24 hours had a perinatal mortality of 50%. In contrast, infants born near term to afebrile mothers without prolonged ruptured membranes or cervical ligature showed no increased morbidity or mortality despite the presence of chorioamnionitis.[220]

Several methods have been proposed to permit a rapid diagnosis of chorioamnionitis and potential infection of the exposed fetus. These include (1) cytology of a gastric aspirate or ear canal fluid, (2) smear of chorion or amnion, (3) whole mount of amnion, and (4) frozen section of the umbilical cord. These techniques attempt to document an inflammatory infiltrate and the presence and type of microorganisms involved. Since many cases of chorioamnionitis are associated with normal healthy neonates, these techniques serve only to alert the clinician to the potential for infection in an exposed neonate.

Hematogenous Infection

In hematogenous infections of the placenta, infectious agents reach the placenta through the maternal blood. In contrast to chorioamnionitis, which is usually a purely local infection, placental involvement in hematogenous infection is usually only one manifestation of maternal systemic disease. The histologic hallmark of this type of infection is villitis, inflammation in the villous parenchyma itself. Villitis is usually but not invariably due to hematogenous spread of organisms. There is some evidence that such placental infection might also spread from a focus of endometrial inflammation or might even result from noninfectious immunologic problems comparable to the graft-vs-host reaction.

Characteristically, hematogenous infections involve the placental villi, not the fetal membranes. Commonly, villitis is discovered incidentally on microscopic examination, with neither clinical suspicion of nor gross pathologic clue to the underlying inflammatory process. In some cases, there may be some subtle gross abnormalities, including placental enlargement, edema, or scattered minute necrotic foci. Histologically, the essential features of villitis are (1) a villous inflammatory infiltrate and (2) vasculitis. Morphologically, the villitides may be subdivided based on the nature of the inflammatory infiltrate (acute or chronic), type of inflammatory cell involved (lymphocyte, histiocyte, plasma cell, neutrophil), distribution of lesions (focal, diffuse, basal), and severity (mild, moderate, severe).[12,44,98,99,222] Altshuler and Russell[13] have divided the villitides into histologic groups based on stages of evolution and repair as follows:

1. Proliferative villitis: Inflammatory cells are present in the villi, but there is no necrosis.
2. Necrotizing villitis: Inflammatory cells and necrosis are present in the villi.
3. Reparative villitis: The inflammatory process is resolving with granulation tissue and fibroblastic proliferation.
4. Stromal fibrosis: The villi are fibrotic but do not show evidence of active inflammation.

These histologic patterns usually do not correlate with specific etiologic agents and may occur in various combinations. An exact diagnosis is reached in only a small number of cases when a specific agent is identified on light or electron microscopy or is cultured from the placental or fetal tissue. Serologic studies of the mother and infant may provide valuable information about etiology. Clinical and microbiologic correlations with the histologic finding of villitis are scant. Available information is based on the study of a relatively small number of cases due to an identifiable agent. Most villitides are of unknown etiology. Many show evidence of both chronic and active infection manifested by the coexistence of fresh and old, healed lesions. Practically speaking, villitis is often mild and focal and, therefore, may be entirely overlooked if a considerable number of sections are not examined.

Specific Variants

Viral Infection

Cytomegalovirus (*CMV*). The pathology of CMV placentitis is the histologic prototype for all viral villitides.* The placenta may be normal in size, small in cases of fetal growth retardation, or large and edematous when associated with fetal anemia. Histologically, the villi may exhibit any or all of a wide spectrum of changes including acute necrotizing villitis, lymphoplasmacytic villous infiltrates that are especially rich in plasma cells, or complete villous fibrosis (Figs. 23.32 and 23.33). Vasculitis and stromal hemosiderin deposition are very characteristic (Fig. 23.34). In old lesions, only the remnants of occluded vessels may remain (Fig. 23.35). Villous histiocytes and stromal cells are usually increased, and foci of stromal calcification may be found. The typical, large, intranuclear and intracytoplasmic eosinophilic inclusions may be found in endothelial cells, Hofbauer cells, or trophoblast (Fig. 23.36). When found, they are diagnostic, but

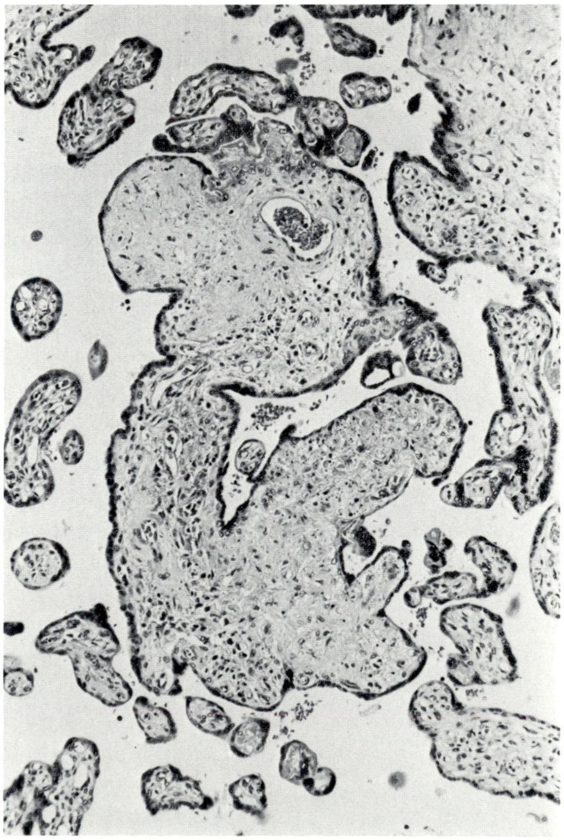

Fig. 23.32. Villitis, cytomegalovirus infection. Lymphoplasmacytic villous infiltrate and focal villous necrosis.

* References 13, 32, 42, 44, 98, 99, 169.

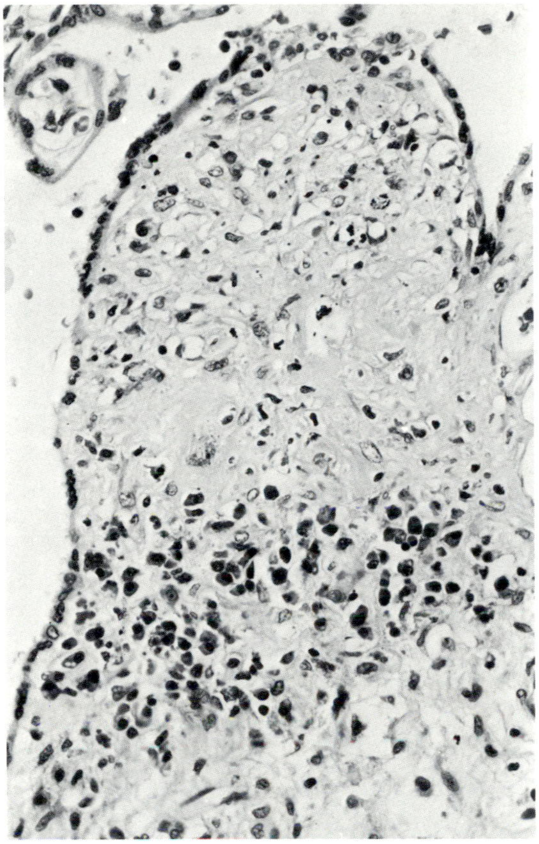

FIG. 23.33. Villitis, cytomegalovirus infection. Villous inflammatory infiltrate, especially rich in plasma cells, is associated with focal necrosis and fibrosis, *top*.

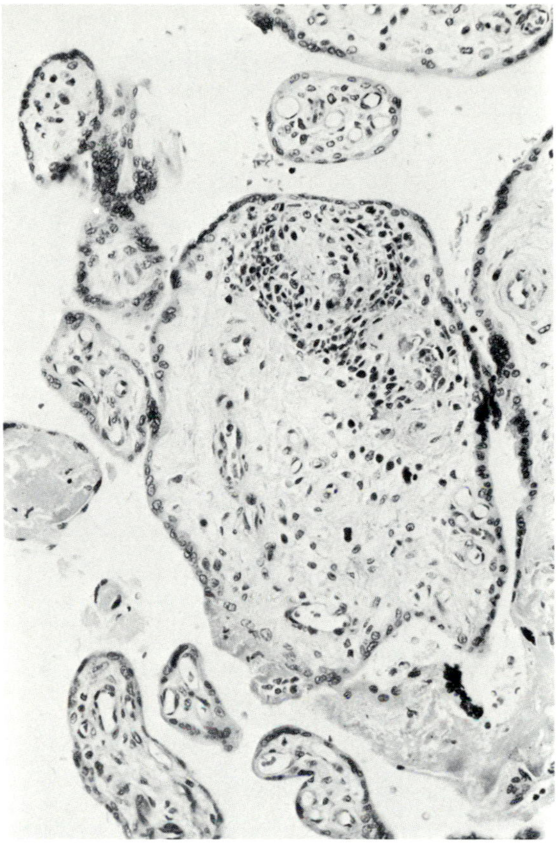

FIG. 23.34. Villitis, cytomegalovirus infection. Segmental vasculitis.

unfortunately they are usually scarce and seldom identified, even after diligent search. Relative villous immaturity and edema are nonspecific changes related to the fetal anemia in some cases.

CMV placentitis is the most commonly identified of all viral placental infections. The incidence of congenital infection ranges from 0.2 to 2.2% among all live births. The natural history of cytomegalovirus infection in pregnancy is complex and not completely understood despite intense investigation.† Epidemiologic data indicate that (1) transmission to the offspring may occur in utero, at birth, or postnatally, (2) intrauterine infection may result from either primary or recurrent maternal infection, the latter despite substantial humoral immunity, (3) infection may be symptomatic at birth (hepatosplenomegaly, microcephaly, petechiae), but in the vast majority of infants, infection is subclinical, (4) late complications, including mental retardation, chorioretinitis, seizures, learning disabilities, and especially neurosensory hearing loss, are most common among the survivors of symptomatic congenital infection but may also occur later in children with no clinical manifestations at birth, and (5) congenital infections resulting from reactivation of latent virus are less likely to produce fetal damage and late sequelae than those resulting from primary maternal infections.

Cytomegaloviruses are common and readily infect the fetus and newborn. They are unique in their ability to cause both acute infection and chronic subtle disease that may not manifest itself for months or years. At this time, CMV is the most commonly recognized infectious cause of developmental impairments. In practical terms, a multifocal lymphoplasmacytic villitis with vasculitis and stromal hemosiderin in the United States is probably a CMV infection. Some authors have found a "fairly good" correlation between the severity of the placental lesions and the clinical outcome.[42]

Rubella. The pathologic findings associated with rubella infection have been described mainly in placentas from first and second trimester abortions[84,194,266] but in a few term deliveries as well.[29,107,194] In placental tissue examined shortly after the acute clinical infection, there may be focal necrotizing villitis and vasculitis that vary mark-

† References 5, 6, 8, 113, 160, 189, 212, 245, 247–249.

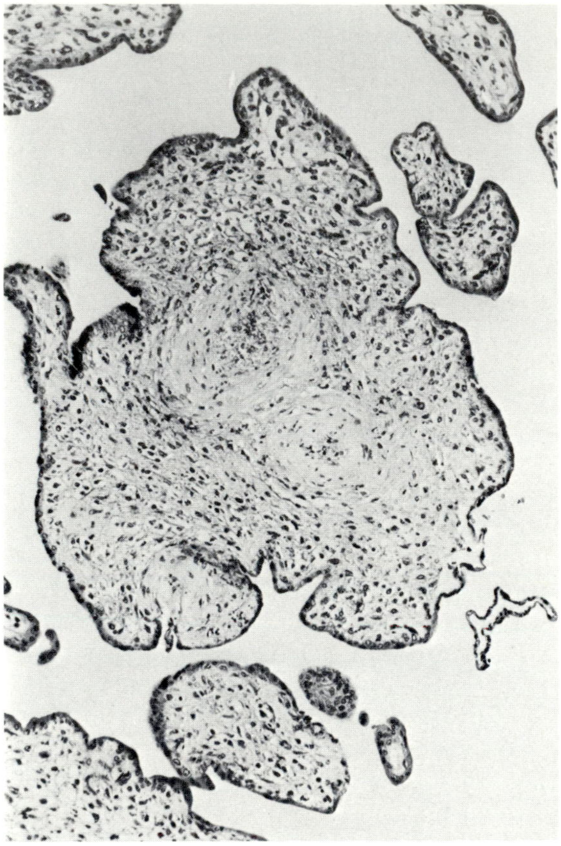

Fig. 23.35. Villitis, cytomegalovirus infection. Villi showing remnants of hyalinized, obliterated vessels.

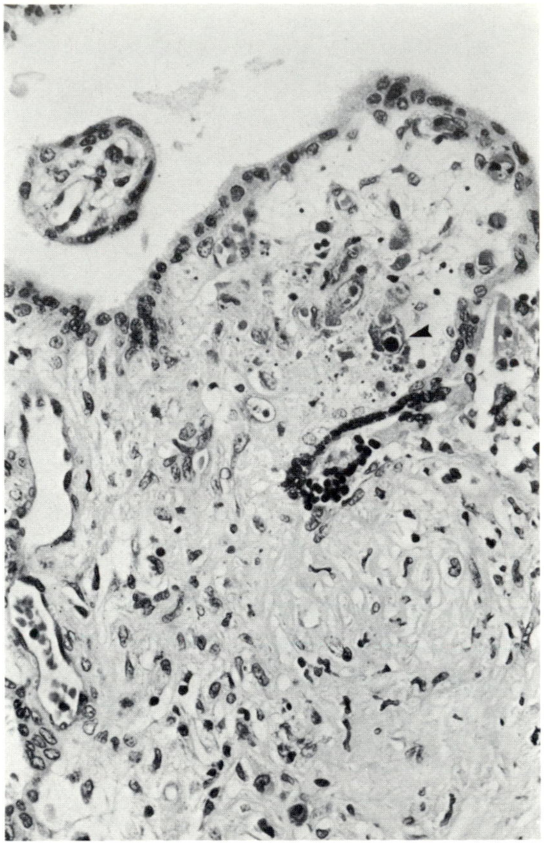

Fig. 23.36. Villitis, cytomegalovirus infection. Typical cytomegalic intranuclear inclusion bodies (*arrow*) associated with focal villous necrosis.

edly in severity and extent. Some villi exhibit only focal trophoblastic necrosis, whereas in others, totally necrotic trophoblast is associated with perivillous fibrin and acute inflammation. Endothelial necrosis, often associated with fragmentation of fetal red cells, is probably the most characteristic finding. There may be an associated chronic perivascular infiltrate. Eosinophilic cytoplasmic viral inclusion bodies may be found in endothelial cells, Hofbauer cells, villous stromal cells, and trophoblast. Identical viral inclusions and perivascular chronic inflammatory infiltrates have been reported in the decidua in some cases.[194] A mild, focal chronic inflammatory infiltrate occurs infrequently in the membranes and cord.[107]

Placentas delivered and examined after the acute stage of the maternal disease may show only scattered, shrunken, avascular villi. In some cases, these healed lesions coexist with more acute changes, as described above. Such placentas may be very small for gestational age. The combination of severe hypoplasia and vascular changes is very characteristic of rubella infection. A number of placentas from which rubella virus has been isolated do not show any inflammatory changes or other morphologic abnormality.[98,194]

The consequences of rubella infection during pregnancy include spontaneous abortion, fetal death, intrauterine growth retardation, congenital malformations, active neonatal infection, and such delayed manifestations as deafness and mental retardation. Fortunately, these are now limited to rare sporadic cases, since epidemics of rubella have been controlled by immunization programs. The exact incidence of fetal damage from maternal rubella infection is unknown, but infection during the first trimester appears to present the greatest risk to the fetus. During past rubella epidemics, microscopic abnormalities have been documented in 33–68% of fetuses infected and aborted in the first trimester, although gross malformations were not evident in these fetuses.[194,266] However, gross malformations, usually multiple, were found in half of the fetuses infected in the first trimester but not aborted until 5–6 months.[194] These malformations involve primarily the eyes (cataract), cardiovascular system (patent ductus arteriosus, ventricular septal defect), and central nervous system (microcephaly) and are postulated to result from a combination of viral inhibition of cell growth, cytolysis, and interference with blood supply.[179] Survivors of congenital rubella infection can also suffer from late sequelae, including panencephalitis[270,276] and diabetes mellitus.[92,131,165]

Herpes Simplex Virus. Disseminated herpes simplex virus infection, once a rare occurrence, has become an increasingly common cause of devastating disease and death in the newborn. Intrapartum transmission of virus from the maternal genital tract is by far the most common mode of fetal infection.[246] In only a very few cases has there been histologic documentation of ascending[11,44] or transplacental dissemination[44,285] or both of the herpes simplex virus. Foci of villous necrosis, agglutination of villi, and fibrinoid necrosis of villous vessels have been documented in the rare cases of hematogenous infection. Chorioamnionitis, of both the necrotizing and chronic lymphoplasmacytic types, has been described in a few cases of ascending infection. An increased frequency of spontaneous abortion and congenital malformation has been reported in patients with primary infection in the first 20 weeks of pregnancy.*

Other Viruses. Pathologic findings in the few placentas with documented infection by other viruses, such as vaccinia, variola, varicella, Coxsackie B, and hepatitis B virus, have been detailed by Fox,[98,99] Blanc,[42,44] and Altshuler and Russell.[13] Unfortunately, the potential effects of many of the most common viruses that must be frequently encountered during pregnancy (enteroviruses, adenoviruses, influenza viruses) are not well known.

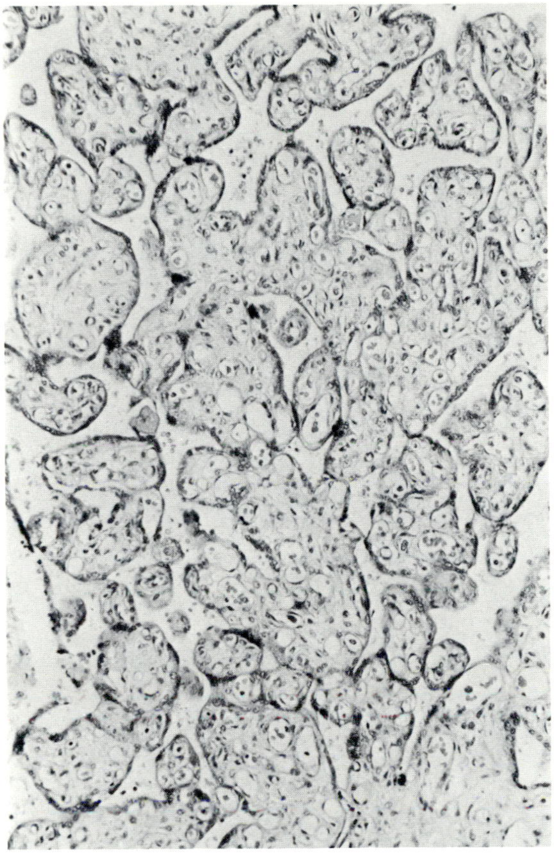

FIG. 23.37. Congenital syphilis at term in a liveborn infant. Large, immature, actively budding villi with pronounced increase in vascularity. Erythroblasts are present in villous capillaries.

Bacterial Infection

Treponema Pallidum. Once a major cause of abortion and stillbirth, congenital syphilis is now uncommon. Grossly, infected placentas tend to be large and bulky. Histologically, the villi are large and relatively immature but not markedly edematous (Fig. 23.37). Villous vessels exhibit subendothelial and perivascular fibrosis, resulting in luminal narrowing and occlusion (Fig. 23.38). A lymphoplasmacytic villous infiltrate and increased numbers of Hofbauer cells may be seen focally (Fig. 23.39). The histologic changes in the placenta are not diagnostic but are highly suggestive, especially in conjunction with the characteristic lesions that occur in the fetal organs (pneumonia alba, pancreatic fibrosis, cirrhosis, osteitis). Definitive diagnosis depends on demonstration of spirochetes in the placental or fetal tissue, which may be accomplished by a Warthin-Starry or Levaditi stain.[223]

The traditional view that congenital syphilis occurs only after infection in the second half of pregnancy has now been disproved. Transplacental transmission of circulating spirochetes may occur at any time during pregnancy.[44,118] Morphologic expression of the placental and fetal lesions of congenital syphilis, however, seems to depend on the fetal inflammatory response, which is not yet developed in the very immature fetus.[25,242]

Listeria Monocytogenes. L. monocytogenes is a significant cause of intrauterine infection, spontaneous abortion, prematurity, and neonatal sepsis, morbidity, and death.† Although *L. monocytogenes* is a well-recognized cause of septic abortion in animals, reports incriminating it as a possible cause of habitual abortion in humans are conflicting.[111,154,207] The epidemiology, mode of spread, and pathogenesis of *L. monocytogenes* infection are still obscure.[126]

In cases of intrauterine infection, the characteristic and relatively specific histologic pattern of placental microabscesses has led to the traditional view of *L. monocytogenes* as a transplacentally acquired infection. In fact, chorioamnionitis and funisitis are also almost invariably

* References 91, 117, 170, 186–188, 244, 246.

† References 17, 116, 126, 201, 209, 288.

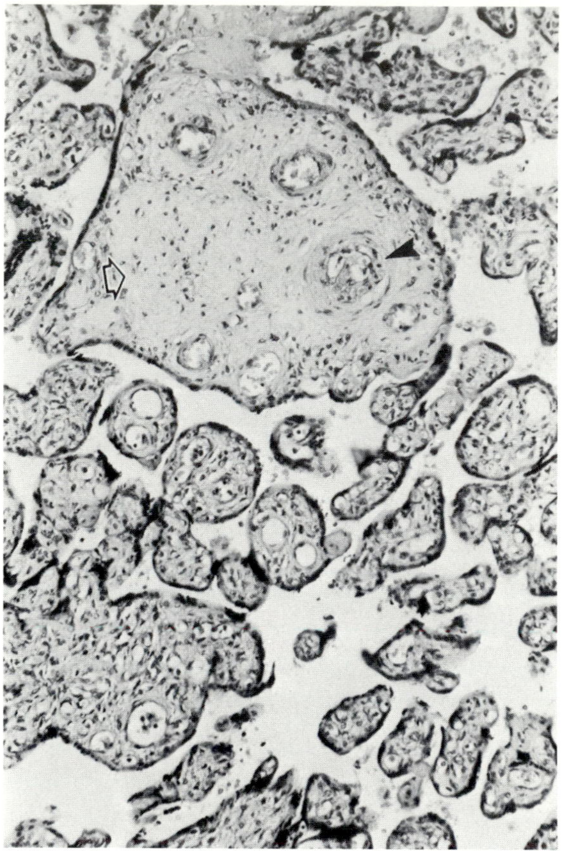

FIG. 23.38. Congenital syphilis at term in a liveborn infant. Perivascular and subendothelial fibrosis resulting in partial (*black arrow*) and complete (*open arrow*) vascular obliteration in a stem villus.

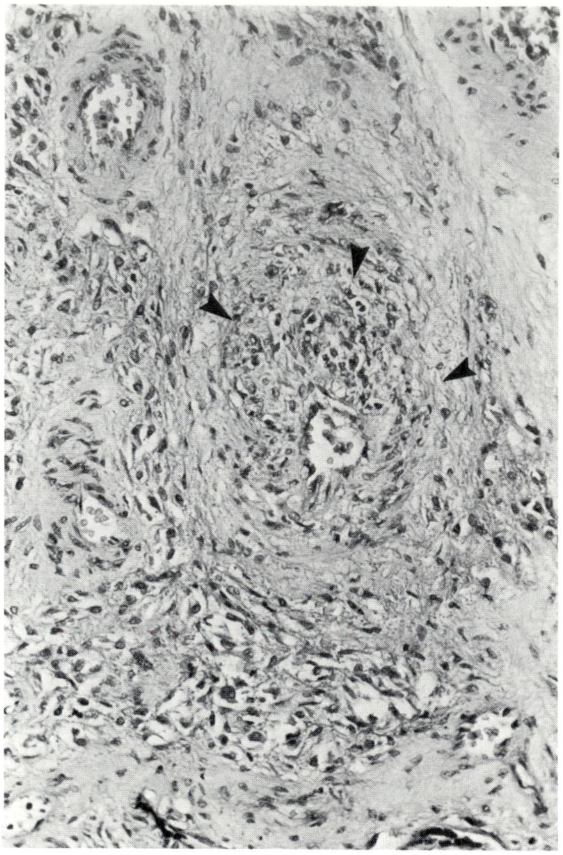

FIG. 23.39. Congenital syphilis at term in a liveborn infant. Stem villus with a lymphohistiocytic infiltrate and vasculitis. *Arrows* indicate a vessel infiltrated by lymphocytes.

present.[44,86,286] Grossly, the placenta may appear normal or, on careful inspection, contain minute, yellow-white necrotic foci that correspond histologically to small foci of purulent villitis in which groups of acutely inflamed villi are enmeshed in fibrin and an acute perivillous and intervillous inflammatory infiltrate. These abscesses may be surrounded by a rim of palisaded histiocytes and occasional giant cells (Fig. 23.40). Typically, in scattered, individual villi, a ring of neutrophils is localized between the trophoblast and villous stroma. Occasionally, macroscopic abscesses are present,[250] and extensive spread into the intervillous space may cause infarction. The coexistence of villitis and chorioamnionitis is consistent with either (1) primary hematogenous dissemination and secondary contamination of the amniotic cavity, (2) primary ascending infection with secondary fetal infection and villitis, or (3) simultaneous dissemination via hematogenous and ascending routes. Microabscesses identical to those found in the placenta may be widely disseminated in the fetal organs as well (granulomatosis infantiseptica).[234] The organism, a small, gram-positive, nonsporulating, microaerophilic, motile bacillus with rounded ends, is difficult to demonstrate in the sections of fetal lesions, placenta, or fetal membranes. Nor is it always easy to isolate the organism in culture, owing, in part, to the fact that its growth favors relatively low temperatures (35–36°C). The diagnosis has been made by amniocentesis.[200]

Other Bacteria. Hematogenous dissemination of other bacteria does occur but is uncommon. The placental lesions of the few documented cases associated with hematogenous spread of organisms, such as pyogenic and enteric bacteria, *Francisella tularensis*, *Brucella*, *Vibrio fetus*, *Mycobacterium tuberculosis*, and *Mycobacterium leprae*, are detailed in the treatises by Fox[98] and Blanc.[44]

Protozoan and Parasitic Infection

Toxoplasma Gondii. The placenta infected with *Toxoplasma gondii* may be grossly normal but is more commonly large and edematous, resembling the hydropic placenta of severe Rh incompatibility.[10,20] Microscopically, there is a low-grade chronic villitis in which a predominantly lymphocytic infiltrate invades single or

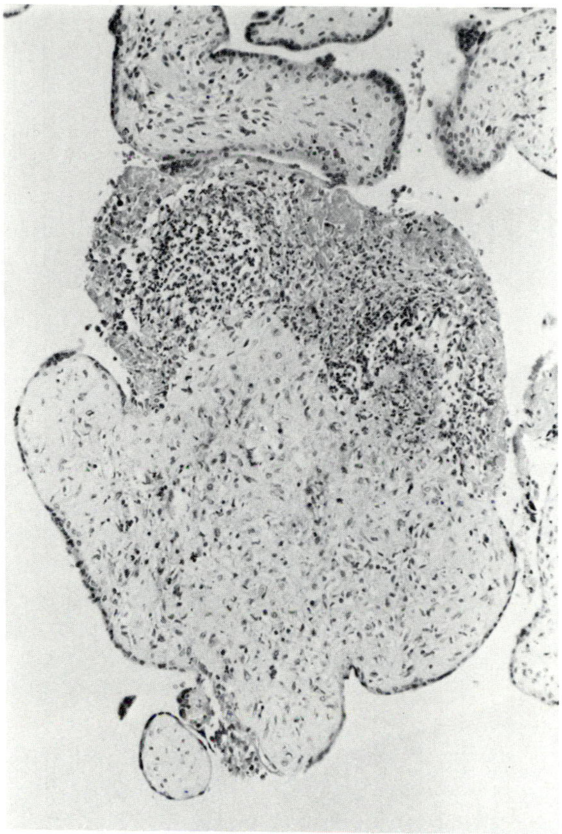

FIG. 23.40. Congenital listeriosis. Massive subtrophoblastic acute villitis with necrosis.

small groups of villi. Endarteritis, focal villous necrosis, or fibrosis may be seen.[87] A chronic inflammatory infiltrate has been reported in the umbilical cord.[192] The organism, usually in the encysted form, is identified rarely in the fetal membranes or chorionic plate, if found at all. It is typically unassociated with any inflammation.[10,29,87] In instances of perinatal death, organisms can be identified readily in the fetal brain.

The epidemiology, clinical features, and laboratory diagnosis of toxoplasma are reviewed in several articles.[73,101] Congenital infection appears to result mainly from maternal infection acquired for the first time early in pregnancy, usually by ingesting undercooked meat or by contact with cat feces. The risk of fetal infection in these circumstances is less than 50%. The clinical spectrum of fetal involvement ranges from severe damage to the central nervous system and eyes to completely asymptomatic infection, recognized only by the development of chorioretinitis after months of follow-up. Antibiotic treatment during pregnancy seems to reduce the frequency of congenital infection.[282] Infection acquired later in pregnancy is less likely to cause overt disease in the newborn, presumably because of the resistance offered by a more mature immune system. In the presence of maternal antibodies from past infections, fetal lesions do not occur.[73]

Villitis of Unknown Etiology (VUE)

Although potentially catastrophic, fetoplacental infections caused by the agents detailed previously (CMV, rubella, *T. gondii*, *T. pallidum*) are infrequent. Far more commonly, a focal chronic villitis, for which no etiology can be established, is discovered incidentally in sections of the placenta. Estimates of this phenomenon vary greatly, but Russell identified chronic villitis of unknown etiology (VUE) in 7.6% of over 7500 consecutively examined single placentas.[221] Knox and Fox identified the same lesion in 13.6% of 1000 randomly selected patients.[145]

The infant associated with such placental changes is generally unaffected, although Russell and others have presented convincing evidence that VUE is associated with intrauterine growth retardation and that the severity of the villitis correlates directly with the degree of growth retardation and the perinatal mortality rate.[145,150,221,222] VUE has a considerable tendency to recur,[221,222,224] but its potential role in repeated pregnancy loss is unknown,

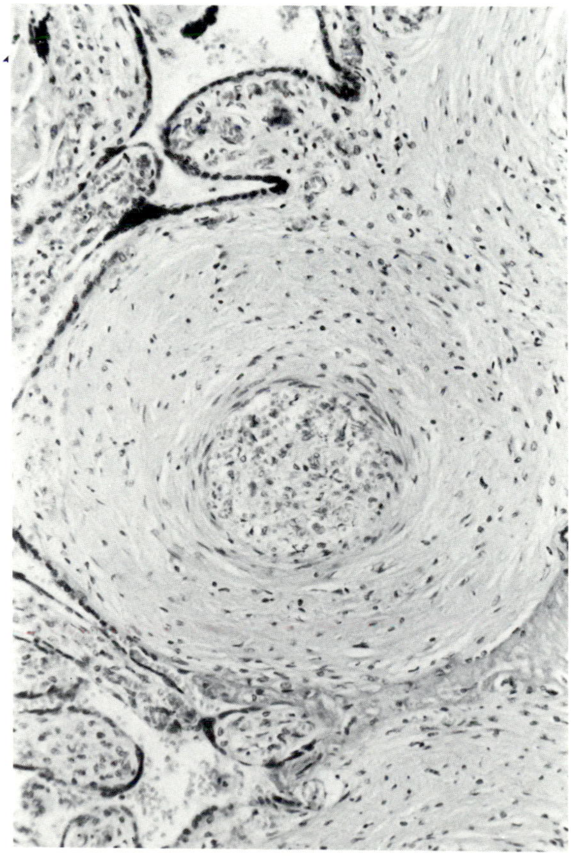

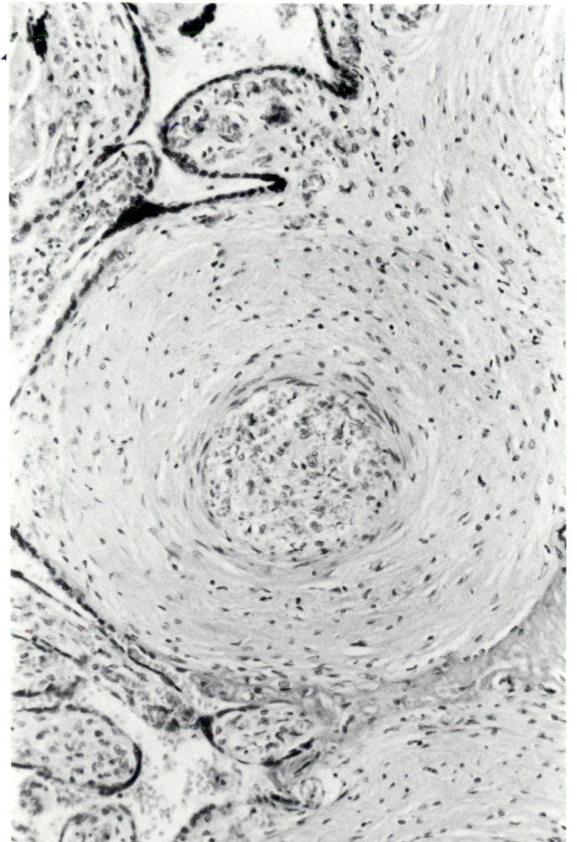

FIG. 23.41. Hemorrhagic endovasculitis. Recent organizing thrombus within a large vessel of a stem villus.

since routine histologic examination of the placenta is not performed in most institutions.

The lesions are always found incidentally in histologic sections of the placenta; there are no macroscopic abnormalities. Histologically, the villitis may resemble any of the previously described morphologic varieties, with predominance of any one of, or combination of, cell types. Russell has subdivided cases of VUE into two groups, lymphocytic and histiocytic, but has shown no difference in clinical significance between the two.[221]

Because of the histologic similarity between these lesions and those caused by known infectious agents, VUE is presumed to be infectious. Attempts to identify a causative agent by microscopic, serologic, or morphologic techniques have failed so far. The possibility that VUE might represent an immunologic, host versus graft response has been considered.

Hemorrhagic endovasculitis is a recently described variant of VUE.[226] Histologically, this condition is distinguished by thrombi in various stages of organization within fetal vessels of all sizes. Fragmentation and diapedesis of fetal red cells, villous stromal hemorrhage and hemosiderin, vascular necrosis, endothelial proliferation, and recanalization of vessels all combine to produce a distinctive pattern (Figs. 23.41, 23.42, and 23.43). Sixty to seventy percent of cases are associated with chronic villitis. An association with significant fetal morbidity and mortality has been established.

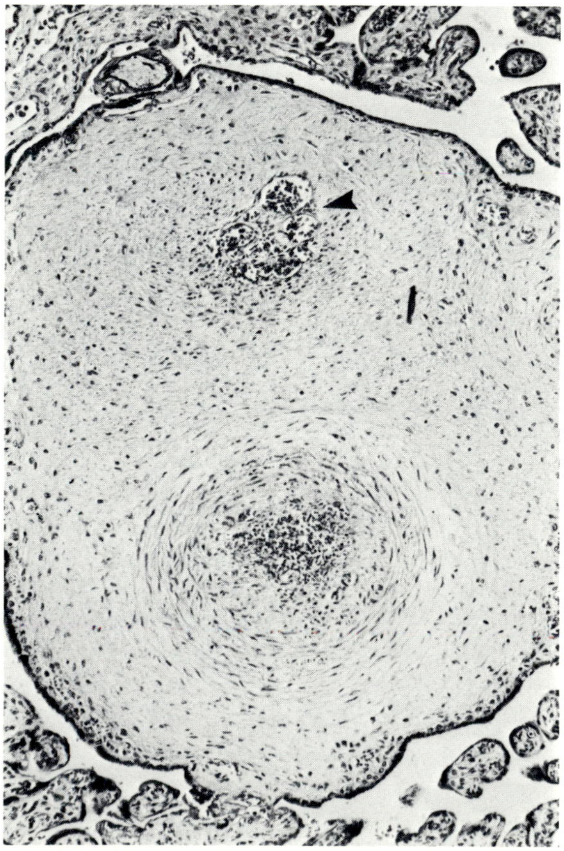

FIG. 23.42. Hemorrhagic endovasculitis. Thrombi in various stages of organization in vessels of stem villi. Recanalized channels are apparent (*arrow*).

Circulatory Disorders

Infarct

An infarct in the placenta, as in any other organ, is an area of ischemic necrosis resulting from obstruction of its blood supply. Because of the unique, dual blood supply to the placenta, there has been some controversy historically about whether infarction is a result of obstruction of the fetal or the maternal circulatory system or both. It is now clear that the villi are sustained by the oxygen and nutrients supplied by the maternal blood in the intervillous space and that most infarcts are due to occlusion of maternal uteroplacental vessels. Occasionally, a retroplacental hematoma may result in an infarct by physically separating the placenta from its maternal blood supply. It may be conceptually difficult to imagine how villi immersed in a pool of blood supplied by numerous maternal arterioles can become ischemic after the occlusion of a single or even a few maternal vessels. Hemodynamically, however, there does not appear to be any significant amount of mixing of blood from the various maternal inflow streams, despite the fact that these are not defined by actual anatomic channels. Functionally, then, the streams or jets of blood from the maternal spiral arteries are as necessary to the tissue they supply as are end arterioles in other organs.

Infarcts may occur in any portion of the placenta but are most common at its periphery. They are often triangular in shape, with the base abutting the basal plate (Fig. 23.44). The gross appearance of the infarct, as in other organs, changes with age. Fresh infarcts are red and might be difficult to distinguish from the surrounding normal placenta were it not for their firm consistency. Infarcts grow progressively firmer and change in color from red to brown and then to yellow or white. The histologic appearance of an infarct also changes with age. In early infarcts, the villi are crowded together, with extreme narrowing or obliteration of the intervillous space (Fig. 23.45). Small amounts of fibrin may accumulate in the intervillous space. The villous vessels are dilated and congested (Fig. 23.46). The syncytiotrophoblast, vascular endothelium, and villous stroma undergo progressive necrosis until eventually the infarct consists of crowded, ghostlike remnants of necrotic villi. A perivillous rim of acidophilic material is all that remains of the syncytiotrophoblast (Figs. 23.47 and 23.48). Eventually, the fetal stem arteries supplying the infarcted villi

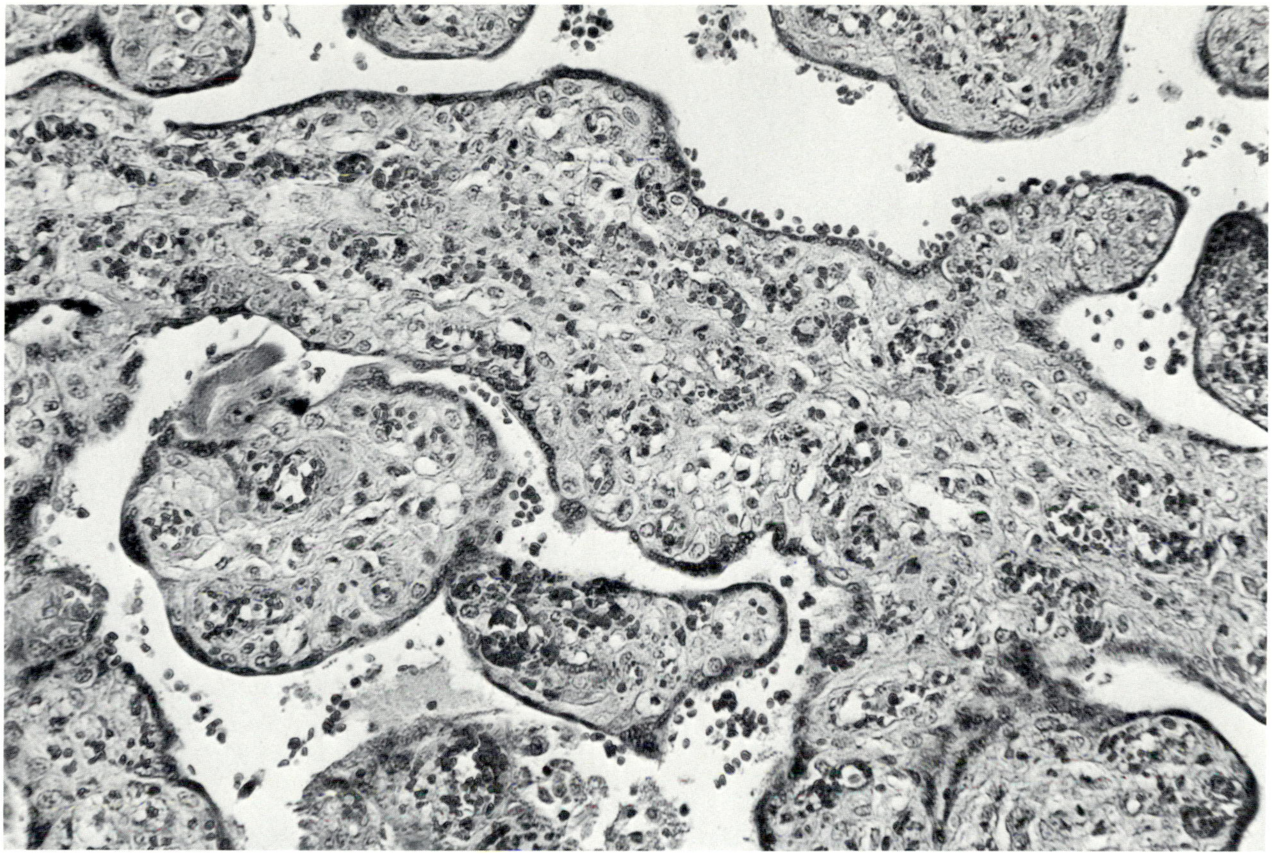

FIG. 23.43. Hemorrhagic endovasculitis. Fragmented red blood cells and nuclear debris are present in the terminal villi. Many of the vessels of these terminal villi have been destroyed.

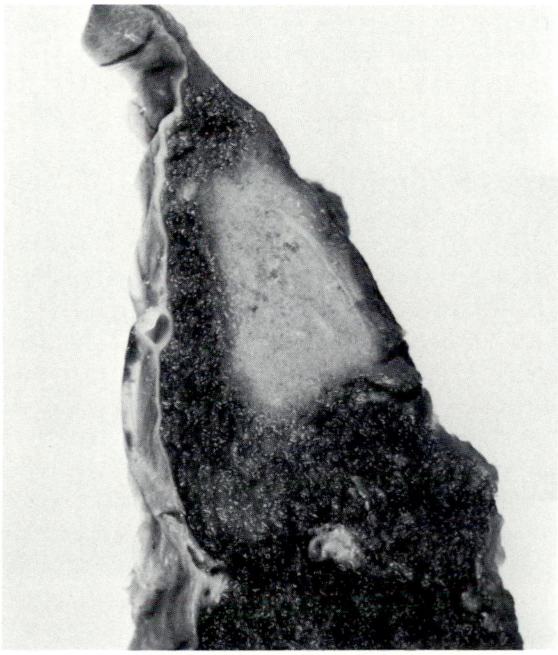

FIG. 23.44. Triangular, white infarct with base abutting the basal plate.

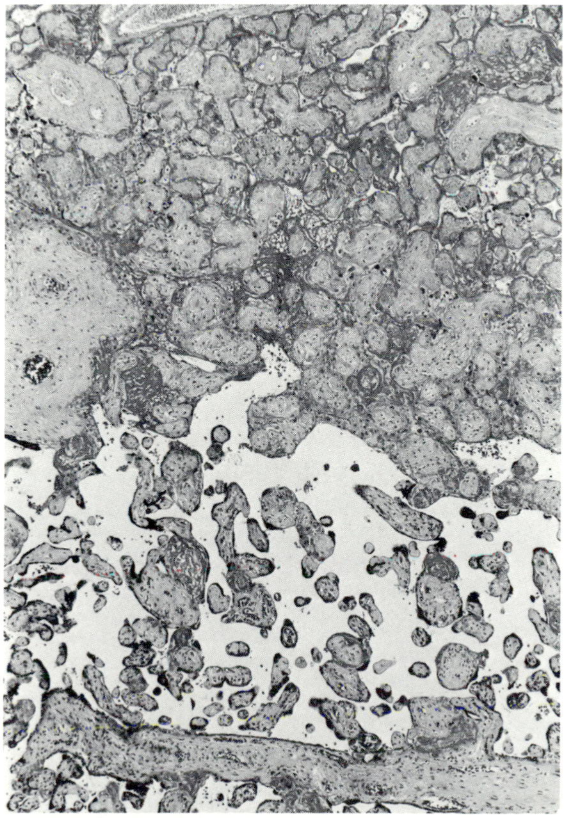

FIG. 23.45. Placental infarct (*top*) with aggregation of villi and obliteration of the intervillous space. Adjacent normal placenta is on the *bottom*.

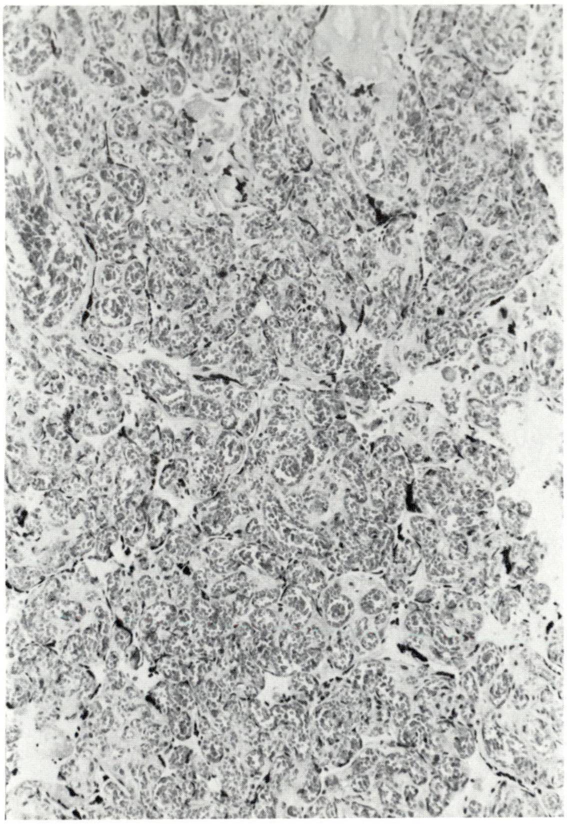

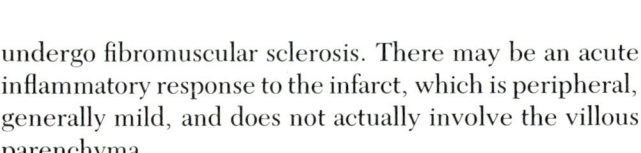

FIG. 23.46. Very early placental infarct. The villous vessels are markedly dilated and congested, but there is little evidence of necrosis.

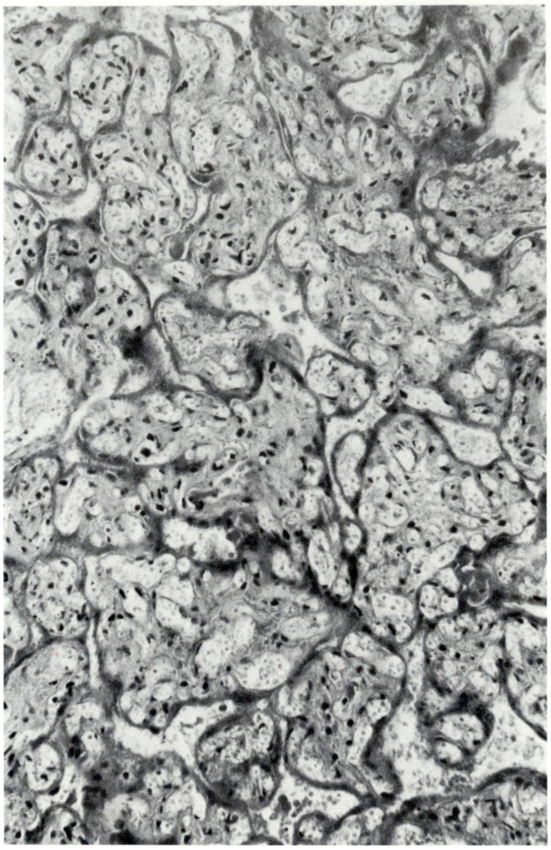

FIG. 23.47. Placental infarct. Much of the villous trophoblast is necrotic in this older infarct. The erythrocytes in the fetal capillaries have undergone hemolysis.

undergo fibromuscular sclerosis. There may be an acute inflammatory response to the infarct, which is peripheral, generally mild, and does not actually involve the villous parenchyma.

Infarcts are common; they occur in about 25% of otherwise normal term placentas.[94] In this situation, they are small, generally involving less than 5% of the villous parenchyma. In women with hypertension (preeclampsia and essential hypertension), the frequency and extent of infarction are increased in proportion to the severity of the underlying maternal disease.[94]

The finding of a small infarct in an otherwise normal placenta is of no clinical significance. Multiple or large infarcts are indicative of significant, underlying maternal vascular disease. Extensive placental infarction of this type is associated with fetal hypoxia, intrauterine growth retardation, and fetal death in utero.[94] These ill effects on the fetus are probably not due simply to the destruction of villous tissue but are the result of the superimposition of infarction on a placenta already compromised by a pathologically altered maternal vascular tree (see section on preeclampsia and essential hypertension).

Perivillous Fibrin Deposition

Grossly, massive deposition of perivillous fibrin may be impossible to distinguish from an infarct. When the process is extensive enough to result in a grossly visible lesion, it forms a hard, white, well-defined plaque often located peripherally in the marginal angle of the placenta.

Microscopically, the intervillous space is distended and obliterated by fibrin, which widely separates the entrapped, fibrotic, avascular villi (Fig. 23.49). Whereas these villi have lost their syncytiotrophoblastic covering, the cytotrophoblast proliferates markedly, forming prominent mantles around the villi and extending into the surrounding fibrin.

Plaques of perivillous fibrin are found in about 20% of normal full-term placentas.[93] The etiology of this condition is unknown, but it is thought to result from localized stasis and thrombosis of the maternal blood in the intervillous space. The fibrin deposition isolates the entrapped villi from their maternal blood supply, and they undergo ischemic necrosis. The process seems to require good maternal blood flow. Perivillous fibrin deposition is actu-

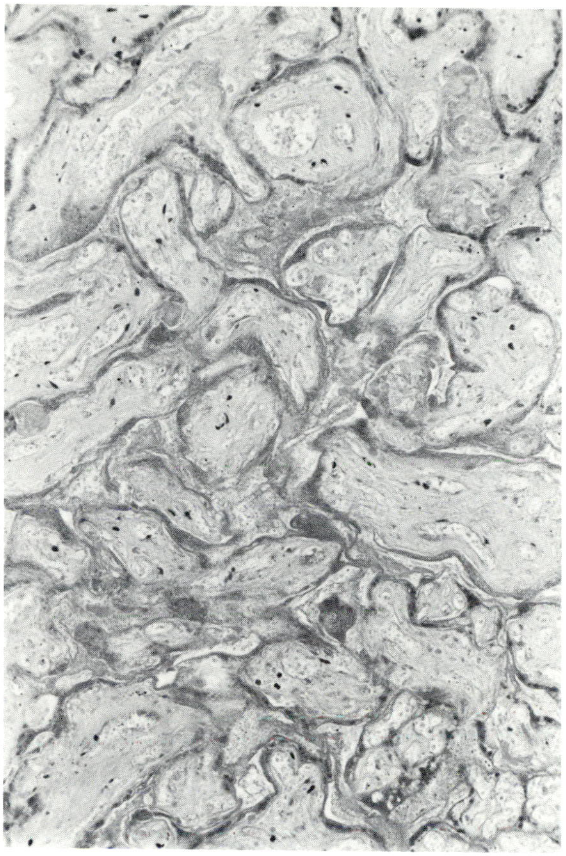

FIG. 23.48. Placental infarct. The villi in this old infarct are ghost-like. A perivillous eosinophilic rim is all that remains of the completely necrotic trophoblast.

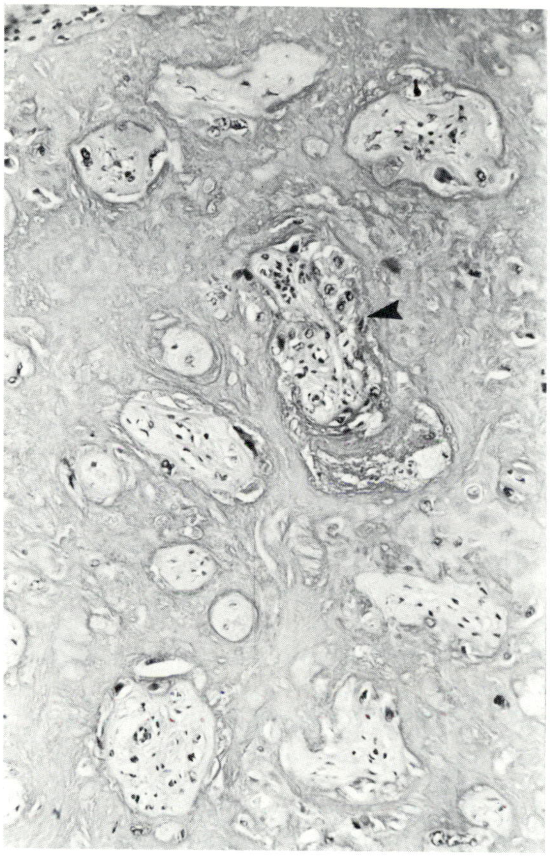

FIG. 23.49. Perivillous fibrin deposition. Villi are separated by and enmeshed in dense perivillous fibrin plaque. The cytotrophoblast proliferates around villi (*arrow*) and extends into surrounding fibrin.

ally less frequent in the placentas of women with preeclampsia.[93]

Perivillous fibrin deposition seems to have no adverse clinical effects, even when sectors of the villous parenchyma rendered nonfunctional by this process reach the size of large infarcts. Specifically, there is no relationship between the occurrence of perivillous fibrin deposition and decreased fetal weight, fetal distress, or intrauterine fetal death. This emphasizes the considerable functional reserve of the placenta under normal conditions. In contrast, when large true infarcts result in the inactivation of a similar or even lesser number of villi, fetal anoxia or growth retardation is much more likely. The difference may be explained by the differing background from which the two lesions arise, placental ischemia and uteroplacental vascular disease in the case of infarction as opposed to healthy maternal vessels and good blood supply in perivillous fibrin deposition.

Subchorionic Fibrin

Subchorionic fibrin plaques are similar to perivillous deposits of fibrin but are distinguished from them by their subchorionic location and complete lack of villi within the laminated fibrin. They are a frequent finding in term placentas and are of no clinical significance. They are thought to have the same pathogenesis as perivillous fibrin deposition, that is, thrombosis of maternal blood or plasma in the subchorionic space.

Massive Subchorial Thrombosis (Breus' Mole)

In contrast to the common occurrence of small subchorial fibrin deposits, a massive thrombohematoma in the subchorionic region is a rare phenomenon. The massive subchorial thrombohematoma has been defined as coagulated blood, at least 1 cm in thickness, which separates the chorionic plate from the underlying villi over much of its area (Fig. 23.50).[236] These are generally relatively fresh, red thrombi that distort the chorionic plate and protrude as nodular or tuberous masses into the amnionic cavity. They may dissect into the chorionic plate itself or extend into the intervillous space, sometimes as far as the basal plate. Histologically, they consist of laminated thrombus devoid of villi.

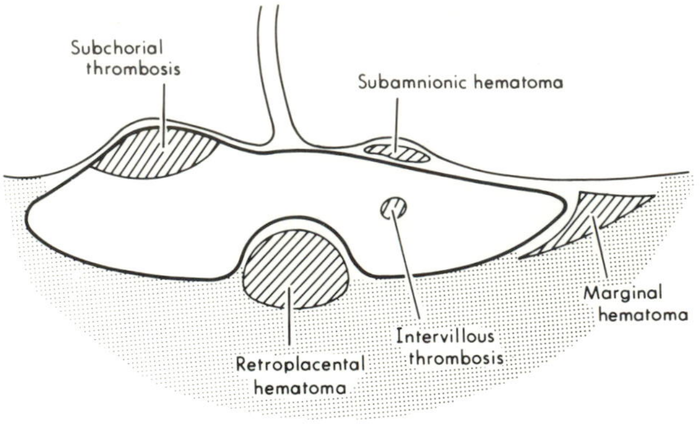

FIG. 23.50. Diagrammatic representation of various placental thrombi and hematomas. (After Fox, Ref. 98.)

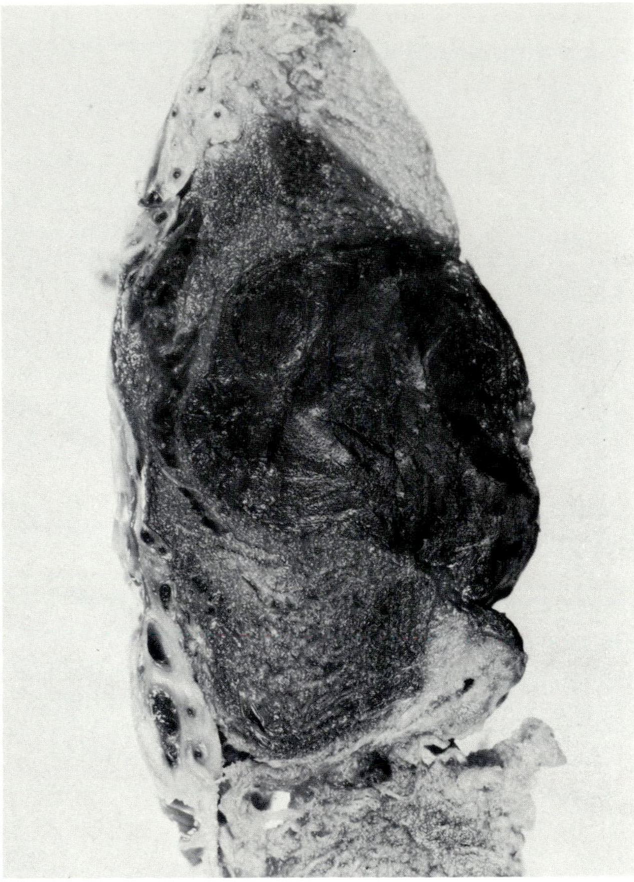

FIG. 23.51. Retroplacental hematoma. Characteristic compression and infarction of the placental parenchyma overlying a large retroplacental hematoma. The surrounding, lighter, normal placenta contrasts with the darker, infarcted tissue.

The incidence of massive subchorial thrombohematoma was estimated to be 0.53 per 1000 deliveries in one large study.[236] The etiology and pathogenesis of the lesion are unknown. The original description by Breus and subsequent reports by others indicated that these thrombi are mainly found in abortions and, therefore, may be a consequence of fetal death. However, the demonstration of massive subchorial thrombohematomas in mature placentas associated with live births refutes the view that fetal death is necessarily the primary event.[236] Rather, it is possible that the hematoma may cause fetal death by distortion and compression of the chorionic plate and fetal vessels. Most authors agree that the thrombi are maternal in origin.[29,98,236]

Retroplacental Hematoma

A retroplacental hematoma is located between the basal plate of the placenta and the uterine wall (Fig. 23.50). Whether large or small, it compresses the overlying placental parenchyma, which is often, but not always, infarcted (Fig. 23.51). This characteristic depression in the maternal surface permits gross recognition and diagnosis of the pathologic process, even when the hematoma itself has been detached from the placenta during delivery (see abruptio placenta). As the name indicates, retroplacental hematomas originate behind the placenta. A large retroplacental hematoma, however, may extend to the placental margin, in which case it must be distinguished from a marginal hematoma. Marginal hematomas, in contrast to retroplacental hematomas, do not cause depression of the basal plate or infarction of villous parenchyma (Fig. 23.50). Their epicenter is at the placental margin, and they generally extend laterally beneath the fetal membranes as well as onto the adjacent maternal surface.

Microscopically, retroplacental hematomas consist of red cells and fibrin, the proportion of fibrin increasing as the lesion ages and the red cells degenerate. The overlying basal plate may be normal but is more commonly necrotic (Fig. 23.52). An acute inflammatory infiltrate and hemosiderin deposits are often present.

The infarcted placenta overlying the hematoma is microscopically identical to the true infarcts described above. Blanc has described an additional, somewhat different pattern in some infarcts associated with retroplacental hematoma. These so-called divergent infarcts are characterized by necrotic villi that are widely separated by a markedly enlarged and congested intervillous space.[41] This particular infarction pattern has been attributed to interruption of both venous and arterial circulations in contrast to true or convergent infarcts, which are secondary to pure maternal artery occlusion. Other infarcts of varying ages may be found elsewhere in the placenta with a retroplacental hematoma.

The overall prevalence of retroplacental hematoma is reportedly about 4.5%,[98] but it is considerably increased in the placentas of women with preeclampsia. The etiology and pathogenesis of retroplacental bleeding

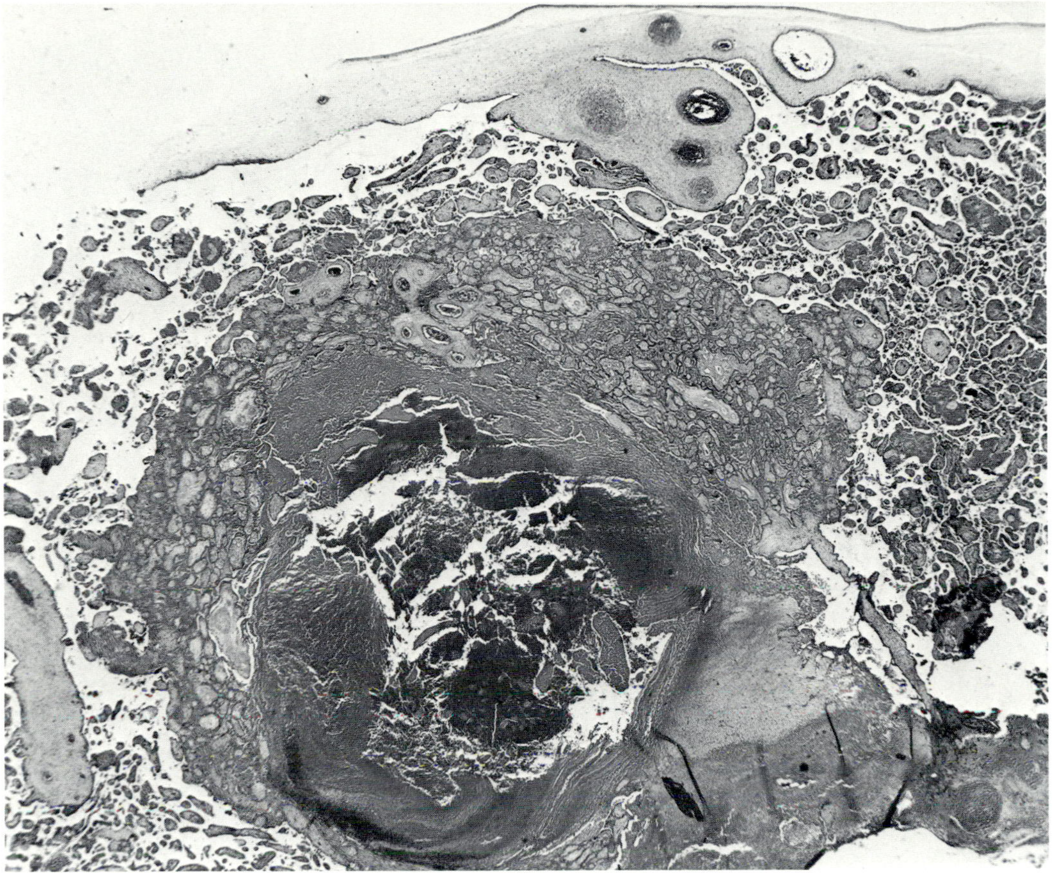

FIG. 23.52. Retroplacental hematoma. Histologic appearance of a retroplacental hematoma showing elevation of the basal plate and infarction of the adjacent placenta.

are uncertain. Rupture of a spiral artery weakened by the pathologic alterations that occur in preeclampsia is the usual explanation, but since retroplacental hematomas are by no means confined to women with preeclampsia, other factors must be involved. Alternative theories include venous outflow obstruction, venous rupture, or primary placental separation. A deficiency of folic acid has been proposed as one factor predisposing to abnormal placental separation.[123]

Retroplacental hematoma, the pathologic lesion, should be distinguished from placental abruption (abruptio placenta), the acute clinical syndrome. Although the two are frequently associated, clinical abruption is often not associated with any discernible placental abnormality, and, conversely, retroplacental hematomas may be found in the absence of physiologic signs or symptoms. In fact, Gruenwald et al. have shown that each of these conditions is present more frequently without than with the other.[115] Placental abruption is an acute clinical situation followed rapidly by delivery. It is not surprising that the authentic clinical syndrome may be associated with a placenta that lacks the expected pathologic changes. A retroplacental hematoma, on the other hand, must have been present for some period of time to be recognizable as such. The frequent association of the two conditions may be explained by postulating that retroplacental hematomas and premature separation may occur in several stages, finally resulting in the clinical syndrome of placental abruption in some patients.

Both abruption and retroplacental hematoma have serious implications for fetal well-being. Individually, each carries the same high risk of premature birth and perinatal mortality. When the two conditions are combined, however, both premature delivery and perinatal mortality are much more likely.[115] The significance of a retroplacental hematoma appears to be related to size.[98] In separating a portion of the placenta from its maternal blood supply, a retroplacental hematoma is responsible for an infarct. The larger the infarct, the more likely it will be to exceed the functional reserve capability of the placenta. Placental abruption complicated by disseminated intravascular coagulation is also responsible for high maternal morbidity and mortality.

Marginal Hematoma

A marginal hematoma is named to specify its location where the external, or lateral, wall of the placenta joins the fetal membranes (Fig. 23.50). Grossly, the marginal hematoma forms a crescent-shaped clot adherent to the lateral margin of the placenta. It may extend beneath the adjacent fetal membranes or for some distance onto the maternal aspect of the placenta. On cut section, the clot is triangular in shape, the apex of the triangle being formed by the junction of the membranous and villous chorion. Microscopically, the blood clot is generally accompanied by an acute inflammatory infiltrate and hemosiderin deposition. The clot usually lies entirely outside the placental disk but may occasionally involve the intervillous space. With this exception, the presence of a marginal hematoma has no effect on the adjacent villi. Microscopic examination allows the distinction between a marginal hematoma and thrombosis of large decidual veins, which would be impossible based on gross examination alone.

Marginal hematomas are thought to result from rupture of uteroplacental veins at the margin of a low-lying placenta. The hematoma is invariably found at the margin of the placenta closest to the site of membrane rupture, which is usually only a few centimeters from the placental margin.[98]

A marginal hematoma is associated with antepartum maternal hemorrhage but does not have any untoward affects on the fetus.

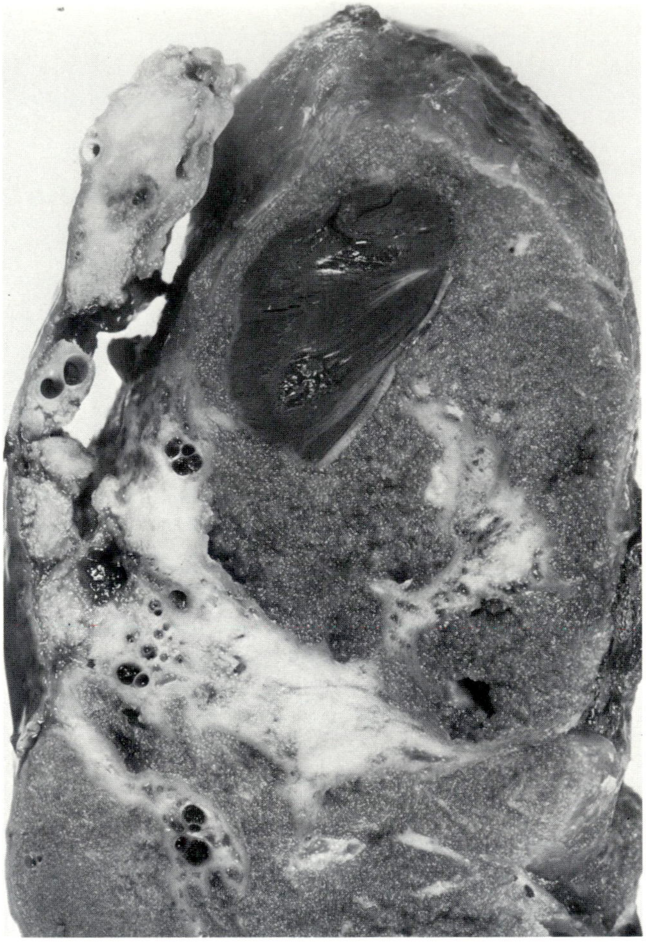

Fig. 23.53. Laminated intervillous thrombus.

Intervillous Thrombus

Intervillous thrombi are round or oval blood clots that may occur anywhere in the intervillous space but are most common midway between the chorionic and basal plates. They begin as red, fluid, or semifluid blood (Kline's hemorrhage) and become progressively laminated and depigmented with age (Fig. 23.53). They may be single, although multiple lesions are very common. Most are 1–3 cm in diameter. Microscopically, the thrombi consist of erythrocytes and fibrin, the proportion of fibrin increasing with the age of the lesion (Fig. 23.54). All villi are displaced to the margins of the clot. Nucleated red blood cells have been identified in these thrombi.[74,98,139]

Recent studies have confirmed that intervillous thrombi do contain a proportion of fetal erythrocytes,[139] although maternal erythrocytes seem to comprise the majority of the lesion. Fetal bleeding into the intervillous space is thought to occur through rupture of the attenuated vasculosyncytial membrane. The mechanism of coagulation is unknown, but there does not appear to be a link between the intervillous thrombus and maternofetal ABO incompatibility.[23]

An intervillous thrombus is significant in that it marks the site of hemorrhage from the fetal to the maternal circulation. Fetomaternal hemorrhages are relatively common in the third trimester of pregnancy, occuring in 15–30% of cases as assessed by the Kleihauer-Betke technique. Intervillous thrombi are also found with increasing frequency in the third trimester. There appears to be good correlation between the number of fetal cells in the maternal circulation and the number of intervillous thrombi.[74,280] The same relationship applies in some other placental lesions, including retroplacental hematomas and infarcts.[280]

Fetomaternal hemorrhage, when massive, may be a cause of fetal anemia or intrauterine demise.[210] Smaller fetomaternal transfusions may initiate the production of maternal antibodies to fetal cells, resulting in hemolytic disease in the fetus. When this occurs before the administration of anti-D gamma-globulin prophylaxis, hemolytic disease may recur in subsequent pregnancies. Factors cited as potential causes of villous damage resulting in fetomaternal transfusion include trauma, amniocentesis, and external version.[210,277]

Subamnionic Hematoma

A subamnionic hematoma lies between the amnion and chorion on the fetal surface of the placenta (Fig. 23.50).

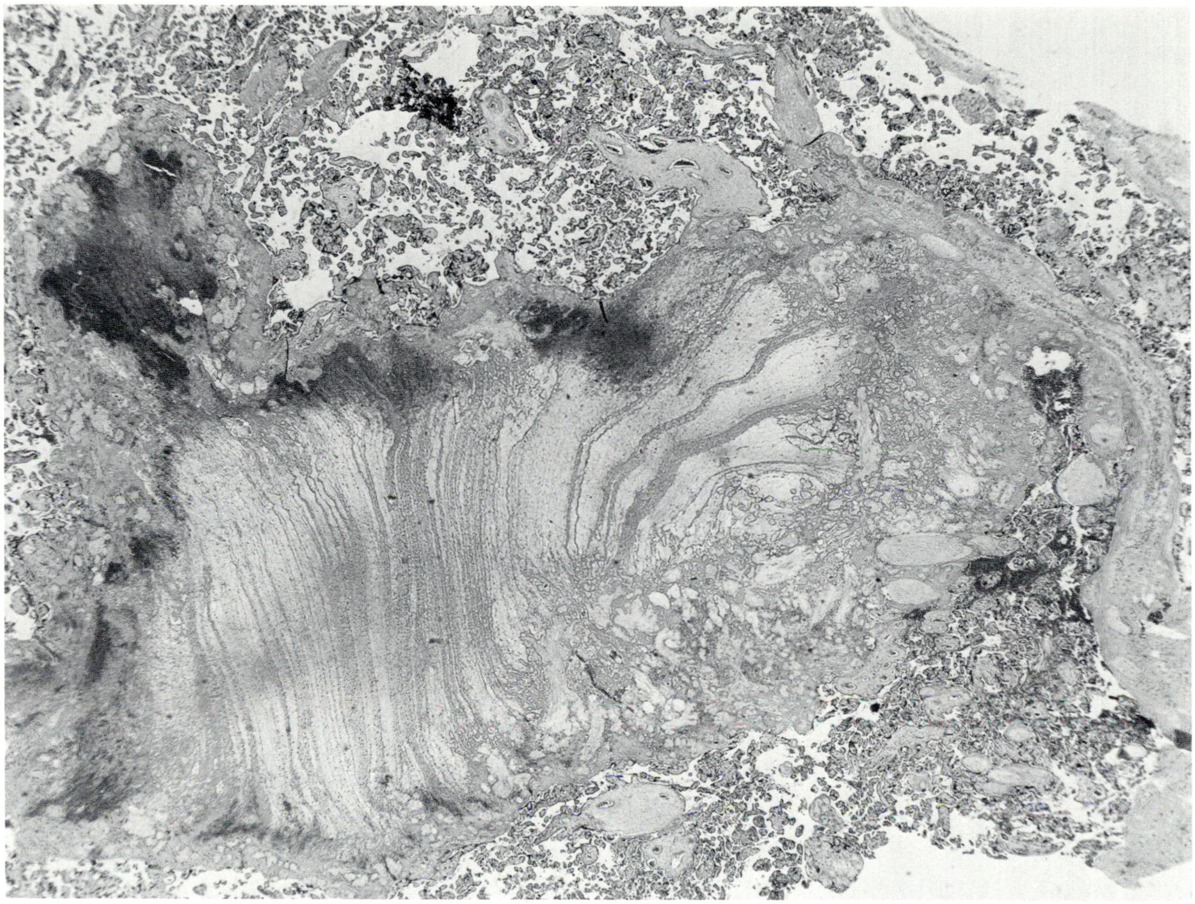

FIG. 23.54. Intervillous thrombus. Histologic appearance of laminated fibrin and erythrocytes in an intervillous thrombus.

Very recent lesions are thought to result from trauma to the chorionic veins during delivery, especially after excessive traction on the umbilical cord. Older chorionic fibrin clots, of unknown pathogenesis, form dome-shaped blisters and contain a mixture of brown-tinged fluid and fibrin. Neither form has significant implications for the fetus.

Fetal Artery Thrombosis

Occlusion of a fetal stem artery results in villous avascularity distal to the lesion. Grossly, the lesion produced is a well-delineated area of pallor without any marked change in consistency as compared to the surrounding normal parenchyma. Microscopically, the villi are avascular, the villous stroma is hyalinized and fibrotic, and the syncytiotrophoblast nuclei cluster extensively to form prominent syncytial knots. The intervillous space is normally patent. The thrombosed fetal stem artery may show some degree of recanalization. There is usually marked fibromuscular sclerosis in the vessels of stem villi distal to the thrombosis.

Isolated thrombosis of a fetal stem artery is uncommon; it occurs in about 4.5% of full-term placentas.[98] The lesion is seen with increased frequency in diabetes mellitus.[82,98] There are no other obvious predisposing conditions.

The Placenta in Maternal and Fetal Disorders

Placentas in pregnancies complicated by any maternal disease should be routinely submitted for pathologic examination with the goal of defining what morphologic effect such diseases have had on the placenta and fetus. Although a large number of studies have focused on these very issues, there is, unfortunately, a great deal of disagreement and direct contradiction about the nature and significance of the lesions or alterations described.

Preeclampsia (Toxemia of Pregnancy) and Eclampsia

A major cause of morbidity and mortality in both the mother and fetus, preeclampsia is defined as the development of hypertension in pregnancy with proteinuria or generalized edema or both after 20 weeks of gestation.

Eclampsia means the occurrence of convulsions in a patient with preeclampsia. The etiology of this condition is not completely understood, but reduced choriodecidual blood flow and uteroplacental ischemia play an important role.[58,59,80] There is an extensive but conflicting literature dealing with the placental lesions associated with preeclampsia. Most investigators agree that, overall, both the number and size of infarcts are larger in placentas from preeclamptic women than in uncomplicated pregnancy.[98,278] The extent of infarction is directly related to the severity of the preeclampsia. Extensive placental infarction is a cardinal sign of preeclampsia, but it is neither specific for nor invariable in that condition. Placental infarcts are common, and their significance in preeclampsia is a quantitative distinction. Retroplacental hematoma is the other gross lesion identified with undue frequency (12–15%) in preeclamptic women.[98] This, of course, is an added factor in the increased frequency of infarction in these placentas. The placenta in preeclampsia has a tendency to be smaller on the average than the placenta from an uncomplicated pregnancy.[98]

Histologically, the infarcts may be old or recent, but there is some indication that recent, or red, infarcts are particularly characteristic of the placentas of severe preeclamptics.[22,278] There are no distinctive gross or microscopic pathologic features of the infarcts and retroplacental hematomas associated with preeclampsia. There are, however, subtle but consistent microscopic changes in the placenta, which include cytotrophoblastic proliferation, thickening and alteration of the trophoblastic basement membrane,[214] relative villous hypovascularity, small, inconspicuous fetal capillaries, and increased prominence of the villous stroma (Fig. 23.55). Villous syncytial sprouts are increased,[152] and there is narrowing and ultimate obliteration of the lumens of the fetal stem arteries.[152,272] Ultrastructural studies have confirmed all these changes and have emphasized the finding of focal syncytiotrophoblastic necrosis, an additional abnormality not appreciated at the light microscopic level.[136] These changes have been attributed to placental ischemia, and they occur in villi cultured under conditions of low oxygen tension[96,157] as well as in the placentas of pregnant animals in whom toxemia has been produced experimentally by ligating the terminal aorta.[1,2]

In addition, well-described, distinctive morphologic abnormalities occur in the maternal arteries of the placental bed in preeclampsia. These arteries differ from their normal counterparts in two important respects: (1) the adaptive and physiologic changes that take place routinely in the vessels of the placental bed are decreased in degree and extent, and (2) some of the vessels exhibit an acute necrotizing arteriopathy termed *acute atherosis*. The identification and characterization of pathologic lesions in the uteroplacental arteries is greatly complicated by the marked morphologic changes that occur in these vessels during the course of normal pregnancy. These physiologic alterations have been described and beautifully illustrated in the work of Robertson et al.[77,216,217]

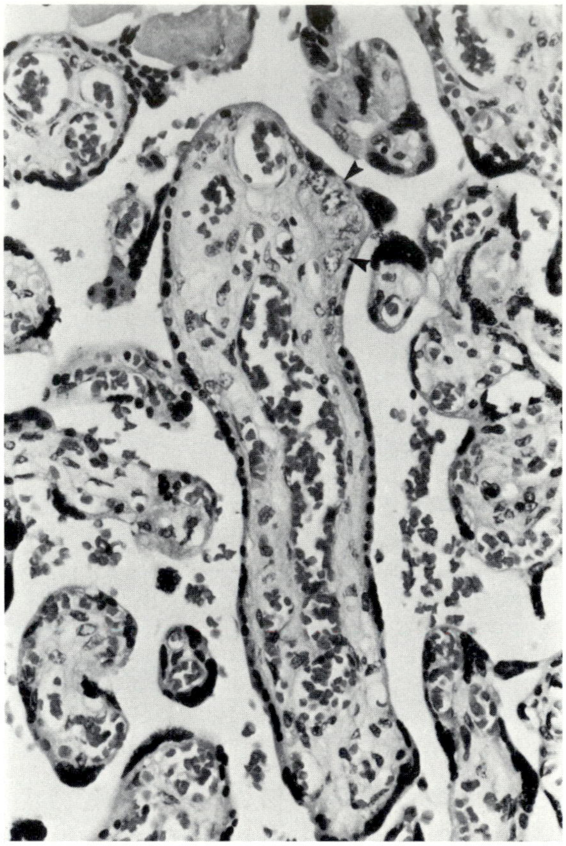

FIG. 23.55. Placenta from a patient with preeclampsia. Villi show prominent syncytial knots, cytotrophoblastic hyperplasia (*arrows*), and focal thickening of the trophoblastic basement membrane.

In the early weeks of normal pregnancy, trophoblast from the trophoblastic shell invades the decidua and intradecidual portions of the spiral arteries. The endovascular trophoblast replaces the maternal endothelium and disrupts the arterial wall. The muscular and elastic tissue of the media is largely replaced by fibrinoid material composed of a complex of maternal fibrin, plasma constituents, and proteinaceous substances produced by the trophoblast (Fig. 23.4). As pregnancy advances, the proliferating interstitial trophoblast extends into the inner myometrium, and sometime between 14 and 20 weeks, a retrograde wave of endovascular trophoblast moves from the decidual segments into the myometrial segments of the spiral arteries. This intravascular trophoblastic migration is associated with the same destruction and fibrinoid replacement of the arterial media as seen in the decidual segments of the spiral arteries. The vessels affected by these physiologic changes undergo progressive distention to funnel-shaped channels that augment the blood flow to the implantation site from 100 ml/minute in the nonpregnant uterus to over 500 ml/ minute in the uterus at term. There is some evidence that additional maternal vascular adaptations in the myometrial segments of the spiral arteries are necessary before endovascular trophoblastic migration can occur. As detailed by Pijnenborg et al., these changes may be effected by the migrating interstitial trophoblast.[202] The physiologic changes as described in these classic articles have all been attributed to cytotrophoblast. Recent evidence indicates that actually the cells currently referred to as *intermediate trophoblast* play this key role in implantation and establishment of the uteroplacental circulation.[148]

In women with preeclampsia, it appears that the second wave of intravascular trophoblastic migration does not occur. The intramyometrial segments of the spiral arteries, therefore, retain their musculoelastic media and do not dilate. The physiologic vascular changes that accompany normal implantation are, therefore, incomplete in women with preeclampsia.

Subsequently, a dramatic vascular lesion termed *acute atherosis*[287] occurs in women with preeclampsia and is characterized by fibrinoid necrosis of vessel walls, accumulation of lipid-containing macrophages, and a perivascular mononuclear infiltrate (Fig. 23.56). The evolution of the lesion, as defined in ultrastructural studies, begins with lipid accumulation in the muscle cells of the intima and media. These cells undergo necrosis and release lipid, which is engulfed by macrophages that accumulate in the damaged vessel wall.[76] According to Robertson et al., acute atherosis is a specific feature of preeclampsia that has a very characteristic distribution: it is limited to those vessels that have not been altered by the normal adaptive processes of implantation, namely, the decidual segments of spiral arteries outside the placental bed, the basal arteries, and the myometrial segments of the spiral arteries in the placental bed that have not undergone physiologic adaptations.[216] Other investigators disagree on both points. Sheppard and Bonnar maintain that acute atherosis may be observed in the spiral arteries of the placental bed in normotensive women with in-

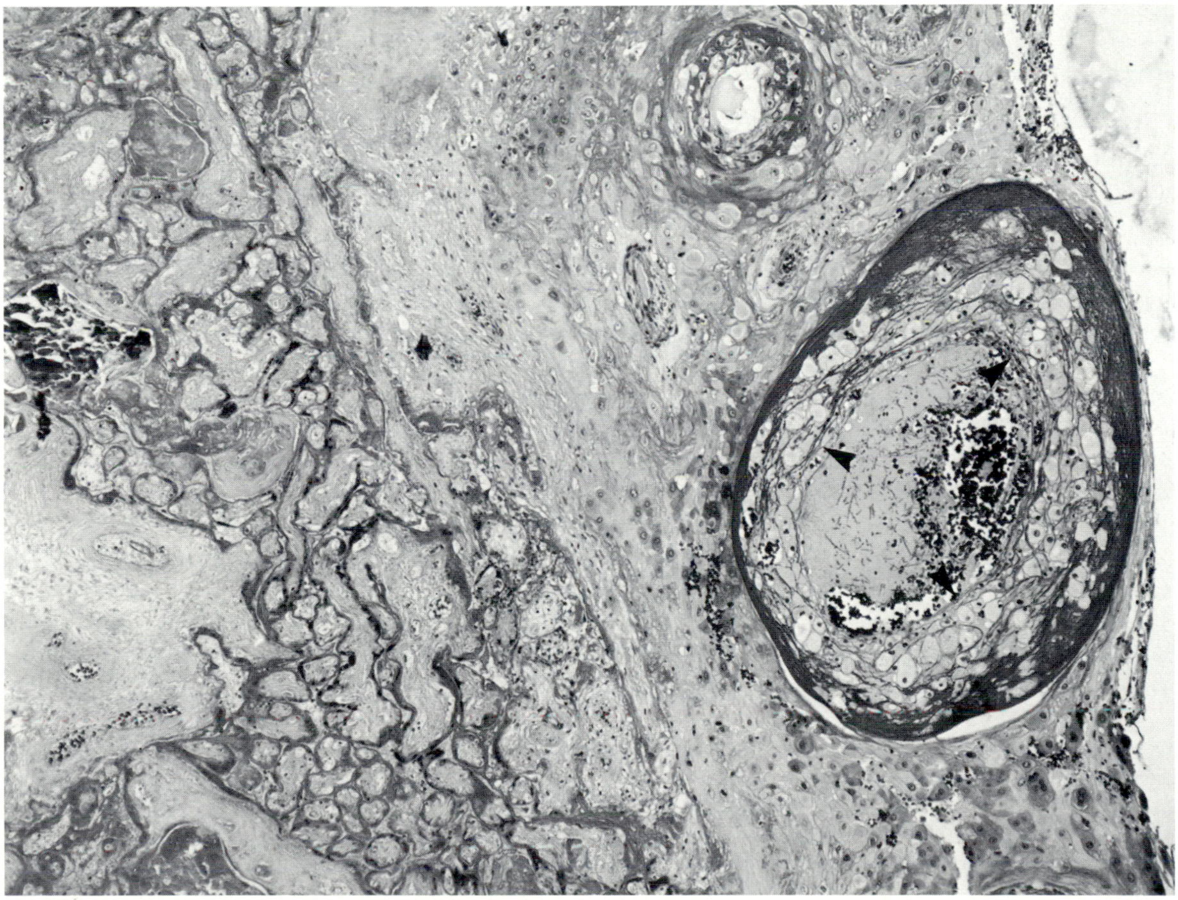

FIG. 23.56. Acute atherosis, preeclampsia. The spiral arteries are distorted by fibrinoid necrosis of the vessel wall and accumulation of lipid-containing macrophages (*arrows*). The largest artery is thrombosed, and there is infarction of the overlying placenta (*left*).

trauterine growth retardation.[237] DeWolf et al. have reported the occurrence of acute atherosis in decidual segments of the placental bed spiral arteries lacking physiologic changes in normotensive or only mildly hypertensive women with intrauterine growth retardation.[75] A similar lesion has been described in the diabetic placenta and in systemic lupus erythematosus.[3,144] All agree that in some cases of growth retarded or small for gestational age babies, the physiologic changes of the placental bed spiral arteries may be limited to their decidual segments.[9,56,237] Placental infarction is thought to be the direct result of these vascular lesions in preeclamptics (Fig. 23.56).[55]

The pathogenesis of the vascular lesions is not known. Their similarity to the pathologic changes in renal transplant rejection has stimulated a search for an immunopathologic basis.[231] Immunoglobulins and complement have been demonstrated in vessels showing acute atherosis, but this is neither a specific nor a constant finding in preeclampsia.[143] How the multitude of pathologic features associated with preeclampsia—acute atherosis, inadequacy of physiologic adaptive processes, increased frequency of infarcts and retroplacental hematoma, ischemic villous changes—relate etiologically to each other and to the reduced uteroplacental blood flow, biochemical abnormalities,[71] and clinical manifestations[232] of preeclampsia is unknown.

Essential Hypertension

The pathology of the placenta in essential hypertension has received little attention. A few studies have shown that morphologic changes in the placenta in this disease are qualitatively very similar to those found in preeclampsia (increased frequency and extent of infarcts, cytotrophoblastic hyperplasia, trophoblastic basement membrane thickening). The similarities extend to the ultrastructural level, although the extent and degree of pathologic changes are less marked in placentas from cases of essential hypertension than in preeclampsia.[137] A maternal vascular abnormality, termed *hyperplastic arteriosclerosis*, characterized by marked thickening of all coats of the vessel wall, intimal hyperplasia, and luminal narrowing, has been described in women with essential hypertension.[216,217,238] These changes are most conspicuous in the myometrial segments of the spiral arteries. When preeclampsia complicates essential hypertension, there may be superimposition of acute atherosis on hyperplastic arteriosclerosis. Surprisingly, the placental changes (presumably reflecting ischemic damage) in cases of essential hypertension complicated by preeclampsia are less marked than those found in the placentas of previously normotensive women who develop preeclampsia of comparable severity.[137]

Diabetes Mellitus

Reports on the pathology of the placenta in diabetes mellitus are numerous but often contradictory. The inconsistency may be explained, in part, by the inclusion of cases with superimposed hypertension or fetal death in utero. Moreover, the category of diabetic pregnant women is not homogeneous. Many are diabetic before pregnancy (overt diabetes), whereas others become diabetic during pregnancy. In the latter group, the diabetes may persist (early diabetes) or regress (gestational diabetes) after pregnancy. Furthermore, a number of normal women may give birth to infants resembling those born to women with established diabetes. When followed, some of these mothers may become diabetic and, in retrospect, may be considered to have had prediabetes during pregnancy.

The placentas from diabetic women are, on the average, heavier than normal controls of the same gestational age.[98,119,193] Some, however, may be of normal weight or even small if the patient is suffering from diabetic vascular disease. Grossly, the placenta may appear to be bulky and edematous. The umbilical cord may be increased in diameter, and there is an increased likelihood of finding a single umbilical artery (3–5%) as compared with the general population (1%).[82,119] Most agree that infarcts are not increased in extent or frequency in the placentas of diabetics, but there has been some debate on this point.[178]

Histologically, there are no specific features allowing absolute distinction of the diabetic placenta from any other. There are, however, a constellation of abnormalities that, when taken together, are fairly characteristic. Some degree of villous immaturity is common, although villous maturation may sometimes be normal or even accelerated. Villous edema is common. Cytotrophoblastic cells are numerous and may contain mitotic figures. The trophoblastic basement membrane often shows focal, marked thickening. Villous vascularity is variable; the villi may be hypovascular, normovascular, or show diffuse hypervascularity (chorangiosis).[82] Proliferative endarteritis and fetal artery thrombosis have been reported.[82,98] Villi showing fibrinoid necrosis, the deposition of fibrinoid material between the trophoblast and basement membrane, are unduly frequent.[133] Extramedullary hematopoiesis in the villous stroma has been described,[82] although we have not encountered it. Some diabetic placentas have significantly more parenchymal and villous tissue than normal placentas when studied by morphometric techniques.[261]

Ultrastructural studies have confirmed these light microscopic observations.[119,134] Patchy focal trophoblastic necrosis, usually involving only the syncytiotrophoblast but occasionally also the cytotrophoblast, is an additional ultrastructural feature. Enlargement and immaturity of the endothelial cells with protrusion into and reduction in the size of the capillary lumen has also been emphasized in ultrastructural studies.[134]

Light and electron microscopic changes qualitatively identical to those found in placentas from women with well-established, overt diabetes mellitus have been documented in women with well-controlled gestational diabetes.[7,134] Although these changes tend to be less marked and occur with lesser frequency in the group with gestational diabetes, there is considerable overlap between the pathologic findings in overt and gestational diabetics.[133,134] Correlation between the severity of the diabetes or degree of metabolic control and the extent of placental changes is poor.[37,262,263]

The status of the uteroplacental vasculature in diabetic women is debated. Some investigators have found no morphologic abnormalities in the maternal vessels.[98,203] Driscoll, however, has described two types of vascular lesions in the decidual vessels: (1) arteriolar medial hypertrophy, hyalinization, and onion skinning in 50% of diabetics and (2) acute atherosis identical to that described in preeclamptic women.[82] The latter change has been reported both in diabetics with superimposed preeclampsia and in normotensive diabetic women.[144]

So far, there has been no good correlation between the presence or extent of the pathologic changes in the placenta and the well-documented increase in congenital fetal malformations, neonatal morbidity, or fetal macrosomia in diabetic pregnancies.[119,128,191,199]

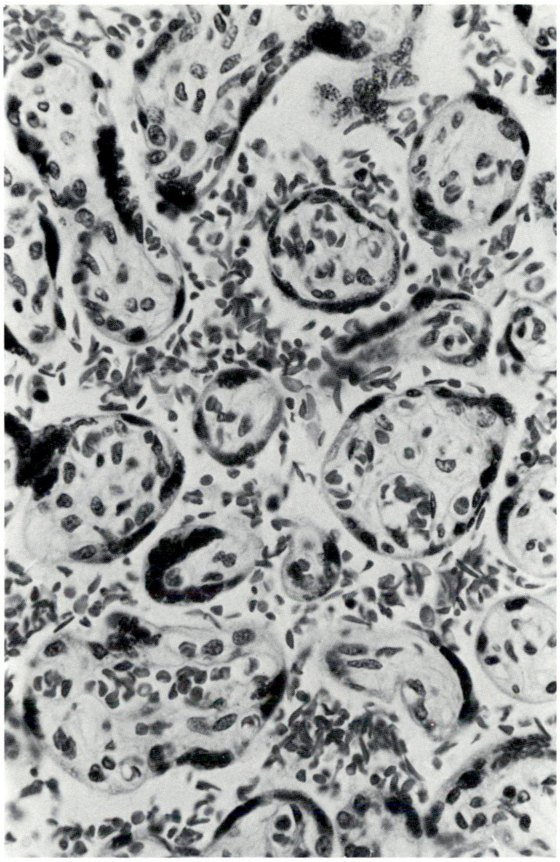

FIG. 23.57. Placenta from a patient with sickle cell trait. Maternal erythrocytes in the intervillous space show marked sickling.

Sickle-Cell Trait

The placenta is actually a sensitive detector of sickle cells.[46,104] The maternal erythrocytes in the intervillous space undergo sickling, and careful placental examination can uncover unsuspected or undiagnosed sickle cell trait in some patients (Fig. 23.57). Other placental abnormalities have not been described. The significance of sickle-cell trait in pregnancy outcome is a matter of debate. Reports range from those showing no evidence of adverse clinical sequelae[45] to others that document increased rates of maternal pyelonephritis, refractory anemia,[213] premature rupture of membranes, prematurity,[213] and increased perinatal mortality[204] in pregnancy associated with sickle-cell trait. Lethal maternal complications are rare.[196]

Maternofetal Rhesus Incompatibility

Before the advent of prevention programs in the 1960s, maternofetal Rh incompatibility was a significant cause of fetal compromise. There is general agreement on the pathologic findings in this condition, and they have been well characterized.[279]

Classically, these placentas are enlarged, bulky, edematous, and strikingly pale, although a proportion may be grossly normal in all respects. Intervillous thrombosis is the only gross lesion that occurs with undue frequency; such thrombi are present in almost 50% of placentas and are often multiple. Septal cysts are more common in edematous placentas and are, therefore, frequently found in cases of maternofetal Rh incompatibility.

Histologically, the villi typically exhibit a combination of nonspecific but characteristic changes. There is a generalized delay in villous maturation, and clumps of markedly immature villi are scattered throughout the placenta. Cytotrophoblastic cells, many containing mitoses, are conspicuous, and there is some degree of thickening of the trophoblastic basement membrane (Fig. 23.58). The villous stroma is edematous and abundant. Hofbauer cells are numerous and prominent. One of the characteristic features of the placenta in Rh incompatibility is the wide variance in the appearance of the villi even in the same field of examination (Fig. 23.59). Nucleated red blood cells and erythoblasts are present within the fetal capillaries (Fig. 23.60). This finding is indicative of fetal anemia and is, therefore, characteristic of mater-

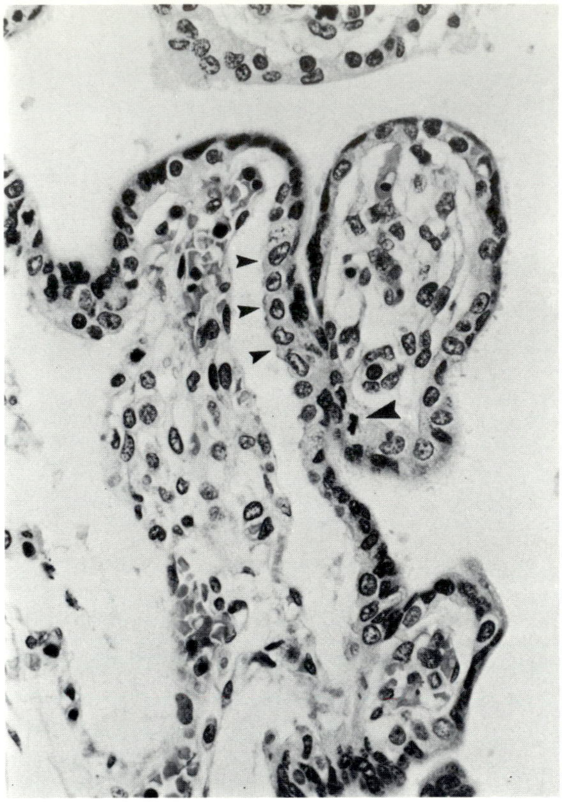

FIG. 23.58. Maternofetal Rh incompatibility, placenta at term. Immature villi with conspicuous cytotrophoblast (*small black arrows*), showing some mitotic activity (*large black arrow*).

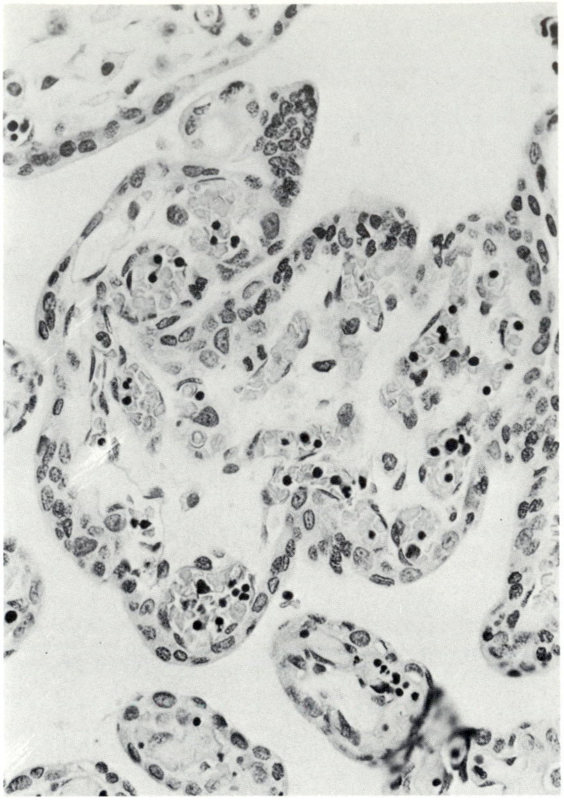

FIG. 23.60. Maternofetal Rh incompatibility, placenta at term. Fetal capillaries are filled with normoblasts and erythroblasts.

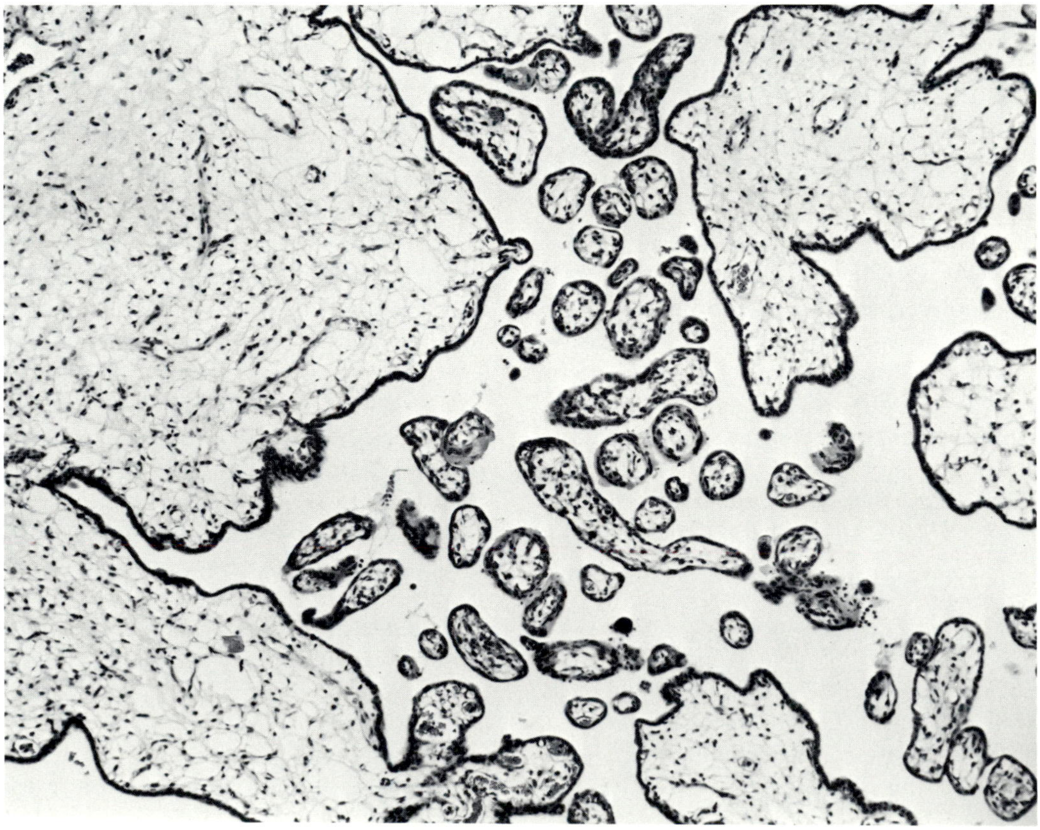

FIG. 23.59. Maternofetal Rh incompatibility, placenta at term. Pronounced variability in villous appearance characterized by markedly immature (*large*) villi interspersed among normal, mature villi.

nofetal Rh incompatibility but may be found in any other situation resulting in severe fetal anemia.

The pathogenesis of the placental changes in maternofetal Rh incompatibility is unknown. Commonly associated with fetal edema (so-called hydrops fetalis), the placental changes have been considered part of a generalized expression of fluid accumulation in the fetus. There is, however, evidence that the increased bulk of the placenta may be due to placental hyperplasia rather than edema.[69] An ultrastructural study of placentas in Rh incompatibility has shown no evidence of immune-mediated damage.[135] It has been demonstrated that the intervillous space is reduced.[15]

The classic constellation of gross and microscopic findings, which includes placental enlargement and pallor, villous dysmaturity and edema, cytotrophoblastic hyperplasia, and eythroblastosis, is common and represents an end-stage picture with a variable pathogenesis. In addition to Rh incompatibility, isoimmunization against other blood group antigens (ABO, Kell antigens), red cell enzyme defects, alpha-thalassemia, cardiac failure (malformations, endocardial fibroelastosis, large arteriovenous shunts), hypoproteinemia (congenital nephrotic syndrome, defects in hepatic protein synthesis), congenital malformations, congenital infections, fetal blood loss (fetomaternal hemorrhage), and other miscellaneous disorders (Gaucher's disease, sacrococcygeal teratoma) may result in identical gross and microscopic changes.[83,88,156,158] When none of these immunologic or nonimmunologic causative factors is identified, the hydrops is considered to be idiopathic. Idiopathic fetal–placental hydrops has been reported to recur in successive pregnancies.[241]

Pathology of the Membranes

Squamous Metaplasia

Foci of squamous metaplasia may be found on the amnionic surface of the fetal membranes and umbilical cord. Grossly, these foci are slightly elevated, pearly white macules that tend to be most numerous at the site of cord insertion (Fig. 23.61). Although they are generally very small, measuring no more than a few millimeters in diameter, they may rarely form larger plaques. Histologically, the foci consist of stratified squamous epithelium, with or without superficial keratinization, that has a sharp transition from the surrounding normal amnion (Fig. 23.62). The frequency of squamous metaplasia is a matter of some dispute. According to Benirschke and Driscoll, it may be found in the majority of placentas if specifically sought.[29] Squamous metaplasia has no clinical significance, and it is not known to be associated with any particular pathologic event. Its only importance is in distinguishing it from amnion nodosum pathologically.

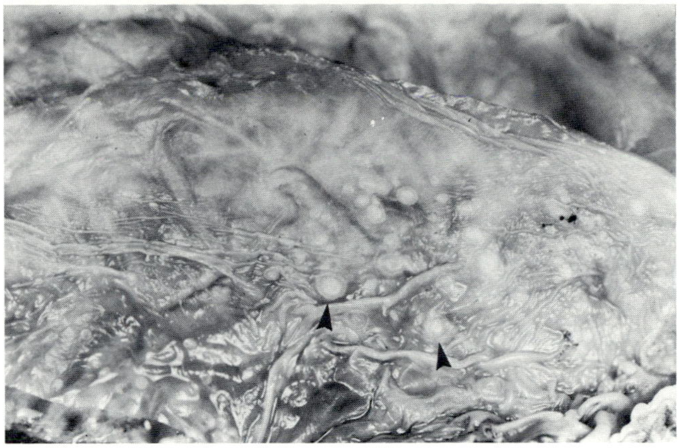

Fig. 23.61. Squamous metaplasia of amnion. Elevated white macules of squamous metaplasia (*arrows*).

Amnion Nodosum

Amnion nodosum is a relatively rare condition in which the surface of the amnion is studded with small (1–5 mm), yellowish, elevated nodules (Fig. 23.63). These are generally concentrated on the portion of amnion

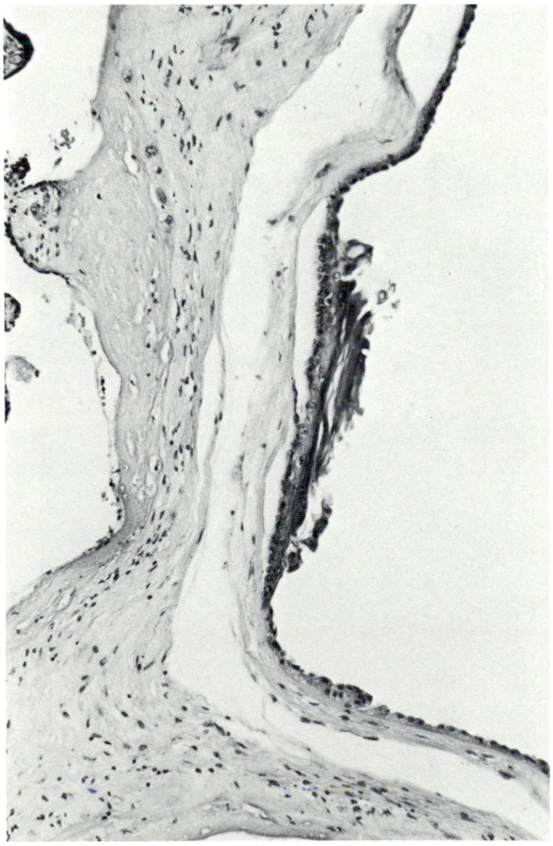

Fig. 23.62. Squamous metaplasia of amnion. Small focus of squamous metaplasia showing keratinization.

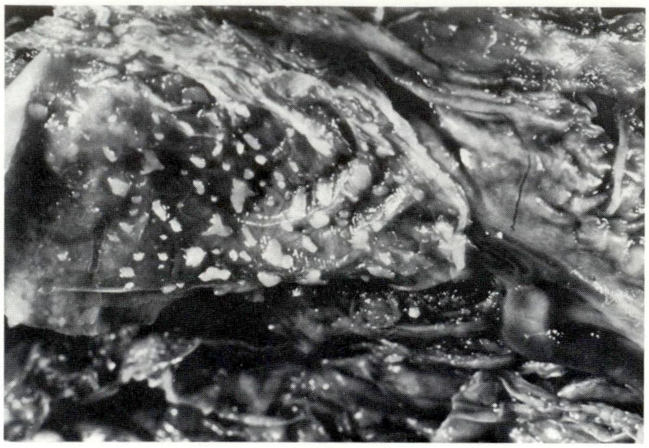

Fig. 23.63. Amnion nodosum. Elevated, irregular nodules on the fetal surface of the placenta.

covering the placenta, particularly around the insertion of the umbilical cord. Rarely, they may occur on the extraplacental amnion as well. By light microscopy, these nodules are composed primarily of amorphous, eosinophilic, and granular material containing scattered cells, degenerating cell fragments, and occasional fragments of hair (Figs. 23.64 and 23.65). The relationship of the nodule to the amnionic epithelium, basement membrane, and underlying connective tissue is disputed somewhat. According to Blanc, the nodules may be infiltrated by the underlying connective tissue cells.[39] In one ultrastructural study of two patients, however, the nodules were separated from the underlying stroma by a well-defined, though often multilaminated basement membrane.[225] A distinct cell type thought to represent amnionic epithelium was found lying on the basement membrane beneath the nodules. By light microscopy, the amnionic epithelium may be totally preserved, partially persistent, or totally absent under the plaques (Fig. 23.65). There is general agreement that a layer of amnion is commonly present over the surface of the nodule.

The nature of the electron-dense fibrillar material that forms the major component of the nodules has not been determined, although Salazar and Kanbour believe that it resembles the material that constitutes the vernix caseosum.[225] The majority of the cells and cell fragments have been identified ultrastructurally as epithelial in nature, consistent with fetal skin origin.[225]

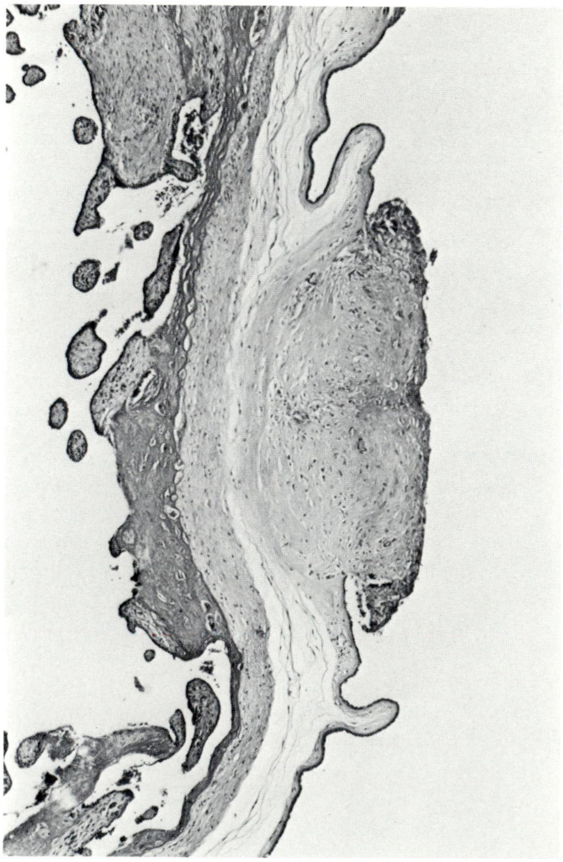

Fig. 23.64. Amnion nodosum. Nodular deposit on the amnionic surface of the placenta.

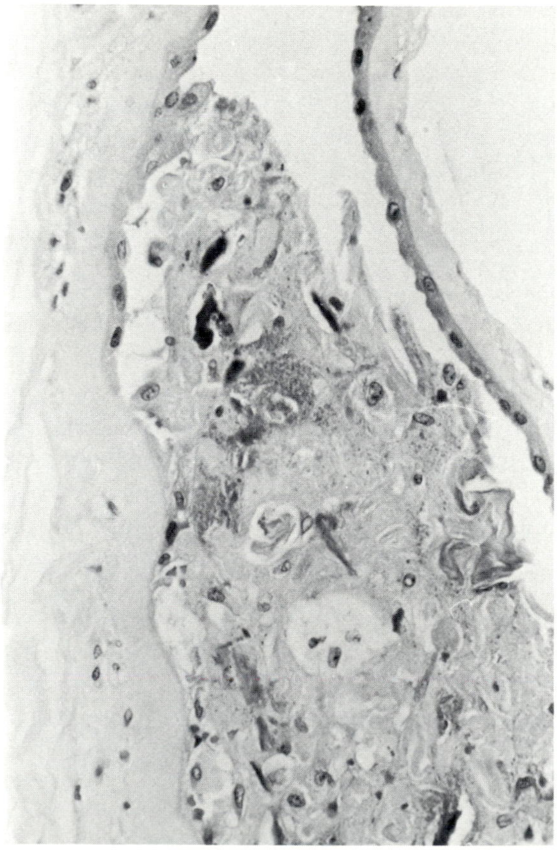

Fig. 23.65. Amnion nodosum. Nodular deposits are composed of degenerating cell fragments and hair embedded in amorphous granular material. Amnionic epithelium is preserved under a portion of this nodule.

The association of amnion nodosum with oligohydramnios is clearly established, but the nature of the link between the two conditions is still debated. Many believe that desquamated elements from the fetal epidermis and possibly oral cavity, urinary tract, or amnion itself are abnormally concentrated in the scant amnionic fluid and are deposited nonspecifically on the amnionic surface. Whether the process requires a primary abnormality of the amnion, antecedent trauma to the amnion, or direct contact and transfer of squamous cells, vernix, and lanugo hair from the fetal skin to the amnion are debated issues.[29,132]

The underlying cause of the oligohydramnios varies. In most cases, a fetal renal urinary tract abnormality is responsible (renal agenesis, urethral obstruction). This is logical given the fact that fetal urine does, in part, form the amnionic fluid. Prolonged amnionic fluid loss or the oligohydramnios associated with an acardiac fetus or the donor twin in the transfusion syndrome[177] may also be accompanied by amnion nodosum. However, amnion nodosum is not invariably present in cases of oligohydramnios.[57] The practical point is that amnion nodosum is a very reliable, if not totally absolute, indication of oligohydramnios and should alert the pediatrician to the possibility of congenital abnormalities in the fetus, especially affecting the urinary tract.

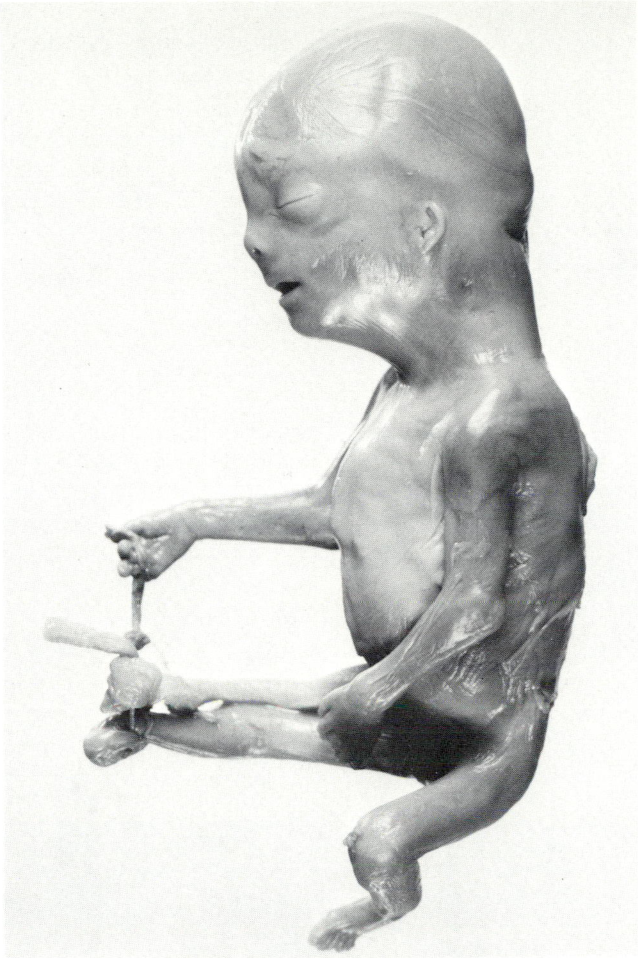

FIG. 23.66. Amnionic bands. Thin fibrous bands encircle and deform the leg and digits of this fetus.

Amnionic Bands

Amnionic bands, strings, and adhesions have been associated with a wide variety of fetal deformities. These vary in distribution and severity from constriction and amputation defects of the limbs and digits to major craniofacial and visceral abnormalities. Torpin strongly espoused the concept that amnionic bands cause the structural defects in this disorder.[269] The bands and strings are thought to result from amnionic rupture early in pregnancy. The ruptured amnion becomes partially or totally detached from the chorion and may fragment, shred, or shrink down to form a collar around the insertion of the umbilical cord. The mesoblastic tissue of the amnion and exposed chorion may form thin fibrous strands that encircle the fetal limbs, digits, neck, or umbilical cord, causing constriction, syndactyly, or amputation (Fig. 23.66). Malformations may also result when a band interferes with the normal sequence of embryonic development, as when interruption of fusion of the facial processes results in cleft lip. Adhesions may form between the placenta and fetus.

Some babies with amnionic band defects have additional structural anomalies that cannot be explained by the amnionic bands alone. These abnormalities, usually severe, include major limb deficiency, body wall defects, clubfeet, open cranial defects, and short umbilical cord.[35,121,122,168,252] It has been hypothesized that these defects are due to fetal compression that occurs secondary to the oligohydramnios produced by the amnionic rupture.[168] This hypothesis is supported by experimental studies in which puncture of the amnion of rats early during gestation produces an identical array of defects.* The widely variable nature and extent of the defects are presumed to be due to the timing of amnionic rupture.[124] Early rupture is thought to result in severe, multiple system defects. These may be difficult to diagnose unless ring constrictions and amputations are also present. Those infants in whom amnionic rupture occurs later in gestation are more mildly affected. Characteristic limb involvement facilitates the correct diagnosis in these fetuses. The recognition and correct diagnosis of amnion rupture and its consequences are important in counseling parents, since the risk of recurrence in this event is negligible. The etiology of amnionic rupture early in

*References 72, 141, 142, 155, 205, 271.

pregnancy is unknown. Some authors ascribe to the other major theory of pathogenesis, that a primary embryologic defect results in the formation of a defective body stalk and amnion.[121,252]

When this syndrome is suspected, examination of the placenta is aided by submersion of the placenta in water. This procedure facilitates recognition of the thin, delicate fibrous strands. Histologic examination of the placental surface will show absence of the amnion.

Meconium Stain

The passage of meconium may result in degenerative changes in the amnion evidenced by heaping, pseudostratification, and nuclear pyknosis of the epithelial cells. When exposure to meconium is prolonged, the amnionic epithelium may undergo complete necrosis. After some time has elapsed, macrophages in the compact layer of the amnion may engulf the meconium and become distended with granular, greenish yellow pigment (Fig. 23.67). Meconium may be distinguished from hemosiderin, which is yellowish, crystalline, and slightly refractile and forms larger granules.

Pathology of the Umbilical Cord

Vestigial Remnants

The normal umbilical cord contains two arteries and one vein surrounded by Wharton's jelly, a loosely structured myxomatous tissue. The cord is covered by a layer of amnion. No other vessels, specifically vasa vasorum, or lymphatics are found in the cord. Occasionally, remnants of the allantoic or omphalomesenteric ducts may be apparent on microscopic examination. Traces of the omphalomesenteric duct are quite infrequent. This duct connects the fetal ileum and the yolk sac of the early embryo. Its remnants are usually discontinuous, are located peripherally, beneath the amnionic surface, and may be lined by nondescript flat or columnar epithelium. Frequently, the lining resembles intestinal epithelium (Fig. 23.68). Rarely, omphalomesenteric remnants have been reported to show remarkable differentiation to gastric or small intestinal mucosa and pancreas. If found at all, the remainder of the original yolk sac, usually only a tiny, yellow-white nodule, is present not in the umbilical cord but beneath the amnion at the periphery

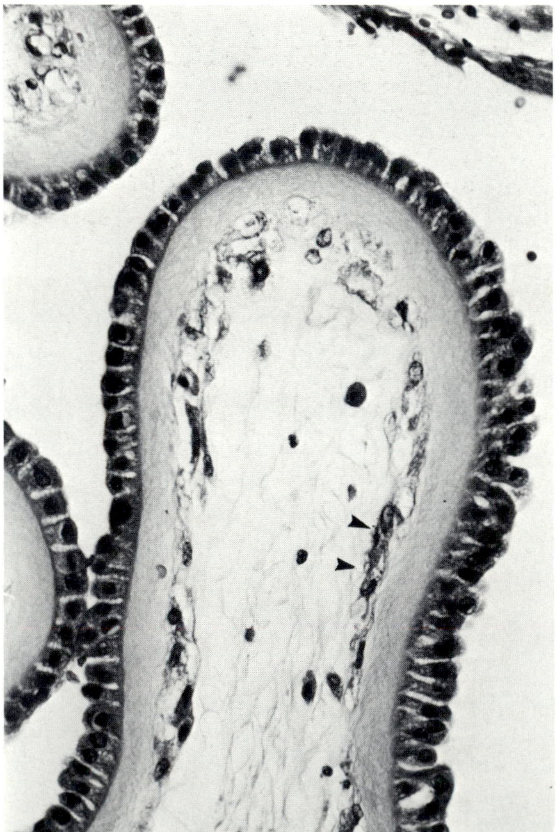

Fig. 23.67. Meconium stain. Accumulation of granular meconium pigment in the amnionic macrophages (*arrows*).

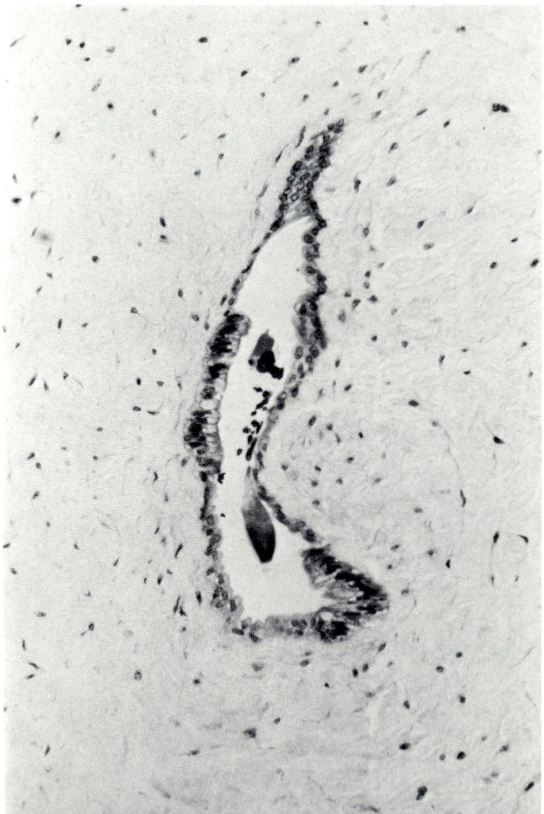

Fig. 23.68. Omphalomesenteric duct remnant, umbilical cord. This omphalomesenteric duct remnant is lined by columnar, mucin-containing epithelium.

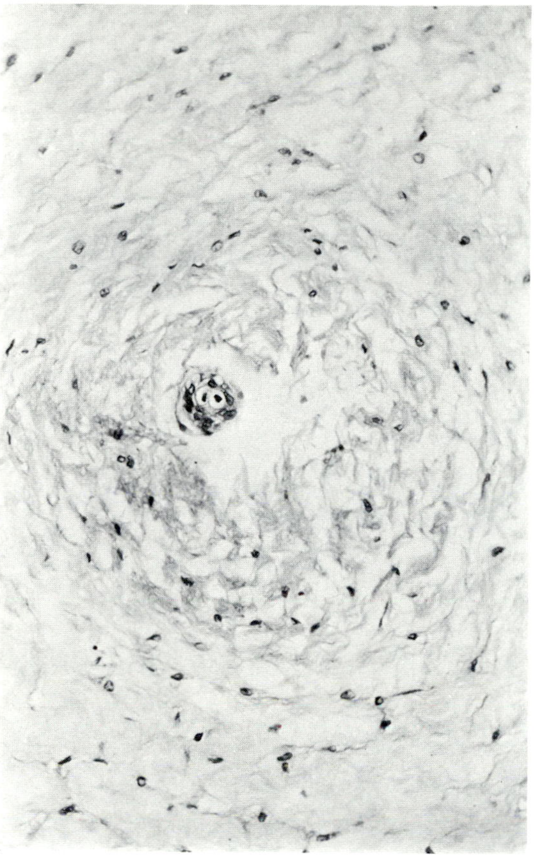

FIG. 23.69. Allantoic duct remnant, umbilical cord. Allantoic duct remnant lined by transitional type cuboidal cells.

of the placenta. Histologically, this consists of an amorphous, subamnionic, basophilic mass.

Remnants of the allantoic duct are more frequently recognized. This duct, the connection between the bladder via the urachus and rudimentary allantois, is lined by flat or cuboidal cells often reminiscent of transitional epithelium (Fig. 23.69). A lumen may or may not be present. Allantoic duct remnants are regularly located between the umbilical arteries.

Insertion of the Cord

Marginal Insertion

The umbilical cord generally inserts into the placenta either centrally or at some distance from the center (eccentric insertion). Insertion onto the peripheral margin of the placenta (marginal, or battledore, insertion) is less common than either central or eccentric insertion, but its reported frequency varies greatly. The significance of a marginal insertion is debated. It has been reported to occur with increased frequency in abortions, with malformed fetuses, and in association with neonatal asphyxia and premature labor. Fox could not confirm any of these reported associations.[98]

Velamentous Insertion

In approximately 1% of all deliveries, the cord inserts into the fetal membranes at some distance from the edge of the placenta. The umbilical vessels run in the chorion from the point of insertion to the main placental mass. During their course, they are unprotected by the connective tissue of the umbilical cord. These vessels are easily injured during labor and delivery, especially if they traverse the internal os (vasa previa). If one or more of these vessels is torn, rapid fetal exsanguination may result.

The frequency of velamentous insertion is definitely increased in multiple pregnancies. Other conditions that have been reported to be associated with velamentous insertion include extrachorial placentation and single umbilical artery. Neither the etiology nor pathogenesis of velamentous insertion is understood.

Abnormal Length

The length of the umbilical cord varies considerably but averages between 54 and 61 cm. Occurrence of longer than average cords is more frequent in series of infants in whom the cord is wound about the neck. Excessive cord length has been associated with knots, torsion, partial or complete vascular occlusion, and cord prolapse during delivery. Abnormally short umbilical cords may predispose to intrauterine distress, neonatal asphyxia, cord rupture and hemorrhage, abruptio placenta, and uterine inversion. In cases of acordia, or total absence of the umbilical cord, the umbilical region of the fetus, often malformed, merges with the placenta. This anomaly is usually found in abortions or stillbirths.

Single Umbilical Artery

The presence of a single umbilical artery (SUA) is a very common anomaly that is frequently associated with other congenital malformations (Fig. 23.70). The reported frequency of SUA varies depending on the type of study. In neonatal autopsies and spontaneous abortions, SUA occurs in about 2.5–3.0%.[120] In prospective studies of consecutive deliveries, the frequency is consistently somewhat less than 1%.[27,60,102] Other factors influence the prevalence of this abnormality. SUA is more common in white infants than in blacks and Orientals.[102,198] There is an excess of SUA in babies of diabetic mothers.[102] Some authors have reported that SUAs are found more commonly in multiple pregnancies,[27,243] but this has been disputed in other series, where the frequency has not been greater and has even been some-

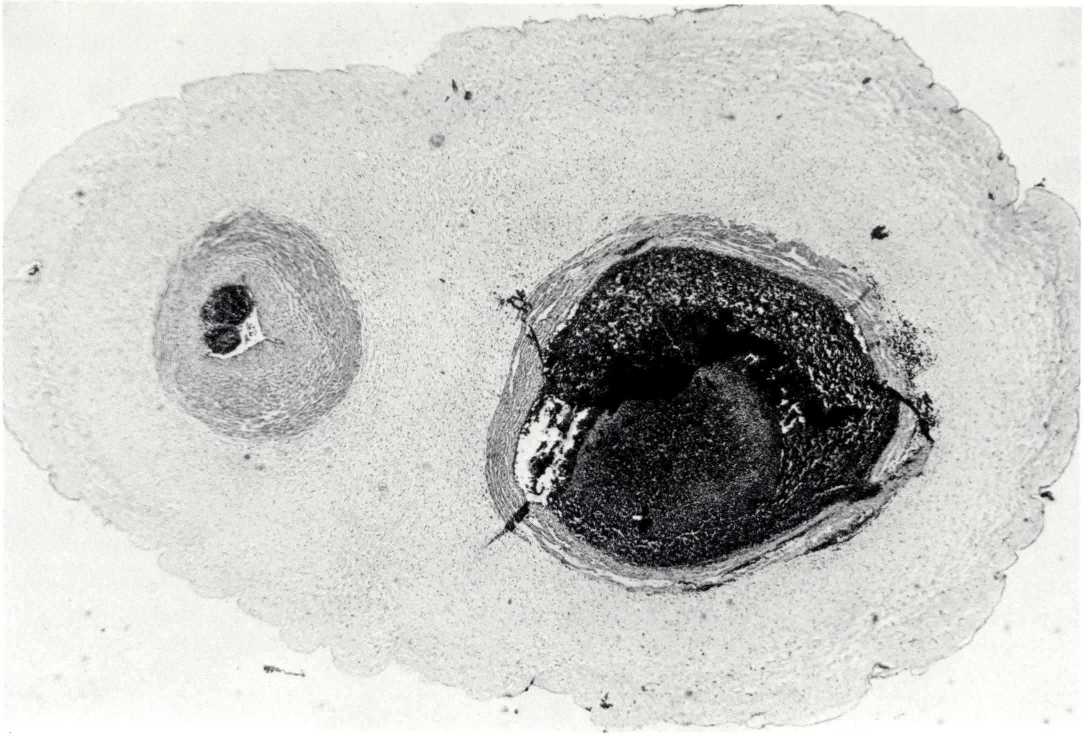

FIG. 23.70. Single umbilical artery; on *left*, umbilical cord.

what less in twins.[60,198] There is no association with maternal age or parity.

There is a definite and well-documented association between fetal malformations and SUA.[27–29,60,102,120,243] The severity of these malformations varies tremendously, and there is no particular organ or specific abnormality characterizing this association. Any organ system may be involved, and genitourinary, musculoskeletal, cardiovascular, central nervous system, and gastrointestinal malformations are encountered most frequently.[60,102,103,243] Malformations are often multiple. The frequency with which these malformations are reported to occur in association with SUA varies considerably, from 17.5% to 97%.[243] This discrepancy largely reflects the much higher malformation rate found in autopsied SUA infants when compared with infants having SUA who survive. This is emphasized in one study where 52.8% of autopsied infants with SUA had associated malformations compared to only 4.1% of SUA survivors.[103] Furthermore, the most severe malformations are predominantly in stillborn fetuses and in infants dying in the first weeks of life.[60,61,102,103] Major malformations are much less common in babies surviving the neonatal period. This suggests that SUA infants with severe abnormalities tend to die in utero or early in the perinatal period. One follow-up study of SUA infants who survived the neonatal period with no clinically detectable malformation at birth showed only an unexplained increase in inguinal hernia.[103] Bryan and Kohler reported the subsequent discovery of malformations in 10 of 98 infants in whom anomalies had not been apparent at birth. These were much less severe than those documented at birth.[61]

SUA is associated with a tendency toward low birth weight. This relationship persists even when infants with major malformations are excluded from analysis.[60,120] The overall perinatal mortality rate of infants with SUA is greatly increased (11–41%). The occurrence of major malformations is the most significant factor in the high perinatal mortality rate, although an increased mortality rate has also been reported among the normal infants with SUA.[60] A remarkable frequency of SUA in chromosomal abnormalities, especially trisomies, has been reported.[243] In some series, SUA has been associated with velamentous insertion of the cord and low placental weight.[102,120]

There has been considerable debate whether a single umbilical artery is due to primary aplasia or secondary atrophy. Certainly, histologic evidence of portions or remnants of a vessel may be documented in the umbilical cord in some cases of SUA, providing support for the theory of secondary atrophy of a formerly present vessel (Figs. 23.71 and 23.72). Evidence of such atrophy was found in 19 of 48 cases of SUA in a study that specifically investigated this point.[14] Whether the SUA actually causes the associated fetal malformations or is just another manifestation of them is a matter of conjecture. The

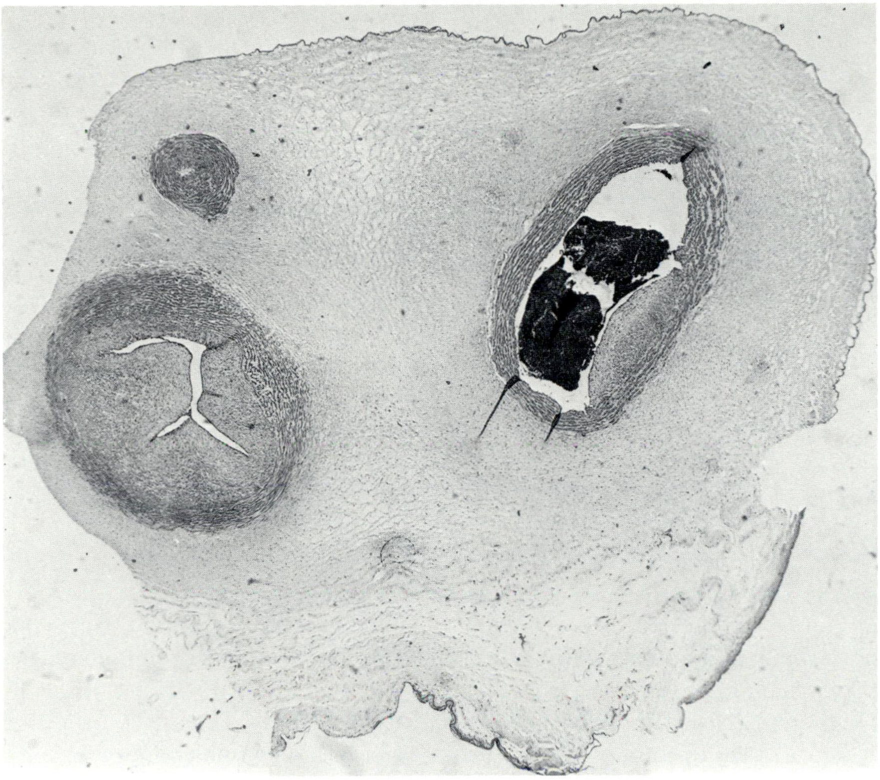

Fig. 23.71. Marked hypoplasia of one umbilical artery. This anomaly was found in conjunction with several congenital malformations in a fetus dying shortly after birth.

practical point is that it is very important for the pathologist to recognize and document the occurrence of SUA. Gross examination of a fresh cord is not sufficient, since a significant number of cases of SUA will be missed. Fixation does aid in gross examination, but sections of the cord should be examined microscopically. If the umbilical cord is sectioned very close to the chorionic plate, fusion of the two umbilical arteries, which often occurs normally in this location, may be misinterpreted as SUA. This source of error may be obviated by taking an additional section at a different level of the cord.

Knots

True knots do occur in the umbilical cord (Fig. 23.73). They are sometimes confused with, and must be distinguished from, false knots resulting from focal accentuation of the vascular spiral, a varicosity, or excess Whar-

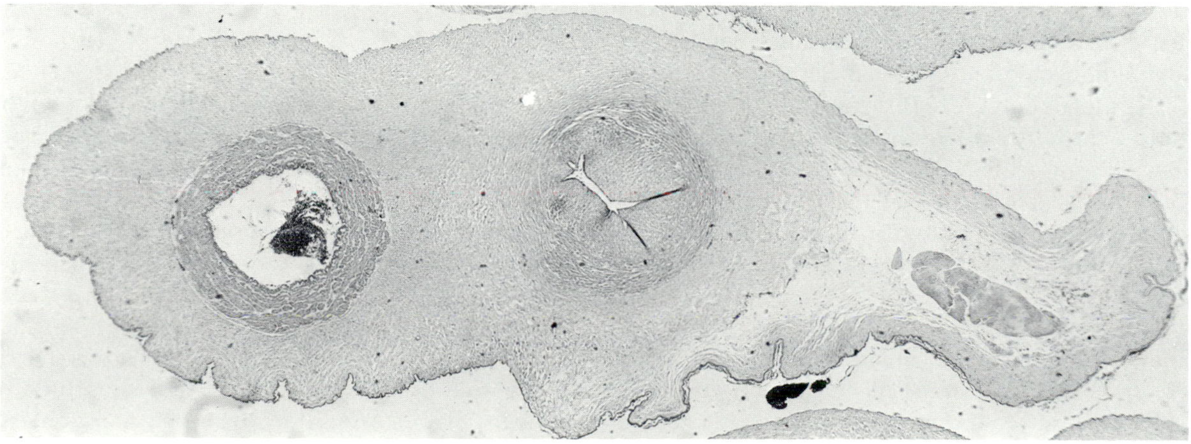

Fig. 23.72. Amorphous remnant of one umbilical artery (*right*).

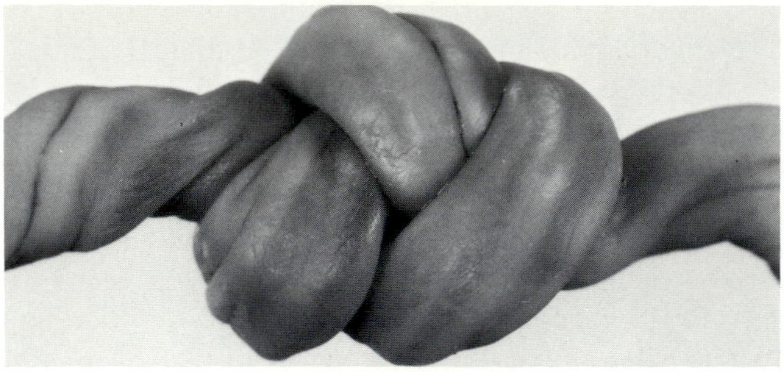

FIG. 23.73. True knot of umbilical cord in a normal liveborn infant.

ton's jelly. True knots are found in fewer than 1% of all deliveries. They are usually a complication of an excessively long umbilical cord. An increased perinatal mortality rate in the range of 8 to 11% is associated with the presence of true knots, presumably due to obstruction of the fetal circulation through a tight knot. The criteria for distinguishing a long-standing knot from one that has undergone acute tightening during labor and delivery include compression and a definite groove at the site of the knot, loss of Wharton's jelly, and persistence of these structural changes after the knot is untied. Knots that have been acutely tightened show edema, venous stasis and congestion distal to the knot, and occlusive thrombi in the vessels. Either an acutely tightened or long-standing knot may be responsible for intrauterine or intrapartum fetal death.

Torsion and Stricture

The normal spiraling of vessels in the umbilical cord creates the impression of twisting. Occasionally, however, excessive torsion of the cord occurs, characteristically at its fetal end. Associated congestion, edema, and vascular thrombi provide evidence that this anomaly is real and may result in interruption of blood flow and fetal death. Strictures of the umbilical cord are rare and are often complicated by torsion. Strictures are usually single, sharply defined, short segments located most commonly at the fetal end of the cord.[275] Microscopically, there may be contraction of the vessels, loss of Wharton's jelly, or fibrosis in the area of the constriction. This anomaly is usually described in stillborn babies.

Hematoma

Hematomas of the umbilical cord are a rare complication of pregnancy.[78,230] They are usually confined to the cord but occasionally may rupture into the amnionic cavity. Grossly, hematomas appear as a red-purple, fusiform swelling of the cord, most often near its fetal end. In some cases, the hemorrhage may be demonstrated to originate from the umbilical vein and much less commonly from an umbilical artery. In most cases, an obvious source of the hemorrhage is not apparent.

The etiology of such hemorrhage is unknown. Included among the proposed possible causes are rupture of a varix, trauma, structural anomalies of the vessel wall, mechanical damage due to traction on a short cord, and inflammation.

The perinatal mortality of infants with an umbilical cord hematoma is in the range of 40 to 50%. The nature of the relationship between this high perinatal mortality and the occurrence of a cord hematoma is unclear, but it has been theorized that the hematoma may result in compression and thrombosis of fetal vessels with cessation of fetal blood flow.

Cysts

Cysts within the umbilical cord may be of several types. Probably the most common type is not a true cyst at all but rather a cavity resulting from degeneration of Wharton's jelly. These lack an epithelial lining. Remnants of either an omphalomesenteric or allantoic duct may undergo cystic dilatation. These can sometimes be distinguished by their resemblance to gastrointestinal-type or transitional-type epithelium. They are generally small and inconsequential. Cystic inclusions of the amnion are uncommon.

Edema

The umbilical cord occasionally appears enlarged and swollen with very loose, edematous Wharton's jelly. Edema has been specifically defined as a visibly edematous cord with a cross-sectional area of 1.3 cm^2 or greater.[68] Edema of the cord is not uncommon in maternal diabetes, Rh incompatibility, and fetal death in utero.

Abortion

Abortion is defined as the spontaneous or operative termination of pregnancy before fetal viability. The legal definition of viability varies from one location to another and may not correspond to the medical definition of viability. Spontaneous abortions are common, and their exact incidence is difficult to assess, since many are clinically inapparent. It has been estimated that as many as 45% of pregnancies abort.

The etiology of spontaneous abortion is diverse but may result from either fetal or maternal factors. In general, the factors associated with early abortion are fetal, primarily chromosomal abnormalities and an ill-defined group of immunologic incompatibilities. Maternal factors (cervical incompetence, developmental abnormalities in the genital tract, infection) are more often associated with midtrimester abortions.

Products of conception submitted for pathologic examination consist of a combination of placental, fetal, and maternal elements, in any state of organization or disarray. Very early in pregnancy, the decidual component predominates. Thereafter, the placental and then the fetal tissues are most conspicuous. At the minimum, intrauterine pregnancy should be documented in any putative early abortion specimen. This requires the definite identification of trophoblast, which is usually found in association with villi but is sometimes limited to the trophoblastic elements infiltrating the endometrium at the implantation site. Occasionally, isolated clumps of trophoblast may be admixed with clotted blood. The presence of decidua or gestational endometrium does not constitute adequate documentation of intrauterine pregnancy, since this change may be associated with ectopic pregnancy or hormonal manipulation. When trophoblastic elements are not found in the initial sections, the entire specimen should be examined microscopically. If trophoblast is still not identified, the clinician is alerted to the consideration of an ectopic gestation. It should be recognized that no combination of findings in the endometrium, including villi, can exclude an ectopic pregnancy. There are numerous reports of simultaneous intrauterine and tubal pregnancy.[284]

The villi, if present, may be normal, show evidence of fetal death in utero, or exhibit other characteristic pathologic changes known to be associated with abortion. Normal chorionic villi are generally punctuated by fine fetal vessels that contain nucleated red blood cells during the first 10–20 weeks of pregnancy. A constellation of morphologic alterations that is the result, not the cause, of fetal death begins about 24 hours after fetal death and is fully established within 5–6 days.[95,129] These changes include sclerosis and obliteration of fetal stem arteries and villous capillaries, progressive villous stromal fibrosis, increased numbers of syncytial knots, increased numbers of cytotrophoblastic cells, and thickening of the trophoblastic basement membrane (Fig. 23.74).

A fetus or embryo, when present in aborted material, also deserves careful study. Fusion defects in the face, ocular anomalies, limb bud deformities, and cervical edema, especially, suggest specific genetically deter-

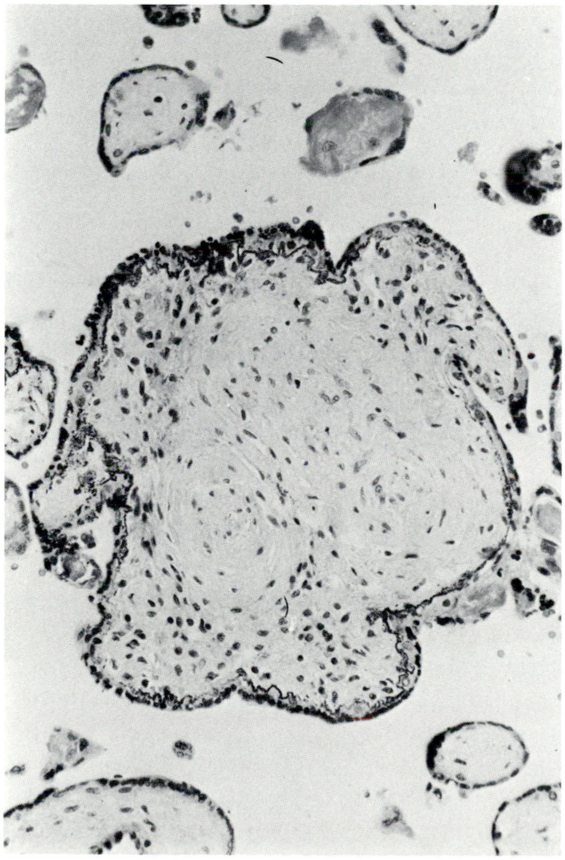

FIG. 23.74. Fetal death in utero. The villous alterations resulting from fetal death in utero include sclerosis and obliteration of the fetal vessels, stromal fibrosis, and prominence of the cytotrophoblast.

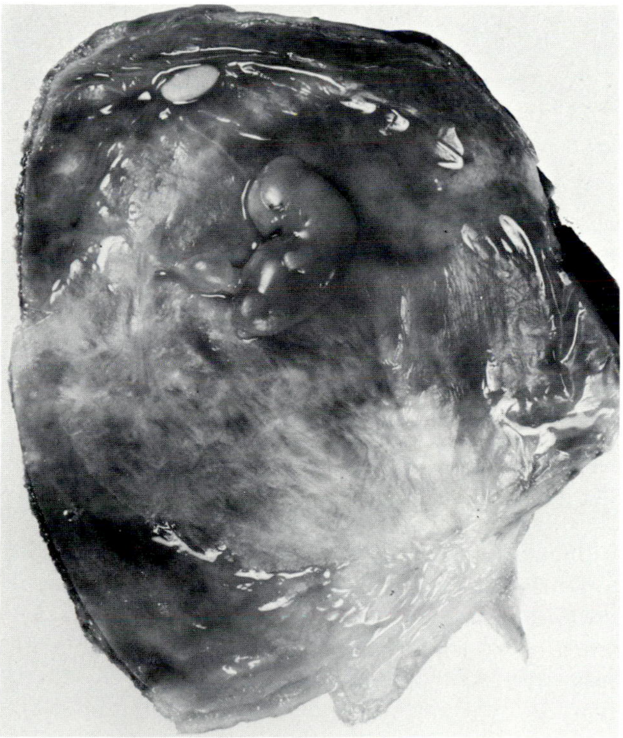

FIG. 23.75. Spontaneous abortion with intact amnion and deformed embryo. The bulbous, amorphous limb buds, distorted facial clefts, constricted body stalk (umbilical cord), and greatly distended amnion all suggest abnormal karyotype, probably a trisomy.

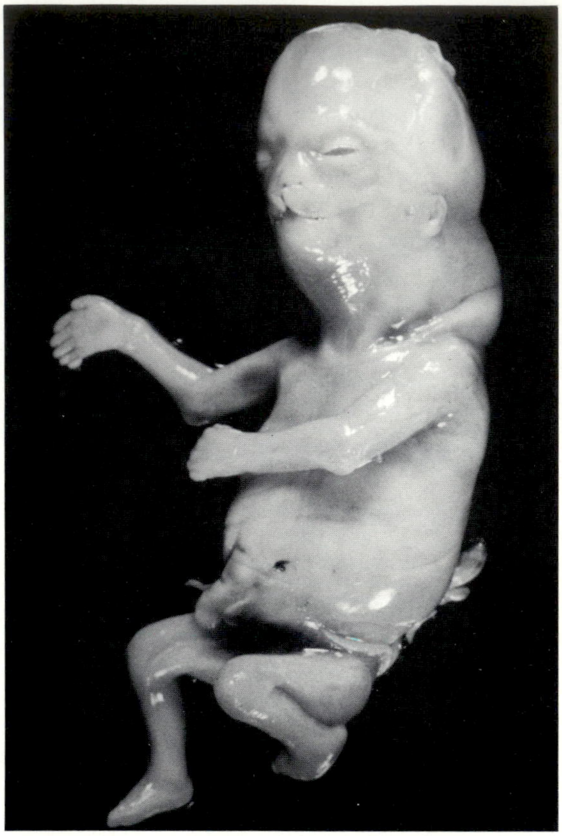

FIG. 23.76. Aborted 47XX (trisomy 13) fetus. Note supernumerary digits, facial fusion defect, cervical swelling, low set ears, and ventral hernia. (Karyotype courtesy of P. Monteleone, M.D., St. Louis, Missouri.)

mined anomalies. Certain combinations can be extremely useful in defining abnormal karyotypes when cytogenetic studies cannot be performed, for instance, in specimens already fixed at the time of examination[138] (Figs. 23.75 and 23.76).

Morphologic Correlations in Spontaneous Abortion

Although morphologic alterations in abortions are not absolutely specific for well-defined etiologies, some abnormalities are sufficiently distinctive to suggest the cause. These observations are important because they may carry serious implications for repeated malformations in subsequent pregnancies. Some immunologic problems are associated with repeated abortions and life-threatening thrombotic problems in the mother. It is clear that dismissing spontaneously aborted tissue as "products of conception" is insufficient in many cases. Detailed studies in many of these areas are lacking, but a number of significant observations are possible.

Immunologic Factors

Blocking Antibodies. Rocklin et al.[218] identified a maternal IgG antibody in normal multigravid women that is absent in some women who experience repeated abortion. The presence of this serum blocking factor is believed to support the fetus and placenta as an allograft. Morphologic changes at the implantation site in these abortions have not been correlated with the immunologic findings. It would be interesting and very desirable to see if placental site trophoblast is altered or absent in women who experience habitual abortion. The absence of vessel changes and intermediate trophoblast is an easily recognized pattern variation in some abortions, but clinical correlations with this deficit are lacking (Fig. 23.77).

Circulating Lupus Anticoagulant. This immunoglobulin (usually IgG but sometimes IgM) that inhibits coagulation derives its name (a misnomer) from the circumstances of its first identification in patients with lupus erythematosus. It has been implicated as a clinical marker for recurrent first trimester spontaneous abortion and for fetal death in later trimesters as well. It prolongs phospholipid-dependent coagulation times but paradoxically is associated with an increased risk of thrombotic disease in the mother.[52,90] Certainly, morphologic studies of the aborted tissues associated with this condition would have practical benefit. Whether any of the circulatory lesions of the placenta described earlier in this chapter could serve as identifiers for this condition remains to be shown.

Defined Genetic Defects

The defects responsible for most spontaneous abortions appear to be genetically determined, and many can be identified by karyotyping fetal or placental tissue.[163] The most common abnormal karyotypes have been trisomies, triploidy, and 45X0 (Table 23.2). In much smaller numbers, tetraploidy and a variety of mosaics have been documented. Karyotyping may be clinically very useful in evaluation of couples distressed by repeated spontaneous abortions.[251] Morphologic correlations, though not absolute, can be distinctive enough in many instances to suggest the nature of the abnormal karyotype. Earlier abortions, occurring before the 8th week of gestation, have the highest percentage of aneuploidy (about 66%), whereas later abortions (23% aneuploid) are more likely to have other causes.

Triploid abortions have the most distinctive morphologic features. About 86% have the gross and microscopic characteristics of partial mole (see Chapter 24, Gestational Trophoblastic Disease). Numerous villi are grossly hydropic (not all as in hydatidiform mole) (Fig. 23.78). A fetus may be identified. The typical histologic features include villi with trophoblastic invaginations, cisterns or empty spaces lined by endothelial cells, and extremely

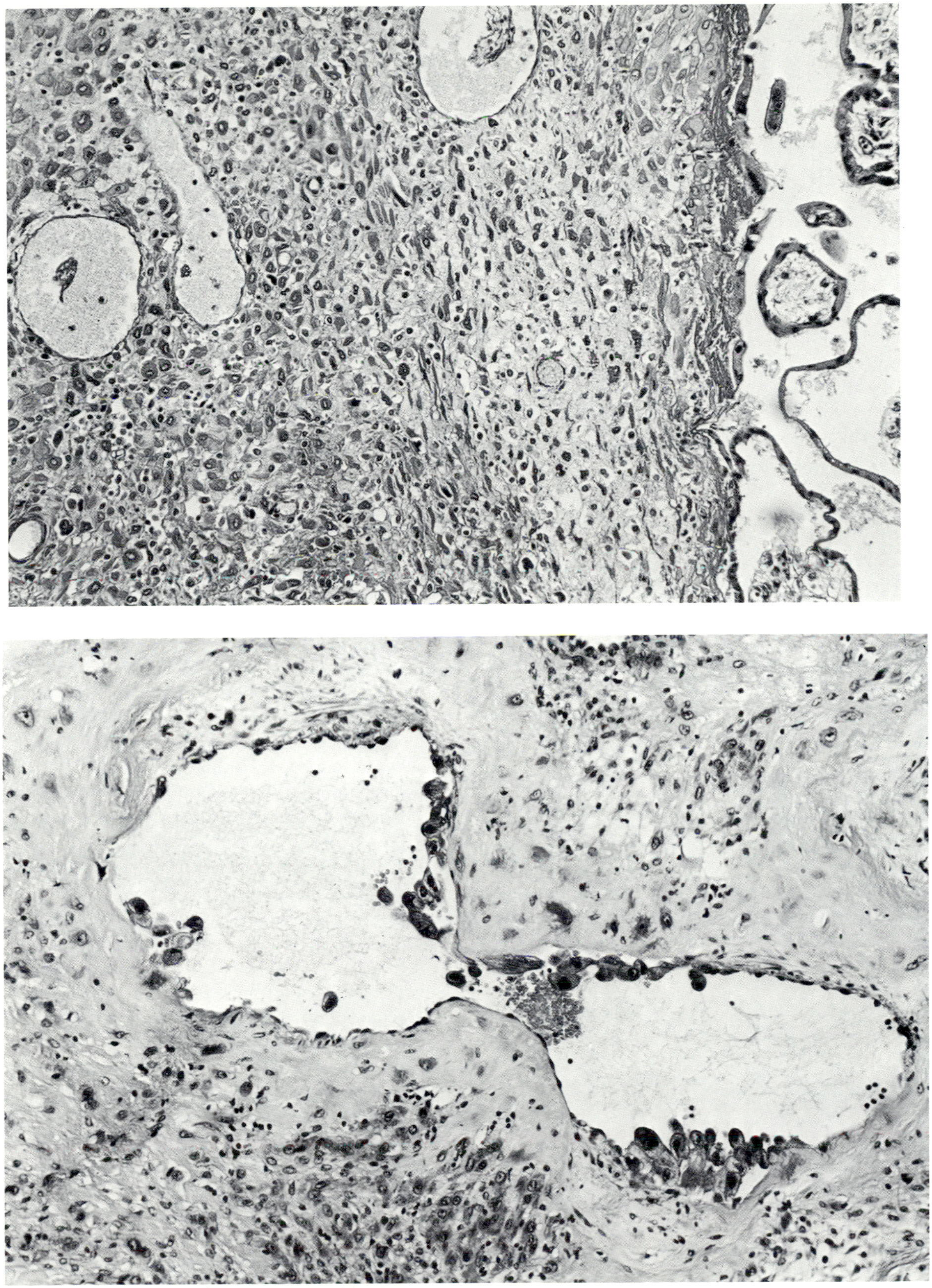

a

b

FIG. 23.77. *a*. Implantation site of spontaneous abortion. Placental site intermediate trophoblast cells are markedly deficient in size and numbers. *b*. Normal appearance of intermediate trophoblast at implantation site. Numerous trophoblast cells replace intima, infiltrate the wall of the large spiral artery at *center*, and cluster irregularly in the surrounding decidua, especially at *bottom center*.

TABLE 23.2. Proportions of abnormal karyotypes in 1500 spontaneous abortions.

Karyotype abnormality	Approximate percentage
Trisomies	52
Triploidy	20
XO	15
Tetraploidy	6
Translocations	4
Double trisomy	2
Mosaics	1

From data of Boue and Boue, modified after Benirschke, Ref. 26.

irregular surfaces, often covered by hyperplastic vacuolated syncytiotrophoblast (Fig. 23.79a).[259] The trophoblastic invaginations form a targetlike arrangement of central space, syncytiotrophoblast, and peripheral cytotrophoblast cells that border upon the villous stroma (Fig. 23.79b). The fetuses, when present, have external dysmorphic features that include hypertelorism, micrognathia, low set ears, camptodactyly, 3–4 syndactyly, and adrenal hypoplasia. Triploid abortions are sporadic, unlikely to be repeated, and not related to abnormal parental karyotypes. The presence of hydropic villi and the expression, mole, seem to cast an ominous shadow on the potential for aggressive trophoblastic disease after triploid partial moles.[34] It is desirable to emphasize, therefore, that morphologically diagnosed choriocarcinoma has not yet been recorded in this setting and that the chromosomes of a hydatidiform mole (usually 46XX, all paternally derived) are very different from partial mole, which is nearly always 69XXY or 69XXX. One example of invasive partial mole has been documented clearly.[106] Until the full biologic potential for triploid partial mole has been defined, it will be important to provide appropriate quantitative gonadotropin follow-up as it is done for a typical 46XX hydatidiform complete mole (see Chapter 24, Gestational Trophoblastic Disease).

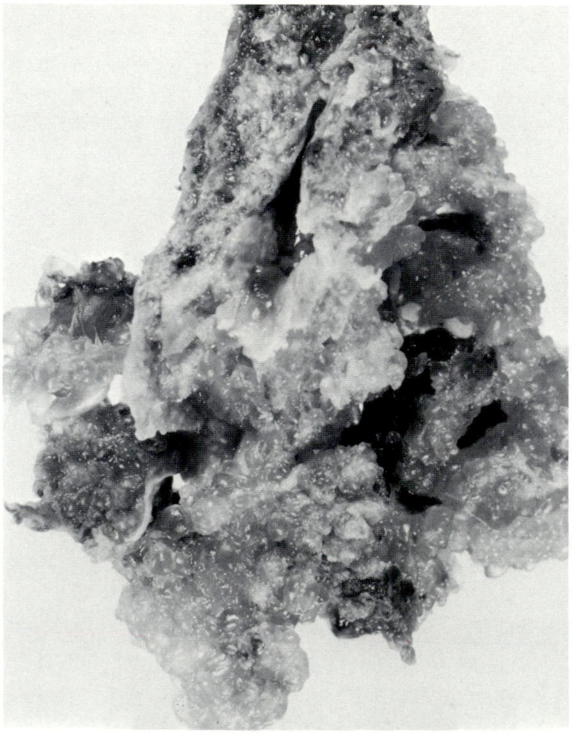

FIG. 23.78. Partial mole. Empty amnionic sac is at top center. Many villi are swollen and hydropic (*at bottom*) but many others (*at top*) are nearly normal. Total mass, in contrast to true hydatidiform mole, is approximately the size of other spontaneous abortions. (Reproduced by permission from Kraus, Frederick T.: Gynecologic Pathology, St. Louis, 1967, The C.V. Mosby Co.)

The villi in trisomic abortions are also usually swollen and avascular, but they are smaller and cisterns are absent. Trophoblast invaginations occur but less commonly. The most characteristic histologic feature may be large, mononuclear cells infiltrating into the villous stroma (Fig. 23.80). These cells are generally believed to represent migratory cytotrophoblast,[138] but altered Hofbauer cells represent a possible alternative.[26] In our experience, some, at least, are marked by antisera to human placental lactogen in immunocytochemical preparations, which suggests but does not prove trophoblastic derivation. Many trisomies result from parental chromosomal anomalies, mostly balanced translocations. When abnormal parental karyotypes are demonstrated, the prospects for future anomalous conceptions are much greater.

The villi of abortions with 45X0 (monosomy X) karyotype may have focal slight swelling in early abortions or scattered large immature villi in later abortions, but the most distinctive morphologic changes affect the fetus itself. Massive edema of the entire fetus is common. Most are dead and macerated, but most characteristic is the pronounced dorsal and lateral swelling of the neck, which may triple the size of the fetal head (Fig. 23.81). Placental villi may be normal or focally enlarged and immature (Fig. 23.82). Monosomy X conceptions are usually not repeated, but they seem to be more commonly associated with young maternal age.[274] The phenotype in those who survive is that of Turner's syndrome.

The clinical importance of these observations must be stressed because some abnormalities, especially trisomies, may occur repeatedly, reflecting chromosomal anomalies in the parents. Balanced translocations are the most common parental karyotypic defects. Although these are not currently treatable, they are of immense importance in genetic counseling as the prospects for future pregnancies are evaluated. The use of a dissecting microscope in examination of aborted fetuses and careful attention to variation in villous morphology are of great

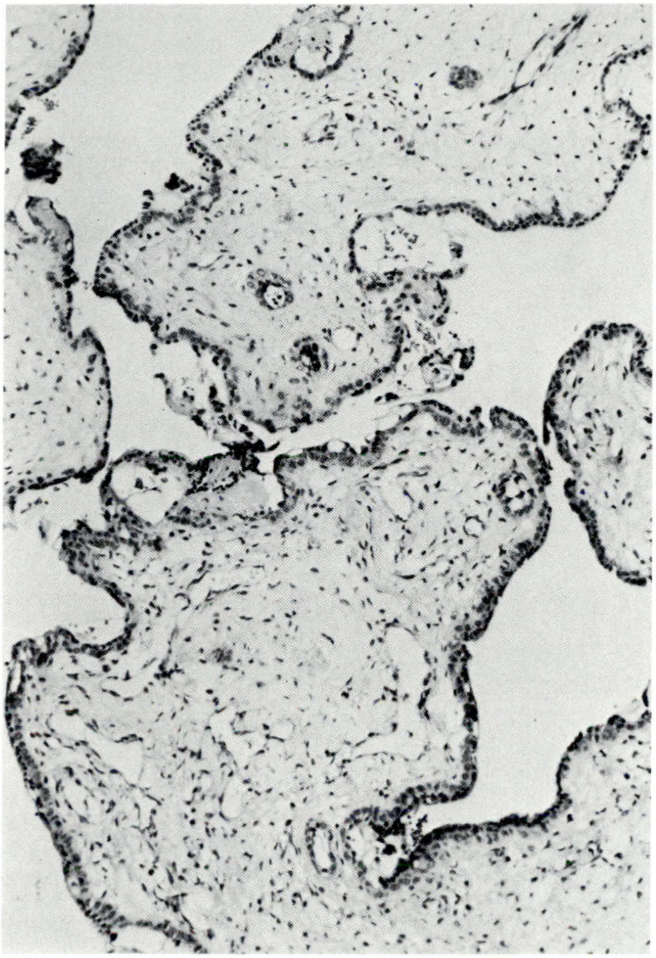

a.

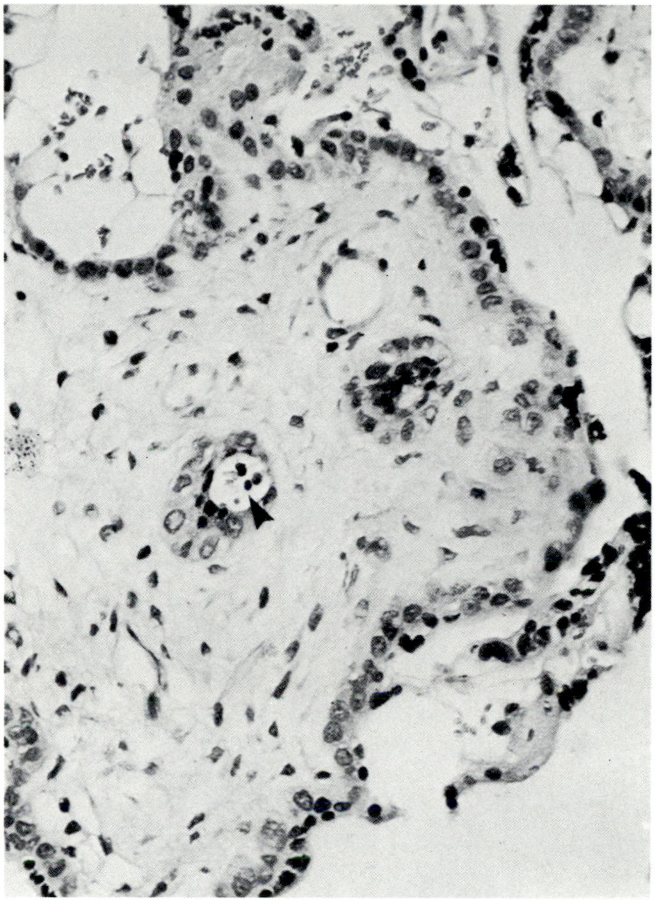

b.

FIG. 23.79. *a*. Partial mole (69XXY). Distinctive features are trophoblastic invaginations that appear circular in cross-section (villus at *top center*), the scalloped, irregular margins, and empty endothelium-lined vascular sinusoids (cisterns) (villus at *bottom*). (Karyotype courtesy of K. Taysi, M.D., St. Louis, Missouri.) *b*. Higher magnification of trophoblastic invaginations. Note the peripheral, pale-staining, larger cytotrophoblast cells and the more central, darker, syncytiotrophoblast nuclei. The central space (*arrow*) communicates with the maternal intervillous space.

potential usefulness as data are accumulated to justify the effort and expense of parental karyotyping. The facial fusion defects, polydactyly, foot deformities, low set ears, and ventral hernia in the fetus shown in Fig. 23.76 should prompt detailed histologic scrutiny of the villi and strong consideration of karyotyping the parents. Balanced translocation may represent the basis for repeated abortion in such cases.[251]

Other Noninflammatory Changes Associated with Abortion or Death In Utero

Villous Edema. Naeye et al. noted that placental villous edema correlated strongly with morbidity and mortality in neonates with chorioamnionitis.[184] The chief morphologic alteration is the presence of open spaces in the interstitium of the villi (Fig. 23.83). Villous edema also occurs in association with maternal hypertension, diabetes mellitus, premature rupture of membranes, abruption, and other states associated with fetal hypoxia. In many instances, no disorder has been identified.

Nonimmune Fetal Hydrops. Fetal hydrops, a syndrome characterized by soft tissue edema and effusion in the fetus, has been classically associated with maternal isoimmunization to fetal erythrocyte antigens, usually Rh sensitization. A variety of other causes are recognized, including viral infections, twin transfusion syndrome, fetomaternal hemorrhage, trisomy, and monosomy X.[172] Because some of the basic lesions carry important prognostic considerations for future gestations, an explanation for all instances of nonimmune fetal hydrops should be sought and identified when possible.

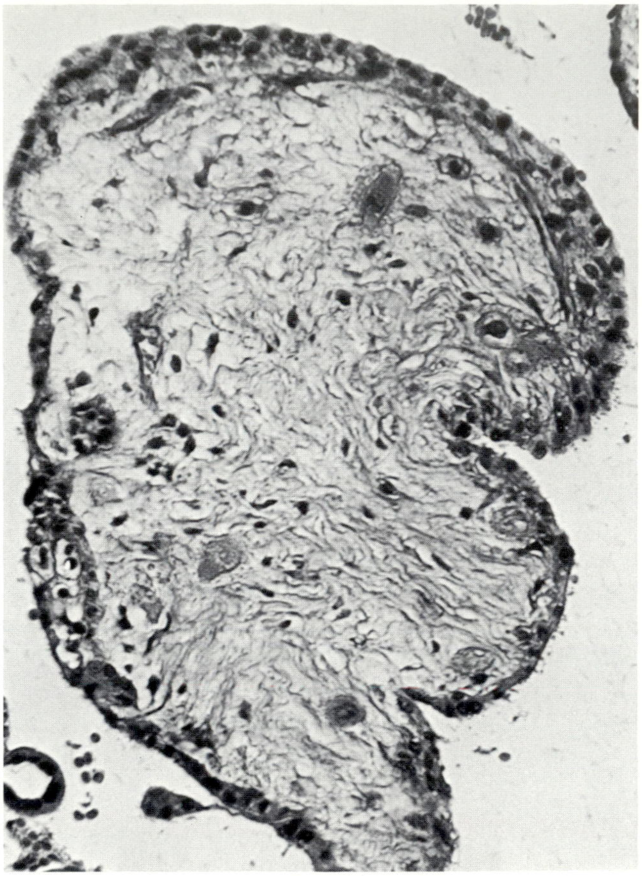

FIG. 23.80. Villus from D-trisomy spontaneous abortion. A few large, irregular cells resembling cytotrophoblast extend into the villous stroma at *top, center,* and *bottom center.*

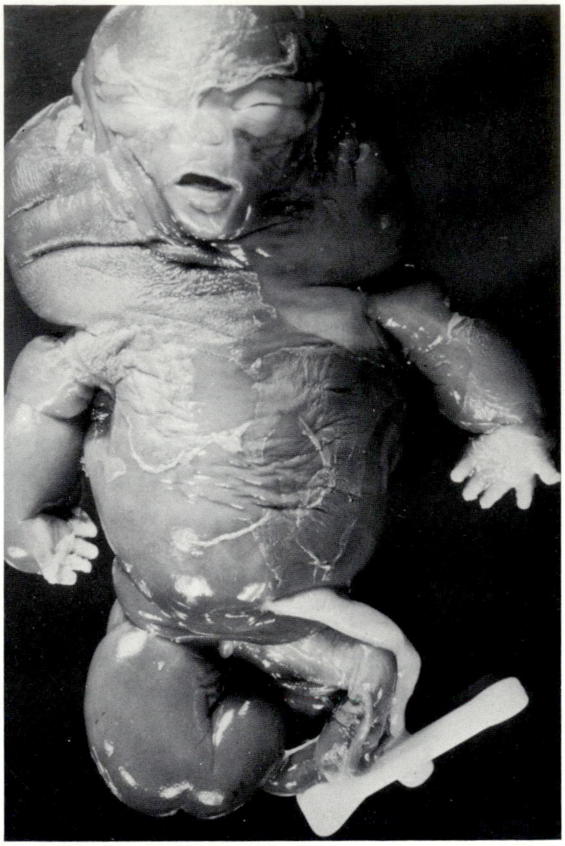

FIG. 23.81. Aborted 45 XO fetus. The large, symmetrical cervical swellings and generalized edema are characteristic features. Cardiovascular anomalies are also common, as in Turner's syndrome. (Karyotype courtesy of K. Taysi, M.D., St. Louis, Missouri.)

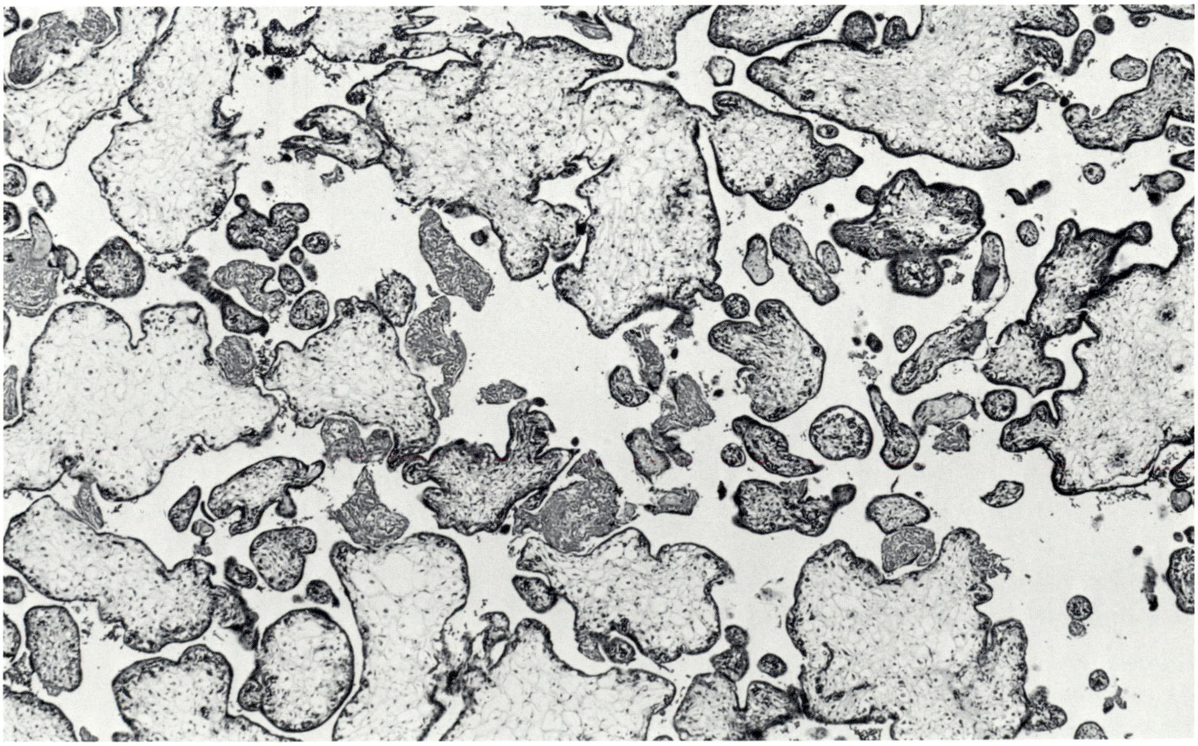

FIG. 23.82. Immature, enlarged villi from a 45XO spontaneous abortion similar to the fetus shown in Figure 23.81, but of longer (26 weeks) gestation. Patchy clusters of larger immature villi with abundant stroma are not specific but suggestive of this and other abnormal placental genotypes, including trisomies. (Karyotype courtesy of K. Taysi, M.D., St. Louis, Missouri.)

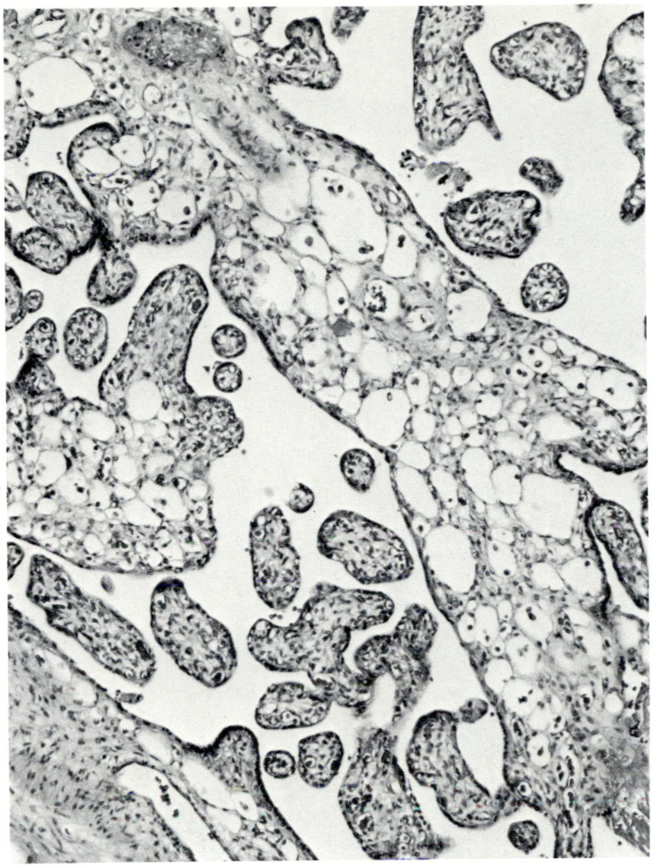

Fig. 23.83. Villous edema, forming clusters of open spaces delimited by attenuated strands of stromal cells and collagen. When associated with amnionitis, the clinical severity is much greater and mortality is more likely.

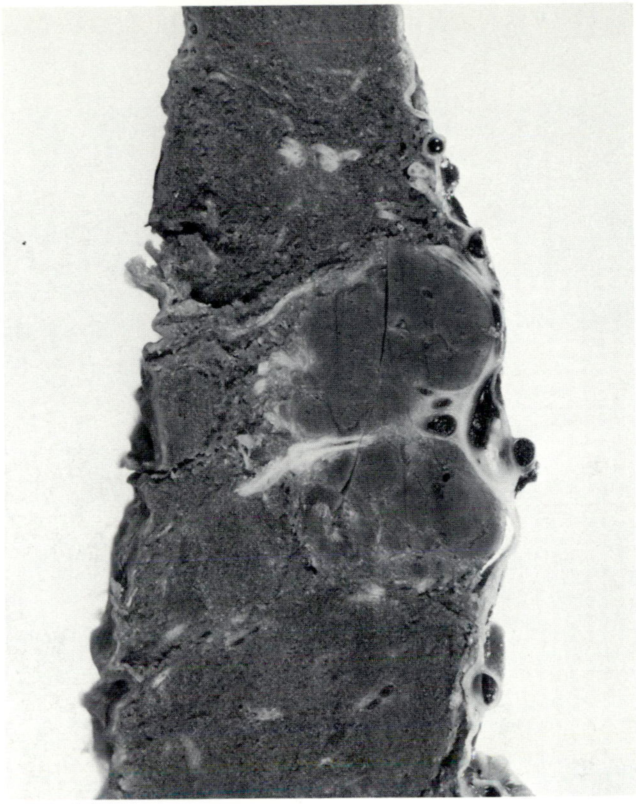

Fig. 23.84. Placental hemangioma. Firm, red hemangioma, well demarcated from the surrounding placental parenchyma.

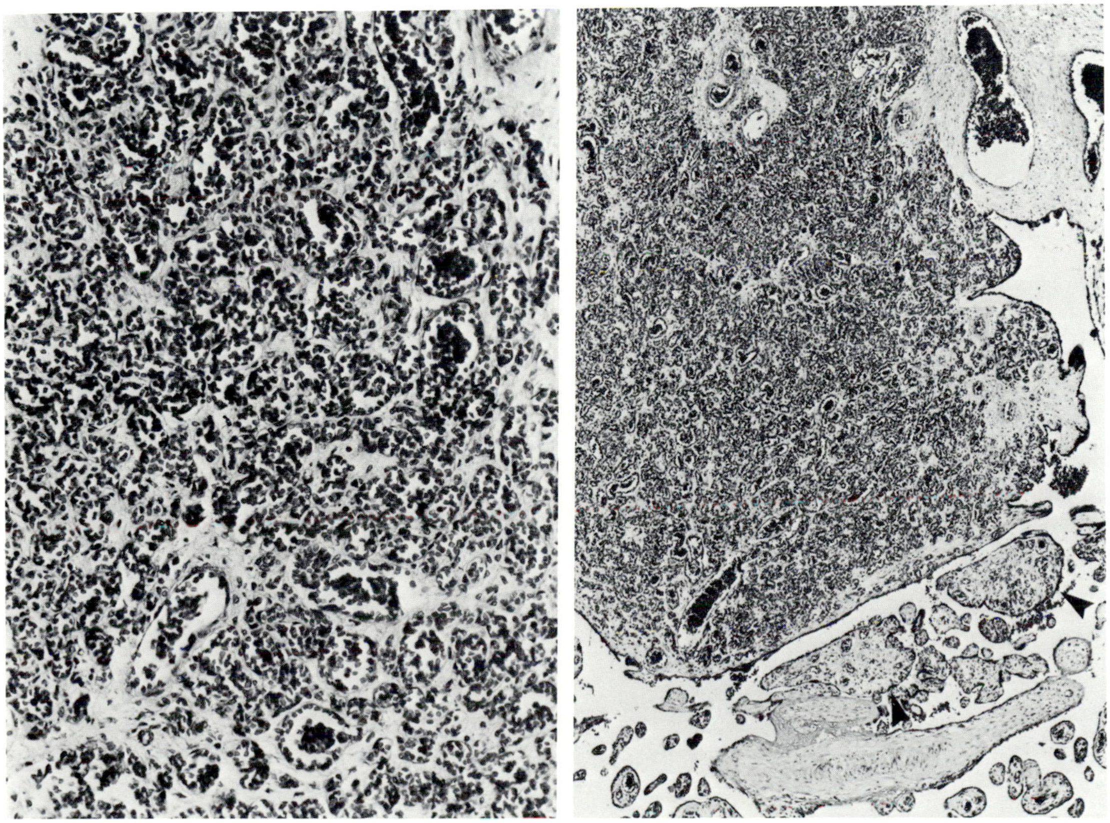

Fig. 23.85. Placental hemangioma. Angiomatous type characterized by numerous capillary-sized vessels separated by inconspicuous stroma (*left*). Adjacent villi show telangiectatic change (*arrows, right*).

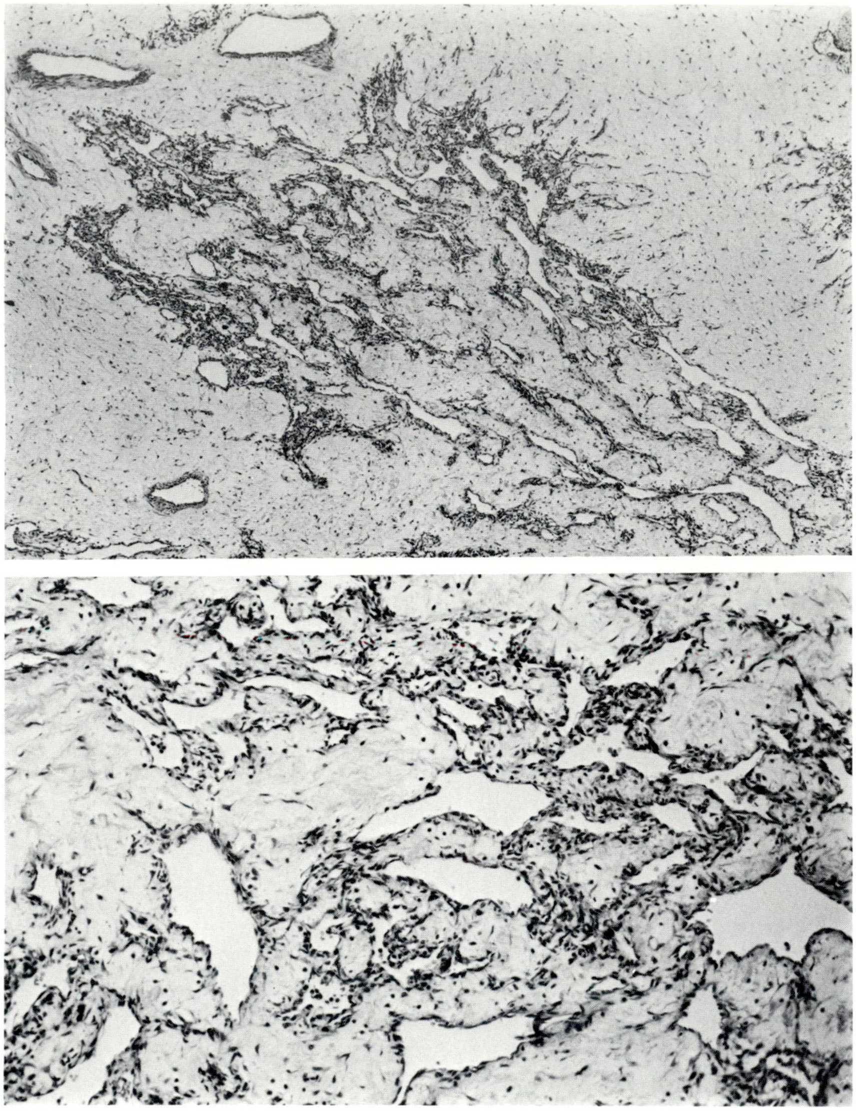

FIG. 23.86. Hemangioma of umbilical cord. Large, cavernous vessels suspended in abundant, myxoid stroma. *Top:* Low power. *Bottom:* High power.

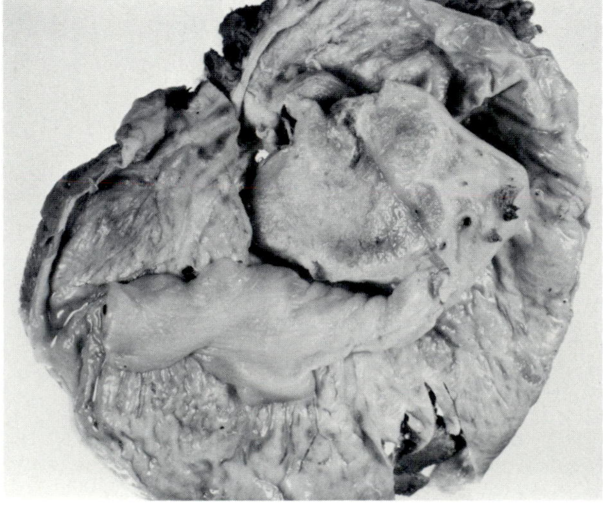

FIG. 23.87. Hemangioma of umbilical cord in a liveborn normal infant. Large hemangioma is located near cord insertion.

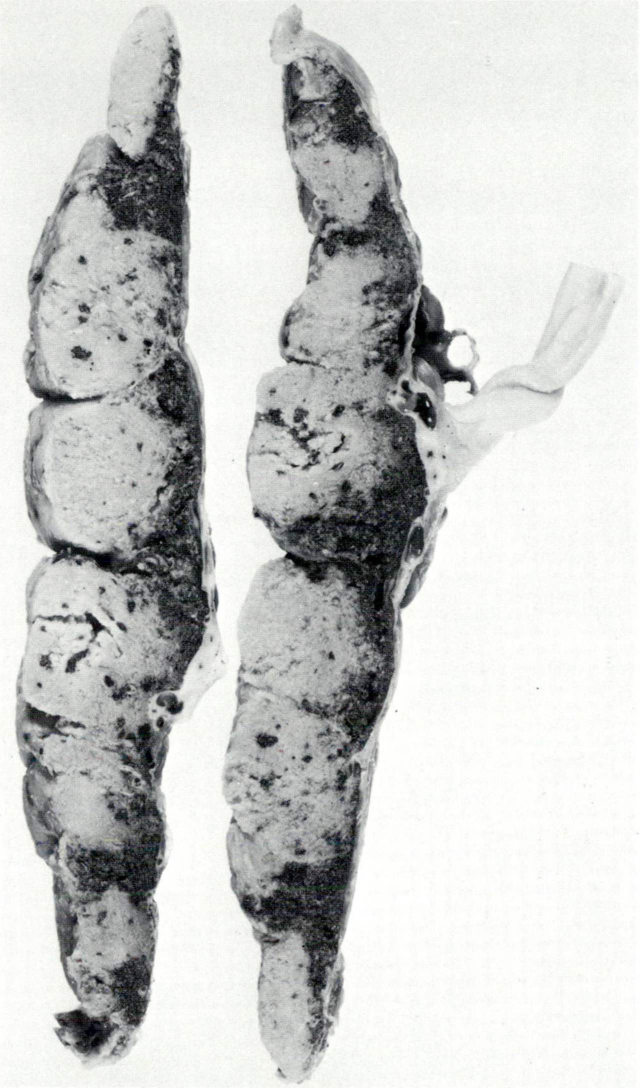

FIG. 23.88. Metastatic malignant melanoma of placenta. Dark areas represent metastatic deposits of malignant melanoma.

Nontrophoblastic Tumors

Hemangioma (Chorangioma)

Hemangiomas occur in about 1% of placentas.[273] They are usually small and entirely intraplacental and will not be discovered on simple external examination. These tumors may be brown, yellow, tan, red, or white and are usually firm and well demarcated from the surrounding parenchyma (Fig. 23.84). Large tumors are rare and may either project above the chorionic plate of the placenta or be visible on the maternal surface. Rarely, a hemangioma is attached to the placenta by a thin pedicle. Usually hemangiomas are solitary, but they may be multiple or, rarely, involve the placenta diffusely.

The microscopic appearance of placental hemangiomas varies depending on the degree of differentiation and distribution of the vascular elements and on the amount of degeneration. Three microscopic types have been described: (1) angiomatous (vascular, mature)—numerous blood vessels, usually capillary but occasionally cavernous in type, supported by inconspicuous, loose stroma (Fig. 23.85), (2) cellular (immature)—compact arrangement of primitive cells, presumably endothelial, and (3) degenerate—prominent myxoid change, hyalinization, necrosis, or calcification (Fig. 23.86). Many tumors have a variable appearance, with gradual transition between the different histologic patterns. Localized groups of large telangiectatic villi are often identified adjacent to the tumor (Fig. 23.85). Although mitotic figures and some degree of nuclear atypicality may be found in occasional tumors,[159] there has yet to be a proven case of angiosarcoma arising in the placenta. The tumor cells have been demonstrated to contain factor VIII antigen[159] and to resemble endothelial cells ultrastructurally.[65] Whether these tumors represent hamartomas or true neoplasms is the subject of debate. Hemangiomas of identical gross and microscopic appearance may also occur in the umbilical cord (Fig. 23.87).[21]

Various clinical complications have been reported in association with hemangiomas of the placenta.[62,65,240,273] The most significant of these are hydramnios and premature delivery; the latter appears to be a consequence of the former. Hydramnios is always associated with larger tumors, but the nature of the link between the two is unclear. Fetal cardiomegaly and congestive heart failure have been attributed to shunting of blood through the hemangioma. Other transitory fetal complications have included edema, anemia, and thrombocytopenia. Skin angiomas have been reported in a few babies with placental hemangiomas.

Teratoma

Placental teratomas are rare. The few tumors reported have been located between the amnion and chorion, usually on the placental surface. Teratomas have been found in the umbilical cord as well. Histologically, they have the usual features of a mature teratoma. They are distinguished from an acardiac fetus by the lack of an umbilical cord and the total disorganization of the component tissues.

Placental Metastases

Metastases to the placenta from either maternal or fetal neoplasms are very rare. Although carcinomas of the cervix and breast are the most frequently encountered malignancies in pregnant women, malignant melanoma

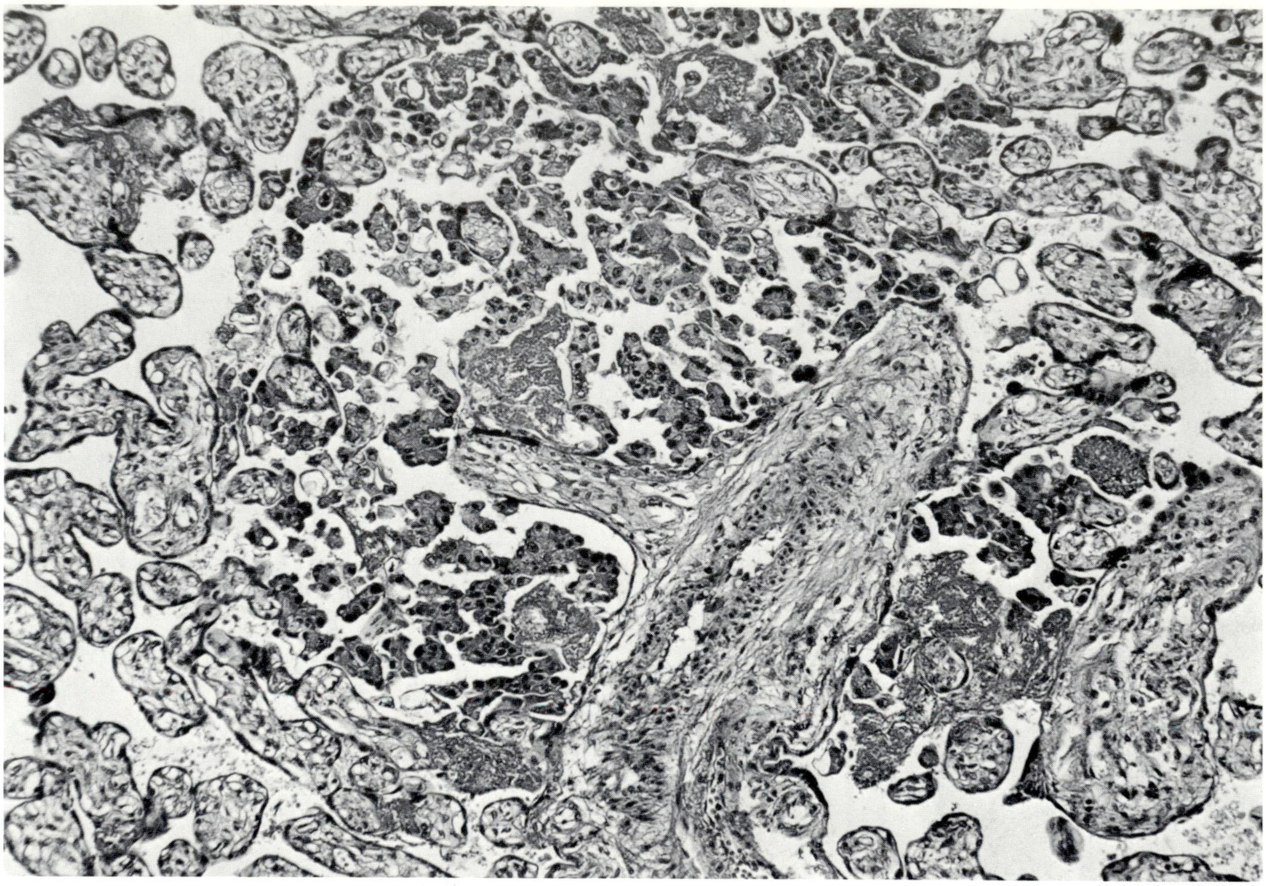

FIG. 23.89. Metastatic breast carcinoma of placenta. Metastatic breast carcinoma is confined to the intervillous space. There is no villous invasion.

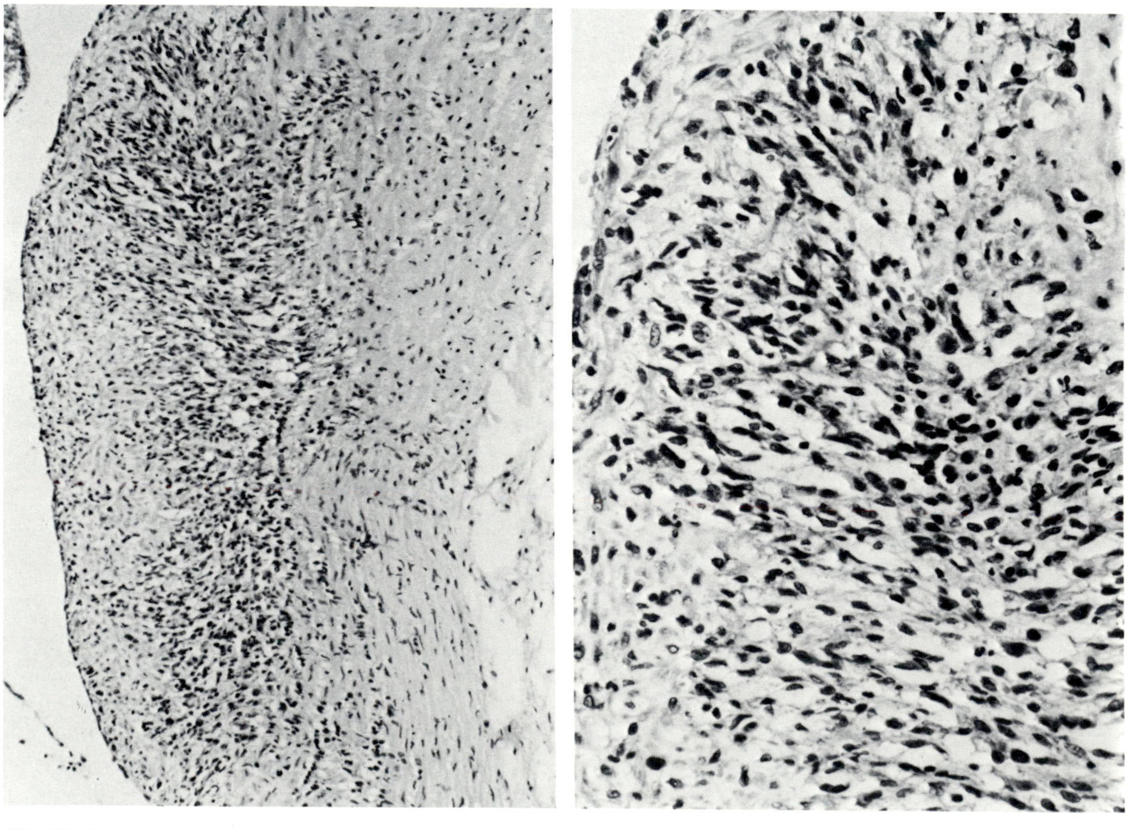

FIG. 23.90. Umbilical artery. Disseminated histiocytosis in subendothelial location. *Left:* Low power. *Right:* High power.

is by far the most common maternal tumor to metastasize to the placenta or spread to the fetus.[206,211,256]

Placentas harboring metastases are usually normal on gross inspection. Tumor deposits may be seen in cases of metastatic melanoma (Fig. 23.88) and have been reported in one recent case of metastatic Ewing's sarcoma.[112] Microscopically, nests of malignant cells are usually confined to the intervillous space. Villous or fetal vascular invasion is very uncommon (Fig. 23.89).

A few cases of dissemination of congenital malignant tumors to the placenta have been reported. There are well-documented cases of placental metastases from neuroblastoma.[36,253] Grossly, these placentas have been pale and bulky, resembling the hydropic placentas of Rh incompatibility. Fetal vessels plugged by clumps of neuroblastoma cells have been found microscopically. Rare cases of fetal leukemic involvement of the placenta have also been illustrated.[29] Disseminated histiocytosis involving the vessels of the umbilical cord may occur (Fig. 23.90).

References

1. Abitbol MM, Driscoll SG, Ober WB (1976) Placental lesions in experimental toxemia in the rabbit. Am J Obstet Gynecol 125: 942–948
2. Abitbol MM, Pirani CL, Ober WB, Driscoll SG, Cohen MW (1976) Production of experimental toxemia in the pregnant dog. Obstet Gynecol 48: 537–548
3. Abramowsky CR, Vegas ME, Swinehart G, Gyves MT (1980) Decidual vasculopathy of the placenta in lupus erythematosus. N Engl J Med 303: 668–672
4. Aherne W, Strong SJ, Corney G (1968) The structure of the placenta in the twin transfusion syndrome. Biol Neonate 12: 121–135
5. Ahlfors K, Forsgren M, Ivarsson S-A, Harris S, Svanberg L (1983) Congenital cytomegalovirus infection: On the relation between type and time of maternal infection and infant's symptoms. Scand J Infect Dis 15: 129–138
6. Ahlfors K, Ivarsson S-A, Harris S, Svanberg L, Holmqvist R, Lernmark B, Theander G (1984) Congenital cytomegalovirus infection and disease in Sweden and the relative importance of primary and secondary maternal infections. Scand J Infect Dis 16: 129–137
7. Aladjem S (1967) Morphologic aspects of the placenta in gestational diabetes seen by phase-contrast microscopy. An anatomicroclinical correlation. Am J Obstet Gynecol 99: 341–349
8. Alford CA, Stagno S, Pass RF (1980) Natural history of perinatal cytomegaloviral infection. Excerpta Medica Ciba Foundation Symposium 77: 125–147
9. Althabe O, LaBarrere C, Telenta M (1985) Maternal vascular lesions in placentae of small-for-gestational-age infants. Placenta 6: 265–276
10. Altshuler G (1973) Toxoplasmosis as a cause of hydranencephaly. Am J Dis Child 125: 251–252
11. Altshuler G (1974) Pathogenesis of congenital herpesvirus infection. Am J Dis Child 127: 427–429
12. Altshuler G (1977) Placentitis, with a new light on and old torch. Obstet Gynecol Annu 6: 197–221
13. Altshuler G, Russell P (1975) The human placental villitides. A review of chronic intrauterine infection. Curr Top Pathol 60: 63–112
14. Altshuler G, Tsang RC, Ermocilla R (1975) Single umbilical artery. Correlation of clinical status and umbilical cord histology. Am J Dis Child 129: 697–700
15. Alvarez H, Sala MA, Benedetti WL (1972) Intervillous space reduction in the edematous placenta. Am J Obstet Gynecol 112: 819–820
16. Amatuzio JC, Gorlin RJ (1981) Conjoined acardiac monsters. Arch Pathol 105: 253–255
17. Anderson GD (1975) *Listeria monocytogenes* septicemia in pregnancy. Obstet Gynecol 46: 102–104
18. Appelbaum PC, Shulman G, Chambers NL, Simon NV, Granados JL, Fairbrother PF, Naeye RL (1980) Studies on the growth-inhibiting property of amniotic fluids from two United States population groups. Am J Obstet Gynecol 137: 579–582
19. Auger P, Marquis G, Dallaire L, Montplaisir S, Ghoubril S (1980) Natural occurrence of a humoral response to *Candida* in human amniotic fluid. Am J Obstet Gynecol 136: 1075–1079
20. Bain AD, Bowie JH, Flint WF, Beverley JKA, Beattie CP (1956) Congenital toxoplasmosis simulating haemolytic disease of the newborn. J Obstet Gynaecol Br Emp 63: 826–832
21. Barry FE, McCoy CP, Callahan, Jr WP (1951) Hemangioma of the umbilical cord. Am J Obstet Gynecol 62: 675–680
22. Bartholomew RA, Colvin ED, Grimes WH Jr, Fish JS, Lester WM, Galloway WH (1961) Criteria by which toxemia of pregnancy may be diagnosed from unlabeled formalin-fixed placentas. Am J Obstet Gynecol 82: 277–290
23. Batcup G, Tovey LAD, Longster G (1983) Fetomaternal blood group incompatibility studies in placental intervillous thrombosis. Placenta 4: 449–454
24. Benirschke K (1961) Examination of the placenta. Obstet Gynecol 18: 309–333
25. Benirschke K (1974) Syphilis—The placenta and the fetus. Am J Dis Child 128: 142–143
26. Benirschke K (1981) Abortions and moles. In: Perinatal diseases, International Academy of Pathology Monograph, Naeye RL, Kissane JM, Kaufman N (eds). Baltimore, Williams & Wilkins
27. Benirschke K, Bourne GL (1960) The incidence and prognostic implication of congenital absence of one umbilical artery. Am J Obstet Gynecol 79: 251–254
28. Benirschke K, Brown WH (1955) A vascular anomaly of the umbilical cord: The absence of one umbilical artery in the umbilical cords of normal and abnormal fetuses. Obstet Gynecol 6: 399–404
29. Benirschke K, Driscoll SG (1967) The pathology of the human placenta. New York, Springer-Verlag
30. Benirschke K, Kim CK (1973) Multiple pregnancy (first of two parts). N Engl J Med 288: 1276–1284
31. Benirschke K, Kim CK (1973) Multiple pregnancy (second of two parts). N Engl J Med 288: 1329–1335
32. Benirschke K, Mendoza GR, Bazely PL (1974) Placental

and fetal manifestations of cytomegalovirus infection. Virchows Arch [B Cell Pathol] 16: 121–139
33. Benson RC, Fujikura T (1969) Circumvallate and circummarginate placenta. Obstet Gynecol 34: 799–804
34. Berkowitz RS, Goldstein DP, Bernstein MR (1983) Natural history of partial molar pregnancy. Obstet Gynecol 66: 677–681
35. Beyth Y, Perlman M, Ornoy A (1977) Amniogenic bands associated with facial dysplasia and paresis. J Reprod Med 18: 83–86
36. Birner WF (1961) Neuroblastoma as a cause of antenatal death. Am J Obstet Gynecol 82: 1388–1391
37. Bjork O, Persson B (1982) Placental changes in relation to the degree of metabolic control in diabetes mellitus. Placenta 3: 367–378
38. Blanc WA (1959) Amniotic infection syndrome. Pathogenesis, morphology, and significance in circumnatal mortality. Clin Obstet Gynaecol 2: 705–734
39. Blanc WA (1961) Vernix granulomatosis of amnion ("amnion nodosum") in oligohydramnios. Lesion associated with urinary abnormalities, retention of dead fetuses, and prolonged leakage of amniotic fluid. NY State J Med 61: 1492–1496
40. Blanc WA (1976) Pathology of placenta accreta. Verh Deutsch Ges Pathol 60: 393–399
41. Blanc WA (1976) Circulatory lesions of the human placenta in abruptio. Verh Deutsch Ges Pathol 60: 386–392
42. Blanc WA (1978) Pathology of the placenta and cord in some viral infections. In: Viral diseases of the fetus and newborn. Major problems in clinical pediatrics, Hanshan JB, Dregeon JA (eds). Philadelphia, Saunders, Vol 17
43. Blanc WA (1980) Pathology of the placenta and cord in ascending and in haematogenous infection. Excerpta Medica Ciba Foundation Symposium 77: 17–38
44. Blanc WA (1981) Pathology of the placenta, membranes, and umbilical cord in bacterial, fungal and viral infections in man. In: Perinatal diseases. International Academy of Pathology Monograph, Naeye RL, Kissane JM, Kaufman N (eds). Baltimore, Williams & Wilkins
45. Blattner P, Dar H, Nitowsky HM (1977) Pregnancy outcome in women with sickle cell trait. JAMA 238: 1392–1394
46. Bloomfield RD, Suarez JR, Malangit AC (1978) The placenta: A diagnostic tool in sickle cell disorders. J Natl Med Assoc 70: 87–88
47. Boronow RC, West RH (1964) Monster acardius parasiticus. Am J Obstet Gynecol 88: 233–237
48. Botha MC (1969) Spontaneous rupture of the uterus due to placenta percreta. S Afr Med J 43: 39–41
49. Boue J, Phillipe E, Girond A, Boue A (1976) Phenotypic expression of lethal chromosomal anomalies in human abortuses. Teratology 14: 3–20
50. Bourne GL (1976) The microscopic anatomy of the human amnion and chorion. Am J Obst Gynecol 79: 1070–1073
51. Boyd JD, Hamilton WJ (1970) The human placenta. Cambridge, W Heffer and Sons
52. Branch DW, Scott JR, Kochenour NK, Hershgold E (1985) Obstetric complications associated with the lupus anticoagulant. N Engl J Med 313: 1322–1326
53. Breen JL, Neubecker R, Gregori CA, Franklin JE (1977) Placenta accreta, increta, and percreta. Obstet Gynecol 49: 43–47
54. Brescia RJ, Kurman RJ, Main C, Surti U, Szulman A (1986) The immunocytochemical localization of human chorionic gonadotropin, human placental lactogen and placental alkaline phosphatase in complete and partial hydatidiform moles. Lab Invest 54: 8A
55. Brosens I, Renaer M (1972) On the pathogenesis of placental infarcts in pre-eclampsia. J Obstet Gynaecol Br Commonw 79: 794–799
56. Brosens I, Dixon HG, Robertson WB (1977) Fetal growth retardation and the arteries of the placental bed. Br J Obstet Gynaecol 84: 656–663
57. Brown DR, Doshi N, Taylor PM (1978) Oligohydramnios and fatal pulmonary hypoplasia without amnion nodosum. J Reprod Med 20: 293–296
58. Browne JC (1958) The uterine circulation in toxemia. Clin Obstet Gynaecol 1: 341–348
59. Browne JC, Veall N (1953) The maternal placental blood flow in normotensive and hypertensive women. J Obstet Gynaecol Br Emp 60: 141–147
60. Bryan EM, Kohler HG (1974) The missing umbilical artery. I. Prospective study based on a maternity unit. Arch Dis Child 49: 844–852
61. Bryan EM, Kohler HG (1975) The missing umbilical artery. II. Paediatric follow-up. Arch Dis Child 50: 714–718
62. Burrows S, Gaines JL, Hughes FJ (1973) Giant chorioangioma. Am J Obstet Gynecol 115: 579–580
63. Butany J, Quinn PA (1986) Correlation between chorioamnionitis and evidence of infection during pregnancy. Lab Invest 54: 8A
64. Cameron AH (1968) The Birmingham twin survey. Proc R Soc Med 61: 229–234
65. Cash JB, Powell DE (1980) Placental chorioangioma. Presentation of a case with electron microscopic and immunochemical studies. Am J Surg Pathol 4: 87–92
66. Cooperman NR, Kasim M, Rajashekaraiah KR (1980) Clinical significance of amniotic fluid, amniotic membranes, and endometrial biopsy cultures at the time of cesarean section. Am J Obstet Gynecol 137: 536–542
67. Corney G, Aherne W (1965) The placental transfusion syndrome in monozygous twins. Arch Dis Child 40: 264–270
68. Coulter JBS, Scott JM, Jordan MM (1975) Oedema of the umbilical cord and respiratory distress in the newborn. Br J Obstet Gynaecol 82: 453–459
69. Crawford JM (1959) A study of human placental growth with observations on the placenta in erythroblastosis foetalis. J Obstet Gynaecol Br Emp 66: 885–896
70. Deacon JS, Machin GA, Martin JME, Nicholson S, Nwankwo DC, Wintemute R (1980) Investigation of acephalus. Am J Med Genet 5: 85–99
71. Demers LM, Gabbe SG (1976) Placental prostaglandin levels in pre-eclampsia. Am J Obstet Gynecol 126: 137–139
72. DeMyer W, Baird I (1969) Mortality and skeletal malformations from amniocentesis and oligohydramnios in rats: Cleft palate, clubfoot, microstomia, and adactyly. Teratology 2: 33–38

73. Desmonts G, Couvreur J (1974) Congenital toxoplasmosis. A prospective study of 378 pregnancies. N Engl J Med 290: 1110–1116
74. Devi B, Jennison RF, Langley FA (1968) Significance of placental pathology in transplacental haemorrhage. J Clin Pathol 21: 322–331
75. DeWolf F, Brosens I, Renaer M (1980) Fetal growth retardation and the maternal arterial supply of the human placenta in the absence of sustained hypertension. Br J Obstet Gynaecol 87: 678–685
76. DeWolf F, Robertson WB, Brosens I (1975) The ultrastructure of acute atherosis in hypertensive pregnancy. Am J Obstet Gynecol 123: 164–174
77. DeWolf F, DeWolf-Peeters C, Brosens I, Robertson WB (1980) The human placental bed: Electron microscopic study of trophoblastic invasion of spiral arteries. Am J Obstet Gynecol 137: 58–70
78. Dippel AL (1940) Hematomas of the umbilical cord. Surg Gynecol Obstet 70: 51–57
79. Dische MR, Quinn PA, Czegledy-Nagy E, Sturgess JM (1979) Genital mycoplasma infection. Am J Clin Pathol 72: 167–174
80. Dixon HG, Browne JCM, Davey DA (1963) Choriodecidual and myometrial blood-flow. Lancet 2: 369–373
81. Dobashi K, Ajika K, Ohkawa T, Okano H, Okinaga S, Arai K (1984) Immunohistochemical localization of pregnancy-associated plasma protein A (PAPP-A) in placentae from normal and pre-eclamptic pregnancies. Placenta 5: 205–212
82. Driscoll SG (1965) The pathology of pregnancy complicated by diabetes mellitus. Med Clin North Am 49: 1053–1067
83. Driscoll SG (1966) Current concepts. Hydrops fetalis. N Engl J Med 275: 1432–1434
84. Driscoll SG (1969) Histopathology of gestational rubella. Am J Dis Child 118: 49–53
85. Driscoll SG (1979) Significance of acute chorioamnionitis. Clin Obstet Gynecol 22: 339–349
86. Driscoll SG, Gorbach A, Feldman D (1962) Congenital listeriosis: Diagnosis from placental studies. Obstet Gynecol 20: 216–220
87. Elliott WG (1970) Placental toxoplasmosis: Report of a case. Am J Clin Pathol 53: 413–417
88. Etches PC, Lemons JA (1979) Nonimmune hydrops fetalis: Report of 22 cases including three siblings. Pediatrics 64: 326–332
89. Evaldson GR, Malmborg AS, Nord CE (1982) Premature rupture of the membranes and ascending infection. Br J Obstet Gynaecol 89: 793–801
90. Feinstein DI (1985) Lupus anticoagulant, thrombosis, and fetal loss. N Engl J Med 313: 1348–1350
91. Florman AL, Gershon AA, Blackett PR, Nahmias AJ (1973) Intrauterine infection with herpes simples virus. Resultant congenital malformations. JAMA 225: 129–132
92. Forrest JM, Menser MA, Burgess JA (1971) High frequency of diabetes mellitus in young adults with congenital rubella. Lancet 2: 332–334
93. Fox H (1967) Perivillous fibrin deposition in the human placenta. Am J Obstet Gynecol 98: 245–251
94. Fox H (1967) The significance of placental infarction in perinatal morbidity and mortality. Biol Neonate 11: 87–105
95. Fox H (1968) Morphological changes in the human placenta following fetal death. J Obstet Gynaecol Br Commonw 75: 839–843
96. Fox H (1970) Effect of hypoxia on trophoblast in organ culture. A morphologic and autoradiographic study. Am J Obstet Gynecol 107: 1058–1064
97. Fox H (1972) Placenta accreta, 1945–1969. Obstet Gynecol 27: 475–486
98. Fox H (1978) Pathology of the placenta. Major problems in pathology. Philadelphia, Saunders, Vol 7
99. Fox H (1981) Placental involvement in maternal systemic infection. In: Perspectives in pediatric pathology. Infectious diseases. Rosenberg HS, Bernstein J (eds). New York, Vol 6 Masson
100. Fox H, Sen DK (1972) Placenta extrachorialis. A clinicopathologic study. J Obstet Gynaecol Br Commonw 79: 32–35
101. Frenkel JK (1971) Toxoplasmosis. Mechanisms of infection, laboratory diagnosis and management. Curr Top Pathol 54: 28–75
102. Froehlich LA, Fujikura T (1966) Significance of a single umbilical artery. Report from the collaborative study of cerebral palsy. Am J Obstet Gynecol 94: 274–279
103. Froehlich LA, Fujikura T (1973) Follow-up of infants with single umbilical artery. Pediatrics 52: 22–29
104. Fujikura T, Froehlich L (1968) Diagnosis of sickling by placental examination. Geographic differences in incidence. Am J Obstet Gynecol 100: 1122–1124
105. Fujikura T, Benson RC, Driscoll SG (1970) The bipartite placenta and its clinical features. Am J Obstet Gynecol 107: 1013–1017
106. Gaber LW, Redline RW, Moustoufi-Zadeh M, Driscoll SG (1986) Invasive partial mole. Am J Clin Pathol 85: 722–724
107. Garcia AGP, Marques RLS, Lobato YY, Fonseca MEF, Wigg MD (1985) Placental pathology in congenital rubella. Placenta 6: 281–295
108. Georgakopoulos P (1974) Placenta accreta following lysis of uterine synechiae (Asherman's syndrome). J Obstet Gynaecol Br Commonw 81: 730–733
109. Gillim DL, Hendricks CH (1953) Holoacardius. Review of the literature and case report. Obstet Gynecol 2: 647–653
110. Gilstrap LC III, Cunningham FG (1979) The bacterial pathogenesis of infection following cesarean section. Obstet Gynecol 53: 545–549
111. Gray ML (1960) Genital listeriosis as a cause of repeated abortion. Lancet 2: 315–317
112. Greenberg P, Collins JD, Voet RL, Jariwala L (1982) Ewing's sarcoma metastatic to placenta. Placenta 3: 191–196
113. Griffiths PD, Baboonian C (1984) A prospective study of primary cytomegalovirus infection during pregnancy: Final report. Br J Obstet Gynaecol 91: 307–315
114. Gruenwald P (1970) Environmental influences on twins apparent at birth. Biol Neonate 15: 79–93
115. Gruenwald P, Levin H, Yousem H (1968) Abruption and premature separation of the placenta. The clinical and

the pathologic entity. Am J Obstet Gynecol 102: 604–610
116. Halliday HL, Hirata T (1979) Perinatal listeriosis—A review of twelve patients. Am J Obstet Gynecol 133: 405–410
117. Hanshaw JB (1973) *Herpesvirus hominis* infections in the fetus and the newborn. Am J Dis Child 126: 546–555
118. Harter CA, Benirschke K (1976) Fetal syphilis in the first trimester. Am J Obstet Gynecol 124: 705–711
119. Haust MD (1981) Maternal diabetes mellitus—Effects on the fetus and placenta. In: Perinatal diseases. International Academy of Pathology monograph No. 22: Baltimore, Williams & Wilkins, pp 201–285
120. Heifetz SA (1984) Single umbilical artery: A statistical analysis of 237 autopsy cases and review of the literature. Perspect Pediatr Pathol 8: 345–378
121. Herva R, Karkinen-Jaaskelainen M (1984) Amnionic adhesion malformation syndrome: Fetal and placental pathology. Teratology 29: 11–19
122. Herva R, Rapola J, Rosti J, Karlson H (1980) Cluster of severe amniotic adhesion malformations in Finland. Lancet 1: 818–819
123. Hibbard BM, Jeffcoate TNA (1966) Abruptio placentae. Obstet Gynecol 27: 155–167
124. Higginbottom MC, Jones KL, Hall BD, Smith DW (1979) The amniotic band disruption complex: Timing of amniotic rupture and variable spectra of consequent defects. J Pediatr 95: 544–549
125. Hood IC, Desa DJ, Whyte RK (1983) The inflammatory response in candidal chorioamnionitis. Hum Pathol 14: 984–990
126. Hood M (1961) Listeriosis as an infection of pregnancy manifested in the newborn. Pediatrics 27: 390–396
127. Hoshina M, Boothby M, Hussa R, Pattillo R, Camel HM, Boime I (1985) Linkage of human chorionic gonadotrophin and placental lactogen biosynthesis to trophoblast differentiation and tumorigenesis. Placenta 6: 163–172
128. Hubbell JP, Muirhead DM, Drorbaugh JE (1965) The newborn infant of the diabetic mother. Med Clin North Am 49: 1035–1052
129. Hustin J, Gaspard U (1977) Comparison of histological changes seen in placental tissue cultures and in placentae obtained after fetal death. Br J Obstet Gynaecol 84: 210–215
130. Irving FL, Hertig AT (1937) A study of placenta accreta. Surg Gynecol Obstet 64: 178
131. Johnson GM, Tudor RB (1970) Diabetes mellitus and congenital rubella infection. Am J Dis Child 120: 453–455
132. Johnstone BH, Benirschke K (1975) Monozygotic twins discordant for urinary tract anomalies and presenting as hydramnios. Obstet Gynecol 47: 610–615
133. Jones CJP, Fox H (1976) Placental changes in gestational diabetes. An ultrastructural study. Obstet Gynecol 48: 274–280
134. Jones CJP, Fox H (1976) An ultrastructural and ultrahistochemical study of the placenta of the diabetic woman. J Pathol 119: 91–99
135. Jones CJP, Fox H (1978) An ultrastructural study of the placenta in materno-fetal Rhesus incompatibility. Virchows Arch [A Pathol Anat] 379: 229–241
136. Jones CJP, Fox H (1980) An ultrastructural and ultrahistochemical study of the human placenta in maternal preeclampsia. Placenta 1: 61–76
137. Jones CJP, Fox H (1981) An ultrastructural and ultrahistochemical study of the human placenta in maternal essential hypertension. Placenta 2: 193–204
138. Kalousek D, Poland BJ (1984) Embryonic and fetal pathology of abortion. In: Pathology of the placenta, Perrin EDVK (ed). New York, Churchill Livingstone, Chap 2
139. Kaplan C, Blanc WA, Elias J (1982) Identification of erythrocytes in intervillous thrombi. A study using immunoperoxidase identification of hemoglobins. Hum Pathol 13: 554–557
140. Keenan WJ, Steichen JJ, Mahmood K, Altshuler G (1977) Placental pathology compared with clinical outcome. Am J Dis Child 131: 1224–1227
141. Kendrick FJ, Feild LE (1967) Congenital anomalies induced in normal and adrenalectomized rats by amniocentesis. Anat Rec 159: 353–356
142. Kennedy LA, Persaud TVN (1977) Pathogenesis of developmental defects induced in the rat by amniotic sac puncture. Acta Anat 97: 23–35
143. Kitzmiller JL, Benirschke K (1973) Immunofluorescent study of placental bed vessels in pre-eclampsia of pregnancy. Am J Obstet Gynecol 115: 248–251
144. Kitzmiller JL, Watt N, Driscoll SG (1981) Decidual arteriopathy in hypertension and diabetes in pregnancy: Immunofluorescent studies. Am J Obstet Gynecol 141: 773–779
145. Knox WF, Fox H (1984) Villitis of unknown aetiology: Its incidence and significance in placentae from a British population. Placenta 5: 395–402
146. Kraemer BB, Kraus FT, Sheldon G (1985) Expression of pregnancy-specific proteins in maternal diabetes. An immunocytochemical study of placental bed biopies and placental tissues. Lab Invest 52: 37A
147. Kundsin RB, Driscoll SG, Monson RR, Yeh C, Biano SA, Cochran WD (1984) Association of *Ureaplasma urealyticum* in the placenta with perinatal morbidity and morality. N Engl J Med 310: 941–945
148. Kurman RJ, Main CS, Chen H-C (1984) Intermediate trophoblast: A distinctive form of trophoblast with specific morphological, biochemical and functional features. Placenta 5: 349–370
149. Kurman RJ, Young RH, Norris HJ, Main CS, Lawrence WD, Scully RE (1984) Immunocytochemical localization of placental lactogen and chorionic gonadotropin in the normal placenta and trophoblastic tumors, with emphasis on intermediate trophoblast and the placental site trophoblastic tumor. Int J Gynecol Pathol 3: 101–121
150. LaBarrere C, Althabe O, Telenta M (1982) Chronic villitis of unknown aetiology in placentae of idiopathic small for gestational age infants. Placenta 3: 309–318
151. Las Heras J, Harding P, Haust MD (1980) The morphology of third order fetal arteries in normal and "toxemic" placentas. Lab Invest 40: 260
152. Las Heras J, Baskerville JC, Harding PGR, Haust MD (1985) Morphometric studies of fetal placental stem arter-

ies in hypertensive disorders ("toxaemia") of pregnancy. Placenta 6: 217–228
153. Lauweryns J, Bernat R, Lerut A, Detournay G (1973) Intrauterine pneumonia. An experimental study. Biol Neonate 22: 301–318
154. Lawler FC, Wood WS, King S, Metzger W (1964) *Listeria monocytogenes* as a cause of fetal loss. Am J Obstet Gynecol 89: 915–923
155. Love AM, Vickers TH (1972) Amniocentesis dysmelia in rats. Br J Exp Pathol 53: 435–444
156. Machin GA (1981) Differential diagnosis of hydrops fetalis. Am J Med Genet 9: 341–350
157. MacLennan AH, Sharp F, Shaw-Dunn J (1972) The ultrastructure of human trophoblast in spontaneous and induced hypoxia using a system of organ culture. A comparison with ultrastructural changes in pre-eclampsia and placental insufficiency. J Obstet Gynaecol Br Commonw 79: 113–121
158. Maidman JE, Yeager C, Anderson V, Makabali G, O'Grady JP, Arce J, Tishler DM (1980) Prenatal diagnosis and management of nonimmunologic hydrops fetalis. Obstet Gynecol 56: 571–576
159. Majlessi HF, Wagner KM, Brooks JJ (1983) Atypical cellular chorangioma of the placenta. Int J Gynecol Pathol 1: 403–408
160. Mar JL (1975) Cytomegalovirus: A major cause of birth defects. Science 190: 1184–1186
161. Martin DH, Koutsky L, Eschenbach DA, Daling JR, Alexander ER, Benedetti JK, Holmes KK (1982) Prematurity and perinatal mortality in pregnancies complicated by maternal *Chlamydia trachomatis* infections. JAMA 247: 1585–1588
162. Maudsley RF, Brix GA, Hinton NA, Robertson EM, Bryans AM, Haust MD (1966) Placental inflammation and infection. A prospective bacteriologic and histologic study. Am J Obstet Gynecol 95: 648–659
163. McConnell HD, Carr DH (1975) Recent advances in the cytogentic study of human spontaneous abortions. Obstet Gynecol 45: 547–552
164. McKeogh RP, D'Errico E (1951) Placenta accreta: Clinical manifestations and conservative management. N Engl J Med 245: 159–165
165. Menser MA, Forrest JM, Bransby RD (1978) Rubella infection and diabetes mellitus. Lancet 1: 57–60
166. Meyer B (1955) Placenta accreta. An analysis based on an unusual case. Acta Obstet Gynecol Scand 34: 189–201
167. Miller JM, Pupkin MJ, Hill GB (1980) Bacterial colonization of amniotic fluid from intact fetal membranes. Am J Obstet Gynecol 136: 796–804
168. Miller ME, Graham JM Jr, Higginbottom MC, Smith DW (1981) Compression-related defects from early amnion rupture: Evidence for mechanical teratogenesis. J Pediatr 98: 292–297
169. Monif GRG, Dische RM (1972) Viral placentitis in congenital cytomegalovirus infection. Am J Clin Pathol 58: 445–449
170. Montgomery JR, Flanders RW, Yow MD (1973) Congenital anomalies and herpesvirus infection. Am J Dis Child 126: 364–366
171. Morison JE (1978) Placenta accreta: A clinicopathologic review of 67 cases. Obstet Gynecol Annu 7: 107–123
172. Mostoufi-Zadeh M, Weiss LM, Driscoll SG (1985) Nonimmune hydrops fetalis. A challenge in perinatal pathology. Hum Pathol 16: 785–789
173. Naeye RL (1975) Causes and consequences of chorioamnionitis. N Engl J Med 293: 40–41
174. Naeye RL (1977) Causes of perinatal mortality in the U.S. Collaborative Perinatal Project. JAMA 238: 228–229
175. Naeye RL (1979) Coitus and associated amniotic-fluid infections. N Engl J Med 301: 1198–1200
176. Naeye RL (1980) Factors in the mother/infant dyad that influence the development of infections before and after birth. Excerpta Medica Ciba Foundation Symposium 77: 3–16
177. Naeye RL (1963) Human intrauterine parabiotic syndrome and its complications. N Engl J Med 268: 804–809
178. Naeye RL (1979) The outcome of diabetic pregnancies: A prospective study. In: Pregnancy, metabolism, diabetes and the fetus. Ciba Foundation Symposium 63: 227–241
179. Naeye RL, Blanc W (1965) Pathogenesis of congenital rubella. JAMA 194: 109–115
180. Naeye RL, Blanc WL (1970) Relation of poverty and race to antenatal infection. N Engl J Med 283: 555–560
181. Naeye RL, Peters EC (1978) Amniotic fluid infections with intact membranes leading to perinatal death: a prospective study. Pediatrics 61: 171–177
182. Naeye RL, Peters EC (1980) Causes and consequences of premature rupture of fetal membranes. Lancet 1: 192–194
183. Naeye RL, Dellinger WS, Blanc WA (1971) Fetal and maternal features of antenatal bacterial infections. J Pediatr 79: 733–739
184. Naeye RL, Maisels J, Lorenz RP, Botti JJ (1983) The clinical significance of placental villous edema. Pediatrics 71: 588–594
185. Naeye RL, Tafari N, Judge D, Gilmour D, Marboe C (1977) Amniotic fluid infections in an African city. J Pediatr 90: 965–970
186. Nahmias AJ, Alford CA, Korones SB (1970) Infection of the newborn with herpesvirus hominis. Adv Pediatr 17: 185–226
187. Nahmias AJ, Josey WE, Naib ZM, Freeman MG, Fernandez RJ, Wheeler JH (1971) Perinatal risk associated with maternal genital herpes simplex virus infection. Am J Obstet Gynecol 110: 825–837
188. Naib ZM, Nahmias AJ, Josey WE, Wheeler JH (1970) Association of maternal genital herpetic infection with spontaneous abortion. Obstet Gynecol 35: 260–263
189. Nankervis GA, Kumar ML, Cox FE, Gold E (1984) A prospective study of maternal cytomegalovirus infection and its effect on the fetus. Am J Obstet Gynecol 149: 435–440
190. Napolitani FD, Schreiber I (1960) The acardiac monster. A review of the world literature and presentation of 2 cases. Am J Obstet Gynecol 80: 582–589
191. Navarrete VN, Torres IH, Rivera IR, Shor VP, Gracia PM (1967) Maternal carbohydrate disorder and congenital malformations. Diabetes 16: 127–130

192. Navarro C, Blanc WA (1977) Chronic viral funisitis. J Pediatr 91: 967–973
193. Nummi S (1972) Relative weight of the placenta and perinatal mortality. A retrospective clinical and statistical analysis. Acta Obstet Gynecol Scand [Suppl] 17: 1–69
194. Ornoy A, Segal S, Nishmi M, Simcha A, Polishuk WZ (1973) Fetal and placental pathology in gestational rubella. Am J Obstet Gynecol 116: 949–956
195. Pankuch GA, Applebaum PC, Lorenz RP, Botti JJ, Schachter J (1983) Placental microbiology in the diagnosis of chorioamnionitis. Abstracts of the Annual Meeting of American Society for Microbiology. Am Soc Microbiol p 319
196. Pastorek JG II, Seiler B (1985) Maternal death associated with sickle cell trait. Am J Obstet Gynecol 152: 295–297
197. Pauls F (1969) Monoamniotic twin pregnancy: A review of the world literature and a report of two new cases. Can Med Assoc J 100: 254–256
198. Peckham CH, Yerushalmy J (1965) Aplasia of one umbilical artery: Incidence by race and certain obstetric factors. Obstet Gynecol 26: 359–366
199. Pedersen LM, Tygstrup I, Pedersen J (1964) Congenital malformations in newborn infants of diabetic women. Correlation with maternal diabetic vascular complications. Lancet 1: 1124–1126
200. Petrilli ES, D'Ablaing G, Ledger WJ (1980) *Listeria monocytogenes* chorioamnionitis: Diagnosis by transabdominal amniocentesis. Obstet Gynecol 55s: 5–8
201. Pezeshkian R, Fernando N, Carne CA, Simanowita MD (1984) Listeriosis in mother and fetus during the first trimester of pregnancy. Case report. Br J Obstet Gynaecol 91: 85–86
202. Pijnenborg R, Bland JM, Robertson WB, Brosens I (1983) Uteroplacental arterial changes related to interstitial trophoblast migration in early human pregnancy. Placenta 4: 397–414
203. Pinkerton JHM (1963) The placental bed arterioles in diabetes. Proc R Soc Med 56: 1021–1022
204. Platt HS (1971) Effect of maternal sickle cell trait on perinatal mortality. Br Med J 4: 334–336
205. Poswillo D (1966) Observations of fetal posture and causal mechanisms of congenital deformity of palate, mandible, and limbs. J Dent Res [Suppl] 45: 584–596
206. Potter JF, Schoeneman M (1970) Metastasis of maternal cancer to the placenta and fetus. Cancer 25: 380–388
207. Rappaport F, Rabinovitz M, Toaff R, Krochik N (1960) Genital listeriosis as a cause of repeated abortion. Lancet 1: 1273–1275
208. Rausen AR, Seki M, Strauss L (1965) Twin transfusion syndrome. A review of 19 cases studied at one institution. J Pediatr 66: 613–628
209. Ray CG, Wedgwood RJ (1964) Neonatal listeriosis. Six case reports and a review of the literature. Pediatrics 34: 378–392
210. Renaer M, Van de Putte I, Vermylen C (1976) Massive feto-maternal hemorrhage as a cause of perinatal mortality and morbidity. Eur J Obstet Gynecol Reprod Biol 6: 125–140
211. Rewell RE, Whitehouse WL (1966) Malignant metastasis to the placenta from carcinoma of the breast. J Pathol 91: 255–256
212. Reynolds DW, Stagno S, Stubbs KG, Dahle AJ, Livingston MM, Saxon SS, Alford AC (1974) Inapparent congenital cytomegalovirus infection with elevated cord IgM levels. N Engl J Med 290: 291–296
213. Rimer BA (1975) Sickle-cell trait and pregnancy: A review of a community hospital experience. Am J Obstet Gynecol 123: 6–11
214. Risteli J, Foidart JM, Risteli L, Boniver J, Goffinet G (1984) The basement membrane proteins laminin and type IV collagen in isolated villi in pre-eclampsia. Placenta 5: 541–550
215. Robertson EG, Neer KJ (1983) Placental injection studies in twin gestation. Am J Obstet Gynecol 147: 170–174
216. Robertson WB (1976) Uteroplacental vasculature. J Clin Pathol [Suppl] 10: 9–17
217. Robertson WB, Brosens I, Dixon G (1975) Uteroplacental vascular pathology. Eur J Obstet Gynecol Reprod Biol 5: 47–65
218. Rocklin RE, Kitzmiller VL, Carpenter CB, Garovoy MR, David JR (1976) Maternal–fetal relation. Absence of an immunologic blocking factor from the serum of women with chronic abortions. N Engl J Med 295: 1209–1213
219. Ross SM, MacPherson T, Wallace J, Khatree MH, Naeye RL, Applebaum PC (1978) Unsuccessful pregnancies—Report on 200 perinatal postmortems. S Afr Med J 53: 828–829
220. Russell P (1979) Inflammatory lesions of the human placenta I. Am J Diagn Gynecol Obstet 1: 127–137
221. Russell P (1979) Inflammatory lesions of the human placenta II. Villitis of unknown etiology in perspective. Am J Diagn Gynecol Obstet 1: 339–346
222. Russell P (1980) Inflammatory lesions of the human placenta. III. The histopathology of villitis of unknown etiology. Placenta 1: 227–244
223. Russell P, Altshuler G (1974) Placental abnormalities of congenital syphilis. A neglected aid to diagnosis. Am J Dis Child 128: 160–163
224. Russell P, Atkinson K, Krishnan L (1980) Recurrent reproductive failure due to severe placental villitis of unknown etiology. J Reprod Med 24: 93–98
225. Salazar H, Kanbour AI (1974) Amnion nodosum. Ultrastructure and histopathogenesis. Arch Pathol 98: 39–46
226. Sander CH (1980) Hemorrhagic endovasculitis and hemorrhagic villitis of the placenta. Arch Pathol Lab Med 104: 371–373
227. Sands J, Dobbing J (1985) Continuing growth and development of the third-trimester human placenta. Placenta 6: 13–22
228. Schlievert P, Johnson W, Galask RP (1976) Bacterial growth inhibition by amniotic fluid. VI. Evidence for a zinc-peptide antobacterial system. Am J Obstet Gynecol 125: 906–910
229. Schindler A-M, Bordignon P, Bischop P (1984) Immunohistochemical localization of pregnancy-associated plasma protein A in decidua and trophoblast: Comparison with human chorionic gonadotropin and fibrin. Placenta 5: 227–236

230. Schreier R, Brown S (1962) Hematoma of the umbilical cord. Report of a case. Obstet Gynecol 20: 798–800
231. Scott JR, Beer AA (1976) Immunologic aspects of preeclampsia. Am J Obstet Gynecol 125: 418–427
232. Scott JS (1958) Pregnancy toxaemia associated with hydrops foetalis, hydatidiform mole and hydramnios. J Obstet Gynaecol Br Emp 65: 689–701
233. Scott JS (1960) Placenta extrachorialis (placenta marginata and placenta circumvallata). A factor in antepartum hemorrhage. J Obstet Gynaecol Br Emp 67: 904–918
234. Sepp AH, Roy TE (1963) *Listeria monocytogenes* infections in metropolitan Toronto. Can Med Assoc J 88: 549–561
235. Severn CB, Holyoke EA (1973) Human acardiac anomalies. Am J Obstet Gynecol 116: 358–365
236. Shanklin DR, Scott JS (1975) Massive subchorial thrombohaematoma. (Breus' mole). Br J Obstet Gynaecol 82: 476–487
237. Sheppard BL, Bonnar J (1976) The ultrastructure of the arterial supply of the human placenta in pregnancy complicated by fetal growth retardation. Br J Obstet Gynaecol 83: 948–959
238. Sheppard BL, Bonnar J (1980) Uteroplacental arteries and hypertensive pregnancy. In: Pregnancy hypertension, Bonnar J, McGilliray I, Symonds E (eds). Lancaster, MTP Press, pp 213–219
239. Shurin PA, Alpert S, Rosner B, Driscoll SG, Lee Y-H, McCormack WM, Santamarina BAG, Kass EH (1975) Chorioamnionitis and colonization of the newborn infant with genital mycoplasmas. N Engl J Med 293: 5–8
240. Sieracki JC, Panke TW, Horvat BL, Perrin EV, Nanda B (1975) Chorioangiomas. Obstet Gynecol 46: 155–159
241. Silverstein AJ, Kanbour AI (1981) Repetitive idiopathic fetal hydrops. Obstet Gynecol [Suppl] 57:18s–21s
242. Silverstein AM (1962) Congenital syphilis and the timing of immunogenesis in the human foetus. Nature 194: 196–197
243. Soma H (1979) Single umbilical artery with congenital malformations. Curr Top Pathol 66: 159–173
244. South MA, Tompkins WAF, Morris CR, Rawls WE (1969) Congenital malformation of the central nervous system associated with genital type (type 2) herpesvirus. J Pediatr 75: 13–18
245. Stagno S, Whitley RJ (1985) Herpesvirus infections of pregnancy. Part I. Cytomegalovirus and Epstein-Barr virus infections. N Engl J Med 313: 1270–1274
246. Stagno S, Whitley RJ (1985) Herpesvirus infections of pregnancy. Part II. Herpes simplex virus and varicella zoster infections. N Engl J Med 313: 1327–1330
247. Stagno S, Pass RF, Dworsky ME, Alford CA (1983) Congenital and perinatal cytomegalovirus infections. Semin Pathol 7: 31–42
248. Stagno S, Reynolds DW, Huang E-S, Thames SD, Smith RJ, Alford CA (1977) Congenital cytomegalovirus infection. Occurrence in an immune population. N Engl J Med 296: 1254–1258
249. Stagno S, Pass RF, Dworsky ME, Henderson RE, Moore EG, Walton PD, Alford CA (1982) Congenital cytomegalovirus infection. The relative importance of primary and recurrent maternal infection. N Engl J Med 306: 945–949
250. Steele PE, Jacobs DS (1979) *Listeria monocytogenes* macroabscesses of placenta. Obstet Gynecol 53: 124–127
251. Stenchever MA, Parks KA, Daines TL, et al. (1977) Cytogenetics of habitual abortion and other reproductive wastage. Am J Obstet Gynecol 127: 143–150
252. Stock RJ, Stock ME (1979) Congenital annular constrictions and intrauterine amputations revisited. Obstet Gynecol 53: 592–598
253. Strauss L, Driscoll SG (1964) Congenital neuroblastoma involving the placenta. Pediatrics 34: 23–31
254. Strong SJ, Corney G (1967) The placenta in twin pregnancy. Oxford, Pergamon
255. Sumawong V, Nondasuta A, Thanapath S, Budthimedhee V (1966) Placenta accreta. A review of the literature and a summary of 10 cases. Obstet Gynecol 27: 511–516
256. Sweet LK, Connerty HV (1941) Congenital melanoma. Report of a case in which antenatal metastasis occurred. Am J Dis Child 62: 1029–1040
257. Szulman AE, Surti U (1978) The syndromes of hydatidiform mole. I. Cytogenetic and morphologic correlations. Am J Obstet Gynecol 131: 665–671
258. Szulman AE, Surti U (1978) The syndromes of hydatidiform mole. II. Morphologic evolution of the complete and partial mole. Am J Obstet Gynecol 132: 20–27
259. Szulman AE, Philippe E, Boue JG, Boue A (1981) Human tripoloidy: Association with partial hydatidiform moles and non-molar conceptuses. Hum Pathol 12: 1016–1021
260. Tafari N, Ross S, Naeye RL, Judge DM, Marboe C (1976) Mycoplasma T strains and perinatal death. Lancet 1: 108–109
261. Teasdale F (1981) Histomorphometry of the placenta of the diabetic woman: Class A diabetes mellitus. Placenta 2: 241–252
262. Teasdale F (1983) Histomorphometry of the human placenta in class B diabetes mellitus. Placenta 4: 1–12
263. Teasdale F (1985) Histomorphometry of the human placenta in class C diabetes mellitus. Placenta 6: 69–82
264. Thadepalli H, Appleman MD, Maidman JE, Arce JJ, Davidson EC (1977) Antimicrobial effect of amniotic fluid against anaerobic bacteria. Am J Obstet Gynecol 127: 250–254
265. Timmons JD, de Alvarez RR (1963) Monoamniotic twin pregnancy. Am J Obstet Gynecol 86: 875–881
266. Tondury G, Smith DW (1966) Fetal rubella pathology. J Pediatr 68: 867–879
267. Torbet TE, Tsoutsoplides GC (1968) Placenta praevia accreta: Conservative management. J Obstet Gynaecol Br Commonw 75: 737–740
268. Tornehave D, Chemnitz J, Teisner B, Folkersen J, Westergaard JG (1984) Immunohistochemical demonstration of pregnancy-associated plasma protein A (PAPP-A) in the syncytiotrophoblast of the normal placenta at different gestational ages. Placenta 5: 427–432
269. Torpin R (1965) Amniochorionic mesoblastic fibrous strings and amnionic bands: Associated constricting fetal malformations of fetal death. Am J Obstet Gynecol 91: 65–75
270. Townsend JJ, Baringer JR, Wolinsky JS, Malamud N,

Mednick JP, Panitch HS, Scott RAT, Oshiro LS, Cremer NE (1975) Progressive rubella panencephalitis. N Engl J Med 292: 990–993
271. Trasler DG, Walker BE, Fraser FC (1956) Congenital malformations produced by amniotic sac puncture. Science 124: 439
272. Van Der Veen F, Walker S, Fox H (1982) Endarteritis obliterans of the fetal stem arteries of the human placenta: An electron microscopic study. Placenta 3: 181–190
273. Wallenburg HCS (1971) Chorioangioma of the placenta. Obstet Gynecol Surv 26: 411–425
274. Warburton D, Kline J, Stein Z, Susser M (1980) Monosomy X: A chromosomal anomaly associated with young maternal age. Lancet 1: 167–169
275. Weber J (1963) Constriction of the umbilical cord as a cause of fetal death. Acta Obstet Gynecol Scand 42: 259–268
276. Weil ML, Itabashi HH, Cremer NE, Oshiro LS, Lennette EH, Carnay L (1975) Chronic progressive panencephalitis due to rubella virus simulating subacute sclerosing panencephalitis. N Engl J Med 292: 994–998
277. Wentworth P (1968) Circumvallate and circummarginate placentas. Am J Obstet Gynecol 102: 44–47
278. Wentworth P (1967) Placental infarction and toxemia of pregnancy. Am J Obstet Gynecol 99: 318–326
279. Wentworth P (1967) The placenta in cases of hemolytic disease of the newborn. Am J Obstet Gynecol 98: 283–289
280. Wentworth P (1964) A placental lesion to account for foetal haemorrhage into the maternal circulation. J Obstet Gynaecol Br Commonw 71: 379–387
281. Wharton B, Edwards JH, Cameron AH (1968) Monoamniotic twins. J Obstet Gynaecol Br Commonw 75: 158–163
282. Wilson CB, Remington JS (1980) What can be done to prevent congenital toxoplasmosis? Am J Obstet Gynecol 138: 357–363
283. Wilson EA (1972) Holoacardius. Obstet Gynecol 40: 740–748
284. Winer AE, Bergman WD, Fields C (1957) Combined intra- and extrauterine pregnancy. Am J Obstet Gynecol 74: 170–178
285. Witzleben CL, Driscoll SG (1965) Possible transplacental transmission of herpes simplex infection. Pediatrics 36: 192–199
286. Yamazaki K, Price JT, Altshuler G (1977) A placental view of the diagnosis and pathogenesis of congenital listeriosis. Am J Obstet Gynecol 129: 703–705
287. Zeek PM, Assali NS (1950) Vascular changes in the decidua associated with eclamptogenic toxemia of pregnancy. Am J Clin Pathol 20: 1099–1109
288. Zervoudakis IA, Cederqvist LL (1977) Effect of *Listeria monocytogenes* septicemia during pregnancy on the offspring. Am J Obstet Gynecol 129: 465–467
289. Zhang J, Kraus FT, Aquino TI (1985) Chorioamnionitis: A comparative histologic, bacteriologic, and clinical study. Int J Gynecol Pathol 4: 1–10

24

Gestational Trophoblastic Disease

Michael T. Mazur, M.D., and Robert J. Kurman, M.D.

Gestational trophoblastic disease (GTD) encompasses a heterogeneous group of lesions, including hydatidiform mole, invasive mole, choriocarcinoma, and placental site trophoblastic tumor, that are characterized by an abnormal proliferation of trophoblastic tissue. Some of these lesions are true neoplasms, whereas others represent abnormally formed placentas that have a predisposition to neoplastic transformation of the trophoblast. The literature on this subject is extensive but confusing because of differences in classification and terminology that have been applied. The necessity of a morphologic classification has been questioned, since the current management is largely medical and often conducted in the absence of a histologic diagnosis. Thus, all trophoblastic lesions are frequently combined under the rubric of gestational trophoblastic disease without applying specific pathologic terms. Recent cytogenetic and immunocytochemical studies have demonstrated profound differences in the etiology, morphology, and clinical behavior of various forms of the disease, underscoring the importance of a uniform histologic classification to facilitate standardized reporting of data and to ensure appropriate clinical management.

This chapter discusses the clinical and pathologic features of each specific form of GTD. In addition, the morphologic and immunohistochemical features of the three types of trophoblastic cells, cytotrophoblast, syncytiotrophoblast, and intermediate trophoblast, are presented, since an awareness of their morphologic and functional characteristics is essential in understanding the pathologic and clinical aspects of the various forms of GTD. Sections on epidemiology, risk factors, behavior, management and therapy of GTD are included to correlate with the pathology, not to provide a comprehensive review of these subjects.

Classification and Definitions

Classification

The World Health Organization Scientific Group on Gestational Trophoblastic Disease[212] recently proposed the following classification that has been adopted by the International Society of Gynecological Pathologists.

- Hydatidiform mole
  - Complete (classic)
  - Partial
- Invasive mole
- Choriocarcinoma
- Placental site trophoblastic tumor

Definitions

Hydatidiform Mole. This lesion is characterized by edematous, vesicular chorionic villi accompanied by a variable amount of proliferative trophoblast. Hydatidiform mole is subdivided into two categories, complete mole and partial mole, based on morphologic, cytogenetic, and clinicopathologic characteristics.

Complete Mole. A hydatidiform mole in which there is hydropic swelling of the majority of villi, associated with a variable degree of trophoblastic proliferation. Fetal tissue usually is not present.

Partial Mole. A hydatidiform mole in which there is an intimate admixture of two populations of villi: enlarged, edematous villi and those of normal size. Evidence of fetal development is often present in partial moles. A previous synonym that is no longer used is *transitional mole.*

Invasive Mole. A hydatidiform mole in which hydropic villi invade the myometrium or blood vessels or, more rarely, are deported to extrauterine sites. In the past, this lesion was referred to as *chorioadenoma destruens*, a term that is no longer used.

Choriocarcinoma. A highly malignant epithelial tumor arising from the trophoblast of any type of gestational event, most often a hydatidiform mole. It consists predominantly of a biphasic proliferation of cytotrophoblast and syncytiotrophoblast that recapitulates the primitive trophoblast of the implanting blastocyst. Chorionic villi are not a component of this tumor. *Chorionepithelioma* is a synonym that is no longer used.

Placental Site Trophoblastic Tumor. A neoplasm composed predominantly of intermediate trophoblast that is generally benign but may be highly malignant. It resembles, in an exaggerated form, the trophoblast that infiltrates the endometrium and myometrium of the placental bed. The neoplasm lacks the biphasic pattern of trophoblast seen in choriocarcinoma. Villi are absent. An earlier term, *trophoblastic pseudotumor*, is no longer used.

Exaggerated Placental Site. This is not a type of GTD. It is a physiologic infiltration of the endometrium and myometrium at the implantation site by trophoblast, predominantly intermediate trophoblast. *Syncytial endometritis*, an earlier term, is a misnomer, since the process is neither inflammatory nor confined to the endometrium.

Gestational Trophoblastic Disease. This refers to all types of abnormal gestational trophoblastic proliferations, including hydatidiform mole, invasive mole, choriocarcinoma, and placental site trophoblastic tumor. The term has clinical utility, since the principles of human chorionic gonadotropin (hCG) monitoring in follow-up and the chemotherapy of metastatic or persistent disease are similar for all these entities.[115]

Epidemiology and Risk Factors

The pathogenesis of trophoblastic tumors is not known. Two mechanisms have been proposed for the development of hydatidiform moles: (1) failure of development of the fetal circulation with resultant hydropic swelling of the villi[82] and (2) overgrowth of the villous trophoblast with secondary hydropic swelling.[150] Neither mechanism adequately explains why moles arise only in a small percentage of abortions, even those with failure of development of the embryo. The etiology of choriocarcinoma is also enigmatic. The trophoblast of a normal gestation grows rapidly after implantation, but this growth is limited and contained. In gestational choriocarcinoma, trophoblast escapes these normal growth and control mechanisms. Although the causes of GTD are not known, epidemiologic and cytogenetic studies have offered some clues to its development.

Age

Both hydatidiform mole and choriocarcinoma are disorders of the reproductive years. Women who are sexually active are at risk for developing GTD, but the incidence is substantially higher in older women. Women over the age of 30[21] and especially those over 40 are at increased risk for GTD,* but the absolute number of cases of mole or choriocarcinoma in women over 40 is smaller

* References 13, 24, 81, 127, 136, 171, 217.

because of their lower fertility. There also is a higher rate of occurrence of hydatidiform mole in teenagers. Thus, there appears to be an increased risk of having a complete mole at both extremes of reproductive age. Paternal age does not seem to have an effect on this risk. Malignant sequelae for hydatidiform mole occur more frequently in older patients.[14,192,193] Maternal age has no effect on the incidence of partial mole.[94,128]

Incidence and Geographic Distribution

The reported incidence of hydatidiform mole and choriocarcinoma varies widely throughout the world, being greatest in Asia, Africa, and Latin America and substantially lower in North America, Europe, and Australia (Table 24.1).[24,37,75] The incidence rate for hydatidiform mole has been reported to be as high as 11.5 per 1000 deliveries in Indonesia[154] and as low as 0.5 per 1000 deliveries in the United States.[82] The incidence rates are difficult to compare, however, because of limitations in the methodology of these studies.[24,75] Among these limitations, failure to define clearly the disease entities and lack of consistent diagnostic criteria are common shortcomings. One series of cases classified as hydatidiform mole was found to show a significant variation in the diagnoses when reviewed by a single pathologist.[97] This problem is further compounded by the recent recognition of partial mole as a relatively frequent type of molar pregnancy.

Some studies of incidence rates have used hospital-based rather than population-based figures, which probably results in overreporting.[75] This is especially true of data from less well developed countries, where uncomplicated deliveries tend to occur at home and patients with abnormal pregnancies, such as hydatidiform mole, are more likely to receive hospital care. Finally, different denominators, such as the total number of pregnancies, deliveries, or live births, have been used to determine incidence rates in different studies (Table 24.1). The incidence rate based on the number of pregnancies would best estimate the risk of GTD in a population, but this figure is extremely difficult to determine, especially in countries where there is less consistent obstetrical care. In addition, since incidence rates by country are not age adjusted, countries with high age-specific pregnancy rates in young and older women, as occurs in underdeveloped countries, have higher crude rates of hydatidiform mole.[37]

The incidence rate for hydatidiform mole in the United States and Europe is between 1 in 1000 and 1 in 2000 pregnancies.[4A,37,57,81,157,217] Women in the United States who were born outside of North America appear to be at increased risk for molar pregnancy, however.[21] In some other geographic regions, especially Asia, the incidence is as high as 1 in 500 pregnancies.[24,57,75] The striking variability in incidence rates even within geographic regions is illustrated by the low incidence of hydatidiform mole in Paraguay (1 in 5000 pregnancies)[159] compared to the high incidence in Mexico (5 in 1000 pregnancies).[126]

Choriocarcinoma occurs with a frequency of 1 in 20,000 to 1 in 40,000 pregnancies in the United States and Europe.[24,57,75,157,217] Estimates for the incidence in Asia, Africa, and Latin America generally have been higher, and incidence rates as high as 1 in 500 to 1000 pregnancies have been reported,[24,57,75,126,154] although marked regional variations occur.[160] In Nigeria, choriocarcinoma is the third most common malignant tumor in women at one institution, ranking behind breast and cervical carcinoma.[102] Again, the studies suffer from problems in methodology, precluding meaningful interpretation of the data. Nonetheless, it appears that choriocarcinoma occurs at a substantially higher rate in some geographic regions than it does in North America and Europe. The differences in geographic distribution of hydatidiform mole and choriocarcinoma also suggest that low socioeconomic conditions or dietary factors may contribute to the development of GTD. A recent case-control study suggested that dietary deficiency of carotene, a vitamin A precursor, may predispose to molar pregnancy.[21] Definitive evidence linking possible etiologic factors with GTD is lacking.

TABLE 24.1 Selected incidences of hydatidiform mole to show geographic variation.

Region	Rate per 1000[a]
Indonesia	9.9 (pregnancies)
Taiwan	8.3 (deliveries)
Phillipines	5.0 (deliveries)
Mexico	4.6 (pregnancies)
Nigeria	2.6 (deliveries)
Japan	1.9 (pregnancies)
Australia	1.4 (pregnancies)
United States	1.1 (pregnancies)
Israel	0.8 (live births)
Sweden	0.6 (pregnancies)
Paraguay	0.2 (pregnancies)

Adapted with permission of Bracken et al., Ref. 24.
[a] Data include population-based and hospital-based studies.

Previous Obstetrical History

Several studies have found that a history of prior spontaneous abortions is more common in patients with GTD, both hydatidiform mole and choriocarcinoma.[13,130,147] Furthermore, women who have had one hydatidiform mole are at greatly increased risk of having another.[18,127,217] Conversely, term pregnancy and live births have a protective effect, with GTD less common in patients who are parous.[147] The protective effect appears to increase with an increased number of live births.

Hydatidiform mole is a significant risk factor for choriocarcinoma. From 2 to 3% of complete molar pregnancies are followed by choriocarcinoma,[33,85] and almost one half of all choriocarcinomas follow a molar pregnancy.[84,122] Other abnormal pregnancies, especially spontaneous abortions, are more commonly followed by choriocarcinoma, although choriocarcinoma may follow any type of gestation, including a term pregnancy.

Blood Groups

An association has been reported between ABO blood groups and the occurrence of choriocarcinoma but not hydatidiform mole. Blood group A is more frequent and group O less common in patients with choriocarcinoma. This association is particularly strong with blood group A women whose husbands are group O and, conversely, for group O women whose husbands are group A.[7,11,43] Patients of blood group B or AB have a worse prognosis, however.[7,43] The significance of these data is difficult to assess, since the children of the gestation associated with the choriocarcinoma show no trend in blood group distribution.[7] Furthermore, some studies have found no association or even a decrease in the frequency of group A among patients with malignant GTD.[132,165] In contrast to ABO blood group interactions, there has been no consistent pattern in HLA distribution between women with choriocarcinoma and their consorts.[7,132,216]

Cytogenetics

Cytogenetic studies of complete and partial hydatidiform mole have shown that chromosomal abnormalities play a role in the development of molar gestations.[49,181] Furthermore, the karyotype patterns of the two types of moles are generally different. Most complete hydatidiform moles have a normal complement at 46XX,[181,201] but both X chromosomes are androgenic, that is, of paternal origin[103,205] (Fig. 24.1). This 46XX karyotype results from duplication of a haploid sperm (23 chromosomes) pronucleus in an empty ovum that lacks functional maternal DNA.[96,206] Duplication of a 23Y sperm results in a nonviable 46YY cell. A smaller proportion (3–13%) of complete moles have a 46XY chromosome complement, but in these moles, too, the chromosomes are androgenetic.[104,151,174,175] In this instance, the 46XY-complete mole is believed to form by dispermy, that is, fertilization of an empty ovum by two sperm pronuclei, one with the X and the other with the Y chromosome.[145,175] The complete mole, being paternally derived, constitutes a total allograft in the mother. This

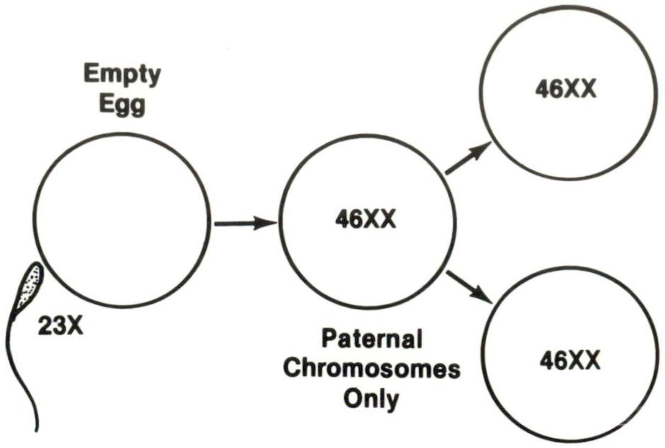

FIG. 24.1. Chromosomal origin of a complete hydatidiform mole. A single sperm fertilizes an empty egg. Reduplication of its 23X set gives a completely homozygous diploid genome of 46XX. A similar process follows fertilization of an empty egg by two sperms with two independently drawn sets of 23X or 23Y. Note that both karyotypes 46XX and 46XY can ensue. (Adapted with permission of Szulman, Ref. 180.)

feature may play some role in the behavior of GTD, such as spontaneous remission.

The karyotypes of partial mole most frequently show triploidy (69 chromosomes)[181] (Fig. 24.2) with a maternal chromosome complement.[10,49] Conversely, the majority (86%) of triploid conceptuses have histologic features of partial mole.[185] Rarely, however, a partial mole with an identifiable fetus will have a 46XX karyotype.[94,181] Rare examples of tetraploidy have also been reported.[176] When triploidy is present in a partial mole, the chromosomal complement is XXY in 70% of cases, XXX in 27%, and XYY in 3%.[181] These abnormal conceptuses result from the fertilization of an egg with a haploid set of chromosomes by either two sperms, each with a set of haploid chromosomes, or by a single sperm with a diploid genome of 46XY.[95] A conceptus with a diploid 46XX maternal genome due to failure of the first meiotic division and a haploid paternal set of chromosomes results in an abnormal, triploid fetus but with generally a nonmolar pregnancy. This is referred to as a *digynic conceptus* and is believed to account for only 15–20% of cases of triploidy.[94] Thus, all well-documented partial moles are triploid, but not all triploid conceptuses are associated with partial moles. Partial molar pregnancies may have a grossly identifiable embryo or fetus with congenital anomalies.[181] Although many partial moles do have a triploid karyotype and evidence of an embryo or fetus, there is no consensus yet that all partial moles have these features. Likewise, not all molar pregnancies with evidence of fetal development need be regarded as partial moles, since fetal development rarely may occur in complete moles.[23,82,94]

The cytogenetic findings indicate that abnormal fertilization plays a key role in the evolution of both complete

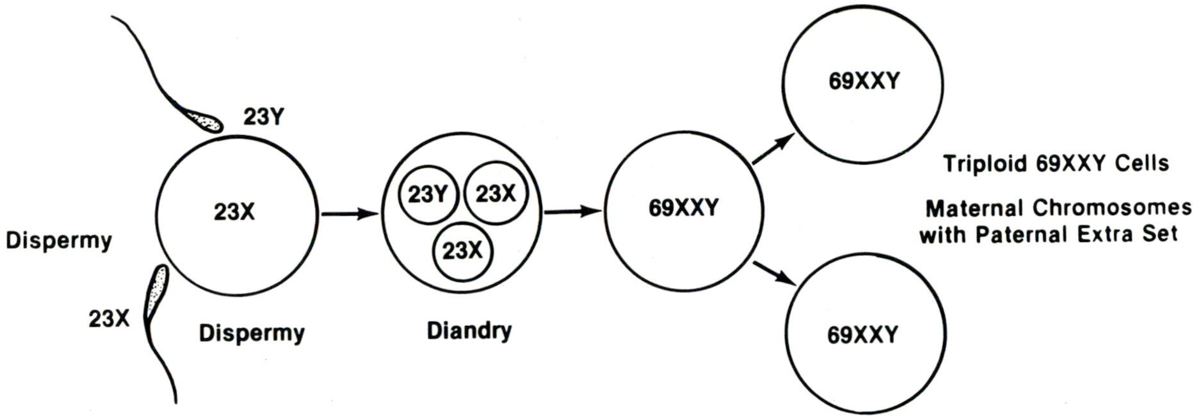

FIG. 24.2. Chromosomal origin of the triploid, partial hydatidiform mole. A normal egg with a 23X haploid set is fertilized by two sperms that carry either sex chromosome, to give a total of 69 chromosomes with a sex configuration of XXY, XXX, or XYY. A similar result can be obtained by fertilization of a sperm carrying the unreduced paternal genome 46XY (resulting sex complement, XXY only). (Adapted with permission from Szulman, Ref. 180.)

and partial hydatidiform moles. Although it is not known why these chromosomal aberrations lead to the formation of a molar pregnancy, recent experimental studies in mice suggest that there may be a relationship between the molar phenotype and the ratio of paternal to maternal haploid sets of chromosomes. The hypothesis has been advanced that the formation of a mole is associated with an excess of paternal compared to maternal haploid contributions.[176] The higher the ratio of paternal to maternal chromosomes, the greater the molar change. Complete moles show a 2:0 paternal to maternal ratio, whereas partial moles show a 2:1 ratio. This hypothesis is supported by experimental evidence in mice in which enucleated eggs are implanted with male or female pronuclei. In a conceptus with two maternal sets of chromosomes, the embryo develops, albeit not beyond a certain stage, but the trophoblast is stunted. In contrast, in a conceptus with two paternal sets of chromosomes, there is much greater trophoblastic development, and the embryo dies earlier.[173]

The chromosomal complements of invasive mole and choriocarcinoma have not been as well studied. In a retrospective analysis, Davis et al. evaluated the presence of Y chromatin using quinacrine fluorescent staining.[42] Fourteen (73%) of 19 choriocarcinomas and 2 (50%) of 4 invasive moles were Y chromatin positive, whereas only 9% of 182 hydatidiform moles contained a Y chromosome.

Morphology and Immunocytochemistry of Trophoblast

The abnormal trophoblastic tissue in GTD recapitulates the trophoblast present in the early developing placenta and the implantation site. In normal placentation, the trophoblast growing in association with chorionic villi is referred to as *villous trophoblast*, whereas the trophoblast in all other locations is termed *extravillous trophoblast*. Three distinct types of trophoblastic cells have been recognized: cytotrophoblast (CT), syncytiotrophoblast (ST), and intermediate trophoblast (IT). Villous trophoblast is composed, for the most part, of CT and ST with small amounts of IT. In contrast, extravillous trophoblast that infiltrates the decidua, myometrium, and spiral arteries of the placental site is composed mostly of IT with a minor component of CT and ST. The CT or Langhans cell is the germinative trophoblastic cell, whereas the ST is the highly differentiated cell that interfaces with the maternal circulation and produces most of the placental hormones. The IT is a distinct form of trophoblastic cell that shares some of the morphologic and functional features of both CT and ST.[109] Each form of trophoblastic cell has specific microscopic, ultrastructural, and immunohistochemical features.

Light Microscopy

In normal gestation, CT is composed of primitive epithelial cells that are uniform and polygonal to oval in shape. They have a single nucleus, clear to granular cytoplasm, and well-defined cell borders (Fig. 24.3a, b). The CT shows mitotic activity. Syncytiotrophoblast is composed of large, multinucleate cells with dense amphophilic cytoplasm containing multiple vacuoles that vary in size, some of which form lacunae (Fig. 24.3a, b). A distinct brush border often lines the cell membrane. The ST does not show mitotic activity.

The cells of IT are generally mononucleate but binucleate, trinucleate, and multinucleate forms are present. The IT cells vary in shape, ranging from round to polyhedral cells to spindle-shaped, bipolar cells with attenuated

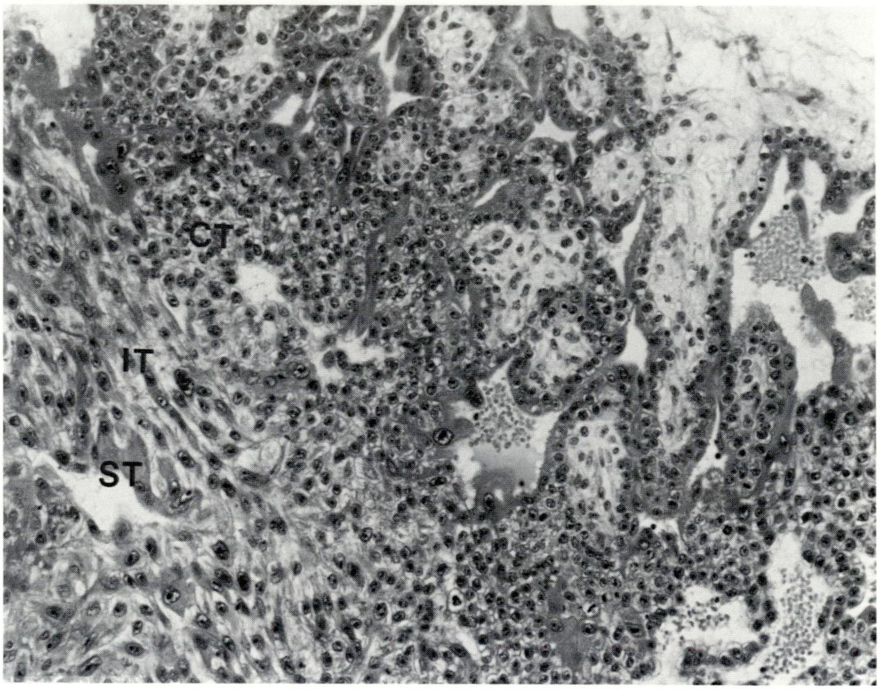

a

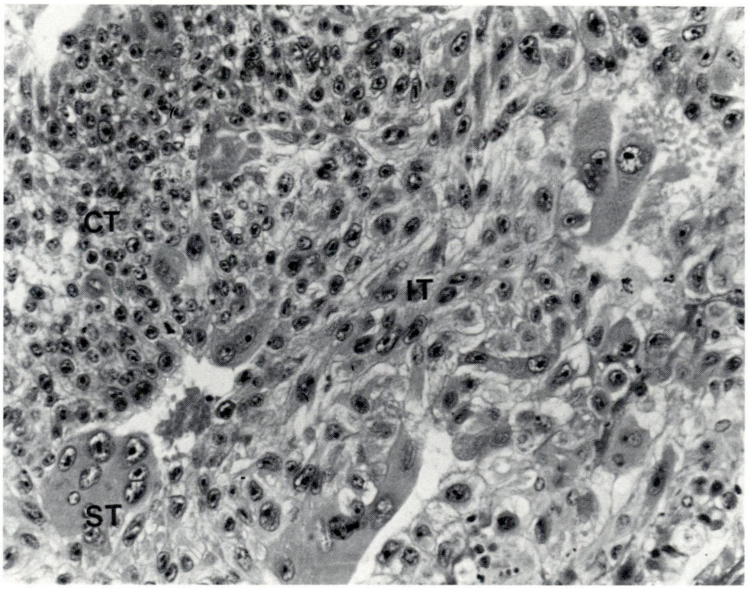

b

FIG. 24.3.*a*. Villous and extravillous trophoblast of a 16-day blastocyst showing cytotrophoblast (CT), intermediate trophoblast (IT), and syncytiotrophoblast (ST). *b*. Cytotrophoblast (CT) is characterized by small, uniform, mononucleate cells with distinct cell membranes, intermediate trophoblast (IT) by larger cells that are mononucleate but show greater pleomorphism, and syncytiotrophoblast (ST) by multinucleate giant cells with much larger nuclei.

cytoplasmic processes. Cytoplasm is abundant and is eosinophilic to amphophilic (Fig. 24.3a, b). Scattered small vacuoles may be present in the IT cytoplasm, and nuclei of IT are irregular and hyperchromatic with coarsely granular chromatin. Often the nuclei will be lobulated. Nucleoli are smaller and less prominent than those seen in CT. Cytoplasmic nuclear invaginations may be seen.

The cytologic features that distinguish IT from CT include the larger size of the IT cell and the abundant amphophilic cytoplasm, which contrasts with the sparse, clear to faintly granular cytoplasm of CT. Cell membranes are less distinct in IT. The IT in contrast to ST is largely mononucleate and lacks the extremely dense eosinophilic cytoplasm of ST. Furthermore, IT does not show the extensive vacuolization of ST.

An intimate mixture of CT, IT, and ST forms the cellular population of hydatidiform moles (Fig. 24.4) and choriocarcinoma. The CT (Fig. 24.5) and IT (Fig. 24.6) in moles and choriocarcinoma tend to grow in clusters and sheets, separated by ST (Fig. 24.7), that line large, angular spaces containing red cells. The patterns of growth recapitulate the relationship of the trophoblast to the maternal–placental circulation of the early implanting blastocyst. These vascular spaces lined by ST are intimately admixed with CT and IT and comprise the plexiform pattern typically associated with hemorrhage and necrosis in many trophoblastic lesions. There may be considerable cytologic atypia in the CT and ST in hydatidiform moles and choriocarcinoma with pleomorphic enlarged nuclei, abnormal mitotic figures, and bizarre cellular configurations. Nuclear chromatin is coarsely granular, with an uneven distribution, and multiple nucleoli may be present. Enlarged, binucleate, and multinucleate IT also occur, and these cells are distinguished from ST by their cytoplasm, which lacks the dense eosinophilia and vacuolization (Fig. 24.8).

IT comprises the predominant cellular population in the placental site trophoblastic tumor. IT in extravillous locations usually grows as large sheets of cells or shows an infiltrative pattern in decidua, myometrium, or blood vessels as the cells dissect between the smooth muscle cells (Figs. 24.9 and 24.10). Typically, this cell infiltrates the wall of large vascular channels until the wall is entirely replaced. This highly infiltrative pattern is a characteristic of IT.

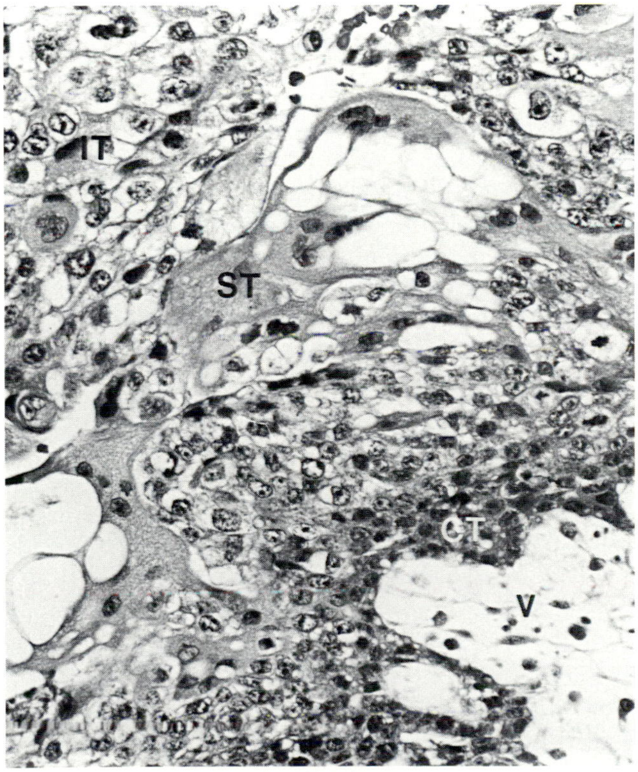

Fig. 24.4. A mixture of cytotrophoblast (CT), intermediate trophoblast (IT), and syncytiotrophoblast (ST) grows from the surface of a villus (V) of a complete mole.

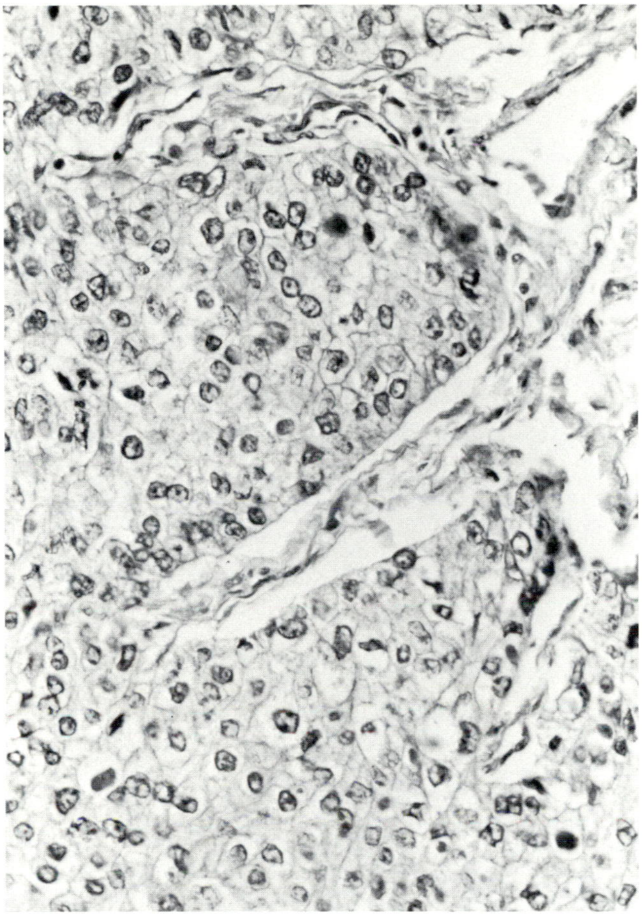

Fig. 24.5. A sheet of cytotrophoblast in a metastatic choriocarcinoma, characterized by a uniform population of small mononucleate cells with sharply defined cell membranes.

Ultrastructure

The fine structure of CT correlates with the functional and light microscopic features of this cell in GTD and the developing placenta.[44,57,58,112] These cells are closely apposed with polygonal outlines (Fig. 24.11). The most striking feature is their simplicity, with electron-lucent cytoplasm containing numerous free cytoplasmic ribosomes and aggregates of particulate glycogen. Other organelles are sparse. Mitochondria, scattered strands of rough endoplasmic reticulum (RER), and Golgi complexes are the other components. A few small electron-dense lysosomes, vesicles, and lipid droplets may be found, but cytoplasmic filaments are not present. The nuclei have smooth, round to oval contours and contain

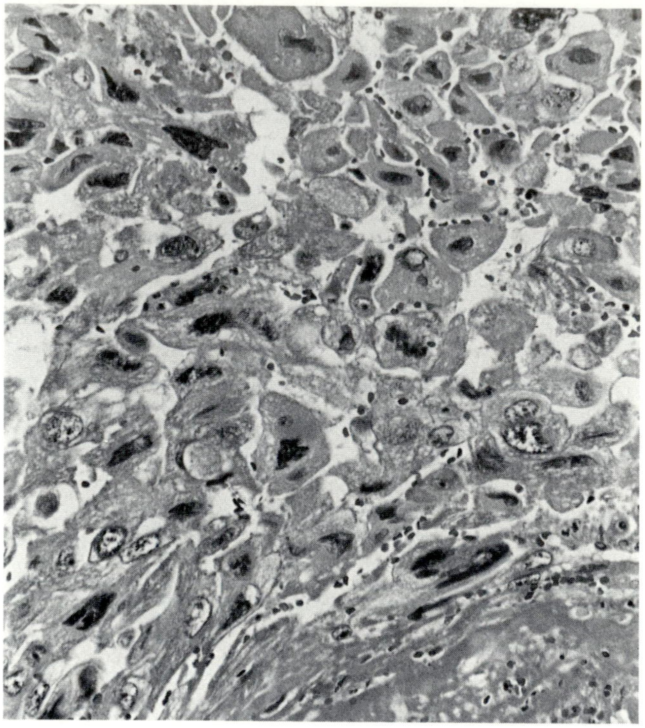

FIG. 24.6. A mass of intermediate trophoblast in a complete hydatidiform mole, characterized by a population of pleomorphic mononucleate cells with abundant amphophilic cytoplasm.

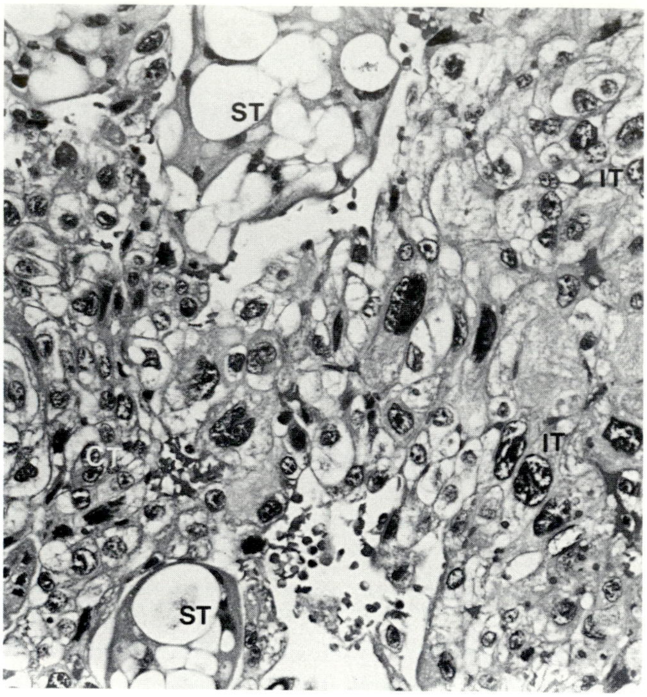

FIG. 24.8. Trophoblast of a complete mole demonstrating cytologic atypia. The intermediate trophoblast (IT) in the *center* and the *right side* of the field has enlarged, irregular nuclei. Cytotrophoblast (CT) is present on the *left*, and vacuolated syncytiotrophoblast (ST) is present in the *upper* and *lower portions* of the micrograph.

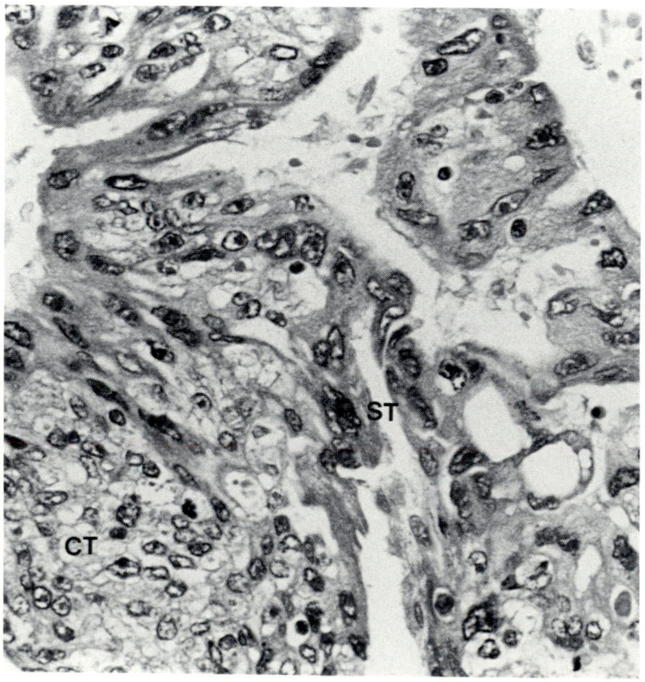

FIG. 24.7. Syncytiotrophoblast (ST) in a choriocarcinoma, lining vascular spaces and capping cytotrophoblast (CT).

a prominent nucleolus. The cells are joined by widely separated, well-formed desmosomes.

The ST contrasts markedly with CT.[44,57,58,112] These highly developed epithelial cells have a complex cytoplasm and cell membrane structure. Often, ST is directly joined to CT by desmosomes, and here the distinction between the two cell types is immediately apparent (Fig. 24.12). In addition to the multiple nuclei, ST demonstrate an electron-dense cytoplasm due to the presence of multiple organelles (Fig. 24.13). RER is abundant and often dilated, giving an appearance of multiple tiny vacuoles within the cytoplasm. In addition, the cytoplasm contains abundant free cytoplasmic ribosomes, many prominent lipid droplets, vesicles, and lysosomes. Another important cytoplasmic constituent is thick bundles of tonofilaments scattered throughout the cell (Fig. 24.14). The ST cell surface is covered with many long microvilli. Infolding of the microvillous surface into the cytoplasm that forms the interconnecting lacunae gives an appearance of multiple intracytoplasmic lumens when viewed in cross-section. Well-formed desmosomes connect the cells. The ST nuclei tend to have highly irregular outlines and coarsely clumped chromatin, which further contribute to the cellular complexity.

Since ST forms by coalescence of CT, transition forms

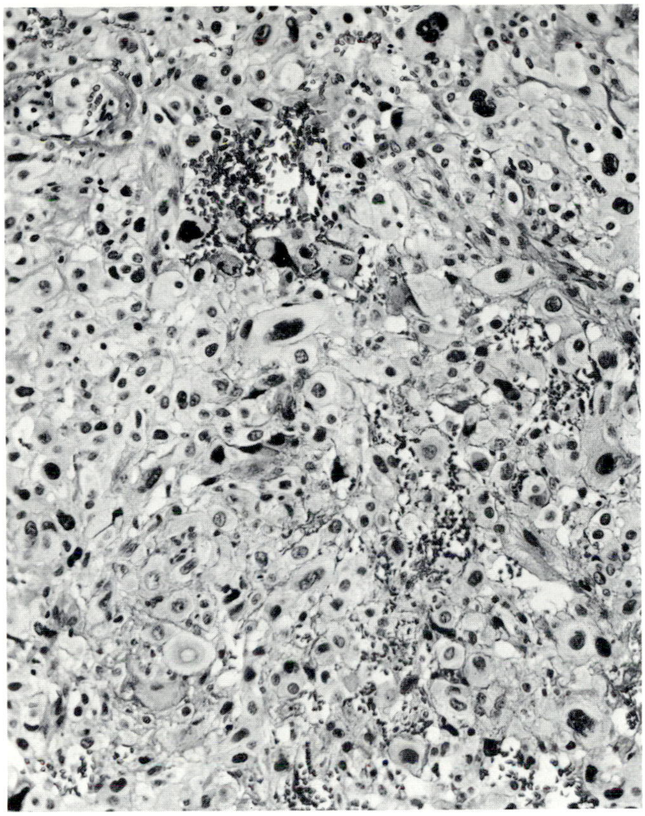

Fig. 24.9. Placental site trophoblastic tumor composed of sheets of intermediate trophoblast characterized by large polyhedral cells with pleomorphic nuclei. (Reprinted with permission of Kurman et al., Ref. 110.)

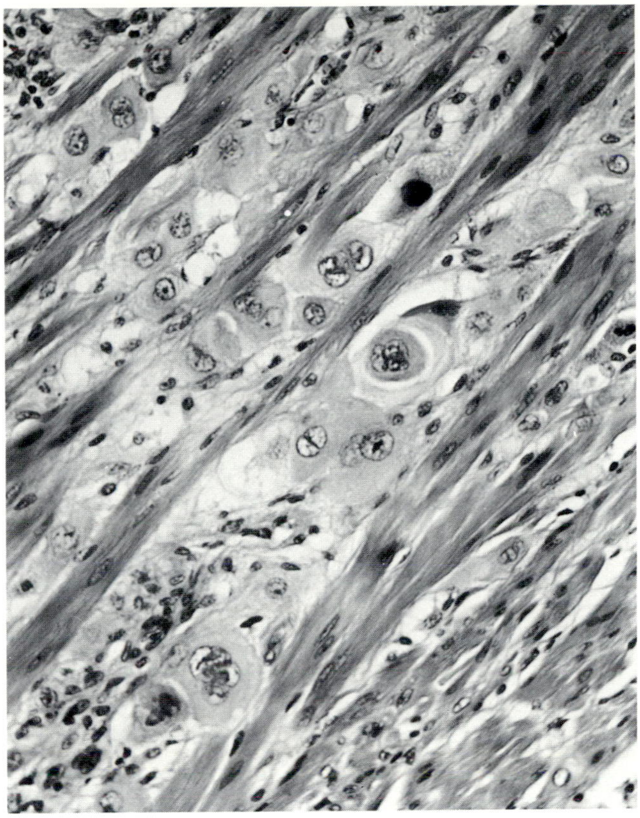

Fig. 24.10. The intermediate trophoblastic cells comprising placental site trophoblastic tumor characteristically separate muscle bundles as they invade myometrium. (Reprinted with permission of Kurman et al., Ref. 110.)

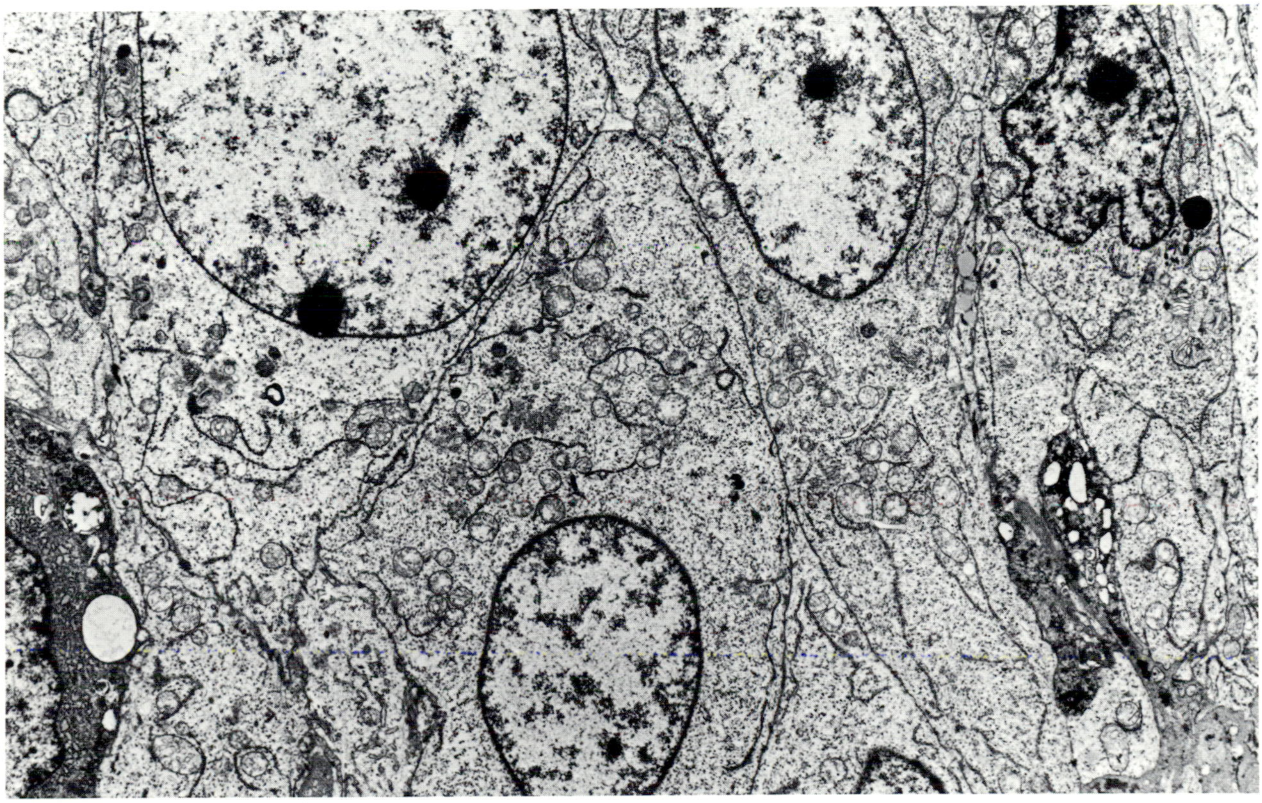

Fig. 24.11. Cytotrophoblastic cells in choriocarcinoma have simple cytoplasm with few organelles except RER and mitochondria. Occasional desmosomes join cells. Nuclei are round to oval. ×4000.

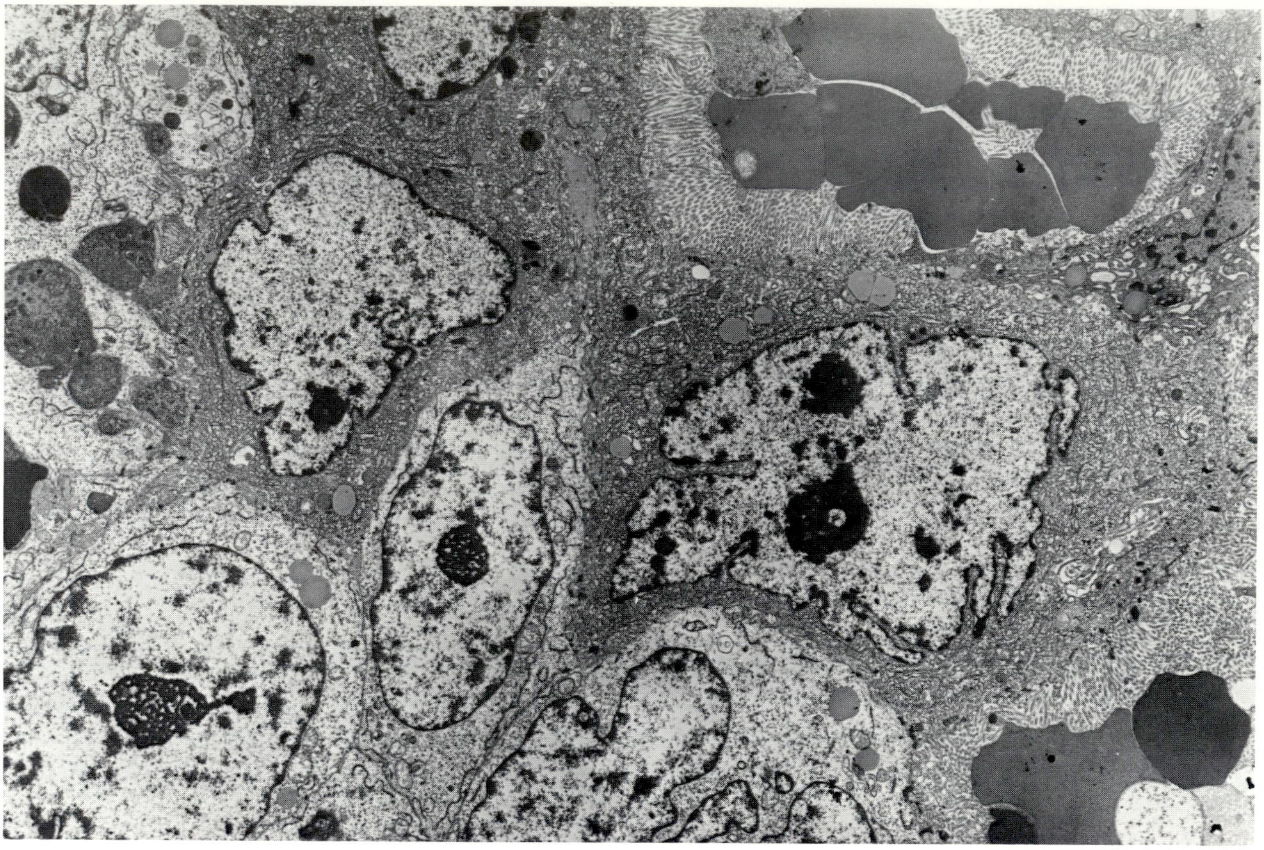

FIG. 24.12. Electron micrograph of trophoblast in choriocarcinoma shows syncytiotrophoblast in *right upper portion,* with dense, complex cytoplasm and multiple nuclei. A vascular lacuna containing red blood cells is present in the *right upper portion.* In contrast, the cytotrophoblast at the *left lower portion* of the micrograph has electron-lucent cytoplasm. ×4000.

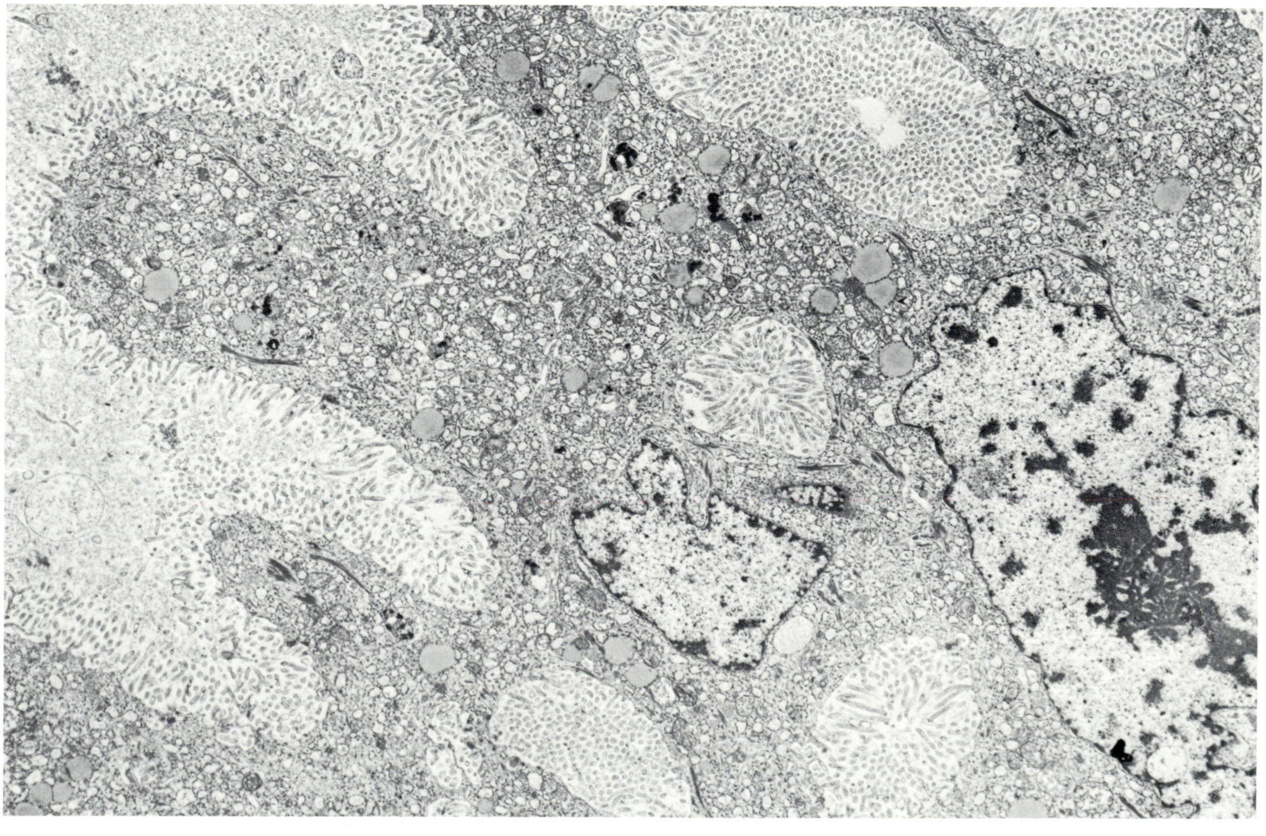

FIG. 24.13. Portion of syncytiotrophoblast from choriocarcinoma demonstrates multiple lacunae lined by slender microvilli. The complex cytoplasm contains dilated RER, lipid vacuoles, and dark granules. The nuclei have irregular contours and clumped chromatin. ×4500.

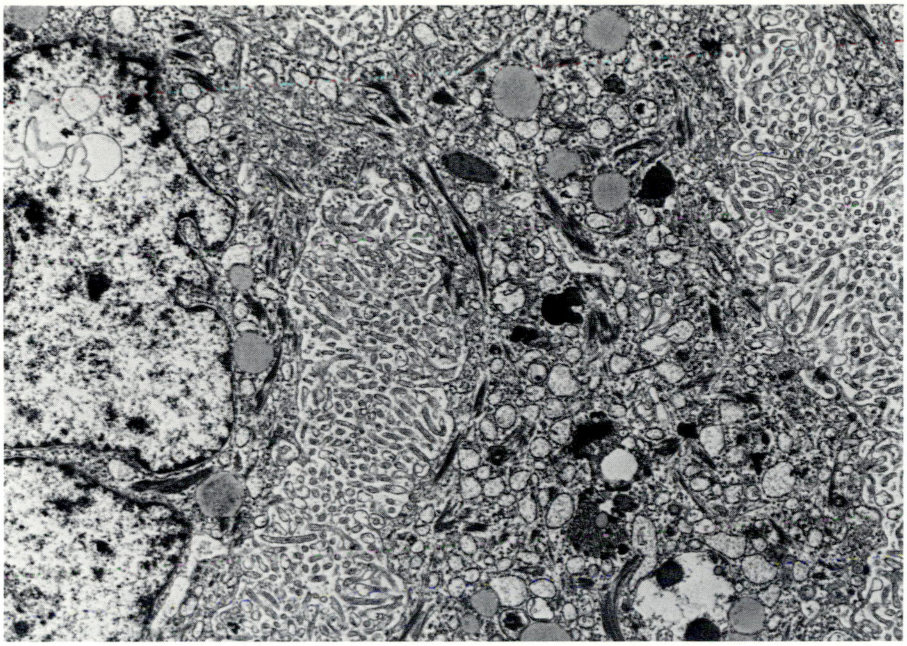

Fig. 24.14. Portion of syncytiotrophoblast shows multiple cytoplasmic organelles including dilated RER, lipid vacuoles, and bundles of tonofilaments. Numerous slender microvilli line the cell surfaces. ×6000.

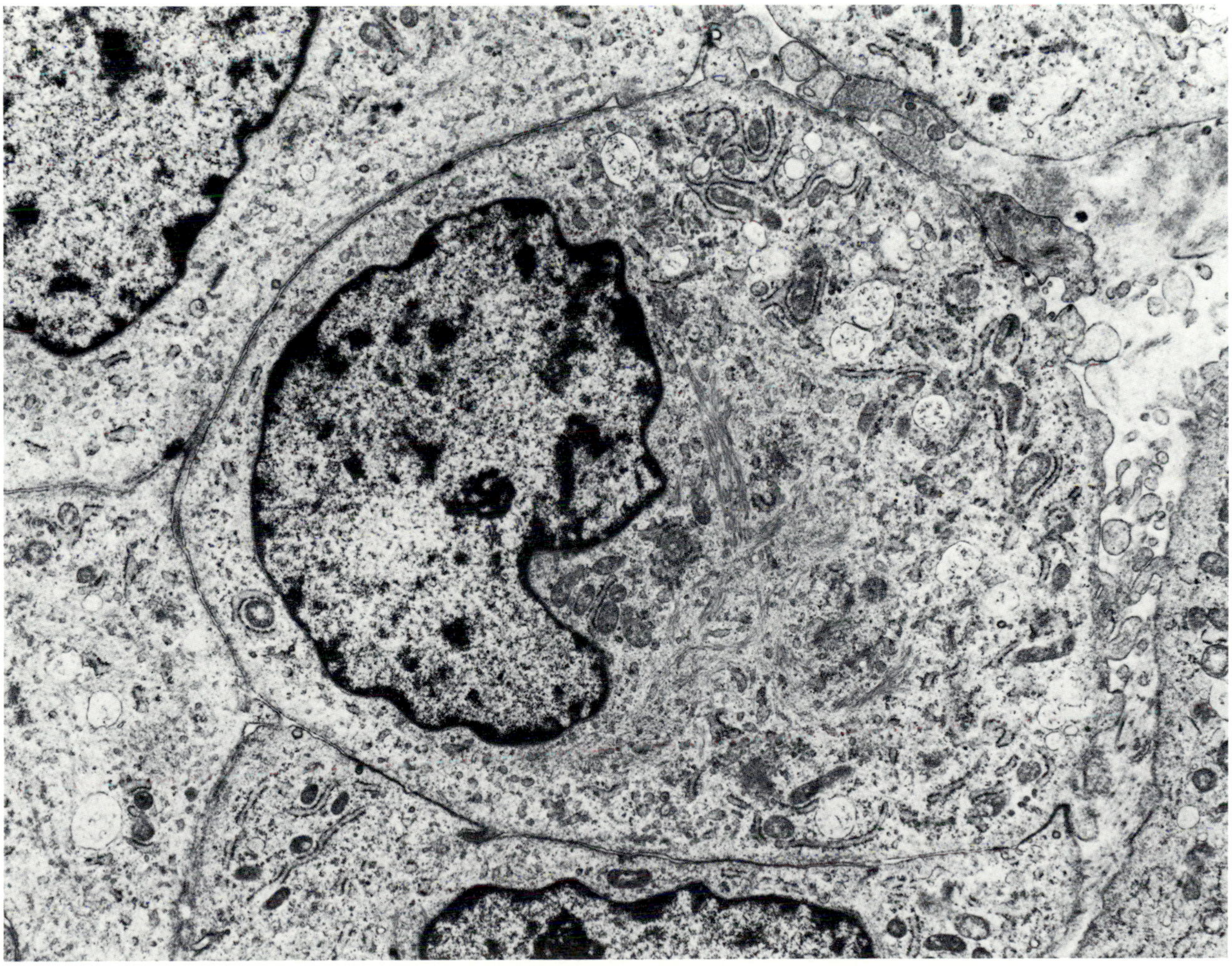

Fig. 24.15. Electron micrograph of intermediate trophoblast (IT) from a placental site trophoblastic tumor showing abundant cytoplasm containing RER, mitochondria, and perinuclear filament bundles. The cell surface to the right contains blunt microvilli. ×6000.

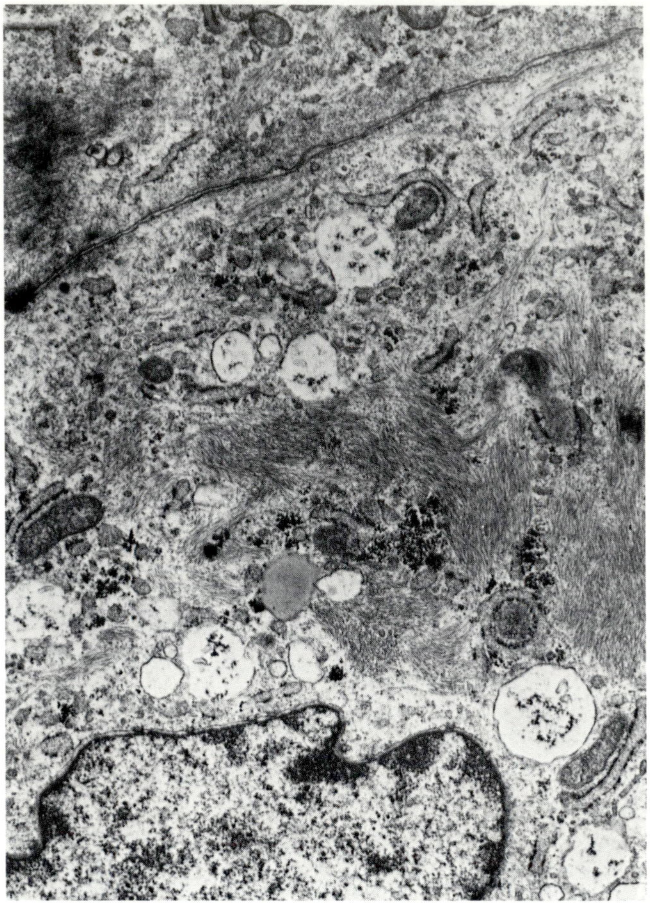

FIG. 24.16. Portion of intermediate trophoblast in placental site trophoblastic tumor shows multiple cytoplasmic organelles including RER, glycogen, and aggregates of filaments. A desmosome is present along the cell membrane. ×14,000.

can be found ultrastructurally that share features of both CT and ST.[153,215] These cells correspond to IT and may have one or more nuclei in a cytoplasm that is more dense and complex than that of CT but less well developed than ST cytoplasm. Occasional aggregates of intracytoplasmic desmosomes can be found where fusion of cell membranes has taken place. The ultrastructural morphology of IT is best demonstrated in the placental site trophoblastic tumor, where specific patterns of fine structure have emerged from isolated case reports.[17,68,87,196] The cells are large and have abundant cytoplasm. The cell outlines are polygonal when the IT cells are closely apposed (Fig. 24.15). Free surfaces show microvilli that are less numerous and more blunt than the microvilli of ST. The cytoplasm of IT is electron-dense and contains numerous organelles although lacking the overall complexity of ST cytoplasm (Fig. 24.16). Typically, moderate numbers of mitochondria, dilated RER, scattered single strands of RER, and free ribosomes are present. Some cells contain vesicles of smooth endoplasmic reticulum, Golgi complexes, and pools of glycogen. One feature described in most of the reported cases is the presence of large bundles of paranuclear intermediate filaments that are apparently distinctive for IT as compared to ST or CT. When IT cells are closely apposed they are joined by well-formed desmosomes.

Immunocytochemistry

A large number of protein hormones, steroid hormones, and enzymes such as hCG, human placental lactogen (hPL), pregnancy specific beta-$_1$-glycoprotein, placental protein 5, pregnancy-associated plasma protein A, estradiol, progesterone, and placental alkaline phosphatase have been localized in the placenta during various stages of development by immunoperoxidase techniques. The majority are confined to the ST. In particular, the localization of hCG and hPL has led to a more complete characterization of the various types of trophoblast,[109,111] and, therefore, this discussion is limited to these two placental hormones.

The immunocytochemical localization of hCG and hPL in the normal placenta according to the gestational age is shown in Table 24.2. Intermediate trophoblast contains abundant hPL, which appears as early as 12 days and reaches a peak at 11–15 weeks of gestation (Fig. 24.17).[109] In contrast, hCG is present only focally in IT (Fig. 24.17), appearing as early as 12 days and remaining until 6 weeks,

TABLE 24.2. Localization of chorionic gonadotropin beta-subunit and placental lactogen in different types of trophoblastic cells in the placenta and the placental site throughout gestation.

Trophoblastic cell type	First trimester		Second trimester		Third trimester	
	hCG	hPL	hCG	hPL	hCG	hPL
Cytotrophoblast	−	−	−	−	−	−
Intermediate trophoblast	+	++	−/+	+++	−	+/++
Syncytiotrophoblast	++++	+	++	+++	+	++++

− → ++++ denotes semiquantitative scoring of the proportion of cells showing a positive reaction: + = 1–24%, ++ = 25–49%, +++ = 50–74%, ++++ = 75–100%.

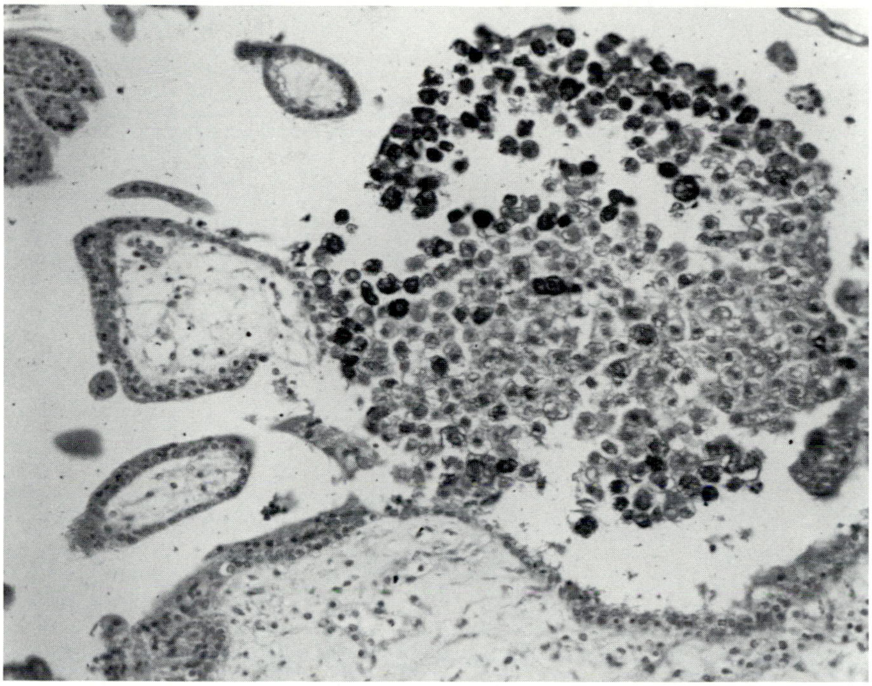

a

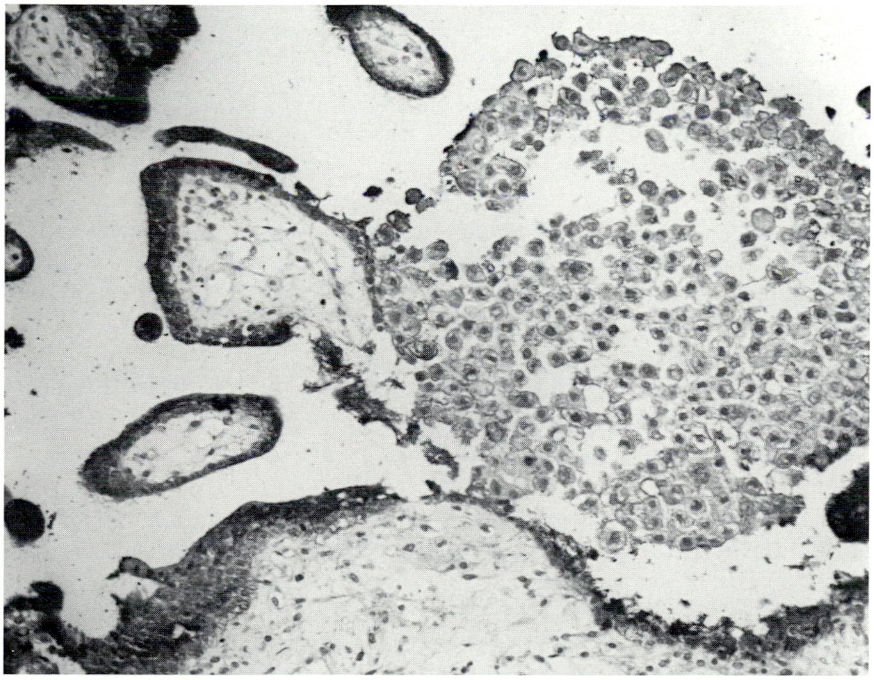

b

FIG. 24.17.*a*. Localization of hPL (*black deposit*) within the cytoplasm of intermediate trophoblastic cells sprouting from a chorionic villus. Note absence of hPL in syncytiotrophoblast. Gestational age is 4 weeks. *b*. Localization of hCG (*black deposit*) within the cytoplasm of syncytiotrophoblast. Note absence of hCG in intermediate trophoblast. (Reprinted with permission of Kurman et al., Ref. 109.)

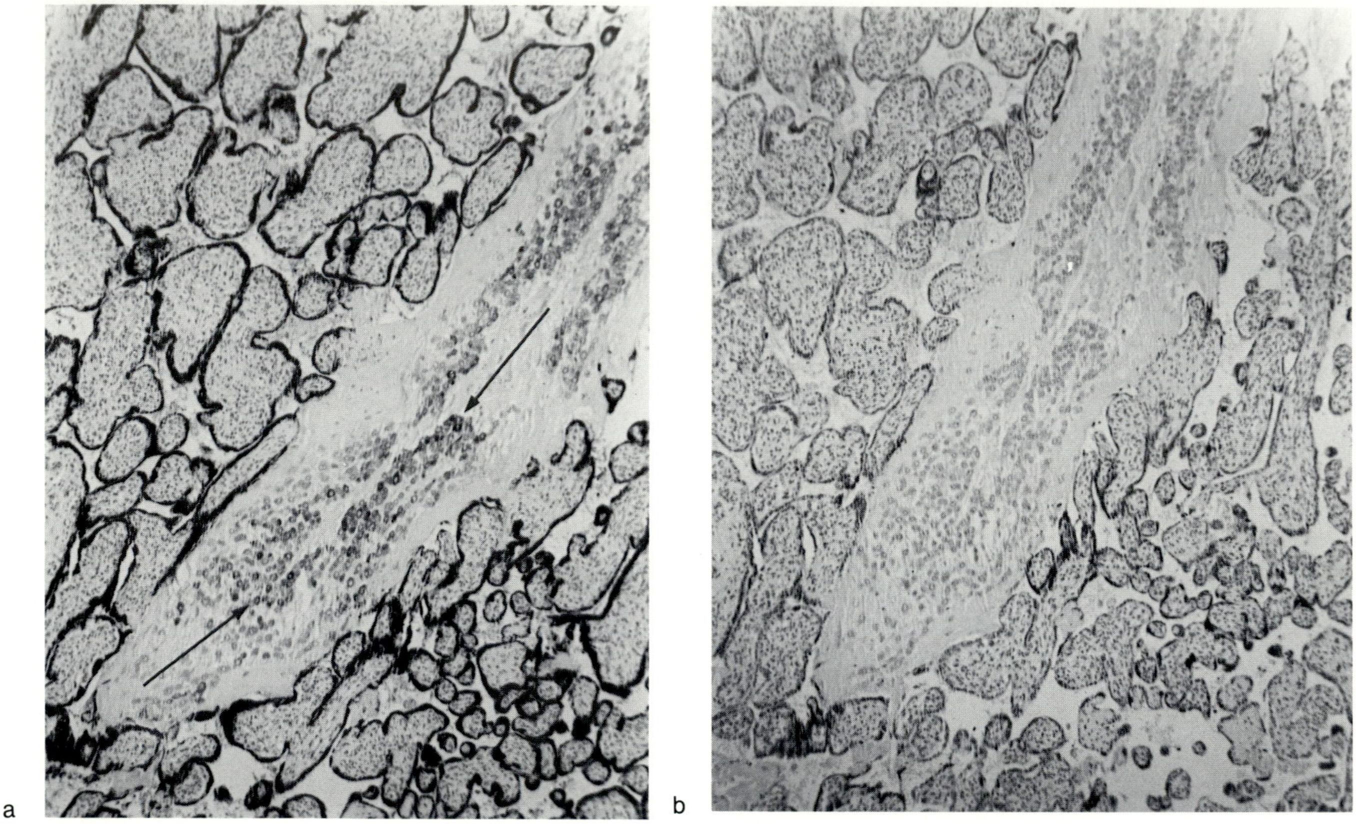

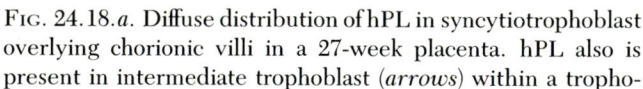

Fig. 24.18. *a*. Diffuse distribution of hPL in syncytiotrophoblast overlying chorionic villi in a 27-week placenta. hPL also is present in intermediate trophoblast (*arrows*) within a trophoblastic column. *b*. hCG is focally distributed in syncytiotrophoblast and is absent in intermediate trophoblast.

after which it disappears. CT does not appear to contain either hCG or hPL. ST contains abundant hCG from at least 12 days of gestation until approximately 8–10 weeks, after which it diminishes. By 40 weeks it is present only focally (Fig. 24.18). Placental lactogen is also localized in ST at 12 days but increases steadily thereafter. From late in the second trimester to term, hPL is diffusely distributed in the ST overlying the chorionic villi (Fig. 24.18).[109]

At the placental site, immunocytochemical reactions for hPL aid in distinguishing IT from decidual and smooth muscle cells because the hormone is not present in either decidua or smooth muscle (Fig. 24.19). The binucleate and trinucleate cells show the same pattern of staining as the mononucleate form of IT.[111] In contrast, although some multinucleate IT contain hPL, a larger proportion of them contain hCG in the first trimester. During the second and third trimesters, hCG progressively decreases in these cells, whereas hPL is present through the second trimester and diminishes in the last trimester. The IT cells that invade the spiral arteries show the same pattern of staining as those within the decidua and myometrium. Typically, they contain hPL and little if any hCG (Fig. 24.20). These findings indicate that the invasive property of trophoblast in normal placentation appears to reside in IT, which, therefore, plays a key role in the development of the uteroplacental circulation.[109,111]

Clinicopathologic Features and Behavior

Complete Hydatidiform Mole

Clinical Aspects. Complete hydatidiform mole, also known as classic hydatidiform mole, is the most frequent form of molar pregnancy and GTD. This disorder typically develops between the 11th and 25th weeks of pregnancy, with a mean gestational age of about 18 weeks.[39,82,133] Patients often have vaginal bleeding or uterine enlargement in excess of that expected for the gestational age.[18,39,71,133] In approximately one-third of patients, however, the uterus is small for dates.[39] Occasionally, the initial clinical manifestation can be the sudden passage of molar vesicles. Preeclampsia (pregnancy-induced hypertension with edema and proteinuria) occurs in up to one-fourth of patients with complete mole.[71] In contrast to nonmolar gestations in which preeclampsia occurs typically in the last trimester, in molar gestations preeclampsia occurs in the first trimester. Thus, early

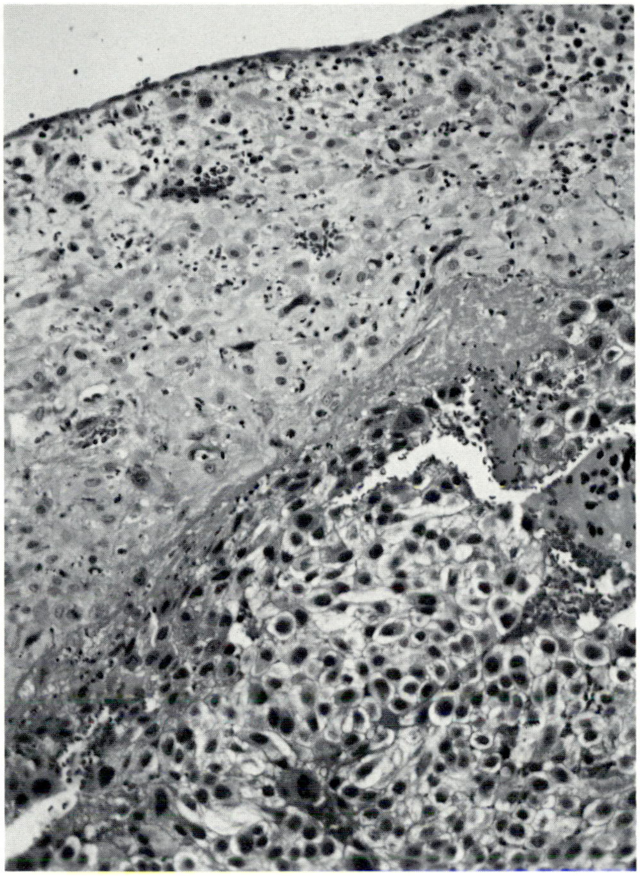

a

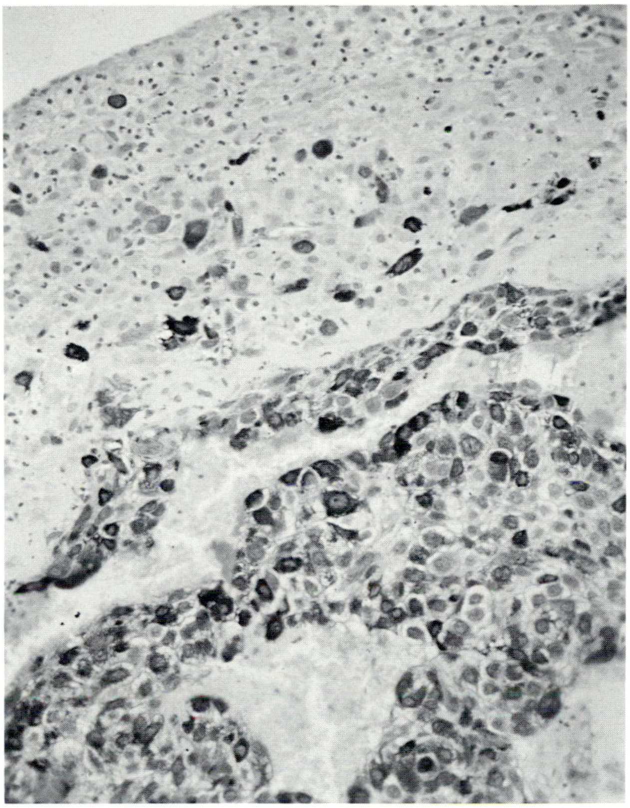

b

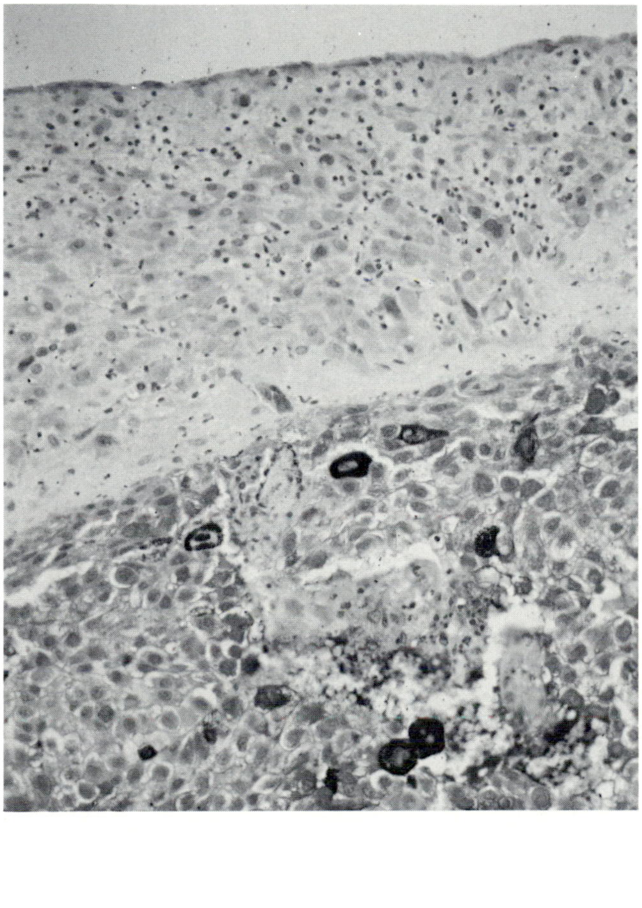

c

FIG. 24.19.*a*. A 12-day blastocyst. The decidua in the upper part of the field contains numerous intermediate trophoblastic cells with enlarged nuclei. These cells may be difficult to distinguish from decidua. *b*. The intermediate trophoblastic cells in the trophoblastic shell (lower half of field) and those infiltrating the decidua contain hPL, but decidual cells do not. *c*. A few intermediate trophoblastic cells in the trophoblastic shell are positive for hCG, but those in the decidua are negative. (Reprinted with permission of Kurman et al., Ref. 111.)

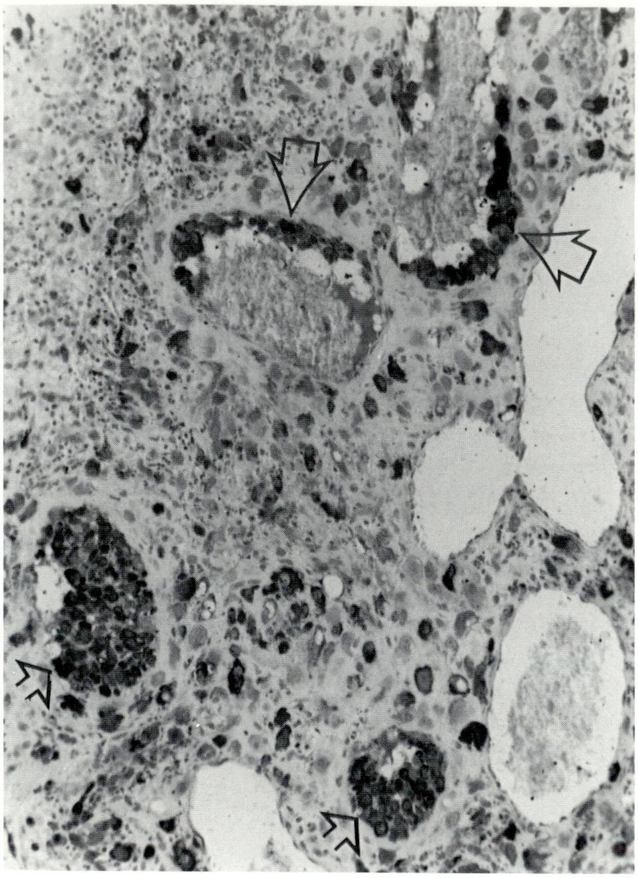

FIG. 24.20. Placental site at 11-weeks gestation. Numerous intermediate trophoblastic cells containing hPL (*black deposit*) infiltrate the decidua and invade spiral arteries. Two arteries are completely plugged with intermediate trophoblast (*small arrows*), and two have the intimal surface partially lined by intermediate trophoblast (*large arrows*).

onset of preeclampsia, especially when coupled with excessive uterine enlargement, suggests the presence of a molar pregnancy. Additional clinical signs of molar pregnancy include hyperemesis gravidarum, occurring in a quarter of patients, and hyperthyroidism in 7%.[71] The cause of hyperthyroidism is not fully known. Intrinsic thyroid-stimulating activity of hCG is one possible mechanism,[71,139] but some investigators suggest that trophoblast produces other undefined substances that cause thyroxicosis.[2] Pulmonary embolization of trophoblast and massive ovarian enlargement due to benign theca–lutein cysts (hyperreactio luteinalis) (see Chapter 16, Nonneoplastic Lesions of Ovary) are other possible clinical manifestations of a hydatidiform mole. The serum or urine hCG titer is markedly elevated. Pelvic ultrasonic examination discloses a snowstorm pattern that is diagnostic of hydatidiform mole, especially when associated with the elevated hCG level.[161]

Although these clinical signs and symptoms permit the diagnosis of a molar pregnancy before evacuation, the clinical presentation is quite variable, and many moles are not recognized before curettage.[94,181] In one study, more than 80% of patients with a molar pregnancy were first diagnosed by histologic study of spontaneously passed or operatively evacuated tissue.[39] Hydatidiform moles can also be found unexpectedly in elective abortion specimens of asymptomatic patients.[220A] In one study, almost 1 in 600 consecutive elective abortions revealed hydatidiform mole, and a quarter of these were not apparent on gross examination.[35]

Gross Appearance. Massively enlarged, edematous villi give the classic grape-like appearance to the placenta (Fig. 24.21). The swollen villi may range from a few

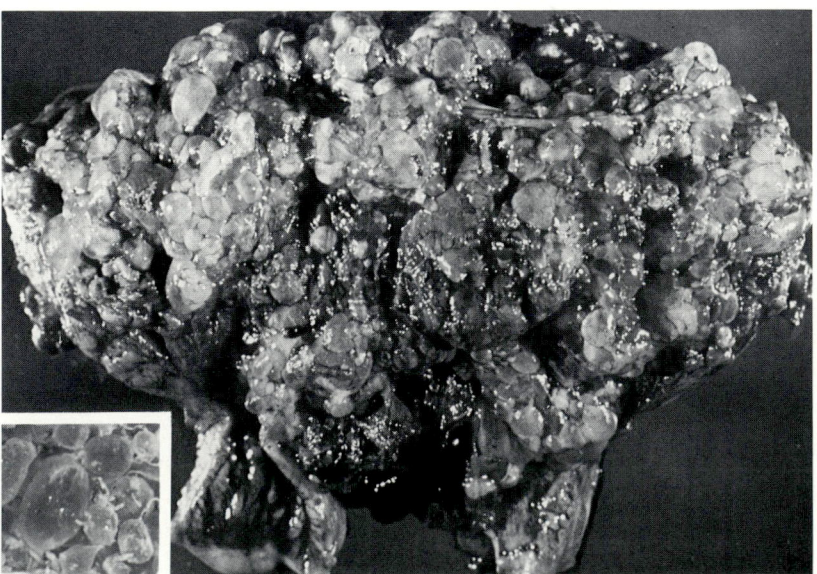

FIG. 24.21. Complete hydatidiform mole in a hysterectomy specimen shows an enlarged uterus with molar placental tissue protruding from the opened specimen. *Inset:* The hydropic villi range from a few millimeters to over 1 cm in diameter.

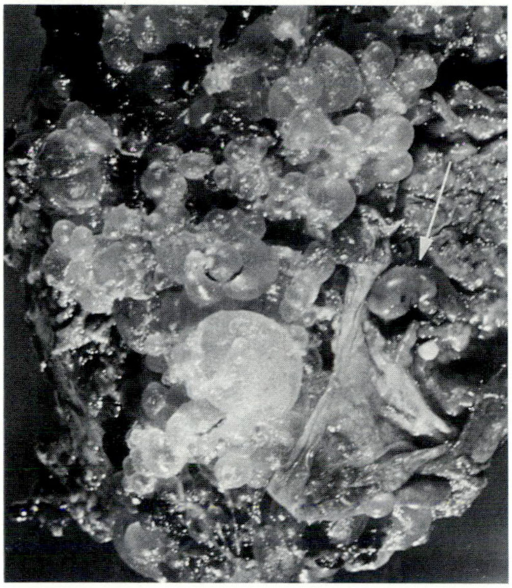

FIG. 24.22. Complete hydatidiform mole in a hysterectomy specimen contains a small, 2.0 cm embryo (*arrow*). Histologically, the villi showed generalized edema, and there was marked proliferation of the trophoblast.

millimeters to as large as 3.0 cm in diameter but usually average about 1.5 cm. Rarely, fetal development may occur in complete mole (Fig. 24.22). Following suction curettage, a large amount of bloody tissue may obscure the edematous villi, especially if a mole is extracted early in pregnancy when villous enlargement is less striking. Suction curettage also can distort molar villi by causing them to collapse. In this instance, there may be no gross evidence of molar enlargement, and histologic evaluation of the material adherent to the gauze used to collect the suctioned uterine contents is necessary to establish the diagnosis.

Microscopic Appearance. Complete moles are characterized by two features: trophoblastic proliferation and villous edema, although a few small villi usually are present. The majority of villi display central cistern formation characterized by a prominent central space that is entirely acellular (Fig. 24.23). The villi usually are avascular, although occasionally attenuated vascular spaces that may contain necrotic debris are found. Typically, patchy villous calcification is present. All hydatidiform moles display some degree of trophoblastic proliferation on the villous surface. This trophoblastic proliferation in hydatidiform mole is haphazard and circumferential around the villus. Columns and streamers of cells composed of a mixture of CT, ST, and IT project randomly from the villous surface (Figs. 24.4 and 24.24). Frequently, the trophoblast shows cytologic atypia (Fig. 24.8). The amount of proliferative trophoblast in moles varies greatly. It may be marked, affecting most villi, or it may be subtle and only focally present, emphasizing the need for thorough sampling. Large sheets of trophoblast appearing to be unattached to villi also may be present. These sheets of trophoblast result from tangential sectioning, or they represent detached fragments of the trophoblast that proliferates at the implantation site.

Partial Hydatidiform Mole

Clinical Aspects. Partial moles account for 25–43% of all molar pregnancies and occur between the 9th and 34th weeks of pregnancy.[40,183,211] Patients with partial moles may have signs and symptoms similar to those seen in complete moles, but usually this is less likely.[20,40,183] Uterine size is generally small for dates. Enlargement in excess of that expected for the gestational age is uncommon.[20,183] Frequently, patients with partial mole appear to have a missed abortion. Preeclampsia tends to occur later than in complete mole but can be equally severe in partial mole.[183] Serum hCG levels are often in the low or normal range for gestational age.[20,168] Only a few patients with partial mole show markedly elevated hCG titers such as those seen in complete mole.[40] A comparison of the clinical features of partial as compared to complete moles is shown in Table 24.3.

Gross Appearance. The volume of tissue is generally small, less than 100 or 200 ml. The villi are frequently grossly enlarged and recognizable as molar, yet are smaller than those found in complete mole[181,182] (Fig. 24.25). Fragments of more normal placental tissue may also be seen. A fetus or fetal membranes can frequently be identified (Fig. 24.26). If a fetus is present, it often shows gross congenital anomalies.[181]

Microscopic Appearance. Partial mole shows features in some villi that are similar to those seen in complete moles, but the molar change is focal[181,182] (Fig. 24.27). When there is evidence of a fetus or embryo as well, the diagnosis is readily apparent. In the absence of fetal tissues, the other morphologic criteria, most importantly the amount of villous involvement, must be carefully evaluated to render the appropriate diagnosis.

By definition, there should be a mixture of edematous villi and small, relatively normal sized villi.[40,181,182] Central cisterns are less conspicuous than in complete moles. Smaller villi may show stromal fibrosis similar to that seen in missed abortions (Fig. 24.28). Trophoblastic hyperplasia is less marked than in complete mole. It is generally more focal and shows little, if any, atypia. Another feature commonly encountered in partial mole is invaginations of trophoblast into the villous stroma, which results in the molar villi having a scalloped appearance.[182] When the invaginations do not show continuity with the surface trophoblast, they appear as inclusions within the stroma (Fig. 24.28). Invaginations are not exclusive for partial moles and may, on occasion, be found in other conditions including complete mole.

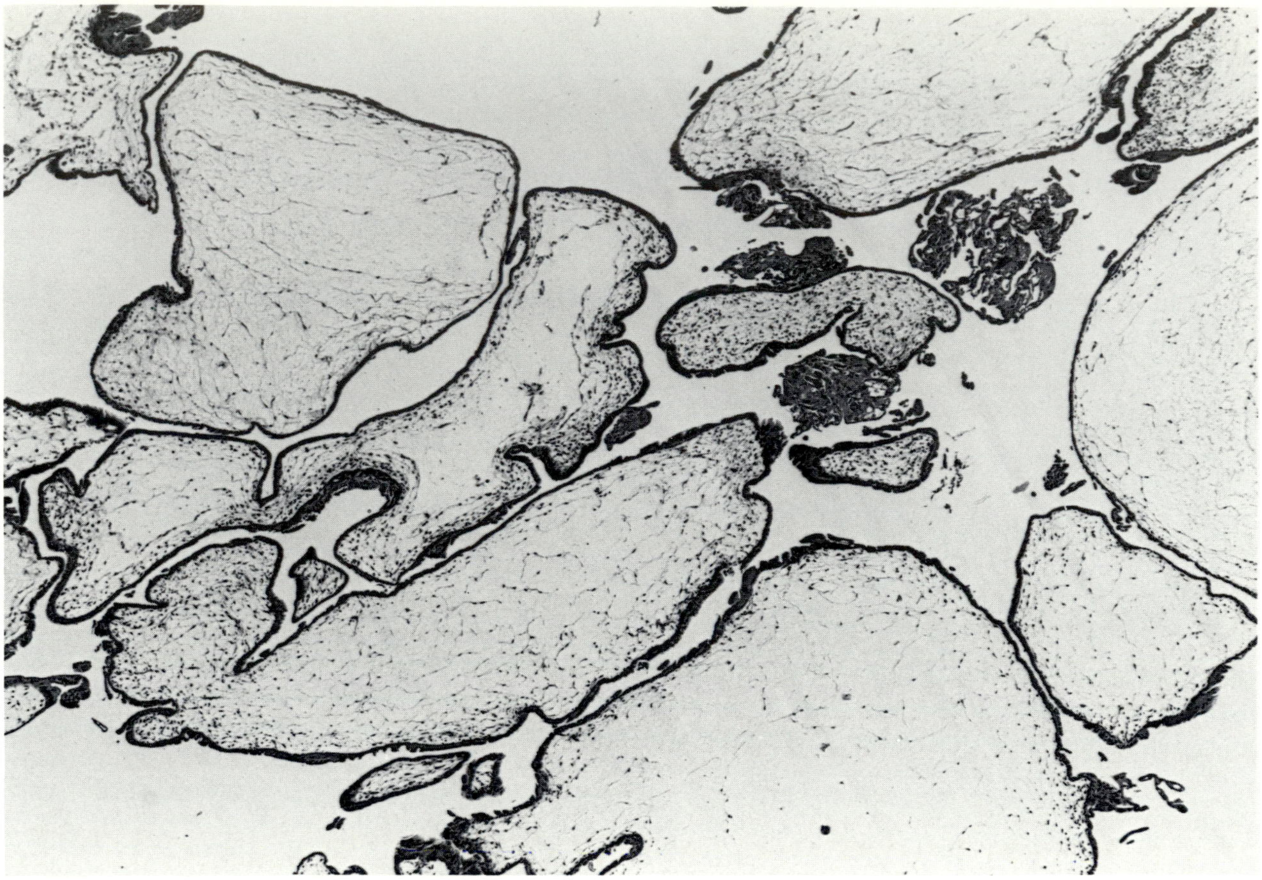

FIG. 24.23. Villi of a complete mole have extensive stromal edema with central cisterns. There is a minimal amount of proliferative trophoblast in this field.

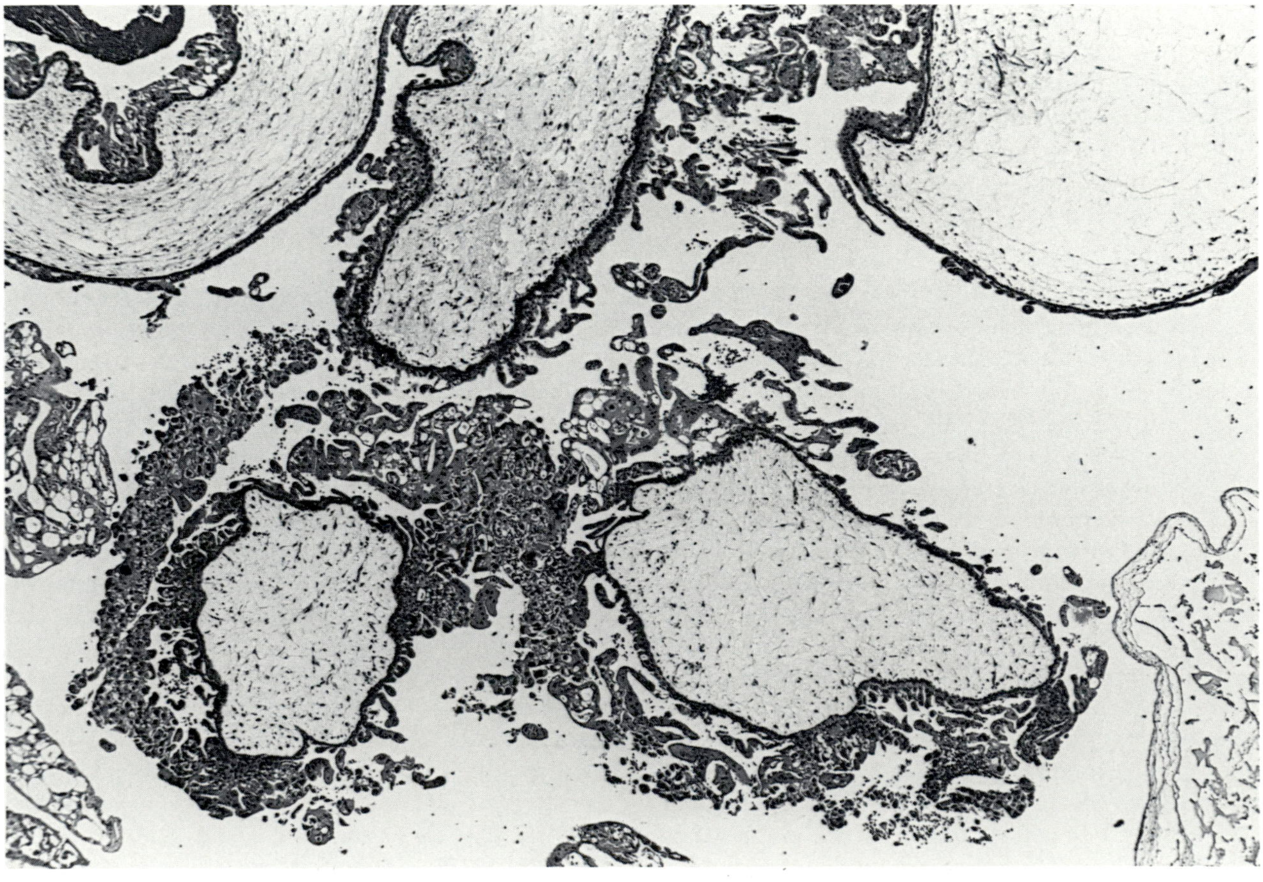

FIG. 24.24. Enlarged villi of complete mole have a circumferential proliferation of trophoblast from the surface of several villi. A portion of a necrotic villus is seen in the *right lower corner*.

TABLE 24.3. Clinical features of complete and partial moles.

Feature	Complete	Partial
Clinical presentation	Spontaneous abortion	Missed or spontaneous abortion
Gestational age	16–18 weeks	18–20 weeks
Uterine size	Often large for dates	Often small for dates
Serum hCG	++++	++
Behavior	10–30% develop persistent GTD	4–11% develop persistent GTD

Partial moles with triploid chromosomes are associated with the presence of a fetus or its amnionic covering, in contrast to the absence of fetal structures in most complete moles. Fetal demise with subsequent degeneration of fetal structures may make identification of fetal development more difficult, however. A subtle clue is the presence of a functioning villous circulation containing nucleated red cells, a feature that requires fetal development.[182] In contrast, the embryo associated with a complete mole usually dies before organogenesis, and, therefore, fetal structures are not present in the specimen. Similarly, fetal erythrocytes are not present within placental vessels. One theoretical concern in the diagnosis of an apparent partial mole is that the specimen represents a twin gestation with a fetus and a complete mole. Such twin pregnancies may occur[15,202A] but probably are a very infrequent occurrence relative to singleton gestations of a partial mole.

Differential Diagnosis. Most hydatidiform moles, complete and partial, are readily identifiable and present little diagnostic difficulty, but some may be extremely difficult to distinguish. The pathologic features of partial as compared to complete moles are shown in Table 24.4. A recent immunocytochemistry study indicates that the distribution of hCG and human placental alkaline phosphase (PLAP) can aid in this distinction. In complete moles, there is a much greater distribution of hCG compared to PLAP (Fig. 24.29), whereas in partial moles the reverse was found (Fig. 24.30).[26]

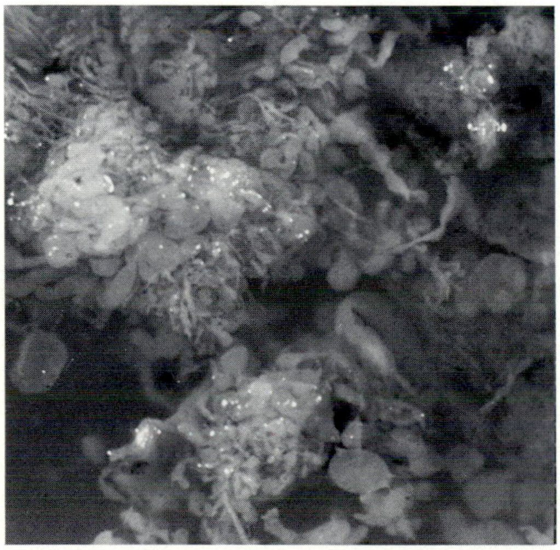

FIG. 24.25. Partial mole shows hydropic villi mixed with smaller villi.

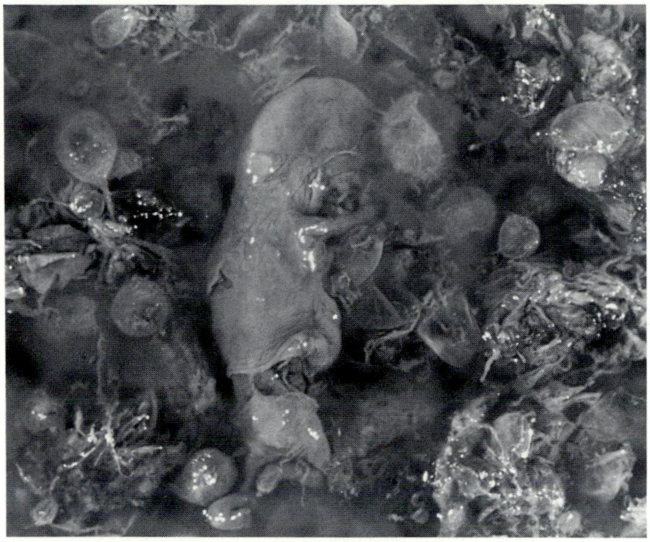

FIG. 24.26. Partial mole with a macerated fetus shows a portion of the villi with visible hydropic change. Often, the fetus in partial mole shows congenital abnormalities.

Distinction of a mole from an abortus with hydropic villi may be a problem.[56] Spontaneous abortions are often associated with failure of development or early demise of the embryo, the so-called blighted ovum. These specimens show some villous edema or hydropic swelling and an absence of villous blood vessels, features shared with molar placentas. Nonetheless, the villi of the blighted ovum are only slightly enlarged and do not assume the large dimensions found in molar gestations, complete or partial. Formation of cisterns does not occur in nonmolar abortions. Clearly, there must be a point when a developing gestation evolves into a molar pregnancy as "the missed abortion of a pathologic ovum,"[82] and the exact point at which the transformation is sufficient to warrant a diagnosis of molar pregnancy is not known. For practical purposes, however, if an abortion specimen shows villous edema that is only evident microscopically and lacks central cisterns, it should not be considered a molar pregnancy. In placentas with hydropic change, there is only focal staining for placental alkaline phosphatase, whereas in partial moles, the staining is significantly more[26] (Fig. 24.31).

The proliferative trophoblast of early pregnancy also must be distinguished from the trophoblastic hyperplasia

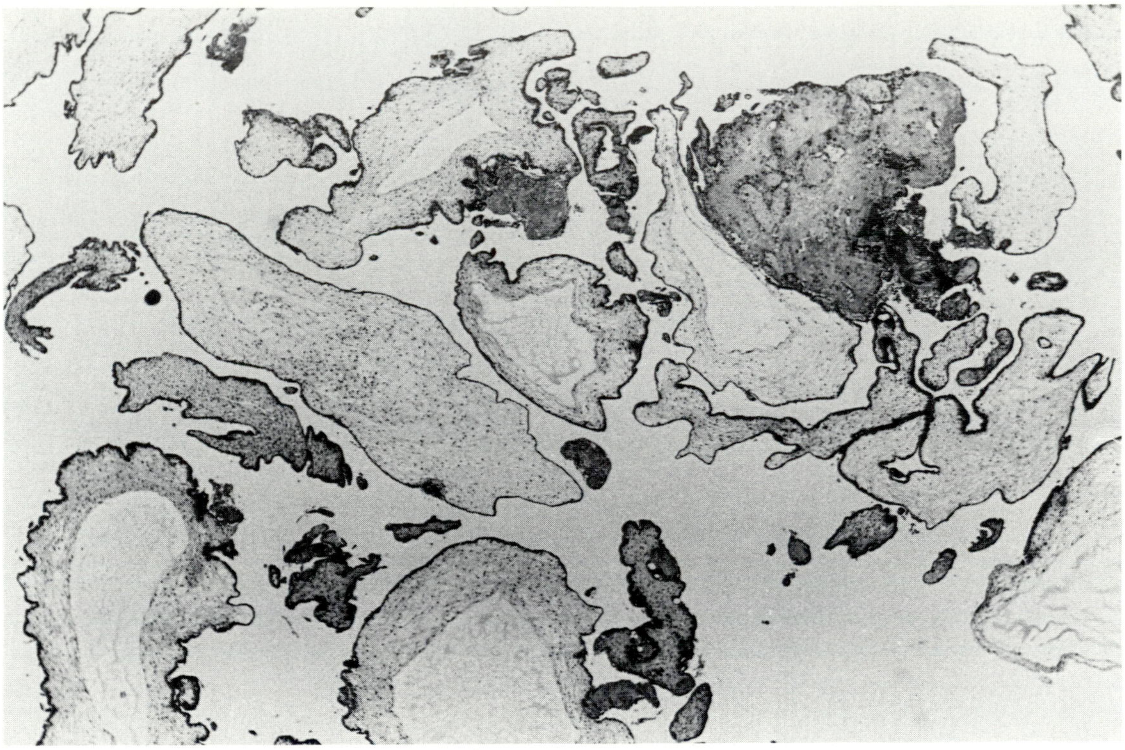

FIG. 24.27. Partial mole shows a mixture of enlarged villi with cisterns and small, normal-sized villi. A small degenerating fetus was present.

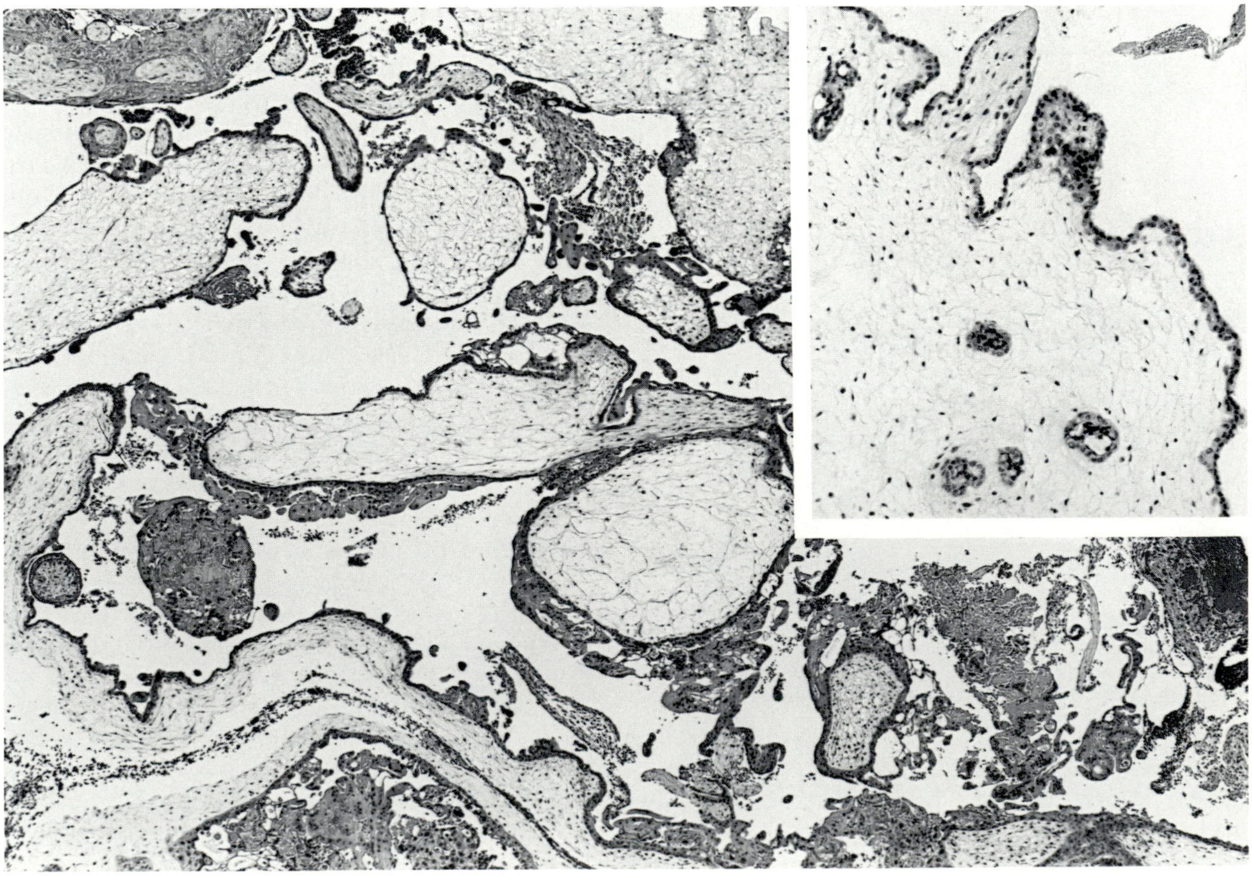

FIG. 24.28. A partial mole demonstrates proliferative trophoblast projecting randomly from the villus surface. Normal-sized, fibrotic villi are present in the left upper corner. This specimen consisted of 50 ml of tissue. There was no evidence of a fetus. *Inset:* Scalloped villous surface with trophoblast infolding forming inclusions.

TABLE 24.4. Pathologic features of complete and partial moles.

	Complete mole	Partial mole
Karyotype	46XX, 46XY	Triploid
Embryo/fetus	Absent	Present
Villus outline	Round	Scalloped
Hydropic swelling	Marked	Less pronounced
	Cisterns present	Cisterns less prominent
	All villi involved	Focal villous involvement
		Villous fibrosis
Trophoblastic proliferation	Circumferential	Focal
	Variable, may be marked	Minimal
Trophoblastic atypia	Often present	Absent
Immunocytochemistry		
hCG	++++	+
PLAP	+	++++

Adapted and reprinted with permission of World Health Organization, Ref. 212.
hCG, human chorionic gonadotropin; PLAP, placental alkaline phosphatase.

of molar pregnancy.[56,60] In very early gestation, masses of ST and CT are normally present at the implantation site. Characteristically, the trophoblast proliferating from the villous surface shows polarity, extending from the villi only in the direction of implantation, which contrasts with the irregular, circumferential proliferation of molar trophoblast. In later pregnancy, however, trophoblastic growth associated with villi is limited, and the finding of sheets of trophoblast should be viewed as abnormal. If the villi are not molar, the rare possibility of choriocarcinoma originating within a placenta should be considered.[27,28,52]

When large aggregates of atypical or proliferating trophoblast are encountered without any villi, the differential diagnosis should include choriocarcinoma or placental site trophoblastic tumor but not hydatidiform mole. Care must be taken to be certain that sampling is adequate. Limited examination of a uterine, vaginal, or pulmonary lesion may show only trophoblast, but further sectioning might reveal the presence of molar villi.[210]

Behavior. Severe respiratory distress may ensue immediately after uterine evacuation of a hydatidiform mole in 2–12% of patients.[71,107,133] This phenomenon is usually attributed to massive deportation of trophoblast to lungs,[107,204] an exaggeration of a physiologic process occurring in normal pregnancy.[51] It has been suggested that other factors, including fluid overload, dilutional edema, preeclampsia, and hyperthyroidism, may also contribute to the pathogenesis of this disease.[36,195] The greatest threat from hydatidiform mole, however, is the risk of persistent or metastatic GTD. Postmolar trophoblastic disease may represent persistent mole in the uterine cavity or it may be invasive mole or choriocarcinoma.

The frequency with which invasive mole or choriocarcinoma occurs after a molar gestation is dependent on the sensitivity of the follow-up hCG assay, length of follow-up, type of primary therapy, and terminology used in reporting sequelae.[33] Hertig and Sheldon,[85] in an early study performed before sensitive assays for hCG and cytotoxic chemotherapy were available, reported that 16% of hydatidiform moles developed into invasive moles and 2.5% into choriocarcinomas. These figures have been confirmed by more recent studies.[123] About 8–30% of patients with hydatidiform mole will require chemotherapy sometime after primary evacuation.[12,39,123,136] The wide range in the percentage of patients treated reflects the different criteria used by various investigators of what constitutes persistent disease.

The clinical correlates of partial mole are not as well known, since it has only recently been identified as a separate entity. Since most partial moles have evidence of development of an embryo or fetus, some authors have viewed all molar gestation with an associated fetus as a partial mole regardless of the morphology of the villi, but this is not correct. Nonetheless, it appears that the risk of persistent or metastatic GTD is less after a partial mole than after a complete mole. Several series have reported that only about 4% of patients with partial mole will have persistent or metastatic GTD that requires chemotherapy,[40,183] but other investigators have found that up to 11% of patients with a diagnosis of partial mole will require chemotherapy.[20,134,211] Invasive mole[66,184] and metastatic pulmonary lesions[172,211] have occurred in association with partial mole. There have been other reports of hydatidiform mole with a fetus that have been called partial mole that were followed by invasive mole and choriocarcinoma, but these reports did not give histologic verification of true partial molar change to the villi.[119,187] These cases emphasize the necessity of applying strict morphologic criteria for a diagnosis of partial mole to ensure exclusion of rare cases of complete mole with a fetus in clinicopathologic studies. Nonetheless, although the diagnosis of partial mole indicates a decreased risk of persistent GTD that requires treatment, patients with this diagnosis need the same follow-up as patients with complete mole until more is known about the behavior of the partial mole.

A number of clinical and pathologic features have been analyzed in an attempt to identify patients who are at increased risk of developing persistent GTD after uterine evacuation of a mole, but most studies have not distinguished complete from partial moles. Important clinical risk factors in over 60% of patients who have required

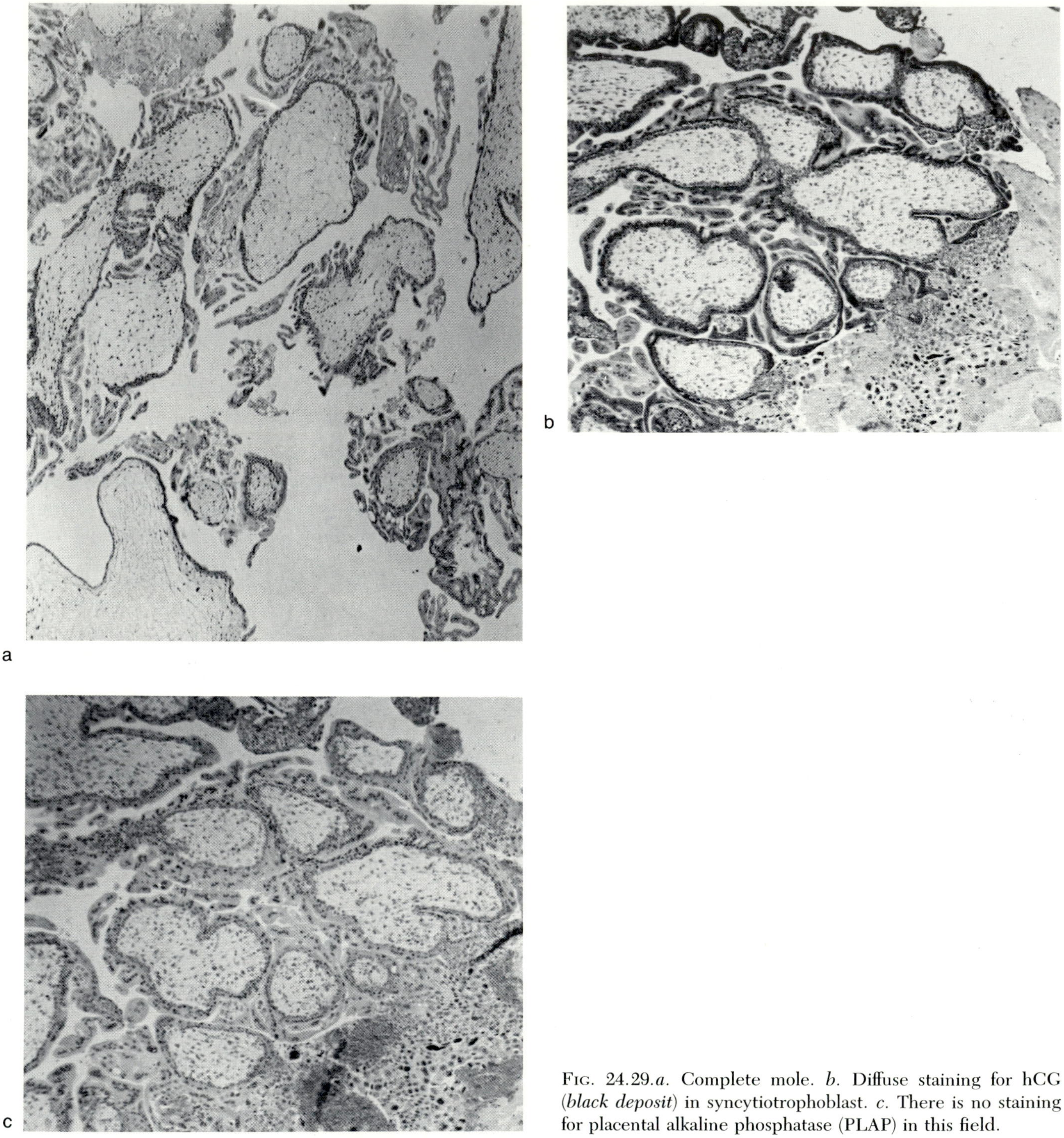

FIG. 24.29.*a*. Complete mole. *b*. Diffuse staining for hCG (*black deposit*) in syncytiotrophoblast. *c*. There is no staining for placental alkaline phosphatase (PLAP) in this field.

subsequent chemotherapy, however, included large-for-dates uteri and ovarian enlargement due to theca–lutein cysts.[39,133]

Morphologic studies have tried to predict the prognosis of moles based on the degree of trophoblastic proliferation and atypia,[53,84,85] but at present it appears that grading of moles has little predictive value, since moles with little trophoblastic proliferation may still develop postmolar disease requiring therapy. Conversely, not all patients with proliferative and atypical trophoblast in moles will require therapy.[39,59,190] Part of the difficulty in grading may be due to the marked variation of the trophoblastic proliferation and atypia in microscopic sections of moles. Although evaluation of the amount of trophoblas-

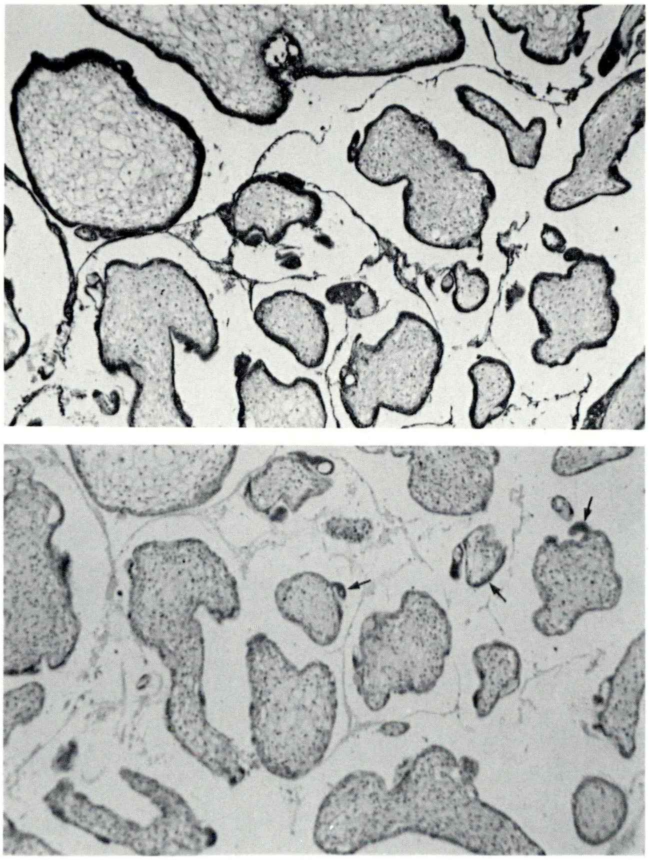

FIG. 24.30. *Bottom* panel shows only focal staining for hCG (*arrows*) in this partial mole. *Top* panel shows diffuse staining (*black deposit*) for PLAP.

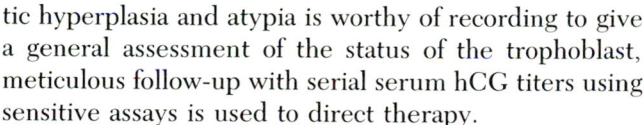

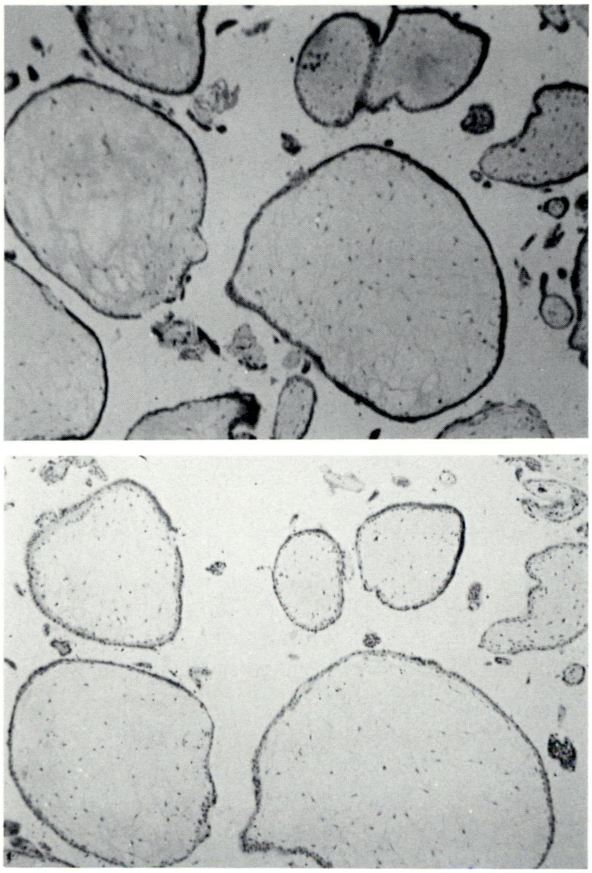

FIG. 24.31. Abortus with hydropic change. *Bottom* panel shows diffuse staining (*black deposit*) for hCG. *Top* panel shows no staining for PLAP. Compare with Figure 24.30.

tic hyperplasia and atypia is worthy of recording to give a general assessment of the status of the trophoblast, meticulous follow-up with serial serum hCG titers using sensitive assays is used to direct therapy.

Between 0.6 and 1.5% of patients who have had a complete hydatidiform mole are at risk of having recurrent molar pregnancies.[64,124] As many as nine consecutive molar pregnancies have been reported.[213] The magnitude of the risk of repeated partial moles is not known. Some reports suggest that recurrent molar pregnancy may show more proliferative trophoblast and that the likelihood of the need for chemotherapy is greater than with the first molar gestation.[64] Successful term pregnancies may occur after recurrent disease, however.[124]

Invasive Mole

Clinical Aspects. Invasive mole is a possible sequela of hydatidiform mole, complete or partial. The diagnosis depends on demonstrating molar villi invading the myometrium, and consequently the diagnosis is almost always made on a hysterectomy specimen. Since hysterectomy is rarely performed in patients with persistent hCG titers after removal of an intrauterine mole and since metastatic lesions of GTD are usually successfully treated with cytotoxic chemotherapy without biopsy, invasive mole is rarely confirmed histologically.[45] It is unusual for invasive mole to present primarily, although invasive mole may be present simultaneously with a molar pregnancy.[90] When metastases occur they generally are found in the lungs, vagina, vulva, or broad ligament.[1,90,99,188,210]

Gross Appearance. In the uterus, an invasive mole is an erosive, hemorrhagic lesion extending from the uterine cavity into the myometrium (Fig. 24.32). Invasion can range from superficial penetration to extension through the wall, with perforation or involvement of the broad ligament. Molar vesicles often are grossly apparent.

Microscopic Appearance. Microscopically, the diagnostic feature is the presence of molar villi along with trophoblast outside of the endometrial cavity (Fig. 24.33). Trophoblastic proliferation with atypia invariably accompanies the enlarged villi and is as variable as in noninva-

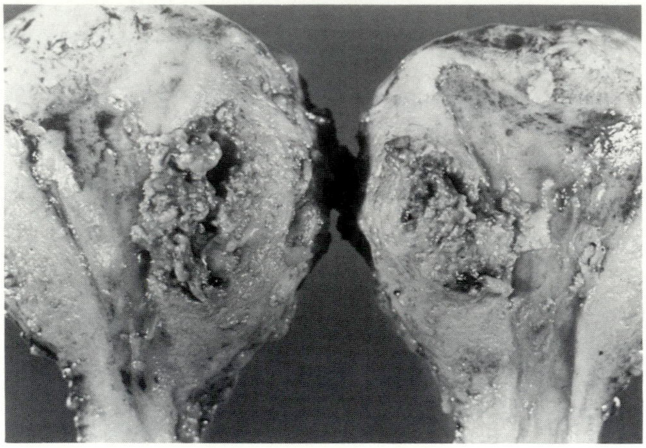

FIG. 24.32. Invasive mole infiltrates deeply into the myometrium, forming a ragged, irregular mass.

sive mole, ranging from slightly proliferative or atypical trophoblast to marked trophoblastic proliferation with extreme atypia. Hydropic swelling tends not to be as marked as in noninvasive mole. Molar villi are usually no more than 4 to 5 mm in diameter. In metastatic sites, the diagnosis is based on the presence of villi. Careful searching may be necessary to identify villi within a lesion seemingly composed entirely of highly proliferative trophoblast. Lesions at distant sites are usually composed of molar villi confined within blood vessels without invasion into adjacent tissue. Some authors prefer to regard this as deportation rather than metastasis.

Behavior. Invasive mole is the most common form of persistent or metastatic GTD following hydatidiform mole, occurring 6–10 times more frequently than choriocarcinoma.[33,85,123] In histologically verified cases, the lesion most often is confined to the uterus, with metastases occurring in 24–40% of cases.[57] Metastases most frequently occur in the lungs, and these may be multiple or localized. Spread to the vagina, vulva, and broad ligament is well recognized.[1,74,210] Metastases to other sites are unusual, but rare examples of histologically verified metastases to regions, such as the paraspinal soft tissue, have been reported.[46,92] Before cytotoxic chemotherapy was available, 4–15% of patients with invasive mole died of disease.[29,57,58,74] Mortality was usually due to local complications, such as uterine perforation with intraperitoneal hemorrhage.[57,58] Death from metastasis occurred less frequently. Most patients, even those with metastases, survived, and untreated metastases frequently showed spontaneous regression.[154,188,210] The risk of progression to choriocarcinoma is no greater than that following complete mole.[143,148] Using modern chemotherapy, death from invasive mole is extremely unusual.[32,122]

Invasive mole must be discriminated from choriocarcinoma, but this is often not possible clinically.[210] Both invasive mole and choriocarcinoma following a hydatidiform mole are manifested by a plateau or elevation in the hCG titer, and both can give rise to metastatic lesions. A repeat curettage may yield more molar tissue, choriocarcinoma, or no trophoblastic tissue. When molar tissue is found, a diagnosis of persistent hydatidiform mole is made, and invasive mole remains an elusive pathologic diagnosis. Invasive mole is the clinical diagnosis given to many patients with metastases or abnormally persistent hCG titers after molar pregnancy and no residual hydatidiform mole within the uterine cavity.[32,122] In such instances, there is a possibility that persistent hCG levels may, however, be due to choriocarcinoma. In these cases, the clinical term *persistent GTD* is used without attempting to discriminate between an invasive mole and choriocarcinoma.

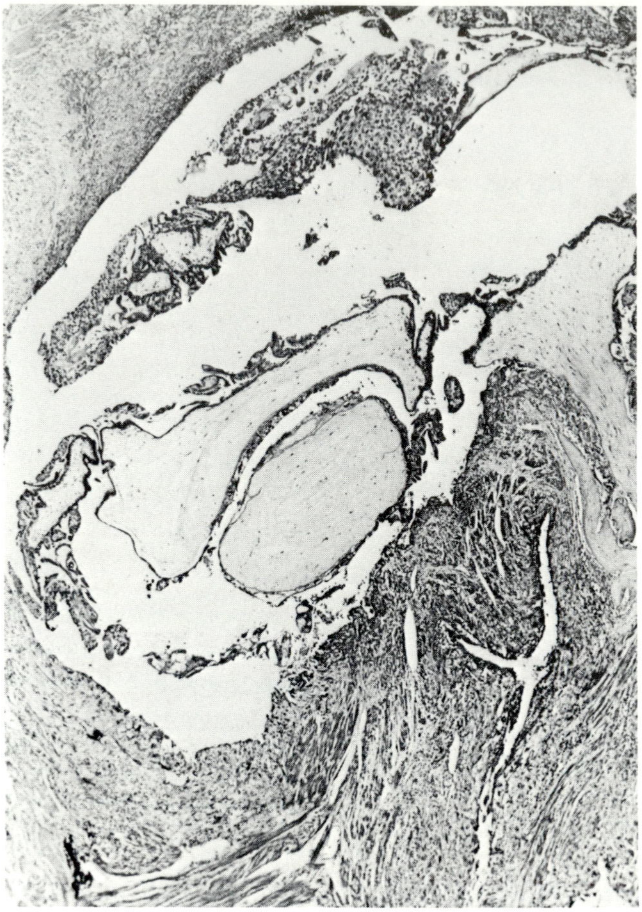

FIG. 24.33. Invasive mole deep within the myometrium shows a hydropic villus within a large vein. Proliferative trophoblast accompanies the villi.

Choriocarcinoma

Clinical Aspects. This highly aggressive neoplasm of trophoblast may be associated with any form of gestation.

Theoretically, choriocarcinoma may arise in the trophoblast of the primitive blastocyst before implantation, but most cases of choriocarcinoma appear to follow a recognizable gestational event. The more abnormal the pregnancy, the more likely that choriocarcinoma may supervene. Hertig and Mansell found an incidence of 1 in 160,000 normal gestations, 1 in 15,386 abortions, 1 in 5,333 ectopic pregnancies, and 1 in 40 molar pregnancies.[84] In that series, one half of the cases of choriocarcinoma were preceded by hydatidiform mole, with 25% following abortion, 22.5% following normal pregnancy, and 2.5% following ectopic pregnancy.[84] Other studies have generally confirmed these figures.[122]

The signs and symptoms of choriocarcinoma are protean, whether it occurs in association with a molar or nonmolar pregnancy.[80,143,146] Abnormal uterine bleeding is one of the most frequent presentations of choriocarcinoma,[146] (Fig. 24.34) but uterine lesions may be restricted to the myometrium and remain asymptomatic (Fig. 24.35). Not all patients will have a demonstrable lesion in the uterus after an intrauterine gestation. Many examples of metastatic choriocarcinoma with no uterine tumor have been described.[33,89,102,129] Apparently the neoplasm either skips the uterus while spreading through the bloodstream or undergoes regression in the uterus.[33,89,150]

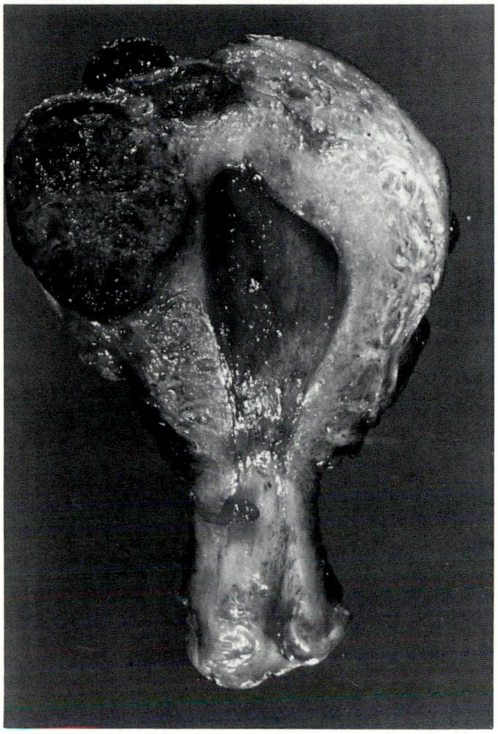

FIG. 24.35. Choriocarcinoma forms a circumscribed mass within the myometrium that does not involve the endometrium. Lesions such as this may be asymptomatic because of their location.

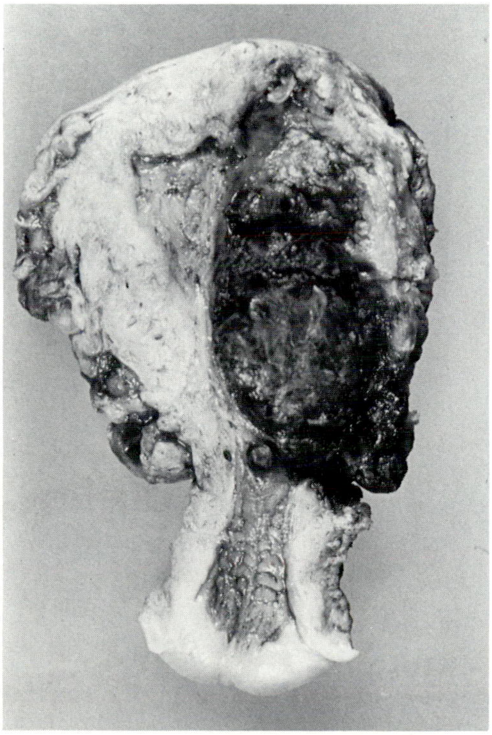

FIG. 24.34. Choriocarcinoma within the uterus forms a large, hemorrhagic mass that involves the endometrium and myometrium.

Sometimes, symptoms related to metastases are the first indication that choriocarcinoma is present.[34,194] The lungs are the most frequent site for bloodborne lesions,[118,129,143] and a patient may have hemoptysis.[191] Symptomatology related to hemorrhagic events in the central nervous system, liver, and gastrointestinal or urinary tracts may also occur[47,73,199] (Figs. 24.36 and 24.37). Choriocarcinoma may have an unusually long latent period,[76,113,150] occurring 10 or more years after hysterectomy or tubal ligation. Rare examples of choriocarcinoma in postmenopausal women have been reported.[50] Thyroxicosis may occur in choriocarcinoma.[139]

Over 90% of patients with extrauterine gestational choriocarcinoma will have lung metastases.* The frequency of involvement of other sites is somewhat variable, depending on whether the data represent autopsy studies or whether the patients have received chemotherapy. Brain and liver metastases frequently are found, occurring in 20–60% of patients.[57,102,129,143] Kidney and abdomen, including intestinal tract, are the other common sites of spread, but almost any organ, including the skin, may be involved.[62,129,143] Lymph nodes will contain tumor on occasion, often as tertiary

* References 89, 102, 118, 129, 143, 150.

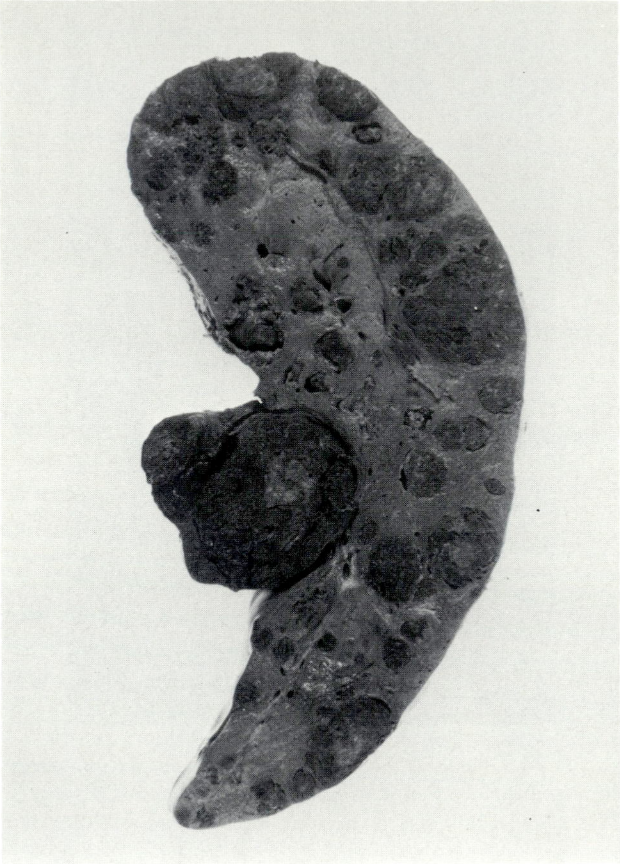

FIG. 24.36. Liver metastases from choriocarcinoma form multiple, circumscribed, hemorrhagic masses.

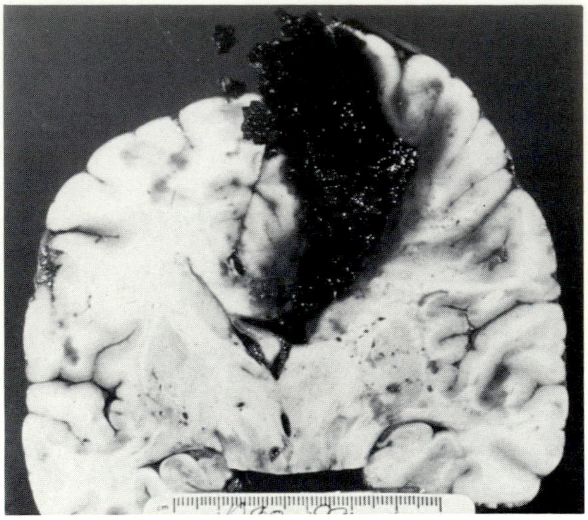

FIG. 24.37. Metastatic choriocarcinoma to the central nervous system with extensive hemorrhage that caused death. At autopsy, the patient had metastases in multiple organs.

lesions from metastases in other organs.[129,143] Vaginal involvement has been reported in 16–32% of patients.[102,129,140,143] There have been a few isolated reports of metastatic choriocarcinoma occurring in the mother and child of a term pregnancy.[3,41] Usually, the infant is free of disease.

Gross Appearance. Uterine choriocarcinoma generally is a dark red, hemorrhagic mass with a shaggy, irregular surface[57,58,140,143] (Figs. 24.34 and 24.35). Occasionally, a lesion may lack significant hemorrhage and appear as a fleshy, tan-gray mass with necrosis. The size of uterine lesions varies greatly, ranging from tiny, microscopic foci to huge, necrotic tumors. Metastases beyond the uterus appear well circumscribed and hemorrhagic[143] (Figs. 24.36 and 24.37). Ill-defined, infiltrative growth is unusual because of the rapid proliferation with hemorrhage and necrosis that characterize the neoplasm.

Microscopic Appearance. Choriocarcinoma usually has a readily identifiable microscopic appearance, with a mixture of CT, IT, and ST[†] (Figs. 24.5, 24.7, 24.38, and

[†] References 45, 53, 56–58, 140, 143, 148.

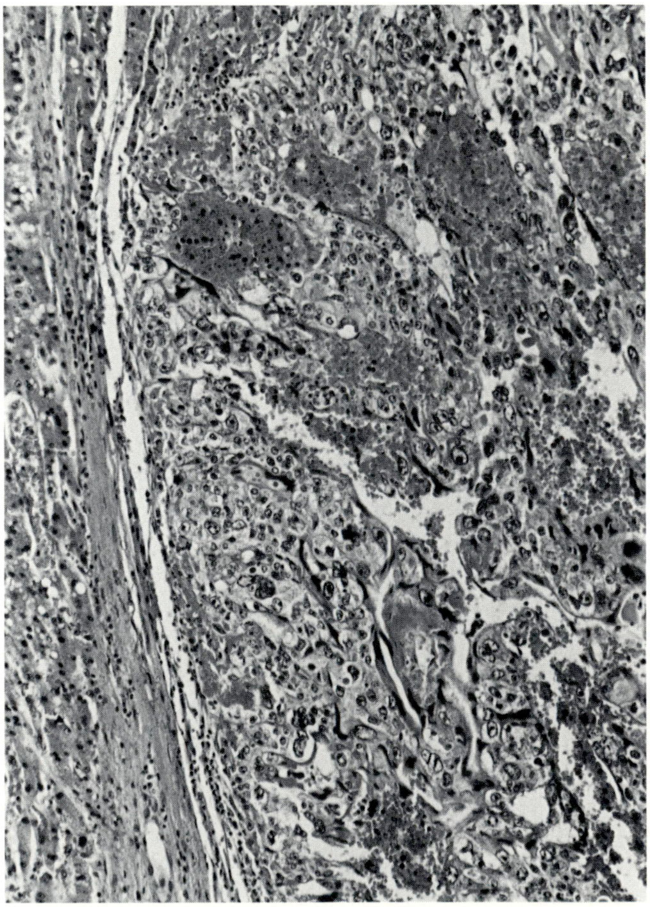

FIG. 24.38. Metastatic choriocarcinoma in the liver shows syncytiotrophoblast, cytotrophoblast, and intermediate trophoblast. Hemorrhage and necrosis are typical of the lesion. On the *left*, the boundary with preserved liver is circumscribed.

24.39). The tumor is characterized by masses and sheets of cells that invade surrounding tissue and permeate vascular spaces. Generally, the pattern of growth recapitulates that of the early previllous trophoblast, but a wide variation in patterns may occur. The interface with normal tissues, if preserved, is circumscribed and appears expansile (Fig. 24.38). Vascular invasion may be prominent in uterine lesions. Often, viable tumor constitutes only a thin rim around a central area of hemorrhage and necrosis. Extensive sectioning may be necessary to identify the typical pattern of choriocarcinoma. The tumor can undergo extensive necrosis so that little or no viable tissue is identified in a lesion. Generally, choriocarcinoma has no intrinsic vascular stroma, the tumor receiving its vascular supply by syncytial cells permeating and replacing host vessels.[45,53,143] Infiltrative growth of normal tissues and blood vessels, however, can add an apparent vascular framework to the pattern.[129]

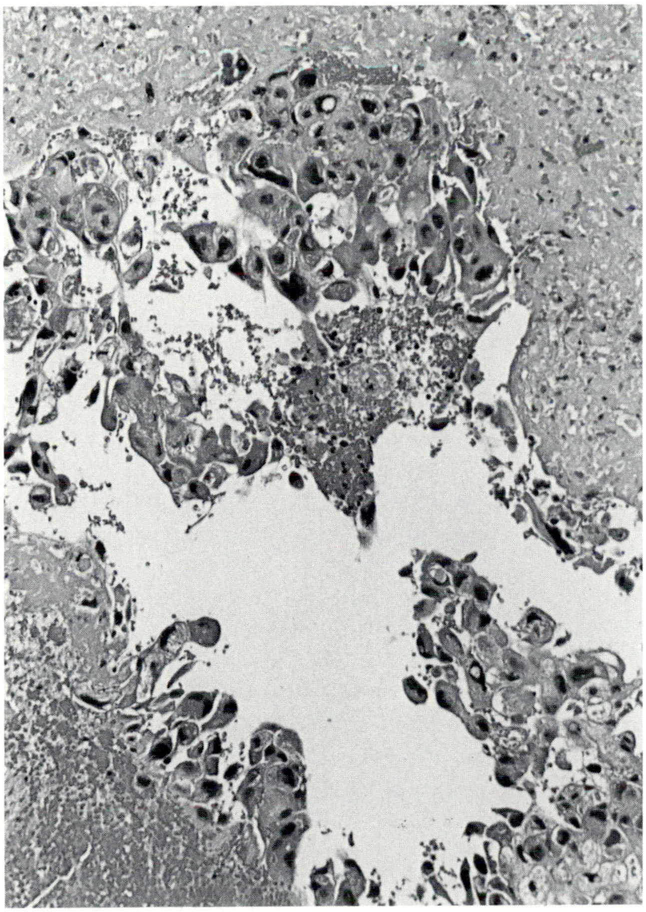

FIG. 24.39. Portion of uterine choriocarcinoma shows predominance of intermediate trophoblast that is composed largely of mononucleate and binucleate cells with amphophilic cytoplasm. In other areas, this tumor showed biphasic cytotrophoblast and syncytiotrophoblast.

Differential Diagnosis. Choriocarcinoma must be distinguished from the normal trophoblast of early gestations, from molar pregnancies, from placental site trophoblastic tumor, and from other forms of epithelial malignancy.[60] Occasionally, normal trophoblast of an early gestation will be found in curettings without associated villi. In this circumstance, the trophoblast should be present only in small quantities. Normal trophoblast of an early gestation, although proliferative, does not show atypical features with the marked cellular enlargement and nuclear abnormalities found in choriocarcinoma. Large amounts of trophoblast showing atypia and no associated villi should be viewed suspiciously for choriocarcinoma. If the diagnosis is in doubt, a chest x-ray and careful monitoring of beta-hCG levels should resolve the problem.

As a general rule, choriocarcinoma should not be diagnosed in the presence of villi.[140] Proliferative trophoblast in association with villi usually indicates either an abortion or hydatidiform mole. The differential diagnosis of these lesions is discussed under hydatidiform mole. Rarely, gestational choriocarcinoma can arise within an otherwise normally developing placenta, with the neoplasm intimately associated with well-formed nonmolar villi[27,28,52,194] (Fig. 24.40), but careful sectioning of other suspected examples of choriocarcinoma with villi is necessary to exclude an abortion or a molar pregnancy.

Discriminating choriocarcinoma from other carcinomas either within the uterus or at other sites usually is not a problem, but on occasion a biopsy or curetting of choriocarcinoma may show only a few ST cells, and the pattern can mimic a poorly differentiated carcinoma (Fig. 24.41).[129] When this differential diagnosis arises, the clinical history may reveal a previous molar pregnancy or another suspicious pregnancy event that can clarify the diagnosis. Serum hCG levels and immunocytochemical localization of hCG are extremely helpful.

Behavior. In the past, gestational choriocarcinoma was usually fatal.[143] Before cytotoxic chemotherapy was available, hysterectomy and, in some instances, irradiation were the only forms of treatment. The absolute 5-year survival for patients treated by hysterectomy before the chemotherapy era was 32%.[30] If metastases were not evident at the time of surgery, the survival rate was 41%, whereas if metastases were present, the survival rate was 19%. Survival rates have improved dramatically since the introduction of cytotoxic chemotherapy combined with accurate and sensitive assays for hCG to monitor the course of the disease. The overall survival now for persistent and metastatic GTD is about 90%.[116,122] When a morphologic diagnosis of choriocarcinoma is established, however, the survival rate is less, declining to 81% of all patients with choriocarcinoma and 71% of patients with metastatic choriocarcinoma.[122]

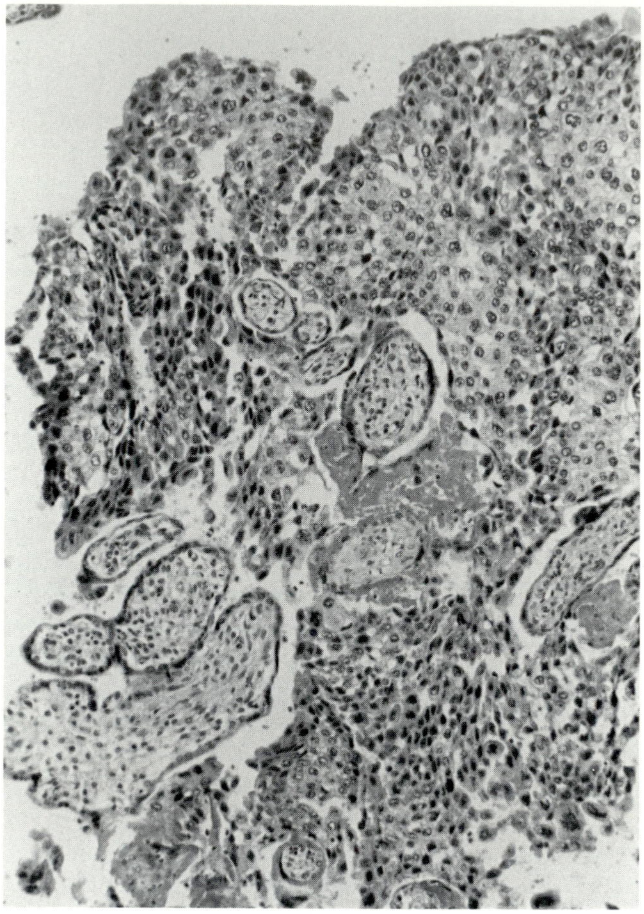

FIG. 24.40. Choriocarcinoma arising in a placenta shows malignant trophoblast arising from the surface of normally formed villi.

There are several clinical features that are useful in predicting the response to treatment. Poor prognostic factors include advanced disease at diagnosis, cerebral or hepatic metastases, symptoms of the disease for more than 4 months, failure of prior chemotherapy, and a pretreatment serum beta-hCG titer of greater than 100,000 mIU/ml.[7,79,115,120] More recently, the critical hCG level has been reduced to 40,000 mIU/ml by some investigators.[177,179,208] Metastatic disease limited to the lungs or vagina is not a poor prognostic sign. Choriocarcinoma following term gestation has a generally worse prognosis than that following a mole. These patients have lower cure rates than other poor prognosis patients, the decreased survival attributed to delay in treatment and metastases beyond the lungs and vagina.[19,131,146] Although it is difficult to assess the precise prognostic significance of extrapulmonary metastases, patients with central nervous system metastases have an approximately 50% remission rate.[4,9,207] Development of central nervous system metastases during the course of treatment has an even worse prognosis.[4,9,122] Patients with hepatic metastases have a poor prognosis,[14A] but multiagent chemotherapy appears to increase the survival rate.[211A]

Histologic features that have been reported to correlate with response to treatment and clinical outcome include a marked lymphoid infiltrate, high mitotic activity, nuclear atypia, vascular invasion, and a compact growth pattern showing minimal differentiation into ST.[48,61,93,101,129,138] These observations may have prognostic value but are based on a small number of cases, and therefore further study is needed to determine if they are significant.

Death from choriocarcinoma most commonly results from hemorrhage or pulmonary insufficiency.[18,121,129] Fatal hemorrhage usually occurs in the CNS or lungs, but intraperitoneal and gastrointestinal hemorrhage also can cause death.[18,129] Exsanguination may occur after biopsy of a vaginal metastasis.[33] Pulmonary insufficiency can be caused either by a large tumor burden or by the effects of irradiation and cytotoxic chemotherapy.[129]

Placental Site Trophoblastic Tumor

The placental site trophoblastic tumor (PSTT) of the uterus is the rarest form of GTD. The tumor was originally termed *atypical chorioepithelioma* by Marchand,[125] but because of its rarity, it never became established as a separate entity distinct from choriocarcinoma. In the century after its initial description, it was periodically rediscovered and renamed. Terms that have been used include *atypical choriocarcinoma*,[149] *syncytioma*,[63] *chorioepitheliosis*,[166,198] and *trophoblastic pseudotumor*,[110] but these are no longer considered appropriate.[167] Occasionally, the tumor has been mistaken for a sarcoma.[68,83,141]

Clinical Aspects. Patients are in the reproductive age group and can have either amenorrhea or abnormal bleeding, often accompanied by uterine enlargement.[54,68,110] These women frequently are thought to be pregnant. The results of pregnancy tests depend on the type of test used, but with a sensitive immunologic assay, they are almost always positive. When progressive uterine enlargement ceases, the diagnosis of a missed abortion is made.[110] In one patient, PSTT was associated with virilization.[135] The clinical features of PSTT as compared to choriocarcinoma are shown in Table 24.5.

Gross Appearance. The lesion varies from one that is only microscopic in size to a diffuse nodular enlargement of the myometrium. Most of the tumors are well circumscribed but sometimes they are ill-defined. The PSTT may be polypoid, projecting into the uterine cavity or predominantly invading the myometrium (Fig. 24.42). The sectioned surface is soft and tan and contains only

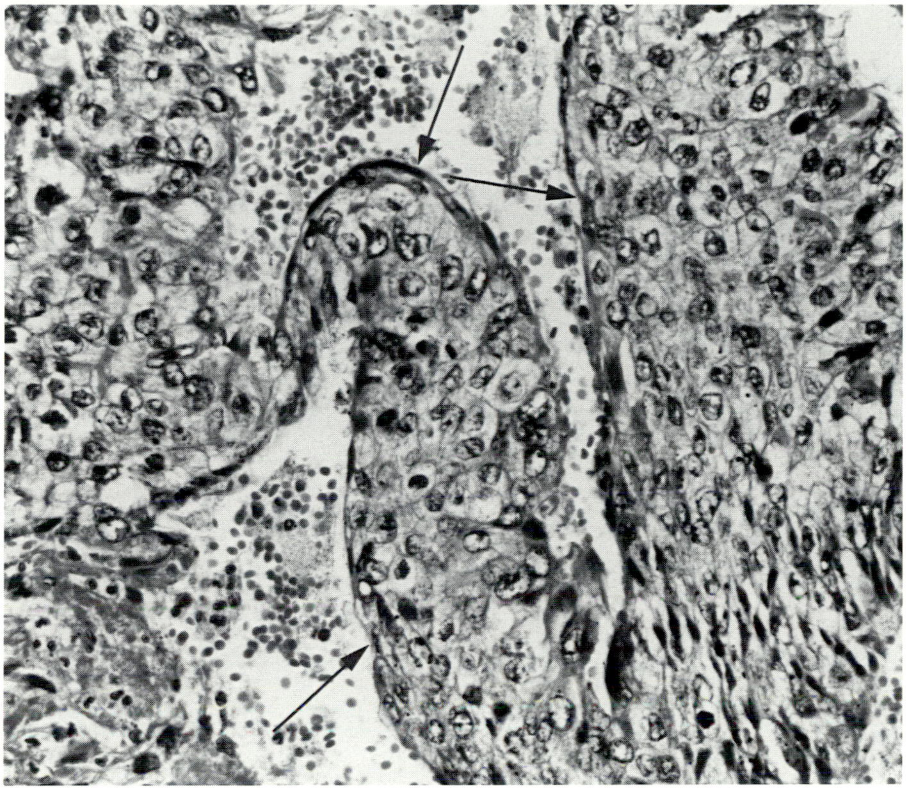

FIG. 24.41. Most of the cells in this choriocarcinoma are cytotrophoblast and may simulate a poorly differentiated carcinoma. Syncytiotrophoblast (*arrows*) is attenuated, forming a thin layer between the cytotrophoblast and vascular spaces.

focal areas of hemorrhage or necrosis. Invasion frequently extends to the uterine serosa and, in rare instances, to the adnexal structures.

Microscopic Appearance. The predominant cell in PSTT is IT.[109,111] The majority of the cellular population is monomorphic in contrast to the mixture of cell types

TABLE 24.5. Clinical features of placental site trophoblastic tumor (PSTT) and choriocarcinoma.

Feature	PSTT	Choriocarcinoma
Clinical presentation	Missed abortion	Persistent GTD after hydatidiform mole
Serum hCG	Low	High
Behavior	Self-limited Persistent or Highly aggressive	Highly aggressive
Response to chemotherapy	Poor	Good
Treatment	Surgery (hysterectomy)	Chemotherapy

GTD, gestational trophoblastic disease; hCG, human chorionic gonadotropin.

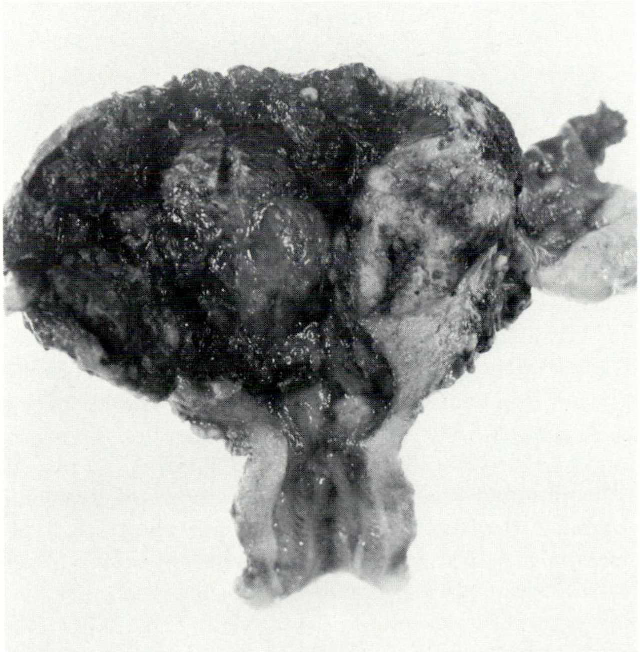

FIG. 24.42. Opened uterus showing a large, erosive placental site trophoblastic tumor involving most of the fundus. The tumor invaded to the serosal surface. The uterus was perforated at curettage.

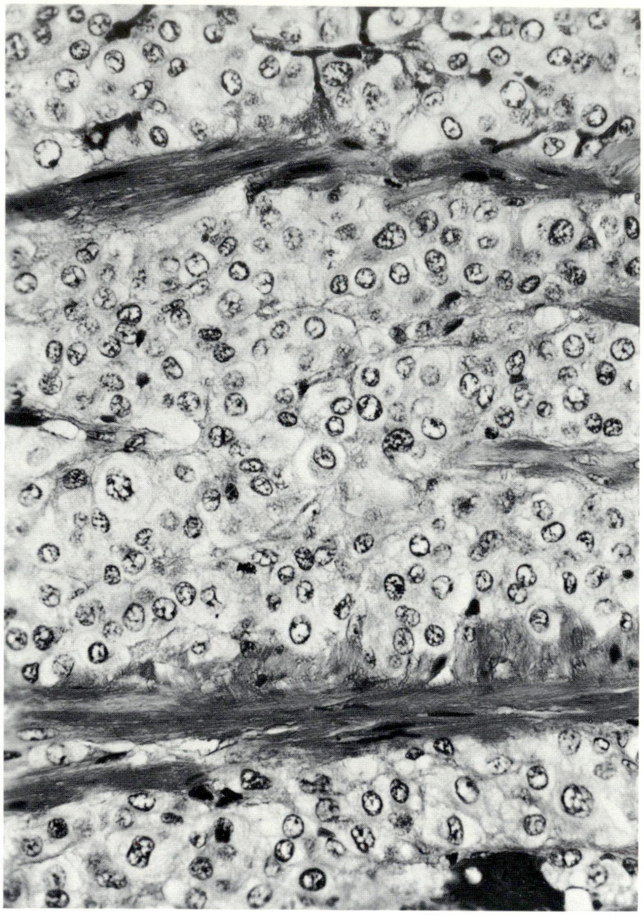

FIG. 24.43. Placental site trophoblastic tumor is composed of a monomorphic population of intermediate trophoblast in contrast to the mixture of cytotrophoblast, syncytiotrophoblast, and intermediate trophoblast in choriocarcinoma.

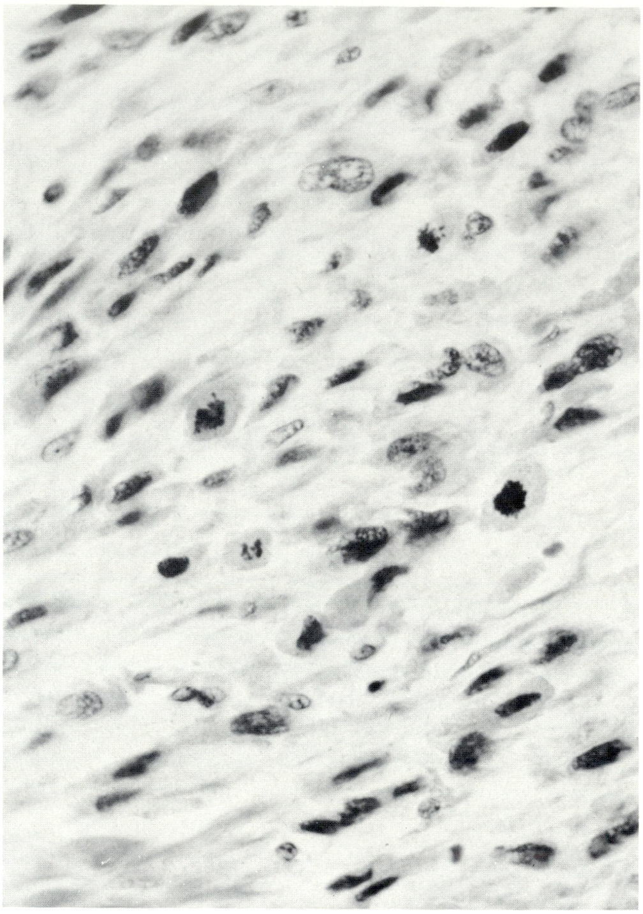

FIG. 24.44. Cells of placental site trophoblastic tumor may assume spindle-shape and may, therefore, be confused with leiomyosarcoma. Four mitotic figures are in center of field. (Reprinted with permission from Kurman et al., Ref. 110.)

in other forms of GTD (Figs. 24.9, 24.10, 24.43, and 24.44). The IT cells invade singly or in cords and sheets, characteristically separating individual muscle fibers and groups of fibers without producing extensive destruction of the muscle. Many of the intermediate trophoblastic cells assume a spindle-shape (Fig. 24.44) and are closely apposed to myometrial cells (Fig. 24.10). The neoplasm has a characteristic form of vascular invasion in which the blood vessel wall appears to be completely replaced by trophoblastic cells or fibrin, as observed near the placental site (Fig. 24.45). Decidua or an Arias-Stella reaction may be present in the adjacent, uninvolved endometrium. Villi are generally not present.

Differential Diagnosis. The PSTT must be distinguished from choriocarcinoma. In contrast to choriocarcinoma, the PSTT lacks the biphasic cell pattern, being composed of a relatively monotonous cell population (Table 24.6). Other neoplasms in the differential diagnosis include sarcomas, especially epithelioid leiomyosarcoma because of the infiltrative pattern within the myometrium, poorly differentiated carcinoma, or even metastatic melanoma because many of the cells have a distinct epithelial appearance. The pattern of prominent blood vessel invasion (Figs. 24.45 and 24.46), characteristic myometrial invasion (Fig. 24.10), and extensive deposition of fibrinoid material (Fig. 24.45) are helpful diagnostic features of PSTT. Immunoperoxidase stains for hPL and hCG can assist in the differential diagnosis.[111] Immunoperoxidase stains for hPL are typically diffusely positive within PSTT and only focally positive for hCG, whereas the reverse staining pattern is seen in choriocarcinoma (Figs. 24.47, 24.48, 24.49, and 24.50). Localization of hPL and hCG in a PSTT showing a prominent spindle cell pattern is helpful in distinguishing the PSTT from sarcomas which are negative (Fig. 24.50).

The PSTT also must be differentiated from a normal but exaggerated placental site. Distinction may be diffi-

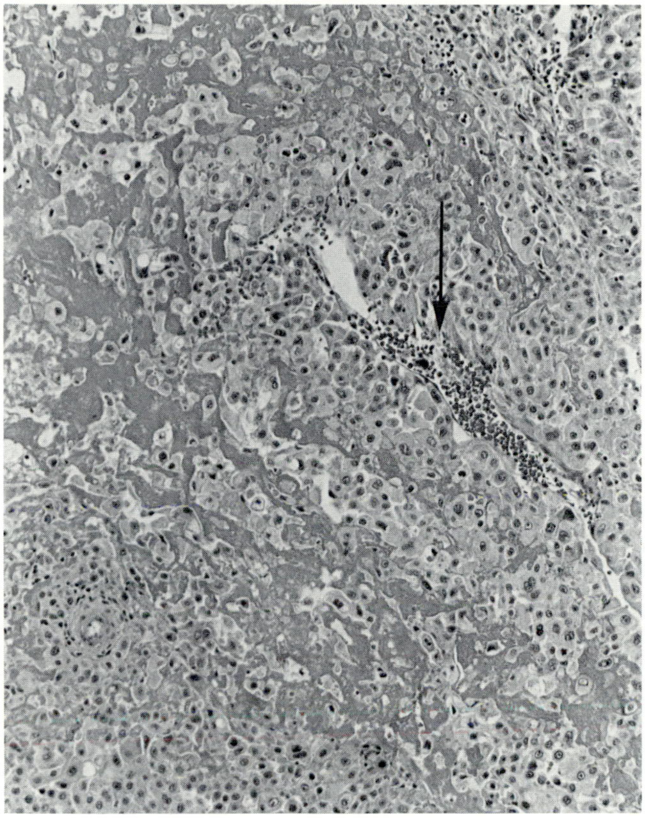

FIG. 24.45. Fibrin and intermediate trophoblast replace the wall of a uterine blood vessel in placental site trophoblastic tumor. The vessel lumen (*arrow*) still contains red cells.

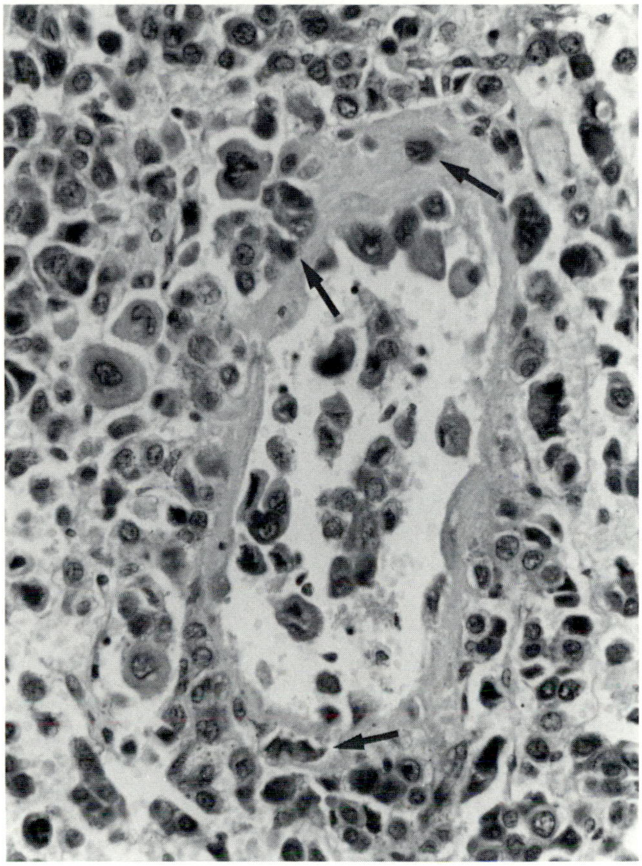

FIG. 24.46. Vascular invasion by intermediate trophoblast in placental site trophoblastic tumor resembles that of the normal implantation site (compare to Fig. 24.20). The neoplastic cells surround and invade (*arrows*) a blood vessel, extending into the vascular lumen. The vessel wall has been replaced by fibrin. The tissue is immunostained for hPL, and all the neoplastic cells in this field contain hPL. (Reprinted with permission of Kurman et al., Ref. 111.)

cult in curettings. Generally, in the placental site the intermediate trophoblastic cells do not form confluent masses, and there is little or no mitotic activity. In addition, other chorionic elements, including villi and spiral arteries, will appear in normal implantations but not in PSTT.

TABLE 24.6. Pathologic features of placental site trophoblastic tumor (PSTT) and choriocarcinoma.

Feature	PSTT	Choriocarcinoma
Cellular population	Monomorphic Intermediate trophoblast	Dimorphic Mainly cytotrophoblast and syncytiotrophoblast
Margin	Infiltrating	Circumscribed
Hemorrhage	Focal and haphazard	Massive and central
Vascular invasion	From periphery to lumen	From lumen to periphery
Fibrinoid change	Present	Absent
Immunocytochemistry		
hCG	+	++++
hPL	++++	+

hCG, human chorionic gonadotropin; hPL, human placental lactogen.

Behavior. Most cases of PSTT are self-limited,* but there have been several reports of malignant behavior.[54,55,69,87,167,196] Among a group of nearly 50 reported and unreported cases, 6 (10%) have resulted in the death of the patient.[219] These tumors often invade through the myometrium to the serosa, causing perforation.[110] Curettage performed for a missed abortion may result in perforation as a result of the deep myometrial invasion.[110,196] In several cases, the tumor invaded into the broad ligament and ovary.[54,110] The few overtly malignant cases have had widely disseminated metastases resembling choriocarcinoma in their distribution and have not responded to multiagent chemother-

* References 17, 68, 110, 135, 137, 162.

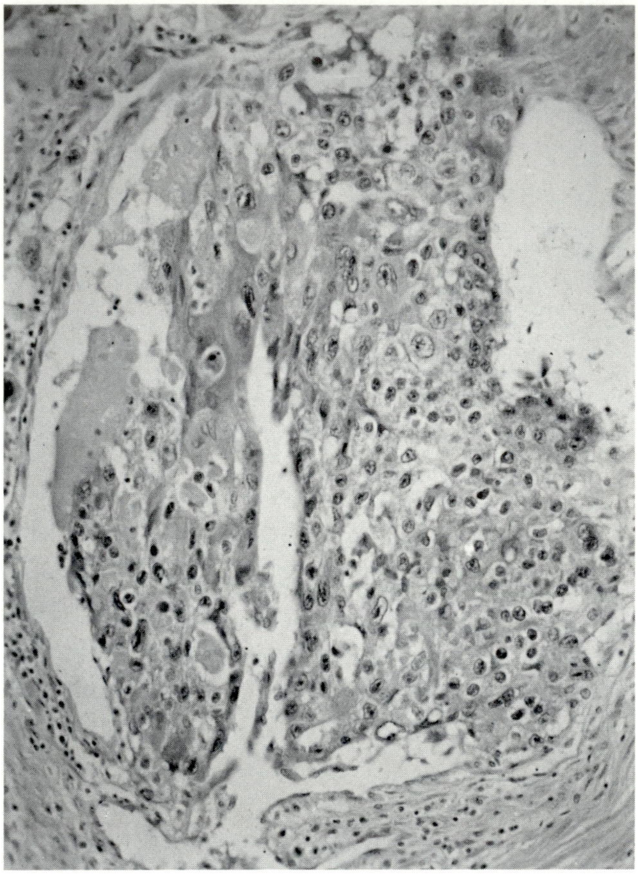
a

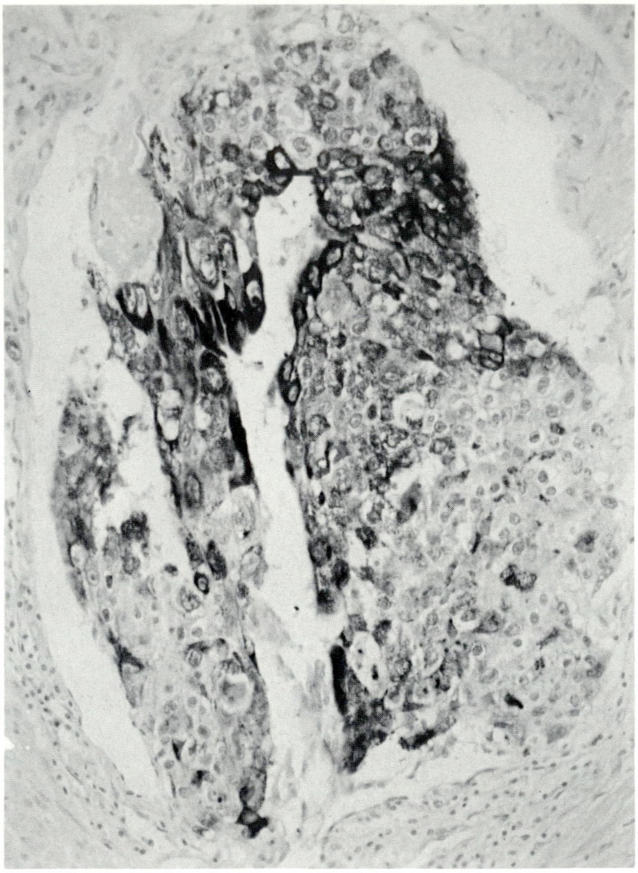
b

FIG. 24.47.*a*. Choriocarcinoma showing no staining for hPL. *b*. Choriocarcinoma showing diffuse staining for hCG in syncytiotrophoblast. Compare to Figures 24.48 and 24.49. (Reprinted with permission of Kurman et al., Ref. 111.)

apy.[54,55,69,87,196] Lung, liver, abdominal cavity, and brain have been involved. Metastases have the same histologic appearance as the primary tumor and may develop rapidly after initial diagnosis, but one fatal case recurred 5 years after hysterectomy that was thought to be curative.[69] Because these tumors are composed of neoplastic IT that contain only small amounts of hCG, the serum levels of hCG are much lower than with choriocarcinoma that is composed predominantly of CT and ST.

Comparison of benign to malignant cases indicates that the malignant lesions generally are composed of larger masses and sheets of cells, many with clear instead of amphophilic cytoplasm, and have more extensive necrosis and higher mitotic activity than the benign lesions.[167,218] In benign lesions, the mean mitotic rate is 2 mitotic figures/10 HPF, with the highest reported being 5 mitotic figures/10 HPF, whereas most of the malignant lesions have displayed greater than 5 mitoses/10 HPF.[167,218] In one fatal case, however, the mean mitotic rate was 2/10 HPF.[69] In addition, there is a tendency for the malignant cases to stain more diffusely for hCG than hPL, that is, more closely resembling the distribution of these hormones in choriocarcinoma.[111,221] Abnormal mitotic figures can be found in either benign or malignant tumors.

An apparently unique form of renal disease has been described in a few patients with PSTT.[54,220] These patients had severe proteinuria and, in one patient, hematuria and were thought to have the nephrotic syndrome. Renal biopsies showed glomerular lesions with prominent eosinophilic deposits in the capillary lumens that stained for fibrinogen and IgM. This lesion has been found in 3 and possibly 4 of more than 40 patients, with the PSTT suggesting that the lesion is specific and not fortuitous.[220] However, its pathogenesis is unknown. Nephrotic syndrome is not observed in association with other forms of GTD.[6]

Gestational Trophoblastic Disease at Ectopic Sites

Hydatidiform mole, choriocarcinoma, and PSTT may rarely occur primarily at ectopic sites, since GTD can arise wherever a gestation implants. Rarely, hydatidiform mole arises in the fallopian tube[72,209] and ovary.[98,170] A true primary mole of the adnexa should be discriminated

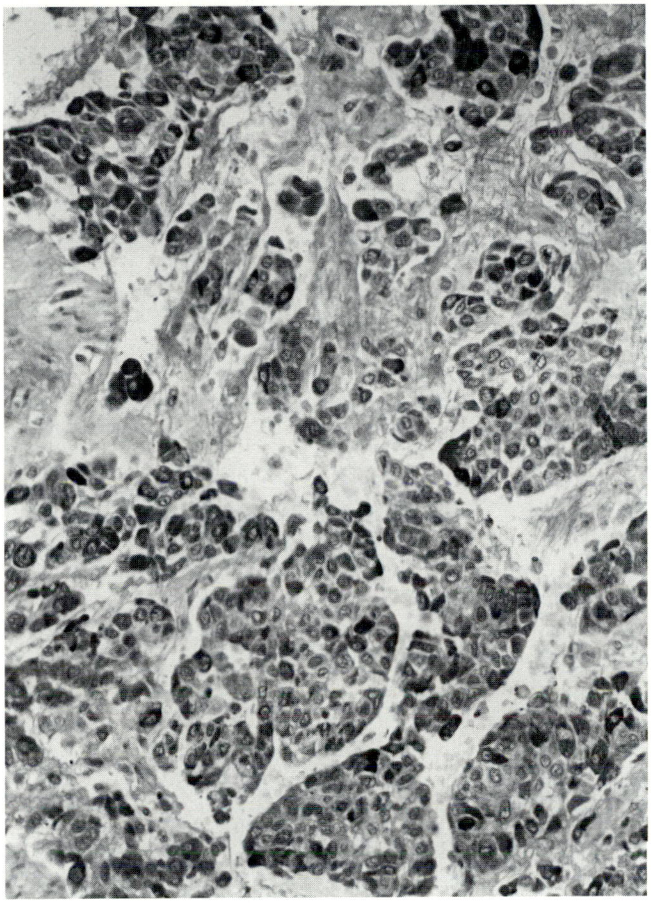

FIG. 24.48. Placental site trophoblastic tumor showing diffuse staining for hPL.

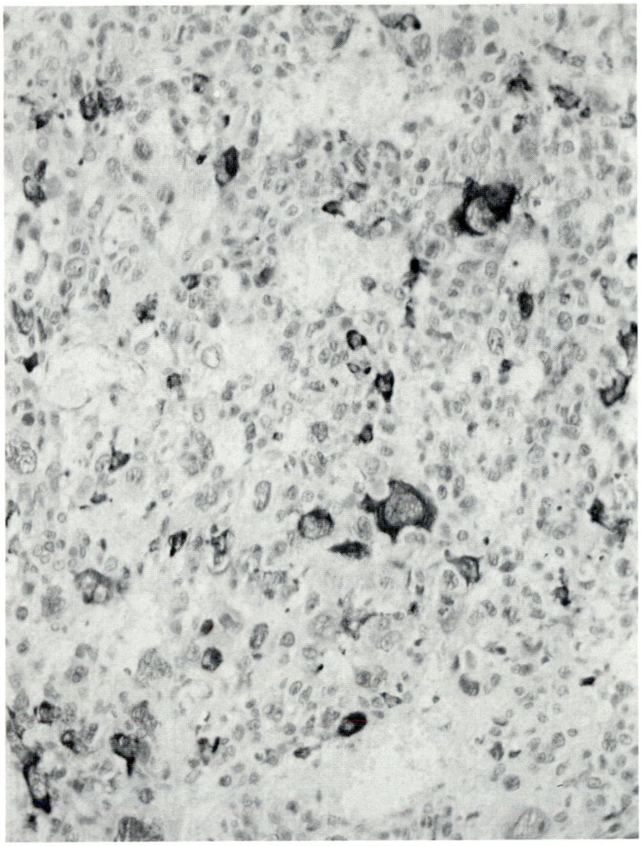

FIG. 24.49. Placental site trophoblastic tumor showing a focal pattern of staining for hCG.

from the hydropic change that can be seen in aborting ectopic pregnancy and from invasive mole with extension to the region of the broad ligaments.

Gestational choriocarcinoma also may be primary in the fallopian tube,[105,142,152] and in this instance, the tumor probably is a sequela to an ectopic pregnancy.[120A] These tumors usually cause symptoms suggesting an ectopic pregnancy or appear as an adnexal mass that mimics an ovarian tumor.[142] With proper diagnosis and therapy, survival rates are similar to those of choriocarcinoma arising as a result of an intrauterine gestation. Primary gestational choriocarcinoma of the ovary is difficult to document but does occur.[16,38,152,203] Most examples of ovarian choriocarcinoma represent metastases from uterine primaries or are germ cell tumors.[5,67,200] In primary germ cell tumors, sufficient sampling often reveals other germ cell elements, thus establishing a diagnosis of mixed germ cell tumor. When pure choriocarcinoma is present in the ovary, the principles of hCG monitoring and chemotherapy remain the same whether it is a gestational or germ cell neoplasm.[5,67]

Choriocarcinoma has been described as a primary tu-

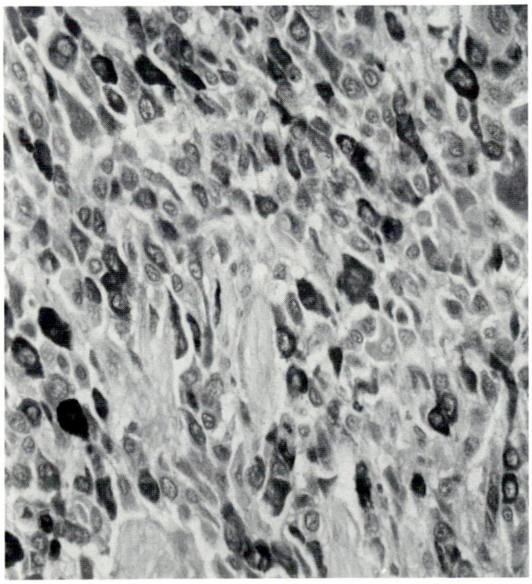

FIG. 24.50. The intermediate trophoblastic cells in this placental site trophoblastic tumor are spindle-shaped. The diffuse staining for hPL (*gray and black intracytoplasmic deposit*) is useful in distinguishing the tumor from a sarcoma, which is negative. (Reprinted with permission of Kurman et al., Ref. 111.)

mor arising in a number of different sites besides the uterus and gonads.[81A,128A] These tumors may be extragonadal germ cell tumors, or they may be derived from dedifferentiation of an ordinary carcinoma.[65,214] In women of reproductive age and rarely in older women choriocarcinoma that appears to be an extrauterine primary tumor probably represents gestational choriocarcinoma in which the index pregnancy was undetected.

Although PSTT is a rare neoplasm even in the uterus, we are aware of one case that occurred in the groin after a cesarean section for a full-term infant. After biopsy the mass disappeared spontaneously.[108]

Management

Chorionic Gonadotropin and Other Tumor Markers

In GTD, human chorionic gonadotropin (hCG) has proven to be an ideal tumor marker and a prototype for all other tumor markers. Produced mainly by ST,[111] it is almost invariably present when trophoblastic tissue exists, and it can now be measured at extremely low levels in the serum. For these reasons, its presence or absence is a critical factor in the diagnosis, follow-up, and therapy of GTD.

hCG is a glycoprotein composed of two polypeptide chains, alpha and beta, attached to a carbohydrate moiety. There is a high content of sialic acid in the molecule.[71,163] The configuration of hCG is similar to other gonadotropins, particularly luteinizing hormone (LH). The alpha-polypeptide chain in all these hormones is identical; it is the difference in the beta chain that gives the hormones their unique immunologic specificity and biologic function.

In normal pregnancy, hCG reaches a peak level of 50,000–100,000 mIU/ml at about 10 weeks gestation and decreases to 10,000–20,000 mIU/ml by 20 weeks, remaining at that level until term.[25,46] Levels as high as 600,000 mIU/ml in early pregnancy have been reported.[46] In molar gestations, hCG levels at diagnosis are variable, but most show a markedly elevated hCG titer, which is a useful diagnostic feature.[29,46] Levels greater than 2 million mIU/ml have been reported. Markedly elevated hCG titers are more common in complete as compared to partial molar pregnancies.[40,168,183]

It has been possible to assess the presence of hCG qualitatively and semiquantitatively for many years using bioassays[31,33,46] and immunoassays.[71,114] These methods were sufficient to detect hCG at higher concentrations but lacked sensitivity to detect hCG at lower concentrations and were not specific, measuring LH as well. The development of the radioimmunoassay (RIA) lowered the sensitivity to the normal level of LH but still did not discriminate between LH and hCG.[12]

RIA for the beta-subunit of hCG developed in 1972[197] is sufficiently sensitive and specific to permit follow-up to complete disappearance of trophoblastic tissue. Disappearance of hCG from the serum as measured by half-life shows two components, one with a half-life of 6 hours and a slower component with a half-life of about 30 hours.[158,163] With the serum RIA for beta-hCG, it is possible to measure hCG to a level of 1.6–5 mIU/ml, depending on the lowest level of sensitivity measured in the laboratory performing the test. Normally, the values do not reach zero. The assay is sufficiently sensitive to determine hCG production from as few as 1000 trophoblast cells.[71] Rarely, however, choriocarcinoma may be associated with undectable levels of hCG.[114A] Cerebral spinal fluid can also be assayed for the presence of hCG in patients at risk of central nervous system involvement by choriocarcinoma. A serum to cerebral spinal fluid ratio of less than 60 usually is suggestive but not diagnostic of CNS metastases.[9,22,169]

Measurement of other pregnancy-specific proteins in conjunction with hCG may be useful in the follow-up of patients with GTD. Measurement of the alpha-hCG subunit can help identify patients at risk of recurrences after successful initial chemotherapy.[155] hPL is produced by trophoblastic tissues, but it has a rapid half-life and, therefore, may be undetectable in the serum despite the presence of metastases.[88] Goldstein reported that hPL levels are inversely correlated with the histologic grade of hydatidiform moles, suggesting that patients with low hPL levels along with high hCG levels represent a high-risk group.[70] Furthermore, since the majority of cells in the PSTT contain hPL as compared to hCG, hPL may be useful as a marker for this neoplasm.[111]

Pregnancy-specific beta-$_1$-glycoprotein (SP1) is often present in GTD.[88,186] This protein is less sensitive than hCG in monitoring GTD, but in a few patients with recurrent disease, elevated levels of SP1 have been present when hCG was undetectable.[186] It is also suggested that the ratio between SP1 and beta-hCG may reflect the degree of differentiation of trophoblastic cells, lower levels being found in choriocarcinoma than in hydatidiform mole.[88,144,164] Other markers, including placental protein 5 (PP5) and pregnancy-associated plasma protein-A (PAPP-A) appear to offer no advantages over monitoring hCG.[88,91]

Treatment

The basic principles of treatment of GTD include identifying, when possible, the specific histologic type of GTD, monitoring serum hCG titers, and instituting chemotherapy when appropriate.[39,77,116] Molar pregnancy, complete or partial, is generally first treated by suction curettage of the uterus. Some investigators advocate prophylactic chemotherapy with dactinomycin coincident with suction evacuation for patients at high risk of persistent disease, especially those with large-for-dates uteri and ovarian enlargement due to theca–lutein cysts.[71] In patients in whom preservation of fertility is not a consideration, abdominal hysterectomy is an effective alternative approach as an initial treatment of molar pregnancy, but careful follow-up is mandatory.[71] Regardless of the initial method of removal of the hydatidiform mole, a chest radiograph before treatment and 4 weeks later should be performed to exclude metastases.

In the follow-up of GTD, serial hCG titers are mandatory until titers fall and remain within the normal range. A typical regimen for follow-up of a molar pregnancy is serial hCG levels at 10, 20, 30, 45, and 60 days after termination of the gestation and every 2 weeks thereafter until undetectable.[123] Plateauing or rising titers can be the first sign of persistent GTD. The titers will fall to normal between 10 and 170 days after evacuation of a mole, and the majority of patients will have normal titers by 60 days postevacuation.[123] After hCG levels reach normal values, monthly assays are performed for 6 months, and pregnancy must be avoided.[71,123] If the values remain normal, chances of recurrence are slight. Occasional late recurrences of GTD more than 1 year after therapy have been reported, however.[100,178,202]

Persistent GTD after molar pregnancy is heralded by plateauing hCG titers for 2–4 weeks,[71,106] rising hCG titers, persistent uterine disease, or evidence of metastases. Depending on clinical criteria for treatment, between 8 and 30% of patients with mole who are carefully followed will require therapy for persistent or metastatic GTD.[12,31,33,39,123,136] Either invasive mole or choriocarinoma may be present, but in the absence of histologic confirmation, the disorder is regarded clinically as postmolar GTD. When disease appears to be confined to the uterus, hysterectomy may be curative in patients who do not wish to preserve fertility. All other patients with persistent or metastatic GTD after moles require chemotherapy. In addition, hCG monitoring is necessary until titers fall to normal whether patients are treated surgically or medically. Thereafter, titers are followed weekly for 3 consecutive weeks and then monthly for at least 12 months to ensure no recurrence.[71] Contraception is necessary during the entire follow-up period.

Methotrexate, a folic acid antagonist, was the first drug reported to be successful in the therapy of choriocarcinoma.[86,117] Subsequently, numerous other chemotherapeutic agents have been used, especially dactinomycin and an alkylating agent (cyclophosphamide or chlorambucil).[120] Initial therapy for persistent disease after a molar pregnancy usually consists of methotrexate or dactinomycin or a combination of the two.[71,122] High-risk GTD is treated with a combination of dactinomycin, methotrexate, and an alkylating agent.[122] Alternatively, a multiagent chemotherapy program with seven drugs—hydroxyrea, dactinomycin, vicristine, methotrexate, cyclophosphamide, folinic acid, and doxdrubicin—has been developed by Bagshawe[8] and appears to offer an increased rate of sustained remissions for high-risk patients and for those who have not benefited from other conventional forms of chemotherapy.[177,208] Other chemotherapeutic agents have been used successfully to treat GTD.[179]

GTD without a preceding molar pregnancy represents choriocarcinoma or, rarely, PSTT. The principles of management of choriocarcinoma are similar to those for GTD after hydatidiform mole; hCG monitoring and chemotherapy are essential.[28,122] Hysterectomy can reduce hospitalization and the amount of chemotherapy needed to induce remission.[78] Resection of pulmonary metastases may have therapeutic value in patients with persistent but limited pulmonary disease, no evidence of tumor at other sites, and a low hCG titer.[189] Irradiation combined with chemotherapy will give a 50% remission rate for cerebral metastases,[4,207] but irradiation to other sites generally is not useful.[122]

Once the diagnosis of a PSTT is established microscopically, continued close surveillance with frequent serologic measurements of the hCG level using an RIA specific for the beta-subunit is essential. Curettage may be therapeutic, but if uterine disease persists, as evidenced by persistently elevated serum hCG levels, hysterectomy is indicated to remove the tumor.[110,218] Limited experience with tumors behaving in a clinically malignant fashion suggests that they may secrete relatively low levels of hCG and may not be as responsive to the usual chemotherapeutic agents that have proved successful with other forms of trophoblastic disease.[167] Immunocytochemical staining in some of the aggressive tumors has shown a reversal of the usual hPL:hCG ratio, with hCG predominating,[111,221] suggesting that serum measurement of hPL along with hCG may prove to be valuable in monitoring these tumors. However, a larger number of cases must be studied.

References

1. Acosta-Sison H (1960) Chorioadenoma destruens. A report of 41 cases. Am J Obstet Gynecol 80: 176
2. Amir SM, Osathanondh R, Berkowitz RS, Goldstein DP (1984) Human chorionic gonadotropin and thyroid function in patients with hydatidiform mole. Am J Obstet Gynecol 150: 723
3. Aozasa K, Ito H, Kohro T, Ha K, Nakamura M, Okada A (1981) Choriocarcinoma in infant and mother. Acta Pathol Jpn 31: 317

4. Athanassiou A, Begent RHJ, Newlands ES, Parker D, Rustin GJS, Bagshawe KD (1983) Central nervous system metastases of choriocarcinoma. Cancer 52: 1728

4A. Atrash HK, Hogue CJR, Grimes DA (1986) Epidemiology of hydatidiform mole during early gestation. Am J Obstet Gynecol 154: 906

5. Axe SR, Klein VR, Woodruff JD (1985) Choriocarcinoma of the ovary. Obstet Gynecol 66: 111

6. Bagshawe KD Personal communication

7. Bagshawe KD (1976) Risk and prognostic factors in trophoblastic neoplasia. Cancer 38: 1373

8. Bagshawe KD (1976) Treatment of trophoblastic tumors. Ann Acad Med 5: 273

9. Bagshawe KD, Harland S (1976) Immunodiagnosis and monitoring of gonadotrophin-producing metastases in the central nervous system. Cancer 38: 112

10. Bagshawe KD, Lawler SD (1982) Unmasking moles. Br J Obstet Gynaecol 89: 255

11. Bagshawe KD, Rawlins GJ, Pike MC, Lawler SD (1971) ABO blood groups in trophoblastic neoplasia. Lancet 1: 553

12. Bagshawe KD, Wilson H, Dublon P, Smith A, Baldwin M, Kardana A (1973) Follow-up after hydatidiform mole: Studies using radioimmunoassay for urinary human chorionic gonadotrophin (hCG). J Obstet Gynaecol Br Commonw 80: 461

13. Baltazar JC (1976) Epidemiological features of choriocarcinoma. Bull WHO 54: 523–532

14. Bandy LC, Clarke-Pearson DL, Hammond CB (1984) Malignant potential of gestational trophoblastic disease at the extreme ages of reproductive life. Obstet Gynecol 64: 395

14A. Barnard DE, Woodward KT, Yancy SG, Weed JC, Hammond CB (1986) Hepatic metastases of choriocarcinoma: A report of 15 patients. Gynecol Oncol 25: 73

15. Beischer NA, Fortune DW (1968) Significance of chromatin patterns in cases of hydatidiform mole with an associated fetus. Am J Obstet Gynecol 100: 276

16. Benjamin F, Rorat E (1978) Primary gestational choriocarcinoma of the ovary. Am J Obstet Gynecol 131: 343

17. Berger G, Verbaere J, Feroldi J (1984) Placental site trophoblastic tumor of the uterus: An ultrastructural and immunohistochemical study. Ultrastruct Pathol 6: 319

18. Berkowitz RS, Goldstein DP (1981) Pathogenesis of gestational trophoblastic neoplasms. Pathobiol Annu 11: 391

19. Berkowitz RS, Goldstein DP, Bernstein MR (1984) Choriocarcinoma following term gestation. Gynecol Oncol 17: 52

20. Berkowitz RS, Goldstein DP, Bernstein MR (1985) Natural history of partial molar pregnancy. Obstet Gynecol 66: 677

21. Berkowitz RS, Cramer DW, Bernstein MR, Cassells S, Driscoll SG, Goldstein DP (1985) Risk factors for complete molar pregnancy from a case-control study. Am J Obstet Gynecol 152: 1016

22. Berkowitz RS, Osathanondh R, Goldstein DP, Martin PM, Mallampati SR, Datta S (1981) Cerebrospinal fluid human chorionic gonadotropin levels in normal pregnancy and choriocarcinoma. Surg Gynecol Obstet 153: 687

23. Block MF, Merrill JA (1982) Hydatidiform mole with coexistent fetus. Obstet Gynecol 60: 130

24. Bracken MB, Brinton LA, Hayashi K (1984) Epidemiology of hydatidiform mole and choriocarcinoma. Epidemiol Rev 6: 52

25. Braunstein GD, Rasor J, Adler D, Danzer H, Wade ME (1976) Serum human chorionic gonadotropin levels throughout normal pregnancy. Am J Obstet Gynecol 126: 678

26. Brescia RJ, Kurman RJ, Main C, et al. (1987) Immunocytochemical localization of chorionic gonadotropin, placental lactogen, and placental alkaline phosphatase in the diagnosis of complete and partial hydatidiform moles. Int J Gynecol Pathol (In press)

27. Brewer JI, Gerbie AL (1966) Early development of choriocarcinoma. Am J Obstet Gynecol 94: 692

28. Brewer JI, Mazur MT (1981) Gestational choriocarcinoma: Its origin in the placenta during seemingly normal pregnancy. Am J Surg Pathol 5: 267

29. Brewer JI, Tamimi HK (1976) Gestational trophoblastic disease. Obstet Gynecol Annu 5: 367

30. Brewer JI, Smith RT, Pratt GB (1963) Choriocarcinoma. Absolute 5-year survival rates of 122 patients treated by hysterectomy. Am J Obstet Gynecol 85: 841

31. Brewer JI, Torok EE, Webster A, Dolkart RE (1968) Hydatidiform mole. A follow-up regimen for identification of invasive mole and choriocarcinoma and for selection of patients for treatment. Am J Obstet Gynecol 101: 557

32. Brewer JI, Eckman TR, Dolkart RE, Torok EE, Webster A (1971) Gestational trophoblastic disease. A comparative study of the results of therapy in patients with invasive mole and with choriocarcinoma. Am J Obstet Gynecol 109: 335

33. Brewer JI, Torok EE, Kahan BD, Stanhope CR, Halpern B (1978) Gestational trophoblastic disease: Origin of choriocarcinoma, invasive mole and choriocarcinoma associated with hydatidiform mole, and some immunologic aspects. Adv Cancer Res 27: 89

34. Carlson JA, Day Jr TG, Kuhns JG, Howell RS, Masterson BJ (1984) Endoarterial pulmonary metastasis of malignant trophoblast associated with a term intrauterine pregnancy. Gynecol Oncol 17: 241

35. Cohen BA, Burkman RT, Rosenshein NB, Antienza MF, King TM, Parmley TH (1979) Gestational trophoblastic disease within an elective abortion population. Am J Obstet Gynecol 135: 452

36. Cotton DB, Bernstein SG, Read JA, Benedetti TJ, D'Ablaing G, Miller FC, Morrow CP (1980) Hemodynamic observations in evacuation of molar pregnancy. Am J Obstet Gynecol 138: 6

37. Craighill MC, Cramer DW (1984) Epidemiology of complete molar pregnancy. J Reprod Med 29: 784

38. Cunanan RG Jr, Lippes J, Tancinco PA (1980) Choriocarcinoma of the ovary with coexisting normal pregnancy. Obstet Gynecol 55: 669

39. Curry SL, Hammond CB, Tyrey L, Creasman WT, Parker RT (1975) Hydatidiform mole: Diagnosis, management, and long-term follow-up of 347 patients. Obstet Gynecol 45: 1

40. Czernobilsky B, Barash A, Lancet M (1982) Partial moles: A clinicopathologic study of 25 cases. Obstet Gynecol 59: 75
41. Daamen CBF, Bloem GWD, Westerbeek AJ (1961) Chorionepithelioma in mother and child. J Obstet Gynecol Br Commonwlth 68: 144
42. Davis JR, Surwit EA, Garay JP, Fortier KJ (1984) Sex assignment in gestational trophoblastic neoplasia. Am J Obstet Gynecol 148: 722
43. Dawood MY, Teoh ES, Ratnam SG (1971) ABO blood group in trophoblastic disease. J Obstet Gynaecol Br Commonw 78: 918
44. Dearden L, Ockleford CD, Gupta M (1983) Structure of human trophoblast: Correlation with function. In: Biology of Trophoblast. Luke YW, Whyte A (eds). New York, Elsevier, pp 70–110
45. Dehner LP (1980) Gestational and nongestational trophoblastic neoplasia. A historic and pathobiologic surgery. Am J Surg Pathol 4: 43
46. Delfs E (1957) Quantitative chorionic gonadotrophin: Prognostic value in hydatidiform mole and chorionepithelioma. Obstet Gynecol 9: 1
47. Deligdisch L, Waxman J (1984) Metastatic gestational trophoblastic neoplasm. A study of two cases in unusual clinical settings and review of the literature. Gynecol Oncol 19: 323
48. Deligdisch L, Driscoll SG, Goldstein DP (1978) Gestational trophoblastic neoplasms: Morphologic correlates of therapeutic response. Am J Obstet Gynecol 130: 801
49. Dodson MG (1983) New concepts and questions in gestational trophoblastic disease. J Reprod Med 28: 741
50. Dougherty CM, Cunningham C, Mickal A (1978) Choriocarcinoma with metastasis in a postmenopausal woman. Am J Obstet Gynecol 132: 700
51. Douglas GW, Thomas L, Carr M, Cullen NM, Morris R (1959) Trophoblast in the circulating blood during pregnancy. Am J Obstet Gynecol 78: 960
52. Driscoll SG (1963) Choriocarcinoma: An "incidental finding" within a term placenta. Obstet Gynecol 21: 96
53. Driscoll SG (1977) Gestational trophoblastic neoplasms: Morphologic considerations. Hum Pathol 8: 529
54. Eckstein RP, Paradinas FJ, Bagshawe KD (1982) Placental site trophoblastic tumour (trophoblastic pseudotumour): A study of four cases requiring hysterectomy, including one fatal case. Histopathology 6: 211
55. Eckstein RP, Russell P, Friedlander ML, Tattersall MHN, Bradfield A (1983) Metastasizing placental site trophoblastic tumor: A case study. Hum Pathol 16(6): 632
56. Elston CW (1976) The histopathology of trophoblastic tumors. J Clin Pathol 29 [Suppl] (Roy Coll Pathol) 10: 111
57. Elston CW (1978) Trophoblastic tumors of the placenta. In: Pathology of the Placenta. Fox H (ed). Philadelphia, Saunders, pp 368–425
58. Elston CW (1983) Development and structure of trophoblastic neoplasms. In: Biology of Trophoblast. Luke YW, Whyte A (eds). New York, Elsevier, pp 188–232
59. Elston CW, Bagshawe KD (1972) The value of histological grading in the management of hydatidiform mole. J Obstet Gynaecol Br Commonw 79: 717
60. Elston CW, Bagshawe KD (1972) The diagnosis of trophoblastic tumours from uterine curettings. J Clin Pathol 25: 111
61. Elston CW, Bagshawe KD (1973) Cellular reaction in trophoblastic tumours. Br J Cancer 28: 245
62. Ertungealp E, Axelrod J, Stanek A, Boyce A, Sedlis A (1982) Skin metastases from malignant gestational trophoblastic disease: Report of two cases. Am J Obstet Gynecol 143: 843
63. Ewing J (1910) Chorioma. Surg Gynecol Obstet 10: 366
64. Federschneider JM, Goldstein DP, Berkowitz RS, Marean AR, Bernstein MR (1980) Natural history of recurrent molar pregnancy. Obstet Gynecol 55: 457
65. Fukuda Y, Sakurai M, Matsuura N (1985) Primary gastric choriocarcinoma. Report of an autopsy case with immunohistochemical study. Acta Pathol Jpn 35: 655
66. Gaber LW, Redline RW, Mostoufi-Zadeh M, Driscoll SG (1986) Invasive partial mole. Am J Clin Pathol 85: 722
67. Gerbie MV, Brewer JI, Tamimi H (1975) Primary choriocarcinoma of the ovary. Obstet Gynecol 46: 720
68. Gloor E, Hurlimann J (1981) Trophoblastic pseudotumor of the uterus. Clinicopathologic report with immunohistochemical and ultrastructural studies. Am J Surg Pathol 5: 5
69. Gloor E, Dialdas J, Hurlimann J, Ribolzi J, Barrelet L (1983) Placental site trophoblastic tumor (trophoblastic pseudotumor) of the uterus with metastases and fatal outcome. Am J Surg Pathol 7: 483
70. Goldstein DP (1979) Gestational neoplasms. In: Endocrinology. DeGroot LJ, Cahill GF, Martini L, Nelson DH, Odell WD, Potts JT, Steinberger E, Winegard AI (eds). New York, Grune & Stratton, Vol 3, pp 1629–1648.
71. Goldstein DP, Berkowitz RS (1982) Gestational Trophoblastic Neoplasms. Clinical Principles of Diagnosis and Management. Philadelphia, Saunders
72. Govender NSK, Goldstein DP (1977) Metastatic tubal mole and coexisting intrauterine pregnancy. Obstet Gynecol 49 [Suppl]: 67s
73. Greene JB, McCue SA (1978) Choriocarcinoma with cerebral metastases coexistent with a first pregnancy. Am J Obstet Gynecol 131: 253
74. Greene RR (1959) Chorioadenoma destruens. Ann NY Acad Sci 80: 143
75. Grimes DA (1984) Epidemiology of gestational trophoblastic disease. Am J Obstet Gynecol 150: 309
76. Guvener S, Kazancigil A, Erez S (1972) Long latent development of trophoblastic disease. Am J Obstet Gynecol 114: 679
77. Hammond CB, Parker RT (1970) Diagnosis and treatment of trophoblastic disease. A report from the Southeastern Regional Center. Obstet Gynecol 35: 132
78. Hammond CB, Weed JC, Currie JL (1980) The role of operation in the current therapy of gestational trophoblastic disease. Am J Obstet Gynecol 136: 844
79. Hammond CB, Borchert LG, Tyrey L, Creasman WT, Parker RT (1973) Treatment of metastatic trophoblastic disease. Good and poor prognosis. Am J Obstet Gynecol 115: 451

80. Hammond CB, Hertz R, Ross GT, Lipsett MB, Odell WD (1967) Diagnostic problems of choriocarcinoma and related trophoblastic neoplasms. Obstet Gynecol 29: 224
81. Hayashi K, Bracken MB, Freeman DH, Hellenbrand K (1982) Hydatidiform mole in the United States (1970–1977): A statistical and a theoretical analysis. Am J Epidemiol 115: 67
81A. Heaton GE, Matthews TH, Christopherson WM (1986) Malignant trophoblastic tumors with massive hemorrhage presenting as liver primary. A report of two cases. Am J Surg Pathol 10:342
82. Hertig AT, Edmonds HW (1940) Genesis of hydatidiform mole. Arch Pathol 30: 260
83. Hertig AT, Gore H (1960) Tumors of the female sex organs, Part 2, Tumors of the vulva, vagina and uterus. In: Atlas of Tumor Pathology, Section IX, Fascicle 33. Armed Forces Institute of Pathology, Washington, D.C., pp. 329–333.
84. Hertig AT, Mansell (1956) Tumors of the female sex organs. Part 1. Hydatidiform mole and choriocarcinoma. In: Atlas of Tumor Pathology, Section 9, Fascicle 33. Washington, D.C., Armed Forces Institute of Pathology
85. Hertig AT, Sheldon WH (1947) Hydatidiform mole. A pathologicoclinical correlation of 200 cases. Am J Obstet Gynecol 53: 1
86. Hertz R, Lewis J Jr, Lipsett MB (1961) Five years' experience with the chemotherapy of metastatic choriocarcinoma and related trophoblastic tumors in women. Am J Obstet Gynecol 82: 631
87. Hopkins M, Nunez C, Murphy JR, Wentz WB (1985) Malignant placental site trophoblastic tumor. Obstet Gynecol 66(3): 95S
88. Horne CHW, Rankin R, Bremner RD (1984) Pregnancy-specific proteins as markers for gestational trophoblastic disease. Int J Gynecol Pathol 3: 27
89. Hou PC, Pang SC (1956) Chorionepithelioma: An analytical study of 28 necropsied cases with special reference to the possibility of spontaneous retrogression. J Pathol Bacteriol 72: 95
90. Hsu CT, Huang LC, Chen TY (1962) Metastases in benign hydatidiform mole and chorioadenoma destruens. Am J Obstet Gynecol 84: 1412
91. Inaba N, Ishige H, Ijichi M, Satoh N, Katoh T, Sekiya S, Shirotake S, Ohkawa R, Takamizawa H, Nitoh A, Renk T, Bohn H (1982) Possible new markers in trophoblastic diseases. Am J Obstet Gynecol 143: 973
92. Ishizuka N (1967) Chemotherapy of chorionic tumors. In: Choriocarcinoma. UICC Monograph Series. Holland JF, Hreshchyshyn MM (eds). New York, Springer-Verlag, Vol 3, pp 116–118
93. Ito H, Sekine T, Komuro N, Tanaka T, Yokoyama S, Hosokawa T (1981) Histologic stromal reaction of the host with gestational choriocarcinoma and its relation to clinical stage classification and prognosis. Am J Obstet Gynecol 140: 781
94. Jacobs PA, Hunt PA, Matsuura JS, Wilson CC, Szulman AE (1982) Complete and partial hydatidiform mole in Hawaii: Cytogenetics, morphology and epidemiology. Br J Obstet Gynaecol 89: 258
95. Jacobs PA, Szulman AE, Funkhouser J, Matsuura JS, Wilson CC (1982) Human triploidy: Relationship between parental origin of the additional haploid complement and development of partial hydatidiform mole. Ann Hum Genet 46: 223
96. Jacobs PA, Wilson CM, Sprenkle JA, Rosenshein NB, Migeon BR (1980) Mechanism of origin of complete hydatidiform moles. Nature 286: 714
97. Javey H, Borazjani G, Behmard S, Langley FA (1979) Discrepancies in the histological diagnosis of hydatidiform mole. Br J Obstet Gynaecol 86: 480
98. Jock DE, Schwartz PE, Portnoy L (1981) Primary ovarian hydatidiform mole: Addition of a sixth case to the literature. Obstet Gynecol 58: 657
99. Johnson TR, Comstock CH, Anderson DG (1979) Benign gestational trophoblastic disease metastatic to pleura: Unusual case of hemothorax. Obstet Gynecol 53: 509
100. Jones WB, Lewis JL (1985) Late recurrence of gestational trophoblastic disease. Gynecol Oncol 20: 83
101. Junaid TA, de V Hendrickse JP, Williams AO, Osunkoya BO (1976) Choriocarcinoma in Ibadan: Clinicopathologic studies. Hum Pathol 7: 215
102. Junaid TA, de V Hendrickse JP, Oladiran B, Edington GM, Williams AO (1974) Choriocarcinoma in Ibadan, Nigeria: Epidemiologic aspects. J Natl Cancer Inst 53: 1597
103. Kajii T, Ohama K (1977) Androgenetic origin of hydatidiform mole. Nature (London) 268: 633
104. Kajii T, Kurashige H, Ohama K, Uchino F (1984) XY and XX complete moles: Clinical and morphologic correlations. Am J Obstet Gynecol 150: 57
105. Kay S, Schneider V, Litt J (1983) Choriocarcinoma of the mesosalpinx masquerading as congestive heart failure: Ultrastructural observations of the tumor. Int J Gynecol Pathol 2: 72
106. Kohorn EI (1982) Criteria toward the definition of nonmetastatic gestational trophoblastic disease after hydatidiform mole. Am J Obstet Gynecol 142: 416
107. Kohorn EI, McGinn RC, Gee JBL, Goldstein DP, Osathanondh R (1978) Pulmonary embolization of trophoblastic tissue in molar pregnancy. Obstet Gynecol 51 [Suppl]: 16S
108. Kurman RJ Personal observation
109. Kurman RJ, Main CS, Chen HC (1984) Intermediate trophoblast: A distinctive form of trophoblast with specific morphological, biochemical and functional features. Placenta 5: 349
110. Kurman RJ, Scully RE, Norris HJ (1976) Trophoblastic pseudotumor of the uterus. An exaggerated form of "syncytial endometritis" simulating a malignant tumor. Cancer 38: 1214
111. Kurman RJ, Young RH, Norris HJ, Main CS, Lawrence WD, Scully RE (1984) Immunocytochemical localization of placental lactogen and chorionic gonadotropin in the normal placenta and trophoblastic tumors, with emphasis on intermediate trophoblast and the placental site trophoblastic tumor. Int J Gynecol Pathol 3: 101
112. Larsen JF (1973) Ultrastructure of abnormal human trophoblast. Acta Anat 86 [Suppl 1]: 47
113. Lathrop JC, Wachtel TJ, Meissner GF (1978) Uterine choriocarcinoma fourteen years following bilateral tubal ligation. Obstet Gynecol 51: 477

114. Lau HL, Jones GS, Schwartz CM (1965) Immunoassay of serum human chorionic gonadotropin by quantitative complement fixation and its comparison with Delfs bioassay and two international standard preparations. Am J Obstet Gynecol 92: 483

114A. Lemonnier M-C, Glezerman M, Vauclair R, Audet-Lapointe P (1986) Choriocarcinoma associated with undetectable levels of human chorionic gonadotropin. Gynecol Oncol 25: 48

115. Lewis JL (1979) Classification of trophoblastic neoplasia. Ann Clin Lab Sci 9: 387

116. Lewis JL (1980) Treatment of metastatic gestational trophoblastic neoplasms. A brief review of developments in the years 1968 to 1978. Am J Obstet Gynecol 136: 163

117. Li MC, Hertz R, Spencer DB (1956) Effect of methotrexate therapy upon choriocarcinoma and chorioadenoma. Proc Soc Exp Biol Med 93: 361

118. Libshitz HI, Baber CE, Hammond CB (1977) The pulmonary metastases of choriocarcinoma. Obstet Gynecol 49: 412

119. Looi LM, Sivanesaratnam V (1981) Malignant evolution with fatal outcome in a patient with partial hydatidiform mole. Aust NZ J Obstet Gynaecol 21: 51

120. Lurain JR, Brewer JI (1985) Treatment of high-risk gestational trophoblastic disease with methotrexate, actinomycin D, and cyclophosphamide chemotherapy. Obstet Gynecol 65: 830

120A. Lurain JR, Sand PK, Brewer JI (1986) Choriocarcinoma associated with ectopic pregnancy. Obstet Gynecol 68: 286

121. Lurain JR, Brewer JI, Mazur MT, Torok EE (1982) Fatal gestational trophoblastic disease: An analysis of treatment failures. Am J Obstet Gynecol 144: 391

122. Lurain JR, Brewer JI, Torok EE, Halpern B (1982) Gestational trophoblastic disease: Treatment results at the Brewer Trophoblastic Disease Center. Obstet Gynecol 60: 354

123. Lurain JR, Brewer JI, Torok EE, Halpern B (1983) Natural history of hydatidiform mole after primary evacuation. Am J Obstet Gynecol 145: 591

124. Lurain JR, Sand PK, Carson SA, Brewer JI (1982) Pregnancy outcome subsequent to consecutive hydatidiform moles. Am J Obstet Gynecol 142: 1060

125. Marchand F (1895) Uber die sogenannten "decidualen" Geschwulste im Anschloss an normale Geburt, Abort, Blasenmole, und Extrauterin Schwangerschaft. Monatsschr Geburtshilfe Gynaekol 1: 419

126. Marquez-Monter H, De La Vega GA, Ridaura C, Robles M (1968) Gestational choriocarcinoma in the general hospital of Mexico. Cancer 22: 91

127. Matalon M, Modan B (1972) Epidemiologic aspects of hydatidiform mole in Israel. Am J Obstet Gynecol 112: 107

128. Matsurra J, Chin D, Jacobs PA, et al. (1984) Complete hydatidiform mole in Hawaii: An epidemiologic study. Genet Epidemiol 1: 271

128A. Matthews TH, Heaton GE, Christopherson WM (1986) Primary duodenal choriocarcinoma. Arch Pathol Lab Med 110: 550

129. Mazur MT, Lurain JR, Brewer JI (1982) Fatal gestational choriocarcinoma. Clinicopathologic study of patients treated at a trophoblastic disease center. Cancer 50: 1833

130. Messerli ML, Lilienfeld AM, Parmley T, Woodruff JD, Rosenshein NB (1985) Risk factors for gestational trophoblastic neoplasia. Am J Obstet Gynecol 153: 294

131. Miller JM, Surwit EA, Hammond CB (1979) Choriocarcinoma following term pregnancy. Obstet Gynecol 53: 207

132. Mittal KK, Kachru RB, Brewer JI (1975) The HL-A and ABO antigens in trophoblastic disease. Tissue Antigens 6: 57

133. Morrow CP, Kletzky OA, Disaia PJ, Townsend DE, Mishell DR, Nakamura RM (1977) Clinical and laboratory correlates of molar pregnancy and trophoblastic disease. Am J Obstet Gynecol 128: 424

134. Mostoufi M, Driscoll SG (1985) Persistence of partial hydatidiform mole. Lab Invest (Abst) 52: 45A

135. Nagelberg SB, Rosen SW (1985) Clinical and laboratory investigation of a virilized woman with placental site trophoblastic tumor. Obstet Gynecol 65: 527

136. Nakano R, Sasaki K, Yamoto M, Hata H (1980) Trophoblastic disease: Analysis of 342 patients. Gynecol Obstet Invest 11: 237

137. Nickels J, Risberg B, Melander S (1978) Trophoblastic pseudotumor of the uterus. Acta Pathol Microbiol Immunol Scand [A]86: 14

138. Nishikawa Y, Kaseki S, Tomoda Y, Ishizuka T, Asai Y, Suzuki T, Ushijima H (1985) Histopathologic classification of uterine choriocarcinoma. Cancer 55: 1044

139. Nisula BC, Taliadouros GS (1980) Thyroid function in gestational trophoblastic neoplasia: Evidence that the thyrotropic activity of chorionic gonadotropin mediates the thyrotoxicosis of choriocarcinoma. Am J Obstet Gynecol 138: 77

140. Novak E, Seah CS (1954) Choriocarcinoma of the uterus. A study of 74 cases from the Mathieu Memorial Chorionepithelioma Registry. Am J Obstet Gynecol 67: 933

141. Ober WB (1970) Gestational choriocarcinoma. Immunologic aspects, diagnosis and treatment. In: Gynecological Oncology—A Comprehensive Review and Evaluation. Proceedings of the Lenox Hill Hospital Symposium, New York, May 19–23, 1969. Amsterdam, New York, Excerpta Medica Foundation 304–315. Excerpta Medica International Congress Series No. 203

142. Ober WB, Maier RC (1981) Gestational choriocarcinoma of the fallopian tube. Diagn Gynecol Obstet 3: 213

143. Ober WB, Edgcomb JH, Price EB (1971) The pathology of choriocarcinoma. Ann NY Acad Sci 179: 299

144. O'Brien TJ, Engvall E, Schlaerth JB, Morrow CP (1980) Trophoblastic disease monitoring: Evaluation of pregnancy-specific B_1-glycoprotein. Am J Obstet Gynecol 138: 313

145. Ohama K, Kajii T, Okamoto E, Fukuda Y, Imaizumi K, Tsukahara M, Kobayashi K, Hagiwara K (1981) Dispermic origin of XY hydatidiform moles. Nature 292: 551

146. Olive DL, Lurain JR, Brewer JI (1984) Choriocarcinoma associated with term gestation. Am J Obstet Gynecol 148: 711

147. Parazzini F, LaVecchia C, Pampallona S, Franceschi S

(1985) Reproductive patterns and the risk of gestational trophoblastic disease. Am J Obstet Gynecol 152: 866
148. Park WW (1971) Choriocarcinoma. A Study of Its Pathology. Philadelphia, Davis
149. Park WW (1981) Pathology and classification of trophoblastic tumors. In: Gynecologic Oncology. Coppleson W (ed). Edinburgh, Churchill-Livingstone, Vol 2, pp 745–756
150. Park WW, Lees JC (1936) Choriocarcinoma. A general review with an analysis of 516 cases. Arch Pathol 160: 205
151. Pattillo RA, Sasaki S, Katayama KP, Roesler M, Mattingly RF (1981) Genesis of 46, XY hydatidiform mole. Am J Obstet Gynecol 141: 104
152. Patton GW, Goldstein DP (1973) Gestational choriocarcinoma of the tube and ovary. Surg Gynecol Obstet 137: 608
153. Pierce GB Jr, Midgley AR Jr (1963) The origin and function of human syncytiotrophoblastic giant cells. Am J Pathol 43: 153
154. Poen HJ, Djojopranoto M (1965) The possible etiologic factors of hydatidiform mole and choriocarcinoma. Am J Obstet Gynecol 92: 510
155. Quigley MM, Tyrey L, Hammond CB (1980) Utility of assay of alpha-subunit of human chorionic gonadotropin in management of gestational trophoblastic malignancies. Am J Obstet Gynecol 138: 545
156. Ring AM (1972) The concept of benign metastasizing hydatidiform moles. Am J Clin Pathol 58: 111
157. Ringertz N (1970) Hydatidiform mole, invasive mole and choriocarcinoma in Sweden 1958–1965. Acta Obstet Gynecol Scand 49: 195
158. Rizkallah T, Gurpide E, Van de Wiele RL (1969) Metabolism of hCG in man. J Clin Endocrinol 29: 92
159. Rolon PA, de Lopez BH (1977) Epidemiological aspects of hydatidiform mole in the Republic of Paraguay (South America). Br J Obstet Gynaecol 84: 862
160. Rolon PA, de Lopez BH (1979) Malignant trophoblastic disease in Paraguay. J Reprod Med 23: 94
161. Romero R, Horgan JG, Kohorn EI, Kadar N, Taylor KJW, Hobbins JC (1985) New criteria for the diagnosis of gestational trophoblastic disease. Obstet Gynecol 66: 553
162. Rosenshein NB, Wijnen H, Woodruff JD (1980) Clinical importance of the diagnosis of trophoblastic pseudotumors. Am J Obstet Gynecol 136: 635
163. Ross GT (1977) Clinical relevance of research on the structure of human chorionic gonadotropin. Am J Obstet Gynecol 129: 795
164. Sakuragi N (1982) Serum SPI and hCG β-subunit (hCG-β) levels in choriocarcinoma, invasive mole and hydatidiform mole—Clinical significance of SPI/hCG-β ratio. Gynecol Oncol 13: 393
165. Sasaki K, Hata H, Nakano R (1985) ABO blood group in patients with malignant trophoblastic disease. Gynecol Obstet Invest 20: 23
166. Schopper W, Pliess G (1949) Uber chorioepitheliosis. Ein beitrag zur genese, diagnostik und bewertung ektopischer chorionepithelialer wurcherungen. Virchows Arch [Pathol Anat] 317: 347
167. Scully RE, Young RH (1981) Trophoblastic pseudotumor (Editorial). Am J Surg Pathol 5: 75
168. Smith EB, Szulman AE, Hinsaw W, Tyrey L, Surti U, Hammond CB (1984) Human chorionic gonadotropin levels in complete and partial hydatidiform moles and in nonmolar abortuses. Am J Obstet Gynecol 149: 129
169. Soma H, Takayama M, Tokoro K, Kikuchi K, Saegusa H (1980) Radioimmunoassay of hCG as an early diagnosis of cerebral metastases in choriocarcinoma patients. Acta Obstet Gynecol Scand 59: 445
170. Stanhope CR, Stuart GCE, Curtis KL (1983) Primary ovarian hydatidiform mole: Review of the literature and report of a case. Am J Obstet Gynecol 145: 886
171. Stone M, Bagshawe KD (1979) An analysis of the influences of maternal age, gestational age, contraceptive method, and the mode of primary treatment of patients with hydatidiform moles on the incidence of subsequent chemotherapy. Br J Obstet Gynaecol 86: 782
172. Stone M, Bagshawe KD (1976) Hydatidiform mole: Two entities. Lancet 1: 535
173. Surani MAH, Barton SC, Norris ML (1984) Development of reconstituted mouse eggs suggests imprinting of the genome during gametogenesis. Nature 308: 548
174. Surti U, Szulman AE, O'Brien S (1979) Complete (classic) hydatidiform mole with 46,XY karyotype of paternal origin. Hum Genet 51: 153
175. Surti U, Szulman AE, O'Brien S (1982) Dispermic origin and clinical outcome of three complete hydatidiform moles with 46,XY karyotype. Am J Obstet Gynecol 144: 84
176. Surti U, Szulman AE, Wagner K, et al. (1986) Tetraploid partial moles: Two cases with a triple paternal contribution and a 92,XXXY karyotype. Hum Genet 72: 15
177. Surwit EA, Hammond CB (1980) Treatment of metastatic trophoblastic disease with poor prognosis. Obstet Gynecol 55: 565
178. Surwit EA, Hammond CB (1981) Recurrent gestational trophoblastic disease. Gynecol Oncol 12: 177
179. Surwit EA, Alberts DS, Christian CD, Graham VE (1984) Poor-prognosis gestational trophoblastic disease: An update. Obstet Gynecol 64: 21
180. Szulman AE (1984) Syndromes of hydatidiform moles. Partial vs complete. J Reprod Med 29: 788
181. Szulman AE, Surti U (1978) The syndromes of hydatidiform mole. I. Cytogenetic and morphologic correlations. Am J Obstet Gynecol 131: 665
182. Szulman AE, Surti U (1978) The syndromes of hydatidiform mole. II. Morphologic evolution of the complete and partial mole. Am J Obstet Gynecol 132: 20
183. Szulman AE, Surti U (1982) The clinicopathologic profile of the partial hydatidiform mole. Obstet Gynecol 59: 597
184. Szulman AE, Ma HK, Wong LC, Hsu C (1981) Residual trophoblastic disease in association with partial hydatidiform mole. Obstet Gynecol 57: 392
185. Szulman AE, Philippe E, Boue JG, Boue A (1981) Human triploidy: Association with partial hydatidiform moles and nonmolar conceptuses. Hum Pathol 12: 1016
186. Tatarinov YS, Sokolov AV (1977) Development of a radioimmunoassay for pregnancy-specific beta-globulin and its measurement in serum of patients with trophoblastic and non-trophoblastic tumors. Int J Cancer 19: 161
187. Teng NNH, Ballon SC (1984) Partial hydatidiform mole

with diploid karyotype: Report of three cases. Am J Obstet Gynecol 150: 961
188. Thiele RA, de Alvarez RR (1962) Metastasizing benign trophoblastic tumors. Am J Obstet Gynecol 84: 1395
189. Tomoda Y, Arii Y, Kaseki S, Asai Y, Gotoh S, Suzuki T, Kondoh T, Imaizumi M (1980) Surgical indications for resection in pulmonary metastasis of choriocarcinoma. Cancer 46: 2723
190. Tow WSH, Yung RH (1967) The value of histological grading in the prognostication of hydatidiform mole. J Obstet Gynaecol Br Commonw 74: 292
191. Tsao MS, Schraufnagel D, Wang NS (1981) Pulmonary metastasis of choriocarcinoma with a miliary roentgenographic pattern (Letter to the Editor). Arch Pathol Lab Med 105: 557
192. Tsuji K, Yagi S, Nakano R (1981) Increased risk of malignant transformation of hydatidiform moles in older gravidas: A cytogenetic study. Obstet Gynecol 58: 351
193. Tsukamoto N, Iwasaka T, Kashimura Y, Uchino H, Kashimura M, Matsuyama T (1985) Gestational trophoblastic disease in women aged 50 or more. Gynecol Oncol 20: 53
194. Tsukamoto N, Kashimura Y, Sano M, Saito T, Kanda S, Taki I (1981) Choriocarcinoma occurring within the normal placenta with breast metastasis. Gynecol Oncol 11: 348
195. Twiggs LB, Morrow CP, Schlaerth JB (1979) Acute pulmonary complications of molar pregnancy. Am J Obstet Gynecol 135: 189
196. Twiggs LB, Okagaki T, Phillips GL, Stroemer JR, Adcock LL (1981) Trophoblastic pseudotumor—Evidence of malignant disease potential. Gynecol Oncol 12: 238
197. Vaitukaitis JL, Braunstein GD, Ross GT (1972) A radioimmunoassay which specifically measures human chorionic gonadotropin in the presence of human luteinizing hormone. Am J Obstet Gynecol 113: 751
198. Van Bogaert L-J, Staguet J-P (1977) Chorionepitheliosis: A rare benign trophoblastic disease. Acta Obstet Gynecol Scand 56: 69
199. Van Der Werf AJM, Broeders GHB, Vooys GP, Mastboom JL (1970) Metastatic choriocarcinoma as a complication of pregnancy. Obstet Gynecol 35: 78
200. Vance RD, Geisinger KR (1985) Pure nongestational choriocarcinoma of the ovary. Report of a case. Cancer 56: 2321
201. Vassilakos P, Riotton G, Kajii T (1977) Hydatidiform mole: Two entities. A morphologic and cytogenetic study with some clinical considerations. Am J Obstet Gynecol 127: 167
202. Vaughn TC, Surwit EA, Hammond CB (1980) Late recurrences of gestational trophoblastic neoplasia. Am J Obstet Gynecol 138: 73
202A. Vejerslev LD, Dueholm M, Hassing N (1986) Hydatidiform mole: Cytogenetic marker analysis in twin gestation. Report of two cases. Am J Obstet Gynecol 155: 614
203. Veridiano NP, Gal D, Delke I, Rosen Y, Tancer ML (1980) Gestational choriocarcinoma of the ovary. Gynecol Oncol 10: 235
204. Wagner D (1967) Trophoblastic cells in the blood stream in normal and abnormal pregnancy. Acta Cytol 12: 137
205. Wake N, Takagi N, Sasaki M (1978) Androgenesis as a cause of hydatidiform mole. J Natl Cancer Inst 60: 51
206. Wallace DC, Surti U, Adams CW, Szulman AE (1982) Complete moles have paternal chromosomes but maternal mitochondrial DNA. Hum Genet 61: 145
207. Weed Jr JC, Hammond CB (1980) Cerebral metastatic choriocarcinoma: Intensive therapy and prognosis. Obstet Gynecol 55: 89
208. Weed Jr JC, Barnard DE, Currie JL, Clayton LA, Hammond CB (1982) Chemotherapy with the modified Bagshawe protocol for poor prognosis metastatic trophoblastic disease. Obstet Gynecol 59: 377
209. Westerhout FC (1964) Ruptured tubal hydatidiform mole. Report of a case. Obstet Gynecol 23: 138
210. Wilson RB, Hunter Jr JS, Dockerty MB (1961) Chorioadenoma destruens. Am J Obstet Gynecol 81: 546
211. Wong LC, Ma HK (1984) The syndrome of partial mole. Arch Gynecol 234: 161
211A. Wong LC, Choo YC, Ma HK (1986) Hepatic metastases in gestational trophoblastic disease. Obstet Gynecol 67: 107
212. World Health Organization Scientific Group on Gestational Trophoblastic Disease (1983) Gestational trophoblastic diseases. Technical Report Series 692. Geneva, WHO
213. Wu FYW (1973) Recurrent hydatidiform mole: A case report of nine consecutive molar pregnancies. Obstet Gynecol 41: 200
214. Wurzel J, Brooks JJ (1981) Primary gastric choriocarcinoma: Immunohistochemistry, postmortem documentation, and hormonal effects in a postmenopausal female. Cancer 48: 2756
215. Wynn RM (1972) Cytotrophoblastic specializations: An ultrastructural study of the human placenta. Am J Obstet Gynecol 114: 339
216. Yamashita K, Nakamura T, Shimizu T (1984) Absence of major histocompatibility complex antigens in choriocarcinoma. AM J Obstet Gynecol 150: 896
217. Yen S, MacMahon B (1968) Epidemiologic features of trophoblastic disease. Am J Obstet Gynecol 101: 126
218. Young RH, Scully RE (1984) Placental-site trophoblastic tumor: Current status. Clin Obstet Gynecol 27: 248
219. Young RH, Kurman RJ, Scully RE Unpublished data
220. Young RH, Scully RE, McCluskey RT (1985) A distinctive glomerular lesion complicating placental site trophoblastic tumor: Report of two cases. Hum Pathol 16(1): 35
220A. Yuen BH, Callegari PB (1986) Occurence of molar pregnancy in patients undergoing elective abortion: Comparison with other clinical presentations. Am J Obstet Gynecol 154: 273
221. Zhang J, Kraus FT (1986) Placental site trophoblastic tumor. Immunocytochemical correlations. Lab Invest 54: 73A

25

Cytology of the Female Genital Tract

Rita Leff Blaustein, M.D.

Diagnostic cytology is based on the fact that cells exfoliated or collected from the cervix and the vagina reflect features of the tissue from which they arise. The main application of cytology to the female genital tract is in the early diagnosis of precancerous and cancerous lesions. Patients who have been treated for cervical cancer can be followed cytologically for response to radiation and recurrence of the disease.

Assessment of hormonal function is possible if the specimen is obtained properly and if the limitations of cytology are understood by the cytologist and the clinician.

Normal Components of the Routine Smear

Epithelial Cells

The components of a smear are related to age, phase of the menstrual cycle, such exogenous influences as inflammation or therapy, and the site from which the material is obtained.[26] The term "normal," therefore, carries the connotation of "compatible with the clinical data." An atrophic smear in a 70-year-old woman is compatible with her age. An atrophic smear in a 20-year-old is not compatible with her age. Yet both smears contain "normal" parabasal cells.

The most prominent epithelial cells of the routine cervical–vaginal smear are squamous cells originating from the pars vaginalis of the cervix and from the vagina. Essentially there are three types of squamous cells to be identified.

The parabasal cells (Fig. 25.1), as their name implies, originate from the zone immediately above the basal layer of the stratum germinativum. They are round or oval and small, ranging in size from 12 to 30 μm. Their cytoplasm is opaque and usually basophilic and may show vacuolization. Occasionally, when they are in a group, tails of cytoplasm may be seen. The nucleus is round and vesicular, and the nucleocytoplasmic ratio is high.

The intermediate cells (Fig. 25.2) are polygonal, and their cytoplasm is transparent and usually basophilic,

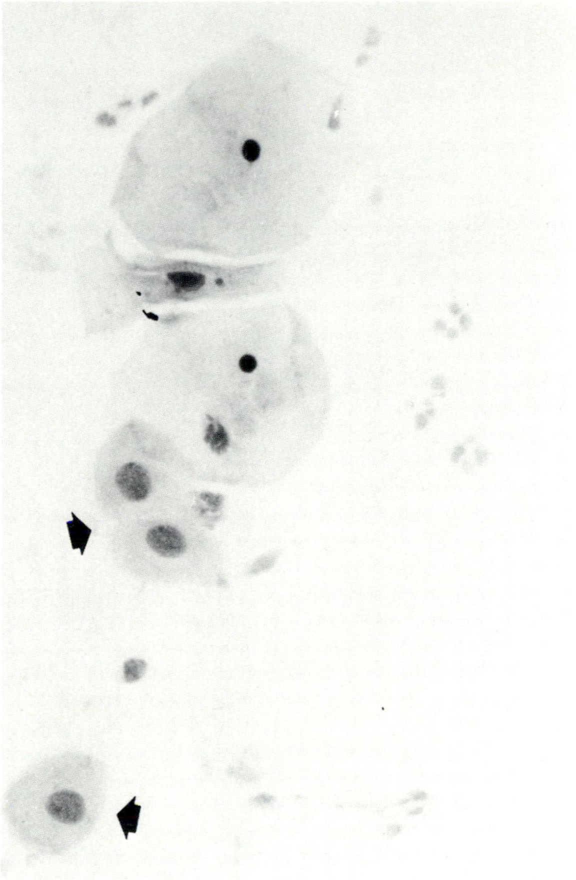

FIG. 25.1. Parabasal cells. The parabasal cells (*arrows*) are small, round or oval squamous cells with opaque cytoplasm and vesicular nuclei. The nucleocytoplasmic ratio is high. Occasionally, these cells may have cytoplasmic tails. Contrast the pyknotic nucleus and abundant transparent cytoplasm of the superficial cells in the same field.

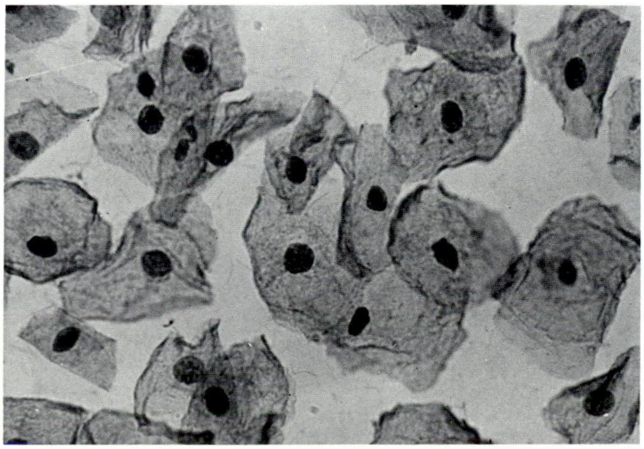

FIG. 25.2. Intermediate cells. This group of intermediate cells shows the vesicular nuclei and transparent, abundant cytoplasm that characterize them. Many of the cells show folding of the cytoplasm.

but it can be eosinophilic. They are large, measuring up to 50 μm. The nucleus is centrally located, and the chromatin is finely distributed, producing a vesicular pattern. Navicular cells are glycogen-containing intermediate cells that characteristically show folding and rolling of their cytoplasmic borders and areas of yellow-orange staining (Papanicolaou stain technique).

The superficial cells (Fig. 25.3) originate from the outermost layers of the epithelium. They are large, polyhedral, flat, and waferlike but occasionally may be rolled and appear thin and spindly. The cytoplasm is usually eosinophilic but can be basophilic. It may contain very small, dark granules, so-called keratohyaline granules. The nucleus is small, measuring less than 6 μm in diameter, with no discernible nuclear structure. This is the "ink dot," karyopyknotic nucleus characteristic of the superficial cell. It is this pyknosis of the nucleus that distinguishes the superficial cell from the large intermediate cell.

In addition to the three types of cells described above, two other types of squamous cells may be noted. If procidentia is present, anucleated and keratinized cells may appear in the smear as flat, orange-staining squamous cells. They may contain a pyknotic nucleus or the nucleus may be absent.[29]

Basal cells may sometimes be seen in a smear, as

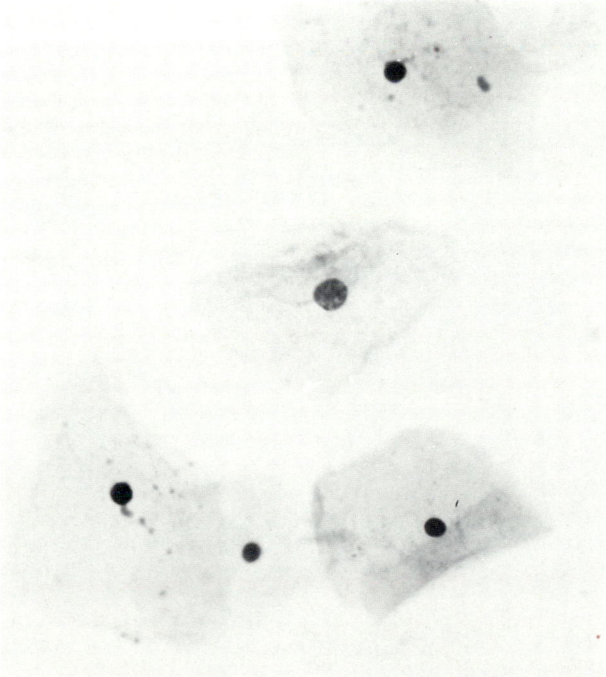

FIG. 25.3. Superficial cells and an intermediate cell. Pyknotic nucleus and abundant, transparent cytoplasm are the characteristics of these large polyhedral superficial cells. The single intermediate cell in the center of the group displays the vesicular nucleus that differentiates the intermediate cell from the superficial cells.

the result of inflammation or trauma. They are uniform in size, are rounded, and show densely basophilic, opaque cytoplasm. The nuclei appear hyperchromatic, and the nucleocytoplasmic ratio is high. It is important to recognize the benign nature of these cells and not confuse them with malignant cervical cells, which may also exhibit nuclear hyperchromatism and a high nucleocytoplasmic ratio. The basal cells display a uniformity of appearance that the malignant cells lack.

The endocervical cells (Figs. 25.4 and 25.5) appear as tall columnar cells arranged usually in characteristic groupings, either in parallel rows or, in cross-section, forming a honeycomb pattern with clearly defined cell borders. Individual columnar cells are basophilic, and their nuclei are basal in position. At the free or luminal edge of the cell, pink-staining cilia and a terminal bar can occasionally be identified (Papanicolaou stain). The nuclei of these cells are finely granular and round or oval in shape, and they can show considerable variation in size. Small nucleoli may be present. Evidence of secretory activity, in the form of cytoplasmic vacuoles and flattening of a nuclear border, is common. During the height of estrogenic stimulation, a nipplelike nuclear protrusion may be seen.

The endometrial cells are smaller than endocervical cells and when single are difficult to detect in the cervical–vaginal smear. Endometrial cells, occurring as cell balls or clusters (Fig. 25.6), can be seen from day 1 to days 10–12. These cells usually exhibit a marked degree of degeneration and necrosis. Vacuoles in the cytoplasm of the glandular cells may be seen. Fine chromatin granules are present in the nuclei. The appearance of endometrial cells in the cervicovaginal smear at times other than the first half of the menstrual cycle is abnormal and requires further evaluation, whether the cells show atypia or not.[26]

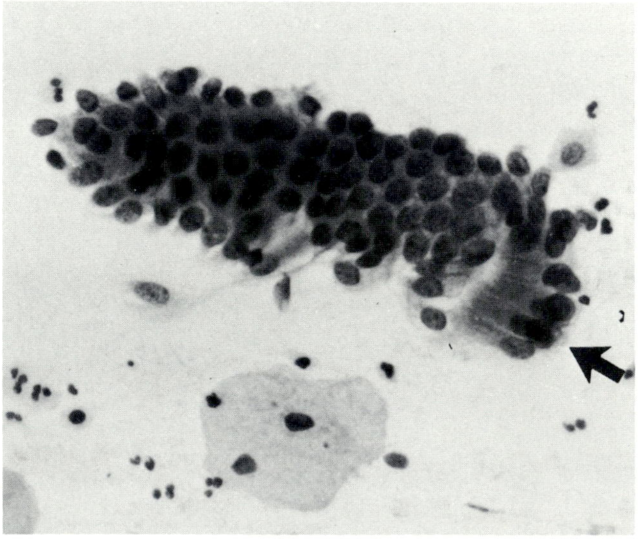

Fig. 25.4. Endocervical cells. This sheet of endocervical cells shows both the characteristic picket fence arrangement of columnar cells (*arrow*) and the honeycomb appearance, wherein the cell borders can be discerned and cytoplasm can be seen surrounding each nucleus.

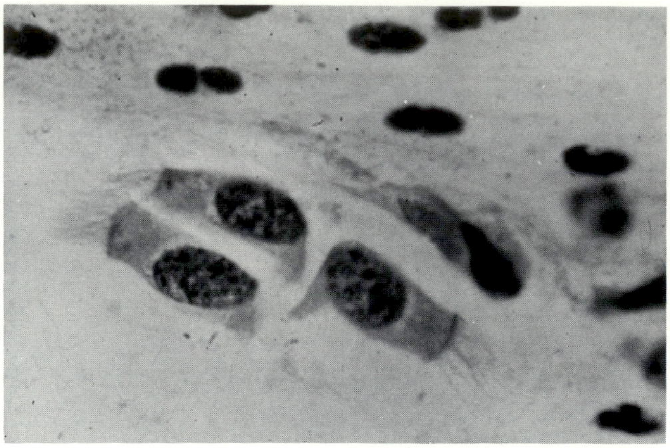

Fig. 25.5. Endocervical cells. Cilia and terminal plates are clearly seen. The chromatin is somewhat coarse but it is distributed uniformly in all of the patient's endocervical cells.

Nonepithelial Components

Histiocytes are often found in the normal smear. Small histiocytes (Fig. 25.7), singly or in clusters, are normally seen during the exodus phase, occurring during the first 10 days after menstruation. Their cytoplasm is finely vacuolated or foamy and may contain phagocytosed particulate matter, cellular debris, and blood cells. Larger histiocytes and multinucleated giant cells can measure

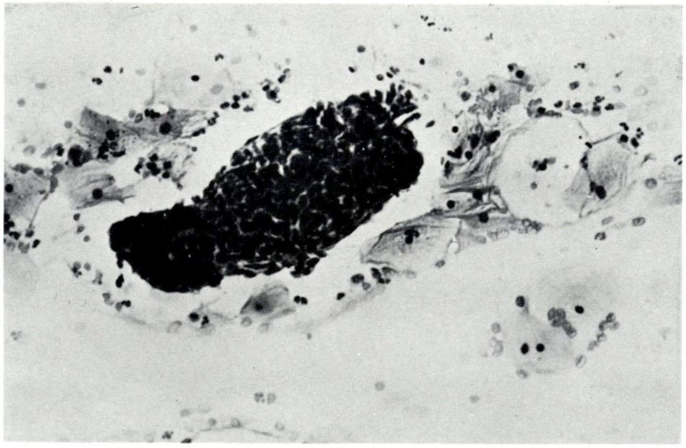

Fig. 25.6. Endometrial cells, day 8 of the menstrual cycle. Against a background of superficial and intermediate cells and polymorphonuclear leukocytes, a cluster of overlapping and partly degenerated endometrial cells is seen. The presence of clusters of endometrial cells up to the 10th to 12th day of the cycle is a normal finding.

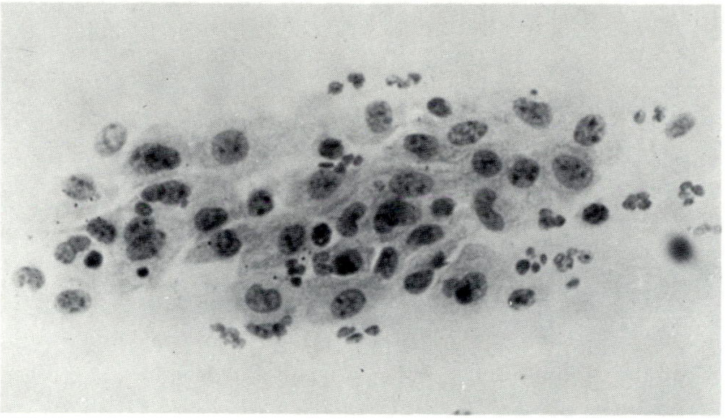

Fig. 25.7. Histiocytes. A loosely arranged group of small histiocytes with foamy cytoplasm and poorly delineated cell borders is seen. There is nuclear pleomorphism, but the chromatin pattern is quite uniform from cell to cell. Several of the histiocytes exhibit reniform nuclei.

in excess of 100 μm. Histiocytes frequently exhibit kidney-shaped nuclei with fine or coarse, well-distributed chromatin and occasionally, karyosomes. Multinucleated histiocytes (Fig. 25.8) must be distinguished from multinucleated malignant cells. Characteristically, the multiple nuclei of histiocytes resemble each other, whereas in multinucleated malignant cells, there is marked variation from nucleus to nucleus.

Erythrocytes are often seen in the cervical–vaginal smear at times other than menstrual. Frequently, their presence results from slight trauma during gynecologic exploration or from energetic cervical scraping. When bleeding is profuse or the blood is lysed, the possibility of a pathologic process should be kept in mind. The presence of an increased number of leukocytes just before or after menstruation is physiologic. With the Papanicolaou stain, it is not possible to distinguish the several types of leukocytes because cytoplasmic granules do not stain. Spermatozoa can be seen in the smear after coitus, often permitting a good evaluation of their morphology (Fig. 25.9).

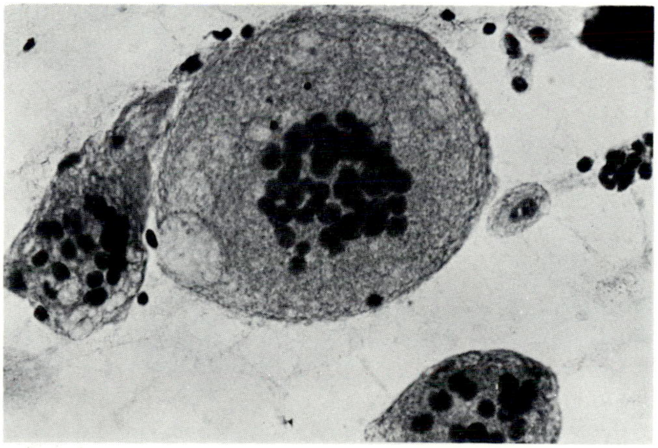

Fig. 25.8. Multinucleated histiocyte. Multinucleated histiocytes must be distinguished from multinucleated malignant cells. Typically, the multiple nuclei of histiocytes resemble each other, whereas in the malignant cell, there is marked variation from nucleus to nucleus, in chromatin distribution, hyperchromasia, size, and shape.

Powder from surgical gloves, a variety of crystals from unfiltered stains and fixatives, cotton fibers, and pollen granules are frequent contaminants of the smear. Lubricant and anticonceptual jellies produce a deep blue haze so dense at times that they may obscure the cellular components of the smear, thus rendering the material unsatisfactory for evaluation.

Nonmalignant Disorders

The term *cytologic atypia* is used to denote those alterations of the squamous and columnar epithelia that may be induced by infection, trauma, and physical or chemical stimuli. Most of these benign, cellular changes are nonspecific. However, at times, the alteration may be specific enough to permit a presumptive cytologic diagnosis. The primary importance of recognizing atypia is to avoid mistaking it for the more serious cellular changes seen in premalignant disorders of the cervix.

The presence of a few inflammatory cells in the smear does not necessarily reflect a pathologic condition, partic-

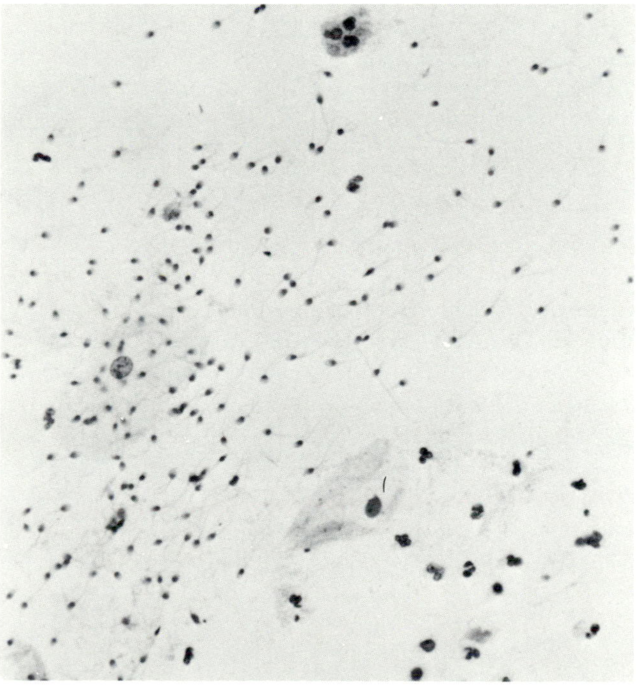

Fig. 25.9. Spermatozoa. These are readily recognizable when well preserved. The portion of the head at the flagellar pole appears darker than the opposite pole.

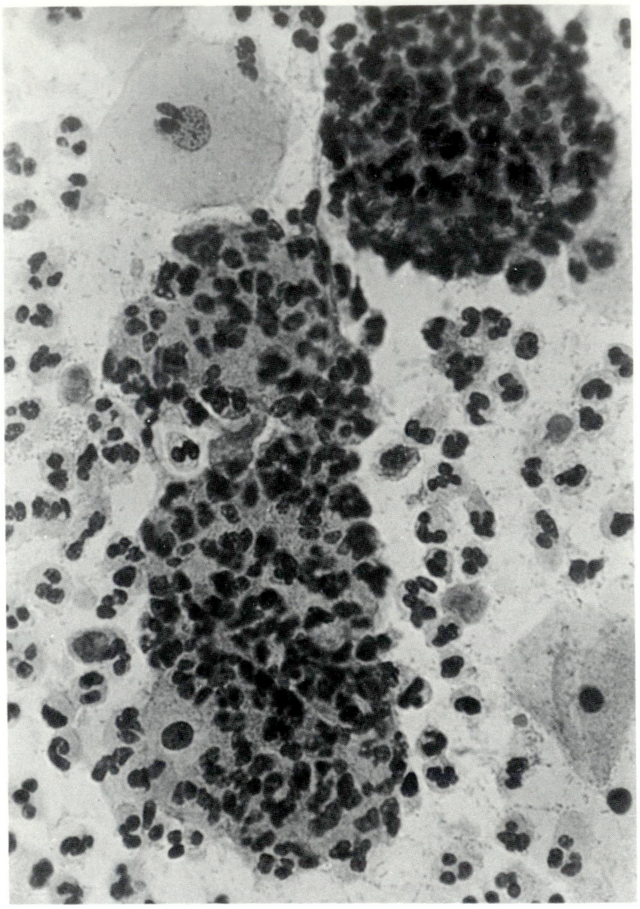

FIG. 25.10. Inflammatory exudate. Large numbers of polymorphonuclear leukocytes are present, as well as bacteria and cellular debris. When the exudate is so dense as to obscure the epithelial elements, the smear must be considered unsatisfactory, and a repeat smear, after the inflammation has cleared, should be requested.

ularly when the inflammatory cells are seen immediately before, during, or immediately after menstruation. During acute or chronic inflammation, there is usually an increased desquamation of epithelial cells, abundant production of mucus, and varying numbers of leukocytes and histiocytes. The inflammatory exudate (Fig. 25.10) may be so dense as to obscure the presence of the epithelial elements. When this occurs, the smear may be considered unsatisfactory for reliable evaluation, and a repeat smear, after the inflammation has cleared, should be requested. In response to inflammation, the epithelial elements may exhibit changes in the overall cellular pattern and also in alterations within the individual cells.[49]

Changes in Cellular Pattern

The proportions of parabasal, intermediate, and superficial cells can be altered by inflammation. The general effect is a wider distribution of the three cell types. In a postmenopausal patient whose smear prior to the occurrence of the inflammation has revealed parabasal cells exclusively, parabasal, intermediate, and superficial cells may all be present simultaneously in varying proportions. Similarly, parabasal cells may appear in the smear of a woman in the childbearing age where previously only superficial and intermediate cells have been expected. Because inflammation can alter the characteristic cytologic patterns that are associated with normal physiologic changes from birth to the postmenopausal phase, hormonal assessment should not be undertaken on a smear in which an inflammatory process is noted.

Changes Within Epithelial Cells

The epithelial cells may exhibit changes in both nucleus and cytoplasm. The importance of recognizing inflammation-associated changes is twofold: It enables the cytologist to report to the physician the presence of inflammation, often identifying the offending agent, and it enables the cytologist to differentiate between benign abnormalities and malignant changes.

Nucleopyknosis, which is normal in superficial cells, may occur in intermediate and parabasal cells in the presence of inflammation. Some nuclei may exhibit karyorrhexis (Fig. 25.11); the condensation of chromatin into coarse, rounded, darkly staining masses around the periphery of the nucleus. This change must be distinguished from the irregular, coarse, often angular clumping of chromatin, which is the most reliable evidence of malignancy. Some nuclei may undergo karyolysis. Nuclear enlargement, binucleation, some coarsening of the chromatin, and hyperchromatism can also be seen with inflammation. Occasionally, a small nucleolus may appear in the nucleus of squamous cells. Degenerative changes within the cytoplasm may include a poorly defined cell border that is ragged, changes in the staining reaction to an eosinophilia or polychromatia, and the appearance of coarse vacuoles.

In columnar cells of the endocervix, nuclei can show considerable variation in size but usually exhibit a uniformity from nucleus to nucleus in chromatin pattern and in shape. The nucleolus may be more prominent. Multinucleation may be seen. Perinuclear vacuolation may also occur. Denuded nuclei are common, and although these nuclei may vary considerably in size, they are usually uniform in shape and chromatin distribution (Fig. 25.12).

Cytolysis (Fig. 25.13) of intermediate cells by the enzymes of Döderlein bacilli–a heterogeneous group of lactobacilli—is seen in those situations where intermediate cells predominate, such as pregnancy, the premenarche, or the second half of the menstrual cycle.

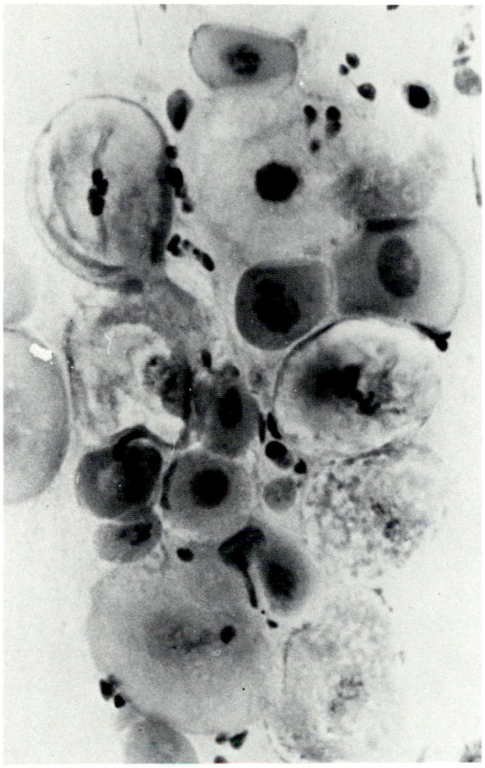

FIG. 25.11. Benign atypia. This group of epithelial cells shows cytoplasmic preservation and considerable variation in size and shape. Several nuclei are moderately hyperchromatic, whereas others have undergone karyolysis. Some nuclei show karyorrhexis. The benign nature of these cells is apparent; the even distribution of chromatin within the nuclei and the normal nucleocytoplasm ratio are maintained.

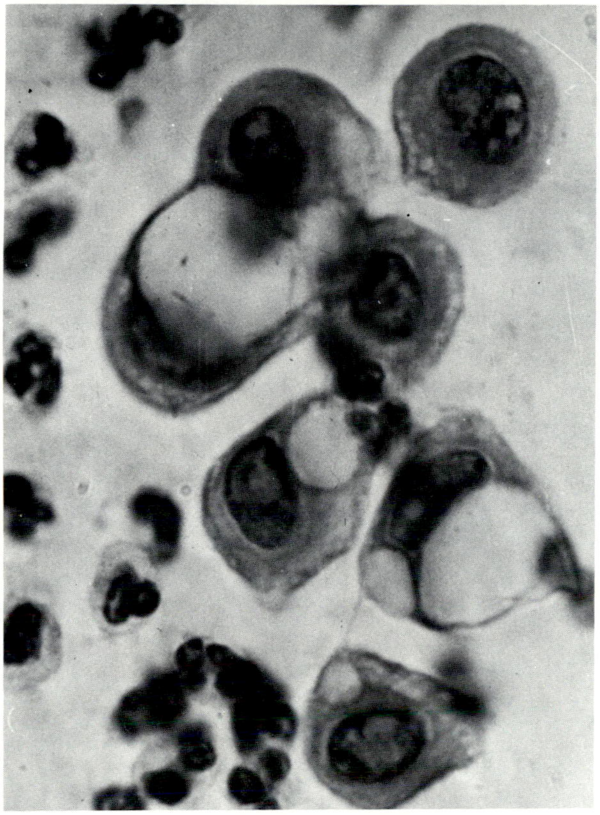

FIG. 25.12. Acute cervicitis. A group of endocervical cells shows changes caused by inflammation. There are large intracytoplasmic vacuoles, which have pushed the nucleus toward the periphery in some of the cells. Perinuclear halos are visible. The individual cells retain abundant cytoplasm. Polymorphonuclear leukocytes are present. These cellular changes should not be confused with endocervical malignancy. The nuclear chromatin pattern remains uniform, and no prominent nucleoli are present.

Squamous Metaplasia

Squamous metaplasia (Figs. 25.14 and 25.15), another nonmalignant change often encountered in smears from the cervix, may accompany inflammation. It can also be found in cervices where no evidence of inflammation is discernible. Koss[26] has defined metaplasia as "the replacement of one type of epithelium by another that is not normally present in a given location." He explains that "the basis of the process is the ability of the germinative or reserve cells of the endocervix to produce either the typical columnar glandular epithelium or, under abnormal circumstances, squamous epithelium."[26] The metaplastic cells may appear in cervical smears as sheets of elongated and angular cells, often with finely vacuolated cytoplasm. The nuclei are uniformly ovoid, with a delicate chromatin network and often prominent nucleoli. At times, metaplastic cells (Fig. 25.15) may present as a group, comparable in size to parabasal cells, with opaque cytoplasm that shows some vacuolation and occasional infiltration by polymorphonuclear leukocytes. Attenuated tails of cytoplasm are common.

Effects of Folic Acid and Vitamin B_{12} Deficiency

Patients with megaloblastic anemia caused by folic acid or vitamin B_{12} deficiency may exhibit both nuclear and cellular enlargement of epithelial cells. Occasionally, abnormalities in chromatin pattern and the presence of nucleoli may be seen in these enlarged cells, giving rise to diagnostic difficulty. Women who develop megaloblastic anemia during the course of their pregnancy may display these alterations.

Specific Inflammations

Bacteria are common components of smears from the cervix and vagina. Their presence does not necessarily

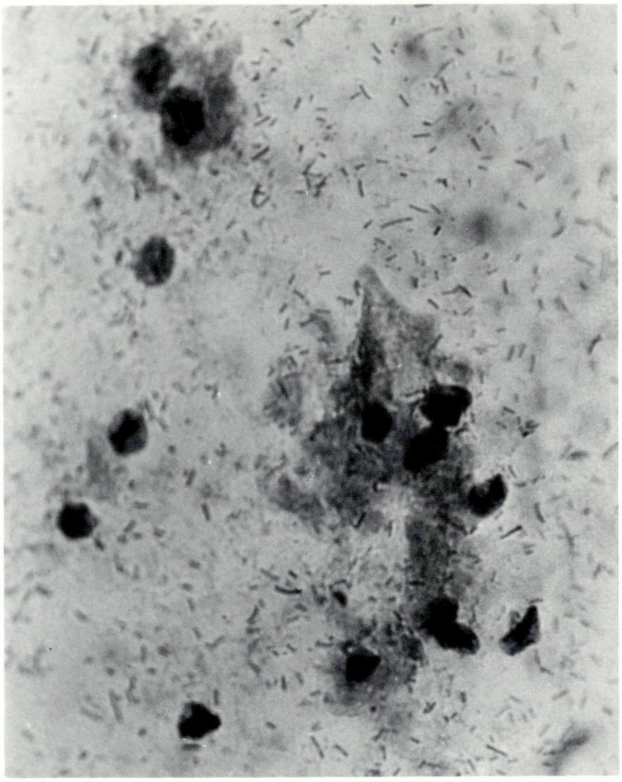

FIG. 25.13. Cytolysis. Denuded nuclei, fragments of cytoplasm, and large numbers of Döderlein bacilli are present. In the smear from a pregnant woman, cytolysis of intermediate cells can be marked. In an atrophic smear, the parabasal cells may also exhibit cytolysis, and numerous denuded nuclei are present.

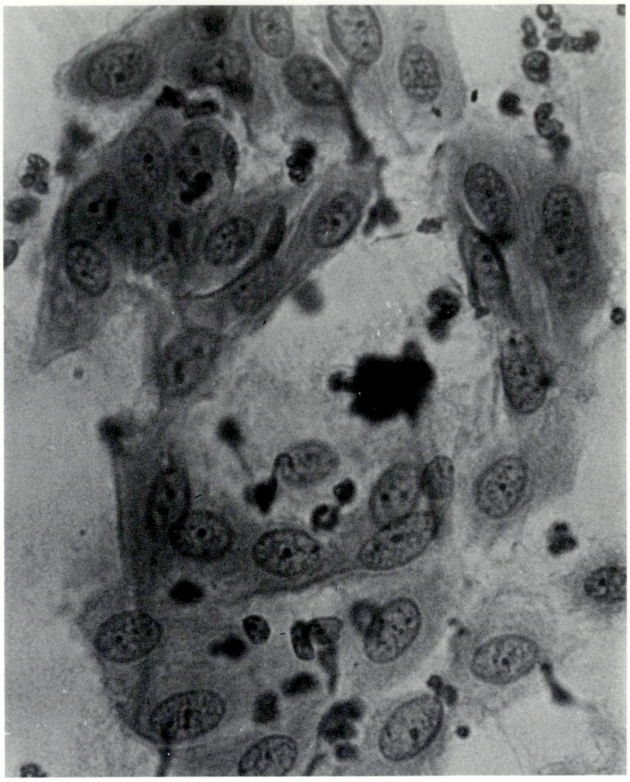

FIG. 25.14. Squamous metaplasia. This sheet of elongated cells with vacuolated cytoplasm and large vesicular nuclei represents squamous metaplasia of the reserve cells in the endocervical epithelium. Note the prominent nucleoli. Some inflammatory cells are also present.

signify the presence of infection. Coccoid bacteria may be present in large numbers, but specific identification can only be made by culture. Among the rod forms, *Escherichia coli* is often implicated in the vaginitis of girls and postmenopausal women. *Haemophilus vaginalis* (*Corynebacterium vaginale*), as the causative agent in some cases of vaginitis, may be suspected when epithelial cells covered by numerous rods are observed. These cells have been termed *clue cells* (Fig. 25.16).

Four specific etiologic agents that are important clinically and that merit special consideration are: (1) *Trichomonas vaginalis*, a protozoon, (2) *Candida albicans*, a fungus, (3) herpes simplex, a virus, and (4) human papillomavirus (condyloma).

Trichomonas

Cervicitis and vaginitis caused by *Trichomonas vaginalis* are a common clinical occurrence. In the Papanicolaou-stained smear, the protozoa appear as oval or pear-shaped structures and range in size from a small histiocyte to that of a parabasal cell. The flagella are rarely discernible. Therefore, the proper identification of the organism is accomplished by recognition of the small, eccentric, pale-staining nucleus. Tiny eosinophilic granules are often seen in the cytoplasm.

In some cases, numerous well-preserved trichomonads (Fig. 25.17a) can be seen in the smear, with no discernible inflammatory reaction or cellular atypia. Usually, however, in cases of trichomonal cervicovaginitis, the presence of the organism is accompanied by abundant epithelial desquamation, inflammatory exudate, and epithelial atypia. The atypia may be seen in both the squamous and the columnar cells, which show cytolysis, nuclear enlargement, perinuclear halos, and eosinophilia of the cytoplasm. At times trichomonads are seen parasitizing superficial squamous cells. Vacuolated parabasal cells, either from areas of ulceration or from metaplasia, may be numerous (Fig. 25.17b).

Candida

The fungus *Candida albicans* appears in smears as long eosinophilic filaments or hyphae and small conidia or

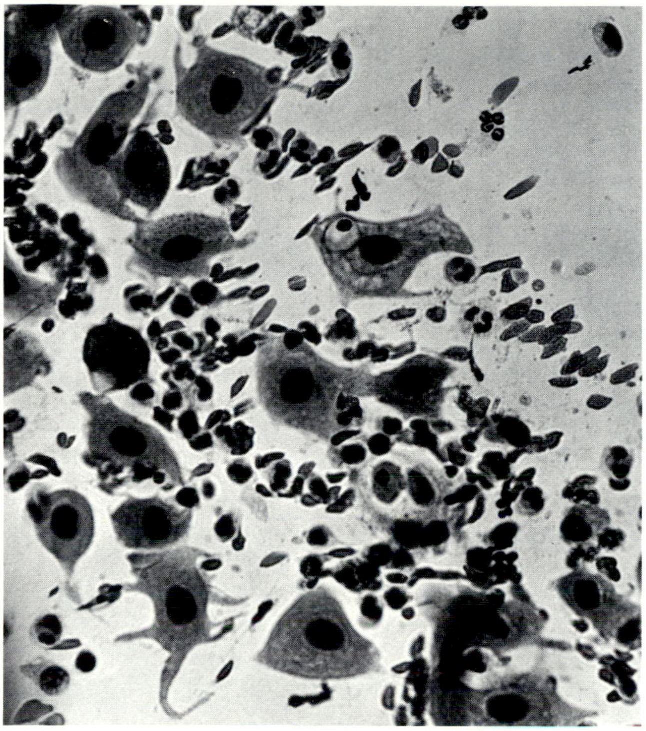

FIG. 25.15. Squamous metaplasia. This is a group of metaplastic cells, comparable in size to parabasal cells, with cytoplasm showing some vacuolation. Attenuated tabs of cytoplasm are prominent.

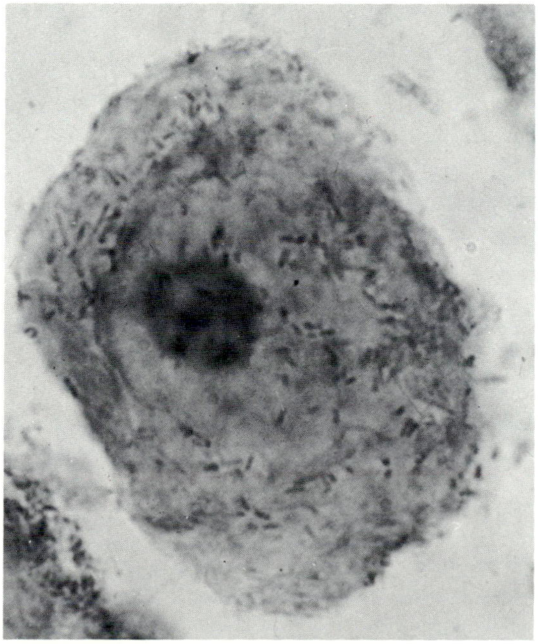

FIG. 25.16. Clue cell. This large squamous cell is covered with numerous small rods of *Haemophilus vaginalis*, an organism that is responsible for some instances of vaginitis.

yeast bodies (Fig. 25.18). Degeneration of polymorphonuclear leukocytes is often striking.

Herpes Simplex

The cytologic findings in *herpes simplex* infection are very characteristic.[24] In the early phase of the infection, there is a striking enlargement of the nucleus of the squamous cells, with a ground-glass appearance. Multinucleation occurs with a molding of adjacent nuclei (Fig. 25.19). The cytoplasm also enlarges, producing very large cells. In recurrent herpes, large inclusions (Fig. 25.20) may be seen within the nucleus. They are larger than nucleoli and lack the smooth, rounded outline of a nucleolus. A clear halo around the inclusion is usually evident.

Genital herpes inflammations[24] are self-limited. Their importance, from a clinical standpoint, is that the virus may be transmitted to the newborn during delivery if the mother has contracted a herpetic infection near term. The infant may develop fatal encephalitis and meningitis. Delivery by cesarean section is, therefore, undertaken.

Human Papillomavirus (HPV)—Condyloma[23,30,31,41]

The possibility that the viruses associated with condylomata of the cervix contribute to the development of uterine cervical carcinoma is considered in Chapter 7, Cervical Intraepithelial Neoplasia, and Chapter 8, Cervical Carcinoma. Meisels et al. have suggested that the atypical condyloma represents a more advanced step toward possible malignant transformation.[30,31]

The cytologic findings in typical condyloma of the cervix are seen in the squamous cells, where nuclear enlargement and multinucleation occur. The background is generally clear. Groups or sheets of cells exhibit orangeophilic staining and hyperchromatic nuclei. The pathognomonic koilocytotic cell is one in which there is a large zone of perinuclear clearing and dense cytoplasm in the periphery of the cell (Figs. 25.21, 25.22, 25.23, and 25.24). Nuclei may show degenerative changes.

Other Agents[32,33]

Chlamydia trachomatis, an obligatory, intracellular organism, has been implicated as a common causative agent in nongonococcal genital infections. In routine Papanicolaou-stained material, the chlamydial organisms cannot be identified with certainty. The detection of inclusions is an insensitive method for making the diagnosis of chlamydial infection. It has been recommended that the inflammatory cell pattern, that is, increased numbers of histiocytes and polymorphonuclear leukocytes, and the presence of transformed lymphocytes may be used

a

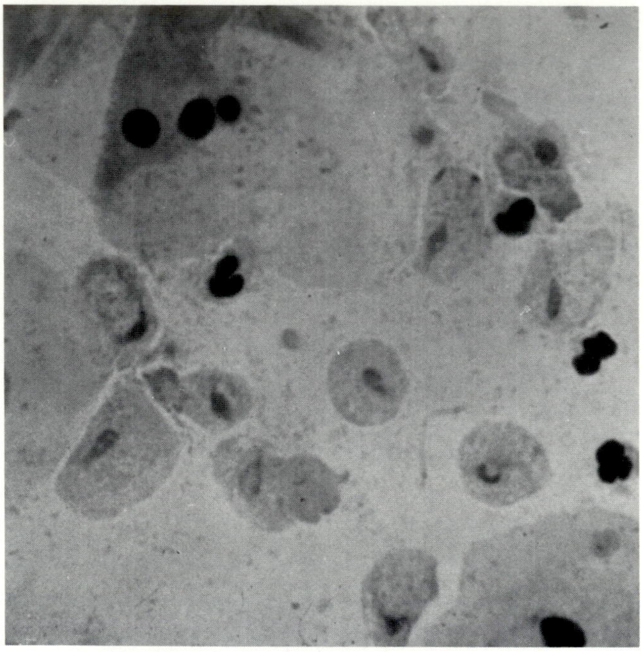

b

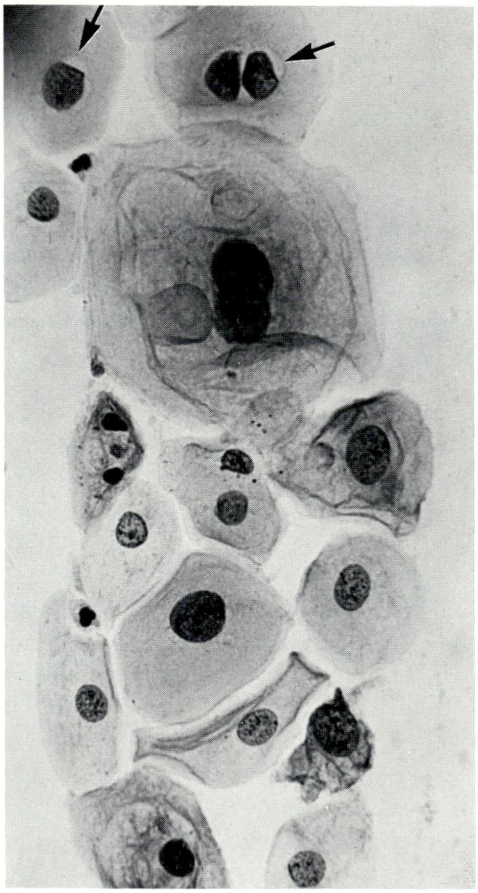

FIG. 25.17.*a*. Trichomonads. These pear-shaped or ovoid protozoa range in size from that of a small histiocyte to that of a parabasal cell. The nucleus is tiny and usually eccentric. *b*. Changes in squamous cells secondary to trichomoniasis. This group of cells reveals a variety of changes secondary to *Trichomonas* infection. Perinuclear haloes are seen (*arrows*), as well as hyperchromatism, binucleation, and prominent nuclear borders. There is considerable variation in size and chromatin intensity, but none of the nuclei exhibits the strikingly abnormal distribution of chromatin seen in malignant cells. These changes are compatible with the diagnosis of *benign atypia*.

to identify a group of women who are at high risk for *C. trachomatis* infection and who should have immunodiagnostic tests[44] for detection of the organisms (see Chapter 6, Benign Lesions of Cervix).

Actinomyces israelii in a smear[15] is most often associated with the presence of a foreign body, commonly an intrauterine device (IUD). Typically, isolated, woolly, fuzzy masses of actinomycetes are noted, which under high power reveal delicate filamentous organisms that branch at acute angles, so-called sulfur granules. Cellular changes induced by IUDs include vacuolation and polymorphonuclear leukocytes within the cytoplasm of endocervical cells and degenerative cell changes in clusters of shed endometrial cells in a background of inflammation (see Chapter 10, Benign Diseases of Endometrium).

Aberrant genital vaccinia has been described following vaccination or by contact contamination. Cytologic diagnosis depends on the finding of large, eosinophilic, intracytoplasmic inclusions.[22]

In the detection of cytomegalovirus infection,[22] a prominent, single, basophilic intranuclear inclusion surrounded by a clear halo is sought. The term *owl eye* has been given to this finding.

With adenovirus infection, multiple intranuclear inclusions suggest the diagnosis. Other organisms, including *Entamoeba histolytica*, *Enterobius vermicularis*, *Ascaris lumbricoides*, and vinegar eels, have been observed occasionally in smears from the female genital tract.[8]

Intraepithelial Neoplasia of the Cervix

The main objective in cytologic diagnosis is to detect those cellular abnormalities that are the precursors of cervical cancer. A number of terms have been used to designate those intraepithelial changes that have been considered precancerous. One may subscribe to the International Agreement of 1962,[21] which, following its definitions of invasive carcinoma and carcinoma in situ, defines dysplasia as "all other disturbances of differentiation of the squamous epithelial lining of surface and glands." Koss[26] has proposed that intraepithelial precancerous changes form a progressive spectrum of abnormalities ranging from slight changes (early borderline lesions

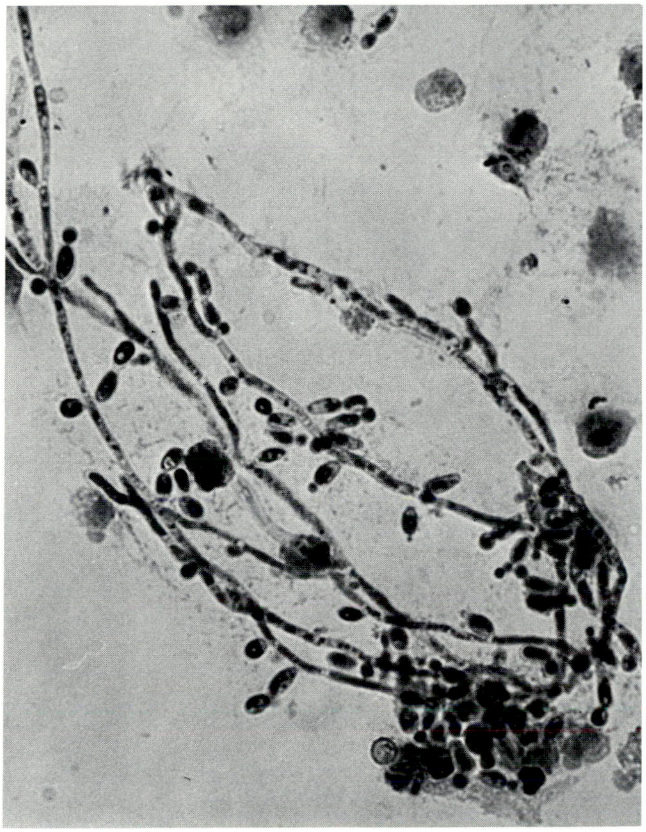

FIG. 25.18. *Candida albicans* and trichomonads. Both hyphae and conidia are present. The hyphae are eosinophilic filaments; the conidia appear as small ovoid structures. Trichomonads are also present, a not uncommon combination of pathogens in the lower genital tract.

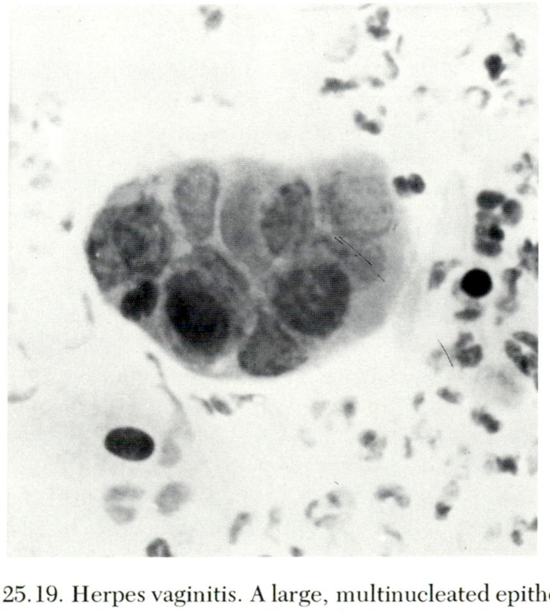

FIG. 25.19. Herpes vaginitis. A large, multinucleated epithelial cell showing characteristic molding of adjacent nuclei is seen.

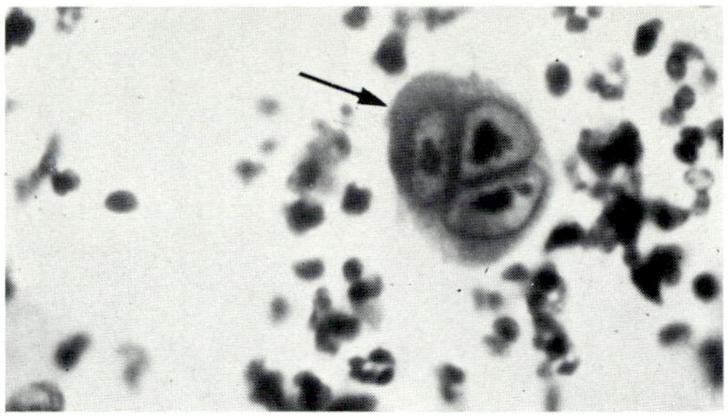

FIG. 25.20. Herpes vaginitis. Against a background of inflammatory cells, an epithelial cell with several nuclei is visible. There are intranuclear inclusions (*arrow*), each of which is surrounded by a halo.

or mild dysplasia) to severe changes (carcinoma in situ). Richart[38] has used the term *cervical intraepithelial neoplasia* (CIN) to designate all precursors to invasive cervical cancer. For a thorough review of the nature and natural history of cervical intraepithelial lesions, the

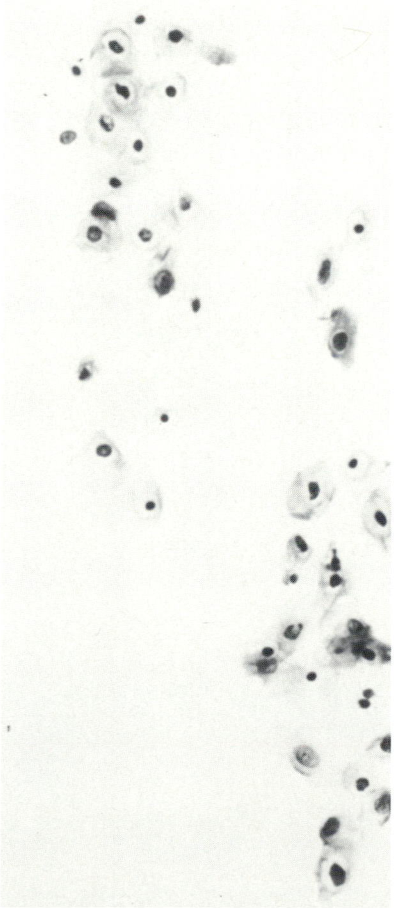

FIG. 25.21. Condyloma of cervix. Many of the squamous cells have large perinuclear areas of clearing, producing the almost pathognomonic balloon cell. Generally, the background is clear, as in this example.

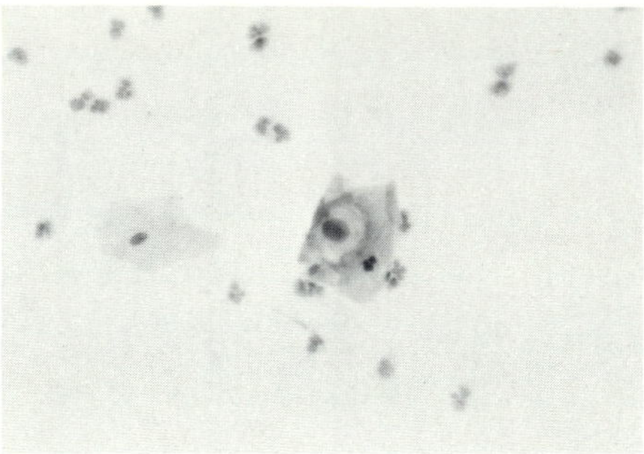

FIG. 25.22. Condyloma of the cervix. The high power view of a koilocytotic cell reveals the nuclear enlargement (compare it to the nucleus of the adjacent intermediate cell) and the denser cytoplasm in the periphery of the cell.

reader is referred to Chapter 7, Cervical Intraepithelial Neoplasia.

The cytologist can make a major contribution toward eradicating cervical cancer by directing his or her efforts to the detection of abnormalities in the cervical epithelium as they manifest themselves in the cervical smear. Whether the cells under scrutiny are labeled dysplastic, borderline lesions, or intraepithelial neoplasm, the crucial point is that they be recognized and appropriate follow-up measures be instituted.

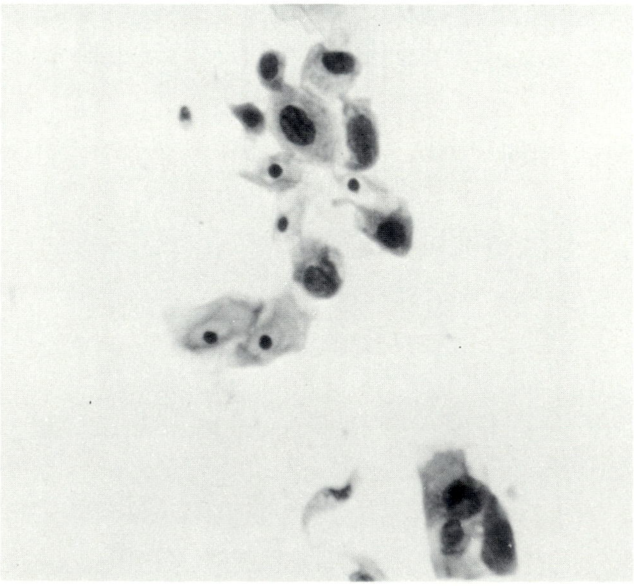

FIG. 25.23. Condyloma. The nuclear atypia can be so prominent that the diagnosis of dysplasia or CIS might be considered on cytologic material. The large, darkly stained nuclei show a smudged appearance, which helps to distinguish them from dysplastic nuclei, in which the chromatin details are well preserved, albeit irregular in distribution.

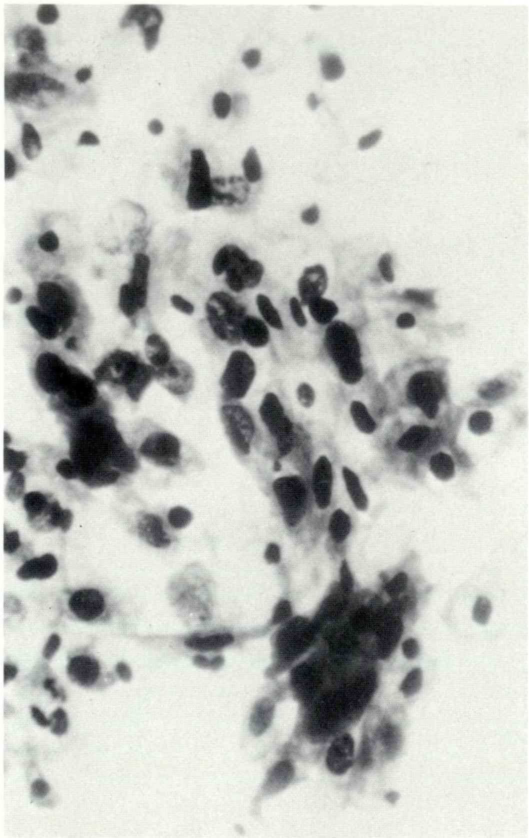

FIG. 25.24. Condyloma. The aggregate of cells with enlarged, dark-staining nuclei could be misinterpreted as invasive squamous carcinoma. The indistinct, smudged chromatin structure helps to distinguish it from carcinoma. The irregular, generally well preserved chromatin clumping, angularity, and abnormal distribution of the malignant cells are not seen in condyloma.

Mild Dysplasia and Dyskaryosis (CIN 1)

The smear shows predominantly polygonal superficial and intermediate cells with abundant eosinophilic or basophilic transparent cytoplasm. The cells lie singly or in clusters. There is nuclear enlargement, occasional multinucleation, and slight hyperchromasia (Fig. 25.25). The term *dyskaryosis* has been applied to those cells in which the nucleus exhibits abnormal morphology but in which the cytoplasm is abundant and the nucleocytoplasmic ratio is low. Nucleoli are rarely seen. The background of the smear is usually clean. Although the cytologic findings show minimal departures from the norm, a follow-up smear is mandatory because sufficient evidence has been accumulated that a proportion of such lesions progresses to more severe forms of intraepithelial neoplasia.

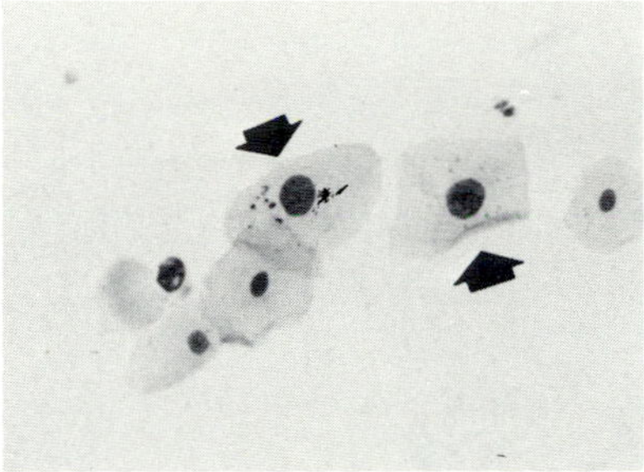

FIG. 25.25. Mild dysplasia, dyskaryosis (Grade 1 CIN). Two squamous cells (*arrows*) exhibit abnormal morphology within the nucleus including chromatin clumping and hyperchromatism. The cytoplasm, however, is abundant. These cells, although exhibiting a minimal departure from the norm, signal the need for follow-up.

Moderate Dysplasia (CIN 2)

The smear in moderate dysplasia shows predominantly round or oval cells with basophilic cytoplasm. The nuclei are moderately hyperchromatic. The nucleocytoplasmic ratios may be more strikingly altered, but the cytoplasmic width exceeds the diameter of the nucleus (Fig. 25.26). A greater number of abnormal cells than in a mild dysplasia are observed. Characteristically, the cells are arranged singly, although loosely arranged groups may be present.

Severe Dysplasia and Carcinoma in Situ (CIN 3)

Histologic differentiation between severe dysplasia and carcinoma in situ has been based on the finding of a layer of flattened cells on the surface of the epithelium in the former, whereas in the latter no differentiation takes place throughout the entire thickness of the epithelium. In the light of studies by Richart[38,39] and others, this appears to be an arbitrary distinction. The cytologic findings in severe dysplasia are indistinguishable from the cytologic findings in carcinoma in situ.

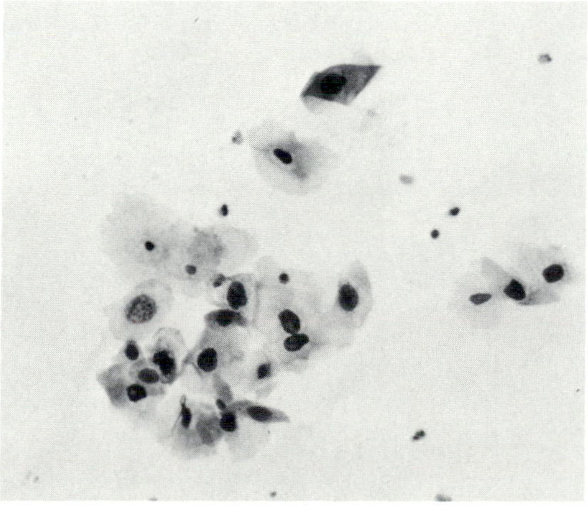

FIG. 25.26. Moderate dysplasia (Grade 2, CIN). The nuclei are hyperchromatic and the nucleocytoplasmic is more obviously altered, but the cytoplasmic width exceeds the diameter of the nucleus.

The distribution and basic morphology of the cellular content of smears from carcinoma in situ may vary with the method of collection and the anatomic location of the tumor, as well as with the presence of cells from coexistent areas of metaplasia. In general, three smear patterns can be recognized. One pattern is composed mainly of differentiated malignant cells, suggesting origin from squamous epithelium, and another pattern consists mainly of smaller malignant cells, the origin of which is primarily from areas of endocervical metaplasia. Occasionally, it is possible to recognize the highly differentiated keratinizing carcinoma in situ.

A smear from the differentiated squamous type of carcinoma in situ (Fig. 25.27a,b,c,d) shows a predominance of round cells with a large nucleus and a narrow rim of cytoplasm. The nuclei reveal those characteristics that are the hallmarks of malignancy: the abnormal distribution of chromatin, irregular, often angular outline, variation in size and configuration, and often hyperchromatism. These malignant cells are usually termed *third-type* malignant cells, distinguishing them from the other two types, which are more bizarre morphologically but are seen less often. The tadpole cell is one in which the head contains an enlarged malignant nucleus, and the remainder of the cytoplasm appears as an attenuated tail. A fiber cell is an elongated cell in which a malignant nucleus is present (Fig. 25.27c,d).

The cytologic findings in the small-cell, anaplastic carcinoma in situ consist of small, poorly differentiated cells, present singly or in loosely arranged linear groups. The nuclei occupy most of the cell. Often the cytoplasm may appear merely as an incomplete rim. Nucleoli may be present.

Invasive Neoplasms of the Cervix

Invasive Squamous Carcinoma

Paradoxically, the cytologic diagnosis of invasive epidermoid carcinoma of the cervix may often prove more difficult than that of the in situ lesions (Figs. 25.28, 25.29, and 25.30). Blood, necrotic material, and leukocytes may obscure the malignant cells, which are frequently poorly preserved. The malignant cells are of a heterogeneous mixture, with many extreme abnormalities in both nucleus and cytoplasm. Differentiated malignant squamous cells and undifferentiated malignant cells may coexist throughout the smear. Multinucleated malig-

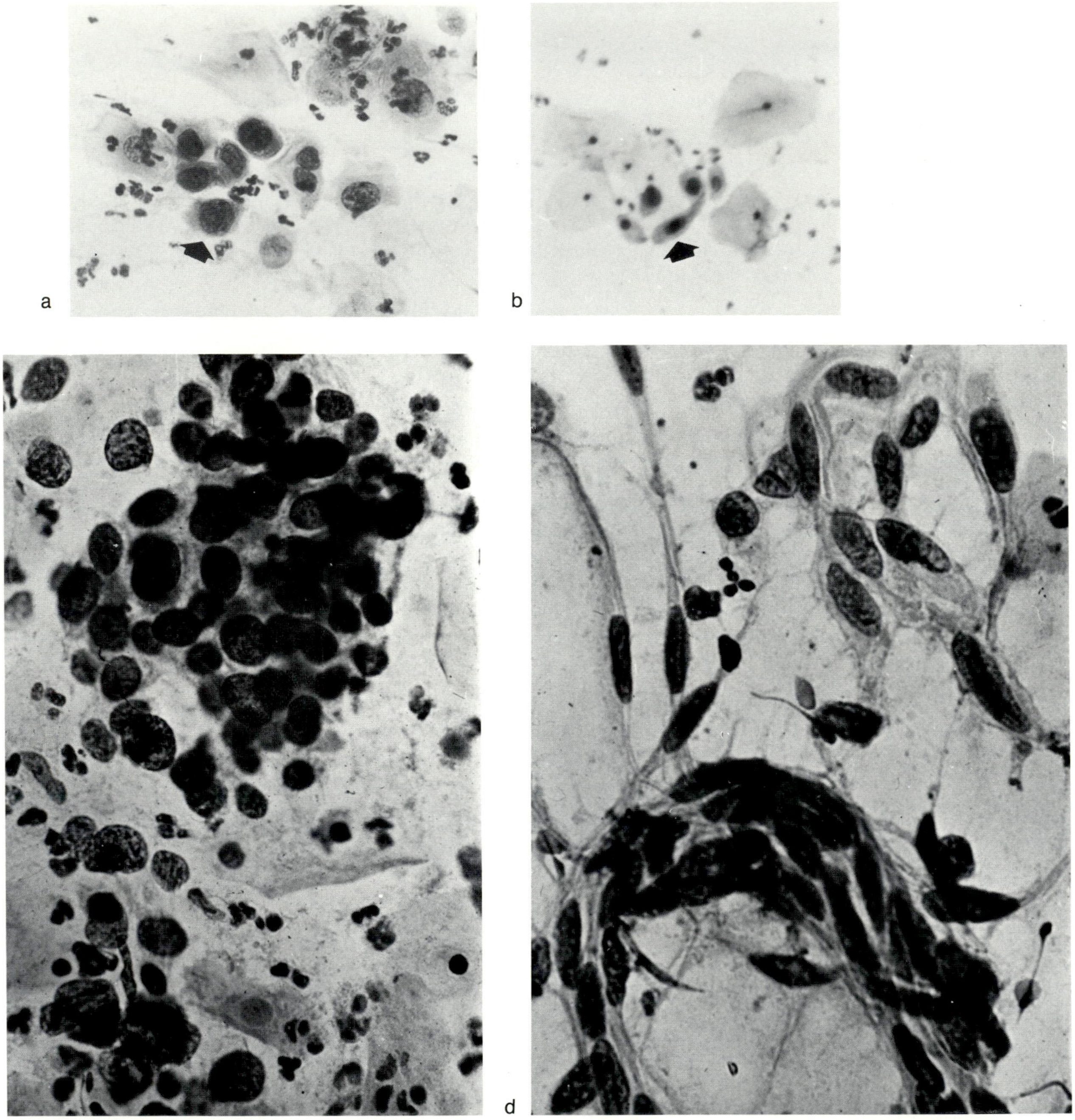

FIG. 25.27.*a*. Severe dysplasia/carcinoma in situ (Grade 3 CIN). The nuclei are large, in proportion to the overall cell size; some have a narrow rim of cytoplasm around them (*arrow*). The chromatin is irregularly distributed. Many of the nuclear membranes show uneven thickening. *b*. One of the dysplastic cells in the central cluster of abnormal cells displays the tadpole configuration (*arrow*). *c*. Carcinoma in situ. This smear reveals a group of relatively small anaplastic cells with hyperchromatic nuclei that vary somewhat in size and shape but are mainly round or oval. Many of these cells have scant cytoplasm, which occurs as a partial rim or fragment. Most of the nuclei are denuded. *d*. Fiber cells from carcinoma in situ. This smear reveals a group of elongated fiber cells, the nuclei of which show varying degrees of hyperchromatism and variation in size, as well as irregular chromatin clumping.

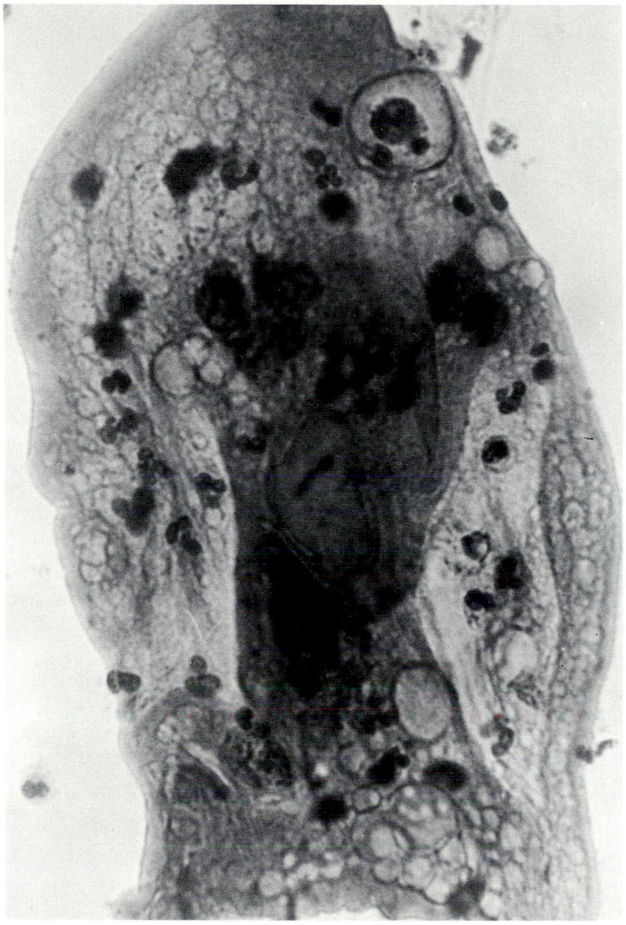

FIG. 25.33. Radiation response. The striking cytoplasmic vacuolation that occurs following radiation can produce bizarre morphology.

recurrent malignancy. The negative smear, by which is meant the smear that ultimately proves to be negative for malignancy, may appear abnormal at first glance. Degenerative changes, cytoplasmic vacuolation, multinucleation, cytoplasmic and nuclear enlargement, and the rare bizarre shape may be present in the epithelial cells. However, nuclear chromatin distribution is normal. Commonly, the cellular pattern may be atrophic or consist of parabasal and intermediate cells. Large numbers of histiocytes, often multinucleated, are seen and frequently show considerable nuclear activity. Polymorphonuclear leukocytes are also present.

Positive postradiation smears, that is, those containing malignant cells, are seen in patients with persistent disease or in patients in whom the disease has recurred after variable lengths of time. Graham[12] has pointed out that the patient with persistent disease is difficult from a cytologic standpoint. If the smear exhibits a predominance of intermediate and superficial cells showing no radiation effect, if histiocytes are absent or few in number, if the background is clean, a very careful search must be made for small, undifferentiated malignant cells. The abnormal chromatin pattern of their nuclei makes it possible to identify them. The smear from a patient with recurrent malignancy usually contains differentiated and undifferentiated malignant cells, often in large numbers.

Cryosurgery

In recent years, cryosurgery has been used in the treatment of cervicitis. It is incumbent on the cytologist to be familiar with the changes produced by this modality and incumbent on the clinician to inform the cytologist that cryosurgery has been used. Two weeks after treatment, the cervical smear contains cells showing enlargement of nuclei, multinucleation, and karyorrhexis. Micro- and macrovacuoles are present in the cytoplasm. If a smear is taken about 3 months after treatment, dysplasialike changes may be present, particularly parakeratotic changes. Cytoplasmic vacuolation may persist for up to 6 months.

Alkylating Agents

Koss et al.[28] have described the alterations in cervical squamous epithelium that may develop in the course of long-term administration of busulfan (Myleran), an alkylating agent used in the treatment of chronic myelogenous leukemia. These changes closely resemble spontaneously occurring precancerous conditions of the cervix. It is not clear as to whether these are cancer-mimetic cellular abnormalities or whether they may represent the early stages of drug-induced human cancer.

Laser treatment produces changes in squamous and columnar epithelial cells similar to those induced by electrocautery, dehydration and elongation of both the cell and its nucleus.[19] Regeneration and repair follow rapidly. Subsequent, follow-up cytology in patients who have been treated with laser does not appear to be compromised; within approximately 3 weeks, cytology returns to normal.

Exposure to Diethylstilbestrol

It has been recommended that cytology,[17,40,43] with biopsy of abnormal appearing areas of vagina and cervix, be used in studying patients exposed prenatally to diethylstilbestrol (DES) because neither cytology nor biopsy alone is uniformly reliable. In properly obtained cellular specimens, vaginal adenosis, as well as dysplastic and neoplastic lesions, may be detected cytologically. However, the absence of columnar or metaplastic squamous cells in a vaginal smear cannot be construed as ruling it out (see Chapter 4, Diseases of Vagina). Five types of abnormal cells can be identified in smears from cases of vaginal adenosis: columnar cells, metaplastic squamous cells, metaplastic squamous cells with cytoplasmic mucinous droplets, dysplastic squamous cells, and atypical glandular cells.

Oral Contraceptives

The overall effect of progestagen on the vaginal smear is the absence of the orderly cyclic changes that accompany a normal menstrual cycle.[37] A predominance of intermediate cells early in the cycle is seen. Folded intermediate cells persist throughout the cycle. Often cytolysis is prominent and Döderlein bacilli are present. Inflammatory changes are common.

Intrauterine Devices

Gupta has studied the IUD-related cytologic changes and has grouped them into (1) reparative and healing changes resulting from inflammation or infection and (2) changes interpreted to represent specific IUD usage.[14] Atypical columnar cells can be misinterpreted as adenocarcinoma. A helpful diagnostic feature is the lack of a continuous spectrum of atypical epithelial changes, as opposed to the spectrum commonly seen in in situ carcinoma.

Neoplasms of the Female Genital Tract Other than Cervical

The cytologic detection of endometrial carcinoma in the asymptomatic female does not approach the accuracy or dependability with which cervical neoplasms are diagnosed.[4–6,35,46,48] When aspiration of the vaginal pool is performed, the yield of diagnostically significant material is greater than that obtained from cervical smears, which are a rather poor source of endometrial cells. Hofmeister[18] has emphasized the important point that in investigating lesions of the endometrium, any technique is of value only when positive or atypical cells are identified and if it alerts the clinician that adequate additional procedures should be carried out. If the technique, be it endometrial biopsy, jet wash, or endometrial aspiration,[13,18,25,28,47] is negative and symptoms persist, dilatation and curettage is mandatory.

In premenopausal women, a vaginal smear that contains endometrial cells, singly or more commonly in clusters, after the 10th or 12th day of the cycle is usually interpreted as an abnormal finding, although not necessarily one suggesting the presence of endometrial cancer. In the smear of an asymptomatic postmenopausal woman, endometrial cells, normal or abnormal, are to be considered an abnormal finding, and further investigation is warranted. The finding of marked histiocytic activity or striking maturation of squamous cells similarly signals the necessity for further investigation. In the postmenopausal woman with a history of spotting or bleeding, a careful scrutiny of the smear for abnormal endometrial cells must be carried out. Small cells (Figs. 25.34 and 25.35), lying singly or in small clusters, may be detected. The nuclei are slightly enlarged and show abnormal chromatin clumping and clear areas in the karyolymph.[26] Large, prominent, eosinophilic nucleoli, often angular in shape, are a helpful clue to the malignant nature of the cell. The eccentric position of the nucleus is a characteristic feature of adenocarcinoma (Fig. 25.36a,b). Much of the cytoplasm may be absent in the more undifferentiated tumor cells.

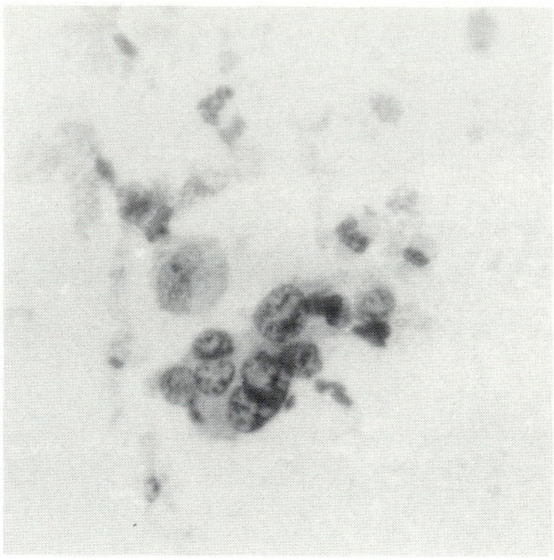

FIG. 25.34. Endometrial carcinoma. An aggregate of small, overlapping cells is present. Chromatin clumping, nuclear enlargement, and areas of clearing are seen.

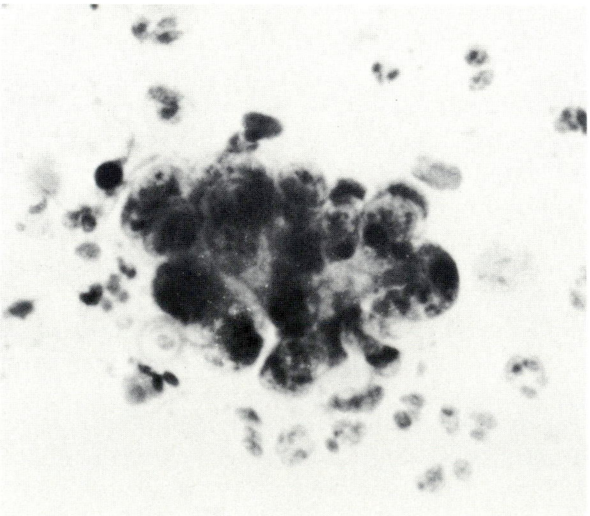

FIG. 25.35. The cluster of cells forms a three-dimensional grouping in which the chromatin abnormalities are visible. Prominent nucleoli are present in some of these cells. Many of the nuclei are located peripherally.

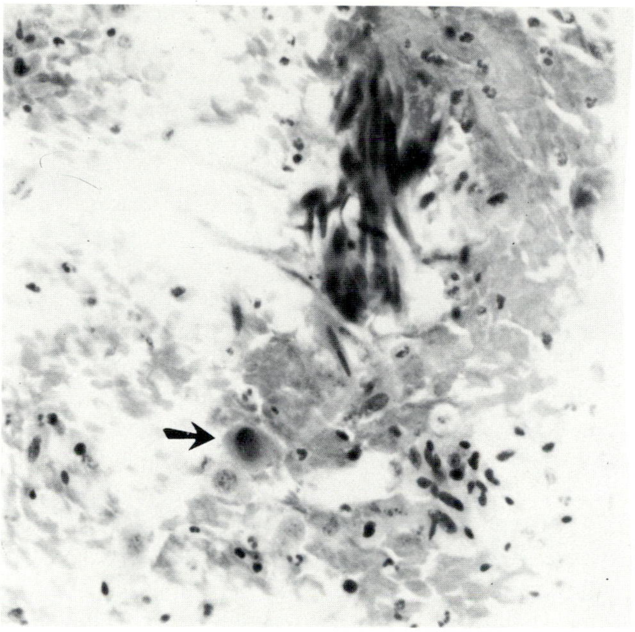

FIG. 25.28. Invasive squamous carcinoma of the cervix. Against a background of blood and cellular debris, groups of malignant cells are seen. There is marked variation in the size and shape of the nuclei. The cells in the right lower field are small and many are devoid of cytoplasm. Contrast these cells with the extremely large cell (*arrow*). The cells in the center of the field contain elongated nuclei (fiber cells).

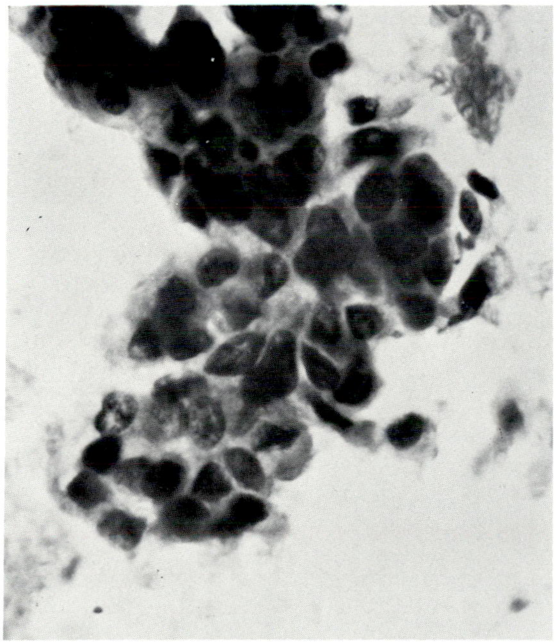

FIG. 25.29. Invasive squamous carcinoma of the cervix. The field reveals a loosely arranged group of malignant cells, both differentiated and undifferentiated. Many of the nuclei are markedly hyperchromatic, and nuclear detail is difficult to evaluate. However, in a few of the nuclei, the abnormal chromatin is discernible.

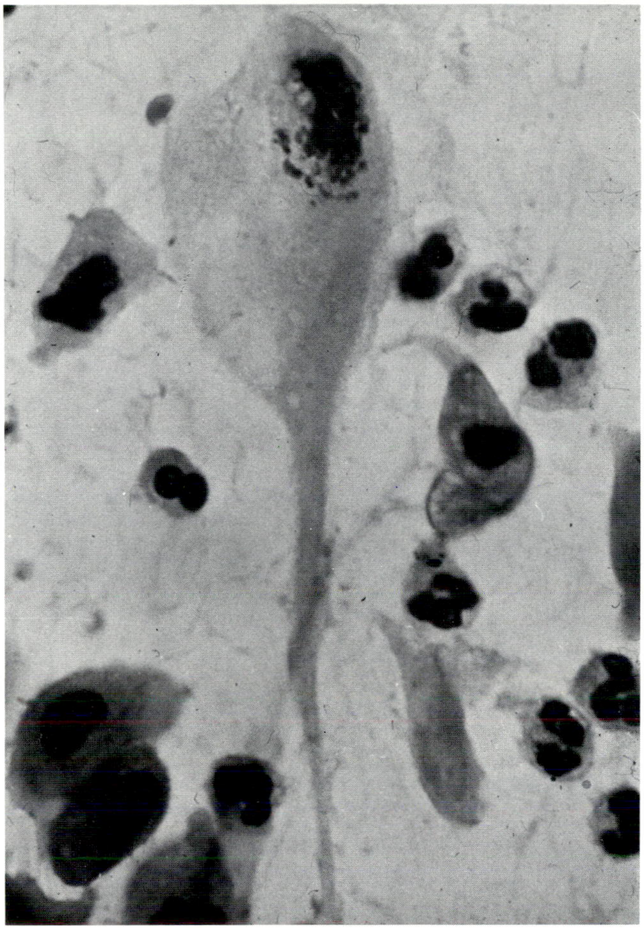

FIG. 25.30. Tadpole cell from an invasive squamous carcinoma of the cervix. The nucleus has undergone karyorrhexis. The nuclear membrane is no longer discernible. Several smaller malignant cells and polymorphonuclear leukocytes are present.

nant cells exhibit variation in size and shape and abnormal chromatin patterns from nucleus to nucleus. Fiber cells, with elongated irregular hyperchromatic nuclei, may be found, as well as large, bizarre cells similar to tadpole cells but often exhibiting more extreme nuclear and cytoplasmic aberrations (Fig. 25.30). When undifferentiated cells predominate, the smear may be composed mainly of small cells with little cytoplasm. Dysplastic and dyskaryotic cells may be present in the smears of invasive epidermoid carcinoma, a not surprising finding because areas of dysplasia and areas of carcinoma in situ may lie adjacent to the frankly invasive lesion.

Adenocarcinoma

Adenocarcinoma is a relatively uncommon malignancy of the cervix as compared to the intraepithelial neoplasms of the squamous epithelium.[45] Abnormal distribution of chromatin is the most significant feature. The chromatin

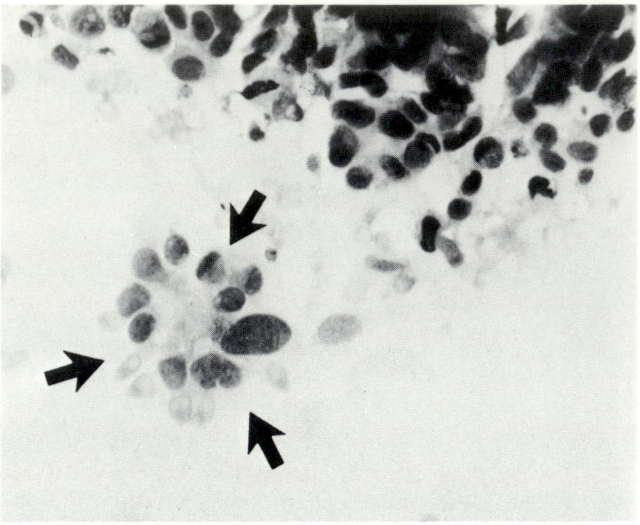

FIG. 25.31. Adenocarcinoma of the cervix. The pseudoacinar arrangement of the cells (*arrows*), the variation in size and shape of the nuclei, and their peripheral location in the cell suggest the diagnosis of adenocarcinoma.

shows clumping, often as irregular and angular masses. Condensation at the nuclear margins may produce an irregularly thickened nuclear border. Prominent large, pink-staining nucleoli may be present. An eccentric peripheral malignant nucleus within a cytoplasm displaying coarse vacuolation or an elongated columnar form suggests the adenocarcinomatous nature of the lesion. When a group of malignant cells is observed, the nuclei are frequently located peripherally, producing a pseudoacinar appearance (Fig. 25.31). The malignant cells may be undifferentiated, with almost total loss of cytoplasm. Differentiation of endocervical adenocarcinoma from endometrial adenocarcinoma may not always be possible on a cytologic specimen.

Changes in Epithelia Secondary to Therapy

A thorough familiarity with the marked cellular changes that radiation produces in both benign and malignant cells is vital.[12] In the follow-up smears of patients who have been treated by radiotherapy for cervical cancer, the cytologist must be able to distinguish among benign cells showing radiation effect, malignant cells altered by radiation, and malignant cells unaffected by radiation. The nonspecific degenerative changes of pyknosis, karyorrhexis, and karyolysis are seen initially, in both benign and malignant cells, and signify cell destruction. In many of the benign cells that retain their structure, that is, cells that have not degenerated, there may be a striking enlargement of both nucleus and cytoplasm (Fig. 25.32) with maintenance of the nucleocytoplasmic ratio. At times, cytoplasmic enlargement occurs, but the nucleus does not enlarge; consequently the nucleus appears smaller than normal. Within the enlarged nuclei, structure remains normal, but, as a consequence of the enlargement, the nuclear membrane may appear wrinkled. This wrinkling and folding must be distinguished from malignant intranuclear changes. Multinucleation is also seen.

Vacuolation, both coarse and fine, is seen in the cytoplasm of the benign cells that have responded to radiation (Fig. 25.33). Bizarrely shaped benign cells are occasionally seen, but the normal structure of their nuclei makes it possible to distinguish them from the bizarrely shaped malignant cells. Malignant cells can also respond to radiation with nuclear and cytoplasmic enlargement, but, in these cells, the features that are diagnostic of malignancy are usually still recognizable.

After radiation therapy has been completed, ongoing cytologic studies are essential in detecting residual and

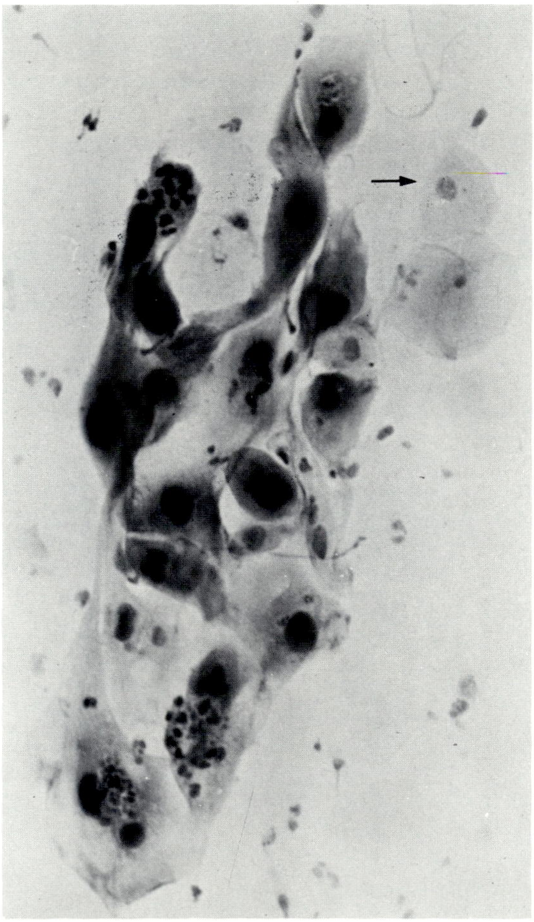

FIG. 25.32. Radiation response. There is enlargement of nucleus and cytoplasm. For comparison, observe the normal intermediate cell (*arrow*). Cytoplasmic vacuolation is present in some of the cells.

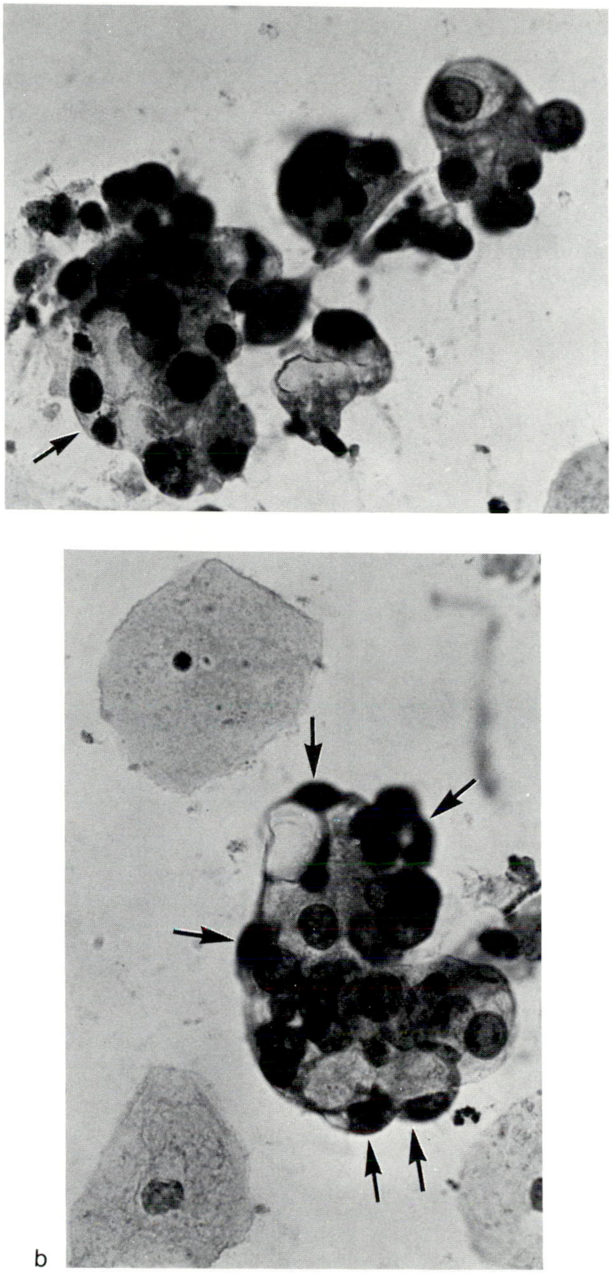

a

b

Fig. 25.36.*a*. Endometrial adenocarcinoma. This grouping of malignant cells suggests an attempt to form an acinar structure (*arrow*). Prominent nucleoli are visible in some of the cells. *b*. Endometrial adenocarcinoma. This aggregate of malignant cells illustrates the peripheral position of many of the nuclei (*arrows*), a characteristic finding in adenocarcinoma.

Adenocarcinoma of the fallopian tube is a rare tumor of the female genital tract. Exfoliated tumor cells may be present in a vaginal smear, where they may be indistinguishable from an endometrial adenocarcinoma.

Rarely, an adenocarcinoma originating in the ovary may shed malignant cells that appear in the vaginal smear.[24] If endometrial curettings do not reveal adenocarcinoma, the possibility of an ovarian tumor must be considered (Fig. 25.37).

In clear cell adenocarcinoma of the genital tract,[43] a lesion that has been described in young females whose mothers have been administered DES during pregnancy, vaginal smears may reveal tumor cells occurring singly and in clumps. In general, they resemble endocervical cells, and nuclear atypia may be seen.

Squamous cell carcinoma of the vagina occurs mainly in elderly women. A smear taken from the vaginal wall, if there is a suspicious area, or from the vaginal pool occasionally yields material that permits a definitive diagnosis to be made. Differentiated and undifferentiated malignant cells may be present, and some of the malignant cells may be keratinized.

Occasionally, a cytologic diagnosis of vulvar epidermoid carcinoma may be made. However, the diagnosis is usually made by biopsy of a suspicious site.

Aspiration and Peritoneal Cytology

The contribution of aspiration cytology to determining the nature of ovarian masses has received considerable attention.[5,7,10,11,16,27,34,42] Transabdominal, transvaginal,

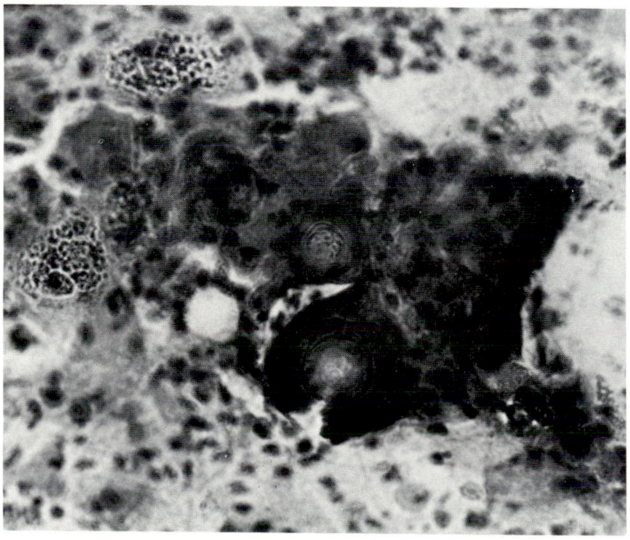

Fig. 25.37. Psammoma bodies. These lamellated, calcific granules, so-called psammoma bodies, were found in the vaginal smear of a patient with serous cystadenocarcinoma.

and transrectal needle aspiration have been recommended as a means of investigating pelvic masses. Positive cytologic evidence of malignancy, on aspiration, does not preclude laparotomy. Adequate clinical management requires laparotomy for histologic typing, grading, and staging. Negative results do not connote the absence of malignancy in the lesion under investigation. Geier and Strecker[11] would limit the indications for aspiration of ovarian tumors to recurrence of previously diagnosed and treated ovarian cancer and to those cases where the poor physical condition of patients does not allow laparotomy.

The presence of malignant cell fluid specimens from the peritoneal cavity collected at laparotomy from patients with ovarian or endometrial carcinoma is an important factor in prognosis. In the absence of an increase in the peritoneal fluid, peritoneal washings, at the time of laparotomy, as an adjunct procedure, are indicated. The presence of malignant cells is generally regarded as an unfavorable prognostic factor for both types of tumors (see Chapter 12, Endometrial Carcinoma).

Hormonal Cytology

Cytohormonal evaluation can be useful in investigating disturbances of endocrine function and in assessing the effects of hormone therapy,[24,51] however, it is essential that the material be suitable and that adequate clinical data be available. The specimen should be taken from the upper third of the vagina or the posterior fornix. The patient's age, menstrual history, and pertinent clinical history, including administration of exogenous hormones and prior surgical or radiation therapy must be supplied if a valid assessment is to be made.

The vaginal smear reflects the interaction of several hormones, namely, estrogens, progesterone, and androgens. Therefore, at times, it may not be possible to assess whether the changes seen in a smear result from a specific hormonal alteration or from multihormonal factors. Nonhormonal factors, such as inflammation, may also influence the content of the smear. A smear in which there is evidence of inflammation is not suitable for hormonal assessment.

In general, under estrogenic stimulation, the vaginal epithelium undergoes proliferation and maturation. Consequently, the vaginal smear consists of superficial and intermediate cells. When there is unopposed estrogenic stimulation, the smear consists of superficial cells that lie flat and singly on a clean background. Because only estrogens can produce this epithelial maturation, such a smear may be taken as evidence of estrogen stimulation, whether endogenous or exogenous.

Progesterone produces proliferation and maturation of the squamous cells, but, by itself, it does not produce maturation to superficial cells. The smear, under the influence of progesterone, contains folded intermediate cells, desquamated in large clumps. It is this pattern of exfoliation that is most characteristic of a progesterone effect (Fig. 25.38).

Androgens also produce proliferation and maturation of squamous cells to the intermediate cell stage. However, the exfoliated pattern is one of single cells or small groups of folded or flat intermediate cells.

Basically, there are two significant extremes in the main patterns of hormonal cytology. If the smear consists of abundant, single, flat, superficial cells, this can be interpreted as definite estrogenic stimulation. If the smear contains only parabasal cells, it can be interpreted as a lack of estrogenic stimulation. Patterns containing superficial intermediate and parabasal cells may not be used for hormonal assessment because nonhormonal factors may produce this pattern.

Numerical Indices

Several numerical indices have been proposed to express hormonal cytologic patterns.[26,51] Their major usefulness

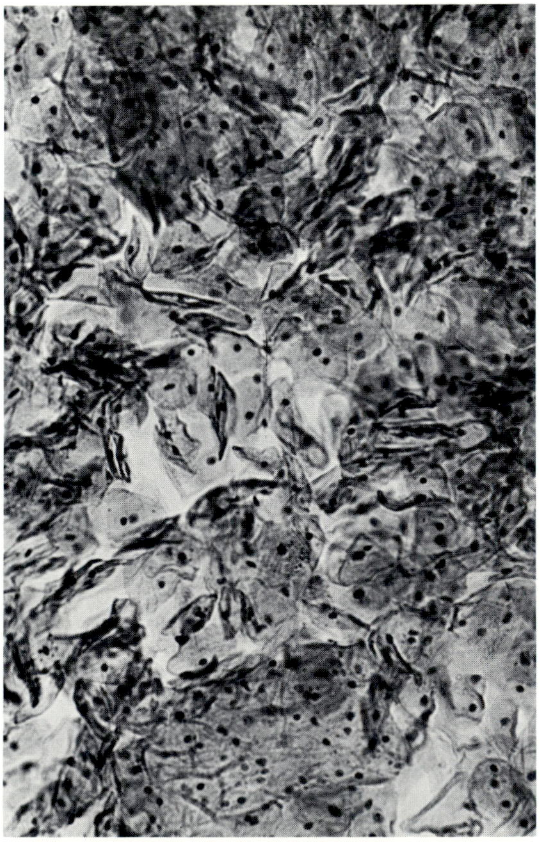

FIG. 25.38. Vaginal smear, day 22 of the menstrual cycle. Crowded sheets of overlapping intermediate cells are present. The cytoplasmic borders are folded. Some superficial cells are discernible; they lie flat and show no folding.

is in assessing estrogenic activity. The indices are often of questionable value in assessing progesterone effect.

The eosinophilic index measures the relation of mature eosinophilic squamous cells to mature cyanophilic squamous cells, regardless of nuclear appearance.

The karyopyknotic index measures the relation of superficial cells to intermediate cells, regardless of cytoplasmic staining.

The folded index measures the percentage of folded mature squamous cells to flat mature squamous cells, regardless of cytoplasmic staining or of nuclear appearance.

The crowded cell index measures the relation of mature squamous cells in groups or clusters of four or more cells to mature squamous cells lying singly or in clusters of fewer than four cells, regardless of staining reaction or nuclear appearance.

The maturation index[9] measures the relation of superficial, intermediate, and parabasal cells (S/I/P).

Meisels has recommended the use of an assigned numerical value to the different cell types[51] to facilitate communication between cytologists and to make easier the use of digital computers for statistical evaluation in large series. The assigned values are:

Superficial eosinophilic cell	1.0
Superficial cyanophilic cell	0.8
Large intermediate cell	0.6
Small intermediate cell	0.5
Parabasal cell	0.0

When the percentage of each of these cells is multiplied by the corresponding numerical factor and the results are added up, a number between 0 and 100 is obtained. This is designated the *maturation value.* To compare maturation indices, for example, the newborn is 60–70, the menstrual cycle 60–90, pregnancy is 60–69, and menopause is 0–40.

The interpretation of a vaginal smear, regardless of which index is used, ultimately depends on the correlation by the cytologist of the clinical data provided by the clinician and the data obtained from the smear, the proportions of cells present, and their appearance in the smear. The final cytologic report should be in the form of a statement. For example: "The cytohormonal pattern is consistent with . . ." or "The cytohormonal pattern is not compatible with . . ." or "The cytohormonal pattern suggests the possibility of. . . ." It should not be in the form of an isolated numerical index.

The Vaginal Smear

Birth and Childhood

At birth, the vaginal smears of mother and child are quite similar, because they are under similar hormonal stimulation. Intermediate cells, usually in groups, predominate, with some admixture of superficial cells. During the next few weeks, these cells disappear gradually from the smear. Parabasal cells become the predominant cell type. Leukocytes and some erythrocytes may be present.

This smear pattern in childhood is stable. It alters only in response to infection, to which the thin epithelium is vulnerable, or to endogenous production of estrogens, as from an estrogen-producing ovarian tumor.

Premenarcheal

The early premenarcheal period is quite variable. There is a gradually increased steroid stimulation reflected in the vaginal smear by a reduction in the proportion of parabasal cells and increased intermediate cells. During this transitional period, considerable variation may exist until the normal cycle patterns are established.

Menstrual Cycle

The follicular or proliferative phase extends from the fourth or fifth day to the fourteenth day of a 28-day cycle (in prolonged cycles, the extended phase is the preovulatory one). During the first few days, the smear is composed chiefly of intermediate cells, histiocytes, and clumps of endometrial cells. Gradually, the smear shows an increasing number of single, flat, eosinophilic, karyopyknotic, superficial cells, reflecting the increased growth and maturation of the vaginal epithelium. Histiocytes and polymorphonuclear leukocytes gradually disappear from the smear.

The so-called ovulatory smear pattern consists almost exclusively of flat superficial cells. The background is clean. It should be emphasized that this type of smear, screened as an isolated specimen, cannot be used as definitive evidence that ovulation has occurred. Unopposed estrogen stimulation also produces this type of smear.

During the ensuing secretory phase, there is a gradual decrease in the number of superficial cells and a progressive increase in the number of intermediate cells, which are arranged in clumps and show a fraying or wrinkling of their cytoplasm.

In the premenstrual phase, the number of polymorphonuclear leukocytes increases. Prior to overt menstruation, clumps of endometrial cells may be identified. The vaginal smear in the menstrual phase consists of compact clumps of endometrial cells in a background of blood, leukocytes, and histiocytes.

If vaginal smears are to be used to investigate disturbances in the menstrual cycle, serial specimens must be studied, preferably for two or more cycles. Evidence of cycling is sought, and this can only be determined by looking for the changing patterns that are associated with the menstrual cycle.

Pregnancy

In pregnancy, the cyclic changes are absent and the smear consists almost wholly of clumps of intermediate cells that characteristically show folding and thickening of their cytoplasmic borders.[50] The term *navicular* has been used to describe these intermediate cells. Their cytoplasm is rich in glycogen and, with the Papanicolaou stain, shows areas of yellow-orange staining. The nuclei are frequently elongated.

Superficial cells may be present in small numbers. Parabasal cells are rare. A smear in which superficial cells predominate may indicate placental insufficiency.

It must be emphasized that the pattern described is compatible with pregnancy, not diagnostic of pregnancy. Other conditions, such as menopause, can produce a similar pattern.

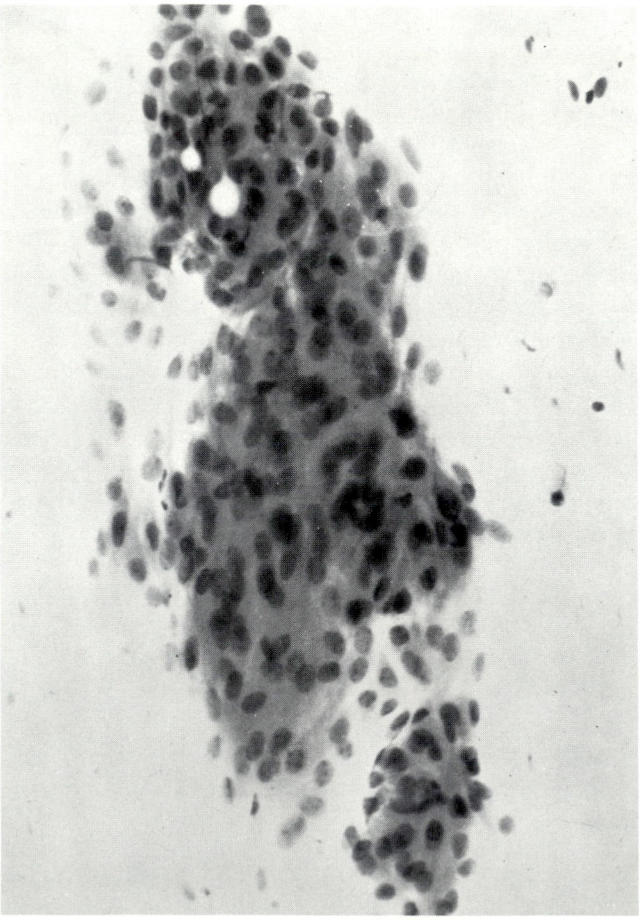

FIG. 25.39. Crowding in an atrophic smear. Sheets of parabasal cells are seen. The nuclei are regular; no chromatin abnormalities are seen. The denuded nuclei around these sheets are readily identified as parabasal in origin.

The Menopause and Postmenopausal Period

Marked individual variations, both clinical and cytologic, are found in the menopause and postmenopausal period. In some women, cessation of menstruation may have occurred, yet some cyclic changes persist in the smears. Anovulation marked by periods of unopposed estrogen production may often occur. Serial smears may reveal a pattern of flat superficial cells. Evidence of cycling is absent.

The general cytologic progression of events is toward a decrease and then disappearance of superficial cells in the vaginal smear. The patterns that emerge eventually are of two types. Intermediate cell predominance consists of intermediate cells showing clumping and cytoplasmic folding, a pattern that may be indistinguishable from the one seen in pregnancy. The administration of small doses of estrogen can resolve this diagnostic problem. In pregnancy, the intermediate cell pattern persists. In the menopausal or postmenopausal woman, a maturation to superficial cells ensues.

The atrophic or parabasal predominant smear reveals sheets of parabasal cells (Fig. 25.39) in which some eosinophilic staining of cytoplasm and crowding of nuclei are evident. Parabasal cells may show cytolysis and, occasionally, denuded nuclei appear hyperchromatic and may raise the suspicion of malignancy, however, the uniformity of the nuclear chromatin should dispel this impression. Numerous histiocytes are often present in these smears, and giant multinucleated histiocytes are not uncommon. The latter must not be confused with multinucleated malignant cells.

Endocrinopathies

Primary Amenorrhea

In gonadal dysgenesis (Turner's syndrome), the smear is atrophic. Examination of well-preserved nuclei in intermediate cells fails to reveal sex chromatin bodies unless mosaicism is present, in which case sex chromatin bodies may be seen.

In testicular feminization, a disorder in which the patients are genetic males (XY), epithelial maturation is present because female hormones are produced by the undescended testes. Sex chromatin bodies are absent (see Chapter 2, Abnormal Sexual Development).

In congenital absence of the uterus, ovarian function is present and epithelial maturation occurs.

Secondary Amenorrhea

Aside from the physiologic amenorrhea of pregnancy, secondary amenorrhea is indicative of impairment of ovarian function. The Stein-Leventhal syndrome (polycystic ovarian disease) includes a group of disorders in which follicles persist and become enlarged and cystic.[1] The vaginal smears are generally composed of folded and clustered intermediate cells and superficial cells. Navicular cells with glycogen deposits within the cytoplasm are often seen.

Occasionally, in young girls, periodic vaginal bleeding may occur. Serial vaginal smears in the precocius puberty syndrome often reveal evidence of cycling.

In a child or in a postmenopausal woman whose vaginal smear reveals a high degree of maturation, the possibility of a granulosa cell tumor must be considered. These tumors may produce estrogenlike substances, which act on the vaginal epithelium.

In the Chiari-Frommel syndrome, a condition in which normal lactation continues over a prolonged period, amenorrhea is accompanied by atrophy of the vaginal epithelium. The smear mirrors this atrophy; it is composed of parabasal cells.

Methods of Obtaining Cellular Samples from the Female Genital Tract

Cervical Smear

The cervical smear is the method of choice for diagnosis of intraepithelial neoplasms of the cervix:

1. Do not lubricate the speculum. The lubricant can contaminate the smear, producing a basophilic background that can obscure cellular detail.
2. A cotton swab or wooden scraper is applied to the entire portio of the cervix and into the external os so that material is collected from the endocervical canal.
3. The material is immediately and quickly spread onto clean glass slides.
4. The smear must be fixed immediately in order to prevent cellular distortion. Immersion in 95% alcohol or the use of a coating fixative, either dropped on or sprayed on, are acceptable procedures.
5. Proceed to Papanicolaou staining method.

Vaginal Smear

The vaginal smear is useful for assessment of hormonal status if the guidelines described in the text are followed:

1. Material is obtained from the lateral wall of the upper third of the vagina.
2. Subsequent handling of the material is as in cervical smear.

Posterior Fornix Aspiration

The posterior fornix aspiration may be useful in the detection of endometrial cancer. It is a poor method for the detection of cervical lesions. A pipette with a suction bulb is used.

Endometrial Aspiration

Endometrial aspiration permits a sampling of material from the endometrium directly. Neither the cervical nor the vaginal smear is sufficient in the detection of endometrial cancer. Endometrial aspiration, jet wash, vabra suction, or variants of these techniques are directed to obtaining material directly from the endometrium.

References

1. Bamford SB, Mitchell GW Jr, Bardawil WA, Casin CM (1965) Vaginal cytology in polycystic ovarian disease. Acta Cytol 9: 332
2. Benson PA (1973) Psammoma bodies found in cervical–vaginal smear. Acta Cytol 17: 64
3. Beyer-Boon ME (1974) Psammoma bodies in cervical–vaginal smears: An indicator of the presence of ovarian carcinoma. Acta Cytol 18: 41
4. Burk JR, Lehman HF, Wolf FS (1974) Inadequacy of Papanicolaou smears in the detection of endometrial cancer. N Engl J Med 291: 191
5. Christopherson WW (1983) Cytologic detection and diagnosis of cancer: Its contributions and limitations. Cancer 51: 1201
6. Creasman WT, Weed JC Jr (1976) Screening technique in endometrial cancer Cancer 38: 436
7. Di Saia PJ, Creasman WT (1984) Clinical Gynecologic Oncology, 2nd ed. St. Louis, MO CV Mosby
8. Fentanes de Torres E, Benitez-Bribiesca L (1973) Cytologic detection of vaginal parasitosis. Acta Cytol 17: 252
9. Frost JK (1967) Exfoliative cytology. In: Gynecologic and Obstetric Pathology, 6th ed. Novak ER, Woodruff JD (eds). Philadelphia, Saunders
10. Ganjei P, Nadji M (1984) Aspiration cytology of ovarian neoplasms—A review. Acta Cytol 28: 329
11. Geier GR, Strecker JR (1981) Aspiration cytology and E2 content in ovarian tumors. Acta Cytol 25: 401
12. Graham RM (1963) The Cytologic Diagnosis of Cancer, 2nd ed. Philadelphia, Saunders
13. Gravlee LC Jr (1969) Jet irrigation method for the diagnosis of endometrial adenocarcinoma. Its principle and accuracy. Obstet Gynecol 34: 168
14. Gupta PK (1982) Intrauterine contraceptive devices—Vaginal cytology, pathologic changes and clinical implications. Acta Cytol 26: 571
15. Gupta PK, Woodruff JD (1982) Actinomyces in vaginal smears. JAMA 247: 1175
16. Hajdu ST, Melamed MR (1984) Limitations of aspiration cytology in the diagnosis of primary neoplasms. Acta Cytol 28: 337
17. Hart WR, Zaharov I, Kaplan BJ, Townsend DE, Aldrick JO, Henderson BE, Ray M, Benton B (1976) Cytologic findings in stilbestrol-exposed females with emphasis on detection of vaginal adenosis. Acta Cytol 20: 7

18. Hofmeister FJ (1974) Endometrial biopsy: Another look. Am J Obstet Gynecol 118: 773
19. Holmquist ND, Bellina JH, Danos ML (1976) Vaginal and cervical cytologic changes following laser treatment. Acta Cytol 20: 290
20. Hughes RR (1972) Errors in the use of the Pap smear. South MJ 65: 575
21. International agreement on histological terminology for the lesions of the uterine cervix (1962) Acta Cytol 6: 255
22. Josey YW, Nahmias A, Naib ZM (1969) Viral and virus-like infections of the female genital tract. Clin Obstet Gynecol 12: 161
23. Kaufman R, Koss LG, Kurman RJ, et al. (1983) Guest editorial. Statement of caution in the interpretation of papilloma-associated lesions of the epithelium of uterine cervix. Am J Obstet Gynecol 146: 125
24. Keebler CM, Wied GL (1974) The estrogen test: An aid in differential cyto-diagnosis. Acta Cytol 18: 483
25. Kohl GC, Larson CP (1974) Office endometrial biopsies. Am J Obstet Gynecol 118: 406
26. Koss LG (1979) Diagnostic Cytology and Its Histopathologic Bases, 3rd ed. Philadelphia, Lippincott
27. Koss LG (1980) Thin needle aspiration biopsy. Acta Cytol 24: 1
28. Koss LG, Melamed MR, Mayer K (1965) The effect of busulfan on human epithelia. Am J Clin Pathol 44: 385
29. Lui W (1959) An Introduction to Gynecological Exfoliative Cytology. Springfield, IL, Charles C Thomas
30. Meisels A, Fortin R, (1976) Condylomatous lesions of the cervix and vagina: I. Cytological patterns. Acta Cytol 20: 505
31. Meisels A, Fortin R, Roy M (1977) Condylomatous lesions of the cervix: II. Cytologic, colposcopic and histopathologic study. Acta Cytol 21: 379
32. Monif GRG (1982) Infectious Diseases in Obstetrics and Gynecology, 2nd ed. New York, Harper and Row
33. Nayar M, Chandra M, Chitraratha K, Das SK, Chowhardy GR (1985) Incidence of actinomycetes infection in women using intra-uterine contraceptive devices. Acta Cytol 29: 111
34. Nordqvist SRB, Sevin B, Nadji M, Greening SE, Ng ABP (1979) Fine needle aspiration cytology in gynecologic oncology. Obstet Gynecol 54: 719
35. Reagan JW (1980) Cytologic aspects of endometrial neoplasia. Acta Cytol 24: 488
36. Reagan JW, Patten SF Jr (eds) (1967) The female reproductive tract. In: The Manual for the Atlas of Cytology. Chicago, American Society for Clinical Pathology
37. Reyniak JV, Sedlis A, Stone D, Connell E (1969) Cytohormonal findings in patients using various forms of contraception. Acta Cytol 13: 315
38. Richart RM (1967) Natural history of cervical intraepithelial neoplasia. Clin Obstet Gynecol 10: 748
39. Richart RM, Vaillant HW (1965) The irrigation smear: False negative rates in a population with cervical neoplasia. JAMA 192: 199
40. Robboy SJ, Friedland LM, Welch WR, Keh PC, Taft PD, Barnes AB, Scully, RE, Herbst AL (1976) Cytology of 575 young women with prenatal exposure to diethylstilbestrol. Obstet Gynecolo 48: 511
41. Syrjanen KJ, Heinonen U, Kauraniemi T (1981) Cytologic evidence of the association of condylomatous lesions with dysplastic and neoplastic changes in the uterine cervix. Acta Cytol 25: 17
42. Szpak CA, Creasman WT, Vollmer RT, Johnston WW (1981) Prognostic value of cytologic examination of peritoneal washings in patients with endometrial carcinoma. Acta Cytol 25: 640
43. Taft PD, Robboy S, Herbst AL, Scully RE (1974) Cytology of clear cell adenocarcinoma of genital tract in young females: Review of 95 cases from the registry. Acta Cytol 18: 279
44. Tam MR, Stamm WE, Handsfield HH, Stephens R, Kuo CC, Holmes KK, Ditzenberger K, Krieger M, Nowinski RC (1984) Culture-independent diagnosis of *Chlamydia trachomatis* using monoclonal antibodies. N Engl J Med 310: 1146
45. Tasker JT, Collins JA (1974) Adenocarcinoma of the uterine cervix. Am J Obstet Gynecol 118: 344
46. Te Linde RW (1973) Demonstration of the relationship of carcinoma-in-situ to invasive carcinoma of the cervix. Am J Obstet Gynecol 115: 1022
47. Torres JE, Holmquist ND, Danos ML (1969) The endometrial irrigation smear in the detection of adenocarcinoma of the endometrium. Acta Cytol 13: 163
48. Weiss NS, Szekely DR, Austin DL (1976) Increasing incidence of endometrial cancer in the United States. N Engl J Med 294: 1259
49. Wied GL (1957) Interpretation of inflammatory reactions in vagina, cervix and endocervix by means of cytologic smears. Am J Clin Pathol 28: 233
50. Wied GL (1960) Cytology during pregnancy. In: Yearbook of Obstetrics and Gynecology. Greenhill JP (ed). Chicago, Year Book Medical Publishers, pp 15–33
51. Wied GL (ed) (1968) Symposium: Hormonal cytology. Acta Cytol 12: 87

26

Animal Models for Tumors of the Female Genital Tract

June Marchant, Ph.D.

The ultimate objective of animal studies of cancer is to achieve a better understanding of factors responsible for human disease in the hope that it may be eliminated or controlled. Information about spontaneously occurring tumors comes largely from veterinary records of tumors in domesticated animals, but also from wild animals and animals in zoos and laboratories. Study of the commonly occurring tumors in animals can provide epidemiologic and other clues to their etiology, as well as material for biologic and therapeutic investigation.

Although counterparts of most human genital tumors have been found to occur spontaneously in animals, they tend to do so infrequently. For a detailed review of spontaneous tumors of the uterus and ovaries in animals see Chapter 38 of the first edition of this book or the special edition of Chapters 38 and 39 by Cotchin.[43]

Some tumors of importance to humans, such as cancer of the uterine cervix and choriocarcinoma, are rarely seen in animals, and this may indicate that the etiologic factors causing them are specific to humans. Conversely, other tumors, such as ovarian tubular adenoma of rats and mice and venereal sarcoma of the dog, are not seen in the human species.

It is important to realize the great interspecies variations in the gross anatomy of the female reproductive tract in mammals. They are matched by complementary variations in the anatomy of the penile structure of the male. This lock-and-key principle is probably one of nature's ways of keeping closely related species distinct from one another.

Some of the features of the female reproductive tract are illustrated in Figure 26.1 and may have bearing on the species tumor susceptibility at certain sites.

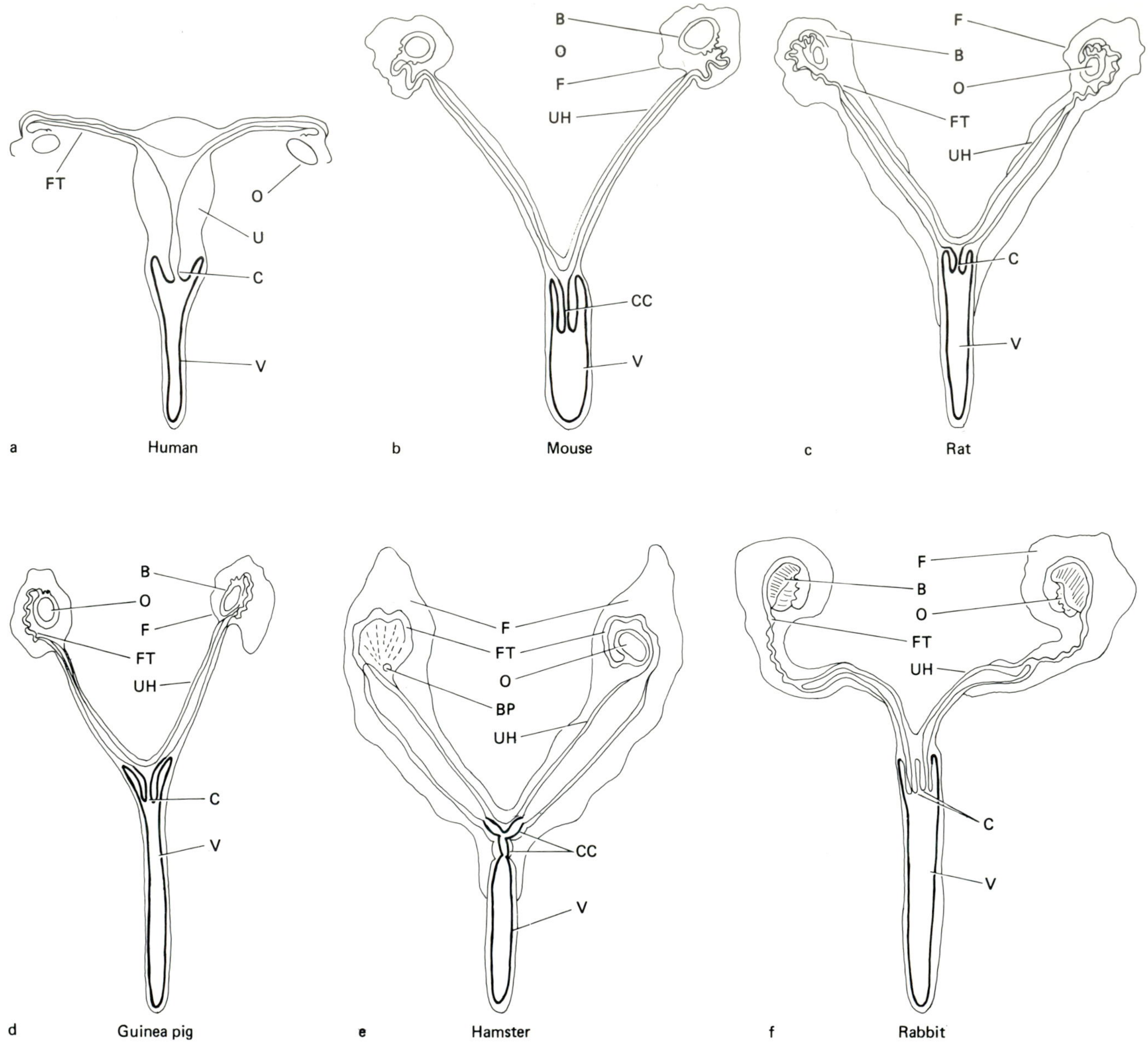

FIG. 26.1. Comparative aspects of female reproductive tract of human and laboratory animal species. B, ovarian bursa; BP, blind pore; C, cervix; CC, cervical canal; F, fat; FT, fallopian tube; O, ovary; U, uterus; UH, Uterine horn; and V, vagina. Note complete (mouse and hamster), almost complete (rat, guinea pig), or partial (rabbit) enclosure of the ovary in a bursa, or pouch, whereas the human ovary remains free in the peritoneum. Also note different proportions of various anatomic sites, as well as different extent of vaginal squamous epithelium (heavy line) in cervical region. (Redrawn and adapted with permission from Hafez ESE (1973) The comparative anatomy of the mammalian cervix, Mossman, HW (1973) The embryology of the cervix. In: *The Biology of the Cervix.* Blandau RJ, Moghissi K (eds). Chicago, University of Chicago Press.

Tumors of the Ovary

Spontaneous Ovarian Tumors in Animals

Domesticated Animals

Ovarian neoplasms in domesticated animals have been seen most frequently in the cow, dog,[104] and domestic fowl, less frequently in the mare and cat, and rarely in the ewe, sow, goat, and buffalo.[20,43]

Some idea of the frequency of bovine ovarian tumors was obtained from postmortem examination of 6286 genital tracts of cows of the Swedish Highland breed. Only 13 ovarian tumors were found, the commonest type being granulosa cell tumors.[155] However, in an abattoir survey in Denver, Colorado, five of the six ovarian tumors recorded in cows were carcinomas,[4] and carcinomas seem to have predominated over granulosa cell tumors in other reports.

In adult swine, 2–5 years old, the occurrence of ovarian hemangiomas during a 3-year survey was 14 (around $1.6/10^5$), whereas granulosa cell tumors occurred in 2 sows and 2 gilts (around $0.4/10^5$).[283] In a recent examination of 1445 elderly sows in Holland, tumor-like lesions were detected in the ovary of 56 animals, 3 of which were bilateral. The ovarian tumors showed proliferation of granulosa cells and blood vessels and were five times more frequent than uterine tumors.[1]

Surveying reports of 196 canine ovarian tumors, Cotchin[43] found that 83 were of the papilloma–adenoma–carcinoma group, 74 of the granulosa cell–sertoliform group, and 25 of the seminoma–teratoma group. Most tumors showed signs of endocrine activity leading to such conditions as cystic endometrial hyperplasia, pyometra, and vaginal hemorrhage. The papillary and adenomatous types of tumors appear to be derived mainly from surface epithelium, showing hormone-dependent proliferation on administration of stilbestrol. They are most commonly seen in the pointer breed, whereas granulosa cell tumors are commonest in the English bulldog.[222]

Equine ovarian tumors appear to be granulosa cell type,[40] but, curiously, none of the seven reported by Norris et al.[220] was known to cause endocrine abnormality. Teratomas are occasionally seen in mares.

In feline species, few ovarian tumors are reported, probably because of the common practice of spaying female cats. In those that have been observed, the granulosa cell-type predominates, but there is an absence of the sertoliform pattern, and they do not appear to secrete estrogen.[219]

In domestic fowl, ovarian tumors of the granulosa–theca–lutein type are not uncommon in broiler chickens aged 10 weeks or less.[30] Adenocarcinomas are common in old hens and are serous or mucus secreting. Theca cell tumors, Brenner tumors, lipoid cell tumors, and hemangiomas have also been seen. Oviduct carcinoma has been seen in laying hens.[88]

Wild and Zoo Animals

Ovarian tumors have occasionally been observed in species ranging from whales to the fruit fly, *Drosophila*.[43]

Spontaneous ovarian tumors have been found in subhuman primates. One case of ovarian adenocarcinoma with extensive peritoneal implantation was seen in a *Cebus albifrons* monkey in a series of 1065 postmortem examinations.[248] Others have been observed in rhesus monkeys[176] and in aged chimpanzees.[92]

Ovarian cysts filled with jelly or greasy sebaceous material were found in 48 of 1176 ovaries from hares shot in New Zealand, 6 of which had true teratomas containing bone, teeth, or hair. It was suggested that a genetic effect might be involved because only a few hares were liberated in New Zealand in 1851, or it might possibly have been caused by DDT spraying.[66]

Postmortem examination of wild house mice demonstrated 7 granulosa-cell tumors in 99 breeding females and 2 in virgin females.[5]

For other species of wild animals, see the bibliography by Halloran.[101]

Laboratory Animals

In outbred laboratory rodents, ovarian tumors have rarely been seen. The early report of postmortem examinations of 22,000 laboratory mice mentions 46 solid ovarian tumors, together with a few simple cysts.[260] An ovarian teratoma has been seen in a mouse.[279]

Three ovarian tumors, one granulosa cell, one cystadenoma, and one anaplastic carcinoma, were found in about 300 Chester Beattie stock rats.[31] In a survey of 5903 elderly rats of two Sprague-Dawley strains kept as untreated control animals, 116 tubular adenomas of the ovary were found, as well as 24 granulosa cell tumors (7 malignant), 9 theca cell tumors, and smaller numbers of other types.[97] Spontaneous ovarian tumors reported in the guinea pig have included granulosa cell tumors and teratomas.[297,299] Thecomas have been seen in ovaries of the Syrian hamster.[103] Granulosa cell tumors, cystadenoma, and leiomyoma have been reported in gerbils.[237] Bilateral ovarian thecomas were noted in a stock of female ferrets aged over 1 year,[34] and malignant granulosa cell tumors are said to occur frequently in *Praeomys* (*Mastomys*) *natalensis*, a small rodent found in Eastern Europe.[161]

Table 26.1 summarizes the distribution of histologic types of spontaneous ovarian tumors in different species.[20] It can be seen that spontaneous ovarian tumors in animals occur sporadically in many species, but they are neither predictable in histologic type nor reproducible in substantial numbers. Although tumors resembling virtually all human histologic types have been found, their infrequent occurrence makes them poor animal models and contributes little to our understanding of factors responsible for human disease.

For good animal models that are both predictable and reproducible, we have to turn to inbred strains of laboratory species, mainly mice and rats selected and mated brother to sister for 20 generations or more. Each strain has its own characteristic susceptibility to disease, and spontaneous ovarian tumors are seen quite frequently in research institutes holding certain strains of animals allowed to live out their normal life span if they do not die from competing diseases, for example, those caused by mammary tumor or leukemia viruses.

TABLE 26.1 Classification of spontaneous primary tumors reported in human and other mammalian species

Species	Total ovarian tumors classified	Cystadenoma	Carcinoma	Granulosa series	Dysgerminoma	Teratoma	Other	No. of reports
Rodents (five species)	82	4	2	65	1	4	6	4
Guinea pig	3	0	0	1	0	2	0	2
Hamster	5	0	0	5	0	0	0	1
Equine	55	11	3	26	0	5	10	4
Sheep	1	0	0	0	0	1	0	1
Swine	31	11	3	4	2	2	9	4
Bovine	227	9	46	146	4	7	15	18
Feline	14	1	1	6	2	3	1	3
Canine	194	61	16	73	33	4	7	12
Monkey	13	4	1	3	0	2	3	2
All mammalian[a]	624	101 (16)	72 (12)	329 (52)	42 (7)	29 (5)	51 (8)	51
Human (two series)[a]	482	252 (52)	88 (18)	13 (3)	4 (1)	67 (14)	58 (12)	1

Data condensed with permission from Bonser and Jull.[20]
[a] Numbers in parentheses are percentages.

The Ovary as an Experimental Model

The ovary has many advantages as a model for disease. It is a well-defined entity that can be completely removed without the problem of residual rests. In the mouse, it is often small enough to be transplanted *in toto* back into the ovarian capsules from which it originated (orthotopic transplantation), or it can be exchanged for the ovary of another animal of histocompatible genotype with a high degree of functional success. With larger ovaries, vascularization of the complete organ is not achieved by this means. However, in such cases, the organ can be cut into several fragments, each containing a full representation of all the different cell types present in the normal organ. These may be transplanted to a variety of different sites, including the anterior chamber of the eye, where they may become vascularized and remain under constant observation. Function of the transplants can be monitored by taking vaginal smears.

Of the thousands of oocytes present in the normal mouse ovary at birth, only a few are destined for release during reproductive life. However, reduction in their numbers occurs by degeneration, and this atresia continues throughout life, its rate varying in different mouse strains.

The rate of oocyte atresia is retarded when the pituitary is removed[127] and is speeded up by neonatal thymectomy, suggesting that growth and maturation of follicles in postnatal ovarian development may be controlled by a dual mechanism.[212] Atretic follicles in the stroma probably comprise the interstitial cells in the aging ovary, which are capable of responding to stimulation by pituitary hormones.

The number of oocytes present in the ovaries of mice at birth can vary considerably according to strain, as can the rate of atresia.[128] Oocyte deficiency, the prime effect of aging, can lead to tumor development without further intervention, as will be seen.

The following discussion examines the evidence in detail and looks at just how far the present ovarian tumor models of the mouse or other species of laboratory animals can satisfy the criteria of predictability, reproducibility, and resemblance to the human counterpart. Because the literature is rather cumbersome, the reader requiring a more comprehensive reference list is referred to the excellent reviews by Jull[132] and Murphy.[202]

Methods of Induction of Ovarian Tumors in Experimental Animals

Many methods have been devised to induce ovarian tumors in animals. Some, employing known or suspected carcinogenic agents, for example, chemical carcinogens, irradiation, or viruses, have a direct deleterious effect on the ovary, bringing about premature aging and tumor development. Others do not have so marked an initial effect on the ovary but have a chronic effect on its internal environment, eventually leading to tumor development. The following discussion considers the different methods of induction of tumor in the mouse and indicates those that also apply to other species.

Genetic Selection

Pure strains of mice have been established that are genetically identical and will accept skin grafts from one another. Strains particularly susceptible to the development of spontaneous ovarian tumors include CBA,[272]

CE,[53] C3H freed from mammary tumor-inducing virus,[52] RIII,[265] Han:NMRA,[234] and several strains of New Zealand mice.[15] In females of these strains reaching 18 months of age or more, the incidence of ovarian tumors may be very high.

After 28 ovarian tumors had been found postmortem in 3032 SWR/J female mice aged 100 to 150 days, further selection of family lines resulted in one line with 45 tumors in 537 mice. Neoplastic growth in these mice begins at puberty while follicles are still in the ovary, and the tumors are grossly identifiable as early as 5 weeks of age. Oocytes disappear after 90 days from the tumorous ovaries. The tumors, which are usually unilateral, may approach 2 cm in diameter by 150 days. They are granulosa-celled, and no evidence of any virus can be seen in them on electron microscopic examination.[11]

Mutant Genes

Mutant genes, causing true hermaphroditism, have been observed in four sublines of BALB/c mice, and in the BALB/cWt line a high incidence of granulosa cell tumors occurs in the ovotestis after 8–20 months.[11]

Other mutant genes of the W series can lead to a high incidence of spontaneous ovarian tumors in mice carrying them.[202,239] The gonads of W^vW^v mice are deficient in oocytes at birth because of a failure of the primordial germ cells to multiply between the 8th and 12th days of fetal life. The animals are sterile, and the females develop a 95% incidence of bilateral tubular adenomas of the ovary at about 7 months of age. F_1 hybrid (C57B1 × C3H) mice with W^xW^v genes develop bilateral complex tubular adenomas, which are locally invasive in 95% of females by 5 months of age.[203] They are derived from tubular ingrowth of the germinal epithelium and are preceded and accompanied by fourfold increases in gonadotropic follicle-stimulating hormone (FSH) and luteinizing hormone (LH).[205] Granulosa cell tumors frequently arise in them at a later stage.[204]

Genes of the steel (*Sl*) series have similar effects.[202] Some of the homozygotes are not viable because of severe macrocytic anemia, but a high proportion of the less severely affected genotypes, such as Sl^d/Sl^d and Sl/Sl^d, survive to adulthood and develop ovarian tumors in old age.

There is a mutant gene nude (*nu*) in mice, among the pleiotrophic effects of which are the absence of a thymus and infertility in both sexes.[225]

It appears that there is a relationship between the thymus and gonad during postnatal differentiation of the latter, which can be manipulated to give rise to ovarian tumors by the following technique.

Neonatal Thymectomy

It was shown (for three different mouse strains and four hybrid genotypes) that thymectomy performed before 4 days of age, but not at 7 days or later, leads to arrest in ovarian growth in about one-half of females.[211] It was later observed in two of the hybrid genotypes thymectomized at 3 days of age and allowed to live out their full life span that unilateral ovarian tumors of the granulosa cell or tubular adenomatous types developed in 40% of them.[214] The early ovarian lesion seen in these mice was first described as *dysgenesis*,[211] but in more recent investigations, it has been termed *oophoritis* because of its pathogenesis.[213] Two months after thymectomy on day 3, female BALB/c mice develop a lymphocytic oophoritis, as well as losing all stages of follicles and corpora lutea.[211] Although this lesion was never seen in nude mice, it could be induced in BALB/c-*nu*/*nu* mice by incompletely reconstituting them with specific numbers of syngeneic spleen or lymph node cells. Spleen cells (10^7) from neonatally thymectomized males or females were by far the most effective in inducing the oophoritis and also the gastritis and occasional thyroiditis seen together in these animals. There is good evidence to suggest that the condition brought about by thymectomy of mice at 3 days of age is an autoimmune one[213] that results in early sterility caused by oocyte depletion, thereby disturbing the endocrinologic homeostasis of the ovary. In a few mice, pituitary tumors develop and mammary ducts become hypertrophic and filled with milky substances, indicating prolactin secretion.[147]

The results of lymphoid cell transfer experiments suggest that thymectomy at 2–4 days of age prevents establishment of immunity to specific oocyte or parietal cell antigens, which first appear between 3 and 7 days of age.[146]

In thymectomized (C3H × 129) F_1 hybrid mice, ovarian tumors developed in 29% of females. Of these, granulosa cell tumors made up 70% and cystadenomas 20%.[147]

Ovarian Transplantation

As mentioned in the discussion of the mouse ovary as a tumor model, transplantation has been much used in the study of ovarian tumorigenesis. However, it cannot be regarded as an innocuous procedure. When a mouse ovary is transplanted, even back into its own ovarian capsule, substantial tissue breakdown occurs. If vascularization occurs, the grafted organ becomes reconstituted but never fully. There is an early decrease in the number of oocytes and ripening follicles, associated with a shortening of reproductive life. The diminished amount of functional ovarian tissue may also lead to an imbalance of ovarian and pituitary hormones, which can contribute to ovarian tumorigenesis. When ovaries of DBA mice were transplanted orthotopically into normal F_1 (DBA × C3H) hybrid hosts, five of nine animals killed 12–24 months later had ovarian tumors.[117]

Tumors have also developed in normal mouse ovaries

transplanted subcutaneously into castrated hosts of the same genotype.[132] Few tumors were seen if the hosts were castrated females, but up to 80% were seen in some genotypes when the hosts were castrated males, suggesting an influence of the noncycling male pituitary, which produces constant LH and no FSH. Almost all of these tumors were tubular adenomas. In experiments with rats, ovarian fragments transplanted to the anterior chamber of the eye of gonadectomized hosts all became vascularized after 1 year. Many developed into granulosa cell tumors.[152]

Ovarian Vasoligation

In the rat, abnormal ovarian activity can be brought about by temporarily ligating its blood supply. A continuous estrus is established that fails to control the hypophysis, the histology of which becomes similar to that of a castrated animal.[63] A ligature of only 30 minutes duration was required to produce lasting changes, and ovarian tumors followed 20 months later.[64] This simple method of ovarian tumor induction does not seem to have been exploited further.

Intrasplenic Ovarian Grafting to a Castrated Host

Ovaries transplanted to the spleens of castrated rats were found to develop tumors with great regularity.[17] A similar operation in mice was soon shown to have the same effect.[73] It was postulated that steroid hormones from the grafts would be destroyed in the liver and unable to exert normal feedback inhibition of the pituitary gonadotropins. The latter would be secreted chronically, at an elevated level that would heighten the stimulation of the ovarian graft in the spleen, giving rise to hyperplasia and eventually neoplasia.

Support for this hypothesis came when it was found that if one ovary remained in situ, no tumors developed in intrasplenically grafted ovaries[19] and also when it was shown that tumorigenesis could be inhibited by high systemic levels of estrogens or androgens, even when their administration was delayed for 3 or 4 months after transplantation.[158] Ovaries grafted into the pancreas were also shown to become tumorous, demonstrating the significance of transplanting into the hepatic portal drainage system. Furthermore, repeated injections of luteotropin or of pregnant mare's serum were found to accelerate tumor appearance.[18] In rats bearing intrasplenic ovary grafts without vascular adhesions, levels of both progestins and LH were found to be high, and tumors developed in all animals. However, these consequences were avoided when the animals were given an Eck fistula, which produces hepatic bypass of the hormones from the intrasplenic ovary by a portacaval shunt.[157] Recent direct measurements of hormones during the early stages of ovarian neoplasm development after intrasplenic ovary grafts into castrated rats showed an immediate significant rise in gonadotropin levels, which persisted throughout the 6-month study. Plasma estrone and estradiol were lowered significantly after 3 months, but, paradoxically, the progestins were raised, presumably secondary to extraovarian (adrenal) progestin secretion.[156] In mice with intrasplenic grafts, receptors for hCG–LH have been demonstrated and their numbers per cell shown to increase 17-fold, relating to the degree of graft luteinization.[138]

Intrasplenic grafting of an ovary to a castrated rat or mouse leads to the disappearance of oocytes and follicles and the luteinization of interstitial cells to form a benign luteoma. Granulosa cell tumors appear within the luteoma after 6 months in mice[73] and after 10 months in rats.[17] In rabbits, they have been seen after about 18 months[227] but not before 5 years in guinea pigs.[175] They do not appear to develop in golden hamsters.[144]

Intrasplenic transplants of testes in castrated ACI rats develop into granulosa cell tumors.[148]

Exposure to Constant Bright Illumination

Ovaries of mice exposed to constant illumination from a 100 W electric bulb over their cage for 10 months showed cystic follicles, absence of corpora lutea, downgrowths of germinal epithelium, and occasional tubular adenomas.[206]

A polycystic ovarian disease also developed in rats exposed to continual illumination by electric light,[258] and the incidence of tumors arising in rats with ovarian arterial ligatures was enhanced.[64]

Brown Leghorn hens in a constant climatic chamber exposed to 12 hours of fluorescent lighting daily, with no natural daylight, had no seasonal cycle of egg laying. Egg production was continuous, gradually falling off, and hatchability declined. After 3.5–6.8 years, all 19 fowl died, and adenocarcinoma involving the ovary, oviduct, mesentery, and intestine was found on necrospy. Only three such tumors and one sarcoma developed in a control group in an intensive house with 12 hours of light daily provided by a 100 W electric bulb in up to 12.5 years. These hens had the usual cycle phase of molting and decline of egg laying in the winter months.[96]

Chronic Exposure to Hormones

Chronic exposure to a variety of hormones—both male and female—can lead to ovarian tumor induction in laboratory animals.

Estrogens. Regular administration of estrogens to adult mice leads to hydronephrosis, but when strain CD-1 female mice were exposed prenatally to diethylstilbestrol (DES) on the 1st and 17th days of fetal life and later mated to unexposed males, 5 ovarian cystadenocarcinomas developed in 40 mice (in addition to 10 uterine adenocarcinomas).[295] In hamsters, it leads to kidney tumors.[144] Daily doses of DES to prepubertal rats led to the development of huge cysts in the ovaries filled with yellow caseous material, and to pyometra and uterine metaplasia.[100] However, in adult female black-hooded rats implanted with subcutaneous pellets of estriol or DES, some ovarian thecomas were seen, although the most commonly observed changes were pituitary enlargement, eventually leading to tumor, mammary fibroadenomas in the second year, and adrenal carcinomas.[215] DES administered to bitches caused proliferative lesions derived mainly from the surface of the ovary in which sialic acid-containing mucinous secretions were detected, and the lesions were interpreted as metastasizing carcinomas.[123]

Progestagens. During chronic treatment of mice with synthetic progestins used as contraceptive agents in women, it was noted that subcutaneous pellets of 19-norprogesterone led to ovarian tumors in 4 of 18 BALB/c mice after 13 months or more.[164] A small incidence was seen after implantation of progesterone itself and in 2 of 24 mice that received norethynodrel, but ovarian tumors occurred in 13 of 45 mice receiving implants of norethinodrone.[165,167]

Androgens. Normal ovaries grafted subcutaneously or intratesticularly into male mice of the same genotype frequently develop tumors, whereas subcutaneous grafts into intact females do not.[70] However, the rate of ovarian tumor induction is also high when ovaries are grafted to castrated males. Tumor induction occurs more frequently in ovarian grafts in castrated males than in castrated females.[131] These differences may be caused by androgen influence on sexual differentiation of the hypothalamus that occurs during the neonatal period in mice and rats, giving rise to a continuous pattern of gonadotropin secretion in males and a cyclic release in females.[89,162]

Administration of testosterone propionate daily to female rats from ages 3 days to 21 months led to hypertrophy of the clitoris, and theca-cell ovarian tumors developed in 3 of 10 animals surviving 16 months or more.[113]

Thyroid Hormone. Thyroid function affected the incidence of tumors developing in intrasplenic ovarian grafts in mice. Addition of thyroid powder to the diet resulted in fewer tumors, but thyroid inhibition with thiouracil or limitation of food intake had no effect.[188]

Proliferative and neoplastic changes have been reported in ovaries of hamsters treated with ^{131}I and methylthiouracil.[36]

Gonadotropins. One method of achieving a persistently high level of gonadotropins is side-by-side suturing of an intact female with a histocompatible castrated partner. This technique is known as *parabiosis.* Excess gonadotropins circulating in the castrated male readily pass over into the circulation of the intact partner, stimulating its ovaries to produce larger amounts of estrogens readily detectable by vaginal smears.

When an attempt was made to induce mouse ovarian tumors by this method, the high estrogen levels reached led to hydronephrosis and early death. However, in one pair that survived 9 months, an ovarian tumor was observed.[197]

Better survival occurs in parabiotic triplets with one intact partner joined to two castrated partners on the same side. In this situation, the estrogens passing from the normal triplet are metabolized before they can reach the farthest castrated partner, whose pituitary remains stimulated. The excess gonadotropins produced by this triplet are less readily metabolized than are the estrogens, and they succeed in reaching the intact triplet in elevated amounts.

When parabiosis was combined with other methods, such as irradiation or intrasplenic ovary grafting into a castrated animal, parabiosis to one or two castrated partners accelerated the appearance of ovarian tumors.[198] Parabiosis also acted synergistically with the administration of 2-fluorenlyacetamide (FAA) to induce ovarian tumors in rats, when neither agent alone was effective.[16]

Transplants of a pituitary tumor secreting FSH and LH produced granulosa-cell tumors in 8 of 146 female F_1 (A × C) rats at a much earlier age than the 7 spontaneous tumors found in 1812 old females of this genotype. Two of the tumors were transplanted and showed some dependence on gonadotropins. These ovarian tumors, in turn, produced estrogenic effects, for example, enlarged uterus, pituitary, and mammary glands, as well as androgenic effects, for example, enlarged clitoris and paraurethral glands. The pituitary hyperplasia led to the production of excessive prolactin, which, together with estrogen from the granulosa cell tumors, stimulated the mammary glands to become neoplastic. Because of the more rapid growth of the latter, the full chain reaction could occur in a single individual.[119]

A recent attempt to induce ovarian tumors in BALB/c mice by administration of gonadotropins for 11 months proved unsuccessful.[185]

Ionizing Irradiation

Whole-body irradiation with x-rays leads to ovarian tumorigenesis in both mice[71] and rats. The minimum dose required is around 25 R, and the tumor incidence rises with the radiation dose.[69]

Three types of tumor have been seen: tubular adenoma, granulosa cell tumor, and luteoma. The two latter types are believed to be capable of hormone secretion, since they almost doubled the incidence of coexisting mammary tumors in mice of strain A containing mammary tumor virus, but this did not occur with tubular adenomas.[70] Thirteen of 21 attempts to transplant granulosa cell tumors and luteomas succeeded, and on serial transplantation some of them gained vigor and metastasized.[68] A luteoma appeared to be associated with secondary changes indicative of progestin secretion.[72]

Practically all Bagg albino female mice developed bilateral ovarian tumors after 200 R whole-body x-rays if they survived 16 months, but it was found that no tumors developed if only one ovary was given contact irradiation while leaving the other ovary unirradiated.[159]

When adult (L × A) F_1 mice were subjected to 300 R whole-body x-rays and their ovaries were implanted intramuscularly into irradiated or nonirradiated histocompatible host mice that had been spayed, many grafts became granulosa cell tumors or luteomas, whereas unirradiated ovarian grafts did not.[76] However, ovarian grafts from irradiated mice did not become tumors in host mice retaining their own ovaries whether or not the hosts had themselves been irradiated, that is, tumor development in an irradiated ovary depended on its being in a host whose pituitary hormonal balance had been disturbed by castration.[139]

At birth, mouse oocytes are extremely resistant to irradiation damage, but by 10 days of age, a dose of only 25 rad reduced them to zero at between 200 and 300 days of age, whereas unirradiated mice had several hundred remaining at 600 days.[221] Radiation sensitivity was maximal at 21 days, after which it declined.[228]

The first change seen in the ovaries of adult mice after irradiation was the degeneration of oocytes. Small oocytes disappeared within 2 days when most of the larger ones were degenerating. After 5 weeks, 75% had no oocytes remaining.[23] Irradiated females rapidly become sterile because the supply of oocytes becomes exhausted, whereas unirradiated animals eventually become sterile even when an ample supply of oocytes still remains in the ovary.

Preneoplastic ovarian changes induced by irradiation were found to be speeded up in the 16th generation offspring of x-irradiated mothers,[223] suggesting an effect of irradiation on the germ line.

Other forms of irradiation have been found effective in inducing ovarian tumors in mice. Some dose–responses have been reported for gamma-rays and neutrons in mice exposed to an atomic bomb detonation.[287] Comparison of single doses of protons with x-rays showed similar effects over a range of 0–400 rad, with doses of 50–100 rad yielding the optimum numbers of tumors in the RF strain of mice used. Tubular adenomas were the predominant type of tumor seen at the lowest doses, with the proportion of luteomas increasing up to 100 rad and granulosa cell tumors remaining at 15–20% at all doses. Metastases were very rare. Among the 2400 ovarian tumors examined histologically, only 6 locally invasive adenocarcinomas were seen.[37]

Whole-body irradiation of BALB/c mice with fission-spectrum neutrons induced ovarian tumorigenesis at dosage below 50 rad, and the responses after split doses and a single high dose were similar. Lowering the dose rate reduced the incidence.[286]

Chemical Carcinogens

During investigations of mammary carcinogenesis with polycyclic hydrocarbon carcinogens, it was noted that 7,12-dimethylbenz[a]anthracene (DMBA) skin paintings in oily solution gave rise to ovarian tumors in mice.[115] Administration of DMBA was also effective when given by other routes: intragastric,[13] intraperitoneal,[150] intravenous,[154] subcutaneous neonatal injection,[256] direct application to the ovary,[151] as well as after a brief exposure in vitro.[135] There is evidence of a dose–response effect in vitro and in vivo.[134] A single exposure was sufficient.[81]

Tumor incidence rates and induction time are influenced by age and strain of mice. Administration of DMBA to immature mice of two strains induced tumors in all treated mice by 6 months.[150] DMBA treatment of adults of the C3H or IF strains, which have large ovaries with numerous corpora lutea, yielded more tumors than treatment of mice of the C57B1 strain, which have small ovaries and few corpora lutea.[154,172]

With treatment of adult (C57B1 × IF) F_1 hybrid mice, which have larger ovaries than do IF, the first tumor nodules appeared after 3 months, and the number of mice affected increased rapidly from then on, but there were competing mortality risks from the more rapidly growing mammary tumors, which prevented the ovarian tumors from reaching large size. However, when ovaries were transplanted orthotopically into the emptied ovarian capsules of untreated mice of the same genotype, no mammary tumors developed and the granulosa cell tumors that developed in the transplanted ovaries grew huge and showed a marked degree of luteinization.[173]

Experiments in which tumors have developed in ovaries reimplanted after exposure to DMBA in vitro suggest that DMBA is itself the effective carcinogen, rather than some metabolite formed by the liver. Nevertheless, one of three such metabolites, 12-hydroxymethyl-7-methylbenz[a]anthracene, was found to be effective in vitro.[134] It has also been shown that the related chemical, 7,8,12-trimethyl-benz[a]anthracene (TMBA) has ovarian tumor-inducing potential comparable to that of DMBA.[285]

Other polycyclic hydrocarbon carcinogens are relatively poor in inducing ovarian tumors in mice. 3-Methylcholanthrene (MC) is much less effective than DMBA, and benzo[a]pyrene (BP) has only weakly carcinogenic action on the mouse ovary,[13,190] yet a single injection of BP has a dose-related destructive effect on primary oocytes.[178]

Other chemical methods of inducing ovarian tumors in adult mice included intraperitoneal injection of the chemotherapeutic agent, triethylene melamine.[174]

Treatment of pregnant (C57B1/J × C3HB/FeJ) F_1 mice with injections of ethylnitrosourea on the 12th–18th prenatal days caused tumors (predominantly tubular adenomas) of the ovary to appear in the offspring, the maximal incidence being seen after injection on the 14th day. Injection of the young postnatally also produced ovarian tumors, but they were predominantly granulosa cell, the maximal incidence being seen after injection on day 1, gradually diminishing to about 50% by 6 weeks.[293]

Cystadenomas have been induced in ICR/J mice whose mothers were injected with the cancer initiator urethane on days 11 and 13 of pregnancy, but they were induced more frequently in young mice injected when 64 days old.[216] Transplacental carcinogenesis by urethane was enhanced if mothers were also injected with urethane during lactation.[217]

Chemical induction of ovarian epithelial cancer in mice has been reviewed recently.[124]

DMBA does not give rise to ovarian tumors in guinea pigs or rabbits. In Syrian hamsters, a low incidence has been seen after treatment with DMBA or MC and occasionally after BP or o-aminoazotoluene.[111]

Rats respond to systemic administration of DMBA in a different manner from mice, developing severe adrenal necrosis and vascular tumors.[114,116] Both rats and mice frequently develop mammary tumors, and ^{14}C-DMBA is taken up in similar fashion by the adrenals and ovaries of both species,[133] so the different susceptibilities of the organs are not attributable to a particularly high ability to concentrate the carcinogen. It has been shown, however, that synergism between DMBA treatment and intrasplenic ovary grafting to a castrated animal could cause benign tumors to become malignant and to metastasize.[109] Implanting DMBA-coated threads in rat ovaries has been successful in inducing adenocarcinoma, which seemed to arise from surface epithelial proliferations in the hilar region.[140,251]

Another chemical with tumorigenic potential for the rat ovary is 2-fluorenylacetamide (FAA), which has induced granulosa cell tumors in intact rats parabiosed to a castrated rat. The latter procedure enhances the gonadotropin stimulation in the intact animal. No tumors occurred either in single females or in untreated parabionts given FAA.[16] Clear cell adenomas, which seem to be of a type that is different from other experimental ovarian tumors, occurred in about 10% of Sprague–Dawley rats given *n*-butylnitrosourea by stomach tube or intramuscular injection.[67] Benign mesovarial leiomyomas have been induced in Charles River CD rats by high and middle doses of mesuprine hydrochloride and sotonerol hydrochloride, which are chemically similar and are long-acting, potent, beta-adrenergic receptor stimulants.[209]

Tumors of Fetal Origin (Teratomas and Yolk Sac Tumors)

Spontaneous Teratomas

Spontaneous teratomas are rarely seen in animals, but they have occurred occasionally in guinea pigs[294,299] and have been reported in hares.[66] Several have been found in the C3H strain of mice, one of which was found to be transplantable.[62] They have also been seen in the CBA and DBA strains,[182] and bilateral teratomas were found in a Swiss albino mouse.[61] Recent research has resulted in some excellent tumor models in rats and mice.

Methods of Induction of Teratomas in Experimental Animals

Genetic Selection

An inbred mouse strain, *LT/Sv*, has been derived in which histologically recognizable ovarian teratomas are first seen in females only 1 month old. By 3 months, 40% have grossly recognizable tumors containing many different types of differentiated tissues, in addition to undifferentiated embryonal cells and trophoblastic giant cells. The most commonly observed tissue is neural tissue. Frequently, there is movement within them, indicating the presence of muscle tissue.[271]

It has been found that these ovarian teratomas are derived from ovarian oocytes that begin to develop parthenogenetically after they have completed the first meiotic division.[60] Cleaved eggs are present in ovaries of mature *LT/Sv* mice, and, much less frequently, blastocysts indistinguishable from normal ones are seen. After the stage seen in normal 6-day embryos, most parthenogenetic embryos become disorganized but occasionally may reach the 7- or 8-day stage, and rarely a primitive streak is formed.

About 10% of *LT/Sv* virgin females are found to be pregnant. Eggs cleave and implant in the uterus, where most die at 5–7 days. The *LT/Sv* ovarian teratomas are mostly benign because their stem cells differentiate and cease to proliferate. However, two such ovarian teratomas composed of stem cells and immature tissues have been transplanted successfully. One, maintained by intraperitoneal transfer, makes structures that resemble early mouse embryos.[270]

The *LT/Sv* ovarian teratomas appear to be excellent models of human ovarian teratomas. Like the human variety, these tumors appear at an early age. Human teratomas form nearly half the ovarian tumors seen before the age of 20.[105] Chromosome analyses and enzyme studies indicate that the human variety may also have a parthenogenetic origin.[160]

Extrauterine Transplantation of Early Embryos

Transplantation of 8-day-old egg cylinders under the kidney capsules of C3H mice resulted in huge tumors 2–8 months later. They caused blood to appear in the ascitic fluid but were not invasive.[263] Transplantation of such early embryos to various other sites of the body, for example, the testes, can give rise to teratocarcinomas if they contain sufficient undifferentiated embryonic cells. They can be obtained only from presomitic embryos and not from 8-day-old mouse embryos, which are post-gastrulation. They are commonly obtained (around 50%) from egg cylinder isografts in C3H,A or CBA strain mice but not in C57B1.[48]

Grafted under the kidney capsule, these early embryos grow very rapidly and in 2 months may reach 5–6 cm in diameter and weigh 15 g, penetrating the kidney and abdominal muscles but seldom metastasizing. These teratomas are composed of haphazard somatic tissues, with foci of undifferentiated (embryonal carcinoma) stem cells showing high alkaline phosphatase activity. They have a high degree of transplantability, leading to splenomegaly in their recipients, possibly attributable to tumor-specific transplantation antigens expressed on embryonal cells.[47]

In rats, also, transplantation of 7.5–9-day-old embryonic shields from pregnant Fischer or random-bred rats under kidney capsules grew into teratomas, the largest ones being seen after 4–6 months, one weighing 800 mg. They contained well-differentiated tissues and were not malignant.[259]

Yolk sac carcinomas can be grown from the embryonic but not from the extraembryonic portion of mouse egg cylinders[46] and also from 8-day rat egg cylinders transplanted under kidney capsules.[44,45]

Chemical Induction

An ovarian teratoma was found in a mouse of the ICR/Jcl strain whose mother had been treated with urethane on day 9 of pregnancy.[218]

Methods of Induction of Yolk Sac Tumors in Experimental Animals

Fetectomy

Yolk sac tumors developed in the uterus of one third of R-strain pregnant rats after fetectomy on the 12th gestational day and injection of mouse sarcoma virus (MSV) into the placenta, intraperitoneally or intravenously, followed by treatment with medroxyprogesterone. The tumors metastasized to the peritoneal cavity, kidney, lungs, and axillary lymph nodes. Four of five were transplanted successfully into syngeneic hosts, provided they had not been inoculated with MSV at birth. These yolk sac tumors could not be induced in nonpregnant R-strain rats inoculated in utero or intravenously with MSV, nor in R-strain rats pregnant by BN strain males.[289] The MSV virus is not necessary to induce yolk sac tumors. In WKA rats, fetectomy on the seventh day of gestation leaving fetal membranes attached to placentas in situ protruding into the peritoneal cavity induced extrauterine tumors in 80% of rats. Alpha-fetoprotein in serum was elevated in 80% and was always associated with yolk sac tumor elements.[241]

Yolk sac tumors have been induced in R-strain pregnant rats by removal of the fetuses together with the amnion from both uterine horns of pregnant females, and pulling the visceral yolk sac through the incision to the outside of the uterine wall. When killed at intervals from 2–60 days later, small nodules were found from the sixth day, increasing in size from 3 mm to 3 cm by day 22. In these yolk sac teratomas, well-differentiated tissues of all types appeared in the same time sequence as in normal embryogenesis, but nests of undifferentiated carcinoma cells, trophoblast, or neuroepithelium, which are frequent constituents of teratocarcinomas, were not seen.[262] Teratoid yolk sac tumors have also been induced in BALB/c mice fetectomized on the 12th and 15th gestational days.[141] It is intriguing that visceral yolk sac, composed only of endoderm and mesoderm, can give rise to teratomas containing ectodermal tissues, such as skin and neural tissues.

Tumors of Placental Origin

Spontaneous Choriocarcinomas

These tumors have not been reported as occurring spontaneously in domestic or laboratory animals, but chorionic epithelioma and choriocarcinoma have been seen in porcupines.[101]

Induction of Placental Tumors

Fetectomy Plus Chemical Carcinogen

Four months after the removal of a 2-week-old rat fetus and dusting of benzo[a]pyrene powder into the gestational sac, vaginal bleeding was noted, and at 5 months a large tumor was palpated, after which the animal was killed. The firm, white tumor was 60 mm and had metastasized freely in the abdominal cavity. It proved to have both "sarcomatous and decidual elements," was highly anaplastic with numerous metastases, and was 100% transplantable subcutaneously, killing the hosts in 7–10 days.[267]

When Long-Evans rats were fetectomized on the 10th–12th days of pregnancy and beeswax pellets containing DMBA were inserted in the gestational sacs, many uterine tumors appeared, among which were seven choriocarcinomas. These choriocarcinomas appeared 3 weeks after the insertion of the pellets and were composed of trophoblastic giant cells as well as trophoblasts proper. They invaded uterine muscle extensively, producing necrosis and hemorrhage; lung metastases were found in three animals.[254] Luteomammotropic hormone, but no gonadotropic activity, was detected in these tumors.[255]

Choriocarcinomas have also been induced in Wistar rats fetectomized between the 15th and 20th days of pregnancy and injected with DMBA in fat emulsion into each placental site, one fetus being left at the top of each uterine horn, and the lower end of the uterus ligated. Next, 17-hydroxyprogesterone capronate was injected once weekly for 20 weeks. After 8 months, 4 of 30 animals developed large abdominal tumors with thick walls composed of two types of cells, multinucleated protoplasmic and trophoblastic with a few mitoses. These tumors invaded the uterine muscle extensively but did not metastasize. They contained soft, green, smudgy material as well as some remnants of bone.[189]

Tumors histologically resembling human chorioadenoma destruens have been induced in Japanese Hartley guinea pigs after fetectomy at 4–5 weeks gestation. The placental mass was left in situ, and a suspension of *N*-butyl-*N*-nitrosourea in carboxymethyl cellulose was instilled into the uterus. Some animals also received intramuscular injections of hCG. The tumors were composed of bizarre cells that invaded the myometrium and were also seen as perivascular infiltrates. Pleomorphic cells resembled malignant cytotrophoblasts. The changes were much more striking in the animals not given hCG.[253]

In female ICR/Jcl mice injected with urethane on days 11–13 of pregnancy, the rapidly proliferating blood vessels of the placenta and decidua were sensitive to induction of cavernous hemangiomas.[216]

Destruction of the Hypothalamic Nucleus during Pregnancy

Tumors resembling human choriocarcinoma were induced in 2 of 15 pregnant rabbits that survived destruction of the hypothalamic nucleus by means of electrocoagulation carried out on the ninth day postcopulation. Fifty-five animals were treated, but 10 died rapidly and 30 failed to show pregnancy. No macroscopic metastases were found, but vascular tumor emboli were seen in the lungs of one animal.[153]

Tumors of the Uterine Corpus

Cancer of the body of the uterus, one of the leading causes of female cancer mortality in developed countries, is geographically associated with various indicators of affluence. Cancer of the uterine cervix, which occurs in the region of the junction of the columnar epithelium of the uterine corpus with the squamous epithelium of the vagina, shows a quite different geographic distribution and is generally associated with low socioeconomic status. It would seem that they should be regarded as two quite distinct diseases having different causative factors. This discussion of tumor models attempts to make the distinction but includes discussion of the vulva and of the vagina, which are lined by squamous epithelium similar to the cervix, together under one heading.

Spontaneous Tumors of the Uterine Fundus or Cornua

Spontaneous tumors of the uterine fundus or cornua are rare in most species, but there have been a few reports in wild and zoo animals[101] and in domestic[180] or laboratory animals.[42,43] Although sporadic cases have been reported in the mare, ewe, goat, sow, bitch, and cat, significant numbers occur only in the cow, and the data come largely from American abattoirs. Of 737 bovine tumors of all kinds (253 benign and 484 malignant) submitted for histologic examination, uterine carcinoma was diagnosed in 166 and was second in frequency to lymphosarcoma.[24] In 1445 uneconomic sows, only 11 tumors of the uterus were seen, 6 of which were leiomyomas.[1]

In fowl, the oviduct differs structurally and functionally from the mammalian uterus. It is single and is found on the left side. Adenocarcinoma of this structure has been found to occur spontaneously in more than one-third of laying Light Sussex hens about 15 months old.[82]

In laboratory animals, uterine tumors have been observed occasionally in primates.[248] In guinea pigs, leiomyomas are the most frequent type reported.[168,236] A variety of uterine tumors has been seen in aging gerbils.[237] In a colony of Chinese hamsters, adenocarcinomas that always involved the cervical area were found in 30 of 120 females. They occurred during the second year of life, showing extensive stromal fibrosis, and they frequently implanted on the peritoneum. In 3 animals, lung metastases developed.[296] In another colony of Chinese hamsters, 21 endomyometrial neoplasms were seen among 93 nulliparous noninbred aging females surviving 93–1040 days.[25]

Of the more common laboratory animals, the rabbit seems to be the most sensitive species. Uterine tumors usually of epithelial nature have been observed in several colonies and in different breeds.[8,28,94,121,298] They increase in frequency with age.

Spontaneous uterine tumors have been seen in rats and are particularly frequent in certain strains.[27] Nearly two thirds of females of the Fischer 344 strain and one-third of the Marshall 520 strain over age 20 months had endometrial tumors, whereas only a few were seen in OM, ACI, or BUF rats, and none was found in WN animals. Most tumors were adenomatous polyps, a few were angiosarcomas, and occasionally other types were seen.[261] Old Fischer rats had a high incidence of polypoid glandular structures covered with endometrium and with sarcomatous changes in some. These structures were transplantable.[125] Other strains have been reported as showing endometrial polyps that were adenomatous. In female Wistar rats, the uterus was the commonest site of tumor. One half of the tumors seemed to be fibroadenomas, whereas the next most common was highly malignant adenocarcinoma. Endometrial adenocarcinomas have been seen in about 14% of old NIH (Bethesda) black rats.[257]

There have been a few reports of spontaneous uterine sarcomas in mice,[35] and age-related uterine leiomyomas or leiomyosarcomas have been observed.[171] Adenocarcinomas have been seen in mice of the BALB/c strain, as well as in C3H free from mammary tumor virus and their first-generation hybrids. Some of these tumors were transplantable.[56]

In the Pybus Miller (PM) mouse strain, spontaneous tumors of the uterus and vagina were found in 13 of 56 exbreeding females. Females often had imperforate vaginas, and males had few mammary rudiments, which suggest that a hormonal imbalance probably existed during fetal life. Unfortunately, this strain showed a high degree of sterility and was later lost.[79]

In summary, it would seem that, whereas counterparts of human cancer of the uterine fundus do occur spontaneously in laboratory animals, their infrequency makes them unacceptable as models of human disease, except in the case of aged rabbits[8,257,298] and of certain rat strains. Methods of inducing them in more substantial numbers are available.

Induction of Tumors of the Uterine Fundus or Cornua

Hormones

Estrogens. Many attempts to induce uterine tumors in rats and mice with estrogens have been made, but they usually result in glandular hyperplasia, squamous cell metaplasia, hydrometra, and pyometra, rarely going on to malignancy. However, in hybrid (PM × C3H) mice backcrossed to PM and in CBA mice and their F_1 hybrids, adenomas or adenocarcinomas, as well as infiltrative uterocervical epidermoid lesions (some of which were considered to be carcinomas), were seen after treatment with various estrogens.[78] Hybrid (BALB/c × C3H) mice have given a similar range of tumors after injection of estradiol benzoate.[10] Occasional tumors occurred in the uterus of black-hooded NB rats that were estrogen dependent when transplanted, but tumors also appeared in many other organs.[215]

In guinea pigs, prolonged treatment with estrogen injections, beginning in early life, caused cystic glandular hyperplasia, which spread from the uterine horns to the upper part of the fundus. After 200 days of treatment, fibromyomas were found in the uterus and at other abdominal sites, some of which were invasive.[210] Other experiments have shown that when the estrogen stimulus was withdrawn, fibromyomas began to regress, undergoing hyalinization and ossification.[163]

DES injected intravenously into 16-day pregnant mice appeared in the fetal plasma within 0.5 hours and was associated with a low incidence of cancer of the uterus and cervix and vagina in the female offspring.[276] Strain CD-1 female mice exposed to DES on day 0 and day 17 of fetal life developed uterine adenocarcinomas in 10 of 40 mice as well as 5 ovarian cystadenocarcinomas.[295]

DES given by stomach tube to female Syrian golden hamsters on the 14th to 15th days of pregnancy resulted in multiple reproductive tract neoplasms developing in the female offspring. Multiple uterine lesions, usually with squamous metaplasia, were found in more than one half of the animals. Virtually all animals showed endometrial hyperplasia and increase in glands. Some were adenomatous with cystic dilation. Others were villous, polypoid projections containing stroma and glands and sometimes invaginating through the myometrium. At 35 weeks, a well-differentiated adenocarcinoma was seen.[240] Female hamsters that had received prenatal exposure to DES on the 8th–11th day of fetal life and later received a DES pellet when 50 days old and another every 30 days later developed hypertrophied uteri with fingerlike polyps extending into the lumen with cystic glandular structures not opening into the lumen. In older animals, the polyps were often hemorrhagic and invaded by inflammatory tissues and fibrous material sometimes firm fibrous or chondromatous.[83]

In rabbits, some malignant growths have been described after administration of estrogens.[231] The high incidence of cystic endometrial hyperplasia and uterine tumors seen in old breeding females in some colonies after toxemia of pregnancy is believed to be caused by an excessive concentration of estrogen, resulting from impaired liver function.[93]

When rabbits were injected with DES, cervical

polyps, endometrial hyperplasias and carcinomas, adenomyosis, endometriosis, and fibroids were observed but were not enhanced by alloxan-induced diabetes.[184] Examination of the endocrine organs led to the conclusions that estrogens had both direct and indirect uterine effects mediated through stimulation of the pituitary basophils as well as consequent ovarian stimulation. Cancerous animals showed hypertrophy of the pituitary, adrenals, and ovaries, with indications of adrenocortical hyperactivity.[264]

Prolonged treatment of 10 squirrel monkeys with DES led to malignant uterine mesotheliomas originating from the serosa, sometimes in glandular or papillary form, in 7 of the treated animals. The other 3 showed early lesions of the serosa.[179] This species would seem particularly sensitive to uterine tumor induction by estrogen.

Estrogen Plus Androgen. In all female Syrian hamsters given pellets containing both DES and testosterone propionate, cystic glandular hyperplasia of the uteri occurred, and multiple foci of nodular hyperplasia were observed in the muscle of both horns. In addition, 6 of 10 had multiple leiomyomas in one or both uterine horns that were indistinguishable from the lyomyomas of the epididymes seen in 5 of 11 males similarly treated.[9] Hormone dependency and progress toward autonomy after serial transplantation of similarly induced tumors has been demonstrated.[145]

Progesterones. In an investigation of progesterone and 19-nor contraceptives in mice, tumors of the endometrial stroma, varying between fibrosarcoma and sarcoma, were produced by progesterone and by norethinodrone. Another 19-nor contraceptive, norethynodrel, produced metaplasia of the endometrium and glandular epithelium.[166] The effect of progesterone on cell division in chemically-induced endometrial and adenocarcinoma in mice has been described.[143]

Oral Contraceptives. In a review of estrogens and oral contraceptives, it was concluded that there are no animal or human data to indicate that combination oral contraceptives cause endometrial cancer.[54]

Testicular Grafts. Leiomyomas arose in female rats that had received testicular grafts (usually 2) from littermates when newborn. By sexual maturity, most animals had constant estrus, and pyometra appeared after 6 months. The uterus usually ulcerated into the body cavity through the digestive tract or through the body wall to the exterior, and the animals died. Only 16 of 185 survived more than 3 years, 4 of which had uterine leiomyomas similar to fibromyomas that frequently occur in women.[229] One rat showing continuous estrus died at 2.5 years with a huge typical adenocarcinoma in the left uterine horn and numerous metastases. The pituitary of this animal was enlarged and hemorrhagic.[230]

Pituitary Growth Hormone. Daily intraperitoneal injections of pituitary growth hormone in gradually increasing doses caused hypertrophy of the myometrium in all 15 Long-Evans rats and glandular cystic hyperplasia in 2 (1 with a polyp). In 1 animal, the entire right horn of the uterus was replaced by a tumor that adhered to the bowel and infiltrated the myometrium extensively.[191]

Pituitary Isografts. The onset of the benign condition, uterine adenomyosis, occurred within 2 months of transplantation of an anterior pituitary isograft into one uterine horn of young adult mice of the SHN, SLN, C3H, and C57BL strains, associated with significantly elevated levels of circulating prolactin. Ovariectomy after transplantation completely eliminated the adenomyosis, but continuous treatments with combined estrogen and progesterone reversed the effect of ovariectomy.[193] Similar lesions were induced in F_1 hybrid C3H × BALB/c female mice grafted with a single ectopic pituitary, indicating that chronic hyperprolactinemia was a major endocrine factor in its genesis. The grafting of the pituitary induced adenomyosis whether it was done to 1-day-old or 4-week-old mice.[118]

Ovarian Fragmentation. Uterine tumors have been induced in the guinea pig by subtotal castration. When one ovary was completely removed and only a fragment of the other left behind, an irregular sexual cycle reestablished itself, with prolonged estrus and diestrus phases. The uterus sometimes increased up to 10-fold or even 20-fold its normal weight, showing cystic glandular hyperplasia and metaplasia of the endometrium, as well as polyps filling the uterine cavity. Uterine glands were frequently seen in the myometrium, where some animals showed subserous adenofibromyomas. After 3 years or so, multifocal adenocarcinomas were seen in the small number of survivors.[162]

As with prolonged estrogen treatment, other abdominal fibroids were seen. There was also nodular hyperplasia of the adrenal cortex, and a Brenner-type ovarian tumor occurred in one instance. The ovarian fragment contained lutein cysts that were sometimes blood filled, as well as hemorrhagic follicles.[26] These observations and other experimental evidence led to the assumption that the ovarian remnant lost the faculty to control the gonadotropic function of the hypophysis.

Antiprolactin. Administration of the antiprolactin drug, bromocriptine, inhibited progesterone, preventing pseudopregnancy periods and inducing an unopposed high estrogen state when administered to rats. When given in increasing doses, it caused a decrease in mortality from mammary cancer and adrenal tumors but a dose-related time-related increase in uterine neoplasia—some being frank tumors—in long-term studies.[280] Mutagenic studies indicated no direct carcinogenic potential, and the effects were not seen in mice.[98]

Chemical Carcinogens

There have been many reports of the induction of tumors of the uterus in rats and mice by polycyclic hydrocarbon carcinogens, certain fluorenyl derivatives, and various polyvinyl substances.

3-Methylcholanthrene. Large tumors of the mouse uterus were induced by implantation of MC crystals, 1% MC in lard, or 1% MC plus estradiol propionate. The mice used were CBA strain or outbred white animals, and the implants were secured by ligatures above and below. In all, 14 of 109 developed fibromyosarcomas that were mostly locally invasive and tended to appear earlier than tumors in the 20 mice developing endometrial carcinomas. Immature CBA mice were particularly susceptible to uterine tumor development by this method (12 of 15 mice).[21]

Another method of MC application involved using cotton thread, part of which was impregnated with a 1:3 mixture of MC in beeswax. At laparotomy, the thread was inserted with a needle through the lateral wall of one uterine horn and pulled through the tip until the impregnated part lay in contact with the endometrium. Endometrial hyperplasia appeared after 7 weeks, along with fibrous proliferation of stromal tissue. Of a total of 110 mice of the na2 strain, 32 developed adenocarcinoma of the endometrium, 3 adenoacanthoma, 2 sarcoma, and 2 squamous cell carcinoma.[276] In NIH black rats, insertion of strings saturated with a 20% solution of MC also yielded endometrial tumors, which were squamous cell carcinomas.[6] Tampons of cotton tape or silk strings impregnated with MC in polyvinylchloride and melted paraffin wax induced adenocarcinomas in rabbit uteri and squamous cell carcinoma in rats and mice.[7]

In 161 female survivors of Syrian hamsters given MC by stomach tube, there were 55 uterine tumors in addition to 82 ovarian and 123 mammary tumors.[111]

Cotton strings impregnated with MC in beeswax and placed in the right uterine horn with beeswax only strings in the left horn of young adult rabbits led to cancer in all seven animals surviving 11 months. Six carcinomas developed in right horns and one small focus in a left horn. Repeated laparotomies for biopsy specimens showed the sequence of lesions to be cystic and adenomatous hyperplasia—carcinoma in situ—cancer.[186] It would seem that the approximation of MC to the uterine lining of mouse, rat, or rabbit is an effective method of inducing tumors and that the hamster uterus is also sensitive to this carcinogen.

7,12-Dimethylbenz[a]anthracene. In mice, DMBA administration by most methods leads to ovarian tumors and mammary tumors and in rats to adrenal necrosis and mammary tumors. However, when applied locally by sticks impregnated with DMBA in paraffin wax, a high yield of endometrial carcinomas in rats was obtained. Stratified squamous epithelium spread and denuded the endometrium, invading the underlying smooth muscle. Within 4 or 5 months, invasive squamous cell carcinoma developed, often accompanied by atypical growths of small uterine glands.[249] Later, the carcinomas metastasized to the abdominal viscera and peritoneum.[33]

Uterine adenocarcinoma, squamous carcinoma and sarcoma have also been induced in Sprague–Dawley rats by implanting strings coated with DMBA in beeswax locally in the endometrial cavity. Various ablative operations and hormone estimations have indicated that it is doubtful whether endometrial cancer can be produced in the absence of endogenous estrogenic hormones.[250] Similar tumors were also produced by implantation of pellets of DMBA in beeswax into the uteri of pregnant females.[249]

Benzo[a]pyrene. When injected intraperitoneally into rats, this polycyclic hydrocarbon carcinogen induced endometrial adenocarcinomas.[226]

Fluorenyl Derivatives. There are several reports that oral administration of certain fluorenyl derivatives to rats induces endometrial carcinomas.[14,187,195,235,274]

Procarbazine Hydrochloride. When administered to newborn or young Fischer 344/N rats either by injection or by mouth, this chemical produced endometrial polyps and stromal sarcoma among a miscellany of other tumors.[142]

4-Nitroquinoline-1-Oxide. Weekly injections of female Buffalo rats for 10 weeks led to development of uterine tumors in 7 of 25 animals, together with many subcutaneous sarcomas and lung neoplasms. The uterine tumors were 3 leiomyosarcomas, 2 squamous metaplasias of glands, and 2 adenocarcinomas.[192]

N-Nitroso Compounds. Various *N*-nitroso compounds given orally to BD rats produced endometrial adenocarcinomas and, when given by intravenous injection, produced uterine sarcomas.[55]

1,2-Dimethylhydrazine. This chemical has induced uterine sarcomas in CBA mice.[284]

Urethane. Urethane has multipotential carcinogenicity and has produced tumors in the endometrial cavity of rats.[277] When given to ICR/JCL female mice on the 13th and 19th days of pregnancy, it induced endometrial hyperplasia in one-third of the mothers, and uterine hemangiomas appeared in two-thirds when they were maintained unmated and further treated after delivery.[216]

Organic Polymer. Cotton tampons coated with vinyl copolymer and paraffin wax, when inserted into one uterine horn of NIH black rats, induced marked inflammation of the endometrium and moderate enlargement with pyometra after 4–10 months and marked epithelial dysplasia at 10–12 months. At 10–18 months, 5 of 12 animals had squamous cell carcinoma. Controls with strings coated only with paraffin had similar changes over a much longer period of time, and no carcinoma, whereas strings coated with MC produced them in a much shorter time.[7]

Other Chemicals. Other chemicals with carcinogenic potential for the rat uterus include biphenyl derivatives,[32,194] aflatoxin,[29] elaiomycin,[247] and epoxy resin hardener.[246]

Intrauterine Devices

Stainless steel or polyethylene loops or springs inserted into both horns of the uteri of virgin female Wistar rats led to the appearance of malignancy. Sarcomas came earliest and epidermoid carcinoma later, their appearance being more rapid with the steel devices than with the plastic.[41]

Irradiation

In rabbits, uterine tumors are common in old animals. Chronic exposure to low doses (8.8 R) of gamma-rays caused them to appear in a very much shorter time.[170]

Implantation of ^{60}Co wires in the pelvis of female rats for periods from 10 to 200 days induced adenocarcinoma of the uterus in 14 of 32 animals. The tumors were composed of dilated glands with scanty stroma, and the longer exposures increased the yield. It was calculated that the uterus received about 16,000–961,000 rad, most of these doses being much too high to induce tumors in the ovary, which was often reduced to scar tissue.[112]

Viruses. Eight endometrial sarcomas and one leiomyosarcoma (37%) developed in F_1 (C57B1 × DBA) female mice reaching 18 months of age. These sarcomas were readily transplantable but did not respond to either endogenous or exogenous progesterone. Seven of the eight mice had been inoculated with either Friend or Rauscher leukemia virus.[51]

When athymic nude mice were inoculated with polyoma virus at birth or at 3–15 weeks of age and the experiment terminated after 4.5 months, spindle-cell sarcomas of the uterus were found in a ratio of 6:0 when compared with uninoculated controls.[288]

Tumors of the Uterine Cervix, Vagina, and Vulva

The cervix is defined as "the caudal, nongestational portion of the mammalian uterus whose epithelial lining is continuous with that of the vagina."[196] The extent of this lining into the uterine horns varies considerably between different species, as shown in Figure 26.1.

Although little attention has been paid to uterine growth in fetal animals, it is known that the human uterus undergoes a rapid spurt of growth during the last trimester of pregnancy under the influence of maternal (possibly placental) hormones. Sudden removal of these hormones at birth causes very rapid involution of the organ during the first 2 postnatal weeks. These postnatal decreases in growth rate occur mainly in the cervix and vagina.[49,108] At this early stage in life, the sensitivity of the human cervix and vagina to female sex hormones is much greater than that of the uterine fundus.

In mammals, it is also known that in adult life there are definite cyclic changes in the histology of the cervix[59] (of the mouse,[90] rat,[102] and guinea pig[136]). With increasing age in the mouse, processes from the surface epithelium of vagina and cervix penetrate increasingly into the underlying connective tissue, and this is accelerated by estrogen.[273]

Spontaneous Tumors of the Uterine Cervix, Vagina, and Vulva

Cervical cancer has rarely been reported to occur spontaneously in animals. Isolated cases have been seen in the Macacca monkey, the mare, the cow, and the rat. However, they were commonly seen, along with cancer of the vagina, in mice of the Pybus Miller strain after 200 days of age. Unfortunately, this strain was later lost.[79] Vaginal fibropapillomas have been seen in cows,[180] epidermoid carcinomas of vagina, vulva, and clitoris in mares,[278] and occasional tumors have been seen in dogs, goats, and other species. In rabbits, the cervix is lined with columnar epithelium, but spontaneous epidermoid cancer has been reported at the squamocolumnar epithelial junction some way down the vaginal wall.[95]

Induction of Tumors of the Cervix, Vagina, and Vulva

Hormones

Estrogens. In view of the great sensitivity of the cervix and vagina to female sex hormones, it is not surprising that many reports from the 1930s onward have shown the carcinogenic action of estrogens on these sites of the genital tract in mice. A few key reports are worth mentioning.

The reactions of mouse uterus, cervix, and vagina to injections of estrogens have been found to vary greatly with age at injection. If begun in adult life, there is often hypertrophy of the uterus and pyometria. If begun on the day of birth, the entire uterine epithelium becomes stratified, but not cornified, with metaplasia extending into the uterine ends of the fallopian tubes. The vagina becomes greatly enlarged, with rapid growth of epithelial tissues.[80]

When weekly injections of estrogen were continued for more than 1 year, carcinoma of the cervix developed in 50–60% of animals.[2] Mice of all genotypes used in this investigation responded in this way if they survived long enough, the highest tumor incidence being seen at 450–600 days. After cornification, the epithelium sometimes atrophied before the earliest invasive lesions were seen. On gross examination, the cervices appeared firm and white, with deficient blood supply.[74]

The effectiveness of injections of estrogens on the day of birth was shown in mice of three strains. Astonishing vaginal concretions appeared in 12 of 30 mice after 13 months, as well as cancer of the cervix and vagina.[58] The antifertility drug mestranol (Enovid) fed to newborn BALB/c mice produced similar endometrial changes to estrogens, and some animals developed cervical cancer after 2 years.[57]

Transplacental administration of diethylstilbestrol on the 9th–16th day of fetal life led to a low incidence of cancer of the vagina, cervix, and uterus in mice.[181] When DES was fed continuously to pregnant female F_1 hybrid C3H × BALB/c mice from the seventh day of pregnancy until the morning after delivery, two benign lesions of the genital tract occurred frequently in the exposed offspring. The most frequent striking abnormality was a uterine lesion resembling human adenomyosis and similar to those induced by intrauterine pituitary isografts.[183] The other was an enlargement of the cervix, accumulation of mucoid material, and almost complete disappearance of recognizable smooth muscle.[118] Other mammalian species that respond to the transplacental administration of DES and related synthetic estrogens with cervical and vaginal lesions and neoplasms include the rat,[208] golden hamster,[240] and human.[106]

In adult mice, local application of estrogens to the cervix and vagina can lead to cancer of these sites. A number of methods have been devised for this purpose: (1) the introduction of estrogen solutions intravaginally through an eyedropper several times a week, (2) the application of estrogen or cholesterol pellets to the cervix with forceps, or (3) the use of knotted threads dipped in such mixtures and pulled through the vagina, cervix, and one horn of the uterus and secured there at laparotomy. With the last technique, half of the adult BC mice developed lesions in the upper vagina, fornices, and cervix when DES was the estrogen used. None were seen when estrone or progesterone was used, but the addition of testosterone to DES also yielded lesions in half of the animals.[75]

Progesterone. When cervicovaginal tracts of 2-year-old female BALB/c mice exposed neonatally to progesterone were cut into small segments and transplanted into syngeneic hosts, some tumors developed with squamous and glandular components, whereas those from estrogen-treated mice were squamous cell carcinomas. One derived from a mouse that had received estrogen and progesterone was of a basal cell type. They were maintained for 2 years and did not show hormone dependency when transplanted.[129]

Androgen. When female F_1 (C57B1 × dba) mice were implanted subcutaneously with pellets of testosterone twice a week starting at age 6–13 weeks and continuing until they had to be killed, uterine tumors were found, mostly in the cervix and unpaired uterine part in 26 of 42 animals treated for 10 months or more, and 10 of these 26 animals had lung metastases. Two of the primary tumors were transplanted and showed testosterone dependence, but one became autonomous after the sixth generation transplant. Nodules considered to be preneoplastic lesions developed in the stroma of the uterine epithelium, leaving muscle layers and epithelium intact, first appearing after 2 months and present in all animals after 9 months.[290] At 11 months, the last nodules and first tumors were seen. Histologically, they showed highly developed organization consisting of large trabeculae of cells, locally forming branched papillae inside large sinuses, with no evidence of dedifferentiation.[12]

Androgen Plus Estrogen. In C3H mice receiving estradiol and testosterone simultaneously, malignant and nonmalignant tumors were seen in the cervix and upper vagina in half the treated animals.[77]

Chemical Carcinogens

A high incidence of vaginal tumors or cervical tumors or both can be obtained by local application of polycyclic hydrocarbon carcinogens to these sites.

Benzo[a]pyrene. BP, used as a 5% solution in cholesterol broken into tiny fragments sufficient to induce subcutaneous tumors and poked into the vagina of 10 mice two or three times weekly, produced tumors in the vagina in all mice in 10–14 months. All were squamous cell carcinomas with varying degrees of keratinization. Similar applications of human smegma from elderly institutionalized men was ineffective.[65]

Other methods devised for reaching the mouse cervix included painting of acetone solutions of the carcinogen with cotton-tipped wire loops, later aided by the use of an infant-sized optic speculum[149] and the use of knotted threads impregnated with BP and threaded through the vagina, cervix, and one uterine horn and stitched in place.[232] These were removed later if limited exposure was desired. The cervices of rats painted with a lumbar puncture needle covered with cotton wool soaked in 1% BP in acetone solution yielded a low incidence of cancer and polyps of the cervix.[268]

3-Methylcholanthrene. MC crystals inserted into uteri removed from mice and transplanted subcutaneously on the abdomen of other mice of the same strain produced 61 tumors among 55 of 104 mice of 10 genetic types (32 were carcinomas, which included epidermoid, adenocarcinomas, adenoacanthomas, and carcinomas, whereas 29 developed sarcomas). Most tumors arose from the cervices, rather than from the uterine horns, and most appeared by the eighth week.[224]

In later studies, the mouse cervix was painted with a saturated solution of MC in acetone, or a thread impregnated with crystalline MC was suspended in the endocervical canal. A comparison of these two methods demonstrated that the latter gave the highest yield and halved the latent period.[200] The MC string method is also effective in rabbits.[3] Comparison of BP and MC by painting or string method in C3H mice showed that the highest yield (85%) was with the MC string method, followed by BP string, MC painting, and lowest (50%) with BP paintings.[244,245]

Dimethylbenz[a]anthracene. DMBA was first used by the knotted string method to induce carcinoma of the cervix in rats. Eleven of 39 adult Wistar rats surviving the operation developed gross tumors, and 2 more had microtumors. The endocervix of 12 of the 13 rats with neoplasia became dilated and filled with keratin. In the walls, papillomas appeared that ultimately transformed to epidermoid carcinoma. Sometimes, local invasion was seen, but no metastases.[291] Direct painting of DMBA in acetone solution intravaginally has also been used to induce cervical cancer in rats[85] and in mice.[86]

Induction of cervical cancer by the direct application of polycyclic chemical carcinogens to the cervices of adult animals has been used to study the histogenesis of the lesions,[91,120,238,301] and as a model for testing anticancer drugs.[275] It has also been widely used to study the effects of sex steroid hormones on cervical cancer induction.[85,86,137,183] These studies may be complicated, however, by the fact that the polycyclic carcinogens have hormone-mimetic action themselves. MC and DMBA have progesterone-like effects, and BP has estrogen-like effects on the mammary tissue of mice.[130] Also, cocarcinogenic effects may be seen when the carcinogen is used with the appropriate mimetic hormone.[233]

General conclusions about cervical carcinogenesis in rats were that the effects of hormones and radiation on the carcinogenic process differed from their effects on the normal target tissue. For example, estrogens stimulate the normal growth of the cervicovaginal stroma, but they inhibit development of sarcomas in a dose-dependent way. Conversely, testosterone, cortisone, methylthiouracil, L-thyroxine, and x-rays do not stimulate normal stromal growth or epithelial keratinization, but they were found to increase the rate of growth of DMBA-induced tumors in rats.

With limited exposure of the mouse cervix to MC threads, a promoting effect of estrogen has been observed.[201] A cocarcinogenic effect of progesterone and MC has also been seen.[233]

When the painting method of applying carcinogenic solutions to the cervix has been used, contamination of the vulva has occurred. With DMBA paintings in rats, squamous cell papillomas increased in numbers and rate of appearance with the number of paintings given. Castration promoted progression of vulval papillomas to carcinomas.[87]

N,N′-*Dimethyl*-N-*nitrosurea.* DMNU injected subcutaneously into adult Syrian hamsters once a week induced adenoacanthomas of the uterine cervix in 86% of animals, in addition to producing a high incidence of mammary tumors and smaller numbers of cholangiocarcinomas of the liver, as well as other tumors.[110]

Carbowax 1000 (Polyethylene Glycol). In testing spermicidal contraceptives for possible carcinogenesis in mice, test substances were dissolved in Carbowax 1000 and introduced into the vagina twice a week using a syringe with a blunt needle. Eighteen months later, tumors of the cervix and vagina were seen in almost one half of the control animals that had received only the Carbowax. When DMBA was used in this medium, 9 tumors developed in 10 animals over a 12-month period.[22]

Virus

Herpesvirus Type 2 (HSV-2). Attempts to induce cervical cancer in animals with this virus have been made. The animals were infected by applying the virus on cotton-wool swabs to the cervix. Rabbits treated in this way were reported to have died with paralysis and encephalitis.[252]

BALB/c mice treated with hormones (estrogen, progesterone, or Enovid) and with HSV-2 intravaginally (twice at the beginning and again after 10 months) showed characteristic cytologic changes of herpes infection in 40%. In 2 mice of 19 having HSV-2 alone, 1 precancerous lesion and 1 transplantable cancer developed. Addition of hormones made no significant difference.[199]

Treatment of nonhuman primates with HSV-2 has also been tried. Rhesus and squirrel monkeys could not be infected. Baboons could be but did not show lesions. Marmosets could be infected but soon died. However, *Cebus* monkeys (*C. albifrons* or *C. apella*) were susceptible to genital infection and survived. Of 12 strains of HSV-2 used, each on at least two monkeys, 11 strains caused genital infection and 5 strains produced tumors. In a total of 89 female *Cebus* monkeys exposed to HSV-2 infection, 50% developed lesions on the vulva, on the cervix, and occasionally on the mouth. Nineteen males were exposed to the infected females, and venereal cross-infection by two animals was noted. One of these had penile lesions similar to those found in humans.[169]

Mucosal Abrasion and Spermatozoal Penetration

The uterine mucosas of young Wistar rats were curetted with a ribbed probe, and spermatozoa from minced epididymes were injected into a uterine horn just above the bifurcation and loosely ligated to delay evacuation. As a result, the sperm penetrated into the submucosal tissue and the cervical epithelium showed varying degrees of hyperplastic and dysplastic change not always reflected in vaginal smears. The changes occurred much more rapidly than after carcinogen treatment, and at 4 months there was proliferation and downgrowth of basal cells, after which loss of stratification with large foci of densely packed basal cells was seen.[269] These changes were not seen after curettage alone or after artificial insemination alone. It was suggested that, because rodents mate only during the estrus phase of the cycle when the uterine epithelium is high and multilayered, they may be protected against penetration of the cervix by spermatozoa, whereas humans mating at any time during the estrous cycle would not always be protected. This might explain the comparative rarity of spontaneous cervical cancer in animals.

Venereal Sarcoma of the Dog

This animal tumor, which has no human counterpart, is a naturally occurring, coitally transmitted tumor that affects the genitalia of both sexes. It grows from single or multiple nodules, often developing a cauliflower-like shape that can reach more than 10 cm in size and may metastasize. It evokes an immune response, and spontaneous regressions may occur. This unusual tumor seems to be an implant of undifferentiated round cells regarded to be of reticuloendothelial origin. It has evolved into a tumor that is autonomous from the original host and has become a neoplastic cell that is a parasite.[38,39]

Laboratory Animals as Hosts for Human Tumors

The experimentally minded gynecologic oncologist may be interested in using laboratory animals as hosts for human tumor transplants, enabling studies of their hormone dependence or drug sensitivity to be made. Two types of systems permit this to be done: the immunologically privileged site and the immunologically suppressed animal.

Immunologically Privileged Sites

Hamster Cheek Pouch

Xenografts of trophoblastic tumors have been grown in this site and have shown profound inhibition by methotrexate (MTX).[107]

Other Sites

Successful xenographs of human tumors have been made in the brain and the anterior chamber of the eye of laboratory species.

Immunologically Suppressed Hosts

Nude Mice and Rats

An animal currently popular as a host for human tumor xenografts is the genetically determined, athymic nude mouse. These naturally immunosuppressed animals have been used to show the hormone requirements of a variety of different human gynecologic tumors,[84,122,302] as well as the effects of human interferon on human yolk sac tumors[242] and of chemotherapeutic agents.[50,177,281,300] Nude rats allow tumors to grow to a larger size than in nude mice, where they may not always be adequate for studies involving surgery, intraarterial tubing or sampling of blood.[243]

Other Hosts

Other hosts for human tumor xenografts are animals artificially immunosuppressed by x-rays, cortisone treatment, neonatal thymectomy, or antilymphocyte serum.[269]

Relevance of Animal Tumor Models to Human Disease

Although spontaneous tumors of the female genital tract are by and large uncommon in laboratory species, this chapter indicates that tumors of all sites have been successfully induced in one species or another, either by induction of hormonal imbalance or by the systemic or local direct effect of a carcinogen, for example, chemical, radiation, or virus, or by ectopic transplantation of tissues.

The importance of genetic factors has been shown by the selective inbreeding of strains of animals particularly likely to develop cancer of specific sites, either spontaneously or when carcinogen treated.

In many instances, age at time of exposure to hormonal or carcinogenic agents or fetal age at time of tissue misplacements has been shown to be essential to determining the sensitivity of a particular tissue to cancer induction. These vital periods seem to be those of rapid cell multiplication.[292]

Oogonia of mice and rats divide rapidly during the mid and late stages of fetal life, and there is accumulating evidence that offspring of mothers treated with carcinogenic agents during pregnancy show a greater susceptibility to cancer, or to carcinogenesis by the same agent,[199,267,282] suggesting a transplacental effect of the agents.

In humans, the chemical carcinogen BP is a common urban pollutant and a constituent of cigarette smoke. BP has been shown to have a dose-related ovotoxicity in mice, and a dose-dependent relationship exists between smoking and early onset of the menopause in women,[178] which might indicate a similar toxicity of BP on human oocytes, although other toxins in cigarette smoke may be involved.

It seems possible that if a woman smokes, she might damage the oocytes in her own ovaries. If she smokes during pregnancy, she could damage the oogonia of her unborn child, who might receive further carcinogenic doses from suckling the smoking mother's milk. In all cases, the germ line could be affected and could lead to greater sensitivity of offspring in subsequent generations to cancers induced by BP or possibly to other carcinogens to which 20th-century urbanized societies have been increasingly exposing themselves.

It is hoped that this review of the reports of animal tumors of the female genital tract will lead to a better understanding of human disease and that such models will encourage society's health leaders to take more effective steps toward eliminating known and suspected carcinogenic agents. Methods of counteracting carcinogenic agents must be found. A few are known for specific agents, but much more needs to be done in this sphere.

The gynecologic oncologist could contribute greatly by directing attention to the effect of such factors as smoking on the germ line, which might influence the health of generations to come, as well as by focusing on the transplacental effect of such factors as smoking and using drugs, for example, DES, which affect the unborn child. Some human cancers are known to be influenced by less direct factors, which include, dietary deficiencies or excesses. The animal experimenter might be rewarded by putting more effort into studying these nutritional aspects of cancer.

References

1. Alkermans JPWM, Van Beusekom WJ (1984) Tumors and tumor-like lesions in the genitalia of sows. Vet Q 6: 90
2. Allen E, Gardner WU (1941) Cancer of the cervix of the uterus in hybrid mice following long-continued administration of estrogen. Cancer Res 1: 359
3. Alvizouri M, De Pita VR (1964) Experimental carcinoma of the cervix. Hormonal influences. Am J Obstet Gynecol 89: 940
4. Anderson LJ, Sandison AT, Jarrett WFH (1969) A British abbatoir survey of tumors in cattle, sheep and pigs. Vet Rec 84: 547
5. Andervont HB, Dunn TB (1962) Occurrence of tumors in wild house mice. J Natl Cancer Inst 28: 1153
6. Baba N, Haam E von (1967) Experimental carcinoma of the endometrium. Prog Exp Tumor Res Basel 9: 192
7. Baba N, Haam E von (1971) Squamous cell carcinoma of the rat endometrium produced by insertion of strings coated with paraffin and polymer. J Natl Cancer Inst 47: 675
8. Baba N, Haam E von (1972) Spontaneous carcinoma in aged rabbits. Am J Pathol 68: 653
9. Bacon RR (1952) Tumors of the epididymus and of the uterus in hamsters treated with diethylstilbestrol and testosterone propionate. Cancer Res 12: 246
10. Barbieri G, Olivi M, Sacco O (1958) Lesioni microscopiche nel' uteri di topi (BALB/Cf, C3H/CB/Se substrain) trattati con benzoato di estradiolo. Lav Inst Anat Istol Patol Perugia 18: 165
11. Beamer WG (1980) Endocrine aspects of ovarian tumours. In: Biology of Ovarian Neoplasia, UICC Technical Report Series. Murphy ED, Beamer WG (eds). Geneva, Union Internationale Contre le Cancer, Vol 50, p 82
12. Benedetti EL, van Nie R (1962) On the histology and fine structure of uterine tumours induced by testosterone in mice. Acta Un Contr Cancr 18: 197
13. Biancifiori C, Bonser GM, Caschera F (1961) Ovarian and mammary tumours in intact C3Hb virgin mice following a limited dose of four carcinogenic chemicals. Br J Cancer 15: 270
14. Bielschowsky F (1944) Distant tumours produced by 2-aminofluorene and 2-acetyl aminofluorene. Br J Exp Pathol 25: 1
15. Bielschowsky M, D'Ath EF (1973) Spontaneous granulosa cell tumours of mice of strain NZC-Bi, NZO-Bi, NZY-Bi and NZB-Bi. Pathology 5: 303
16. Bielschowsky F, Hall WH (1951) Carcinogenesis in parabiotic rats joined to gonadectomised litter mates and the reaction of their pituitaries to endogenous estrogens. Br J Cancer 5: 331
17. Biskind GR, Biskind MS (1949) Experimental ovarian tumors in rats. Am J Clin Pathol 19: 501
18. Biskind GR, Bernstein DE, Gospe SM (1953) The effect of exogenous gonadotrophins on the development of ovarian tumors in rats. Cancer Res 13: 216
19. Biskind GR, Kordan B, Biskind MS (1950) Ovary transplanted to spleen in rats. The effect of unilateral castration, pregnancy and subsequent castration. Cancer Res 10: 309
20. Bonser GM, Jull JW (1974) Tumors of the ovary. Personal communication
21. Bonser GM, Robson JM (1950) The induction of tumours following the direct implantation of 20-methylcholanthrene in the uterus of mice. Br J Cancer 4: 196
22. Boyland E, Charles RT, Gowing NFC (1961) The induction of tumours in mice by intravaginal application of chemical compounds. Br J Cancer 15: 252
23. Brambell FWR, Fielding U, Parkes AS (1927) Changes in the ovary of the mouse following exposure to x-rays. Part III. Irradiation of the non-parous adult. Proc R Soc Lond [Biol] 101: 316
24. Brandly PJ, Migaki G (1963) Types of tumors found by federal meat inspectors in an eight-year survey. Ann NY Acad Sci 108: 872
25. Brownstein DG, Brooks AL (1980) Spontaneous endomyo-

metrial neoplasms in aging Chinese hamsters. J Natl Cancer Inst 64: 1209
26. Bruzzone S, Lipschutz A (1954) Endometrial adenocarcinoma and extragenital tumours in guinea-pigs with "ovarian fragmentation." Br J Cancer 8: 613
27. Bullock FD, Curtis MR (1930) Spontaneous tumors of the rat. J Cancer Res 14: 1
28. Burrows H (1940) Spontaneous uterine and mammary tumours in the rabbit. J Pathol Bacteriol 51: 385
29. Butler WH, Barnes JM (1968) Carcinogenic action of groundnut meal containing aflatoxin in rats. Food Cosmet Toxicol 6: 135
30. Campbell JG (1951) Some unusual gonadal tumours of the fowl. Br J Cancer 5: 69
31. Carter RL (1968) Pathology of ovarian neoplasms in rats and mice. Eur J Cancer 3: 537
32. Castro HF, Fechner RE, Spjut HJ (1968) Induced mesenchymal tumors of the rat genital tract. Arch Pathol 86: 475
33. Charkviani LI (1961) [Experimental cancer of the uterus produced in rats by 9,10-dimethyl-1,2-benzanthracene]. Vopr Onkol 7: 52
34. Chesterman FC, Pomerance A (1965) Spontaneous neoplasms in ferrets and polecats. J Pathol Bacteriol 89: 529
35. Chouroulinkov I, Guillon JC, Guerin M (1969) Endometrial sarcomas in mice: A survey of 130 cases. J Natl Cancer Inst 42: 593
36. Christov K, Raichev R (1973) Proliferative and neoplastic changes in the ovaries of hamsters treated with 131-iodine and methylthiouracil. Neoplasma 20: 511
37. Clapp NK (1978) Ovarian tumor types and their incidence in intact mice following whole-body exposure to ionising radiation. Radiat Res 74: 405
38. Cohen D (1978) The transmissible venereal tumor of the dog. A naturally occurring allograft? A review. Isr J Med Sci 14: 14
39. Cohen D (1985) Canine transmissable venereal tumor: A unique result of tumor progression. Adv Canc Res 43: 75
40. Cordes DO (1969) Equine granulosa tumours. Vet Rec 85: 186
41. Corfman PA, Richart RM (1967) Induction in rats of uterine epidermoid carcinomas by plastic and stainless steel intrauterine devices. Am J Obstet Gynecol 98: 987
42. Cotchin E (1964) Spontaneous uterine tumours in animals. Br J Cancer 18: 209
43. Cotchin E (1977) Spontaneous tumors of the uterus and ovaries in animals. In: Animal Tumors of the Female Reproductive Tract: Spontaneous and Experimental. Cotchin E, Marchant J. New York, Springer-Verlag
44. Damjanov I (1980) Yolk sac carcinoma (endodermal sinus tumor). Animal model: Parietovisceral yolk sac carcinoma in the rat. Am J Pathol 98: 569
45. Damjanov I, Sell S (1977) Yolk-sac carcinoma grown from rat egg cylinder. J Natl Cancer Inst 58: 1523
46. Damjanov I, Solter D (1973) Yolk-sac carcinoma grown from mouse egg cylinder. Arch Pathol. 95: 182
47. Damjanov I, Solter D (1974) Experimental teratoma. Curr Top Pathol 59: 69
48. Damjanov I, Solter D (1976) Animal models of human disease: Embryo-derived teratomas and teratocarcinomas in mice. Am J Pathol 83: 241
49. Davies J, Kusama H (1962) Developmental aspects of the human cervix. Ann NY Acad Sci 97: 534
50. Davy M, Mossige J, Johannessen JV (1977) Heterologous growth of human ovarian cancer. A new in vivo testing system. Gynecol Scand 56: 55
51. Dawson PJ, Brooks RE, Fieldsteel AH (1974) Unusual occurrence of endometrial sarcomas in hybrid mice. J Natl Cancer Inst 52: 207
52. Deringer MK (1959) Occurrence of tumors, particularly mammary tumors, in agent-free strain C_3HeB mice. J Natl Cancer Inst 22: 995
53. Dickie MM (1954) The use of F_1 hybrid and backcross generations to reveal new and/or uncommon tumor types. J Natl Cancer Inst 15: 791
54. Drill UA (1980) Relationship of estrogens and oral contraceptives to endometrial cancer in animals and women. J Reprod Med 24: 7724
55. Druckrey H, Preussman R, Ivankovic S, Schmahl D (1967) Organotrope carcinogene Wirkungen bei 65 verscheidenen N-Nitroso- Verbindungen an BD-Ratten. Z Krebsforsch 69: 103
56. Dunn TB (1954) The importance of differences in morphology in inbred strains. J Natl Cancer Inst 15: 573
57. Dunn TB (1969) Cancer of the uterine cervix in mice fed a liquid diet containing anti-fertility drug. J Natl Cancer Inst 46: 671
58. Dunn TB, Green AW (1963) Cysts of the epididymus, cancer of the cervix, granular myoblastoma, and other lesions after estrogen injection in newborn mice. J Natl Cancer Inst 31: 425
59. El-Banna AA, Hafez ESE (1971) The uterine cervix in mammals. Am J Obstet Gynecol 112: 145
60. Eppig JJ, Kozac LP, Eicher EM, Stevens LC (1977) Ovarian teratomas in mice are derived from oocytes that have completed the first meiotic division. Nature 269: 517
61. Fawcett DW (1950) Bilateral ovarian teratomas in a mouse. Cancer Res 10: 705
62. Fekete E, Ferringo MA (1952) Studies on a transplantable teratoma of the mouse. Cancer Res 12: 438
63. Fels E (1954) Effet de la ligature tubaire sur la fonction ovarienne chez le rat. CR Soc Biol 148: 1666
64. Fels E (1956) Aspectos morfologicos y functionales de los tumores experimentales del ovario. Rev Arg Endocrinol Metab 2: 1
65. Fishman M, Shear MJ, Friedman HF, Stewart HL (1941–1942) Studies in carcinogenesis. XVII. Local effect of repeated application of 3,4-benzpyrene and of human smegma to the vagina and the cervix of mice. J Natl Cancer Inst 2: 361
66. Flux JEC (1965) Incidence of ovarian tumors in hares in New Zealand. J Wildl Mgmnt 29: 622
67. Fukunishi R, Wang H, Yoshida A, Yoshida H, Hirota N (1975) Induction of ovarian tumor in rats with *N*-butylnitrosourea. Gann 66: 323
68. Furth J (1946) Transplantability of induced granulosa cell tumors and of luteoma in mice. Secondary effects of these growths. Proc Soc Exp Biol Med 61: 212

69. Furth J, Boon MC (1947) Induction of ovarian tumors in mice by x-rays. Cancer Res 7: 241
70. Furth J, Butterworth JS (1936) Neoplastic diseases occurring among mice subjected to general irradiation with x-rays. II. Ovarian tumors and associated lesions. Am J Cancer 28: 66
71. Furth J, Furth OB (1936) Neoplastic diseases produced in mice by general irradiation with x-rays. Am J Cancer 28: 54
72. Furth J, Sobel H (1947) Transplantable luteoma in mice and associated secondary changes. Cancer Res 7: 246
73. Furth J, Sobel H (1947) Neoplastic transformations of granulosa cells in grafts of normal ovaries into spleens of gonadectomised mice. J Natl Cancer Inst 8: 7
74. Gardner WU (1947) Studies on steroid hormones in experimental carcinogenesis. Rec Prog Horm Res 1: 127
75. Gardner WU (1959) Experimental induction of uterine, cervical and vaginal cancer in mice. Cancer Res 19: 170
76. Gardner WU (1961) Tumorigenesis in transplanted irradiated and nonirradiated ovaries. J Natl Cancer Inst 26: 829
77. Gardner WU, Allen E (1939) Malignant and non-malignant uterine and vaginal lesions in mice receiving estrogens and androgens simultaneously. Yale J Biol Med 12: 213
78. Gardner WU, Ferrigno M (1956) Unusual neoplastic lesions in the uterine horns of estrogen-treated mice. J Natl Cancer Inst 17: 601
79. Gardner WU, Pan SC (1948) Malignant tumors of the uterus and vagina in untreated mice of the PM stock. Cancer Res 8: 241
80. Gardner WU, Allen E, Strong LC (1936) Atypical uterine and vaginal changes in mice receiving large doses of estrogenic hormone (Abstr). Anat Rec 64: 17 [Suppl 3]
81. Geary CP (1984) Carcinogen-induced granulosa cell tumors in NZC/BL mice. Pathology 16: 131
82. Gellatly JBM (1967) Normal and pathological anatomy and histology of the genital tract of rats and mice. In: Pathology of Laboratory Rats and Mice. Cotchin E, Roe FCJ (eds). Oxford and Edinburgh, Blackwell Scientific Publications, p 498
83. Gilloteaux J, Paul RJ, Steggles AW (1982) Upper genital tract abnormalities in the Syrian hamster as a result of in utero exposure to diethylstilbestrol. I. Uterine cystadenomatous papilloma and hypoplasia. Virchows Arch 398: 163
84. Giovanella BC, Stehlin JS (1974) Influence of the host's sex on the growth of human tumors heterotransplanted in "nude" thymusless mice (Abstr). Am Assoc Cancer Res 15: 92
85. Glucksman A (1971) Some effects of steroid hormones on carcinogenesis in rats: Effects of oestrogens on the induction of tumours in the cervico-vaginal tract and in the salivary glands. In: Some Implications of Steroid Hormones in Cancer. Williams DC, Briggs MC (eds). London, Heinemann, p 70
86. Glucksman A, Cherry CP (1962) The effect of castration and of additional hormone treatments on the induction of cervical and vulval tumours in mice. Br J Cancer 16: 634
87. Glucksman A, Cherry CP (1970) The effect of increased numbers of carcinogenic treatments on the induction of cervico-vaginal and vulval tumors in intact and castrate rats. Br J Cancer 24: 333
88. Goodchild WM, Cooper DM (1968) Oviduct adenocarcinoma in laying hens. Vet Rec 82: 389
89. Gorski RA, Wagner JW (1965) Gonadal activity and sexual differentiation of the hypothalamus. Endocrinology 76: 226
90. Graham CE (1966) Cyclic changes in the squamocolumnar junction of the mouse cervix uteri. Anat Rec 155: 251
91. Graham CE (1971) Histogenesis of methylcholanthrene-induced murine cervical cancer. Oncology 25: 269
92. Graham CE, McKlure HM (1977) Ovarian tumors and related lesions in aged chimpanzees. Vet Pathol 14: 380
93. Greene HSN (1959) Adenocarcinoma of the uterine fundus in the rabbit. Ann NY Acad Sci 75: 535
94. Greene HSN (1965) Diseases of the rabbit. In: The Pathology of Laboratory Animals. Ribelin WE, McCoy JR (eds). Springfield, IL, Charles C Thomas, p 330
95. Greene HSN, Newton BL, Fisk AA (1947) Carcinoma of the vaginal wall in the rabbit. Cancer Res 7: 502
96. Greenwood AW (1967) Controlled environments and cancer incidence in the domestic fowl. In: Racial and Geographical Factors in Tumour Incidence. Shivas AA (ed). Medical Monograph 2. Edinburgh, University Press, p 241
97. Gregson RL, Lewis DJ, Abbott DP (1984) Spontaneous ovarian neoplasms of the laboratory rat. Vet Pathol 21: 292
98. Griffith RW (1977) Bromocriptine and uterine neoplasia. Br Med J 2: 1605
99. Hafez ESE (1973) The comparative anatomy of the mammalian cervix. In: The Biology of the Cervix. Blandau RJ, Moghissi K (eds). Chicago, University of Chicago Press, Chap 3
100. Hale HB, Weichert CK (1944) Ovarian tumors in adult rats following prepuberal administration of estrogens. Proc Soc Exp Biol Med 55: 201
101. Halloran P O'C (1955) A Bibliography of references to diseases in wild mammals and birds. Am J Vet Res 16(12): 1
102. Hamilton CE (1947) The cervix uteri of the rat. Anat Rec 97: 47
103. Handler AH (1965) Spontaneous lesions of the hamster. In: The Pathology of Laboratory Animals. Ribelin WE, McCoy JR (eds). Springfield, Ill, Charles C Thomas, p 210
104. Hayes HM, Young JL (1978) Epidemiologic features of canine ovarian neoplasms. Gynecol Oncol 6: 348
105. Hecht F, McCaw BK, Patil S (1976) Ovarian teratomas and genetics of germ-cell formation. Lancet 2: 131
106. Herbst AL, Kurman RJ, Scully RE, Poskanzer DC (1972) Clear-cell adenocarcinoma of the genital tract in young females. N Engl J Med 287: 1259
107. Hertz R (1971) Biological aspects of gestational neoplasms derived from trophoblast. Ann NY Acad Sci 172: 279
108. Hiersche HD (1970) Funktionelle Morphologie des fetalen und kindlichen cervical Drusenfeldes in Uterus. Adv Anat Embryol Cell Biol 43: 1

109. Hilfrich J (1973) A new model for inducing malignant ovarian tumors in rats. Br J Cancer 28: 46
110. Hiraki S (1971) Carcinogenic effect of N,N′-dimethylnitrosourea in Syrian hamsters. Gann 62: 321
111. Homburger F (1972) Chemical carcinogenesis in Syrian hamsters. Prog Exp Tumor Res 16: 152
112. Hori CG, Warren S, Patterson WB, Chute RN (1971) Gamma ray induction of malignant tumors in rats. Am J Pathol 65: 279
113. Horning ES (1958) Carcinogenic action of androgens. Br J Cancer 64: 414
114. Howell JS (1963) The experimental production of vascular tumours in the rat. Br J Cancer 17: 663
115. Howell JS, Marchant J, Orr JW (1954) The induction of ovarian tumours in mice with 9:10-dimethyl-1:2-benzanthracene. Br J Cancer 8: 635
116. Huggins CB, Sugiyama T (1965) Production and prevention of two distinctive kinds of destruction of the adrenal cortex. Nature 206: 1310
117. Hummel KP (1954) Induced ovarian tumors. J Natl Cancer Inst 15: 711
118. Huseby RA, Thurlow S (1982) Effects of prenatal exposure of mice to "low dose" diethylstilbestrol and the development of adenomyosis associated with evidence of hyperprolactinemia. Am J Obstet Gynecol 144: 939
119. Iglesias R (1974) Newer concepts in pathogenesis. Secondary endocrine and mammary malignancies as main signs of hormonal syndromes produced by endocrine tumors. Ann NY Acad Sci 230: 500
120. Iijima H, Nasu K, Taki I (1964) Comparative study of carcinogenesis in squamous and columnar epithelium of mouse uterus by string method of producing cervical carcinoma. Am J Obstet Gynecol 89: 946
121. Ingalls TH, Adams WM, Lurie MP, Ipsen J (1964) Natural history of adenocarcinoma of the uterus in the Phipps rabbit colony. J Natl Cancer Inst 33: 799
122. Ishiwata L, Udagawa Y, Okumura H, Nozawa S (1978) Effects of progesterone on human endometrial carcinoma cells in vivo and in vitro. J Natl Cancer Inst 60: 947
123. Jabara AG (1962) Induction of canine ovarian tumours by diethylstilbestrol and progesterone. Aust J Exp Biol Med Sci 40: 139
124. Jacobs AJ, Curtis GL, Newland JR, Wilson RB, Ryan WL (1984) Chemical induction of ovarian epithelial carcinoma in mice. Gynecol Oncol 18: 177
125. Jacobs BB, Huseby RA (1967) Neoplasms occurring in aged Fischer rats, with special reference to testicular, uterine and thyroid tumors. J Natl Cancer Inst 39: 303
126. Jick H, Porter J, Morrison AS (1977) Relation between smoking and age at natural menopause. Lancet 1: 1354
127. Jones EC, Krohn PL (1959) Influence of the anterior pituitary on the aging process in the ovary. Nature 183: 1155
128. Jones EC, Krohn PL (1961) The relationships between age, numbers of oocytes and fertility in virgin and multiparous mice. J Endocrinol 21: 469
129. Jones LA, Pacillas-Verjan R (1979) Transplantability and sex hormone responsiveness of cervicovaginal tumor derived from female BALB/cCrgl mice neonatally treated with ovarian steroids. Cancer Res 39: 2591
130. Jull JW (1956) Hormones as promoting agents in mammary carcinogenesis. Acta Un Intl Cancer (Louvain) 12: 653
131. Jull JW (1969) Mechanism of induction of ovarian tumors in the mouse by 7,12-dimethylbenz[a]anthracene. VI. Effect of normal ovarian tissue on tumor development. J Natl Cancer Inst 42: 967
132. Jull JW (1973) Ovarian tumorigenesis. Methods Cancer Res 7: 131
133. Jull JW, Jellink PH (1968) Mechanism of induction of ovarian tumors in the mouse by 7,12-dimethylbez[a]anthracene. IV. Uptake and retention of C^{14}-DMBA by mouse and rat tissues. J Natl Cancer Inst 40: 707
134. Jull JW, Russell A (1970) Mechanism of induction of ovarian tumors in the mouse by 7,12-dimethylbez[a]anthracene. VII. Relative activities of parent carcinogen and some of its metabolites. J Natl Cancer Inst 44: 841
135. Jull JW, Hawryluk A, Russell A (1968) Mechanism of induction of ovarian tumors in the mouse by 7,12-dimethylbenz[a]anthracene. III. Tumor induction in tissue culture. J Natl Cancer Inst 40: 687
136. Jurow HN (1943) Cyclic variations in the cervix of the guinea-pig. Am J Obstet Gynecol 45: 762
137. Kaminetzky HA (1966) Methylcholanthrene-induced cervical dysplasia and the sex steroids. Obstet Gynecol 27: 489
138. Kammerman S, Demopoulos RI, Ross J (1977) Gonadotropin receptors in experimentally induced ovarian tumors in mice. Cancer Res 37: 2578
139. Kaplan HS (1950) Influence of ovarian function on incidence of radiation-induced ovarian tumors in mice. J Natl Cancer Inst 11: 125
140. Kato T, Yakashigi M, Tsunawaki A, Ide K (1974) Studies on experimental ovarian tumors developed in rats receiving chemical carcinogen 9,10-dimethyl-1,2 benzanthracene. Kurume Med J 21: 11
141. Katsuse K, Kakudo K, Sakurai M, Kitamura H (1978) Experimental teratoid tumor after fetectomy in mice. Gann 69: 447
142. Kelly MG, O'Gara RW, Yancey ST, Botkin C (1958) Induction of tumors in rats with procarbazine hydrochloride. J Natl Cancer Inst 40: 1027
143. Kimura J (1978) Effect of progesterone on cell division in chemically induced endometrial hyperplasia and adenocarcinoma in mice. Cancer Res 38: 78
144. Kirkman H (1972) Hormone-related tumors in Syrian hamsters. Prog Exp Tumor Res 16: 201
145. Kirkman H, Algard FT (1970) Characteristics of an androgen/estrogen-induced uterine smooth muscle tumor of the Syrian hamster. Cancer Res 30: 794
146. Kojima A, Taguchi O, Nishizuka A (1980) Induced oophoritis and gastritis in nude mice: A new approach to the localized type of autoimmunity. In: Proceedings of the 3rd International Workshop on Nude Mice. Reed ND (ed), New York, Gustav Fischer
147. Kojima A, Taguchi O, Sakakura T, Nishizuka Y (1979) Prevalent types of tumors developing in neonatally thymectomized mice. Gann 70: 839
148. Kojima A, Yamashita K, Tsutsui K, Ishii S (1984) Development of "granulosa" cell tumors from intrasplenic testicular transplants in castrated NCI rats. Gann 75: 159
149. Koprowska I, Bogacz J, Pentikas C, Stypulkowski W (1958)

Induced cervical carcinoma of the mouse. A quantitative cytological method for evaluation of the neoplastic process. Cancer Res 18: 1186
150. Krarup T (1967) 9,10-Dimethyl-1,2-benzanthracene-induced ovarian tumours in mice. Acta Pathol Microbiol Scand 70: 241
151. Krarup T (1969) Oocyte destruction and ovarian tumorigenesis after direct applications of a chemical carcinogen (9,10-dimethyl-1,2-benzanthracene) to the mouse ovary. Int J Cancer 4: 61
152. Kullander S (1960) On tumor formation in gonadal and hypophyseal transplants into the anterior eye chambers of gonadectomised rats. Cancer Res 20: 1079
153. Kushima K, Noda K, Makita M (1967) Experimental production of chorionic tumor in rabbits. Tohuko J Exp Med 91: 209
154. Kuwahara I (1967) Experimental induction of ovarian tumors in mice treated with a single administration of 7,12-dimethylbenz[a]anthracene and its pathological observation. Gann 58: 253
155. Lagerlof N, Boyd H (1953) Ovarian hypoplasia and other abnormal conditions in the sexual organs of cattle of the Swedish Highland breed: Results of postmortem examination of over 6000 cows. Cornell Vet 43: 64
156. Lee S, Chandler JG, Broelsch CE, Ehara Y, Yen SS, Charters AC, Orloff MJ (1975) Intrasplenic ovarian neoplasm formation; direct measurement of FSH, LH, estrogens and progestins. Surg Forum 26: 149
157. Lee S, Condon JK, Chandler JG, Koopmans H, Ehara Y, Yen SS, Orloff MJ (1972) The effect of Eck fistula upon intrasplenic ovarian neoplasm formation. Surg Forum 23: 110
158. Li MH, Gardner WU (1949) Further studies on the pathogenesis of ovarian tumors in mice. Cancer Res 9: 35
159. Lick L, Kirschbaum A, Mixer H (1949) Mechanisms of induction of ovarian tumors by x-rays. Cancer Res 9: 532
160. Linder D, McCaw BK, Hecht F (1975) Parthenogenic origin of benign ovarian teratomas. N Engl J Med 292: 63
161. Lingeman CH (1974) Etiology of cancer of the human ovary: A review. J Natl Cancer Inst 53: 1603
162. Lipschutz A (1957) Steroid Homeostasis, Hypophysis and tumorigenesis. Cambridge, Heffer and Sons
163. Lipschutz A, Vargas L (1941) Structure and origin of uterine and extragenital fibroids induced experimentally in the guinea pig by prolonged administration of estrogens. Cancer Res 1: 236
164. Lipschutz A, Iglesias R, Panasevich VI (1966) Experimental conditions under which contraceptive steroids may become toxic. Nature 212: 686
165. Lipschutz A, Iglesias R, Panasevich VI, Salinas S (1967) Granulosa cell tumours induced in mice by progesterone. Br J Cancer 21: 144
166. Lipschutz A, Iglesias R, Panasevich VI, Salinas S (1967) Pathological changes induced in the uterus of mice with the prolonged administration of progesterone and 19-nor-contraceptives. Br J Cancer 21: 160
167. Lipschutz A, Iglesias R, Panasevich VI, Socorro S (1967) Ovarian tumours and other ovarian changes induced in mice by two 19-nor-contraceptives. Br J Cancer 21: 153
168. Lipschutz A, Iglesias R, Rojas G, Cerisola H (1959) Spontaneous tumorigenesis in aged guinea pigs. Br J Cancer 13: 486
169. London WT, Nahmias AJ, Naib ZM, Fucillo DA, Ellenberg JH, Sever JL (1974) A nonhuman primate model for the study of cervical oncogenic potential of herpes simplex virus type 2. Cancer Res 34: 1118
170. Lorenz E (1950) Some biologic effects of long continued radiation. AJR 63: 176
171. Malinin GI, Malinin IM (1972) Age-related spontaneous uterine lesions in mice. J Gerontol 27: 193
172. Marchant J (1957) The chemical induction of ovarian tumours in mice. Br J Cancer 11: 452
173. Marchant J (1959) Breast and ovarian tumours in F_1 C57B1 × IF hybrid mice after reciprocal exchange of ovaries between normal females and females pretreated with 9,10-dimethyl-1,2-benzanthracene. Acta Un Int Contr Cancrum 15: 196
174. Marchant J (1960) Personal observation
175. Mardones E, Iglesias R, Lipschutz A (1955) Granulosa cell tumours in intrasplenic ovarian grafts with intrahepatic metastases, in guinea pigs at five years after grafting. Br J Cancer 9: 409
176. Martin CB Jr, Misenhimer HR, Ramsey EM (1970) Ovarian tumors in rhesus monkeys (*Macaca mulatta*): Report of three cases. Lab Anim Sci 20: 686
177. Mattern J, Wayss K, Volm M (1984) Effect of five antineoplastic agents on tumor xenografts with different growth rates. J Natl Cancer Inst 72: 1335
178. Mattison DR, Thorgeirsson SS (1978) Smoking and industrial pollution and their effects on menopause and ovarian cancer. Lancet 1: 187
179. McClure HM, Graham CE (1973) Malignant uterine mesotheliomas in squirrel monkeys following diethylstilbestrol administration. Lab Anim Sci 23: 493
180. McEntee K, Nielson SW (1976) Tumours of the female genital tract. Bull WHO 53: 203
181. McLachlan JA (1979) Transplacental effects of diethylstilbestrol in mice. Natl Cancer Inst Monog 51: 67
182. Meier H, Myers DD, Fox RR, Laird CW (1970) Occurrence, pathological features, and propagation of gonadal teratomas in inbred mice and rabbits. Cancer Res 30: 30
183. Meisels A (1966) Effect of sex hormones on the carcinogenic action of dimethylbenzanthracene on the uterus of intact and castrated mice. Cancer Res 26: 757
184. Meissner WA, Sommers SC, Sherman G (1957) Endometrial hyperplasia, endometrial carcinoma and endometriosis produced experimentally by estrogen. Cancer 10: 500
185. Menczer J, Komarov H, Shenbaum M, Insler V, Czernobilsky B (1977) Attempted induction of granulosa cell tumors in BALB/c mice with gonadotropin administration. Gynecol Invest 8: 314
186. Merriam J, Easterday C, McKay DG, Hertig AT (1960) Experimental production of endometrial carcinoma in the rabbit. Obstet Gynecol 16: 253
187. Miller EC, Fletcher TL, Margreth A, Miller JA (1962) The carcinogenicities of derivatives of fluorene and bi-

phenyl:fluoro derivatives as probes for active sites in 2-acetylaminofluorene. Cancer Res 22: 1002
188. Miller OJ, Gardner WU (1954) The role of thyroid function and food intake in experimental ovarian tumorigenesis in mice. Cancer Res 14: 220
189. Miyamoto M (1971) Experimental induction of choriocarcinoma in rats. Gann 62: 55
190. Mody JK (1960) The action of four carcinogenic hydrocarbons on the ovaries of IF mice and the histogenesis of induced tumours. Br J Cancer 14: 256
191. Moon HD, Simpson ME, Li CH, Evans HM (1950) Neoplasms in rats and mice treated with pituitary growth hormone. III. Reproductive organs. Cancer Res 10: 549
192. Mori K (1964) Induction of pulmonary and uterine tumors in rats by subcutaneous injections of 4-nitroquinoline-1-oxide. Gann 55: 277
193. Mori T, Nagasawa H, Takahashi S (1981) The induction of adenomyosis in mice by intrauterine pituitary isografts. Life Sci 29: 1277
194. Morris HP, Velat CA, Wagner BP (1957) Carcinogenicity of some ingested acetylated mono- and diaminobiphenyl compounds in the rat. J Natl Cancer Inst 18: 101
195. Morris HP, Wagner BP, Ray FE, Stewart HL, Snell KC (1963) Carcinogen effects of N,N′-2,7-fluorenylenebis-2,2,2-trifluoroacetamide (2,7-FAA-F) administered orally to Buffalo strain rats. J Natl Cancer Inst 30: 143
196. Mossman HW (1973) The embryology of the cervix. In: The Biology of the Cervix. Blandau RJ, Moghissi K (eds). Chicago, University of Chicago Press, Chap 2
197. Muhlbock O (1953) Ovarian tumours in mice in parabiotic union. Acta Endocrinol (Copenh) 12: 105
198. Muhlbock O (1954) On the genesis of ovarian tumours. Experiments with mice in parabiotic union. Acta Un Int Cancr (Louvain) 10: 141
199. Munoz N (1973) Effect of herpesvirus type 2 and hormone imbalance on the uterine cervix of the mouse. Cancer Res 33: 1504
200. Murphy ED (1953) Studies on carcinogen-induced carcinoma of the cervix in mice. Am J Pathol 29: 608
201. Murphy ED (1961) Carcinogenesis of the uterine cervix in mice: Effect of diethylstilbestrol after limited application of 3-methylcholanthrene. J Natl Cancer Inst 27: 611
202. Murphy ED (1966) Characteristic tumors. In: Jackson Laboratory. Biology of the Laboratory Mouse, 2nd ed. Green EL (ed). New York, McGraw-Hill, Chap 27
203. Murphy ED (1972) Hyperplastic and early neoplastic changes in the ovaries of mice after genic deletion of germ cells. J Natl Cancer Inst 48: 1283
204. Murphy ED (1980) Major experimental models: Histogenesis and evaluation. In: Biology of Ovarian Neoplasia. UICC Technical Report Series, Murphy ED, Beamer WG (eds). Geneva, Union Internationale Contre le Cancer, Vol 50, p 6
205. Murphy ED, Beamer WG (1973) Plasma gonadotropin levels during early stages of ovarian tumorigenesis in mice of the W^x/W^v genotype. Cancer Res 33: 721
206. Murthy ASK, Russfield AB (1970) Endocrine changes in two strains of mice exposed to constant illumination. Endocrinology 86: 914
207. Napalkov NP, Alexandrov VA (1968) On the effects of blastomogenic substance on the organism during embryogenesis. Z Krebsforsch 71: 32
208. Napalkov NP, Anisimov VN (1979) Transplacental effect of diethylstilbestrol in female rats. Cancer Lett 6: 107
209. Nelson LW, Kelly WA, Weikel JH (1972) Mesovarial leiomyomas in rats in a chronic toxicity study of mesuprine hydrochloride. Toxicol Appl Pharmacol 23: 731
210. Nelson WO (1939) Atypical uterine growths produced by prolonged adminstration of estrogenic hormones. Endocrinology 24: 50
211. Nishizuka Y, Sakakura T (1971) Ovarian dysgenesis induced by neonatal thymectomy in the mouse. Endocrinology 89: 886
212. Nishizuka Y, Sakakura T (1971) Effect of combined removal of thymus and pituitary on post-natal ovarian follicular development in the mouse. Endocrinology 89: 902
213. Nishizuka Y, Sakakura T, Taguchi O (1979) Mechanism of ovarian tumorigenesis in mice after neonatal thymectomy. Natl Cancer Inst Monog 51: 89
214. Nishizuka Y, Tanaka Y, Sakakura T, Kojima A (1972) Frequent development of ovarian tumors from dysgenetic ovaries of neonatally thymectomised mice. Gann 63: 139
215. Noble RL, Hochachka BC, King D (1975) Spontaneous and estrogen-produced tumors in NB rats and their behavior after transplantation. Cancer Res 35: 766
216. Nomura T (1976) Comparison of tumour susceptibility among various organs of foetal, young and adult ICR/Jcl mice. Br J Cancer 33: 521
217. Nomura T (1973) Carcinogenesis by urethane via mother's milk and its enhancement of transplacental carcinogenesis in mice. Cancer Res 33: 1677
218. Nomura T, Okamoto E (1972) Transplacental carcinogenesis by urethane in mice; teratogenesis and carcinogenesis in relation to organogenesis. Gann 63: 731
219. Norris HJ, Gardner FM, Taylor HB (1969) Pathology of feline ovarian neoplasms. J Pathol 97: 138
220. Norris JH, Taylor HB, Gardner FM (1968) Equine ovarian granulosa tumours. Vet Rec 82: 419
221. Oakberg EF (1966) Effect of 25R of x-rays at 10 days of age on oocyte numbers and fertility of female mice. In: Radiation and Aging. Lindop PJ, Sacher GA (eds). London, Taylor and Francis, p 293
222. O'Shea JD, Jabara AG (1971) Proliferative lesions of serous membranes in ovariectomised female and entire male dogs after stilboestrol administration. Vet Pathol 8: 81
223. Palayoor T, Batra UK, Batra BK (1977) Radiation-induced pathogenesis in the progeny of x-irradiated female mice. Indian J Exp Biol 15: 163
224. Pan SC, Gardner WU (1948) Induction of malignant tumors by methycholanthrene in transplanted uterine cornua and cervixes of mice. Cancer Res 8: 337
225. Pantelouris EM (1973) Athymic development in the mouse. Differentiation 1: 437
226. Payne S (1958) The pathological effects of the intraperitoneal injection of 3,4-benzopyrene into rats and mice. Br J Cancer 12: 65
227. Peckham BM, Greene RR (1952) Experimentally produced granulosa cell tumors in rabbits. Cancer Res 12: 654
228. Peters H (1969) Effects of radiation in early life on the

morphology and reproductive function of the mouse ovary. Adv Reprod Physiol 4: 149

229. Pfeiffer CA (1949) Development of leiomyomas in female rats with an endocrine imbalance. Cancer Res 9: 277
230. Pfeiffer CA (1949) Adenocarcinoma in the uterus of an endocrine imbalance female rat. Cancer Res 9: 347
231. Pierson H (1934) Experimental production of uterine enlargement with cancer through ovarian hormones. Z Krebsforsch 41: 103
232. Reagen JW, Wentz BW, Hachicao N (1955) Induced cancer of the cervix uteri of the mouse. Arch Pathol 6: 451
233. Reboud S, Pageaut G (1973) Co-carcinogenic effect of progesterone on 20-methylcholanthrene-induced cervical carcinoma in mice. Nature 241: 398
234. Rehm S, Dierksen D, Deerberg F (1984) Spontaneous ovarian tumors in Han:NMR1 mice: Histologic classification, incidence and influence of food restriction. J Natl Cancer Inst 72: 1383
235. Reuber MD (1960) Endometrial sarcomas of the uterus and carcinosarcomas of the submaxillary salivary glands in castrated A × C strain female rats receiving N,N'-fluorenyldiacetamide and norethandrolone. J Natl Cancer Inst 25: 1141
236. Rogers JB, Blumenthal HT (1960) Studies of guinea pig tumors. I. Report of fourteen spontaneous guinea pigs tumors with a review of the literature. Cancer Res 20: 191
237. Rowe SE, Simmons JL, Ringler DH, Lay DM (1974) Spontaneous neoplasms in aging Gerbillinae. A summary of forty-four neoplasms. Vet Pathol 11: 38
238. Rubio CA, Lagerlof B (1974) Studies on the histogenesis of experimentally induced cervical carcinoma. Acta Pathol Microbiol Scand [A] 82: 153
239. Russell ES, Fekete E (1968) Analysis of W-series pleiotropism in the mouse: Effect of W^vW^v substitution on definitive germ cells and on ovarian tumorigenesis. J Natl Cancer Inst 21: 365
240. Rustia M (1979) Role of hormone imbalance in transplacental carcinogenesis in Syrian golden hamsters by sex hormones. Natl Cancer Inst Monog 51: 77
241. Sakashita S, Tsukada Y, Nakamura K, Tsuji I, Hirai H (1977) Experimental yolk sac tumors produced by fetectomy without virus infection in rats. Int J Cancer 20: 83
242. Sawada M, Matsui Y, Okudaira Y (1983) Effect of human lymphoblastoma interferon on human yolk sac tumors in nude mice. Biken J 26: 169
243. Sawada M, Matsui Y, Hayakawa K, Nishiura H, Okudaira Y, Taki L (1982) Human gynecologic cancers hetero transplanted into athymic nude rats. Gynecol Oncol 13: 220
244. Scarpelli DG, Haam E von (1955) Experimental carcinoma of the cervix: A comparative cytologic and histologic study. Cancer Res 15: 449
245. Scarpelli DG, Haam E von (1957) Experimental carcinoma of the cervix in the mouse. Am J Pathol 33: 1059
246. Schoental R (1968) Pathologic lesions, including tumors, in rats after 4,4'-diaminodiphenylmethane and alpha-butyrolactone. Isr J Med Sci 4: 1146
247. Schoental R (1969) Carcinogenic action of elaiomycin in rats. Nature 221: 765
248. Seibold HR, Wolf RH (1973) Neoplasms and proliferative lesions in 1065 nonhuman primate necropsies. Lab Anim Sci 23: 53
249. Sekiya S, Takamizawa H, Wang F, Takane T, Kuwata T (1972) In vivo and in vitro studies on uterine adenocarcinoma of the rat induced by 7,12-dimethlybenz[a]anthracene. Am J Obstet Gynecol 111: 691
250. Sekiya S, Kikuchi Y, Katoh T, Kobavashi W, Takeda B, Takamizawa H (1979) Effect of ovariectomy, adrenalectomy, and hypophysectomy on carcinogenesis of the endometrium by 7,12-dimethlybenz[a]anthracene in rats. Gynecol Oncol 7: 281
251. Sekiya S, Endoh N, Kikuchi Y, Katoh T, Matsura A, Iwasawa H, Takeda B, Takamizawa H (1979) In vivo and in vitro studies of experimental ovarian adenocarcinoma in rats. Cancer Res 39: 1108
252. Sever JL (1973) Herpes virus and cervical cancer studies in experimental animals. Cancer Res 33: 1509
253. Shen CN (1971) Experimental induction of placental tumor in the guinea pig. Nagoya Med J 17: 33
254. Shintani S, Glass LE, Page EW (1966) Studies of induced malignant tumors of placental and uterine origin in the rat. II. Induced tumors and their pathogenesis with special reference to choriocarcinoma. Am J Obstet Gynecol 95: 550
255. Shintani S, Glass LE, Page EW (1966) Studies of induced malignant tumors of placental and uterine origin in the rat. III. Identification of experimentally induced choriocarcinoma by detection of placenta hormone. Am J Obstet Gynecol 95: 559
256. Shisa H, Nishizuka Y (1968) Unilateral development of ovarian tumor in thymectomized Swiss mice following a single injection of 7,12-dimethlybenz[a]anthracene at neonatal stage. Br J Cancer 22: 70
257. Shulze F (1960) Spontantumoren der Schadelhohle und Genitalorgane bei Sprague-Dawley und Bethesda-black Ratten. Z Krebsforsch 64: 78
258. Singh KB (1969) Induction of polycystic ovarian disease in rats by continuous light. I. The reproductive cycle, organ weights and histology of the ovaries. Am J Obstet Gynecol 103: 1078
259. Skreb N, Svajger A, Levak-Svajger B (1971) Growth and differentiation of rat egg cylinders under the kidney capsule. J Embryol Exp Morphol 25: 47
260. Slye M, Holmes MF, Wells HG (1920) Primary spontaneous tumors of the ovary in mice. J Cancer Res 5: 205
261. Snell K (1925) Spontaneous lesions of the rat. In: The Pathology of Laboratory Animals. Ribelin WE, McCoy JP (eds). Springfield, Ill, Charles C Thomas, p 241
262. Sobis H, Vandeputte M (1975) Sequential morphological study of teratomas derived from displaced yolk sac. Dev Biol 45: 276
263. Solter D, Sreb N, Damjanov I (1970) Extrauterine growth of mouse egg-cyclinders results in malignant teratoma. Nature 227: 503
264. Sommers SC, Meissner WA (1957) Host relationship in experimental endometrial carcinoma. Cancer 10: 510
265. Staats J (1964) Standardised nomenclature for inbred strains of mice. Third listing. Cancer Res 24: 147
266. Steel GG, Courtenay VD, Roston AY (1978) Improved

immunosuppression techniques for the xenografting of human tumors. Br J Cancer 37: 224
267. Stein-Werblowsky R (1960) Induction of a choriocarcinoma in the rat. Nature 186: 980
268. Stein-Werblowsky R (1960) Induction of cancer in the cervix uteri in relation to the oestrus cycle. Br J Cancer 14: 300
269. Stein-Werblowsky R (1977) The induction of precancerous changes in the uterine epithelium of the rat: The role of spermatozoa. Gynecol Oncol 5: 251
270. Stevens LC (1980) The origin and development of ovarian teratomas in mice. In: Biology of Ovarian Neoplasia. UICC Technical Report Series, Geneva, UICC, Vol 50, p 74
271. Stevens LC, Varnum DS (1974) The development of teratomas from parthenogenetically activated ovarian mouse eggs. Dev Biol 37: 369
272. Strong LC, Gardner WU, Hill RT (1937) Production of estrogenic hormone by a transplantable ovarian carcinoma. Endocrinology 21: 268
273. Suntzeff V, Burns EL, Moskop M, Loeb L (1938) On proliferative changes taking place in the epithelium of vagina and cervix of mice with advancing age and under influence of experimentally administered estrogenic hormones. Am J Cancer 32: 256
274. Symeonidis A (1954) Tumors induced by 2-acetylaminofluorene in virgin and breeding females of five strains of rats and their offspring. J Natl Cancer Inst 15: 539
275. Takamizawa H, Wong K (1973) Effect of anticancer drugs on uterine carcinogenesis. Obstet Gynecol 41: 701
276. Taki I, Iijima H (1963) A new method of producing endometrial cancer in mice. Am J Obstet Gynecol 87: 926
277. Tannenbaum A, Vessilinovitch SD, Maltoni C, Mitchell DS (1962) Multipotential carcinogenicity of urethan in the Sprague-Dawley rat. Cancer Res 22: 1362
278. Teutscher R (1959) Ein Plattenepithelkrebs der Schamlippe der Stute. Deutsch Tierarztl Wachenschr 66: 567
279. Thiery M (1936) Ovarian teratoma in the mouse. Br J Cancer 17: 231
280. Thorpe P, Isaac P (1977) Long-term use of bromocriptine. Med J Aust 2: 721
281. Tokita H, Tanaka N, Sekimoto K, Heno T, Okamoto K, Fugimura S (1980) Experimental model for combination chemotherapy with metronidazole using human uterine cervical carcinomas transplanted into nude mice. Cancer Res 40: 4287
282. Tomatis L (1979) Prenatal exposure to chemical carcinogens and its effect on subsequent generations. Natl Cancer Inst Monog 51: 159
283. Tsutae K, Saito T, Hura I, Abe N, Shinoda M, Miyashita I, Nomura Y, Shirota K, Saito Y (1982) Primary ovarian tumors in swine. Bull Azabu Univ Vet Med 3: 147
284. Turusov VS, Bazlova LS, Lanko NS (1977) Nonepithelial uterine tumours induced in CBA mice by 1,2-dimethylhydrazine. Cancer Lett 3: 37
285. Uematsu K, Huggins CB (1968) Induction of leukaemia and ovarian tumors in mice by pulse-doses of aromatic hydrocarbons. Mol Pharmacol 4: 427
286. Urich RL (1984) Tumor induction in BALB/c mice after fractionated or protracted exposure to fission-spectrum neutrons. Radiat Res 97: 587
287. Upton AC, Kimball AW, Furth J, Christenberry KW, Benedict WH (1960) Some delayed effects of atom-bomb radiations in mice. Cancer Res 20(8) 1
288. Vandeputte M, Eyssen H, Sobis H, DeSomer P (1974) Induction of polyoma tumors in athymic nude mice. Cancer 14: 445
289. Vandeputte M, Sobis H, Billiau A, van de Maele B, Leyter R (1973) In utero tumor induction by murine sarcoma virus (Moloney) in the rat. I. Biological characteristics. Int J Cancer 11: 536
290. Van Nie R, Smit GMJ, Muhlbock O (1962) The induction of uterine tumors in mice treated with testosterone. Acta Un Contr Cancr 18: 194
291. Vellios F, Griffin J (1955) The pathogenesis of dimethylbenz[a]-anthracene-induced carcinoma of the cervix in rats. Cancer Res 17: 364
292. Vesselinovich SD, Rao KUN, Mihailovich N (1979) Neoplastic response of mouse tissues during perinatal age periods and its significance in chemical carcinogenesis. Natl Cancer Inst Monog 51: 239
293. Vesselinovich SD, Mihailovich N, Rao KV, Itze L (1971) Perinatal carcinogenesis by urethane. Cancer Res 31: 2143
294. Vink HH (1970) Ovarian teratomas in guinea pigs: A report of ten cases. J Pathol 102: 180
295. Walker BE (1984) Tumors of female offspring of mice exposed prenatally to diethylstilbestrol. J Natl Cancer Inst 73: 133
296. Ward BC, Moore W Jr (1969) Spontaneous lesions in a colony of Chinese hamsters, *Cricetulus griseus*. Lab Anim Sci 19: 516
297. Warren S, Gates O (1941) Spontaneous and induced tumors of the guinea pig. Cancer Res 1: 65
298. Weisbroth SH (1974) Neoplastic diseases. In: The Biology of the Laboratory Rabbit. Weisbroth SH, Flatt RE, Kraus AL (eds). New York, Academic Press, p 331
299. Willis RA (1962) Ovarian teratomas in guinea pigs. J Pathol Bacteriol 84: 237
300. Yeh SDJ, Woo SK (1980) Gallium uptake in heterotransplanted human choriocarcinoma and ovarian carcinoma in nude mice. Proc Soc Exp Biol Med 165: 361
301. Yong HY, Campbell JS (1965) Evolution of dysplasia of the uterine cervix and vagina induced by low dosages of carcinogen in mice. Obstet Gynecol 26: 91
302. Zaino RJ, Satyaswaroop PG, Mortel R (1984) Morphology of human uterine cancer in nude mice. Effects of hormone and antihormone treatment. Arch Pathol Lab Med 108: 571

27

Gross Description, Processing, and Reporting of Gynecologic and Obstetric Specimens

Stanley J. Robboy, M.D., Frederick T. Kraus, M.D., and Robert J. Kurman, M.D.

The surgical pathology report provides the histopathologic diagnosis and specific information relating to prognosis and treatment. Accordingly, the surgical pathologist must have sufficient familiarity with the management of gynecologic and obstetric disorders that clinically relevant information is the focus of the report. This chapter provides an approach to the processing of gynecologic and obstetric tissue specimens. The techniques of the gross examination and the method of reporting the pathologic findings are guided by the clinical principles on which patient management is based.

The types of gynecologic tissue specimens that are submitted to the surgical pathology laboratory can be divided into two categories: (1) biopsy specimens and (2) therapeutic resections. Obstetric tissue specimens include placentas and sometimes uterine curettings. Although some biopsies are therapeutic, the main purpose of the biopsy is to provide a histologic diagnosis that will guide management. Biopsy specimens should, therefore, be processed expeditiously. The gross description must be precise and brief. There should be correlation between the microscopic tissue section and the gross specimen with regard to the number of specimens and the approximate size of each or aggregate size of the total. This is especially important when it appears that a slide or block may have been mislabeled. Two examples of appropriate description are "3 ovoid fragments 2 to 4 mm in diameter" and "multiple shreds of tissue 5 cm in aggregate diameter."

For operative specimens, particularly those containing a tumor, information in the surgical pathology report should include a description of the extent of the tumor and specific features that are related to prognosis. The adequacy of the surgical treatment as well as the need for additional therapy depend on these findings. Since the gynecologic surgeon has seen the pathology in vivo, it is important that he communicate the operative findings, since these will bear directly on how the pathologist processes the specimen. For example, adequacy of resection margins requires an appreciation of the orientation of the specimen to certain anatomic landmarks that are obvious to the surgeon but cannot always be reconstructed by the pathologist in the laboratory.

The gross description and final diagnosis must be clearly written. A good gross description enables the reader to reconstruct an image that corresponds to the specimen and its lesion. Since the histologic diagnosis for many tumors has been made previously by a biopsy, the gross description of an operative specimen should focus on the size and extent of the lesion and its relationship to adjacent structures. In this sense the gross description is analogous to the provisional anatomic diagnosis of a postmortem examination in which the microscopic examination confirms the gross anatomic findings. It should be uncommon to have significant findings discovered unexpectedly on the microscopic examination. A careful gross examination and description is mandatory to ensure that the appropriate microscopic sections are obtained.

The final diagnosis of a tumor should include the cell type, grade, location, extent, adequacy of the resection margins, presence of lymphatic or vascular invasion, and status of the regional lymph nodes. It is one thing to report a "squamous cell carcinoma of the cervix" but far better to add that "It is a small cell type with extensive lymphatic invasion, penetration of tumor to within 0.2 mm of the margin of a 1.0 cm thick uterine wall, and 6 of 24 lymph nodes contain tumor." The former merely reaffirms what was known before the operation, whereas the latter presents information that helps to predict prognosis and plan further treatment.

General Procedures

Gross Description

Specimens received in the fresh state should be described before fixation, since formalin alters the natural color and consistency of tissue. The opening sentence of the gross description should be a statement of whether the tissue is fresh or fixed and how it is labeled. Note whether the specimen received corresponds with how it is labeled. For example, "Received fresh is a specimen labeled 'uterus, tubes, and ovaries,' however, only the uterus and right ovary and tube are identified." State the overall measurements and weight of the entire specimen as well as the individual components.

The gross description should proceed in an organized fashion, with the focus on the primary lesion. For example, in a radical hysterectomy, describe the cervical cancer before describing the normal ovaries, incidental appendectomy, and multiple lymph nodes. Emphasize the pathology and avoid elaborate descriptions of incidental organs, for example, a normal incidental appendix can be described as "5 cm long" and "normal" rather than as a "5 cm long, 4 mm in diameter, vermiform appendix with a tan, unremarkable serosa, a 1 mm thick wall, and a lumen without identifiable abnormality." The gross description should conclude with a statement of whether all of the tissue has been processed for microscopic examination or whether tissue remains.

Drawings

The description of a specimen with complicated relationships may be simplified by including a drawing as part of the surgical pathology report. This permits orientation of the tumor to the remainder of the specimen, especially surgical resection margins, and visual identification of section codes.

Section Codes

A key at end of the gross description is more clearly seen than a key included in the text of the gross description. Blocks are labeled consecutively in alphabetical order. After Z, proceed to AA. After AZ, proceed to BA and continue in this way.

Formalin Fixation

Neutral buffered formalin is generally the most practical and commonly used fixative. A specimen to be submitted for microscopic examination should be cut into blocks no more than 3 mm in thickness. Thicker specimens will autolyze at the center. It is much easier and efficient to cut blocks from tissue that have been fixed for several hours instead of attempting to cut 3 mm blocks directly from the fresh specimen. Large specimens should be bread-loafed or alternatively cut into slabs, 5–7 mm in thickness, to permit adequate penetration by formalin and then trimmed to 3 mm blocks after 2–3 hours of fixation. Frequently, fixation of only parts of the specimen may be desirable, allowing preservation of a semi-intact specimen for gross teaching.

Other Types of Fixatives

Bouin's fixative provides superior cellular detail and is practical for the fixation of biopsies and curettings. Endometrial biopsies should be fixed in Bouin's fixative because most of the relevant literature on dating is based on this technique. It can be used for large specimens as well, but its slow penetration requires more meticulous handling and is, therefore, more time consuming. Consequently, Bouin's fixative is less practical than formalin.

Although not always feasible in a busy surgical pathology laboratory, it is useful to fix some tissue from all tumors in glutaraldehyde for possible electron microscopic examination. A portion of the tumor should be snap frozen for immunocytochemical analysis, since some antibodies do not bind to antigens that have been altered by formalin fixation, for example, monoclonal antibodies to estrogen receptor protein and immunoglobulin antibodies to lymphomas.

Specific Procedures

Biopsies and Curettings

Vulvar Biopsy

Excisional biopsies should be handled like skin biopsies. Resection margins, deep as well as lateral, can be marked with India ink to facilitate their recognition on microscopic examination. Sections should be perpendicular to the surface and should be obtained from the longitudinal axis and perpendicular to it across the shorter axis. In a complicated specimen that the surgeon has oriented carefully, multiple colors of ink can be used to locate specific surfaces.

Smaller punch biopsies are submitted totally. To assist the histotechnologist in orienting the specimen correctly, bisect the specimen, cutting it perpendicular to the mucosal surface, and mark the cut surface with mercurochrome. Instruct the histotechnologist to embed the specimen with the mercurochrome-marked surface facing up. It is often useful to request at the time of submission that the paraffin block be cut at multiple levels. This shortens the turnaround time, since small biopsies frequently are not adequately sectioned the first time they are cut. Remounting the block and cutting again takes more time then obtaining multiple levels at the outset.

Vaginal Biopsy

Most vaginal biopsies are small punch biopsies and should be handled similar to vulvar punch biopsies.

Cervical Punch Biopsy

Colposcopically directed punch biopsies should be handled in the same manner as small vulvar and vaginal biopsies. A technique to facilitate orientation is to sandwich the biopsy specimen between blue Gelfoam sponges that fit into the cassette. Another effective technique is to have the gynecologist place the biopsy on its side on a piece of paper towel and then place the specimen and attached paper into fixative (Fig. 27.1). The paper must be removed by the surgical pathologist before processing.

Endocervical Curettings

The endocervical curettage is performed either to evaluate the presence of cervical neoplasia in the endocervical canal or to determine whether endometrial carcinoma has spread into the cervix. Clinical management depends on the presence or absence of disease in the curettings, and, therefore, considerable care must be exercised in handling these specimens, which are typically scant and composed mostly of blood and mucus.

The specimen should be transferred directly from the curette by the gynecologist to a Telfa pad. Sponges should be avoided, since tissue becomes enmeshed in the sponge and is difficult to retrieve. After the curettage is completed, the curette can be passed through the fixative to dislodge small fragments of tissue that otherwise might remain adherent to the curette. In the laboratory, the entire specimen should be wrapped in filter paper or a tea bag before placing it into a cassette to avoid losing small fragments of tissue during processing.

Cervical Cone Biopsy

This procedure can be either diagnostic or therapeutic. In either case, besides the microscopic diagnosis, it is essential to determine whether the surgical resection margins, especially the endocervical margin, are free of the neoplastic process.

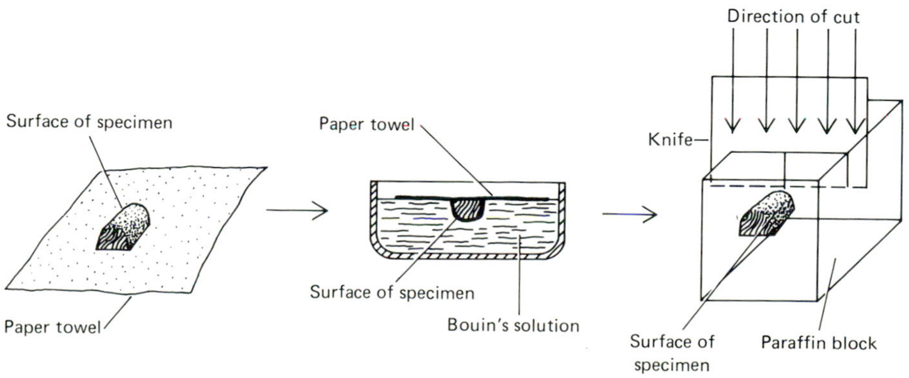

FIG. 27.1. Orientation, fixation, and microtome sectioning of a cervical punch biopsy. (Courtesy of Alex M. Ferenczy, M.D.)

The gynecologist should remove the cone biopsy intact. If a laser is used, the endocervical margin should be resected with scissors in order that the tissue at this crucial site can be evaluated microscopically in the absence of vaporization artifact. Another method to assess the endocervical margin is to amputate the endocervical margin and send it as a separate specimen labeled "apical margin." A suture, conventionally placed through the cervical stroma at 12 o'clock, is useful to orient the specimen. Avoid manipulation of the surface epithelium, since it is easily denuded. The specimen, wrapped in saline-soaked gauze, should be transported immediately to the surgical pathology laboratory.

The surgical pathologist can limit the gross description to the measurements of the specimen and any obvious lesion. The endocervical margin is marked with India ink, opened at 12 o'clock, and pinned on a corkboard with the mucosa facing up (Fig. 27.2). Intraepithelial neoplasia of the cervix is usually found on the anterior and posterior aspects of the cervix of the region of the squamocolumnar junction. Since it may be difficult to obtain optimally oriented specimens once the cone biopsy is opened, Schmidt[5] recommends opening the specimen at 3 o'clock, where lesions are less frequently encountered. The pins should not pass through the epithelium. Three hours of fixation before cutting is adequate. The specimen should be sectioned serially at 1–3 mm intervals. Each block should be marked with mercurochrome or eosin to orient embedding. Serially cut blocks should be submitted in separate cassettes numbered consecutively. When there are many blocks, it is often more convenient and economical to place two blocks in each cassette.

Endometrial Biopsy and Curettings

All tissues should be submitted from diagnostic procedures, whereas selected samples should be submitted from therapeutic procedures in which a large volume of tissue is received. In general, one cassette for every 5 g of tissue is adequate. Endometrial biopsies and diagnostic curettings should be processed in the same manner as endocervical curettings. The gross description should include a measurement of the aggregate specimen. The specimen should be wrapped in fine filter paper or a tea bag and submitted in its entirety. For therapeutic abortions, evaluate the completeness of removal of the fetus and placenta when possible. Single small samples of fetal parts and placenta should suffice for sectioning. In cases of saline abortion, where a fetus or fetal parts can be identified grossly, microscopic sampling of the specimen is not necessary if there is no gross abnormality. For spontaneous abortions, attempt to find the fetus or chorionic tissues, since their presence confirms that the chorionic sac is passed intact. Note the length and configuration of the fetus if present. Initially, blood clot need not be sampled. If microscopic examination does not reveal villi, only then should additional tissue be processed. In the appropriate clinical setting, for example, habitual abortion or previous newborn with multiple congenital malformations, some tissue should be transported to a cytogenetics laboratory in the appropriate transfer medium (see section on placental examination).

Curettings from a hydatidiform mole come in two parts: (1) the suction curettage and (2) the sharp curettage. The former should be carefully examined for the presence of fetal parts and areas of necrosis. Tissue from the sharp curettage should be processed entirely, since it must be evaluated for the presence of myometrial invasion.

Ovarian Biopsy

Biopsies of the ovary are diagnostic, since wedge resection for the treatment of polycystic ovarian disease is now rarely performed. A biopsy of a normal-appearing ovary may be submitted for frozen section interpretation when unilateral salpingo-oophorectomy is contemplated as definitive therapy in a child or young woman with an ovarian neoplasm. After the specimen has been measured and any obvious abnormality described, the biopsy should be sectioned into smaller pieces and submitted entirely.

Large Operative Specimens

Vulva

Superficial Vulvectomy. Most specimens are variable in their composition, since the procedure is tailored to the extent of the lesion. Generally, the operative specimen includes the labia minora, labia majora, clitoris, perineal body, and perianal tissue without subcutaneous fat. The procedure is performed for widespread, multifocal, intraepithelial lesions, for example, carcinoma in situ, and therefore only the epithelium, devoid of underlying subcutaneous tissue, is removed.

The gross description should specify the features and extent of the lesion as well as the anatomic structures involved. Since intraepithelial lesions are subtle, careful attention must be paid to coloration and surface texture. The lesions are typically red, brown, or white and are often roughened. They should be measured, and distances from the lesion to the resection margin should be recorded.

Because the disease process is multicentric and difficult to discern with the naked eye, all surgical resection margins must be examined microscopically. This requires sections through all obvious lesions to rule out invasive carcinoma and sections from all the lateral resection mar-

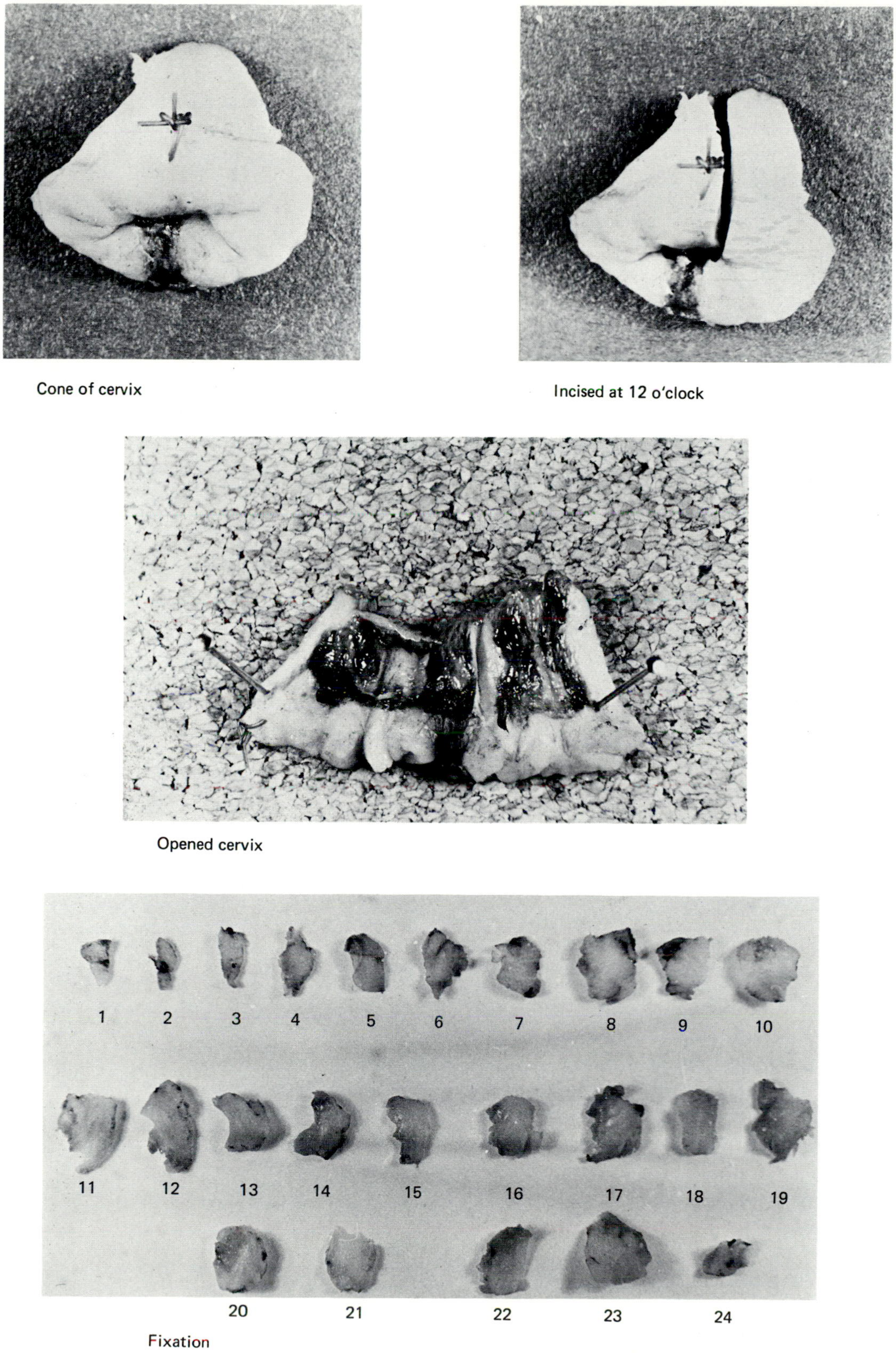

FIG. 27.2. Method of sectioning a cone biopsy of the cervix. In this case the specimen has been opened at 12 o'clock.

gins. Sections parallel to the surgical margins are often taken to completely evaluate the excision lines, a method which uses fewer sections than those taken perpendicular to the line of resection. Multiple perpendicular sections, however, have the advantage that the central lesion, margin, and intervening areas can be included in one slide. To facilitate sectioning, pin the specimen on a corkboard or a block of paraffin and fix for 2–3 hours before sectioning.

The surgical pathology report should include microscopic diagnosis, extent of the involvement, and adequacy of the surgical resection margins.

Total Vulvectomy. The specimen includes the entire vulva and subcutaneous fat, since the surgical dissection is carried down to the deep fascia. This procedure is usually performed for extramammary Paget's disease.

The gross description is similar to that outlined for the superficial vulvectomy. Although Paget's disease of the vulva is usually also an intraepithelial lesion, it may be associated with an underlying sweat gland carcinoma, and, therefore, the underlying subcutaneous tissue is removed. The specimen should be pinned, fixed, and then sectioned at approximately 0.5 cm intervals in order to evaluate the underlying dermis adequately for an associated sweat gland carcinoma. Typically, microscopic involvement of Paget's disease exceeds laterally the visible extent of the lesion on gross examination. Occult foci of Paget's disease may also be present within normal-appearing skin, and consequently deep and lateral resection margins must be thoroughly evaluated in a similar manner as that described for the superficial vulvectomy specimen.

The surgical pathology report should include the microscopic diagnosis, extent of involvement, adequacy of the resection margins, and whether an underlying sweat gland carcinoma is present.

Radical Vulvectomy. The specimen consists of the vulva, inguinal skin, subcutaneous tissue, femoral and inguinal lymph nodes, and portions of the saphenous veins. The procedure is performed for invasive squamous carcinoma.

The gross description should include the size, location, and depth of penetration of the primary lesion, as well as the status of the circumferential skin, deep clitoral stumps, and perirectal and vaginal margins of resection. After the gross description, the specimen can be dissected fresh or pinned, fixed, and then sectioned. Sections should include the primary site, showing the depth of invasion, sections of the labium majora and minora, appropriate resection margins, the clitoris, the vaginal margin, and all the inguinal lymph nodes. Separation of lymph nodes into superficial and deep groups requires communication with the gynecologic surgeon. Invasive vulvar neoplasms, in contrast to intraepithelial lesions, tend to be solitary, and, consequently, evaluation of resection margins can be limited to the margins near the tumor. Because the specimen contains a considerable amount of fatty tissue, identification of lymph nodes may be difficult. In the fresh state, lymph nodes are recognized by palpation. Alternatively, xerography[4] (Fig. 27.3) or Bouin's fixation may assist in locating lymph nodes.

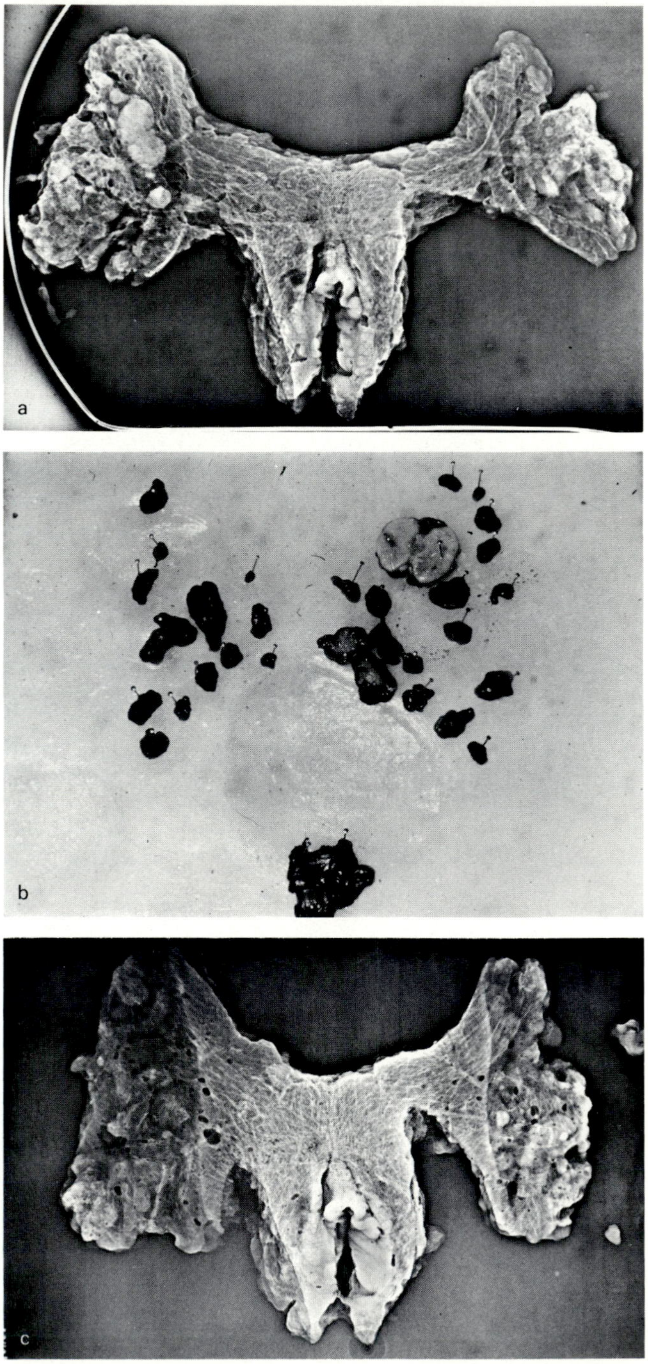

Fig. 27.3.*a*. Xerogram of radical vulvectomy specimen before dissection. Nodes can be clearly seen. *b*. Lymph nodes dissected from specimen. *c*. Xerogram of postdissection specimen. (Courtesy of J. Milbrath, M.D., and Edward J. Wilkinson, M.D., University of Florida.)

The fatty tissue should be bread loafed at 1–2 cm intervals to allow adequate penetration of the fixation. After a few hours in Bouin's fixation, fat remains yellow but lymph nodes appear white. Location of lymph nodes is facilitated by an understanding of the lymphatic drainage of the vulva (Fig. 27.4).

The surgical pathology report should include the microscopic diagnosis, tumor grade, dimensions, location and maximum depth of invasion, presence of lymphatic invasion, and the number and location of the involved lymph nodes.

Vagina

Vaginectomy and Pelvic Exenteration. The vaginectomy specimen consists of the vagina as well as the cervix and uterus, since the procedure is an en bloc resection for invasive carcinoma of the vagina. Depending on the location and extent of the tumor, the urinary bladder and rectum may also be removed. The procedure is termed an *anterior exenteration* if the urinary bladder is included and a *posterior exenteration* if the rectum is included. Pelvic exenteration is infrequently performed today. The most common indication is for a central recurrence of a cervical carcinoma.

The vagina should be opened longitudinally opposite from the tumor. The total length of the vagina is measured, and the distances between the tumor, the cervix, and the resection margins are recorded. The tumor mass should be described and measured and the maximum depth of invasion noted. The extent of involvement should be described, in particular, the relationship of the tumor to the cervix and the urinary bladder or rectum if the latter organs have been removed. In order to evaluate these features, the rectum and bladder must be opened, the specimen fixed, and sections taken perpendicular to the mucosa directly overlying the tumor in the vagina. A good method, which provides excellent orientation of the tumor to adjacent structures for exenteration specimens, is to inflate the urinary bladder and rectum with formalin and fix the specimen for several hours. The entire specimen can then be hemisected through the neoplasm, and the appropriate sections can be obtained (Fig. 27.5). Sections from the surgical resection margins and any lymph nodes identified in the attached soft tissue should be obtained. India ink marking of all resection margins and a diagram describing the specimen, tumor, and the section code is useful for orientation and correlation of the microscopic sections and the gross findings.

The surgical pathology report should include the microscopic diagnosis, tumor grade, dimensions, location and relationship to adjacent structures, presence of lymphatic invasion, number of involved lymph nodes, and adequacy of the surgical resection margins.

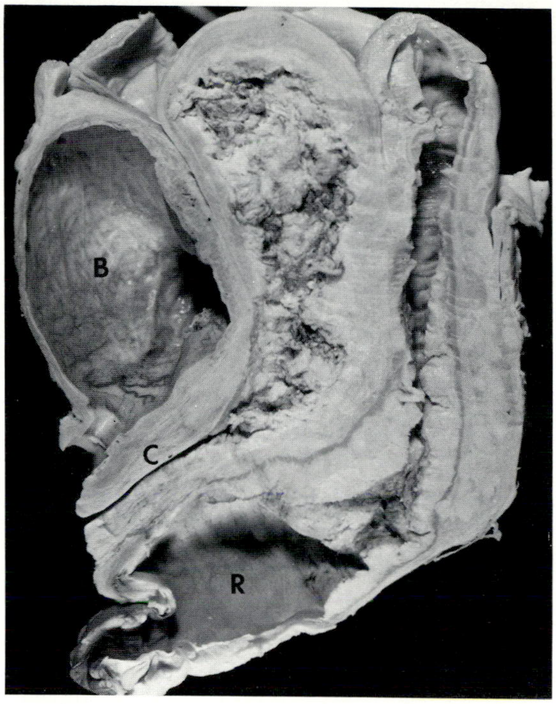

FIG. 27.5. Hemisection of bladder (B), uterus with cervix (C), rectum (R), and sigmoid colon. (Courtesy of Dennis O'Connor, M.D., Georgetown University, Washington, D.C.)

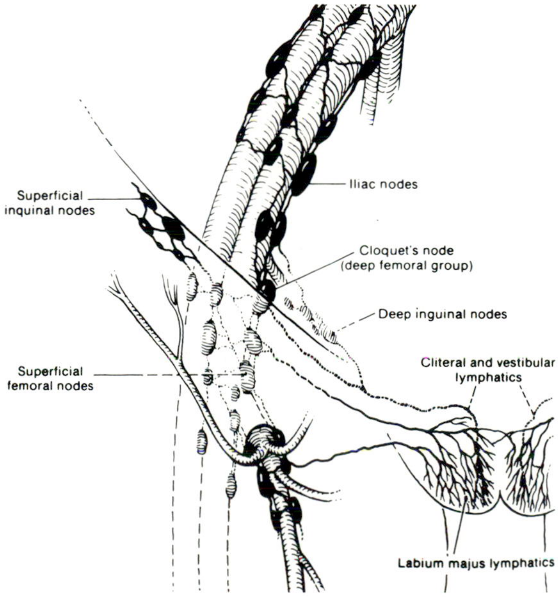

FIG. 27.4. Lymphatics of the vulva. (Reprinted with permission of Schmidt, Ref 5.)

Cervix and Uterus

Total Hysterectomy. The total hysterectomy specimen consists of the cervix and the uterine corpus. Supracervical hysterectomy in which the uterus is amputated at the internal cervical os is now rarely performed. Removal of the cervix and uterus is treatment for a variety of benign and malignant diseases. Because of the diverse nature of the disease processes for which a hysterectomy is performed, the approach to processing the specimen as well as the hysterectomy procedure itself vary accordingly. The different pathologic techniques used are, therefore, considered according to the surgical indication.

Hysterectomy for Benign Functional Uterine Disease. Included in this category are hysterectomies for persistent abnormal bleeding, uterine prolapse, or intractable pelvic pain. The last may sometimes be due to unrecognized organic causes, such as adenomyosis or endometriosis, that are only recognized after thorough pathologic examination.

Begin the description by listing the specimens received, including whether the cervix or adnexae are attached or separate. The specimen is oriented (Fig. 27.6) by identifying the round ligaments that insert anterior to the fallopian tubes. In addition, on the posterior surface of the uterus, the peritoneum covers a larger area and extends farther down toward the cervix than anteriorly, where it is reflected high over the bladder (Fig. 27.7). The specimen should then be weighed after the adnexae have been removed. The parous uterus is heavier (premenopausal adult 75–100 g) than the nulliparous uterus (premenopausal adult 30–40g), and weight increases with increasing parity. After eight pregnancies a weight of 240 g is normal.[3] The postmenopausal uterus, because of the diminished amount of muscle, weighs 20–40 g. The following measurements should then be taken: (1) top of the fundus to the exocervix (premenopausal adult 5–8 cm), (2) cornu to cornu (premenopausal adult 3–5 cm), (3) thickness from anterior to posterior surface (premenopausal adult 2–4 cm), (4) length and diameter of the cervix (premenopausal adult 3 cm each), and (5) sounding depth from the external os to the inside of the top of the fundus (premenopausal adult 7–8 cm). The last measurement is important in the staging of endometrial cancer.

The outer surface of the uterus should be examined and described. The posterior surface of the uterine serosa

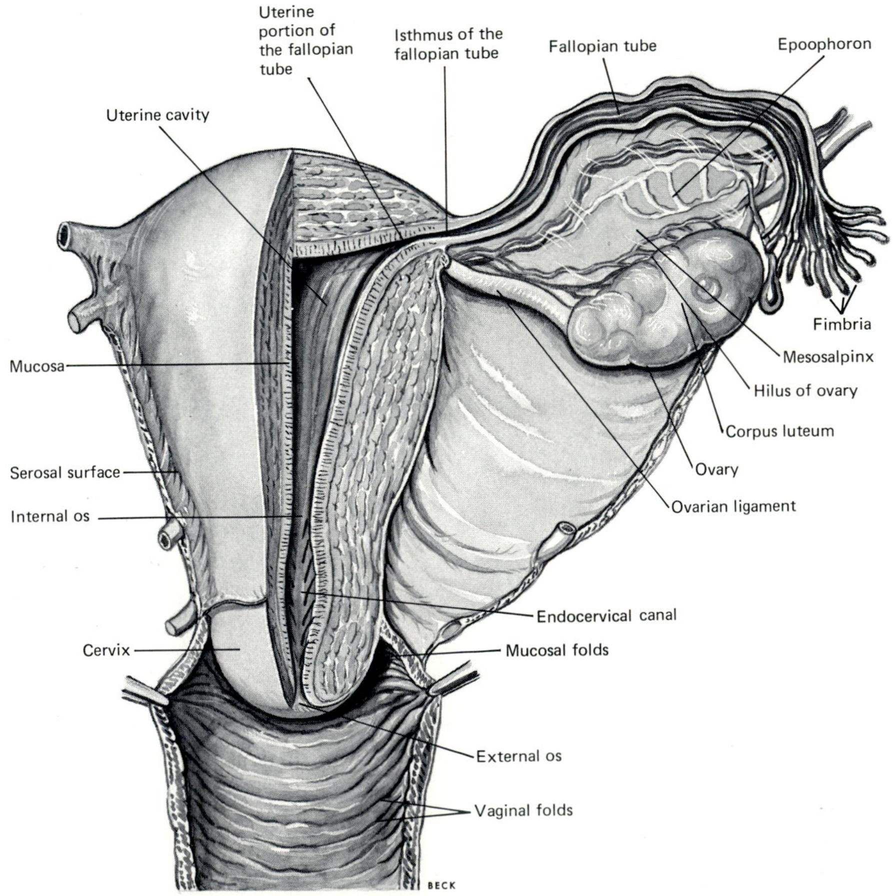

FIG. 27.6. The uterus, vagina and adnexa. [Modified from Gray's Anatomy, 30th ed. (C.D. Clemente, ed.), 1985. Courtesy of Lea & Febiger.]

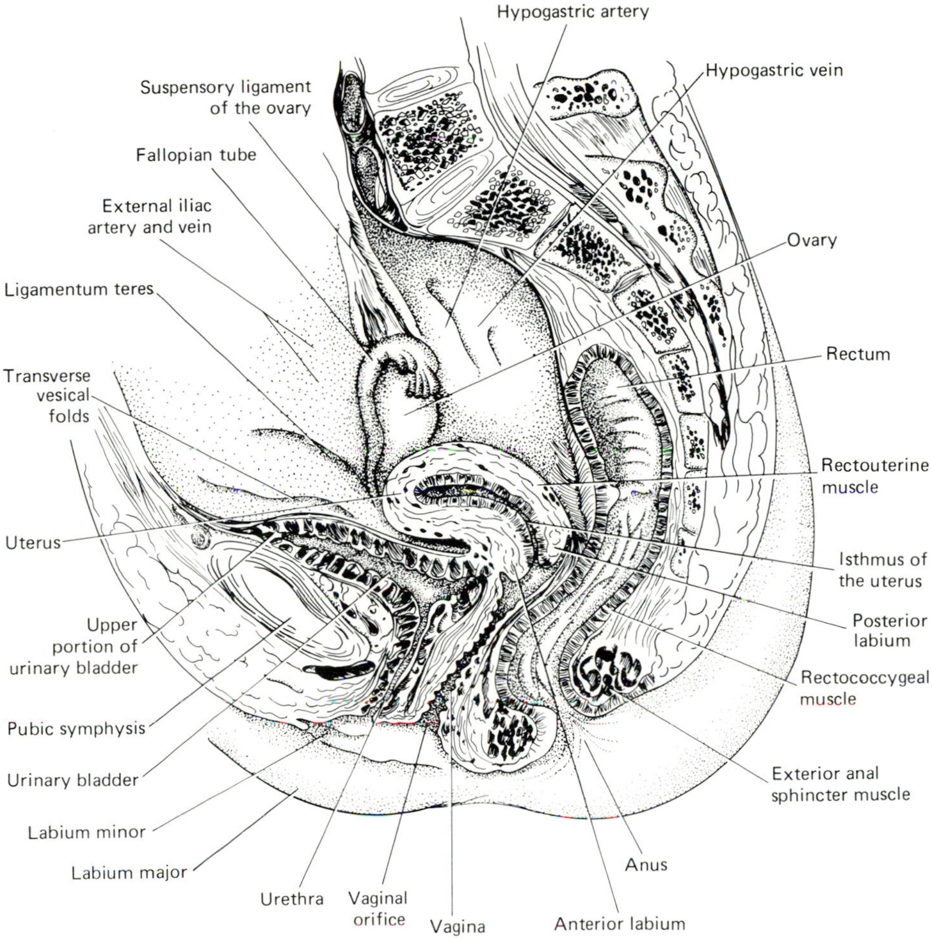

FIG. 27.7. Sagittal section through the pelvis illustrating the anterior and posterior peritoneal reflections on the uterus. [Modified from Gray's Anatomy, 30th ed. (C.D. Clemente, ed.), 1985. Courtesy of Lea & Febiger.]

should be carefully examined for adhesions and brown hemosiderin deposits, so-called powder burns, if endometriosis is suspected. The exocervix should be examined for lacerations, scarring, ulcerations, and cysts.

Before opening of the uterus, the cervical canal and endometrial cavity should be probed. This establishes the patency of the endocervical canal and facilitates opening the uterus. An incision is made with a scalpel or scissors along the probe extending from the cervical os to the cornu along one lateral margin to the fundus and then along the other lateral margin (Fig. 27.8). The average thickness of the endometrium should be measured and a statement made whether it is atrophic, polypoid, or hemorrhagic. Polyps should be measured and their location specified. The myometrium is evaluated when sections through the full thickness of the anterior and posterior walls of the uterus are obtained. The maximum thickness of the myometrium should be measured. A thickened myometrium showing small cystic or focal areas of hemorrhage is suggestive of adenomyosis. If the cervix is normal, sections including the endocervix and portio at 6 and 12 o'clock are adequate. The section of the cervix should include the entire wall to involve the endocervix, squamocolumnar junction, exocervix, and paracervical soft tissue. The section through the endometrium, if the lesion is benign, should be up to 2 cm long and should include the full thickness of the endometrium and a wedge of myometrium. In routine cases, four microscopic sections, one each from the anterior and posterior cervix and one each from the anterior and posterior endomyometrium, suffice.

Hysterectomy for Benign Organic Uterine Disease. This includes hysterectomies performed for leiomyomas and endometrial hyperplasia. In addition to the routine processing described previously, more detailed examination is required in these cases.

In a specimen removed for leiomyomas, the number of leiomyomas present, their location (submucosal, intramural, subserosal) and size (e.g., "ten less than 1 cm and two measuring 13 and 18 cm in diameter") should be noted. If submucous, whether the tumor distorts

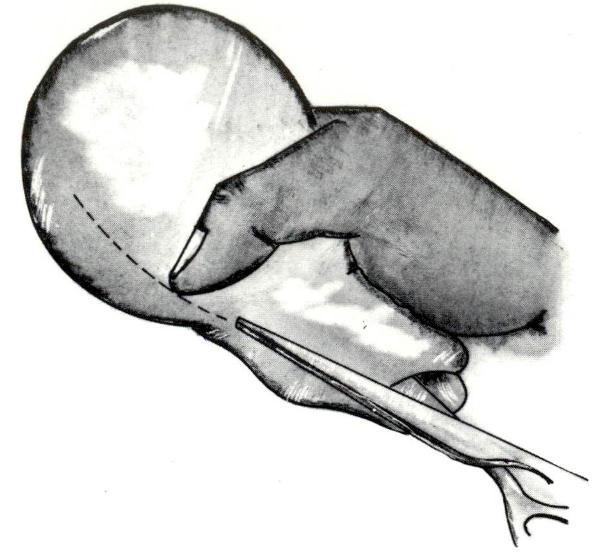

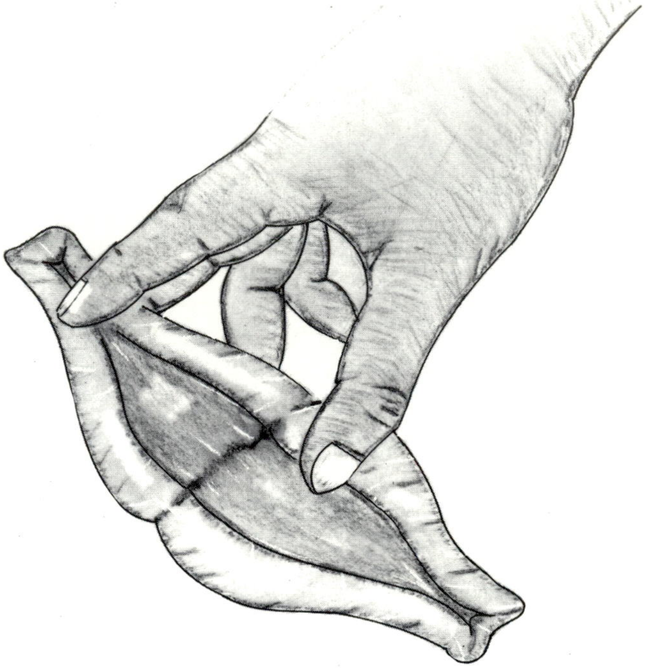

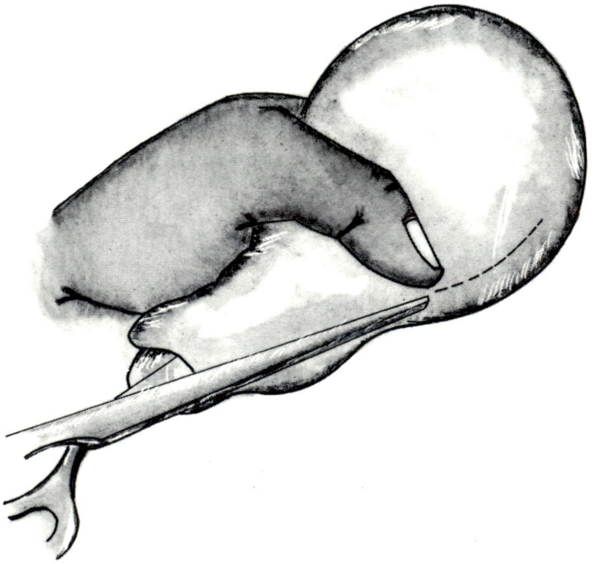

FIG. 27.8. Bivalve opening of the uterus.

the endometrial cavity or whether it protrudes into the lower uterine canal or cervix, should be stated. Each leiomyoma should be sectioned and examined grossly but not necessarily microscopically. If all are white, firm, and whorled and do not contain areas that are soft, necrotic, or hemorrhagic, usually 2–3 blocks in toto are sufficient. Since leiomyomas tend to be multiple and leiomyosarcomas single, solitary tumors that are soft, degenerating, or in any way suspicious should be sampled more extensively. As a rule of thumb, one microscopic section per centimeter of the greatest tumor diameter is recommended. For myomectomy specimens, each leiomyoma should be transected and a section taken from each. Additional sections should be taken if suspicious areas are present.

Uteri removed for endometrial hyperplasia should have multiple full-thickness sections of the endomyometrium in order to rule out the presence of carcinoma. Six sections (three sections, each 2 cm long, of each wall) should sample nearly all the endometrium adequately for most cases.

Hysterectomy for Malignant Uterine Disease. This includes uteri removed for endometrial carcinoma and sarcomas of the uterus. Hysterectomy specimens received with a preoperative diagnosis of carcinoma must be evaluated for residual carcinoma. If present, the maximum depth of myometrial invasion and involvement of the cervix must be determined. Uterine sarcomas should be evaluated in a similar fashion.

The gross description should include whether the tumor is focal or diffuse, sessile or polypoid. The uninvolved endometrium should be described. The dimensions and location of the tumor should be noted, and the gross depth of myometrial invasion should be recorded. Sections must be submitted in an effort to determine maximum depth of myometrial invasion and involvement of the cervix.

The surgical pathology report should include the microscopic diagnosis, tumor grade, depth of myometrial invasion, involvement of the cervix, presence of vascular invasion, and the number of positive lymph nodes with their location specified, that is, pelvic or para-aortic.

Hysterectomy for Malignant Cervical Disease. For intraepithelial neoplasms, a simple hysterectomy often with a vaginal cuff is performed. For microinvasive squamous carcinoma, a simple hysterectomy or a modified radical hysterectomy (inclusion of some paracervical soft tissue) is performed depending on the depth of invasion and the institutional criteria, which may vary. For stage I squamous carcinomas, depending on size and configuration of the tumor in the endocervical canal, and for stage IIa tumors, depending on the extent of vaginal involvement, a radical hysterectomy (Wertheim hysterectomy) and pelvic lymphadenectomy is performed. Para-aortic lymph nodes are also frequently sampled.

For uteri removed for intraepithelial neoplasms, the cervix should be amputated approximated 0.5 cm above the level of the internal os and processed as a cone biopsy. If a vaginal cuff has been submitted, the distance from the exocervix to the line of resection should be measured. Sections should be obtained from the surgical resection line in order to determine the adequacy of the margin. As with the vulva, sections may be circumferential or perpendicular as long as the blocking process is thorough and complete. This information, along with the microscopic diagnosis, should appear in the surgical pathology report.

A radical hysterectomy differs from a simple hysterectomy by virtue of the presence of attached paracervical tissues, which extend to and around the ureter and iliac artery and vein. Accompanying the specimen is a cuff of vagina and pelvic lymph nodes. The gross description should include the dimensions of the tumor, its location, relation to the vaginal margin, depth of invasion, and an impression of whether the lymph nodes appear normal or contain metastases. The cervix can be either processed as a cone biopsy or selectively sampled to demonstrate the maximum depth of invasion and relationship to the surgical margins. The vaginal resection margin is evaluated as described previously. In addition, since the lymphatic drainage of the uterus is lateral toward the parametrium, these areas are especially important in defining the extent of lymphatic permeation. The parametrial tissue should be completely processed, since this represents the lateral and most significant resection margin. The outer surface of the cervix overlying the tumor anteriorly and posteriorly should be marked with India ink to delineate the extent of the tumor in relationship to the bladder and rectum. Lymph nodes should be grouped according to areas. Right and left should be separated and internal iliac, external iliac, obturator, and so on should be separately grouped. Lymph nodes can often be better evaluated when they are fresh, at which time they are firm and nodular. Alternatively, Bouin's fixation, by turning lymph nodes white, whereas fat remains yellow, can be used to facilitate detection.

The surgical pathology report should include the microscopic diagnosis, maximum size, location, and extent of the tumor, as well as the presence of lymphatic invasion, number of involved lymph nodes, and adequacy of the resection margins, especially lateral margins, adjacent to the uterine arteries.

Hysterectomy Performed During Obstetrical Procedures. Hysterectomy at the time of delivery is performed for intractable hemorrhage, placenta accreta, uterine rupture, or cervical neoplasia. For the last, processing of the specimen should be as described previously. For the other conditions, the gross description and sectioning should focus on the relationship of the placenta and membranes to the uterus. Lacerations should be carefully described as to location, extent, and depth of penetration. Sections should be obtained from these sites. If the patient has had a previous cesarean section, the old scar, usually in the anterior lower uterine segment, should be sampled. In instances of placenta previa, the zone of the internal os should be sampled carefully to indicate associated placenta accreta.

Fallopian Tube

Salpingectomy. Removal of the fallopian tube (salpingectomy) often accompanies removal of the ovary (oophorectomy). Removal of both fallopian tubes and ovaries (bilateral salpingo-oophorectomy) is often performed in conjunction with a hysterectomy, especially in older women in whom it is no longer necessary to preserve fertility. In these cases, there is typically no pathologic condition in the fallopian tubes, and the gross examination and sampling are routine. The overall length and diameter of the tube should be measured. The patency of the fimbriated end can be determined with a blunt-tipped probe. If a lesion is present, it should be measured, its location (cornual, isthmic, infundibular, or ampullary) noted, and its relationship to the lumen and serosa described. If no lesion is present, transverse sections from the isthmic, infundibular, and ampullary portions of the tube can be placed into one cassette and labeled "right" or "left" (Fig. 27.9).

Total or Partial Salpingectomy for Tubal Ectopic Pregnancy or Sterilization. If the tubal pregnancy is apparent, its size and location should be noted as described previously. A rupture site if present should be described and sampled. If the ectopic pregnancy is not obvious, a focal enlargement or swelling of the tube should be searched for. Blood distending the lumen of the fallopian tube is so unlikely to result from any other cause that it is worth documenting. It may be necessary to section the area extensively. Even a tubal abortion leaves foci of trophoblast at the implantation site. Blood clot in the tube, sometimes submitted as a separate specimen, should be carefully examined for gray-white tissue and sampled for microscopic examination to identify trophoblast or chorionic villi. Rarely does the entire specimen

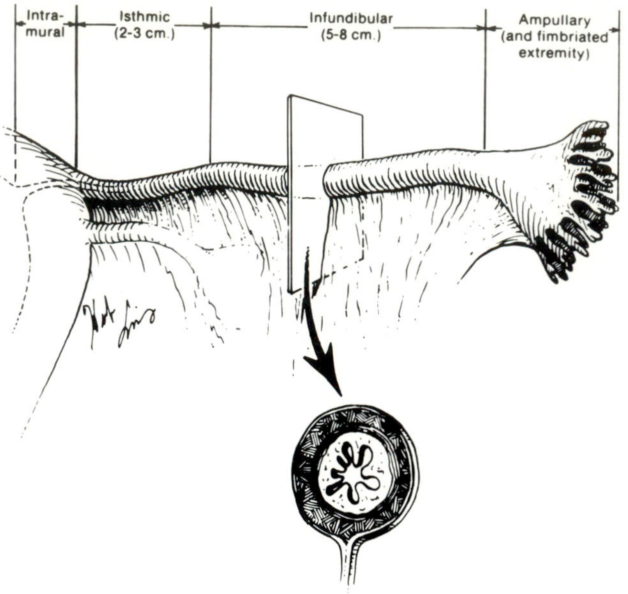

FIG. 27.9. Technique for sectioning the fallopian tube in the absence of abnormalities. Representative transverse sections are obtained from the isthmic, infundibular, and ampullary regions. (Reprinted with permission of Schmidt, Ref. 5.)

need to be sectioned to identify trophoblastic tissues.

Segments of fallopian tube removed for sterilization should be received labeled "right" and "left," and they should be maintained separately throughout processing. The portion of tube submitted should be measured, and a transverse section from each side should be obtained and separately submitted to confirm that the specimen represents a segment from the fallopian tube. Epithelium needs to be present to confirm the presence of fallopian tube.

Salpingectomy for a Tubal Neoplasm. Tubal carcinoma is rare, and its behavior and management are similar to ovarian carcinoma. Typically, a total abdominal hysterectomy and bilateral salpingo-oophorectomy are performed. The size of the tumor, location, and extent, with reference to other pelvic structures, should be described. Transverse sections through the full thickness of the tube permit determination of the depth of penetration. All of this information as well as the grade of the tumor should be included in the microscopic diagnosis of the surgical pathology report.

Ovary

Oophorectomy. The ovaries, like the fallopian tubes, are frequently removed at the time of hysterectomy in older women even if there is no apparent pathology. Routine processing of this type of specimen includes weighing and measuring the ovary in three dimensions. The normal ovary in the reproductive years weighs approximately 8–12 g, is ovoid, and measures approximately $4 \times 2.5 \times 1.5$ cm. The external surface should be inspected for stigmata of ovulation, adhesions, excresences, hemorrhage, or hemosiderin (powder burns), indicative of possible endometriosis. The hilus and broad ligament should be examined, and any suspicious lesion should be submitted for microscopic examination. Each ovary should be sectioned sagittally through its greatest dimension to include the hilus and submitted in a single cassette labeled "right" or "left" (Fig. 27.10).

Cystectomy or Oophorectomy for a Neoplasm. Cystectomy is usually performed for a dermoid cyst. After weighing and measuring the specimen in three dimensions, the external surface should be examined and the cyst opened. The sebum within the cyst can be removed by washing with hot water. The water must be hot to liquefy the sebum. Short exposure to hot water does not destroy the epithelial lining. Identify and serially block the knobby protuberance in the wall, so-called Rokitansky's tubercle, teat, or mammilla, and any other areas where the wall is thickened.

Except for obvious benign paraovarian and functional ovarian cysts, all other cystic and solid ovarian neoplasms are treated by a unilateral salpingo-oophorectomy or a hysterectomy and bilateral salpingo-oophorectomy. The hysterectomy specimen and normal-appearing contralateral ovary and fallopian tube should be processed and reported as described previously. The ovarian tumor should be weighed and measured in three dimensions. The fallopian tube is generally removed with the ovary but may be draped over the tumor and difficult to identify. If present, it should be measured and its relationship to the ovary noted. Similarly, if a tumor appears to have largely replaced the ovary, any residual ovary should be identified and its relationship to the tumor noted. Not uncommonly, the only portion of residual ovary in

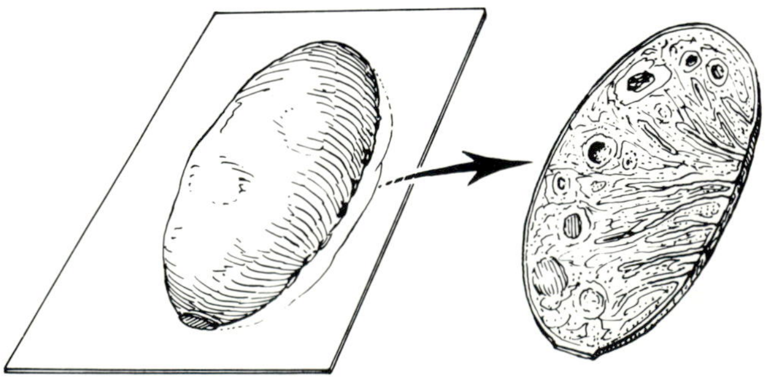

FIG. 27.10. Technique for sectioning the ovary in the absence of abnormalities. (Reprinted with permission of Schmidt, Ref. 5.)

a tumor is that portion of the gonad immediately adjacent to the fallopian tube.

The gross description should state whether the specimen is received intact or fragmented. The capsule should be examined for rents, adhesions, implants, or extension and penetration of the underlying tumor. The tumor is then hemisected, and the cut surfaces are examined. Each cyst of a cystic tumor should be examined for papillary excresences and solid foci, since these may reveal areas of low malignant potential or frankly malignant tumor on microscopic examination. If a solid ovarian tumor is small, identify its location, that is, cortical, medullary, or hilar.

Microscopic sections should be obtained from the external surface of the neoplasm, especially in areas of adhesions, to document whether tumor involves the surface. In particular, penetration of underlying tumor through the capsule should be documented, since this plays a role in staging. It is important to demonstrate invasion microscopically. Blocks cut to show the interface between the tumor and the adjacent tube are especially useful. All solid and hemorrhagic areas should be sampled, and a minimum of one block per centimeter of the greatest tumor dimension should be submitted.

The microscopic diagnosis should include the cell type and, for epithelial tumors, whether benign, of low malignant potential, or frankly malignant. For frankly malignant tumors, include tumor grade, whether the capsule is invaded, the extent of the tumor, and the site and number of involved lymph nodes.

Placental Examination

Routine Processing

Since most newborns and their mothers are normal and healthy, detailed pathologic examination of all placentas is not warranted. The obstetrician must select for examination those placentas that may help in the diagnosis of illness in parent or newborn. The pathologist must respond with an informative report.[2]

Examination of the placenta can provide information useful in patient management, especially infections, and identify instances in which karyotyping is indicated. Further, in the current litiginous environment, placental examination may define types of birth injury that lie outside the control of the obstetrician. Documentation of twinning relationships may be useful in later life, for example, in patients evaluated for organ transplantation.

Placentas selected for examination should be sent fresh to the laboratory with a requisition that states the questions the pathologist is expected to answer. Placentas not selected can be labeled and stored in plastic bags, either frozen or refrigerated, for retrieval if problems develop in the neonatal period.

Indications for placental examination and a format suitable for transmission of the placenta and necessary data to the laboratory are listed in Table 27.1. The list begins with the mother's name and age. It can be used as a checklist sufficient to provide the pathologist with enough clinical data to start the examination.

TABLE 27.1. Request for placental examination.

	Circle appropriate indications
	Mother's name ____________ Age ____ M.D. ____________
	Cesarean section/vaginal delivery
1.	Specific maternal disease: Diagnosis ____________
2.	High-risk pregnancy: Diagnosis ____________
3.	Death: Antepartum Intrapartum Neonatal
4.	Baby small for date: Baby anemic
5.	Postmature
6.	Premature rupture of membranes
7.	Possible intrauterine infection: viral (specify) ____________
	toxoplasma ________ chorioamnionitis ________ other ________
8.	Isoimmunization: Rh ________ Other ________
9.	Malformations of baby or placenta ________ Single umbilical artery ________
10.	Evaluate antepartum intrauterine procedures (specify) ____________
11.	Gestational bleeding: 1st 2nd 3rd trimester ____________
12.	Placenta previa-vasa previa ____________
13.	Premature separation ____________
14.	Toxemia, eclampsia ____________
15.	Maternal diabetes mellitus ____________
16.	Maternal anemias (sickle cell, megaloblastic, other ____________
17.	Other disease ____________
18.	History of habitual abortion ____________
19.	Cord entanglements, amniotic bands, or adhesions. Membrane tears, defects

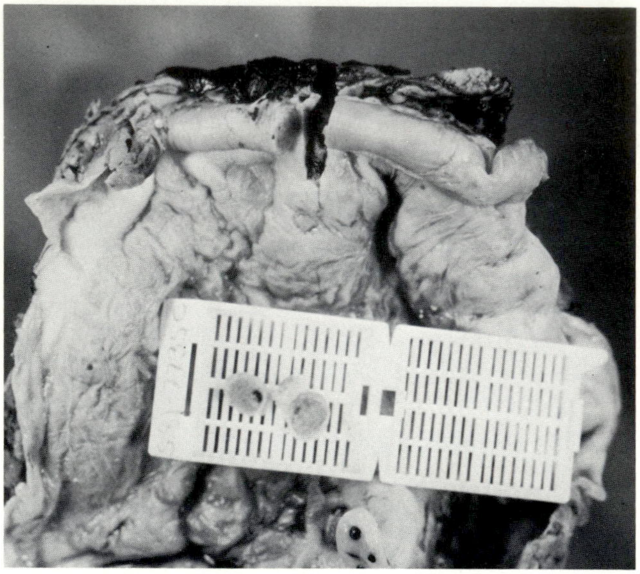

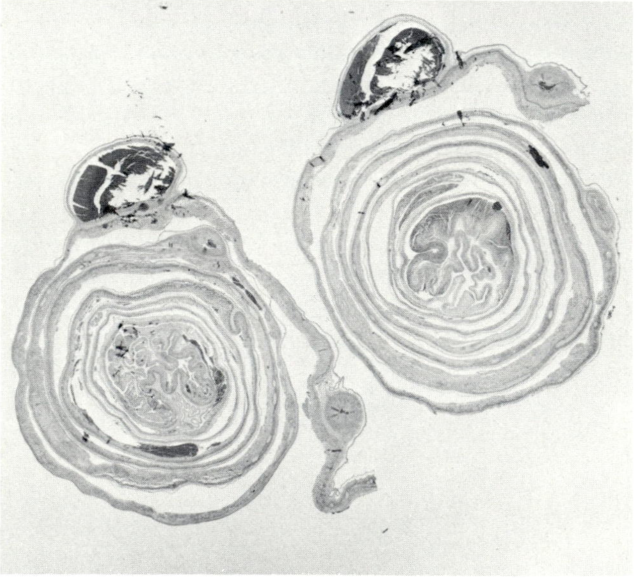

FIG. 27.11. *Top:* A placenta with membrane roll attached at top before fixation. The resulting spiral in cassette retains its tight coil after the block has been processed. *Bottom:* Margin of membrane opening is always at the center of the spiral. This consistent orientation helps demonstrate the ascending route of infections.

The membrane of the specimen should be translucent, and the fetal surface should be shiny, dark purple. Reconstruct the membranous sac, noting its narrowest margin between placental edge and site of rupture. The absence of a margin may explain bleeding; any margin excludes placenta previa. Record tears or bands. Cut a strip of membrane about 5 cm wide, roll it toward the placental margin, and affix it with a pin (Fig. 27.11). Cut away the rest of the membranes from the rest of the placental margin with scissors. Next, examine the fetal surface. Note exudate, discoloration (green-brown) from meconium staining, and adherent extraneous material that does not easily wipe away. The umbilical cord must be carefully examined and measured. Record knots, hemorrhages, and number of vessels on cross-section cut away from the placenta near the fetal surface. Insertion of the cord near the narrowest membrane margin may be a cause of intrapartum fetal distress (vasa previa). The inspection should conclude with an examination of the maternal surface. Cotyledons should be intact. Note any adherent clot, especially clots that compress the placenta or have become indurated and laminated.

Weigh the placenta and record the maximum dimensions. Cut sections at 1–3 cm intervals with a sharp knife; this is accomplished most easily with the maternal surface up. The cut surface should have a uniform granu-

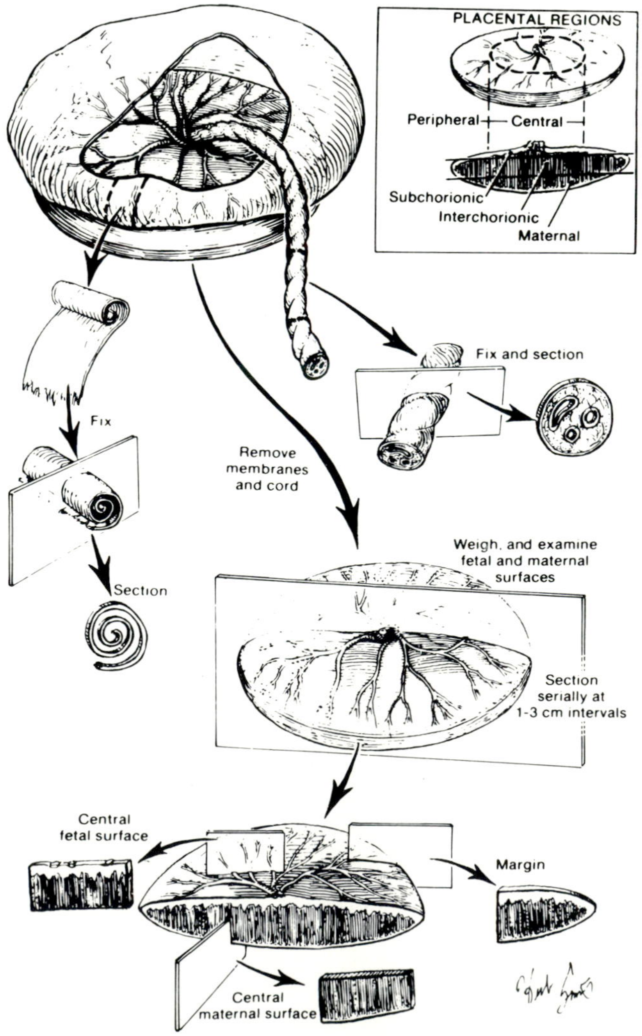

FIG. 27.12. Adequate sampling for histologic study includes membrane roll, cross-section of cord, and specific placental regions, specifically cut to display fetal and maternal surfaces. (Reprinted with permission of Schmidt, Ref. 5.)

lar surface and a bright red color. Record clots, infarcts, and other lesions.

After the specimen has been fixed for several hours in 10% buffered neutral formalin, blocks can be cut for histologic sections (Fig. 27.12) to include a cross-section of the cord, membrane roll, fetal surface with amnion attached, and lesions identified on cross-section.

Special Studies

Twins and Other Multiple Gestations. The amnionic septum between two amnionic cavities serves to define identical or fraternal relationships insofar as placental examination allows. The dividing membrane of dichorionic placentas is thicker and opaque because of the intervening chorionic tissue. Attach a roll of this membrane also, as described for single placentas, affixing it to the placental surface with a pin. After fixation, cut a cross-section from this roll and the T zone, where it attaches to the fetal surface of the placenta (Fig. 27.13). After stripping both amnions away, a ridge or layer of chorion persists in fused dichorionic twin placentas, but the site of the septum vanishes without a trace in monochorionic twin placentas.

Culture Methods. Aerobic and anaerobic bacterial cultures, when performed by swabbing the fetal surface, introduce so many contaminants that the procedure has little value. To reduce the frequency of contaminants, the subchorionic zone is best cultured with a swab after the surface has been seared and incised with a heated scalpel[1] (Fig. 27.14).

Cytogenetic Studies. These studies require a fragment of villous tissue or skin or pericardium if perinatal death has occurred. Death of the fetus does not necessarily preclude successful culture. The tissue should be placed

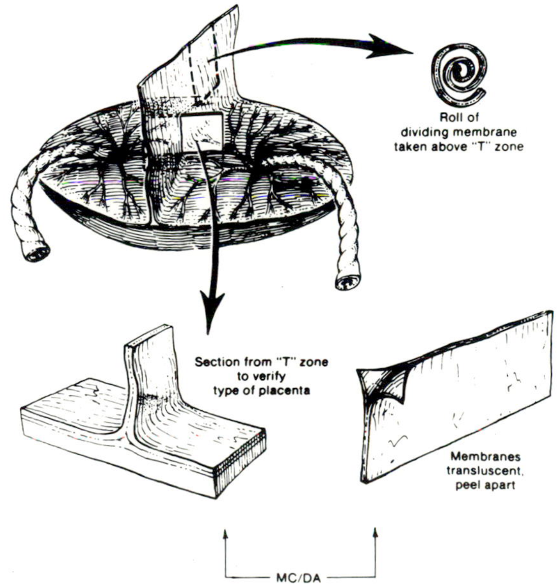

Fig. 27.13. Sampling of a twin placenta includes a section of septal membrane dividing the amnionic cavities, cut to display the T zone, where the septal membrane attaches to the placental surface. (Reprinted with permission of Schmidt, Ref. 5.)

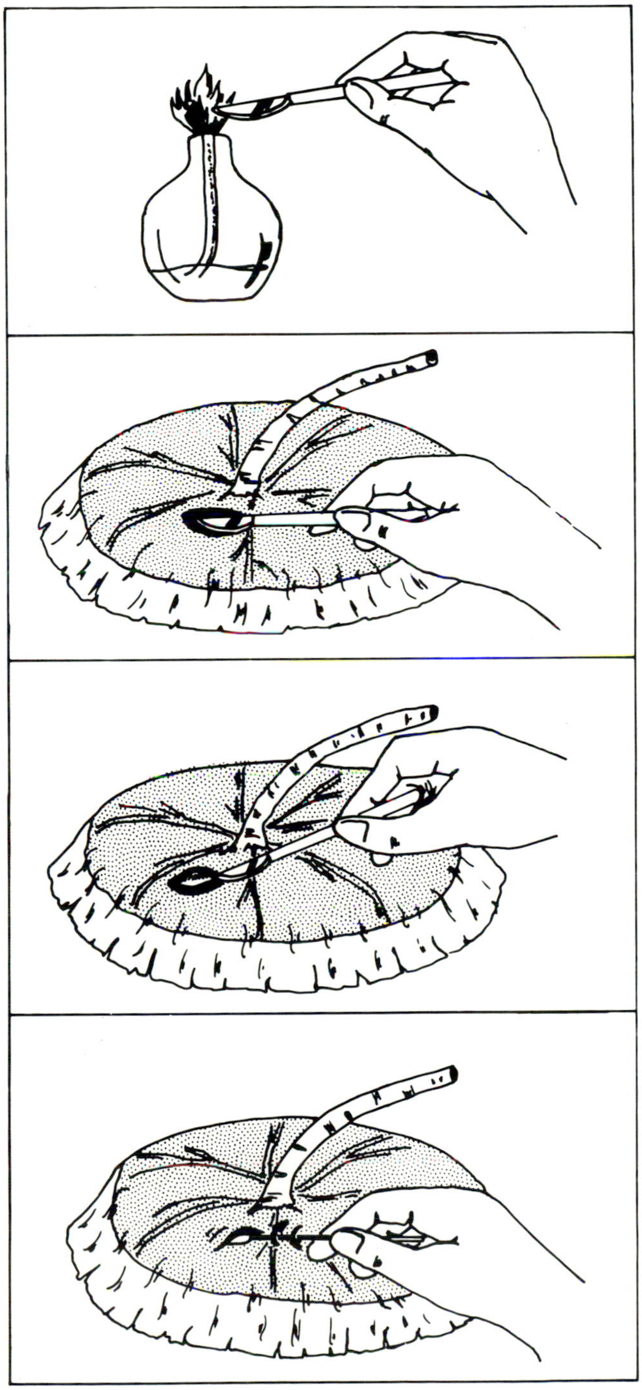

Fig. 27.14. Culture technique to sample subchorionic fibrin layer. This method reduces surface contamination.

TABLE 27.2. Cytogenetic studies for curretted and miscarried material.

Curettings
1. Call laboratory for sterile media containers and to notify that a specimen is coming.
2. Cytogenetics needs 2–3 cm of sterile material for culture. Put the material into the bottle, cap tightly, label and send to the laboratory with the appropriate request form.
Miscarriage
1. Call laboratory for two sterile media and two sodium heparin Vacutainers. Also notify the laboratory that a specimen is coming.
2. If the miscarriage is small, put the material into the containers and cap tightly. Draw maternal blood into sodium heparin Vacutainer and send with miscarriage material and the appropriate forms to the laboratory.
3. If the miscarriage is term (stillborn baby) and large:
a. Cut a skin sample and/or pericardium and put into one media container (sterile).
b. Draw fetal blood (intracardiac puncture with heparinized syringe) and put into sodium heparin Vacutainer.
c. Cut a small piece of placenta and put into second media bottle.
d. Draw maternal blood into a sodium heparin Vacutainer.
4. Label all specimens and send to the laboratory with the appropriate form.

Cytogenetics Lab, St. John's Mercy Medical Center.

in sterile media containers provided by the cytogenetics laboratory. Tissue obtained properly may be shipped to a distant facility if desired. (See Table 27.2 for directions for preparation and transmission of tissue.)

Dissecting Microscope. A dissecting microscope should be available for adequate study of many small abortuses. Some anomalies, including fusion defects of the facial clefts, fused or supernumerary digits, partial limb reduction, and such ocular defects as coloboma, are too minute to evaluate adequately with the unaided eye, but alone or in combination they may be sufficiently suggestive of trisomy to indicate the need for karyotypes of the conceptus and possibly the parents.

References

1. Aquino TI, Zhang J, Kraus FT, et al. (1984) Subchorionic fibrin cultures for bacteriologic study of the placenta. Am J Clin Pathol 81: 482
2. Benirschke K, Driscoll SG (1967) The Pathology of the Human Placenta. New York, Springer-Verlag
3. Langlois PL (1970) The size of the normal uterus. J Reprod Med 4: 220
4. Milbrath JR, Wilkinson EJ, Friedrich EG (1975) Xerographic evaluation of radical vulvectomy specimens. AJR 125: 486
5. Schmidt WA (1983) Principles and Techniques of Surgical Pathology. Butterworths, Stoneham, Massachusetts.

Index